# Textbook of
# Malignant Hematology

# Textbook of Malignant Hematology

## Second Edition

**Edited by**

**Laurent Degos, MD, PhD**
Institute of Haematology University Paris 7
Saint-Louis Hospital
Paris
France

**David C Linch, FRCP, FRCPath, FMedSci**
Department of Haematology
University College London Medical School
London
UK

**Bob Löwenberg, MD, PhD**
Department of Hematology
Erasmus University Medical Center
Rotterdam
The Netherlands

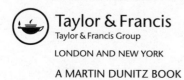 Taylor & Francis
Taylor & Francis Group

LONDON AND NEW YORK

A MARTIN DUNITZ BOOK

© 1999, 2005 Taylor & Francis, an imprint of the Taylor & Francis Group

First published in the United Kingdom in 1999 by
Martin Dunitz Ltd

This edition published in 2005 by Taylor & Francis Medical Books, part of the
Taylor & Francis Group, 2 Park Square, Milton Park, Abingdon, Oxon OX14 4RN

Tel.:      +44 (0)1235 828600
Fax.:      +44 (0)1235 829000
E-mail:    info@dunitz.co.uk
Website: http://www.dunitz.co.uk

Although every effort has been made to ensure that all owners of copyright
material have been acknowledged in this publication, we would be glad to
acknowledge in subsequent reprints or editions any omissions brought to our
attention.

Although every effort has been made to ensure that drug doses and other
information are presented accurately in this publication, the ultimate responsibility
rests with the prescribing physician. Neither the publishers nor the authors can be
held responsible for errors or for any consequences arising from the use of
information contained herein. For detailed prescribing information or instructions
on the use of any product or procedure discussed herein, please consult the
prescribing information or instructional material issued by the manufacturer.

A CIP record for this book is available from the British Library.

Library of Congress Cataloging in Publication Data available on application.

ISBN 1 84184 145 5


Distributed in North and South America by

Taylor & Francis
2000 NW Corporate Blvd
Boca Raton, FL 33431, USA

Within Continental USA
Tel:       800 272 7737;       Fax:      800 374 3401
Outside Continental USA
Tel:       561 994 0555;       Fax:      561 361 6018
E-mail:   orders@crcpress.com


Distributed in the rest of the world by
Thomson Publishing Services
Cheriton House
North Way
Andover, Hampshire SP10 5BE, UK
Tel.:      +44 (0)1264 332424
E-mail:   salesorder.tandf@thomsonpublishingservices.co.uk


Composition by Phoenix Photosetting, Chatham, Kent
Printed and bound in Italy by Printer Trento

# Contents

## PART SIX: LATE EFFECTS OF THERAPY

## PART SEVEN: SUPPORTIVE CARE

## APPENDICES

# Contributors

**Kenneth C Anderson, MD**
Jerome Lipper Multiple Myeloma Center
Dana Farber Cancer Institute
Boston
Massachusetts
USA

**Lionel Ades, MD**
Hôpital Saint-Louis University Paris 7
Paris
France

**Fanny Baran-Marszak, MD, PhD**
Laboratory of Hematology and Immunology
Cytogenetics
CHU Bicêtre
France

**Giovanni Barosi, MD**
Laboratorio di Informatica Medica
IRCCS Policlinico S Matteo
Pavia
Italy

**Tiziano Barbui, MD**
Divisione di Ematologia
Ospedale Riuniti
Bergamo
Italy

**Karolin Behringer, MD**
First Department of Internal Medicine
University Hospital Cologne
Cologne
Germany

**Alan K Burnett, MD**
Department of Haematology
University of Wales College of Medicine
Cardiff
UK

**William T Bellamy, PhD**
Department of Pathology
University of Arizona Health Sciences Center
Tucson
Arizona
USA

**Malcolm Brenner, MD**
Centre for Cell and Gene Therapy
Department of Immunology
Baylor College of Medicine
Houston
Texas
USA

**Anne Cambiaggi, PhD**
Centre d'Immunologie de Marseille-Luminy
Marseille
France

**Jonathan Cebon, MB, BS, PhD**
Joint Medical Oncology Unit
Melbourne Tumour Biology Branch
Ludwig Institute for Cancer Research
Royal Melbourne Hospital
Melbourne
Victoria
Australia

**Michael A Chapman**
Department of Haematology
Cambridge Institute for Medical Research
Cambridge
UK

**Catherine Cordonnier, MD**
Service d'Hématologie Clinique
Hôpital Henri Mondor
Créteil
France

**Peter T Daniel, MD, PhD**
Clinical and Molecular Oncology
University Medical Center Charlté
Humboldt University
Berlin
Germany

**Marloes LH de Bruijn, MD**
Leiden University Medical Center
Leiden
The Netherlands

**Najet Debili, MD**
INSERM U362
Institut Gustave Roussy
Villejuif
France

**Laurent Degos, MD, PhD**
Institute of Haematology University Paris 7
Saint-Louis Hospital
Paris
France

**Stephen Devereux, FRCPath**
Department of Haematological Medicine
King's College Hospital
London
UK

**Volker Diehl, MD**
First Department of Internal Medicine
University Hospital Cologne
Cologne
Germany

**Elaine A Dzierzak, MD**
Department of Cell Biology and Genetics
Erasmus University Medical Center
Rotterdam
The Netherlands

**Andreas Engert, MD**
First Department of Internal Medicine
University Hospital Cologne
Cologne
Germany

**Pierre Fenaux, MD**
Université Paris XIII and Service d'Hématologie clinique
Hôpital Avicenne
Bobigny
France

**Willem E Fibbe, MD, PhD**
Department of Hematology
Leiden University Medical Center
Leiden
The Netherlands

**Guido Finazzi, MD**
Division of Haematology
Ospedali Riuniti di Bergamo
Bergamo
Italy

**Michel Forgereau, Dr Sc, DVM**
Centre d'Immunologie de Marseille-Luminy
Marseille
France

**Rosemary E Gale, MD**
Department of Haematology
University College London Medical School
London
UK

**Claude Gardin, MD**
Université Paris XIII and Service d'Hématologie clinique
Hôpital Avicenne
Bobigny
France

**Antoine Gessain, MD**
Chef d'Unité
Bâtiment Lwoff
Unité d'Epidémiologie et Physiopathologie des Virus
Oncogénes
Institut Pasteur
Paris
France

**Nicola Gökbuget, MD**
JW Goethe University Hospital
Frankfurt
Germany

**Marcos González, MD**
Department of Hematology
University Hospital of Salamanca
Salamanca
Spain

**Anthony R Green, PhD, FRCP, FRCPath, FMedSci**
Department of Haematology
Cambridge Institute for Medical Research
Cambridge
UK

**François Guilhot, MD**
Department of Oncology Hematology and Cell Therapy
Centre Hospitalier Universitaire de Poitiers
Poitiers
France

**Torsten Haferlach, MD, PhD**
Labor für Leukämie-Diagnostik
University Hospital Grosshadern
Marchioninstr
Munich
Germany

**Anne Hagemeijer, MD**
Center for Human Genetics
University of Leeuven
Herestraat 49
Leuven
Belgium

**Anton Hagenbeek, MD, PhD**
University Medical Center Utrecht
Utrecht
The Netherlands

**Dieter Hoelzer, MD**
JW Goethe University Hospital
Frankfurt
Germany

**Stephen P Hunger, MD**
Children's Cancer Chair and Chief
Division of Pediatric Hematology/Oncology
University of Florida College of Medicine
Gainesville
Florida
USA

**Balkrishna N Jahagirdar, MD**
Division of Hematology-Oncology
VA Medical Center
Minneapolis
Minnesota
USA

**Roland Kanaar, MD**
Department of Cell Biology and Genetics
Erasmus University Medical Center
Rotterdam
The Netherlands

**Gertjan JL Kaspers, MD, PhD**
Department Pediatric Oncology/Hematology
VU University Medical Center
Amsterdam
The Netherlands

**Wolfgang Kern, MD**
Laboratory for Leukemia Diagnostics
University Hospital Grosshadern
Ludwig-Maximilians-University
Munich
Germany

**Asim Khwaja, MD, MRCP, MRCPath**
Department of Haematology
University College London Medical School
London
UK

**Philip M Kluin, MD**
Department of Pathology and Laboratory Medicine
Academic Hospital Groningen
Groningen
The Netherlands

**Alexander Kohlmann, MD**
Laboratory for Leukemia Diagnostics
University Hospital Grosshadern
Ludwig-Maximilians-University
Munich
Germany

**Peter M Lansdorp, MD, PhD**
Terry Fox Laboratory
British Columbia Cancer Agency
Vancouver, BC
Canada

**Anton W Langerak, PhD**
Department of Immunology
Erasmus University Medical Center
Rotterdam
The Netherlands

**Gill Levitt, MRCP**
Department of Haematology/ Oncology
Great Ormond Street
London
UK

**David C Linch, FRCP, FRCPath, FMedSci**
Department of Haematology
University College London Medical School
London
UK

**Bob Löwenberg, MD, PhD**
Department of Hematology
Erasmus University Medical Center
Rotterdam
The Netherlands

**Stephen Mackinnon, MD, FRCP**
Department of Haematology
Royal Free and University College
London Medical School
London
UK

**Andrew K McMillan, PhD, FRCP, FRCPath**
Department of Haematology
Nottingham City Hospital
Nottingham
UK

**Renaud Mahieux, PhD**
Unité d'Epidémiologie et Physiopathologie des Virus
Oncogènes
Institut Pasteur
Paris
France

**Eugene Maraskovsky, MD**
Joint Medical Oncology Unit
Melbourne Tumour Biology Branch
Ludwig Institute for Cancer Research
Royal Melbourne Hospital
Melbourne
Victoria
Australia

**Jean-Pierre Marie, MD**
Department of Hematology and Medical Oncology
Hospital Hôtel-Dieu
Paris
France

**Cristina Mecucci, MD, PhD**
Hematology and Bone Marrow Transplantation Unit
Hematology University of Perugia
Policlinico Monteluce
Perugia
Italy

**Cornelius JM Melief, MD**
Department of Immunohematology and Blood
Transfusion,
Leiden University Medical Center
Leiden
The Netherlands

**Emilio Montserrat, MD**
Institute of Hematology and Oncology Hospital Clinic
Villarroel, 170
Barcelona
Spain

**Stuart Mucklow, MRCP**
Department of Haematology/ Oncology
Great Ormond Street
London
UK

**Nikhil C Munshi, MD**
Jerome Lipper Multiple Myeloma Center
Dana Farber Cancer Institute
Boston
Massachusetts
USA

**Rienk Offringa, MD**
Department of Immunohematology and Blood
Transfusion,
Leiden University Medical Center
Leiden
The Netherlands

**Jørgen H Olsen, MD**
Institute of Cancer Epidemiology
Danish Cancer Society
Copenhagen
Denmark

**Richard J O'Reilly, MD**
Marrow Transplantation Service
Memorial Sloan-Kettering Cancer Center
New York
USA

**Alberto Orfao, MD**
Department of General Cytometry
University Hospital of Salamanca
Salamanca
Spain

**Antonio Pagliuca, MA, FRCP, FRCPath**
Department of Haematological Medicine
King's College Hospital
London
UK

**Esperanza B Papadopoulos, MD**
Department of Medicine
Memorial Sloan-Kettering Cancer Center
New York
USA

**Rob E Ploemacher, MD**
Department of Hematology
Erasmus University Medical Center
Rotterdam
The Netherlands

**Ching-Hon Pui, MD**
Hematology/Oncology
St Jude Children's Research Hospital
Memphis
Tennessee
USA

**Martin Pulè, MD**
Center for Cell and Gene Therapy
Deparment of Immunology
Baylor College of Medicine
Houston
Texas
USA

**Hélène A Poirel, MD**
Laboratory of Hematology and Immunology
Cytogenetics
CHU Bicêtre
France

**Martine Raphaël, MD, PhD**
Laboratory of Hematology and Immunology
Cytogenetics
CHU Bicêtre
France

**Yaddanapudi Ravindranath, MBBS**
Georgie Ginopolis Chair for Pediatric Cancer and
Hematology
Wayne State University School of Medicine
Detroit
Michigan
USA

**Maaike E Ressing, MD**
Department of Medical Microbiology,
Immunohematology and Blood Transfusion, and
Pediatrics
Leiden University Medical Center
Leiden
The Netherlands

**Raul C Ribeiro, MD**
Hematology/Oncology
St Jude Children's Research Hospital
Memphis
Tennessee
USA

**Paul-Hénri Roméo, PhD**
INSERM Cochin U567
Maternité Port-Royal
Paris
France

**Lydia Roy, MD**
Department of Oncology Hematology and Cell Therapy
Centre Hospitalier Universitaire de Poitiers
Poitiers
France

**Jesús Fernando San Miguel, MD**
Department of Hematology
University Hospital of Salamanca
Salamanca
Spain

**Claudine Schiff, MD**
Immunology Center of Marseille-Luminy
Marseille
France

**Susanne Schnittger, MD**
Laboratory for Leukemia Diagnostics
University Hospital Grosshadern
Ludwig-Maximilians-University
Munich
Germany

**Claudia Schoch, MD**
Laboratory for Leukemia Diagnostics
University Hospital Grosshadern
Ludwig-Maximilians-University
Munich
Germany

**Max Schnurr, MD**
Joint Medical Oncology Unit
Melbourne Tumour Biology Branch
Ludwig Institute for Cancer Research
Royal Melbourne Hospital
Melbourne
Victoria
Australia

**William B Slaytor, MD**
Division of Pediatric Hematology/Oncology
University of Florida College of Medicine
Health Science Center
Gainesville
Florida
USA

**Trudy N Small, MD**
Department of Pediatrics
Memorial Sloan-Kettering Cancer Center
New York
USA

**Gérard Socié, MD, PhD**
Hôpital Saint-Louis University Paris 7
Paris
France

**Anthony J Swerdlow, MD**
Section of Epidemiology
Institute of Cancer Research
Sutton
UK

**Tomasz Szczepañski, MD**
Department of Immunology
Erasmus University Medical Center
Rotterdam
The Netherlands

**N Shaun B Thomas, MD**
Guy's, King's and St Thomas' School of Medicine and
Dentistry
The Rayne Institute
London
UK

**Rene EM Toes, MD**
Department of Rheumatology
Leiden University Medical Center
Leiden
The Netherlands

**Ivo P Touw, MD**
Department of Hematology
Erasmus University Medical Center
Rotterdam
The Netherlands

**Sophie Ugolini, PhD**
Laboratory of NK cells and Innate Immunity
Centre d'Immunologie de Marseille-Luming
Marseille
France

**William Vainchenker, MD**
INSERM U362
Institut Gustave Roussy
Villejuif
France

**Thamar B van Dijk, MD**
Department of Hematology
Erasmus University Medical Center
Rotterdam
The Netherlands

**Jacques JM van Dongen, MD**
Department of Immunology
Erasmus University Medical Center
Rotterdam
The Netherlands

**DC van Gent, MD**
Department of Cell Biology and Genetics
Erasmus University Medical Center
Rotterdam
The Netherlands

**Flora E van Leewen, MD**
Department of Epidemiology
Netherlands Cancer Institute
Amsterdam
The Netherlands

**Lieneke R van Veelen, MD**
Department of Radiation Oncology
Erasmus University Medical Center-Daniel den Hoed
Rotterdam
The Netherlands

**VHJ van der Velden, MD**
Department of Immunology
Erasmus University Medical Center
Rotterdam
The Netherlands

**Catherine M Verfaillie, MD**
Stem Cell Institute
Division of Hematology, Oncology, and Transplantation
University of Minneapolis
Minnesota
USA

**Eric Vivier, MD, PhD**
Immunology
Centre d'Immunologie de Marseille-Luminy
Marseille
France

**Françoise Wendling, MD**
INSERM U363
Institut Gustave Roussy
Villejuif
France

# Preface

The hematological malignancies as a whole are the fourth most common form of cancer in men and the third most common in women. By the age of 75 years, nearly 1 in 20 individuals will have developed a hematological malignancy if they have not died of something else beforehand. The importance of the hematological malignancies far exceeds their frequency, however. The repeated accessibility of hematological tissue has facilitated rapid advances in the understanding of the molecular pathogenesis of the hematological malignancies and their diagnostic implications. From a therapeutic perspective, the hematological malignancies have been the test-bed for the development of the principles of therapy, which apply to most other forms of cancer. This includes combination chemotherapy, chemotherapy dose escalation and, most recently, immuno-chemotherapy and the use of biological therapies.

The first edition of this book emphasized the recent insights into the pathophysiology of the hematological malignancies and focussed on the scientific principles underlying current therapy. This approach has been maintained in the second edition, and it has required considerable revision of some chapters and the addition of new chapters, including stem cell plasticity, DNA repair, senescence and telomeres, angiogenesis and tumor development, microarray analysis, and expression profiling. There has also been a major increase in the emphasis given to late effects of therapy and there are now three chapters devoted to this topic.

Many authors from the first edition have been retained, but numerous new authors have also been recruited to maintain an up-to-date international perspective from experts in their fields.

Laurent Degos
David C Linch
Bob Löwenberg

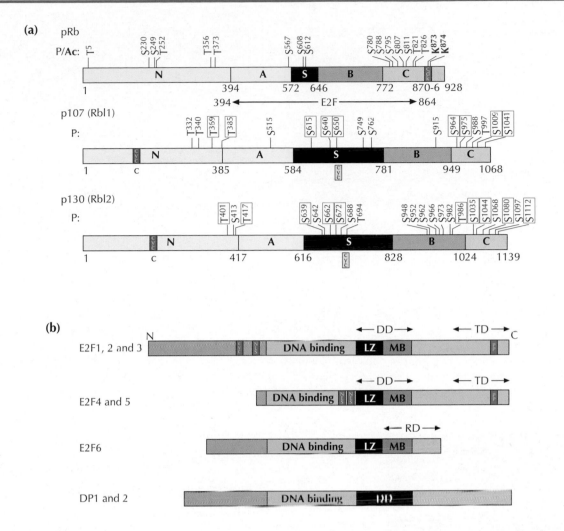

**Figure 4.7** (a) The pRb family. The schemaata depicting each member of the pRb family show phosphorylation sites and acetylation sites (in red). The phosphorylation sites that are conserved in p130 and p107 are boxed.[162] The A and B domains (separated by a spacer domain, S) make up the 'pocket' that binds proteins with LXCXE motifs. The 'large pocket' (domains A, B, and C) binds E2F–DP factors. The C-terminal domain also binds MDM2 and c-ABL. cyc is the cyclin–cdk binding site (KXLKXL). Numbers indicate amino acids (N→C terminus). (b) The E2F and DP families. The domains shown allow the E2F and DP proteins to dimerize as E2F–DP heterodimers (DD, comprising leucine zipper (LZ) and marked box (MB) domains), to bind pRb, p130, or p107 'pocket proteins' (pp), to bind E2F-binding sequences in the promoters of genes (DNA binding), and to transactivate (TD) or repress (RD) transcription. E2F1, 2, and 3 have nuclear localization signals (NLS) and E2F4 and 5 have nuclear export signals (NES). Cyclin A binds E2F1, 2, and 3 (cyc). The schema is shown with N→C terminus, left to right.

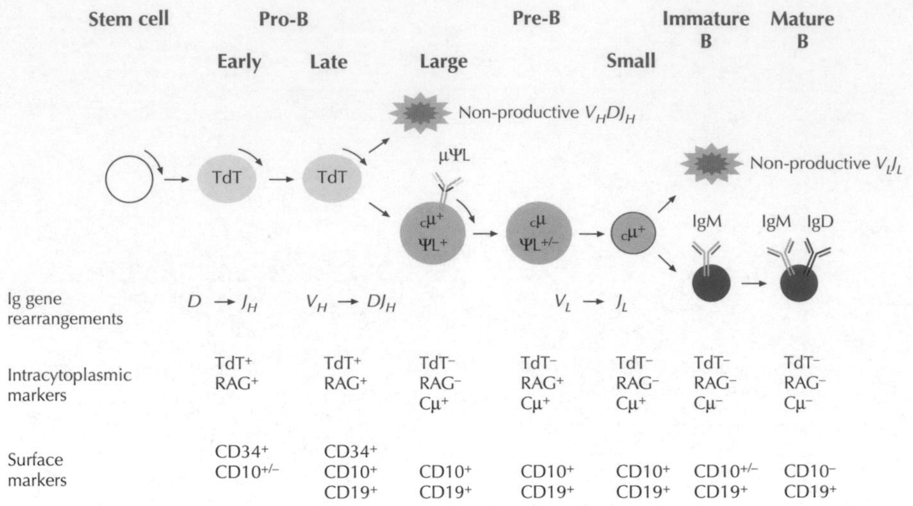

| | Stem cell | Pro-B | | | Pre-B | | Immature B | Mature B |
|---|---|---|---|---|---|---|---|---|
| | | Early | Late | Large | | Small | | |

Non-productive $V_HDJ_H$

μΨL

Non-productive $V_LJ_L$

cμ⁺ ΨL⁺ — cμ ΨL⁺/⁻ — cμ⁺ — IgM — IgM IgD

| Ig gene rearrangements | | $D \rightarrow J_H$ | $V_H \rightarrow DJ_H$ | | | $V_L \rightarrow J_L$ | | |
|---|---|---|---|---|---|---|---|---|
| Intracytoplasmic markers | | TdT⁺ RAG⁺ | TdT⁺ RAG⁺ | TdT⁻ RAG⁻ Cμ⁺ | TdT⁻ RAG⁺ Cμ⁺ | TdT⁻ RAG⁻ Cμ⁺ | TdT⁻ RAG⁻ Cμ⁻ | TdT⁻ RAG⁻ Cμ⁻ |
| Surface markers | | CD34⁺ CD10⁺/⁻ | CD34⁺ CD10⁺ CD19⁺ | CD10⁺ CD19⁺ | CD10⁺ CD19⁺ | CD10⁺ CD19⁺ | CD10⁺/⁻ CD19⁺ | CD10⁻ CD19⁺ |

**Figure 6.2** The early steps of B-cell differentiation take place in the bone marrow and are antigen-independent. The main discrete steps that lead from the hematopoietic stem cell to the immature B lymphocyte are identified by the successive Ig gene rearrangements, by the presence of intracytoplasmic markers, and by the expression of characteristic markers at the cell surface. The very early stages that go from the stem cell to the early pro-B cell encompass several precursors that are not completely defined to date. TdT, terminal deoxynucleotidyl transferase, responsible for including N diversity; ΨL, surrogate light chain that combine with the Ig μ chain to form the pre-B receptor; RAG, recombination activating genes, which encode for the recombinase enzyme.

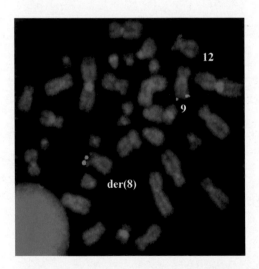

**Figure 17.2** Double-color metaphase FISH in a patient with a cryptic *ETV6–ABL1* fusion gene and only a t(8;12)(p12;p13) translocation on classical cytogenetics. Red signals mark the *ETV6* gene both in the abnormal 12p and in the abnormal 8 derived from the chromosomal translocation. Green signals label the *ABL1* gene in both the normal chromosome 9 and the abnormal 8.

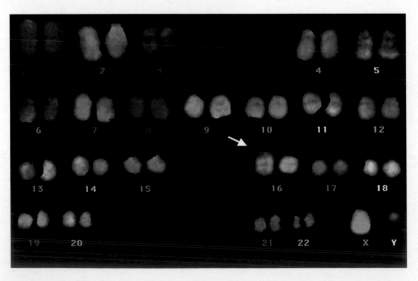

**Figure 17.3** AML with extra material in the short arm of chromosome 16 derived from chromosome 1 (arrow), as revealed by multicolor FISH karyotype.

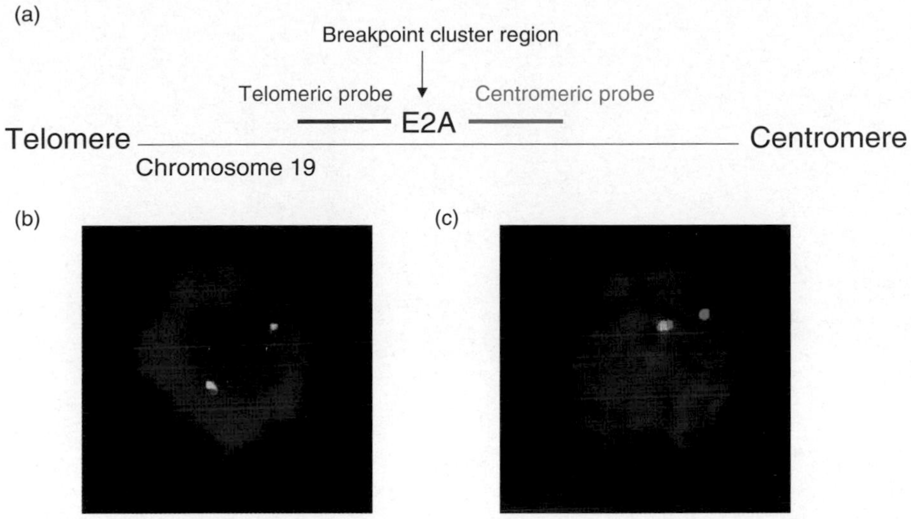

(a)

Breakpoint cluster region

Telomeric probe    Centromeric probe

Telomere ——————————— E2A ——————————— Centromere

Chromosome 19

(b)        (c)

**Figure 18.1** Detection of *E2A* translocations in interphase cells via two-color 'split apart' FISH. (a) Schematic depiction of the *E2A* gene on chromosome 19 and location of probes centromeric (green) and telomeric (red) to *E2A*. (b) Interphase FISH of a normal cell shows two fused red/green or yellow signals from the adjacent signals on each chromosome 19 homologue. (c) Interphase FISH of a cell with a t(1;19)(q23;p13) shows one fused red/green signal from the normal chromosome 19, and single red and green signals from the der(1) and der(19) chromosomes, respectively.

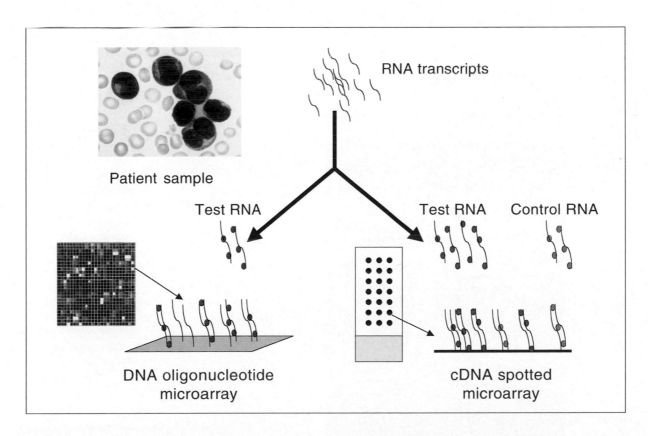

**Figure 20.1** Schematic illustration of microarray technology. For DNA oligonucleotide microarrays, one sample is hybridized per experiment. The detection is accomplished by a fluorescent dye, and results in an absolute expression level for each gene. The oligonucleotides are synthesized in situ onto the array surface. For spotted microarrays, the test RNA is co-hybridized with control RNA. Following detection of the signals, the ratio of differentially tagged test and control RNA is calculated.

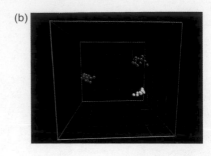

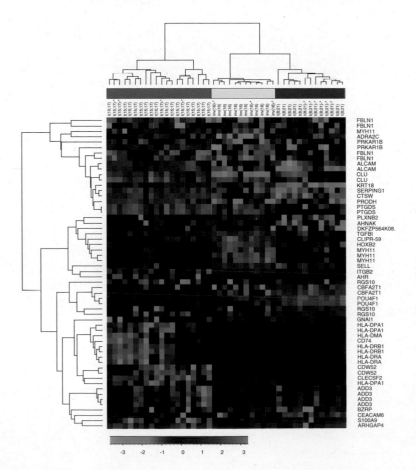

**Figure 20.3** Principal component analysis (PCA) is a classical analysis technique to reduce the dimensionality of the data set. New uncorrelated variables summarize characteristical features of the original data. Two-dimensional hierarchical clustering orders primary expression data. Genes with similar expression patterns are grouped together. Displayed graphically, the relationship amoung genes can be explored intuitively.

**Figure 20.6** Hierarchical clustering based on U133A expression data of 45 AML samples (columns) comprising the subgroups t(15;17) (*n* = 20), t(8;21) (*n* = 13), and inv(16) (*n* = 12) versus 36 informative genes represented by 58 U133A chip design probesets (rows). New patient samples, which were not previously hybridized to U95Av2 microarrays are marked by asterisks. The normalized expression value for each gene is coded by color, with the scale shown at the lower left (standard deviation from mean). Red cells represent high expression and green cells low expression. The previously published set of diagnostic markers is given by respective gene symbols.

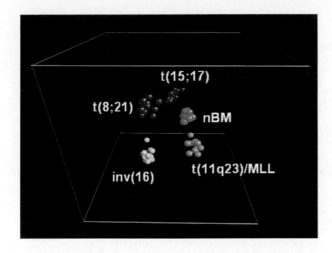

**Figure 20.7** Principal component analysis based on U133A expression data of WHO-classified AML subtypes with recurrent chromosome aberrations and normal bone marrow mononuclear cells from healthy volunteers. Sixty AML samples comprising the color-coded subgroups t(15;17) ($n$ = 20), t(8;21) ($n$ = 13), inv(16) ($n$ = 12), and t(11q34)/*MLL* gene rearrangement-positive samples ($n$ = 15) can be discriminated accurately, and are different from normal bone marrow nBM ($n$ = 9).

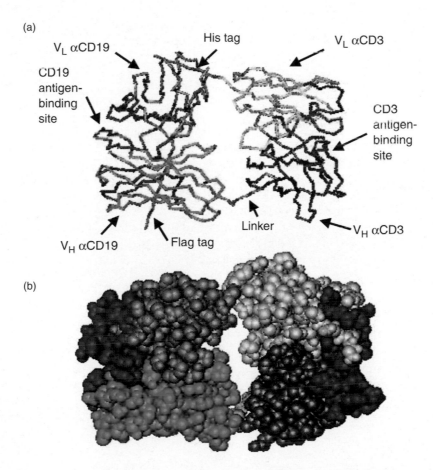

**Figure 25.15** Three-dimensional (3D) structure of a recombinant bispecific single-chain antibody (diabody). An scFv antibody against CD19 was fused by a linker to an scFv against CD3. This diabody construct is highly efficient in activating resting T cells and inducing a CTL response and target cell lysis of CD19+ malignant B cells.[158] (a) Backbone of the peptide chain. (b) Rendering of the 3D surface structure. Green, $V_H$ of the anti-CD19 scFv; purple, $V_L$ of the anti-CD19 scFv; gray, $V_H$ of the anti-CD3 scFv; light blue, $V_L$ of the anti-CD3 scFv; yellow, linker peptide; orange, His tag; darker blue, Flag tag (employed for detection and purification of the recombinant protein).

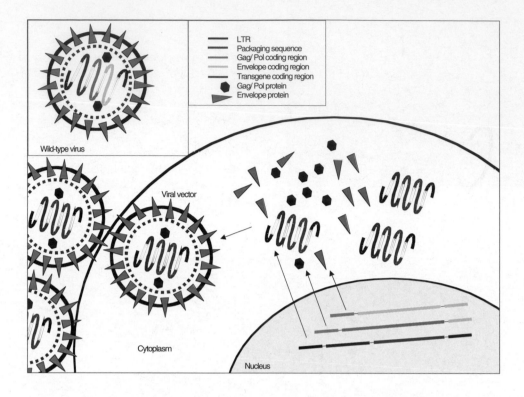

**Figure 28.1** Creation of a replication incompetent retroviral vector with a split packaging cell line. Wild-type retrovirus is shown in inset upper-left corner. Virus is composed of gag/pol and env proteins and a RNA genome. This genome codes for gag/pol and env proteins, hence upon infecting a host cell, all retroviral elements can be generated and virus can replicate. Split packaging line provides coding regions for gag/pol and env elements in trans. Coding region for our transgene (red) is preceded by a packaging signal (blue). Packaging signal has been removed from gag/pol and envelope coding regions. Hence virus is assembled as normal but our transgene replaces usual genome. Upon infecting a cell, our transgene is expressed but no gag/pol or env can be generated, and virus cannot replicate. For replication competent virus to be generated, packaging sequence, gag/pol and env elements would have to coincidentally recombine.

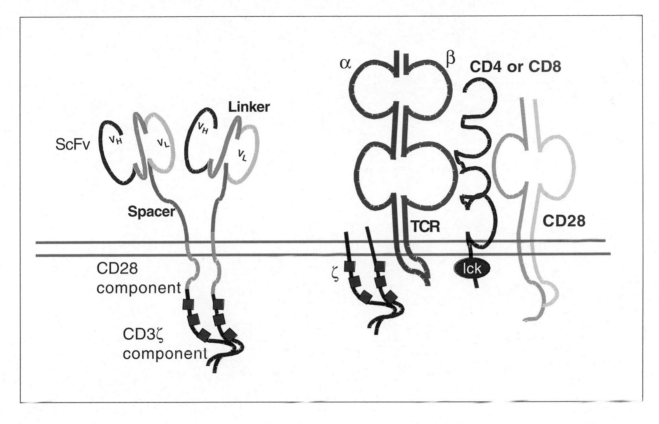

**Figure 20.2** Artificial TCR (dimer) and native TCR. Artificial receptor components can be divided into two groups. External section is involved with antigen recognition. This is usually composed of a Single Chain Variable Fragment (ScFv) derived from a monoclonal antibody. This is connected to the internal section of the receptor via a flexible spacer which allows the receptor multiple orientations. The internal section transmits signal. In this figure we show a signaling domain composed of a fusion of signaling portions of CD28 and CD3ζ. This receptor is capable of transmitting a CD3ζ signal and CD28 co-stimulatory signal upon antigen recognition. Simplicity of artificial receptor is contrasted to the complexity of the native TCR which requires an aggregate of multiple proteins to transmit a similar signal.

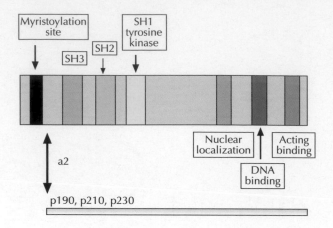

**Figure 41.2** Structure of *ABL*, with its domains.

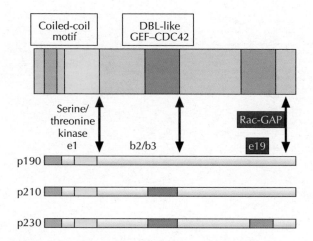

**Figure 41.3** Structure of *BCR*, with its domains.

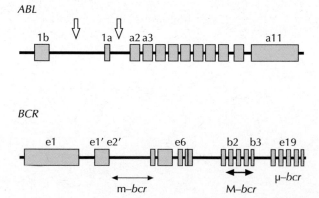

**Figure 41.5** Structure of the *ABL* and *BCR* genes, with their exons and introns.

# 1 The stem cell

**Rob E Ploemacher and Elaine A Dzierzak**

## Introduction

The hematopoietic stem cell (HSC) compartment is composed of primitive cells that maintain blood cell production throughout the lifetime of an individual. In the adult, most of the HSC are located in the bone marrow. They are able to migrate in a highly regulated fashion via the bloodstream between the widely dispersed areas of blood cell formation. The HSC compartment is heterogeneous in various aspects, possibly as a result of different mitotic histories of the individual stem cells. It is generally accepted that the majority of HSC have a very low turnover rate and/or extended $G_1$ cell cycle phase, while potentially possessing considerable capability to both self-renew and differentiate into at least eight hematolymphoid lineages. The activation of cycling activity is probably regulated by stochastic mechanisms.[1,2]

By analogy to the situation in the mouse, the human HSC compartment most likely represents a hierarchy of primitive cells. This is based on their decreasing ability to generate new HSC, decreasing pluripotentiality and proliferative potential, and increasing turnover rate.[3–9] When bone marrow is used for transplantation, its heterogeneity may be reflected in the different time periods that individual stem cell clones contribute to long-term reconstitution of a conditioned host, irrespectively of whether this includes all hematopoietic lineages.[10–15] Because of this heterogeneity, the question may arise as to what one should denote as a 'stem cell'.

## Lifetime conservation of stem cell activity

Many research papers have focused on the topic of HSC 'self-maintenance' and the current high expectations of 'ex vivo expansion of HSC'. Moreover, gene therapy for the hematopoietic system is based on the general acceptance of HSC immortality. However, there is no extensive evidence for unlimited HSC self-renewal, and it should be questioned whether such a cell would not endanger the integrity of life because it has qualities of neoplasia. Secondly, immortality could be interpreted in a semantic manner, so that a future of 50 cell divisions meets conditions of virtual self-maintenance. For example, the recent demonstration that lymphomyeloid-repopulating HSC can expand their numbers more than 300-fold following their transplantation into a conditioned recipient is impressive indeed, but this takes a mere 8–10 cell divisions with full self-renewal.[16] Thirdly, a clear distinction should be made between maintenance of an individual stem cell and that of the HSC population as a whole. The well-known cartoon of an individual stem cell that divides and produces two distinct daughter cells – one remaining 'stem cell' and the other committing itself towards differentiation – may not be commonplace. Rather, one should use operational terms that apply to the whole population and characterize the HSC compartment as a cell population with a probability of self-renewal that approaches 0.5. Alternatively, a population can be structured in a way that it uses a (small) number of cells from a reserve compartment, while the largest part is responsible for the daily supply of differentiated progeny. This structure can be recognized in many tissues. There is ample evidence for a metabolically quiescent HSC population with relatively low turnover that harbors a high proliferative potential and probability to give multilineage offspring. Many observations have suggested that in the steady state, only a few stem cell clones at the same time display clonogenic expansion and contribute to daily blood cell production.[10,11,17–20] In a transplant setting, it has been shown that many different clones contribute to the initial phase of hematopoietic reconstitution. However, within weeks, only a few remain (and some arise in delayed manner) to provide for the body's demand of blood cells over the longer term. In contrast, the work of Harrison and colleagues supports a model wherein HSC function continuously.[15,21] The ultimate self-renewal capacity of a single HSC is unknown, but serial transplantation studies in mice and reports on chromosome telomere shortening in human HSC suggest that human HSC self-replication is limited to around 50 cell divisions.[22] Extinction of individual clones may then feed back into the quiescent HSC compartment and trigger proliferation of other HSC.

## Adult stem cell plasticity

Until recently, HSC have been regarded as being committed, to give rise exclusively to hematopoietic progeny. This concept is now being challenged in a variety of experimental settings, and the available evidence suggests that adult HSC are flexible in their differentiation repertoires and can be reprogrammed, both in vivo and in vitro. Such observations suggest that under certain conditions HSC are able to produce cells with specialized structural and metabolic features of tissues distinct from the bone marrow, such as liver, gastrointestinal tract, pancreas, kidney, skin, skeletal and heart muscle, brain, or adult endothelium. The reprogramming most likely occurs within the organ to which HSC have been transplanted but would not have migrated to under normal conditions. A further prerequisite would be that the specific site should have extensive damage or a deficiency that attracts and stimulates the grafted or migrating stem cells to reprogram and produce adaptations commensurate with their new location.

To date, many studies suggesting stem cell plasticity have not used highly purified HSC, but rather crude bone marrow cell populations. Therefore, not all findings of plasticity may have to be attributed to HSC, but rather mesenchymal stem cells (MSC) or endothelial precursors could be responsible in part for these findings. Indeed, the scientific community has asked for more stringent proof of stem cell plasticity, such as a clonal approach[23] or sustained functional activity.[24] Among the few studies meeting or approaching these criteria is the demonstration that highly purified murine HSC infused into mice with a congenic liver disease (hereditary tyrosinemia type I) contributed not only to the hematopoietic system but to some of the recipient's liver parenchymal cells.[25] More recently, Jiang et al[26] reported that murine bone marrow-derived cells co-purifying with mesenchymal stem cells differentiate at the single-cell level not only into mesenchymal cells but also into cells with visceral mesoderm, neurectoderm, and endoderm characteristics in vitro. On transplantation into a non-irradiated host, these cells – termed multipotent adult progenitor cells (MAPC) – engraft and differentiate into the hematopoietic lineage and in addition into the epithelium of liver, lung, and gut. These MAPC may therefore represent a more primitive precursor of HSC and many other somatic cells.

## Ontogeny of the HSC

The origin of the hematopoietic system is within the mesodermal cell layer of the gastrulating embryo. Once the founding cells are generated within the conceptus, it is thought that these cells migrate and colonize the liver during the fetal stage and subsequently migrate and colonize the bone marrow, where they reside throughout the adult stage.[27] Using the mouse embryo as a model, the earliest observed hematopoietic cells (primitive erythrocytes) are found within the yolk sac blood islands. Both the hematopoietic cells and closely associated endothelial cells of the yolk sac vasculature are thought to arise from a common mesodermal precursor, the hemangioblast.[28] It was recently demonstrated that rigorously selected endothelial cells sorted by flow cytometry from the human yolk sac and embryonic aorta yielded a progeny of myelolymphoid cells in culture, strongly suggesting that HSC may develop directly from endothelium.[29] While other hematopoietic cells and progenitors can be detected shortly thereafter, HSC that are the basis of the adult mouse hematopoietic hierarchy and defined by their adult repopulating properties are not found until midgestation.[30, 31] The first and most active embryonic site involved in HSC generation is the aorta–gonad–mesonephros (AGM) region.[31,32] Extensive studies in many vertebrate species, including mouse and human, strongly support two independent origins of hematopoiesis: an initial wave of transient, embryonic hematopoiesis in the yolk sac and a second wave in which the adult hematopoietic system emerges in the AGM.[33] In the midgestation mouse embryo, the first adult repopulating HSC have been localized to the dorsal aorta[34] and are included in the emergent hematopoietic clusters and endothelium along the ventral aortic wall.[35] Interestingly, some AGM HSC possess surface characteristics of the endothelial lineage,[36] suggesting that some of the cells of the major vasculature are 'hemogenic endothelium' and perhaps act as a specialized type of hemangioblast.[37]

Human embryos have also been studied for the presence of hematopoietic cells in the AGM region. During the fourth week of human ontogeny, hematopoietic clusters emerge from the vascular endothelium of the aorta and vitelline artery.[38] Functional analyses reveal that adult-type, multilineage hematopoietic and presumably adult-repopulating hematopoietic stem cells (some of which exhibit a vascular endothelial phenotype) are present in the aorta and vitelline artery at this time.[38] Moreover, such hemogenic endothelial cells have also been found in the human embryonic liver and fetal bone marrow.[38] These data, taken together with the observation that the number of HSC in the mouse AGM region increases during ex vivo explant culture,[01] suggest that it may be possible to manipulate human HSC growth and expansion in vivo by inducing HSC from non-hematopoietic precursors (fate determination) and/or by expansion of a single founder HSC (proliferation without differentiation). Hence, further studies into the emergence of the first HSC during ontogeny should lead to the identification of the cells and molecules involved in these processes and may result in novel opportunities to induce and/or expand human HSC from fetal and/or adult sources for blood-related therapies.

## Regulation of HSC quiescence and proliferation

It is generally accepted that the bone marrow stromal elements, together with their extracellular matrix molecules, are involved in regulating HSC cycling activity. Many of the cytokines that have been cloned in recent years are actually elaborated and presented by the hematopoietic organ stroma through, for example, membrane-bound glycosaminoglycan species. This local regulation serves to gain specificity and avoid pleiotropic and thus undesired side-effects. In addition, cell adhesion molecules may be directly involved in this regulation, or may contribute to specific interactions between HSC and stromal elements.

The molecular mechanisms regulating cycle activity and facilitating undifferentiated proliferation of HSC are not completely understood, and many cytokines have been shown in recent years to synergize in inducing the proliferation of candidate HSC. These factors may, or may not, have growth factor activity when used alone, and their action may therefore be explained by a series of assumptions, including (a) competence acquisition, i.e. they induce $G_0 \rightarrow G_1$ transition in HSC without being able to drive cells through S phase and $G_2$ to mitosis;[39] (b) induction or upregulation of receptor expression for other cytokines that can activate HSC; (c) downregulation of receptors for negative regulators of HSC; or (d) the downstream targets of receptor–ligand complexes, the transcription molecules, act in concert to affect molecular processes that are essential for regulation. Many small molecules have been proposed to be HSC-specific. However, none has reportedly lived up to its promises thus far. The most studied hematopoietic inhibitors are transforming growth factor β1 (TGF-β1), tumor necrosis factor α (TNF-α), interferon-γ (IFN-γ), and macrophage inflammatory protein 1a (MIP-1α). They are considered pleiotropic factors that may have both stimulatory and inhibitory properties on different cell populations. As an example, TGF-β1 stimulates monocyte cluster formation but at the same time is the most active inhibitor at the stem cell level.[40–44]

Cytokines that are effective in the regulation of HSC proliferation – most likely in a redundant or overlapping fashion and often in synergy – are stem cell factor (SCF, a ligand for the c-Kit receptor), Fms-like tyrosine kinase receptor 3 ligand (Flt3-L), thrombopoietin (Tpo, a ligand for c-Mpl), interleukin-6 (IL-6), IL-11, IL-3, leukemia inhibitory factor (LIF), and granulocyte colony-stimulating factor (G-CSF). The sources of these factors vary and can be autocrine, paracrine (e.g. elaborated by stromal cells in the bone marrow environment, or by T cells or monocytes), or endocrine. The above molecules certainly do not act exclusively on HSC proper, and therefore specificity requires local presentation in context with other signals, possibly cell–cell and cell–extracellular matrix contact mediated by cell adesion molecules (CAM).

In addition to soluble factors elaborated by stromal cells and HSC, there could exist other more intimate levels of regulation of HSC. Rather than exclusively determining HSC sublocalization in the hematopoietic organs, CAM could have direct regulatory effects on HSC. For example, it has been reported that an antibody against LFA-1 inhibits the generation of progenitor cells by a fraction of human HSC in stroma-supported cultures.[45] Maybe the most well-studied CAM interaction is that of c-Kit and its ligand, SCF.[46] SCF is expressed on stromal cells in, for example, the bone marrow, the reproductive organs (Sertoli cells in the testis and follicular cells in the ovary), the skin, and the cerebellum, whereas c-Kit is the SCF receptor expressed on immature cells, including HSC, spermatides, oogonia, and melanocytes.[47–50] Loss of SCF from the stromal cell membrane leads to a pleiotropic phenotype in mice (the Steel phenotype – hence the alternative name for SCF: Steel factor), that includes macrocytic anemia, decreased fertility, and coat color defects. This condition largely develops as a result of a defective stem cell migration during embryogenesis, while the anemia in adult mice cannot be normalized by infusion of the soluble receptor, i.e. SCF. Yet we know that the soluble receptor SCF acts as a survival factor and a growth factor and has potent synergistic activity in vitro.

From embryogenesis it has become evident that genuine cell–cell communication may be even more intimate and involves coupling of intracellular compartments of adjacent cells via gap junctions (GJ). The connexin-43 (Cx43) type GJ can be detected immunohistologically in bone marrow and its expression increases 80–100-fold in murine bone marrow during the neonatal period and shortly after cytoreductive treatment of adult mice during the period when active regeneration is beginning.[51] We have recently reported that functional blocking of all GJ intercellular communication (GJIC) between mutual stromal cells, and stromal cells and hematopoietic cells, in LTC and CAFC cultures (see below) substantially inhibits hematopoietic activity. This inhibition could be fully abrogated by restoring GJIC within the first two weeks of culture.[52] Reintroduction of the

Cx43 gene into Cx43-deficient fetal liver-derived stromal cells was able to restore their diminished intercellular communication as well as their decreased ability to support stem cells in a CAFC culture.[53]

It cannot be excluded that there exist systemic or endocrine signals that regulate or overrule this complex local signaling network if decisive action is required following, for example, blood loss, infection, or cytoreductive therapy.

## Characterization of stem cells

In the last four decades, the description of HSC characteristics has been largely a reflection of the methods, techniques, and hardware that were available to investigators. From these efforts, HSC have emerged as typically small 'blast' cells with a relatively low buoyant density and sedimentation velocity, few and small mitochondria, and a nucleus with several nucleoli and little condensed chromatin. In agreement with these properties, they concentrate in a region of relatively low side and forward light scatter in a flow cytometer. Physical isolation studies using fluorescence-activated cell sorting (FACS) have shown that human HSC express on their surface CD34, c-Kit, IL-6R (brightly), Thy-1, CD45RA and Flt3 (weakly), but not lineage-specific markers, HLA-DR, CD71, CD38, or CD33.

HSC share part of the aforementioned characteristics with other cells, and therefore phenotypical identification and enumeration of HSC is still not truly feasible. In addition, expression of such antigens may depend on the proliferative status of HSC and progenitor cells. A good example of this is the expression of the sialomucin CD34 on progenitor cells, which is extensively used in enumeration, isolation and clinical transplantation of HSC. CD34 is highly expressed on HSC, including cells providing long-term marrow repopulation, and is downregulated as cells differentiate and mature. However, it is not exclusively expressed on hematopoietic progenitor cells but also on vascular endothelial cells[54,55] and some fibroblasts.[56,57] It has been shown that human CD34⁻ cells contained within the bone marrow cell population depleted for cells expressing mature lineage antigens (Lin⁻) could induce long-term repopulation and multilineage differentiation in sheep[58] and murine NOD/SCID[59] xenograft models. As the transplanted cells produced many CD34⁺ stem cells in these in vivo models and little or no clonogenic (CFU-C) or LTC-IC activity was observed in vitro, there is reason to suggest that Lin⁻CD34⁻ cells represent primitive precursors of CD34⁺ cells. Further studies revealed that HSC from the fetus express CD34 at late stages and continue to express it in neonates and adults, but that this expression decreases with aging.[60,61] When older recipients were engrafted with neonatal Lin⁻c-Kit⁺

CD34⁺ cells, containing all HSC activity, the HSC activity shifted to the Lin⁻c-Kit⁺ CD34⁻ bone marrow cell population.[60] Ogawa et al[61] showed that CD34⁻ stem cells from adult bone marrow stimulated in vivo by 5-fluorouracil (5-FU) injection or in vitro by a combination of IL-11 and SCF became CD34⁺. The activated CD34⁺ stem cells reverted to CD34⁻ when the recipients' marrow achieved steady state. The majority of G-CSF-mobilized HSC also were CD34⁺ and reverted to CD34⁻ under steady-state conditions. These observations therefore strongly suggest that the proliferative activity or activation status of HSC determines expression of CD34 by stem cells from fetal, neonatal, and adult mice, and that CD34⁻ HSC are not more primitive than CD34⁺ cells.

The nucleic acid dye Hoechst 33342, which hardly stains the most quiescent HSC, has been extremely helpful in HSC isolation. Similarly useful has been the vital fluorochrome rhodamine-123 (Rh123). Rh123 accumulates in mitochondria and is a substrate of the *MDR1* gene product, the membrane pump P-glycoprotein,[62,63] which is highly expressed in quiescent HSC. For these reasons, primitive HSC hardly stain with Rh123,[64–67] but within the HSC compartment Rh123 retention increases dramatically so that the murine day-12 spleen colony-forming cells are among the brightest Rh123-stained cells in the bone marrow.[64]

Because of their relative quiescence, primitive HSC have been shown to be especially resistant to antimitotic agents (e.g. hydroxyurea and vincristine) and 5-FU,[5,8,66] and this property has been exploited to enrich HSC by exclusion of all other cells.[68] In contrast, the most primitive and in vivo long-term repopulating HSC, as well as CAFC wk5, are extremely sensitive to the alkylating agent busulfan and a number of its derivatives.[69,70] It has been long held that HSC in general represented one of the most radiosensitive cell types in the body, with a $D_0$ of about 0.75 Gy and no sublethal damage (SLD) repair. This notion has resulted from the circumstance that radiation studies were carried out using the CFU-S day 7–9 assay and animal survival as endpoints. However, current views are more in line with the realization that both these methods are a measure of transient repopulating HSC.[6,7,64] The recognition of heterogeneity in the HSC compartment and the development of the CAFC assay allowing the estimation of HSC subset frequencies, and thus radiation survival, has led to a more balanced appraisal of the HSC compartment's radiosensitivity. It is the CFU-S day 7/CAFC day 7–10 population that shows high radiation sensitivity and lack of SLD repair.[71–73] But, with increasing primitivity, CAFC subsets are far more radioresistant and display high levels of SLD repair, matching that of lung tissue.[74] All of the above-mentioned characteristics have emerged from studies on HSC from adult donors and may, or may not, apply to HSC from other developmental stages.

# Measurement of stem cell activity

Because of their low frequencies and lack of truly distinctive physical characteristics, measurements of HSC rely on functional assays. HSC have been defined as cells that have high proliferation potential, are able to self-renew, and give rise to multipotential lineage development. HSC assays commonly use these characteristics as an endpoint. In vivo, spleen colony formation,[75] animal survival, competitive repopulation,[15,21] serial transplantation,[10,76] and engraftment of mice having a congenital immune suppression,[77] anemia,[12,78,79] or polymorphism in an enzyme[69] or cell surface epitope[16,80] have been used to detect HSC and their descendants. In vitro, clonogenic potential[81,82] with particular attention to multipotential or blast colony formation[83] and replating efficiency, short-term liquid (delta) cultures,[84–87] and long-term progenitor cell production on stromal cells[66,88–92] have been employed.

The effectiveness and reliability of such assays depends on many parameters, including (a) HSC seeding efficiency to a specific hematopoietic organ in vivo, (b) knowledge about, and availability of, growth factor combinations that are required to activate the most quiescent HSC to cycle in vitro, (c) insight into the context in which cytokines should be presented to HSC (e.g. bound to stromal cell surfaces or extracellular matrix molecules), (d) knowledge of inhibitors that maintain quiescence of HSC, and methods to neutralize or counteract their activities, (e) the time required to activate the most quiescent HSC, and (f) stochastic mechanisms operating at the HSC level that determine quiescence/cycling ratio, or commitment to specific differentiation lineages. The latter issue clearly demonstrates the limitation of HSC techniques, in that HSC may not always behave according to their ascribed ability for multipotential differentiation and self-renewal capacity. As has been discussed by Lemischka[11] on the basis of extensive transplantation experiments with provirus-marked HSC, analysis of a reconstituted hematopoietic system at a single point in time merely defines a grafted HSC in terms of its minimal differentiation and proliferation potential. Therefore, estimation of HSC self-renewal should preferentially be done by analysis at multiple points in time and transplantation into secondary hosts.

A last matter of concern is the circumstance that human in vitro assays are difficult to validate, so that assumptions have to be made on the basis of single case histories and through extrapolation of the better characterized murine and large animal models.

# Stem cell assays

In the course of time, various assays have been claimed to exclusively detect HSC and even allow their enumeration. It should be realized that a genuine assay should (a) allow frequency assessment independently of the accompanying cells in the sample or of the HSC purity, (b) be validated using in vivo endpoints, and (c) permit indisputable identification of these endpoints. There is perhaps no assay that meets these requirements. The first issue touches on the presence or absence of progenitor cells and bystander cells. As an example, although properly stimulated HSC from various sources may form colonies in semisolid media, such colonies would be outnumbered by progenitor-derived colonies by a factor of $5\times10^2$–$5\times10^5$. These figures are based on the observation that one detects 300–500 colony-forming units in culture (CFU-C) per $10^5$ bone marrow cells (BMC), while primitive HSC have been reported to have a frequency of $10–20/10^5$ BMC, as estimated using LTC-IC week 5 and CAFC week 6 (see below) in stroma-supported long-term cultures,[66,90] or even $1/10^8$, using repopulation of cytokine-treated NOD/SCID mice as an endpoint.[93] In addition, both progenitor cells and accessory cells elaborate cytokines and inhibitors and consequently will affect the outcome of the HSC assay.

The second requirement – one that is underrated and unpopular – is that of proper assay validation. In the past 50 years, it has been proposed that hematopoietic rescue from radiation-inflicted death could be induced by transfusion of body fluids, spleen homogenates, spleen or bone marrow cells, CFU-S (cells that can form hematopoietic nodules in the spleen of an irradiated mouse), or long-term repopulating HSC that have extremely low CFU-S quality. As mentioned above, many types of in vitro methods claim to score 'stem cell quality'. The proof of such statements depends on the acceptance of a stem cell definition and the ability to sort the target cells to high purity and show that the cells comply with the spirit of such a definition.

Thirdly, the most relevant assays for HSC enumeration are those that have a unique endpoint, which is characteristic for HSC, and thus discriminate HSC from accompanying progenitors in the sample. In practice, this includes all assays that detect long-term (multilineage) activity of HSC in vivo or in vitro.

## Long-term cultures

One of these methods is the stroma-dependent long-term culture (LTC) of hematopoietic cells, which is routinely performed in 25 cm² flasks.[88] LTC measures the capacity of a complement of inoculated cells to generate hematopoietic progenitor cells over a number of weeks, typically 5–8 weeks. Progenitor cells can be detected in the non-adherent cell fraction that is weekly harvested during medium changes, and in the adherent layer that can be harvested by trypsinization. The LTC thus gives an insight in the capacity of a graft to produce progenitor cells,[94] while it remains unknown how many HSC and progenitors contribute to it. The latter issue is highly relevant when differences are anticipated in the progenitor cell-generating capacity of HSC, for example on the basis of disease, chemotherapy, or following ex vivo strategies for physical or chemical purging or selection. In order to allow such HSC enumeration, limiting dilution-type miniaturized LTC have been reported that use either CFU-C production (LTC-initiating cells, LTC-IC)[90] or stroma-associated clone formation (cobblestone area-forming cells, CAFC)[8,66,95] as an endpoint for frequency calculation.

The CAFC assay is assumed to detect frequencies of the various HSC subsets with 'transient repopulating' and/or 'long-term repopulating' properties and has been developed as an extrapolation from the murine CAFC assay.[8,9] Extensive studies using physically sorted BMC have allowed regression analysis on the applicability of the murine CAFC assay as an in vitro equivalent of in vivo assays for a series of HSC subsets. These studies have indicated that, both in vivo and in vitro, early developing, short-lived clones are initiated by the transient repopulating spleen colony-forming cells (CFU-S day 12), whereas later-developing and more permanent clones are descendants of more primitive, so-called long-term repopulating, HSC, that induce stable chimerism for more than a year.[8,9,12,13] There is increasing evidence that the human CAFC assay may also detect transiently and long-term repopulating normal and leukemic stem cell subsets.[96–101] A good correlation has been found between CAFC week 7 and cells that repopulate SCID-hu mouse bone implants 8 weeks post engraftment using human mobilized peripheral blood Thy-1$^+$CD34$^+$Lin$^-$ cells.[102] In addition, early detectable CAFC have the characteristics of the more differentiated and transiently repopulating HSC (5-FU-sensitive, CD34$^{medium}$, CD38$^{medium/high}$, HLA-DR$^{high}$), whereas late CAFC meet the phenotype routinely employed for primitive HSC (5-FU-resistant, CD34$^{high}$, CD38$^{negative/medium}$, HLA-DR$^{low/dim}$).[66]

Both the flask LTC and the CAFC assay propagate successive clonal amplification of HSC subsets at their own expense.[103,104] This property renders the CAFC assay useful in assessing the full hematopoietic potential of a marrow specimen in a relatively short period, and in presenting a quantitative cross-section of the heterogeneous stem cell compartment.

Extended stroma-dependent LTC (ELTC; 8–14 weeks) have been described[105] that appear to reveal an even more primitive human HSC population than that detected in regular LTC (5 weeks) and CAFC (6–8 weeks) assays. ELTC-initiating cells (ELTC-IC) differ from LTC-IC in several respects. Firstly, ELTC-IC produce most CFU-C after 60 days, whereas LTC-IC do so before. Currently, it is not clear whether these differences are realistic or merely result from the use of different stromal support layers, cytokine combinations, sera, or the serial replating required for the ELTC. Secondly, in contrast to LTC-IC, which show a high level of gene marking,[93,105] only about 1% of ELTC-IC can be transduced. The latter characteristic is reminiscent of the low transduction efficiency of long-term repopulating cells in human clinical gene therapy trials and most large-animal models.[63,106–109] Finally, ELTC-IC are exclusively found in the CD38$^-$ fraction of CD34$^+$ cells, as are human SCID-repopulating cells (SRC).[93] In contrast, part of LTC-IC and CAFC week 6 are CD38$^{medium}$ (unpublished observations).

## SCID mouse assay

The propagation of human hematopoietic progenitors in mice with a severe combined immune deficiency syndrome (SCID) has dramatically extended our insight into the repopulating abilities and frequencies of primitive human HSC.[77,93,110–112] Grafted human HSC proliferate in SCID mice and differentiate in the murine bone marrow, producing large numbers of LTC-IC, CFU-C, immature CD34$^+$Thy1$^+$ and CD34$^+$CD38$^-$ cells, as well as mature myeloid and erythroid cells. Relatively large numbers of lymphoid cells are produced in the bone marrow, and the human engraftment of the murine thymus and spleen is almost exclusively lymphoid. Reported frequencies of the primitive cells that initiate the graft in sublethally irradiated NOD/SCID mice, the SCID-repopulating cells (SRC), are extremely low: there is about 1 human SRC in 10$^6$ umbilical cord blood (UCB) cells, 1 in 3×10$^6$ mobilized normal BMC and only 1 in 6×10$^6$ peripheral blood (PB) cells.[113,114] These frequencies are far lower than estimated by the LTC-IC and CAFC assays: average CAFC week 8 numbers in all of these specimens are between 1 and 10 per 10$^5$ nucleated cells. We have found that these low apparent HSC frequencies result mainly from extremely low seeding efficiencies of the human HSC in these mice. Indeed, of all infused CAFC subtypes, only 1–5% could be retrieved from the whole NOD/SCID bone marrow within 24 hours following lethal conditioning and cell infusion.[115] In support of these data were our previous observations in SCID mice, which showed a 5–10-fold higher engraftment with human AML cells following pretreatment of the recipients with macrophage-depleting Cl$_2$MDP liposomes.[97] In light of these data, the human HSC frequencies are apparently far higher than those of the reported SRC. A correction with a factor 20–100 thus leads to comparable frequencies of SRC and CAFC/LTC-IC. Different growth requirements of these cells may also affect the apparent frequencies in NOD/SCID mice. UCB cells grow spontaneously in SCID mice, but PB and BM stem cells need continuous cytokine support following their transplantation.

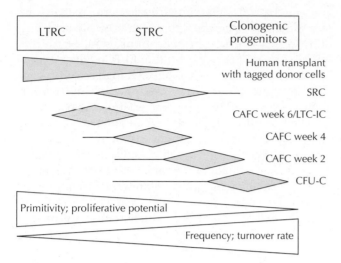

**Figure 1.1** Schematic diagram of the hierarchy in the hematopoietic stem/progenitor cell compartment. Functionally defined assays have been ordered here on the basis of the primitivity of the endpoint detected. LTRC (STRC), long-term (short-term) repopulating cells in vivo; SRC, NOD/SCID mouse repopulating cell; CAFC, cobblestone area-forming cell; LTC-IC, long-term culture-initiating cell; CFU-C, colony-forming unit in culture. Note that these populations probably represent a continuous array of stem cell subsets, differing in mitotic history, that are either able to establish stable chimerism in vivo (LTRC), or induce short-term (1–3 months) hematopoietic repopulation (STRC), or merely give rise to size-restricted clones (clonogenic progenitors).

As opposed to LTC-IC, SRC have been reported to show low transfection efficiencies.[93] Again, seeding of the SRC in vivo could play a role in this observation. It has been shown that cycling CFU-S show a 50% decreased splenic seeding,[116] and a similar loss in seeding and repopulating ability has been demonstrated to be induced by incubations as short as 3 hours.[117] As stable gene integration requires cycling of HSC in a transfection protocol, it is conceivable that transfected cells are preferentially sequestrated following their in vivo transplantation.

The tentative position of the progenitor subsets, as detected by the assays described here, is shown in Figure 1.1.

# Ex vivo expansion of stem cells

The enrichment and in vivo expansion of HSC using a variety of techniques and cytokine cocktails have created novel areas of applied research. The possible therapeutic applications for primitive HSC are many and varied. HSC and progenitor cells have become attractive vehicles for administering certain genes therapeutically, including genes to treat metabolic disorders, inherited immune and hematological diseases, and acquired immune deficiency syndromes. Yet, although experimental data on efficient gene transfer and long-term gene expression in mice have boosted expectations for clinical application of gene therapy, the human data have been extremely disappointing. Low transduction rates of hematopoietic cells, limited lineage expression, and diminishing numbers of transduced cells observed after transplantation have necessitated additional basic research.

With the increasing information on the number, quality, and characteristics of HSC in umbilical cord and placental blood, this material has been found to be efficacious as an alternative source of HSC for transplantation in children.[118] Transplants with UCB have utilized about 10-fold smaller numbers of nucleated cells than comparable transplants with BMC. However, it is held that UCB contains a greater proportion of progenitors than BM and that their proliferative capacity as determined by colony replating, stroma-supported growth in LTC, and SCID mouse engraftment is high.[93,112,119–121] These data suggest that a single UCB collection should suffice for repopulation of the hematopoietic system of an adult. Such transplants in adults have shown long postgrafting intervals to platelet and neutrophil recovery. Although this could have resulted from the transfusion of too few primitive HSC, an alternative explanation could be merely that the number of transient repopulating HSC and progenitors is limited in UCB grafts. These observations therefore present a rationale for the growing number of studies in which ex vivo 'expansion' of true HSC and transient repopulating progenitor cells is investigated. Although impressive increases in CD34+ cells and progenitor cells have been reported, there have been limited reports on net increases in the LTC-IC and CAFC week 6–8 content of cultures initiated with BM stem cells or mobilized stem cells from leukapheresis products (PBSC).[101,122–125] Thus, while modest numerical HSC expansion seems possible in short-term liquid cultures, we have documented a concomitant dramatic loss of the ability of individual HSC to generate progeny if the cells are propagated in the absence of stromal cell layers and Flt3-L.[101,126–128]

It remains unclear why various investigators report different successes in expanding HSC even though often similar cytokine species and concentrations are included and culture periods are comparable. Such cultures generally contain IL-3, SCF, and IL-6, and in addition often a variety of cytokines such as G-CSF granulocyte–macrophage CSF (GM-CSF), and erythropoietin. Likely, undefined factors, including serum batches and medium ingredients, may have profound effects on the results. In addition, the roles of stromal cells, or stroma-conditioned media, and the design of the ex vivo culture vessel (static versus flow-through reactors), have been demonstrated to be of importance.

More recently, it has been reported that umbilical cord stem cells capable of repopulating NOD/SCID mice could be 2–4-fold expanded in 4-day liquid cultures.[129] In 10–12-week cultures, up to a 1000-fold expansion of human stem cells measured as CAFC week 6 was observed on stromal cell lines generated from murine midgestational AGM regions[130,131] in the presence of at least exogenous Tpo.[132] An extraordinary finding has been that HSC from umbilical cord and placental blood can be maintained and expanded for over 20 weeks ex vivo, with a total calculated 200 000-fold numerical expansion of LTC-IC if they were exposed only to Flt3-L and Tpo.[133] During that extended culture period, the HSC still maintained the capacity to differentiate into various lineages, including the B- and T-lymphocytic lineages. However, at present, there is insufficient reproducible evidence that a net increase in long-term in vivo repopulating HSC can be achieved by short-term bulk culture of a graft. Such evidence should come from the demonstration that ex vivo expanded stem cells still possess their long-term in vivo repopulating ability in immune-deficient mice or, better, in a human transplantation setting. In addition, we do not know how ex vivo propagation will affect the behavior of HSC in the recipient, including their post-transplantation homing to hematopoietic organs or in the aging process. The identification of more primitive precursors of hematopoietic stem cells[26] that proliferate extensively ex vivo without obvious senescence or loss of differentiation potential holds promise for an ideal source of stem cells for clinical use.

## REFERENCES

1. Korn AP, Henkelman RM, Ottensmayer FP et al. Investigations of a stochastic model of haematopoiesis. *Exp Hematol* 1973; **1**: 362–75.

2. Nakahata T, Gross AF, Ogawa M. A stochastic model of the primitive hemopoietic stem cells in culture. *J Cell Physiol* 1982; **113**: 455–8.

3. Rosendaal M, Hodgson GS, Bradley TR. Organization of hemopoietic stem cells: The generation-age hypothesis. *Cell Tissue Kinet* 1979; **12**: 17–29.

4. Mauch P, Greenberger JS, Botnick L. Evidence for structured variation in self-renewal capacity within long-term bone marrow cultures. *Proc Natl Acad Sci USA* 1980; **77**: 2927–30.

5. Hodgson GS, Bradley TR. In vivo kinetic status of hematopoietic stem and progenitor cells as inferred from labeling with bromodeoxyuridine. *Exp Hematol* 1984; **12**: 683–7.

6. Ploemacher RE, Brons NHC. Separation of CFU-S from primitive cells responsible for reconstitution of the bone marrow hemopoietic stem cell compartment following irradiation: evidence for a pre-CFU-S cell. *Exp Hematol* 1989; **17**: 263–6.

7. Ploemacher RE, Brons NHC. In vivo proliferative and differential properties of murine bone marrow cells separated on the basis of rhodamine-123 retention. *Exp Hematol* 1989; **16**: 903–7.

8. Ploemacher RE, Van der Sluijs JP, Van Beurden CAJ et al. Use of limiting dilution type long-term marrow cultures in frequency analysis of marrow-repopulating and spleen colony-forming hematopoietic stem cells in the mouse. *Blood* 1991; **78**: 2527–33.

9. Ploemacher RE, Van der Loo JCM, Van Beurden CAJ et al. Wheat germ agglutinin affinity of murine hemopoietic stem cell subpopulations is an inverse function of their long-term repopulating ability in vitro and in vivo. *Leukemia* 1993; **7**: 120–30.

10. Lemischka IR, Raulet DH, Mulligan RC. Developmental potential and dynamic behavior of hematopoietic stem cells. *Cell* 1986; **45**: 917–27.

11. Lemischka IR. What we have learned from retroviral marking of hematopoietic stem cells. In: Muller-Sieburg C, Torok-Storb B, Visser J, Storb R (eds) *Current Topics in Microbiology and Immunology*, Vol 177. *Hematopoietic Stem Cells*. Heidelberg: Springer-Verlag, 1992: 59–71.

12. Van der Loo JCM, Van den Bos C, Baert MRM et al. Stable multilineage hematopoiesis chimerism in alpha-thalassemic mice induced by a bone marrow subpopulation that excludes the majority of day-12 spleen colony-forming units. *Blood* 1994; **83**: 1769–77.

13. Ploemacher RE. Cobblestone area forming cell (CAFC) assay. In: Freshney RI, Pragnell IB, Freshney MG (eds) *Culture of Specialised Cells*, Vol 2. *Culture of Haemopoietic Cells*. New York: Wiley-Liss, 1994: 1–21.

14. Capel B, Hawley RG, Mintz B. Long- and short-lived murine hematopoietic stem cell clones individually identified with retroviral integration markers. *Blood* 1990; **75**: 2267–70.

15. Harrison DE. Evaluating functional abilities of primitive hematopoietic stem cell populations. In: Muller-Sieburg C, Torok-Storb B, Visser J, Storb R (eds) *Current Topics in Microbiology and Immunology*, Vol 177. *Hematopoietic Stem Cells*. Heidelberg: Springer-Verlag, 1992: 13–30.

16. Pawliuk R, Eaves C, Humphries RK. Evidence of both ontogeny and transplant dose-regulated expansion of hematopoietic stem cells in vivo. *Blood* 1996; **88**: 2852–8.

17. Snodgrass R, Keller G. Clonal fluctuation within the hematopoietic system in mice reconstituted with retrovirus-infected cells. *EMBO J* 1987; **6**: 3955–60.

18. Capel B, Hawley R, Covarrubias L et al. Clonal contributions of small numbers of retrovirally marked hematopoietic stem cells engrafted in unirradiated neonatal W/Wv mice. *Proc Natl Acad Sci USA* 1989; **86**: 4564–8.

19. Jordan CT, Lemischka IR. Clonal and systemic analysis of long-term hematopoiesis in the mouse. *Genes Devel* 1990; **4**: 220–32.

20. Abkovitz JL, Linenberger ML, Newton MA et al. Evidence for the maintenance of hematopoiesis in a large animal by the sequential activation of stem-cell clones. *Proc Natl Acad Sci USA* 1990; **87**: 9062–6.

21. Harrison DE, Astle CM, Lerner C. Number and continuous proliferation pattern of transplanted primitive immunohemopoietic stem cells. *Proc Natl Acad Sci USA* 1988; **85**: 822–6.

22. Vaziri H, Dragowska W, Allsopp RC et al. Evidence for a

mitotic clock in humann hematopoietic stem cells: loss of telomeric DNA with age. *Proc Natl Acad Sci USA* 1994; **91**: 9857–60.

23. Lemischka I. The power of stem cells reconsidered? *Proc Natl Acad Sci USA* 1999; **96**: 14193–5.

24. Anderson DJ, Gage FH, Weissman IL. Can stem cells cross lineage boundaries? *Nat Med* 2001; **7**: 393–5.

25. Lagasse E, Connors H, Al-Dhalimy M et al. Purified hematopoietic stem cells can differentiate into hepatocytes in vivo. *Nat Med* 2000; **6**: 1229–34.

26. Jiang Y, Jahagirdar BN, Reinhardt RL et al. Pluripotency of mesenchymal stem cells derived from adult marrow. *Nature* 2002; **418**: 41–9.

27. Moore MA, Metcalf D. Ontogeny of the haemopoietic system: yolk sac origin of in vivo and in vitro colony forming cells in the developing mouse embryo. *Br J Haematol* 1970; **18**: 279–96.

28. Murray P. The development in vitro of the blood of the early chick embryo. *Proc Soc Lond* 1932; **11**: 497–521.

29. Oberlin E, Tavian M, Blazsek I, Peault B. Blood-forming potential of vascular endothelium in the human embryo. *Development* 2002; **129**: 4147–57.

30. Muller AM, Medvinsky A, Strouboulis J et al. Development of hematopoietic stem cell activity in the mouse embryo. *Immunity* 1994; **1**: 291–301.

31. Medvinsky A, Dzierzak E. Definitive hematopoiesis is autonomously initiated by the AGM region. *Cell* 1996; **86**: 897–906.

32. Cumano A, Dieterlen-Lievre F, Godin I. Lymphoid potential, probed before circulation in mouse, is restricted to caudal intraembryonic splanchnopleura. *Cell* 1996; **86**: 907–16.

33. Dzierzak E, Medvinsky A, de Bruijn M. Qualitative and quantitative aspects of haemopoietic cell development in the mammalian embryo. *Immunol Today* 1998; **19**: 228–36.

34. de Bruijn MRTR, Speck NA, Peeters MCE, Dzierzak E. Definitive hematopoietic stem cells first develop within the major arterial regions of the mouse embryo. *EMBO J* 2000; **19**: 2465–74.

35. de Bruijn M, Ma X, Robin C et al. HSC localize to the endothelial layer in the midgestation mouse aorta. *Immunity* 2002; **16**: 673–83.

36. North T, de Bruijn M, Stacy T et al. Runx1 expression marks long-term repopulating HSC in the midgestation mouse embryo. *Immunity* 2002; **16**: 661–72.

37. Nishikawa SI, Nishikawa S, Kawamoto H et al. In vitro generation of lymphohematopoietic cells from endothelial cells purified from murine embryos. *Immunity* 1998; **8**: 761–9.

38. Tavian M, Robin C, Coulombel L, Peault B. The human embryo, but not its yolk sac, generates lympho-myeloid stem cells: mapping multipotent hematopoietic cell fate in intraembryonic mesoderm. *Immunity* 2001; **15**: 487–95.

39. Suda T, Suda J, Ogawa M. Proliferative kinetics and differentiation of murine blast cell colonies in culture: evidence for variable $G_0$ periods and constant doubling rates of early pluripotent hemopoietic progenitors. *J Cell Physiol* 1983; **117**: 308–18.

40. Ottmann OG, Pelus LM. Differential proliferative effects of transforming growth factor-β on human hematopoietic progenitor cells. *J Immunol* 1988; **140**: 2661–7.

41. Hampson J, Ponting ILO, Cook N et al. The effects of TGFβ on haemopoietic cells. *Growth Factors* 1989; **1**: 193–202.

42. Hatzfeld J, Li M-L, Brown E et al. Release of early human hematopoietic progenitors from quiescence by antisense transforming growth factor β1 or Rβ oligonucleotides. *J Exp Med* 1991; **174**: 925–9.

43. Ruscetti FW, Dubois C, Falk LA et al. In vivo and in vitro effects of TGF-β1 on normal and neoplastic haemopoiesis. *Ciba Found Symp* 1991; **157**: 212–27.

44. Ploemacher RE, Van Soest PL, Boudewijn A. Autocrine transforming growth factor-β1 blocks colony formation and progenitor cell generation by hemopoietic stem cells stimulated with steel factor. *Stem Cells* 1993; **11**: 336–47.

45. Gunji Y, Nakamura M, Hagiwara T et al. Expression and function of adhesion molecules on human hematopoietic stem cells: CD34+LFA-1− cells are more primitive than CD34+LFA1+ cells. *Blood* 1992; **80**: 429–36.

46. Kodama H, Nose M, Niida S et al. Involvement of the c-kit receptor in the adhesion of hematopoietic stem cells to stromal cells. *Exp Hematol* 1994; **22**: 979–84.

47. Nishikawa S, Kusakabe M, Yoshinaga K. In utero manipulation of coat color formation by a monoclonal anti-c-kit antibody: two distinct waves of c-kit-dependency during melanocyte development. *EMBO J* 1991; **10**: 2111–18.

48. Ogawa M, Nishikawa S, Yoshinaga HS. Expression and function of c-Kit in fetal hemopoietic progenitor cells: transition from the early c-Kit-independent to the late c-Kit-dependent wave of hemopoiesis in the murine embryo. *Development* 1993; **117**: 1089–98.

49. Hirata T, Morii E, Morimoto M et al. Stem cell factor induces outgrowth of c-kit-positive neurites and supports the survival of c-kit-positive neurons in dorsal root ganglia of mouse embryos. *Development* 1993; **119**: 49–56.

50. Packer AI, Hsu YC, Besmer P et al. The ligand of the c-kit receptor promotes oocyte growth. *Devel Biol* 1994; **161**: 194–205.

51. Rosendaal M, Green CR, Rahman A et al. Up-regulation of the connexin43+ gap junction network in haemopoietic tissue before the growth of stem cells. *J Cell Sci* 1994; **107**: 29–37.

52. Rosendaal M, Mayen AEM, De Koning A et al. Does transmembrane communication through gap junctions enable stem cells to overcome stromal inhibition? *Leukemia* 1997; **11**: 1281–9.

53. Cancelas JA, Koevoet WLM, de Koning AE et al. Connexin-43 gap junctions are involved in multi-connexin-expressing stromal support of hemopoietic progenitors and stem cells. *Blood* 2000; **96**: 498–505.

54. Fina L, Molgaard HV, Robertson D et al. Expression of the CD34 gene in vascular endothelial cells. *Blood* 1990; **75**: 2417–26.

55. Baumhueter S, Dybdal N, Kyle C et al. Global vascular expression of murine CD34, a sialomucin-like endothelial ligand for L-selectin. *Blood* 1994; **84**: 2554–65.

56. Brown J, Greaves MF, Molgaard HV. The gene encoding the stem cell antigen, CD34, is conserved in mouse and expressed in haemopoietic progenitor cell lines, brain, and embryonic fibroblasts. *Int Immunol* 1991; **3**: 175–84.

57. Greaves MF, Brown J, Molgaard HV et al. Molecular features of CD34: a hemopoietic progenitor cell-associated molecule. *Leukemia* 1992; **6** (Suppl 1): 31–6.

58. Zanjani ED, Almeida-Porada G, Livingston AG et al. Human bone marrow CD34− cells engraft in vivo and undergo multilineage expression that includes giving rise to CD34+ cells. *Exp Hematol* 1998; **26**: 353–60.

59. Bhatia M, Bonnet D, Murdoch B et al. A newly discovered

class of human hematopoietic cells with SCID-repopulating activity. *Nat Med* 1998; **4**: 1038–45.

60. Matsuoka S, Ebihara Y, Xu M et al. CD34 expression on long-term repopulating hematopoietic stem cells changes during developmental stages. *Blood* 2001; **97**: 419–25.

61. Ogawa M, Tajima F, Ito T et al. CD34 expression by murine hematopoietic stem cells. Developmental changes and kinetic alterations. *Ann NY Acad Sci* 2001; **938**: 139–45.

62. Chaudhari PM, Roninson IB. Expression and activity of P-glycoprotein, a multidrug efflux pump, in human hematopoietic stem cells. *Cell* 1991; **66**: 748–55.

63. Fruehauf S, Breems DA, Knaan-Shanzer S et al. Frequency analysis of multidrug resistance-1 gene transfer into human primitive hemopoietic progenitor cells using the cobblestone area forming cell assay and detection of vector-mediated P-glycoprotein expression by rhodamine-123. *Hum Gene Ther* 1996; **7**: 1219–31.

64. Ploemacher RE, Brons NHC. Cells with marrow and spleen repopulating ability and forming spleen colonies on day 16, 12, and 8 are sequentially ordered on the basis of increasing rhodamine 123 retention. *J Cell Physiol* 1988; **136**: 531–6.

65. Craig W, Kay R, Cutler R et al. Expression of Thy-1 on human hematopoietic progenitor cells. *J Exp Med* 1993; **177**: 1331–42.

66. Breems DA, Blokland EAW, Neben S et al. Frequency analysis of human primitive haematopoietic stem cell subsets using a cobblestone area forming cell assay. *Leukemia* 1994; **8**: 1095–104.

67. Leemhuis T, Yoder MC, Grigsby S et al. Isolation of primitive human bone marrow hematopoietic progenitor cells using Hoechst 33342 and Rhodamine 123. *Exp Hematol* 1996; **24**: 1215–24.

68. Berardi AC, Wang A, Levine JD et al. Functional isolation and characterization of human hematopoietic stem cells. *Science* 1995; **267**: 104–8.

69. Down JD, Ploemacher RE. Transient and permanent engraftment potential of murine hemopoietic stem cell subsets: differential effects of host conditioning with gamma radiation and cytotoxic drugs. *Exp Hematol* 1993; **21**: 913–21.

70. Down JD, Boudewijn A, Dillingh JH et al. Relationships between ablation of distinct haematopoietic subsets and the development of donor bone marrow engraftment following recipient pretreatment with different alkylating drugs. *Br J Cancer* 1994; **70**: 611–16.

71. Meijne EIM, Van der Winden-Van Groenenwegen AJM. The effects of X-irradiation on hematopoietic stem cell compartments in the mouse. *Exp Hematol* 1991; **19**: 617–23.

72. Meijne EIM, Ploemacher RE, Vos O et al. The effects of graded doses of 1 MeV fission neutrons or X-rays on the murine hematopoietic stroma. *Radiat Res* 1992; **31**: 302–8.

73. Ploemacher RE, Van Os R, Van Beurden CAJ et al. Murine hemopoietic stem cells with long term engraftment and marrow repopulating ability are more resistant to gamma radiation than are spleen colony forming cells. *Int J Radiat Biol* 1992; **61**: 489–99.

74. Down JD, Boudewijn A, Van Os R et al. Variations in radiation dose-survival among different bone marrow hemopoietic cell subsets following fractionated irradiation. *Blood* 1995; **86**: 122–7.

75. Till JE, McCulloch EA. A direct measurement of the radiation sensitivity of normal mouse bone marrow cells. *Radiat Res* 1961; **14**: 213–22.

76. Spangrude G, Brooks DM, Tumas DB. Long-term repopulation of irradiated mice with limiting numbers of purified hematopoietic stem cells: in vivo expansion of stem cell phenotype but not function. *Blood* 1995; **85**: 1006–16.

77. Lapidot T, Pflumio F, Doedens M et al. Cytokine stimulation of multilineage hematopoiesis from immature human cells engrafted in scid mice. *Science* 1992; **255**: 1137–41.

78. Boggs DR, Bogs SS, Saxe DF et al. Hematopoietic stem cells with high proliferative potential. Assay of their concentration in marrow by the frequency and duration of cure of W/Wv mice. *J Clin Invest* 1982; **70**: 242–53.

79. Van den Bos C, Kieboom D, Van der Sluijs JP et al. Selective advantage of normal erythrocyte production after bone marrow transplantation of alpha-thalassemic mice. *Exp Hematol* 1994; **22**: 441–6.

80. Szilvassy SJ, Lansdorp PM, Humphries RK et al. Isolation in a single step of a highly enriched murine hematopoietic stem cell population with competitive long-term repopulating ability. *Blood* 1989; **74**: 930–9.

81. Pluznik DH, Sachs L. The cloning of normal 'mast' cells in tissue culture. *J Cell Physiol* 1965; **66**: 319–24.

82. Bradley TR, Metcalf D. The growth of mouse bone marrow cells in vitro. *Austr J Exp Biol Med Sci* 1966; **44**: 287–99.

83. Tsuji K, Zsebo KM, Ogawa M. Enhancement of murine blast cell colony formation in culture by recombinant stem cell factor (rrSCF), ligand for c-kit. *Blood* 1991; **78**: 1223–9.

84. Muench MO, Moore MA. Accelerated recovery of peripheral blood cell counts in mice transplanted with in vitro cytokine-expanded hematopoietic progenitors. *Exp Hematol* 1992; **20**: 611–18.

85. Moore MAS, Hoskins I. Ex vivo expansion of cord blood-derived stem cells and progenitors. *Blood Cells* 1994; **20**: 468–81.

86. Srour EF, Bregni M, Traycoff CM et al. Long-term hematopoietic culture-initiating cells are more abundant in mobilized peripheral blood grafts than in bone marrow but have a more limited ex vivo expansion potential. *Blood Cells Mol Dise* 1996; **22**: 68–81.

87. Petzer AL, Zandstra PW, Piret JM et al. Differential cytokine effects on primitive (CD34$^+$CD38$^-$) human hematopoietic cells: novel responses to Flt3-ligand and thrombopoietin. *J Exp Med* 1996; **183**: 2551–8.

88. Dexter TM, Allen TD, Lajhta LG. Condition controlling the proliferation of haemopoietic stem cells in vitro. *J Cell Physiol* 1977; **91**: 335–42.

89. Gartner S, Kaplan HS. Long-term culture of human bone marrow cells. *Proc Natl Acad Sci USA* 1980; **77**: 4756–9.

90. Sutherland HJ, Lansdorp PM, Henkelman DH et al. Functional characterization of individual human hematopoietic stem cells cultured at limiting dilution on supportive marrow stromal layers. *Proc Natl Acad Sci USA* 1990; **87**: 3584–8.

91. Sutherland HJ, Eaves CJ, Lansdorp PM et al. Differential regulation of primitive human hematopoietic cells in long-term cultures maintained on genetically engineered murine stromal cells. *Blood* 1991; **78**: 666–72.

92. Sutherland HJ, Eaves CJ, Lansdorp PM et al. Kinetics of committed and primitive blood progenitor mobilization after chemotherapy and growth factor treatment and their use in autotransplants. *Blood* 1994; **83**: 3808–14.

93. Larochelle A, Vormoor J, Hanenberg H et al. Identification of primitive human hematopoietic cells capable of repopulating NOD/SCID mouse bone marrow: implications for gene therapy. *Nat Med* 1996; **2**: 1329–37.

94. Van Hennik PB, Breems DA, Kusadasi N et al. Stroma-supported progenitor production as prognostic tool for graft failure following autologous stem cell transplantation. *Br J Haematol* 2000; **111**: 674–84.

95. Pettengell R, Luft T, Henschler R. Direct comparison by limiting dilution analysis of long-term culture-initiating cells in human bone marrow, umbilical cord blood, and blood stem cells. *Blood* 1994; **84**: 3653–9.

96. Winton EF, Colenda KW. Use of long-term human marrow cultures to demonstrate progenitor cell precursors in marrow treated with 4-hydroperoxycyclophosphamide. *Exp Hematol* 1987; **15**: 710–14.

97. Terpstra W, Ploemacher RE, Prins A et al. Fluorouracil spares AML cells with long term abilities in immunodeficient mice and in stromal culture. *Blood* 1996; **88**: 1944–50.

98. Terpstra W, Prins A, Ploemacher RE et al. Long term leukemia initiating capacity of a CD34 negative subpopulation of acute myeloid leukemia. *Blood* 1996; **87**: 2187–94.

99. Cornelissen JJ, Wognum AW, Ploemacher RE et al. Efficient long-term maintenance of chronic myeloid leukemic cobblestone area forming cells on a murine stromal cell line. *Leukemia* 1997; **11**: 126–33.

100. Breems DA, van Hennik PB, Kusadasi N et al. Individual stem cell quality in leukapheresis product is related to the number of mobilized stem cells as determined using long-term culture and cobblestone area forming cell assays. *Blood* 1996; **87**: 5370–8.

101. Breems DA, Blokland EAW, Ploemacher RE. Stroma-conditioned media improve expansion of human primitive hematopoietic stem cells and progenitors. *Leukemia* 1997; **11**: 142–50.

102. Murray L, Chen B, Galy A et al. Enrichment of human hematopoietic stem cell activity in the CD34⁺ Thy⁺Lin⁻ subpopulation from mobilized peripheral blood. *Blood* 1995; **85**: 368–78.

103. Fraser CC, Eaves CJ, Szilvassy SJ et al. Expansion in vitro of retrovirally marked totipotent hematopoietic stem cells. *Blood* 1990; **76**: 1071–6.

104. Van der Sluijs JP, Van den Bos C, Baert MRM et al. Loss of long-term repopulating ability in long-term bone marrow culture. *Leukemia* 1993; **7**: 725–32.

105. Hao Q-L, Thiemann FT, Petersen et al. Extended long-term culture reveals a highly quiescent and primitive human hematopoietic progenitor population. *Blood* 1996; **88**: 3306–13.

106. Dunbar CE, Cuttler-Fox M, O'Shaughnessy JA et al. Retrovirally marked CD34-enriched peripheral blood and bone marrow cells contribute to long-term engraftment after autologous transplantation. *Blood* 1995; **85**: 3048–57.

107. Hoogerbrugge PM, van Beusechem VW, Fischer A et al. Bone marrow gene transfer in three patients with adenosine deaminase deficiency. *Gene Ther* 1996; **3**: 179–83.

108. Kohn DB, Weinber KI, Nolta JA et al. Engraftment of gene-modified umbilical cord blood cells in neonates with adenosine deaminase deficiency. *Nat Med* 1995; **1**: 1017–23.

109. Bordignon C, Notarangelo L, Nobili N. Gene therapy in peripheral blood lymphocytes and bone marrow for ADA-immunodeficient patients. *Science* 1995; **270**: 470–5.

110. Baum CM, Weissman CL, Tsukamoto AS et al. Isolation of a candidate human hematopoietic stem-cell population. *Proc Natl Acad Sci USA* 1992; **89**: 2804–8.

111. Nolta JA, Hanley MB, Kohn DB. Sustained human hematopoiesis in immunodeficient mice by cotransplantation of marrow stroma expressing human interleukin-3: analysis of gene transduction of long-lived progenitors. *Blood* 1994; **83**: 3041–51.

112. Vormoor J, Lapidot T, Pflumio F et al. Immature human cord blood progenitors engraft and proliferate to high levels in immune-deficient SCID mice. *Blood* 1994; **83**: 2489–97.

113. Dick J. Normal and leukemic human stem cells assayed in SCID mice. *Semin Immunol* 1996; **8**: 197–206.

114. Gan OI, Murdoch B, Larochelle A et al. Differential maintenance of primitive human SCID-repopulating cells, clonogenic progenitors, and long-term culture-initiating cells after incubation on human bone marrow stromal cells. *Blood* 1997; **90**: 641–50.

115. Van Hennik PB, de Koning A, Ploemacher RE. Seeding efficiency of primitive human hematopoietic cells in nonobese diabetic/severe combined immune deficiency mice: implications for stem cell frequency assessment. *Blood* 1999; **94**: 3055–61.

116. Monette FC, DeMello JB. The relationship between stem cell seeding efficiency and position in cell cycle. *Cell Tissue Kinet* 1979; **12**: 161–75.

117. Van der Loo JCM, Ploemacher RE. Marrow and spleen seeding efficiencies of all murine hematopoietic stem cell subsets are decreased by preincubation with hematopoietic growth factors. *Blood* 1995; **85**: 2598–606.

118. Broxmeyer HE, Lu L, Gaddy J et al. Human umbilical cord blood transplantation: the immunology, expansion, and therapeutic applications of hematopoietic stem and progenitor cells. In: Levitt D, Mertelsmann R (eds) *Hematopoietic Stem Cells, Biology and Therapeutic Applications*. New York: Marcel Dekker, 1995: 297–317.

119. Broxmeyer HE, Hangoc G, Cooper S et al. Growth characteristics and expansion of human umbilical cord blood and estimation of its potential for transplantation in adults. *Proc Natl Acad Sci USA* 1992; **89**: 4109–13.

120. Hows JM, Bradley BA, Marsh JCW et al. Growth of human umbilical cord blood in long term haematopoietic cultures. *Lancet* 1992; **340**: 73–6.

121. Lansdorp PM, Dragowska W, Mayani H. Ontogeny-related changes in proliferative potential of human hematopoietic cells. *J Exp Med* 1993; **178**: 787–91.

122. Koller MR, Emerson SG, Palsson BO. Large-scale expansion of human stem and progenitor cells from bone marrow mononuclear cells in continuous perfusion cultures. *Blood* 1993; **82**: 378–84.

123. Zandstra PW, Eaves CJ, Piret JM. Expansion of hematopoietic progenitor cell populations in stirred suspension bioreactors of normal human bone marrow cells. *BioTechnology* 1994; **12**: 909–14.

124. Traycoff CM, Kosak ST, Grigsby S et al. Evaluation of ex vivo expansion potential of cord blood and bone marrow hematopoietic progenitor cells using cell tracking and limiting dilution analysis. *Blood* 1995; **85**: 2059–68.

125. Petzer AL, Hogge DE, Lansdorp PM et al. Self-renewal of primitive human hematopoietic cells (long-term-culture-initiating cells) in vitro and their expansion in defined medium. *Proc Natl Acad Sci USA* 1996; **93**: 1470–4.

126. Breems DA, Blokland EAW, Siebel KE et al. Stroma-contact prevents the loss of hematopoietic stem cell quality during ex vivo expansion of CD34-positive mobilized peripheral blood stem cells. *Blood* 1998; **91**: 111–17.

127. Kusadasi N, Van Soest PL, Ploemacher RE. Successful ex vivo maintenance and expansion of NOD/SCID repopulating cells and CAFC week 6 from umbilical cord blood in 2-week cultures. *Leukemia* 2000; **14**: 1944–53.

128. Kusadasi N, Koevoet JLM, Van Soest PL et al. Stromal support augments extended long-term ex vivo expansion of hemopoietic stem/progenitor cells. *Leukemia* 2001; **15**: 1347–58.

129. Bhatia M, Bonnet D, Kapp U et al. Quantitative analysis reveals expansion of human hematopoietic repopulating cells after short-term ex vivo culture. *J Exp Med* 1997; **186**: 619–24.

130. Oostendorp RAJ, Harvey KN, Kusadasi N et al. Stromal cells from mouse aorta-gonad-mesonephros subregions are potent supporters of hematopoietic stem cell activity. *Blood* 2002; **99**: 1183–9.

131. Oostendorp RA, Medvinsky AJ, Kusadasi N et al. Embryonal subregion-derived stromal cell lines from novel temperature-sensitive SV40 T antigen transgenic mice support hematopoiesis. *J Cell Sci* 2002; **115**: 2099–108.

132. Kusadasi N, Oostendorp RAJ, Koevoet WJLM et al. Stromal cells from murine embryonic aorta–gonad–mesonephros region, liver and gut mesentary expand human umbilical cord blood-derived CAFC$_{week6}$ in extended long-term cultures. *Leukemia* 2002; **16**: 1782–90.

133. Piacibello W, Sanavio F, Garetto L et al. Extensive amplification and self-renewal of human primitive hematopoietic stem cells from cord blood. *Blood* 1997; **89**: 2644–53.

# 2 Stem cell plasticity

Balkrishna N Jahagirdar and Catherine M Verfaillie

## Introduction

For many years, it was thought that embryonic stem (ES) cells were the only pluripotent cells[1] and that somatic stem cells found in postnatal life have a differentiation potential that is limited to a single organ system, as the result of a number of specification and commitment steps during development. For instance, hematopoietic stem cells (HSC), which are part of the splanchnic mesoderm, differentiate[2] to the myeloid and lymphoid hematopoietic lineages, but not cell types outside of the hematopoietic system, in the mesoderm or other germ layers. However, several recent reports have challenged this concept: at least 30 reports have suggested that the stem cells residing in one postnatal organ can differentiate to cells of an entirely different organ system and can therefore cross lineage and even germ layer boundaries.[3] This phenomenon of presumed wider differentiation potential of postnatal stem cells has been termed 'stem cell plasticity'. Although this greater potential has caused significant excitement in the scientific and non-scientific community, the reports have also been viewed with skepticism. This arises from several factors, including the low levels of transdifferentiation observed, the fact that some studies could not be repeated, and most of all the fact that this phenomenon would contradict the dogma that somatic stem cells have been lineage-primed and committed early during development. Several theories have been proposed to explain the apparent plasticity of postnatal stem cells, most of which can be supported with scientific observations. In this chapter, we will first review the criteria that are used to characterize stem cells and that thus should be used to characterize the plasticity of stem cells, discuss the evidence for stem cell plasticity, and then review potential mechanisms that may explain this plasticity.

## The concept of the stem cell

Stem cells are defined by their biological function (Figure 2.1). Stem cells are undifferentiated cells that self-renew,[2] which is critical for maintaining the stem cell pool. Stem cells differentiate to give rise to, in general, at least two mature functional progeny cells, and this occurs in a clonal manner, i.e. a single stem cell should differentiate into two or more different cell types. In addition, a stem cell should be capable of replacing a damaged organ or tissue for the lifetime of the recipient. Some would argue that stem cells should also be capable of functionally integrating into non-damaged tissues.[3]

A fertilized egg is considered a totipotent stem cell, as it gives rise to both intra- and extra-embryonic cells.

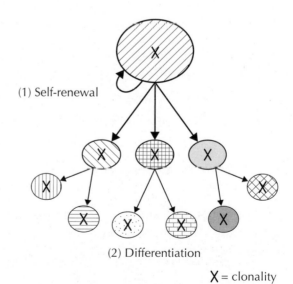

(1) Self-renewal

(2) Differentiation

X = clonality

**Figure 2.1** Definition of a stem cell. Stem cells are defined by their biologic function. They are undifferentiated cells that (1) self-renew, which is critical for maintaining the stem cell pool and (2) differentiate to give rise to, in general, at least two mature functional progeny cells. The stem cell differentiation occurs in a clonal manner, i.e. a single stem cell should differentiate into two or more different cell types. In addition, a stem cell should be capable of replacing a damaged organ or tissue for the lifetime of the recipient.

The inner cell mass of the pre-implantation embryo is considered pluripotent, as these cells give rise to all somatic stem cells, progenitors, and mature cells, as well as germ cells, but not the trophoblast. When removed from the blastocyst and cultured ex vivo, cells from the inner cell mass are termed embryonic stem (ES) cells. ES cells were first described for the mouse, and more recently for non-human primates and humans.[4–8] ES cells spontaneously differentiate into embryoid bodies, which contain cells of the ectodermal, mesodermal, and endodermal lineages. When injected under the skin, in muscle, or under the kidney capsule, ES cells will create teratomas that again contain differentiated cells from all three germ layers. Finally, when injected into a developing blastocyst, ES cells contribute to all tissues of all three germinal layers as well as the gametes. ES cells have proven to be a powerful tool for understanding the normal development and pathogenesis of several diseases. Because ES cells differentiate into relatively homogeneous populations of differentiated ectodermal, mesodermal, and endodermal cells[9–17] under specific inductive ex vivo culture conditions, they have great therapeutic potential. However, their embryonic origin has raised several ethical concerns.

In postnatal life, stem cells maintain the integrity and function of organ systems by replacing the cells that are lost due to normal wear and tear, apoptosis, or injury. Stem cells have been identified in several postnatal organs. Despite extensive investigations, the phenotype of most somatic stem cells remains ill defined, with no single phenotypic marker unique to any stem cell. Many stem cells efflux Hoechst 33342 dye, due to presence of the ABC transporter, BCRP1,[18] and distinctly form a 'side population' (SP) on fluorescence-activated cell sorter (FACS) analysis.[19,20] However, the SP phenotype is not unique to stem cells and is also shared by malignant and multidrug-resistant cells, as well as more mature cells such as natural killer (NK) cells. Several laboratories have used the SP phenotype to isolate stem cells, as described below. Other markers found on stem cells include CD34, AC133, c-Kit, Sca1, and Thy-1.[21–24] However, not all stem cells are positive, and cells other than stem cells also express these markers. Therefore, identification of stem cells requires functional assays, to demonstrate their self-renewal potential and clonal multilineage differentiation potential.

## Hematopoietic stem cells

HSC are by far the best-characterized postnatal stem cells, with extensive in vitro and in vivo data. They can be found in the SP population.[19,20] They are (at least in humans), CD34+ and AC133+, do not express lineage commitment markers, and express Sca1 (mouse),[21–25] low levels of Thy-1, and c-Kit. HSC provide a constant supply of hematopoietic cells in normal individuals. Several studies have elegantly shown that a single murine HSC can repopulate the myeloid and lymphoid lineages following transplantation, and can rescue animals[26] from lethal irradiation. In humans, single-cell transplantation is not possible. However, retroviral marking studies have shown that a single human HSC can contribute to all hematopoietic lineages after transplantation.[27]

## Neural stem cells

The discovery of neural stem cells (NSC) in adults was initially unexpected, as it was thought that in postnatal life, nervous tissue could not be repaired. However, more recently, stem cells for the central nervous system (CNS) have been identified in postnatal brain, including the olfactory bulb and the periventricular zone.[28,29] A recent study has shown that NSC can be purified from neurogenic areas of human brain using antibodies against the stem cell antigen AC133.[23] Rodent and human NSC can be expanded ex vivo for many population doublings when cultured as neurospheres. Single NSC differentiate in vitro and in vivo into neurons, astrocytes, and oligodendrocytes, and migrate in vivo to specific sites of damage.[30] Likewise, stem cells for the peripheral nervous system have been found in the spinal cord.[31]

## Mesenchymal stem cells

In bone marrow (BM)[32–36] and also fat tissue,[37] mesenchymal stem cell (MSC) have been identified, which differentiate into osteoblasts, chondroblasts, adipocytes, fibroblasts, and skeletal muscle. MSC do not express classical stem cell antigens such as CD34 and AC133.[35,36] It is not known whether they purify in the SP fraction of fat or BM cells. MSC can be culture-expanded for several passages without losing their differentiation potential. Ring cloning studies have suggested that such differentiated progeny is indeed derived from single MSC.[35]

## Epithelial stem cells

'Oval cells' that reside in the canals of Herring are thought to be the stem cells for hepatocytes and biliary epithelial cells. Oval cells can be found in the CD34+, c-Kit+, and Thy-1+ fraction of liver cells.[38,39] It is not known whether they can be selected based on an SP phenotype. In response to liver injuries, oval cells proliferate and eventually differentiate into liver and biliary epithelial cells.[38] When cultured ex vivo, oval cells can be induced to differentiate into these two cell types.[40,41] Because terminally differentiated hepatocytes have extensive proliferative potential, they are usually responsible for liver regeneration.[42] The exact role of oval cells in liver regeneration is unclear at present, except under those circumstances where mature hepatocytes are incapable of mounting a proliferative response.[43,44]

The constantly shed epithelium of the skin is replaced by epithelial stem cells present in the bulge zone of the follicular epithelium, which give rise to skin epithelium as well as to hair and other skin appendages.[45] Stem cells for the different types of epithelial cells lining the gastric, duodenal, jejunal, ileal, and colonic epithelia have been identified,[46] residing in the crypts.

## Muscle progenitor cells

Satellite cells are thought to be the progenitors for skeletal myoblasts. Satellite cells are mononuclear cells present under the basal lamina that surrounds multinucleated skeletal muscle fibers.[47] They form myotubes in vitro and contribute to skeletal muscle fibers in response to muscle damage in vivo.[47] In contrast to the cell types described above, satellite cells only give rise to a single mature progeny cell, and are therefore not 'classical' stem cells.

## Other stem/progenitor cells

Angioblasts are progenitors for endothelial cells. Like satellite cells, angioblasts do not fulfill all criteria for a stem cell, as differentiation to endothelium only has been described. Angioblasts can be found in the CD34[+] and AC133[+] fraction of blood and BM.[48] [50] Stem cells have also been identified for many other tissues, including the retina, the cornea, and the skin, even though the phenotype of the latter cells is less well defined.

# Evidence for stem cell plasticity

The traditionally held view of stem cell differentiation – linear and irreversible lineage restriction – is challenged by several recent reports, which suggest that stem cells residing in one postnatal organ can differentiate into cells of an entirely different organ system and therefore have much wider differentiation potential – or are much more plastic – than previously thought (Figure 2.2). Since the initial report of in vivo myogenic differentiation of BM-derived cells by Ferrari et al,[51] over 50 studies claiming stem cell plasticity have been published.

The majority of studies have identified donor-derived non-hematopoietic cells, based on identification of the Y chromosome in recipients of sex-mismatched BM transplants, whereas others have demonstrated plasticity based on transgenic expression of LacZ or enhanced green fluorescent protein (eGFP) in the donor cells. Few studies have shown that lineage switch occurs even in the absence of tissue damage, whereas most studies showed lineage switch in animals with injury to a specific organ. These studies vary widely in the criteria used to define and select stem cells as well as in the details of the experimental

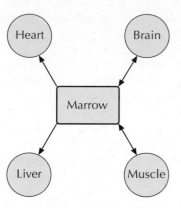

**Figure 2.2** Stem cell plasticity. Several recent reports suggest that stem cells residing in one postnatal organ can give rise to cells from an entirely different organ. This phenomenon of apparent wider potential of the adult stem cells is called 'stem cell plasticity'. Persistence of pleuripotent stem cells in postnatal organs, somatic cell fusion, and dedifferentiation and transdifferentiation of organ-specific stem cells have all been proposed as mechanisms underlying this phenomenon.

designs. In the following section, we will discuss a selection of representative studies.

## Plasticity of BM-derived stem cells

BM is an attractive source of stem cells for several reasons. First, large numbers of BM cells can be harvested without harming the donor and with relative ease. Second, BM transplantation (BMT) is a well-established procedure in the mouse, which is often the first experimental animal, as well as in humans. Third, BM-derived cells may have 'natural' access to the circulation and therefore may be able to correct damage to a 'distant organ'.

For decades, it has been known that BM contains HSC. More recent studies have shown that BM contains MSC and angioblasts. Recent stem cell plasticity studies have suggested that BM may also contain cells that differentiate in vitro and/or in vivo in other cell types of endodermal and ectodermal origin.

### Skeletal muscle from BM-derived cells

The growth and regeneration of skeletal muscle fibers in postnatal life is considered to be the function of satellite cells.[47] However, the number of resident satellite cells in the adult muscle is significantly lower than the number of committed myogenic precursors that populate the muscle tissue after muscle injury. Migration of myogenic precursors from the adjacent fibers, or recruitment of resident non-myogenic cells, such as fibroblasts and MSC, have been proposed to explain this paradox. Ferrari et al,[51] for the first time, demonstrated that BM-derived cells contribute to skeletal muscle myogenesis following muscle injury. Following cardiotoxin-induced tibialis anterior muscle damage in *scid/bg* mice (which lack T- and B-lymphocyte and NK-cell function), unfractionated BM from *C57/MlacZ* transgenic mice (which express nuclear β-galactosidase enzyme under the control of the muscle-specific myosin light-chain promoter) was injected into the damaged muscle. Alternatively, tibialis anterior muscles of *scid/bg* mice that had stable hematopoietic engraftment following BMT from *C57/Mlacz* mice were chemically damaged. In both sets of recipient animals, donor BM-derived cells formed immature centrally nucleated and mature peripherally nucleated myofibers in the damaged muscle. BM-derived myogenesis occurred 7–10 days later than satellite cell-derived myogenesis, suggesting that the satellite cells may represent a committed muscle progenitor, whereas cells in BM may precede the satellite cells in ontogeny. However, the investigators did not show that BM-derived cells contributed to the satellite cell pool. The population of BM cells that does not adhere to plastic had less in vivo myogenic potential than plastic-adherent cells. It is therefore possible that the myogenic cell is derived from MSC, which are plastic-adherent, and not from HSC, which are not plastic-adherent. The exact phenotype of the myogenic cell in BM was not defined. In addition, the investigators did not demonstrate that BM-derived myocytes displayed normal muscle function.

Gussoni et al[52] intravenously injected 2000–5000 BM-derived SP cells from male *C57/MlacZ* mice into lethally irradiated female *mdx* mice, a model of Duchenne muscular dystrophy.[52] Aside from hematopoietic recovery from donor origin, they also showed the presence of up to 4% LacZ-positive, dystrophin-positive muscle fibers at 12 weeks post transplant in the tibialis anterior muscle, with 10–30% of these containing Y-chromosome-positive donor nuclei. The phenotype of the SP cells is Sca1+c-Kit+Lin−CD45+CD34−, consistent with an HSC phenotype. In another set of experiments, these investigators injected *C57/MlacZ* skeletal muscle-derived SP cells into lethally irradiated *mdx* mice and showed that the muscle-derived SP cells reconstitute hematopoiesis and contribute to skeletal myogenesis. Unlike BM-derived SP cells, the muscle-derived SP cells were Sca1+c-Kit−Lin+/−CD45−, suggesting that the stem cell population derived from these two organs may be distinct but shares the SP phenotype. However, as was shown in subsequent studies by McKinney-Freeman et al[53] and Kawada et al,[54] it cannot be ruled out that hematopoietic engraftment was due to HSC present in muscle. Two additional points regarding this study merit consideration. First, a proportion of myocytes from the *mdx* mouse are known to spontaneously revert to synthesize dystrophin and the immunohistochemical methods do not distinguish between donor-derived and native *mdx* dystrophin. Hence, identification of donor-derived myocytes based on dystrophin expression in the *mdx* model may overestimate the number of donor-derived cells. In the *mdx4cv* mouse model, which has almost no spontaneous synthesis of dystrophin, donor-BM-derived cells contributed to a maximum of 1% skeletal muscle fibers.[55] Second, donor-derived cells formed maximally 4% myocytes at 12 weeks post transplantation. The low level of donor-derived myogenesis seen in this study may not be expected to functionally correct the myopathy, although muscle function was not formally assessed here.

These studies thus suggest that BM contains myogenic progenitors, which may have an MSC or an HSC phenotype. Whether the same cell gives rise to myoblasts and hematopoietic cells, or myoblasts and other mesenchymal cell types – a prerequisite for 'stem cell plasticity' – is not known. From a therapeutic standpoint, the current level of BM-derived myogenesis is probably not sufficient to correct myopathy. Here, it should be stressed that in the *mdx* mouse model the native myogenic precursors regenerate muscle throughout life. Hence, the low degree of donor-derived myogenesis in the *mdx* mouse model could be explained by the lack of selective growth advantage to the donor over the native myogenic precursors.[56] However, in Duchenne muscular dystrophy patients, where the degenerating muscles undergo fibrosis, it is possible that the donor-derived myogenic precursors may have a selective growth advantage and progressively replace the diseased muscle with functional muscle fibers.[57] Future studies are expected to address this issue.

### Myocardium from BM-derived cells

Until recently, it was believed that adult cardiomyocytes do not replicate.[58] Following coronary artery occlusion, cardiomyocytes undergo ischemic necrosis, which eventually heals with fibrosis and often results in ventricular failure, although this notion has recently been challenged.[59] The high prevalence of cardiomyopathy from ischemic and non-ischemic causes has led several investigators to search for non-cardiac sources of stem cells that can regenerate cardiomyocytes and revert ventricular dysfunction. Orlic et al,[60] for the first time, demonstrated that c-Kit+Lin− BM mononuclear cells may generate cells with cardiomyoblast features when injected in the peri-infarct myocardium. They demonstrated that about 50% of regenerating cardiomyocytes in the female heart were donor-derived male cells with cardiomyocyte, vascular smooth muscle cell, and endothelial phenotype. This translated into improvement by 36% of left ventricular (LV) diastolic function – the LV end-diastolic pressure in the study animals. c-Kit− BM cells did not contribute to the regenerating myocardium. Although the c-Kit+Lin− cell population contains HSC, it is not known whether a single cell gives rise to hematopoietic progeny and cells with cardiac myocyte characteristics. HSC express c-Kit on their cell membrane.[61] It is thought that membrane-bound stem cell factor (SCF, Steel factor, c-Kit ligand) mediates the migration of HSC and other primitive cells to their target organs.[61] Because SCF and granulocyte colony-stimulating factor (G-CSF) mobilize c-Kit+ BM cells into the circulation,[62] Orlic et al[63] also treated mice with SCF and G-CSF between 5 days before and 3 days after experimental induction of acute LV myocardial infarction. The cytokine-treated animals showed significant improvement in ventricular hemodynamics and mortality at 28 days (approximately 80% survival in treated versus approximately 20% in control animals), which could be attributed to increased cardiomyocyte, endothelium, and vascular smooth muscle regeneration. However, whether the mobilized BM cells contributed to the regeneration or the cytokines had a direct effect on the area of infarction could not be determined by this study.

Jackson et al[64] transplanted BM-derived SP cells into lethally irradiated murine hosts. After hematopoiesis was re-established, a LV infarct was induced by coronary artery occlusion for 50 minutes. Donor-derived cardiomyocytes (0.02–0.3%) could be detected, even though the frequency was significantly lower than what was reported by Orlic et al, after in situ delivery of BM cells or mobilization with SCF and G-CSF. The degree of chimerism seen in the study by Jackson et al is unlikely to be of functional importance, even though this was not directly tested.

### Endothelium from BM-derived cells

Vasculogenesis and angiogenesis are the mechanisms responsible for the development of blood vessels. Vasculogenesis refers to in situ differentiation and growth of blood vessels from mesodermal-derived hemangioblasts that give rise to the heart and the first primitive vascular plexus inside the embryo and in its surrounding membranes, as the yolk sac circulation.[65] Angiogenesis is responsible for the remodeling and expansion of this network. The most important positive regulators of vasculogenesis and angiogenesis are vascular endothelial growth factor (VEGF) and its receptors fetal liver kinase 1 (Flk1) and Fms-like tyrosine kinase (Flt1), the angiopoietin/tie system, and the ephrin-B/EpH-B system.[65] In postnatal life, angiogenesis is essential for a variety of physiological processes, such as female reproduction, wound healing, and neovascularization of ischemic tissue. Until recently, it was thought that blood vessel formation in postnatal life was entirely the process of angiogenesis and not vasculogenesis. However, recent studies have suggested that endothelial stem cells may persist into adult life and contribute to neoangiogenesis, so that the neoangiogenesis in the adult may be at least in part from vasculogenesis.[66–68] Precursors of endothelial

cells, angioblasts, have been isolated from BM and peripheral blood.[66–69] Lin et al[69] showed that in recipients of sex-mismatched BMT who had 100% donor hematopoietic engraftment, most of the circulating endothelial cells (CEC) isolated from fresh blood had recipient genotype. In contrast, blood-outgrowth endothelial cells (BOEC), thought to represent angioblasts, were mostly of donor genotype. The recipient-genotype endothelial cells expanded only about 20-fold over this period, whereas donor-genotype endothelial cells expanded about 1000-fold. These data suggest that most CEC in fresh blood originate from vessel walls and have limited growth capability and that BOEC is mostly derived from transplantable marrow-derived cells. Because these cells had more delayed outgrowth but a greater proliferative rate, they were likely to be derived from circulating angioblasts.[69] Lyden et al[67] showed that BM-derived angioblasts are responsible for tumor angiogenesis. These investigators used angiogenic-defective, tumor-resistant Id-mutant mice to show that transplantation of wild-type BM or VEGF-mobilized stem cells restores tumor angiogenesis and growth. Donor-derived circulating endothelial precursors were detected throughout the tumor neovasculature.[67] Although the exact phenotype of angioblasts is not completely known, they are CD34, VE-cadherin-, AC133-, and Flk1-. Reyes et al[68] have shown that rare multipotent cells in human and murine postnatal BM, called multipotent adult progenitor cells (MAPC) exist that are CD34, VE-cadherin-, AC133-, and Flk1-. When cultured with VEGF, MAPC differentiate into CD34+VE-cadherin+Flk1+ cells – a phenotype that would be expected for angioblasts, and ultimately differentiate into mature functional endothelial cells that contribute to tumor and wound-healing angiogenesis in vivo.[68] MAPC may be the putative progenitor for angioblasts. Given these studies, it is not surprising that unfractionated BM mononuclear cells can give rise to endothelium when implanted into non-hematopoietic tissue, such as infarcted myocardium.[60,63,64]

### Neural cells from BM-derived cells

Developmentally, neurons are derived from the embryonic neuroectoderm, whereas glial cells can be derived from either myeloid cells (microglia) or NSC (astroglia and oligodendrocytes). Recent studies have suggested that BM can give rise to cells with neuronal markers in vivo. Eglitis et al[70] were the first to show that BM-derived cells can give rise to both microglia and macroglia in the brains of adult mice. Since then, Mezey et al and Brazelton et al have found Y-chromosome-containing NeuN+ cells in the brains of female mice that received BM from male donors after lethal irradiation[71] and in newborn PU.1 murine recipients.[72] Whether a single cell gave rise to neuron-like cells and HSC was not addressed. In addition, full characterization of BM-derived neuron-like cells and glia-like cells in terms of their integration into host tissue (e.g. ability to form synapses) and function in vivo is lacking at this point. Several groups have now shown that BM MSC and MAPC can differentiate in vitro into cells that have morphological and phenotypic markers of neurons, astrocytes and oligodendrocytes.[73,74] Again, functional characterization of the neuron-like progeny has yet to be done.

### Liver from BM-derived cells

Initial experiments testing hepatocyte regeneration from BM-derived cells involved transplantation of male BM into myeloablated female recipients and demonstrating the presence of donor-derived cells, containing a Y chromosome, by fluorescence in situ hybridization (FISH) and bearing hepatocyte antigens in the recipient's liver.[75–78] As will be discussed below, these results could be explained by the coexistence of hepatocyte progenitors and HSC within BM.[79]

The strongest evidence for generation of hepatocytes from BM-derived HSC comes from Lagasse et al.[80] These investigators systemically infused as few as 50 c-Kit+Thy$^{low}$Lin−Sca1+ (KTLS) cells derived from the BM of *lacZ* transgenic mice into lethally irradiated FAH$^{-/-}$ mice (fumarylacetoacetate hydroxylase mutant mice – a model of hereditary tyrosinemia). FAH$^{-/-}$ mice die from hepatic failure, unless they are fed NTBC, a substance that blocks the production of fumaryl acetoacetate, which is a substrate for FAH. The recipient animals were maintained on an interrupted course of NTBC for 7 months. The interruptions in NTBC were designed to give a selective growth advantage to the donor cells. After 7 months, when the NTBC was completely stopped, the KTLS cell-transplanted animals survived, and had donor-cell-derived clusters of hepatocytes and marked improvement in biochemical markers of hepatocyte function, indicating that the donor-KTLS cell-derived hepatocytes were functional. Neither study has shown that a single HSC could also differentiate into hepatocytes.

### Plasticity of NSC

After transplantation of genetically labeled NSC into irradiated mice, NSC differentiated into myeloid, lymphoid, and early progenitor cells,[81] indicating that adult NSC can adopt a hematopoietic fate in vivo. However, a more recent study indicated that such a phenomenon may be rare.[82] Clarke et al[83] injected adult mouse brain-derived NSC into the amniotic cavity of early chick embryos and found that the NSC contributed to the formation of tissues from all the germ layers. However, in this study no embryos were allowed to be born.

### Plasticity of skeletal muscle-derived cells

Jackson et al[84] initially reported that postnatal skeletal muscle-derived cells can adopt a hematopoietic fate and rescue a lethally irradiated host. However, subsequently using Ly5.1/5.2 mismatch transplant, Kawada et al[54] have shown that the cells with hematopoietic potential that reside in the skeletal muscle are hematopoietic stem cells. A more recent study by McKinney-Freeman et al[53] also demonstrated that the cell in skeletal muscle that contributes to hematopoietic recovery is CD45+, indicating that HSC lodge in muscle.

### Pitfalls in plasticity studies

Several factors merit consideration when evaluating studies regarding changes in stem cell fate. First, as true stem cell plasticity should be defined as a single tissue-committed stem cell being capable of differentiating into that tissue and a second unrelated tissue, studies using unselected populations of cells (e.g. unfractionated BM) are difficult to interpret. Indeed, as will be discussed below, most tissues are heterogeneous and may contain multiple stem cells. Even within a population of cells that is selected based on the expression of certain markers, there may be heterogeneity. Therefore, true plasticity can only be defined by transplanting a single cell[78] or by retroviral marking.[74,85]

Second, acquisition of a different fate by the stem cell is mostly based on the detection of a donor marker in the cells that express markers of the differentiated cell. Several difficulties may occur in interpreting results. A common method used to identify the donor origin of cells is demonstration of a Y chromosome by FISH in male–female transplantation studies. A false impression of colocalization of the Y chromosome in the cell that expresses a tissue-specific cytoplasmic or cell membrane marker can be created by overlap of the nucleus from an adjacent cell, such as a circulating hematopoietic cell. Somewhat less problematic is the use of transgenically expressed tracers, even though this too may lead to a false impression of engraftment and differentiation. Optimally, the tracer should be activated by a tissue-specific promoter, as this then demonstrates engraftment and activation of a tissue-specific genetic program.[52]

Third, the mere presence of one or two markers consistent with differentiation into a lineage different from the lineage of origin does not suffice to demonstrate true lineage switch. There should be functional characterization of the new lineage. Most studies to date, with a few exceptions,[68,74,80,85] have fallen short in demonstrating functional 'plasticity'.

## Potential mechanisms underlying stem cell plasticity

Why, then, should cells residing in one postnatal organ acquire the fate of cells from another organ?

Several theories have been proposed to explain the plasticity of postnatal stem cells.

## Multiple tissue-specific stem cells are present in different organs

HSC exit the BM space, circulate in the peripheral blood, and 'home' in on different organs – a concept used clinically in peripheral blood transplantations.[86] Recent studies have also shown that HSC reside within muscle,[53,54] and that such muscle HSC can contribute to the hematopoietic system when transplanted in lethally irradiated animals. Aside from HSC, BM contains MSC and endothelial progenitors. More recently, a study has shown that BM may also contain cells with characteristics of oval cells, the progenitors for hepatic and biliary epithelial cells.[79] Thus, liver regeneration following BMT could be the results of infusion of hepatic oval cells present in the BM sample.

## Plasticity is the result of fusion of the donor cell with resident cells in an organ

It has long been known that cellular fusion can change the fate of a cell, as heterokaryon studies were already performed early in the 20th century and a number of studies have shown that cell fate can be changed upon heterokaryon formation. These studies have shown that cytoplasm of one cell has factors that induce a new fate upon the cell with which it fuses.[87] That this may occur in stem cell studies was suggested in two recent studies documenting that coculture of adult tissue cells with ES cells leads to cell fusion and imposition of the ES fate on the fused, tetraploid resulting cell. Terada et al[88] cocultured murine BM cells with ES cells and Ying et al performed similar studies with fetal and adult murine NSC murine fetal or adult NSC.[89] Both groups demonstrated that such coculture yields what appeared initially to be 'transdifferentiated' BM cells or NSC that had acquired ES characteristics. The apparent switch was caused by fusion of an ES cell with $1/10^5$–$1/10^6$ BM cells or NSC, yielding cells with ES characteristics that were tetraploid. The authors of these papers pointed out correctly that this mechanism may underlie at least some of the apparent 'plasticity', even though studies were only done using ES/adult cell coculture, and were only done in vitro.

## Cells undergo dedifferentiation and redifferentiation

'Dolly' the sheep has taught us that genetic information of a cell can be reprogrammed, and that somatic cells can dedifferentiate into pluripotent cells.[90] Even before Dolly, it was known from studies in amphibians such as Urodeles, which can regenerate whole limbs, that differentiated somatic cells can dedifferentiate and generate multiple cell types required for regeneration of whole body parts. The mechanisms underlying this dedifferentiation are not totally understood, although the homeobox gene Msx1, expressed in the regenerating blastema, appears to play an important role. It has been demonstrated that overexpression of this homeobox gene in myotubes derived from the C2C12 cell line causes myotubes to regress into multiple mononuclear cells, which now proliferate and gain the ability to differentiate not only into myoblasts but also into osteoblasts, chondrocytes, and adipocytes.[91] Other examples of possible dedifferentiation include the capability of oligodendrocyte progenitors from the optical nerve, maintained in serum-free and low-density culture conditions, to acquire what appear to be NSC characteristics,[92] pancreatic epithelium to acquire a hepatic phenotype,[93] and hepatocytes to acquire a pancreatic fate.[94,95]

## True multi/pluripotent stem cells persist

Finally, there is mounting evidence that cells with greater multipotency may persist beyond gastrulation. Suzuki et al[96] isolated what appears to be an endodermal stem cell from murine fetal liver at e14. They demonstrated that a VLA6+c-Met+CD34−Thy1−c-Kit− cell can be purified by FACS and culture-expanded, and that upon transplantation into postnatal animals it differentiates not only into liver and biliary epithelial cells but also into epithelium of the pancreas and the gastrointestinal tract. As discussed above, muscle can generate hematopoietic cells. Although two groups have now shown that this is at least in part due to resident HSC in muscle, there is also evidence from mouse genetics that a progenitor may exist in muscle that can differentiate into either muscle or hematopoietic cells – a process governed by the transcription factor Pax7.[97] Finally, Jiang et al[74] showed that cells copurifying with MSC can differentiate into most, if not all, somatic cell types. As these cells are maintained in culture, the verdict is open as to whether this represents resident multipotent cells or dedifferentiation of MSC in vitro. These studies suggest therefore that cells that precede the known somatic stem cells may persist, and, depending on the milieu, differentiate into cells different than the organ of origin.

# Conclusions and future directions

The traditionally held view of stem cell differentiation is that of linear and irreversible lineage restriction. Several recent reports have suggested that stem cells residing in one postnatal organ can differentiate into cells of an entirely different organ system and therefore have much wider differentiation potential – or are much more plastic – than was previously thought. Although such greater potential has caused significant excitement in the scientific and non-scientific community, the reports have also been viewed with skepticism. This arises from several factors, including the low levels of transdifferentiation observed, the fact that some studies could not be repeated, and most of all the fact that this phenomenon would contradict the dogma that somatic stem cells have been lineage-primed and committed early during development. Future studies are expected to explore the molecular mechanisms underlying stem cell fate change, and to use them to optimize the number of derived differentiated cells. If a substantial number of cells of therapeutic interest can indeed be derived from an alternative organ source, especially from an autologous source, and these cells can be used to improve the function of a diseased organ, this will bring about a revolution in the medical field.

## REFERENCES

1. Thomson JA, Itskovitz-Eldor J, Shapiro SS et al. Embryonic stem cell lines derived from human blastocysts. *Science* 1998; **282**: 1145–7.

2. Weissman IL. Translating stem and progenitor cell biology to the clinic: barriers and opportunities. *Science* 2000; **287**: 1442–6.

3. Anderson DJ, Gage FH, Weissman IL. Can stem cells cross lineage boundaries? *Nat Med* 2001; **7**: 393–5.

4. Evans MJ, Kaufman MH. Establishment in culture of pluripotential cells from mouse embryos. *Nature* 1981; **292**: 154–6.

5. Thomson J, Kalishman J, Golos T et al. Isolation of a primate embryonic stem cell line. *Proc Natl Acad Sci USA* 1995; **92**: 7844–8.

6. Thomson JA, Odorico JS. Human embryonic stem cell and embryonic germ cell lines. *Trends Biotechnol* 2000; **18**: 53–7.

7. Reubinoff BE, Pera MF, Fong CY et al. Embryonic stem cell lines from human blastocysts: somatic differentiation in vitro. *Nat Biotechnol* 2000; **18**: 399–404.

8. Pera MF, Reubinoff B, Trounson A. Human embryonic stem cells. *J Cell Sci* 2000; **113**: 5–10.

9. Brustle O, Jones K, Learish R et al. Embryonic stem cell-derived glial precursors: a source of myelinating transplants. *Science* 1999; **285**: 754–6.

10. Lee SH, Lumelsky N, Studer L et al. Efficient generation of midbrain and hindbrain neurons from mouse embryonic stem cells. *Nat Biotechnol* 2000; **18**: 675–9.

11. Hamazaki T, Iiboshi Y, Oka M et al. Hepatic maturation in differentiating embryonic stem cells in vitro. *FEBS Lett* 2001; **497**: 15–19.

12. Soria B, Roche E, Berna G et al. Insulin-secreting cells derived from embryonic stem cells normalize glycemia in streptozotocin-induced diabetic mice. *Diabetes* 2000; **49**: 157–62.

13. Lumelsky N, Blondel O, Laeng P et al. Differentiation of embryonic stem cells to insulin-secreting structures similar to pancreatic islets. *Science* 2001; **292**: 1389–94.

14. Wobus AM, Wallukat G, Hescheler J. Pluripotent mouse embryonic stem cells are able to differentiate into cardiomyocytes expressing chronotropic responses to adrenergic and cholinergic agents and $Ca^{2+}$ channel blockers. *Differentiation* 1991; **48**: 173–82.

15. Kehat I, Kenyagin-Karsenti D, Snir M et al. Human embryonic stem cells can differentiate into myocytes with structural and functional properties of cardiomyocytes. *J Clin Invest* 2001; **108**: 407–14.

16. Hirashima M, Kataoka H, Nishikawa S et al. Maturation of embryonic stem cells into endothelial cells in an in vitro model of vasculogenesis. *Blood* 1999; **93**: 1253–63.

17. Kaufman DS, Hanson ET, Lewis RL et al. Hematopoietic colony-forming cells derived from human embryonic stem cells. *Proc Natl Acad Sci USA* 2001; **98**: 10716–21.

18. Zhou S, Schuetz JD, Bunting KD et al. The ABC transporter Bcrp1/ABCG2 is expressed in a wide variety of stem cells and is a molecular determinant of the side-population phenotype. *Nat Med* 2001; **7**: 1028–34.

19. Goodell M, Brose K, Paradis G et al. Isolation and functional properties of murine hematopoietic stem cells that are replicating in vivo. *J Exp Med* 1996; **183**: 1797–806.

20. Goodell M, Rosenzweig M, Kim H et al. Dye efflux studies suggest that hematopoietic stem cells expressing low or undetectable levels of 34 antigen exist in multiple species. *Nat Med* 1997; **3**: 1337–45.

21. Krause D, Fackler M, Civin C, May W. CD34: structure, biology, and clinical utility. *Blood* 1996; **87**: 1–13.

22. Yin AH, Miraglia S, Zanjani ED et al. AC133, a novel marker for human hematopoietic stem and progenitor cells. *Blood* 1997; **90**: 5002–12.

23. Uchida N, Buck DW, He D et al. Direct isolation of human central nervous system stem cells. *Proc Natl Acad Sci USA* 2000; **97**: 14720–5.

24. Spangrude G, Heimfeld S, Weissman I. Purification and characterization of mouse hematopoietic stem cells. *Science* 1988; **241**: 58.

25. Sutherland H, Eaves C, Eaves A et al. Characterization and partial purification of human marrow cells capable of initiating long-term hematopoiesis in vitro. *Blood* 1989; **74**: 1563–70.

26. Ogawa M, Hanada K, Hamada H, Nakauchi H. Long-term lymphohematopoietic reconstitution by a single CD34[low/−] hematopoietic stem cell. *Science* 1996; **273**: 242–5.

27. Nolta J, Dao M, Wells S et al. Transduction of pluripotent human hematopoietic stem cells demonstrated by clonal analysis after engraftment in immune-deficient mice. *Proc Natl Acad Sci USA* 1996; **93**: 2414–19.

28. Gage FH, Kempermann G, Palmer TD et al. Multipotent progenitor cells in the adult dentate gyrus. *J Neurobiol* 1998; **36**: 249–66.

29. Johansson CB, Momma S, Clarke DL et al. Identification of a neural stem cell in the adult mammalian central nervous system. *Proc Natl Acad Sci USA* 1999; **96**: 25–34.

30. Gage FH. Mammalian neural stem cells. *Science* 2000; **287**: 1433–8.

31. Kalyani AJ, Rao MS. Cell lineage in the developing neural tube. *Biochem Cell Biol* 1998; **76**: 1051–68.

32. Fridenshtein A. Stromal bone marrow cells and the hematopoietic microenvironment. *Arkh Patol* 1982; **44**: 3–11.

33. Haynesworth SE, Barber MA, Caplan IA. Cell surface antigens on human marrow-derived mesenchymal cells are detected by monoclonal antibodies. *Bone* 1992; **13**: 69–80.

34. Prockop D. Marrow stromal cells as stem cells for non-hematopoietic tissues. *Science* 1997; **276**: 71–4.

35. Pittenger MF, Mackay AM, Beck SC et al. Multilineage potential of adult human mesenchymal stem cells. *Science* 1999; **284**: 143–7.

36. Gronthos S, Graves S, Ohta S, Simmons P. The STRO-1+ fraction of adult human bone marrow contains the osteogenic precursors. *Blood* 1994; **84**: 4164–73.

37. Zuk PA, Zhu M, Mizuno H et al. Multilineage cells from human adipose tissue: implications for cell-based therapies. *Tissue Eng* 2001; **7**: 211–28.

38. Paku S, Schnur J, Nagy P, Thorgeirsson SS. Origin and structural evolution of the early proliferating oval cells in rat liver. *Am J Pathol* 2001; **158**: 1313–23.

39. Alison M, Sarraf C. Hepatic stem cells. *J Hepatol* 1998; **29**: 678–83.

40. Tateno C, Yoshizato K. Growth and differentiation in culture of clonogenic hepatocytes that express both phenotypes of hepatocytes and biliary epithelial cells. *Am J Pathol* 1996; **149**: 1593–605.

41. Gordon GJ, Butz GM, Grisham JW, Coleman WB. Isolation, short-term culture, and transplantation of small hepatocyte-like progenitor cells from retrorsine-exposed rats. *Transplantation* 2002; **73**: 1236–43.

42. Fausto N. Liver regeneration: from laboratory to clinic. *Liver Transplant* 2001; **7**: 835–44.

43. Paolucci F, Mancini R, Marucci L et al. Immuno-histochemical identification of proliferating cells following dimethylnitrosamine-induced liver injury. *Liver Growth Repair* 1990; **10**: 278–81.

44. Yin L, Lynch D, Ilic Z et al. Proliferation and differentiation of ductular progenitor cells and littoral cells during the regeneration of the rat liver to CCl4/2-AAF injury. *Histol Histopathol* 2002; **17**: 65–81.

45. Pellegrini G, Bondanza SG, De Luca M. Cultivation of human keratinocyte stem cells: current and future clinical applications. *Med Biol Eng Comput* 1998; **36**: 778–90.

46. Potten C. Stem cells in gastrointestinal epithelium: numbers, characteristics and death. *Philos Trans R Soc Lond B Biol Sci* 1998; **353**: 821–30.

47. Goldring K, Partridge T, Watt D. Muscle stem cells. *J Pathol* 2002; **197**: 457–67.

48. Rafii S, Shapiro F, Rimarachin J et al. Isolation and characterization of human bone marrow microvascular endothelial cells: hematopoietic progenitor cell adhesion. *Blood* 1994; **84**: 10.

49. Peichev M, Naiyer AJ, Pereira D et al. Expression of VEGFR-2 and AC133 by circulating human CD34+ cells identifies a population of functional endothelial precursors. *Blood* 2000; **95**: 952–8.

50. Asahara T, Murohara T, Sullivan A et al. Isolation of putative progenitor endothelial cells for angiogenesis. *Science* 1997; **275**: 964–967.

51. Ferrari G, Cusella-De Angelis G, Coletta M et al. Muscle regeneration by bone marrow-derived myogenic progenitors. *Science* 1998; **279**: 528–30.

52. Gussoni E, Soneoka Y, Strickland C et al. Dystrophin expression in the *mdx* mouse restored by stem cell transplantation. *Nature* 1999; **401**: 390–4.

53. McKinney-Freeman SL, Jackson KA, Camargo FD et al. Muscle-derived hematopoietic stem cells are hematopoietic in origin. *Proc Natl Acad Sci USA* 2002; **99**: 1341–6.

54. Kawada H, Ogawa M. Bone marrow origin of hematopoietic progenitors and stem cells in murine muscle. *Blood* 2001; **98**: 2008–13.

55. Ferrari G, Stornaiuolo A, Mavilio F. Failure to correct murine muscular dystrophy. *Nature* 2001; **411**: 1014–15.

56. Nonaka I. Animal models of muscular dystrophies. *Lab Anim Sci* 1998; **48**: 8–17.

57. Blake DJ, Weir A, Newey SE, Davies KE. Function and genetics of dystrophin and dystrophin-related proteins in muscle. *Physiol Rev* 2002; **82**: 291–329.

58. Soonpaa MH, Koh GY, Klug MG, Field LJ. Formation of nascent intercalated disks between grafted fetal cardiomyocytes and host myocardium. *Science* 1994; **264**: 98–101.

59. Quaini F, Urbanek K, Beltrami AP et al. Chimerism of the transplanted heart. *N Engl J Med* 2002; **346**: 5–15.

60. Orlic D, Kajstura J, Chimenti S et al. Bone marrow cells regenerate infarcted myocardium. *Nature* 2001; **410**: 701–5.

61. Lyman S, Jacobsen S. c-kit ligand and Flt3 ligand: stem/progenitor cell factors with overlapping yet distinct activities. *Blood* 1998; **91**: 1101.

62. Glaspy JA, Shpall EJ, LeMaistre CF et al. Peripheral blood progenitor cell mobilization using stem cell factor in combination with filgrastim in breast cancer patients. *Blood* 1997; **90**: 2939–51.

63. Orlic D, Kajstura J, Chimenti S et al. Mobilized bone marrow cells repair the infarcted heart, improving function and survival. *Proc Natl Acad Sci USA* 2000; **98**: 10344–9.

64. Jackson K, Majka SM, Wang H et al. Regeneration of ischemic cardiac muscle and vascular endothelium by adult stem cells. *J Clin Invest* 2001; **107**: 1395–402.

65. Conway EM, Collen D, Carmeliet P. Molecular mechanisms of blood vessel growth. *Cardiovasc Res* 2001; **49**: 507–21.

66. Asahara T, Masuda H, Takahashi T et al. Bone marrow origin of endothelial progenitor cells responsible for postnatal vasculogenesis in physiological and pathological neovascularization. *Circ Res* 1999; **85**: 221–8.

67. Lyden D, Hattori K, Dias S et al. Impaired recruitment of bone-marrow-derived endothelial and hematopoietic precursor cells blocks tumor angiogenesis and growth. *Nat Med* 2001; **7**: 1194–201.

68. Reyes M, Dudek A, Jahagirdar B et al. Origin of endothelial progenitors in human post-natal bone marrow. *J Clin Invest* 2002; **109**: 337–46.

69. Lin Y, Weisdorf DJ, Solovey A, Hebbel RP. Origins of circulating endothelial cells and endothelial outgrowth from blood. *J Clin Invest* 2000; **105**: 71–7.

70. Eglitis MA, Mezey E. Hematopoietic cells differentiate into both microglia and macroglia in the brains of adult mice. *Proc Natl Acad Sci USA* 1997; **94**: 4080–5.

71. Mezey E, Chandross KJ, Harta G et al. Turning blood into brain: cells bearing neuronal antigens generated in vivo from bone marrow. *Science* 2000; **290**: 1779–82.

72. Brazelton TR, Rossi FMV, Keshet GI, Blau HE. From marrow to brain: expression of neuronal phenotypes in adult mice. *Science* 2000; **290**: 1775–9.

73. Phinney DG, Kopen G, Isaacson RL, Prockop DJ. Plastic adherent stromal cells from the bone marrow of commonly used strains of inbred mice: variations in yield, growth, and differentiation. *J Cell Biochem* 1999; **72**: 570–85.

74. Jiang Y, Jahagirdar B, Reyes M et al. Pluripotent nature of adult marrow derived mesenchymal stem cells. *Nature* 2002; **418**: 41–9.

75. Petersen BE, Bowen WC, Patrene KD et al. Bone marrow as a potential source of hepatic oval cells. *Science* 1999; **284**: 1168–70.

76. Theise ND, Badve S, Saxena R et al. Derivation of hepatocytes from bone marrow cells in mice after radiation-induced myeloablation. *Hepatology* 2000; **31**: 235–40.

77. Theise ND, Nimmakayalu M, Gardner R et al. Liver from bone marrow in humans. *Hepatology* 2000; **32**: 11–16.

78. Krause DS, Theise ND, Collector MI et al. Multi-organ, multi-lineage engraftment by a single bone marrow-derived stem cell. *Cell* 2001; **105**: 369–77.

79. Oh SH, Miyazaki M, Kouchi H et al. Hepatocyte growth factor induces differentiation of adult rat bone marrow cells into a hepatocyte lineage in vitro. *Biochem Biophys Res Commun* 2000; **279**: 500–4.

80. Lagasse E, Connors H, Al-Dhalimy M et al. Purified hematopoietic stem cells can differentiate into hepatocytes in vivo. *Nat Med* 2000; **6**: 1229–34.

81. Bjornson C, Rietze R, Reynolds B et al. Turning brain into blood: a hematopoietic fate adopted by adult neural stem cells in vivo. *Science* 1999; **283**: 354–7.

82. Morshead CM, Benveniste P, Iscove NN, van Der Kooy D. Hematopoietic competence is a rare property of neural stem cells that may depend on genetic and epigenetic alterations. *Nat Med* 2002; **8**: 268–73.

83. Clarke DL, Johansson CB, Wilbertz J et al. Generalized potential of adult neural stem cells. *Science* 2000; **288**: 1660–3.

84. Jackson K, Mi T, Goodell MA. Hematopoietic potential of stem cells isolated from murine skeletal muscle. *Proc Natl Acad Sci USA* 1999; **96**: 14482–6.

85. Schwartz RE, Reyes M, Koodie L et al. Multipotent adult progenitor cells from bone marrow differentiate into functional hepatocyte-like cells. *J Clin Investigation* 2002; **96**: 1291–302.

86. Andrews RG, Briddell RA, Knitter GH et al. Rapid engraftment by peripheral blood progenitor cells mobilized by recombinant human stem cell factor and recombinant human granulocyte colony-stimulating factor in nonhuman primates. *Blood* 1995; **85**: 1995–2006.

87. Kikyo N, Wolffe AP. Reprogramming nuclei: insights from cloning, nuclear transfer and heterokaryons. *J Cell Sci* 2000; **113**: 11–20.

88. Terada N, Hamazaki T, Oka M et al. Bone marrow cells adopt the phenotype of other cells by spontaneous cell fusion. *Nature* 2002; **416**: 542–5.

89. Ying QY, Nichols J, Evans EP, Smith AG. Changing potency by spontaneous fusion. *Nature* 2002; **416**: 545–8.

90. Wolf DP, Mitalipov S, Norgren RB Jr. Nuclear transfer technology in mammalian cloning. *Arch Med Res* 2001; **32**: 609–13.

91. Odelberg SJ, Kollhoff A, Keating MT. Dedifferentiation of mammalian myotubes induced by msx1. *Cell* 2000; **103**: 1099–109.

92. Tang DG, Tokumoto YM, Apperly JA et al. Lack of replicative senescence in cultured rat oligodendrocyte precursor cells. *Science* 2001; **291**: 868–71.

93. Shen CN, Slack JM, Tosh D. Molecular basis of transdifferentiation of pancreas to liver. *Nat Cell Biol* 2000; **2**: 879–87.

94. Yang L, Li S, Hatch H et al. In vitro trans-differentiation of adult hepatic stem cells into pancreatic endocrine hormone-producing cells. *Proc Natl Acad Sci USA* 2002; **99**: 8078–83.

95. Ferber S, Halkin A, Cohen H et al. Pancreatic and duodenal homeobox gene 1 induces expression of insulin genes in liver and ameliorates streptozotocin-induced hyperglycemia. *Nat Med* 2000; **6**: 568–72.

96. Suzuki A, Zheng YY, Kaneko S et al. Clonal identification and characterization of self-renewing pluripotent stem cells in the developing liver. *J Cell Biol* 2002; **156**: 173–84.

97. Seale P, Sabourin LA, Girgis-Gabardo A et al. Pax7 is required for the specification of myogenic satellite cells. *Cell* 2000; **102**: 777–86.

# 3 Cytokine receptors and signal transduction

Ivo P Touw and Thamar B van Dijk

## Introduction

A complex network of signals, provided by the bone marrow microenvironment and by soluble polypeptide growth factors or cytokines, tightly regulates the balance between proliferation, differentiation, and survival of hematopoietic precursor cells. Hematopoietic cytokines include colony-stimulating factors (CSFs), erythropoietin (EPO), thrombopoietin (TPO), stem cell factor (SCF), Flt3 ligand, and certain interleukins (ILs). Cytokines exert their function by binding to their cognate transmembrane receptors on the surface of target cells. Some receptors, like those for granulocyte CSF (G-CSF-R), EPO (EPO-R), and TPO (TPO-R, also known as Mpl), form homodimeric or -oligomeric complexes. Many other receptor systems, however, are heteromers composed of two or three different receptor subunits. Notably, these heteromeric receptors may share subunits. Examples of such common receptor subunits are the γ chain shared by a number of IL-Rs, the gp130 shared by, for example, IL-6R and IL-11R, and the β common chain shared by IL-3R, IL-5R, and GM-CSF-R (Figure 3.1).[1,2]

The interaction between growth factors and their receptors causes either the oligomerization of receptor components or a conformational change of pre-existing receptor dimers.[3,4] This subsequently results in the activation of intracellular protein tyrosine kinase activity and the generation of intracellular signals.[5] Two major groups of tyrosine kinase-linked receptors can be distinguished that act in this way: the cytokine receptor superfamily introduced above, which associate with intracellular tyrosine kinases, and the receptor tyrosine kinases (RTKs), which have an intrinsic tyrosine kinase activity. The receptor for macrophage CSF (M-CSF-R, also referred to as c-Fms or CSF-1R), FLT3 (Fms-like tyrosine kinase receptor), and the receptor for SCF (SCF-R, also known as c-Kit) belong to this latter category of RTKs.[6] As we will see later, transforming mutations contributing to malignant transformation of hematopoietic cells occur most frequently in this group of receptors. These mutations induce growth factor-independent multimerization, affect autoinhibitory regions, or directly affect the tyrosine kinase domain itself. Invariably, these defects lead to uncontrolled and increased tyrosine kinase activity. Activating mutations in the receptors of the cytokine receptor superfamily are less prominent, probably because these receptors do not contain an intrinsic tyrosine kinase domain.[7] However, several hematopoietic disorders have been associated with mutations that alter the signaling

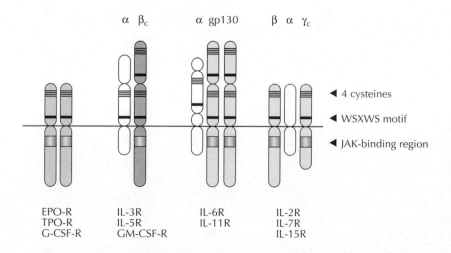

**Figure 3.1** Homodimeric and heteromeric composition of class I cytokine receptors. The four cysteines and WSXWS motif are characteristic of this receptor superfamily. Heteromeric receptors within different clusters may share common receptor subunits (see text).

function of these receptors in a qualitative and/or quantitative manner. In this chapter, we will first summarize the major features of normal cytokine signal transduction and its subsequent downregulation. Then we will discuss some of the consequences of receptor abnormalities and the resulting signaling defects for the pathogenesis of hematological diseases, including leukemia.

# Cytokine receptor signaling

## The JAK–STAT pathway

As explained above, the first intracellular event in cytokine-mediated signal transduction is the initiation of tyrosine kinase activity. Cytokine receptors lack intrinsic tyrosine kinase activity and rely for their function on cytoplasmic tyrosine kinases, in particular of the Janus kinase (JAK) family (Figure 3.2a). The JAK family comprises four mammalian members: JAKs 1–3 and TYK2. Upon their activation via transphosphorylation on tyrosines, JAKs phosphorylate the tyrosine residues in the intracellular domain of the receptor. The phosphorylated tyrosines in both the receptor and JAKs then provide docking sites for signaling proteins with an Src-homology 2 (SH2) domain. The STAT (signal transducer and activator of transcription) proteins form a major group of signaling molecules activated in this way (Figure 3.2a). Once phosphorylated on specific tyrosine residues, STATs dimerize or oligomerize and translocate to the nucleus, where they bind to specific DNA sequences (TTCN$_{2-4}$GAA) in promoter regions, thereby regulating transcription of cytokine-responsive genes.[8–10]

Seven mammalian STAT proteins have been identified (STATs 1–6, STAT5A, and STAT5B). Studies in STAT knockout mice have shown that STATs 1, 2, 4, and 6 have specialized functions: STATs 1 and 2 are crucial in the antiviral response induced by interferons;[11–13] STATs 4 and 6 are exclusively activated by IL-12 and IL-4 respectively and therefore play decisive roles in T helper cell (Th1/Th2) development.[14–17] In contrast, STATs 3 and 5 are activated by multiple receptors and play a more general role in controlling the cell cycle by regulation of the expression, for example, c-*myc*, *p21*, *p27*, and *cyclin D1* and cell survival by regulation of, for example, bcl-x$_L$.[18,19]

It becomes increasingly clear that uncontrolled activity of JAKs and STATs may contribute to malignant transformation of hematopoietic cells. This is most directly exemplified by the cases of human leukemia with chromosomal translocations resulting in oncogenic fusion proteins comprising JAK2 (TEL–JAK2) or STAT5 (STAT5B–RARα).[20–23] Additional evidence comes from studies showing that constitutively active mutants of STATs 3 and 5 are transforming in a variety of models, whereas dominant-negative STAT5 can block the transforming activity of the TEL–JAK2 oncoprotein.[24,25] Finally, the observation that STATs 3 and 5 are often constitutively phosphorylated in leukemia, lymphoma, multiple myeloma as well as in various solid tumors further supports the notion that abnormal activation of these STAT proteins can contribute to tumor cell growth.

## Other signaling pathways

The JAK–STAT pathway is the most direct and potentially most selective route to the regulation of gene

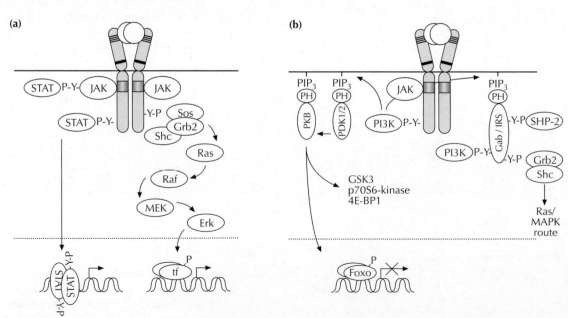

**Figure 3.2** Schematic representations of (a) JAK–STAT and Ras and (b) PI3K/PKB signaling pathways, the latter involving recruitment of signaling molecules with pleckstrin homology (PH) domains to the cell membrane through binding to phosphoinositides (PIP$_3$).

expression, since the SH2-containing target recruited to the receptor complex is the transcription factor itself. Other signals from cytokine receptors take a more tortuous path to the nucleus, providing more opportunity for crosstalk and branching. For example, there are several distinct mechanisms for the activation of the Ras signaling pathway, which may differentially involve the adapter proteins Shc (Figure 3.2a) and docking proteins such as Gab, and IRS (Figure 3.2b). Via binding of an additional adapter protein, Grb2, the nucleotide exchange factor son-of-sevenless (Sos) is recruited, leading to activation of the Ras protein. Ras, in its turn, stimulates the Raf, MEK, and subsequently the MAPK (mitogen-activated protein kinase) protein serine/threonine kinases. Finally, the MAPKs Erk1 and Erk2, JNK, and p38 regulate transcription by phosphorylating several transcription factor complexes involved in controlling the cell cycle, cell survival, and differentiation.[26,27] Other examples of signaling substrates activated in this more complex manner include tyrosine kinases of the Src and Tec families, phospholipid kinases, and phospholipases (PLCγ).[28]

Another important signaling cascade is initiated via recruitment of p85, the SH2-containing regulatory subunit of phosphatidylinositol 3′-kinase (PI3K). This lipid kinase catalyzes the generation of phosphatidylinositol 3,4,5-trisphosphate (PI-3,4,5-$P_3$, or $PIP_3$ for short), which serves as a docking site for proteins with a pleckstrin homology (PH) domain, for instance the docking proteins Gab and IRS, the serine/threonine kinases PDK1 and PDK2 and protein kinase B (PKB/c-Akt) (Figure 3.2b). Apart from its regulatory function in cellular metabolism, by phosphorylating glycogen synthase kinase 3 (GSK3) and phosphofructokinase 2 (PFK2), and protein synthesis, by phosphorylating 4E-binding protein 1 (4E-BP1) and p70S6-kinase, activated PKB plays a major role in controlling cellular survival and growth. PKB directly phosphorylates the Bcl-2 family member Bad and caspase-9, thereby inhibiting their pro-apoptotic activities. Furthermore, PKB negatively regulates the expression of the cell cycle inhibitors p27 and p130 and the pro-apoptotic factor Bim. This involves inhibition of the activity of the Forkhead transcription factors Foxo1, Foxo3A, and Foxo4 through phosphorylation of these proteins, leading to their retention in the cytoplasm[29-31] (Figure 3.2b).

It should be noted that the above description of signaling mechanisms is simplified and far from complete. It is particularly important to realize that, rather than acting in linear pathways, signaling proteins are increasingly seen to form interactive networks at almost every step of the signaling process. As a consequence, activation of distinct signaling routes often converges on a set of target genes.

# Mechanisms that switch off receptor activation

Continuous activation of receptors would eventually lead to uncontrolled responses of the target cells. Therefore, different feedback mechanisms exist to ensure that cytokine receptors act transiently. These mechanisms, depicted in Figure 3.3, include (1) dephosphorylation of phosphotyrosines and $PIP_3$ by phosphatases or inactivation of Ras-like proteins by GTPase accellerating proteins (GAPs), (2) masking phosphotyrosines by CIS/SOCS proteins, and (3) internalization and degradation of receptor complexes.

## Phosphatases and GAPs

Inherent to the fact that the JAK tyrosine kinases are crucial for the cytokine response is that protein tyrosine phosphatases (PTPases) can downmodulate receptor function. Currently, SHP-1 and, to a lesser extent, SHP-2 and CD45 are examples of PTPases whose inhibitory effects on the JAK–STAT pathway have been demonstrated.[32-34] SHP-1, also known as hematopoietic cell phosphatase (HCP), binds to phosphorylated tyrosine residues of the receptors via its SH2 domains. Such a direct interaction of SHP-1 with receptor proteins has been demonstrated for the common β chain of the IL-3/IL-5/GM-CSF receptors, the EPO-R, and c-Kit.[35] The importance of this mechanism is supported by the phenotype of motheaten mice, which lack Shp-1. These mice suffer from a disease characterized by autoimmunity and inflammation.[36] In addition, a human hematological condition, benign

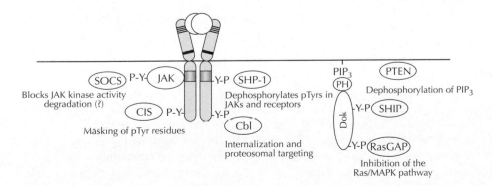

**Figure 3.3** Major mechanisms involved in 'switch-off' of receptor signaling.

erythrocytosis, has been linked to a reduced ability of a cytokine receptor to recruit SHP-1 (see below).

Analogous to phosphotyrosine regulation, dephosphorylation of $PIP_3$ is crucial to silence PI3K signaling. SHIP (SH2-containing inositol-5-phosphatase) is recruited to a number of cytokine receptor complexes and converts PI-3,4,5-$P_3$ to phosphatidylinositol 3,4-bisphosphate (PI-3,4-$P_2$). SHIP$^{-/-}$ mice display a chronic progressive hyperplasia of myeloid cells, associated with increased PKB phosphorylation and reduced apoptosis.[37] The tumor suppressor PTEN (phosphatase and tensin homolog deleted on chromosome 10) dephosphorylates the 3 position of both PI-3,4,5-$P_3$ and PI-3,4-$P_2$, and is therefore a more complete antagonist of PI3K than SHIP. Strikingly, many cell lines and cells from solid tumors show deletions or mutations in the *PTEN* locus, suggesting an important role of this protein in normal growth control. PTEN$^{-/-}$ cells have an extremely high phospho-PKB level, associated with increased survival and proliferation.[38]

As will be explained in more detail in Chapter 27, proteins of the Ras family are inactivated by a group of enzymes that accelerate the GTPase activity of these proteins, thereby reverting the GTP-bound (active) state of Ras-like proteins to their inactive GDP-bound state. These RasGAP proteins can be recruited into the receptor complexes, for example, via interaction with docking proteins such as Dok (Figure 3.3).

### CIS/SOCS/JAB/SSI proteins

Shortly after the cytokine inducible SH2-containing protein CIS (cytokine-inducible substrate) was cloned in 1995, it turned out to be the prototype of a new family of proteins with negative regulatory functions in cytokine receptor signaling.[39] The CIS family comprises eight members that bear the alternative names SOCS (suppressor of cytokine signaling), JAB (JAK-binding protein), and SSI (STAT-induced STAT inhibitor). The principle mode of action of these proteins is that the SH2 domains block critical phosphotyrosines in either receptors or JAKs. CIS is a direct target of STAT5, while SOCS1 and SOCS3 are STAT1,3-responsive genes. Upon induction, they bind to the phosphorylated EPO-R, the common β chain of the IL-3/IL-5/GM-CSF receptors (CIS), or the G-CSF-R (SOCS3) and thereby prevent recruitment and activation of other signaling molecules. The SH2 domain of SOCS1/JAB1, on the other hand, specifically binds to phosphorylated Y1007 in the activation loop of JAK2 and is thought to prevent the access of substrates and/or ATP to the catalytic pocket of JAK2.[40,41]

### Internalization and degradation of receptor complexes

After activation, receptors are rapidly internalized into (early) endosomes. The mechanisms involved in the internalization of cytokine receptors are still poorly characterized. For intrinsic tyrosine kinase receptors, a major mechanism controlling receptor endocytosis has been unveiled.[42,43] An important step in this process is the recruitment of the oncoprotein Cbl, again via a phosphotyrosine–SH2 domain interaction. Cbl attracts a complex that contains the Cbl-interacting protein CIN85 and endophilin. The latter protein is probably involved in the invagination and scission of the vesicle. Furthermore, Cbl recruits an enzymatic machinery that covalently tags receptor, adapter, and/or signaling proteins with ubiquitin, a peptide of 76 amino acids. The level of ubiquitination then serves as a signal for lysosomal degradation or for recycling to the cell surface.[44] Although this is still controversial, the CIS/SOCS proteins are also thought to recruit a ubiquitin ligase complex via their 'SOCS box', a conserved region in the C terminus. In this situation, the JAKs are supposedly the main target for polyubiquitination.[45]

## Involvement of cytokine receptor mutations in hematological disease

The first evidence for the involvement of cytokine receptors in hematological disorders was obtained in mouse models, in which it was shown that mutations in the genes encoding receptors for EPO and GM-CSF were causally involved in the development of erythroid and myeloid leukemia, respectively.[7,46] In addition, after the cloning and structural characterization of the members of the cytokine receptor family, it was readily recognized that the transforming gene of the myeloproliferative leukemia virus (MPLV) coded for a truncated form of a cytokine receptor, which was later identified as the receptor for thrombopoietin (TPO).[47] These mutations resulted in growth factor-independent activation of the receptors, leading to uncontrolled cell proliferation. Although comparable mutations in the EPO, GM-CSF, and TPO receptors have not been detected in human leukemia, there are several other examples of mutations in cytokine receptor genes involved in human hematological diseases. These mutations appear to affect specific signaling functions of the involved receptor complexes.

### Severe combined immunodeficiency (SCID)

While the underlying molecular defects of SCID, a condition characterized by the almost complete absence of functional B and T lymphocytes, are heterogeneous, at least three types have been identified that are caused by defects in the signaling function of interleukin receptors. For instance, in X-SCID, the affected gene located on Xq13.1 encodes the common interleukin receptor γ chain, required for the formation of, for example, functional receptor complexes for IL-2, IL-7 and IL-15, the major cytokines involved in B- and T-cell development[48-50] (Figure 3.1). The essential contribution of this common γ receptor chain to signaling is its unique ability to recruit JAK3 kinase into the receptor complexes. It is not surprising, therefore, that individuals lacking functional JAK3 suffer from clinical symptoms that are identical to X-SCID.[51,52] Individuals with mutations disrupting the function of the IL-7R α chain also suffer from SCID, although with slightly distinct clinical features, due to the fact that natural killer (NK) cells are still formed in these patients.[53] X-SCID is the first human disease that has been successfully corrected with gene therapy. The basis of this success lies in the fact that the genetically corrected lymphoid cells have a proliferative advantage over the noncorrected cells.[54,55] Unfortunately, a recent follow-up of these cases revealed that two patients developed T-cell malignancies.[55a]

## Benign erythrocytosis

Benign erythrocytosis is characterized by enhanced EPO sensitivity of erythroid progenitors and an absolute increase in red cell mass. Similar to SCID, the underlying disease mechanisms are diverse and only partly understood. Familial erythrocytosis with autosomal dominant inheritance is a specific form of benign erythrocytosis that has been associated with mutations in the gene encoding the EPO receptor (EPO-R).[56] Among different families, frameshift mutations and point mutations in the EPO-R gene have been reported, which all lead to truncations of the receptor C terminus.[57-61] Tyr 449, the principle docking site for SHP-1, is invariably deleted due to this truncation. In view of the fact that SHP-1-deficient mice (motheaten; me$^v$/me$^v$) demonstrate an increased sensitivity to EPO, it is now generally believed that the failure of truncated EPO-R to recruit SHP-1, leading to reduced downregulation of JAK2 kinase activity, is the principle underlying signaling defect. Thus far, not a single case of benign familial erythrocytosis with truncated EPO-R has been reported to progress towards (erythroid) leukemia, suggesting that this defect does not confer a strong predisposition to neoplastic transformation. A mouse model has been developed in which a mutant human EPO-R gene derived from one of the affected families was introduced by homologous recombination.[62] These mice show the expected EPO hyperresponsiveness and erythrocytosis and thus provide a good model to further investigate the molecular and cellular pathology of the disease.

## Congenital amegakaryocytic thrombocytopenia (CAMT)

CAMT is a rare disease presenting with isolated thrombocytopenia and a severe paucity of megakaryocytes in the bone marrow. Often, a more generalized cytopenia develops in later childhood. Several cases of CAMT have been reported with frameshift or nonsense mutations in the c-mpl gene that disrupt the expression of a functional TPO-R.[63-66] Because TPO is the main regulator of thrombocytopoiesis and has also been demonstrated to be an important factor in early hematopoiesis, c-mpl mutations are being considered the single cause of both the thrombocytopenia and the progression into pancytopenia seen in patients with CAMT.

## Severe congenital neutropenia (SCN)

SCN is characterized by the almost complete absence of peripheral neutrophils due to a myeloid maturation block in the bone marrow. The disease presents with a variable genetic background and comprises both familial and sporadic cases. While the cellular mechanism(s) involved in the pathogenesis of SCN are still unknown, recent studies have implicated mutations in the gene encoding neutrophil elastase as a major underlying genetic defect in SCN.[67] The disease management of SCN, characterized in the pre-growth factor therapy era by a high mortality due to opportunistic bacterial infections, has improved dramatically upon the introduction of G-CSF in the clinic, with over 90% of the patients responding favorably to G-CSF treatment.[68]

Along with the prolonged lifetime expectancy, a predisposition to develop myelodysplastic syndrome (MDS) and/or acute myeloid leukemia (AML) was unmasked in a subgroup of patients.[69] Progression of SCN to MDS/AML correlates strongly with the presence of acquired mutations in a critical stretch in the coding region of the G-CSF-R gene, resulting in C-terminal truncations of the G-CSF-R protein. Typically, clones harboring such mutations can already be detected in the neutropenic phase of the disease in approximately 20% of cases. In some cases, affected myeloid cells descend from minority clones, originally making up only 1–2% of the myeloid progenitor cell compartment. However, clones harboring G-CSF-R mutations become overt in more than 80% of the SCN cases upon progression to MDS and AML, suggesting that truncated forms of G-CSF-R commonly contribute to the expansion of the (pre-)leukemic clones that arise in SCN. Studies in knock-in mouse models with equivalent targeted mutations have established that the truncated G-CSF-R confers a hyperproliferative response of myeloid progenitor cells to G-CSF.[70,71] The truncated G-CSF-R displays multiple defects that can be linked to its perturbed signaling properties. These abnormalities include defective receptor internalization, increased and sustained activation of STAT5 and PI3K/PKB and the loss of specific docking sites for the negative regulators SOCS3 and SHIP.[72-77]

# Kit mutations in AML and mastocytosis

Kit is a receptor tyrosine kinase encoded by the c-*kit* gene, the cellular homolog of the viral oncogene v-*kit*.[78,79] Different cell types, including hematopoietic precursor cells, mast cells, melanocytes, germ cells, and the interstitial cells of Cajal, express c-Kit. Together with Flt3 and the receptors for M-CSF and platelet-derived growth factor (PDGF), c-Kit belongs to the type III family of RTKs. These receptors have five immunoglobulin-like repeats in the extracellular domain, a single transmembrane region, and a cytoplasmic kinase domain that is interrupted by a kinase insert sequence.[6] In normal situations, the kinase activity of c-Kit is tightly regulated by its ligand, stem cell factor (SCF; also called Steel factor, mast cell growth factor, and c-Kit ligand). Ligand binding induces receptor oligomerization and subsequent auto/transphosphorylation, followed by recruitment and activation of cytoplasmic target proteins, such as members of the MAPK and PI3K pathways, Src tyrosine kinases, and several docking proteins.[80]

## Activating mutations

c-Kit has been implicated in the pathophysiology of a wide variety of human malignancies. These include solid tumors – gastrointestinal stromal tumors (GIST), germ cell tumors, small cell lung, ovarian, and breast carcinomas, neuroblastoma, and melanoma – as well as mastocytosis/mast cell leukemia, sinonasal NK/T-cell lymphoma (SNK/TCL), and AML. Autocrine and/or paracrine stimulation of c-Kit appear to be important for the proliferation of several tumors, but the acquisition of activating mutations is the main cause of aberrant Kit activity in blood cell progenitors.[81]

Mutations associated with human disease have been identified in several different exons of the c-*kit* gene (Figure 3.4). Although the functional significance of some mutations remains to be determined, two different mechanisms of receptor activation can be distin-

guished. 'Enzymatic pocket'-type mutations, represented by codon 816 substitutions (D816V, D816Y, D816F), affect the activation loop at the entrance to the enzymatic pocket (exon 17). The D816V mutation characteristic of mastocytosis results in a higher specific activity and an almost 10-fold increase in ATP affinity.[82] Furthermore, changes in substrate specificity have been reported for codon 816 mutants: (1) STATs 1 and 3 are strongly and constitutively activated, whereas activation of these STATs in normal c-Kit signaling is moderate or absent, depending on the cell type studied, (2) the PI3K pathway is constitutively activated, while activation of the MAPK pathway still requires stimulation with SCF.[83,84]

'Regulatory' mutations do not affect the enzymatic site, but alter regions of the protein that are crucial for the regulation of kinase activity. For example, an $\alpha$ helix in the intracellular juxtamembrane domain (exon 11) suppresses autoactivation, by sterically blocking the activation loop and/or by functioning as an antidimerization domain.[85,86] Small in-frame deletions/insertions or point mutations in this sequence release this inhibitory regulation, resulting in SCF-independent activation.

The distinction between enzymatic and regulatory mutations has major therapeutic implications. To date, most of the small-molecule compounds that have been developed to target tyrosine kinases exhibit their inhibitory effect by binding to the enzymatic site of the kinase. For example, SU9529 and imatinib (STI571) bind to the catalytic site of c-Kit, thereby inhibiting the activity of the wild-type protein. The enzymatic mutations often alter the structure in such a way that the drug no longer obstructs the function of the enzymatic site. This accounts for the fact that these compounds have no effect on the codon 816 mutants of c-Kit, but still inhibit the regulatory c-Kit mutant V560G, which contains a nonmutated kinase domain. These observations have opened new avenues for the development of therapeutic compounds with specific affinity to the mutated enzymatic pocket.[81,87] Furthermore, several new inhibitors have been identified (e.g. SU4984 and SU6577), that

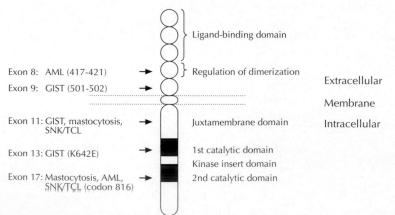

**Figure 3.4** c-*kit* mutations in human disease.

block the activity of wild-type c-Kit, as well as enzymatic and regulatory mutants.

## Mastocytosis and acute myeloid leukemia

SCF is essential for mast cell development. Mutations of codon 816 (most commonly D816V) of c-*kit* are found in neoplastic mast cells in essentially all cases of adult sporadic mastocytosis.[88] As noted above, imatinib does not inhibit the kinase activity of the D816V mutant and would not be predicted to be useful in the treatment of mastocytosis patients with this mutation. Mast cell lines expressing codon 816 mutants are killed when they are cultured in the presence of the compounds SU4984 or SU6577.[89] This indicates that the mutations in c-*kit* are indeed a cause of mastocytosis and that these inhibitors may be clinically useful in treating diseases associated with codon 816 mutations.

In contrast to blast cells in acute lymphoblastic leukemia (ALL), cell surface expression of c-Kit is observed in the neoplastic cells of approximately 80% of AML patients, with a greater prevalence in the M0 and the M1 subtypes than in the M5 subtype.[90,91] Other observations that suggest that c-Kit may be involved in the pathogenesis of AML are (1) the addition of SCF results in the proliferation of some human leukemic cell lines and AML blasts and (2) in a proportion of AML cases, c-Kit phosphorylation was observed in the absence of exogenous SCF, implicating an autocrine loop and/or activating c-*kit* mutations.[81] Recent reports have indeed identified two major classes of c-*kit* mutations in AML. Surprisingly, mutations were only found in patients with core binding factor (CBF) leukemias. The first type of c-*kit* mutation is again the codon 816 substitution, found in 6 of 15 patients with t(8;21) or inv(16).[92] The other class of c-*kit* mutation is the loss or replacement of D419 (exon 8). This type of mutation was found in one-third of cases of AML with the inv(16) karyotype, giving an overall incidence of around 2% in AML.[93] The reason for the association between a translocation of CBF and mutations of c-*kit* is unclear. Also, the functional significance of the codon 419 mutations has not yet been determined. When the D418 mutation is indeed activating, it is most likely a regulatory-type mutation. If this proves correct, inhibitors that act on wild-type c-Kit are expected to block the kinase activity of Kit D418 as well.

## *FLT3* mutations in human AML

Flt3 is by far the most frequently affected receptor in human AML. Mutations in the *FLT3* gene are found in approximately 30% of AML patients and occur in all FAB types and cytogenetic subgroups. Most often, the mutations are small internal tandem duplications (ITD) in the juxtamembrane (JM) domain of the receptor. Similar to the JM mutations in the c-Kit receptor, the *FLT3* JM length mutations affect the kinase autoinhibitory function of the JM domain, resulting in constitutive activation of *FLT3* kinase. Alternatively, but less frequently, mutations affect a critical Asp residue in the activating loop, equivalent to the D816 mutations in c-Kit described above. It has now been firmly established that *FLT3* mutations are indicative of a poor prognosis in AML, independent of other risk parameters, such as specific cytogenetic abnormalities. It is plausible, therefore, that *FLT3* mutations confer a more 'aggressive' phenotype on AML cells, which makes *FLT3* important for the development of kinase inhibitors, along the same lines as the development of imatinib. The significance of *FLT3* mutations in leukemia and their impact on diagnosis/prognosis and therapy development has recently been reviewed[94,95] and is discussed in more detail in Chapter 38.

## REFERENCES

1. Arai K, Watanabe S, Koyano N et al. Cytokine network: control of allergic response and hemopoiesis by hemopoietic growth factors. *J Dermatol* 1992; **19**: 575–83.

2. Theze J. Cytokine receptors: a combinative family of molecules. *Eur Cytokine Netw* 1994; **5**: 353–68.

3. Livnah O, Stura EA, Middleton SA et al. Crystallographic evidence for preformed dimers of erythropoietin receptor before ligand activation. *Science* 1999; **283**: 987–90.

4. Remy I, Wilson IA, Michnick SW. Erythropoietin receptor activation by a ligand-induced conformation change. *Science* 1999; **283**: 990–3.

5. Stahl N, Yancopoulos GD. The alphas, betas, and kinases of cytokine receptor complexes. *Cell* 1993; **74**: 587–90.

6. Ullrich A, Schlessinger J. Signal transduction by receptors with tyrosine kinase activity. *Cell* 1990; **61**: 203–12.

7. Gonda TJ, D'Andrea RJ. Activating mutations in cytokine receptors: implications for receptor function and role in disease. *Blood* 1997; **89**: 355–69.

8. Ihle JN. The Janus protein tyrosine kinase family and its role in cytokine signaling. *Adv Immunol* 1995; **60**: 1–35.

9. Darnell JE Jr. STATs and gene regulation. *Science* 1997; **277**: 1630–5.

10. Aaronson DS, Horvath CM. A road map for those who know JAK–STAT. *Science* 2002; **296**: 1653–5.

11. Meraz MA, White JM, Sheehan KC et al. Targeted disruption of the *Stat1* gene in mice reveals unexpected physiologic specificity in the JAK–STAT signaling pathway. *Cell* 1996; **84**: 431–42.

12. Durbin JE, Hackenmiller R, Simon MC, Levy DE. Targeted disruption of the mouse *Stat1* gene results in compromised innate immunity to viral disease. *Cell* 1996; **84**: 443–50.

13. Park C, Li S, Cha E, Schindler C. Immune response in *Stat2* knockout mice. *Immunity* 2000; **13**: 795–804.

14. Thierfelder WE, van Deursen JM, Yamamoto K et al. Requirement for Stat4 in interleukin-12-mediated responses of natural killer and T cells. *Nature* 1996; **382**: 171–4.

15. Kaplan MH, Sun YL, Hoey T, Grusby MJ. Impaired IL-12 responses and enhanced development of Th2 cells in Stat4-deficient mice. *Nature* 1996; **382**: 174–7.

16. Takeda K, Tanaka T, Shi W et al. Essential role of Stat6 in IL-4 signalling. *Nature* 1996; **380**: 627–30.

17. Shimoda K, van Deursen J, Sangster MY et al. Lack of IL-4-induced Th2 response and IgE class switching in mice with disrupted *Stat6* gene. *Nature* 1996; **380**: 630–3.

18. Igaz P, Toth S, Falus A. Biological and clinical significance of the JAK–STAT pathway; lessons from knockout mice. *Inflamm Res* 2001; **50**: 435–41.

19. Touw IP, De Koning JP, Ward AC, Hermans MH. Signaling mechanisms of cytokine receptors and their perturbances in disease. *Mol Cell Endocrinol* 2000; **160**: 1–9.

20. Maurer AB, Wichmann C, Gross A et al. The Stat5–RARα fusion protein represses transcription and differentiation through interaction with a corepressor complex. *Blood* 2002; **99**: 2647–52.

21. Dong S, Tweardy DJ. Interactions of STAT5b–RARα, a novel acute promyelocytic leukemia fusion protein, with retinoic acid receptor and STAT3 signaling pathways. *Blood* 2002; **99**: 2637–46.

22. Nguyen MH, Ho JM, Beattie BK, Barber DL. TEL–JAK2 mediates constitutive activation of the phosphatidylinositol 3′-kinase/protein kinase B signaling pathway. *J Biol Chem* 2001; **276**: 32704–13.

23. Carron C, Cormier F, Janin A et al. TEL–JAK2 transgenic mice develop T-cell leukemia. *Blood* 2000; **95**: 3891–9.

24. Coffer PJ, Koenderman L, de Groot RP. The role of STATs in myeloid differentiation and leukemia. *Oncogene* 2000; **19**: 2511–22.

25. Schwaller J, Parganas E, Wang D et al. Stat5 is essential for the myelo- and lymphoproliferative disease induced by TEL/JAK2. *Mol Cell* 2000; **6**: 693–704.

26. Su B, Karin M. Mitogen-activated protein kinase cascades and regulation of gene expression. *Curr Opin Immunol* 1996; **8**: 402–11.

27. Shaulian E, Karin M. AP-1 as a regulator of cell life and death. *Nat Cell Biol* 2002; **4**: E131–6.

28. Pawson T, Saxton TM. Signaling networks – Do all roads lead to the same genes? *Cell* 1999; **97**: 675–8.

29. Cantley LC. The phosphoinositide 3-kinase pathway. *Science* 2002; **296**: 1655–7.

30. Kops GJ, Burgering BM. Forkhead transcription factors: new insights into protein kinase B (c-akt) signaling. *J Mol Med* 1999; **77**: 656–65.

31. Leevers SJ, Vanhaesebroeck B, Waterfield MD. Signalling through phosphoinositide 3-kinases: the lipids take centre stage. *Curr Opin Cell Biol* 1999; **11**: 219–25.

32. Jiao H, Berrada K, Yang W et al. Direct association with and dephosphorylation of Jak2 kinase by the SH2-domain-containing protein tyrosine phosphatase SHP-1. *Mol Cell Biol* 1996; **16**: 6985–92.

33. You M, Yu DH, Feng GS. Shp-2 tyrosine phosphatase functions as a negative regulator of the interferon-stimulated Jak/STAT pathway. *Mol Cell Biol* 1999; **19**: 2416–24.

34. Irie-Sasaki J, Sasaki T, Matsumoto W et al. CD45 is a JAK phosphatase and negatively regulates cytokine receptor signalling. *Nature* 2001; **409**: 349–54.

35. Kile BT, Nicola NA, Alexander WS. Negative regulators of cytokine signaling. *Int J Hematol* 2001; **73**: 292–8.

36. Tsui FW, Tsui HW. Molecular basis of the motheaten phenotype. *Immunol Rev* 1994; **138**: 185–206.

37. Rohrschneider LR, Fuller JF, Wolf I et al. Structure, function, and biology of SHIP proteins. *Genes Dev* 2000; **14**: 505–20.

38. Maehama T, Dixon JE. PTEN: a tumour suppressor that functions as a phospholipid phosphatase. *Trends Cell Biol* 1999; **9**: 125–8.

39. Yoshimura A, Ohkubo T, Kiguchi T et al. A novel cytokine-inducible gene *CIS* encodes an SH2-containing protein that binds to tyrosine-phosphorylated interleukin 3 and erythropoietin receptors. *EMBO J* 1995; **14**: 2816–26.

40. Alexander WS. Suppressors of cytokine signalling (SOCS) in the immune system. *Nat Rev Immunol* 2002; **2**: 410–16.

41. Kile BT, Alexander WS. The suppressors of cytokine signalling (SOCS). *Cell Mol Life Sci* 2001; **58**: 1627–35.

42. Petrelli A, Gilestro GF, Lanzardo S et al. The endophilin–CIN85–Cbl complex mediates ligand-dependent downregulation of c-Met. *Nature* 2002; **416**: 187–90.

43. Soubeyran P, Kowanetz K, Szymkiewicz I et al. Cbl-CIN85-endophilin complex mediates ligand-induced downregulation of EGF receptors. *Nature* 2002; **416**: 183–7.

44. Oved S, Yarden Y. Signal transduction: molecular ticket to enter cells. *Nature* 2002; **416**: 133–6.

45. Kile BT, Schulman BA, Alexander WS et al. The SOCS box: a tale of destruction and degradation. *Trends Biochem Sci* 2002; **27**: 235–41.

46. Longmore GD, Lodish HF. An activating mutation in the murine erythropoietin receptor induces erythroleukemia in mice: a cytokine receptor superfamily oncogene. *Cell* 1991; **67**: 1089–102.

47. Vigon I, Mornon JP, Cocault L et al. Molecular cloning and characterization of *MPL*, the human homolog of the v-*mpl* oncogene: identification of a member of the hematopoietic growth factor receptor superfamily. *Proc Natl Acad Sci USA* 1992; **89**: 5640–4.

48. Puck JM, Deschenes SM, Porter JC et al. The interleukin-2 receptor γ chain maps to Xq13.1 and is mutated in X-linked severe combined immunodeficiency, SCIDX1. *Hum Mol Genet* 1993; **2**: 1099–104.

49. Noguchi M, Yi H, Rosenblatt HM et al. Interleukin-2 receptor gamma chain mutation results in X-linked severe combined immunodeficiency in humans. *Cell* 1993; **73**: 147–57.

50. Voss SD, Hong R, Sondel PM. Severe combined immunodeficiency, interleukin-2 (IL-2), and the IL-2 receptor: experiments of nature continue to point the way. *Blood* 1994; **83**: 626–35.

51. Russell SM, Tayebi N, Nakajima H et al. Mutation of Jak3 in a patient with SCID: essential role of Jak3 in lymphoid development. *Science* 1995; **270**: 797–800.

52. Mella P, Schumacher RF, Cranston T et al. Eleven novel JAK3 mutations in patients with severe combined immunodeficiency-including the first patients with mutations in the kinase domain. *Hum Mutat* 2001; **18**: 355–6.

53. Puel A, Ziegler SF, Buckley RH, Leonard WJ. Defective IL7R expression in T⁻B⁺NK⁺ severe combined immunodeficiency. *Nat Genet* 1998; **20**: 394–7.

54. Cavazzana-Calvo M, Hacein-Bey S, de Saint Basile G et al. Gene therapy of human severe combined immunodeficiency (SCID)-X1 disease. *Science* 2000; **288**: 669–72.

55. Hacein-Bey-Abina S, Le Deist F, Carlier F et al. Sustained correction of X-linked severe combined immunodeficiency by ex vivo gene therapy. *N Engl J Med* 2002; **346**: 1185–93.

55a. Hacein-Bey-Abina S, Von Kalle C, Schmidt M, et al. LMO2-associated clonal T cell proliferation in two patients after gene therapy for SCID-X1. *Science* 2003; **302**: 415–9.

56. Prchal JT, Sokol L. 'Benign erythrocytosis' and other familial and congenital polycythemias. *Eur J Haematol* 1996; **57**: 263–8.

57. Arcasoy MO, Degar BA, Harris KW, Forget BG. Familial erythrocytosis associated with a short deletion in the erythropoietin receptor gene. *Blood* 1997; **89**: 4628–35.

58. Arcasoy MO, Karayal AF, Segal HM et al. A novel mutation in the erythropoietin receptor gene is associated with familial erythrocytosis. *Blood* 2002; **99**: 3066–9.

59. de la Chapelle A, Traskelin AL, Juvonen E. Truncated erythropoietin receptor causes dominantly inherited benign human erythrocytosis. *Proc Natl Acad Sci USA* 1993; **90**: 4495–9.

60. Sokol L, Luhovy M, Guan Y et al. Primary familial polycythemia: a frameshift mutation in the erythropoietin receptor gene and increased sensitivity of erythroid progenitors to erythropoietin. *Blood* 1995; **86**: 15–22.

61. Kralovics R, Indrak K, Stopka T et al. Two new EPO receptor mutations: truncated EPO receptors are most frequently associated with primary familial and congenital polycythemias. *Blood* 1997; **90**: 2057–61.

62. Divoky V, Liu Z, Ryan TM et al. Mouse model of congenital polycythemia: homologous replacement of murine gene by mutant human erythropoietin receptor gene. *Proc Natl Acad Sci USA* 2001; **98**: 986–91.

63. Ihara K, Ishii E, Eguchi M et al. Identification of mutations in the c-mpl gene in congenital amegakaryocytic thrombocytopenia. *Proc Natl Acad Sci USA* 1999; **96**: 3132–6.

64. Ballmaier M, Germeshausen M, Schulze H et al. c-mpl mutations are the cause of congenital amegakaryocytic thrombocytopenia. *Blood* 2001; **97**: 139–46.

65. Tonelli R, Scardovi AL, Pession A et al. Compound heterozygosity for two different amino-acid substitution mutations in the thrombopoietin receptor (c-mpl gene) in congenital amegakaryocytic thrombocytopenia (CAMT). *Hum Genet* 2000; **107**: 225–33.

66. van den Oudenrijn S, Bruin M, Folman CC et al. Mutations in the thrombopoietin receptor, Mpl, in children with congenital amegakaryocytic thrombocytopenia. *Br J Haematol* 2000; **110**: 441–8.

67. Dale DC, Person RE, Bolyard AA et al. Mutations in the gene encoding neutrophil elastase in congenital and cyclic neutropenia. *Blood* 2000; **96**: 2317–22.

68. Dale DC, Bonilla MA, Davis MW et al. A randomized controlled phase III trial of recombinant human granulocyte colony-stimulating factor (filgrastim) for treatment of severe chronic neutropenia. *Blood* 1993; **81**: 2496–502.

69. Freedman MH, Bonilla MA, Fier C et al. Myelodysplasia syndrome and acute myeloid leukemia in patients with congenital neutropenia receiving G-CSF therapy. *Blood* 2000; **96**: 429–36.

70. Hermans MH, Ward AC, Antonissen C et al. Perturbed granulopoiesis in mice with a targeted mutation in the granulocyte colony-stimulating factor receptor gene associated with severe chronic neutropenia. *Blood* 1998; **92**: 32–9.

71. McLemore ML, Poursine-Laurent J, Link DC. Increased granulocyte colony-stimulating factor responsiveness but normal resting granulopoiesis in mice carrying a targeted granulocyte colony-stimulating factor receptor mutation derived from a patient with severe congenital neutropenia. *J Clin Invest* 1998; **102**: 483–92.

72. Hunter MG, Avalos BR. Deletion of a critical internalization domain in the G-CSFR in acute myelogenous leukemia preceded by severe congenital neutropenia. *Blood* 1999; **93**: 440–6.

73. Ward AC, van Aesch YM, Schelen AM, Touw IP. Defective internalization and sustained activation of truncated granulocyte colony-stimulating factor receptor found in severe congenital neutropenia/acute myeloid leukemia. *Blood* 1999; **93**: 447–58.

74. Hermans MH, Antonissen C, Ward AC et al. Sustained receptor activation and hyperproliferation in response to granulocyte colony-stimulating factor (G-CSF) in mice with a severe congenital neutropenia/acute myeloid leukemia-derived mutation in the G-CSF receptor gene. *J Exp Med* 1999; **189**: 683–92.

75. Dong F, Larner AC. Activation of Akt kinase by granulocyte colony-stimulating factor (G-CSF): evidence for the role of a tyrosine kinase activity distinct from the Janus kinases. *Blood* 2000; **95**: 1656–62.

76. Hunter MG, Avalos BR. Phosphatidylinositol 3'-kinase and SH2-containing inositol phosphatase (SHIP) are recruited by distinct positive and negative growth-regulatory domains in the granulocyte colony-stimulating factor receptor. *J Immunol* 1998; **160**: 4979–87.

77. Hortner M, Nielsch U, Mayr LM et al. Suppressor of cytokine signaling-3 is recruited to the activated granulocyte-colony stimulating factor receptor and modulates its signal transduction. *J Immunol* 2002; **169**: 1219–27.

78. Besmer P, Murphy JE, George PC et al. A new acute transforming feline retrovirus and relationship of its oncogene v-kit with the protein kinase gene family. *Nature* 1986; **320**: 415–21.

79. Yarden Y, Kuang WJ, Yang-Feng T et al. Human proto-oncogene c-kit: a new cell surface receptor tyrosine kinase for an unidentified ligand. *EMBO J* 1987; **6**: 3341–51.

80. Broudy VC. Stem cell factor and hematopoiesis. *Blood* 1997; **90**: 1345–64.

81. Longley BJ, Reguera MJ, Ma Y. Classes of c-KIT activating mutations: proposed mechanisms of action and implications for disease classification and therapy. *Leuk Res* 2001; **25**: 571–6.

82. Lam LP, Chow RY, Berger SA. A transforming mutation enhances the activity of the c-Kit soluble tyrosine kinase domain. *Biochem J* 1999; **338**: 131–8.

83. Ning ZQ, Li J, Arceci RJ. Signal transducer and activator of transcription 3 activation is required for Asp(816) mutant c-Kit-mediated cytokine-independent survival and proliferation in human leukemia cells. *Blood* 2001; **97**: 3559–67.

84. Chian R, Young S, Danilkovitch-Miagkova A et al. Phosphatidylinositol 3 kinase contributes to the transformation of hematopoietic cells by the D816V c-Kit mutant. *Blood* 2001; **98**: 1365–73.

85. Huse M, Kuriyan J. The conformational plasticity of protein kinases. *Cell* 2002; **109**: 275–82.

86. Ma Y, Cunningham ME, Wang X et al. Inhibition of spontaneous receptor phosphorylation by residues in a putative α-helix in the KIT intracellular juxtamembrane region. *J Biol Chem* 1999; **274**: 13399–402.

87. Heinrich MC, Blanke CD, Druker BJ, Corless CL. Inhibition of KIT tyrosine kinase activity: a novel molecular approach to the treatment of KIT-positive malignancies. *J Clin Oncol* 2002; **20**: 1692–703.

88. Longley BJ Jr, Metcalfe DD, Tharp M et al. Activating and dominant inactivating c-KIT catalytic domain mutations in distinct clinical forms of human mastocytosis. *Proc Natl Acad Sci USA* 1999; **96**: 1609–14.

89. Ma Y, Carter E, Wang X et al. Indolinone derivatives inhibit constitutively activated KIT mutants and kill neoplastic mast cells. *J Invest Dermatol* 2000; **114**: 392–4.

90. Ikeda H, Kanakura Y, Tamaki T et al. Expression and functional role of the proto-oncogene c-*kit* in acute myeloblastic leukemia cells. *Blood* 1991; **78**: 2962–8.

91. Kanakura Y, Ikeda H, Kitayama H et al. Expression, function and activation of the proto-oncogene *c-kit* product in human leukemia cells. *Leuk Lymphoma* 1993; **10**: 35–41.

92. Beghini A, Peterlongo P, Ripamonti CB et al. c-*kit* mutations in core binding factor leukemias. *Blood* 2000; **95**: 726–7.

93. Gari M, Goodeve A, Wilson G et al. c-*kit* proto-oncogene exon 8 in-frame deletion plus insertion mutations in acute myeloid leukaemia. *Br J Haematol* 1999; **105**: 894–900.

94. Gilliland DG, Griffin JD. Role of FLT3 in leukemia. *Curr Opin Hematol* 2002; **9**: 274–81.

95. Gilliland DG, Griffin JD. The roles of FLT3 in hematopoiesis and leukemia. *Blood* 2002; **100**: 1532–42.

# 4 Cell cycle regulation

**N Shaun B Thomas**

## Introduction

Cells of all hematopoietic lineages are derived from a small number of stem cells in the bone marrow. On a population basis, when stem cells divide, it is thought that one of the daughter cells remains as a stem cell (self-renewal) while the other proliferates many times and differentiates to produce a fully functional end-stage cell[1] (see Chapter 1). For an individual stem cell, the decision to self-renew or to differentiate along a particular lineage may be stochastic, but the probabil-

ity of committing to a particular lineage is changed by extrinsic (growth) factors (reviewed in references 2 and 3, and see Chapter 46) which are needed for survival and stimulate cell proliferation. The correct numbers of mature hematopoietic and non-hematopoietic cells of each lineage are produced by a balance between cell division, programmed cell death (apoptosis),[4] replicative senescence, and differentiation governed by the appropriate growth factors. A schema depicting these cell fates during normal hematopoiesis is shown in Figure 4.1(a).

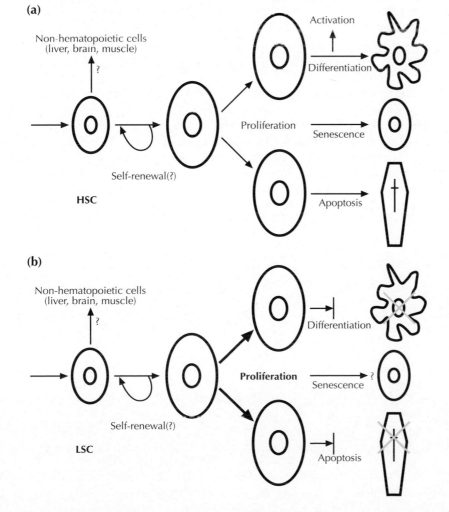

**Figure 4.1** (a) A schema of normal hematopoiesis, highlighting the main processes that govern the fates of hematopoietic cells. The most primitive cells are on the left and mature cells on the right. (HSC, hematopoietic stem cell.) (b) A schema of abnormal hematopoiesis in a patient with leukemia. (LSC, leukemic stem cell.)

Over the past 20 years, many of the basic molecular mechanisms within cells that control each of these processes have been identified. Furthermore, we are beginning to understand how activation of individual molecular mechanisms can have different consequences depending on which other molecular pathways are also activated in the cell. At a given moment in time, a cell has 'molecular circuitry' that interprets the input signal of, for example, *ras* activation, the readout of which may be to cause cell proliferation or to induce replicative senescence. Such complexities enable any given cell to react appropriately and to ensure the production of the correct numbers of mature hematopoietic cells of the appropriate lineage.

In this chapter, I will review what is known about proteins that are involved in regulating cell division, but I will also highlight where they have also been shown to affect other processes such as apoptosis or differentiation. Many of the genes involved in cell proliferation are commonly mutated, deleted, or deregulated in a variety of different malignancies. This, together with inhibition of apoptosis and an aberrant differentiation program, may be sufficient to alter a stem cell so that its progeny predominate and cause leukemia (Figure 4.1b).

This chapter covers what we know about the control of cell division during the mitotic cell cycle. Many of the basic molecular mechanisms are conserved in different cell types and sometimes between organisms that are separated by millions of years of evolution. However, wherever possible, I will concentrate on studies that have been carried out with human hematopoietic cells. The chapter is divided into four sections. The first will cover the principal phases of the cell cycle and where the control points lie. The second reviews those proteins that regulate the cell cycle, concentrating on the cyclin-dependent kinases. The substrates of these kinases will be discussed in the third section, and finally, in the fourth section, I will review what we know about abnormalities in these proteins in hematological malignancies.

## Cell division

In order for a cell to proliferate, an orderly series of processes must be carried out whereby DNA is duplicated and the chromosomes are then segregated accurately to each daughter cell. These processes occur during S (DNA synthesis) phase and mitosis respectively. The mechanisms involved in DNA synthesis and mitosis will not be discussed in this chapter, but there are a number of reviews that cover these topics in detail.[5–8] Although the molecular processes that occur during S and M phases are tightly controlled, responses to extracellular stimuli or to DNA damage that lead to a pause in the cell cycle normally occur during two 'gap' phases, called $G_1$ and $G_2$. These phases precede S phase and M phase respectively (Figure 4.2a). The net result is that when a cell has progressed through all four phases, two genetically identical daughter cells are produced from one original cell.

Certain cells, such as CD34+Lin− stem/early progenitor cells or non-activated peripheral blood T cells are in a quiescent state termed $G_0$ (Figure 4.2a).[9] These are non-dividing cells that will enter the cell cycle ($G_0$→early $G_1$ ($G_{1A}$)) and divide in response to mitogenic growth factors. For example, human T cells require CD3/CD28 costimulation for >2–5 hours to cause them to enter $G_{1A}$, otherwise they remain in $G_0$.[10] A cell that is in $G_0$ will take longer to enter S phase than a proliferating cell that is in $G_{1A}$. In addition, cells in $G_0$ lack many of the proteins that are necessary for S phase to occur. Examples of proteins that are not present in $G_0$ are Cdc6 and the minichromosome maintenance proteins Mcm2 to Mcm7. The Cdc6 and MCM proteins collectively bind DNA at specific sites that define where DNA replication will originate. Binding of these proteins 'licenses' DNA replication at those sites.[11] Enzymes required for DNA synthesis are also not present in $G_0$, including thymidine kinase, ribonucleotide reductase, and DNA polymerase-$\alpha$. These proteins are induced as cells progress from $G_{1A}$ to late $G_1$ ($G_{1B}$).

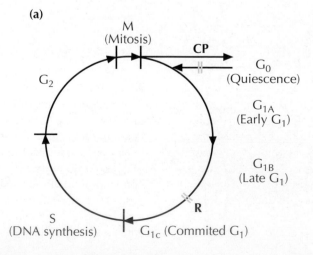

**(a)**

**Figure 4.2** (a) The main phases of the mitotic cell cycle. (R, restriction point; CP, $G_0$→$G_1$ commitment point.)

**(b)**

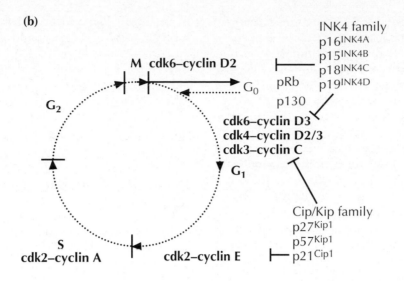

**(c)**

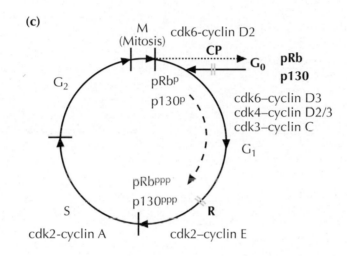

**(d)**

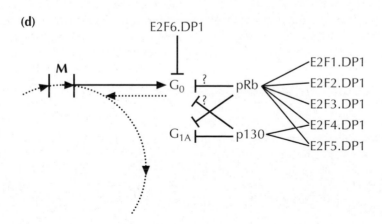

**Figure 4.2** (b) Quiescence ($G_0$). Members of the INK4 and Cip/Kip families of cdk inhibitors prevent the activation of cdk6, cdk4, and cdk2 and maintain cells in a quiescent state. See Figure 4.5 for more details. (A–B indicates that protein A inhibits protein B.) (c) Proliferation. Resorting of cdk–CK1 complexes and down regulation of INK4 and Cip/Kip proteins allows the cdks to be activated by the relevant cyclins. These phosphorylate and inactivate the pRb and p130 proteins and allow cells to progress from $G_0$ through $G_1$ into S phase. (d) pRb, p130, and E2F6 inhibit E2F-dependent transcription. pRb and p130 proteins bind the E2F.DP1 proteins shown and inhibit their activation in $G_0$ or $G_{1A}$. E2F6.DP1 binds to E2F sites in the promoters of several genes in $G_0$ and prevents their activation. See Figure 4.9 for more detail.

Cell size and protein and RNA content also increase markedly as cells progress through $G_1$.[9,12] Entry into the cell cycle and the cellular growth cycle are normally coordinated,[9] and cell size continues to increase as cells progress through the remainder of the cell cycle. This is necessary since cells must ultimately divide to produce two daughter cells that maintain the same characteristic size. Shortening the time taken for a cell to traverse a cell cycle phase such as $G_1$ without also increasing biosynthetic rates to increase cell size would result in smaller cells. Mutations that in vitro reduce the time taken to progress through a given cell cycle phase will not necessarily increase the rate of cell proliferation, as the time taken to traverse through other phases of the cell cycle may be increased to maintain cell size. Homeostatic mechanisms exist to maintain a given cell type at a characteristic size, although the sensing mechanisms in higher eukaryotic cells are poorly understood.[13]

Cell proliferation is controlled at a number of different stages: first, to determine when cells should enter the cell cycle ($G_0 \rightarrow G_1 \rightarrow S$ phase), secondly in proliferating cells ($M \rightarrow G_1 \rightarrow S \rightarrow G_2$), for example to ensure that mitosis follows S phase, and thirdly to control exit from the cell cycle ($M \rightarrow (G_1) \rightarrow G_0$) without inducing apoptosis. For T cells, entry into the cell cycle is regulated by progression through the $G_0 \rightarrow G_1$ commitment point (CP).[10] This is the point beyond which costimulation via the T-cell receptor (CD3) and CD28 are no longer required for progression into $G_{1A}$. There is then a point in $G_{1B}$ called the restriction point (R) beyond which cells become committed to entering S phase (Figure 4.2a) (reviewed in references 9 and 14). The restriction point was defined using fibroblasts, and if these cells are deprived of mitogenic growth factors before R, they will not divide, whereas deprivation after this point (i.e. in $G_{1C}$) has no effect on progression into S phase.

During active proliferation, the cell cycle in progress can be arrested during either $G_1$ or $G_2$ if, for example, DNA has to be repaired. Arrest can also occur when a susceptible cell is exposed to negative growth factors such as interferon-$\alpha$ (IFN-$\alpha$) or transforming growth factor $\beta$ (TGF-$\beta$) that cause cells to exit the cell cycle. However, in the absence either of survival factors or of negative growth factors, growth factor deprivation will trigger some hematopoietic cells to undergo apoptosis.

It is also crucial to maintain the order in which individual cell cycle phases are carried out. Failure to maintain the temporal order between DNA replication and mitosis, i.e. $G_1 \rightarrow S \rightarrow G_2 \rightarrow M \rightarrow G_1$, results in a change in ploidy. This can occur if cell cycle control mechanisms go awry, for example if the *cdc2* gene is deleted experimentally.[15] There are natural situations in which mitosis and cell division do not follow S phase, resulting in the formation of polyploid cells but with no increase in cell number. For example, megakaryocytes are polyploid and one cell can contain hundreds of copies of each chromosome. Experiments that established the basic principles of feedback control governing cell cycle S and M phases include cell fusion experiments of cells in different cell cycle phases,[16,17] and the genes involved are reviewed in references 9, 18, and 19.

# Proteins that regulate the cell cycle

There are certain key proteins within a cell that play a crucial role in responding to a mitogenic stimulus. Cells are maintained in a non-dividing state by members of the INK4 and Cip/Kip families of cyclin-dependent kinase inhibitor (CKI) proteins (Figure 4.2b). Activation of mitogenic signaling pathways in a quiescent cell lead to re-sorting of CKI–cdk–cyclin complexes and activation of cdk4 by D-type cyclins. Some cells also contain cdk6, which is also activated by the D-type cyclins. These kinases then phosphorylate proteins such as the members of the retinoblastoma family (Figure 4.2c). The retinoblastoma protein (pRb), together with its relative, p130, bind E2F transcription factors in non-dividing cells and repress the activity of E2F-responsive genes by recruiting chromatin-remodeling proteins, such as histone deacetylases (HDAC) (Figure 4.2d). This occurs when pRb and p130 are in a hypophosphorylated state. When pRb and p130 are fully (hyper-)phosphorylated during $G_1$ by cdk6–cyclin D, cdk4–cyclin D, and cdk2–cyclin E, they release E2F factors to activate the transcription of a number of different genes that encode proteins required for cells to enter S phase. The E2F family members E2F1 to E2F5 are regulated in this way. However, there is a sixth E2F protein that does not act in the same way as the others. The factor composed of E2F6–DP1 does not bind pRb or p130 but acts as a transcriptional repressor itself when cells are in $G_0$ (Figure 4.2d). In addition to repressing E2F-regulated genes, this factor also inhibits the activities of genes that are activated by c-Myc. Certain cdks are also needed once cells are cycling to coordinate the intricate mechanisms involved in mitosis. The role played by each of these proteins is discussed in detail below, beginning with the cdks.

### Cyclin-dependent kinases

Identification of cell division cycle (*cdc*) yeast mutants by Leland Hartwell, *cdc2* by Paul Nurse, and cyclins by Tim Hunt formed the basis for their shared 2001 Nobel Prize in Medicine (for further details, see the website[20]). These studies provide excellent examples where the power of yeast genetics and biochemical studies of appropriate, simpler eukaryotic organisms have identified evolutionarily conserved mechanisms that also operate in mammalian cells.

The cyclin-dependent kinases (cdks) are a family of serine/threonine kinases that in general control the transitions between successive phases of the cell cycle in eukaryotic cells. Each is the catalytic subunit of a kinase that is activated, as their name suggests, by binding to a cyclin regulatory subunit (reviewed in reference 21). The *cdc2* gene from the budding yeast *Schizosaccharomyces pombe*[22] encodes a protein, p34[cdc2] that is activated by cyclin B and is crucial for regulating mitosis.[5,6,18,23] p34[cdc2] is also important in yeast for ensuring that cells only enter into M phase on completion of the previous S phase.[18,19,22,24,25] If this mitotic kinase is active then the cell is identified as being in $G_2$ and proceeds to M phase. If it is inactive then the cells are redirected into $G_1$ and undergo S phase.

The function of p34[cdc2] in mitosis has been conserved through millions of years of evolution. This was shown by using the human *CDC2* cDNA to functionally replace the yeast *cdc2* gene.[26] However, care should be taken in extrapolating specific details between species. For example, p34[cdc2] has additional roles in higher eukaryotic cells. It can induce apoptosis in terminally differentiated cells but inhibits apoptosis via the survivin pathway during mitosis.[27] Furthermore, whereas the yeast *S. pombe* only needs one cdk, to date 11 kinases homologous to *CDC2* have been identified and cloned from mammalian cells (cdc2 (cdk1) and cdk2–cdk11).[28–34] There is evidence that cdks 7–10 regulate transcription and that cdk11 regulates translation and may also be involved in apoptosis. However, the functions of cdks 1–6 have been studied in most detail and their roles in mammalian cells are discussed below.

Cyclins were originally identified as two proteins (A and B), which were synthesized and degraded in a cyclical fashion during the cell cycle of the surf clam *Spissula* and sea urchin eggs.[35–37] At least 15 cyclins have since been identified in mammalian cells, but not all are synthesized and degraded in this manner.[21] The cyclins do, however, contain a consensus sequence of 100 amino acids, known as the 'cyclin box', which is required for binding the cdk partner.

The mitotic cyclins A, B1, B2, and B3 accumulate during S and $G_2$ phases and are destroyed at a discrete point in mitosis.[20] Degradation requires a small sequence motif (the destruction box) near the N terminus and involves the ubiquitin-dependent proteolytic machinery. Cyclins C, D1, D2, D3, and E accumulate during entry into $G_1$ from $G_0$, and so they are called $G_1$ cyclins (reviewed in reference 38). These $G_1$ cyclins are short-lived proteins, and a sequence, Pro-Glu-Ser-Thr (PEST), within their C terminus is

correlated with their rapid turnover, also probably via a ubiquitin-mediated pathway.[39]

The gene encoding cyclin D1 (*CCND1*) is induced via the ras, Raf, MAPK pathway in some cell types[40,41] and this provides a direct link between growth factor signal transduction (detailed in Chapter 3) and entry into the cell cycle. All three of the D-type cyclins initiate activation of cdk(s) required for progression through $G_1$ into S phase (reviewed in reference 42). They associate primarily with cdk4 and cdk6 but can also bind cdk5.[38,43] Cdk6 activity is detected prior to cdk4 kinase activity in T lymphocytes[10,44,45] and both kinases are involved in early cell cycle events during the $G_0 \rightarrow G_1$ transition. Indeed, suppression of cdk6 by the INK4 protein p18[INK4C] controls the proliferation of murine T cells.[46] Furthermore, inhibition of cdk6/4–cyclin D2 by introducing p16[INK4A] during the first 5 hours of anti-CD3/CD28 stimulation maintains human T cells in $G_0$.[10] In vivo, cyclin D3 is required for the production of CD4+CD8+ double-positive T cells. Thymocytes from *cyclin D3*[-/-] mice fail to proliferate during the DN-3 to DN-4 transition that is required for the maturation of CD4-CD8- to CD4+CD8+ cells.[47,48] Interestingly, cdk6, but not cdk4 or cdk2, also has a role in cell differentiation. Downregulation of cdk6 is required for erythroid differentiation of a mouse erythroleukemia (MEL) cell model and the *CDK6* gene is regulated at least in part by the transcription factor PU.1.[49,50]

In parallel with cyclin association, phosphorylation and dephosphorylation reactions are required for cdks to become active (reviewed in reference 51) (Figure 4.3). For example, although cyclin B accumulates and associates with p34[cdc2] (cdk1) during S and $G_2$/M phases, this complex does not become active until the onset of mitosis. This is because cdk1 is inhibited by phosphorylation of threonine 14 ($T^{14}$) and tyrosine 15 ($Y^{15}$). The crystal structure of cdk2 in active and inactive forms has been solved and the roles of phosphorylation in controlling access to the active site have been determined (reviewed in reference 52). The inhibitory phosphates must be removed in order for the cdk–cyclin complex to become active. This is carried out by cdc25C, which is a member of the cdc25 family of dual-specificity phosphatases (reviewed in reference 51). Furthermore, as an added level of regulation, $T^{161}$ must be phosphorylated by a kinase, which is a complex of cdk7–cyclin H and a p32 protein (reviewed in reference 53). Dephosphorylation of $T^{161}$ occurs at the end of mitosis once the cyclin has been degraded.

Another member of the cdc25 family, cdc25A, forms complexes with the Raf1 kinase in somatic mammalian cells, and Raf1 activates the cdc25A phosphatase in vitro.[54] Thus, this interaction provides another link between mitogenic signal transduction and the cell cycle machinery. As is the case for cdk1,

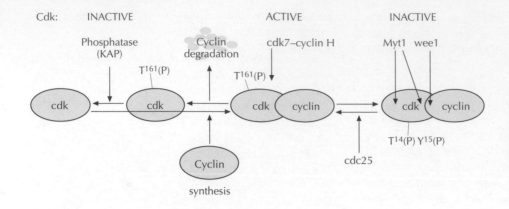

**Figure 4.3** Cdk activation. The cdks are activated by cyclins and by phosphorylation and dephosphorylation of specific amino acids. (Y, tyrosine; T, threonine.)

both cdk4 and cdk2 are phosphorylated on $Y^{15}$, which is a target for cdc25A phosphatase activity. If cdc25A is a substrate in vivo for Raf1 then cdk–cyclin complexes could be activated in $G_1$ in response to growth factors and their activity would then depend only on the balance between relevant cyclins, cdks, and cdk inhibitors (see below). Therefore, withdrawal of growth factors in $G_1$ preceding the restriction point could abort the cell cycle via rapid inactivation of cdc25A and depletion of cyclin D.

Cdk2–cyclin E is active during late $G_1$ and early S phase and is a good candidate for controlling entry into S phase, once cells have passed the restriction point in late $G_1$.[55] It also has a role in centrosome duplication during mitosis.[56] The abundance of cyclin E in the cell has to be regulated within tight limits – too little and cells arrest in $G_1$, whereas too much causes premature entry into S phase and genomic instability (see the section below on abnormalities in malignant cells).

Both c-Myc and Ras pathways can activate cdk2–cyclin E.[57] Activation of cdk2–cyclin E occurs in two steps: the first, induced by c-Myc, involves the release of cdk2–cyclin E from a high-molecular-weight complex, and the second, induced by growth factors, requires cdc25 phosphatase activity[58] (discussed below). However, cdk2–cyclin E is maintained in an inactive state by the cdk inhibitor p27[Kip1] (see the next subsection). Initial activation of cdk2–cyclin E phosphorylates p27[Kip1] and causes its degradation via the ubiquitin pathway (Figure 4.4). This process activates more and more cdk2–cyclin E, which peaks in late $G_1$, allowing cells to enter S phase. It is thought that cdk2 controls its own activity by phosphorylating cyclin E at threonines 62 and 380. An F-box protein hCdc4 (or Fbw7) binds cyclin E when it is phosphorylated at these positions. hCdc4/Fbw7 is an adaptor protein that also binds a ubiquitin ligase complex called SCF (made up of Skp1, Cul1, Rbx1, and E2 proteins). The amount of cyclin E, and hence cdk2 activity, is then reduced by ubiquitination and degradation of cyclin E by the 26S proteasome (Figure 4.4). The papers that delineated these mechanisms provide excellent examples of the power of genetic screens in

model organisms – yeast and fruitflies – to isolate genes whose products carry out similar functions in human cells (reviewed in references 59 and 60).

In spite of such intricate control, genes that encode cdk2 or cyclins E1 and E2 (*CCNE1* and *CCNE2*) are not required for cell proliferation and development in the mouse.[61–64] However, cdk2–cyclin E1/E2 is needed for germ cell development and meiosis. Also, loss of cdk2 affects the timing of S phase, suggesting that cdk2 has a regulatory role in progression through the mitotic cell cycle. Data from a cell-free system suggest that cdk2–cyclin E and cdk2–cyclin A indeed have distinct roles during DNA replication complex assembly and activation. Cdk2–cyclin E stimulates replication complex assembly, making nuclei isolated from cells in $G_1$ competent to replicate DNA. Cdk2–cyclin A then activates DNA synthesis by pre-existing replication complexes and inhibits assembly of new complexes, thereby preventing re-initiation of DNA replication until the next cell cycle.[65]

Cdk2–cyclin A associates with proliferating cell nuclear antigen (PCNA, a cofactor of DNA polymerase δ), as cells enter S phase from $G_1$.[38] Similarly, cdk5 binds PCNA, and so both cdk2 and cdk5 may be involved in DNA synthesis. On the other hand, cdk5 has been detected in terminally differentiated neuronal cells that are incapable of dividing. In non-neuronal cells, cdk5 plays a role in replicative senescence by repressing Rac1 activity and blocking actin polymerization.[66] Cdk5 also phosphorylates proteins called dephosphins that are necessary for synaptic vesicle endocytosis.[67] In hematopoiesis, cdk5 has a role in monocyte differentiation. The cdk5 activator p35[Nck5a] is expressed in monocytes but not in granulocytes or lymphocytes. Activation of cdk5 in HL60 cells causes an increase of markers of monocyte differentiation, such as CD14 and non-specific esterase.[68]

Transfection experiments with dominant-negative mutants have shown that cdk3 as well as cdk2 are required for progression through $G_1$.[69] In addition to inhibiting cell cycle progression dominant-negative cdc2 (cdk1), cdk2, or cdk3 also suppressed apoptosis

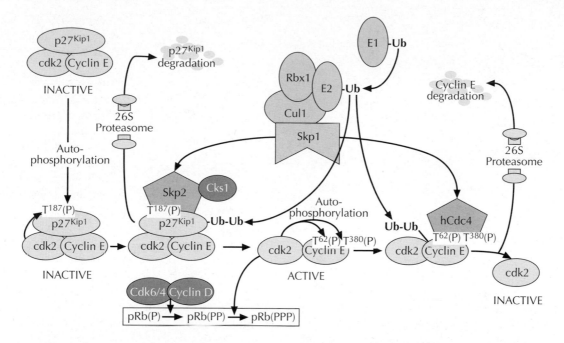

**Figure 4.4** Regulation of cdk2. Cdk2 is activated by cyclin E and inhibited by p27$^{Kip1}$. Both cyclin E and p27$^{Kip1}$ are regulated by ubiquitination and 26S proteasome-mediated degradation. Phosphorylation of p27$^{Kip1}$ by cdk2–cyclin E at T$^{187}$ causes it to be recognized by Skp2 and ubiquitinated by the E2 ligase of the Skp1 complex. Similarly, phosphorylation of cyclin E by cdk2 at T$^{62}$ and T$^{380}$ causes binding of hCdc4 and ubiquitination by the Skp1 complex. Ubiquitinated p27$^{Kip1}$ and cyclin E are degraded by the 26S proteasome.

triggered either by staurosporine or tumor necrosis factor α (TNF-α).[70] Cdk3 is activated by cyclin C, promotes pRb-dependent exit from G$_0$,[71,72] and contributes to the activation of a component of the E2F transcription factor family[73] (the E2F family is reviewed in detail in the section below on substrates of the cdks).

### Cyclin-dependent kinase inhibitors

During G$_1$, cdks are activated by G$_1$ cyclins and inhibited by specific cdk inhibitors (reviewed in reference 74). The cyclin kinase inhibitors (CKI) identified in mammalian cells are proteins that associate either with a cdk or a cyclin–cdk complex and by their association can inhibit kinase activity, leading to cell cycle arrest (Figure 4.5). The CKIs are divided into two groups based both on sequence similarities and on their target proteins. The first group are the inhibitors of cyclin-dependent kinase 4 (INK4). These proteins – p16$^{INK4A}$, p15$^{INK4B}$, p18$^{INK4C}$, and p19$^{INK4D}$ – all have 32-amino-acid ankyrin motifs, inhibit cdk4 and cdk6 specifically, and are potential tumor suppressors. The second group comprises the p21$^{Cip1}$, p27$^{Kip1}$, and p57$^{Kip2}$ proteins, which have homologies in their N-terminal cdk-interacting domain and C-terminal nuclear localization sequence. These are general cdk inhibitors, but they may also be required for activating cdk4–cyclin D (discussed below).

The earliest CKI to be discovered was p16$^{INK4A}$ (encoded by the *CDKN2A* gene; also known as *MTS1* and *Cdk4i*). This protein binds to cdk4 and cdk6, thereby inhibiting their interaction with D-type cyclins.[75] The crystal structure shows that p16$^{INK4A}$ distorts the cyclin-binding site of cdk6 and promotes ATP binding.[76] Inhibition by p16$^{INK4A}$ prevents cdk phosphorylation of the retinoblastoma protein (pRb) (see the section below on substrates of the ckds), halting cell cycle progression from G$_1$ into S phase.[51,77] In contrast, loss of p16$^{INK4A}$ function (see the section below on abnormalities in malignant cells) may result in unscheduled cdk activity, leading to phosphorylation and inactivation of pRb. This in turn can lead to dysregulated progression into the cell cycle[78,79] and may affect other processes such as differentiation and apoptosis (see the section on cdk substrates). p16$^{INK4A}$ expression is high in senescent cells, but it also peaks during S phase, which suggests that it may be required at the G$_1$→S transition to inhibit cdk4 and cdk6 when their activity is no longer necessary.

The p19$^{ARF}$ protein in mice, p14$^{ARF}$ in humans (reviewed in reference 80), is encoded by the same DNA locus as p16$^{INK4A}$. The p19/14$^{ARF}$ protein is produced from an alternative reading frame, which spans exons 2 and 3 of *CDKN2A*[81] (Figure 4.6a). Therefore, the p16$^{INK4A}$ and p19/14$^{ARF}$ proteins are not homologous and p19/14$^{ARF}$ can induce cell cycle arrest without directly inhibiting any of the known cdks.[74]

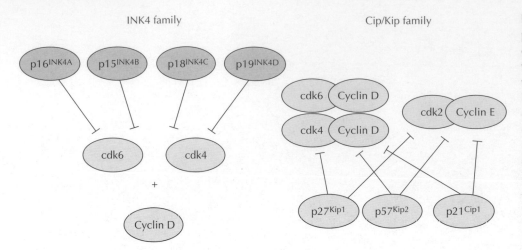

INK4 family

Cip/Kip family

**Figure 4.5** Cdk inhibitor proteins. There are two classes of cdk inhibitors, which act in different ways. The INK4 proteins bind and inhibit cdk4 and ckd6 subunits. The Cip/Kip proteins bind and inhibit the cdk6–cyclin D, cdk4–cyclin E, and cdk2–cyclin E/A complexes. However, the Cip/Kip proteins may also be required for formation of active cdk complexes.

p19/14$^{ARF}$ is induced by mitogenic stimuli, including E1A, c-Myc, activated Ras, v-Abl, and E2F1. The p19/14$^{ARF}$ protein then binds MDM2/HDM2 and sequesters it in the nucleolus where it cannot bind p53.[82] MDM2/HDM2 has E3 ubiquitin ligase activity and causes p53 degradation.[83] Inhibition of MDM2/HDM2 by p19/p14$^{ARF}$ stabilizes p53, leading to growth arrest or apoptosis. Interestingly, p19$^{ARF}$ also binds E2F1, 2, and 3, targets them to the nucleolus, and causes their degradation in a proteasome-dependent manner.[84] Therefore, p19/14$^{ARF}$ can cause cell cycle arrest by more than one mechanism. This is shown schematically in Figure 4.6(b).

p15$^{INK4B}$ (encoded by *CDKN2B*; also known as *MTS*) is highly homologous to p16$^{INK4A}$ (82% protein sequence identity), and the *CDKN2B* gene exists alongside *CDKN2A* on chromosome 9p21. Like p16$^{INK4A}$, p15$^{INK4B}$ binds and inhibits only cdk6 and cdk4, and growth inhibition by TGF-β is mediated in part by the induction of p15$^{INK4B}$. For example, culturing CD34$^+$ long-term culture-initiating cells (LTC-IC) with a neutralizing antibody to TGF-β causes downregulation of p15$^{INK4B}$. When p27$^{Kip1}$ is also depleted by antisense methods, this causes the proliferation of pluripotent hematopoietic progenitor cells that can be retrovirally transduced and engrafted long term in immunocompromised mice.[85] Such data implicate p15$^{INK4B}$ and p27$^{Kip1}$ in maintaining human hematopoietic stem/long-term pluripotent progenitor cells in a quiescent state. In mice, in contrast, p21$^{Cip1}$ is implicated in maintaining stem cells in a quiescent state[86] and p27$^{Kip1}$ regulates the quiescence of early progenitor cells.[87] p15$^{INK4B}$ can also bind other proteins such as NF-κB via ankyrin-binding motifs towards the N terminus, and this may be important for inhibiting cell proliferation independent of the pRb pathway.[88] The role of p15$^{INK4B}$ in hematopoiesis is important, as illustrated by the fact that the *CDKN2B* gene is silenced by promoter hypermethylation in a high percentage of patients with late-stage MDS or AML (see the section on abnormalities in malignant cells).

p18$^{INK4C}$ (encoded by *CDKN2C*; also known as *Ink6A*) and p19$^{INK4D}$ (encoded by *CDKN2D*; *Ink6B*) share some homology with p16$^{INK4A}$ (~40%) and inhibit both cdk4 and cdk6.[51,74] p18$^{INK4C}$, but not p19$^{INK4D}$, is implicated in the cell cycle arrest that occurs during myogenic differentiation.[89] Furthermore, p18$^{INK4C}$ preferentially binds cdk6 in murine T cells, and deleting the *CDKN2C* gene causes T-cell proliferation in response to CD3 that does not require CD28 costimulation.[46] In addition, deletion of *CDKN2C* increases the self-renewal capacity of hematopoietic stem cells.[90]

p21$^{Cip1}$ was discovered in several laboratories using different approaches and is encoded by the *CDKN1A* gene (also known as *WAF1*, *Pic1* and *SDI1*[91]). In whole cells, DNA damage induces the production of p53, which in turn activates the transcription of *CDKN1A*, leading to transient cell cycle arrest by inhibiting cdk activity. p21$^{Cip1}$ can inhibit cell proliferation by two independent mechanisms: cdk inhibition is mediated by sequences towards the N terminus of p21$^{Cip1}$, but p21$^{Cip1}$ also binds proliferating cell nuclear antigen (PCNA) via a sequence at its C terminus, thereby inhibiting PCNA-dependent DNA replication.[92] The importance of these mechanisms is highlighted by the fact that inhibition of p21$^{Cip1}$ by the human papillomavirus (HPV-16) E7 protein uncouples differentiation and proliferation in keratinocytes.[93,94]

Although p21$^{Cip1}$ is a general cyclin-dependent kinase inhibitor, it has greater selectivity for cdks 2, 3, 4 and 6.[95] In normal fibroblasts, inactive cdks exist predominantly in p21$^{Cip1}$–PCNA–cyclin–cdk quarternary complexes and the active kinases exist in cyclin–cdk binary states. The modes of action of members of the two groups of cdk inhibitors have been compared by binding assays in vitro: p21$^{Cip1}$ (and p27$^{Kip1}$ – see below) bind to cyclins even in the absence of the relevant cdk, whereas p15$^{INK4B}$ and p16$^{INK4A}$ bind cdk4 and cdk6 in the absence of cyclins[75] (Figure 4.5). Thus, the inhibitors differ in that p15$^{INK4B}$ and p16$^{INK4A}$ interfere with the formation of cyclin D-dependent kinase complexes, whereas p21$^{Cip1}$ and p27$^{Kip1}$ inhibit by binding

**(a)**

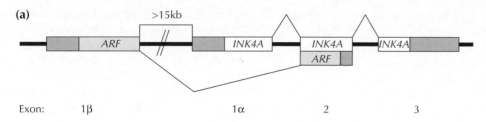

**(b)**

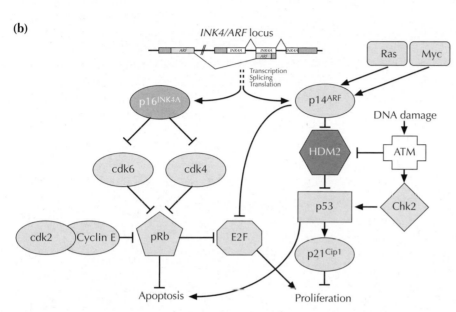

**Figure 4.6** (a) The *INK4A/ARF* locus. The INK4A and ARF proteins are encoded by the same locus. They only use exon 2 in common but the reading frames are different. Therefore, p14[ARF] and p16[INK4A] proteins do not share amino acid sequences in common. (b) The *INK4A/ARF* locus encodes proteins that regulate both the p53 and pRb pathways. p16[INK4A] inhibits cdk4 and cdk6 and so prevents the phosphorylation and inactivation of pRb. This in turn inhibits proliferation and apoptosis. p14[ARF] binds HDM2 (the human homolog of mouse MDM2) and causes its degradation. This in turn allows the activation of p53, which can inhibit proliferation by inducing p21[Cip1] and causes apoptosis.

to cyclin–cdk complexes. Cdks can exist in both active and inactive states in complexes containing p21[Cip1], and the stoichiometry of the complexes is important for determining whether the cdk is active.

p27[Kip1] is homologous to p21[Cip1], binds to cyclin E–cdk2, cyclin A–cdk2, and cyclin D–cdk4, and inhibits the activity of these kinases in vitro in a stoichiometric manner.[74] It also inhibits cdk2, cdk4, and cdk6 by preventing their phosphorylation. In whole cells, p27[Kip1] inhibits cdk2–cyclin E more effectively than cdk4–cyclin D[96,97] and arrests cells in $G_1$. p27[Kip1] is probably involved in a number of mechanisms that cause cell cycle arrest in $G_1$ since its abundance in the cell is elevated following treatment of cells with TGF-β, cAMP, drugs such as tamoxifen, rapamycin, and lovastatin, through cell–cell contact, and during differentiation (reviewed in references 98 and 99). However, the level of mRNA encoding p27[Kip1] does not change markedly under any of these circumstances. Rather, p27[Kip1] is predominantly regulated by degradation via the ubiquitin pathway.[100] p27[Kip1] ubiquitinating activity is more pronounced in cycling cells than in quiescent cells; hence, p27[Kip1] is more abundant during quiescence. However, p27[Kip1] can also be regulated by transcriptional[101] and translational[102] mechanisms.

Degradation of p27[Kip1] is regulated by phosphorylation. It is phosphorylated on serine 10 by human kinase interacting stathmin (hKIS).[103] Phosphory-

lation at p27[Kip1]($S^{10}$) occurs in $G_0/G_1$ after mitogen stimulation and causes p27[Kip1] to be exported from the nucleus to the cytoplasm in association with CRM1.[104] p27[Kip1] can be degraded during $G_1$,[105] although the mechanisms involved have yet to be elucidated. p27[Kip1] is also phosphorylated in the nucleus by cdk2–cyclin E/A at threonine 187 during S and $G_2$ phases of the cell cycle. This allows binding of the Skp2–E3 ubiquitin protein ligase SCF and leads to degradation of p27[Kip1] by the proteasome (reviewed in reference 106). These mechanisms cause p27[Kip1] degradation during transition of cells into the cell cycle (Figure 4.4), but also allow p27[Kip1] levels to be regulated during S and $G_2$.[107] The latter may be important for inhibiting cell proliferation, as elevating p27[Kip1] would then cause cell cycle arrest when they next entered $G_1$. Thus, protein degradation can either inhibit or activate cdk activity: cdk activity is inhibited by ubiquitin-mediated cyclin degradation and can also be activated by ubiquitin-mediated p27[Kip1] degradation.

The mechanisms of action of p27[Kip1] are complex and there is conflicting evidence as to whether p27[Kip1] (or p21[Cip1]) is required for the formation of stable and active cdk4–cyclin D.[108–110] In non-dividing cells, nuclear p27[Kip1] binds cdk–cyclin complexes through its N terminus and in particular it prevents cdk2–cyclin E activation. Mitogenic stimulation causes the formation and activation of cdk6–cyclin D and cdk4–cyclin D complexes in early to mid $G_1$. This causes resorting of cdk–cyclin–CKI complexes, so that some of the p27$^{Kip1}$ binds and stabilizes cdk4–cyclin D, allowing activation of cdk2–cyclin E in late G$_1$ and phosphoryation and degradation of the remaining p27$^{Kip1}$. Mitogen stimulation also causes p27$^{Kip1}$ to be exported from the nucleus to the cytoplasm by stathmin/CRM1. Cytoplasmic p27$^{Kip1}$ can then bind RhoA and regulate cell migration.[111]

p57$^{Kip2}$ is another p21$^{Cip1}$ and p27$^{Kip1}$ homolog, although with a more restricted tissue expression pattern. Its function as a candidate tumor suppressor gene[112,113] is discussed in the section on abnormalities in malignant cells.

# Substrates of the cyclin-dependent kinases

During mitosis, many changes occur in the nucleus, including chromatin condensation, reduction of DNA transcription, inhibition of membrane and vesicular traffic, reorganization of microtubules to form the mitotic spindle apparatus, breakdown of the nuclear envelope, and rearrangement of the actomyosin cytoskeleton for cell rounding and cytokinesis. Many of these changes are regulated by cdk1–cyclin B (reviewed in references 21 and 23). The consensus site that is phosphorylated by cdk1–cyclinB is ($^K/_R$)-$^S/_T$-P-X-K and about 200 potential substrates have been identified that are involved in each of these processes.[51,114] The substrate specificity of each cdk is dependent on its expression in the correct cell cycle phase and in the right place in the cell. For example cdk2–cyclin A cannot phosphorylate substrates in early or mid G$_1$, since cyclin A is only synthesized at the G$_1$/S border. Cyclin B1 translocates to the nucleus at the start of mitosis and cyclin B2 associates with the Golgi, implying that they must cause the phosphorylation of different substrates in each location.

The cdk substrate in G$_1$ that has been studied in most detail is the protein encoded by the *RB1* gene, pRb.[115] pRb is a nuclear phosphoprotein, which is involved in regulating progression through G$_1$ into S phase (reviewed in references 42, 51, and 115). The human protein can be phosphorylated on 15 different sites, all of which are serines or threonines (Figure 4.7a, see Plate 1). This occurs progressively as quiescent cells progress through G$_1$, and pRb is present in a hyperphosphorylated form by the time cells reach the G$_1$/S border. The pRb protein may be inactive when it is completely dephosphorylated in quiescent cells and becomes active when phosphorylated at a few sites by cdk6– or cdk4–cyclin D (so-called hypophosphorylated form) as cells progress into G$_1$.[116] The hypophosphorylated form of pRb binds E2F transcription factors and thereby represses genes encoding proteins that are required for cell cycle progression (see below). Hyperphosphorylation inactivates pRb, allowing cells to enter S phase.

pRb is also acetylated by p300/CBP as cells enter the cell cycle, in response to differentiation signals (e.g. U937 cells plus phorbol ester (PMA)) or in the presence of adenovirus E1A.[117] Acetylation of pRb occurs at lysines 873 and 874, and acetylation of these residues reduces pRb phosphorylation. Thus, acetylation or phosphorylation are two ways of regulating pRb so that the same molecule can potentially operate in different pathways. Acetylation of pRb enhances its ability to bind the MDM2 protein, which indicate that this post-translational modification may also be involved in regulating protein–protein interaction. This may be important in light of the fact that pRb can form a trimeric complex with p53 and MDM2 that is involved in apoptosis.[118]

The pRb protein binds many other proteins and over a hundred have been described.[119,120] Some of the interactions are based on yeast two-hybrid screens and in vitro biochemical binding ('pull-down') assays. However, several have been analyzed in more detail, and these are involved in a number of cellular processes. Some are involved in entry into the cell cycle, while others are important in apoptosis, differentiation, and replicative senescence (Figure 4.8). Space constraints preclude a description of most of these proteins and discussion of the processes that they regulate. However, some are described below and the reader is directed to references 119 and 120 for further references.

Data on the timing of cyclin–cdk activation would suggest that pRb may be phosphorylated by a succession of cdks that are activated at different times during G$_1$: for example, cdk6– and cdk4–cyclin D in early/mid G$_1$, followed by cdk2–cyclin E in late G$_1$ (reviewed in reference 51). Based on sequences around the sites that are phosphorylated in pRb, the consensus sequences that are phosphorylated by cdk2–cyclin E and cdk4–cyclin D have been determined as $^S/_T$-P-X-$^K/_R$ for cdk2 and either P-L-$^S/_T$-P-X-$^K$/R/$_H$ or P-L-$^S/_T$-P-I-P-$^K$/R/$_H$ for cdk4.[121] Phosphorylation-site specificity may be mediated by cyclins; for example, D-type cyclins are nuclear during G$_1$, bind pRb, and target cdk4 to carry out phosphorylation (reviewed in reference 122). pRb is hyperphosphorylated by the time cells reach the G$_1$/S border, which allows progression from late G$_1$ into S phase (reviewed in reference 42). During continuous proliferation of hematopoietic cells, pRb becomes transiently dephosphorylated to several partially phosphorylated forms in early G$_1$ and is hyperphosphorylated from late G$_1$ through the remainder of the cell cycle.[123] Experiments in which individual pRb phosphorylation sites were mutated and these mutants expressed in fibroblast or osteosarcoma cell lines showed that phosphorylation of pRb at specific

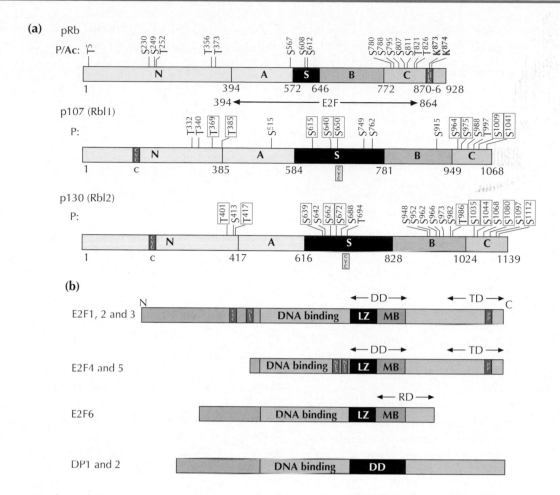

**Figure 4.7** (a) The pRb family. The schema depicting each member of the pRb family show phosphorylation sites in yellow and acetylation sites in red. The phosphorylation sites that are conserved in p130 and p107 are boxed.[162] The A and B domains (separated by a spacer domain, S) make up the 'pocket' that binds proteins with LXCXE motifs. The 'large pocket' (domains A, B, and C) binds E2F–DP factors. The C-terminal domain also binds MDM2 and c-ABL. cyc is the cyclin–cdk binding site (KXLKXL). Numbers indicate amino acids (N→C terminus). (b) The E2F and DP families. The domains shown allow the E2F and DP proteins to dimerize as E2F–DP heterodimers (DD, comprising leucine zipper (LZ) and marked box (MB) domains), to bind pRb, p130, or p107 'pocket proteins' (pp), to bind E2F-binding sequences in the promoters of genes (DNA binding), and to transactivate (TD) or repress (RD) transcription. E2F1, 2, and 3 have nuclear localization signals (NLS) and E2F4 and 5 have nuclear export signals (NES). Cyclin A binds E2F1, 2, and 3 (cyc). The schema is shown with N→C terminus, left to right. See Plate 1.

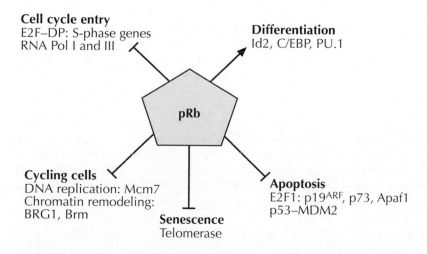

**Figure 4.8** pRb regulates a number of cellular processes. The pRb protein is directly involved in inhibiting (–|) cell cycle progression, apoptosis, and senescence, and induces (→) differentiation. It does so by binding to the proteins shown. Inhibition of E2F1 prevents induction of the pro-apoptotic proteins p19[ARF], p73, and Apaf1.

sites is also necessary for the completion of S phase as well as the transition through $G_1$.[124,125]

Hypophosphorylated pRb prevents cell cycle progression in part by binding E2F transcription factors through the so-called pRb 'pocket' domain and represses their activities. Conversely, hyperphosphorylation of pRb releases E2Fs to activate transcription of genes encoding proteins that are required for DNA synthesis (e.g. DHFR, TK, and DNA Pol $\alpha$) as well as for regulating the cell cycle (e.g. cdk1 and cyclin A) (reviewed in reference 126). pRb can also bind a number of other cellular proteins, such as MDM2–p53,[127] c-Jun, ATF-2, Sp1, Elf-1, C/EBP, PU.1, c-ABL, and PML (reviewed in references 119, 120, and 128–130). PML, which is crucial in the pathogenesis of acute promyelocytic leukemia,[131] is important for the proliferation and differentiation of hematopoietic precursors to erythroid or granulocytic lineages and also has a role later in erythropoiesis.[129,130,132] Phosphorylation of pRb at $S^{780}$ is required to prevent E2F binding, $S^{807}$ and $S^{811}$ phosphorylation inhibits binding to c-Abl but not to E2F, whereas phosphorylation at $T^{826}$ and $T^{821}$ inhibits binding to proteins that contain an LXCXE motif, such as the transcription factor Elf-1, as well as virally encoded E7 and Lg T-antigen proteins.[124,125,133] The phosphorylation site(s) that regulate binding to the myriad of other proteins have not yet been characterized.

Site-specific phosphorylation can regulate binding to specific cellular proteins and, by implication, must be important for controlling a variety of different cellular functions. For example, pRb represses apoptosis (reviewed in references 134 and 135), which is mediated in part through its interaction with MDM2–p53.[127] Cleavage of pRb towards its C terminus by caspase-3 is thought to inhibit its anti-apoptotic function.[136] When the caspase site was mutated in mice such that pRb could no longer be cleaved, this rendered certain tissues resistant to apoptosis triggered via the tumor necrosis factor $\alpha$ (TNF-$\alpha$) receptor, but did not protect against apoptosis induced by DNA damage.[137] pRb also controls muscle, adipocyte, and neuronal differentiation through interacting with specific proteins expressed in these cells, such as MyoD and C/EBP (reviewed in reference 138). Binding to E2F is not necessary for pRb to activate myogenic differentiation or muscle-specific transcription, so the functions of pRb in regulating proliferation and differentiation are separable.[139] Downregulation of pRb with antisense oligodeoxynucleotides increased the number of CFU-E and BFU-E colonies produced from cord blood CD34+ cells in vitro in the presence of interleukin-3 (IL-3) and erythropoietin (EPO), suggesting that pRb may control the proliferation of erythroid cells.[140] Similar experiments with CD34+ cells cultured with Flt3 ligand and IL-3 show that pRb is required for monocytic differentiation.[141] In addition, abnormalities of pRb are fre-

quent in myeloid leukaemias (reviewed in reference 142) and may be prognostic of poor survival[143,144] (discussed in the next section). The $RB1^{-/-}$ mice die at embryonal day 14.5 with neuronal abnormalities, defects in the terminal stages of erythroid differentiation, and unscheduled cell proliferation and apoptosis.[145–149] These observations were thought to support a direct role for pRb in cellular proliferation, apoptosis, and differentiation in vivo. However, ablation of the $RB1$ gene also led to excessive proliferation of trophoblast cells and disruption of placental architecture. This was accompanied by decreased vascularization and reduced placental transport function. Furthermore, a wild-type placenta rescued the neurological and erythroid abnormalities thought to be responsible for the embryonic lethality of $RB1^{-/-}$ animals, but the rescued animals died at birth with severe skeletal muscle defects.[150,151] These data show that pRb has cell-autonomous as well as non-cell-autonomous roles in development.

In addition to having roles in proliferation, differentiation, and apoptosis, pRb is also thought to be involved in replicative senescence.[152] The cdk inhibitor proteins p16INK4A and p21Cip1 are elevated in senescent cells and such cells contain hypophosphorylated pRb. However, the downstream mechanisms are not understood, although it seems that the role of pRb in inducing replicative senescence is independent of its ability to bind E2F or PML.[153] The pRb pathway also has a role in regulating telomerase activity. Expression of full-length pRb but not pRb mutants downregulates telomerase activity.[154] Furthermore, expression of p16INK4A or p15INK4B can inhibit telomerase activity[155] and the E2F1 transcription factor inhibits the $hTERT$ gene.[156] However, mice deficient for $RB1$ did not have elongated telomeres, but combined pRb family knockouts ($RB1^{-/-}p107^{-/-}$ or $RB1^{-/-}p107^{-/-}p130^{-/-}$) did.[157] Thus, although the full picture has yet to emerge, the connections between the pRb family and telomerase activity are important for cellular senescence, and may contribute to the development of cancers in which the pRb pathway is abnormal.

The pRb protein shares regions of homology with two other proteins, p107 and p130 (Rb-like proteins 1 and 2: Rbl1 and Rbl2). Like pRb, they are phosphoproteins that have consensus sites for phosphorylation by cdks. In particular, 22 different serines and threonines are phosphorylated in p130[158] (Figure 4.7a, see color plate). The p130 protein can be separated into at least four forms by one-dimensional polyacrylamide gel electrophoresis. It is present in two distinct forms (forms 1 and 2) in non-dividing cells, and these forms bind proteins such as E2F transcription factors.[159,160] Fully phosphorylated p130 (form 3) is present in actively dividing cells, albeit at lower levels. This form of the protein does not bind E2F4 but does bind E2F1.[161] Twelve of the phosphorylation sites in p130 are not necessary for repressing E2F activity,[158] but it is not clear what other regulatory roles they fulfill. The p107 protein can also be phosphorylated on multiple sites. Seventeen different serine and threonine sites have been identified[162] (Figure 4.7a), and some of these are phosphorylated in whole cells by cyclin D1–cdk4.[163] For each member of the pRb family, there are many different possible phosphorylated forms that could be present in a cell. We know that certain phosphorylation sites in pRb and p130 are required to regulate E2F activity, but it is not known how the vast number of other proteins that bind members of the pRb family are regulated. No doubt, proteome analyses and investigation by protein : protein interaction screens (see e.g. reference 164) will shed light on the complexity of the cellular mechanisms that are controlled by particular forms of each of these proteins.

Hypophosphorylated pRb binds members of the E2F transcription factor family (reviewed in reference 165), and p130 and p107 function in a similar way (Figure 4.2d) (reviewed in reference 166). E2F was named for the factor that regulated the transcription of the *E2* gene of adenovirus. The nomenclature for E2F factors and their protein components can be a little confusing. Each member of the E2F transcription factor family is composed of a heterodimer of an E2F protein (E2F1 to E2F5 are known to bind the pRb family) together with a member of the DP (dimerization partner) family (DP1 and DP2) (Figure 4.7b) (reviewed in reference 167). Different members of the pRb family have some specificity for binding different E2Fs: E2F1, 2, and 3 bind pRb rather than p107, whereas E2F4 and 5 bind p130 and p107 in preference to pRb[51] (Figure 4.2d). The functional consequences are that E2F1 overexpression preferentially overcomes cell cycle arrest by pRb, and E2F4/DP1 overcomes arrest caused by p130. Thus, the balance between particular E2Fs and pRb or p130 is important in determining whether a cell proliferates or remains quiescent. The major E2F complex in primary, CD34+ hematopoietic progenitor cells,[168] quiescent primary T cells,[160,169] B cells, and monocytes is composed of E2F4–DP1 bound to p130.[170] In cycling cells, E2F4 either binds both pRb and p107 or p107 alone.[171] It has been suggested that the presence of the p130–E2F4–DP1 complex defines the non-dividing state,[172] as this complex is not present in proliferating cells. However, E2F6 was identified after these studies were done, and it may also play a role in regulating E2F activity during quiescence.[173]

E2F6 has a truncated C terminus compared with other E2F proteins (Figure 4.7b), and cannot bind pRb, p130, or p107. It also lacks a transcription activation domain, and so does not induce E2F-regulated genes. E2F6–DP1 binds to the promoter of a target gene when cells are in G$_0$ and represses transcription by the assembly of a complex of proteins that alters chromatin structure. This complex contains histone methyltransferase

(HMTase) activity that methylates lysine 9 of histone H3. There are two methyltransferases, NG36/G9A and a newly described Eu-HMTase 1. The roles of histone methylation and other post-translational modifications are reviewed in reference 174. The complex also contains the transcriptional repressor protein HP1γ and polycomb group (PcG)-related proteins (RING1, RING2, MBLR, h-1(3)mbt-like protein, and YAF2). As depicted in Figure 4.9(a) and reviewed in reference 175, E2F6–DP1 binds to the E2F site in the promoter of genes such as *E2F1*, c-*myc*, *cdc25A*, and *TK* (thymidine kinase) in quiescent cells. The histone methyltransferases present in the complex methylate lysine 9 of histone H3 and allow binding of HP1γ. This protein, together with PcG proteins, then cause long-term repression of the chromatin structure, and hence gene activity, at that site. However, the E2F6 complex also contains the Max and Mga proteins and is able to bind to Myc sites in the promoters of target genes. This is important, as this complex therefore has the ability to bind to more than one DNA-binding site. Many E2F and c-Myc-regulated genes are involved in cell proliferation, and it is important that they be repressed effectively on a long-term basis in quiescent cells. Several genes encoding proteins such as E2F1, cdc2, cyclin E, Mcm7, and TK have both E2F and Myc sites in their promoters, and the complex may occupy both sites in these genes. This study was carried out with fibroblasts that were contact-inhibited and serum starved. It is not yet known whether such mechanisms also repress gene transcription long-term in quiescent hematopoietic cells.

Chromatin immunoprecipitation studies have been used to determine which proteins bind to specific sites in the promoters of E2F-regulated genes. Such experiments showed that E2F sites in the promoters of several genes are occupied by the E2F6–DP1 complex when cells are in G$_0$.[173] Complexes containing E2Fs 1 to 4 occupy these sites when cells are in G$_1$. Therefore, it is thought that pRb and p130 take over from E2F6–DP1 and regulate E2F-dependent transcription as cells enter and progress through G$_1$. p130, pRb, and p107 bind individual E2Fs at different stages during entry into the first cell cycle (see reference 171 and references therein), so in theory transcription controlled by specific E2Fs could be repressed at different times. Furthermore, expression of E2F1, 2, or 3 alone, or E2F4 in combination with DP-1, causes quiescent cell lines to progress through G$_1$ into S phase.[176,177] Different genes can be induced preferentially by different E2Fs.[172,178] For example, *DHFR* and *TK* are induced by transfecting E2F2, *CCNA2*, and *CDC2* by both E2F1 and 2 and *CDK2* by E2F3.[172] Thus, activation of specific E2Fs at particular times during G$_1$ may orchestrate the timely activation of individual genes with specific E2F-binding sites in their promoters as cells progress through G$_1$ and into S phase.

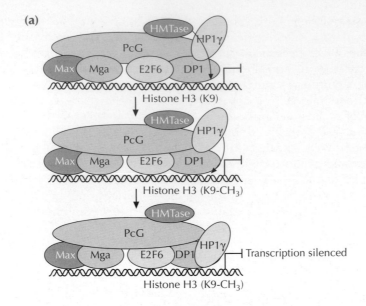

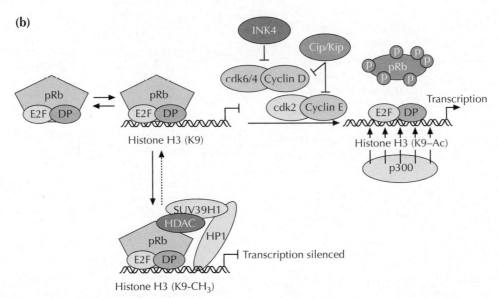

**Figure 4.9** (a) Inhibition of transcription by E2F6. The E2F6–DP1 heterodimer binds to E2F sites in genes such as thymidine kinase (*TK*) and recruits a complex of proteins that lead to gene inactivation. The complex contains several polycomb group-related proteins (PcG) as well as two histone methyltransferases (HMTase). The latter methylate lysine 9 (K9) of histone H3, and this allows the HP1γ transcriptional repressor to silence transcription. The complex also contains Max and Mga proteins that direct binding to Myc and T-box DNA-binding sites. (b) Inhibition of E2F activity by pRb. Hypophosphorylated pRb binds E2F–DP proteins that direct binding to E2F sites in the promoters of genes such as *TK* and DNA POLA. Lysine 9 (K9) of histone H3 is deacetylated by histone deacetylases (HDACs) recruited by pRb, and transcription is inhibited. Deacetylation of histone H3 K9 allows methylation by SUV39H1 and binding by the transcriptional repressor protein HP1. Gene activation involves hyperphosphorylation of pRb by cdk6/4–cyclin D and cdk2–cyclin E, which releases pRb from E2F–DP and allows acetylation of histone H3 K9 by p300.

The p130 and pRb proteins also repress gene activity, which causes cells to exit the cell cycle. This occurs by a mechanism that is similar to E2F6–DP1. p130 or pRb bound to the appropriate E2F–DP heterodimer forms a complex containing histone deacetylase (HDAC).[179,180] This in turn alters chromatin conformation and represses gene activity. Indeed, deacetylation at a specific nucleosome of the CCNE1 gene (encoding cyclin E) may be sufficient to repress its transcription.[181] However, histones can also be replaced in chromatin rather than necessarily being methylated or acetylated.[182] In addition to HDACs, pRb binds a histone methyltransferase (SUV39H1) that methylates lysine 9 of histone H3[183] and targets binding of the repressor HP1[184] (Figure 4.9b). In essence, members of the pRb family act as adaptor proteins that bring together specific combinations of proteins. Therefore, binding of individual E2F–DP combinations by different pRb family members may target these repressor complexes to the promoters of specific groups of genes. This provides a mechanism for turning the transcription of these genes off at specific times during exit from the cell cycle. Understanding such detail is very important, as there are pRb abnormalities or abnormalities in proteins such as p16[INK4A] that regulate the pRb pathway in a number of malignancies, including leukemias (see the next section).

Cells driven to proliferate by experimental overexpression of E2F1 die later by apoptosis; however, this is not necessarily true for E2F2 or E2F3.[185] This has led to the suggestion that E2F1 but not E2F2 or E2F3 specifically induces genes that trigger apoptosis and that a proliferating cell is therefore primed for apoptosis unless rescued by the presence of antiapoptotic proteins, such as pRb[186] or p53.[177] Indeed, overproducing E2F1 in cells containing a temperature-sensitive p53 protein causes apoptosis at the permissive but not at the non-permissive temperature.[187,188] It is important to note that E2F1[-/-] mice have an excess of mature T cells due to a defect in thymocyte apoptosis. The phenotype of the E2F1[-/-] mice is, however, complex (reviewed in reference 189), and suggests that E2F1 can act both as a tumor suppressor and as an oncogene under different circumstances.

E2F1 is a phosphoprotein that can be phosphorylated in vitro only by certain cdks: cdk1–cyclin A > cdk2–cyclin A or cdk1–cyclin B > cdk2–cyclin E, and not at all by cdk4–cyclin D1.[51] Cyclin A is only present from the $G_1$/S border onwards, and the timing of cdk activation by cyclin A correlates with the timing of E2F1 phosphorylation, which occurs during S phase. It is likely that E2F1 phosphorylation during S phase switches off its transcriptional activation, thereby downregulating certain E2F-dependent genes that were activated at the $G_1$/S border when the unphosphorylated E2F was released from repression by pRb. Indeed, there is a checkpoint during S phase that requires E2F1 phosphorylation by cyclin A–cdk. Cells in which this occurs progress through S phase, and if this is disrupted then the cells die by apoptosis.[190] Thus, this mechanism links transcription, DNA replication, and cell cycle progression. Although E2F1 can be phosphorylated by cdk2–cyclin A in the absence of pRb or p107, p107 may provide a link between the cdk and E2F1, which could regulate the timing or specificity of the phosphorylation. In contrast to E2F1, E2F4 is phosphorylated on many different sites and the hyperphosphorylated form is predominant in human quiescent primary CD34+ progenitor cells.[168] This form is lost as cells progress through $G_1$, and this may be required for activation of E2F4. In addition to being phosphorylated, 'free'

E2F1, 2, and 3 that are not bound to pRb, p130, or p107 can also be acetylated.[191,192] Acetylation occurs by CBP/p300-associated P/CAF, and causes increased DNA-binding ability, activation potential, and protein half-life.

The pRb protein regulates transcription of specific genes through suppressing E2F activity, as described above. pRb also regulates rRNA transcription via RNA Pol I and tRNA and 5S rRNA transcription via Pol III. Thus pRb regulates the activity of all three classes of RNA polymerases (reviewed in reference 193). However, suppression of cell proliferation by p107 and pRb are not the same. There are two domains in p107, either of which will prevent proliferation.[194] One domain binds E2F and also HDAC1, and so in this respect the mechanism of growth inhibition may be similar to that of pRb. The second growth-inhibitory domain of p107 binds cdk2–cyclin A or cdk2–cyclin E and this domain does not have a counterpart in pRb. pRb and p107 may also differ in that the c-Myc protein, which is important in driving proliferation, is inhibited by binding to p107.[195] The structure and functions of p130 and p107 proteins are reviewed in reference 196.

From what has been described above, it is clear that regulation of cell cycle entry is complex and involves a coordinated series of phosphorylations of key cell cycle proteins and the activation of a number of genes. Cell cycle exit is also a complicated process, and this is illustrated by the way in which IFN-α causes cell cycle arrest. IFN-α was thought to exert its antiproliferative effect in part via the pRb pathway.[197–200] However, the cytostatic effect of IFN-α may be mediated by a more complicated series of mechanisms that lead to orderly cell cycle arrest rather than triggering apoptosis. We know about some of the processes involved. Cdk activity is decreased,[200–204] which may be due in part to decreases in cdc25A and cyclins D3, E, and H, and an increase in p18[INK4C], in Daudi B cells,[203,205] and induction of the cdk inhibitors p15[INK4B], p16[INK4A], p21[Cip1], and p27[Kip1] in other cell types.[206–209] The initial phosphorylation of pRb during $G_{1A}$ is prevented[198] and free E2F binding to DNA is reduced.[210,211] The latter may in part be due to the induction of the gene 200 cluster (Ifi 200 genes), in particular the p202[212] and p204[213] proteins that bind directly to pRb. IFN-α also causes depletion of the c-Myc protein[200,211,214] by transcriptional and post-transcriptional mechanisms,[211] mediated by the double-stranded RNA-activated kinase PKR,[215] and also causes downregulation of the Oct-1 and Oct-2 transcription factors.[216] Thus, entry into and exit from the cell cycle are complex, orderly processes that involve cdks, the pRb family, and proteins (e.g. the E2Fs), with which they interact. It is not surprising, therefore, that abnormalities in many of these proteins occur in a range of malignancies.

# Abnormalities in malignant cells

## Introduction

Carcinogenesis is thought to be a multistep process involving changes in the expression or abnormalities in the function of proteins encoded by a number of genes within the same cell (reviewed in references 217–219). Such abnormalities affect the balance between cell proliferation, apoptosis, and differentiation, and in hematopoietic malignancies this leads to an expansion of the malignant clone (Figure 4.1b). In at least some malignancies, such as acute myeloid leukemia (AML), this is aided in turn by immune suppression. This is caused in part by inhibition of the proliferation and activity of normal cells by cells of the malignant clone (see reference 220 and references therein). Deregulation of or inactivating mutations in cell cycle proteins contribute to the malignant phenotype. However, as illustrated in the previous section, aberrant expression of a gene that causes cells to proliferate when they should not may lead to apoptosis rather than uncontrolled cell proliferation. Therefore, it is envisaged that abnormalities in numerous genes are needed to deregulate cell proliferation and also to bypass controls that would normally trigger apoptosis, differentiation, or senescence (reviewed in reference 221). The need for multiple mutations to deregulate proliferation without apoptosis is illustrated by the fact that proliferation and apoptosis occur in $RB1^{-/-}$ mouse lens cells but comparable cells lacking both $RB1$ and $TP53$ genes do not undergo apoptosis.[222] Thus, it is not surprising that there are abnormalities in p53 as well as pRb in a large number of different tumors. Many other tumors have mutations, which affect proteins that are necessary for pRb and p53 function. The pRb and p53 proteins are also key targets for inactivation by DNA tumor viruses, including adenovirus (E1A and E1B proteins), simian virus (SV) 40 (large T antigen), and human papillomavirus (HPV E6 and E7 proteins) (reviewed in reference 223).

Studies have been carried out to determine the minimum number of abnormalities that are necessary to cause a cell to become transformed. The classic assay for cooperating oncogenes is the NIH-3T3-transformation assay.[224] However, as NIH-3T3 cells have an unknown number of genetic abnormalities, this assay does not define the minimum number of genetic 'hits' needed. The assay simply defines the number of additional oncogenes that are required to cause anchorage-independent growth in soft agar and tumors in nude mice. Many studies have investigated combinations of oncogenes that transform mouse cells, and transgenic models of various maligancies have been established.[225] Similarly, gene knockout, knock-in, and conditional knockout studies have established that certain genes predispose mice to specific malignan-cies. As an example, the need for cyclins D1 and D2 in cancers caused by aberrant expression of *myc*, *ras*, *neu* and *wnt-1* is discussed in reference 226. Experiments have also been conducted in which gene expression or protein function can be switched on or off at will. These studies investigated the requirement for proteins such as c-Myc and p53 in the establishment and, importantly, in the maintenance of cancers (reviewed in reference 227).

The studies described above relate to mouse models of carcinogenesis. However, mice and humans are not the same, and there are differences in the way the cells respond to genetic abnormalities in both species.[228] Put simply, genes that transform cells in mice do not necessarily do so in humans, and so the implications of such studies for human diseases have to be treated with caution. Studies have investigated whether deregulation of the controls exerted by a combination of pathways, namely Ras, pRb, p53, and telomerase, are sufficient to transform human cells.[229,230] The aim was to produce an immortal human cell that could survive without growth factors and did not need to be anchored to a solid support in order to proliferate. This was achieved in the first study[229] using human embryonic kidney and early-passage normal human fibroblast cells. SV40 large T antigen was introduced to abrogate the functions of both p53 and pRb, and the telomerase catalytic subunit (hTERT) was used to prevent telomere shortening, and the cells were also transfected with an activated *ras* gene (H-*ras*V12). Introduction of H-*ras*V12 alone caused replicative senescence, which was shown previously for murine cells.[231] This is now known to be dependent on p53: caused by acetylation of p53, induction of PML, and formation of PML–p53–CBP chromosomal complexes.[232] hTERT and large T antigen caused immortalization, but only the combination of hTERT, large T antigen, and H-*ras*V12 allowed growth in soft agar and tumors in nude mice. However, in a second study[230] using the same fibroblast line, abrogation of p53 and pRb this time with human papillomavirus 16 E6 and E7 proteins, together with hTERT and H-*ras*V12, was not sufficient to cause growth in soft agar. There are two possible explanations for differences between these studies. First, it is known that large T antigen affects other proteins in addition to pRb and p53,[233] and so other pathways, such as those involving protein phosphatase 2A, may also be involved in transformation;[234] or, secondly, that the order in which the pathways are deregulated is important. In the first paper, a plasmid expressing large T antigen was transfected first, whereas in the second study, cells expressing hTERT were used. However, notwithstanding the differences in outcomes, there is proof of the principle that human cells can be transformed with a limited number of well-defined molecules. This was confirmed by studies on breast[235] and airway epithelial cells.[236] Such studies beg the question whether

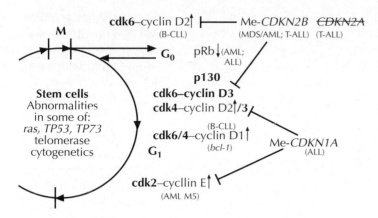

**Figure 4.10** Abnormalities of cell cycle proteins in leukemias. A number of abnormalities in the expression or activities of components of the CKI/cdk/pRb pathway exist in different leukemias. Some of these are illustrated, together with the leukemias in which they are found. The effects of such abnormalities are dependent on the context of abnormalities in other genes such as *ras* and *TP53*, as discussed in the text. (Me-*CDKN2B*: hypermethylation of the *p15^INK4B* gene; *CDKN2A*: deletion in the *CDKN2A* gene; ↑ or ↓: upregulation or downregulation of the protein.)

similar mechanisms that inactivate those pathways are important in the development of a variety of cancers, including leukemias and whether such studies relate to the formation of human cancers in vivo.

This section of the chapter will discuss how overexpression, absence, or mutations of key cell cycle proteins, normally involved in $G_1$ phase of the cell cycle, can result in bypassing control points, which would otherwise induce cell cycle arrest, apoptosis, senescence, or differentiation (Figure 4.1b). I will concentrate on the CKI–cdk–pRb–E2F pathway (Figure 4.2b–d), and the key abnormalities in these molecules in leukemias are summarized in Figure 4.10. At the beginning of this chapter, I alluded to the fact that the molecular circuitry of cells can be important for determining the way in which an abnormal protein acts, and this has been highlighted by recent studies described above (reviewed in reference 237). Therefore, where possible, I will describe what is known of the action of a particular abnormality in the context of other abnormalities that are known to exist in the disease. More generally, there are several excellent reviews of the ways in which cell cycle deregulation contributes to cancer.[238–243] They contain more detail and bibliography than can be covered here.

## pRb, p130, and p107

Abnormalities in the *RB1* gene[244] are responsible for the childhood tumor retinoblastoma.[245] In many other malignancies, *RB1* mutations and deletions[115] are likely to be involved in disease progression. This is true of the invasive phase of bladder cancer and non-small cell lung cancer and in high-grade sarcomas with poor prognosis. pRb is also involved in hematological malignancies (reviewed in references 246–248). Loss of pRb is common in acute lymphoblastic leukemia (ALL), but abnormalities in either pRb or p53 have no prognostic significance.[249] In Hodgkin lymphoma, 16% of patients had loss of pRb and high expression correlated with better survival.[250,251] Abnormalities in the pRb protein also occur in 20–55% of cases of AML, and in three of four

studies this was prognostic of poor remission or survival (reviewed in references 246 and 252). In some cases, pRb may control the proliferation of AML blasts by regulating the *IL-6* gene, and absence of pRb in these cells or suppression of pRb production in vitro with antisense oligodeoxynucleotides causes increased proliferation.[253,254] No mutations, deletions, or promoter hypermethylation of *RB1* have been reported in AML, and no *RB1* mutations have been detected in myelodysplastic syndromes (MDS).[255] However, *RB1* mutations do occur in chronic myeloid leukemia (CML) during accelerated phase and blast crisis, but these may not be the crucial events responsible for CML progression (reviewed in reference 246). In addition, many other genes that regulate pRb have been implicated in carcinogenesis, including the D-type cyclins and the cdk inhibitors, discussed below.

Some abnormalities have also been reported for p130 and p107, although these have not been studied as extensively as pRb. The nuclear localization signal of p130 was mutated in T-ALL and Burkitt lymphoma cell lines as well as in half of primary samples from patients with Burkitt lymphoma.[256,257] This caused p130 to be localized to the cytoplasm rather than the nucleus, where it would be expected to be inactive. Abnormalities in p107 were reported in one T-ALL and one diffuse large cell lymphoma cell line.[258] However, the functional consequences of these abnormalities in p130 and p107 are unclear. Mouse knock-out studies have shown that the other members of the pRb family can compensate for loss of one family member. However, the functional consequences may depend on the other abnormalities that exist in the cells. It is also possible that these are bystander effects that do not contribute to the disease, but cosegregate with other abnormalities that do.

## Cyclins

The gene encoding cyclin D1 (*CCND1*) was identified as the *PRAD1* oncogene of parathyroid adenoma as well as the *bcl-1* oncogene in human B-cell lymphomas (reviewed in reference 122). Amplification of the CCND1 locus occurs in up to 50% of squamous cell, liver, and breast carcinomas. Mice carrying a CCND1 transgene driven by the promoter of the mouse mammary tumor virus develop mammary hyperplasia and adenocarcinoma, providing further evidence that connects overexpression of cyclin D1 and tumorigenesis. When cyclin D1 overexpression is targeted to the lymphoid system and coupled with c-Myc overexpression, the transgenic mice develop lymphomas[259] indicating that cyclin D1 cooperates with other proto-oncogenes in transformation. The hallmark of mantle cell lymphoma (MCL) is the t(11;14) translocation that fuses the immunoglobulin heavy-chain enhancer/promoter to the CCND1 gene. This constitutively activates the CCND1 gene, disrupting its normal regulation. Importantly, gene expression profiling of MCL expressing cyclin D1 identified 20 'proliferation signature' genes that were prognostic of the duration of survival.[260] Those rare MCL cases lacking cyclin D1 expression produce higher levels of cyclins D2 and D3, which are presumed to compensate for its function.

Overexpression of cyclin D1 in mammalian cell lines results in a shortening of $G_1$ phase of the cell cycle,[261] which leads to the appearance of hyperphosphorylated pRb.[51] As mentioned in the section above on cell division, premature entry into S phase that shortens the time taken to progress through the cell cycle would lead to a reduction in cell mass upon cell division, with the result that the cells would be smaller. However, other cell cycle phases are prolonged when cyclin D1 is overexpressed, so the time taken to complete a cell cycle does not change. Other factors associated with cyclin D1 overexpression may contribute to malignancy, such as promotion of growth factor independence or escaping replicative senescence (see below).

Female mice lacking the CCND2 gene have defects in the production of granulosa cells, and so are infertile.[262] This specificity is important, since even though cyclin D2 is expressed in a variety of cell types in the body, it is absolutely necessary for the FSH-driven proliferation of granulosa lutein cells. A possible role in cancer is indicated by the fact that cells from patients with granulosa cell malignancies contain elevated cyclin D2 levels. Furthermore, the CCND2 gene is amplified in a colorectal cancer. There is also a critical role for cyclin D2 in the action of BCR–ABL. Elevated cyclin D2 correlates with BCR–ABL activity,[263,264] and bone marrow cells from cyclin D2$^{-/-}$ mice do not proliferate when transduced with a vector expressing BCR–ABL.[264] These data indicate that cyclin D2 is a necessary downstream target of BCR–ABL in CML. Overexpression of cyclin D2 is a common feature of B-CLL.[265–267] In one patient who transformed to non-Hodgkin lymphoma, a translocation disrupted a negative element in the CCND2 pro-

moter, which would be expected to elevate CCND2 transcription.[268] Cyclin D2 also cooperates with H-Ras, and, in the presence of a low serum concentration, the cells continue to increase their cell mass up to ten times their normal size but do not enter S phase.[269] Thus, they engage the cellular growth cycle[9] without being able to enter the cell cycle.

In normal B lymphocytes, engagement of the B-cell antigen receptor (BCR) induces a cascade of signaling events that culminate in B-cell proliferation and activation. In leukemias and lymphomas, these signaling pathways are dysregulated, which could lead to unscheduled proliferation, survival, and deregulated differentiation. In B-CLL, this allows CD5$^+$ B cells to predominate. In splenic mature B cells, cyclin D2 is essential for BCR-induced hyperphosphorylation of pRb, p130, and p107, regulation of E2F activity, and S-phase entry.[270–272] Furthermore, genetic ablation of the cyclin D2 gene causes a depletion of the B1 (CD5$^+$) population of B cells, but not the conventional CD5$^-$ B2 B cells or other hematopoietic cells.[273] Cyclin D1 is not present in normal B cells, and the existence of normal B cells in cyclin D2 null mice is due to the fact that cyclin D3 can compensate for the function of cyclin D2 in conventional B2 cells.[270]

The cdk inhibitor p27$^{Kip1}$ is a potential downstream target of cyclin D2–cdk4/6, and there is a reciprocal relationship between cyclin D2 and p27$^{Kip1}$ expression.[270,274,275] Furthermore, forced p27$^{Kip1}$ expression causes cell cycle arrest in $G_1$ and induces B-cell apoptosis.[274] In B-CLL, cyclin D2 is overexpressed in CD5$^+$ B cells,[265–267] but cyclin D3 and p27$^{Kip1}$ are also expressed in a higher proportion of CD5$^+$CD19$^+$ B-CLL cells than in normal controls.[268] Cyclin D2–cdk4 and cyclin D3–cdk4 complexes are present in B-CLL cells stimulated to proliferate in vitro, whereas cyclin D3–cdk6 complexes predominate in normal B lymphocytes.[276] In addition to cyclin D2, B-CLL cells also contain high levels of Bcl-2[277,278] and express survivin upon stimulation with CD40L.[279] It has been proposed that the expression of Bcl-2 and survivin protect the CD5$^+$ B cells in B-CLL from undergoing apoptosis. In addition to its role in cell proliferation, cyclin D2 may also have a role in protecting lymphoid and myeloid cells from undergoing apoptosis.[263,266,268] These data indicate that the molecular controls of cell cycle proteins are aberrant in B-CLL,[276] and since this pathway is crucial for the development of CD5$^+$ B cells, individual components of the pathway potentially offer opportunities for therapeutic intervention.

As described above, the third D-type cyclin, cyclin D3, is necessary for the production of CD4$^+$CD8$^+$ double-positive T cells. Cyclin D3 is also necessary for development of mouse models of T-ALL that are induced by Notch1 or p56$^{lck}$. Furthermore, depletion of cyclin D3 by RNAi methods caused $G_0$/$G_1$ arrest of human T-ALL cell lines, indicating that cyclin D3 is necessary for maintaining T-ALL proliferation.[47] The *CCND3* gene is also dysregulated by translocation to immunoglobulin loci in multiple myeloma (MM).[280,281]

The D-type cyclins activate cdk6 and cdk4, and aberrant activation of one or both of these kinases could be responsible for the abnormalities caused by dysregulation of cyclin D1, D2, or D3. Indeed, the gene encoding cdk6 is also dysregulated or forms a fusion gene as a result of chromosomal translocations in several hematopoietic diseases. These include T-ALL, infant ALL (t(7;11)(q22–23)), T-cell lymphoblastic lymphoma with leukemia (t(2;7)(p12;q21–22) juxtaposes the *CDK6* and *Igκ* genes), and B-cell splenic lymphoma with villous lymphocytes (t(2;7)(q21–22)). In-frame *CDK6–MLL* fusion genes have been detected in ALL, and in one case a three-way *MLL, AF4, CDK6* fusion occurred.[282–284] In contrast, *CDK6* is disrupted in splenic marginal zone lymphoma (t(7;21)).[283] Overexpression of cdk6, but not cdk4, blocks erythroid differentiation in vitro,[50] and inhibition of cdk6 and cdk2, but not cdk4 and cdk2, leads to differentiation of erythroleukemia (MEL) cells.[49] Taken together, these data indicate that cdk6 and cdk4 have different roles and implicate cdk6 in regulating cell fates (cell cycle and differentiation).

Overexpression of the D-type cyclins may also affect cell fate decisions by mechanisms that are not dependent on activating cdk6 or cdk4. Most of the evidence (reviewed in reference 285) stems from studies on the role of cyclin D1 in non-hematopoietic cells, such as breast epithelium. Cyclin D1 expression does not correlate with cdk4 activity or other markers of cell proliferation. Cyclin D1 can effect the transcription of several genes, including those encoding chaperone proteins. This occurs at least in part by binding C/EBPβ, and the transcription factors affected include DMP1, androgen receptor, STAT3, BETA2/NeuroD, and thyroid receptors. Cyclin D1 also binds the estrogen receptor. However, it is not yet known to what extent some of these functions are also carried out by cyclins D2 and D3 in hematopoietic cells.

Cyclin E is also elevated in a number of cancers, including cervical and breast cancers (reviewed reference 286). This can occur by gene amplification but also by mutation of *hCDC4*.[287] hCDC4 is an F-box protein that normally regulates cyclin E levels by targeting the cyclin E protein for poly-ubiquitination and proteolysis (Figure 4.4). In hematological malignancies, cyclin E protein is overexpressed in 27% of patients with AML, and in particular in 60% of patients with the M5 subtype.[288] Furthermore, rates of complete remission and disease-free survival were low in patients with M4 or M5 AML with high levels of cyclin E. Cyclin E overexpression is also associated with CLL as well as Hodgkin and non-Hodgkin lymphomas (reviewed in reference 289). The role played by elevated cyclin E is unclear. Elevated expression of cyclin E by transfection shortens $G_1$ phase of the cell cycle, as does elevating cyclin D1, and expression of both cyclins has an additive effect of shortening $G_1$.[261] However, it is not known whether this mechanism operates in AML or CLL. Cyclin E overexpression also leads to changes in chromosome ploidy.[290] This seems to be specific to cyclin E, as neither cyclin D1 nor cyclin A have the same effect. However, it is not known whether cyclin E contributes to malignant transformation in vivo by promoting changes in chromosome ploidy or by affecting the control of cell proliferation.

## CKIs

Abnormalities in cyclin-dependent kinase inhibitors are implicated in a variety of malignancies (reviewed in reference 291). Specific *CDKN2A* mutations, which produce defective p16[INK4A] protein, as well as deletions of the gene, have been detected in a wide range of malignancies.[78,79,292] These include a high proportion of patients with T-ALL,[293] some precursor B-ALL,[293,294] and high-grade and transformed non-Hodgkin lymphoma.[292] In general, cancer-associated mutations in the *CDKN2A* locus do not affect the expression or function of p14[ARF].[295] However, some changes in p14[ARF] in human hematological malignancies have been noted, especially in diffuse large B-cell lymphoma.[296]

Although p14[ARF] is not a CKI, abnormalities in the *INK4/ARF* locus must be considered both in the context of the roles of p14[ARF] as well as p16[INK4A] in malignancy. *Arf* is induced by oncogenes such as *myc*, *ras* and v-*abl*. As discussed in the section on CKIs earlier in this chapter, this causes p53 activation and cell cycle arrest or replicative senescence (Figure 4.6b). Losing the function of p14[ARF] or p53 leads to a breakdown in this mechanism and potentially allows oncogenes such as *myc* to induce proliferation. This is supported by the fact that animals that contain Eµ-*myc* and aberrantly express c-Myc from an immunoglobulin promoter develop B-cell lymphomas in which there are also abnormalities in *Arf* or *TP53*. Furthermore, Eµ-*myc*, *Arf*-/- animals develop rapid and aggressive disease (reviewed in reference 241). These examples show that the consequences of *Arf* abnormalities are complex and dependent on the molecular circuitry that is present in the cell (reviewed in reference 297). Furthermore, the functions of p14/19[ARF] and p16[INK4A] may be different in human and mouse cells (reviewed in reference 298). Such differences in function complicate our analysis and understanding of the functions of p14[ARF] and p16[INK4A]. They also indicate that any basic biological mechanisms that we may consider pertinent to human diseases must be validated with primary human cells rather than necessarily extrapolating from experiments with mice or other organisms.

Another mechanism of *CDKN2A* inactivation is by gene silencing caused by hypermethylation of 5′ CpG islands. Silencing *CDKN2A* occurs in a number of different primary neoplasms and cell lines,[299] including lymphomas, but is rare in leukemias (reviewed in references 248 and 300). Similarly, hypermethylation of $p14^{Arf}$ is rare in leukemias and lymphomas but common in cancers such as colon and stomach (25% and 38%). Genes such as *CDKN2B* (encoding p15$^{INK4B}$), *DAPK*, *CDH1*, and *TP73* are more commonly hypermethylated in leukemias (62%, 9%, 40%, and 31% respectively of patients tested).[301] It should be noted that more than one gene is silenced by aberrant hypermethylation in different cancers and these differ depending on the cancer concerned. As mentioned in the earlier discussion of CKIs, both p16$^{INK4A}$ and p15$^{INK4B}$ prevent cdk4 and cdk6 phosphorylating pRb, and so loss of a functional p16$^{INK4A}$ or p15$^{INK4B}$ would be expected to remove the constraints on cdk6/4–cyclin D activity, thereby promoting cell cycle progression. This view is supported by studies where microinjection of p16$^{INK4A}$ into cell lines deficient for pRb failed to inhibit progression into S phase, whereas elevated levels of p16$^{INK4A}$ in cells containing functional pRb inhibited proliferation.[45,51,177] Cells lacking in pRb have in fact been shown to overexpress p16$^{INK4A}$, and a negative feedback loop between p16$^{INK4A}$ and pRb has been postulated (reviewed in reference 122). However, analysis of blasts from patients with AML showed that this reciprocal relationship occurs only in a subset of cases.[302]

The products of other cell cycle genes implicated in malignancy include cdk4 and p15$^{INK4B}$. The *CDK4* gene is amplified in some tumors, and deletions of *CDKN2B* have been reported in non-small cell lung cancer and in hematological malignancies. *CDKN2B* is abnormal in a high percentage of T-ALL cases, and about half of the cases were reported to have alterations in both *CDKN2B* and *CDKN2A*.[293,303] Deletion of *CDKN2B* also occurs in precursor B-ALL, but at a low frequency.[293]

The importance of silencing of the *CDKN2B* gene comes from an analysis of the myelodysplastic syndromes (MDS). These are a group of hematological disorders that have been described as preleukemic, since many transform to acute leukemia (reviewed in reference 304 and see Chapter 40). Several molecular abnormalities in MDS have been described (reviewed in reference 305), for example *ras* mutations (48% in chronic myelomonocytic leukemia (CMML)),[306,307] Ras overexpression (30%),[308] *p53* (8%), *fms* (5–10%),[309] *IRF1* exon skipping and nucleophosmin overexpression,[310,311] fusion genes (<1%) and increased telomerase activity (×10–50 in refractory anemia with excess blasts in transformation (RAEB-t))[312–314] As mentioned above, the gene encoding the CKI p15$^{INK4B}$ is silenced by promoter hypermethylation in the later stages of MDS in up to 80% of cases.[315–319] This is associated with poor prognosis, increased transformation rates to aggressive subtypes of MDS and AML, and resistance to standard combination chemotherapy regimens, such as those used in de novo AML. This underscores the importance of *CDKN2B* hypermethylation during the transformation of MDS to AML. Furthermore, a randomized trial of the DNA methyltransferase inhibitor 5-azacytidine increased the time taken for transformation to AML, although overall survival was unaffected.[320] *CDKN2B* is also hypermethylated in de novo AML (79%) and in acute promyelocytic leukemia (APL) (73%).[321]

The role of p15$^{INK4B}$ in normal myeloid development is unclear and the effect of losing the p15$^{INK4B}$ protein in the progression of MDS is not understood. Knocking out murine *CDKN2B* alone leads to lymphoproliferative disorders rather than myelodysplasia.[322] As detailed above in the section on proteins that regulate the cell cycle, p15$^{INK4B}$ inhibits cdk6–cyclin D and cdk4–cyclin D activities, which would be expected to cause cell cycle arrest in $G_1$ via pRb- and p130-dependent pathways. However, p15$^{INK4B}$ can also inhibit proliferation by a mechanism independent of pRb.[323] Studies on the function of p15$^{INK4B}$ have been carried out with cell lines or in mice, and not in primary cells from patients that contain other abnormalities that will affect the cellular phenotype. This is crucial since, for example, H-*ras*V12 causes replicative senescence in a normal genetic background[231] but transformation of cells in which the functions of pRb, p53, and telomerase are abrogated.[324] Furthermore, *CDKN2B*$^{-/-}$ mouse embryo fibroblasts, but not *CDKN2B*$^{+/+}$ controls, undergo transformation and grow in soft agar when transfected with H-*ras*V12.[322] The reason why some wild-type cells are resistant to H-*ras*V12 may be that *CDKN2B* can be induced by *ras* activation and p15$^{INK4B}$ expression is sufficient to stop transformation by H-*ras*V12.[325] Taken together, these data would suggest that silencing *CDKN2B* could contribute to leukemic progression by allowing activated *ras* to cause deregulated growth without inducing replicative senescence, by shortening the time taken to progress from $G_0$ to $G_1$, by preventing full differentiation, or by a combination of these. However, several other proteins (p16$^{INK4A}$, p21$^{Cip1}$, and p57$^{Kip2}$) suppress transformation by *ras* or other oncogenes, and studies show that p19$^{ARF}$ and p53 are required for *ras*-induced senescence.[326,327] Thus, the expression of these proteins, as well as abnormalities such as N-*ras*V12 or pRb, will affect the cellular phenotype produced. Several studies have suggested that abnormalities or hypermethylation of *CDKN2A* or *CDKN2B* have prognostic significance. However, to date the data are equivocal (reviewed in reference 248).

Abnormalities in other CKI proteins are uncommon in hematological malignancies. Tissue microarray studies of samples from 316 Hodgkin lymphoma patients showed absence of p18[INK4C] immunostaining in nearly half of the patients studied. The *CDKN2C* gene promoter was hypermethylated in 5 of 26 patients analyzed.[328] Silencing of the *CDKN2C* gene may give the abnormal stem cell a proliferative advantage as studies on *CDKN2C*[-/-] mice show increased stem cell self-renewal.[90] Furthermore, haploinsufficiency in *CDKN2C* sensitizes the mice to carcinogen-induced tumors.[329] In contrast to other INK4 proteins, no abnormalities in *CDKN2D* (encoding p19[INK4D]) were found in a range of hematological malignancies.[330]

A mutation in *CDKN1A* was detected in a cell line derived from a patient with Burkitt lymphoma.[331] The mutated p21[Cip1] protein may function by being less able to suppress cell proliferation than the normal p21[Cip1] protein. *CDKN1A* was silenced by hypermethylation in 41% of ALL patients, and was an independent prognostic factor in predicting disease-free survival in children and adults.[332]

Abnormalities in the gene encoding p27[Kip1] are uncommon,[333] but a mutation in *CDKN1B* was reported in a child with ALL.[334] However, p27[Kip1] expression may be a prognostic indicator of survival in a number of cancers, particularly in combination with cyclin E.[335–337] The abundance of p27[Kip1] in the cell is controlled in part by Skp2 (see the earlier section on CKIs and Figure 4.4). Skp2 is elevated in a number of transformed cell lines[338] and elevating Skp2 in fibroblasts prevents cell cycle exit upon serum withdrawal and causes entry into S phase even in the absence of serum.[339] This provides a mechanism for deregulating the cell cycle, although a role in leukemogenesis has not been investigated. Haploinsufficiency in *CDKN1B*[340] is also important, and animals lacking one copy of *CDKN1B* develop tumors late in life and are very sensitive to chemical carcinogenesis. In humans, hemizygous loss of *CDKN1B* indicates poor prognosis.[341]

p57[Kip2] is a candidate tumor suppressor, as mentioned earlier in this chapter. The *CDKN1C* gene is located at chromosome 11p15.5 and this region is implicated in a number of human cancers, including breast, liver, and bladder cancers, rhabdomyosarcoma, as well as Beckwith–Wiedemann syndrome and Wilms' tumor.[113] Indeed, mice lacking *CDKN1C* exhibit a range of cellular differentiation and proliferation defects reminiscent of Beckwith–Wiedemann syndrome in humans.[112] The *CDKN1C* gene was reported to be silenced by hypermethylation in AML patients, exclusively in those exhibiting a CpG methylator phenotype.[342] However, in another study, *CDKN1C* hypermethylation was detected neither in 14 AML patients nor in MDS or adult T-ALL, but it was hypermethylated in diffuse large B-cell lymphoma (55%) and follicular lymphoma (44%).[343] The functional significance of *CDKN1C* silencing in different hematopoietic cell types remains to be determined.

## Clinical implications of the analyses of pRb/cyclin–cdk/CKI families

Abnormalities in molecules that cause or are normally associated with a particular cancer provide markers that could be used for identifying and categorizing the disease as well as potentially being prognostic indicators. For example, abnormalities in the INK4 and Cip/Kip families have been analyzed in sufficient numbers of patients, so the prognostic significance of such CKI abnormalities can be evaluated. p27[Kip1] is a predictor of poor prognosis in breast, prostate, gastric, and colon cancers (reviewed in reference 337). As described in the preceding subsection, silencing *CDKN1A* by promoter hypermethylation is a prognostic factor in ALL[325] as well as other non-hematological malignancies.[337] Abnormalities in the *CDKN2A* and *CDKN2B* genes are also common in ALL, but to date their prognostic value is controversial.[248,337]

A number of studies have used 'global' gene expression profiling to identify genes that are characteristically expressed in a particular disease. Such analyses have been used to identify known diseases, such as correctly identifying samples from patients with AML, B-ALL, and T-ALL.[344] Microarray studies have also enabled the subclassification of diffuse large B-cell lymphoma[345] and to predict those patients who are more likely to respond to treatment.[346] In each case, the expression of genes encoding proteins responsible for regulating cell proliferation were part of the cohort of 'predictive' genes. For example, the expressions of cyclin *CCND3*, *RBBP4* (a pRb regulator), and *MCM3* (part of the DNA replication origin recognition complex) were all low in AML and high in ALL.[344] High levels of cyclin D2 were characteristic of Philadelphia chromosome-positive cells.[264] Expressions of *CCNB1* and *CDC47* were high in DLBCL relative to follicular lymphoma,[347] and a 'proliferation signature' of 20 genes predicted survival duration in mantle cell lymphoma.[260]

The cell cycle proteins that are abnormal or are aberrantly expressed in hematological malignancies are potential targets for new drugs. One goal is to target the molecules involved in DNA CpG methylation in order to re-express genes such as *CDKN2B* that are silenced by hypermethylation. The drugs 5-azacytidine and 5-aza-2'-deoxycytidine are effective in reactivating a number of silenced genes (reviewed in reference 348), including *CDKN2B* in MDS.[349] Administration of 5-aza-2'-deoxycytidine at lower doses in combination with an HDAC inhibitor (TSA) synergistically cause gene re-expression.[350] These drugs globally change the expression of silenced genes in the cell that may induce apoptosis or cause normal differentiation. However, in some cases, it may be more effective to target specific proteins, such as cdks, that are active in malignant cells. As described earlier in this section, a variety of cdk regulators have been shown to be abnormal in hematological malignancies. These include activating abnormalities such as the expression of cyclins D2 and E, as well as removal of cdk inhibitors such as p16[INK4A]. In addition, the chaperone protein hsp90 is elevated in MDS, AML and chronic lymphocytic leukemia (CLL),[351–353] and this would be expected to stabilize active cdk4–cyclin D, as well as other kinases.

One criterion of carcinogenesis, as described by Hanahan and Weinberg,[240] is that proliferation should become independent of external mitogenic stimuli. Therefore, inhibition of cdk activity should arrest these malignant cells and may induce apoptosis. However, it may also be possible to induce leukemic cells to differentiate by inhibiting cdk2 and cdk6.[354] The active ingredient in a Chinese antileukemia medicine, indirubin, is a cdk inhibitor.[355] The medicine has been used for hundreds of years, and indirubin is currently being tested in clinical trials for CML and chronic granulocytic leukemia (CGL). Flavopiridol and UCN-01 are both cdk inhibitors that have been tested in phase I and II clinical trials in non-Hodgkin lymphoma and non-hematopoietic cancers,[356] and other cdk inhibitors are under development. Drugs that target hsp90, such as geldanamycin and derivatives (e.g. 17AAG), inhibit cdk4–cyclin D, as well as other kinases in the cell.[357] There is much to be done to determine to what extent abnormalities in the CKI–cdk–pRb–E2F pathways are necessary for the maintenance of human leukemic cells and in particular for the survival of leukemic stem cells that can exist in a quiescent state for prolonged periods. Over the coming years, new drugs that target specific components of these pathways may come to the forefront in treating hematological malignancies.

## Conclusions

The control of cell proliferation is a complex process, involving a number of key proteins in the cell. Many of these are part of a pathway that involves pRb, either directly or indirectly. In addition, pRb or one of a number of proteins with which it interacts is abnor-mal in a wide range of malignancies. pRb is also pivotal as it has a role in regulating cell proliferation, apoptosis, and differentiation, as well as replicative senescence. The roles of many of the proteins that are known to bind to or regulate pRb have been studied and we know a great deal about their modes of action. Similarly, defining combinations of proteins that are mutated or that are not expressed in various malignancies is giving us clues as to how they function in a coordinated way to affect the fates of various cell types. In particular, we are beginning to understand that the molecular circuitry is important for determining what consequence a mutation in a given gene will have on that cell. In particular, the molecular abnormalities in each malignancy may differ, but certain pathways are commonly deregulated. This is important as our knowledge is leading to therapies directed at abnormalities in specific cancers that should be more effective, with fewer side-effects on normal cells. However, our increasing knowledge of the mechanisms involved in carcinogenesis also highlights the fact that we cannot simply extrapolate from studies on mice or on cell lines to inform us of the role that specific abnormalities have in particular diseases, such as human leukemias. We know least about which abnormality initiates normal hematopoietic stem cells to become leukemic and which abnormality is necessary to maintain their leukemic potential. Such information would provide targets for early diagnosis and treatment. Obtaining this information presents a considerable challenge for the future, but meeting this challenge is crucial if disease-specific drug therapies are to be effective in eliminating leukemic stem cells from the body.

## Acknowledgments

I thank my colleagues in Leukaemia Sciences at King's College London for critical comments on the manuscript. Work in my laboratory on cell cycle regulation is funded by the Charles Wolfson Charitable Trust, the Leukaemia Research Fund, and the UK Medical Research Council.

**REFERENCES**

1. Morrison SJ, Shah NM, Anderson DJ. Regulatory mechanisms in stem cell biology. *Cell* 1997; **88**: 287–98.

2. Metcalf D, Nicola NA. *The Hemopoietic Colony-Stimulating Factors*. Cambridge: Cambridge University Press, 1995.

3. Devalia V, Linch D. Haemopoietic regulation by growth factors. In: Newland A (ed) *Cambridge Medical Reviews: Haematological Oncology 1*. Cambridge: Cambridge University Press, 1991: 1–28.

4. McKenna SL, Cotter TG. *Adv Cancer Res* 1997: 121–64.

5. Murray A, Hunt T. *The Cell Cycle: An Introduction*. New York: WH Freeman, 1993.

6. Norbury C, Nurse P. Animal cell cycles and their control. *Annu Rev Biochem* 1992; **61**: 441–70.

7. Heichman KA, Roberts JM. Rules to replicate by. *Cell* 1994; **79**: 577–62.

8. King RW, Jackson PK, Kirschner MW. Mitosis in transition. *Cell* 1994; **79**: 563–71.

9. Zetterberg A. Cell growth and cell cycle progression in mammalian cells. In: Thomas NSB (ed) *Apoptosis and Cell Cycle Control in Cancer 2*. Oxford: Bios, 1996: 17–36.

10. Lea NC, Orr SJ, Stoeber K et al. Commitment point during

$G_0 \rightarrow G_1$ that controls entry into the cell cycle. *Mol Cell Biol* 2003; **23**: 2351–61.

11. Blow JJ, Hodgson B. Replication licensing-defining the proliferative state? *Trends Cell Biol* 2002; **12**: 72–8.

12. Morley SJ. Regulation of components of the translational machinery by protein phosphorylation. In: Clemens MJ (ed) *Protein Phosphorylation in Cell Growth Regulation*. Amsterdam: Harwood, 1996: 197–224.

13. Fingar DC, Blenis J. Target of rapamycin (TOR): an integrator of nutrient and growth factor signals and co-ordinator of cell growth and cell cycle progression. *Oncogene* 2004; **23**: 3151–71.

14. Pardee AB. A restriction point control of normal animal cell proliferation. *Proc Natl Acad Sci USA* 1974; **71**: 1286–90.

15. O'Connor DS, Wall NR, Porter AC, Altieri DC. A p34cdc2 survival checkpoint in cancer. *Cancer Cell* 2002; **2**: 43–54.

16. Johnson RT, Rao PN. Mammalian cell fusion: induction of premature chromosome condensation in interphase nuclei. *Nature* 1970; **226**: 717–22.

17. Rao PN, Johnson RT. Mammalian cell fusion: studies on the regulation of DNA synthesis and mitosis. *Nature* 1970; **225**: 159–64.

18. Nurse P. Ordering S phase and M phase in the cell cycle. *Cell* 1994; **79**, 545–50.

19. O'Connell MJ, Nurse P. How cells know they are in $G_1$ or $G_2$. *Curr Opin Cell Biol* 1994; **6**: 867–71.

20. http://www.nobel.se/medicine/laureates/2001/index.html

21. Pines J. Cyclins and cyclin dependent kinases. *Biochem J* 1995; **308**: 697–711.

22. Nurse P, Thuriaux P, Nasmyth K. Genetic control of the cell division cycle in the fission yeast *Schizosaccharomyces pombe*. *Mol Gen Genet* 1976; **146**: 167–78.

23. Nurse P. Universal control mechanism regulating onset of M phase. *Nature* 1990; **344**: 503–8.

24. Hayles J, Fisher D, Woolard A, Nurse P. Temporal order of S phase and mitosis in fission yeast is determined by the state of the p34cdc2–mitotic B cyclin complex. *Cell* 1994; **78**: 813–22.

25. Murray AW. The cell cycle as a *cdc2* cycle. *Nature* 1989; **342**: 14–15.

26. Lee MG, Nurse P. Complementation used to clone a human homologue of the fission yeast cell cycle control gene *cdc2*. *Nature* 1987; **327**: 31–5.

27. O'Connor DS, Wall NR, Porter AC, Altieri DC. A p34cdc2 survival checkpoint in cancer. *Cancer Cell* 2002; **2**: 43–54.

28. Nigg EA. Cyclin-dependent protein kinases: key regulators of the eukaryotic cell cycle. *Bioessays* 1995; **17**: 471–9.

29. Tassan JP, Jaquenoud M, Leopold P et al. Identification of human cyclin-dependent kinase 8, a putative protein kinase partner for cyclin C. *Proc Natl Acad Sci USA* 1995; **92**: 8871–5.

30. Napolitano G, Majello B, Lania L. Role of cyclinT/Cdk9 complex in basal and regulated transcription. *Int J Oncol* 2002; **21**: 171–7.

31. Kasten M, Giordano A. Cdk10, a Cdc2-related kinase, associates with the Ets2 transcription factor and modulates its transactivation activity. *Oncogene* 2001; **20**: 1832–8.

32. Liu Y, Kung C, Fishburn J et al. Two cyclin-dependent kinases promote RNA polymerase II transcription and formation of the scaffold complex. *Mol Cell Biol* 2004; **24**: 1721–35.

33. Mikolajczyk M, Shi J, Vaillancourt RR et al. The cyclin-dependent kinase 11 (p46) isoform interacts with RanBPM. *Biochem Biophys Res Commun* 2003; **310**: 14–18.

34. Shi J, Feng Y, Goulet AC et al. The p34cdc2-related cyclin-dependent kinase 11 interacts with the p47 subunit of eukaryotic initiation factor 3 during apoptosis. *J Biol Chem* 2003; **278**: 5062–71.

35. Evans T, Rosenthal ET, Youngblom J et al. Cyclin: a protein specified by maternal mRNA in sea urchin eggs that is destroyed at each cleavage division. *Cell* 1983; **33**: 389–96.

36. Doree M, Hunt T. From Cdc2 to Cdk1: when did the cell cycle kinase join its cyclin partner? *J Cell Sci* 2002; **115**: 2461–4.

37. Hunt T. The discovery of cyclin (I). *Cell* 2004; **116**: S63–4.

38. Sherr CJ. Mammalian $G_1$ cyclins. *Cell* 1993; **73**: 1059–65.

39. Brandeis M, Hunt T. The proteolysis of mitotic cyclins in mammalian cells persists from the end of mitosis until the onset of S phase. *EMBO J* 1996; **15**; 5280–9.

40. Lavoie JN, L'Allemain G, Brunet A et al. Cyclin D1 expression is regulated positively by the p42/p44MAPK and negatively by the p38/HOGMAPK pathway. *J Biol Chem* 1996; **271**: 20608–16.

41. Peeper DS, Upton TM, Ladha MH et al. Ras signalling linked to the cell cycle machinery by the retinoblastoma protein. *Nature* 1997; **386**: 177–81.

42. Weinberg R. The retinoblastoma protein and cell cycle control. *Cell* 1995; **81**: 323–30.

43. Bates S, Bonetta L, MacAllan D et al. CDK6 (Plstire) and CDK4 (Psk-j3) are distinct subset of the cyclin-dependent kinases that associate with cyclin D1. *Oncogene* 1994; **9**: 71–9.

44. Meyerson M, Harlow E. Identification of $G_1$ kinase activity for cdk6, a novel cyclin D partner. *Mol Cell Biol* 1994; **14**: 2077–86.

45. Lukas J, Parry D, Aagaard L et al. Retinoblastoma-protein-dependent cell-cycle inhibition by the tumour suppressor p16. *Nature* 1995; **375**: 503–6.

46. Kovalev GI, Franklin DS, Coffield VM et al. An important role of CDK inhibitor p18INK4c in modulating antigen receptor-mediated T cell proliferation. *J Immunol* 2001; **167**: 3285–92.

47. Sicinska E, Aifantis I, Le Cam L et al. Requirement for cyclin D3 in lymphocyte development and T cell leukemias. *Cancer Cell* 2003; **4**: 451–61.

48. Weng AP, Aster JC. No T without D3: a critical role for cyclin D3 in normal and malignant precursor T cells. *Cancer Cell* 2003; **4**: 417–18.

49. Matushansky I, Radparvar F, Skoultchi AI. Reprogramming leukemic cells to terminal differentiation by inhibiting specific cyclin-dependent kinases in $G_1$. *Proc Natl Acad Sci USA* 2000; **97**: 14317–22.

50. Matushansky I, Radparvar F, Skoultchi AI. CDK6 blocks differentiation: coupling cell proliferation to the block to differentiation in leukemic cells. *Oncogene* 2003; **22**: 4143–9.

51. Tiwari S, Jamal R, Thomas NSB. Protein kinases and phosphatases in cell cycle control. In: Clemens MJ (ed) *Protein Phosphorylation in Cell Growth Regulation*. Amsterdam: Harwood, 1996: 255–82.

52. Pines J. Confirmation change. *Nature* 1995; **376**: 294–5.

53. Morgan DO. Principles of CDK regulation. *Nature* 1995; **374**: 131–4.

54. Galaktionov K, Jessus C, Beach D. Raf1 interaction with

cdc25 phosphatase ties mitogenic signal transduction to cell cycle activation. *Genes Dev* 1995; **9**: 1046–58.

55. Ekholm SV, Zickert P, Reed SI, Zetterberg A. Accumulation of cyclin E is not a prerequisite for passage through the restriction point. *Mol Cell Biol* 2001; **21**: 3256–65.

56. Ekholm SV, Reed SI. Regulation of G$_1$ cyclin-dependent kinases in the mammalian cell cycle. *Curr Opin Cell Biol* 2000; **12**: 676–84.

57. Leone G, DeGregori J, Sears R et al. Myc and Ras collaborate in inducing accumulation of active cyclin E/Cdk2 and E2F. *Nature* 1997; **387**: 422–6.

58. Steiner P, Philipp A, Lukas J et al. Identification of a Myc-dependent step during the formation of active G$_1$ cyclin–cdk complexes. *EMBO J* 1995; **14**: 4814–26.

59. Bartek J, Lukas J. Cell cycle. Order from destruction. *Science* 2001; **294**: 66–7.

60. Schwab M, Tyers M. Cell cycle. Archipelago of destruction. *Nature* 2001; **413**: 268–9.

61. Aleem E, Berthet C, Kaldis P. Cdk2 as a master of S phase entry: fact or fake? *Cell Cycle* 2004; **3**: 35–7.

62. Berthet C, Aleem E, Coppola V et al. Cdk2 knockout mice are viable. *Curr Biol* 2003; **13**: 1775–85.

63. Mendez J. Cell proliferation without cyclin E–CDK2. *Cell* 2003; **114**: 398–9.

64. Ortega S, Prieto I, Odajima J et al. Cyclin-dependent kinase 2 is essential for meiosis but not for mitotic cell division in mice. *Nat Genet* 2003; **35**: 25–31.

65. Coverley D, Laman H, Laskey RA. Distinct roles for cyclins E and A during DNA replication complex assembly and activation. *Nat Cell Biol* 2002; **4**: 523–8.

66. Alexander K, Yang HS, Hinds PW. Cellular senescence requires CDK5 repression of Rac1 activity. *Mol Cell Biol* 2004; **24**: 2808–19.

67. Tan TC, Valova VA, Malladi CS et al. Cdk5 is essential for synaptic vesicle endocytosis. *Nat Cell Biol* 2003; **5**: 701–10.

68. Chen F, Studzinski GP. Expression of the neuronal cyclin-dependent kinase 5 activator p35$^{Nck5a}$ in human monocytic cells is associated with differentiation. *Blood* 2001; **97**: 3763–7.

69. Van den Heuvel S, Harlow E. Distinct roles for cyclin-dependent kinases in cell cycle control. *Science* 1993; **262**: 2050–4.

70. Meikrantz W, Schlegel R. Suppression of apoptosis by dominant negative mutants of cyclin-dependent protein kinases. *J Biol Chem* 1996; **271**: 10205–9.

71. Ren S, Rollins BJ. Cyclin C/cdk3 promotes Rb-dependent G$_0$ exit. *Cell* 2004; **117**: 239–51.

72. Sage J. Cyclin C makes an entry into the cell cycle. *Dev Cell* 2004; **6**: 607–8.

73. Hofmann F, Livingston DM. Differential effects of cdk2 and cdk3 on the control of pRb and E2F function during G$_1$ exit. *Genes Dev* 1996; **10**: 851–61.

74. Sherr CJ, Roberts JM. Inhibitors of mammalian G$_1$ cyclin-dependent kinases. *Genes Dev* 1995; **9**: 1149–63.

75. Hall M, Bates S, Peters G. Evidence for different modes of action of cyclin-dependent kinase inhibitors: p15 and p16 bind to kinases, p21 and p27 bind to cyclins. *Oncogene* 1995; **11**: 1581–8.

76. Russo AA, Tong L, Lee JO et al. Structural basis for inhibition of the cyclin-dependent kinase Cdk6 by the tumour suppressor p16$^{INK4a}$. *Nature* 1998; **395**: 237–43.

77. Serrano M, Gomez-Lahoz E, DePinho RA et al. Inhibition of ras-induced proliferation and cellular transformation by p16$^{INK4}$. *Science* 1995; **267**: 249–52.

78. Koh J, Enders G, Dynlacht B, Harlow E. Tumour-derived p16 alleles encoding proteins defective in cell-cycle inhibition. *Nature* 1995; **375**: 506–10.

79. Serrano M, Lee H-W, Chin L et al. Role of the *INK4a* locus in tumour suppression and cell mortality. *Cell* 1996; **85**: 27–37.

80. Sharpless NE, DePinho RA. The INK4A/ARF locus and its two gene products. *Curr Opin Genet Dev* 1999; **9**: 22–30.

81. Quelle DE, Zindy F, Ashmun RA, Sherr CJ. Alternative reading frames of the *INK4a* tumor suppressor gene encode two unrelated proteins capable of inducing cell cycle arrest. *Cell* 1995; **83**: 993–1000.

82. Weber JD, Taylor LJ, Roussel MF et al. Nucleolar Arf sequesters Mdm2 and activates p53. *Nat Cell Biol* 1999; **1**: 20–6.

83. Zhang Y, Xiong Y. Control of p53 ubiquitination and nuclear export by MDM2 and ARF. *Cell Growth Differ* 2001; **12**: 175–86.

84. Martelli F, Hamilton T, Silver DP et al. p19$^{ARF}$ targets certain E2F species for degradation. *Proc Natl Acad Sci USA* 2001; **98**: 4455–60.

85. Dao MA, Taylor N, Nolta JA. Reduction in levels of the cyclin-dependent kinase inhibitor p27$^{kip-1}$ coupled with transforming growth factor beta neutralization induces cell-cycle entry and increases retroviral transduction of primitive human hematopoietic cells. *Proc Natl Acad Sci USA* 1998; **95**: 13006–11.

86. Cheng T, Rodrigues N, Shen H et al. Hematopoietic stem cell quiescence maintained by p21$^{cip1/waf1}$. *Science* 2000; **287**: 1804–8.

87. Cheng T, Rodrigues N, Dombkowski D et al. Stem cell repopulation efficiency but not pool size is governed by p27$^{kip1}$. *Nat Med* 2000; **6**: 1235–40.

88. Aytac U, Konishi T, David H et al. Rb independent inhibition of cell growth by p15$^{INK4B}$. *Biochem Biophys Res Commun* 1999; **262**: 534–8.

89. Franklin DS, Xiong Y. Induction of p18$^{INK4c}$ and its predominant association with CDK4 and CDK6 during myogenic differentiation. *Mol Biol Cell* 1996; **7**: 1587–99.

90. Yuan Y, Shen H, Franklin DS et al. In vivo self-renewing divisions of haematopoietic stem cells are increased in the absence of the early G$_1$-phase inhibitor, p18$^{INK4C}$. *Nat Cell Biol* 2004; **6**: 436–42.

91. El-Deiry WS. p53, p21$^{WAF1/CIP1}$ and the control of cell proliferation. In: Thomas NSB (ed) *Apoptosis and Cell Cycle Control in Cancer 2* Oxford: Bios, 1996: 55–76.

92. Luo Y, Hurwitz J, Massague J. Cell cycle inhibition by independent CDK and PCNA domains in p21$^{CIP1}$. *Nature* 1995; **375**: 159–61.

93. Funk JO, Waga S, Harry JB et al. Inhibition of CDK activity and PCNA-dependent DNA replication by p21 is blocked by interaction with the HPV-16 E7 oncoprotein. *Genes Dev* 1997; **11**: 2090–100.

94. Jones DL, Alani RM, Munger K. The human papillomavirus E7 oncoprotein can uncouple cellular differentiation and proliferation in human keratinocytes by abrogating p21$^{Cip1}$-mediated inhibition of cdk2. *Genes Dev* 1997; **11**: 2101–11.

95. Harper JW, Ellege SJ, Keyomarsi K et al. Inhibition of cyclin-dependent kinases by p21. *Mol Cell Biol* 1995; **6**: 387–400.

96. Blain SW, Montalvo E, Massague J. Differential interaction of the cyclin-dependent kinase (Cdk) inhibitor p27$^{Kip1}$ with cyclin A–Cdk2 and cyclin D2–Cdk4. *J Biol Chem* 1997; **272**: 25863–72.

97. Soos TJ, Kiyokawa H, Yan JS et al. Formation of p27-CDK complexes during the human mitotic cell cycle. *Cell Growth Differ* 1996; **7**: 135–46.

98. Alessandrini A, Chiaur DS, Pagano M. Regulation of the cyclin-dependent kinase inhibitor p27 by degradation and phosphorylation. *Leukaemia* 1997; **11**: 342–5.

99. Durand B, Gao F-B, Raff M. Accumulation of the cyclin-dependent kinase inhibitor p27/Kip1 and the timing of oligodendrocyte differentiation. *EMBO J* 1997; **16**: 306–17.

100. Pagano M, Tam SW, Theodoras AM et al. Role of the ubiquitin-proteasome pathway in regulating abundance of the cyclin-dependent kinase inhibitor p27. *Science* 1995; **269**: 682–5.

101. Servant MJ, Coulombe P, Turgeon B, Meloche S. Differential regulation of p27$^{Kip1}$ expression by mitogenic and hypertrophic factors: Involvement of transcriptional and posttranscriptional mechanisms. *J Cell Biol* 2000; **148**: 543–56.

102. Hengst L, Reed SI. Translational control of p27$^{Kip1}$ accumulation during the cell cycle. *Science* 1996; **271**: 1861–4.

103. Boehm M, Yoshimoto T, Crook MF et al. A growth factor-dependent nuclear kinase phosphorylates p27$^{Kip1}$ and regulates cell cycle progression. *EMBO J* 2002; **21**: 3390–401.

104. Ishida N, Hara T, Kamura T et al. Phosphorylation of p27$^{Kip1}$ on serine 10 is required for its binding to CRM1 and nuclear export. *J Biol Chem* 2002; **277**: 14355–8.

105. Malek NP, Sundberg H, McGrew S et al. A mouse knock-in model exposes sequential proteolytic pathways that regulate p27$^{Kip1}$ in G$_1$ and S phase. *Nature* 2001; **413**: 323–7.

106. Amati B, Vlach J. Kip1 meets SKP2: new links in cell-cycle control. *Nat Cell Biol* 1999; **1**: E91–3.

107. Hara T, Kamura T, Nakayama K et al. Degradation of p27$^{Kip1}$ at the G$_0$–G$_1$ transition mediated by a Skp2-independent ubiquitination pathway. *J Biol Chem* 2001; **270**: 48937–43.

108. Bagui TK, Mohapatra S, Haura E, Pledger WJ. p27$^{Kip1}$ and p21$^{Cip1}$ are not required for the formation of active D cyclin–cdk4 complexes. *Mol Cell Biol* 2003; **23**: 7285–90.

109. Cheng M, Olivier P, Diehl JA et al. The p21$^{Cip1}$ and p27$^{Kip1}$ CDK 'inhibitors' are essential activators of cyclin D-dependent kinases in murine fibroblasts. *EMBO J* 1999; **18**: 1571–83.

110. Olashaw N, Bagui TK, Pledger WJ. Cell cycle control: a complex issue. *Cell Cycle* 2004; **3**: 263–4.

111. Besson A, Gurian-West M, Schmidt A et al. p27$^{Kip1}$ modulates cell migration through the regulation of RhoA activation. *Genes Dev* 2004; **18**: 862–76.

112. Matsuoka S, Edwards M, Bai C et al. p57$^{KIP2}$, a structurally distinct member of the p21 (CIP1) cdk inhibitor family, is a candidate tumour suppressor gene. *Genes Dev* 1995; **9**: 650–62.

113. Zhang P, Liegeois NJ, Wong C et al. Altered cell differentiation and proliferation in mice lacking p57$^{KIP2}$ indicates a role in Beckwith–Wiedemann syndrome. *Nature* 1997; **387**: 151–8.

114. Ubersax JA, Woodbury EL, Quang PN et al. Targets of the cyclin-dependent kinase Cdk1. *Nature* 2003; **425**: 859–64.

115. Goodrich DW, Lee W-H. Molecular characterisation of the retinoblastoma susceptibility gene. *Biochim Biophys Acta* 1993; **1155**: 43–61.

116. Ezhevsky SA, Ho A, Becker-Hapak M et al. Differential regulation of retinoblastoma tumor suppressor protein by G$_1$ cyclin-dependent kinase complexes in vivo. *Mol Cell Biol* 2001; **21**: 4773–84.

117. Chan HM, Krstic-Demonacos M, Smith L et al. Acetylation control of the retinoblastoma tumour-suppressor protein. *Nat Cell Biol* 2001; **3**: 667–74.

118. Hsieh JK, Chan FS, O'Connor DJ et al. RB regulates the stability and the apoptotic function of p53 via MDM2. *Mol Cell* 1999; **3**: 181–93.

119. Taya Y. RB kinases and RB-binding proteins: new points of view. *TIBS* 1997; **22**: 14–17.

120. Morris EJ, Dyson NJ. Retinoblastoma protein partners. *Adv Cancer Res* 2001; **82**: 1–54.

121. Kitagawa M, Higashi H, Jung H-K et al. The consensus motif for phosphorylation by cyclin D1–Cdk4 is different from that for phosphorylation by cyclin A/E–Cdk2. *EMBO J* 1997; **15**: 7060–9.

122. Peters G, Bates S, Pary D. The D-cyclins, their kinases and their inhibitors. In: Thomas NSB (ed) *Apoptosis and Cell Cycle Control in Cancer 2*. Oxford: Bios, 1996: 37–54.

123. Burke LC, Bybee A, Thomas NSB. The retinoblastoma protein is partially phosphorylated during early G$_1$ in cycling cells but not in G$_1$ cells arrested with α-interferon. *Oncogene* 1991; **7**: 782–8.

124. Chew YP, Ellis M, Wilkie S, Mittnacht S. pRB phosphorylation mutants reveal role of pRB in regulating S phase completion by a mechanism independent of E2F. *Oncogene* 1998; **17**: 2177–86.

125. Knudsen ES, Buckmaster C, Chen T-T et al. Inhibition of DNA synthesis by RB: effects on G$_1$/S transition and S-phase progression. *Genes Dev* 1998; **12**: 2278–92.

126. Lavia P, Jansen-Durr P. E2F target genes and cell-cycle checkpoint control. E2F target genes and cell cycle checkpoints. *Bioessays* 1999; **21**: 221–30.

127. Hsieh J-K, Chan FSG, O'Connor DJ et al. RB regulates the stability and the apoptotic function of p53 via MDM2. *Mol Cell* 1999; **3**: 181–93.

128. Grana X, Garriga J, Mayol X. Role of the retinoblastoma protein family, pRB, p107 and p130 in the negative control of cell growth. *Oncogene* 1998; **17**: 3365–83.

129. Labbaye C, Valtieri M, Grignani F et al. Expression and role of *PML* gene in normal adult hematopoiesis: functional interaction between PML and Rb proteins in erythropoiesis. *Oncogene* 1999; **18**: 3529–40.

130. Alcalay M, Tomassoni L, Colombo E et al. The promyelocytic leukemia gene product (PML) forms stable complexes with the retinoblastoma protein. *Mol Cell Biol* 1998; **18**: 1084–93.

131. Grignani F, Fagioli M, Alcalay M et al. Acute promyelocytic leukemia: from genetics to treatment. *Blood* 1994; **83**: 10–25.

132. Wang ZG, Delva L, Gaboli M et al. Role of PML in cell growth and the retinoic acid pathway. *Science* 1998; **279**: 1547–51.

133. Knudsen ES, Wang JYJ. Differential regulation of retinoblastoma protein function by specific Cdk phosphorylation sites. *J Biol Chem* 1996; **271**: 8313–20.

134. Tan X, Wang JY. The caspase-RB connection in cell death. *Trends Cell Biol* 1998; **8**: 116–20.

135. Dou QP, An B. RB and apoptotic cell death. *Front Biosci* 1998; **3**: 419–30.

136. Katsuda K, Kataoka M, Uno F et al. Activation of caspase-3 and cleavage of Rb are associated with p16-mediated apoptosis in human non-small cell lung cancer cells. *Oncogene* 2002; **21**: 2108–13.

137. Chau BN, Borges HL, Chen TT et al. Signal-dependent protection from apoptosis in mice expressing caspase-resistant Rb. *Nat Cell Biol* 2002; **4**: 757–65.

138. Yee AS, Shih HH, Tevosian SG. New perspectives on retinoblastoma family functions in differentiation. *Front Biosci* 1998; **3**: 532–47.

139. Sellers WR, Novitch BG, Miyake S et al. Stable binding to E2F is not required for the retinoblastoma protein to activate transcription, promote differentiation, and suppress tumor cell growth. *Genes Dev* 1998; **12**: 95–106.

140. Mahdi T, Alcalay D, Brizard A et al. Role of p53 and RB on in vitro growth of normal umbilical cord blood cells. *Exp Haematol* 1996; **24**: 702–12.

141. Bergh G, Ehinger M, Olsson I et al. Involvement of the retinoblastoma protein in monocytic and neutrophilic lineage commitment of human bone marrow progenitor cells. *Blood* 1999; **94**: 1971–8.

142. Jamal R, Gale RE, Shaun N et al. The retinoblastoma gene (rb1) in acute myeloid leukaemia: analysis of gene rearrangements, protein expression and comparison of disease outcome. *Haematology* 1996; **2**: 342–51.

143. Kornblau SM, Andreff M, Hu SX et al. Low and maximally phosphorylated levels of the retinoblastoma protein confer poor prognosis in newly diagnosed acute myelogenous leukemia: a prospective study. *Clin Cancer Res* 1998; **4**: 1955–63.

144. Jamal R, Gale RE, Thomas NSB, Linch DC. The retinoblastoma gene (*rb1*) in acute myeloid leukaemia: analysis of gene rearrangements, protein expression and comparison of disease outcome. *Br J Haematol* 1994; **94**: 324–51.

145. Lee EY-HP, Chang C-Y, Hu N et al. Mice deficient for Rb are nonviable and show defects in neurogenesis and haematopoiesis. *Nature* 1992; **359**: 288–94.

146. Jacks T, Fazeli A, Schmitt EM et al. Effects of an Rb mutation in the mouse. *Nature* 1992; **359**: 295–300.

147. Clarke AR, Maandag ER, van Roon M et al. Requirement for a functional *Rb-1* gene in murine development. *Nature* 1992; **359**: 328–30.

148. Hu N, Gulley ML, Kung JT, Lee EY. Retinoblastoma gene deficiency has mitogenic but not tumorigenic effects on erythropoiesis. *Cancer Res* 1997; **57**: 4123–9.

149. Harlow E. Retinoblastoma. For our eyes only. *Nature* 1992; **359**: 270–1.

150. de Bruin A, Wu L, Saavedra HI et al. Rb function in extraembryonic lineages suppresses apoptosis in the CNS of Rb-deficient mice. *Proc Natl Acad Sci USA* 2003; **100**: 6546–51.

151. Wu L, de Bruin A, Saavedra HI et al. Extra-embryonic function of Rb is essential for embryonic development and viability. *Nature* 2003; **421**: 942–7.

152. Campisi J. Cellular senescence as a tumor-suppressor mechanism. *Trends Cell Biol* 2001; **11**: S27–31.

153. Fang W, Mori T, Cobrinik D. Regulation of PML-dependent transcriptional repression by pRB and low penetrance pRB mutants. *Oncogene* 2002; **21**: 5557–65.

154. Nguyen DC, Crowe DL. Intact functional domains of the retinoblastoma gene product (pRb) are required for down-regulation of telomerase activity. *Biochim Biophys Acta* 1999; **1445**: 207–15.

155. Fuxe J, Akusjarvi G, Goike HM et al. Adenovirus-mediated overexpression of p15INK4B inhibits human glioma cell growth, induces replicative senescence, and inhibits telomerase activity similarly to p16INK4A. *Cell Growth Differ* 2000; **11**: 373–84.

156. Crowe DL, Nguyen DC, Tsang KJ, Kyo S. E2F-1 represses transcription of the human telomerase reverse transcriptase gene. *Nucleic Acids Res* 2001; **29**: 2789–94.

157. Garcia-Cao M, Gonzaldo S, Dean D, Blasco MA. A role for the Rb family of proteins in controlling telomere length. *Nat Genet* 2002; **32**: 415–19.

158. Hansen K, Farkas T, Lukas J et al. Phosphorylation-dependent and -independent functions of p130 cooperate to evoke a sustained G$_1$ block. *EMBO J* 2001; **20**: 422–32.

159. Grana X, Garriga J, Mayol X. Role of the retinoblastoma protein family, pRB, p107 and p130 in the negative control of cell growth. *Oncogene* 1998; **17**: 3365–83.

160. Thomas NS, Pizzey AR, Tiwari S et al. p130, p107, and pRb are differentially regulated in proliferating cells and during cell cycle arrest by α-interferon. *J Biol Chem* 1998; **273**: 23659–67.

161. Calbo J, Parreno M, Sotillo E et al. G$_1$ cyclin/CDK coordinated phosphorylation of endogenous pocket proteins differentially regulates their interactions with E2F4 and E2F1 and gene expression. *J Biol Chem* 2002; **52**: 50263–74.

162. Farkas T, Hansen K, Holm K et al. Distinct phosphorylation events regulate p130- and p107-mediated repression of E2F-4. *J Biol Chem* 2002; **277**: 26741–52.

163. Beijersbergen RL, Carlee L, Kerkhoven RM, Bernards R. Regulation of the retinoblastoma protein-related p107 by G$_1$ cyclin complexes. *Genes Dev* 1995; **9**: 1340–53.

164. von Mering C, Krause R, Snel B et al. Comparative assessment of large-scale data sets of protein–protein interactions. *Nature* 2002; **417**: 399–403.

165. Lam EW-F, LaThangue NB. DP and E2F proteins: coordinating transcription with cell cycle progression. *Curr Opin Cell Biol* 1994; **6**: 859–66.

166. Whyte P. The retinoblastoma family of proteins. In: Thomas NSB (ed) *Apoptosis and Cell Cycle Control in Cancer 2*. Oxford: Bios, 1996: 77–92.

167. LaThangue NB. DP and E2F proteins: components of a heterodimeric transcription factor implicated in cell cycle control. *Curr Biol* 1994; **6**: 443–50.

168. Williams CD, Linch DC, Watts MJ, Thomas NSB. Characterization of cell cycle status and E2F complexes in mobilised CD34+ cells before and after cytokine stimulation. *Blood* 1997; **90**: 194–203.

169. Vario G, Livingston DM, Ginsberg D. Functional interaction between E2F-4 and p130: evidence for distinct mechanisms underlying growth suppression by different retinoblastoma protein family members. *Genes Dev* 1995; **9**: 869–81.

170. Williams CD, Linch DC, Sorensen TS et al. The predominant E2F complex in human primary haemopoietic cells and in AML blasts contains E2F-4, DP-1 and p130. *Br J Haematol* 1997; **96**: 688–96.

171. Moberg K, Starz MA, Lees JA. E2F-4 switches from p130 to p107 and pRB in response to cell cycle reentry. *Mol Cell Biol* 1996; **16**: 1436–49.

172. Smith EJ, Leone G, DeGregori J et al. The accumulation of an E2F-p130 transcriptional repressor distinguishes a G$_0$ cell state from a G$_1$ cell state. *Mol Cell Biol* 1996; **16**: 6965–76.

173. Ogawa H, Ishiguro K, Gaubatz S et al. A complex with chromatin modifiers that occupies E2F- and Myc-responsive genes in G$_0$ cells. *Science* 2002; **296**: 1132–6.

174. Turner BM. Cellular memory and the histone code. *Cell* 2002; **111**: 285–91.

175. La Thangue NB. Chromatin control – a place for E2F and Myc to meet. *Science* 2002; **296**: 1034–5.

176. DeGregori J, Leone G, Miron A et al. Distinct roles for E2F

proteins in cell growth control and apoptosis. *Proc Natl Acad Sci USA* 1997; **94**: 7245–50.

177. Lukas J, Petersen BO, Holm K et al. Deregulated expression of E2F family members induces S-phase entry and overcomes p16^INK4A-mediated growth suppression. *Mol Cell Biol* 1996; **16**: 1047–57.

178. Muller H, Bracken AP, Vernell R et al. E2Fs regulate the expression of genes involved in differentiation, development, proliferation, and apoptosis. *Genes Dev* 2001; **15**: 267–85.

179. Lai A, Lee JM, Yang WM et al. RBP1 recruits both histone deacetylase-dependent and -independent repression activities to retinoblastoma family proteins. *Mol Cell Biol* 1999; **19**: 6632–41.

180. Ferreira R, Naguibneva I, Mathieu M et al. Cell cycle-dependent recruitment of HDAC-1 correlates with deacetylation of histone H4 on an Rb–E2F target promoter. *EMBO Rep* 2001; **2**: 794–9.

181. Morrison AJ, Sardet C, Herrera RE. Retinoblastoma protein transcriptional repression through histone deacetylation of a single nucleosome. *Mol Cell Biol* 2002; **22**: 856–65.

182. Goll MG, Bestor TH. Histone modification and replacement in chromatin activation. *Genes Dev* 2002; **16**: 1739–42.

183. Vandel L, Nicolas E, Vaute O et al. Transcriptional repression by the retinoblastoma protein through the recruitment of a histone methyltransferase. *Mol Cell Biol* 2001; **21**: 6484–94.

184. Nielsen SJ, Schneider R, Bauer UM et al. Rb targets histone H3 methylation and HP1 to promoters. *Nature* 2001; **412**: 561–5.

185. DeGregori J, Leone G, Miron A et al. Distinct roles for E2F proteins in cell growth control and apoptosis. *Proc Natl Acad Sci USA* 1997; **94**: 7245–50.

186. Haas-Kogan DA, Kogan SC, Levi D et al. Inhibition of apoptosis by the retinoblastoma gene. *EMBO J* 1995; **14**: 461–72.

187. Qin X-Q, Livingston DM, Kaelin WG, Adams PD. Deregulated transcription factor E2F-1 expression leads to S-phase entry and p53-mediated apoptosis. *Proc Natl Acad Sci USA* 1994; **91**: 10918–22.

188. Wu X, Levine AJ. p53 and E2F-1 cooperate to mediate apoptosis. *Proc Natl Acad Sci USA* 1994; **91**: 3602–6.

189. Weinberg RA. E2F and cell proliferation: a world turned upside down. *Cell* 1996; **85**: 457–9.

190. Krek W, Xu G, Livingston DM. Cyclin A-kinase regulation of E2F-1 DNA binding function underlies suppression of an S phase checkpoint. *Cell* 1995; **83**: 1149–58.

191. Marzio G, Wagener C, Gutierrez MI et al. E2F family members are differentially regulated by reversible acetylation. *J Biol Chem* 2000; **275**: 10887–92.

192. Martinez-Balbas MA, Bauer UM, Nielsen SJ et al. Regulation of E2F1 activity by acetylation. *EMBO J* 2000; **19**: 662–71.

193. Nasmyth K. Retinoblastoma protein. Another role rolls in. *Nature* 1996; **382**: 28–9.

194. Zhu L, Enders G, Lees JA et al. The pRB-related protein p107 contains two growth suppression domains: independent interactions with E2F and cyclin/cdk complexes. *EMBO J* 1995; **14**: 1904–13.

195. Beijesbergen RL, Hijmans EM, Zhu L, Bernards R. Interaction of c-Myc with the pRb-related protein p107 results in inhibition of c-Myc-mediated transactivation. *EMBO J* 1994; **13**: 4080–6.

196. Classon M, Dyson N. p107 and p130: versatile proteins with interesting pockets. *Exp Cell Res* 2001; **264**: 135–47.

197. Thomas NSB, Burke LC, Bybee A, Linch DC. The phosphorylation state of the retinoblastoma (RB) protein in $G_0/G_1$ is dependent on growth status. *Oncogene* 1991; **6**: 317–22.

198. Burke LC, Bybee A, Thomas NSB. The retinoblastoma protein is partially phosphorylated during early $G_1$ in cycling cells but not in $G_1$ cells arrested with α-interferon. *Oncogene* 1992; **7**: 783–8.

199. Resnitzky D, Teifbrun N, Berissi H, Kimchi A. Interferons and interleukin 6 suppress phosphorylation of the retinoblastoma protein in growth-sensitive hematopoietic cells. *Proc Natl Acad Sci USA* 1992; **89**: 402–6.

200. Arany I, Rady P, Tyring SK. Interferon treatment enhances the expression of underphosphorylated (biologically-active) retinoblastoma protein in human papilloma virus-infected cells through the inhibitory TGF β1/IFN β cytokine pathway. *Antiviral Res* 1994; **23**: 131–41.

201. Thomas NSB. Regulation of the product of a possible human cell cycle control gene CDC2Hs in B-cells by α-interferon and phorbol ester. *J Biol Chem* 1989; **264**: 13697–700.

202. Yamada H, Ochi K, Nakada S et al. Changes of cell cycle-regulating genes in interferon-treated Daudi cells. *Mol Cell Biochem* 1994; **136**: 117–23.

203. Yamada H, Ochi K, Nakada S et al. Interferon modulates the messenger RNA of $G_1$-controlling genes to suppress the $G_1$-to-S transition in Daudi cells. *Mol Cell Biochem* 1995; **152**: 149–58.

204. Zhang K, Kumar R. Interferon-α inhibits cyclin E and cyclin D1-dependent CDK2 kinase activity associated with RB protein and E2F in Daudi cells. *Biochem Biophys Res Commun* 1994; **200**: 522–8.

205. Tiefbrun N, Melamed D, Levy N et al. α-Interferon suppresses the cyclin D3 and cdc25A genes, leading to a reversible $G_0$-like arrest. *J Biol Chem* 1996; **16**: 3934–44.

206. Kuniyasu H, Yasui W, Kitahara K et al. Growth inhibitory effect of interferon-β is associated with the induction of cyclin-dependent kinase inhibitor p27^Kip1 in human gastric carcinoma cell line. *Cell Growth Diff* 1997; **8**: 47–52.

207. Subramaniam PS, Johnson HM. A role for the cyclin-dependent kinase inhibitor p21 in the $G_1$ cell cycle arrest mediated by the type I interferons. *J Interferon Cytokine Res* 1997; **17**: 11–15.

208. Hobeika AC, Subramaniam PS, Johnson HM. IFNα induces the expression of the cyclin-dependent kinase inhibitor p21 in human prostate cancer cells. *Oncogene* 1997; **14**: 1165–70.

209. Sangfelt O, Erickson S, Eindhorn S, Grander D. Induction of Cip/Kip and Ink4 cyclin dependent kinase inhibitors by interferon-α in hemopoietic cell lines. *Oncogene* 1997; **14**: 415–23.

210. Melamed D, Tiefenbrun N, Yarden A, Kimchi A. Interferons and interleukin-6 suppress the DNA-binding activity of E2F in growth-sensitive hematopoietic cells. *Mol Cell Biol* 1993; **13**: 5255–65.

211. Iwase S, Furukawa Y, Kikuchi J et al. Modulation of E2F activity is linked to interferon-induced growth suppression of haemopoietic cells. *J Biol Chem* 1997; **272**: 12406–14.

212. Choubey D, Li SJ, Datta B et al. Inhibition of E2F-mediated transcription by p202. *EMBO J* 1996; **15**: 5668–78.

213. Hertel L, Rolle S, De Andrea M et al. The retinoblastoma protein is an essential mediator that links the interferon-inducible 204 gene to cell-cycle regulation. *Oncogene* 2000; **19:** 3598–608.

214. Einat M, Resnitzky D, Kimchi A. Close link between reduction of c-*myc* expression by interferon and $G_0/G_1$ arrest. *Nature* 1985; **313:** 597–600.

215. Raveh T, Hovanessian AG, Meurs EF et al. Double-stranded RNA-dependent protein kinase mediates c-*Myc* suppression induced by type I interferons. *J Biol Chem* 1996; **271:** 25479–84.

216. Dent CL, Lillycrop KA, Bybee A et al. Interferon-α treatment of Daudi cells down-regulates the Octamer binding transcription/DNA replication factors Oct-1 and Oct-2. *J Biol Chem* 1991; **266:** 20888–92.

217. Knudson AG, Strong LC. Mutation and cancer: statistical study of retinoblastoma. *Proc Natl Acad Sci USA* 1971; **68:** 820–3.

218. Pitot H, Dragan Y. Facts and theories concerning the mechanisms of carcinogenesis. *FASEB J* 1991; **5:** 2280–6.

219. Vogelstein B, Kinzler KW. The multistep nature of cancer. *Trends Genet* 1993; **9:** 138–41.

220. Buggins AG, Milojkovic D, Arno MJ et al. Microenvironment produced by acute myeloid leukemia cells prevents T cell activation and proliferation by inhibition of NF-κB, c-Myc, and pRb pathways. *J Immunol* 2001; **167:** 6021–30.

221. Green DR, Evan GI. A matter of life and death. *Cancer Cell* 2002; **1:** 19–30.

222. Morgenbesser SD, Williams BO, Jacks T, DePinho RA. p53-dependent apoptosis produced by Rb-deficiency in the developing mouse lens. *Nature* 1994; **371:** 72–4.

223. Marston NJ, Vousden KH. Interactions of HPV E6 and E7 with regulators of cell cycle and proliferation. In: Thomas NSB (ed) *Apoptosis and Cell Cycle Control in Cancer 2.* Oxford: Bios, 1996: 93–108.

224. Land H, Parada LF, Weinberg RA. Tumorigenic conversion of primary embryo fibroblasts requires at least two cooperating oncogenes. *Nature* 1983; **304:** 596–602.

225. Jackson-Grusby L. Modeling cancer in mice. *Oncogene* 2002; **21:** 5504–14.

226. Bartek J, Lukas J. Are all cancer genes equal? *Nature* 2001; **411:** 1001–2.

227. Pelengaris S, Khan M, Evan G. c-Myc: more than just a matter of life and death. *Nat Rev Cancer* 2002; **2:** 764–76.

228. Drayton S, Peters G. Immortalisation and transformation revisited. *Curr Opin Genet Dev* 2002; **12:** 98–104.

229. Hahn WC, Counter CM, Lundberg AS et al. Creation of human tumour cells with defined genetic elements. *Nature* 1999; **400:** 464–8.

230. Morales CP, Holt SE, Ouellette M et al. Absence of cancer-associated changes in human fibroblasts immortalized with telomerase. *Nat Genet* 1999; **21:** 115–18.

231. Serrano M, Lin AW, McCurrach ME et al. Oncogenic ras provokes premature cell senescence associated with accumulation of p53 and p16[INK4a]. *Cell* 1997; **88:** 593–602.

232. Pearson M, Carbone R, Sebastiani C et al. PML regulates p53 acetylation and premature senescence induced by oncogenic Ras. *Nature* 2000; **406:** 207–10.

233. Bryan TM, Reddel RR. SV40-induced immortalization of human cells. *Crit Rev Oncog* 1994; **5:** 331–57.

234. Hahn WC, Dessain SK, Brooks MW et al. Enumeration of the simian virus 40 early region elements necessary for human cell transformation. *Mol Cell Biol* 2002; **22:** 2111–23.

235. Elenbaas B, Spirio L, Koerner F et al. Human breast cancer cells generated by oncogenic transformation of primary mammary epithelial cells. *Genes Dev* 2002; **15:** 50–65.

236. Lundberg AS, Randell SH, Stewart SA et al. Immortalization and transformation of primary human airway epithelial cells by gene transfer. *Oncogene* 2002; **21:** 4577–86.

237. Hahn WC, Weinberg RA. Modelling the molecular circuitry of cancer. *Nat Rev Cancer* 2002; **2:** 331–41.

238. Hartwell LH, Kastan MB. Cell cycle control and cancer. *Science* 1994; **266:** 1821–8.

239. Sherr CJ. Cancer cell cycles. *Science* 1996; **274:** 1672–7.

240. Hanahan D, Weinberg RA. The hallmarks of cancer. *Cell* 2000; **100:** 57–70.

241. Evan GI, Vousden KH. Proliferation, cell cycle and apoptosis in cancer. *Nature* 2001; **411:** 342–8.

242. Sherr CJ. Principles of tumor suppression. *Cell* 2004; **116:** 235–46.

243. Sherr CJ, McCormick, F. The RB and p53 pathways in cancer. *Cancer Cell* 2002; **2:** 103–12.

244. Friend SH, Bernards R, Rogelj S et al. A human DNA segment with properties of the gene that predisposes to retinoblastoma and osteosarcoma. *Nature* 1986; **323:** 643–6.

245. Godbout R, Dryja TP, Squire J et al. Somatic inactivation of genes on chromosome 13 is a common event in retinoblastoma. *Nature* 1993; **304:** 451–3.

246. Jamal R. The retinoblastoma gene in myeloid leukaemias. *Hematology* 1996; **1:** 43–51.

247. Zhu YM, Haynes AP, Keith FJ, Russell NH. Abnormalities of retinoblastoma gene expression in hematological malignancies. *Leuk Lymphoma* 1995; **18:** 61–7.

248. Krug U, Ganser A, Koeffler HP. Tumor suppressor genes in normal and malignant hematopoiesis. *Oncogene* 2002; **21:** 3475–95.

249. Tsai T, Davalath S, Rankin C et al. Tumor suppressor gene alteration in adult acute lymphoblastic leukemia (ALL). Analysis of retinoblastoma (*Rb*) and *p53* gene expression in lymphoblasts of patients with de novo, relapsed, or refractory ALL treated in Southwest Oncology Group studies. *Leukaemia* 1996; **10:** 1901–10.

250. Sanchez-Beato M, Martinez-Montero JC, Doussis-Anagnostopoulou TA et al. Anomalous retinoblastoma protein expression in Sternberg–Reed cells in Hodgkin's disease: a comparative study with p53 and Ki67 expression. *Br J Cancer* 1996; **74:** 1056–62.

251. Morente MM, Piris MA, Abraira V et al. Adverse clinical outcome in Hodgkin's disease is associated with loss of retinoblastoma protein expression, high Ki67 proliferation index, and absence of Epstein–Barr virus-latent membrane protein 1 expression. *Blood* 1997; **90:** 2429–36.

252. Sauerbrey A, Stammler G, Zintl F, Volm M. Expression of the retinoblastoma tumor suppressor gene (*RB-1*) in acute leukemia. *Leuk Lymphoma* 1998; **28:** 275–83.

253. Zhu YM, Bradbury DA, Russell N. Decreased retinoblastoma protein expression in acute myeloblastic leukaemia is associated with the autonomous proliferation of clonogenic blasts. *Br J Haematol* 1994; **86:** 533–9.

254. Zhu YM, Bradbury DA, Keith FJ, Russell N. Absence of retinoblastoma protein expression results in autocrine production of interleukin-6 and promotes the autonomous growth of acute myeloid leukaemia blast cells. *Leukaemia* 1994; **8:** 1982–8.

255. Preudhomme C, Vachee A, Lepelley P et al. Inactivation of the retinoblastoma gene appears to be very uncommon in myelodysplastic syndromes. *Brit J Haematol* 1994; **87:** 61–7.

256. Cinti C, Claudio PP, Howard CM et al. Genetic alterations disrupting the nuclear localization of the retinoblastoma-related gene *RB2/p130* in human tumor cell lines and primary tumors. *Cancer Res* 2000; **60**: 383–9.

257. Cinti C, Leoncini L, Nyongo A et al. Genetic alterations of the retinoblastoma-related gene *RB2/p130* identify different pathogenetic mechanisms in and among Burkitt's lymphoma subtypes. *Am J Pathol* 2000; **156**: 751–60.

258. Takimoto H, Tsukuda K, Ichimura K et al. Genetic alterations in the retinoblastoma protein-related *p107* gene in human hematologic malignancies. *Biochem Biophys Res Commun* 1998; **251**: 264–8.

259. Bodrug S, Warner B, Bath M et al. *Cyclin D1* transgene impedes lymphocytic maturation and collaborates in lymphomagenesis with the *myc* gene. *EMBO J* 1994; **13**: 2124–30.

260. Rosenwald A, Wright G, Wiestner A et al. The proliferation gene expression signature is a quantitative integrator of oncogenic events that predicts survival in mantle cell lymphoma. *Cancer Cell* 2003; **3**: 185–97.

261. Resnitzky D, Reed SI. Different roles for cyclins D1 and E in regulation of the $G_1$-to-S transition. *Mol Cell Biol* 1995; **15**: 3463–9.

262. Sicinski P, Donaher JL, Geng Y et al. *Cyclin D2* is an FSH-responsive gene involved in gonadal cell proliferation and oncogenesis. *Nature* 1996; **384**: 470–4.

263. Deininger MW, Vieira SA, Parada Y et al. Direct relation between BCR–ABL tyrosine kinase activity and cyclin D2 expression in lymphoblasts. *Cancer Res* 2001; **61**: 8005–13.

264. Jena N, Deng M, Sicinska E et al. Critical role for cyclin D2 in BCR/ABL-induced proliferation of hematopoietic cells. *Cancer Res* 2001; **62**: 535–41.

265. Caligaris-Cappio F. Cellular interactions, immunodeficiency and autoimmunity in CLL. *Hematol Cell Ther* 2000; **42**: 21–5.

266. Dighiero G, Binet JL. When and how to treat chronic lymphocytic leukemia. *N Engl J Med* 2000; **343**: 1799–801.

267. Wolowiec D, Ciszak L, Kosmaczewska A et al. Cell cycle regulatory proteins and apoptosis in B-cell chronic lymphocytic leukemia. *Haematologica* 2001; **86**: 1296–304.

268. Qian L, Gong J, Liu J et al. *Cyclin D2* promoter disrupted by t(12;22)(p13;q11.2) during transformation of chronic lymphocytic leukaemia to non-Hodgkin's lymphoma. *Br J Haematol* 1999; **106**: 477–85.

269. Kerkhoff E, Ziff EB. Cyclin D2 and Ha-Ras transformed rat embryo fibroblasts exhibit a novel deregulation of cell size control and early S phase arrest in low serum. *EMBO J* 1995; **14**: 1892–903.

270. Lam EW, Glassford J, Banerji L et al. Cyclin D3 compensates for loss of cyclin D2 in mouse B-lymphocytes activated via the antigen receptor and CD40. *J Biol Chem* 2000; **275**: 3479–84.

271. Lam EW, Glassford J, van der Sman J et al. Modulation of E2F activity in primary mouse B cells following stimulation via surface IgM and CD40 receptors. *Eur J Immunol* 1999; **29**: 3380–9.

272. van der Sman J, Thomas NS, Lam EW. Modulation of E2F complexes during $G_0$ to S phase transition in human primary B-lymphocytes. *J Biol Chem* 1999; **274**: 12009–16.

273. Solvason N, Wu WW, Parry D et al. Cyclin D2 is essential for BCR-mediated proliferation and CD5 B cell development. *Int Immunol* 2000; **12**: 631–8.

274. Banerji L, Glassford J, Lea NC et al. BCR signals target p27$^{Kip1}$ and cyclin D2 via the PI3-K signalling pathway to mediate cell cycle arrest and apoptosis of WEHI 231 B cells. *Oncogene* 2001; **20**: 7352–67.

275. Parada Y, Banerji L, Glassford J et al. BCR–ABL and interleukin 3 promote haematopoietic cell proliferation and survival through modulation of cyclin D2 and p27$^{Kip1}$ expression. *J Biol Chem* 2001; **276**: 23572–80.

276. Decker T, Schneller F, Hipp S et al. Cell cycle progression of chronic lymphocytic leukemia cells is controlled by cyclin D2, cyclin D3, cyclin-dependent kinase (cdk) 4 and the cdk inhibitor p27. *Leukemia* 2002; **16**: 327–34.

277. Pezzella F, Jones M, Ralfkiaer E et al. Evaluation of bcl-2 protein expression and 14;18 translocation as prognostic markers in follicular lymphoma. *Br J Cancer* 1992; **65**: 87–9.

278. Schena M, Larsson LG, Gottardi D et al. Growth- and differentiation-associated expression of bcl-2 in B-chronic lymphocytic leukemia cells. *Blood* 1992; **79**: 2981–9.

279. Granziero L, Ghia P, Circosta P et al. Survivin is expressed on CD40 stimulation and interfaces proliferation and apoptosis in B-cell chronic lymphocytic leukemia. *Blood* 2001; **97**: 2777–83.

280. Barille-Nion S, Barlogie B, Bataille R et al. Advances in biology and therapy of multiple myeloma. *Hematology (Am Soc Hematol Educ Program)* 2003: 248–78.

281. Shaughnessy J Jr, Gabrea A, Qi Y et al. Cyclin D3 at 6p21 is dysregulated by recurrent chromosomal translocations to immunoglobulin loci in multiple myeloma. *Blood* 2001; **98**: 217–23.

282. Brito-Babapulle V, Gruszka-Westwood AM, Platt G et al. Translocation t(2;7)(p12;q21–22) with dysregulation of the *CDK6* gene mapping to 7q21–22 in a non-Hodgkin's lymphoma with leukemia. *Haematologica* 2002; **87**: 357–62.

283. Corcoran MM, Mould SJ, Orchard JA et al. Dysregulation of cyclin dependent kinase 6 expression in splenic marginal zone lymphoma through chromosome 7q translocations. *Oncogene* 1999; **18**: 6271–7.

284. Raffini LJ, Slater DJ, Rappaport EF et al. Panhandle and reverse-panhandle PCR enable cloning of der(11) and der(other) genomic breakpoint junctions of *MLL* translocations and identify complex translocation of *MLL, AF-4,* and *CDK6*. *Proc Natl Acad Sci USA* 2002; **99**: 4568–73.

285. Ewen ME, Lamb J. The activities of cyclin D1 that drive tumorigenesis. *Trends Mol Med* 2004; **10**: 158–62.

286. Donnellan R, Chetty R. Cyclin E in human cancers. *FASEB J* 1999; **13**: 773–80.

287. Reed SE, Spruck CH, Sangfelt O et al. Mutation of *hCDC4* leads to cell cycle deregulation of cyclin E in cancer. *Cancer Res* 2004; **64**: 795–800.

288. Iida H, Towatari M, Tanimoto M et al. Overexpression of cyclin E in acute myelogenous leukemia. *Blood* 1997; **90**: 3707–13.

289. Erlanson M, Landberg G. Prognostic implications of p27 and cyclin E protein contents in malignant lymphomas. *Leuk Lymphoma* 2001; **40**: 461–70.

290. Spruck CH, Won KA, Reed SI. Deregulated cyclin E induces chromosome instability. *Nature* 1999; **401**: 297–300.

291. Hirama T, Koeffler HP. Role of the cyclin-dependent kinase inhibitors in the development of cancer. *Blood* 1995; **86**: 841–54.

292. Siebert R, Willers CP, Opalka B. Role of the cyclin-dependent kinase 4 and 6 inhibitor gene family *p15, p16, p18*

and *p19* in leukemia and lymphoma. *Leuk Lymphoma* 1996; **23**: 505–20.

293. Takeuchi S, Bartram CR, Serui T et al. Analysis of a family of cyclin-dependent kinase inhibitors: *p15/MTS2/INK4B*, *p16/MTS1/INK4A*, and *p18* genes in acute lymphoblastic leukemia of childhood. *Blood* 1995; **86**: 755–60.

294. Stranks G, Height SE, Mitchell P et al. Deletions and rearrangement of *CDKN2* in lymphoid malignancy. *Blood* 1995; **85**: 893–901.

295. Quelle DE, Cheng M, Ashmun RA, Sherr CJ. Cancer-associated mutations at the *INK4a* locus cancel cell cycle arrest by p16INK4a but not by the alternative reading frame protein p19ARF. *Proc Natl Acad Sci USA* 1997; **94**: 669–73.

296. Taniguchi T, Chikatsu N, Takahashi S et al. Expression of p16INK4A and p14ARF in hematological malignancies. *Leukemia* 1999; **13**: 1760–9.

297. Sherr CJ. The INK4a/ARF network in tumour suppression. *Rev Mol Cell Biol* 2001; **2**: 731–7.

298. Drayton S, Peters G. Immortalisation and transformation revisited. *Curr Opin Genet Dev* 2002; **12**: 98–104.

299. Merlo A, Herman JG, Mao L et al. 5′ CpG island methylation is associated with transcriptional silencing of the tumour suppressor *p16/CDKN2/MTS1* in human cancers. *Nat Med* 1995; **1**: 686–93.

300. Drexler HG. Review of alterations of the cyclin-dependent kinase inhibitor *INK4* family genes *p15*, *p16*, *p18* and *p19* in human leukemia–lymphoma cells. *Leukemia* 1998; **12**: 845–59.

301. Esteller M, Corn PG, Baylin SB, Herman JG. A gene hypermethylation profile of human cancer. *Cancer Res* 2001; **61**: 3225–9.

302. Jamal R, Thomas NSB, Gale RE, Linch DC. Variable expression of p16 protein in patients with acute myeloid leukaemia without gross rearrangements at the DNA level. *Leukaemia* 1996; **10**: 629–36.

303. Batova A, Diccianni MB, Yu JC et al. Frequent and selective methylation of p15 and deletion of both p15 and p16 in T-cell acute lymphoblastic leukemia. *Cancer Res* 1997; **57**: 832–6.

304. Mufti GJ, Galton DA. Myelodysplastic syndromes: natural history and features of prognostic significance. *Clin Haematol* 1986; **15**: 953–71.

305. Padua RA, McGlynn A, McGlynn H. Molecular cytogenetics and genetics of MDS and secondary AML. In: Raza A, Mundle S (eds) *Myelodysplastic Syndromes and Secondary Acute Myelogenous Leukemia – Directions for the New Millenium*. Dordrecht: Kluwer, 2001: 111–57.

306. Parker J, Mufti GJ. Ras and myelodysplasia: lessons from the last decade. *Semin Hematol* 1996; **33**: 206–24.

307. Paquette RL, Landaw EM, Pierre RV et al. N-*ras* mutations are associated with poor prognosis and increased risk of leukemia in myelodysplastic syndrome. *Blood* 1993; **82**: 590–9.

308. Gallagher A, Padua RA, Al-Sabah AI et al. Aberrant expression of p21RAS but not p120GAP is a common feature of myelodysplasia. *Leukemia* 1995; **9**: 1833–40.

309. Padua RA, Guinn BA, Al-Sabah AI et al. *RAS*, *FMS* and *p53* mutations and poor clinical outcome in myelodysplasias: a 10-year follow-up. *Leukemia* 1998; **12**: 887–92.

310. Harada H, Kondo T, Ogawa S et al. Accelerated exon skipping of IRF-1 mRNA in human myelodysplasia/leukemia; a possible mechanism of tumor suppressor inactivation. *Oncogene* 1994; **9**: 3313–20.

311. Kondo T, Minamino N, Nagamura Inoue T et al. Identification and characterization of nucleophosmin/ B23/numatrin which binds the anti-oncogenic transcription factor IRF-1 and manifests oncogenic activity. *Oncogene* 1997; **15**: 1275–81.

312. Counter CM, Gupta J, Harley CB et al. Telomerase activity in normal leukocytes and in hematologic malignancies. *Blood* 1995; **85**: 2315–20.

313. Ohyashiki JH, Iwama H, Yahata N et al. Telomere stability is frequently impaired in high-risk groups of patients with myelodysplastic syndromes. *Clin Cancer Res* 1999; **5**: 1155–60.

314. Li B, Yang J, Andrews C et al. Telomerase activity in preleukemia and acute myelogenous leukemia. *Leuk Lymphoma* 2000; **36**: 579–87.

315. Herman JG, Jen J, Merlo A, Baylin SB. Hypermethylation-associated inactivation indicates a tumor suppressor role for p15INK4B. *Cancer Res* 1996; **56**: 722–7.

316. Herman JG, Civin CI, Issa JP et al. Distinct patterns of inactivation of p15INK4B and p16INK4A characterize the major types of hematological malignancies. *Cancer Res* 1997; **57**: 837–41.

317. Uchida T, Kinoshita T, Nagai H et al. Hypermethylation of the *p15INK4B* gene in myelodysplastic syndromes. *Blood* 1997; **90**: 1403–9.

318. Quesnel B, Fenaux P. *P15INK4b* gene methylation and myelodysplastic syndromes. *Leuk Lymphoma* 1999; 35, 437–443.

319. Tien HF, Tang JL, Tsay W et al. Methylation of the *p15INK4B* gene in myelodysplastic syndrome: it can be detected early at diagnosis or during disease progression and is highly associated with leukaemic transformation. *Br J Haematol* 2001; **112**: 148–54.

320. Silverman LR, Demakos EP, Peterson BL et al. Randomized controlled trial of azacytidine in patients with the myelodysplastic syndrome: a study of the Cancer and Leukemia Group B. *J Clin Oncol* 2002; **20**: 2429–40.

321. Chim CS, Liang R, Tam CY, Kwong YL. Methylation of *p15* and *p16* genes in acute promyelocytic leukemia: potential diagnostic and prognostic significance. *J Clin Oncol* 2001; **19**: 2033–40.

322. Latres E, Malumbres M, Sotillo R et al. Limited overlapping roles of p15INK4b and p18INK4c cell cycle inhibitors in proliferation and tumorigenesis. *EMBO J* 2000; **19**: 3496–506.

323. Aytac U, Konishi T, David H et al. Rb independent inhibition of cell growth by p15INK4B. *Biochem Biophys Res Commun* 1999; **262**: 534–8.

324. Hahn WC, Counter CM, Lundberg AS et al. Creation of human tumour cells with defined genetic elements. *Nature* 1999; **400**: 464–8.

325. Malumbres M, Perez De Castro I, Hernandez MI et al. Cellular response to oncogenic ras involves induction of the Cdk4 and Cdk6 inhibitor p15INK4b. *Mol Cell Biol* 2000; **20**: 2915–25.

326. Palmero I, Pantoja C, Serrano M. p19ARF links the tumour suppressor p53 to Ras. *Nature* 1998; **395**: 125–6.

327. Sherr CJ. Tumor surveillance via the ARF–p53 pathway. *Genes Dev* 1998; **12**: 2984–91.

328. Sanchez-Aguilera A, Delgado J, Camacho FI et al. Silencing of the *p18INK4c* gene by promoter hypermethylation in Reed–Sternberg cells in Hodgkin lymphomas. *Blood* 2004; **103**: 2351–7.

329. Bai F, Pei XH, Godfrey VL, Xiong Y. Haploinsufficiency of p18INK4c sensitizes mice to carcinogen-induced tumorigenesis. *Mol Cell Biol* 2003; **23**: 1269–77.

330. Shiohara M, Spirin K, Said JW et al. Alterations of the cyclin-dependent kinase inhibitor p19$^{INK4D}$ is rare in hematopoietic malignancies. *Leukaemia* 1996; **10**: 1897–900.

331. Bhatia K, Fan S, Spragler G et al. A mutant p21 cyclin-dependent kinase inhibitor isolated from a Burkitt's lymphoma. *Cancer Res* 1995; **55**: 1431–5.

332. Roman-Gomez J, Castillejo JA, Jimenez A et al. 5′ CpG island hypermethylation is associated with transcriptional silencing of the *p21$^{CIP1/WAF1/SDI1}$* gene and confers poor prognosis in acute lymphoblastic leukemia. *Blood* 2002; **99**: 2291–6.

333. Kawamata N, Morosetti R, Miller CW et al. Molecular analysis of the cyclin-dependent kinase inhibitor gene *p27/Kip1* in human malignancies. *Cancer Res* 1995; **55**: 2266–9.

334. Takeuchi C, Takeuchi S, Ikezoe T et al. Germline mutation of the *p27/Kip1* gene in childhood acute lymphoblastic leukemia. *Leukemia* 2002; **16**: 956–8.

335. Yokozawa T, Towatari M, Iida H et al. Prognostic significance of the cell cycle inhibitor p27$^{Kip1}$ in acute myeloid leukemia. *Leukemia* 2000; **14**: 28–33.

336. Vrhovac R, Delmer A, Tang R et al. Prognostic significance of the cell cycle inhibitor p27$^{Kip1}$ in chronic B-cell lymphocytic leukemia. *Blood* 1998; **91**: 4694–700.

337. Tsihlias J, Kapusta L, Slingerland J. The prognostic significance of altered cyclin-dependent kinase inhibitors in human cancer. *Annu Rev Med* 1999; **50**: 401–23.

338. Zhang H, Kobayashi R, Galaktionov K, Beach D. p19$^{Skp1}$ and p45$^{Skp2}$ are essential elements of the cyclin A–CDK2 S phase kinase. *Cell* 1995; **82**: 915–25.

339. Sutterluty H, Chatelain E, Marti A et al. p45$^{SKP2}$ promotes p27$^{Kip1}$ degradation and induces S phase in quiescent cells. *Nat Cell Biol* 1999; **1**: 207–14.

340. Fero ML, Randel E, Gurley KE et al. The murine gene *p27$^{Kip1}$* is haplo-insufficient for tumour suppression. *Nature* 1998; **396**: 177–80.

341. Blain SW, Scher HI, Cordon-Cardo C, Koff A. p27 as a target for cancer therapeutics. *Cancer Cell* 2003; **3**: 111–15.

342. Kikuchi T, Toyota M, Itoh F et al. Inactivation of p57$^{KIP2}$ by regional promoter hypermethylation and histone deacetylation in human tumors. *Oncogene* 2002; **21**: 2741–9.

343. Li Y, Nagai H, Ohno T et al. Aberrant DNA methylation of *p57$^{KIP2}$* gene in the promoter region in lymphoid malignancies of B-cell phenotype. *Blood* 2002; **100**: 2572–7.

344. Golub TR, Slonim DK, Tamayo P et al. Molecular classification of cancer: class discovery and class prediction by gene expression monitoring. *Science* 1999; **286**: 531–7.

345. Davis RE, Staudt LM. Molecular diagnosis of lymphoid malignancies by gene expression profiling. *Curr Opin Hematol* 2002; **9**: 333–8.

346. Rosenwald A, Wright G, Chan WC et al. The use of molecular profiling to predict survival after chemotherapy for diffuse large-B-cell lymphoma. *N Engl J Med* 2002; **346**: 1937–47.

347. Shipp MA, Ross KN, Tamayo P et al. Diffuse large B-cell lymphoma outcome prediction by gene-expression profiling and supervised machine learning. *Nat Med* 2002; **8**: 68–74.

348. Christman JK. 5-Azacytidine and 5-aza-2′-deoxycytidine as inhibitors of DNA methylation: mechanistic studies and their implications for cancer therapy. *Oncogene* 2002; **21**: 5483–95.

349. Daskalakis M, Nguyen TT, Nguyen C et al. Demethylation of a hypermethylated *p15/INK4B* gene in patients with myelodysplastic syndrome by 5-aza-2′-deoxycytidine (decitabine) treatment. *Blood* 2002; **100**: 2957–64.

350. Cameron EE, Bachman KE, Myohanen S et al. Synergy of demethylation and histone deacetylase inhibition in the re-expression of genes silenced in cancer. *Nat Genet* 1999; **21**: 103–7.

351. Chant ID, Rose PE, Morris AG. Analysis of heat-shock protein expression in myeloid leukaemia cells by flow cytometry. *Br J Haematol* 1995; **90**: 163–8.

352. Xiao K, Liu W, Qu S et al. Study of heat shock protein HSP90α, HSP70, HSP27 mRNA expression in human acute leukemia cells. *J Tongji Med Univ* 1996; **16**: 212–16.

353. Yufu Y, Nishimura J, Nawata H. High constitutive expression of heat shock protein 90α in human acute leukemia cells. *Leuk Res* 1992; **16**: 597–605.

354. Matushansky I, Radparvar F, Skoultchi AI. Reprogramming leukemic cells to terminal differentiation by inhibiting specific cyclin-dependent kinases in G$_1$. *Proc Natl Acad Sci USA* 2000; **97**: 14317–22.

355. Hoessel R, Leclerc S, Endicott JA et al. Indirubin, the active constituent of a Chinese antileukaemia medicine, inhibits cyclin-dependent kinases. *Nat Cell Biol* 1999; **1**: 60–7.

356. Senderowicz AM. The cell cycle as a target for cancer therapy: basic and clinical findings with the small molecule inhibitors flavopiridol and UCN-01. *Oncologist* 2002; **7** (Suppl 2): 12–19.

357. Workman P. Altered states: selectively drugging the Hsp90 cancer chaperone. *Trends Mol Med* 2004; **10**: 47–51.

# 5 Transcription factors in hematopoietic differentiation and leukemia

**Michael A Chapman and Anthony R Green**

## Introduction

One of the central issues of developmental biology concerns the molecular mechanisms whereby a multipotent cell gives rise to distinct differentiated progeny. Differences between specialized cell types reflect variations in patterns of gene expression. The regulation of transcription is an important control point for gene expression, and it is therefore not surprising that transcription factors play a pivotal role in mammalian development and differentiation.

Hematopoiesis, the process of blood cell formation, is a powerful experimental model for studies of these processes. During embryonic development, hematopoiesis occurs in sequential phases. Early hematopoiesis, and particularly erythropoiesis, is observed in the yolk sac, but later moves to the fetal liver and finally to the bone marrow. It has long been thought that stem cells formed in the yolk sac migrate to the fetal liver, but more recently it has become clear that stem cells can also arise independently at an early stage of development within the embryo in the region of the dorsal aorta.[1,2] In an adult, pluripotent stem cells give rise to a hierarchy of multi- and oligopotent progenitor cells, which, in turn, differentiate into at least nine specialized and very different cell types. The scale of the process is staggering. Over $10^{11}$ differentiated cells are produced each day.

How is hematopoiesis regulated? First, it should be made clear that different regulatory mechanisms are likely to operate in the different phases of hematopoiesis. The early embryo has very different requirements from an adult individual, and hence yolk sac and adult hematopoiesis are likely to be regulated differently. However, there are two broad views of how any stem cell gives rise to its various progeny. One possibility is that signals arising from growth factor/growth factor receptor interactions positively 'instruct' a multipotent cell to differentiate along a particular lineage.[3] Alternatively, growth factors may allow the survival of daughter cells that have already become committed to a particular lineage. In the latter case, the decision to differentiate may represent a stochastic intracellular event independent of environmental cues. Cells subsequently finding themselves in an appropriate growth factor environment would then be 'selected' to survive and proliferate, whereas less fortunate cells would undergo apoptotic cell death. The stochastic or selective model is favored by evidence that growth factors are not essential for hematopoietic differentiation.[4] Furthermore, exchanging the cytoplasmic signaling domains of the erythropoietin (EPO), thrombopoietin (TPO), and granulocyte colony-stimulating factor (G-CSF) receptors does not appear to alter their function, a finding that does not fit easily with the 'instructive' model of cell signaling.[5,6] Regardless of which model is invoked, transcription factors represent the final common pathway that drives differentiation, and differences between cell types reflect the operation of distinct patterns of transcription factor expression.

## Transcription factors and normal hematopoiesis

### Combinations of transcription factors drive lineage-specific gene expression

One major route to identifying transcription factors important for individual hematopoietic lineages is to study the regulatory regions of lineage-specific genes. Studies of promoter and enhancer elements that control expression of globin and other erythroid genes have identified three recurrent motifs in various combinations: a GATA motif, an AP-1-like sequence and a CACC-like sequence.[7] The implication is that transcription factors binding to these three motifs are likely to be important for erythroid differentiation, and subsequent work has identified the critical transcription factors as GATA-1, NF-E2 (which binds to an AP-1-like sequence) and EKLF (which binds to the CACC motif). Indeed, it is possible to synthesize an artificial promoter that exhibits erythroid-specific activity by combining these three binding sites.[8] See also Chapter 10 on erythropoiesis.

As shown in Table 5.1, analogous observations have been made in myeloid and lymphoid cells. Binding sites for PU.1, CBFα and C/EBP transcription factors are found in the regulatory elements of most genes expressed in myeloid cells. Similarly, binding sites for Ikaros, NF-κB, OCT-1, OCT-2, E2A, LEF-1, and TCF-1 have all been identified in the regulatory elements of genes expressed in various categories of lymphoid cells.

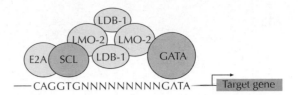

**Figure 5.1** SCL and GATA proteins form part of a multiprotein complex implicated in erythroid differentiation and T-cell tumorigenesis.

### Table 5.1  Transcription factor motifs commonly found in regulatory elements of lineage-specific genes

| Lineage | Transcription factor motifs | Refs |
|---|---|---|
| Erythroid | GATA, NF-E2, CACC | 113 |
| Megakaryocyte | GATA, ETS | 114 |
| Mast | GATA | 115 |
| Myeloid | PU.1, RUNX1, C/EBP | 19, 116, 117 |
| Lymphoid | Ikaros, NF-κB, OCT-1, OCT-2 | 118–120 |
| | E2A, LEF-1, TCF-1 | 121–123 |

The fact that no single transcription factor-binding motif is sufficient to direct lineage-specific expression suggests that combinations of transcription factors are required. Indeed, all 'lineage-restricted' hematopoietic transcription factors are expressed in more than one lineage – an observation that again implies that combinations of transcription factors are needed to provide true lineage-specific gene expression. A third and more tangible line of evidence also supports the combinatorial concept of gene regulation. In many instances, individual transcription factors form part of multicomponent transcription factor complexes. Thus, the helix–loop–helix protein SCL not only binds to other helix–loop–helix proteins encoded by the *E2A* gene, but also forms part of an oligomeric, DNA-binding complex that contains SCL, E2A, LMO-2, GATA-1, and LDB-1 proteins.[9] As indicated in Figure 5.1, the SCL, E2A, and GATA-1 proteins bind directly to DNA, and presumably recruit the LMO-2 and LDB-1 proteins. Recent evidence suggests that the complex can be recruited to DNA via the zinc finger protein SP1.[10] Important target genes included the stem cell factor receptor, c-Kit, the promoter of which is activated by the complex.[10] The complex has been best studied in erythroid cells – in other cell types, variations in individual components (e.g. replace-

ment of GATA-1 by GATA-2) may result in specificity for a distinct pattern of target genes.

## Knockout studies identify transcription factors with important roles in vivo

A large number of transcription factors are now known to be expressed in various hematopoietic cell types. Their detailed patterns of expression give some clues as to where the transcription factors are likely to be important, but devising experiments to ascertain specific functions can be difficult. The most powerful approach has been a genetic one – the generation of targeted mutations in mice using homologous recombination (Figure 5.2). This technology has provided numerous insights into the transcriptional control of hematopoiesis.[11]

## Transcription factors critical for stem cells

Homologous recombination studies have led to the identification of a small number of transcription factors that are essential for normal stem cell behavior. The *SCL* gene was first identified by virtue of its disruption by chromosome rearrangements in T-cell acute lymphoblastic leukemia (T-ALL). These rearrangements (both translocations and deletions) result in SCL expression in T cells, a lineage normally lacking SCL protein. SCL is normally expressed in erythroid, mast, and megakaryocytic cells, as well as in multipotent progenitors. Early experiments in cell lines suggested that SCL controls the proliferation of primitive multipotent cells,[12] as well as acting as a positive regulator or erythroid differentiation.[13,14] When *SCL*-knockout mice were generated, their phenotype was dramatic[15,16] – mice lacking SCL protein were completely unable to produce any hematopoietic cells (Figure 5.3). Subsequent experiments showed that stem cells responsible for both primitive (yolk sac) and adult (fetal liver) hematopoiesis were affected. Moreover, embryonic stem (ES) cells null for SCL protein were unable to undergo differentiation in vitro to produce hematopoietic cells.[17,18] These data suggest that the SCL protein is vital for the development or behavior of pluripotent hematopoietic stem cells. The nature of the target genes regulated by SCL is now clearly an important issue, as is the question of what regulates *SCL* itself.

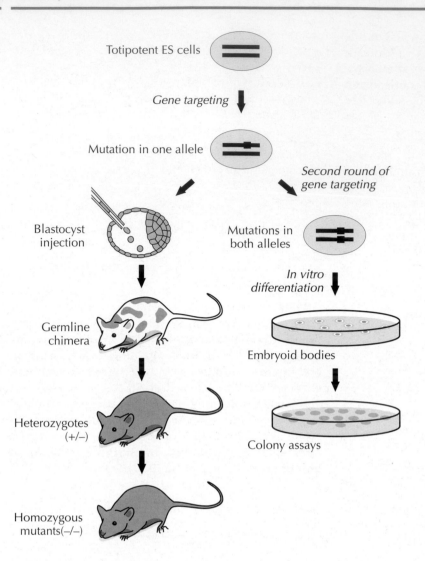

Totipotent ES cells

*Gene targeting*

Mutation in one allele

*Second round of gene targeting*

Blastocyst injection

Mutations in both alleles

*In vitro differentiation*

Germline chimera

Embryoid bodies

Heterozygotes (+/–)

Colony assays

Homozygous mutants(–/–)

**Figure 5.2** Use of homologous recombination in embryonic stem (ES) cells to 'knock out' target genes. Once one allele has been mutated, the ES cells can be injected into blastocysts to generate chimeric mice; subsequent breeding generates heterozygous and homozygous mutants. Alternatively, homozygous mutant ES cells can be generated and used to assess the effect of the mutation on hematopoietic differentiation in vitro.

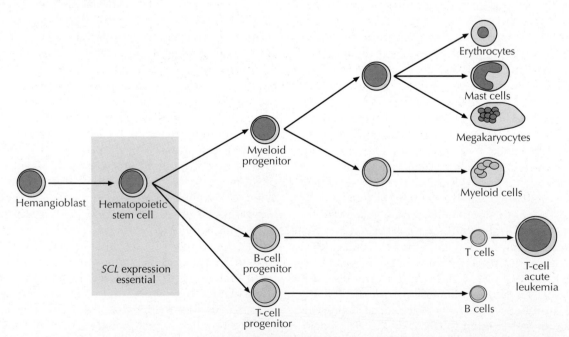

Hemangioblast

Hematopoietic stem cell

*SCL* expression essential

Myeloid progenitor

B-cell progenitor

T-cell progenitor

Erythrocytes

Mast cells

Megakaryocytes

Myeloid cells

T cells

B cells

T-cell acute leukemia

**Figure 5.3** The *SCL* gene is essential for the development of all hematopoietic lineages. A dark nucleus indicates lineages/cell types expressing the *SCL* gene. *SCL* is expressed in the pluripotent hematopoietic stem cell. Its expression is maintained following commitment to the erythroid, mast, and megakaryocytic lineages, but not following commitment to other lineages. Ectopic expression resulting from chromosome rearrangements in a T-cell precursor results in T-cell acute leukemia. Adapted from Green.[60]

*RUNX1* (also known as *AML1*, *PEBPA2B*, or *CBFA2*) is another gene that was identified on the basis of its involvement in a leukemia-associated translocation.[19] It too was subsequently demonstrated to have a critical role in the hematopoietic system following the generation of knockout mice. *RUNX1⁻/⁻* embryos die at embryonic day 12.5–13.5, with a profound block in definitive hematopoiesis. There is necrosis and hemorrhaging within the central nervous system and a lack of definitive hematopoietic progenitors, definitive enucleated erythrocytes, and mature myeloid-lineage cells.[20,21] Like their *SCL⁻/⁻* counterparts, ES cells homozygous for the *RUNX1* deletion do not contribute to any adult hematopoietic cells in chimeric mice.[21] However, in contract to *SCL*, *RUNX1* does not appear to be necessary for primitive hematopoiesis.[20,21]

A number of other transcription factors have knockout phenotypes almost as dramatic as those of *SCL* and *RUNX1*, indicating a role in multipotent progenitors (Figure 5.4). The phenotype of the *LMO-2* knockout is similar to that of *SCL*, although small numbers of hematopoietic cells may still be found.[22] Similarly, *LMO-2⁻/⁻* embryonic stem cells do not contribute to any hematopoietic lineage in adult chimeric mice.[23] The similarity between the *SCL* and *LMO-2* knockout phenotypes is particularly provocative, since these two proteins have been shown to physically interact in vivo (see above), and, like *SCL*, *LMO-2* is a T-cell oncogene. These data suggest that a complex containing SCL and LMO-2 may be crucial for both stem cell behavior and T-cell tumorigenesis.

The zinc finger protein GATA-2 also affects the production of all hematopoietic lineages, but small numbers of hematopoietic cells can be produced by *GATA-2*-null mice and also by in vitro differentiation of *GATA-2*-null ES cells.[24] These results raise the possibility that *GATA-2* may be necessary for the expansion of early hematopoietic cells, but that its absence may not prevent at least some differentiation.[24]

## Transcription factors critical for the formation or function of specific lineages

GATA motifs known to bind GATA-1 are prominent in the regulatory elements of all erythroid-specific genes, and so it is reassuring that the absence of GATA-1 blocked erythropoiesis at the pro-erythroblast stage.[25–27] *GATA-1* therefore seems to be particularly important for survival and terminal maturation of erythroid progenitors. By contrast, mice null for a different zinc finger protein, EKLF, exhibited a thalassemic syndrome resulting from the specific inhibition of β-globin transcription. Defects of other single lineages have also been observed. Mice lacking NF-E2 protein failed to produce megakaryocytes,[28] whereas mice with no Fos protein developed osteopetrosis as a result of a specific lack of osteoclasts.[29] Similarly, in lymphoid development, OCT-2 is reported to be essential for functional maturation of mature B cells,[30] and TCF-1 for the differentiation of immature CD8⁺ precursors into more mature CD4⁺CD8⁺ thymocytes.[31]

However, some transcription factors present a more complex picture. Mice null for the PU.1 protein lack B

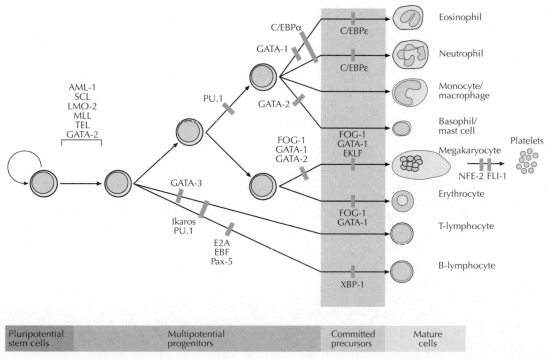

**Figure 5.4** Homologous recombination experiments reveal roles for transcription factors in hematopoiesis. Knockout studies have identified a number of transcription factors important for the formation or function of specific hematopoietic cells. Adapted from Cantor and Orkin.[163]

cells, macrophages, and neutrophils.[32,33] This result could represent a defect of a multipotent myelo-lymphoid progenitor that results in restricted lineage commitment options. Alternatively, the data are also consistent with postcommitment differentiation defects in several independent lineages.

## Caveats and limitations

Although a powerful approach to analyzing transcription factor function in vivo, homologous recombination experiments are subject to a number of limitations. First, if loss of function blocks an early step in differentiation, this will compromise the analysis of later stages of development. Thus, the death of mouse embryos at an early stage of development because of the failure of hematopoiesis has precluded analysis of SCL function in other tissues where it is expressed, such as in endothelium and in developing brain. Regulatable or conditional knockouts are being developed and should circumvent this problem. Second, the lack of an obvious phenotype may mean that the targeted transcription factor is superfluous, or that we are not looking in the right way to detect the phenotype, or that compensatory mechanisms are operating. Thus, the *SCL* gene is normally expressed in endothelial cells, but these appear to develop normally in *SCL*-null embryos. The possible function of SCL in endothelial cells therefore remains an open question. Finally, the phenotype observed in a given knockout mouse will reflect the net result of a complex interplay of direct and indirect effects. These may be influenced by the genetic background of the mouse, and so details of the knockout phenotype may vary between mouse strains.

## Chromatin structure

It has been increasingly clear over the past decade that chromatin structure plays a vital role in regulating transcription.[34,35] If placed end-to-end, the DNA packaged into the chromosomes of a single cell would stretch for over a meter. In order to accommodate this length of DNA within an individual nucleus, the DNA is wrapped around histone proteins and then folded into a complex higher-order structure termed chromatin. This solves the packaging issue, but raises a second problem: How do transcription factors gain access to DNA-binding sites buried within such chromatin structures? We still do not have all the answers, but is is clear that chromatin exists in a number of different states. Heterochromatin is densely packaged, and the genes within it are transcriptionally silent. In other regions, the chromatin structure is looser. Transcription factors can access the DNA in these regions, and so genes are potentially active if the appropriate transcription factors are present.

The basic building block of chromatin is the nucleosome, which consists of DNA wrapped around a cylinder of eight core histone proteins (two each of H2A, H2B, H3, and H4).[36] Individual nucleosomes are linked by intervening stretches of DNA, and can be unfolded to resemble 'beads on a string'. However, in the nucleus, the nucleosomes are stacked closely together in higher-order structures that are dependent on a large number of non-histone proteins. The precise structures found in different regions of the genome dictate whether genes in those regions are potentially active. Moreover, a form of molecular memory is needed to ensure that daughter cells inherit the same patterns of gene expression as a parent cell. Experiments in *Drosophila* have identified a number of non-histone proteins important for this molecular memory, including the Polycomb and Su(var) families, which play a role in maintaining inactive chromatin, and the Trithorax and E(var) families, which appear to maintain regions of active chromatin.[36–38]

The products of these genes appear to interact with eight N-terminal histone tails that protrude from the nucleosome (reviewed by Jenuwein and Allis[36] and Spotswood and Turner[39]). They are capable of covalently modifying specific residues on the tails, by acetylation (and de-acetylation), methylation, and phosphorylation. These modifications can be recognized by a number of highly conserved domains found within 'effector' proteins (including Polycomb, Trithorax, Su(var), and E(var) themselves), which can remodel the chromatin to a more open (active) or condensed (inactive) state. This complex interplay provides a mechanism for the spreading of active or inactive chromatin, and has given rise to the concept of the 'chromatin code', the idea that modifications of the histone tails can determine the transcriptional activity of regions of DNA. The turnover of these covalent modifications may be rapid (half-lives of a few minutes to hours),[40] as might be expected in the control of genes that need to be up- or downregulated quickly, such as hormone- and growth factor-responsive genes. Alternatively, the modifications may be very stable. This can provide the basis of longer-term 'molecular memory', including phenomena such as X-inactivation and imprinting.[41]

## Stem cells, lineage commitment, and plasticity

The mechanisms responsible for lineage commitment of stem cells remain among the central mysteries of hematopoiesis. It is tempting to speculate that some transcription factors function as 'master regulators' capable of switching on lineage-specific programs of gene expression. However, direct evidence is sparse. Knockout data showing that individual transcription factors are essential for the development of certain lineages are consistent with, but do not prove, a role for those transcription factors in lineage commitment. More convincing evidence comes from studies in which specific transcription factors are overexpressed and shown to influence lineage choice.

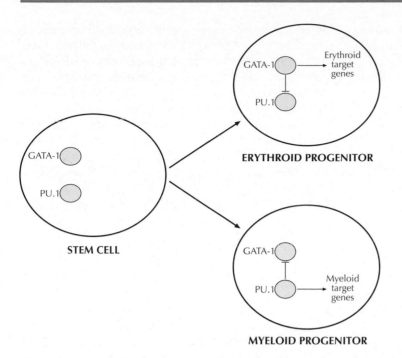

**ERYTHROID PROGENITOR**

**STEM CELL**

**MYELOID PROGENITOR**

**Figure 5.5** Reciprocal repression between PU.1 and GATA-1. At the stem cell stage, neither transcription factor is dominant. However, following lineage commitment, each factor promotes its lineage choice whilst downregulating the other by protein–protein interactions.

Overexpression of *GATA-1* in a primitive myeloid cell line resulted in the acquisition of megakaryocytic features.[42] This result is consistent with the observation that loss of *GATA-1* expression in megakaryocytes in vivo resulted in dysregulation of megakaryocyte development.[43] Even more convincing are elegant results from Graf and colleagues using chicken cell lines. Overexpression of *GATA-1* in myeloblasts resulted in a switch to erythroid cells, thromboblasts (equivalents of megakaryocytes), or eosinophils.[44] The level of *GATA-1* expression was crucial, with erythroid or thromboblast fates being favored by levels of GATA-1 only fourfold greater than the levels favoring eosinophil formation.

The same avian system has also provided evidence of another emerging principle – that of reciprocal repression. This refers to the situation where a given transcription factor may be important for directing the transcriptional program of one lineage while at the same time downregulating genes important for the program of a different lineage. The ETS-1 transcription factor is expressed in both erythroid and myeloid cells, whereas the MafB transcription factor is only expressed in myeloid cells. MafB appears to direct the expression of myeloid genes, but also inhibits the action of ETS-1 on target genes important for erythropoiesis.[45] A more complex example is provided by the transcription factors GATA-1 and PU.1. Each antagonizes the other by protein–protein interactions. The result is a cross-inhibition, in which the dominant factor promotes its lineage choice at the expense of the other (Figure 5.5).[46]

Several important principles governing the role of transcription factors in hematopoiesis are therefore becoming clear, and are outlined in Figure 5.6. Lineage commitment of stem cells is likely to involve

upregulation (by mechanisms that remain unclear) of one or more critical transcription factors. GATA-1 and PU.1 are prime candidates for erythroid and myeloid differentiation respectively. Activation of these pivotal transcription factors has multiple consequences, including autoregulation of the transcription factor gene itself, upregulation of receptors for lineage-specific growth factors, activation of lineage-specific

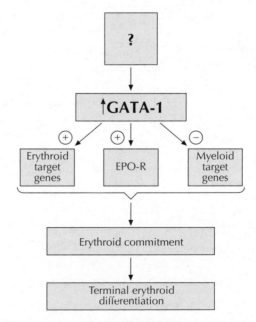

**Figure 5.6** A model for erythroid lineage commitment of a multipotent stem cell. Upregulation of GATA-1 (by mechanisms that remain obscure) results in autoregulation of the *GATA-1* gene, activation of erythroid target genes, including the erythropoietin receptor (EPO-R), and repression of target genes normally expressed in other lineages (reciprocal repression). The net effect is commitment to terminal erythroid differentiation.

programs of gene expression, and reciprocal repression of genes expressed in other lineages. The net effect of these multiple changes is to produce a progenitor that has become committed to differentiate along a particular lineage.

The data presented above suggest that hematopoietic differentiation may not be as irreversible as previously thought, but instead exhibits a remarkable degree of plasticity. Pax5 is a transcription factor essential for the normal development of B lymphocytes. Pro-B cells derived from *Pax5*$^{-/-}$ mice demonstrate a striking ability to differentiate not only into non-B lymphocytes (T cells and natural killer (NK) cells), but also into cells of other hematopoietic lineages, including macrophages, dendritic cells, and neutrophils. Moreover, restoration of *Pax5* expression induces differentiation into B cells.[47,48] Lineage switches involving other cell types have been demonstrated in vitro, and are not limited to knockout or other mutant cell lines.[49] More striking still are data from a number of transplantation experiments that suggest an ability of hematopoietic cells to differentiate into non-hematopoietic cells (reviewed by Graf,[49] and see Chapter 2 on stem cell plasticity). Examples of cell types shown to arise from bone marrow cells include endothelium, parenchymal liver cells, neuronal and glial cells, and skeletal and cardiac muscle cells. However, in many cases, clonal analysis has not been performed, and it remains an open question whether these represent true plasticity of hematopoietic stem cells or the presence of non-hematopoietic stem cells in the bone marrow.[49,50] Furthermore, as is the case with intrahematopoietic lineage switches, the *in vivo* significance is unknown.

It is clear that transcription factors play a central role in regulating proliferation and differentiation of multipotent hematopoietic progenitors. It is therefore not surprising that perturbation of transcription factor function has dire consequences and that transcription factor genes are common targets for leukemogenic mutations.

# Transcription factors and leukemia

## Genetic changes associated with leukemia

A multitude of acquired genetic alterations associated with leukemia have been characterized at a molecular level. This wealth of information has arisen largely as a result of the relative ease with which leukemias can be characterized at a cytogenetic level.[51] Unlike cells of solid tumors, leukemia cells are readily accessible, and can be encouraged to divide in culture and so generate metaphases.

There are three main cytogenetic changes associated with leukemia: translocations, inversions, and deletions. Changes consistently found in particular leukemia types are highly likely to contribute to the pathogenesis of those leukemias. Translocations and inversions are the most informative abnormalities, since identification of the breakpoints is likely to lead directly to the location of critical target genes. The Human Genome Project is providing a massive increase in the molecular tools available for characterized rearrangements, and the past decade has seen an exponential rise in the number of leukemia genes identified.

However, despite this rapid increase in the identification of target genes, it is likely that we are still only scratching the surface. Deletions are commonly seen in various forms of hematological malignancy, but in most cases the tumor suppressor genes that they harbor have not been successfully identified. This is because most deletions are large and frequently contain hundreds of genes. In addition to cytogenetically visible changes, more subtle alterations can perturb the function of critical target genes: point mutations can activate or disable proteins; small deletions will be below the resolution of cytogenetic analysis; and even some translocations are not detectable using standard G-banding techniques. Moreover, most leukemias are likely to reflect acquired alterations in several target genes; and, to further add to the complexity, these acquired genetic changes are likely to interact with inherited polymorphisms – interactions that are likely to account for the varying degrees of inherited predisposition to leukemia.

## Target cells for transformation

One view of the origin of different types of hematological malignancy is that they represent transformation of distinct progenitor cells. To some extent, this may be true. Lymphoid tumors are thought to result from transformation of committed lymphoid cells, perhaps reflecting the innate ability of lymphocytes to undergo self-renewal when stimulated. However, in the context of myeloid malignancies, this concept may be misleading. Thus, it has been suggested that acute myeloid leukemia (AML) with promyelocytic or megakaryocytic features may represent the transformation of normal progenitors committed to promyelocytic or megakaryocytic differentiation. However, this concept is not consistent with recent evidence that suggests that all forms of AML arise from transformation of a primitive multipotent stem cell. Thus, cytogenetic abnormalities associated with specific types of AML have been identified in a small population of primitive CD34$^+$ 'leukemic stem cells' as well as in the bulk of the more differentiated leukemia cells.[52,53]

Furthermore, these primitive 'leukemic stem cells' have been shown to be capable of initiating leukemia in immunodeficient mice.[54] These data suggest that

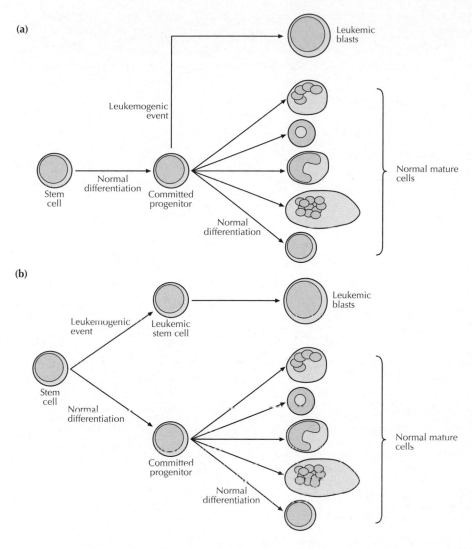

(a)

(b)

**Figure 5.7** Models for the origin of acute myeloid leukemia (AML). (a) The leukemogenic event occurs in a committed progenitor, and the phenotype of the resultant leukemic blasts reflects the phenotype of the committed progenitor. (b) The leukemogenic event occurs in a stem cell. The transformed stem cell can still undergo limited differentiation. The choice of lineage and degree of differentiation depend on the nature of the transforming event. As discussed in the text, current evidence favors model (b).

the different phenotypes exhibited by distinct types of AML reflect the effect of diverse mutations on the differentiation capacity of the transformed stem cell (Figure 5.7).

## Mechanisms responsible for target gene activation in leukemia

Numerous different target genes have now been implicated in the genesis of leukemia. In most cases, they have been identified by virtue of their presence at translocation or inversion breakpoints. Two broad conclusions can be drawn. First, transcription factor genes are common targets in leukemia. Second, translocations perturb target genes by two main mechanisms: dysregulation of a target gene or the generation of a fusion gene.

## Transcription factor genes are common targets in leukemia

As summarized in Table 5.2, a large number of transcription factors have been implicated in human hematological malignancies (see also Table 17.1 in Chapter 17 on acquired genetic changes in myeloid

malignancies). However, our existing knowledge is biased by the way in which these have been identified – namely by the characterization of chromosome rearrangements. It should be remembered that a point mutation can also perturb transcription factor function, the *p53* gene being a classic example. Similarly, tumor suppressor genes include those encoding transcription factors (e.g. *WT-1*). It remains to be seen whether the deletions associated with hematological malignancies will prove to harbor additional critical transcription factors. However, despite our incomplete knowledge, it is already clear that transcription factor genes are common targets for leukemogenic mutations. Why should transcription factors play such a central role in leukemogenesis? The neoplastic behavior of a malignant cell reflects altered patterns of transcription factor activity. One can speculate that mutations affecting cytoplasmic and cell surface components of signal transduction pathways may be vulnerable to a series of physiological checks and balances, which would tend to limit significant downstream alterations of nuclear transcription factor activity. By contract, mutations that directly affect transcription factor activity may be less open to such regulation, and hence be more potently oncogenic.

**Table 5.2  Transcription factor genes adjacent to the breakpoints of translocations associated with hematological malignancies. At least one of the two genes disrupted by each translocation encodes a transcription factor[93,120–165]**

| Lineage | Malignancy[a] | Translocation | Gene(s) | Refs |
|---|---|---|---|---|
| T-cell | T-cell ALL | t(1;14), t(1;7), t(1;3) | *SCL* | 128–132 |
| | | t(7;9) | *TAL-2* | 133 |
| | | t(6;11) | *MLL, AF6* | 162 |
| | | t(7;19) | *LYL-1* | 134 |
| | | t(11;14) | *LMO-1* | 135, 136 |
| | | t(11;14), t(7;11) | *LMO-2* | 137, 138 |
| | | t(10;14), t(7;10) | *HOX11* | 139–142 |
| | | t(8;14) | *MYC* | 143 |
| | ALL | t(1;19) | *PBX-1, E2A* | 144, 145 |
| | | t(4;11) | *MLL, AF4* | 163 |
| | | t(9;12) | *TEL, JAK2* | 160 |
| | | t(17;19) | *HLF, E2A* | 146, 147 |
| | | t(12;21) | *TEL, RUNX1* | 148, 149 |
| B-cell | Burkitt lymphoma | t(8;14), t(2;8), t(8;22) | *MYC* | 143 |
| | NHL, CLL | t(2;14) | *BCL11A* | 164 |
| | | t(8;14) | *PAX5* | 165 |
| | | t(10;14) | *LYT-10* | 150 |
| | | t(14;19) | *BCL-3* | 165 |
| | | 3q27 rearrangements | *BCL-6* | 151 |
| Myeloid | AML | t(1;11) | *NUP98, PMX1* | 162 |
| | | t(1;12) | *TEL, ARNT* | 160 |
| | | t(2;11) | *NUP98, HOXD13* | 162 |
| | | t(3;3) | *EVI-1* | 162 |
| | | t(3;21) | *RUNX1, EVI-1* | 64 |
| | | t(6;9) | *DEK/CAN* | 162 |
| | | t(7;11) | *NUP98, HOXA9* | 162 |
| | | t(16;16) | *CBFβ, MYF11* | 162 |
| | | t(16;21) | *RUNX1, MTG16* | 162 |
| | | t(16;21) | *TLS, ERG* | 160 |
| | | t(15;17) | *PML, RARAα* | 152, 153 |
| | | t(17;17) | *STAT5b, RARAα* | 162 |
| | | t(11;17) | *PLZF, RARAα* | 154 |
| | | t(5;17) | *NPM, RARAα* | 155 |
| | | t(8;21) | *RUNX1, ETO* | 124, 125 |
| | | t(9;12) | *ABL, TEL* | 94 |
| | | t(12;22) | *TEL, MN1* | 156 |
| | | t(8;16) | *MOZ, CBP* | 157 |
| | | Inv 16 | *CBFβ, SMMHC* | 158 |
| | | 11q23 rearrangements | *MLL* | 159 |
| | MDS | t(3;21) | *RUNX1, MDS-1* | 126 |
| | CMML | t(3;21) | *RUNX1, EAP* | 160 |
| | | t(5;12) | *TEL, PDGFR* | 97 |
| | CML (atypical) | t(9;15;12) | *TEL, JAK2* | 160 |
| | CML (myeloid blast crisis) | t(2;11) | *NUP98, HOXD13* | 162 |
| | | t(3;21) | *RUNX1, EVI-1* | 127 |
| | | t(7;11) | *NUP98, HOXA9* | 162 |
| | | t(16;21) | *TLS, ERG* | 160 |

[a] ALL, acute lymphoblastic leukemia; NHL, non-Hodgkin lymphoma; CLL, chronic lymphocytic leukemia; AML, acute myeloid leukemia; MDS, myelodysplastic syndrome; CMML, chronic myelomonocytic leukemia; CML, chronic myeloid leukemia.

## Dysregulated expression of a normal protein

Normal lymphoid cells undergo genetic rearrangement of their antigen receptor genes. Errors in this process of recombination result in chromosome translocations that involve immunoglobulin and T-cell receptor loci. Such translocations may result in powerful regulatory elements from the antigen receptor loci being relocated to the vicinity of potential oncogenes. The net effect is dysregulated expression of the potential oncogene in lymphoid progenitors.

The classic example of this mechanism is activation of the MYC transcription factor in Burkitt lymphoma and other B-cell tumors by the t(2;8), t(8;14), and t(8;22) translocations involving the immunoglobulin heavy- or light-chain loci (reviewed by Rabbitts[55]). More recently the SCL gene has provided a complementary example of transcription factor that is activated by translocations involving the T-cell reception loci. Translocations involving SCL account for approximately 3% of T-ALL. However, the SCL gene is also activated by cytogenetically invisible deletions that bring the promoter of the SIL gene (usually 90 kb upstream of SCL) into the immediate vicinity of the SCL promoter. In both translocation and deletion cases, the net effect is ectopic expression of SCL in T-cell progenitors, which do not normally express SCL (Figure 5.3). The two types of SCL rearrangements are found in up to one-third of pediatric T-ALL, and so rearrangement of the SCL locus is perhaps the commonest molecular pathology associated with this disease. It has also been reported that SCL is expressed in a further third of T-ALL cases that lack evidence of DNA rearrangement, and both cis- and trans-acting mechanisms have been implicated.[56]

Transgenic experiments have confirmed that overexpression of the SCL protein in T-cell progenitors can result in T-cell tumors.[57–59] However, the precise mechanism by which ectopic SCL expression is leukemogenic remains unclear. SCL may directly activate or inhibit transcription of target genes in T-cell progenitors. Alternatively, overexpressed SCL protein may bind to and sequester other transcription factors, thus producing an indirect effect on target genes regulated by those factors.[60] Whichever of these mechanisms is true, the consequences may include inhibition of apoptosis.[61]

## Generation of fusion proteins

The second major mechanism by which chromosome rearrangements generate tumorigenic genes involves the formation of fusion proteins. Many proteins, and especially transcription factors, exhibit a modular structure – that is, they contain a number of domains that can function independently of each other.

Fusion proteins contain functional domains from two different proteins unnaturally welded together. The consequences will depend on the precise functions of the various domains in each case. When transcription factors are involved, several scenarios can be envisaged: abnormal DNA binding; normal DNA binding but abnormal transactivation; sequestration of other proteins by protein–protein interaction; and ectopic expression driven by the promoter of the fusion gene's upstream component.

The number of fusion genes identified in human leukemia (and solid tumors) is rapidly increasing.[55] This category of oncogene is particularly tantalizing from the therapeutic point of view, because each fusion protein forms a tumor-specific molecule. Such molecules provide the substrate for powerful polymerase chain reaction (PCR)-based methods to monitor residual disease. They also represent an attractive target for tumor-specific therapies targeted at DNA, RNA, or protein levels.

## Leukemogenic alterations may target distinct steps in common signaling pathways

A recently emerging theme is that leukemias, like cancers, result from molecular alterations that interfere with signal transduction pathways regulating normal cell proliferation, differentiation, or death. It is becoming apparent that different genetic events in independent leukemias may prove to target distinct steps in a common pathway. Three examples will now be used to illustrate this principle: first, translocations involving 21q22 and inversion 16, which target different components of the core binding factor (CBF) complex; second, disruption of the CCAAT enhancer binding protein α (C/EBPα) leading to a block in granulopoiesis; and third, leukemogenic changes that perturb tyrosine kinase signaling pathways.

## Translocations involving 21q22 and inversion 16

The CBF gene family consists of three α subunits, encoded by RUNX1, RUNX2, and RUNX3, each of which heterodimerizes with CBFβ, encoded by the CBFβ gene (reviewed by Speck and Gilliland[62]). The RUNX1–CBFβ protein complex is essential for definitive hematopoiesis, as illustrated by the RUNX1 knockout mouse,[20,21] described above. RUNX1, like the other CBFα proteins, has DNA-binding properties. The exact role of the CBFβ subunit is unclear. It does not contact DNA directly, but may either stabilize the RUNX1 protein, or act as a recruitment moiety for other proteins in the complex.[63–66] Whatever its precise role, it is essential for RUNX1 activity; CBFβ knockout mice have an identical phenotype to RUNX1−/− mice.[67,68]

The RUNX1 gene is located on chromosome 21, and is involved in a number of cytogenetic abnormalities commonly associated with leukemia. Translocations t(8;21), t(12;21), and t(3;21) result in the generation of the fusion proteins RUNX1–ETO, TEL–RUNX1, and RUNX1–EVI1 respectively (Figure 5.8a). Inv(16) results in fusion of the smooth muscle myosin heavy chain (SMMHC) to the CBFβ subunit. The net result of all of these cytogenetic abnormalities is thought to be a fusion protein, which inhibits normal RUNX1 function (Figure 5.8b). This dominant negative effect has been demonstrated for the RUNX1–ETO and CBFβ–SMMHC products by the generation of knock-in mice, in which the fusion protein is expressed under control of the endogenous *RUNX1* promoter. Despite the presence of one fully functional *RUNX1* allele, the mutation results in a near phenocopy of the *RUNX1* knockout, and death during embryogenesis.[69–71]

In some cases, the mechanism of the dominant negative activity may be mediated through aberrant recruitment of a nuclear transcriptional complex by the fusion protein. RUNX1–ETO recruits SIN3 and various histone de-acetylases,[72,73] and TEL–RUNX1 recruits nuclear cofactor R (N-CoR).[74] The mechanism of the dominant negative activity of CBFβ–SMMHC is as yet undetermined, but may involve sequestration of RUNX1 or introduction of a repressor domain into CBFβ.[62]

Abrogation of RUNX1 function is not limited to the dominant negative effect of fusion proteins. Point mutations in the *RUNX1* gene are found in families with a familial platelet disorder and a propensity to develop AML (FPD/AML syndrome; reviewed by Speck and Gilliland[62]). Heterozygosity for the mutation appears to be sufficient for development of thrombocytopenia. However, progression to leukemia seems to require further genetic abnormalities, including mutations in the second *RUNX1* allele. Point

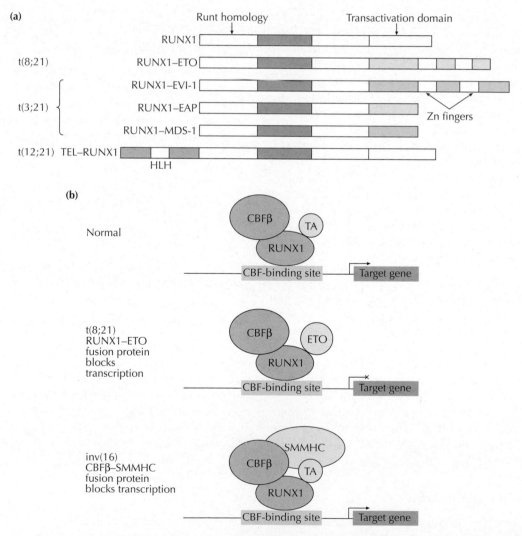

**Figure 5.8** Fusion proteins involving the *RUNX1* and *CBFβ* genes perturb normal transcription factor function. (a) Fusion proteins arising from t(8;21) and t(3;21) translocations result in loss of the *RUNX1* transactivation domain and its replacement by domains from several different genes. By contrast, the fusion protein created by the t(12;21) translocation fuses part of the TEL protein to the N-terminal end of the RUNX1 protein. (b) RUNX1 normally forms part of a multiprotein complex that includes CBFβ and that regulates the expression of target genes with CBF-binding sites in their regulatory elements. The RUNX1–ETO and CBFβ–SMMHC fusion proteins both perturb transcriptional regulation of normal target genes. Adapted from Sawyers.[157]

mutations in *RUNX1* have also been found in 3–5% of sporadic leukemias. The majority of these involve biallelic mutations.

## Disruption of the C/EBPα transcription factor

The transcription factor C/EPBα is expressed in many tissues, but within the hematopoietic system is largely confined to the granulocytic lineage.[75] It binds to the sequence CCAAT, or slight variations thereof, and is necessary for granulocytic lineage development.[76] It is expressed in the earliest myeloid cells, and other family members (C/EBPβ and C/EBPε) are induced later as differentiation proceeds.[75,77] *C/EBPα* knockout mice develop all hematopoietic lineages normally, apart from the granulocytic lineage, which is subject to maturation arrest with an accumulation of early granulocytic blasts.[78] Cell lines derived from these mice can be induced to differentiate by conditional expression of C/EBPα.[79]

It has recently become clear that inhibition of C/EBPα function by a number of different mechanisms is associated with distinct forms of AML (reviewed by Tenen[76]). First, in a subset of patients with AML (M1 or M2) and no cytogenetic abnormalities, mutations in the *C/EBPα* gene itself are seen.[80] Most of the mutations are heterozygous, suggesting a dominant negative function, and this is supported by in vitro studies.[81] Second, in t(8;21) AML, it has been demonstrated that the RUNX1–ETO fusion protein inhibits C/EBPα function and downregulates its expression.[82] Third, in acute promyelocytic leukemia (APL, also known as AML M3), *C/EBPα* is neither downregulated nor mutated. However, the PML–RAR fusion protein found in APL interacts with C/EBPα and inhibits its DNA-binding activity. All-*trans*-retinoic acid (ATRA), an effective therapeutic agent in APL, reverses this interaction and restores DNA binding.

## Tyrosine kinase and RAS signaling pathways

The t(9;22) translocation associated with chronic myeloid leukemia (CML) was the first tumor-specific abnormality to be described,[83,84] and results in generation of the *BCR–ABL* fusion gene (reviewed by Melo[85]). The N-terminal half of the BCR protein is fused to the majority of the ABL protein (Figure 5.9). The ABL protein contains a tyrosine kinase domain, and activity of this enzyme is dysregulated in the fusion protein.[86] The tumorigenic properties of the fusion protein depend on several other features: the ABL and BCR portions interact with adaptor proteins (CRKL and GRB-2 respectively), which connect the fusion protein to positive regulators of the RAS/MAPK signal transduction pathway.[87,88] The BCR–ABL kinase therefore mimics the activity of receptor tyrosine kinases and of cytokine receptors, both of which respond to ligand stimulation by activating the RAS pathway.[89–91] In many cases, it has been shown that ligand–receptor interaction results in dimer formation, which is essential for proper signaling. It is therefore probably no coincidence that the BCR portion of the BCR–ABL fusion protein contains a coiled-coil motif that can mediate dimer or tetramer formation.[92]

A number of other examples of tyrosine kinase fusion proteins have been described in leukemias and lymphomas. The *TEL* gene on chromosome 12 is fused to the PDGF receptor by the t(5;12) translocation associated with a subset of patients with chronic myelomonocytic leukemia (CMML).[93] The *TEL* gene is also fused to the *ABL* gene in a small number of patients with AML or undifferentiated acute leukemia.[94] In the

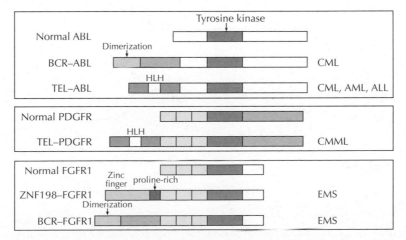

**Figure 5.9** Tyrosine kinase fusion proteins. The BCR–ABL fusion protein contains a tyrosine kinase motif (from ABL) and a coiled-coil dimerization motif (from BCR). In the TEL–ABL and TEL–PDGFR fusion proteins, the TEL helix–loop–helix (HLH) motif provides a dimerization domain. CML, chronic myeloid leukemia; AML, acute myeloid leukemia; ALL, acute lymphoblastic leukemia; CMML, chronic myelomonocytic leukemia; EMS, 8p11 myeloproliferative syndrome. Adapted from Sawyers.[157]

8p11 myeloproliferative syndrome (EMS), the fibroblast growth factor receptor 1 (*FGFR1*) gene is fused to one of a number of partners, including *ZNF198*, *CEP110*, *FOP*, and *BCR*, following various translocations involving chromosome 8.[95]

Comparison of the structures of these different tyrosine kinase fusion genes suggests some common principles (Figure 5.10a). All are potentially linked to the RAS pathway: TEL–PDGFR and the FGFR1 fusions by a GRB-2-binding site in the PDGFR portion; TEL–ABL by CRKL-binding sites in the ABL portion; and BCR–ABL by both GRB-2 and CRKL motifs. All contain oligomerization motifs: BCR–ABL and FGFR1–BCR contain the coiled-coil motif in their BCR portions; FGFR1–ZNF198 contains a proline-rich domain; and TEL–PDFGR and TEL–ABL contain a helix–loop–helix protein interaction domain in the TEL portion of the fusion protein. In the latter two cases, a transcription factor gene (*TEL*) is involved, but it merely contributes a protein-dimerization domain to the resultant fusion protein, which does not appear to function as a transcription factor itself.

Finally, downstream components of the RAS pathway have also been implicated in hematological malignancies. Activating mutations in *RAS* genes are found in numerous tumors, including myelodysplastic syndromes (MDS) and AML.[96–98] RAS activity is normally regulated by a molecule called GAP (GTPase activating protein), which returns the activated RAS to an inactive form (Figure 5.10b). Neurofibromatosis type 1 is an inherited condition in which a GAP molecule termed NF-1 is inactive. Intriguingly, children with neurofibromatosis type 1 have an increased risk of developing MDS, particularly juvenile myelomonocytic leukemia (JMML), and the wild-type *NF-1* allele is frequently deleted in the malignant bone marrow cells.[99–101] Mutations in both *RAS* and *NF-1* are not seen in the same tumor, suggesting that they represent alternative ways of activating the same pathway. A causal role for *NF-1* mutations is strongly suggested by the observation that mice lacking NF-1 protein develop a disease closely resembling JMML.[101,102]

## Genes influencing chromatin structure may be targets for leukemogenic rearrangements

Two lines of evidence suggest that proteins that regulate chromatin structure may also be targets for leukemogenic rearrangement. The *MLL* gene (also

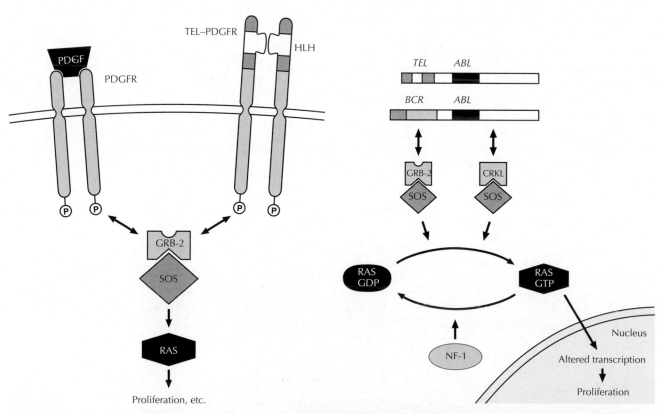

**Figure 5.10** Aberrant activation of the RAS pathway. (a) PDGF induces receptor dimerization and phosphorylation. Subsequent binding of the adaptor protein GRB-2 results in activation of SOS and stimulation of RAS. The TEL helix–loop–helix (HLH) domain results in analogous dimerization, with subsequent activation of the RAS pathway. (b) BCR and TEL contribute a dimerization domain to their respective fusion proteins. Subsequent binding of adaptor proteins (GRB-2 and CRKL) results in activation of SOS, which in turn mediates activation of RAS. Conversion of the active RAS-GTP to the inactive RAS-GDP is regulated by NF-1.

called *HRX* or *ALL-1*) forms a large number of different fusion genes in distinct forms of acute leukemia. Thirty fusion genes have been cloned,[103] all involving different partner genes, and cytogenetic data predict the existence of several more. The subtype of leukemia correlates with the particular MLL fusion protein. Thus, t(4;11) is found in ALL and acute undifferentiated leukemia, whereas t(9;11) is found mainly in AML.

The *MLL* gene encodes a large protein with homology to the *Drosophila Trithorax* family of genes. Like its *Drosophila* homologs, the *MLL* gene regulates genes encoding homeobox transcription factors, and is crucial for determining body structures during development. It is thought to act by creating regions of active chromatin, thus permitting gene transcription in that locality. The molecular basis of the leukemogenic effect of MLL fusion proteins is not yet clear. It seems likely that they interfere with the normal regulation of chromatin structures at specific regions of the genome. Perhaps different fusion partners influence which precise regions are affected, and hence the phenotype of the resultant leukemia.

The second line of evidence comes from murine experimental systems. The *BMI* gene was identified as an oncogene that cooperates with *MYC* in the generation of murine B-cell tumors.[104,105] Proviral insertions adjacent to the *BMI* gene upregulated *BMI* expression and accelerated the formation of B-cell tumors. The *BMI* gene is homologous with the *Polycomb* gene family. Whilst no examples of human leukemias with *BMI* rearrangements have been reported to date, the *BMI* gene has been mapped to human chromosome location 10p13, a region involved in translocations and rearrangements in infant leukemias and T-cell lymphomas.[106]

Genes regulating chromatin structure are likely to have a particularly powerful effect on cellular transcription programs, since they exert a dominant effect on the transcriptional activity of large numbers of target genes. Therefore, rearrangements involving such genes might be particularly leukemogenic. However, it is also possible that such rearrangements might be too potent and result in the death of the host cell.

## Therapeutic significance

The clinical relevance of all this apparently arcane detail is considerable. PCR-based and fluorescence in situ hybridization (FISH)-based technologies already allow us to detect many of the molecular abnormalities. This in turn provides more accurate diagnostic and prognostic information. It seems highly likely that therapy will be more and more individualized as it becomes tailored to reflect the molecular profile exhibited by individual leukemias. The same molecular techniques are also permitting quantitation and monitoring of residual disease, with major implications for autografting as well as the early treatment of relapse.

Above all, treatments tailored to the molecular basis of a given leukemia are fast becoming a reality. Two current examples are the use of ATRA in APL (see above, and Chapter 39 on APL) and the specific BCR–ABL kinase inhibitor imatinib (STI571, Gleevec/Glivec) in CML.[107,108] With the description of large numbers of molecular defects and the likelihood that many more will be described over the next few years, we shall have a wide range of potential therapeutic targets. Of these, the fusion proteins are particularly attractive in view of their tumor specificity. However, two important hurdles remain to be overcome. Transcription factors and many other leukemia oncoproteins are nuclear or cytoplasmic proteins, and so access to these targets is difficult. Second, not all molecular changes will prove useful therapeutic targets. Leukemia is likely to involve several sequential genetic events, some of which may no longer be required for the continued growth of leukemia cells. It will therefore be important to identify and concentrate on those genetic changes that are still necessary for tumor growth.

## REFERENCES

1. Dzierzak E, Medvinsky A. Mouse embryonic hematopoiesis. *Trends Genet* 1995; **11**: 359–66.

2. Medvinsky A, Dzierzak E. Definitive hematopoiesis is autonomously initiated by the AGM region. *Cell* 1996; **86**: 897–906.

3. Metcalf D. Hematopoietic regulators: redundancy or subtlety? *Blood* 1993; **82**: 3515–23.

4. Fairbairn LJ, Cowling BJ, Reipert BM et al. Suppression of apoptosis allows differentiation and development of a multipotent haemopoietic cell line in the absence of added growth factors. *Cell* 1993; **74**: 823–32.

5. Socolovsky M, Lodish HF, Daley GQ. Control of hematopoietic differentiation: lack of specificity in signalling by cytokine receptors. *Proc Natl Acad Sci USA* 1998; **95**: 6573–5.

6. Stoffel R, Ziegler S, Ghilardi N et al. Permissive role of thrombopoietin and granulocyte coloystimulating factor receptors in hematopoietic cell fate decisions in vivo. *Proc Natl Acad Sci USA* 1999; **96**: 698–702.

7. Orkin SH. Transcription factors and hematopoietic development. *J Biol Chem* 1995; **270**: 4955–8.

8. Walters M, Martin DIK. Functional erythroid promoters created by interaction of the transcription factor GATA-1 with CACCC and AP-1/NFE-2 elements. *Proc Natl Acad USA* 1992; **89**: 10444–8.

9. Wadman IA, Osada H, Grutz GG et al. The LIM-only pro-

tein Lmo2 is a bridging molecule assembling an erythroid, DNA-binding complex which includes the TAL1, E47, GATA-1 and Ldb1/NL1 proteins. *EMBO J* 1997; **16**: 3145–57.

10. Lecuyer E, Herblot S, Saint-Denis M et al. The SCL complex regulates c-*kit* expression in hematopoietic cells through functional interaction with Sp1. *Blood* 2002; **100**: 2430–40.

11. Shivdasani RA, Orkin SH. The transcriptional control of hematopoiesis. *Blood* 1996; **87**: 4025–39.

12. Green AR, De Luca E, Begley CG. Antisense *SCL* suppresses self-renewal and enhances spontaneous erythroid differentiation of the human leukaemic cell line K562. *EMBO J* 1991; **10**: 4153–8.

13. Green AR, Salvaris E, Begley CG. Erythroid expression of the 'helix–loop–helix' gene, *SCL*. *Oncogene* 1991; **6**: 475–9.

14. Aplan PD, Nakahra K, Orkin SH et al. The *SCL* gene product: a positive regulator of erythroid differentiation. *EMBO J* 1992; **11**: 4073–81.

15. Shivdasani RA, Mayer EL, Orkin SH. Absence of blood formation in mice lacking T-cell leukaemia oncoprotein tal-1/SCL. *Nature* 1995; **373**: 432–4.

16. Robb L, Lyons I, Li R et al. Absence of yolk sac hematopoiesis from mice with a targeted disruption of the *scl* gene. *Proc Natl Acad Sci USA* 1995; **92**: 7075–9.

17. Robb L, Elwood NJ, Elefanty AG et al. The *T SCL* gene product is required for the generation of all hematopoietic lineages in the adult mouse. *EMBO J* 1996; **15**: 4123–9.

18. Porcher C, Swat W, Rockwell K et al. The T cell leukaemia oncoprotein SCL/tal-1 is essential for development of all hematopoietic lineages. *Cell* 1996; **86**: 47–57.

19. Miyoshi H, Shimizu K, Kozu T. t(8;21) breakpoints on chromosome 21 in acute myeloid leukaemia are clustered within a limited region of a single gene, *AML1*. *Proc Natl Acad Sci USA* 1991; **88**: 10431–4.

20. Wang Q, Stacy T, Binder M et al. Disruption of the *Cbfa2* gene causes necrosis and hemorrhaging in the central nervous system and blocks definitive hematopoiesis. *Proc Natl Acad Sci USA* 1996; **93**: 3444–9.

21. Okuda T, van Deursen J, Hiebert SW et al. *AML1*, the target of multiple chromosomal translocations in human leukaemia, is essential for normal fetal liver hematopoiesis. *Cell* 1996; **84**: 321–30.

22. Warren AJ, Colledge WH, Carlton MB et al. The oncogenic cysteine-rich LIM domain protein Rbtn2 is essential for erythroid development. *Cell* 1994; **78**: 45–57.

23. Yamada Y, Warren AJ, Dobson C et al. The T cell leukaemia LIM protein Lmo2 is necessary for adult mouse hematopoieses. *Proc Natl Acad Sci USA* 1998; **95**: 3890–5.

24. Tsai F-Y, Keller G, Kuo FC et al. An early haemopoietic defect in mice lacking the transcription factor GATA-2. *Nature* 1994; **371**: 221–6.

25. Weiss MJ, Keller G, Orkin SH. Novel insights into erythroid development revealed through in vitro differentiation of GATA-1 embryonic stem cells. *Genes Dev* 1994; **8**: 1184–97.

26. Simon MC, Pevny L, Wiles MV et al. Rescue of erythroid development in gene targeted GATA-1-mouse embryonic stem-cells. *Nat Genet* 1992; **1**: 92–8.

27. Pevny L, Simon MC, Robertson E et al. Erythroid differentiation in chimeric mice blocked by a targeted mutation in the gene for the GATA-1 transcription factor. *Nature* 1991; **349**: 257–60.

28. Shivdasani RA, Rosenblatt MF, Zucker-Franklin D et al. Transcription factor NF-E2 is required for platelet formation independent of the actions of thrombopoietin/MGDF in megakaryocyte development. *Cell* 1995; **81**: 695–704.

29. Grigoriadis AE, Wang Z-Q, Cecchini MG et al. c-Fos: a key regulator of osteoclast–macrophage lineage determination and bond remodelling. *Science* 1994; **266**: 443–8.

30. Corcoran LM, Karvelas M, Nossal GJV et al. Oct-2, although not required for early B-cell development, is critical for later B-cell maturation and for postnatal survival. *Genes Dev* 1993; **7**: 1598.

31. Verbeek S, Izon D, Jofhuis F et al. An HMG-box-containing T-cell factor required for thymocyte differentiation. *Nature* 1995; **374**: 70–4.

32. Scott EW, Simon MC, Anastasi J et al. Requirement of transcription factor PU-1 in the development of multiple hematopoietic lineages. *Science* 1994; **265**: 1573–7.

33. McKercher SR, Torbett BE, Anderson KL et al. Targeted disruption of the *PU.1* gene results in multiple hematopoietic abnormalities. *EMBO J* 1996; **15**: 5647–58.

34. Lewin B. Chromatin and gene expression: constant questions, but changing answers. *Cell* 1994; **79**: 397–406.

35. Felsenfeld G, Boyes J, Chung J et al. Chromatin structure and gene expression. *Proc Natl Acad Sci USA* 1996; **93**: 9384–8.

36. Jenuwein T, Allis CD. Translating the histone code. *Science* 2001; **293**: 1074–80.

37. Kennison JA. The polycomb and trithorax group proteins of *Drosophila*: *trans*-regulators of homeotic gene function. *Annu Rev Genet* 1995; **29**: 289–303.

38. Orlando V, Paro R. Chromatin multiprotein complexes involved in the maintenance of transcription patterns. *Curr Opin Genet Dev* 1995; **5**: 174–9.

39. Spotswood HT, Turner BM. An increasingly complex code. *J Clin Invest* 2002; **110**: 577–82.

40. Covault J, Chalkley R. The identification of distinct populations of acetylated histone. *J Biol Chem* 1980; **255**: 9110–16.

41. Gregory RI, O'Neill LP, Randall TE et al. Inhibition of histone deacetylases alters allelic chromatin conformation at the imprinted Uaf1–rs1 locus in mouse embryonic stem cells. *J Biol Chem* 2002; **277**: 11728–34.

42. Visvader JE, Elefanty AG, Strasser A et al. GATA-1 but not SCL induces megakaryocytic differentiation in any early myeloid line. *EMBO J* 1992; **11**: 4557–64.

43. Shivdasani RA, Fujiwara Y, McDevitt MA et al. A lineage-selective knockout establishes the critical role of transcription factor GATA-1 in megakaryocyte growth and platelet development. *EMBO J* 1997; **16**: 3965–73.

44. Kulessa H, Frampton J, Graf T. GATA-1 reprograms avian myelomonoytic cell lines into eosinophils, thromboblasts, and erythroblasts. *Genes Dev* 1995; **9**: 1250–62.

45. Sieweke MH, Tekotte H, Frampton J et al. MafB is an interaction partner and repressor of Ets-1 that inhibits erythroid differentiation. *Cell* 1996; **85**: 49–60.

46. Orkin SH, Diversification of haematopoietic stem cells to specific lineages. *Nat Rev Genet* 2001; **1**: 57–64.

47. Rolink AG, Nutt SL, Melchers F et al. Long-term in vivo reconstitution of T-cell development by Pax5-deficient B-cell progenitors. *Nature* 1999; **401**: 603–6.

48. Nutt SL, Heavey B, Rolink AG et al. Commitment to the B-lymphoid lineage depends on the transcription factor Pax5. *Nature* 1999; **401**: 556–62.

49. Graf T. Differentiation plasticity of hematopoietic cells. *Blood* 2002; **99**: 3089–101.

50. Lemischka I. A few thoughts about the plasticity of stem cells. *Exp Hematol* 2002; **30**: 848–52.

51. Mitelman F, Mertens F, Johansson B. A breakpoint map of recurrent chromosomal rearrangements in human neoplasia. *Nat Genet* 1997; **15**: 417–74.

52. Mehrotra B, George TI, Kavanau K et al. Cytogenetically aberrant cells in the stem cell compartment (CD341lin2) in acute myeloid leukaemia. *Blood* 1995; **86**: 1139–47.

53. Haase D. Evidence for malignant transformation in acute myeloid leukaemia at the level of early hematopoietic stem cells by cytogenetic analysis of CD341 subpopulations. *Blood* 1995; **86**: 2906–12.

54. Bonnet D, Dick JE. Human acute myeloid leukaemia is organised as a hierarchy that originates from a primitive hematopoietic cell. *Nat Med* 1997; **3**: 730–7.

55. Rabbitts TH. Chromosomal translocations in human cancer. *Nature* 1994; **372**: 143–9.

56. Bash RO, Hall S, Timmons CF et al. Does activation of the *TAL1* gene occure in a majority of patients with T cell acute lymphoblastic leukaemia? A Pediatric Oncology Group study. *Blood* 1995; **86**: 666–76.

57. Kelliher MA, Seldin DC, Leder P. *Tal-1* induces T cell acute lymphoblastic leukaemia accelerated by casein kinase II α. *EMBO J* 1996; **15**: 5160–6.

58. Larson RC, Lavenir I, Larson TA et al. Protein dimerization between Lmo2 (Rbtn2) and Tal1 alters thymocyte development and potentiates T cell tumorigenesis in transgenic mice. *EMBO J* 1996; **15**: 1021–7.

59. Aplan PD, Jones CA, Chervinsky DS et al. An *scl* gene product lacking the transactivation domain induces bony abnormalities and cooperates with LMO1 to generate T-cell malignancies in transgenic mice. *EMBO J* 1997; **16**: 2408–19.

60. Green T. Hematopoiesis: master regulator unmasked. *Nature* 1996; **383**: 575–7.

61. Leroy-Viard K, Vinit M-A, Lecointe N et al. Loss of TAL-1 protein activity induces premature apoptosis of Jurkat leukemic T cells upon medium depletion. *EMBO J* 1995; **14**: 2341–9.

62. Speck NA, Gilliland DG. Core-binding factors in haematopoiesis and leukaemia. *Nat Rev Cancer* 2002; **2**: 502–13.

63. Ogawa E, Inuzuka M, Maruyama M et al. Molecular cloning and characterization of PEBP2β, the heterodimeric partner of a novel *Drosophila* Runt-related DNA binding protein PEBP2α. *Virology* 1993; **194**: 314–31.

64. Wang S, Wang Q, Crute BE et al. Cloning and characterization of subunits of the T-cell receptor and murine leukaemia virus enhancer core-binding factor. *Mol Cell Biol* 1993; **13**: 3324–39.

65. Li LH, Gergen JP. Differential interactions between Brother proteins and Runt domain proteins in the *Drosophila* embryo and eye. *Development* 1999; **126**: 3313–22.

66. Sakuma T, Li QL, Jin Y et al. Cloning and expression pattern of a novel PEBP2β-binding protein (charged amino acid rich leucine zipper-1[Crl-1]) in the mouse. *Mech Dev* 2001; **104**: 151–4.

67. Sasaki K, Yagi H, Bronson, RT et al. Absence of fetal liver hematopoiesis in mice deficient in transcriptional coactivator core binding factor β. *Proc Natl Acad Sci USA* 1996; **93**: 12359–63.

68. Wang Q, Stacy T, Miller JD et al. The CBFβ subunit is essential for CBFα2 (AML1) function in vivo. *Cell* 1996; **87**: 697–708.

69. Okuda T, Cai Z, Yang S et al. Expression of a knocked-in *AML1–ETO* leukaemia gene inhibits the establishment of normal definitive hematopoiesis and directly generates dysplastic hematopoietic progenitors. *Blood* 1998; **91**: 3134–43.

70. Yergeau DA, Hetherington CJ, Wang Q et al. Embryonic lethality and impairment of haematopoiesis in mice heterozygous for an *AML1–ETO* fusion gene. *Nat Genet* 1997; **15**: 303–6.

71. Castilla LH, Wijmenga C, Wang Q et al. Failure of embryonic hematopoiesis and lethal hemorrhages in mouse embryos heterozygous for a knocked-in leukaemia gene *CBFB–MYH11*. *Cell* 1996; **87**: 687–96.

72. Gelmetti V, Zhang J, Fanelli M et al. Aberrant recruitment of the nuclear receptor corepressor–histone deacetylase complex by the acute myeloid leukaemia fusion partner ETO. *Mol Cell Biol* 1998; **18**: 7185–91.

73. Lutterback B, Westendorf JJ, Linggi B et al. ETO, a target of t(8;21) in acute leukaemia interacts with the N-CoR and mSin3 corepressors. *Mol Cell Biol* 1998; **18**: 7176–84.

74. Fenrick R, Amann JM, Lutterback B et al. Both TEL and AML-1 contribute repression domains to the t(12;21) fusion protein. *Mol Cell Biol* 1999; **19**: 6566–74.

75. Scott LM, Civin CI, Rorth P et al. A novel temporal expression pattern of three C/EBP family members in differentiating myelomonocytic cells. *Blood* 1992; **80**: 1725–35.

76. Tenen DG. Abnormalities of the CEBPα transcription factor: a major target in acute myeloid leukaemia. *Leukaemia* 2001; **15**: 688–9.

77. Radomska HS, Huettner CS, Zhang P et al. CCAAT/enhancer binding protein α is a regulatory switch sufficient for induction of granulocytic development from bipotential myeloid progenitors. *Mol Cell Biol* 1998; **18**: 4301–14.

78. Zhang DE, Zhang P, Wang ND et al. Absence of granulocyte colony-stimulating factor signalling and neutrophil development in CCAAT enhancer binding protein α-deficient mice. *Proc Natl Acad Sci USA* 1997; **94**: 569–74.

79. Zhang P, Nelson E, Radomska HS et al. Induction of granulocytic differentiation by two pathways. *Blood* 2002; **99**: 4406–12.

80. Pabst T, Mueller BU, Zhang P et al. Dominant-negative mutations of CEBPA, encoding CCAAT/enhancer binding protein-α (C/EBPα), in acute myeloid leukemia. *Nat Genet* 2001; **27**: 263–70.

81. Zhang P, Iwama A, Datta MW et al. Upregulation of interleukin 6 and granulocyte colony-stimulating factor receptors by transcription factor CCAAT enhancer binding protein α (C/EBPα) is critical for granulopoiesis. *J Exp Med* 1998; **188**: 1173–84.

82. Pabst T, Mueller BU, Harakawa N et al. AML1–ETO downregulates the granulocytic differentiation factor C/EBPα in t(8;21) myeloid leukemia. *Nat Med* 2001; **7**: 444–51.

83. Nowell PC, Hungerford DA. A minute chromosome in human chronic granulocytic leukemia. *Science* 1960; **132**: 1497–500.

84. Rowley JD. A new consistent chromosomal abnormality in chronic myelogenous leukaemia identified by quinacrine fluorescence and Giemsa staining. *Nature* 1973; **243**: 290–3.

85. Melo JV. The diversity of BCR–ABL fusion proteins and

their relationship to leukemia phenotype. *Blood* 1996; **88**: 2375–84.

86. Davis RL, Konopka JB, Witte ON. Activation of the c-*abl* oncogene by viral transduction or chromosomal translocation generates altered c-Abl proteins with similar in vitro kinase properties. *Mol Cell Biol* 1985; **5**: 204–13.

87. Prendergast AM, Quilliam LA, Cripe LD. BCR–ABL-induced oncogenesis is mediated by direct interaction with the SH2 domain of the GRB-2 adaptor protein. *Cell* 1993; **75**: 175–85.

88. Senechal K, Halpern J, Sawyers CL. The CRKL adaptor protein transforms fibroblasts and functions in transformation by the *Bcr–Abl* oncogene. *J Biol Chem* 1996; **271**: 23255–61.

89. Schlessinger J. SH2/SH3 signaling proteins. *Curr Opin Genet Dev* 1994; **4**: 25–30.

90. Taniguchi T. Cytokine signaling through nonreceptor protein tyrosine kinases. *Science* 1995; **268**: 251–5.

91. Ihle JN, Kerr LM. JAKs and STATs in signaling by the cytokine receptor superfamily. *Trends Genet* 1995; **11**: 69–74.

92. McWhirter JR, Galasso DL, Wang YL. A coiled-coil oligomerization domain of Bcr is essential for the transforming function of Bcr–Abl oncoproteins. *Mol Cell Biol* 1993; **13**: 7587–95.

93. Golub TR, Barker GF, Lovett M et al. Fusion of PDGF receptor β to a novel *ets*-like gene, *tel*, in chronic myelomonocytic leukemia with t(5;12) chromosomal translocation. *Cell* 1994; **77**: 307–16.

94. Papadopoulous P, Ridge SA, Boucher CA et al. The novel activation of *ABL* by fusion to an *ets*-related gene, *TEL*. *Cancer* 1995; **55**: 34–8.

95. Cross NC, Reiter A. Tyrosine kinase fusion genes in chronic myeloproliferative diseases. *Leukemia* 2002; **16**: 1207–12.

96. Bos JL, Verlaan-de Vries M, Van der Eb AJ et al. Mutations in N-*ras* predominate in acute myeloid leukemia. *Blood* 1987; **69**: 1237–41.

97. Lyons J, Janssen JWG, Bartram CR et al. Mutation of Ki-*ras* and N-*ras* oncogenes in myelodysplastic syndromes. *Blood* 1988; **71**: 1707–12.

98. Janssen JWG, Steenvoorden ACM, Lyons J et al. *ras* gene mutations in acute and chronic myelocytic leukemias, chronic myeloproliferative disorders and myelodysplastic syndromes. *Proc Natl Acad Sci USA* 1987; **84**: 9228–32.

99. Shannon KM, O'Connell P, Martin GA et al. Loss of the normal *NF1* allele from the bone marrow of children with type 1 neurofibromatosis and malignant myeloid disorders. *N Engl J Med* 1994; **330**: 597–601.

100. Arico M, Biondi A, Pui C-H. Juvenile myelomonocytic leukemia. *J Am Soc Hematol* 1997; **90**: 479–88.

101. Bollag G, Clapp DW, Shih S et al. Loss of *NF1* results in activation of the Ras signaling pathway and leads to aberrant growth in haematopoietic cells. *Nat Genet* 1996; **12**: 144–8.

102. Largaespada DA, Brannan CL, Jenkins NA et al. Nf1 deficiency causes Ras-mediated granulocyte–macrophage colony stimulating factor hypersensitivity and chronic myeloid leukaemia. *Nat Genet* 1996; **12**: 137–43.

103. Ayton PM, Cleary ML. Molecular mechanisms of leukemogenesis mediated by MLL fusion proteins. *Oncogene* 2001; **20**: 5695–707.

104. Haupt Y, Alexander WS, Barri G et al. Novel zinc finger gene implicated as *myc* collaborator by retrovirally accelerated lymphomagenesis in Eμ-*myc* transgenic mice. *Cell* 1991; **65**: p. 753–63.

105. van Lohuizen M, Frasch M, Wientjens E et al. Sequence similarity between the mammalian *bmi-1* proto-oncogene and the *Drosophila* regulatory genes *Psc* and *Su(z)2*. *Nature* 1991; **353**: 353–5.

106. Bea S, Tort F, Pinyol M et al. *BMI-1* gene amplification and overexpression in hematological malignancies occur mainly in mantle cell lymphomas. *Cancer Res* 2001; **61**: 2409–12.

107. Druker BJ, Talpaz M, Resta DJ et al. Efficacy and safety of a specific inhibitor of the BCR–ABL tyrosine kinase in chronic myeloid leukemia. *N Engl J Med* 2001; **344**: 1031–7.

108. Druker BJ, Tamura S, Buchdunger E et al. Effects of a selective inhibitor of the Abl tyrosine kinase on the growth of Bcr–Abl positive cells. *Nat Med* 1996; **2**: 561–6.

109. Crossley M, Orkin SH. Regulation of the β-globin locus. *Curr Opin Genet Dev* 1993; **3**: 2327.

110. Lemarchandel V, Ghysdael J, Mignotta V et al. GATA and Ets *cis*-acting sequences mediate megakaryocyte specific expression. *Mol Cell Biol* 1993; **13**: 668–76.

111. Liao Y, Yi T, Hoit BD et al. Selective reporter expression in mast cells using a chymase promoter. *J Biol Chem* 1997; **272**: 2969–76.

112. Klemsz MJ, McKercher SR, Celada A et al. The macrophage and B cell-specific transcription factor PU-1 is related to the *ets* oncogene. *Cell* 1990; **61**: 113–24.

113. Katz S, Kowenz LE, Muller C et al. The NF-M transcription factor is related to C/EBP β and plays a role in signal transduction, differentiation and leukemogenesis of avian myelomonocytic cells. *EMBO J* 1993; **12**: 1321–32.

114. Georgopoulos K, Moore DD, Defler B. Ikaros, an early lymphoid-specific transcription factor and a putative mediator for T cell commitment. *Science* 1992; **258**: 808–12.

115. Clerc RG, Corcoran LM, LeBowitz JH et al. B-cell-specific-Oct-2 protein contains POU box- and homeo box-type domains. *Genes Dev* 1988; **2**: 1570–81.

116. Sturm RA, Das G, Herr W. The ubiquitous octamer-binding protein Oct-1 contains a POU domain with a homeo box subdomain. *Genes Dev* 1988; **2**: 1582–99.

117. Murre C, McCaw PS, Baltimore D. A new DNA binding and dimerization motif in immunoglobulin enhancer binding, daughterless, MyoD and myc proteins. *Cell* 1989; **56**: 777–83.

118. Oosterwegel M, van de Wetering M, Dooijes D et al. Cloning of murine TCF-1, a T cell-specific transcription factor interacting with functional motifs in the CD3-ε and T cell receptor α enhancers. *J Exp Med* 1991; **173**: 1133–42.

119. Travis A, Amsterdam A, Belanger C et al. *LEF-1*, a gene encoding a lymphoid-specific protein with an HMG domain, regulates T-cell receptor α enhancer function. *Genes Dev* 1991; **5**: 880–94.

120. Erickson P, Gao J, Chang K-S. Identification of breakpoints in t(8;21) AML and isolation of a fusion transcript with similarity to *Drosophila* segmentation gene *runt*. *Blood* 1992; **80**: 1825–31.

121. Miyoshi H, Shimizu K, Kozu T. The t(8;21) breakpoints in chromosome 21 in acute myeloid leukemia clustered within a limited region of a novel gene. *Proc Natl Acad Sci USA* 1993; **88**: 10431–5.

122. Nucifora G, Begy CR, Kobayashi H et al. Consistent inter-

genic splicing and production of multiple transcripts between *AML1* at 21q22 and unrelated genes at 3q26 in (3;21)(q26;q22) translocations. *Proc Natl Acad Sci USA* 1994; **91**: 4004–8.

123. Mitan K, Ogawa S, Tanaka T et al. Generation of *AML1/EVI1* fusion gene in the t(3;21)(q26;q22) causes blastic crisis in chronic myelocytic leukemia. *EMBO J* 1994; **13**: 504–10.

124. Begley CG, Aplan PD, Denning SM et al. The gene, *SCL*, is expressed during early hematopoiesis and encodes a differentiation-related DNA-binding motif. *Proc Natl Acad Sci USA* 1989; **86**: 10128–32.

125. Chen Q, Cheng JT, Tsai LH et al. The *tal* gene undergoes chromosome translocation in T cell leukemia and potentially encodes a helix–loop–helix protein. *EMBO J* 1990; **9**: 415–24.

126. Bernard O, Guglielmi P, Jonveaux P et al. Two distinct mechanisms for the *SCL* gene activation in the t(1;14) translocation of T-cell leukemias. *Genes Chromosomes Cancer* 1990; **1**: 194–208.

127. Fitzgerald TJ, Geoffrey AM, Neale SC et al. c-tal, a helix–loop–helix protein, is juxtaposed to the T-cell receptor-β chain gene by a reciprocal chromosomal translocation: t(1;7)(p32;q35). *Blood* 1991; **78**: 2686–95.

128. Aplan PD, Raimondi SC, Kirsch IR. Disruption of the *SCL* gene by a t(1;3) translocation in a patient with T cell acute lymphoblastic leukemia. *J Exp Med* 1992; **176**: 1303–10.

129. Xia Y, Brown L, Yang CY-C et al. *TAL-2*, a helix–loop–helix gene activated by the (7;9)(q34;q32) translocation in human T cell leukemia. *Proc Natl Acad Sci USA* 1991; **88**: 11416–20.

130. Mellentin JD, Smith SD, Cleary ML. *Lyl-1*, a novel gene altered by chromosomal translocation in T cell leukemia, codes for a protein with a helix–loop–helix DNA binding motif. *Cell* 1989; **58**: 77–83.

131. Boehm T, Baer R, Lavenir L et al. The mechanism of chromosomal translocation t(11;14) involving the T-cell receptor δ locus on human chromosome 14q11 and a transcribed region of chromosome 11p15. *EMBO J* 1988; **7**: 385–94.

132. McGuire EA, Hockett RD, Pollock KM et al. The t(11;14)(p15;q11) in a T-cell acute lymphoblastic leukemia cell line activates multiple transcripts including *TTG-1*, a gene encoding a potential zinc finger. *Mol Cell Biol* 1989; **9**: 2124–32.

133. Boehm T, Foroni L, Kaneko Y et al. The rhombotin family of cysteine-rich LIM-domain oncogenes: distinct members are involved in T-cell translocations to human chromosomes 11p15 and 11p13. *Proc Natl Acad Sci USA* 1991; **88**: 4367–71.

134. Royer-Pokora B, Loos U, Ludwig W-D. *TTG-2*, a new gene encoding a cysteine-rich protein with the LIM motif, is overexpressed in acute T cell leukaemia with the (11;14)(p13;q11). *Oncogene* 1991; **6**: 1887–93.

135. Dube LD, Kanel-Reid S, Yuan CC et al. A novel human homeobox gene lies at the chromosome 10 breakpoint in lymphoid neoplasias with chromosomal translocation t(10;14). *Blood* 1991; **78**: 2996–3003.

136. Hatano M, Roberts CWM, Minden M et al. Deregulation of a homeobox gene, *HOX 11*, by the t(10/14) in T cell leukemia. *Science* 1991; **253**: 79–82.

137. Lu M, Gong Z, Sher W et al. The *tcl-3* proto-oncogene altered by chromosomal translocation in T-cell leukemia codes for a homeobox protein. *EMBO J* 1991; **10**: 2905–10.

138. Kennedy MA, Gonzalez-Sarmiento R, Kees UR et al. *Hox 11*, a homeobox-containing T-cell oncogene on human chromosome 10q24. *Proc Natl Acad Sci USA* 1991; **88**: 8900–4.

139. Spencer CA, Groudine M. Control of c-*myc* regulation in normal and neoplastic cells. *Adv Cancer Res* 1991; **56**: 1–48.

140. Kamps MP, Murre C, Sun XHB et al. A new homeobox gene contributes the DNA binding domain of the t(1;19) translocation protein in pre-B ALL. *Cell* 1990; **60**: 547–55.

141. Nourse J, Mellentin JD, Galili N et al. Chromosomal translocation t(1;19) results in synthesis of a homeobox fusion mRNA that codes for a potential chimeric transcription factor. *Cell* 1990; **60**: 535–45.

142. Inaba T, Roberts WM, Shapiro LH et al. Fusion of the leucine zipper gene *HLF* to the *E2A* gene in human acute B-lineage leukemia. *Science* 1992; **257**: 531–4.

143. Hunger SP, Ohyashiki K, Toyama K et al. Hlf, a novel hepatic bZIP protein, shows altered DNA-binding properties following fusion to E2A in t(17;19) acute lymphoblastic leukemia. *Genes Dev* 1992; **6**: 1608–20.

144. Golub TR, Barker GF, Bohlander SK et al. Fusion of the *TEL* gene on 12p13 to the *AML1* gene on 21q22 in acute lymphoblastic leukemia. *Proc Natl Acad Sci USA* 1995; **92**: 4917–21.

145. Romana SP, Poirel H, Leconiat M et al. High frequency of t(12;21) in childhood B-lineage acute lymphoblastic leukemia. *Blood* 1995; **86**: 4263–9.

146. Neri A, Chang C, Lombardi L et al. B cell lymphoma-associated chromosomal translocation involves candidate oncogene *Lyt-10*, homologous to *NF-kB p50*. *Cell* 1991; **67**: 1075–87.

147. Kluin PM, *bcl-6* in lymphoma – Sorting out a wastebasket? *N Engl J Med* 1994; **331**: 116–19.

148. de Thé H, Lavau C, Marchio A et al. The *PML–RARα* fusion mRNA generated by the t(15;17) translocation in acute promyelocytic leukemia encodes a functionally altered RAR. *Cell* 1991; **66**: 675–84.

149. Kakizuka A, Miller WH, Umesono K et al. Chromosomal translocation t(15;17) in human acute promyelocytic leukemia fuses RARα with a novel putative transcription factor, PML. *Cell* 1991; **66**: 663–74.

150. Chen Z, Brand NJ, Chen A et al. Fusion between a novel Kruppel-like zinc finger gene and the retinoic acid receptor-α locus due to a variant t(11;17) translocation associated with acute promyelocytic leukaemia. *EMBO J* 1993; **12**: 1161–7.

151. Redner RL, Rush EA, Faas S et al. The t(5;17) variant of acute promyelocytic leukaemia expresses a nucleophosmin–retinoic acid receptor fusion. *Blood* 1996; **87**: 882–6.

152. Buijs A, Sherr S, van Baal S et al. Translocation (12;22)(p13;q11) in myeloproliferative disorders results in fusion of the *ETS*-like *TEL* gene on 12p13 to the *MN1* gene on 22q11. *Oncogene* 1995; **10**: 1511–19.

153. Borrow J, Stanton VP, Andresen JM et al. The translocation t(8;16)(p11;p13) of acute myeloid leukaemia fuses a putative acetyltransferase to the CREB-binding protein. *Nat Genet* 1996; **14**: 33–41.

154. Liu P, Tarle SA, Hajra A. Fusion between transcription factor CBFβ/PEBP2β and a myosin heavy chain in acute myeloid leukemia. *Science* 1993; **261**: 1041–4.

155. Canaani E, Nowell PC, Croce CM. Molecular genetics of 11q23 chromosome translocations. *Adv Cancer Res* 1995; **66**: 213–34.

156. Nucifora G, Begy CR, Erickson P et al. The 3;21 transloca-tion in myelodysplasia results in a fusion transcript between the *AML* gene and the gene for EAP, a highly con-served protein associated with the Epstein–Barr virus small RNA EBER 1. *Proc Natl Acad Sci USA* 1993; **90**: 7784–8.

157. Sawyers CL. Molecular genetics of acute leukaemia. *Lancet* 1997; **349**: 196–200.

158. Scandura JM, Boccuni P, Cammenga J et al. Transcription factor fusions in acute leukemia: variations on a theme. *Oncogene* 2002; **21**: 3422–44.

159. Hrusak O, Porwit-MacDonald A. Antigen expression pat-terns reflecting genotype of acute leukemias. *Leukemia* 2002; **16**: 1233–58.

160. Crans HN, Sakamoto KM. Transcription factors and translocations in lymphoid and myeloid leukemia. *Leukemia* 2001; **15**: 313–31.

161. Dyer MJ, Oscier DG. The configuration of the immunoglobulin genes in B cell chronic lymphocytic leukemia. *Leukemia* 2002; **16**: 973–84.

162. Falini B, Mason DY. Proteins encoded by genes involved in chromosomal alterations in lymphoma and leukemia: clinical value of their detection by immunocytochemistry. *Blood* 2002; **99**: 409–26.

163. Cantor AB, Orkin SH. Transcriptional regulation of ery-thropoiesis: an affair involving multiple partners. *Oncogene* 2002; **21**: 3368–76.

164. Dyer MJ, Oscier DG. 'The configuration of the immuno-globulin genes in B cell chronic lymphocytic leukemia'. *Leukemia* 2002; **16**: 973–84.

165. Barr FG. 'Chromosomal translocations involving paired box transcription factors in human cancer.' *Int J Biochem Cell Bid* 1997; **29**: 1449–61.

# 6 Cellular aspects of lymphoid differentiation: B cells

Claudine Schiff and Michel Fougereau

## Introduction

Specific recognition by the immune system, often referred to as self–non-self discrimination, is essentially mediated by B and T lymphocytes, as opposed to innate immunity, basically supported by natural killer (NK) cells. These cells derive from hematopoietic stem cells through discrete differentiation pathways, although both originate in the bone marrow (and in the liver during embryonic and fetal life). T cells mature in the thymus, whereas B cells continue to differentiate in the bone marrow itself. A second feature that distinguishes B and T cells is their distinctive ways of recognizing antigens, due to the different nature of the recognition molecules that are expressed at their surface. B cells express immunoglobulins (Ig) that interact directly with native epitopes, i.e. subregions of the antigen that have a well-defined three-dimensional structure. Surface immunoglobulins are also the recognition module of the B-cell receptor (BCR), analogous to the TCR found on T cells. In contrast to the BCR, TCR do not interact directly with native epitopes, but identify peptides derived from the original antigen as presented by molecules encoded by genes of the major histocompatibility complex (MHC). Cleavage of the protein antigen into peptides is known as the 'antigen processing', and takes place within antigen-presenting cells (APC) before 'presentation' to T cells in association with an MHC molecule at the APC cell surface.

Both B and T cells have to face the repertoire problem, i.e. how to generate an extremely large number of different immunoglobulins and TCR to allow the recognition of an extraordinarily large number of discrete epitopes. A theoretical approach suggests that this number might be as large as $10^{17}$. Since the total number of lymphocytes in a human adult averages $10^{12}$ (roughly divided into one-fifth B cells and four-fifths T cells), and taking their clonal organization into account, the numbers of BCR and/or TCR expressed at a given time appear to be well below this estimate, which implies some basic degeneracy in the immune recognition system. Nevertheless, the number of different structures must still be quite large, which therefore raises the problem of how to generate such a large repertoire with, necessarily, a limited number of genes. This is the main challenge faced by B and T cells, which is achieved during their respective differentiation processes. The second problem that the immune system has to face is the fact that self-recognition should be controlled so that harmful consequences do not occur. This implies that once the repertoire is at hand, it must be appropriately selected. In this chapter, we shall focus on the B-cell compartment, the T-cell case being discussed in Chapter 7.

During fetal life, B lymphocytes differentiate in the liver and then in the bone marrow. After birth, the first steps of B-cell differentiation take place in the bone marrow, which is a primary lymphoid organ, and drive precursors derived from the hematopoietic stem cells to become immature B lymphocytes. This period of differentiation is antigen-independent and is essentially devoted to generate the basic Ig repertoire, which is the result of a complex sequence of events involving multiple gene rearrangements. Immature B lymphocytes migrate to secondary lymphoid organs, namely the spleen, lymph nodes, tonsils, mucosa-associated lymphoid tissues (MALT), and gut-associated lymphoid tissues (GALT), including Peyer's patches. Further differentiation necessitates antigen encounter and a number of complex cellular interactions, among which T–B cooperation plays a major role. A second level of diversity is then generated, which mostly results from somatic mutations, and the final steps of differentiation, including isotype switching, lead to the emergence of plasma cells and memory B cells. Plasma cells secrete Igs in the bloodstream, which are also referred to as circulating antibodies.

## Generation of immature B cells

The early steps of B-cell differentiation take place in the bone marrow, and are antigen-independent.

All differentiation events that drive the emergence of the various lineages (granulocytes, erythrocytes, monocytes, megakaryocytes, lymphocytes, etc.) derive from a common hematopoietic stem cell, which originates in the bone marrow.[1,2] Emergence of the B lineage is initiated from a precursor common to the B, T, and NK lymphocytes.[3] Evidence for this was first based on the phenotype of mutants of the *Ikaros* gene, encoding a transcription factor that is indispensable for the occurrence of the different lineages.[4,5] Further engagement towards the B-cell lineage is driven by sequential expression of several transcription factors, including E2A, EBF, and Pax5.[6] This engagement correlates with the selective inhibition of the pathways leading to pro-NK and pro-T cells, which necessitate the expression of Id2 and Notch1, respectively (Figure 6.1).

The main features of the molecular and cellular events that take place in the bone marrow[7-12] and lead to B-cell commitment are shown in Figure 6.2. The use of various nomenclatures encountered in the literature may be somehow confusing; therefore we shall only consider three major subpopulations defining the B lineage: the pro-B, pre-B, and immature B cells. The successive steps of differentiation proceed towards the center of the bone marrow,[13] and may be followed in several ways:

- acquisition and/or loss of surface antigens (CD markers; see Table 6.1), identified by monoclonal antibodies;
- identification of intracytoplasmic proteins and/or mRNA transcripts;
- analysis of the gene rearrangement status for each of the three Ig loci: H, κ and λ;

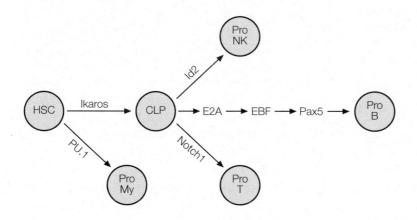

**Figure 6.1** Transcription factors involved in the early stages of lymphopoiesis. The common lymphoid progenitor (CLP) and the common myeloid progenitor (Pro My) are derived from hematopoietic stem cells (HSC). CLP gives rise to progenitors of the different lymphocyte lineages (Pro B, Pro T, and Pro NK). Cooperation of E2A and EBF conditions the engagement of CLP towards the B lineage, which becomes definitively committed upon Pax5 expression.

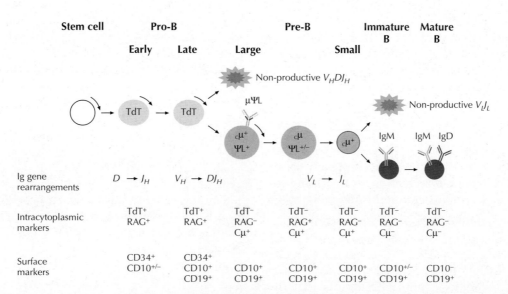

**Figure 6.2** The early steps of B-cell differentiation take place in the bone marrow and are antigen-independent. The main discrete steps that lead from the hematopoietic stem cell to the immature B lymphocyte are identified by the successive Ig gene rearrangements, by the presence of intracytoplasmic markers, and by the expression of characteristic markers at the cell surface. The very early stages that go from the stem cell to the early pro-B cell encompass several precursors that are not completely defined to date. TdT, terminal deoxynucleotidyl transferase, responsible for including N diversity; ΨL, surrogate light chain that combine with the Ig μ chain to form the pre B receptor; RAG, recombination activating genes, which encode for the recombinase enzyme. See Plate 2.

**Table 6.1 Cell surface molecules of central interest expressed at various stages of the B-cell lineage (this is not exhaustive)**

| Molecules | Localization[a] | Function |
|---|---|---|
| BCR | | |
| IgM | Immature B cells | Antigen recognition |
| IgM + IgD | Mature B cells | " |
| IgG | " | " |
| IgA | " | " |
| IgE | " | " |
| Igα/Igβ (CD79a/79b) | | Signaling module |
| Pre-BCR | | |
| μ + ΨL | Pre-B cells | Regulation of early B-cell differentiation Control of allelic exclusion. |
| Igα/Igβ (CD79a/79b) | | Signaling module |
| CD5 | B1 cells | Minor population of B cells Role in autoimmunity? |
| CD10 (CALLA) | Pro-B to immature B cells and GC-B[b] | Neutral endopeptidase |
| CD19 | Pan B | Regulation of activation |
| CD20 | Pre-B and B cells | Regulation of activation? |
| CD21 | T2, mature follicular and marginal zone B cells | C3d/EBV receptor. With CD19 and CD81 forms coreceptor for B cells |
| CD22 | Mature B cells | Adhesion of B cells to monocytes, T cells |
| CD23 | T2, mature follicular B cells | Low-affinity IgE receptor (FcεRIIa), ligand for CD19/CD21/CD81 coreceptor |
| CD24 | Pan B | B-cell growth? |
| CD27 | Memory B cells | ? |
| CD38 | Early B and GC-B[b] | ? |
| CD40 | B cells | B-cell activation. Switch. Binds CD40L |
| CD45 | Hematopoietic cells | PhosphoTyr-phosphatase. Signaling |
| CD77 | GC-B[b] | Apoptosis? |
| CD79a (Igα) | Pre-B and B cells | *mb1* gene-encoded. See above, BCR |
| CD79b (Igβ) | Pre-B and B cells | *B29* gene-encoded. See above, BCR |
| CD138 | Plasma cells | Ligand for collagen type 1 |

[a] Most indicated CDs are also expressed on other cell types. CD19, CD20, CD21, CD22, CD23, and CD24 are mostly expressed on the B lineage, although some of them (CD19, CD21, and CD23) may be expressed on follicular dendritic cells (FDC). CD23 is found on eosinophils, platelets, and other cells. Therefore expression of only one marker is not sufficient to assign a cell a given phenotype.
[b] GC, germinal center.

- localization of blockage points resulting from mutations leading to primary immune deficiency.

**Interaction of B-cell progenitors with stromal cells in the bone marrow**

The first steps of differentiation involve a sequence of direct interactions of the precursors with the stromal cells,[14] ensured by various sets of cellular adhesion molecules (CAMs). The VLA-4 integrin expressed at the cell surface of the precursors interacts with stromal VCAM-1,[15] and the resulting early pro-B cells now express c-Kit,[16] a receptor that binds the stem cell

factor (SCF, Steel factor) of stromal cells. This interaction triggers proliferation of the pro-B cells, which continue to differentiate through other stimuli. Late pro-B cells are stimulated by a soluble growth factor, also from stromal origin, interleukin-7 (IL-7),[17] which drives proliferation of pre-B cells.

As these steps of differentiation proceed, cells are cycling and Ig-gene rearrangements that generate the basic repertoire take place in a sequential fashion. One way to characterize the various populations at each stage of differentiation relies on the identification of a number of CD markers (Figure 6.2, see Plate 2). CD34, which is already expressed in hematopoietic stem cells,[18] remains present at the surface of precursors and pro-B cells. Late pro-B cells can be characterized by the coexpression of CD34 with CD19,[7] which is a very specific marker of the B lineage, as it is found on all subsequent stages, with the exception of plasma cells. CD10, also known as the common acute lymphoblastic leukemia antigen (CALLA), is expressed up to the immature B-cell stage, and seems to be expressed slightly before CD19.[19,20] Other markers are expressed as differentiation proceeds, including CD20, CD21, CD22, CD23, and CD24.

## Development of the basic Ig repertoire in the bone marrow as B cells differentiate

As already stated, the main feature of the early steps of differentiation is the acquisition of the basic repertoire of immunoglobulins, which becomes expressed as surface IgM (sIgM) on immature B cells. Immunoglobulins are symmetrical molecules composed of two heavy (H) chains and two light (L) chains ($\kappa$ or $\lambda$). Depending upon the nature of the H chain, immunoglobulins exist as discrete classes or isotypes, termed IgM, IgG, IgA, IgD, and IgE, corresponding to the $\mu$, $\gamma$, $\alpha$, $\delta$, and $\varepsilon$ heavy chains, respectively. All classes may exist as surface or secreted immunoglobulins. When expressed at the surface of B cells, immunoglobulin molecules are associated with the Ig$\alpha$–Ig$\beta$ heterodimer, encoded by the *mb1* and *B29* genes respectively, to form the so-called B-cell receptor (BCR).[21] Each of the H and L chains has a variable and a constant region. The variable regions of the H and L chains interact in the antibody-combining site, which is responsible for specific antigen recognition. Heavy and light chains are encoded by genes that are localized on three discrete gene clusters, *H*, $\kappa$, and $\lambda$, located on chromosomes 14, 2, and 22, respectively.

The unique feature of the organization of Ig genes is that they must be rearranged before becoming functional.[22] These rearrangements allow the immune system to generate a very large repertoire by recombination and random association of a limited number of gene segments (between 200 and 300 in humans), leading to at least 10 million discrete Igs, thus having different specificities. In the light chains, the variable region results from the random association of *V* and *J* genes. The heavy chains are more complex, since their diversity results from the random association of $V_H$, *D*, and $J_H$ genes. Immunoglobulin genes are rearranged exclusively in the B lineage, and these events constitute the hallmark of B-cell differentiation in the bone marrow.

Ig gene rearrangements necessitate a precise signaling on the DNA, known as 'recombination signal sequences' (RSS), which flank each of the *V*, *D*, and *J* gene segments, and that are recognized by highly specific recombinases encoded by two genes, termed *RAG-1* and *RAG-2*.[23,24] In addition to the RAG proteins, other molecules such as DNA-PKcs and Artemis play a critical role in the ultimate steps of DNA rearrangements, mostly by cleaving and repairing double-stranded DNA elements.[25] The first recombination event, $D_H$ to $J_H$, takes place in early pro-B cells (see Figure 6.2) and is rapidly followed by the rearrangement of one of the $V_H$ segments to $DJ_H$. Another enzyme, terminal deoxynucleotidyl transferase (TdT), is also active in pro-B cells, for which it represents an additional intracytoplasmic marker. This enzyme adds nucleotides in a random fashion, during the joining of *D* to $J_H$, and $V_H$ to $DJ_H$ rearrangements.[26] The addition of these non-germline-encoded nucleotides is known as N-diversity and obviously amplifies the repertoire. Pro-B cells are cycling, and it seems likely that at least some molecules that drive the differentiation are cell cycle-dependent, as is the case for RAG-2.

Pro-B cells that have rearranged the *IGVH* locus must 'make' two decisions. One is to remain 'monoclonal' with respect to H-chain production, the second is to activate the rearrangement of the light-chain genes. Both events are regulated by the $\mu$ chain itself, which must be in its membrane form. Once the first allele of the *IGH* locus has completed the rearrangement process, the resulting gene may be functional or not, depending on whether the recombination has generated a sequence of nucleotides with an open reading frame. Because of the triplet organization of the genetic code, this happens only once every three rearrangements. If the first rearrangement is out of frame, the second allele will recombine, with the same probability of success. A new failure will lead to cell death. Conversely, once a functional gene has been obtained, the resulting heavy chain will exert a negative feedback on a further rearrangement of the *IGH* locus, ensuring 'monoclonal' expression of the $\mu$ chain.[27] The negative feedback presumably results in the turning off of the *TdT* and *RAG* genes.[8]

There is considerable evidence suggesting that the heavy chain must be expressed at the cell surface to regulate these events. Expression of the $\mu$ chain at the cell surface requires that it associate with another partner, which resembles the light chain and is therefore termed the $\Psi$L or surrogate light chain. First described by Melchers in the mouse[28] and then identified in humans,[29,30] the surrogate light chain is composed of two polypeptides, encoded by the *$\lambda$-like* (or $\lambda5$ in the mouse) and the *Vpre-B* genes,[31] which pertain to the regular *IGL* locus. The $\mu$–$\Psi$L complex becomes expressed at the surface of what is now a large pre-B cell, which also expresses CD10 and CD19, but no longer CD34. It is of note that $\mu$–$\Psi$L is associated with the Ig$\alpha$–Ig$\beta$ heterodimer to form the pre-B cell receptor (pre-BCR).[32–34] Expression of the pre-BCR is required for further progression along the B-cell differentiation pathway. Recent identification of galectin-1 as a physiological ligand of the pre-BCR has provided the first experimental basis for the mode of interaction of pre-B cells with stromal cells.[35] The next step of differentiation involves light-chain gene rearrangements, which occur in the order $\kappa \rightarrow \lambda$. The recombination process is regulated in the same manner as for the heavy chains, so that there is only one light chain that is expressed in any given cell, either $\kappa$ or $\lambda$. The negative feedback on further rearrangements of the light-chain genes is exerted by the complete IgM, which is expressed on the surface of the immature B cell and has now replaced the pre-BCR.

## Selection of immature B cells before leaving the bone marrow

Before leaving the bone marrow, immature B cells that express surface IgM are confronted to the local 'self' antigenic environment. They are particularly sensitive to triggering by multivalent antigens, resulting in their clonal deletion by apoptosis. Alternately, soluble self-antigens will not cause death of the immature B cells, but instead will induce an anergic state, which does not seem to prevent the cells from migrating to the periphery.[36] At this point, cells that have uncounted self-antigen may also escape cell death or anergy by changing their specificities. This is achieved by the so-called 'receptor editing' phenomenon, which allows the cells to replace one light chain by another one, or induces secondary rearrangement on both the heavy- and light-chain loci. It should be noted, however, that this negative selection has a threshold that leaves a fraction of autoreactive cells going to the periphery. These cells are responsible for the presence in the bloodstream of natural autoantibodies that must be of some physiological relevance.

Once validated by this 'quality control', immature B cells circulate to the periphery, through blood vessels and the lymphatic system, colonize the secondary lymphoid organs, and actively recirculate.

# Generation of plasma cells and memory B cells

The final steps of B-cell differentiation take place in the periphery and are antigen-dependent.

## Germinal center formation and the acquisition of somatic mutations

As recently described, bone marrow immature B lymphocytes emigrate to the spleen, as transitional T1 (IgM$^{high}$IgD$^{low}$) and T2 (IgM$^{high}$IgD$^{high}$CD21$^+$CD23$^+$) B cells.[37,38] Depending upon the stimulating conditions, transitional T2 cells will progress either to mature follicular or to marginal zone B cells, the former being preferentially involved in T-cell-dependent responses (Figure 6.3). Within the first days after antigenic stimulation and T-cell help involving molecules such as CD40L and various monocytic-derived factors, such as BAFF (B-cell activating factor of the tumor necrosis factor family) or APRIL, another member of the TNF superfamily,[39] the activated B cells may differentiate into plasma cells and memory B cells, which are the terminal stages of B-cell differentiation (Figures 6.3 and 6.4). Plasma cells are large cells that have an abundant endoplasmic reticulum and secrete immunoglobulins. After a primary stimulation, the first antibodies that are produced belong to the IgM isotype. Alternatively, some stimulated B cells may

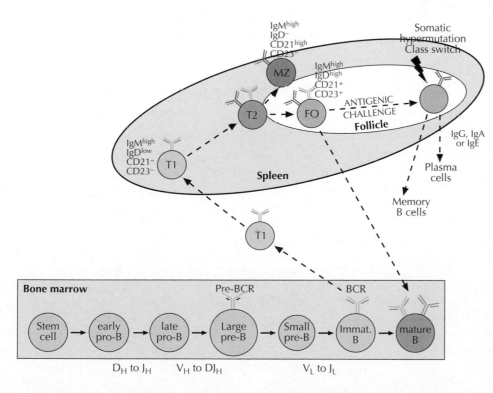

**Figure 6.3** Late events of B-cell differentiation, which take place in the periphery, are antigen-dependent. Immature B cells produced in the bone marrow migrate as transitional T1 and T2 cells to the spleen. T2 cells may evolve either to marginal zone B cells (MZ) or to follicular B cells (FO). Upon antigenic challenge and T-cell help, the latter develop in the germinal center, where somatic hypermutations and isotype switching take place. Ultimate steps of differentiation lead to plasma cells that produce circulating antibodies, and memory B cells that will be available for secondary responses.

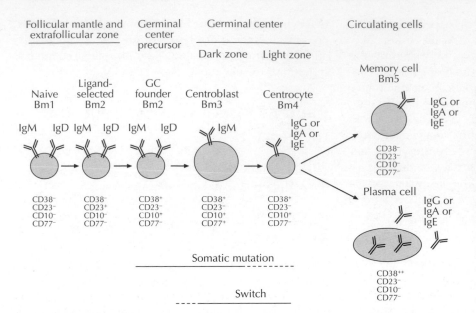

Figure 6.4 Last stages of B-cell differentiation. The germinal center organization plays a key role in mounting a T-dependent B-cell response, during which affinity is tuned upon the acquisition of somatic mutations, and the biological functions of the antibodies are adapted by isotype switching. Each step of differentiation may be followed by cell surface markers, which define classes denoted Bm1 to Bm5, according to Liu and Arpin.[40]

colonize the primary follicles of a lymph node and generate a germinal center,[40] where they interact with follicular dendritic cells (Figure 6.5).[41] B cells divide rapidly, giving rise to a clonal amplification in situ. They present a blastic morphology and are termed centroblasts, which delimitate the so-called dark zone of the germinal center. As the centroblasts actively divide, they accumulate somatic mutations, which occur at a very high rate (i.e. $10^{-3}$) and which are mostly localized in the regions of the $V_H$ and $V_L$ segments that interact with the antigen. This mechanism, which underlies a specialized machinery found only in B cells (see below), considerably amplifies the antibody diversity. As a result of these mutations, the array of affinities is largely increased, and the organization of the germinal center permits the antigen to

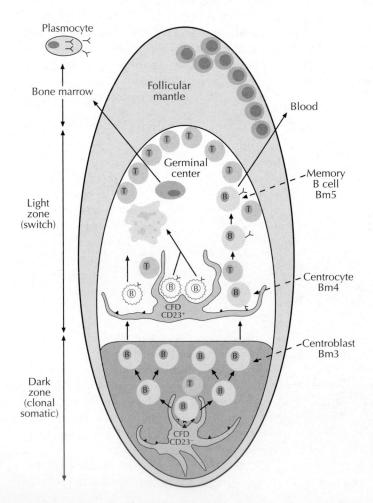

Figure 6.5 Schematic organization of a germinal center. As a result of antigenic stimulation, centroblasts develop as discrete clones in the dark zone, where they actively divide and start to accumulate somatic mutations. As they migrate to the light zone, they stop dividing and enter the centrocyte stage, where isotype switching takes place. They migrate through the germinal center and recirculate, either as plasma cells or as memory B cells. Adapted from Banchereau and Rousset.[41]

positively select the B cells that express at their surface the immunoglobulins with the highest affinities.[42] At this stage, centroblasts cease to divide, and become small non-dividing centrocytes that accumulate in the light zone of the germinal center, where they actively interact with numerous follicular dendritic cells. There is evidence that these cells play a major role in the selection of centrocytes with the highest affinity because they retain antigen at their surface. As a result of this interaction, the selected centrocytes can now either proceed towards plasma cell differentiation or become long-lived memory B cells.[43]

## Isotype switching

It has long been known that, upon antigenic stimulation, circulating antibodies first belong to the IgM isotype, before being replaced by immunoglobulins of another class (most frequently an IgG in the bloodstream). This phenomenon is known as isotype switching (or switch), and is the consequence of a new type of gene rearrangement, which takes place in the centrocytes, located in the light zone of the germinal center (Figure 6.5). As a result, the VDJ rearranged region of the mature B cell, which was initially associated with a constant $C_\mu$ to make a complete $\mu$ chain, now becomes associated with the constant region of another isotype.[44] This gene rearrangement involves recognition sequences termed 'switch regions', which are located 5′ of each constant $C_H$ gene (with the exception of the δ-chain gene). These regions present high levels of homology and are recognized by an enzymatic system that does not involve the Rag proteins (see below). As a result of this recombination event, the portion of DNA localized between the two switch regions concerned is deleted. The light-chain genes are not affected by isotype switching, so the antibody-combining site remains unaffected. In other words, isotype switching changes the Ig isotype without modifying the specificity of the antibody. It simply confers on the antibody a distinct biological function, which can amplify the physiological action of the immune system in a number of ways, such as to enable a more appropriate fight against pathogens, to ensure fetal protection through transplacental transfer, or to be expressed in secretions, depending upon the selected isotype. Isotype switching is another example of a mechanism that necessitates interaction between T and B lymphocytes and makes use of two molecular signals. One involves CD40 ligand (CD40L) and CD40, expressed at the cell surface of T helper ($T_H$) and B lymphocytes respectively and ensuring direct contact between the cells.[45] The second signal is provided by the $T_H$ cell, and is a cytokine that is released as a soluble factor in the immediate proximity of the B cell. Depending upon the nature of the cytokine, and therefore on the type of interacting T cell, the switch mechanism will address a discrete

isotype. For instance, secretion of IL-4 will favor a switch towards the IgE class,[46] whereas transforming growth factor β1 (TGF-β1) will induce switching to IgA.[47]

## Isotype switching and somatic mutations may be driven by the same basic mechanisms

A major breakthrough in the understanding of the mechanisms that drive isotype switching and generation of somatic hypermutations has recently been reported,[48] with the identification of mutations in the gene encoding activated induced deaminase (AID). As a result of these mutations, identified both in mice[49] and in human patients suffering from a type 2 hyper IgM syndrome,[50] absence of isotype switching coexisted with the absence of somatic mutations, leading to the exclusive expression of IgM germline genes in the bloodstream. AID is a deaminase enzyme that transforms a cytidine into a uracil in the RNA. Thus it may play a major role in the so-called mechanism of RNA editing, which operates at the mRNA level, by changing one nucleotide as a consequence of the $C \rightarrow U$ replacement. This is expected to change the nature of the messenger, one interesting possibility being the transformation of an inactive mRNA into a new species that now encodes for an active protein. Furthermore, recent data demonstrate that the AID protein is also able to perform the $C \rightarrow U$ replacement directly at the DNA level.[51] In that case, uracil is excised by uracil-DNA glycosidase (UNG) and replaced by any of the other deoxyribonucleotides under the action of the cell DNA repair machinery.[52]

For isotype switching, the general scheme would be as follows: (i) opening of the chromatin in the S regions upon the specific action of cytokines; (ii) transitional transcription of the region of DNA that is now accessible; (iii) cleavage of the appropriate S regions by the newly generated endonuclease, specifically expressed in germinal centers; (iv) ligation of the new constant heavy-chain region gene, with a concomitant looping out of the intervening section of DNA. Since the absence of switching correlated with the absence of somatic mutations in AID-mutant mice and in patients suffering from the type 2 hyper IgM syndrome, it was proposed that this endonuclease was also at hand for the generation of somatic mutations.

# Conclusions

Differentiation of B cells is a highly sophisticated process, which takes place continuously in the bone marrow and results in the constant emergence of a very large repertoire of immunoglobulins, expressed both as membrane B-cell receptors (BCR) and soluble antibodies. The numerous molecular events that lead from the hematopoietic stem cell to the mature B cell are under constant selective pressure, implying a high level of cell death. Therefore the available repertoire appears, at any given time, as a compromise between the necessary economy in gene number, compensated by the recombination processes, and an unavoidable wastage due to the stochastic aspects of gene rearrangements and to negative selection of clones having a high affinity for self components.

Alterations in the differentiation of B cells either in the bone marrow or in secondary lymphoid organs could lead to pathological situations such as B-cell malignancies. These disorders may be considered as amplification – frequently clonal – of one B-cell subpopulation 'frozen' at a given stage of differentiation, as a result of malignant transformation. The second group of disorders relates to inherited primary immune deficiencies, which are very rare diseases resulting from mutations of genes encoding various factors necessary to ensure the B-cell differentiation pathway.[53–56] Finally, defects in selection processes may also lead to the generation of self-reactive B cells and thus to autoimmune diseases.[57]

# REFERENCES

1. Morrison SJ, Wright DE, Cheshier SH, Weissman IL. Hematopoietic stem cells: challenges to expectations. *Curr Opin Immunol* 1997; **9**: 216–21.

2. Galy A, Travis M, Cen D, Chen B. Human T, B, natural killer, and dendritic cells arise from a common bone marrow progenitor cell subset. *Immunity* 1995; **3**: 459–73.

3. Schebesta M, Heavey B, Busslinger M. Transcriptional control of B-cell development. *Curr Opin Immunol* 2002; **14**: 216–23.

4. Georgopoulos K, Bigby M, Wang JH et al. The *Ikaros* gene is required for the development of all lymphoid lineages. *Cell* 1994; **79**: 143–56.

5. Wang JH, Nichogiannopoulou A, Wu L et al. Selective defects in the development of the fetal and adult lymphoid system in mice with an *Ikaros* null mutation. *Immunity* 1996; **5**: 537–49.

6. Busslinger M, Nutt SL, Rolink AG. Lineage commitment in lymphopoiesis. *Curr Opin Immunol* 2000; **12**: 151–8.

7. Uckun FM. Regulation of human B-cell ontogeny. *Blood* 1990; **76**: 1908–23.

8. Ghia P, ten Boekel E, Sanz E et al. Ordering of human bone marrow B lymphocyte precursors by single-cell polymerase chain reaction analyses of the rearrangement status of the immunoglobulin H and L chain loci. *J Exp Med* 1996; **184**: 2217–29.

9. Lassoued K, Nunez CA, Billips L et al. Expression of surrogate light chain receptors is restricted to a late stage in pre-B cell differentiation. *Cell* 1993; **73**: 73–86.

10. Guelpa-Fonlupt V, Tonnelle C, Blaise D et al. Discrete early pro-B and pre-B stages in normal human bone marrow as defined by surface pseudo-light chain expression. *Eur J Immunol* 1994; **24**: 257–64.

11. Nunez C, Nishimoto N, Gartland GL et al. B cells are generated throughout life in humans. *J Immunol* 1996; **156**: 866–72.

12. Meffre E, Fougereau M, Argenson J-N et al. Cell surface expression of surrogate light chain (ΨL) in the absence of μ on human pro-B cell lines and normal pro-B cells. *Eur J Immunol* 1996; **26**: 2172–80.

13. Jacobsen K, Osmond DG. Microenvironmental organization and stromal cell associations of B lymphocyte precursor cells in mouse bone marrow. *Eur J Immunol* 1990; **20**: 2395–404.

14. Kincade PW, Lee G, Pietrangeli CE et al. Cells and molecules that regulate B lymphopoiesis in bone marrow. *Annu Rev Immunol* 1989; **7**: 111–43.

15. Springer TA. Traffic signals for lymphocyte recirculation and leukocyte emigration: the multistep paradigm. *Cell* 1994; **76**: 301–14.

16. Galli SJ, Zsebo KM, Geissler EN. The kit ligand, stem cell factor. *Adv Immunol* 1994; **55**: 1–96.

17. Namen AE, Lupton S, Hjerrild K et al. Stimulation of B-cell progenitors by cloned murine interleukin-7. *Nature* 1988; **333**: 571–3.

18. Law CL, Clark EA. Cell–cell interactions that regulate the development of B-lineage cells. *Curr Opin Immunol* 1994; **6**: 238–47.

19. Uckun FM, Ledbetter JA. Immunobiologic differences between normal and leukemic human B-cell precursors. *Proc Natl Acad Sci USA* 1988; **85**: 8603–7.

20. Pontvert-Delucq S, Breton-Gorius J, Schmitt C et al. Characterization and functional analysis of adult human bone marrow cell subsets in relation to B-lymphoid development. *Blood* 1993; **82**: 417–29.

21. Reth M. The B-cell antigen receptor complex and co-receptors. *Immunol Today* 1995; **16**: 310–13.

22. Alt FW, Oltz EM, Young F et al. VDJ recombination. *Immunol Today* 1992; **13**: 306–14.

23. Oettinger MA, Schatz DG, Gorka C, Baltimore D. *RAG-1* and *RAG-2*, adjacent genes that synergistically activate V(D)J recombination. *Science* 1990; **248**: 1517–23.

24. Gellert M. Recent advances in understanding V(D)J recombination. *Adv Immunol* 1997; **64**: 39–64.

25. Bassing CH, Swat W, Alt FW. The mechanism and regulation of chromosomal V(D)J recombination. *Cell* 2002; **109** (Suppl): S45–55.

26. Alt FW, Baltimore D. Joining of immunoglobulin heavy chain gene segments: implications from a chromosome with evidence of three D–JH fusions. *Proc Natl Acad Sci USA* 1982; **79**: 4118–22.

27. Alt FW, Blackwell TK, Yancopoulos GD. Development of the primary antibody repertoire. *Science* 1987; **238**: 1079–87.

28. Sakaguchi N, Melchers F. λ5, a new light-chain-related locus selectively expressed in pre-B lymphocytes. *Nature* 1986; **324**: 579–82.

29. Schiff C, Milili M, Fougereau M. Isolation of early immunoglobulin lambda-like gene transcripts in human fetal liver. *Eur J Immunol* 1989; **19**: 1873–8.

30. Hollis GF, Evans RJ, Stafford-Hollis JM et al. Immunoglobulin λ light-chain-related genes 14.1 and 16.1 are expressed in pre-B cells and may encode the human

immunoglobulin ω light-chain protein. *Proc Natl Acad Sci USA* 1989; **86**: 5552–6.

31. Karasuyama H, Kudo A, Melchers F. The proteins encoded by the *VpreB* and *λ5* pre-B cell-specific genes can associate with each other and with μ heavy chain. *J Exp Med* 1990; **172**: 969–72.

32. Melchers F, Karasuyama H, Haasner D et al. The surrogate light chain in B-cell development. *Immunol Today* 1993; **14**: 60–8.

33. Bossy D, Milili M, Zucman J et al. Organization and expression of the λ-like genes that contribute to the μ–Ψ light chain complex in human pre-B cells. *Int Immunol* 1991; **3**: 1081–90.

34. Bossy D, Salamero J, Olive D et al. Structure, biosynthesis, and transduction properties of the human μ–Ψ L complex: similar behavior of preB and intermediate preB–B cells in transducing ability. *Int Immunol* 1993; **5**: 467–78.

35. Gauthier L, Rossi B, Roux F et al. Galectin-1 is a stromal cell ligand of the pre-B cell receptor (BCR) implicated in synapse formation between pre-B and stromal cells and in pre-BCR triggering. *Proc Natl Acad Sci USA* 2002; **99**: 13014–19.

36. Nemazee DA, Bürki K. Clonal deletion of B lymphocytes in a transgenic mouse bearing anti-MHC class I antibody genes. *Nature* 1989; **337**: 562–6.

37. Su TT, Rawlings DJ. Transitional B lymphocyte subsets operate as distinct checkpoints in murine splenic B cell development. *J Immunol* 2002; **168**: 2101–10.

38. Loder F, Mutschler B, Ray RJ et al. B cell development in the spleen takes place in discrete steps and is determined by the quality of B cell receptor-derived signals. *J Exp Med* 1999; **190**: 75–89.

39. Mackay F, Schneider P, Rennert P, Browning J. BAFF and APRIL: A tutorial on B cell survival. *Annu Rev Immunol* 2003; **21**: 231–64.

40. Liu YJ, Arpin C. Germinal center development. *Immunol Rev* 1997; **156**: 111–26.

41. Banchereau J, Rousset F. Human B lymphocytes: phenotype, proliferation, and differentiation. *Adv Immunol* 1992; **52**: 125–262.

42. Kuppers R, Zhao M, Hansmann ML, Rajewsky K. Tracing B cell development in human germinal centres by molecular analysis of single cells picked from histological sections. *EMBO J* 1993; **12**: 4955–67.

43. Liu YJ, Zhang J, Lane PJ et al. Sites of specific B cell activation in primary and secondary responses to T cell-dependent and T cell-independent antigens. *Eur J Immunol* 1991; **21**: 2951–62.

44. Harriman W, Volk H, Defranoux N, Wabl M. Immunoglobulin class switch recombination. *Annu Rev Immunol* 1993; **11**: 361–84.

45. Aruffo A, Farrington M, Hollenbaugh D et al. The CD40 ligand, gp39, is defective in activated T cells from patients with X-linked hyper-IgM syndrome. *Cell* 1993; **72**: 291–300.

46. Pene J, Rousset F, Briere F et al. IgE production by normal human B cells induced by alloreactive T cell clones is mediated by IL-4 and suppressed by IFN-γ. *J Immunol* 1988; **141**: 1218–24.

47. Islam KB, Nilsson L, Sideras P et al. TGF-β1 induces germ-line transcripts of both IgA subclasses in human B lymphocytes. *Int Immunol* 1991; **3**: 1099–106.

48. Honjo T, Kinoshita K, Muramatsu M. Molecular mechanism of class switch recombination: linkage with somatic hypermutation. *Annu Rev Immunol* 2002; **20**: 165–96.

49. Muramatsu M, Sankaranand VS, Anant S et al. Specific expression of activation-induced cytidine deaminase (AID), a novel member of the RNA-editing deaminase family in germinal center B cells. *J Biol Chem* 1999; **274**: 18470–6.

50. Revy P, Muto T, Levy Y et al. Activation-induced cytidine deaminase (AID) deficiency causes the autosomal recessive form of the hyper-IgM syndrome (HIGM2). *Cell* 2000; **102**: 565–75.

51. Petersen-Mahrt SK, Harris RS, Neuberger MS. AID mutates *E. coli*, suggesting a DNA deamination mechanism for antibody diversification. *Nature* 2002; **418**: 99–103.

52. Rada C, Williams GT, Nilsen H et al. Immunoglobulin isotype switching is inhibited and somatic hypermutation perturbed in UNG-deficient mice. *Curr Biol* 2002; **12**: 1748–55.

53. Rosen FS, Cooper MD, Wedgwood RJ. The primary immunodeficiencies. *N Engl J Med* 1995; **333**: 431–40.

54. Schiff C, Lemmers B, Deville A et al. Autosomal primary immunodeficiencies affecting human bone marrow B cell differentiation. *Immunol Rev* 2000; **178**: 91–8.

55. Conley ME, Rohrer J, Rapalus L et al. Defects in early B-cell development: comparing the consequences of abnormalities in pre-BCR signaling in the human and the mouse. *Immunol Rev* 2000; **178**: 75–90.

56. Durandy A, Honjo T. Human genetic defects in class-switch recombination (hyper-IgM syndromes). *Curr Opin Immunol* 2001; **13**: 543–8.

57. Gauld SB, Dal Porto JM, Cambier JC. B cell antigen receptor signaling: roles in cell development and disease. *Science* 2002; **296**: 1641–2.

# 7 Cellular aspects of lymphoid differentiation: T and NK cells

**Anna Cambiaggi, Sophie Ugolini, and Eric Vivier**

## Introduction

Cells belonging to the lymphoid lineages ensure the protection of their hosts against an enormous variety of (potential pathogenic) microorganisms as well as against alterations of self tissues (e.g. tumor cells). T and B cells are the most studied type of lymphocytes: their recognition of foreign antigens through rearranged T-cell receptors (TCR) and B-cell receptors (BCR) has been extensively investigated. TCR and BCR are generated by gene rearrangement, providing T and B cells with a virtually infinite capacity to recognize antigens. T and B lymphocytes comprise the cellular component of adaptive immunity and provide the lifelong immunity that can follow exposure to disease or vaccination. The third type of lymphocytes, natural killer (NK) cells, do not express rearranged antigen receptors on their surface; they are effector lymphocytes contributing to host defense against viral infections and to immune surveillance against the establishment of primary tumors through cytolytic activity and cytokine secretion.

All hematopoietic cells originate from one pluripotent stem cell that has the ability of self-renewal. The existence of a common progenitor cell that should be able to differentiate only into cells of the lymphoid lineages is generally accepted, but this common lymphoid progenitor has not yet been identified. Evidence for this model is provided by mice deficient for the Ikaros transcription factor, which lack B, T, NK, and dendritic cells, but not the myeloid and erythroid compartments.[1] Further, it has been shown that T and NK cells are more closely related to each others than to B cells, supporting the existence of a bipotential T/NK precursor.[2]

T lymphocytes and NK cells can be defined via morphological, phenotypical, and functional criteria. Mature circulating T lymphocytes are small cells with condensed chromatin in the nucleus and few cytoplasmic organelles; upon antigen recognition and activation, the T-cell volume increases, the chromatin in the nucleus becomes less dense, and abundant mitochondria and rough endoplasmic reticulum are present in the cytoplasm. Circulating NK cells are large granular lymphocytes with abundant cytoplasm containing granules loaded with molecules involved in the execution phase of the cytolytic mechanisms. Phenotypically, T cells are characterized by the surface expression of the TCR/CD3 complex that is totally absent on NK cells. Otherwise, the two cell types share the expression of numerous differentiation antigens, as shown in Table 7.1. The cell surface markers commonly utilized to define human NK cells (CD16 and CD56) can also be expressed by discrete subpopulations of T lymphocytes. Activation markers such as CD69 and CD25 are also shared between activated T and activated NK cells.[3] T lymphocytes can be subdivided into two subsets on the basis of their phenotype and function. CD4+ T helper (Th) lymphocytes are specialized in the activation of other immune effectors (B cells and macrophages) with cytokine secretion upon recognition of pathogen antigens in the context of major histocompatibility complex (MHC) class II molecules. CD8+ cytotoxic T lymphocytes (CTL) recognize antigenic peptides in the context of MHC class I molecules and exert their function in one of two ways: cytolytic activity and cytokine secretion. CTL are commonly considered as counterparts of Th cells, but a comparison of CTL and NK cells on the basis of functional parameters reveals striking similarities.[4] Both T and NK cells lyse their target using both perforin-dependent mechanisms and Fas/Fas-ligand interactions. They also respond to the same cytokines both for proliferation and for increase of cytolytic activity, and they produce a similar set of lymphokines – interferon-$\gamma$ (IFN-$\gamma$), granulocyte–macrophage colony-stimulating factor (G-CSF), and tumor necrosis factor $\alpha$ (TNF-$\alpha$) – shown in Table 7.2. Despite these similarities, CTL and NK cells' effector mechanisms are triggered by distinct molecular pathways. After recognition of the specific MHC class I/antigenic peptide complex, T lymphocytes proliferate, acquire an effector potential, and also become memory T cells. NK cells are also able to

## Table 7.1 Expression of surface molecules by human T and NK cells

| Surface molecule[a] | NK | T |
|---|---|---|
| TCR | − | + |
| CD1 | − | +[b] |
| CD2 | + | + |
| CD3 γ δ ε (cy) | +[b] | + |
| CD3 γ δ ε (m) | − | + |
| CD3 ζ/FcεRI-γ | + | + |
| CD4 | − | +[c] |
| CD5 | − | + |
| CD7 | + | + |
| CD8 | +[c] | +[c] |
| CD11a/CD18 | + | + |
| CD11b/CD18 | + | +[d] |
| CD11c/CD18 | + | +[d] |
| CD16 (FcγRIII) | + | +[c] |
| CD25 (IL-2Rα) | +[d] | +[d] |
| CD38 | + | +[d] |
| CD44 | + | + |
| CD56 | + | +[c] |
| CD57 | +[c] | +[c] |
| CD69 | +[d] | +[d] |
| CD122 (IL-2Rβ) | + | +[d] |
| PEN5 | + | [e] |

[a]cy, cytoplasmic; m, membrane surface expression. Expression of surface antigens on T and NK cells: + indicates expression of the indicated molecule and − its absence; [b] Expressed by thymocytes or immature NK cells, [c] Expressed by a subpopulation of T or NK cells, [d] expressed by activated cells only. [e] A discrete subset of T cells (<2%) may express PEN5 at their surface.

## Table 7.2 Functional comparison of CTL and NK cells

| Functions | CTL | NK cells |
|---|---|---|
| *Cytotoxicity* | | |
| Adaptive | + | − |
| Natural cytotoxicity | − | + |
| ADCC | − | + |
| Perforin-dependent | + | + |
| Fas-mediated | + | + |
| *Cytokines produced* | | |
| IFN-γ | + | + |
| GM-CSF | + | + |
| TNF-α | + | + |
| *Response to cytokines* | | |
| IL-2-induced proliferation | ++ | + |
| IL-2- and IL-12-induced cytokine production | + | + |
| IFN-α-, IFN-β-, IL-2-, and IL-12-induced cytotoxicity increase | + | + |
| IL-4- and TGF-β-induced cytotoxicity reduction | + | + |

ADCC, antibody-dependent cell-mediated cytotoxicity; IFN, interferon; GM-CSF, granulocyte–macrophage colony-stimulating factor; TNF, tumor necrosis factor; IL, interleukin; TGF, transforming growth factor.

interact with MHC class I molecules, but through NK receptors for MHC class I molecules (NKR), and this recognition results in the inhibition of NK cells' effector functions. Downregulation or absence of MHC class I molecules on target cells induces lysis by NK cells; as a consequence, NK cells can eliminate cells that, through lack of MHC class I molecules, evade CTL recognition. Total or partial loss of MHC class I expression is a common feature of viral infections and malignant transformations. NK cells are also able to participate in the adaptive response through the expression of the FcγRIIIA (CD16) receptor complex, which allows them to perform antibody-dependent cell-mediated cytotoxicity (ADCC) against antibody-coated target cells.

# T- and NK-cell development

Hematopoietic cells originate in the yolk sac, then migrate to the fetal liver, which is the major hematopoietic organ during fetal life. T-cell precur-

sors and mature NK cells can be identified in the fetal liver starting from week 6 of gestation. A rudiment of thymus of epithelial origin, the thymic anelage, is formed at week 7 of gestation, but only at week 9 of gestation is it colonized by dendritic cells, macrophages, and thymic precursors. After birth, bone marrow becomes the major hematopoietic organ and is likely to be the development site for NK cells, whereas the vast majority of T cells mature in the thymus. The importance of the thymus in T-cell development can be observed in the DiGeorge syndrome in humans, as well as in nude mutant mice. In these cases, as the thymus fails to form, the affected individuals lack the vast majority of T lymphocytes, but produce normal B lymphocytes and NK cells. Recent evidence indicates that some T cells can have an extrathymic differentiation in the gut mucosa or in the liver, but these cells differ from thymic T lymphocytes in phenotype and function.[5] Within the thymus, T-cell precursors proceed to differentiation and education. As shown in Figure 7.1, the more immature precursors lack TCR/CD3, CD4, and CD8 molecules and are defined as triple-negative (TN). The earliest thymic precursors are CD34+CD33+CD45RA+; then they acquire the expression of CD7 and CD38 at the cell surface and of CD3 molecules in the cytoplasm. These cells are still able to generate both T and NK cells. The first committed T cells acquire the

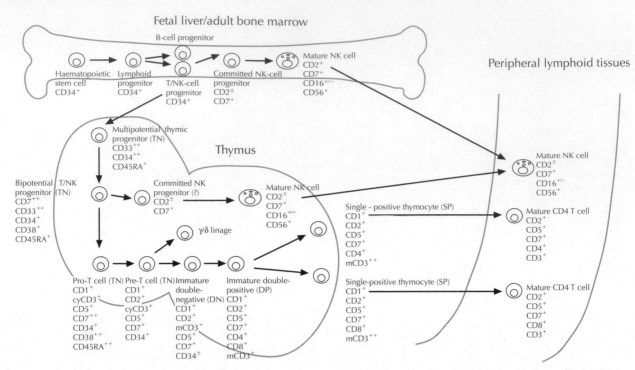

**Figure 7.1** Schematic representation of human T- and NK-cell development. The development of T and NK lymphocytes from hematopoietic precursors (fetal liver/adult bone marrow) is shown here schematically. m, membrane (cell surface expression); cy, cytoplasm (cytoplasmic expression).

expression of CD1, an MHC class I-like protein associated with $\beta_2$-microglobulin, CD2, and CD5; at this stage, TCRβ-chain rearrangement starts.[6] Probably, at this point, T-cell precursors for the TCRγδ T-cell lineage differentiate from TCRαβ-committed thymocytes. The rearranged TCRβ chain is expressed at the cell surface associated with a pre-TCRα (pTα) chain and with CD3 molecules (Figure 7.2) (double-negative stage, DN). Expression of the pre-TCR complex prevents further rearrangements at the TCRβ locus, controls the initiation of TCRα-chain rearrangement and is required for the expression of CD4 and CD8 molecules on the thymocytes (double-positive stage, DP).[7] In the mouse, the most immature thymocytes express c-Kit and CD44, but not CD25 (Figure 7.3). Concomitant with CD25 surface expression, DN thymocytes proliferate strongly. The downregulation of c-Kit and CD44 that follows indicates a stage of fully T-cell commitment as well as the initiation of TCRα rearrangement. The availability of genetically modified mice has allowed the identification of the molecules involved in early T-cell maturation as well as major checkpoints of T-cell thymic development. The first checkpoint occurs at the transition from TN to DN cells and is blocked by the absence of RAG-1 and RAG-2, enzymes involved in TCR rearrangements. Thymocytes isolated from TCRβ[-/-]×TCRδ[-/-] or CD3ε[-/-] mice are blocked at the CD25[+]CD44[+] stage: in these mice, TCRβ rearrangement is unaltered, but the pre-TCR is not expressed on the surface and cannot transduce further development signals. Evidence for the role of pre-TCR in allelic exclusion at the TCRβ locus

was documented with the introduction of a rearranged TCRβ gene into the mouse genome: the transgenic receptor prevents any rearrangement at the endogenous TCRβ locus. The rearrangement of TCR genes occurs during early stages of thymocyte maturation, and allows the generation of a large number of immature T cells bearing a single specificity. It has been estimated that the repertoire of thymocytes before selection ranges between $10^{10}$ to $10^{15}$ distinct specificities. The mechanisms of TCR chain rearrangement are similar to those that occur in B cells to generate immunoglobulins (Igs), and the genomic organization of TCR genes resembles the organization of Ig genes. Each TCR locus consists of variable ($V$), joining ($J$), and constant ($C$) region genes, TCRβ and TCRγ chain loci also contain diversity ($D$) segment genes. The β-chain locus is on chromosome 7; it consists of two $C_\beta$ regions associated with a 5′ cluster of five $J_\beta$ segments and one $D_\beta$ segment, most of the $V_\beta$ segments are 5′ of $C_\beta$ and $J_\beta$ clusters. The α locus is on chromosome 14, there is a single $C_\alpha$ segment associated with a 5′ cluster of up to 50 $J_\alpha$ segments; 5′ from the cluster, there are around 75 $V_\alpha$ segments. The TCRδ locus is located between $V_\alpha$ and $J_\alpha$ genes. The TCRγ chain locus is on chromosome 7 and has an organization similar to that of the TCRβ chain locus. We will discuss in detail TCRβ and TCRα chain rearrangement. The TCRβ chain locus rearranges first with the joining between a $D_\beta$ and a $J_\beta$ segment; the $D_\beta J_\beta$ segment is joined to a $V_\beta$ segment to form a $V_\beta D_\beta J_\beta$ gene (Figure 7.4). If the rearrangement is productive, a long mRNA also containing some intronic sequences

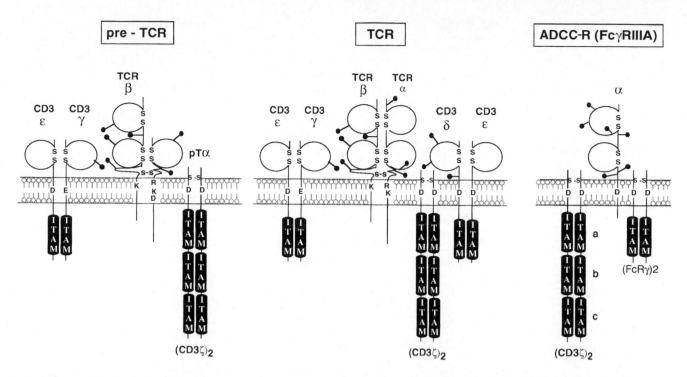

**Figure 7.2** Schematic representation of the pre-TCR/CD3, TCR/CD3, and ADCC-R complexes. The oligomeric pre-TCR/CD3, TCR/CD3, and ADCC-R (CD16) complexes are represented according to their canonical stochiometry. Immunoreceptor tyrosine-based activation motifs (ITAM) are shown as black cylinders; the three CD3$\zeta$ ITAMs are indicated by a, b, and c respectively. Ig-like domains and carbohydrate moieties are also indicated. The charged amino-acid residues in the transmembrane domains are represented by the single-letter code.

is synthesized and spliced out to obtain a mature mRNA. Once the TCR$\beta$ has been produced and associated with pT$\alpha$ on the cell surface, the cell undergoes active proliferation and CD4 and CD8 molecules are expressed on the cell surface. With the end of the proliferative phase, the TCR$\alpha$ locus starts its rearrangement, with the production first of a $V_\alpha J_\alpha$ segment. The large number of $V_\alpha$ and $J_\alpha$ segments allows the cell to undergo successive rearrangements, in the case of initial non-productive rearrangements. The allelic exclusion at the TCR$\alpha$ locus is less stringent than at the TCR$\beta$ locus, and a single T cell can express on its surface two distinct TCR$\alpha\beta$.[8]

When both TCR$\beta$ and TCR$\alpha$ loci are rearranged, the thymocyte undergo selective processes: positive selection assures that only thymocytes that recognize self MHC molecules progress in their maturation, and the thymocytes that cannot interact with any self MHC molecule die by neglect; negative selection eliminates potentially self-reactive cells that have been generated during random rearrangement of $V_\beta D_\beta J_\beta / V_\alpha J_\alpha$ segments. It has been calculated that more than 95% of thymocytes are eliminated during the positive and negative selection processes. Most of the evidence for positive selection comes from animal models, in particular when lethally irradiated mice were injected with bone marrow cells from mice of

another MHC haplotype. In the host mice, all the bone marrow-derived cells are of donor origin; these mice are known as bone marrow chimeras. In the experiment depicted in Figure 7.5, donor cells are derived from $F_1$ of MHC$^a$ and MHC$^b$ parents (MHC$^{axb}$) and the irradiated hosts are mice of the parental strains (either MHC$^a$ or MHC$^b$) in which only radioresistant thymic epithelial cells survive. When MHC$^{axb}$ cells develop in an MHC$^a$ mouse, the mature T cells are able to recognize antigens presented only by MHC$^a$ antigen-presenting cells (APC), but not by MHC$^b$ APC, showing that the T cells had been restricted by the MHC$^a$ molecules that they encountered during thymic maturation. The use of TCR transgenic mice has provided another model to investigate positive selection processes. These mice were created by injecting into their genome DNA coding for the $\alpha$ and $\beta$ chains of a TCR of defined MHC restriction. Mature T cells were found only in mice of the appropriate MHC haplotype, but not in mice of other MHC haplotypes.[9] During positive selection, the thymocytes undergo transition from a DP to an SP stage: cells restricted for MHC class I molecules will express CD8 on their surface, while cells restricted for MHC class II molecules will express CD4 (Figure 7.1). Again, TCR transgenic mice turned out to be a good model to investigate the role of TCR/MHC interactions and the expression of CD4 or CD8 coreceptors. In mice with a TCR restricted

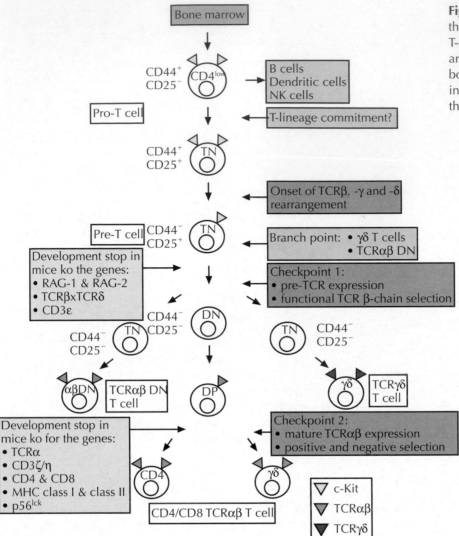

**Figure 7.3** T-cell development in the thymus. The major stages of T-cell development in the thymus are schematized. The large shaded boxes on the left show the blocks in T-cell development observed in the indicated knockout (ko) mice.

for MHC class I molecules, all the peripheral lymphocytes are CD8+; when the TCR is specific for MHC class II molecules, the mature T cells express CD4 on their membrane. The same TCR transgenic mice mentioned above to demonstrate the requirement of TCR/MHC interactions during positive selection were also useful to study negative selection. Injection of the antigenic peptide recognized by the transgenic TCR results in the apoptotic death of developing thymocytes because the peptide is then presented as self antigen in the thymus and autoreactive cells are thus deleted.[9] Only recently has the answer to the central question of selective events been obtained: How does TCR engagement lead to cell maturation during positive selection and to cell death during negative selection? The 'avidity hypothesis' is now accepted and supported by experimental evidence. It postulates that the strength of the interaction between TCR and peptide/MHC complexes and the density of the complexes are responsible for the selective events. If the signal is weak, the thymocytes are selected to mature, but if the signal is too low, the thymocytes will die of neglect; if the signal is strong, the thymocytes are driven to programmed cell death and negatively selected.[10]

As discussed above, there are several lines of evidence indicating that T and NK cells derive from a common progenitor.[11] Most of the indications for the existence of a bipotential progenitor derive from studies of human thymic precursors. In particular, one report showed that immature CD34high thymocytes are able to develop in T cells in fetal thymic organ culture (FTOC) and to generate NK cells when cultured in the presence of stem cell factor (SCF, Steel factor, c-Kit ligand), interleukin-3 (IL-3), and IL-7. To demonstrate directly that CD34high cells retained a bipotential capacity, they were single-cell-sorted, expanded for a short period with SCF, IL-2, and IL-7 on feeder cells, and then pooled together. Half of these were cultured in FTOC and matured into T cells; the other half were cultured with SCF, IL-3, and IL-7 in the absence of a thymic environment, and almost all the cells developed into NK cells.[12]

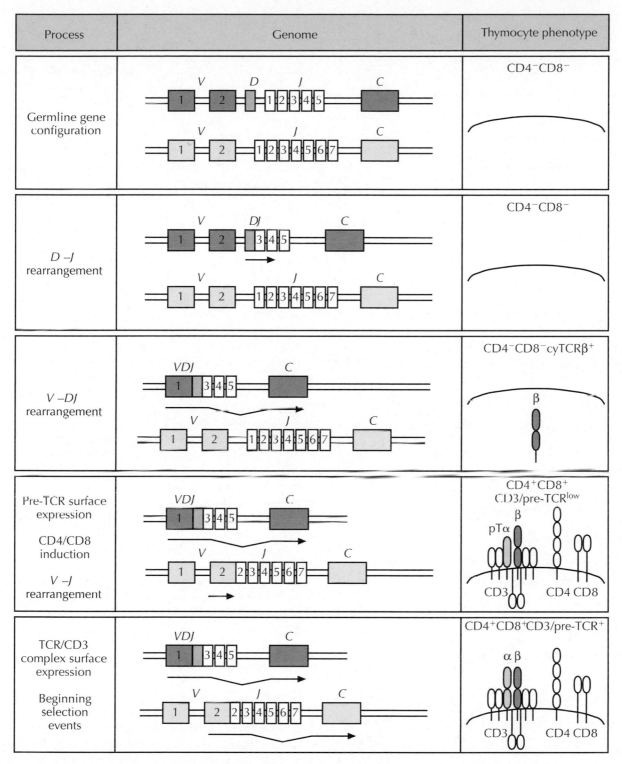

**Figure 7.4** TCR gene rearrangements in TCRαβ cells. *V*, *D*, and *J* segments on homologous chromosomes are depicted. The cell surface phenotype of thymocytes is indicated at each stage of development.

The demonstration that there exists a T/NK bipotential precursor in the thymus indicates that NK cells can develop in the thymus; however, the thymus is not required for normal NK-cell development, since athymic nude mice have normal NK cells. The main site of NK-cell development is likely to be the bone marrow (Figure 7.1). In humans, a bone marrow origin for NK cells is supported by experience with aplastic patients transplanted with allogeneic bone marrow. In these patients, the emergence of a wave of NK cells of donor origin is reported 2–3 weeks after transplant. Early studies with murine models showed that an intact bone marrow environment is necessary for NK-cell development. Mice treated with the radioisotope strontium-89 ($^{89}$Sr) are characterized by the destruction of bone marrow and present a marked decrease in

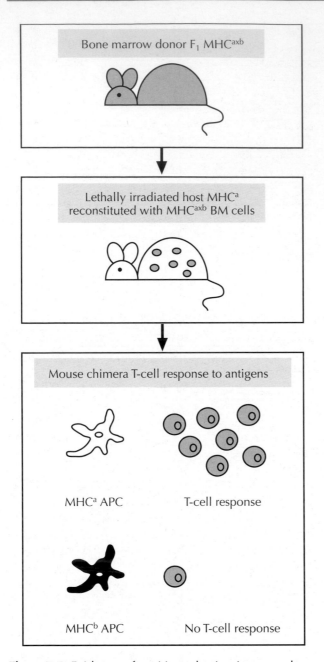

**Figure 7.5** Evidence of positive selection in mouse bone marrow chimeras. T cells from MHC$^{axb}$ F$_1$ mice are able to respond in vitro to antigens presented by antigen-presenting cells (APC) of both MHC$^a$ and MHC$^b$ origin. If bone marrow cells from these mice are transferred to lethally irradiated mice of MHC$^a$ (or MHC$^b$) parental haplotype, the T cells mature and are positively selected in the host thymus. T lymphocytes isolated from these bone marrow chimeras are able to respond in vitro to antigens presented only by APC of recipient MHC (bottom panel).

NK-cell activity. Moreover, bone marrow grafts from normal mice to [89]Sr-treated mice failed to reconstitute the NK-cell compartment, indicating the need of stromal and/or humoral signals provided by an intact bone marrow environment to support NK-cell maturation.[13]

# Mature T and NK cells

Mature naive T cells leave the thymus and migrate through the bloodstream into the peripheral lymphoid organs. Then, in the presence of specific antigens, T cells proliferate and differentiate into effector T cells, which are able to participate in the adaptive immune response. All mature T lymphocytes express on their surface the TCR/CD3 complex (Figure 7.2). TCRα and TCRβ chains have two Ig-like domains in the extracytoplasmic portion, two or one positively charged amino-acid residues in the transmembrane portion respectively, and a short intracellular domain. They are associated with the CD3 complex, which consists of three distinct IgSF proteins, CD3γ, CD3δ and CD3ε, and a dimer of CD3ζ polypeptides. Molecules of the CD3 complex contain in their intra-cytoplasmic portion immunoreceptor tyrosine-based activation motifs (ITAMs), which are responsible for the transduction of activating signals upon TCR engagement. The CD3 proteins are also required for the assembly and cell surface expression of TCR.[14]

The activation of naive T cells in the lymph nodes requires the engagement of TCR (signal 1) and also of costimulatory molecules such as CD28 (signal 2). Only professional APC (macrophages, dendritic cells, and B lymphocytes) express on their surface, together with MHC class I and class II molecules, B7.1 (CD80) and B7.2 (CD86), which serve as CD28 ligands. Antigen recognition by naive T lymphocytes without costimulatory signals induces a state of anergy in the cell (signal 1 only). This mechanism helps to ensure tolerance of T lymphocytes to self antigens. Indeed, negative selection in the thymus is not totally efficient; some tissue-specific proteins are not presented to T cells during their thymic maturation. Once T cells encounter the antigen presented by a professional APC, they rapidly proliferate and differentiate into progenies of effector and memory T cells. CD8+ T lymphocytes are predominantly cytotoxic effectors, while CD4+ T cells can differentiate into inflammatory T cells (Th1) and helper T cells (Th2). Upon activation, Th1 lymphocytes produces cytokines (IFN-γ, GM-CSF, and TNF-α) that activate macrophages to more efficiently eliminate intracellular microorganisms. Th2 lymphocytes secrete a different set of cytokines (mainly IL-4, IL-5, and IL-6) that regulate B-cell activation programs to differentiate and to produce immunoglobulins.

Mature NK cells migrate from the bone marrow to the blood, where they constitute around 4–15% of peripheral blood mononuclear cells (PBMC); the spleen also constitutes a source of NK cells (which represent 3–4% of splenic lymphocytes). In healthy individuals, rare NK cells are barely detectable in non-inflammatory lymph nodes. The presence of NK cells has also been demonstrated in the gut mucosa.[15]

All mature NK cells have a high density of adhesion molecules, such as CD2 and the three $\beta_2$ integrins (CD11a/CD18, CD11b/CD18, and CD11c/CD18); in humans, NK cells also express at their surface CD56, an isoform of neural cell adhesion molecule (NCAM), whose function on NK cells is still unknown. Around 10% of NK cells express a high density of CD56 (CD56[bright]); these cells constitutively express the trimeric high-affinity IL-2 receptor (IL-2R), together with the intermediate-affinity IL-2R. The remaining 90% of NK cells have a lower expression of CD56 (CD56[dim]) and express only the intermediate-affinity IL-2R. IL-2 stimulation of CD56[bright] NK cells results in a proliferative response and an increase in their cytolytic function, whereas IL-2 stimulation of CD56[dim] NK cells only results in an enhancement of their cytolytic activity. Therefore CD56[bright] NK cells resemble immature NK cells with poor cytolytic activity but high proliferative capacity; while CD56[dim] cells have the attributes of more differentiated cells.[16] The vast majority (>90%) of NK cells express the low-affinity receptor for the Fc portion of immunoglobulins (Fc$\gamma$RIII or CD16), which is part of the ADCC receptor (ADCC-R) complex and mediates the lysis of antibody-coated cells. The elucidation of ADCC-R molecular structure revealed striking structural and functional homologies with the TCR/CD3 complex (Figure 7.2). CD16 is non-covalently associated with CD3$\zeta$ and FcRI disulfide-linked dimers. Similarly to TCR$\alpha\beta$ (and TCR$\gamma\delta$) chains, the signaling properties of the ADCC-R complex are dependent upon the association between CD16 and polypeptide subunits specialized in transducing activating signals. CD3$\zeta$ and FcR$\gamma$ express in their intracytoplasmic domain three and one ITAM respectively; this motif is necessary and sufficient for transducing activating signals. Irrespective of their role in coupling to the transduction pathway, that is dependent upon the integrity of their ITAM domains, CD3$\zeta$ and FcR$\gamma$ are also required for the assembly and the surface expression of the ADCC-R complex via a charged amino-acid residue present in their intracytoplasmic portion.[17] PEN5 is a highly glycosylated molecule selectively expressed on CD56[dim]CD16+ human NK cells and thus represents a useful phenotypic marker of a large proportion of NK cells.[18]

Whereas T cells are MHC-restricted (i.e. they only recognize antigens presented by self MHC molecules), NK cells are *not MHC-restricted*. However, their function is *controlled* by the MHC. Indeed, human and mouse mature NK cells express on their surface inhibitory receptors for MHC class I molecules (natural killer cell receptors, NKR); engagement of NKR with their MHC class I ligands transduces a negative signal that leads to the inhibition of NK cell activation programs. In humans, NKR belong to two distinct families: IgSF and type C lectins[19] (Figure 7.6 and Table 7.3). In mice, only type C lectin NKR have been

described.[20] During maturation, NK cells acquire the expression of at least one inhibitory receptor for self MHC class I alleles, the engagement of which prevents the killing of autologous cells. IgSF NKR are defined as killer-cell Ig-like receptors (KIR), they belong to a multigenic and multiallelic family and all the genes are localized on chromosome 19 (at 19q13.4). KIR are characterized by two or three Ig-like domains in their extracytoplasmic portion, a transmembrane portion, and a long intracellular domain that contains two immunoreceptor tyrosine-based inhibitory motifs (ITIM). The integrity of ITIM sequences is necessary for the recruitment of intracytoplasmic effector substrates involved in the inhibition of NK-cell activity (i.e. the protein tyrosine phosphatases SHP-1 and SHP-2). In humans, the lectin-like NKR are heterodimers between the CD94 molecule and members of the NKG2 family. In mice, NKR are constituted by homodimers of lectins belonging to the Ly49 family, as well as CD94/NKG2 heterodimers.

Inhibitory recognition of MHC class I molecules accounts only in part for the target cell specificity of NK cells. Indeed, some sensitive target cells express normal level of MHC class I molecules while some others are not sensitive to lysis by NK cells despite low or absent class I expression. These observations imply the existence of activating receptors on NK cells. Several activating molecules, such as CD2, CD28, CD40L, 2B4, and leukocyte function-associated antigen (LFA)-1, are expressed on NK cells. However, we shall not focus here on these structures, which appear to 'co-activate' rather than directly stimulate NK cells. Several stimulatory structures expressed on NK cells have been identified.[21] As with inhibitory receptors, these activating receptors include members of the KIR, Ly49, and CD94/NKG2 families (Table 7.4). Activating receptors are highly homologous to the inhibitory molecules in their extracytoplasmic

**Table 7.3 Human MHC class I specific inhibitory receptors expressed on NK cells**

| Inhibitory receptors | CD antigen | Ligands |
|---|---|---|
| KIR2DL1 | CD158a | HLA Cw4 and related alleles (Asn 80) |
| KIR2DL2/3 | CD158b1/b2 | HLA Cw3 and related alleles (Lys 80) |
| KIR2DL4 | CD158d | HLA-G |
| KIR2DL5 | CD158f | Unknown |
| KIR3DL1 | CD158e1 | HLA-Bw4 |
| KIR3DL3 | CD158z | Unknown |
| KIR3DL2 | CD158k | HLA-A3/A11 |
| CD94/NKG2A | CD94/CD159a | HLA-E |

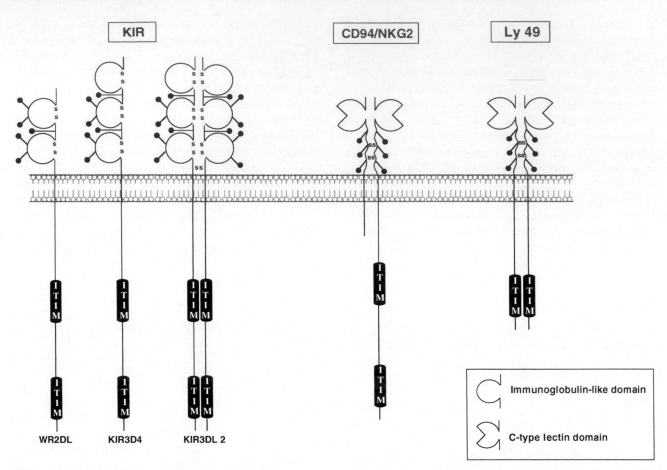

**Figure 7.6** Schematic representation of NK inhibitory receptors for MHC class I molecules (NKR). NKR belong either to the immunoglobulin superfamily (IgSF) or to the type C lectin-like family. Members of the IgSF NKR are defined as killer-cell inhibitory receptors (KIR), whereas the lectin-like receptors are heterodimers including an invariant CD94 molecule and various members of the NKG2 family. Mouse NKR are homodimers of the Ly49 molecular family. ITIM are indicated as black cylinders; Ig-like domains and lectin-like domains are also indicated.

domain, but are devoid of intracytoplasmic ITIM. The ligands of activating receptors are not always the same as those of their inhibitory counterparts. Indeed, the ligand of the activating receptor Ly49H is an MHC-like protein (m157) encoded by mouse cytomegalovirus (MCMV).[22] In mice and humans, NKG2D is another stimulatory receptor is expressed on a wide range of other effector cells, including NKT cells, γδ T cells,

## Table 7.4 Activating receptors on NK cells

| Activating receptors | CD antigen | Adapter | Ligand | Species |
|---|---|---|---|---|
| KIR2DS 1,2,4,5,6 | CD158h, j, i, g, c | KARAP/DAP12 | Unknown | Human |
| KIR3DS1 | CD158e2 | KARAP/DAP12 | Unknown | Human |
| NKG2C, NKG2E | | KARAP/DAP12 | HLA-E, Qa-1 | Human, mouse |
| Ly49D | | KARAP/DAP12 | H2-D$^d$ | Mouse |
| Ly49H | | KARAP/DAP12 | m157 (MCMV) | Mouse |
| NKG2D | | DAP10 | MICA, MICB | Human |
| | | | ULBP1,2,3 | Human |
| | | KARAP/DAP12 | Rae1α,β,γ | Mouse |
| | | and DAP10 | H60 | Mouse |
| NKp46 | | CD3ζ, FcRγ | Viral hemagglutinin | Human, mouse |
| NKp44 | | KARAP/DAP12 | Unknown | Human |
| NKp30 | | CD3ζ, FcRγ | Unknown | Human |
| NKR-P1 | | FcRγ | Unknown | Human, mouse |

and CD8[+] αβ T cells. NKG2D forms a homodimeric structure, in contrast with other receptors of the NKG2 family, which form heterodimeric receptors with CD94. Two structurally distinct families of molecules, MIC and ULBP (UL16-binding proteins), have been identified as ligands of human NKG2D. The extracellular portions of ULBP and MIC proteins share weak homology with MHC class I molecules. Mouse NKG2D ligands are the glycosyl-phosphatidylinositol (GPI)-anchored membrane proteins of the Rae (retinoic acid early inducible 1) family and the transmembrane protein H60, both of which are also distantly related to MHC molecules. Interestingly, these human and mouse NKG2D ligands are induced and/or upregulated upon cellular distress. Finally, in humans, three natural cytotoxicity receptors (NCR) have been described – NKp30, NKp44, and NKp46 – whose engagement, alone or in combination, accounts for an important part of NK-cell natural cytotoxicity against multiple types of tumors in vitro.[21] Their ligands on tumor cells are unknown but it has been reported that NKp46 and NKp44 can recognise viral hemagglutinins.[24]

A common feature of all stimulatory receptors resides in the presence of a charged amino-acid residue in their transmembrane domains that is required for association with adapter signaling proteins (Table 7.4). The adapter proteins – FcRγ, CD3ζ, and the killer cell activating receptor-associated protein (KARAP/DAP12) – have very short extracellular domains but contain ITAM in their cytoplasmic domains, which allows them to associate with the signaling ZAP 70 and/or Syk protein tyrosine kinases. NKG2D is included in an oligomeric complex with the transducing polypeptide DAP10/KAP10 that contains a cytoplasmic YINM motif allowing the recruitment of the p85 subunit of the phosphatidylinositol 3'-kinase (PI3K).[25] In the mouse, two alternative splice products of the NKG2D gene have been described: NKG2D-L and NKG2D-S. Whereas mouse NKG2D-L associates selectively with DAP10, NKG2D-S is more promiscuous and associates with KARAP/DAP12 and DAP10.[26]

NK cells thus appear to have evolved at least two complementary mechanisms that ensure self-tolerance and elimination of pathogens: recognition of infectious non-self and stressed-induced self by activating receptors, as well as recognition of constitutive self by inhibitory receptors. If it holds true for other activating and inhibitory NK receptors, this strategy of NK-cell recognition is of major importance in the development of novel immunotherapeutic approaches based on NK-cell manipulation.[27]

## REFERENCES

1. Wang JH, Nichogiannopoulou A, Wu L et al. Selective defects in the development of the fetal and adult lymphoid system in mice with an ikaros null mutation. *Immunity* 1996; **5**: 537–49.

2. Spits H, Lanier LL, Phillips JH. Development of human T and natural killer cells. *Blood* 1995; **85**: 2654–70.

3. Lanier LL, Spits H, Phillips JH. The developmental relationship between NK cells and T cells. *Immunol Today* 1992; **13**: 392–5.

4. Valiante NM, Parham P. NK cells and CTL: opposite sides of the same coin. *Chem Immunol* 1996; **64**: 146–63.

5. Rocha B, Guy-Grand D, Vassali P. Extrathymic T cell differentiation. *Curr Opin Immunol* 1995; **7**: 235–42.

6. Spits H. Early stages in human and mouse T-cell development. *Curr Opin Immunol* 1994; **6**: 212–21.

7. von Boehmer H, Fehling HJ. Structure and function of the pre-T cell receptor. *Annu Rev Immunol* 1997; **15**: 433–52.

8. Malissen M, Trucy J, Jouvin-Marche E et al. Regulation of *TCR α* and *β* gene allelic exclusion during T-cell development. *Immunol Today* 1992; **13**: 315–22.

9. von Boehmer H. Developmental biology of T cells in T cell-receptor transgenic mice. *Annu Rev Immunol* 1990; **8**: 531–56.

10. Ashton-Rickardt PG, Bandeira A, Delaney JR et al. Evidence for a differential avidity model of T cell selection in the thymus. *Cell* 1994; **76**: 651–63.

11. Rodewald HR, Moingeon P, Lucich JL et al. A population of early fetal thymocytes expressing FcγRII/III contains precursors of T lymphocytes and natural killer cells. *Cell* 1992; **69**: 139–50.

12. Sánchez MJ, Muench MO, Roncarolo MG et al. Identification of a common T/natural killer cell progenitor in human fetal thymus. *J Exp Med* 1994; **180**: 569–76.

13. Puzanov IJ, Williams NS, Schatzle J et al. Ontogeny of NK cells and the bone marrow microenvironment: Where does IL15 fit in? *Res Immunol* 1997; **148**: 195–201.

14. Malissen B, Schmitt-Verhulst AM. Transmembrane signalling through the T-cell-receptor–CD3-complex. *Curr Opin Immunol* 1993; **5**: 324–33.

15. Trinchieri G. Biology of natural killer cells. *Adv Immunol* 1989; **47**: 187–376.

16. Carson W, Caligiuri M. Natural killer cell subsets and development. *Methods* 1996; **9**: 327–43.

17. Vivier E, Rochet N, Kochan J-P et al. Structural similarities between Fc receptors and T cell receptors: expression of the γ subunit of FcεRI in human T cells, NK cells and thymocytes. *J Immunol* 1991; **147**: 4263–70.

18. Vivier E, Sorrell JM, Ackerly M et al. Developmental regulation of a mucinlike glycoprotein selectively expressed on natural killer cells. *J Exp Med* 1993; **178**: 2023–33.

19. Moretta A, Biassoni R, Bottino C et al. Major histocompatibility complex class I-specific receptors on human natural killer and T lymphocytes. *Immunol Rev* 1997; **155**: 105–17.

20. Takei F, Brennan J, Mager DL. The Ly-49 family: genes, proteins and recognition of class I MHC. *Immunol Rev* 1997; **155**: 67–77.

21.  Diefenbach A, Raulet D. Strategies for target cell recognition by natural killer cells. *Immunol Rev* 2001; **181**: 170–84.

22.  Vivier E, Biron CA. A pathogen receptor on natural killer cells. *Science* 2002; **296**: 1248–9.

23.  Vivier E, Tomasello E, Paul P. Lymphocyte activation via NKG2D : towards a paradigm in immune recognition? *Curr Opin Immunol* 2002; **14**: 306–11.

24.  Arnon TI, Lev M, Katz G et al. Recognition of viral hemagglutinins by NKp44 but not by NKp30. *Eur J Immunol* 2001; **31**: 2680–9.

25.  Lanier L. On guard-activating NK cell receptors. *Nat Immunol* 2001; **2**: 23–7.

26.  Diefenbach A, Tomasello E, Lucas M et al. Stimulatory and costimulatory functions of the immunoreceptor NKG2D are determined by selective adaptor usage. *Nat Immunol* (in press).

27.  Ruggeri L, Capanni M, Urbani E et al. Effectiveness of donor natural killer cell alloreactivity in mismatched hematopoietic transplants. *Science* 2002; **295**: 2097–100.

# 8 Dendritic cell development

M Schnurr, Eugene Maraskovsky, and Jonathan Cebon

## Introduction

The immune system has evolved to protect the host from invasion by pathogens. Dendritic cells (DC) are a heterogeneous family of rare, phagocytic leukocytes, which form sentinel networks throughout the body, particularly at sites of potential pathogen entry such as epithelial and mucosal surfaces. Sentinel DC normally exist in an 'immature state', sampling the local environment for evidence of pathogens, tissue damage, or inflammation. These immature DC are particularly effective at antigen capture, uptake, and processing, but less efficient at antigen presentation. DC are rapidly activated in response to environmental stimuli, which signal 'danger', such as microbial products and cytokines found at inflammatory sites. Activation initiates a coordinated sequence of processes, which in their sum are termed 'maturation'. Mature DC switch off their capacity to capture antigen, and increase the expression of antigen-presenting molecules (major histocompatibility complex (MHC) molecule–peptide complexes and costimulatory molecules) on their cell surface. In addition, they gain the ability to migrate into T-cell areas of draining lymphoid tissue. This uniquely enables DC to present antigens to lymphocyte populations, thereby priming naive antigen-specific T cells, which recognize immunogenic peptides presented on MHC molecules. In this way, DC regulate the proliferation and differentiation of effector T cells. There is also evidence that DC can play a complimentary, yet paradoxically opposing, role in downregulating immunity in order to maintain tolerance toward self antigens. In addition to initiating and regulating T-cell responses, DC play roles in the activation of B cells and in innate immunity.

DC are not a homogeneous population of cells. As well as displaying heterogeneity in relation to activation or maturation state, they also derive from different hematopoietic lineages, although the common source is the marrow-derived multipotential CD34+ hematopoietic progenitor cell. The 'lineage model' proposes that different DC types emerge from distinct lineage pathways, each with distinct functions that regulate immune responses, such as helper T-cell differentiation. However, DC function is strongly influenced by the local environment. Environmental effects are mediated by cytokines and chemokines, through the activation of pattern recognition receptors by microbial products and through interaction with other leukocyte populations. The 'instruction model' proposes that the diversity of immune outcomes results from environmental instruction of DC. Most of our knowledge to date about DC has been gained from studying the murine system and from culturing human DC in vitro. DC research has gained momentum from the discovery that DC can be exploited as adjuvants in the immunotherapy of cancer and infectious disease. In this chapter, we shall discuss the heterogeneity of DC based on their development from hematopoietic precursors and their functional diversity due to environmental influences. Finally, we shall provide a clinical perspective for using DC in the immunotherapy of human disease.

## Development of DC from hematopoietic precursors

### DC origins and differentiation pathways

DC represent a heterogeneous population of antigen-presenting cells, which appear to develop via multiple differentiation pathways (Figure 8.1).[1-3] The life cycle of DC involves the differentiation from CD34+ progenitor cells into blood-borne DC precursors that seed peripheral tissues. Seminal work by Steinman and Cohn[4] in 1973 suggested that DC are myeloid in origin. This was based upon similarities with monocytes and macrophages in their tissue distribution, morphology, phenotype, and enzymatic and phagocytic capacities. Further evidence that DC have a myeloid origin derives from in vitro differentiation assays, in which DC were generated from monocytes or from intermediate precursors that retained the

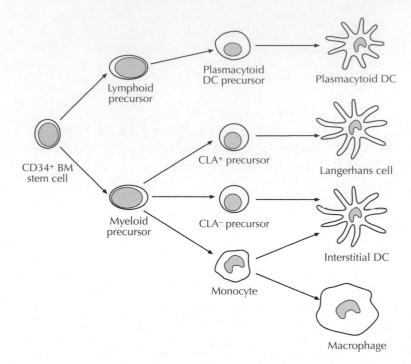

**Figure 8.1** Differentiation pathways for dendritic cells (DC). BM, bone marrow; CLA, (cutaneous lymphocyte-associated antigen)

capacity to generate macrophages.[5–7] However, DC may also derive from early thymic progenitors[8–11] or from lymphoid progenitors.[12–14]

## Human DC populations

Human DC are found throughout the body, being present in most organs except for the brain, parts of the eye, and the testes.[20] Despite their widespread distribution, it was not possible to study their function adequately until the discovery of effective tissue culture conditions and the determination of appropriate cell sorting techniques to enable sufficient numbers of DC to be isolated for functional studies. Most of our understanding of DC biology has been gained by studying DC derived from monocytes in vitro. Nonetheless, it is unclear whether monocyte-derived DC (MoDC) have a physiological counterpart, and two recent reports from our own group have demonstrated striking functional differences between MoDC and physiologic DC types in the blood.[21,22] Two DC populations are present in the peripheral blood, expressing a myeloid and a lymphoid/myeloid phenotype respectively. Epidermal DC or Langerhans cells are the prototype of tissue-resident DC and have also been generated in vitro using various precursor populations and cytokines. These DC types are discussed below.

### DC derived from CD34+ hematopoietic progenitors

Caux et al[5,23] produced landmark experimental evidence that DC could be generated from CD34+ progenitors. These progenitors, which can be derived from cord blood, bone marrow, or peripheral blood, differentiate into DC when cultured with granulocyte–macrophage colony-stimulating factor (GM-CSF) and

tumor necrosis factor (TNF)-α. Differentiation proceeds through two independent, immature DC progenitors, defined by their mutually exclusive expression of CD1a and CD14. When cultured with GM-CSF and TNF-α, CD14+CD1a– precursors become E-cadherin-negative mature DC, with a dermal or lymphoid-organ DC phenotype. By contrast, CD14–CD1a+ intermediates generate E-cadherin-positive Langerhans cell-like DC. DC can also be generated from human bone marrow CD34+ CD10+ Lin– precursors with combinations of interleukin (IL)-1β, IL-7, GM-CSF, stem cell factor (SCF, Steel factor, c-Kit ligand) and Flt3 ligand (FL).[12,17,18]

### Monocyte-derived DC

The best-studied model for human DC biology is the MoDC. A variety of techniques have been used to isolate monocytes and to generate DC in vitro. Generally, monocytes are cultured for 5–7 days with GM-CSF and IL-4,[6,24] although modifications of this cytokine combination have been reported. For example, MoDC could be generated using GM-CSF and interferon (IFN)-α,[25] GM-CSF and IL-13,[7] or IL-3 and IFN-β.[26] Of note, the majority of culture systems generate MoDC that are functionally immature. These immature MoDC can rapidly mature in response to microbial and other stimuli. Evidence that monocytes can differentiate into DC in vivo has been provided by a study from Randolph et al.[27] The same group also demonstrated that a subset of human monocytes is able to differentiate into DC-like cells in vitro during transendothelial migration, particularly following a phagocytic stimulus such as ingestion of latex beads.[28,29] Further studies are required to determine whether this pathway is the primary mechanism for differentiation of DC in vivo.

## Peripheral blood DC

At least two human DC subsets exist in the peripheral blood (PBDC),[30–32] collectively representing less than 1% of all mononuclear cells. PBDC express CD4 and high levels of MHC II molecules, but lack lineage markers such as CD3, CD14, CD16, CD19, CD20, and CD56. When isolated from blood, PBDC have an immature appearance and lack dendrites. Following appropriate in vitro tissue culture, they rapidly acquire dendritic processes and potent T-cell stimulatory capacity. The two PBDC populations differ in their expression of various cell surface markers (Table 8.1). One population expresses the myeloid markers CD11b, CD11c, CD13, CD33, and GM-CSFRα (CD116),

### Table 8.1 Expression of surface molecules and function of human dendritic cells (DC)

|  | Myeloid DC | Plasmacytoid DC |
| --- | --- | --- |
| **Surface markers** | | |
| CD1a | – | – |
| CD1c | + | – |
| CD4 | + | + |
| CD11c | ++ | – |
| CD11b | ++ | – |
| CD13 | + | – |
| CD25 | + | – |
| CD33 | ++ | – |
| CD40 | + | + |
| CD45RO | + | – |
| CD45RA | – | + |
| CD54 | ++ | ++ |
| CD62L | – | + |
| CD80 | +/– | +/– |
| CD83 | +/– | +/– |
| CD86 | +/– | +/– |
| CD116 (GM-CSFR) | + | – |
| CD123 (IL-3R) | – | + |
| MHC I | ++ | ++ |
| MHC II | ++ | ++ |
| Neuropilin 1 | – | ++ |
| pTα | – | + |
| **Pattern-recognition receptors** | | |
| TLR2 and 4 | + | – |
| TLR7 | + | + |
| TLR9 | – | + |
| MMR | + | – |
| DEC205 | + | – |
| BDCA2 | – | + |
| **Function** | | |
| Phagocytosis | + | – |
| Type I IFN | – | ++ |
| IL-12p70 | + | – |
| Th1/Th2 | +/+ | +/+ |

as well as the MHC-like molecules CD1b, c and d, but exhibits low expression of IL-3Rα (CD123w). This population is referred to as 'myeloid' or CD11c+ PBDC. The second population is known as plasmacytoid DC (formerly also called plasmacytoid T cells or plasmacytoid monocytes due to their distinct plasmacytoid morphology).[33,34] Plasmacytoid DC have very different cell surface molecules when compared with myeloid PBDC, expressing high levels of IL-3Rα, low levels of GM-CSFRα, and low levels of the above myeloid markers. Plasmacytoid DC can also be distinguished by the expression of BDCA-2 (a novel C-type lectin) and BDCA-4 (neuropilin-1).[35]

While it is generally accepted that CD11c+ PBDC are myeloid in origin, the lineage origin of plasmacytoid DC is less clear.[10,36–39] Plasmacytoid DCs are functionally distinct from CD11c+ PBDC. They depend on IL-3, whereas CD11c+ PBDC depend on GM-CSF for in vitro survival.[37,40,41] The two PBDC populations differ also in their sensitivity to microbial stimuli. Lipopolysaccharide (LPS) is a potent stimulus for CD11c+ PBDC.[42] In contrast, plasmacytoid DC are highly sensitive to certain viruses or unmethylated CpG DNA motifs and produce large amounts of IFN-α in response to these stimuli.[43,44] These differences are due to distinct expression of receptors for microbial products known as Toll-like receptors (TLR). CD11c+ PBDC express the LPS-receptor TLR4 and plasmacytoid DC express TLR9, a receptor recognizing unmethylated CpG DNA, which is characteristic of bacteria.[45,46] Plasmacytoid DC also appear to skew the T helper cell cytokine response differently to CD11c+ PBDC.[47,48] However, this seems to depend on the maturational stimuli that they encounter,[49] demonstrating that both lineage and environmental instruction play roles in T helper cell regulation. A new tissue culture technique that allows the in vitro generation of plasmacytoid DC from blood CD34+ CD45RA– IL-3Rα– cells[14,36] is likely to facilitate the study of this rare DC type.

## Langerhans cells and dermal DC

Epidermal DC, or Langerhans cells (LC), together with dermal DC, form an immune surveillance network in the skin. LC possess unique trilaminar cytoplasmic structures known as Birbeck granules and express langerin, a type II lectin that can bind mannose, a sugar that is rarely displayed as a terminal sugar residue on mammalian cell surfaces although it is ubiquitous on the surfaces of lower organisms. The induction of Birbeck granules is a consequence of the antigen-capture function of langerin,[50] Additionally, LC may be identified by their expression of CD1a, MHC II and Fc-IgG receptors type II (CD32), Fc-IgE receptors type I, and C3bi receptor (CD11b). LC may be generated from CD34+ progenitors. Exposure of CD34+ progenitors to GM-CSF and TNF-α gives rise to a population of cells that possess Birbeck granules and are CD1a[+] and E-cadherin-positive.[23,51] Langerhans cell-like cells have also been generated in vitro from monocytes[52,53] or from blood CD11c[+] PBDC[54] by culturing these cells with the cytokine combination of GM-CSF, IL-4, and transforming growth factor (TGF)-β.

Dermal DC may also be generated from CD34[+] progenitors when cultured with GM-CSF and TNF-α via an alternative differentiation pathway involving CD1a⁻ CD14[+] intermediates.[5] These dermal DC possess factor XIIIa, lack Birbeck granules, and do not stain for E-cadherin. The functions of both LC and dermal DC can be modulated by a range of cytokines produced by keratinocytes.[55] Pathogens may also activate LC directly. Functional differences between LC and dermal DC remain to be clearly defined.

## DC differentiation from multipotential thymic precursors

Although most studies examining the origins of DC indicate that they are of myeloid lineage, they may also arise from lymphoid-committed precursors. This has best been described in the mouse, where CD8α[+] thymic DC appear to be derived from lymphoid-committed progenitors that lack myeloid potential.[13] Although CD8α[+] DC are also found in the spleen and lymph nodes, it is less clear whether these DC subsets (which are phenotypically similar to their thymic counterparts) are derived from lymphoid-committed precursors. Traver et al[15] demonstrated that both CD8α[+] and CD8α⁻ DCs could arise from common lymphoid and myeloid progenitors in thymus and spleen.[15] Thus, CD8α expression may not reflect lineage derivation but more likely maturation or differentiation stage and perhaps functional commitment of the DC. Studies by Wu et al[16] further clarified these findings by demonstrating that myeloid precursors give rise to both CD8α⁻ and CD8α[+] DC, whereas lymphoid precursors predominantly give rise to CD8α[+] DC.[16] Therefore, the hematopoietic precursor origin of DC may bias but not dictate the phenotype of the DC produced.

In the human, evidence for a lymphoid origin of DC relies predominantly on in vitro studies. Bone marrow CD34[+] CD10[+] Lin⁻ precursors with T-, B-, and NK-cell potential, but lacking myeloid differentiation capacity, can generate DC after culture with IL-1β, IL-7, GM-CSF, SCF, and FL.[12] Putative lymphoid-derived DC may also be generated from CD34[+] CD1a⁻ lymphoid-committed thymic precursors after culture with IL-7, TNF-α, SCF, and FL.[17,18] Importantly, the myeloid growth factor GM-CSF was dispensable in these culture systems. Despite their apparent lymphoid commitment, these thymic precursors retained myeloid capacity, as they could give rise to monocytes when cultured with macrophage colony-stimulating factor (M-CSF). More recently, it has been shown that the thymus contains a DC precursor population with lymphoid and myelomonocytic potential.[19] It was found that intrathymic DC are myeloid in origin, since they arise from CD34[+] early thymic progenitors that display myelomonocytic differentiation potential. Furthermore, phenotypically and functionally equivalent myeloid precursors devoid of T-cell potential were shown to exist in vivo in the postnatal thymus. Although these studies seem to contradict each other, they demonstrate that DC precursors are capable of considerable plasticity. They also indicate that the differentiation pathways are not exclusive or irreversible. Thus, apparent commitment to 'myeloid' or 'lymphoid' pathways may be contingent on the context in which DC develop.

## Cytokines that expand DC numbers in vivo

Several cytokines are known to expand DC numbers in vivo, including granulocyte colony-stimulating factor (G-CSF),[56,57] GM-CSF,[58] FL,[59,60] and a synthetic G-CSF–FL fusion protein called progenipoietin (ProGP).[61] FL stimulates the proliferation of stem and progenitor cells by binding to the FL-receptor (Flt3), which is a type III receptor tyrosine kinase member of the platelet-derived growth factor (PDGF) family. Although FL is expressed by many different cell types and in many tissues, its receptor Flt3 is restricted to hematopoietic progenitors, early B cells, and myeloid cells.[62] Daily subcutaneous injections of recombinant human FL for 10 days in healthy volunteers resulted in a 40-fold increase in the numbers of circulating CD11c[+] PBDC.[60] These DC were phenotypically immature, expressing low levels of CD80, CD83, and CD86 and intermediate levels of HLA-DR. Following in vitro culture, these markers were rapidly upregulated. While FL expands both CD11c[+] PBDC and plasmacytoid DC, G-CSF only expands plasmacytoid DC.[57] A recent study in mice compared the effect of all of the above DC-expanding cytokines on DC generation in vivo.[61] The study found not only that different cytokines expanded different DC subpopulations, but that DC populations that appeared to be identical at the phenotypic level functioned differently depending on the cytokines that were used to generate them. This suggests that the use of certain cytokines in vivo could be used to generate DC with distinct functions.

## Cytokines inhibiting DC differentiation

The study of culture conditions leading to DC development from precursors has provided insight into cytokine environments that can interfere with DC differentiation. A number of inhibitory cytokines have been found to act during early phases of DC differentiation, including vascular endothelial growth factor (VEGF),[63] TGF-β,[64] IL-10,[65–67] IL-6,[68,69] M-CSF,[69] and prostaglandin (PG)E₂.[70] Interestingly, tumor cells can produce these factors. It therefore appears that tumors may be able to inhibit DC function, and deploy this as a mechanism for evading immune surveillance.

# Maturation and functional development of DC

DC display extraordinary plasticity, transforming from one form to another in order to perform a variety of distinct and highly specialized functions. Immature DC are extremely efficient in the uptake and processing of antigen, but are poor inducers of T-cell proliferation. Upon maturation, DC develop characteristic cytoplasmic processes (dendrites), lose their capacity to take up antigens, and upregulate molecules for DC–T-cell interaction, such as costimulatory and MHC molecules (Figure 8.2). Furthermore, DC upregulate certain chemokine receptors, enabling them to migrate from peripheral tissues to lymph nodes, which is a prerequisite for interaction with T cells.[1] To control these transformations, complex regulation is required throughout the DC life cycle. Soluble and membrane-associated signals enable fine control of phenotype and function through maturation and migration and, finally, orchestrate immune responses.

## Signals inducing DC maturation

The tissue environment plays a major role in the differentiation of DC and provides an important link between the innate and adaptive immune system. DC mature in response to four classes of stimuli found at sites of infection or inflammation: (1) pro-inflammatory mediators, (2) pathogen-derived signals, (3) T-cell-derived signals, and (4) mediators of cell stress and damage. These factors generally accumulate only under pathological conditions and are recognized by the DC as 'danger' signals.[71]

Pro-inflammatory mediators that induce DC maturation include prostaglandins and cytokines, such as IFN-$\alpha/\beta$, TNF-$\alpha$, and IL-1$\beta$. These factors can be released by monocytes[72] and keratinocytes.[73] Microbes (bacteria, viruses, and parasites) and their products, such as LPS, double-stranded RNA, and bacterial DNA motifs, are recognized through TLR on DC.[74] Other potent DC stimuli are members of the TNF family, such as CD40 ligand (CD40L), which is present on activated T helper cells[75–77] and mediates DC activation when T cells and DC engage in lymphoid tissues. CD40L is also present on other immune and tissue cells, so this mechanism is also likely to be important in peripheral tissues. Mediators released during cell stress and damage, such as nucleotides[78] and heat-shock proteins,[79] also have the potential to

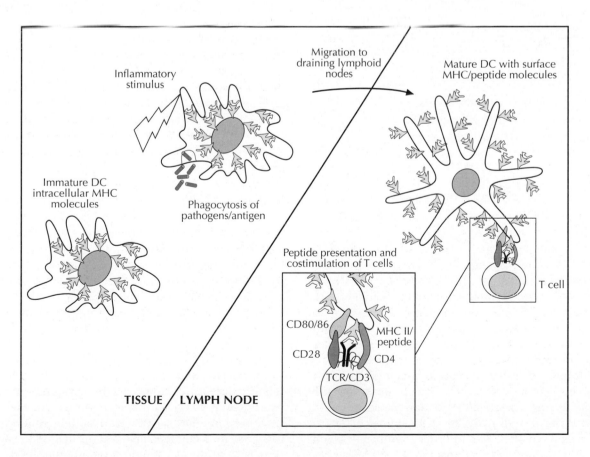

**Figure 8.2** Maturation and functional development of dendritic cells (DC). MHC, major histocompatibility complex; TCR, T-cell receptor.

activate DC. Stimulation by these various mediators alone or in combination results in qualitative and quantitative differences in DC maturation. This is reflected in differences in the levels of various DC surface molecules, T-cell stimulatory capacity, and cytokine production. As a result, the final immune outcome depends on the net composition of the stimuli experienced by the DC. This in turn reflects the context in which activation occurs.

## Regulation of antigen uptake, processing, and presentation

Immature DC take up antigens very efficiently by macropinocytosis and receptor-mediated endocytosis using a variety of receptors such as integrins, C-type lectins and Fc receptors, which bind to immune complexes. Integrins such as $\alpha_v\beta_5$ also mediate the uptake of apoptotic cells.[80] Examples of C-type lectin receptors that are expressed by DC are the mannose macrophage receptor (MMR) and DEC205, which bind to molecules that have distinguishing carbohydrate structures (reviewed in reference 81). Following internalization, antigen is transported to the late endosomes and lysosomes of the endocytic system of the MHC II compartment. In immature DC, MHC II molecules are almost entirely located within intracellular endocytic vacuoles, colocalizing with lysosomal-associated membrane proteins. Under these conditions, internalized antigens are loaded onto MHC molecules. Upon maturation, antigen uptake is rapidly downregulated and MHC II molecules are redistributed to the cell surface over 12–24 hours for antigen presentation.[82] In addition, MHC II levels are regulated by their rate of turnover. In immature DC, MHC II molecules are constantly degraded, whereas in mature DC, a lower rate of degradation results in a longer half-life and surface accumulation.[82,83] These mechanisms contribute to the highly efficient presentation of antigen to CD4 T cells by mature DC (Figure 8.2). In addition to presentation on MHC II molecules, DC are also capable of stimulating CD8+ T-cell responses by presenting exogenous antigen on MHC I molecules, a phenomenon termed 'cross-presentation'. Processing of antigen for the MHC I pathway involves an intracellular proteolytic enzyme complex known as the proteasome; however, the precise mechanisms regulating cross-presentation are not fully understood. For clinical vaccine purposes, targeting antigens to DC surface receptors, such as DEC205 or $\alpha_v\beta_5$ integrin, can enhance MHC I antigen processing, but productive T-cell immunity only occurs if an associated maturation stimulus is included in the strategy.[80,84] The ability of DC to cross-prime naive T cells in order to induce the generation of tumor antigen-specific T cells provides the rationale for clinical vaccination trials using DC (see the final section of this chapter).

## Regulation of migratory function

Both immature and mature DC are mobile cell populations, migrating to peripheral sites and lymphoid tissue respectively. DC homing is regulated by migration in response to chemokine gradients. It has been proposed that DC migration occurs in a stepwise fashion in which each distinct step is regulated by a particular chemokine–receptor pair.[85] For homing to peripheral inflammatory sites, immature DC migrate towards chemokines such as macrophage inflammatory protein (MIP)-1α (CCL3), monocyte chemoattractant protein (MCP)-1 (CCL2), and RANTES (regulated upon activation normal T-cell expressed and secreted, CCL5). Upon maturation, DC upregulate chemokine receptors in order to then migrate to lymphoid tissue. Here, the homing chemokines include the CCR7-binding chemokines, 6Ckine (CCL21) and MIP-3β (CCL19).[85–87] Mature DC can express chemokine receptors for (and migrate towards) both of these chemokine classes. The trafficking outcome may therefore depend on which gradient is strongest at any given tissue location in which the DC resides.

## T-cell activation by DC

The interaction between DC and T cells involves the binding of cell surface receptors and their ligands, which are responsible for (i) specificity, (ii) adhesion, and (iii) the regulation of T-cell proliferation through costimulatory and inhibitory signaling molecules. In addition, soluble mediators stimulate the proliferation and polarization of the T-cell response. The antigen, presented as MHC–peptide complexes, determines the specificity of the T-cell response. These are present on DC at densities 10- to 100-fold higher than on other antigen-presenting cells, such as B cells and monocytes.[88] Physical contact between DC and T cells is facilitated by adhesion molecules, such as integrins and members of the immunoglobulin superfamily (CD54 and CD58).[1] DC-SIGN is a C-type lectin abundantly expressed on DC that mediates adhesion to T cells and stabilizes DC–T-cell contact.[89,90] Costimulatory molecules, such as CD86,[91,92] amplify the T-cell response. This is potentially countered by regulatory inhibitors such as CTLA4 (reviewed in references 93 and 94). In addition to specificity signals provided through the MHC–peptide complexes and regulatory signals via the costimulatory factors, DC provide a 'third signal', which reflects information concerning the local environment. This signal polarizes the T helper (Th) repertoire toward a Th1 or Th2 response.[95] Th1 cell polarization is favored by several cytokines produced by DC, such as IL-12, IFN-α, IL-18, IL-23, and IL-27 (reviewed in reference 96). Additionally, the cytokine response by T cells may be determined by the activation stage of the DC, the dose of antigen, the strength of DC–T-cell interaction, the ratio of DC to T cells, and the type of DC (these are reviewed in reference 97).

## DC and the induction of tolerance

In addition to stimulating immunity, DC also present antigens in order to maintain tolerance to 'self' and suppress autoimmune responses. This process requires the silencing of self-reactive T cells. This probably takes place in two separate sites; in both, however, DC play the critical role.[98,99] Central tolerance occurs in the thymus, where DC present self antigens to developing T cells with the specific purpose of deleting those that are self-reactive.[100] However, this mechanism has limitations: self-reactive T and B cells may escape deletion, some antigens may not access the thymus, and others may only be expressed in later life after the lymphocyte repertoire has been established. In addition, lymphocyte receptors specific for foreign antigens may also cross-react with self-antigens. As a result, a separate mechanism known as 'peripheral tolerance' appears to exist. Here, DC are able to silence self-reactive T cells in tissues, outside the thymus. The switch between maintaining tolerance and stimulating immunity appears to depend on the maturation state of the DC. Steinman and Nussenzweig[99] suggest that DC in the steady state (i.e. in the immature stage in the absence of danger signals) define immunological self and tolerize T cells. In contrast, activation and maturation of DC converts them into cells that stimulate immunity. This hypothesis is supported by investigations that used either immature or mature DC to vaccinate healthy volunteers against an influenza antigen. A single injection of peptide-pulsed mature DC rapidly expanded peptide-specific immunity.[101] In contrast, the injection of immature peptide-pulsed DC resulted in inhibition of peptide-specific IFN-$\gamma$-secreting T cells and the appearance of peptide-specific IL-10-secreting T cells.[102] IL-10 is a cytokine produced by 'regulatory' T cells, which are able to suppress the responses of other T cells.[103]

## Clinical perspectives

The ability of DC to rapidly induce T-cell immunity has been demonstrated in normal human volunteers and cancer patients. Several clinical trials using DC-based anticancer vaccine therapy have been published to date, some with promising results (reviewed in references 104 and 105). The study protocols for DC preparation and the choice of antigen and vaccination routes as well as schedules have varied considerably, making it difficult to compare different strategies. In most protocols, DC are expanded in vivo with growth factors or derived from cultured monocytes or CD34+ progenitor cells. DC are then pulsed with antigen in the form of peptides, proteins, tumor RNA, or tumor cell lysates, exposed to maturation-inducing stimuli, and subsequently injected into the patient's skin, blood, or lymph nodes. The production of such a DC vaccine is shown in Figure 8.3. The optimization of DC vaccination protocols will require a better understanding of DC biology. Several critical variables are currently under preclinical and clinical investigation, such as the identification of new tumor antigens, choice of DC type and antigen source, DC maturation stimuli, use of adjuvants, and routes of vaccine delivery, as well as the dose and timing of vaccinations. Strategies to manipulate DC function genetically in order to improve vaccine delivery and the subsequent induction of a powerful immune response are also being developed. In parallel approaches, DC are also being developed in strategies that seek to delete autoreactive T cells. Clinical trials for the treatment of autoimmune disease have not yet been reported. Considerable progress has been made in recent years in monitoring rare antigen-specific lymphocytes in the peripheral blood of cancer patients. Ongoing trials should be helpful in correlating immune with clinical responses and to identify subgroups of patients who

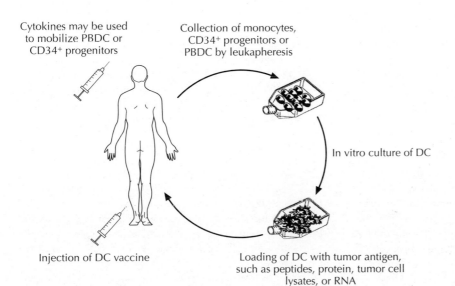

Cytokines may be used to mobilize PBDC or CD34+ progenitors

Collection of monocytes, CD34+ progenitors or PBDC by leukapheresis

In vitro culture of DC

Injection of DC vaccine

Loading of DC with tumor antigen, such as peptides, protein, tumor cell lysates, or RNA

**Figure 8.3** Production of a dendritic cell (DC) vaccine. PBDC, peripheral blood DC.

might benefit from such a treatment. Results from controlled clinical trials have to be awaited to assess the value of DC vaccination in the treatment of cancer, infectious disease, and autoimmunity.

## REFERENCES

1. Banchereau J, Steinman RM. Dendritic cells and the control of immunity. *Nature* 1998; **392**: 245–52.

2. Ardavin C, Martinez del Hoyo G, Martin P et al. Origin and differentiation of dendritic cells. *Trends Immunol* 2001; **22**: 691–700.

3. Shortman K, Liu YJ. Mouse and human dendritic cell subtypes. *Nat Rev Immunol* 2002; **2**: 151–61.

4. Steinman RM, Cohn ZA. Identification of a novel cell type in peripheral lymphoid organs of mice. I. Morphology, quantitation, tissue distribution. *J Exp Med* 1973; **137**: 1142–62.

5. Caux C, Vanbervliet B, Massacrier C et al. CD34+ hematopoietic progenitors from human cord blood differentiate along two independent dendritic cell pathways in response to GM-CSF + TNFα. *J Exp Med* 1996; **184**: 695–706.

6. Sallusto F, Lanzavecchia A. Efficient presentation of soluble antigen by cultured human dendritic cells is maintained by granulocyte/macrophage colony-stimulating factor plus interleukin 4 and downregulated by tumor necrosis factor α. *J Exp Med* 1994; **179**: 1109–18.

7. Romani N, Reider D, Heuer M et al. Generation of mature dendritic cells from human blood. An improved method with special regard to clinical applicability. *J Immunol Meth* 1996; **196**: 137–51.

8. Ardavin C, Wu L, Li CL, Shortman K. Thymic dendritic cells and T cells develop simultaneously in the thymus from a common precursor population. *Nature* 1993; **362**: 761–3.

9. Res P, Martinez-Caceres E, Cristina Jaleco A et al. CD34+CD38dim cells in the human thymus can differentiate into T, natural killer, and dendritic cells but are distinct from pluripotent stem cells. *Blood* 1996; **87**: 5196–206.

10. Res PC, Couwenberg F, Vyth-Dreese FA, Spits H. Expression of pTα mRNA in a committed dendritic cell precursor in the human thymus. *Blood* 1999; **94**: 2647–57.

11. Spits H, Blom B, Jaleco AC et al. Early stages in the development of human T, natural killer and thymic dendritic cells. *Immunol Rev* 1998; **165**: 75–86.

12. Galy A, Travis M, Cen D, Chen B. Human T, B, natural killer, and dendritic cells arise from a common bone marrow progenitor cell subset. *Immunity* 1995; **3**: 459–73.

13. Wu L, Li CL, Shortman K. Thymic dendritic cell precursors: relationship to the T lymphocyte lineage and phenotype of the dendritic cell progeny. *J Exp Med* 1996; **184**: 903–11.

14. Spits H, Couwenberg F, Bakker AQ et al. Id2 and Id3 inhibit development of CD34+ stem cells into predendritic cell (pre-DC)2 but not into pre-DC1. Evidence for a lymphoid origin of pre-DC2. *J Exp Med* 2000; **192**: 1775–84.

15. Traver D, Akashi K, Manz M et al. Development of CD8α-positive dendritic cells from a common myeloid progenitor. *Science* 2000; **290**: 2152–4.

16. Wu L, D'Amico A, Hochrein H et al. Development of thymic and splenic dendritic cell populations from different hemopoietic precursors. *Blood* 2001; **98**: 3376–82.

17. Dalloul AH, Patry C, Salamero J et al. Functional and phenotypic analysis of thymic CD34+CD1a− progenitor-derived dendritic cells: predominance of CD1a+ differentiation pathway. *J Immunol* 1999; **162**: 5821–8.

18. Kelly KA, Lucas K, Hochrein H et al. Development of dendritic cells in culture from human and murine thymic precursor cells. *Cell Mol Biol (Noisy-le-grand)* 2001; **47**: 43–54.

19. de Yebenes VG, Carrasco YR, Ramiro AR, Toribio ML. Identification of a myeloid intrathymic pathway of dendritic cell development marked by expression of the granulocyte macrophage-colony-stimulating factor receptor. *Blood* 2002; **99**: 2948–56.

20. Hart DN. Dendritic cells: unique leukocyte populations which control the primary immune response. *Blood* 1997; **90**: 3245–87.

21. Luft T, Jefford M, Luetjens P et al. Functionally distinct dendritic cell (DC) populations induced by physiologic stimuli: prostaglandin $E_2$ regulates the migratory capacity of specific DC subsets. *Blood* 2002; **100**: 1362–72.

22. Schnurr M, Toy T, Stoitzner P et al. ATP gradients inhibit the migratory capacity of specific human dendritic cell types: implications for P2Y11 receptor signaling. *Blood* 2003; **102**: 613–20.

23. Caux C, Dezutter-Dambuyant C, Schmitt D, Banchereau J. GM-CSF and TNF-α cooperate in the generation of dendritic Langerhans cells. *Nature* 1992; **360**: 258–61.

24. Romani N, Gruner S, Brang D et al. Proliferating dendritic cell progenitors in human blood. *J Exp Med* 1994; **180**: 83–93.

25. Santini SM, Lapenta C, Logozzi M et al. Type I interferon as a powerful adjuvant for monocyte-derived dendritic cell development and activity in vitro and in Hu-PBL-SCID mice. *J Exp Med* 2000; **191**: 1777–88.

26. Buelens C, Bartholome EJ, Amraoui Z et al. Interleukin-3 and interferon β cooperate to induce differentiation of monocytes into dendritic cells with potent helper T-cell stimulatory properties. *Blood* 2002; **99**: 993–8.

27. Randolph GJ, Inaba K, Robbiani DF et al. Differentiation of phagocytic monocytes into lymph node dendritic cells in vivo. *Immunity* 1999; **11**: 753–61.

28. Randolph GJ, Beaulieu S, Lebecque S et al. Differentiation of monocytes into dendritic cells in a model of transendothelial trafficking. *Science* 1998; **282**: 480–3.

29. Randolph GJ, Sanchez-Schmitz G, Liebman RM, Schakel K. The CD16+ (FcγRIII+) subset of human monocytes preferentially becomes migratory dendritic cells in a model tissue setting. *J Exp Med* 2002; **196**: 517–27.

30. O'Doherty U, Steinman RM, Peng M et al. Dendritic cells freshly isolated from human blood express CD4 and mature into typical immunostimulatory dendritic cells after culture in monocyte-conditioned medium. *J Exp Med* 1993; **178**: 1067–76.

31. O'Doherty U, Peng M, Gezelter S et al. Human blood contains two subsets of dendritic cells, one immunologically mature and the other immature. *Immunology* 1994; **82**: 487–93.

32. Robinson SP, Patterson S, English N et al. Human

peripheral blood contains two distinct lineages of dendritic cells. *Eur J Immunol* 1999; **29**: 2769–78.

33. Facchetti F, Candiago E, Vermi W. Plasmacytoid monocytes express IL3-receptor α and differentiate into dendritic cells. *Histopathology* 1999; **35**: 88–9.

34. Vollenweider R, Lennert K. Plasmacytoid T-cell clusters in non-specific lymphadenitis. *Virchows Arch B Cell Pathol Incl Mol Pathol* 1983; **44**: 1–14.

35. Dzionek A, Fuchs A, Schmidt P et al. BDCA-2, BDCA-3, and BDCA-4: three markers for distinct subsets of dendritic cells in human peripheral blood. *J Immunol* 2000; **165**: 6037–46.

36. Blom B, Ho S, Antonenko S, Liu YJ. Generation of interferon α-producing predendritic cell (Pre-DC)2 from human CD34+ hematopoietic stem cells. *J Exp Med* 2000; **192**: 1785–96.

37. Olweus J, BitMansour A, Warnke R et al. Dendritic cell ontogeny: a human dendritic cell lineage of myeloid origin. *Proc Natl Acad Sci USA* 1997; **94**: 12551–6.

38. Strobl H, Scheinecker C, Riedl E et al. Identification of CD68+lin- peripheral blood cells with dendritic precursor characteristics. *J Immunol* 1998; **161**: 740–8.

39. Banchereau J, Pulendran B, Steinman R, Palucka K. Will the making of plasmacytoid dendritic cells in vitro help unravel their mysteries? *J Exp Med* 2000; **192**: F39–44.

40. Grouard G, Rissoan MC, Filgueira L et al. The enigmatic plasmacytoid T cells develop into dendritic cells with interleukin (IL)-3 and CD40-ligand. *J Exp Med* 1997; **185**: 1101–11.

41. Kohrgruber N, Halanek N, Groger M et al. Survival, maturation, and function of CD11c- and CD11c+ peripheral blood dendritic cells are differentially regulated by cytokines. *J Immunol* 1999; **163**: 3250–9.

42. Willmann K, Dunne JF. A flow cytometric immune function assay for human peripheral blood dendritic cells. *J Leukoc Biol* 2000; **67**: 536–44.

43. Cella M, Jarrossay D, Facchetti F et al. Plasmacytoid monocytes migrate to inflamed lymph nodes and produce large amounts of type I interferon. *Nat Med* 1999; **5**: 919–23.

44. Siegal FP, Kadowaki N, Shodell M et al. The nature of the principal type 1 interferon-producing cells in human blood. *Science* 1999; **284**: 1835–7.

45. Hemmi H, Takeuchi O, Kawai T et al. A Toll-like receptor recognizes bacterial DNA. *Nature* 2000; **408**: 740–5.

46. Hornung V, Rothenfusser S, Britsch S et al. Quantitative expression of Toll-like receptor 1–10 mRNA in cellular subsets of human peripheral blood mononuclear cells and sensitivity to CpG oligodeoxynucleotides. *J Immunol* 2002; **168**: 4531–7.

47. Rissoan MC, Soumelis V, Kadowaki N et al. Reciprocal control of T helper cell and dendritic cell differentiation. *Science* 1999; **283**: 1183–6.

48. Liu YJ, Kadowaki N, Rissoan MC, Soumelis V. T cell activation and polarization by DC1 and DC2. *Curr Top Microbiol Immunol* 2000; **251**: 149–59.

49. Ito T, Amakawa R, Kaisho T et al. Interferon-α and interleukin-12 are induced differentially by Toll-like receptor 7 ligands in human blood dendritic cell subsets. *J Exp Med* 2002; **195**: 1507–12.

50. Valladeau J, Ravel O, Dezutter-Dambuyant C et al. Langerin, a novel C-type lectin specific to Langerhans cells, is an endocytic receptor that induces the formation of Birbeck granules. *Immunity* 2000; **12**: 71–81.

51. Strunk D, Rappersberger K, Egger C et al. Generation of human dendritic cells/Langerhans cells from circulating CD34+ hematopoietic progenitor cells. *Blood* 1996; **87**: 1292–302.

52. Mohamadzadeh M, Berard F, Essert G et al. Interleukin 15 skews monocyte differentiation into dendritic cells with features of Langerhans cells. *J Exp Med* 2001; **194**: 1013–20.

53. Geissmann F, Prost C, Monnet JP et al. Transforming growth factor β1, in the presence of granulocyte/macrophage colony-stimulating factor and interleukin 4, induces differentiation of human peripheral blood monocytes into dendritic Langerhans cells. *J Exp Med* 1998; **187**: 961–6.

54. Ito T, Inaba M, Inaba K et al. A CD1a+/CD11c+ subset of human blood dendritic cells is a direct precursor of Langerhans cells. *J Immunol* 1999; **163**: 1409–19.

55. Luger TA, Bhardwaj RS, Grabbe S, Schwarz T. Regulation of the immune response by epidermal cytokines and neurohormones. *J Dermatol Sci* 1996; **13**: 5–10.

56. Arpinati M, Green CL, Heimfeld S et al. Granulocyte-colony stimulating factor mobilizes T helper 2-inducing dendritic cells. *Blood* 2000; **95**: 2484–90.

57. Pulendran B, Banchereau J, Burkeholder S et al. Flt3-ligand and granulocyte colony-stimulating factor mobilize distinct human dendritic cell subsets in vivo. *J Immunol* 2000; **165**: 566–72.

58. Daro E, Pulendran B, Brasel K et al. Polyethylene glycol-modified GM-CSF expands CD11bhighCD11chigh but not CD11blowCD11chigh murine dendritic cells in vivo: a comparative analysis with Flt3 ligand. *J Immunol* 2000; **165**: 49–58.

59. Maraskovsky E, Brasel K, Teepe M et al. Dramatic increase in the numbers of functionally mature dendritic cells in Flt3 ligand-treated mice: multiple dendritic cell subpopulations identified. *J Exp Med* 1996; **184**: 1953–62.

60. Maraskovsky E, Daro E, Roux E et al. In vivo generation of human dendritic cell subsets by Flt3 ligand. *Blood* 2000; **96**: 878–84.

61. O'Keeffe M, Hochrein H, Vremec D et al. Effects of administration of progenipoietin 1, Flt-3 ligand, granulocyte colony-stimulating factor, and pegylated granulocyte–macrophage colony-stimulating factor on dendritic cell subsets in mice. *Blood* 2002; **99**: 2122–30.

62. Rasko JE, Metcalf D, Rossner MT et al. The flt3/flk-2 ligand: receptor distribution and action on murine haemopoietic cell survival and proliferation. *Leukemia* 1995; **9**: 2058–66.

63. Gabrilovich DI, Chen HL, Girgis KR et al. Production of vascular endothelial growth factor by human tumors inhibits the functional maturation of dendritic cells. *Nat Med* 1996; **2**: 1096–103.

64. Bonham CA, Lu L, Banas RA et al. TGF-β1 pretreatment impairs the allostimulatory function of human bone marrow-derived antigen-presenting cells for both naive and primed T cells. *Transplant Immunol* 1996; **4**: 186–91.

65. Buelens C, Verhasselt V, De Groote D et al. Human dendritic cell responses to lipopolysaccharide and CD40 ligation are differentially regulated by interleukin-10. *Eur J Immunol* 1997; **27**: 1848–52.

66. D'Amico G, Frascaroli G, Bianchi G et al. Uncoupling of inflammatory chemokine receptors by IL-10: generation of functional decoys. *Nat Immunol* 2000; **1**: 387–91.

67. Allavena P, Piemonti L, Longoni D et al. IL-10 prevents the differentiation of monocytes to dendritic cells but pro-

motes their maturation to macrophages. *Eur J Immunol* 1998; **28**: 359–69.

68. Chomarat P, Banchereau J, Davoust J, Palucka AK. IL-6 switches the differentiation of monocytes from dendritic cells to macrophages. *Nat Immunol* 2000; **1**: 510–14.

69. Menetrier-Caux C, Montmain G, Dieu MC et al. Inhibition of the differentiation of dendritic cells from CD34+ progenitors by tumor cells: role of interleukin-6 and macrophage colony-stimulating factor. *Blood* 1998; **92**: 4778–91.

70. Kalinski P, Hilkens CM, Snijders A et al. IL-12-deficient dendritic cells, generated in the presence of prostaglandin E2, promote type 2 cytokine production in maturing human naive T helper cells. *J Immunol* 1997; **159**: 28–35.

71. Gallucci S, Matzinger P. Danger signals: SOS to the immune system. *Curr Opin Immunol* 2001; **13**: 114–19.

72. Jonuleit H, Kuhn U, Muller G et al. Pro-inflammatory cytokines and prostaglandins induce maturation of potent immunostimulatory dendritic cells under fetal calf serum-free conditions. *Eur J Immunol* 1997; **27**: 3135–42.

73. Kock A, Schwarz T, Kirnbauer R et al. Human keratinocytes are a source for tumor necrosis factor α: evidence for synthesis and release upon stimulation with endotoxin or ultraviolet light. *J Exp Med* 1990; **172**: 1609–14.

74. Takeda K, Kaisho T, Akira S. Toll-like receptors. *Annu Rev Immunol* 2003; **21**: 335–76.

75. Ridge JP, Di Rosa F, Matzinger P. A conditioned dendritic cell can be a temporal bridge between a CD4+ T-helper and a T-killer cell. *Nature* 1998; **393**: 474–8.

76. Bennett SR, Carbone FR, Karamalis F et al. Help for cytotoxic-T-cell responses is mediated by CD40 signalling. *Nature* 1998; **393**: 478–80.

77. Schoenberger SP, Toes RE, van der Voort EI et al. T-cell help for cytotoxic T lymphocytes is mediated by CD40–CD40L interactions. *Nature* 1998; **393**: 480–3.

78. Schnurr M, Then F, Galambos P et al. Extracellular ATP and TNF-α synergize in the activation and maturation of human dendritic cells. *J Immunol* 2000; **165**: 4704–9.

79. Srivastava P. Roles of heat-shock proteins in innate and adaptive immunity. *Nat Rev Immunol* 2002; **2**: 185–94.

80. Albert ML, Pearce SF, Francisco LM et al. Immature dendritic cells phagocytose apoptotic cells via α$_v$β$_5$ and CD36, and cross-present antigens to cytotoxic T lymphocytes. *J Exp Med* 1998; **188**: 1359–68.

81. Figdor CG, van Kooyk Y, Adema GJ. C-type lectin receptors on dendritic cells and Langerhans cells. *Nat Rev Immunol* 2002; **2**: 77–84.

82. Pierre P, Turley SJ, Gatti E et al. Developmental regulation of MHC II transport in mouse dendritic cells. *Nature* 1997; **388**: 787–92.

83. Cella M, Engering A, Pinet V et al. Inflammatory stimuli induce accumulation of MHC II complexes on dendritic cells. *Nature* 1997; **388**: 782–7.

84. Bonifaz L, Bonnyay D, Mahnke K et al. Efficient targeting of protein antigen to the dendritic cell receptor DEC-205 in the steady state leads to antigen presentation on major histocompatibility complex class I products and peripheral CD8+ T cell tolerance. *J Exp Med* 2002; **196**: 1627–38.

85. Sallusto F, Palermo B, Lenig D et al. Distinct patterns and kinetics of chemokine production regulate dendritic cell function. *Eur J Immunol* 1999; **29**: 1617–25.

86. Forster R, Schubel A, Breitfeld D et al. CCR7 coordinates the primary immune response by establishing functional microenvironments in secondary lymphoid organs. *Cell* 1999; **99**: 23–33.

87. Gunn MD, Kyuwa S, Tam C et al. Mice lacking expression of secondary lymphoid organ chemokine have defects in lymphocyte homing and dendritic cell localization. *J Exp Med* 1999; **189**: 451–60.

88. Inaba K, Pack M, Inaba M et al. High levels of a major histocompatibility complex II-self peptide complex on dendritic cells from the T cell areas of lymph nodes. *J Exp Med* 1997; **186**: 665–72.

89. Geijtenbeek TB, Torensma R, van Vliet SJ et al. Identification of DC-SIGN, a novel dendritic cell-specific ICAM-3 receptor that supports primary immune responses. *Cell* 2000; **100**: 575–85.

90. Geijtenbeek TB, Krooshoop DJ, Bleijs DA et al. DC-SIGN–ICAM-2 interaction mediates dendritic cell trafficking. *Nat Immunol* 2000; **1**: 353–7.

91. Caux C, Vanbervliet B, Massacrier C et al. B70/B7-2 is identical to CD86 and is the major functional ligand for CD28 expressed on human dendritic cells. *J Exp Med* 1994; **180**: 1841–7.

92. Inaba K, Witmer-Pack M, Inaba M et al. The tissue distribution of the B7-2 costimulator in mice: abundant expression on dendritic cells in situ and during maturation in vitro. *J Exp Med* 1994; **180**: 1849–60.

93. Egen JG, Kuhns MS, Allison JP. CTLA-4: new insights into its biological function and use in tumor immunotherapy. *Nat Immunol* 2002; **3**: 611–18.

94. Greenwald RJ, Latchman YE, Sharpe AH. Negative co-receptors on lymphocytes. *Curr Opin Immunol* 2002; **14**: 391–6.

95. Liu YJ, Kanzler H, Soumelis V, Gilliet M. Dendritic cell lineage, plasticity and cross-regulation. *Nat Immunol* 2001; **2**: 585–9.

96. Brombacher F, Kastelein RA, Alber G. Novel IL-12 family members shed light on the orchestration of Th1 responses. *Trends Immunol* 2003; **24**: 207–12.

97. Pulendran B, Banchereau J, Maraskovsky E, Maliszewski C. Modulating the immune response with dendritic cells and their growth factors. *Trends Immunol* 2001; **22**: 41–7.

98. Heath WR, Carbone FR. Cross-presentation, dendritic cells, tolerance and immunity. *Annu Rev Immunol* 2001; **19**: 47–64.

99. Steinman RM, Nussenzweig MC. Avoiding horror autotoxicus: the importance of dendritic cells in peripheral T cell tolerance. *Proc Natl Acad Sci USA* 2002; **99**: 351–8.

100. Matzinger P, Guerder S. Does T-cell tolerance require a dedicated antigen-presenting cell? *Nature* 1989; **338**: 74–6.

101. Dhodapkar MV, Steinman RM, Sapp M et al. Rapid generation of broad T-cell immunity in humans after a single injection of mature dendritic cells. *J Clin Invest* 1999; **104**: 173–80.

102. Dhodapkar MV, Steinman RM, Krasovsky J et al. Antigen-specific inhibition of effector T cell function in humans after injection of immature dendritic cells. *J Exp Med* 2001; **193**: 233–8.

103. Shevach EM. Certified professionals: CD4+CD25+ suppressor T cells. *J Exp Med* 2001; **193**: F41–6.

104. Jefford M, Maraskovsky E, Cebon J, Davis ID. The use of dendritic cells in cancer therapy. *Lancet Oncol* 2001; **2**: 343–53.

105. Davis ID, Jefford M, Parente P, Cebon J. Rational approaches to human cancer immunotherapy. *J Leukoc Biol* 2003; **73**: 3–29.

# 9 Granulomonopoiesis

**Willem E Fibbe and Rob E Ploemacher**

## Introduction

An appropriate inflammatory response requires the recruitment of large numbers of leukocytes to sites of injury or infection. These cells are produced in the bone marrow, which serves as the major hematopoietic organ during adult life. Mature myeloid blood cells have a relatively limited lifespan and are incapable of further cell division. Therefore, large numbers of cells have to be replaced each day. For instance, an adult human being must produce an average of about 120 million neutrophils per minute.[1] In steady state, the levels of mature cells in the blood are maintained within relatively narrow limits. In response to hematological stress such as occurs during infection, the numbers of circulating cells can increase significantly. These considerations indicate the requirement for a complex control system that regulates hematopoietic cell production. In this chapter, the function of granulocytes and mononuclear phagocytes as well as the regulation of their production will be discussed.

Monocytes, macrophages, and neutrophils provide the phagocytic defence against microbial invasion. Under most circumstances, neutrophils are more efficient phagocytic cells than monocytes and macrophages. But when the particle is large, or when the load of particles increases, mononuclear phagocytes are more effective. The antimicrobial capacity of macrophages is markedly enhanced upon activation by activating substances such as bacterial endotoxin. Activated cells may kill ingested microorganisms by generating toxic metabolites.

## Granulocytes and mononuclear phagocytes

Both mononuclear phagocytes and neutrophils are able to phagocytose and kill bacteria in sites of infection. They exhibit chemotaxis (i.e. directed movements towards sites of infection) in response to various stimuli. This movement is influenced by chemotactic factors, which include complement (C5a) and substances derived from bacteria, cells, and connective tissue proteins. Chemokines form a novel class of small (92–99 amino acids) chemotactic cytokines that have the ability to activate leukocytes as mediators of inflammation.[2-4] Two subfamilies are distinguished by the arrangement of the first two cysteines, resulting in the family of so-called C-X-C chemokines, in which either cysteine is separated by one amino acid, or the C-C chemokines, where they are adjacent. While the C-C chemokines, including monocyte chemotactic (chemoattractant) proteins (McP-1, -2, and 3) predominantly stimulate monocytes, the C-X-C chemokine family, consisting of interleukin-8 (IL-8) and a number of related molecules (e.g. macrophage inflammatory protein 1α, MIP-1α), is mainly active on neutrophils. In response to the primary pro-inflammatory cytokines IL-1 and tumor necrosis factor α (TNF-α), fibroblasts, endothelial cells, epithelial cells, smooth muscle cells, and a variety of more specialized cells are able to produce monokines as well as IL-8. Under specific conditions, IL-8 can also be produced by neutrophils. Heparin-binding sites on chemokines provide a mechanism for their retention in the extracellular matrix and may serve to enhance concentration gradients.

### Granulocytes

#### Polymorphonuclear neutrophils

Neutrophil production in the adult occurs exclusively in the bone marrow. The life cycle of the neutrophil comprises phases in the bone marrow, blood, and tissues. Polymorphonuclear neutrophils in the blood are fully differentiated cells that remain in the circulation for only 6–7 hours before migrating into the tissues. Neutrophils circulate at a lower limit of approximately 1800 cells/μl.[5] During infection, these numbers may increase 10- to 30-fold within hours. These numbers illustrate the requirement for relatively large storage compartments, enabling the rapid release of mature cells into the circulation. In addition to the large storage compartment in the bone marrow, a portion of the neutrophils in the blood are found in the marginating granulocyte pool comprising cells that adhere to the endothelial walls of post-capillary venules. There is a continuing exchange between these two compartments and the circulating blood granulocyte pool, until neutrophils migrate from the blood into the tissues.

Morphologically recognizable myeloid precursor cells are only found in the bone marrow under steady-state conditions. They include myeloblasts, promyelocytes, and myelocytes that are still capable of cell division and that comprise the *mitotic compartment*. The cells that mature in the bone marrow no longer have the capacity of cell division: these are the metamyelocytes, band forms, and mature neutrophils, which form the *maturation compartment*. Mature neutrophils remain for several days in the bone marrow and form the maturation *storage compartment*. During infection, and also during treatment with granulocyte colony-stimulating factor (G-CSF), the marrow transit time can be significantly reduced, thereby allowing rapid increments in circulating neutrophil concentrations during infection. The mechanisms controlling the release of mature neutrophils from the marrow into the blood are not fully understood, but it is clear that bacterial endotoxins or pro-inflammatory cytokines such as IL-1 and TNF-$\alpha$ induced by endotoxins are able to induce rapid migration through endothelial cells. This involves a highly regulated process mediated by cell adhesion molecules.

Polymorphonuclear neutrophils play a crucial role in host defense against bacterial infections, their primary function being phagocytosis. Impaired neutrophil function or a reduction in their number are directly associated with an increased risk of infections, for example bacterial sepsis in newborn infants and chronic bacterial infections in older children and adults. The dysfunction may result from inborn errors (e.g. congenital neutrophilia) or from neutropenia induced by chemotherapy or following conditioning for stem cell transplantation. Both the duration and the severity of neutropenia will increase the likelihood of infections. In particular, severe neutropenia (i.e. a neutrophil count < 500/µl) is likely to be associated with the development of recurrent bacterial infections.

### Eosinophilic and basophilic granulocytes

Neutrophilic, eosinophilic, and basophilic granulocytes follow similar patterns in their development in the bone marrow and their release into the blood. Using standard staining techniques, only the more mature stages can be distinguished morphologically.

The association of eosinophilic granulocytes with some parasitic infections is well known. Their major function relates to hypersensitivity reactions and to host defence mechanisms against the larval states of parasitic infections. Basophils and tissue mast cells are capable of phagocytosis, but their major function may be associated with their high content of histamine, present in basophilic granules. Histamine is released from the granules in response to a variety of stimuli, including antigen exposure (IgE) in sensitized subjects,[6] and also (a variety of) cytokines (e.g. IL-3 and granulocyte–macrophage colony-stimulating factor, GM-CSF).

## Monocytes and macrophages

The mononuclear phagocyte system comprises monocytes, macrophages, and their precursor cells. The bone marrow is the major site of de novo mononuclear phagocyte production. Cells of the monocyte–macrophage series and neutrophilic granulocytes are derived from a common progenitor cell, i.e. the colony-forming unit granulocyte–monocyte (CFU-GM, see below). This progenitor cell matures into promonocytes and monocytes that are released into the blood. Monocytes remain in the blood for approximately 12 hours before they migrate into the tissues, to become tissue macrophages. Resident tissue macrophages do not re-enter the circulation; these include Kupffer cells in the liver, alveolar macrophages in the lung, dermal Langerhans cells, peritoneal and pleural macrophages, reticular dendritic cells in lymphatic tissues, and possibly osteoclasts and chondroclasts. The pool of resident macrophages is largely self-sustaining.

### Function of mononuclear phagocytes

In addition to their function as phagocytic cells, mononuclear phagocytes are also essential for the development of cellular and humoral immune responses. The recognition of antigens by T lymphocytes is usually preceded by phagocytosis and processing of antigens by macrophages. Mononuclear phagocytes may thus act as antigen-presenting cells (APC). In particular, dendritic cells (which are phenotypically different from macrophages) act as professional antigen-presenting cells. These cells also secrete IL-1,[7] which enhances T- and B-lymphocyte proliferation. Mononuclear phagocytes secrete a number of other soluble factors that promote the proliferation of other cell types. In addition to IL-1, macrophages are able to produce TNF-$\alpha$ as well as a number of myeloid colony-stimulating factors (i.e. G-CSF, GM-CSF, and macrophage colony-stimulating factor (M-CSF).[8] They also produce factors that inhibit hematopoiesis (e.g. interferon-$\alpha$ (IFN-$\alpha$) and MIP-1$\alpha$).[9]

Mononuclear phagocytes may also exhibit antitumor activities. Activated macrophages may recognize tumor cells in a non-antigen-dependent way. This cytotoxic activity requires cell–cell contact and a number of mediators, including nitric oxide (NO). Mononuclear phagocytes may also kill tumor cells through a mechanism termed antibody-dependent cellular cytotoxicity (ADCC), which involves the killing of antibody-coated tumor cells.

## The hematopoietic precursor cells

Mononuclear phagocytes and granulocytes are derived from a common precursor cell, committed to differentiation into the granulocytic or mononuclear phagocytic lineage (CFU-GM). In contrast to true pluripotent stem cells, committed progenitor cells are restricted to differentiation into one or various lineages, and are limited in their capacity for self-renewal. Committed progenitor cells are recognized by the ability to form colonies of mature cells in semi-solid culture media in vitro in the presence of designated hematopoietic growth factors. Therefore, hematopoietic committed progenitor cells are referred to as colony-forming cells (CFC) or colony-forming units (CFU). Different types of mature cells can be recognized in these colonies. For instance, myeloid progenitor cells (CFU-GM) are capable of differentiation into aggregates of mature granulocytes and/or monocytes/macrophages. Similarly, CFU-G, CFU-M, CFU-Eo refer to cells forming colonies of granulocytes, macrophages, or eosinophils respectively. The large majority of the myeloid bone marrow cells belongs to the heterogeneous population of post-progenitor cells, ranging from cells that still have some proliferative capacity to those becoming morphologically recognizable to mature, fully functional end cells.[10]

## Hematopoietic growth factors

The formation and development of in vitro colonies by hematopoietic progenitor cells requires the presence of specific regulatory molecules. In early experiments, colony growth was dependent on the presence of feeder cell layers that could later be replaced by media conditioned by a variety of cell populations, including peripheral blood leukocytes, spleen cells, vascular endothelial cells, and lung and placental cells. These conditioned media were referred to as colony-stimulating activity and contained combinations of growth factors. Over the past decade or so, a large number of distinct human hematopoietic colony-stimulating factors and interleukins have been purified and their cDNA has been cloned. Cytokine receptors are found in many tissues, and specificity results mainly from local production of cytokines and specific localizations of target cells at the site of cytokine presentation. The major cytokine activities include enhancement of cell survival and proliferation, induction of cell differentiation, and functional activation of mature cells (Table 9.1). In this chapter, emphasis will be placed on growth factors regulating the production of granulocytes and macrophages (Table 9.2). These include the colony-stimulating factors (M-CSF, G-CSF, and GM-CSF), IL-3 and IL-5, stem cell factor (SCF), and Flk2/Flt3 ligand (Flk2/Flt3-L (Fms-like tyrosine kinase receptor)).

### Table 9.1  General activities of hematopoietic growth factors

- Enhancement of cell survival
- Enhancement of cell proliferation
- Induction of cellular differentiation
- Activation of mature effector cells

### Table 9.2  The myeloid growth factors

| Factor | Chromosome locus | Cellular source | Target cells |
|---|---|---|---|
| GM-CSF | 5q23–31 | Monocytes, fibroblasts, endothelial cells, T cells, mast cells | CFU-G, CFU-M, CFU-GM, CFU-GEMM, CFU-Mk, CFU-GE, BFU-E, neutrophils, eosinophils |
| G-CSF | 17q11.2–21 | Monocytes, fibroblasts, endothelial cells, mesothelial cells | CFU-G, neutrophils |
| M-CSF | 1p13–21 | Monocytes, fibroblasts, endothelial cells | CFU-M, mononuclear phagocytes |
| IL-3 | 5q23–31 | T cells, mast cells, monocytes | CFU-G, CFU-M, CFU-GM, CFU-Eo, CFU-GEMM, CFU-Mk, CFU-GE, BFU-E |
| SCF | 12q22–24 12q14.3–12qter | Stromal cells, endothelial cells, monocytes | Mast cells, CFU-E, BFU-E, CFU-Mk, CFU-GEMM |
| IL-5 | 5q23–31 | T cells | Eosinophils, B cells |

GM, granulocyte–macrophage; G, granulocyte; M, macrophage; GEMM, granulocyte–erythroid–macrophage–megakaryocyte; Mk, megakaryocyte; GE, granulocyte–erythroid; E, erythroid; Eo, eosinophil; CSF, colony-stimulating factor; IL, interleukin; SCF, stem cell factor (Steel factor, c-Kit ligand); CFU, colony-forming unit; BFU, burst-forming unit.

## Physiological role of myeloid growth factors

### Inducible hematopoiesis

Hematopoietic growth factors play an important role in the body's response to trauma or infection by initiating its repair and defense mechanisms. The acute phase response to most infectious diseases is usually accompanied by increased numbers of peripheral blood neutrophils, in particular band forms. This neutrophilia is attributed to premature and accelerated release of mature neutrophils from the bone marrow reservoir. Under these circumstances, the production of hematopoietic growth factors is induced by endotoxin or by pro-inflammatory cytokines such as IL-1 and TNF-α. For example, IL–1 induces fibroblasts, endothelial cells, and marrow stromal cells to synthesize G-CSF, GM-CSF, M-CSF, IL-6, and TNF-α, as well as IL-1 itself.[11–13] In vivo, a single injection of IL-1 itself induces a rapid neutrophilia within several hours,[14] and in mice, administration of IL-1 accelerates myelopoiesis following cyclophosphamide-induced neutropenia.[15] Furthermore, increased production of colony-stimulating factors induced by these pro-inflammatory cytokines may contribute to the leukocytosis observed during infection.

### Steady-state hematopoiesis – growth factors act at a local level

Since hematopoietic cytokines exert their effect in a paracrine or autocrine fashion rather than acting as classical hormones, most factors (e.g. GM-CSF and IL-3) are undetectable in the serum of healthy human subjects. SCF and Flk2/Flt3-L are produced constitutively. Through alternative splicing, M-CSF[16,17] and Flk2/Flt3-L[18] are expressed in a soluble form and in a biologically active transmembrane form on stromal cells. Healthy individuals have serum concentrations of M-CSF in the range of 2–7 ng/ml[19] and soluble SCF concentrations of approximately 3 ng/ml.[20] The transmembrane form of SCF expressed on stromal cells may serve as a cell adhesion molecule that binds hematopoietic progenitor cells expressing C-Kit, the receptor for SCF.[17] Soluble growth factors (e.g. GM-CSF) can also be retained in the microenvironment and presented to hematopoietic stem cells through binding to glycosaminoglycans such as heparin sulfate in the extracellular matrix.[21] G-CSF is found in serum at detectable concentrations in a minority of healthy persons. During neutropenia, however, there is a direct relationship between serum concentrations of G-CSF and the absolute neutrophil count.[22] During chemotherapy-induced neutropenia, G-CSF levels may rise to concentrations that are close to the levels observed following therapeutic administration of G-CSF. Following bone marrow recovery, levels decrease to baseline. A similar inverse correlation between G-CSF levels and neutrophil counts has been reported for patients with aplastic anemia or cyclic neutropenia.[23] Such an inverse correlation is not observed for the other myeloid growth factors, with the exception of thrombopoietin. These data are consistent with G-CSF being a physiological feedback regulator of neutrophil production. Finally, increased serum levels of Flk2/Flt3-L have been reported in patients with aplastic anemia, supporting a possible role in the development of primitive hematopoietic cells.[24]

### Growth factor-deficient animals

Much insight in the role of growth factors in regulating steady-state hematopoiesis has been derived from mice deficient for the gene encoding the growth factor or the growth factor receptor. In these experiments, targeting constructs are designed to eliminate exons of the gene of interest in embryonic stem cell clones undergoing homologous recombination. These mutations will result in the removal of one or several critical regions of the protein and lead to functional inactivation. Following injection of targeted clones into blastocysts, chimeric animals are generated that will transmit the mutant allele through the germline. Homozygous mutant animals are generated by mating of heterozygous mutants. GM-CSF-deficient mice exhibit completely normal peripheral blood hematocrits, platelet, and white blood cell counts, while differential counts reveal similarly normal proportions of lymphocytes, neutrophils, eosinophils, and monocytes.[25] The numbers of granulocyte–macrophage (CFU-GM) as well as multipotent (granulocyte–erythroid–macrophage–megakaryocyte: CFU-GEMM) progenitor cells in bone marrow and spleen are also normal. Mutant bone marrow cells can engraft lethally irradiated mice, although the rate of reconstitution is somewhat delayed in comparison with animals transplanted with bone marrow from normal littermates. The only abnormality observed in GM-CSF-deficient mice is an accumulation of surfactant in the lungs reminiscent of human pulmonary alveolar proteinosis.[25] These data do not support the major role initially attributed to GM-CSF as a critical regulator of hematopoiesis.

Mice lacking the gene for G-CSF are viable, and fertile, and although they appear healthy, they have chronic neutropenia.[26] Blood neutrophil counts are in the range of 20–30% of wild-type mice. Similar defects have recently been reported in mice deficient for the G-CSF receptor (G-CSFR). Mature neutrophils are still present in G-CSF-deficient mice, indicating that other growth factors are able to support neutrophil production in vivo. G-CSF-deficient mice also have a markedly impaired ability to control infection with *Listeria monocytogenes*, with diminished neutrophil and delayed monocyte increases in the blood in response to infection. In the bone marrow, the numbers of early (myelocyte and promyelocyte) and late (metamyelocyte) neutrophil precursors are reduced. The frequency of total marrow progenitor cells responsive to a variety of growth factor combinations is consistently reduced. This includes not only granulocytic precursor cells in the eosinophilic, megakaryocytic, and erythroid lineages, but also blast colony-forming cells. Following G-CSF administration, neutrophil levels in the blood return to normal and the bone marrows are morphologically indistinguishable from those of control mice. These data indicate that G-CSF is indispensable for maintenance of normal neutrophil production during steady-state hematopoiesis and also indicate an important role for G-CSF in inducible granulopoiesis during infections.

In humans, no defects in the G-CSF gene have been reported. However, mutations in the gene encoding the G-CSFR have been reported in patients with acute myeloid leukemia (AML) preceded by severe congenital neutropenia (Kostmann syndrome).[27] Kostmann syndrome comprises a heterogeneous group of disorders characterized by severe chronic neutropenia and recurrent bacterial infections. The bone marrow of affected patients shows an arrest of granulocytic maturation at the stage of promyelocytes or myelocytes. Patients with Kostmann syndrome are at an increased risk of developing AML. The in vitro response to G-CSF of myeloid progenitor cells is often reduced. Following administration of pharmacological doses of G-CSF, neutrophil counts increase in the majority of Kostmann syndrome patients. In some patients, a truncated G-CSFR lacking the C-terminal maturation domain has been observed as a result of a point mutation.[27] In addition, point mutations have also been found in patients with AML secondary to severe congenital neutropenia. In one of these patients, the mutation was already present during the neutropenic phase of the disease. However, mutations have not been found in all patients with congenital neutropenia, indicating that the disorder is heterogeneous in its pathogenesis. Collectively, these findings indicate that mutations in the genes encoding G-CSFR, or molecules involved in intracellular signaling, may induce a block in maturation that can be associated with the progression to AML. Recent evidence has implicated a possible role for thrombopoietin (TPO) in the regulation of myelopoiesis.[28] TPO-deficient mice exhibit a substantial reduction in the size of the bone marrow stem and progenitor cell pool of 60–80%. In spite of this, TPO-deficient mice display thrombocytopenia only and have normal numbers of circulating red blood cells and neutrophils. Mice that are deficient for both TPO and G-CSFR exhibit excessive neutropenia – far greater than that observed in either TPO-deficient or G-CSFR-deficient mice.[28] Not only do these data suggest that TPO plays a role in the regulation of myelopoiesis, but they also support the hypothesis that G-CSF may compensate for the deficiency in marrow stem and progenitor cells, by expansion of the pool of relatively mature myeloid progenitors, in particular the mature stages of granulopoiesis.[28]

As an experiment of nature the *M-CSF* gene is deleted in the naturally occurring osteopetrotic (*op*) mice that lack functional osteoclasts.[29] This mutation was demonstrated to be due to an alteration in the *M-CSF* gene resulting in the introduction of a stop codon and the production of a truncated and biologically inactive protein.[30] In addition to osteopetrosis, these mice exhibit severe deficiencies in mononuclear phagocyte subpopulations, including blood monocytes and macrophages in serosal cavities and in the bone marrow.[29] They develop skeletal abnormalities, have low birthweight, and have a reduced life expectancy.[29,31] Administration of M-CSF to new born *op/op* mice cures osteopetrosis and corrects the numbers of blood monocytes and macrophages in the bone marrow, but not the numbers of macrophages in the serosal cavity.[31] These data support the crucial role of M-CSF in macrophage development and function.

Mutations at the *Steel* locus encoding SCF or in its receptor, which is the product of the dominant *White spotting* (*W*) locus, in the mouse, have also been described.[32,33] These animals develop similar abnormalities in multiple organs, including marrow hypoplasia, reduced fertility, and diminished or even lack of skin pigmentation. The hematopoietic defects comprise macrocytic anemia, reduced production of granulocytes and megakaryocytes, and a severe deficiency in tissue mast cells. Mice carrying mutations at the *W* locus have a reduced number of multipotent stem cells, including CFU-GEMM, in the bone marrow that can be entirely corrected by transplantation of bone marrow from unaffected littermates. Mutations at the *Steel* locus result in a deficient microenvironment, which can be restored by transplanting marrow stromal cells. These observations led to the discovery of the human c-Kit tyrosine kinase receptor and its ligand SCF (also known as c-Kit ligand, Steel factor, or mast cell growth factor). A related gene defect in men has been described that affects hair pigmentation (piebald trait).[34]

## Biological effects of hematopoietic growth factors in vitro

### Enhancement of cell survival

The culture of hematopoietic progenitor cells in the absence of exogenously added growth factors and under conditions that exclude the endogenous production of growth factors by accessory cells results in rapid initiation of the process of programmed cell death (apoptosis).[35] Apoptotic cell death starts shortly after withdrawal of growth factors. It is associated with distinct morphological changes, including nuclear condensation and cleavage of nuclear DNA by endonucleases. This results in the formation of small pieces of DNA appearing as a characteristic laddered fragmentation pattern on gel electrophoresis. Not only progenitor cells but also mature cells are subject to apoptosis.[36] Thus, apoptosis may account for the normal physiological destruction of neutrophils. Similarly, monocytes undergo apoptosis unless their survival is promoted by the action of IL-1, GM-CSF, or M-CSF.[37] The concentrations of these factors required for maintaining cell viability are usually considerably lower than those required for the proliferation and functional activation of cells.[38] Promotion of cell survival appears to occur at all stages of differentiation. Following clearance of infection, apoptosis may thus be a physiological mechanism to rapidly reduce the number of cells in a population that has been expanded by stimulatory cytokines.

### Enhancement of cell proliferation

Proliferation of hematopoietic progenitor cells requires the continuous presence of hematopoietic growth factors. Induction of cycling is mediated by 'competence' factors (e.g. G-CSF, SCF, IL-6, Flt3-L, or IL-11) that support the transition from $G_0$ to the $G_1$ phase of the cell cycle. To enter $S$–$G_2$ phases of the cell cycle, the cell then needs 'progression' factors (e.g. GM-CSF, IL-3, or M-CSF). Upon exposure to higher concentrations of the factors, the cell cycle time of progenitor cells progressively decreases, thereby increasing the number of progeny cells generated.[39] Individual growth factors affect multiple hematopoietic lineages, and each lineage may be regulated by various hematopoietic growth factors. For instance, neutrophil production is stimulated by GM-CSF, G-CSF, SCF, IL-3, and IL-6. Even the relatively lineage-restricted factors such as G-CSF and M-CSF, which induce a selective proliferation for neutrophils or macrophage precursor cells respectively, stimulate other cell types at higher concentrations. At high concentrations, G-CSF also stimulates macrophage and granulocyte–macrophage progenitor cells, while M-CSF stimulates granulocyte–macrophage and granulocyte progenitor cells.[40]

The response of progenitor cells to hematopoietic growth factors also depends on the stage of maturation of the responding cell. IL-3 and GM-CSF both initiate the proliferation of granulocyte–macrophage precursor cells. During maturation, however, the number of receptors for IL-3 decreases, whereas receptor numbers for GM-CSF are maintained.[41] As a result, the proliferative response on GM-CSF is maintained while the IL-3 response decreases.

Another property of many hematopoietic growth factors is their synergistic interaction. The maximal production of eosinophils in vitro requires the combined presence of IL-3, GM-CSF, and IL-5.[42] Synergy is particularly evident when early-acting cytokines such as IL-3, IL-6, or SCF are combined with factors affecting committed progenitor cells (i.e. GM-CSF, G-CSF, or M-CSF). Other interactions between growth factors are even more complex, since they may influence the differentiation lineage of the progeny cells. IL-4 represents an example of a cytokine that as a single factor has no colony-stimulating activity. However, it may profoundly affect colony formation in the presence of other hematopoietic growth factors. In both murine and human bone marrow cultures, addition of IL-4 enhances granulocyte colony formation in the presence of G-CSF[43] and erythroid colonies in the presence of erythropoietin (EPO). Inclusion of IL-4 in cultures stimulated with GM-CSF results in almost complete disappearance of macrophage colonies.[44] Thus, in the presence of G-CSF and GM-CSF, IL-4 will favor the formation of neutrophils over macrophages. In contrast, IL-6 will favor differentiation into macrophages over neutrophils.

### Activation of mature effector cells

In addition to their proliferative effects, colony-stimulating factors stimulate the function of mature end cells. G-CSF promotes the survival of neutrophils, and also enhances their function by stimulating adhesion to endothelium and by enhancing the ability to respond to microorganisms with a respiratory burst.[45] G-CSF also enhances antibody-dependent cell killing,[46] IgA-mediated phagocytosis,[47] and generation of superoxide anions.[48]

GM-CSF is also directly chemotactic for neutrophils[49] and inhibits cell migration.[50] GM-CSF primes neutrophils for oxidative bursts,[51] enhances phagocytosis, and increases the expression of certain adhesion molecules.[52] It also increases the capacity of neutrophils to phagocytose and to kill intracellular yeasts, parasites, and bacteria, in particular in antibody-dependent cell killing.

The action of hematopoietic growth factors on mature cells that circulate or that reside in tissues will enhance their ability to overcome infections and to promote tissue repair. The release of growth factors at local sites of infection attracts effector cells to the site of infection, and directly activates the cells for enhanced ingestion and killing of bacteria. The recruitment of other inflammatory cells to the site of infection will be promoted by the induction of other cytokines. Thus, the functional activation of granulocytes and other phagocytic cells is an important activity of hematopoietic growth factors in addition to their growth-promoting properties.

### GM-CSF

GM-CSF is the product of T lymphocytes, macrophages, endothelial cells, fibroblasts, and a variety of neoplastic cells.[53] It acts as a growth factor on a number of cells belonging to hematopoietic as well as non-hematopoietic lineages.[54] GM-CSF is a multilineage colony-stimulating factor that promotes the growth of progenitor cells belonging to the granulocyte, macrophage, eosinophil, and basophil lineages.[55] In enriched monocyte-depleted cultures of CD34+ cells, GM-CSF stimulates the colony formation development of eosinophil (CFU-Eo), erythroid (BFU-E), and multipotent (CFU-GEMM) progenitor cells, but not the formation of granulocyte–macrophage (CFU-GM), granulocyte (CFU-G), or macrophage (CFU-M) colonies.[56] However, following the addition of monocytes, development of CFU-GM, CFU-G, and CFU-M is observed. Most likely, growth factor release from monocytes in response to GM-CSF is responsible for this effect.[57] Nevertheless, it is widely accepted that GM-CSF directly affects the growth of granulocytes and monocyte/macrophage progenitor cells.[58] In addition, GM-CSF has been reported to stimulate the growth of megakaryocytic colonies in vitro.[59] GM-CSF has a number of synergistic interactions with other growth factors. GM-CSF and G-CSF act synergistically on the growth of CFU-GM.[60] GM-CSF synergizes with M-CSF in the formation of CFU-M.[56-58] It has some burst-promoting activity in the presence of EPO.[61] In addition, GM-CSF and IL-3 increase the number of multipotent progenitor cells in the presence of EPO.[62]

## G-CSF

G-CSF is produced by a variety of normal and neoplastic cells. Mouse and human G-CSF exhibit more than 70% homology at a protein level and are highly cross-species reactive.[63,64] G-CSF is a primary stimulator of the proliferation and differentiation of committed progenitor cells into the neutrophil–granulocytic lineage. It primarily acts as a lineage-restricted late-acting colony-stimulating factor for committed neutrophilic progenitor cells.[65] In addition, it is a potent activator of mature neutrophils, inducing enhanced phagocytosis and chemotaxis.[66,67] Although G-CSF is relatively specific for cells belonging to the neutrophil lineage, at higher cell concentrations it has some effect on multipotent progenitor cells. In this way, it may induce resting stem cells to enter the cell cycle, rendering the cells responsive to the action of other growth factors.[68-70] In addition to having a colony-stimulating effect on late committed neutrophilic progenitors, G-CSF may thus be considered as a competence factor for primitive hematopoietic progenitor cells.

## M-CSF

M-CSF is a lineage-specific factor for progenitor cells and mature cells belonging to the monocyte–macrophage lineage.[71] Similar to other growth factors, M-CSF has potent effects on the function of mature monocytes.[72] It enhances the antibody-mediated anti-tumor cytotoxicity of monocytes. It is also believed to be a survival factor for these cells, explaining its

presence in the serum of healthy subjects.[73] At higher cell concentrations, M-CSF stimulates other cell lineages and promotes the formation of neutrophil colonies. In addition to a soluble form of M-CSF, a membrane-bound biologically active form of this molecule has been reported.[16] The soluble isoform may be important as a survival and developmental factor for monocytes and macrophages, whereas its glycosaminoglycan chain may aid in the specific binding to extracellular matrix molecules.[74,75] The cell-associated form may be involved in cell–cell interaction. The M-CSF receptor is identical to the product of the proto-oncogene c-*fms*. This receptor has also been detected in placental tissues and in human choriocarcinoma cell lines established from malignant placental trophoblasts.[76] These data suggest a possible role for M-CSF in placental development.

## IL-3

IL-3 is primarily produced by activated T lymphocytes, but also by mast cells.[77] It stimulates the growth and differentiation of multiple lineages, including granulocytes, macrophages, megakaryocytes, erythrocytes, eosinophils, and mast cells. It is also a factor promoting the growth of relatively primitive stem cells. It synergizes with a number of other factors, including SCF, Flt3-L, GM-CSF, G-CSF, EPO, and IL-6 and IL-11, thus promoting the formation of granulocyte macrophage, neutrophile, erythroid, and megakaryocyte colonies.[78-80] As a single factor, it has relatively little activity and it does not fully support development into a single lineage. IL-3 is one of the factors that has independent stimulatory activity on the in vitro growth of megakaryocytic progenitor cells.[59] However, later-acting factors, such as IL-6 and TPO, are required for full maturation into megakaryocytes. IL-3 potentiates the functional activities of eosinophils, basophils, and monocytes, but not of neutrophils, since IL-3 receptors decrease in number along the neutrophilic maturation pathway and matured neutrophils have no receptors for IL-3.[41,80] In conjunction with GM-CSF and the eosinophil-specific factor IL-5, IL-3 is involved in the regulation of eosinophils.[81] Mast cells and P cells (persistant cells in long-term culture) both produce histamine and persist for a considerable time (months) in long-term cultures in the presence of IL-3 as a single factor.[82]

## SCF

SCF is the ligand for the receptor c-Kit encoded by the c-*kit* proto-oncogene. It is a highly pleiotropic cytokine with multiple activities on myeloid and lymphoid cells as well as on non-hematopoietic cells.[83-85] It is expressed in a variety of organs, this expression being especially high in the cerebellum. SCF plays a role in the development and migration of germ cells, neural crest cells, and mast cells, as well as hematopoietic cells, where it preferentially promotes the growth of relatively primitive progenitor cells.[86] By alternative splicing, SCF is produced as a membrane-bound form and as a soluble form. The importance of the membrane-bound form is clearly illustrated by the presence of hematopoietic defects in mice with a mutation in the *Steel* locus, resulting in the absence of the membrane-bound isoform of SCF but normal levels of the soluble form.[17] As a soluble factor, it has limited activities on myeloid colony formation. However, it enhances the formation of myeloid and erythroid colonies when combined with other factors, such as GM-CSF, G-CSF, IL-3, and EPO.[83–86] In synergy with IL-3 and GM-CSF, SCF stimulates the formation of megakaryocytes.[87] Primitive hematopoietic progenitor cells do not express detectable levels of c-Kit. This receptor is downregulated by cytokines such as IL-3 and GM-CSF[88] – a phenomenon that may play a role in the release of stem cells from the bone marrow microenvironment.

### Flt3-L

The identification of Flk2/Flt3-L was directly derived from the discovery of its receptor: Flk2 in mice[89] and Flt3[90] in humans. This receptor belongs to the immunoglobulin superfamily of tyrosine kinase receptors and is similar to the receptors for SCF, M-CSF, and platelet-derived growth factor (PDGF) $\alpha$ and $\beta$. It has five extracellular immunoglobulin-like domains and split tyrosine kinase catalytic domains in its cytoplasmic region. In the mouse, Flt2 is reported to be expressed in a variety of different organs, including (fetal) liver, ovary, skin, thymus, spleen, lymph node, testis, kidney, and brain,[90] although others have found a more limited expression.[89,91] The human receptor was found to be expressed in bone marrow, thymus, spleen, liver, and lymph nodes.[92] Flt3 was found to be expressed on monocytes in bone marrow and blood, but not on granulocytes.[93] Primitive multilineage progenitor cells have been reported to express low levels of Flt3, while high levels have been found on myelomonocytic precursors.[93] Flt3-L is expressed in virtually all murine and human tissues studied. As a single factor, Flt3-L has a modest proliferative effect on c-Kit-positive mouse bone marrow cells and it synergizes with IL-3.[94] It had no activity on purified mouse stem cells, but colony formation is synergistically enhanced in combination with IL-3 or IL-6. Similarly, Flt3-L promotes the formation of secondary colonies of mouse Thy-1 $^{low}$Sca-1$^+$ stem cells in combination with G-CSF, SCF, IL-3, or IL-6. In combination with IL-6, it expands the numbers of CFU,[95] and combinations with G-CSF, IL-11, or IL-12 expand the numbers of cells with an immature blast cell appearance.[96] Flt3-L alone has relatively little activity on colony formation

of high-proliferative-potential colony-forming cells of purified CD34$^+$CD33$^-$Lin$^-$ cells derived from human fetal liver, but synergizes with IL-3 and GM-CSF.[94] In contrast to SCF and IL-3, Flt3-L has no effect on the growth or activation of mast cells. These data indicate a role for Flt3-L as a synergistic factor for primitive hematopoietic progenitor cells.

## Role of adhesion molecules

Cell adhesion molecules have been identified as mediators of cellular and cell–matrix interactions in immune responses and tissue repair. More recently, they have also been implicated in the regulation of hematopoiesis, and are considered to play an important role in the proliferation and differentiation of progenitor cells. Studies in long-term bone marrow cultures have indicated that primitive progenitor cells are preferentially bound to the extracellular matrix in the stromal layer.[97]

Two major families of adhesion molecules have been identified, namely selectins and integrins.[98] L-selectin is expressed on all circulating leukocytes except for a subpopulation of memory lymphocytes. P-selectin is stored in the Weibel–Palade bodies of endothelial cells and the $\alpha$ granules of platelets. E-selectin is induced on vascular endothelial cells by cytokines such as IL-1 and TNF-$\alpha$. All selectins recognize a sialylated carbohydrate determinant on their counter-receptors. Selectins mediate the attachment of circulating leukocytes to the vessel wall through labile adhesions that permit the leukocytes to roll in the direction of flow. Shedding of neutrophil L-selectin is rapidly induced by IL-8 and is associated with demargination of granulocytes from the endothelial vessel wall and subsequent tissue invasion.

Integrins are mediators of the cellular interactions between hematopoietic cells and stromal cells and components of the extracellular matrix in the bone marrow microenvironment. They also mediate the second step in leukocyte accumulation, which involves firm adhesion of the granulocyte to the vessel wall. Integrins are heterodimers composed of an $\alpha$ subunit non-covalently associated with a $\beta$ subunit. Eight different $\beta$ subunits and 14 different $\alpha$ subunits have been identified thus far. Several distinct $\alpha$ subunits can associate with only one $\beta$ subunit. Based on the $\beta$ subunits, several families can be distinguished within the family of integrins. The $\beta_1$ integrins are also called very late antigens (VLA) and consist of receptors for cell matrix components such as fibronectin, laminin, and collagen. VLA are expressed on a variety of cells, including hematopoietic cells. Human CD34$^+$ progenitor cells have been found to express the integrin $\beta_1$ chain (CD29) as well as VLA-4$\alpha$ and VLA-5$\alpha$.[99]

Expression of the $\beta_2$ integrins is mainly restricted to leukocytes, i.e. T and B lymphocytes, monocytes, and granulocytes. This group of integrins consists of three members: LFA-1 (leukocyte function antigen), CR3 (Mac-1), and P150,95. These members have distinct $\alpha$ subunits (CD11a, b, and c respectively) but share a common $\beta$ subunit (CD18). LFA-1 (CD11a/CD18)-mediated cell–cell interaction involves the binding of one of its three counter-receptors belonging to the immunoglobulin superfamily, called intracellular adhesion molecules 1, 2, and 3 (ICAM-1, -2, and -3). LFA-1 is expressed on all leukocytes. It is involved in functions such as T-cell-mediated killing and leukocyte adhesion to endothelial cells. LFA-1 is also expressed on the majority of hematopoietic progenitor cells. Altered cytoadhesion of CD34+ progenitor

cells induced by (stimulatory) anti-CD34 antibodies is associated with activation of the $\beta_2$-integrin pathway and can be inhibited by LFA-1 or ICAM-1 antibodies.[100] Very primitive hematopoietic progenitor cells seem to lack LFA-1 expression,[101] suggesting that expression of LFA-1 on CD34+ cells identifies an intermediate stage in the differentiation of progenitor cells, and may therefore be used to characterize progenitor cell subsets. The differences between bone marrow-derived and peripheral blood-derived progenitor cells with respect to the expression levels of cytoadhesion molecules has not yet been fully studied, but the selective recruitment of specific types of leukocytes into various tissues has been suggested to result from the use of various combinations of selectins, leukocyte-activating factors, and integrins.

## REFERENCES

1. Dexter TM. The message in the medium. *Nature* 1984; **309**: 746–7.

2. Van Damme J. Interleukin-8 and related molecules. In: Thomsom AW (ed) *The Cytokine Handbook*, 1st edn. San Diego: Academic Press, 1991: 201–14.

3. Oppenheim JJ, Zachariae COC, Mukaida N, Matsushima K. Properties of the novel proinflammatory supergene intercrine cytokine family. *Annu Rev Immunol* 1991; **9**: 617–48.

4. Rollins BJ. Chemokines. *Blood* 1997; **90**: 909–28.

5. Athens JW. Granulocytes and neutrophils. In: Lee GR, Bithell TC, Foerster J et al (eds) *Wintrobe's Clinical Hematology*. Philadelphia: Lea & Febiger, 1993: 223–66.

6. Jukkin L, Shelley WB. A new test for detecting anaphalytic sensitivity: the basophilic reaction. *Nature* 1961; **191**: 1056–8.

7. Flynn A, Finke JH, Hilfiker ML. Placental mononuclear phagocytes as a source of interleukin-1. *Science* 1982; **218**: 475–7.

8. Fibbe WE, Van Damme J, Billiau A et al. Interleukin-1 (22-K factor) induces release of granulocyte–macrophage colony-stimulating activity from human mononuclear phagocytes. *Blood* 1986; **68**: 1316–21.

9. Wright EG, Pragnell IB. Stem cell proliferation inhibitors. *Baillières Clin Hematol* 1992; **5**: 723–39.

10. Juttner CA, Fibbe WE, Nemunaitis J et al. Blood cell transplantation: report from an International Consensus Meeting. *Bone Marrow Transplant* 1994; **14**: 689–93.

11. Zuculi JR, Dinarello CA, Oblon DJ et al. Interleukin-1 stimulates fibroblasts to produce granulocyte-macrophage colony-stimulating activity and protaglandin E$_2$. *J Clin Invest* 1986; **77**: 1857–63.

12. Bagby GC Jr, Dinarello CA, Wallace P et al. Interleukin 1 stimulates granulocyte macrophage colony-stimulating activity release by vascular endothelial cells. *J Clin Invest* 1986; **78**: 1316–23.

13. Fibbe WE, Van Damme J, Billiau A et al. Interleukin-1 induces human marrow stromal cells in long-term culture to produce G-CSF and M-CSF. *Blood* 1998; **71**: 430–5.

14. Van Damme J, Opdenakker G, De Ley M et al. Pyrogenic and haematological effects of the interferon-inducing 22K factor (interleukin-1) from human leukocytes. *Clin Exp Immunol* 1986; **66**: 303–11.

15. Fibbe WE, van der Meer JWM, Falkenburg JHF et al. A single low dose of human recombinant interleukin-1 accelerates the reconstitution of neutrophils in mice with cyclophosphamide-induced neutropenia. *Exp Hematol* 1989; **17**: 805–8.

16. Rettenmier CW, Roussel MF, Ashmun RA et al. Synthesis of membrane-bound colony-stimulating factor 1 (CSF-1) and downmodulation of CSF-1 receptors in NIH 3T3 cells transformed by cotransfection of the human *CSF-1* and *c-fms* (CSF-1 receptor) genes. *Mol Cell Biol* 1987; **7**: 2378–87.

17. Flanagan JG, Chan DC, Leder P. Transmembrane form of kit ligand growth factor is determined by alternative splicing and is missing in the Sld mutant. *Cell* 1991; **64**: 1025–35.

18. Lyman SD, James L, Vanden Bos T et al. Molecular cloning of a ligand for the flt3/flk-2 tyrosine kinase receptor: a proliferative factor for primitive hematopoietic cells. *Cell* 1993; **75**: 1157–67.

19. Bartocci A, Mastrogiannis DS, Migliorati G et al. Macrophages specifically regulate the concentration of their own growth factor in the circulation. *Proc Natl Acad Sci USA* 1987; **84**: 6179–83.

20. Langley KE, Bennett LC, Wypych J et al. Soluble stem cell factor in human serum. *Blood* 1993; **81**: 656–60.

21. Gordon MY, Riley GP, Watt SM et al. Compartmentalization of a hematopoietic growth factor (GM-CSF) by glycosaminoglycans in the bone marrow microenvironment. *Nature* 1987; **326**: 403–4.

22. Cairo MS, Suen Y, Sender L et al. Circulating granulocyte colony-stimulating factor (G-CSF) levels after allogeneic and autologous bone marrow transplantation: endogenous G-CSF production correlates with myeloid engraftment. *Blood* 1992; **79**: 1869–73.

23. Kawakami M, Tsutsumi H, Kumakawa T et al. Levels of serum granulocyte colony-stimulating factor in patients with infections. *Blood* 1990; **76**: 1962–4.

24. Lyman SD, Seaberg M, Hanna R et al. Plasma/serum levels of flt3 ligand are low in normal individuals and highly elevated in patients with Fanconi anemia and acquired aplastic anemia. *Blood* 1995; **86**: 4091–6.

25. Dranoff G, Crawford AD, Sadelain M et al. Involvement of

granulocyte–macrophage colony-stimulating factor in pulmonary homeostasis. *Science* 1994; **264**: 713–16.

26. Lieschke GJ, Grail D, Hodgson G et al. Mice lacking granulocyte colony-stimulating factor have chronic neutropenia, granulocyte and macrophage progenitor cell deficiency, and impaired neutrophil mobilization. *Blood* 1994; **84**: 1737–46.

27. Dong F, Brynes RK, Tidow N et al. Mutations in the gene for the granulocyte colony-stimulating-factor receptor in patients with acute myeloid leukemia preceded by severe congenital neutropenia. *N Engl J Med* 1995; **333**: 487–93.

28. Kaushanski K, Fox N, Lin NL, Liles WC. Lineage specific growth factors can compensate for stem and progenitor cell deficiencies at the post progenitor cell level: an analysis of double TPO- and G-CSF receptor deficient mice. *Blood* 2002; **99**: 3573–8.

29. Marks SC, Lane PW. Osteopetrosis: a new recessive skeletal mutation on chromosome 12 of the mouse. *J Hered* 1976; **67**: 11–18.

30. Yoshida H, Hayashi S, Kunisada T et al. The murine mutation osteopetrosis is in the coding region of the macrophage colony stimulating factor gene. *Nature* 1990; **345**: 442–4.

31. Stanley ER, Berg KL, Einstein DB et al. The biology and action of colony-stimulating factor-1. *Stem Cells* 1994; **12**(Suppl 1):15–25.

32. Zsebo KM, Williams DA, Geissler EN et al. Stem cell factor is encoded at the *Sl* locus of the mouse and is the ligand for the c-kit tyrosine kinase receptor. *Cell* 1990; **63**:213–24.

33. Russell ES. Hereditary anemias of the mouse: a review for geneticists. *Adv Genet* 1979; **20**: 357–459.

34. Fleischmann RA, Saltman DL, Stastny V, Zneimer S. Deletion of the c-*kit* protooncogene in the human developmental defect piebald trait. *Proc Natl Acad Sci USA* 1991; **88**: 10885–9.

35. Williams GT, Smith CA, Spooncer E et al. Hematopoietic colony-stimulating factors promote cell survival by suppressing apoptosis. *Nature* 1990; **343**: 76–9.

36. Savill J, Wyllie AH, Henson JE et al. Macrophage phagocytosis of aging neutrophils in inflammation: programmed cell death of neutrophils leads to its recognition by macrophages. *J Clin Invest* 1989; **83**: 865–75.

37. Mangal DF, Wahl SM. Differential regulation of human monocyte programmed cell death (apoptosis) by chemotactic factors and proinflammatory cytokines. *J Immunol* 1991; **147**: 3408–12.

38. Begley CG, Lopez AF, Nicola NA et al. Purified colony-stimulating factors enhance the survival of human neutrophils and eosinophils in vitro: a rapid and sensitive microassay for colony-stimulating factors. *Blood* 1986; **68**: 162–6.

39. Metcalf D. Clonal analysis of proliferation and differentiation of paired daughter cells: action of granulocyte–macrophage colony-stimulating factor on granulocyte–macrophage precursors. *Proc Natl Acad Sci USA* 1980; **77**: 5327–30.

40. Metcalf D. *The Molecular Control of Blood Cells.* Cambridge: Harvard University Press, 1988.

41. Koike K, Ihle JN, Ogawa M. Declining sensitivity to interleukin 3 of murine multipotential hemopoietic progenitors during their development. *J Clin Invest* 1986; **77**: 894–9.

42. Warren DJ, Moore MA. Synergism among interleukin 1, interleukin 3, and interleukin 5 in the production of eosinophils from primitive hemopoietic stem cells. *J Immunol* 1988; **140**: 94–9.

43. Jansen JH, Fibbe WE, Wientjens GJHM et al. Differential stimulatory and inhibitory effects of interleukin-4 on granulocytic and monocytic colony formation in human bone marrow cultures. *Int J Cell Cloning* 1991; **9**: 570–8.

44. Jansen JH, Wientjes GJ, Fibbe WE et al. Inhibition of human macrophage-colony formation by interleukin-4. *J Exp Med* 1989; **170**: 577–82.

45. Wang SY, Ho CK, Chen LY et al. The effect of lipopolysaccharide on the production of GM-EA, GM-CSA, and $PGE_2$ by human monocyte-derived lipid-containing macrophages. *Exp Hematol* 1988; **16**: 349–54.

46. Lopez AF, Begley CG, Williamson DJ et al. Murine eosinophil differentiation factor. An eosinophil-specific colony-stimulating factor with activity for human cells. *J Exp Med* 1986; **163**: 1085–99.

47. Weisbart RH, Kacena A, Shuh A, Golde DW. GM-CSF induces neutrophil IgA-mediated phagocytosis by an IgA Fc receptor activation mechanism. *Nature* 1988; **332**: 647–8.

48. Yuo A, Kitagawa S, Okabe T et al. Recombinant human granulocyte colony-stimulating factor repairs the abnormalities of neutrophils in patients with myelodysplastic syndromes and chronic myelogenous leukemia. *Blood* 1987; **70**: 404–11.

49. Wang JM, Colella S, Allavena P, Mantovani A. Chemotactic activity of human recombinant granulocyte–macrophage colony-stimulating factor. *Immunology* 1987; **60**: 439–44.

50. Weisbart RH, Golde DW, Clark SC et al. Human granulocyte–macrophage colony-stimulating factor is a neutrophil activator. *Nature* 1985; **314**: 361–3.

51. Weisbart RH, Kwan L, Golde DW, Gasson JC. Human GM-CSF primes neutrophils for enhanced oxidative metabolism in response to the major physiological chemoattractants. *Blood* 1987; **69**: 18–21.

52. Arnaout MA, Wang EA, Clark SC, Sieft CA. Human recombinant granulocyte–macrophage colony-stimulating factor increases cell-to-cell adhesion and surface expression of adhesion-promoting surface glycoproteins on mature granulocytes. *J Clin Invest* 1986; **78**: 597–601.

53. Wong GG, Wites JS, Temple PA et al. Human GM-CSF: molecular cloning of the complementary DNA and purification of the natural end recombinant proteins. *Science* 1985; **228**: 810–15.

54. Dedhar S, Gaboury L, Galloway P, Eaves C. Human granulocyte colony-stimulating factor is a growth factor active on a variety of cell types of non-hematopoietic origin. *Proc Natl Acad Sci USA* 1988; **85**: 9253–7.

55. Rapoport AP, Abboud CN, DiPersio JF. Granulocyte–macrophage colony-stimulating factor (GM-CSF) and granulocyte colony-stimulating factor (G-CSF): receptor biology, signal transduction, and neutrophil activation. *Blood Rev* 1992; **6**: 43–57.

56. Bot FJ, van Eijk L, Schipper P, Löwenberg B. Human granulocyte–macrophage colony-stimulating factor (GM-CSF) stimulates immature marrow precursors but no CFU-GM, CFU-G, or CFU-M. *Exp Hematol* 1989; **17**: 292–5.

57. Namiki M, Hara H. Enhancement of colony-forming activity of granulocyte–macrophage colony-stimulating factor by monocytes in-vitro. *Blood* 1989; **74**: 918–24.

58. Williams DE, Straneva JE, Cooper S et al. Interactions between purified murine colony-stimulating factors (nat-

ural CSF-1, recombinant GM-CSF, and recombinant IL-3) on the in vitro proliferation of purified murine granulocyte–macrophage progenitor cells. *Exp Hematol* 1987; **15**: 1007–12.

59. Hoffman R. Regulation of megakaryocytopoiesis. *Blood* 1989; **74**: 1196–212.

60. McNiece I, Andrews R, Stewart M et al. Action of interleukin-3, G-CSF, and GM-CSF on highly enriched human hematopoietic progenitor cells: synergistic interaction of GM-CSF plus G-CSF. *Blood* 1989; **74**: 110–14.

61. Migliaccio AR, Bruno M, Miglicaccio G. Evidence for direct action of human biosynthetic (recombinant) GM-CSF in erythroid progenitors in serum-free culture. *Blood* 1987; **70**: 1867–71.

62. Sieff CA, Emerson SG, Donahue RE et al. Human recombinant granulocyte–macrophage colony-stimulating factor: a multilineage hematopoietin. *Science* 1985; **230**: 1171–3.

63. Nagata S, Tsuchiya M, Asano S et al. Molecular cloning and expression of cDNA for human granulocyte colony-stimulating factor. *Nature* 1986; **319**: 415–18.

64. Tsuchiya M, Asano S, Kaziro Y, Nagata S. Isolation and characterization of the cDNA for murine granulocyte colony-stimulating factor. *Proc Natl Acad Sci USA* 1986; **83**: 7633–7.

65. Souza LM, Boone TC, Gabrilove J et al. Recombinant human granulocyte colony-stimulating factor: effects on normal and leukemic myeloid cells. *Science* 1986; **232**: 61–5.

66. Bronchud MH, Potter MR, Morgenstern G et al. In vitro and in vivo analysis of the effects of recombinant human granulocyte colony-stimulating factor in patients. *Br J Cancer* 1988; **58**: 64–9.

67. Lindemann A, Herrmann F, Oster W et al. Hematologic effects of recombinant human granulocyte colony-stimulating factor in patients with malignancy. *Blood* 1989; **74**: 2644–51.

68. Ikebuchi K, Clark SC, Ihle JN et al. Granulocyte colony-stimulating factor enhances interleukin 3-dependent proliferation of multipotent hemopoietic progenitors. *Proc Natl Acad Sci USA* 1988; **85**: 3445–9.

69. Ikebuchi K, Ihle JN, Hirai Y et al. Syngergistic factors for stem cell proliferation: further studies of the target stem cells and the mechanisms of stimulation by interleukin-1, interleukin-6, and granulocyte colony-stimulating factor. *Blood* 1988; **72**: 2007–14.

70. Leary AG, Hirai Y, Kishimoto T et al. Survival of hemopoietic progenitors in the $G_0$ period of the cell cycle does not require early hemopoietic regulators. *Proc Natl Acad Sci USA* 1989; **86**: 4535–8.

71. Stanley ER, Guilbert LJ, Tushinski RJ, Bartelmez SH. CSF-1 – a mononuclear phagocyte lineage-specific hemopoietic growth factor. *J Cell Biochem* 1983; **21**: 151–9.

72. Stanley ER. Colony stimulating factor-1 (macrophage colony stimulating factor). In: Thomson AW (ed) *The Cytokine Handbook*, 2nd edn. San Diego: Academic Press, 1994: 387–418.

73. Bartocci A, Mastrogiannis DS, Migliorati G et al. Macrophages specifically regulate the concentration of their own growth factor in the circulation. *Proc Natl Acad Sci USA* 1987; **84**: 6179–83.

74. Price LK, Choi HU, Rosenberg L, Stanley ER. The predominant form of secreted colony stimulating factor-1 is a proteoglycan. *J Biol Chem* 1992; **267**: 2190–9.

75. Suzu S, Ohtsuki T, Yanai N et al. Identification of a high molecular weight macrophage colony-stimulating factor as a glycosaminoglycan-containing species. *J Biol Chem* 1992; **267**: 4345–8.

76. Pollard JW, Bartocci A, Arceci R et al. Apparent role of the macrophage growth factor, CSF-1, in placental development. *Nature* 1987; **330**: 484–6.

77. Guba SC, Stella G, Turka LA et al. Regulation of interleukin 3 gene induction in normal T cells. *J Clin Invest* 1989; **84**: 1701–6.

78. Ogawa M, Clark SC. Synergistic interaction between interleukin-6 and interleukin-3 in support of stem cell proliferation in culture. *Blood Cells* 1988; **14**: 329–37.

79. Ottmann OG, Abboud M, Welte K et al. Stimulation of human hematopoietic progenitor cell proliferation and differentiation by recombinant human interleukin 3. Comparison and interactions with recombinant human granulocyte–macrophage and granulocyte colony-stimulating factors. *Exp Hematol* 1989; **17**: 191–7.

80. Emerson SG, Yang YC, Clark SC, Long MW. Human recombinant granulocyte–macrophage colony stimulating factor and interleukin 3 have overlapped but distinct hematopoietic activities. *J Clin Invest* 1988; **82**: 1282–7.

81. Lu L, Lin ZH, Shen RN et al. Influence of interleukin 3, 5, and 6 on the growth of eosinophils progenitors in highly enriched human bone marrow in the absence of serum. *Exp Hematol* 1990; **18**: 1180–5.

82. Schrader JW, Lewis SJ, Clark-Lewis I, Culvenor JG. The persisting (P) cell: histamine content, regulation by a T cell-derived factor, origin from a bone marrow precursor, and relationship to mast cells. *Proc Natl Acad Sci USA* 1981; **78**: 323–7.

83. Heyworth CM, Whetton AD, Nicholls S et al. Stem cell factor directly stimulates the development of enriched granulocyte-macrophage colony-stimulating cells and promotes the effects of other colony-stimulating factors. *Blood* 1992; **80**: 2230–6.

84. McNiece IK, Langley KE, Zsebo KM. Recombinant human stem cell factor synergizes with GM-CSF, G-CSF, IL3 and Epo to stimulate human progenitor cells of the myeloid and erythroid lineages. *Exp Hematol* 1991; **19**: 226–30.

85. Williams N, Bertoncello I, Kavnoudias H et al. Recombinant rat stem cell factor stimulates the amplification and differentiation of fractionated mouse stem cell populations. *Blood* 1992; **79**: 58–64.

86. Carow CE, Hangoc G, Cooper SH et al. Mast cell growth factor (c-kit ligand) supports the growth of human multipotential progenitor cells with a high replating potential. *Blood* 1991; **78**: 2216–21.

87. Avraham H, Vannier E, Cowley S et al. Effect of stem cell factor, c-kit ligand on human megakaryocytic cells. *Blood* 1992; **79**: 365–71.

88. Welham M, Schrader JW. Modulation of c-kit mRNA and protein by hemopoietic growth factors. *Mol Cell Biol* 1991; **11**: 2901–4.

89. Matthews W, Jordan CT, Wiegand GW et al. A receptor tyrosine kinase specific to hematopoietic stem and progenitor cell-enriched populations. *Cell* 1991; **65**: 1143–52.

90. Rosnet O, Marchetto S, deLapeyriere O, Birnbaum D. Murine *Flt-3*, a gene encoding a novel tyrosine kinase receptor of the PDGF/CSF1R family. *Oncogene* 1991; **6**: 1641–50.

91. Lyman SD, Brasel K, Rousseau AM, Williams DE. The Flt-3 ligand: a hematopoietic stem cell factor whose activities are distinct from steel factor. *Stem Cells* 1994; **12** (Suppl 1): 99–110.

92. Rosnet O, Schiff C, Pebusque MJ et al. Human *Flt-3/Flk-2* gene: cDNA cloning and expression in hematopoietic cells. *Blood* 1993; **82**: 1110–19.

93. Rappold I, Ziegler BL, Kohler I et al. Functional and phenotypic characterization of cord blood and bone marrow subsets expressing flt3 (CD135) receptor tyrosine kinase. *Blood* 1997; **90**: 111–25.

94. Lyman SD, James L, VandenBos T, et al. Molecular cloning of a ligand for the flt3/flk-2 tyrosine kinase receptor: a proliferative factor for primitive hematopoietic cells. *Cell* 1993; **75**: 1157–67.

95. Hudak S, Hunte B, Culpepper J et al. Flt-3/Flk-2 ligand promotes the growth of murine stem cells and the expansion of colony-forming cells and spleen colony-forming units. *Blood* 1995; **85**: 2747–2755.

96. Jacobsen SE, Okkenhaug C, Myklebust J et al. The Flt-3 ligand potently and directly stimulates the growth and expansion of primitive murine bone marrow progenitor cells in-vitro: synergistic interactions with IL-11, IL-12 and other hematopoietic growth factors. *J Exp Med* 1995; **181**: 1357–63.

97. Coulombel L, Eaves AC, Eaves CJ. Enzymetic treatment of long-term marrow cultures reveals the preferential location of primitive progenitor cells in the adherent layer. *Blood* 1983; **62**: 291–7.

98. Springer TA. Traffic signals for lymphocyte recirculation and leukocyte emigration: the multistep paradigm. *Cell* 1994; **76**: 301–14.

99. Liesveld J, Winslow WM, Frediani KE et al. Expression of integrins and examination of their adhesive function in normal and leukemic hematopoietic progenitor cells. *Blood* 1993; **81**: 112–21.

100. Majdic O, Stockl J, Pickl WF et al. Signaling induction of enhanced cytoadhesiveness via the hematopoietic progenitor cell surface molecule CD34. *Blood* 1993; **83**: 1226–34.

101. Gunji Y, Nakamura M, Hagiwara T et al. Expression and function of adhesion molecules on human hematopoietic stem cells CD34+LFA-1- cells are more primitive than CD34+LFA-1+ cells. *Blood* 1992; **80**: 429–36.

# 10 Erythropoiesis

**Paul-Henri Roméo**

## Introduction

Erythropoiesis is the pathway that produces mature red blood cells from hematopoietic stem cells. This cellular process is characterized by a series of commitment and differentiation steps that restrict the proliferative capacity and differentiation potential of the cells as the erythroid-specific program of gene expression is established. Like the other hematopoietic lineages, erythropoiesis is regulated by the combined effects of growth factors that promote the survival, proliferation, or differentiation of hematopoietic progenitor cells and nuclear regulators, mostly transcription factors, that activate erythroid-specific genes. Presently, no single transcription factor has been shown to induce erythropoiesis from hematopoietic stem cells or even from early hematopoietic progenitors, and it is quite possible that the erythrocytic phenotype is controlled by a combination of cell-specific and widely expressed transcription factors that integrate the proliferation, survival, and differentiation signals driving the pluripotent hematopoietic stem cell towards mature red blood cells.

Among the different hematopoietic lineages, erythropoiesis is one of the best studied and might be considered as a major model system for hematopoietic differentiation for two main reasons. First, adult erythropoiesis is completely dependent on the presence of a growth factor, erythropoietin (EPO), owing to the tissue-specific expression of its receptor (EPO-R), and this EPO/EPO-R association is one of the best studied systems for signal transduction and regulation of a hematopoietic lineage. Second, the globin genes, which are exclusively expressed during erythropoiesis, represent a model system for gene activation during cellular differentiation. This chapter summarizes our present knowledge on erythropoiesis at the cellular level, including the function of the EPO/EPO-R association and at the transcription level, with a focus on how study of the regulators of erythropoiesis addresses questions of hematopoietic lineage selection and commitment.

## Adult erythropoiesis at the cellular level

During mammalian development, erythropoiesis takes place successively in the visceral yolk sac, the fetal liver, and the bone marrow. Many features of primitive erythropoiesis are completely different from the fetal and adult erythropoiesis, indicating at least two separate waves of erythroid cells, and the properties of primitive erythropoiesis will only be indicated here when differences might be of biological interest.

At the cellular level, committed erythroid progenitors are detected by the formation of erythroid colonies after in vitro culture in methylcellulose, and are called the burst-forming unit erythroid (BFU-E) and the colony-forming unit erythroid (CFU-E).[1,2] BFU-E are the most immature hematopoietic cells already committed to the erythrocyte lineage. These cells represent 0.02% of bone marrow hematopoietic cells, and only 30% of BFU-E are cycling.[3] CFU-E represent 0.2% of bone marrow hematopoietic cells, and most of them are cycling.[4] There is a continuous cellular process from the earliest BFU-E to the latest CFU-E,[1,2] but the growth factor requirement defines mainly these two cellular entities. CFU-E will differentiate into the first morphologically identified cell of the erythrocyte lineage, the proerythroblast; erythrocytic differentiation will then produce the basophilic erythroblast, the polychromatophilic erythroblast, and the acidophilic erythroblast, which is the last nucleated cell of the mammalian erythrocyte lineage. Enucleation of the acidophilic erythroblast occurs only during fetal and adult mammalian erythropoiesis, giving rise to reticulocytes and finally red blood cells (Figure 10.1). Some of the known human antigens used to characterize the different steps of erythropoiesis are shown in Figure 10.1. The early-expressed erythrocytic antigens (e.g. CD33) are also expressed by precursors of other hematopoietic lineages, while most of the late antigens are erythrocyte-specific.

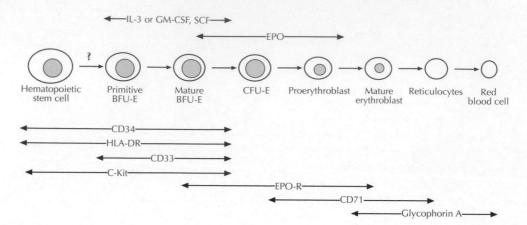

**Figure 10.1** Growth factor requirement and expression of different surface markers and growth factor receptor during erythrocytic differentiation. The primitive burst-forming units erythroid (BFU-E) are at present the most immature known hematopoietic cells already committed to the erythrocytic lineage. Interleukin-3 (IL-3), granulocyte–macrophage colony-stimulating factor (GM-CSF), and stem cell factor (SCF) are required, in addition to erythropoietin (EPO), for efficient differentiation of BFU-E. CD34, HLA-DR, and CD33 are present on BFU-E and are not detected on colony-forming units erythroid (CFU-E), and c-Kit and EPO-R have overlapping expression during erythropoiesis. Glycophorin A is just one of the final surface markers that is specific to red blood cells.

The formation of BFU-E in cell culture is regulated by EPO and other growth factors, including stem cell factor (SCF), interleukin-3 (IL-3), insulin-like growth factor I (IGF-I) and granulocyte–macrophage colony-stimulating factor (GM-CSF),[5] while the formation of CFU-E is highly dependent on low concentrations of EPO alone.[4] EPO is necessary for erythrocytic differentiation until the late basophilic erythroblast stage, and then the erythroid cells are no longer dependent on EPO for final maturation.[6] Genetic analyses of mice with a null mutation in the genes encoding GM-CSF or IL-3[7,8] have indicated that these factors are not crucial for erythropoiesis or that other factors can compensate for their function, while mice lacking SCF or its receptor c-Kit,[9] or lacking EPO or EPO-R,[10] exhibit a dramatic reduction of CFU-E progenitors or erythroid cells derived from CFU-E. Thus this chapter will mainly review the functions of the SCF/c-Kit and EPO/EPO-R associations in erythropoiesis.

## Stem cell factor and its receptor

SCF (also called Steel factor, mast cell growth factor, and c-Kit ligand) is a pleiotropic growth factor. Studies of mice with mutations at the locus that encodes SCF, the *Steel* locus (*Sl*), have shown that SCF is absolutely required during adult hematopoiesis to maintain an adequate output of mature red cells and tissue mast cells.[11,12] SCF is synthesized by bone marrow stromal cells as a transmembrane glycoprotein,[13] which can be proteolytically processed by matrix metalloproteinase-9 (MMP-9) to produce a soluble factor that enables bone marrow-repopulating cells to translocate to a permissive niche favoring differentiation and reconstitution of the hematopoietic stem/progenitor cell pool.[14] Membrane-anchored SCF (mSCF) not only is a precursor of the soluble form (sSCF) but also has its own biological activity, which is necessary in vivo as mice that produce only the soluble SCF isoform die from severe anemia.[15]

SCF interacts with a specific receptor, c-Kit, which is a growth factor receptor with ligand-dependent tyrosine kinase activity.[16] Signaling mediated by c-Kit involves homodimerization of SCF-bound receptor, activation of the intrinsic receptor kinase, autophosphorylation, and association of the phosphorylated receptor with intracellular signaling molecules.[17,18] Briefly, the phosphorylated c-Kit receptor binds the Grb2 protein, phospholipase $C\gamma_1$ (PLC$\gamma_1$), and the regulatory subunit (p85) of phosphatidylinositol 3′-kinase (PI3K).[17,18] These bindings turn on four different intracellular pathways: (i) Raf-1/MAPK, (ii) Src kinase, (iii) Akt kinase, and (iv) the Janus family of protein tyrosine kinases. The activation of these pathways ultimately results in cell proliferation, survival, and adhesion. Inactivation of the c-Kit pathway is mediated by association of the hematopoietic protein tyrosine phosphatase SHP-1 (also called HCP and PTP1C) with phosphorylated tyrosine of the SCF-activated c-Kit receptor[19] and by a ligand-dependent ubiquitination followed by internalization of the c-Kit receptor.[20] This inactivation is modulated differentially, depending on the nature of the c-Kit ligand. In the case of sSCF, the tyrosine phosphorylation of c-Kit is rapid and is followed by a decrease in phosphorylation, while mSCF-induced c-Kit phosphorylation is more durable, likely due to prevention of c-Kit internalization and inactivation.[21,22]

## Erythropoietin and its receptor

EPO is a 34 kDa glycoprotein hormone secreted mainly by the kidney, where its synthesis is regulated, at the transcriptional level, by hypoxia.[23] This regulation of EPO production by hypoxia is controlled by a hypoxia-inducible transcription factor called HIF-1α.[24] EPO is not required for primitive erythropoiesis, but is the crucial growth factor for definitive erythropoiesis as *EPO*–/– mice generated committed BFU-E and CFU-E but died around embryonic day 13 from severe anemia due to the absence of erythrocytic terminal differentiation.[10] EPO specifically interacts with a receptor (EPO-R) that is mainly expressed in cells of the erythrocyte lineage, making EPO highly specific for erythroid progenitors.[25]

EPO-R is a member of the cytokine receptor superfamily, which are type I membrane-spanning glycoproteins with extracellular and cytoplasmic domains of varying sizes. The EPO-R extracellular domain consists of two fibronectin III-like subdomains (D1 and D2) separated by a hinge. In the D2 region, there is a conserved Trp-Ser-X-Trp-Ser motif, which has been shown to be important for EPO-R folding. The EPO-R cytoplasmic domain contains no intrinsic catalytic activity and contains two regions (Box 1 and Box 2) conserved in the membrane-proximal portion of several of these cytokine receptors and a negative regulatory domain present in its membrane-distal portion[26] (Figure 10.2).

Despite the lack of a catalytically active region in the cytoplasmic tail of EPO-R, binding of EPO induces rapid and transient phosphorylation of eight EPO-R cytoplasmic tyrosines.[27] These phosphorylations are mediated by a kinase, Janus kinase 2 (JAK2), whose activity is dependent on EPO stimulation.[28] Actually, JAK2 is bound to the region of EPO-R that contains Box 1 and Box 2 segments, but is inactive in the absence of EPO. Until recently, EPO was assumed to induce dimerization of EPO-R, but investigation of crystal structures has shown that EPO-R in the unliganded state exists as a dimer.[29,30] In response to EPO, this dimer undergoes a dramatic conformational change,[31,32] which is believed to be translated to the cytoplasmic domain, where it brings associated JAK2 into proximity and thus enables them to auto- or *trans*-phosphorylate each other (Figure 10.3). Phosphorylation of JAK2 dramatically activates its kinase activity and leads to tyrosine phosphorylation of eight EPO-R tyrosines as well as other substrates. This JAK2 pathway plays a pivotal role in the EPO-R signaling pathway, as kinase-deficient JAK2 protein or mutations in the Box 1/Box 2 region block signaling by EPO.[33] Among the other JAK2 substrates, a member of the STAT (signal transducers and activators of transcription) family, STAT5, is phosphorylated and then translocates, as a homo- or heterodimer, to the nucleus, where it can activate transcription[34] (Figure

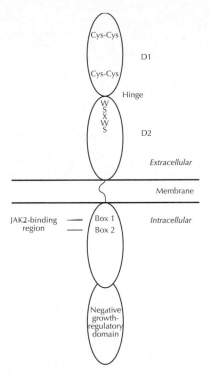

**Figure 10.2** Structure of the erythropoietin receptor (EPO-R). The extracellular domain of EPO-R contains one hematopoietin domain characterized by two fibronectin III-like subdomains (D1 and D2) linked by a hinge. The first subdomain contains four conserved cysteine residues linked two by-two by disulfide bonds, while a second subdomain contains the WSXWS (Trp-Ser-X-Trp-Ser) sequence. This extracellular domain is linked to the intracellular domain by a single transmembrane domain. The intracellular domain consists of a proximal domain characterized by two conserved regions (Box 1 and Box 2), which are involved in JAK2 binding to EPO-R, and a distal domain that acts like a negative growth-regulatory domain.

10.3). More than 20 signal transduction factors are recruited and activated after EPO-R phosphorylation.[35] In addition to STAT5, they include Cis1, SHP-1 and -2, PI3K p85 subunit, PLCγ, Grb2, Shc, Cbl, Gab1 and 2, Vav, and mSOS.[35] Recruitment of these molecules to the EPO-R/JAK2 complex leads to the activation of several signaling cascades, including the Ras and the PI3K pathways.[36,37] Inactivation of EPO-R signaling seems to occur by a direct interaction between EPO-R and the phosphatase SHP-1 via the phosphorylated tyrosine residue 429 (Figure 10.3). After binding to EPO-R, SHP-1 dephosphorylates JAK2 and thus terminates EPO-R signaling.[38] The role of SHP-1 in EPO-R signaling is emphasized by the fact that mice with defects in the *motheaten* locus, encoding SHP-1, have CFU-E that are hypersensitive to EPO in vitro[39] and by the study of two families with dominant benign erythrocytosis. In these two families, a stop codon or a frameshift results in an EPO-R C-terminal truncation that completely suppresses the SHP-1-binding site,

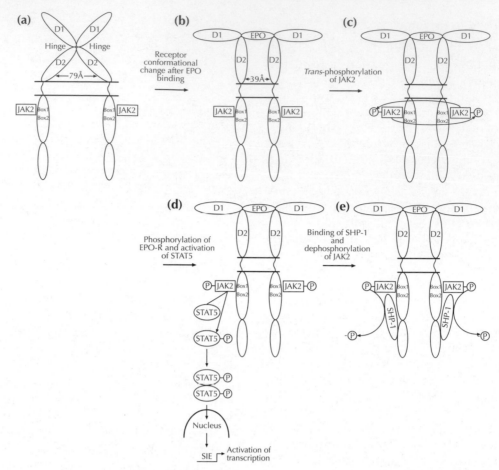

**Figure 10.3** Activation, signal transduction via the STAT pathway, and inactivation of EPO-R. In the absence of EPO, EPO-R is dimeric, but the two JAK2 which are associated with this EPO-R through the Box 1/Box 2 region are kept away (a). Binding of EPO to EPO-R induces a dramatic conformational change of EPO-R. This EPO-induced conformational change of the EPO-R extracellular domains is translated to the cytoplasmic domains, puts the two JAK2 into close proximity, and thus allows *trans*-phosphorylation of these two kinases (b, c). These phosphorylations increase JAK2 activity and lead to phosphorylation of numerous tyrosines in EPO-R as well as in other substrates, including STAT5 (d). Once STAT5 has been phosphorylated, it can form homo- or heterodimers, which are translocated to the nucleus, where they can activate transcription through binding to specific sequences known as c-Sis-inducible elements (SIE). Indeed, JAK2 activity also leads to phosphorylation and activation of proteins involved in other mitogenic pathways, such as the Ras and PI3K pathways, but for simplicity these pathways are not indicated in the figure. JAK2 also phosphorylates tyrosine 429 of EPO-R (e). This phosphotyrosine becomes a docking site for SHP-1, a hematopoietic phosphatase that dephosphorylates JAK2 and thus terminates EPO-R signaling.

and erythroid progenitors from these individuals are also hypersensitive to EPO in vitro.[40,41]

## Synergy between EPO and SCF during adult erythropoiesis; role of the glucocorticoid receptor

During erythrocytic differentiation, c-Kit and EPO-R have an overlapping expression that is indeed biologically relevant. c-Kit is highly expressed at the BFU-E stage, after which its expression decreases until the CFU-E stage, where it is weakly detectable.[42] Conversely, early BFU-E have very little EPO-R on their surface and are not responsive to EPO. Mature BFU-E express a low level of EPO-R and become responsive to EPO; EPO-R expression then increases until the CFU-E stage.[43] CFU-E express more than

1000 EPO-R on their surface, and EPO alone can sustain the terminal erythrocytic differentiation from the CFU-E stage.

These expression patterns are correlated with growth factor requirements during erythropoiesis. SCF is crucial for proliferation and/or differentiation of BFU-E progenitor cells to the CFU-E stage, since mice lacking SCF (*Sl* mutants) or c-Kit (*W* mutants) exhibit a normal number of BFU-E but a significant reduction of CFU-E progenitors. During the transition from BFU-E to CFU-E, there is a synergy between SCF and EPO, SCF increasing EPO sensitivity more than 100-fold and inducing EPO-R phosphorylation.[44] This synergy is mediated by a direct interaction between c-Kit and EPO-R through the EPO-R cytoplasmic region that contains Box 2, and might induce mitogenic and/or differentiation signals that enhance the JAK2 pathway.[45] Thus, before but close to the CFU-E stage, the interaction between c-Kit and EPO-R may be important for triggering subsequent cell proliferation and/or differentiation. After the CFU-E stage, erythropoiesis becomes absolutely dependent on EPO for survival, proliferation, and/or terminal differentiation, since mice lacking EPO or EPO-R produce committed BFU-E and CFU-E progenitors but die from severe anemia as these CFU-E cannot proliferate and terminally differentiate.

Finally, glucocorticoids together with SCF and EPO contribute to stress erythropoiesis in hypoxic mice.[46] In humans, glucocorticoids cooperate with EPO and SCF to induce erythroid progenitors to undergo 15–22 cell divisions corresponding to a $5 \times 10^5$-fold amplification of erythroid cells.[47] This glucocorticoid-dependent amplification may involve the maintenance of c-Kit expression, and is of the greatest interest for molecular and cellular studies of erythropoiesis.

# Adult erythropoiesis at the transcriptional level

From the BFU-E stage to the erythrocyte, the expression pattern of erythroid-specific genes follows a precise timing that is mainly regulated at the transcriptional level. Studies of (i) the regulatory regions of terminally expressed erythroid-specific genes, (ii) the perturbations of erythropoiesis in pathologies such as leukemias, and (iii) the experimental animal models established by gene disruption have greatly increased our knowledge on the cis- and trans-acting elements involved in erythroid-restricted gene expression and have pinpointed erythroid-restricted and pleiotropic trans-acting factors specifically involved in erythrocytic differentiation.

## Cis-acting sequences involved in the regulation of erythroid-specific genes

Functional analysis of erythroid-specific genes, such as the globin genes, the porphobilinogen deaminase gene, the glycophorin A and B genes, and the EPO-R receptor gene, have shown the importance of a sequence 5' A/T GATA A/G 3', now called the GATA motif, in the regulated expression of these genes.[48] This sequence is often associated with a GT or CACC-like sequence, and the GATA/GT or CACC association is presently considered as a hallmark of an erythroid-specific regulatory region.[48] Another motif occurs in the core region of erythroid-expressed gene promoters, enhancers, or locus control region (LCR). This motif, 5' TGA C/G TCAGCA 3' is an AP1-like sequence that seems to be necessary for efficient erythroid-specific gene expression.[49] No other motif has been repeatedly found in regulatory regions of erythroid-specific genes, and, for example, the cis-acting elements involved in the timing of the expression of these genes during erythropoiesis are yet to be characterized. For each type of binding motif identified as recurrent in the regulatory regions of erythroid-specific genes, the nuclear factor(s) that recognizes the motif has been identified and cloned. None of these lineage-specific factors is restricted to a single cell type, showing that specificity of gene expression in erythropoiesis, as in the other hematopoietic lineages, is established by a specific combination of nuclear factors rather than by specific factors (Figure 10.4).

## Trans-acting factors that are required for setting up erythropoiesis

In the mouse, targeted disruption of many different genes (including RB1 and AML1) results in death at the fetal stage from severe anemia.[50–52] These mutant mice have a normal primitive erythropoiesis, indicating again that yolk sac (primitive) and fetal liver (definitive) erythropoiesis are regulated by two distinct

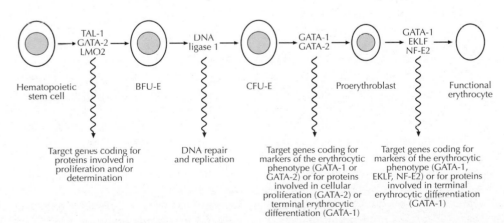

**Figure 10.4** Regulation of the different stages of erythropoiesis by *trans*-acting factors. Nuclear factors that are necessary for the different steps of erythropoiesis are shown and the function of their target genes in erythropoiesis is indicated. Rbtn-2/LMO2 and TAL-1/SCL are also necessary for primitive erythropoiesis. The potential interregulation of GATA-1 and GATA-2 during terminal erythropoiesis is indicated.

genetic programs. Analysis of most of these gene-knockout mice shows a block in the development of all of the definitive hematopoietic lineages, indicating that these gene products are not specifically involved in erythrocytic differentiation but in the proliferation and/or commitment of hematopoietic progenitors, including erythroid ones. However, these targeted disruptions have indicated the importance of two widely expressed genes, DNA ligase I[53] and DNase II,[54] for setting up erythropoiesis. DNA ligase I is central to DNA replication and repair, and a patient with altered DNA ligase I displayed growth retardation and immunodeficiency similar to Bloom's syndrome.[55] Mice lacking DNA ligase I died from anemia at the fetal liver stage, and analysis of the fetal liver hematopoietic cells of these mice indicated only a small decrease in the total number of BFU-E but very few erythrocytes.[53] Since the total number of non-erythroid hematopoietic cells in these *DNA ligase*−/− mice is normal, this knockout pinpoints a major role of this widely expressed enzyme in erythropoiesis at a stage (BFU-E to CFU-E) where an extremely high replicative pressure is exerted on this differentiation (Figure 10.4). DNase II, a lysosomal DNase, degrades DNA of apoptotic cells. *DNase II*−/− mice die in utero due to severe anemia. This defect is non-cell-autonomous, as mutant fetal liver cells transferred into lethally irradiated mice produce mature red blood cells, but is related to abnormal macrophage function in the destruction of the nuclear DNA expelled from erythroid precursor cells.[54] Two other nuclear factors, TAL-1/SCL and Rbtn2/LMO2 play a major role in setting up erythropoiesis. Both TAL-1/SCL and Rbtn2/LMO2 have been identified by the cloning of chromosomal translocation breakpoints associated with human T-cell acute lymphoblastic leukemia (T-ALL).[56,57] The *TAL-1* gene encodes a basic helix–loop–helix (bHLH) transcription factor and the *rbtn2/LMO2* gene encodes a nuclear Lim-domain protein that does not display any sequence-specific DNA binding. During hematopoiesis, TAL-1 and LMO2 are mainly expressed in early hematopoietic progenitors, and then their expression is restricted to the erythrocyte, mastocyte, and megakaryocyte lineages, but not the T-cell lineage.[58] These two proteins are physically linked, as the in vivo immunoprecipitable LMO2 protein is complexed with TAL-1[59] and GATA-1 in erythrocytes, indicating that the TAL-1–LMO2 complex might be important for gene regulation during erythropoiesis. Indeed, while LMO2, TAL-1, and GATA-1 alone have little effect on erythropoiesis in *Xenopus*, their ectopic coexpression in *Xenopus* embryos enlarges the ventral blood islands at the expense of dorsal mesoderm (muscle and notochord) embryogenesis,[60] and LMO2, TAL-1, and GATA-1 overexpression in activin-treated *Xenopus* pole explants further increases the production of hemoglobinized cells.[60]

Mice lacking the Rbtn2/LMO2 or the TAL-1/SCL protein die in utero at day 8.5 with a severe anemia that is thought to be the cause of death.[61,62] These in vivo data indicate that both TAL-1/SCL and Rbtn2/LMO2 are required for primitive erythropoiesis. In vitro differentiation of *tal-1*−/− ES cells have shown an impaired hematopoiesis, and complementation of the lymphoid defect in RAG-2-deficient mice has shown that TAL-1 is also required for adult hematopoiesis.[63] Finally, conditional *tal-1* gene targeting has shown that TAL-1 is essential for the genesis of hematopoietic stem cells but is not essential for the hematopoietic stem cell functions.[64,65] As for erythropoiesis, deletion of the *tal-1* gene results in the complete loss of early progenitors of this lineage, as BFU-E are absent from spleen and bone marrow of these *tal-1*−/− mice.[64,65] Thus, this TAL-1/LMO2 complex might activate target genes involved in proliferation and/or cell death (Figure 10.4), and the identification of these target genes is now an important challenge (Table 10.1).

## *Trans*-acting factors involved in the expression of erythroid-specific genes

The first motif identified in the regulatory regions of erythroid-specific genes is the 5′ A/T GATA A/G 3′ or GATA motif. This sequence is recognized by a family of nuclear proteins called the GATA proteins, whose members are structurally defined by the presence of two highly conserved zinc fingers Cys-$X_2$-Cys-$X_{17}$-Cys-$X_2$-Cys, which display different but cooperative functions. The range of genes regulated by members of the GATA family extends well beyond hematopoietic cells, but only two members of this family, GATA-1 and GATA-2, are expressed during erythropoiesis and play a major role in this hematopoietic lineage[48] (Figure 10.4).

GATA-1 expression is restricted to the erythrocyte, megakaryocyte, and mast cell lineages, and targeted disruption of the mouse *GATA-1* gene has shown that GATA-1 is a key regulator of erythrocytic differentiation. Indeed, GATA-1− embryonic stem (ES) cells contribute to every hematopoietic lineages except the erythrocyte lineage.[66] In vitro differentiation of these GATA-1− ES cells has shown that erythrocytic differentiation was blocked at the proerythroblast stage of development, where the cells die by apoptosis.[67] Interestingly, most of the presumptive GATA-1 target genes in erythroid cells (Table 10.1) are expressed at normal levels in GATA-1− proerythroblast and it is believed that transcription of these genes occur through the action of GATA-2, whose expression is 50-fold upregulated in the GATA-1− ES cells.[67] Thus, survival and terminal differentiation of proerythroblasts appear to be completely dependent on GATA-1. GATA-1 activity is highly regulated by FOG-1 (friend of GATA), a 998-amino-acid nuclear multitype zinc finger protein that interacts with GATA-1 and does not seem to bind to DNA.[68] *FOG-1*−/− mice die in utero at day 10.5–11.5 with severe anemia due to an arrest

**Table 10.1** *Trans*-acting factors involved in erythrocytic differentiation. Their DNA-binding sites, potential target genes, the phenotypes of their genes inactivation, and the human pathologies associated with their genes mutations are indicated

| *Trans*-acting factor | DNA-binding site | Target genes | Phenotype of gene inactivation | Human pathology |
|---|---|---|---|---|
| GATA-1 | 5'A/T GATAA/G3' | Globin; enzymes of the heme biosynthetic pathway; *GATA-1*; *EKLF*; glycophorins; *EPO-R* | Anemia and thrombocytopenia | Familial dyserythropoietic anemia Recessive X-linked thrombocytopenia Megakaryoblastic leukemia of Down syndrome |
| GATA-2 | 5'A/T GATAA/G 3' | *GATA-1* | Absence of multipotent hematopoietic progenitor proliferation | |
| NFE-2 | 5'TGAC/G TCAGCA3' | Globin; enzymes of the heme biosynthesis pathway | Thrombocytopenia | |
| EKLF | 5'CCNCACCC3' | β-Globin gene locus control region | Anemia | β-Thalassemia |
| TAL-1/SCL | 5'AA/C CAGATGG/T T3' | *c-kit* | No hematopoiesis | T-cell acute lymphoblastic leukemia (T-ALL) |

in erythroid maturation that is similar to that observed in the GATA-1⁻ mice, providing a genetic evidence that these two factors act in a common pathway.[69] Erythropoiesis required the GATA-1/FOG-1 interaction, as shown by severe familial X-linked dyserythropoietic anemia found in patients harboring a *GATA-1* missense mutation that impairs the GATA-1/FOG-1 contact.[70]

PU.1, a member of the Ets family of transcription factors, can interact directly with GATA-1 and repress GATA-1-mediated transcriptional activation.[71] Ectopic expression of PU.1 in *Xenopus* embryos blocks erythropoiesis, and exogenous GATA-1 is able to relieve this blockage of erythroid differentiation, suggesting that erythroid commitment is regulated by the relative levels of these two transcription factors.[71]

GATA-2 expression occurs in all the myeloid lineages and in early hematopoietic progenitors, and the role of GATA-2 in erythropoiesis is presently difficult to define since mice lacking GATA-2 exhibit a severe hematopoietic defect where all hematopoietic lineages are affected as no expansion of early hematopoietic progenitors can occur.[72] However, two recent observations have defined a possible role of GATA-2 in erythropoiesis. First, GATA-2 expression is detected in erythroid progenitors and decreases as GATA-1 expression increases during erythrocytic differentiation.[73] Second, forced expression of GATA-2 in chicken erythroid precursors promotes proliferation and blocks differentiation of these cells.[74] Thus GATA-2 might be essential for appropriate expansion of early erythroid progenitors (Figure 10.4) and one attractive hypothesis would be that, just like c-Kit

and EPO-R, GATA-2 and GATA-1 have overlapping functions during erythropoiesis, GATA-2 regulating genes associated with the c-Kit signaling pathway (Table 10.1) and GATA-1 regulating genes associated with the EPO-R signaling pathway (Table 10.1).

The CACCC motif associated with the GATA motif is recognized by erythroid-specific and widely expressed nuclear factors, and the relative contributions of these transcription factors have been the subject of numerous studies. Members of the SP1 family are among the widely expressed nuclear factors that bind the CACCC motif, but targeted disruption of these genes does not impair erythropoiesis. The cloning of erythroid Kruppel-like factor (EKLF), an erythroid-specific CACCC-binding protein, has enlightened the role of this regulatory element.[75] EKLF binds with a very high affinity to the CACCC site found in the human adult β-globin gene promoter and activates this promoter. Mutation of this sequence is found in some patients with β-thalassemia and impairs EKLF binding and transactivation.[76] EKLF-binding sites are also found in the human β-globin LCR, and the transcriptional activity of HS3 is EKLF-dependent.[77] Mice lacking EKLF die at the fetal liver stage with a major thalassemia syndrome due to inefficient β-globin production.[78] Other erythroid-specific genes whose promoters or enhancers contain CACCC sites are expressed at normal level in these *EKLF⁻/⁻* mice, suggesting that EKLF is required principally for the expression of the β-globin gene (Table 10.1). However, a role for EKFL in the coordination of erythroid cell proliferation and hemoglobinization has also been shown by studies on a genetically engineered *EKLF⁻/⁻*

hematopoietic cell line.[79] Despite this function, EKLF is very different from the GATA proteins, as it might only be required for activation of a few erythroid-specific genes that are of the greatest importance for the function of red blood cells (Figure 10.4).

Besides the GATA and CACCC motifs, a third motif recurs in the regulatory regions of erythroid-specific genes. This motif is an AP1-like sequence that is recognized by a nuclear factor designated NF-E2, which is a heterodimer with a hematopoietic-restricted subunit (p45) and a widely expressed subunit (p18) linked by a leucine zipper.[80,81] Although studies in transgenic mice have indicated that globin gene expression requires the NF-E2 DNA-binding motif (Table 10.1), mice lacking p45 NF-E2 have normal erythropoiesis but die from a hemorrhagic diathesis caused by the absence of platelets.[82] This result strongly indicates a redundancy at the level of the p45 subunit during erythropoiesis and does not provide any enlightenment regarding the role of NF-E2 in erythropoiesis.

# Conclusions, unresolved questions, and perspectives

## Regulation of the erythrocytic commitment

The commitment of multipotential hematopoietic progenitors to the erythrocytic pathway is likely to be mediated by a set of transcription factors that promotes erythrocytic differentiation and provides negative signals for differentiation towards the other hematopoietic lineages. These cross-antagonisms between lineage-specific transcription factors have been shown for GATA-1 and PU.1,[71] C/EBPβ and FOG-1,[83] and GATA-2 and PU.1.[84] They occur by direct interaction (GATA-1 and PU.1), by transcription regulation (C/EBPβ and FOG-1), or by both direct interaction and transcription regulation (GATA-2 and PU.1). With regard to erythrocytic commitment in the adult, forced expression of GATA-1 in a murine multipotential cell line does not promote erythrocytic but rather megakaryocytic differentiation,[85] although forced expression can reprogram avian myelomonocytic cell lines towards eosinophils, thromboblasts, and erythroblasts at the expense of the myelomonocytic lineage.[86] As erythrocytes and megakaryocytes are derived from a common precursor, these experiments suggest that GATA-1 may play a major role in the determination of a pluripotent hematopoietic precursor towards the common precursor of these two lineages, differentiation towards the megakaryocyte or the erythrocyte lineage being regulated by other presently unknown factor(s) or, as recently suggested, by the intracellular level of GATA proteins.[86]

## Interplay between growth factors receptors and *trans*-acting factors

Among the genes required for appropriate erythrocytic differentiation and coding for proteins different from transcription factors, growth factors receptor genes such as *EPO-R* and c-*kit* are of major interest. The structure of these genes has been elucidated and potential GATA-, Myb-, Ets-, and SP1-binding sites have been found in their promoter regions.[87] While little is known about the transcriptional regulation of the c-*kit* gene,[88] GATA and SP.1 has been shown to bind specifically to the *EPO-R* promoter in vitro and to transactivate this promoter in vivo.[89] These results indicate how *EPO-R* gene transcription can be maintain during erythropoiesis, but the molecular mechanisms that activate *EPO-R* gene expression during the initial stages of erythropoiesis are presently unknown. On the other hand, the effect of the binding of EPO or SCF to EPO-R or c-Kit on lineage-specific transcription factors such as GATA-1, EKLF, and NF-E2 is presently not explored and might illuminate the interplay between these receptors and major transcription factors.

## Cell cycle, apoptosis, and erythroid-specific *trans*-acting factors

Terminal differentiation of erythroid cells is accompanied by a progressive loss of their proliferative capacity without apoptosis. One attractive hypothesis is that the combination of *trans*-acting factors involved in the regulation of erythroid-specific genes can also reduce cell proliferation without apoptosis. Again, GATA-1 appears to play a major role in a erythroid survival and to be a cell cycle-linked factor, since differentiation of GATA-1⁻ ES cells leads to premature apoptosis[90] and since ectopic expression of this factor in hematopoietic and non-hematopoietic cell lines can lead to alterations in the length of the different phases of the cell cycle.[91] The subset of genes implicated in these phenomena and regulated by GATA-1 are presently unknown and represent a fruitful area for future study.

# REFERENCES

1. Gregory J, Eaves AC. Human marrow cells capable of erythropoietic differentiation in vitro: definition of three erythroid colony responses. *Blood* 1977; **49**: 855–64.

2. Gregory CJ, Eaves AC. Three stages of erythropoietic progenitor cell differentiation distinguished by a number of physical and biologic properties. *Blood* 1978; **51**: 527–37.

3. Iscove NN. The role of erythropoietin in regulation of population size and cell cycling of early and late erythroid precursors in mouse bone marrow. *Cell Tissue Kinet* 1977; **10**: 323–34.

4. Iscove NN, Sieber F, Winterhaltre KH. Erythroid colony formation in cultures of mouse and human bone marrow: analysis of the requirement for erythropoietin by gel filtration and affinity chromatography on agarose-concavalin A. *J Cell Physiol* 1974; **83**: 309–16.

5. Emerson SG, Sieff CA, Wang EA et al. Purification of fetal hematopoietic progenitors and demonstration of recombinant multipotential colony-stimulating activity. *J Clin Invest* 1985; **76**: 1286–90.

6. Koury MJ, Bondurant MC. Maintenance by erythropoietin of viability and maturation of murine erythroid precursor cells. *J Cell Physiol* 1988; **137**: 65–73.

7. Dranoff G, Crawford AD, Sadelain M et al. Involvement of granulocyte–macrophage colony-stimulating factor in pulmonary homeostasis. *Science* 1994; **209**: 713–16.

8. Nishinakamura R, Nakayama N, Hirabayashi Y et al. Mice deficient for the IL-3/GM-CSF/IL-5βc receptor exhibit lung pathology and impaired immune response, while β IL-3 receptor-deficient mice are normal. *Immunity* 1995; **2**: 211–22.

9. Nocka K, Majumder S, Chabot B et al. Expression of c-*kit* gene products in known cellular targets of W mutations in normal and W mutant mice: evidence for an impaired c-kit kinase in mutant mice. *Genes Dev* 1989; **3**: 816–26.

10. Wu H, Liu X, Jaenisch R et al. Generation of committed erythroid BFU-E and CFU-E progenitors does not require erythropoietin or the erythropoietin receptor. *Cell* 1995; **83**: 59–67.

11. Witte ON. *Steel* locus defines new multipotent growth factor. *Cell* 1990; **63**: 5–6.

12. Russel ES. Hereditary anemias of the mouse: a review for geneticists. *Adv Genet* 1979; **20**: 357–459.

13. Anderson DM, Lyman SD, Baird A et al. Molecular cloning of mast cell growth factor, a hematopoietin that is active in both membrane bound and soluble forms. *Cell* 1990; **63**: 235–43.

14. Heissing B, Hattori K, Dias S et al. Recruitment of stem and progenitor cells from the bone marrow niche requires MMP-9 mediated release of kit-ligand. *Cell* 2002; **109**: 625–37.

15. Flanagan JG, Chan DC, Leder P. Transmembrane form of the c-kit ligand growth factor is determined by alternative splicing and is missing in the SLd mutant. *Cell* 1991; **64**: 1025–35.

16. Yarden Y, Kuang WJ, Feng T et al. Human proto-oncogene c-*kit*: a new cell surface receptor tyrosine kinase for an unidentified ligand. *EMBO J* 1987; **6**: 3341–51.

17. Blechman JM, Lev S, Givol D et al. Structure–function analyses of the kit receptor for the steel factor. *Stem Cells* 1993; **11**: 12–21.

18. Smith MA, Court EL, Smith G. Stem cell factor: laboratory and clinical aspects. *Blood Rev* 2001; **15**: 191–7.

19. Yi T, Ihle JN. Association of hematopoietic cell phosphatase with c-kit after stimulation with c-kit ligand. *Mol Cell Biol* 1993; **13**: 3350–8.

20. Miyazawa K, Toyama K, Gotoh A et al. Ligand-dependent polyubiquitination of c-*kit* gene product: a possible mechanism of receptor down modulation in M07e cells. *Blood* 1994; **83**: 137–45.

21. Miyazawa K, Williams DA, Gotoh A et al. Membrane bound steel factor induces more persistant tyrosine kinase activation and longer life span of c-*kit* gene-encoded protein than its soluble form. *Blood* 1995; **85**: 641–9.

22. Gommerman JL, DeSittaro D, Klebasz DA et al. Differential stimulation of c-*kit* mutants by membrane-bound and soluble Steel factor correlates with leukemic potential. *Blood* 2000; **96**: 3734–42.

23. Goldberg MA, Dunning SP, Bunn HF. Regulation of the erythropoietin gene: evidence that the oxygen sensor is a heme protein. *Science* 1988; **242**: 1412–15.

24. Bunn HF, Gu J, Huang LE. Erythropoietin: a model system for studying oxygen-dependent gene regulation. *J Exp Biol* 1998; **201**: 1197–201.

25. D'Andrea A, Lodish H, Wong G. Expression cloning of the murine erythropoietin receptor. *Cell* 1989; **57**: 277–85.

26. D'Andrea AD, Yoshimura A, Youssoufian H et al. The cytoplasmic region of the erythropoietin receptor contains nonoverlapping positive and negative growth-regulatory domains. *Mol Cell Biol* 1991; **11**: 1980–7.

27. Gobert S, Porteu F, Pallu S et al. Tyrosine phosphorylation of the erythropoietin receptor: role for differentiation and mitogenic transduction. *Blood* 1995; **86**: 598–606.

28. Witthuhn BA, Quelle FW, Silvennoinen O et al. JAK2 associates with the erythropoietin receptor and is tyrosine phosphorylated and activated following stimulation with erythropoietin. *Cell* 1993; **74**: 227–36.

29. Livnah O, Stura EA, Middleton SA et al. Crystallographic evidence for preformed dimers of erythropoietin receptor before ligand activation. *Science* 1999; **283**: 987–90.

30. Remy I, Wilson IA, Michnick SW. Erythropoietin receptor activation by a ligand-induced conformational change. *Science* 1999; **283**: 990–3.

31. Constantinescu SN, Keren T, Socolovsky M et al. Ligand-independent oligomerization of cell-surface erythropoietin receptor is mediated by the transmembrane domain. *Proc Natl Acad Sci USA* 2001; **98**: 4379–84.

32. Constantinescu SN, Huang LJS, Nam HS et al. The erythropoietin receptor cytosolic juxtamembrane domain contains an essential, precisely oriented, hydrophobic motif. *Mol Cell* 2001; **7**: 377–85.

33. Zhuang H, Patil SV, He T-C et al. Inhibition of erythropoietin-induced mitogenesis by a kinase-deficient form of Jak2. *J Biol Chem* 1994; **269**: 21411–14.

34. Gouilleux F, Pallard C, Dusanter-Fourt I et al. Prolactin, growth hormone, erythropoietin and granulocyte–macrophage colony stimulating factor induce MGF–Stat5 DNA binding activity. *EMBO J* 1995; **14**: 2005–13.

35. Wojchowski DM, Gregory RC, Miller CP et al. Signal transduction in the erythropoietin receptor system. *Exp Cell Res* 1999; **253**: 143–56.

36. Miura O, Miura Y, Nakamura N et al. Induction of tyrosine phosphorylation of vav and expression of pim-1 correlates

with Jak2-mediated growth signaling from the erythropoietin receptor. *Blood* 1994; **84**: 4135–41.

37. Mayeux P, Dusanter-Fourt I, Muller O et al. Erythropoietin induces the association of phosphatidylinositol 3′-kinase with a tyrosine phosphorylated complex containing the erythropoietin receptor. *Eur J Biochem* 1993; **216**: 821–7.

38. Klingmüller U, Lorenz U, Cantley LC et al. Specific recruitment of SH–PTP1 to the erythropoietin receptor causes inactivation of JAK2 and termination of proliferative signals. *Cell* 1995; **80**: 729–38.

39. van Zant G, Schulz L. Hematologic abnormalities of the immunodeficient mouse mutant, viable motheaten (*me*ᵛ). *Exp Hematol* 1989; **17**: 81–7.

40. de la Chapelle A, Traskelin A-L, Juvonen E. Truncated erythropoietin receptor causes dominantly inherited benign human erythrocytosis. *Proc Natl Acad Sci USA* 1993; **90**: 4495–9.

41. Sokol L, Luhovy M, Guan Y et al. Primary familial polycythemia: a frameshift mutation in the erythropoietin receptor gene and increased sensitivity of erythroid progenitors to erythropoietin. *Blood* 1995; **86**: 15–22.

42. Papayanopoulou T, Brice M, Roudy VC et al. Isolation of c-kit receptor expressing cells from bone marrow, peripheral blood and fetal liver: functional properties and composite antigenic profile. *Blood* 1991; **78**: 1403–12.

43. Broudy VC, Lin N, Brice M et al. Erythropoietin receptor characteristics on primary human erythroid cells. *Blood* 1991; **77**: 2583–90.

44. Jacobs-Helber SM, Penta K, Sun Z et al. Distinct signaling from stem cell factor and erythropoietin in HCD57 cells. *J Biol Chem* 1997; **272**: 6850–3.

45. Wu H, Klingmüller U, Besmer P et al. Interaction of the erythropoietin and stem-cell-factor receptors. *Nature* 1995; **377**: 2422–6.

46. Bauer A, Tronche F, Wessely O et al. The glycocorticoid receptor is required for stress erythropoiesis. *Genes Dev* 1999; **13**: 2996–3002.

47. Linder MV, Zauner W, Mellitzer G et al. The glucocorticoid receptor cooperates with the erythropoietin receptor and c-kit to enhance and sustain proliferation of erythroid progenitors in vitro. *Blood* 1999; **94**: 550–9.

48. Orkin SH. GATA-binding transcription factors in hematopoietic cells. *Blood* 1992; **80**: 575–81.

49. Raich N, Roméo P-H. Erythroid regulatory elements. *Stem Cells* 1993; **11**: 95–104.

50. Shivdasani RA, Orkin SH. The transcriptional control of hematopoiesis. *Blood* 1996; **87**: 4025–39.

51. Cantor AB, Orkin SH. Transcriptional regulation of erythropoiesis: an affair involving multiple partners. *Oncogene* 2002; **21**: 3368–76.

52. Perry C, Soreq H. Transcriptional regulation of erythropoiesis. Fine tuning of combinatorial multi-domain elements. *Eur J Biochem* 2002; **269**: 3607–18.

53. Bentley DJ, Selfridge J, Millar K et al. DNA ligase I is required for fetal liver erythropoiesis but is not essential for mammalian cell viability. *Nat Genet* 1996; **13**: 489–91.

54. Kawane K, Fukuyama H, Kondoh G et al. Requirement of DNase II for definitive erythropoiesis in the mouse fetal liver. *Science* 2001; **292**: 1546–9.

55. Webster ADB, Bames DE, Arlett CF et al. Growth retardation and immunodeficiency in a patient with mutations in the DNA ligase I gene. *Lancet* 1992; **339**: 1508–9.

56. Begley CG, Aplan PD, Davey MP et al. Chromosomal translocation in a human leukemic stem-cell line disrupts the T-cell antigen receptor δ-chain diversity region and results in a previously unreported fusion transcript. *Proc Natl Acad Sci USA* 1989; **86**: 2031–5.

57. Boehm T, Foroni L, Kaneko Y et al. The rhombotin family of cysteine-rich LIM-domain oncogenes: distinct members are involved in T-cell translocations to human chromosomes 11p15 and 11p13. *Proc Natl Acad Sci USA* 1991; **88**: 4367–72.

58. Mouthon M-A, Bernard O, Mitjvila MT et al. Expression of tal-1 and GATA-binding proteins during human hematopoiesis. *Blood* 1993; **81**: 647–55.

59. Valge-Archer VE, Osada H, Warren AJ et al. The LIM protein RBTN2 and the basic helix–loop–helix protein TAL1 are present in a complex in erythroid cells. *Proc Natl Acad Sci USA* 1994; **91**: 8617–22.

60. Mead PE, Deconinck AE, Huber TL et al. Primitive erythropoiesis in the *Xenopus* embryo: the synergistic role of LMO-2, SCL and GATA-binding proteins. *Development* 2001; **128**: 2301–8.

61. Shivdasani RA, Mayer EL, Orkin SH. Absence of blood formation in mice lacking the T-cell leukemia oncoprotein tal-1/SCL. *Nature* 1995; **373**: 432–5.

62. Warren AJ, Colledge WH, Carlton MBL et al. The oncogenic cysteine-rich LIM domain protein Rbtn2 is essential for erythroid development. *Cell* 1994; **78**: 45–58.

63. Porcher C, Swat W, Rockwell K et al. The T cell leukemia oncoprotein SCL/tal-1 is essential for development of all hematopoietic lineages. *Cell* 1996; **86**: 47–57.

64. Hall MA, Curtis DJ, Metcalf D et al. The critical regulator of embryonic hematopoiesis, SCL, is vital in the adult for megakaryopoiesis, erythropoiesis, and lineage choice in CFU-S12. *Proc Natl Acad Sci USA* 2003; **100**: 992–7.

65. Mikkola HKA, Klintman J, Yang H et al. Haematopoietic stem cells retain long-term repopulating activity and multipotency in the absence of stem-cell leukaemia *SCL/tal-1* gene. *Nature* 2003; **421**: 547–51.

66. Pevny L, Simon MC, Robertson E et al. Erythroid differentiation in chimeric mice blocked by a targeted mutation in the gene for transcription factor GATA-1. *Nature* 1991; **349**: 257–62.

67. Weiss MJ, Orkin SH. Transcription factor GATA-1 permits survival and maturation of erythroid precursors by preventing apoptosis. *Proc Natl Acad Sci USA* 1995; **92**: 9623–7.

68. Tsang AP, Visvader JE, Turner CA et al. FOG, a multitype zinc finger protein, acts as a cofactor for transcription factor GATA-1 in erythroid and megakaryocytic differentiation. *Cell* 1997; **90**: 109–19.

69. Tsang AP, Fujiwara Y, Hom DB et al. Failure of megakaryopoiesis and arrested erythropoiesis in mice lacking the GATA-1 transcriptional cofactor FOG. *Genes Dev* 1998; **12**: 1176–88.

70. Nichols KE, Crispino JD, Poncz M et al. Familial dyserythropoietic anaemia and thrombocytopenia due to an inherited mutation in *GATA1*. *Nat Genet* 2000; **24**: 266–70.

71. Rekhtman N, Radparvar F, Evans T et al. Direct interaction of hematopoietic transcription factors PU.1 and GATA-1: functional antagonism in erythroid cells. *Genes Dev* 1999; **13**: 1398–411.

72. Tsai F-Y, Keller G, KLuo FC et al. An early haematopoietic defect in mice lacking the transcription factor GATA-2. *Nature* 1994; **371**: 221–6.

73. Yamamoto M, Ko LJ, Leonard MW et al. Activity and tis-

sue-specific expression of the transcription factor NF-E1 multigene family. *Genes Dev* 1990; **4**: 1650–62.

74. Briegel K, Lim K-C, Plank C et al. Ectopic expression of a conditional GATA-2/estrogen receptor chimera arrests erythroid differentiation in a hormone-dependent manner. *Genes Dev* 1993; **7**: 1097–112.

75. Miller IJ, Bieker JJ. A novel, erythroid cell-specific murine transcription factor that binds to the CACCC element and is related to the Kruppel family of nuclear proteins. *Mol Cell Biol* 1993; **13**: 2776–85.

76. Feng WC, Southwood CM, Bieker JJ. Analyses of β-thalassemia mutant DNA interactions with erythroid Kruppel-like factor (EKLF), an erythroid cell-specific transcription factor. *J Biol Chem* 1994; **269**: 1493–500.

77. Tewari R, Gillemans N, Wijgerde M et al. Erythroid Kruppel-like factor (EKLF) is active in primitive and definitive erythroid cells and is required for the function of 5′HS3 of the β-globin locus control region. *EMBO J* 1998; **17**: 2334–41.

78. Nuez B, Michalovich D, Bygrave A et al. Defective hamatopoiesis in fetal liver resulting from inactivation of the *EKLF* gene. *Nature* 1995; **375**: 316–20.

79. Coghill E, Eccleston S, Fox V et al. Erythroid Kruppel-like factor (EKLF) coordinates erythroid cell proliferation and hemoglobinization in cell lines derived from EKLF null mice. *Blood* 2001; **97**: 1861–8.

80. Andrews NC, Erjument-Bromage H, Davidson MB et al. Erythroid transcription factor NF-E2 is a haematopoietic-specific basic-leucine zipper protein. *Nature* 1993; **362**: 722–7.

81. Andrews NC, Kitkow KJ, Ney PA et al. The ubiquitous subunit of erythroid transcription factor NF-E2 is a small basic-leucine zipper protein related to the v-*maf* oncogene. *Proc Natl Acad Sci USA* 1993; **90**: 11488–93.

82. Shivdasani RA, Rosenblatt MF, Zucker-Franklin D et al. Transcription factor NF-E2 is required for platelet forma-

83. Querfurth E, Schuster M, Kulessa H et al. Antagonism between C/EBPβ and FOG in eosinophil lineage commitment of multipotent hematopoietic progenitors. *Genes Dev* 2000; **14**: 2515–25.

84. Walsh JC, Dekoter RP, Lee HJ et al. Cooperative and antagonistic interplay between PU.1 and GATA-2 in the specification of myeloid cell fates. *Immunity* 2002; **17**: 665–76.

85. Visvader J, Adams JM. Megakaryocytic differentiation induced in 416B myeloid cells by *GATA-2* and *GATA-3* transgenes or 5-azacytidine is tightly coupled to *GATA-1* expression. *Blood* 1993; **82**: 1493–502.

86. Kulessa H, Frampton J, Graf T. GATA-1 reprograms avian myelomonocytic cell lines into eosinophils, thromboblasts, and erythroblasts. *Genes Dev* 1995; **9**: 1250–62.

87. Herbelein C, Fischer K-D, Stoffel et al. The gene for erythropoietin receptor is expressed in multipotential hematopoietic and embryonal stem cells: evidence for differentiation stage-specific regulation. *Mol Cell Biol* 1992; **12**: 1815–21.

88. Lécuyer E, Herblot S, Saint-Denis M et al. The SCL complex regulates c-*kit* expression in hematopoietic cells through functional interaction with Sp1. *Blood* 2002; **100**: 2430–40.

89. Chiba T, Ikawa Y, Todokoro K. GATA-1 transactivates erythropoietin receptor gene, and erythropoietin receptor-mediated signals enhance *GATA-1* gene expression. *Nucleic Acids Res* 1991; **19**: 3843–50.

90. Weiss MJ, Keller G, Orkin SH. Novel insights into erythroid development revealed through in vitro differentiation of GATA-1 embryonic stem cells. *Genes Dev* 1994; **8**: 1184–97.

91. Dubart A, Roméo PH, Vainchenker W et al. Constitutive expression of GATA-1 interferes with the cell-cycle regulation. *Blood* 1996; **87**: 3711–21.

# 11 Megakaryocyte differentiation and regulation

**William Vainchenker, Najet Debili, and Françoise Wendling**

## Introduction

Platelets are anucleate blood cells that play an important role in hemostatis by their adhesion to the endothelium and subendothelial matrix and by the release of the contents of their storage organelles following activation. Platelets are produced by the cytoplasmic fragmentation of their polyploid bone marrow precursors, the megakaryocytes. Understanding of megakaryocytopoiesis has been hampered by the rarity of megakaryocytes in the marrow (< 0.1%). The discovery in 1994 of the physiological regulator of platelet production, thrombopoietin (TPO), has been a major breakthrough in the understanding of the regulation of platelet production and megakaryocyte biology. Whereas, a few years ago, megakaryocytopoiesis was poorly understood, important progress has recently been made that now permits a better understanding of the normal differentiation as well as several pathologies of the megakaryocyte lineage.

In this chapter, we shall focus on the cellular aspects of megakaryocyte differentiation and its regulation by growth factors and particularly by TPO.

## Megakaryocytic cells

The megakaryocyte/platelet lineage is one branch of hematopoiesis, deriving from the differentiation of multipotent hematopoietic stem cells. The megakaryocyte and erythroid lineages have many similarities in their differentiation pathways and in the regulation of their specific genes, and there is evidence for a bipotent progenitor common to the erythroid and megakaryocyte lineages.[1,2]

Megakaryocytopoiesis has many features that distinguish it from all of the other hematopoietic lineages and other cellular differentiation pathways. It can be divided into four steps. In the early stages, megakaryocyte progenitors are capable of proliferation and give rise to in vitro megakaryocyte colonies. These cells undergo a variable number of mitoses (DNA duplication followed by cytokinesis) to differentiate further into transitional cells (promegakaryoblasts, PMKB), which begin to synthesize numerous platelet proteins and enter an endomitotic process (DNA duplication without cytokinesis). This process induces a parallel increase in both nuclear and cytoplasmic volumes and gives rise to a characteristic cell containing a single polylobulated typical nucleus with a $2^xN$ ploidy. After an average of three DNA cycles of duplication (from zero to five or six), cytoplasmic maturation, which had already begun, accelerates and further increases the cytoplasmic volume of the cell. Thereafter, terminal cytoplasmic maturation occurs, leading to proplatelet formation and platelet production (Figure 11.1). Platelet production occurs through a highly regulated process of cytoplasmic fragmentation, each successive stage having increased platelet production, and depends on three parameters the number of megakaryocytes, their sizes, and the efficiency of platelet release.

### Megakaryocyte progenitor cells

Several clonal assays have been developed to investigate megakaryocyte progenitors, and these have usually been coupled with the use of differentiation markers for a precise identification of megakaryocyte colonies. In vitro techniques have shown that, similarly to other hematopoietic cell lineages, megakaryocyte progenitors are heterogenous and represent a continuum of cells. They have been schematically divided into three main types: burst-forming units megakaryocyte (BFU-Mk), colony-forming units megakaryocyte (CFU-Mk), and low-density CFU-Mk (LD-CFU-Mk).

#### BFU-Mk

These progenitors produce colonies (in 12 days in mice and 21 days in humans), which are composed of more than 50 cells organized in subcolonies on the

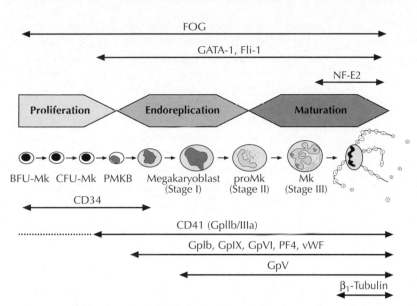

**Figure 11.1** The process of megakaryocyte differentiation. BFU-Mk, burst-forming unit megakaryocyte; CFU-Mk, colony-forming unit megakaryocyte; PMKB, promegakaryoblast; proMK, promegakaryocyte; Mk, megakaryocyte; Gp, glycoprotein; PF4, platelet factor 4; vWF, von Willebrand factor.

same model as BFU erythroid (BFU-E)- derived colonies. BFU-Mk are considered to be very primitive megakaryocyte progenitors. However, megakaryocyte progenitors with even higher proliferative capacities (high-proliferative-potential colony forming cells megakaryocyte, HPP-CFC-Mk) have been found in fetal bone marrow.[4]

### CFU-Mk

These progenitor cells differ from BFU-Mk in their lower proliferative capacities. They give rise to colonies composed of 3–50 cells in 5 days in mice[5] and 12 days in humans.[6] Unlike BFU-Mk, which are in $G_0/G_1$ phase of the cell cycle, CFU-Mk have a high [$^3$H] thymidine suicide rate and are destroyed by chemical agents such as 5-fluorouracil. BFU-Mk and CFU-Mk are also found in fetal tissues, especially in fetal and neonatal blood.

### LD-CFU-Mk

These cells have been identified in the mouse as megakaryocyte progenitors with a density lower than 1.050 g/ml. They give rise within 2–3 days to colonies composed of a few megakaryocytes with a high ploidy.[7] The developmental stage of this progenitor is extremely close to the transitional cell that has switched towards an endomitotic process.

The use of differentiation markers has allowed a more precise delineation of the megakaryocyte progenitors and transitional cell compartments.

### Megakaryocyte precursor cells identified by stage-specific differentiation markers

Initial work used cytochemical markers such as acetylcholinesterase (AChE) in the mouse.[8] Studies have shown the presence in mouse marrow of a compartment of small AChE-positive cells (SACHE) that differentiate into polyploid megakaryocytes in a few

days.[8] A very similar type of cells has been identified in normal human marrow using the platelet peroxidase marker, and has been called a promegakaryoblast (PMKB).[9] Acute megakaryoblastic leukemia corresponds to the proliferation of a cell blocked at this stage of differentiation.

The use of immunological markers has allowed a better characterization of the early steps of megakaryocyte differentiation (Figure 11.1). The initial aspect of these studies involved distinguishing BFU-Mk from CFU-Mk by their immunological phenotype. These two megakaryocyte progenitors express the CD34 antigen, like almost all hematopoietic progenitor cells. In addition, the HLA-DR antigen is detected on CFU-Mk as well as on the majority of hematopoietic progenitors (CFU granulocyte–macrophage (CFU-GM) and immature BFU-E).[10] In contrast, there is a very low expression of HLA-DR on BFU-Mk. CD109 and CD133 are expressed on nearly all types of megakaryocyte progenitors.[11]

Antibodies directed against platelet glycoproteins – for example GpIIb/IIIa ($\alpha_2 \beta_3$ integrin, CD41) GpIb, and different $\alpha$-granule components such as von Willebrand factor (vWF) and platelet factor 4 (PF4) – have been used to monitor megakaryocyte differentiation.[12,13] These studies have indicated that most platelet proteins are expressed by small megakaryocyte precursor cells and all along the differentiation pathway. Among these markers, platelet GpIIb/IIIa seems to be expressed slightly earlier than the others (GpIb, PF4, and vWF). These results have been confirmed more recently by flow cytometry. GpV, a component of the GpIb complex, might be expressed even later than the other markers.[14] However, with the exception of $\beta_1$-tubulin, there is no marker allowing the identification of only post-endomitotic cells. The expression of all the main platelet proteins within a short range of differentiation is probably related to the fact that all these genes have very similar promoters that bind the same transcription factors (see later in this chapter). It has also been shown that immature megakaryocytes express CD4,[15,16] which may be relevant for the mechanisms of thrombocytopenia in HIV infection.

Platelet GpIIb/IIIa is expressed at a high level on late megakaryocyte progenitor cells (equivalent in humans to LD-CFU-MK) and on a fraction of true CFU-Mk.[17] It is also detected at a low level on all myeloid hematopoietic progenitor cells, including CFU granulocyte–erythroid–macrophage–megakaryocyte (CFU-GEMM), and also on lymphoid progenitors in humans, mice, and chickens.[18–20] In humans, GpIIb/IIIa seems to be more widely expressed on cord blood progenitor cells than in adults.[21]

GpIb (CD42) is considered to be a late marker of megakaryocytic differentiation. However, it is also detected on some late megakaryocyte progenitors and on erythroid progenitor cells.[17,21,22]

Thus, most platelet-restricted glycoproteins, especially GpIIb/IIIa, which is not entirely specific, allow the direct identification of late megakaryocyte progenitors and $2N$ cells that are entering endomitosis.

## The endomitotic compartment

Endomitosis is the cellular process that leads to polyploidization and transforms a small megakaryocyte precursor cell into a giant cell, the megakaryocyte. It was considered until recently that megakaryocyte polyploidization was part of megakaryocyte maturation. In fact, there is increasing evidence that polyploidization and megakaryocyte cytoplasmic maturation leading to platelet shedding are two independently regulated processes, since platelet shedding may occur in a $2N$ cell. During this process, the megakaryocyte increases its ploidy and can stop its DNA duplication at any stage between $2N$ and $64N$, and eventually at $128N$. In humans, as well as in the majority of mammals, the modal ploidy is $16N$ (about 50% of megakaryocytes).

The process leading to megakaryocyte polyploidization was initially called endomitosis because it was believed that it was a mitosis occuring without rupture of the nuclear membrane.[23] Description of the endomitotic process has been extremely difficult due to the scarcity of megakaryocytes in the marrow and to the low frequency of megakaryocytes undergoing endomitosis. Initial ultrastructural studies described the endomitotic process and showed that the first steps of endomitosis are identical to mitosis, with chromosome condensation and the presence of a metaphase, suggesting a blockage in the metaphase/anaphase transition.[24,25] More recent studies performed on TPO-stimulated cultures have demonstrated that endomitosis of human and murine megakaryocytes correspond to an abortive mitotic process.[26,27] Mitosis normally occurs until anaphase,

with chromosome condensation and a single multipolar spindle with nuclear membrane breakdown. The first stage of anaphase (anaphase A), characterized by sister chromatid separation, is also observed. However, late stages of anaphase B, consisting of spindle elongation and chromosome movement to the spindle, are not observed. Mitosis ends with the absence of cytokinesis after chromosome decondensation and the formation of a membrane around a single nuclear mass.[28] Thus, megakaryocyte endomitosis is an incomplete multipolar mitosis characterized by skipping of late mitotic stages.

The molecular mechanisms that control the switch from a mitotic to an endomitotic process are presently unknown. The cell cycle of endomitotic megakaryocytes has now been studied in detail, and is characterized by a very high expression of cyclin D3.[29] Transgenic mice overexpressing cyclin D3 have megakaryocytes with higher ploidy than wild-type mice.[30] No evident abnormalities in cell cycle checkpoints have been found, in particular at the metaphase/anaphase transition, although chromosome segregation to each spindle may be asymmetrical.[28] Recent results suggest that the absence of an aurora kinase (AIM1) during the cell cycle may be a key event in the switch from mitosis to endomitosis.[31] At the end of the endomitotic process, megakaryocytes express extremely high levels of p21 and p27, which are members of the Cip/Kip family of cyclin-dependent kinase inhibitors (CKI).[32] p21 and p27 may block the cell cycle and arrest the endomitotic process, permitting synchronization of the end of DNA replication and megakaryocyte terminal differentiation.

Although not directly demonstrated, the major aim of polyploidization is to increase megakaryocyte size and to control platelet production – not by the number of megakaryocytes but by their total mass. Polyploidization consequently induces gene amplification and may thus facilitate parallel increases in cell size and gene expression. In addition, it has been hypothesized that polyploidization contributes to gene regulation during megakaryocyte maturation. There has been much controversy regarding changes in platelet size and function related to increase in megakaryocyte ploidy. In particular, it has been suggested that platelets derived from high-ploidy megakaryocytes are larger and more easily activated.

Polyploidization is regulated by growth factors, especially TPO. An increase in megakaryocyte ploidy is one of the first events occuring after induction of acute severe thrombocytopenia in mice: as early as 24 hours, the modal ploidy increases from $16N$ to $32N$. These changes are maximal at 48 hours and return to normal values within 120 hours.

During human ontogenesis, megakaryocytes increase their ploidy, with the majority of fetal and neonatal megakaryocytes being $2N$ or $4N$ in culture.[33]

## The compartment of cytoplasmic maturation

Following endomitosis, megakaryocyte cytoplasmic maturation accelerates. The synthesis of specific organelles (demarcation membranes and $\alpha$ granules), which began early during megakaryocyte differentiation, increases markedly in post-endomitotic megakaryocytes. Demarcation membranes, an intracytoplasmic membrane system, are invaginations of the surface cell membrane and act as a reservoir of membranes that plays a major role in proplatelet formation.[34,35]

The $\alpha$ granules store the main platelet proteins that are released after platelet activation. They are distinguished at the ultrastructural level by the presence of a dense central core giving the appearance of a 'bull's eye'. Synthesis of most $\alpha$-granule components arise from the Golgi apparatus, such as vWF, PF4, $\beta$-thromboglobulin ($\beta$-TG), platelet-derived growth factor (PDGF), transforming growth factor $\beta1$ (TGF-$\beta1$), basic fibroblast growth factor (bFGF), thrombospondin (TSP), P-selectin (CD62P/GMP 140), osteonectin, clusterin, and serglycin. Other proteins, such as fibrinogen, albumin, and immunoglobulins, are packaged in $\alpha$ granules after endocytosis through clathrin vesicles arising from the cytoplasmic membrane.[36,37] This explains why the main platelet glycoproteins such as GPIIb/IIIa, GpIb, and CD36 are present in $\alpha$ granules. Fibrinogen, one of the main protein of the $\alpha$ granules, is not synthesized by megakaryocytes, but is endocytosed after binding to activated GpIIb/IIIa.[37-39] This process occurs late during megakaryocyte maturation.[40] Inside the $\alpha$ granules, there is a protein compartmentalization, some proteins being localized at the inner face of the $\alpha$-granule membrane and others in the matrix.[41-43]

Proteins packaged in the $\alpha$ granules are involved in platelet aggregation, regulation of fibroblast and endothelial cell proliferation, and regulation of extracellular matrix protein synthesis. Indeed, important cytokines such as TGF-$\beta1$, PDGF, and vascular endothelial growth factor (VEGF), and chemokines such as PF4, are packaged in the $\alpha$ granules and are released either by megakaryocytes in the marrow or by activated platelets. Abnormal release of these mediators in the marrow environment leads to myelofibrosis.

In addition to $\alpha$ granules, other types of granules are present in megakaryocytes, including dense bodies (which contain serotonin, calcium ions, and nucleotides), microperoxisomes, and lysosomal granules. At the ultrastructural level, dense bodies are detected at late stages of megakaryocyte differentiation.[44] However, the serotonin uptake, which occurs by an active mechanism involving specific receptors, begins in small megakaryocyte precursor cells.[45]

## Platelet shedding

At the end of maturation, mature megakaryocytes are large spherical cells of about 50 μm diameter. The large nucleus is polylobulated. The organelles are located in a zone concentric with the nucleus. In contrast, the zone around the plasma membrane is devoid of organelles. In order to shed platelets, profound morphological changes have to occur. The mechanisms of platelet shedding are beginning to be well understood at both the ultrastructural and the molecular level.[34,35,46-48] In contrast to what had been believed for many years, demarcation membranes do not delineate platelet territories, but membranes are evaginated to form long proplatelet extensions. Proplatelet formation leads to pseudopods – which are completely different from cytoplasmic blebs in that they contain all platelet organelles. The cytoskeleton plays an important role in these morphological changes, especially the microtubules. Microtubules are absolutely required for evagination of demarcation membranes.[34,49,50] Proplatelets contain a peripheral bundle of microtubules formed from $\beta_1$-tubulin.[51] This tubulin subtype is synthesized at the end of megakaryocyte maturation and is responsible for both proplatelet formation and the definitive discoid shape of platelets.[51,52] The actin filament also plays an important role in permitting the growth and extension of proplatelets by creating branching on the pseudopods.[53,54] The mechanism of platelet release is still a subject of debate. In the opinion of some, it may occur by breaking off of the long proplatelet extensions at the level of the constrictions, this rupture possibly being due to the mechanical effect of blood flow pressure.[50,55] Platelets are first released into the blood with a longitudinal orientation of the microtubules[55] and are elongated; thereafter, platelets in the circulation acquire their definitive shape. An alternative view is that platelets are formed directly at the end of the proplatelet extensions. Indeed, microtubule coils that are similar to those observed in blood platelets are detected only at the ends of the proplatelet extensions as 'teardrops'.[53]

In normal individuals, platelet shedding occurs not in the marrow but directly in the circulation. In the marrow, megakaryocytes are located in the subendothelial region,[56] in close contact with endothelial cells, which may be involved in megakaryocyte terminal differentiation.[57] Proplatelets may pass through the endothelial barrier and enter the circulation. Alternatively, entire mature megakaryocytes can also migrate through this blood barrier and are detected in the circulation. Several authors have pointed out that megakaryocytes are present in significant numbers in the small vessels of the lung and are trapped in the pulmonary capillary beds, where they release platelets.[58] Thus, the exit of megakaryocytes from the marrow is an important phenomenon regulating platelet production. Regulation of megakaryocyte migration is still poorly understood; it may be controlled by receptors of the extracellular matrix and chemokines.

After platelet shedding, the megakaryocyte (the nucleus surrounded by the remains of the cytoplasm) becomes senescent and dies by apoptosis.[59] The nucleus is engulfed by macrophages.[60] It has been suggested that megakaryocyte fragmentation has many similarities with apoptosis. In favor of this hypothesis is the observation that mice overexpressing the anti-apoptotic Bcl-2 protein or deficient for the apoptotic *bim* gene develop thrombocytopenia with a normal number of megakaryocytes.[61,62]

# Regulation of megakaryocytopoiesis by transcription factors

Analysis of expression patterns of *cis*-regulatory elements important in the regulation of megakaryocyte-specific genes, gene targeting experiments in embryonic stem (ES) cells, and creation of mutant mice have established the essential involvement of a number of transcription factors in megakaryocytopoiesis.[63] These include SCL/TAL-1, c-Myb, the Ets family member Fli-1, GATA-1, GATA-2, FOG, NF-E2, MafG, MafF, and some *Hox* genes.[64] In addition, studies of megakaryocyte-specific gene promoters such as GpIIb, GpIbα, GpIbβ, GpIX, GpV, c-Mpl, and GpVI have shown the existence of binding sites for GATA-1 and members of the Ets family.[65–67] Disruption of these binding sites markedly diminishes the activity of these promoters. Targeted disruption of these transcription factor genes has shown that three of them – FOG, GATA-1, and Fli-1 – are involved in the early stages of megakaryocyte differentiation, including the expression of megakaryocyte-specific genes and polyploidization. In contrast, NF-E2 and its partners (MafG and MafF) play a crucial role in the expression of genes involved in proplatelet formation and platelet activation (Figure 11.1).

Mice with a disruption of *GATA-1* die in utero from anemia.[68] Orkin and co-workers have characterized sites in the *GATA-1* promoter permitting its megakaryocyte-specific expression.[69] Mice with a megakaryocyte-specific disruption of *GATA-1* have an increased number of megakaryocytes, with a severely impaired cytoplasmic maturation in hematopoietic tissues and a profound thrombocytopenia with structurally and functionally abnormal giant platelets.[69] GATA-1-deficient megakaryocytes fail to undergo complete maturation, remain small and immature, and contain markedly reduced levels of all megakaryocytic-specific mRNA.[70] Their small size might be due to their low ploidy. In addition, these small cells have an increased proliferative capacity, which has been related to downregulation of inositol polyphosphate 4-phosphatase type 1.[71] This indicates that GATA-1 is indispensable to the promotion of megakaryocyte

maturation. The *FOG* gene has been isolated as a partner of *GATA-1*.[72] Targeted disruption of the *FOG* gene in mice results in the same phenotype for the erythroid lineage as *GATA-1* gene disruption, with embryonic lethality during mid-gestation due to severe anemia. However, the phenotype of *FOG*- and *GATA-1*-null mice is quite different for the megakaryocyte lineage. FOG-deficient mice have a total absence of megakaryocyte development, including the absence of megakaryocyte progenitor cells. This indicates that FOG is required for the earliest stage of megakaryocyte development and may be associated with a partner other than GATA-1 at these stages of differentiation.[73]

Recent studies have also demonstrated a role of Fli-1 in megakaryocytopoiesis. Target-disruption of the *Fli-1* gene results in an embryonically lethal phenotype with hemorrhage due to disorganization of tissue integrity and disruption of normal hematopoiesis and hemostasis.[74,75] In addition, the megakaryocyte lineage displays important abnormalities similar to those described in GATA-1-deficient mice, with the presence of small immature megakaryocytes.[74] Among the platelet-specific genes, expression of *GpIb* and c-*mpl* are markedly reduced.

The p45[NF-E2] transcription factor was thought to play a crucial role in the regulation of erythroid gene expression such as that of β-globin.[76,77] Unexpectedly, p45[NF-E2]-deficient mice present a profound and lethal thrombocytopenia without any erythroid differentiation defect.[47] This thrombocytopenia is due to a marked dysmegakaryocytopoiesis characterized by an increased number of megakaryocytes associated with an abnormal demarcation membrane distribution and a deficiency in α granules. No proplatelet formation is observed.[48] To explain this phenotype, it has been suggested (i) that the absence of erythroid phenotype in p45[NF-E2]-deficient mice might be due to the presence of a transcription factor redundant with p45[NF-E2] in erythroblasts, and (ii) that p45[NF-E2] regulates as-yet uncharacterized genes in megakaryocytes. By comparing gene expression in normal and p45[NF-E2]-deficient megakaryocytes it has been shown that p45[NF-E2] regulates a set of genes involved in cytoskeletal organization and platelet functions.[52,78] Among them, the $\beta_1$-tubulin gene seems to be the most important because it is expressed only at the end of megakaryocyte maturation in a lineage-specific manner, and its gene disruption leads to thrombocytopenia with non-discoid platelets.[51,52]

p45[NF-E2] is one of two components of the NF-E2 transcription factor and belongs to a subset of bZip proteins termed cap'n collar (CNC). It associates with small Maf proteins to form the heterodimeric NF-E2 protein. In erythroblasts, its predominant partner is the p18/MafK polypeptide,[79] whereas in megakaryocytes, it associates predominantly with MafG and MafF.[80] Recent experiments have shown that MafG-deficient mutant mice have moderate thrombocytopenia with a similar but milder defect in megakaryopoiesis as p45[NF-E2]-deficient mice.[81] MafG- and MafK-deficient mice have the same phenotype as p45[NF-E2]-deficient mice.[82]

# Regulation of megakaryocytopoiesis by growth factors

Although many growth factors act at either early or late stages of megakaryocyte differentiation (Figure 11.2), regulation of megakaryocytopoiesis is dominated by the role of TPO, which is presently the only growth factor involved in homeostatic platelet production.

## Thrombopoietin, a ligand for the Mpl receptor

A factor, called thrombopoietin, able to correct abnormalities of platelet count in a regulated manner and present in plasma from thrombocytopenic rodents and humans, was described in 1958.[83] However, this factor remained elusive for 35 years, despite many attempts to obtain a purified fraction. During the late 1980s, a mutant acutely leukemogenic murine retrovirus (MPLV, for MyeloProliferative Leukemia Virus) was fortuitously isolated from a mouse infected with a Friend helper virus (F-MuLV).[84] This virus isolate had a unique ability to confer growth factor independence and immortalization on progenitor cells from several hematopoietic lineages. Molecular cloning and sequencing demonstrated that the transforming properties of MPLV were related to the presence of a truncated cellular sequence (the viral oncogene v-mpl) inserted in the rearranged envelope region of the retrovirus.[85] Subsequently, the human and murine

proto-oncogene c-mpl was cloned, providing definitive evidence that the product of the c-mpl gene, Mpl, was an orphan type I transmembrane receptor characterized by conserved cysteine residues and a common amino-acid motif (WSXWS) in the extracellular domain and lack of intrinsic tyrosine kinase activity in the intracellular domain.[86,87] Major insights into the physiological role of Mpl arose from several observations. It was demonstrated that its expression was restricted to hematopoietic tissues, progenitor cells included in the CD34+ cell fraction, megakaryocytes, and platelets. c-mpl antisense oligodeoxynucleotides selectively inhibited CFU-Mk colony formation in vitro without affecting the growth of erythroid or myeloid colonies.[88] Disruption of the c-mpl gene in mice resulted in a highly specific loss of megakaryocytes and platelets, leaving other cell lineages unaffected.[89] Together, these results strongly suggested that Mpl and its ligand had key functions in the regulation of megakaryocytopoiesis and platelet production. The c-mpl gene and its encoded proteins is summarized in reference 90.

A ligand capable of binding and activating Mpl was purified in 1994 by five independent groups. Two groups used Mpl-affinity columns to capture the ligand in plasma from thrombocytopenic pigs and dogs. Degenerate oligonucleotides were designed from the N-terminal sequence of the protein and used to screen a human fetal liver cDNA library.[91,92] One group mutagenized a factor-dependent murine cell line expressing Mpl to select mutants for autonomous growth. Among these mutants, one clone produced an activity that could be neutralized by a soluble Mpl form. Breakdown cDNA library pools were prepared and expressed in mammalian cells. A positive clone was identified, from which a full-length cDNA encoding the murine Mpl ligand was isolated.[93] The other two groups directly isolated a thrombocytopoietic factor from the plasma of thrombocytopenic animals using

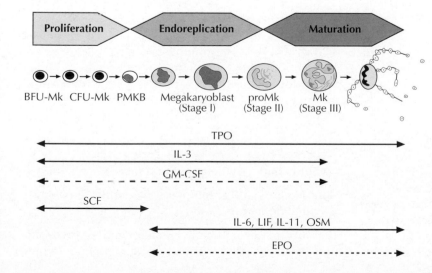

**Figure 11.2** Regulation of megakaryocyte differentiation by growth factors. TPO, thrombopoeitin; IL, interleukin; GM-CSF, granulocyte–macrophage colony-stimulating factor; SCF, stem cell factor; LIF, leukemia inhibitory factor; OSM, oncostatin M; EPO, erythropoietin. For other abbreviations, see the caption to Figure 11.1.

standard purification methods.[94,95] All of these proteins were identical but received different names: Mpl ligand (ML or Mpl-L), or thrombopoietin (TPO), or megakaryocyte growth and development factor (MGDF), or megapoietin. Evidence was rapidly provided that the recombinant molecule had the property to sustain both complete megakaryocytopoiesis and thrombocytopoiesis in vitro and in vivo (reviewed in reference 96).

The human native protein is a 68–85 kDa glycosylated polypeptide comprising 332 amino acids. The molecule can be structurally and functionally divided into two domains: an N-terminal domain of 153 amino acids that shares considerable sequence similarity with erythropoietin (EPO) (the EPO-like domain) and a C-terminal domain that contains all of the potential glycosylation sites. The EPO-like domain is sufficient to fully activate Mpl and to induce the full spectrum of biological responses in vitro and in vivo. The C-terminal domain is required for efficient secretion. Glycosylation increases the stability and potency of the protein in vivo. TPO is mainly produced in the liver and kidneys, but transcripts are also detected in several other organs, including stromal cells from the bone marrow. TPO levels in plasma are inversely correlated with platelet number;[97] however, production of TPO is not regulated by platelet demand or by platelet mass, since no transcriptional regulation of the gene is detected in livers or kidneys from thrombocytopenic or thrombocythemic animals.[98,99] Nevertheless, transcriptional regulation in response to platelet demand has been reported in bone marrow stromal cells.[100,101] The current model for TPO regulation is a constitutive synthesis and a clearance from the circulation by sequestration through binding to Mpl receptors present on the surfaces of both platelets and megakaryocytes, followed by internalization and degradation.[102,103] The contribution of both platelet and megakaryocyte masses to TPO clearance is best demonstrated in murine knockout models. In c-mpl-deficient mice, which have low platelet numbers and high levels of TPO in the plasma, platelet transfusions from normal donors rapidly decrease plasma TPO levels. In NF-E2-knockout mice, which are profoundly thrombocytopenic because megakaryocytes are unable to produce platelets, the predicted elevation of TPO levels is not observed. However, these mice have normal number of megakaryocytes.[47,104] Similarly, high TPO levels are found in thrombocytopenic patients with aplastic anemia,[105] while TPO levels are normal or only mildly elevated in patients with immune thrombocytopenic purpura (ITP).

The potent and lineage-dominant action of the Mpl/TPO system on the regulation of megakaryocytopoiesis and platelet production is clearly demonstrated by the generation of c-mpl- and TPO-knockout mice.[89,106] An identical phenotype is seen in homozygous animals, with a 90% reduction in platelet counts, very low numbers of megakaryocytes with a reduced ploidy in marrow and spleen, but no abnormalities in nucleated cell counts or hematocrit. However, these mice display a 50% reduction in the numbers of all myeloid-committed progenitors,[107,108] and bone marrow stem cells from c-mpl-deficient mice have a significantly reduced self-renewal potential.[109] These murine knockout models highlight the essential physiological role of the Mpl/TPO system in the regulation of megakaryocytopoiesis and platelet production, and clearly indicate that interactions of TPO with Mpl are required to maintain and/or expand early and committed progenitor cells. In vitro, TPO alone has a potent and lineage-specific action on late megakaryocyte progenitor cells, inducing proliferation, ploidization, maturation, and proplatelet formation.[110–113] Several studies have provided evidences that TPO acts in synergy with early-acting cytokines (stem cell factor, interleukin-3, and Flt3 ligand) to sustain the survival and stimulate the proliferation of primitive hematopoietic progenitors by speeding entry of quiescent stem cells into the cell cycle.[114–123] Thus, TPO is not only a lineage-specific cytokine, but also an important cytokine acting on a broad spectrum of primitive stem cells.

Interaction of TPO with Mpl leads to rapid stimulation of multiple intracellular signaling events, including tyrosine phosphorylation and activation of Jak2 (Janus tyrosine kinase 2), Tyk2, STAT1 (signal transducer and activator of transcription 1), STAT3, and STAT5.[124–126] Jak2 and Tyk2 are non-receptor tyrosine kinases that, upon activation, phosphorylate their major target proteins, the STATs. Tyrosine phosphorylation of STATs leads to their translocation from the cytoplasm to the nucleus where they bind to specific DNA motifs and function as transcriptional activators.[127,128] In platelets, megakaryocytes, and the megakaryoblastic UT-7 cell line, other intracellular targets of Mpl activation have been found. They include Shc, Grb2, MAPK, JNK, Raf-1, Cbl, Vav, protein kinase C (PKC), phosphatidylinositol 3′-kinase (PI3K), and the phosphatases SHPTP-1 and SHPTP-2.[129–136] Using mutant receptors containing deletions within the intracytoplasmic domain, it has been shown that the C-terminal 25 amino-acid residues of Mpl are crucial for mitogenic signals,[137] while activation of the MAPK and Ras pathways seem to be involved in megakaryocytic differentiation and polyploidization, especially under conditions of stress.[138,139]

## Other hematopoietic growth factors

### Interleukin-3 and granulocyte–macrophage colony-stimulating factor

The use of recombinant hematopoietic growth factors has revealed that at least two pleiotropic cytokines acting on early stages of hematopoiesis, interleukin-3 (IL-3) and granulocyte–macrophage colony-stimulating factor (GM-CSF), induce megakaryocyte colony formation. Indeed IL-3 was also initially named Mk-CSF.[140] Both cytokines act on CFU-Mk and BFU-Mk.[10] IL-3 is the most effective cytokine on megakaryocyte progenitors after TPO and is capable as a single agent of inducing megakaryocyte colony formation on isolated megakaryocyte progenitors. GM-CSF and IL-3 have additive effects at non-optimal doses. An IL-3/GM-CSF fusion protein (PIXY321) has more effects on in vitro megakaryocytopoiesis than each cytokine used alone, suggesting a true synergy between GM-CSF and IL-3.[141] In primates, injection of IL-3 leads to an enhancement of platelet production, whereas GM-CSF does not result in a significant platelet response.[142] Neither GM-CSF nor IL-3 plays a role in the hemostatic regulation of platelet production.[143]

## Members of the interleukin-6 family

IL-6, leukemia inhibitory factor, (LIF), IL-11, onco-statin M (OSM), and ciliary neurotropic factor (CNTF) have pleiotropic effects on numerous cell types. The redundancy of these cytokines is now explained by the molecular biology of their receptors. All utilize a common signal transducing chain (GP130).[144]

IL-6 was the first cytokine of this family to be demonstrated to act on megakaryocytopoiesis. This cytokine induces an enhancement of (i) megakaryocyte size, (ii) ploidy, (iii) cytoplasmic maturation, including synthesis of platelet proteins, and (iv) number.[145] More recently, it has been shown that IL-6 also induces proplatelet formation by isolated megakaryocytes.[146] Injection of IL-6 in vivo increases platelet production to a greater degree than injection of IL-3 by acting both on CFU-Mk and eventually megakaryocyte numbers, size, and ploidy.[147,148] A synergistic effect between IL-3 and IL-6 on platelet production is also found in vivo in non-human primates. As a consequence, several authors hypothesized that TPO and IL-6 were the same molecule, slowing research on the identification of TPO.[149]

LIF, OSM, and IL-11 have effects very similar to IL-6 on megakaryocytopoiesis.[150–152] IL-11 is considered to be the most potent molecule of this family with regard to platelet production.[152] Injection of IL-11 in mice results in a 1.25-fold increase in platelet counts, mainly due to an increase in $32N$ megakaryocytes. Although the number of CFU-Mk is increased in the spleen, the effects of IL-11 on platelet counts are not abrogated by splenectomy. IL-11 is used in humans to enhance platelet recovery.[153] These different cytokines do not play a significant role in homeostatic platelet production,[154] but are important as mediators of inflammation. They may be responsible for the thrombocytosis observed in inflammatory diseases.

## Stem cell factor

Stem cell factor (SCF; also known as Steel factor and c-Kit ligand) is one of the most potent cytokines, with Flt3 ligand (Flt3-L) acting as a synergistic factor with all hematopoietic growth factors, with the exception of macrophage colony-stimulating factor (M-CSF). Its effect predominates on the erythroid lineage as a costimulator with EPO and on the early stages of hematopoiesis. SCF also plays an important physiological role in megakaryocytopoiesis.[155,156] In in vitro studies, SCF greatly potentiates the effects of IL-3, GM-CSF, IL-6, and TPO on the growth of megakaryocyte progenitors, increasing both cloning efficiency and the size of colonies.[157–159] In the mouse, SCF injection increases the numbers of both CFU-Mk and platelets, especially in immunodeficient mice. SCF in association with TPO plays an important role in the normal regulation of megakaryocytopoiesis.

## Erythropoietin

In mice and humans EPO seems unable by itself to induce megakaryocyte colony formation. However, EPO acts as a costimulator at high concentration and is able to favor terminal differentiation.[160] This effect is also observed on individual transitional cells.[161] Like IL-6, EPO induces proplatelet formation by purified murine megakaryocytes.[146] In vivo, EPO does not appear to be a major regulator of platelet production, but may increase platelet functions. However, EPO injection can increase platelet counts in some human pathologies in the absence of iron deficiency.

## Stromal cell-derived factor 1

Stromal cell-derived factor (SDF-1) is a chemokine having for its only receptor CXCR4, a seven transmembrane receptor coupled to G proteins. SDF-1 plays an important role in the migration and homing of hematopoietic stem cells. It is involved in the retention of hematopoietic cells in the marrow. CXCR4 is expressed all along the megakaryocyte differentiation pathway until platelets, and its expression increases with maturation.[162–164] Surprisingly, the response to SDF-1 decreases with maturation, suggesting that CXCR4 signaling is inhibited at the end of megakaryocytopoiesis.[163,165,166] For this reason, it has been suggested, but not demonstrated, that the loss of SDF-1 signaling in mature megakaryocytes may be involved in the regulation of megakaryocyte exit from the bone marrow. In addition, there is increasing evidence that SDF-1 has a synergistic effect with TPO on megakaryocyte survival, proliferation, polyploidization, and maturation.[167–169]

## Other hematopoietic growth factors

Several other characterized cytokines may also act in vivo or in vitro on megakaryocytopoiesis. Among the most studied cytokines are IL-1α and IL-1β. These two cytokines have marked effects on megakaryocytopoiesis, but most (if not all) of these effects seem to be indirect, by the induction of numerous other cytokines, such as IL-6, GM-CSF, and SCF. IL-1 has been injected into both animals and humans, resulting in an increase in platelet production. However, and as a consequence of its broad effects, IL-1 has major toxic effects, which reduce its interest as a therapeutic agent.[170]

Granulocyte colony-stimulating factor (G-CSF) also has a synergistic effect with IL-3 on the growth of megakaryocyte progenitors, which has been interpreted as a consequence of its proliferative activity on primitive cells. However, it has been shown that platelets are able to bind G-CSF and to respond functionally to this cytokine.[171] In vivo injection of G-CSF has no effect on platelet recovery in humans.

IL-10, a potent immunoregulatory factor, promotes the growth of pure and mixed megakaryocyte colonies in association with IL-3 from Thy$^{low}$ Sca$^+$ murine primitive cells.[172] In contrast, IL-10 induced thrombocytopenia in therapeutic trials.[173]

## Non-hematopoietic growth factors

Basic fibroblast growth factor (bFGF) is a non-hematopoietic growth factor acting on megakaryocytopoiesis, probably by both direct and indirect effects. In humans, the megakaryocyte-stimulating activity of bFGF is totally blocked by antibodies against GM-CSF, IL-3, or IL-6.[174,175] It is noteworthy that megakaryocytes synthesize bFGF and express its receptor.[176] It seems that the effects of bFGF are related to an augmentation of IL-6 secretion by megakaryocytes.[177]

Platelet-derived growth factor (PDGF) increases the expansion of megakaryocyte progenitors in association with other cytokines without inducing maturation.[178] PDGF-B/PDGF-B-receptor-null mice display a lethal phenotype. Embryos have thrombocytopenia, but no abnormalities in megakaryocyte maturation or megakaryocyte progenitor numbers were noted. The thrombocytopenia seems to be related to a decrease in liver size. Thus, most of the effects of PDGF on hematopoiesis and megakaryocytopoiesis seem to be related to the release of cytokines by stromal cells.[179]

In cell therapy, combinations of cytokines are used to expand megakaryocyte progenitors and megakaryocytes from CD34$^+$ cells with the goal of shortening platelet recovery after myeloablative therapy.[180]

## Inhibitory factors

As soon as the megakaryocyte colony assay was available, it became evident that, unlike the erythrocyte or granulocyte lineages, megakaryocyte colony formation was partially inhibited by serum in a dose-dependent manner.[181] In contrast, plasma or serum derived from platelet-poor plasma did not have this inhibitory effect. These results strongly suggested that platelets stored and secreted one or several molecules inhibitory of megakaryocytopoiesis.

It was subsequently demonstrated that these inhibitory proteins are present inside platelets, especially in α granules.[182] Two proteins may be involved in this inhibition: transforming growth factor β1 (TGF-β1) and platelet factor 4 (PF4).

TGF-β1 has an extremely potent inhibitory effect on megakaryocytopoiesis, inhibiting megakaryocyte colony formation, endomitosis, and terminal differentiation.[182–184] Megakaryocytopoiesis is the hematopoietic lineage whose primitive cells are the most sensitive to the inhibitory effect of TGF-β1.[185] TGF-β1 increases the synthesis of TPO by stromal cells. On the other hand, TPO induces an increase in TGF-β receptor expression on megakaryocytes, enhancing in turn their response to TGF-β1.[186] Treatment of mice for 7–14 days with TGF-β1 induces a 95% reduction in platelet counts, as well as anemia and an increase in granulopoiesis.[187] In contrast, TGF-β1-null mice or mice reconstituted with bone marrow cells from TGF-β1-null mice have no thrombocytosis (authors' unpublished data), demonstrating that TGF-β1 is not a physiological negative regulator of platelet production.

PF4, β-thromboglobulin, and CTAP-III belong to the family of chemokines that are capable of binding heparin. In vitro, PF4 inhibits megakaryocyte colony formation.[188,189] In vivo, injection of PF4 into mice induces thrombocytopenia.[190] However, the inhibitory effect of PF4 on megakaryocytopoiesis is non-specific. Like other members of this family, such as macrophage inflammatory protein 1α (MIP-1α), PF4 acts on primitive hematopoietic cells, including all types of hematopoietic progenitors. PF4 may also be used as a hemoprotector.[191] However, it does not seem to be a physiological regulator of megakaryocytopoiesis, because PF4-null mice do not develop thrombocytosis.

As well as these platelet molecules, other cytokines, such as interferons and tumor necrosis factor α (TNF-α), also inhibit megakaryocytopoiesis in vitro.[192] Among the interferons, IFN-α inhibits megakaryocyte colony formation, whereas IFN-γ induces proliferation by a TPO-independent mechanism.[193] The inhibitory effect of IFN-α is related to the induction of SOCS1, an inhibitor of the Jak–STAT pathway activated by TPO.[194]

Finally, there is also evidence that extracellular matrix proteins regulate megakaryocytopoiesis by inhibiting proplatelet formation.

# Megakaryocytopoiesis and human pathology

Recent progress in the understanding of megakaryocytopoiesis has permitted identification of the molecular mechanisms of several human diseases involving platelet production. Three types of molecules have been implicated: (i) TPO/Mpl, (ii) transcription factors, and (iii) molecules involved in the process of proplatelet formation.

## Involvement of TPO/Mpl in human pathology

Mutations and/or deletions of the c-*mpl* and *TPO* genes have been examined to gain insight into the pathophysiology of various thrombocytopenic and thrombocythemic disorders. In congenital amegakaryocytic thrombocytopenia (CAMT), a loss of Mpl function has been demonstrated, due to missense or nonsense mutations in the coding region of c-*mpl* resulting in amino-acid substitutions or the presence of a premature stop codon.[195,196] It is noteworthy that the homozygous mutation in human induces a more profound thrombocytopenia than that observed in c-*mpl*-null mice. In the TAR syndrome (thrombocytopenia and absent radii), megakaryocytes and platelets respond poorly to TPO. No mutation or rearrangement in the c-*mpl* gene or its promoter has been detected, but c-*mpl* mRNA and protein levels are found to be decreased in platelets, suggesting possible abnormal signaling.[197,198] In myeloproliferative disorders, including essential thrombocythemia (ET) and idiopathic myelofibrosis, no mutation in the c-*mpl* gene has been reported so far, although a fraction of CFU-Mk from these patients have the ability to grow autonomously in culture.[199,200] In addition, no aberrant protein tyrosine phosphorylation has been observed in platelets of patients with sporadic ET before TPO activation, indicating that thrombocytosis is not related to a constitutive activation of Mpl signaling. However, expression of Mpl has been found to be strikingly diminished, suggesting that excessive production of platelets might be attributable to the impaired uptake and catabolism of TPO.[201–203] The *TPO* gene is located on human chromosome 3q27–28. Patients with 3q21 or 3q26 rearrangements often develop thrombocytosis or dysmegakaryopoiesis. No transcriptional activation or chromosomal rearrangement of the *TPO* gene has been detected in these patients, excluding involvement of this gene in these malignancies.[204,205] Studies performed on two families with hereditary thrombocythemia in which all affected members had elevated TPO serum levels have demonstrated that single point mutations in the 5′-untranslated region (UTR) of *TPO* mRNA resulted in more efficiently translated transcripts, causing overexpression of TPO.[206,207] However, not all congenital cases of ET are due to increased secretion of TPO.

## Transcription factors and abnormal megakaryocytopoiesis

It has been shown that four transcription factors (GATA-1, FOG, Fli-1, and NF-E2) are essential regulators of megakaryocyte differentiation (Figure 11.1). Mutations in two of them (GATA-1 and Fli-1) cause congenital thrombocytopenia.

X-linked thrombocytopenia (XLT) usually corresponds to mutations in the *WASP* gene and is associated with small platelets.[208,209] Cases of XLT associated with large platelets have been described, but these patients do not carry mutations in the *WASP* gene. These pathologies are associated with mild anemia or dyserythropoiesis. It has been demonstrated in two families that this disorder corresponds to a mutation in the *GATA-1* gene resulting in a loss of FOG binding to GATA-1.[14,210]

Deletion in the locus 11q23.3, where Fli-1 is located, leads to a thrombocytopenia called Jacobsen syndrome or Paris–Trousseau thrombocytopenia. Thrombocytopenia is associated with numerous congenital anomalies, including cardiac defects.[211,212] Platelets in Paris Trousseau thrombocytopenia are characterized by giant granules. In the bone marrow as well as in culture, two populations of megakaryocytes are observed. One is normal, while the other one comprises small immature megakaryocytes that express a low level of platelet glycoproteins and are extremely sensitive to apoptosis.[212] In this syndrome there is a large terminal deletion of 11q that leads to a hemizygous loss of Fli-1 as well as of other genes. *Fli-1*[+/-] mice have normal megakaryocytopoiesis with an absence of thrombocytopenia. Thus, Paris–Trousseau thrombocytopenia may be related to deletions in more than one gene (*Fli-1* plus ?) or to a difference in the regulation of *Fli-1* between human and mouse. This hypothesis is supported by the fact that the abnormal megakaryocytes of Paris–Trousseau thrombocytopenia have the same phenotype as those observed in *Fli-1*[-/-] embryos.[74,212]

More surprisingly, haploinsufficiency of transcription factors, which has not yet been implicated in the regulation of megakaryocytopoiesis, may induce congenital thrombocytopenia. Haploinsufficiency of CBFA2/AML1 leads to a thrombocytopenia associated with a defect in platelet function.[213] The target genes of CBFA2/AML1 in megakaryocytes are presently unknown as are the molecular mechanisms underlying this thrombocytopenia. This haploinsufficiency predisposes to the development of acute myeloid leukemia.[213] In the mouse, haploinsufficiency of CBAF2 does not lead to thrombocytopenia but to alterations in the ontogenic changes of hematopoietic stem cells.[214]

Some thrombocytopenias may be related to mutations in *Hox* genes. A mutation in *HoxA11* has been described, associated with a syndrome similar to the TAR syndrome, i.e. amegakaryocytic thrombocytopenia with radio–ulnar synostosis.[215] However, no mutation in *HoxA10* on *HoxA11* has been found in true TAR syndrome.

The two genes involved in the t(1;22)(p13;q13) translocation and associated with infant acute megakaryoblastic leukemia have been characterized.[216,217] One of these genes, *OTT*, is the human homolog of the *Drosophila spen* gene involved in the *Hox* gene as well as the Ras/MAPK kinase pathways.[218,219] The other MAL is a co-activator of SRF.

### Abnormalities in platelet formation

Up to now, no mutation in NF-E2 associated with thrombocytopenia has been described in humans. In contrast, several congenital thrombocytopenias may be related to genes involved in proplatelet formation, but the molecular mechanisms of most of these thrombocytopenia are still unknown.

Autosomal dominant giant platelet syndromes with or without leukocyte inclusions (Fechtner syndrome, May–Hegglin anomaly, and Sebastian syndrome) are related to mutations in the gene encoding non-muscle myosin heavy chain A.[220–222] It has been suggested that this gene may be involved in proplatelet formation.

Bernard–Soulier syndrome, initially described as an inherited bleeding disorder with mild thrombocytopenia and giant platelets, corresponds to mutations in genes encoding members of the GpIb complex (GpIb or GpIX). Thrombocytopenia is also observed in GpIb-null mice and seems to be related to abnormal proplatelet formation.[223] In humans, the heterozygous form of Bernard–Soulier syndrome seems to be a frequent cause of autosomal dominant macrothrombocytopenia.[224]

Wiskott–Aldrich syndrome (WAS), which associates eczema, immune deficiency, and microthrombocytopenia, and its variant, which only involves microthrombocytopenia (X-linked thrombocytopenia), are due to mutations in the *WASP* gene.[208,209] The WASP protein is involved in actin polymerization. It is a target molecule for activated Cdc42, permitting actin polarization and the formation of filopods.[225] Mutation of *WASP* results in loss of function and induces a cytoskeletal disease. The mechanism of thrombocytopenia is complex and seems to be related essentially to peripheral platelet destruction. Despite divergent results, no marked abnormality in in vitro proplatelet formation from megakaryocytes of WAS patients have been observed, although branching structures have not yet been studied.[226] However, megakaryocytes from WAS patients present abnormal actin filaments, especially after matrix adhesion, which may be responsible for abnormal megakaryocyte exit from the marrow.

# Clinical potentials of TPO

Two different forms of recombinant TPO molecule have been used in clinical trials. One is a full-length glycosylated human protein (rHu-TPO) produced in mammalian cells. The other is a C-terminally truncated version of the human cDNA sequence produced in bacteria and covalently attached to a polyethylene glycol tail to increase in vivo potency (PEG-rHuMGDF).

Treatment of normal animals with glycosylated rHu-TPO or PEG-rHuMGDF potently stimulates the expansion of marrow megakaryocytes and their progenitors, and greatly augments the production of platelets, with only minimal effects on leukocyte and red cell counts.[142,227] Platelets generated in response to PEG-rHuMGDF show normal morphology and hemostatic function. Although PEG-rHuMGDF by itself does not induce aggregation of platelets in vitro, the aggregatory response to ADP or collagen is enhanced in a dose-dependent manner. Nevertheless, in a model of thrombus formation, treatment with PEG-rHuMGDF had no effect.[228] Either of the recombinant molecules used alone markedly expand circulating levels of multiple types of hematopoietic progenitor cells, and this effect is potentiated by G-CSF. A variety of animal models of myelosuppression, including chemotherapy, irradiation or combined treatment, have been used to reveal the effects of rHu-TPO and PEG-rHuMGDF. TPO treatment accelerates multilineage hematopoietic recovery and efficiently improves thrombocytopenia and, in most models, anemia and neutropenia.[229–232] Concurrent administration of PEG-rHuMGDF and G-CSF does not interfere with the in vivo effects of each cytokine, but rather has synergistic effects.[233–235] In bone marrow transplantation (BMT), administration of PEG-rHuMGDF has little or no efficacy.[236,237] However, the use of transplants from TPO-pretreated donors prompts hematopoietic recovery and improves platelet counts.[237,238]

Results of initial clinical trials revealed that the two forms of recombinant molecules were well tolerated, with few adverse events. Phase I trials conducted in patients with advanced cancer have shown that both molecules potently stimulate platelet production when given prior to chemotherapy.[239,240] After chemotherapies that require minimal or no platelet transfusions, administration of TPO alone or in combination with recombinant G-CSF reduces the duration of thrombocytopenia and, in some cases, the platelet nadir.[241,242] TPO given after peripheral blood progenitor cell transplantation (PBPCT) or BMT may not be effective in platelet recovery, since levels are extremely high in the circulation.[105] A placebo-controlled, blinded study was conducted in normal human volunteers to examine the effects of a single bolus administration of PEG-rHuMGDF on platelet production, lifespan, and function.[243] The results show that, within 1 week, megakaryocytopoiesis doubles, leading to a doubling of circulating platelet numbers on day 12. Platelets exhibit normal function and viability during the ensuing 10 days. No increase in thrombotic events was reported in this study. However, the development of PEG-rHuMGDF is presently suspended because of the development of neutralizing antibodies that inactivate endogenous TPO in some individuals after repeated injections.

It is too early to draw definitive conclusions regarding the potential clinical applications of TPO. Nevertheless, TPO in combination with other cytokines remains a key growth factor for cord blood stem cell expansion ex vivo. Encouraging results have suggested that pluripotent stem cells can be expanded for several weeks without loosing pluripotency.[121] Studies with TPO are ongoing to expand CFU-Mk and megakaryocytes ex vivo in order to produce platelets that could be useful for transfusion.[159,180]

## REFERENCES

1. Debili N, Coulombel L, Croisille L et al. Characterization of a bipotent erythro-megakaryocytic progenitor in human bone marrow. *Blood* 1996; **88**: 1284–96.

2. Papayannopoulou T, Brice M, Farrer D, Kaushansky K. Insights into the cellular mechanisms of erythropoietin-thrombopoietin synergy. *Exp Hematol* 1996; **24**: 660–9.

3. Hoffman R. Regulation of megakaryocytopoiesis. *Blood* 1989; **74**: 1196–212.

4. Bruno E, Murray LJ, DiGiusto R et al. Detection of a primitive megakaryocyte progenitor cell in human fetal bone marrow. *Exp Hematol* 1996; **24**: 552–8.

5. Metcalf D, McDonald HR, Odartchenko N, Sordat B. Growth of mouse megakaryocyte colonies in vitro. *Proc Natl Acad Sci USA* 1975; **72**: 1744–8.

6. Vainchenker W, Bouget J, Guichard J, Breton-Gorius J. Megakaryocyte colony formation from human bone marrow precursors. *Blood* 1979; **54**: 940–7.

7. Chatelain C, Debast M, Symann M. Identification of a light density murine megakaryocyte progenitor (LD-CFU-MK). *Blood* 1988; **72**: 1187–92.

8. Jackson CN. Cholinesterase as a possible marker for early cells of the megakaryocytic series. *Blood* 1973; **42**: 413–21.

9. Breton-Gorius J, Guichard J. Ultrastructural localization of peroxidase activity in human platelets and megakaryocytes. *Am J Pathol* 1972; **66**: 277–86.

10. Briddell RA, Brandt JE, Straneva JE et al. Characterization of the human burst-forming unit–megakaryocyte. *Blood* 1989; **74**: 145–51.

11. Murray LJ, Bruno E, Uchida N et al. CD109 is expressed on a subpopulation of CD34+ cells enriched in hematopoietic stem and progenitor cells. *Exp Hematol* 1999; **27**: 1282–94.

12. Rabellino EM, Levene RB, Leung LK, Nachman RL. Human megakaryocytes. II: Expression of platelet proteins in early marrow megakaryocytes. *J Exp Med* 1981; **154**: 85–100.

13. Vinci G, Tabilio A, Deschamps J-F et al. Immunological study of in vitro maturation of human megakaryocytes. *Br J Haematol* 1984; **56**: 589–605.

14. Freson K, Devriendt K, Matthijs G et al. Platelet characteristics in patients with X-linked macrothrombocytopenia because of a novel *GATA1* mutation. *Blood* 2001; **98**: 85–92.

15. Gewirtz AM, Boghosian-Sell L, Catani L et al. Expression of FcγRII and CD4 receptors by normal human megakaryocytes. *Exp Hematol* 1992; **20**: 512–16.

16. Kouri YH, Borkowsky W, Nardi M et al. Human megakaryocytes have a CD4 molecule capable of binding human immunodeficiency virus-1. *Blood* 1993; **81**: 2664–70.

17. Debili N, Issaad C, Masse J et al. Expression of CD34 and platelet glycoproteins during human megakaryocytic differentiation. *Blood* 1992; **80**: 3022–31.

18. Berridge MV, Ralph SJ, Tan AS. Cell lineage antigens of the stem cell–megakaryocyte platelet lineage are associated with the platelet IIb–IIIa glycoprotein complex. *Blood* 1985; **66**: 76–85.

19. Tronik-Le Roux D, Roullot V, Schweitzer A et al. Suppression of erythro-megakaryocytopoiesis and the induction of reversible thrombocytopenia in mice transgenic for the thymidine kinase gene targeted by the platelet glycoprotein αIIβ promoter. *J Exp Med* 1995; **181**: 2141–51.

20. Ody C, Vaigot P, Quéré P et al. Glycoprotein IIb–IIIa is expressed on avian multilineage hematopoietic progenitor cells. *Blood* 1999; **93**: 2898–906.

21. Debili N, Robin C, Schiavon V et al. Different expression of CD41 on human lymphoid and myeloid progenitors from adults and neonates. *Blood* 2001; **97**: 2023–30.

22. Hagiwara T, Kodama I, Horie K et al. Proliferative properties of human umbilical cord blood megakaryocyte progenitor cells to human thrombopoietin. *Exp Hematol* 1998; **26**: 228–35.

23. Therman E, Sarto GE, Stubblefied PA. Endomitosis: a reappraisal. *Hum Genet* 1983; **63**: 13–18.

24. Goyanes-Villaescuca V. Cycles of reduplication in megakaryocyte nuclei. *Cell Tissue Kinet* 1969; **2**: 165–8.

25. Radley JM, Green SL. Ultrastructure of endomitosis in megakaryocytes. *Nouv Rev Fr Hematol* 1989; **31**: 232a.

26. Nagata Y, Muro Y, Todokoro K. Thrombopoietin-induced polyploidization of bone marrow megakaryocytes is due to a unique regulatory mechanism in late mitosis. *J Cell Biol* 1997; **139**: 449–57.

27. Vitrat N, Cohen-Solal K, Pique C et al. Endomitosis of human megakaryocytes are due to abortive mitosis. *Blood* 1998; **91**: 3711–23.

28. Roy L, Coullin P, Vitrat N et al. Asymmetrical segregation of chromosomes with a normal metaphase/anaphase checkpoint in polyploid megakaryocytes. *Blood* 2001; **97**: 2238–47.

29. Zimmet JM, Ladd D, Jackson CW et al. A role for cyclin D3 in the endomitotic cell cycle. *Mol Cell Biol* 1997; **17**: 7248–59.

30. Zimmet JM, Toselli P, Ravid K. Cyclin D3 and megakaryocyte development: exploration of a transgenic phenotype. *Stem Cells* 1998; **16**(Suppl 2): 97–106.

31. Kawasaki A, Matsumura I, Miyagawa J et al. Downregulation of an AIM-1 kinase couples with megakaryocytic polyploidization of human hematopoietic cells. *J Cell Biol* 2001; **152**: 275–87.

32. Taniguchi T, Endo H, Chikatsu N et al. Expression of p21$^{Cip1/Waf1/Sdi1}$ and p27$^{Kip1}$ cyclin-dependent kinase inhibitors during human hematopoiesis. *Blood* 1999; **93**: 4167–78.

33. Hegyi E, Navarro S, Debili N et al. Regulation of human megakaryocytopoiesis: analysis of proliferation, ploidy and maturation in liquid cultures. *Int J Cell Cloning* 1990; **8**: 236–44.

34. Radley JM, Scurfield G. The mechanism of platelet release. *Blood* 1980; **56**: 996–9.

35. Radley JM, Haller CJ. The demarcation membrane system of the megakaryocyte: a misnomer. *Blood* 1982; **60**: 213–19.

36. Handagama P, Rappolee D, Werb Z et al. Platelet α-granule fibrinogen, albumin and immunoglobulin G are not synthetized by rat and mouse megakaryocytes. *J Clin Invest* 1990; **86**: 1364–8.

37. Handagama P, Scarborough R, Shuman M, Bainton DF. Endocytosis of fibrinogen into megakaryocyte and platelets α-granules is mediated by $\alpha_{IIb}\beta_3$ (glycoprotein IIb/IIIa). *Blood* 1993; **82**: 135–8.

38. Harrison P, Wilbourn B, Debili N et al. Uptake of plasma fibrinogen into the α granules of human megakaryocytes and platelets. *J Clin Invest* 1989; **84**: 1320–4.

39. Louache F, Debili N, Cramer E et al. Fibrinogen is not synthesized by human megakaryocytes. *Blood* 1991; **77**: 311–16.

40. Cramer EM, Debili N, Martin JF et al. Uncoordinated expression of fibrinogen compared with thrombospondin and von Willebrand factor in maturing human megakaryocytes. *Blood* 1989; **73**: 1123–9.

41. Breton-Gorius J, Clezardin P, Guichard J et al. Localization of platelet osteonectin at the internal face of the α-granule membranes in platelets and megakaryocytes. *Blood* 1992; **79**: 936–41.

42. Cramer EM, Meyer D, Le Menn R, Breton-Gorius J. Eccentric localization of von Willebrand factor in an internal structure of platelet α-granule resembling that of Weibel–Palade bodies. *Blood* 1985; **66**: 710–13.

43. Stenberg PE, McEver RP, Shuman MA et al. An α granule membrane protein (GMP-140) is expressed on the plasma membrane after activation. *J Cell Biol* 1985; **101**: 880–6.

44. Breton-Gorius J, Vainchenker W. Expression of platelet proteins during the in vitro and in vivo differentiation of megakaryocytes and morphological aspects of their maturation. *Semin Hematol* 1986; **28**: 43–67.

45. Schick PK, Weinstein M. A marker for megakaryocytes: serotonin accumulation in guinea pig megakaryocytes. *J Lab Clin Med* 1981; **98**: 607–15.

46. Thiery JB, Bessis M. Mécanisme de la plaquettogenèse. Etude in vitro par la microcinématographie. *Rev Hematol* 1956; **II**: 162–76.

47. Shivdasani RA, Rosenblatt MF, Zucker-Franklin D et al. Transcription factor NF-E2 is required for platelet formation independent of actions of thrombopoietin/MGDF in megakaryocyte development. *Cell* 1995; **81**: 695–704.

48. Lecine P, Villeval J-L, Vyas P et al. Mice lacking transcription factor NF-E2 provide in vivo validation of the proplatelet model of thrombocytopoiesis and show a platelet production defect that is intrinsic to megakaryocytes. *Blood* 1998; **92**: 1608–16.

49. Becker RP, De Bruyn PPH. The transmural passage of blood cells into myeloid sinusoids and the entry of platelets into the sinusoidal circulation: a scanning microscopic investigation. *Am J Anat* 1976; **145**: 183–206.

50. Cramer E, Norol F, Guichard J et al. Ultrastructure of platelet formation by human megakarocytes cultured with the Mpl ligand. *Blood* 1997; **89**: 2326–46.

51. Schwer HD, Lecine P, Tiwari S et al. A lineage-restricted and divergent β-tubulin isoform is essential for the biogenesis, structure and function of blood platelets. *Curr Biol* 2001; **11**: 579–86.

52. Lecine P, Italiano JEJ, Kim SW et al. Hematopoietic-specific β-1 tubulin participates in a pathway of platelet biogenesis dependent on the transcription factor NF-E2. *Blood* 2000; **96**: 1366–73.

53. Italiano JEJ, Lecine P, Shivdasani RA, Hartwig JH. Blood platelets are assembled principally at the ends of proplatelet processes produced by differentiated megakaryocytes. *J Cell Biol* 1999; **147**: 1299–312.

54. Rojnuckarin P, Kaushansky K. Actin reorganization and proplatelet formation in murine megakaryocytes: the role of protein kinase C. *Blood* 2001; **97**: 154–61.

55. Radley JM, Hartshorn MA. Megakaryocyte fragments and the microtubule coil. *Blood Cells* 1987; **12**: 603–10.

56. Tavassoli M, Aoki M. Migration of entire megakaryocyte through the marrow-barrier. *Br J Haematol* 1981; **48**: 25–9.

57. Avraham H, Cowley S, Chi SY et al. Characterization of adhesive interactions between human endothelial cells and megakaryocytes. *J Clin Invest* 1993; **91**: 2378–84.

58. Trowbridge EA, Martin JF, Slater DN. Evidence for a theory of physical fragmentation of megakaryocytes implying that all platelets are produced in the pulmonary circulation. *Thromb Res* 1982; **28**: 461–75.

59. Zauli G, Vitale M, Falcieri E et al. In vitro senescence and apoptotic cell death of human megakaryocytes. *Blood* 1997; **90**: 2234–43.

60. Radley JM, Holder CJ. Fate of senescent megakaryocytes in the bone marrow. *Br J Haematol* 1983; **53**: 277–87.

61. Ogilvy S, Metcalf D, Print CG et al. Constitutive bcl-2 expression throughout the hematopoietic compartment affects multiple lineages and enhances progenitor cell survival. *Proc Natl Acad Sci USA* 1999; **96**: 14943–8.

62. Bouillet P, Metcalf D, Haung DCS et al. Proapoptotic bcl-2 relative Bim required for certain apoptotic responses, leukocyte homeostasis, and to preclude autoimmunity. *Science* 1999; **286**: 1735–8.

63. Orkin S. Transcription factors and hematopoietic development. *J Biol Chem* 1995; **270**: 4955–61.

64. Shivdasani R, Orkin S. The transcriptional control of hematopoiesis. *Blood* 1996; **87**: 4025–39.

65. Lemarchandel V, Ghysdael J, Mignotte V et al. Gata and Ets cis-acting sequence mediate megakaryocyte-specific expression. *Mol Cell Biol* 1993; **13**: 668–76.

66. Deveaux S, Filipe A, Lemarchandel V et al. Analysis of the thrombopoietin receptor (mpl) promoter implicates GATA and Ets proteins in the coregulation of megakaryocyte-specific genes. *Blood* 1996; **87**: 4678–85.

67. Ravid K, Doi T, Beeler L et al. Transcriptional regulation of the rat platelet factor 4 gene: interaction between an enhancer/silencer domain and the GATA-1 site. *Mol Cell Biol* 1991; **11**: 6116–27.

68. Pevny L, Simon MC, Roberston E et al. Erythroid differentiation in chimeric mice blocked by a targeted mutation in

the gene for transcription factor GATA-1. *Nature* 1991; **349**: 257–61.

69. Shivdasani R, Fujiwara Y, McDevitt M, Orkin S. A lineage-specific knockout establishes the critical role of transcription factor GATA-1 in megakaryocyte growth and platelet development. *EMBO J* 1997; **16**: 3965–73.

70. Vyas P, Ault K, Jackson C et al. Consequences of GATA-1 deficiency in megakaryocytes and platelets. *Blood* 1999; **93**: 2867–75.

71. Vyas P, Norris FA, Joseph R et al. Inositol polyphosphate 4-phosphatase type I regulates cell growth downstream of transcription factor GATA-1. *Proc Natl Acad Sci USA* 2000; **97**: 13696–701.

72. Tsang AP, Visvader JE, Turner CA et al. FOG, a multitype zinc finger protein, acts as a cofactor for transcription factor GATA-1 in erythroid and megakaryocytic differentiation. *Cell* 1997; **90**: 109–19.

73. Tsang A, Fujiwara Y, Hom D, Orkin S. Failure of megakaryopoiesis and arrested erythropoiesis in mice lacking the GATA-1 transcriptional cofactor FOG. *Genes Dev* 1998; **12**: 1176–88.

74. Hart A, Melet F, Grossfeld P et al. Fli-1 is required for murine vascular and megakaryocytic development and is hemizygously deleted in patients with thrombocytopenia. *Immunity* 2000; **13**: 167–77.

75. Spyropoulos D, Pharr P, Lavenburg K et al. Hemorrhage, impaired hematopoiesis, and lethality in mouse embryos carrying a targeted disruption of the fli1 transcription factor. *Mol Cell Biol* 2000; **20**: 5643–62.

76. Mignotte V, Eleouet JF, Raich N, Roméo P-H. *Cis-* and *trans*-acting elements involved in the regulation of the erythroid promoter of the human porphobilinogen deaminase gene. *Proc Natl Acad Sci USA* 1989; **86**: 6548–52.

77. Andrews NC, Erjument-Bromage H, Davidson MB et al. Erythroid transcription factor NF-E2 is a haematopoietic-specific basic-leucine zipper protein. *Nature* 1993; **362**: 722–8.

78. Deveaux S, Cohen-Kaminsky S, Shivdasani RA et al. p45[NF-E2] regulates expression of thromboxane synthase in megakaryocytes. *EMBO J* 1997; **16**: 5654–61.

79. Andrews NC, Kotkow KJ, Ney PA et al. The ubiquitous subunit of erythroid transcription factor NF-E2 is a small basic-leucine zipper protein related to the v-*maf* oncogene. *Proc Natl Acad Sci USA* 1993; **90**: 11488–92.

80. Lecine P, Blank V, Shivdasani R. Characterization of the hematopoietic transcription factor NF-E2 in primary murine megakaryocytes. *J Biol Chem* 1998; **273**: 7572–8.

81. Shavit JA, Motohashi H, Onodera K et al. Impaired megakaryopoiesis and behavioral defects in *mafG*-null mutant mice. *Genes Dev* 1998; **12**: 2164–74.

82. Onodera K, Shavit JA, Motohashi H et al. Perinatal synthetic lethality and hematopoietic defects in compound *MafG/MafK* mutant mice. *EMBO J* 2000; **19**: 1335–45.

83. Kelemen E, Cserhati I, Tanos B. Demonstration and some properties of human thrombopoietin in thrombocythemic sera. *Acta Haematol (Basel)* 1958; **20**: 350–5.

84. Wendling F, Varlet P, Charon M, Tambourin P. MPLV: a retrovirus complex inducing an acute myeloproliferative disorder in mice. *Virology* 1986; **149**: 242–6.

85. Souyri M, Vigon I, Penciolelli J-F et al. A putative truncated cytokine receptor gene transduced by the myeloproliferative leukemia virus immortalizes hematopoietic progenitors. *Cell* 1990; **63**: 1137–47.

86. Vigon I, Mornon J-P, Cocault L et al. Molecular cloning and characterization of *MPL*, the human homolog of the v-*mpl* oncogene: Identification of a member of the hematopoietic growth factor receptor superfamily. *Proc Natl Acad Sci USA* 1992; **89**: 5640–4.

87. Skoda RC, Seldin DC, Chiang M-K et al. Murine c-mpl: a member of the hematopoietic growth factor receptor superfamily that transduces a proliferative signal. *EMBO J* 1993; **12**: 2645–53.

88. Methia N, Louache F, Vainchenker W, Wendling F. Oligodeoxynucleotides antisense to the proto-oncogene c-*mpl* specifically inhibit in vitro megakaryocytopoiesis. *Blood* 1993; **82**: 1395–401.

89. Gurney AL, Carver-Moore K, de Sauvage FJ, Moore MW. Thrombocytopenia in c-mpl-deficient mice. *Science* 1994; **265**: 1445–7.

90. Wendling F, Vainchenker W. Thrombopoietin and its receptor. *Eur Cytofrine Netw* 1998; **9**: 221–31.

91. de Sauvage FJ, Hass PE, Spencer SD et al. Stimulation of megakaryopoiesis and thrombopoiesis by the c-MPL ligand. *Nature* 1994; **369**: 533–8.

92. Bartley TD, Bogenberger J, Hunt P et al. Identification and cloning of a megakaryocyte growth and development factor that its a ligand for the cytokine receptor Mpl. *Cell* 1994; **77**: 1117–24.

93. Lok S, Kaushansky K, Holly RD et al. Cloning and expression of murine thrombopoietin and stimulation of platelet production in vivo. *Nature* 1994; **369**: 564–8.

94. Kato T, Ogami K, Shimada Y et al. Purification and characterization of thrombopoietin. *J Biochem* 1995; **118**: 229–36.

95. Kuter DJ, Beeler DL, Rosenberg RD. The purification of megapoietin: a physiological regulator of megakaryocyte growth and platelet production. *Proc Natl Acad Sci USA* 1994; **91**: 11104–8.

96. Kaushansky K. Thrombopoietin: the primary regulator of platelet production. *Blood* 1995; **86**: 419–31.

97. Kuter DJ, Rosenberg RD. The reciprocal relationship of thrombopoietin (c-Mpl ligand) to changes in the platelet mass during busulfan-induced thrombocytopenia in the rabbit. *Blood* 1995; **85**: 2720–30.

98. Stoffer R, Wiestner A, Skoda RC. Thrombopoietin in thrombocytopenic mice: evidence against regulation at the mRNA level and for a direct regulatory role of platelets. *Blood* 1996; **87**: 567–73.

99. Cohen-Solal K, Villeval J-L, Titeux M et al. Constitutive expression of Mpl ligand transcript during thrombocytopenia and thrombocytosis. *Blood* 1996; **88**: 2578–84.

100. McCarthy JM, Sprugel KH, Fox NE et al. Murine thrombopoietin mRNA levels are modulated by platelet count. *Blood* 1995; **86**: 3668–75.

101. Hirayama Y, Sakamaki T, Matsunaga T et al. Concentrations of thrombopoietin in bone marrow in normal subjects and in patients with idiopathic thrombocytopenic purpura, aplastic anemia, and essential thrombocythemia correlate with its mRNA expression of bone marrow stromal cells. *Blood* 1998; **92**: 46–52.

102. Fielder P, Hass P, Nagel M et al. Human platelets as a model for the binding and degradation of thrombopoietin. *Blood* 1997; **89**: 2782–8.

103. Broudy V, Lin N, Sabath D et al. Human platelets display high-affinity receptors for thrombopoietin. *Blood* 1997; **89**: 1896–904.

104. Shivdasani RA, Fielder P, Keller G-A, Orkin SH, de Sauvage FJ. Regulation of the serum concentration of

thrombopoietin in thrombocytopenic NF-E2 knockout mice. *Blood* 1997; **90**: 1821–7.

105. Emmons RVB, Reid DM, Cohen RL et al. Human thrombopoietin levels are high when thrombocytopenia is due to megakaryocyte deficiency and low when due to increased platelet destruction. *Blood* 1996; **87**: 4068–71.

106. de Sauvage FJ, Carver-Moore K, Luoh S-M et al. Physiological regulation of early and late stages of megakaryocytopoiesis by thrombopoietin. *J Exp Med* 1996; **183**: 651–6.

107. Alexander WS, Roberts AW, Nicola NA et al. Deficiencies in progenitor cells of multiple hematopoietic lineages and defective megakaryocytopoiesis in mice lacking the thrombopoietin receptor c-mpl. *Blood* 1996; **87**: 2162–70.

108. Carver-Moore K, Broxmeyer HE, Luoh S-M et al. Low levels of erythroid and myeloid progenitors in thrombopoietin- and c-*mpl*-deficient mice. *Blood* 1996; **88**: 803–8.

109. Kimura S, Roberts AW, Metcalf D, Alexander WS. Hematopoietic stem cell deficiencies in mice lacking c-Mpl, the receptor for thrombopoietin. *Proc Natl Acad Sci USA* 1998; **95**: 1195–200.

110. Wendling F, Maraskovsky E, Debili N et al. c-Mpl ligand is a humoral regulator of megakaryocytopoiesis. *Nature* 1994; **369**: 571–4.

111. Kaushansky K, Broudy VC, Lin N et al. Thrombopoietin, the Mpl ligand, is essential for full megakaryocyte development. *Proc Natl Acad Sci USA* 1995; **92**: 3234–8.

112. Debili N, Wendling F, Katz A et al. The Mpl-ligand or thrombopoietin or megakaryocyte growth and development factor has both direct proliferative and differentiative activities on human megakaryocyte progenitors. *Blood* 1995; **86**: 2516–25.

113. Choi ES, Hokom M, Bartley T. Recombinant human megakaryocyte growth and development factor (rHuMGDF), a ligand for c-Mpl, produces functional human platelets in vitro. *Stem Cells* 1995; **13**: 317–22.

114. Zeigler FC, de Sauvage F, Widmer HR et al. In vitro megakaryocytopoietic and thrombopoietic activity of c-mpl ligand (TPO) on purified murine hematopoietic stem cells. *Blood* 1994; **84**: 4045–52.

115. Ku H, Yonemura Y, Kaushansky K, Ogawa M. Thrombopoietin, the ligand for the Mpl receptor, synergizes with Steel factor and other early acting cytokines in supporting proliferation of primitive hematopoietic progenitors of mice. *Blood* 1996; **87**: 4544–51.

116. Sitnicka E, Lin N, Priestley GV et al. The effect of thrombopoietin on the proliferation and differentiation of murine hematopoietic stem cells. *Blood* 1996; **87**: 4998–5005.

117. Kobayashi M, Laver JH, Kato T et al. Thrombopoietin supports proliferation of human primitive hematopoietic cells in synergy with Steel factor and/or interleukin-3. *Blood* 1996; **88**: 429–36.

118. Petzer AL, Zanstra PW, Piret JM, Eaves CJ. Differential cytokine effects on primitive (CD34+ CD38–) human hematopoietic cells: novel response to flt-3 ligand and thrombopoietin. *J Exp Med* 1996; **183**: 2551–7.

119. Ramsfjell V, Borge OJ, Veiby OP et al. Thrombopoietin, but not erythropoietin, directly stimulates multilineage growth of primitive murine bone marrow progenitor cells in synergy with early acting cytokines: distinct interactions with the ligands for c-kit and FLT-3. *Blood* 1996; **88**: 4481–92.

120. Ohmizono Y, Sakabe H, Kimura T et al. Thrombopoietin augments ex vivo expansion of human cord blood-derived hematopoietic progenitors in combination with stem cell factor and flt-3 ligand. *Leukemia* 1997; **11**: 524–30.

121. Piacibello W, Sanavio SF, Garetto L et al. Extensive amplification and self-renewal of human primitive hematopoietic stem cells from cord blood. *Blood* 1997; **89**: 2644–53.

122. Ramsfjell V, Borge OJ, Cui L, Jacobsen SEW. Thrombopoietin directly and potently stimulates multilineage growth and progenitor cell expension from primitive (CD34+ CD38–) human bone marrow progenitor cells. *J Immunol* 1997; **158**: 5169–74.

123. Borge OJ, Ramsfjell V, Cui L, Jacobsen SEW. Ability of early acting cytokine to directly promote survival and suppress apoptosis of human primitive CD34+ CD38– bone marrow cells with multilineage potential at the single cell level: key role of thrombopoietin. *Blood* 1997; **90**: 2282–9.

124. Pallard C, Gouilleux F, Bénit L et al. Thrombopoietin activates a STAT5-like factor in hematopoietic cells. *EMBO J* 1995; **14**: 2847–56.

125. Sattler M, Durstin MA, Frank DA et al. The thrombopoietin receptor c-MPL activates JAK2 and TYK2 tyrosine kinases. *Exp Hematol* 1995; **23**: 1040–8.

126. Drachman JG, Griffin JD, Kaushansky K. The c-Mpl ligand (thrombopoietin) stimulates tyrosine phosphorylation of Jak2, Shc, and c-Mpl. *J Biol Chem* 1995; **270**: 4979–82.

127. Ihle JN, Witthuhn BA, Quelle FW et al. Signalling through the hematopoietic cytokine receptors. *Annu Rev Immunol* 1995; **13**: 369–98.

128. Leonard W, O'Shea J. JAKs and STATs: biological implications. *Annu Rev Immunol* 1998; **16**: 293–322.

129. Gurney AL, Wong SC, Henzel WJ, De Sauvage FJ. Distinct regions of c-Mpl cytoplasmic domain are coupled to the JAK–STAT signal transduction pathway and She phosphorylation. *Proc Natl Acad Sci USA* 1995; **92**: 5292–6.

130. Mu SX, Xia M, Elliott G et al. Megakaryocyte growth and development factor and interleukin-3 induce patterns of protein tyrosine phosphorylation that correlate with dominant differentiation over proliferation of mpl-transfected 32D cells. *Blood* 1995; **86**: 4532–43.

131. Miyakawa Y, Oda A, Druker BJ et al. Thrombopoietin induces tyrosine phosphorylation of Stat3 and Stat5 in human blood platelets. *Blood* 1996; **87**: 439–46.

132. Porteu F, Rouyez MC, Cocault L et al. Functional regions of the mouse thrombopoietin receptor cytoplasmic domain: evidence for a critical region which is involved in differentiation and can be complemented by erythropoietin. *Mol Cell Biol* 1996; **16**: 2473–82.

133. Drachman JG, Sabath DF, Fox NE, Kaushansky K. Thrombopoietin signal transduction in purified murine megakaryocytes. *Blood* 1997; **89**: 483–92.

134. Dorsch M, Fan P-D, Danial NN et al. The thrombopoietin receptor can mediate proliferation without activation of the Jak–STAT pathway. *J Exp Med* 1997; **186**: 1947–55.

135. Sattler M, Salgia R, Durstin M et al. Thrombopoietin induces activation of the phosphatidylinositol-3′ kinase pathway and formation of a complex containing p85$^{PI3K}$ and the protooncoprotein p120$^{CBL}$. *J Cell Physiol* 1997; **171**: 28–33.

136. Hong Y, Duménil D, van der Loo B. Protein kinase C mediates the mitogenic action of thrombopoietin in c-Mpl-expressing UT-7 cells. *Blood* 1998; **91**: 813–22.

137. Dorsch M, Danial N, Rothman P, Goff S. A thrombopoietin receptor mutant deficient in Jak–STAT activation

mediates proliferation but not differentiation in UT-7 cells. *Blood* 1999; **94**: 2676–85.

138. Rouyez MC, Bougheron C, Gisselbrecht S et al. Control of thrombopoietin-induced megakaryocytic differentiation by the mitogen-activated protein kinase pathway. *Mol Cell Biol* 1997; **17**: 4991–5000.

139. Matsumura I, Nakajima K, Wakao H et al. Involvement of prolonged Ras activation in thrombopoietin-induced megakaryocytic differentiation of a human factor-dependent hematopoietic cell line. *Mol Cell Biol* 1998; **18**: 4282–90.

140. Mazur EM, Cohen JL, Bogart L et al. Recombinant gibbon interleukin-3 stimulates megakaryocyte colony growth in vitro from human peripheral blood progenitor cells. *J Cell Physiol* 1988; **136**: 439–46.

141. Bruno E, Briddell RA, Cooper RJ et al. Recombinant GM-CSF/IL-3 fusion protein: its effects on in vitro human megakaryocytopoiesis. *Exp Hematol* 1992; **20**: 494–9.

142. Farese AM, Hunt P, Boone T, MacVittie TJ. Recombinant human megakaryocyte growth and development factor stimulates thrombocytopoiesis in normal nonhuman primates. *Blood* 1995; **86**: 54–9.

143. Chen Q, Solar G, Eaton DL, de Sauvage FJ. IL-3 does not contribute to platelet production in c-Mpl-deficient mice. *Stem Cells* 1998; **16**(Suppl 2): 31–6.

144. Kishimoto T, Taga T, Akira S. Cytokine signal transduction. *Cell* 1994; **76**: 253–62.

145. Ishibashi T, Kimura H, Uchida T et al. Human interleukin 6 is a direct promoter of maturation of megakaryocytes in vitro. *Proc Natl Acad Sci USA* 1989; **86**: 5953–7.

146. An E, Ogata K, Kuriya S, Nomura T. Interleukin-6 and erythropoietin act as direct potentiators and inducers of in vitro cytoplasmic process formation on purified mouse megakaryocytes. *Exp Hematol* 1994; **22**: 149–56.

147. Ishibashi T, Kimura H, Shikama Y et al. Interleukin 6 is a potent thrombopoietic factor in vivo in mice. *Blood* 1989; **74**: 1241–4.

148. Zeidler C, Kanz L, Hurkuck F et al. In vivo effects of interleukin-6 on thrombopoiesis in healthy and irradiated primates. *Blood* 1992; **80**: 2740–5.

149. Kishimoto T. The biology of interleukin-6. *Blood* 1989; **74**: 1–10.

150. Metcalf D, Hilton D, Nicola NA. Leukemia inhibitory factor can potentiate murine megakaryocyte production in vitro. *Blood* 1991; **77**: 2150–3.

151. Wallace PM, MacMaster JF, Rillema JR et al. Thrombocytopoietic properties of oncostatin M. *Blood* 1995; **86**: 1310–15.

152. Turner KJ, Neben S, Weich N et al. The role of recombinant interleukin 11 in megakaryocytopoiesis. *Stem Cells* 1996; **14**(Suppl 1): 53–61.

153. Kurzrock R. rhIL-11 for the prevention of dose-limiting chemotherapy-induced thrombocytopenia. *Oncology* 2000; **14**: 9–11.

154. Gainsford T, Nandurkar H, Metcalf D et al. The residual megakaryocyte and platelet production in c-mpl-deficient mice is not dependent on the actions of interleukin-6, interleukin-11, or leukemia inhibitory factor. *Blood* 2000; **95**: 528–34.

155. Ebbe S, Phalen E, Stohlman FJ. Abnormalities of megakaryocytes in *Sl/Sl^d* mice. *Blood* 1973; **42**: 865–9.

156. Ebbe S, Phalen E. Regulation of megakaryocytes in *W/W^v* mice. *J Cell Physiol* 1978; **96**: 73–79.

157. Avraham H, Vannier E, Cowley S et al. Effects of the stem cell factor, c-kit ligand, on human megakaryocytic cells. *Blood* 1992; **79**: 365–71.

158. Debili N, Massé J, Katz A et al. Effects of recombinant hematopoietic growth factors (IL-3, IL6, SCF, LIF) on the megakaryocyte differention of CD34 positive cells. *Blood* 1993; **82**: 84–95.

159. Norol F, Vitrat N, Cramer E et al. Effects of cytokines on platelet production from blood and marrow CD34+ cells. *Blood* 1998; **91**: 830–4.

160. Cardier JE, Erickson-Miller CL, Murphy MJJ. Differential effect of erythropoietin and GM-CSF on megakaryocytopoiesis from primitive bone marrow cells in serum-free conditions. *Stem Cells* 1997; **15**: 286–90.

161. Ishibashi T, Koziol J, Burstein S. Human recombinant erythropoietin promotes differentiation of murine megakaryocytes in vitro. *J Clin Invest* 1987; **79**: 286–9.

162. Hamada T, Mohle R, Hesselgesser J et al. Transendothelial migration of megakaryocytes in response to stromal cell-derived factor 1 (SDF-1) enhances platelet formation. *J Exp Med* 1998; **188**: 539–48.

163. Riviere C, Subra F, Cohen-Solal K et al. Phenotypic and functional evidence for the expression of CXCR4 receptor during megakaryocytopoiesis. *Blood* 1999; **93**: 1511–23.

164. Wang JF, Liu ZY, Groopman JE. The α-chemokine receptor CXCR4 is expressed on the megakaryocytic lineage from progenitor to platelets and modulates migration and adhesion. *Blood* 1998; **92**: 756–64.

165. Kowalska MA, Ratajczak J, Hoxie J Megakaryocyte precursors, megakaryocytes and platelets express the HIV co-receptor CXCR4 on their surface: determination of response to stromal-derived factor-1 by megakaryocytes and platelets. *Br J Haematol* 1999; **104**: 220–9.

166. Mathur A, Hong Y, Martin J, Erusalimsky J. Megakaryocytic differentiation is accompanied by a reduction in cell migratory potential. *Br J Haematol* 2001; **112**: 459–65.

167. Majka M, Janowska-Wieczorek A, Ratajczak J et al. Stromal-derived factor 1 and thrombopoietin regulate distinct aspects of human megakaryopoiesis. *Blood* 2000; **96**: 4142–51.

168. Hodohara K, Fujii N, Yamamoto N. Stromal cell-derived factor-1 (SDF-1) acts together with thrombopoietin to enhance the development of megakaryocytic progenitor cells (CFU-MK). *Blood* 2000; **95**: 769–75.

169. Lataillade JJ, Clay D, Dupuy C et al. Chemokine SDF-1 enhances circulating CD34+ cell proliferation in synergy with cytokines: possible role in progenitor survival. *Blood* 2000; **95**: 756–68.

170. Gordon MS, Hoffman R. Growth factors affecting human thrombocytopoiesis: potential agents for the treatment of thrombocytopenia. *Blood* 1992; **80**: 302–7.

171. Shimoda K, Okamura S, Harada N et al. Identification of a functional receptor for granulocyte colony-stimulating factor on platelets. *J Clin Invest* 1993; **91**: 1310–13.

172. Rennick D, Hunte B, Dang W et al. Interleukin-10 promotes the growth of megakaryocyte, mast cell, and multilineage colonies: analysis with committed progenitors and Thy^lo Sca^+ stem cells. *Exp Hematol* 1994; **22**: 136–41.

173. Sosman JA, Verma A, Moss S et al. Interleukin 10-induced thrombocytopenia in normal healthy adult volunteers: evidence for decreased platelet production. *Br J Haematol* 2000; **111**: 104–11.

174. Bruno E, Cooper RJ, Wilson EL et al. Basic fibroblast growth factor promotes the proliferation of human megakaryocyte progenitor cells. *Blood* 1993; **82**: 430–5.

175. Han ZC, Bellucci S, Wan HY, Caen JP. New insights into the regulation of megakaryocytopoiesis by haematopoietic and fibroblastic growth factors and transforming growth factor-β1. *Br J Haematol* 1992; **81**: 1–5.

176. Bikfavi A, Han ZC, Fuhrmann G. Interaction of fibroblast growth factor (FGF) with megakaryocytopoiesis and demonstration of FGF receptor expression in megakaryocytes and megakaryocyte-like cells. *Blood* 1992; **80**: 1905–13.

177. Avraham H, Banu N, Scadden DT et al. Modulation of megakaryocytopoiesis by human basic fibroblast growth factor. *Blood* 1994; **83**: 2126–32.

178. Su RJ, Li K, Yang M et al. Platelet-derived growth factor enhances ex vivo expansion of megakaryocytic progenitors from human cord blood. *Bone Marrow Transplant* 2001; **27**: 1075–80.

179. Kaminski WE, Lindahl P, Lin NL et al. Basis of hematopoietic defects in platelet-derived growth factor (PDGF)-β and PDGFβ-receptor null mice. *Blood* 2001; **97**: 1990–8.

180. Bertolini F, Battaglia M, Pedrazzoli P et al. Megakaryocytic progenitors can be generated ex vivo and safely administered to autologous peripheral blood progenitor cell transplant recipients. *Blood* 1997; **89**: 2679–88.

181. Vainchenker W, Chapman J, Deschamps JF et al. Normal human serum contains a factor(s) capable of inhibiting megakaryocyte colony formation. *Exp Hematol* 1982; **10**: 650–60.

182. Mitjavila MT, Vinci G, Villeval JL et al. Human platelet α granules contain a non specific inhibitor of megakaryocyte colony formation: its relationship to type β transforming growth factor (TGF-β). *J Cell Physiol* 1988; **134**: 93–100.

183. Ishibashi T, Miller SL, Burstein SA. Type β transforming growth factor is a potent inhibitor of murine megakaryocytopoiesis in vitro. *Blood* 1987; **69**: 1737–41.

184. Kuter DJ, Gminski DM, Rosenberg RD. Transforming growth factor β inhibits megakaryocyte growth and endomitosis. *Blood* 1992; **79**: 619–26.

185. Fortunel NO, Hatzfeld A, Hatzfeld JA. Transforming growth factor β: pleiotropic role in the regulation of hematopoiesis. *Blood* 2000; **96**: 2022–36.

186. Sakamaki S, Hirayama Y, Matsunaga T et al. Transforming growth factor-β1 (TGF-β1) induces thrombopoietin from bone marrow stromal cells, which stimulates the expression of TGF-β receptor on megakaryocytes and, in turn, renders them susceptible to suppression by TGF-β itself with high specificity. *Blood* 1999; **94**: 1961–70.

187. Carlino JA, Higley HR, Creson JR et al. Transforming growth factor β1 systemically modulates granuloid, erythroid, lymphoid, and thrombocytic cells in mice. *Exp Hematol* 1992; **20**: 943–50.

188. Gewirtz AM, Zhang J, Ratajczack M et al. Chemokine regulation of human megakaryocytopoiesis. *Blood* 1995; **86**: 2559–67.

189. Han ZC, Sensebe L, Abgrall JF, Briere J. Platelet factor 4 inhibits human megakacaryocytopoiesis in vitro. *Blood* 1990; **75**: 1234–9.

190. Han ZC, Bellucci S, Bodevin E et al. In vivo inhibition of megakaryocyte and platelet production by platelet factor 4 in mice. *C R Acad Sci III* 1991; **313**: 553–8.

191. Han ZC, Lu M, Li J et al. Platelet factor 4 and other CXC chemokines support the survival of normal hematopoietic cells and reduce the chemosensitivity of cells to cytotoxic agents. *Blood* 1997; **89**: 2328–35.

192. Ganser A, Carlo-Stella C, Greher J et al. Effects of recombinant interferon α and γ on human bone marrow-derived megakaryocytic progenitor cells. *Blood* 1987; **70**: 1173–8.

193. Muraoka K, Tsuji K, Yoshida M et al. Thrombopoietin-independent effect of interferon-γ on the proliferation of human megakaryocyte progenitors. *Br J Haematol* 1997; **98**: 265–73.

194. Wang Q, Miyakawa Y, Fox N, Kaushansky K. Interferon-α directly represses megakaryopoiesis by inhibiting thrombopoietin-induced signaling through induction of SOCS-1. *Blood* 2000; **96**: 2093–9.

195. Ihara K, Ishi E, Eguchi M et al. Identification of mutations in the c-*mpl* gene in congenital amegakaryocytic thrombocytopenia. *Proc Natl Acad Sci USA* 1999; **96**: 3132–6.

196. Ballmaier M, Germeshausen M, Schulze H et al. c-*mpl* mutations are the cause of congenital amegakaryocytic thrombocytopenia. *Blood* 2001; **97**: 139–46.

197. Ballmaier M, Schultze H, Strauss G et al. Thrombopoietin in patients with congenital thrombocytopenia and absent radii: Elevated serum levels, normal receptor expression, but defective reactivity to thrombopoietin. *Blood* 1997; **90**: 612–19.

198. Letestu R, Vitrat N, Massé A et al. Existence of a differentiation blockage at the stage of a megakaryocyte precursor in the thrombocytopenia and absent radii (TAR) syndrome. *Blood* 2000; **95**: 1633–41.

199. Kiladjian JJ, El-Kassar N, Hetet G et al. Study of the thrombopoietin receptor in essential thrombocythemia. *Leukemia* 1997; **11**: 1821–6.

200. Taksin A-L, Le Couedic J-P, Massé A et al. Autonomous megakaryocyte growth in essential thrombocythemia and idiopathic myelofibrosis is not related to a c-*mpl* mutation or to an autocrine stimulation by Mpl-L. *Blood* 1999; **93**: 125–39.

201. Li J, Xia Y, Kuter DJ. Analysis of the thrombopoietin receptor (Mpl) on platelets from normal and essential thrombocythemic (ET) patients. *Blood* 1996; **88**: 545–51.

202. Horikawa Y, Matsumura I, Hashimoto K et al. Markedly reduced expression of platelet c-mpl receptor in essential thrombocythemia. *Blood* 1997; **90**: 4031–8.

203. Moliterno AR, Hankins WD, Spivak JL. Impaired expression of the thrombopoietin receptor by platelets from patients with polycythemia vera. *N Engl J Med* 1998; **338**: 572–80.

204. Bouscary D, Fontenay-Roupie M, Chretien S et al. Thrombopoietin is not responsible for the thrombocytosis observed in patients with acute myeloid leukemias and the 3q21q26 syndrome. *Br J Haematol* 1995; **91**: 425–7.

205. Schnittger S, de Sauvage FJ, Le Paslier D, Fonatsch C. Refined chromosomal localization of the human thrombopoietin gene to 3q27–q28 and exclusion as the responsible gene for thrombocytosis in patients with rearrangements of 3q21 and 3q26. *Leukemia* 1996; **10**: 1891–6.

206. Wiestner A, Schlemper RJ, van der Maas APC, Skoda RC. An activating splice donor mutation in the thrombopoietin gene causes hereditary thrombocythaemia. *Nat Genet* 1998; **18**: 49–52.

207. Ghilardi N, Wiestner A, Kikuchi M et al. Hereditary thrombocythaemia in a japanese family is caused by a novel point mutation in the thrombopoietin gene. *Br J Haematol* 1999; **107**: 310–16.

208. Ochs H. The Wiskott–Aldrich syndrome. *Springer Semin Immunopathol* 1998; **19**: 435–58.

209. Zhu G, Zhang M, Blaese RM et al. The Wiskott–Aldrich syndrome and X-linked congenital thrombocytopenia are caused by mutations of the same gene. *Blood* 1995; **86**: 3797–804.

210. Nichols KE, Crispino JD, Poncz M et al. Familial dyserythropoietic anaemia and thrombocytopenia due to an inherited mutation in *GATA1*. *Nat Genet* 2000; **24**: 266–70.

211. Penny LA, Dell'Aquila M, Jones MC et al. Clinical and molecular characterization of patients with distal 11q deletions. *Am J Hum Genet* 1995; **56**: 676–83.

212. Breton-Gorius J, Favier R, Guichard J et al. A new congenital dysmegakaryopoietic thrombocytopenia (Paris-trousseau) associated with giant platelet α-granules and chromosome 11 deletion at 11q23. *Blood* 1995; **85**: 1805–14.

213. Song WJ, Sullivan MG, Legare RD et al. Haploinsufficiency of *CBFA2* causes familial thrombocytopenia with propensity to develop acute myelogenous leukaemia. *Nat Genet* 1999; **23**: 166–75.

214. Cai Z, de Bruijn M, Ma X et al. Haploinsufficiency of *AML1* affects the temporal and spatial generation of hematopoietic stem cells in the mouse embryo. *Immunity* 2000; **13**: 423–31.

215. Thompson AA, Nguyen LT. Amegakaryocytic thrombocytopenia and radio–ulnar synostosis are associated with *HOXA11* mutation. *Nat Genet* 2000; **26**: 397–8.

216. Ma Z, Morris SW, Valentine V et al. Fusion of two novel genes, *RBM15* and *MKL1*, in the t(1;22)(p13;q13) of acute megakaryoblastic leukemia. *Nat Genet* 2001; **28**: 220–1.

217. Mercher T, Coniat MB, Monni R et al. Involvement of a human gene related to the *Drosophila spen* gene in the recurrent t(1;22) translocation of acute megakaryocytic leukemia. *Proc Natl Acad Sci USA* 2001; **98**: 5776–9.

218. Chen F, Rebay I. Split ends, a new component of the *Drosophila* EGF receptor pathway, regulates development of midline glial cells. *Curr Biol* 2000; **10**: 943–6.

219. Rebay I, Chen F, Hsiao F et al. A genetic screen for novel components of the Ras/mitogen-activated protein kinase signaling pathway that interact with the *yan* gene of *Drosophila* identifies split ends, a new RNA recognition motif-containing protein. *Genetics* 2000; **154**: 695–712.

220. Kelley MJ, Jawien W, Ortel TL, Korczak JF. Mutation of *MYH9*, encoding non-muscle myosin heavy chain A, in May–Hegglin anomaly. *Nat Genet* 2000; **26**: 106–8.

221. The May-Hegglin/Fechtner syndrome consortium. Mutations in *MYH9* results in the May–Hegglin anomaly, and Fechtner and Sebastian syndromes. *Nat Genet* 2000; **26**: 106–8.

222. Kunishima S, Kojima T, Matsushita T et al. Mutations in the *NMMHC-A* gene cause autosomal dominant macrothrombocytopenia with leukocyte inclusions (May–Hegglin anomaly/Sebastian syndrome). *Blood* 2001; **97**: 1147–9.

223. Ware J, Russell S, Ruggeri ZM. Generation and rescue of a murine model of platelet dysfunction: the Bernard–Soulier syndrome. *Proc Natl Acad Sci USA* 2000; **97**: 2803–8.

224. Savoia A, Balduini CL, Savino M et al. Autosomal dominant macrothrombocytopenia in Italy is most frequently a type of heterozygous Bernard–Soulier syndrome. *Blood* 2001; **97**: 1330–5.

225. Symons M, Derry J, Karlak B et al. Wiskott–Aldrich syndrome protein, a novel effector for the GTPase CDC42Hs, is implicated in actin polymerization. *Cell* 1996; **84**: 723–34.

226. Haddad E, Cramer E, Rivière C et al. The thrombocytopenia of Wiskott–Aldrich syndrome is not related to a defect in proplatelet formation. *Blood* 1999; **94**: 509–18.

227. Kaushansky K, Lok S, Holly RD et al. Promotion of megakaryocyte progenitor expansion and differentiation by the c-Mpl ligand, thrombopoietin. *Nature* 1994; **369**: 568–71.

228. Harker LA, Hunt P, Marzec UM et al. Regulation of platelet production and function by megakaryocyte growth and development factor in nonhuman primates. *Blood* 1996; **87**: 1833–44.

229. Kaushansky K, Broudy VC, Grossmann A et al. Thrombopoietin expands erythroid progenitors, increases red cell production, and enhances erythroid recovery after myelosuppressive therapy. *J Clin Invest* 1995; **96**: 1683–7.

230. Grossmann A, Lenox J, Ren HP et al. Thrombopoietin accelerates platelet, red blood cell and neutrophil recovery in myelosuppressed mice. *Exp Hemat* 1996; **24**: 1238–46.

231. Farese A, Hunt P, Boone T, MacVittie T. Combined administration of recombinant human megakaryocyte growth and develpment factor and granulocyte-colony stimulating factor enhances multilineage hematopoietic reconstitution in nonhuman primates after radiation-induced marrow aplasia. *J Clin Invest* 1998; **97**: 2145–51.

232. Shibuya K, Akahori H, Takahashi K et al. Multilineage hematopoietic recovery by a single injection of pegylated recombinant human megakaryocyte growth and development factor in myelosuppressed mice. *Blood* 1998; **91**: 37–45.

233. Farese AM, Hunt P, Grab LB, MacVittie TJ. Combined administration of recombinant human megakaryocyte growth and development factor and granulocyte colony-stimulating factor enhances multilineage hematopoietic reconstitution in nonhuman primates after radiation-induced marrow aplasia. *J Clin Invest* 1996; **97**: 2145–51.

234. Neelis KJ, Dubbelman YD, Qingliang L et al. Simultaneous administration of TPO and G-CSF after cytoreductive treatment of rhesus monkeys prevents thrombocytopenia, accelerates platelet and red cell reconstitution, alleviates neutropenia, and promotes the recovery of immature bone marrow cells. *Exp Hematol* 1997; **25**: 1084–93.

235. Harker LA, Marzec UM, Kelly AB et al. Prevention of thrombocytopenia and neutropenia in a nonhuman primate model of marrow suppressive chemotherapy by combining pegylated recombinant human megakaryocyte growth and development factor and recombinant human granulocyte colony-stimulating factor. *Blood* 1997; **89**: 155–65.

236. Molineux G, Hartley C, McElroy P et al. Megakaryocyte growth and development factor accelerates platelet recovery in peripheral blood progenitor cell transplant recipients. *Blood* 1996; **88**: 366–76.

237. Neelis KJ, Dubbelman YD, Wognum AW et al. Lack of efficacy of thrombopoietin and granulocyte colony-stimulating factor after high dose total-body irradiation and autologous stem cell or bone marrow transplantation in rhesus monkeys. *Exp Hematol* 1997; **25**: 1094–103.

238. Fibbe WE, Heemskerk DPM, Laterveer L et al. Accelerated reconstitution of platelets and erythrocytes after syngeneic transplantation of bone marrow cells derived from thrombopoietin pretreated donor mice. *Blood* 1995; **86**: 3308–13.

239. Basser RL, Rasko JEJ, Clarke K et al. Thrombopoietic

effects of pegylated recombinant human megakaryocyte growth and development factor (PEG-rHuMGDF) in patients with advanced cancer. *Lancet* 1996; **348**: 1279–81.

240. Vadjan-Raj S, Murray LJ, Bueso-Ramos C et al. Stimulation of megakaryocyte and platelet production by a single dose of recombinant human thrombopoietin in patients with cancer. *Ann Intern Med* 1997; **126**: 673–81.

241. Fanucchi MG, Glapsy J, Crawford J et al. Effects of polyethylene glycol-conjugated recombinant human megakaryocyte growth and development factor on platelet counts after chemotherapy for lung cancer. *N Engl J Med* 1997; **336**: 404–9.

242. Basser RL, Rasko JE, Clarke K et al. Randomized, blinded, placebo-controlled phase I trial of pegylated recombinant human megakaryocyte growth and development factor with filgrastim after dose-intensive chemotherapy in patients with advanced cancer. *Blood* 1997; **89**: 3118–28.

243. Harker L, Roskos L, Marzec U et al. Effects of megakaryocyte growth and development factor on platelet production, platelet life span, and platelet function in healthy human volunteers. *Blood* 2000; **95**: 2514–22.

# 12 DNA repair and malignant hematopoiesis

Lieneke R van Veelen, Roland Kanaar, and DC van Gent

## Introduction

Proper maintenance of the genome is crucial for the survival of all organisms. It is of major importance for the functioning of the cell that the information encrypted in the genome be transcribed correctly. However, endogenous and exogenous DNA-damaging agents constantly threaten the integrity of the genome. When a cell detects genome injury, it can arrest the cell cycle at specific checkpoints. The activation of cell cycle checkpoints provides time to repair the DNA lesions before they can be converted into permanent mutations. When DNA damage cannot be repaired, the cell is triggered to go into apoptosis or replicative death (Figure 12.1). Incorrect repair or accumulation of DNA damage results in genome instability, which may lead to impaired functioning of the cell and even to the development of cancer. Therefore, all organisms are equipped with a complex network of DNA repair mechanisms, each of which is able to repair a subset of lesions. The biological significance of DNA repair mechanisms is underlined by the fact that many repair genes are conserved from yeast to humans, which are separated by more than 1.2 billion years of evolution. The importance of the DNA repair pathways is also emphasized by the fact

that defects in DNA repair genes often lead to cancer predisposition in humans.

## DNA repair mechanisms

Different DNA-damaging agents cause a wide variety of lesions in the DNA strands. Depending on the type of injury, a specific DNA repair mechanism will remove the damage (Figure 12.2). Irrespective of the mechanism that is used to repair the lesion, there is a similar succession of events that needs to take place in order to repair the damage. The first step is to recognize the DNA lesion. Subsequently, the lesion is processed, which will eventually lead to its removal. The processing of lesions frequently involves the incision of DNA strands and the removal of the damaged sites, including the surrounding nucleotides. Consequently, the final steps in DNA damage repair are re-incorporation of the missing nucleotides and coupling of the DNA ends by a DNA ligase. Depending on the pathway used to repair the lesion and the stage of the repair reaction, different sets of proteins are required.

There are several pathways available that the cell can use to repair the damage. DNA damage can be

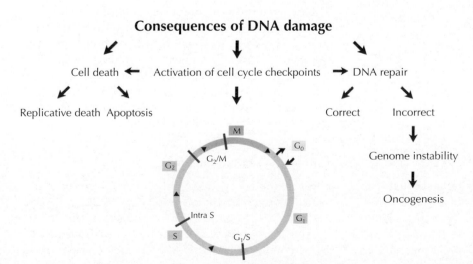

Figure 12.1 Cellular consequences of damage to DNA. DNA damage triggers activation of cell cycle checkpoints. This can lead to cell cycle arrest at $G_1/S$, intra-S, or $G_2/M$ phases. During cell cycle arrest, DNA damage can be repaired. Incorrect repair of DNA may lead to genome instability and oncogenesis. An alternative to repair of DNA damage is the induction of apoptosis or replicative death.

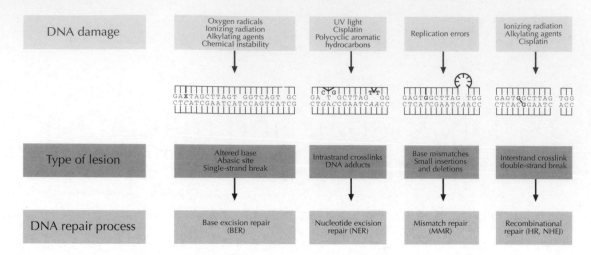

**Figure 12.2** Overview of different DNA repair pathways in mammalian cells. Various types of lesions in DNA can be caused by exogenous or endogenous DNA-damaging agents. They may affect a single strand or both strands of the DNA. Different DNA repair pathways that operate on the various lesions are indicated here.

categorized into two classes: one in which only one of the two strands of the DNA is damaged and a second class of lesions that affects both strands of the DNA. If only one strand is damaged, the DNA repair machinery uses the complementary DNA strand as a template for repair. Examples of this type of repair are base excision repair (BER), nucleotide excision repair (NER), and mismatch repair (MMR) (Figure 12.2).[1,2] Repair of a DNA double-strand break (DSB) cannot be accomplished by using the complementary strand as a template, since both strands are broken at the same site. In this case, the cell can utilize the recombinational repair pathways of non-homologous end-joining (NHEJ) or homologous recombination (HR) (Figure 12.2).[3–5]

An interesting aspect of the hematopoietic system is its unique position in DNA repair: precursor B and T cells are capable of introducing programmed DNA damage in the form of site-specific DSB. Correct repair of these DSB results in functional immunoglobulin and T-cell receptor genes. Occasionally these programmed DSB can be repaired incorrectly, leading to undesirable genomic rearrangements, which might activate oncogenes responsible for the development of leukemia or lymphoma. For this reason, the mechanisms of DSB repair are discussed more extensively in this chapter.

## DNA double-strand break repair

DSB, as well as the less genotoxic single-strand breaks (SSB), can be caused by ionizing radiation, free radicals, and chemicals such as alkylating agents. Furthermore, DSB may arise during replication of a region containing an SSB. Several repair mechanisms

can deal with DSB, emphasizing the importance of repairing this type of DNA damage.

The two major DSB repair pathways are HR and NHEJ. The difference between these two pathways is the use of a homologous sequence. HR uses the sister chromatid or homologous chromosome as a template for repair, whereas NHEJ simply joins the broken ends without the use of a template (Figure 12.3). This difference in repair mechanism leads to a difference in the fidelity of repair. HR restores the original DNA sequence and is therefore a precise type of repair. NHEJ, on the other hand, often leads to addition or deletion of nucleotides at the joining site. In this way, important information may be lost, thus making NHEJ an error-prone repair pathway.

The relative contribution of these pathways to DSB repair likely depends on the cell cycle stage. In $G_1$ phase, when the sister chromatid is absent, a DSB is most likely to be repaired through NHEJ.[6,7] HR is most efficient in S and $G_2$ phases of the cell cycle, when the sister chromatid is available as a template.[8] However, NHEJ may also occur in S and $G_2$ phases.[9,10] The detection, processing, and ligation of the break are organized by a large number of proteins, which are specific for each pathway, although some proteins may be involved in both HR and NHEJ (Figure 12.3). The exact function of many repair proteins involved in these pathways is still unknown.

### Homologous recombination

HR is mediated by the so-called RAD52 group of proteins, which includes RAD50, RAD51, RAD52, RAD54, MRE11, and NBS1.[4,5,11] Recognition of the broken DNA ends may occur by the RAD50/MRE11/NBS1 complex or by RAD52.[12,13] Nucleolytic process-

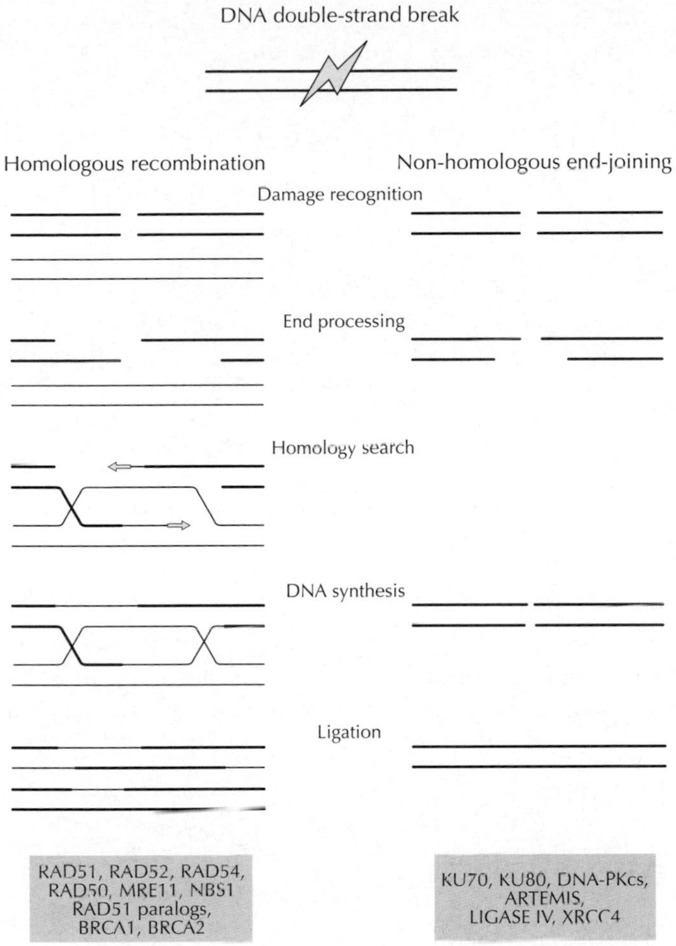

**Figure 12.3** Major repair pathways of DNA double-strand break repair. DNA DSB can be repaired by at least two mechanistically distinct pathways: homologous recombination (HR) and non-homologous end-joining (NHEJ). This figure shows a simplification of the models for DSB repair. During HR, the damaged DNA (thick lines) uses the sister chromatid or homologous chromosome (thin lines) as a template to repair the DNA accurately. NHEJ repairs the damaged DNA by joining the DNA ends in a way that is not necessarily error-free. The succession of events that take place during repair of the damage is presented. A number of proteins involved in each pathway are indicated and discussed in the text.

ing of the broken ends leads to the formation of single-stranded tails (Figure 12.3). RAD51 proteins form a nucleoprotein filament on this single-stranded tail. The RAD51 nucleoprotein filament searches for the homologous piece of DNA.[14] Once the homology has been detected, a joint molecule is generated between the damaged DNA and the undamaged sister chromatid. Several proteins assist RAD51 in this complex reaction, including the breast cancer susceptibility proteins BRCA1 and BRCA2, five RAD51 paralogs, RAD52, and RAD54.[4,15–19] The information that was lost during processing of the DNA ends is restored by DNA polymerases that synthesize new DNA using the undamaged sister chromatid as a template. Finally, the DNA strands are ligated, resulting in accurate repair of the DSB. A putative link between reduced HR efficiency and cancer predisposition is provided by the observation that many carriers of mutations in either BRCA1 or BRCA2 develop breast or ovarian cancer.[20]

### Non-homologous end-joining

Several proteins that are involved in NHEJ have been identified (Figure 12.3). The KU70/KU80 protein complex forms a ring around the DNA ends.[21] End-bound KU70/KU80 activates the DNA-dependent protein kinase catalytic subunit (DNA-PKcs). Together they form a protein complex known as DNA-PK, which is involved in the early recognition of the DSB.[22] Consequently, the DNA can be processed by nucleases or polymerases. Nucleases, such as the ARTEMIS protein, remove nucleotides from the DNA ends.[23] DNA polymerases synthesize new DNA, in order to prepare the DNA ends for ligation. Finally, both ends are joined by the LIGASE IV/XRCC4 complex.[24]

Two groups of patients with defects in NHEJ have been identified. A small subset of patients with severe combined immunodeficiency (SCID) have a mutation in the ARTEMIS gene.[25] Furthermore, patients have been described in which a mutation on one allele of the LIGASE IV gene is detected.[26] The phenotype of these patients is heterogeneous, although most of them suffer from immunodeficiency. It is not clear whether patients with a defect in either ARTEMIS or LIGASE IV display cancer predisposition.

## DNA rearrangements in the immune system

### V(D)J recombination

Not only is the NHEJ repair pathway used to repair DSB that are induced by exogenous factors, but it is also involved in processing the programmed DSB that arise during the generation of immunoglobulin (*Ig*) and T-cell receptor (*TCR*) genes. These programmed DSB are natural intermediates in a specialized recombination event called *V(D)J* recombination.[27] This recombination reaction is required for the creation of functional B and T cells.

Mature *Ig* and *TCR* genes are assembled from separate gene segments in B and T cells, respectively. The lymphoid-specific proteins RAG1 and RAG2 initiate this DNA recombination process. They bind to recombination signal sequences (Figure 12.4a) that flank the variable (*V*), diversity (*D*) and joining (*J*) segments of the *Ig* and *TCR* genes (Figure 12.4b).[27] Subsequently, a DSB is made at the border of the recombination signal sequence and the coding gene segment. The products of this cleavage reaction are blunt DNA ends at the side of the recombination signal sequence. The coding gene segment ends in a hairpin structure, in which the top strand is coupled to the bottom strand. The DNA ends are recombined such that the two coding gene segments form the coding joint, from which the *Ig* or *TCR* genes arise, while the signal sequences are

ligated in the signal joint, which is not used any further (Figure 12.4a). For this joining process, the NHEJ machinery of the cell is used.

*V(D)J* recombination is a highly regulated process. In B-cell development, the *Ig* heavy-chain locus is recombined first. If this yields a functional heavy-chain polypeptide, the cell will start a proliferation phase, after which the *Ig* light-chain loci (κ or λ) are rearranged. These cells enter the circulation as virgin B cells, provided that they produce functional immunoglobulins that are not autoreactive. A similar order of events leads to the formation of virgin T cells.[28] A deficiency in one of the RAG proteins or in one of the components of the NHEJ process severely impairs the capacity to perform *V(D)J* recombination, which results in low levels of mature B and T cells.[29]

### Immunoglobulin class switching

A later step in B-cell development is immunoglobulin heavy-chain class switching. This leads to expression of a different class of antibodies, which are also initiated by programmed DSB formation.[30,31] Most

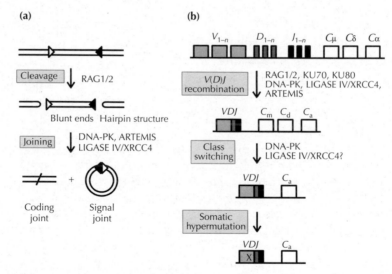

**Figure 12.4** DNA rearrangements in the immune system. (a) The mechanisms of *V(D)J* recombination. DSB are made by the RAG1 and RAG2 proteins at the border of the recombination signal sequences (triangles) that surround the *V*, *D*, and *J* segments of the immunoglobulin (*Ig*) and T-cell receptor (*TCR*) genes. Recombination signal sequences contain motifs separated by a spacer of 12 or 23 base pairs of non-conserved sequence. Recombination always takes place between one signal sequence with a 12 bp spacer and one with a 23 bp spacer (open and closed triangles). The DSB are made in such a way that the ends form a hairpin structure in which the top strand is coupled to the bottom strand. The joining reaction is accomplished by the NHEJ machinery, which involves end recognition by the KU/DNA-PK complex and ligation by the LIGASE IV/XRCC4 complex. The DNA hairpin intermediates are probably opened and processed by the ARTEMIS protein. The coding joint gives rise to the functional *Ig* or *TCR* genes. The signal joint is irrelevant for the further process. (b) Overview of the different types of DNA rearrangements in the immune system. In pre-B cells, the immunoglobulin loci undergo *V(D)J* recombination. As an example, the *IgH* locus is shown. First, one of the *D* segments is coupled to one of the *J* segments, followed by *V* to *DJ* joining. After successful assembly of functional *Ig* genes and stimulation by antigen, a second DNA rearrangement can delete a number of constant regions (indicated by *C* with different subscripts), resulting in expression of a different immunoglobulin isotype. This class switch recombination reaction requires at least the components of the DNA-PK complex, and possibly also the LIGASE IV/XRCC4 complex. Finally, the affinity of the antibodies for the antigen can be modulated by introduction of point mutations into the *VDJ* exon. The mechanism of this somatic hypermutation reaction is not yet clear, although DSB have been found at the site of hypermutation, suggesting that DSB repair mechanisms may be involved.

circulating B cells never encounter antigens that are recognized by the immunoglobulins on their surface. The few B cells that are stimulated by an antigen go into a regulated differentiation scheme. These stimulated B cells are able to change the type of immunoglobulin they produce using a DNA recombination process called immunoglobulin heavy-chain class switching (Figure 12.4b).[30,31] The mechanism of this recombination reaction is less well understood than the process of V(D)J recombination. However, it is clear that class switch recombination requires DNA-PK, which might indicate that DSB are intermediates in this process that may be repaired by the NHEJ proteins.[32-34] After the B cells have undergone the maturation program, they enter the circulation as plasma cells, which produce large amounts of secreted immunoglobulins that recognize the antigen for which they were selected. When the antigen has been removed from the system, some of these plasma cells can develop into memory cells, which survive for a very long time and react very quickly when the organism is invaded for a second time by the same antigen.

### Somatic hypermutation

Somatic hypermutation is another process in the immune system in which the DNA sequence is altered (Figure 12.4b). It changes the binding efficiency of immunoglobulins, by introducing point mutations in the DNA region containing the VDJ segment.[35,36] It has been demonstrated that DSB occur in hypermutating Ig genes, preferentially at mutational hotspots.[35,37] However, the exact function of these DSB is still poorly understood.

## Cell cycle checkpoints

DSB are particularly dangerous lesions when they occur during replication of the genome or during mitosis when the duplicated chromosomes are divided between the daughter cells. When broken chromosomes are carried through mitosis, the chromosome fragments will not distribute evenly between the two daughter cells, thus causing chromosomal aberrations.[38,39] Several checkpoints can stop the cell at different points in the cell cycle when DNA damage is present. The $G_1/S$ checkpoint prevents the cell from starting DNA replication, intra-S checkpoints slow down replication, and $G_2/M$ checkpoints arrest the cell before division.[7] Among the many proteins involved in DNA damage-induced cell cycle arrest are p53, ATM, and the protein complex MRE11/RAD50/NBS1. p53 plays a role in a number of different checkpoints. ATM and the MRE11/ RAD50/NBS1 complex are mainly involved in the intra-S checkpoint.[40,41]

Several human syndromes are associated with defects in these checkpoint genes. Mutations in *ATM* or *MRE11* cause syndromes called ataxia telangiectasia (AT) or AT-like disorder (ATLD), respectively.[42-44] A mutation in *NBS1* leads to the Nijmegen breakage syndrome.[45] These syndromes have a number of overlapping features, such as growth retardation, neurological problems, increased sensitivity to ionizing radiation, and a predisposition to cancer (mainly lymphoma). A heterozygous mutation in *p53* can cause the Li–Fraumeni syndrome, a disorder that is characterized by a high tumor incidence, especially breast cancer, sarcomas, brain tumors, and, to a lesser extent, hematological and adrenocortical neoplasms.[46] Additionally, the *p53* gene is frequently found to be mutated in tumors, which gives an indication of the tumorigenic effects of a defect in *p53*.

## Double-strand breaks and chromosomal aberrations

DSB repair plays a role in the prevention of chromosomal instability and potentially oncogenic translocations.[5,47] Paradoxically, some proteins required for proper DSB repair are likely to be involved in the creation of translocations as well. These translocations arise when a fusion occurs between parts of different chromosomes. A DSB is most probably the initiating DNA lesion that can result in translocations as a consequence of misrepair (Figure 12.5). Since proteins involved in DSB repair are essential for the ligation of DNA ends, this must mean that the generation of translocations requires their activity. Translocations are a characteristic feature of many tumors and have become important markers in diagnosis and prognosis. However, little is known about the relationship between oncogenesis and DSB repair defects in humans.[48] Studies involving mouse models and cell lines with mutations in DNA repair genes have highlighted the relationship between defects in DSB repair pathways and the formation of translocations and oncogenesis (Table 12.1).[49]

### Homologous recombination and chromosomal aberrations

HR uses the sister chromatid or the homologous chromosome as a template for repair of the broken ends. Probably because of its proximity, the sister chromatid is commonly used as the repair template. The preference of the sister chromatid over the homologous chromosome is biologically relevant, since recombination between homologous chromosomes can lead to loss of heterozygosity (LOH).[50] Defects in HR, such as errors in template choice, could even be more harmful when recombination occurs between repetitive sequences, which are present throughout

**Table 12.1  Consequences of homozygous mutations in cell cycle checkpoint genes and genes involved in DSB repair**

| | Genome instability | Mouse knockout: cancer predisposition | Mouse knockout combined with *p53* knockout: cancer predisposition | Refs |
|---|---|---|---|---|
| **Cell cycle checkpoint genes** | | | | |
| *ATM* | Chromosomal aberrations | T-cell lymphomas | Early-onset B- and T-cell lymphomas | 67,68 |
| *p53* | Chromosomal aberrations | T- and B-cell lymphomas | Not applicable | 69–71 |
| **Non-homologous end-joining** | | | | |
| *DNA-PKcs* | Chromosomal aberrations | No overt cancer predisposition | Early-onset pro-B-cell lymphoma | 57,72–74 |
| *Ku70* | Chromosomal aberrations | T-cell lymphomas | ND | 58,59,75,76 |
| *Ku80* | Chromosomal aberrations | No cancer predisposition | Early onset pro-B-cell lymphoma | 77–79 |
| *Artemis* | ND | ND | ND | 25 |
| *XRCC4* | Chromosomal aberrations | Embryonic lethal | Rescues embryonic lethality; early-onset pro-B-cell lymphoma | 60,64 |
| *Ligase IV* | Chromosomal aberrations | Embryonic lethal | Rescues embryonic lethality; early-onset pro-B-cell lymphoma | 49,61,66 |
| **Homologous recombination** | | | | |
| *Rad51* | Chromosomal aberrations | Embryonic lethal | Embryonic lethal | 54,80,81 |
| *Rad52* | ND | No cancer predisposition | ND | 82 |
| *Rad54* | No instability | No cancer predisposition | ND | 83,84 |
| *Brca2* | Chromosomal aberrations | Embryonic lethal | Embryonic lethal | 85,86 |
| **Miscellaneous** | | | | |
| *Brca1* | Chromosomal aberrations | Embryonic lethal | Embryonic lethal | 16,85 |
| *Rad50* | Not viable | Embryonic lethal | ND | 87 |
| *Mre11* | Chromosomal aberrations | Embryonic lethal | ND | 88 |
| *NBS1* | Translocations | Embryonic lethal | ND | 89 |
| **V(D)J recombination genes** | | | | |
| *Rag1* | Translocations | Unknown; mice die at early age | Early-onset T-cell lymphomas | 70,90,91 |
| *Rag2* | Translocations | Unknown; mice die at early age | Early-onset T-cell lymphomas | 70,90,91 |

The influence of a homozygous mutation (knockout mutation) of either of these genes on genomic instability in cells and cancer predisposition in mice is indicated. An additional homozygous mutation of *p53* rescues viability in several embryonic lethal mice and influences the spectrum and time of onset of tumors in these mice. The four rows headed 'Miscellaneous' represent genes that may be involved in more than one of the pathways listed above. ND, not determined.

the genome (Figure. 12.5). This type of ectopic recombination may lead to chromosomal translocations.

The importance of HR is emphasized by the finding that inactivation of genes involved in HR often results in embryonic lethality. Therefore animal models have been designed in which the effect of mutations in specific tissues can be investigated. The role of BRCA1 in genomic instability was studied by creating mice in which the *Brca1* gene was specifically inactivated in epithelial cells.[51] In the mammary tumors that developed, translocations were frequently observed. Additional inactivation of the *p53*

gene accelerated the formation of mammary tumors in these mice. The same results were seen in mice that carry a specific mutation in the *Brca2* gene.[52] *Brca2*-mutant mice have an increased sensitivity to ionizing radiation, growth retardation, infertility, and frequent development of thymic lymphomas, and cells derived from these mice show spontaneous chromosomal aberrations.[53] Chromosomal instability was also observed in a chicken B-cell lymphoma cell line that was conditionally mutated for Rad51.[54] Results from these animal studies suggest a role for HR in the development of chromosomal translocations and oncogenesis.

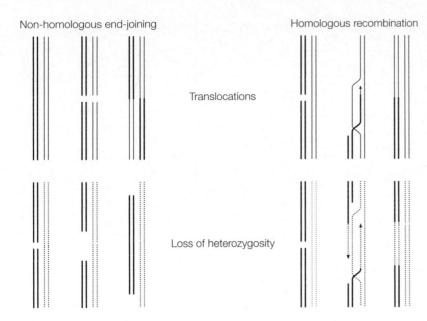

Non-homologous end-joining                          Homologous recombination

Translocations

Loss of heterozygosity

**Figure 12.5** Translocations and loss of heterozygosity during aberrant DSB repair. *Upper left*: Translocations by NHEJ can occur when two DSB on heterologous chromosomes are ligated. Unbroken heterologous chromosomes are depicted by two parallel thick and thin lines, respectively. They are shown to undergo breakage and misligation, resulting in a reciprocal translocation. *Upper right*: Translocations by HR can occur when a DSB is repaired using repetitive sequences located on a heterologous chromosome. *Bottom left*: Loss of heterozygosity (LOH) by NHEJ can occur when DNA sequences around a DSB are degraded before ligation. The sets of thick and dashed lines represent homologous chromosomes. *Bottom right*: LOH during HR can occur when the homologous chromosome instead of the sister chromatid is used for DSB repair.

## Non-homologous end-joining and chromosomal aberrations

The role of NHEJ in oncogenesis has been studied more extensively. Defects in NHEJ not only lead to genomic instability but also to impaired functioning of the V(D)J recombination process. Immunodeficiency is therefore a characteristic feature of humans and mice with defects in one of the NHEJ genes. Mice carrying mutations in NHEJ genes have been studied in more detail. The phenotypes of these mutant mice reveal similarities, such as increased radiation sensitivity and immunodeficiency, but striking differences have also been observed. Mice lacking *Ku70, Ku80*, or *DNA-PKcs* are viable, and *Ku70*-deficient and possibly *DNA-PKcs*-deficient mice develop T-cell lymphomas at late onset.[55–59] This is in contrast with *Xrcc4*- or *Ligase IV*-deficient mice, which die during embryogenesis due to neuronal apoptosis.[60–63] The lethality of the *Xrcc4*- and *Ligase IV*-mutant mice, together with the apoptosis and senescence phenotype of cells derived from the NHEJ-mutant mice, reveal that the NHEJ pathway is critical for the repair of spontaneously occurring DSB. Cells that are deficient in one of the NHEJ genes indeed show genomic instability, particularly spontaneous chromosome and chromatid breaks (Table 12.1).

The main evidence for a role of NHEJ in tumorigenesis is seen in experiments where mice that lack one of the NHEJ genes are crossed with *p53*-deficient mice. Interestingly, the lethality, but not the V(D)J recombination capability, of the *Xrcc4*- and *Ligase IV*-deficient mice is rescued by the absence of *p53*.[61,64]

However, these viable double-mutant mice develop pro-B-cell lymphomas at an early age. Pro-B-cell lymphomas are also observed in other double-mutant mice, which lack *p53* and one of the other NHEJ genes (Table 12.1). A possible explanation for this additional effect of the *p53* mutation can be found in the reduced level of apoptosis in *p53*-deficient mice. Damaged NHEJ-deficient cells, which would normally go into apoptosis, are not eliminated efficiently in this genetic background. The pro-B-cell lymphomas that occur in these mice have a characteristic t(12;15) translocation between the *IgH* locus and the c-*myc* locus.[65] The *IgH* locus is the first target of the RAG endonucleases in the development of B lymphocytes. Most likely, the initiating lesion of the pro-B-cell lymphomas is a RAG-induced DSB. This hypothesis is supported by the fact that triple-mutant *DNA-PK/p53/RAG2* mice do not develop pro-B-cell lymphomas.[65]

The development of mouse models has enabled a detailed analysis of genetic interactions between NHEJ deficiencies and mutations in other genome stability genes. Mice that are deficient for one of the NHEJ genes and heterozygous for *p53* are also prone to get solid tumors, mainly sarcomas. Although this broad spectrum of tumors can also be observed in the heterozygous *p53* mouse, the NHEJ deficiency accelerates this process, leading to development of the tumors at an earlier onset. Complementary to this, heterozygosity for *Ligase IV* also influences tumor development in mice carrying a homozygous deletion in a tumor suppressor gene. These knockout mice are predisposed to get lymphomas, but an additional heterozygous mutation in *Ligase IV* provokes the development of soft tissue sarcomas that possess chromosomal amplifications, deletions, and translocations.[66] This implies that a heterozygous mutation in an NHEJ gene by itself does not lead to an increased cancer risk. However, a combination of such a mutation and a defect in other genes involved in genome stability may accelerate cancer development, emphasizing the importance of the genetic background in oncogenesis. The genetic background on which a mutation in one of the repair genes occurs determines whether a tumor will develop and influences the time of onset. These findings are very important to understand the intricate genetic interactions that may influence the risk for cancer.

# Future perspectives

It is evident that DNA DSB repair proteins play an important role not only in the prevention, but also in the generation of genomic instability. The findings described in this chapter are just the beginning of a deeper understanding of the genetic interactions underlying oncogenic changes. The development of mouse models, which allows investigation of the effects of a combination of two or more mutations, will yield a wealth of information in the near future. In combination with genomics and proteomics, this will lead to a new view on the exact role of the genes involved in DNA repair and their involvement in the etiology of cancer.

## REFERENCES

1. Svejstrup JQ. Mechanisms of transcription-coupled DNA repair. *Nat Rev Mol Cell Biol* 2002; **3**: 21–9.
2. Aquilina G, Bignami M. Mismatch repair in correction of replication errors and processing of DNA damage. *J Cell Physiol* 2001; **187**: 145–54.
3. Karran P. DNA double strand break repair in mammalian cells. *Curr Opin Genet Dev* 2000; **10**: 144–50.
4. Kanaar R, Hoeijmakers JH, van Gent DC. Molecular mechanisms of DNA double strand break repair. *Trends Cell Biol* 1998; **8**: 483–9.
5. van Gent DC, Hoeijmakers JH, Kanaar R. Chromosomal stability and the DNA double-stranded break connection. *Nat Rev Genet* 2001; **2**: 196–206.
6. Dasika GK, Lin SC, Zhao S et al. DNA damage-induced cell cycle checkpoints and DNA strand break repair in development and tumorigenesis. *Oncogene* 1999; **18**: 7883–99.
7. Zhou BB, Elledge SJ. The DNA damage response: putting checkpoints in perspective. *Nature* 2000; **408**: 433–9.
8. Johnson RD, Jasin M. Sister chromatid gene conversion is a prominent double-strand break repair pathway in mammalian cells. *EMBO J* 2000; **19**: 3398–407.
9. Takata M, Sasaki MS, Sonoda E et al. Homologous recombination and non-homologous end-joining pathways of DNA double-strand break repair have overlapping roles in the maintenance of chromosomal integrity in vertebrate cells. *EMBO J* 1998; **17**: 5497–508.
10. Richardson C, Jasin M. Coupled homologous and nonhomologous repair of a double-strand break preserves genomic integrity in mammalian cells. *Mol Cell Biol* 2000; **20**: 9068–75.
11. Paques F, Haber JE. Multiple pathways of recombination induced by double-strand breaks in *Saccharomyces cerevisiae*. *Microbiol Mol Biol Rev* 1999; **63**: 349–404.
12. de Jager M, van Noort J, van Gent DC et al. Human Rad50/Mre11 is a flexible complex that can tether DNA ends. *Mol Cell* 2001; **8**: 1129–35.
13. Van Dyck E, Stasiak AZ, Stasiak A et al. Binding of double-strand breaks in DNA by human Rad52 protein. *Nature* 1999; **398**: 728–31.
14. Baumann P, West SC. Role of the human RAD51 protein in homologous recombination and double-stranded-break repair. *Trends Biochem Sci* 1998; **23**: 247–51.
15. Davies AA, Masson JY, McIlwraith MJ et al. Role of BRCA2 in control of the RAD51 recombination and DNA repair protein. *Mol Cell* 2001; **7**: 273–82.
16. Moynahan ME, Cui TY, Jasin M. Homology-directed DNA repair, mitomycin-C resistance, and chromosome stability is restored with correction of a Brca1 mutation. *Cancer Res* 2001; **61**: 4842–50.
17. Moynahan ME, Pierce AJ, Jasin M. BRCA2 is required for homology-directed repair of chromosomal breaks. *Mol Cell* 2001; **7**: 263–72.
18. Thompson LH, Schild D. Homologous recombinational repair of DNA ensures mammalian chromosome stability. *Mutat Res* 2001; **477**: 131–53.
19. Thacker J. A surfeit of *RAD51*-like genes? *Trends Genet* 1999; **15**: 166–8.
20. Venkitaraman AR. Cancer susceptibility and the functions of BRCA1 and BRCA2. *Cell* 2002; **108**: 171–82.
21. Walker JR, Corpina RA, Goldberg J. Structure of the Ku heterodimer bound to DNA and its implications for double-strand break repair. *Nature* 2001; **412**: 607–14.
22. Jones JM, Gellert M, Yang W. A Ku bridge over broken DNA. *Structure (Camb)* 2001; **9**: 881–4.
23. Ma Y, Pannicke U, Schwarz K et al. Hairpin opening and overhang processing by an artemis/DNA-dependent protein kinase complex in nonhomologous end joining and V(D)J recombination. *Cell* 2002; **108**: 781–94.
24. Lieber MR, Grawunder U, Wu X et al. Tying loose ends: roles of Ku and DNA-dependent protein kinase in the repair of double-strand breaks. *Curr Opin Genet Dev* 1997; **7**: 99–104.
25. Moshous D, Callebaut I, de Chasseval R et al. Artemis, a novel DNA double-strand break repair/V(D)J recombination protein, is mutated in human severe combined immune deficiency. *Cell* 2001; **105**: 177–86.
26. O'Driscoll M, Cerosaletti KM, Girard PM et al. DNA ligase IV mutations identified in patients exhibiting developmental delay and immunodeficiency. *Mol Cell* 2001; **8**: 1175–85.
27. Oettinger MA. V(D)J recombination: on the cutting edge. *Curr Opin Cell Biol* 1999; **11**: 325–9.
28. Schatz DG, Malissen B. Lymphocyte development. *Curr Opin Immunol* 2002; **14**: 183–5.
29. Gennery AR, Cant AJ, Jeggo PA. Immunodeficiency

associated with DNA repair defects. *Clin Exp Immunol* 2000; **121**: 1–7.

30. Chen X, Kinoshita K, Honjo T. Variable deletion and duplication at recombination junction ends: implication for staggered double-strand cleavage in class-switch recombination. *Proc Natl Acad Sci USA* 2001; **98**: 13860–5.

31. Zhang K. Immunoglobulin class switch recombination machinery: progress and challenges. *Clin Immunol* 2000; **95**: 1–8.

32. Rolink A, Melchers F, Andersson J. The *SCID* but not the *RAG-2* gene product is required for Sμ–Sε heavy chain class switching. *Immunity* 1996; **5**: 319–30.

33. Manis JP, van der Stoep N, Tian M et al. Class switching in B cells lacking 3′ immunoglobulin heavy chain enhancers. *J Exp Med* 1998; **188**: 1421–31.

34. Casellas R, Nussenzweig A, Wuerffel R et al. Ku80 is required for immunoglobulin isotype switching. *EMBO J* 1998; **17**: 2404–11.

35. Papavasiliou FN, Schatz DG. Cell-cycle-regulated DNA double-stranded breaks in somatic hypermutation of immunoglobulin genes. *Nature* 2000; **408**: 216–21.

36. Diaz M, Casali P. Somatic immunoglobulin hypermutation. *Curr Opin Immunol* 2002; **14**: 235–40.

37. Bross L, Fukita Y, McBlane F et al. DNA double-strand breaks in immunoglobulin genes undergoing somatic hypermutation. *Immunity* 2000; **13**: 589–97.

38. Myung K, Kolodner RD. Suppression of genome instability by redundant S-phase checkpoint pathways in *Saccharomyces cerevisiae*. *Proc Natl Acad Sci USA* 2002; **99**: 4500–7.

39. Caspari T, Carr AM. Checkpoints: how to flag up double-strand breaks. *Curr Biol* 2002; **12**: R105–7.

40. Falck J, Petrini JH, Williams BR et al. The DNA damage-dependent intra-S phase checkpoint is regulated by parallel pathways. *Nat Genet* 2002; **30**: 290–4.

41. Petrini JH. The Mre11 complex and ATM: collaborating to navigate S phase. *Curr Opin Cell Biol* 2000; **12**: 293–6.

42. Shiloh Y, Kastan MB. *ATM*: genome stability, neuronal development, and cancer cross paths. *Adv Cancer Res* 2001; **83**: 209–54.

43. Lavin MF, Khanna KK. ATM: the protein encoded by the gene mutated in the radiosensitive syndrome ataxia-telangiectasia. *Int J Radiat Biol* 1999; **75**: 1201–14.

44. Stewart GS, Maser RS, Stankovic T et al. The DNA double-strand break repair gene *hMRE11* is mutated in individuals with an ataxia-telangiectasia-like disorder. *Cell* 1999; **99**: 577–87.

45. Carney JP, Maser RS, Olivares H et al. The hMre11/hRad50 protein complex and Nijmegen breakage syndrome: linkage of double-strand break repair to the cellular DNA damage response. *Cell* 1998; **93**: 477–86.

46. Kleihues P, Schauble B, zur Hausen A et al. Tumors associated with *p53* germline mutations: a synopsis of 91 families. *Am J Pathol* 1997; **150**: 1–13.

47. Hoeijmakers JH. Genome maintenance mechanisms for preventing cancer. *Nature* 2001; **411**: 366–74.

48. Pierce AJ, Stark JM, Araujo FD et al. Double-strand breaks and tumorigenesis. *Trends Cell Biol* 2001; **11**: S52–9.

49. Ferguson DO, Alt FW. DNA double strand break repair and chromosomal translocation: lessons from animal models. *Oncogene* 2001; **20**: 5572–9.

50. Thiagalingam S, Foy RL, Cheng KH et al. Loss of heterozy-gosity as a predictor to map tumor suppressor genes in cancer: molecular basis of its occurrence. *Curr Opin Oncol* 2002; **14**: 65–72.

51. Xu X, Wagner KU, Larson D et al. Conditional mutation of *Brca1* in mammary epithelial cells results in blunted ductal morphogenesis and tumour formation. *Nat Genet* 1999; **22**: 37–43.

52. Jonkers J, Meuwissen R, van der Gulden H et al. Synergistic tumor suppressor activity of *BRCA2* and *p53* in a conditional mouse model for breast cancer. *Nat Genet* 2001; **29**: 418–25.

53. Friedman LS, Thistlethwaite FC, Patel KJ et al. Thymic lymphomas in mice with a truncating mutation in *Brca2*. *Cancer Res* 1998; **58**: 1338–43.

54. Sonoda E, Sasaki MS, Buerstedde JM et al. Rad51-deficient vertebrate cells accumulate chromosomal breaks prior to cell death. *EMBO J* 1998; **17**: 598–608.

55. Zhu C, Bogue MA, Lim DS et al. Ku86-deficient mice exhibit severe combined immunodeficiency and defective processing of V(D)J recombination intermediates. *Cell* 1996; **86**: 379–89.

56. Jhappan C, Morse HC 3rd, Fleischmann RD et al. DNA-PKcs: a T-cell tumour suppressor encoded at the mouse scid locus. *Nat Genet* 1997; **17**: 483–6.

57. Kurimasa A, Ouyang H, Dong LJ et al. Catalytic subunit of DNA-dependent protein kinase: impact on lymphocyte development and tumorigenesis. *Proc Natl Acad Sci USA* 1999; **96**: 1403–8.

58. Gu Y, Seidl KJ, Rathbun GA et al. Growth retardation and leaky SCID phenotype of Ku70-deficient mice. *Immunity* 1997; **7**: 653–65.

59. Li GC, Ouyang H, Li X et al. *Ku70*: a candidate tumor suppressor gene for murine T cell lymphoma. *Mol Cell* 1998; **2**: 1–8.

60. Gao Y, Sun Y, Frank KM et al. A critical role for DNA end-joining proteins in both lymphogenesis and neurogenesis. *Cell* 1998; **95**: 891–902.

61. Frank KM, Sharpless NE, Gao Y et al. DNA ligase IV deficiency in mice leads to defective neurogenesis and embryonic lethality via the p53 pathway. *Mol Cell* 2000; **5**: 993–1002.

62. Barnes DE, Stamp G, Rosewell I et al. Targeted disruption of the gene encoding DNA ligase IV leads to lethality in embryonic mice. *Curr Biol* 1998; **8**: 1395–8.

63. Gu Y, Sekiguchi J, Gao Y et al. Defective embryonic neurogenesis in Ku-deficient but not DNA-dependent protein kinase catalytic subunit-deficient mice. *Proc Natl Acad Sci USA* 2000; **97**: 2668–73.

64. Gao Y, Ferguson DO, Xie W et al. Interplay of p53 and DNA-repair protein XRCC4 in tumorigenesis, genomic stability and development. *Nature* 2000; **404**: 897–900.

65. Vanasse GJ, Halbrook J, Thomas S et al. Genetic pathway to recurrent chromosome translocations in murine lymphoma involves V(D)J recombinase. *J Clin Invest* 1999; **103**: 1669–75.

66. Sharpless NE, Ferguson DO, O'Hagan RC et al. Impaired nonhomologous end-joining provokes soft tissue sarcomas harboring chromosomal translocations, amplifications, and deletions. *Mol Cell* 2001; **8**: 1187–96.

67. Xu Y, Yang EM, Brugarolas J et al. Involvement of p53 and p21 in cellular defects and tumorigenesis in *Atm*−/− mice. *Mol Cell Biol* 1998; **18**: 4385–90.

68. Westphal CH, Rowan S, Schmaltz C et al. *atm* and *p53* cooperate in apoptosis and suppression of tumorigenesis,

but not in resistance to acute radiation toxicity. *Nat Genet* 1997; **16**: 397–401.

69. Bouffler SD, Kemp CJ, Balmain A et al. Spontaneous and ionizing radiation-induced chromosomal abnormalities in p53-deficient mice. *Cancer Res* 1995; **55**: 3883–9.

70. Nacht M, Jacks T. V(D)J recombination is not required for the development of lymphoma in p53-deficient mice. *Cell Growth Differ* 1998; **9**: 131–8.

71. Donehower LA, Harvey M, Vogel H et al. Effects of genetic background on tumorigenesis in p53-deficient mice. *Mol Carcinog* 1995; **14**: 16–22.

72. Taccioli GE, Amatucci AG, Beamish HJ et al. Targeted disruption of the catalytic subunit of the *DNA-PK* gene in mice confers severe combined immunodeficiency and radiosensitivity. *Immunity* 1998; **9**: 355–66.

73. Stackhouse MA, Bedford JS. An ionizing radiation-sensitive mutant of CHO cells: irs–20. III. Chromosome aberrations, DNA breaks and mitotic delay. *Int J Radiat Biol* 1994; **65**: 571–82.

74. Nacht M, Strasser A, Chan YR et al. Mutations in the *p53* and *SCID* genes cooperate in tumorigenesis. *Genes Dev* 1996; **10**: 2055–66.

75. Ferguson DO, Sekiguchi JM, Chang S et al. The nonhomologous end-joining pathway of DNA repair is required for genomic stability and the suppression of translocations. *Proc Natl Acad Sci USA* 2000; **97**: 6630–3.

76. Gu Y, Jin S, Gao Y et al. Ku70-deficient embryonic stem cells have increased ionizing radiosensitivity, defective DNA end-binding activity, and inability to support V(D)J recombination. *Proc Natl Acad Sci USA* 1997; **94**: 8076–81.

77. Difilippantonio MJ, Zhu J, Chen HT et al. DNA repair protein Ku80 suppresses chromosomal aberrations and malignant transformation. *Nature* 2000; **404**: 510–14.

78. Lim DS, Vogel H, Willerford DM et al. Analysis of *ku80*-mutant mice and cells with deficient levels of p53. *Mol Cell Biol* 2000; **20**: 3772–80.

79. Vogel H, Lim DS, Karsenty G et al. Deletion of *Ku86* causes early onset of senescence in mice. *Proc Natl Acad Sci USA* 1999; **96**: 10770–5.

80. Tsuzuki T, Fujii Y, Sakumi K et al. Targeted disruption of

81. the *Rad51* gene leads to lethality in embryonic mice. *Proc Natl Acad Sci USA* 1996; **93**: 6236–40.

81. Lim DS, Hasty P. A mutation in mouse *rad51* results in an early embryonic lethal that is suppressed by a mutation in *p53*. *Mol Cell Biol* 1996; **16**: 7133–43.

82. Rijkers T, Van Den Ouweland J, Morolli B et al. Targeted inactivation of mouse *RAD52* reduces homologous recombination but not resistance to ionizing radiation. *Mol Cell Biol* 1998; **18**: 6423–9.

83. Dronkert ML, Beverloo HB, Johnson RD et al. Mouse *RAD54* affects DNA double-strand break repair and sister chromatid exchange. *Mol Cell Biol* 2000; **20**: 3147–56.

84. Essers J, Hendriks RW, Swagemakers SM et al. Disruption of mouse *RAD54* reduces ionizing radiation resistance and homologous recombination. *Cell* 1997; **89**: 195–204.

85. Ludwig T, Chapman DL, Papaioannou VE et al. Targeted mutations of breast cancer susceptibility gene homologs in mice: lethal phenotypes of *Brca1*, *Brca2*, *Brca1/Brca2*, *Brca1/p53*, and *Brca2/p53* nullizygous embryos. *Genes Dev* 1997; **11**: 1226–41.

86. Suzuki A, de la Pompa JL, Hakem R et al. *Brca2* is required for embryonic cellular proliferation in the mouse. *Genes Dev* 1997; **11**: 1242–52.

87. Luo G, Yao MS, Bender CF et al. Disruption of *mRad50* causes embryonic stem cell lethality, abnormal embryonic development, and sensitivity to ionizing radiation. *Proc Natl Acad Sci USA* 1999; **96**: 7376–81.

88. Xiao Y, Weaver DT. Conditional gene targeted deletion by Cre recombinase demonstrates the requirement for the double-strand break repair Mre11 protein in murine embryonic stem cells. *Nucleic Acids Res* 1997; **25**: 2985–91.

89. Zhu J, Petersen S, Tessarollo L et al. Targeted disruption of the Nijmegen breakage syndrome gene *NBS1* leads to early embryonic lethality in mice. *Curr Biol* 2001; **11**: 105–9.

90. Hiom K, Melek M, Gellert M. DNA transposition by the RAG1 and RAG2 proteins: a possible source of oncogenic translocations. *Cell* 1998; **94**: 463–70.

91. Barreto V, Marques R, Demengeot J. Early death and severe lymphopenia caused by ubiquitous expression of the *Rag1* and *Rag2* genes in mice. *Eur J Immunol* 2001; **31**: 3763–72.

# 13 Senescence and telomeres

Peter M Lansdorp

## Introduction

Telomeres are essential genetic elements that consist of specific DNA repeats and associated proteins. Telomeres cap chromosome ends and prevent chromosome fusion and genetic instability. Telomeric DNA is lost with each round of replication and from other causes including (failed repair of) oxidative DNA damage. To compensate for this loss, telomeres are elongated by the reverse transcriptase enzyme telomerase. In most hematopoietic cells, telomerase activity is tightly controlled and present in limiting amounts. As a result, telomeres in leukocytes shorten with age, upon transplantation in vivo, and when cultured in vitro. Progressive telomere shortening eventually results in telomere dysfunction and apoptosis or senescence, but also promotes chromosome instability in hematological disorders such as chronic myeloid leukemia (CML). Here, we review the role of telomeres and telomerase in cells of the hematopoietic system in the context of the emerging concept that telomere shortening represent a tumor suppressor mechanism in long-lived mammals that limits the growth of most (but not all) stem cells and lymphocytes.

## Telomere structure and function

Telomeres or the ends of linear chromosomes consist in all vertebrates of tandem repeats of TTAGGG/CCC-TAA)$_n$ and associated proteins.[1,2] The length of the repeats varies between chromosomes and between species. In humans, the length of telomere repeats varies from 2 to 15 kilobase-pairs, depending on the tissue type, the age of the donor and the replicative history of the cells. Individual chromosome ends also vary in length, and chromosome 17p typically has the shortest track of telomere repeats.[3] Telomeres prevent the ends of linear chromosomes from appearing as DNA breaks and protect chromosome ends from degradation and fusion. Telomeres also play a role in meiosis and the organization of chromosomes within the nucleus.[4] Telomeres contain DNA-binding proteins specific for duplex telomeric DNA, which include TRF1 and TRF2[5] and a protein specific for the single strand overhang that is typically present at the 3′ ends of chromosomes.[6] In addition, many other proteins are known to indirectly bind to telomeres, for example via TRF1 and TRF2 (reviewed in reference 2). The single-strand overhang at the 3′ end of telomeres folds back onto duplex telomeric DNA, forming a protective 'T-loop'.[7] The 3′ overhang associates with telomere repeats via TRF2 in a way that is incompletely understood but which appears to be important for telomere stability.[8,9]

Telomeric DNA is lost in human cells via several mechanisms that are related to DNA replication, remodeling, and repair. Causes of telomere loss include the 'end replication problem',[10,11] nucleolytic processing of 5′ template strands following DNA replication to create a 3′ single-strand overhang,[12,13] and failed repair of oxidative DNA damage to telomeric DNA.[14,15] The relative contributions of these different causes of telomere shortening to the overall decline in telomere length with age are not known and most likely vary between cell types and with age. That telomeres shorten as a result of oxidative damage has only recently been realized. It has been shown that telomeric DNA, with its G-rich repeats, is 5- to 10-fold more vulnerable to oxidative damage than non-telomeric, genomic DNA.[16,17] Repair of oxidative damage to nucleotides is typically achieved using nucleotide excision repair (NER) pathways, which may involve a DNA polymerase template switch.[18] This essential mechanism may fail for lesions near chromosome ends as the repeat nature of target sequences may pose a problem for repair by homologous recombination. In general, the contribution of oxidative damage to telomere shortening and the importance of the redox state in cells to prevent such damage remains to be precisely defined.

The mechanism by which short telomeres signal a DNA damage response is currently not fully understood.[15,19] Recent studies have highlighted the dynamic structure of telomeres (reviewed in reference 20). It now appears that individual telomeres can be either 'on' or 'off' in terms of signaling downstream DNA damage pathways. It seems likely that the terminal 3′ end is involved in generating such signals, but details other than that ATM[21] and p53[22] are likely to be involved are lacking. An important related question is when telomeres signal during the cell cycle. DNA replication inevitably involves remodeling of the telomere structure. Because telomere loss is known to occur during DNA replication, the inability to form functional telomeres following replication is expected to generate a DNA damage signal during S or $G_2$ phase of the cell cycle. However, when diploid human fibroblasts reach replicative senescence, they typically enter an irreversible growth arrest in $G_1$. It has furthermore been shown that disruption of TFR2 binding to telomeres generates a DNA damage signal that is independent of DNA replication.[8] Perhaps telomeres cycle continuously between 'on' and 'off' states even when the cells are in $G_0/G_1$, with the likelihood of the 'on' state being inversely and indirectly correlated with the length of telomere repeats (Figure 13.1). According to this idea, the strength of DNA damage signals generated by telomeres would gradually increase with overall telomere shortening. Anti-apoptotic effects of long telomeres or telomerase expression, as well as increased levels of p53 (and the increased sensitivity to apoptosis) in 'older' cells (with shorter telomeres), are in agreement with this model. Differences between individuals and cells in the telomere length required to activate downstream signaling pathways complicate the use of telomere length as an absolute predictor of cellular responses.[23] Such differences, together with variable heterogeneity in telomere length at individual chromosome arms, help explain the marked variation in telomere length between similar cells from normal individuals of the same age.[24,25]

## Telomere maintenance pathways

To compensate for the loss of telomere repeats, cells require expression of functional telomerase. Telomerase is a ribonucleoprotein containing the reverse transcriptase telomerase protein (hTERT) and the telomerase RNA template (hTERC) as essential components. In addition, a number of proteins have been described that are important for telomerase assembly, nuclear localization, and stability (reviewed in reference 2). Telomerase is capable of extending the 3′ ends of telomeres. Telomerase levels are typically high in immortal cells that maintain a constant telomere length, such as the stem cells of the germline in the testis and embryonic stem cells. For reasons that remain to be precisely defined, telomerase levels are insufficient to maintain the telomere length in hematopoietic stem cells. Nevertheless, telomerase is functionally very important in hematopoietic stem cells, as is highlighted in patients with the disorder dyskeratosis congenita. Patients with the autosomal dominant form of this disease have one normal and one mutated copy of the telomerase RNA template gene. As expected, such patients show a modest reduction in telomerase levels, yet they typically suffer from progressive aplastic anemia, immune deficiencies, or cancer, and rarely live past the age of 50.[2,26–28] These findings are in stark contrast to those in the mouse, where complete lack of telomerase activity is tolerated for up to six generations.[29] Together with the age-related decline in telomere length in leukocytes, these observations have provided strong support for the idea that telomerase levels are extremely tightly regulated and limiting in human hematopoietic stem cells.

The role of so-called alternative ('ALT') pathways[30] in the elongation and/or maintenance of telomeres in hematopoietic cells is not clear. Most likely, such

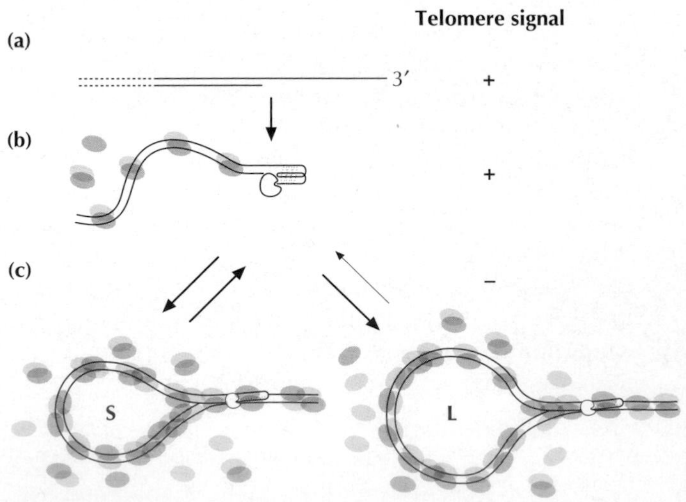

**Figure 13.1** Dynamic model of DNA damage signals generated by short telomeres. (a) Following replication and processing, a chromosome end with a G-rich single-strand overhang is created. (b) This structure is processed and bound by various telomere-binding proteins, including hPOT1[6] (indicated by the small clear circle), which binds to the 3′ single-strand overhang, and TRF1 and TRF2 (indicated by light and dark gray circles), which are capable of folding telomeric DNA.[50] (c) If the length of telomere repeats is sufficiently long (L), double-stranded telomere repeats can easily fold back on to the single-strand overhang, resulting in a relatively stable structure.[7] The stability of the poorly understood foldback structure could be compromised when telomeres are short (S), resulting in a shift of the equilibrium between capped and uncapped telomeres[4] that is independent of DNA replication.

pathways are not very efficient in elongating telomeres in cells that express telomerase. Because telomere lengthening via telomerase and/or ALT appears to be limiting in hematopoietic cells, molecular defects that result in accelerated telomere shortening may result in aplastic anemia. In many cases, it is not possible or straightforward to distinguish direct from indirect causes of telomere shortening. In dyskeratosis, the cause appears to be directly related to telomerase deficiency, whereas in Fanconi anemia,[31] for example, telomere shortening could be caused directly by defective repair of telomeric DNA or indirectly because loss of stem cells (resulting from defective DNA repair) will result in increased (compensatory) proliferation of remaining stem cells.

Following loss of telomere repeats, a DNA damage signal is generated that signals cell cycle arrest, most likely via upregulation of *p53*. When short telomeres are subsequently elongated by 'telomere repair' pathways involving telomerase and/or recombination, the cell cycle arrest will be transient. However, the continued loss of telomeric DNA eventually generates too many short telomeres for the limited capacity of telomere repair pathways (Figure 13.2). At this point, otherwise-normal cells as well as premalignant cells are destined to die by apoptosis or convert to an unresponsive state ('replicative senescence'), depending on the response to high and sustained levels of p53 in a particular cell type. Possibly, the replicative lifespan of cells in long-lived species has been under selective pressure to (1) permit sufficient divisions for the maintenance of cellular function during a normal lifespan while (2) acting as a brake to prevent excessive cellular proliferation and tumor development. It appears that in most hematopoietic cells, the required balance is achieved by regulating telomerase activity at levels that are sufficient to maintain a minimal length in only a proportion of the 92 telomeres in a human cell. Limiting levels of telomerase and the resulting telomere shortening could contribute to organismal aging in at least two ways. First, some increasing proportion of cells could reach the end of their programmed proliferative lifespan in old age. As a result, T-cell responses could be compromised in the elderly. Second, gene expression in cells near or at senescence may be abnormal, resulting in aberrant secretion of molecules, including enzymes and cytokines (see also reference 32). Both factors could contribute to impaired immune responses in old individuals. In general, the study of telomere biology in relation to human aging is in its infancy. Major challenges are difficulties related to longitudinal studies in humans and the limited use of rodent models.

# Telomeres and replicative senescence

In contrast to embryonic stem cells or tumor cell lines, hematopoietic stem cells are not immortal. Forty years ago, Hayflick suggested that most normal human cells are unable to divide indefinitely but are programmed for a given number of cell divisions.[33] In 1990, several papers described loss of telomeres with replication and with age and suggested that progressive telomere shortening could explain Hayflick's original observation.[34–36] This model was confirmed by subsequent studies showing that transfer of the telomerase reverse transcriptase gene could prevent telomere erosion and resulted in immortalizing of the cells that Hayflick studied in most detail: normal diploid human fibroblasts.[37,38] Since then, many papers have appeared that are compatible with the notion that telomere shortening limits the number of times most normal diploid cells can divide (for a review, see reference 39). An emerging consensus is

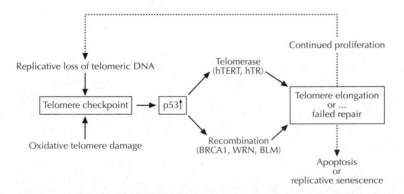

**Figure 13.2** The telomere checkpoint. Loss of telomere repeats following replication and oxidative damage results in activation of a DNA damage signal that triggers DNA repair reactions involving telomerase and/or molecules involved in recombination, such as BRCA1, WRN, and BLM. Following effective repair, cells can go through another round of cell division. However, eventually too many short telomeres accumulate for the limited telomere repair capacity. The resulting high levels of p53 will trigger apoptosis or replicative senescence. Because telomerase levels are limiting in hematopoietic stem cells, such a threshold will be reached earlier in cells that express subnormal levels of telomerase as in, for example, dyskeratosis congenita.

that telomere shortening evolved as a checkpoint mechanism in long-lived mammals that controls unlimited and life-threatening proliferation of organ-specific stem cells and lymphocytes.

Since the important original observation that telomeres in adult blood leukocytes are significantly shorter as compared with germline material (sperm) from the same donor,[40] the decline of somatic telomeres has been documented in three ways. The original observation was confirmed,[36,41] it was shown that telomeres in various tissues were shorter in older donors,[34,35] and telomere shortening was documented during in vitro culture of human cells.[35,42] In the decade that followed these initial reports, a large number of papers have appeared that have greatly refined our understanding of telomere shortening in human nucleated blood cells (reviewed in reference 43). Studies in this general area have been facilitated by the development of quantitative fluorescence in situ hybridization techniques to measure the telomere length in suspension cells using flow cytometry (flow FISH[44]). With these techniques, it was shown that the age-related decline in telomere length in lymphocytes is much more pronounced than in granulocytes and that rapid telomere shortening early in life is followed by a much more gradual decline thereafter.[25] The telomere length in granulocytes can be used as a surrogate marker for the telomere length in hematopoietic stem cells if one assumes that the number of cell divisions between stem cells and granulocytes is relatively constant throughout life and that telomere shortening in stem cells is (1) primarily resulting from replication and (2) relatively constant with each cell division. This approach has been used to model the turnover of human hematopoietic stem cells on the basis of telomere length data.[45]

A striking observation is that telomere length at any given age in humans is very heterogeneous.[24,44] This variation appears to be primarily genetic.[46] For example, monozygous twins of over 70 years of age were shown to have very similar telomere length in both granulocytes and lymphocytes, whereas dizygotic twins differed more but not as much as unrelated individuals.[25] Using further refinements in the flow FISH method (GM Baerlocher and PM Lansdorp, unpublished observations), it was recently shown that the rapid decline early in life is followed by a slow decline until the age of 50–60 years, after which the decline again accelerates (Figure 13.3). The decline in both granulocytes and lymphocytes is non-linear and fits a cubic curve. The pronounced decline in T-cell telomere length could activate the telomere checkpoint in specific T and natural killer (NK) cells during a normal lifetime and as a result compromise immune responses in the elderly.

In view of the modest age-related decline in telomere length in granulocytes, it seems unlikely that hematopoietic stem cells during normal hematopoiesis encounter irreversible cell cycle arrest or undergo apoptosis as a result of telomere shortening. Most likely, the total production of blood cells from a single hematopoietic stem cell is primarily determined by differentiation of stem and progenitor cells and not by replicative senescence. Furthermore, the occasional loss of individual stem cells via telomere shortening is not expected to impact on overall hematopoiesis (or overall telomere length in granulocytes) in the presence of a variable 'reserve' of additional hematopoietic stem cells. That normal hematopoietic stem cells and tissues have extensive replicative potential is also in agreement with extensive experience using allogeneic and autologous stem cell transplantation. Nevertheless, the telomere checkpoint does appear to operate in hematopoietic stem cells, as is indicated by the age-related loss of telomeres in granulocytes (Figure 13.3), the (modest) loss of telomeres following allogeneic transplantation,[43,47] and the aplastic anemia that follows partial telomerase deficiency.[2] Recent studies have shown that the number of hematopoietic stem cells can be altered by manipulating decisions that control self-renewal and differentiation.[48] Indeed, the number of mature 'end' cells such as granulocytes produced by individual stem cells is most likely highly variable and primarily determined by the processes that regulate self-renewal versus differentiation at the level of individual stem

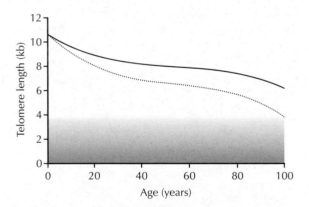

**Figure 13.3** The decline in telomere length with age in lymphocytes (dotted line) is more pronounced than in granulocytes (full line). The mean telomere length is shown for both cell types extracted from several hundred measurements over the entire age range (GM Baerlocher and PM Lansdorp, unpublished observations). Not shown is the considerable variation in telomere length values between individuals at any given age.[25] The gray bar at the bottom represents non-telomeric DNA contributing to the telomere length measurements (flow FISH measurements were calibrated using Southern blot analysis in which on average 2–4 kb of subtelomeric DNA between restriction sites and start of telomere repeats is included in the measurement). Both granulocytes and lymphocytes show a highly significant decline, which is best described by a cubic function.

cells. Even a limited number of additional self-renewal divisions in a stem cell will greatly increase cell output. As a result, individual stem cells can produce staggering numbers of cells. This is illustrated in clonal proliferative disorders such as paroxysmal nocturnal hemoglobinuria (PNH) and CML. However, even in CML, clonally expanded Philadelphia-positive stem cells eventually appear to encounter the telomere checkpoint.[49] Unfortunately, with a large number of cells to select from, the genetic instability triggered by the loss of functional telomeres appears to favor the selection of a subclone with additional genetic abnormalities and more malignant properties.

Not all cells in the hematopoietic system are programmed to encounter the telomere checkpoint. B cells appear to be a particularly interesting exception, as the telomere length in B cells is increasingly heterogenous with age (Figure 13.4). Apparently, some B cells express sufficient telomerase (and presumably other factors) to effectively elongate telomeres. Perhaps the many cell divisions required for effective selection, 'affinity maturation', and maintenace of antibody responses favored inactivation of the telomere checkpoint. It is tempting to speculate that B cells are, as a result, at a higher risk for tumor development, which could explain the much higher incidence of B-versus T-cell lymphomas in the human population.

## Conclusions

Based on observations from several areas, telomeres have emerged as important regulatory elements that control the number of times normal human somatic cells can divide. Activation of the telomere checkpoint results from loss of telomeric DNA with replication and from oxidative damage to telomeric DNA (Figure 13.2). The DNA damage response that is triggered by activation of the telomere checkpoint can be resolved by telomere elongation pathways that involve telomerase or recombination. However, in most somatic cells, including hematopoietic stem cells, the capacity of such telomere repair pathways appears to be limiting, and telomere shortening effectively limits the proliferative potential of such cells. Most likely, the telomere checkpoint evolved as a tumor suppressor mechanism in long-lived species. The function of the telomere checkpoint may help explain poorly understood aspects of stem cell biology, including stem cell 'exhaustion' in aplastic anemia and other proliferative disorders. Cells may bypass the telomere checkpoint by expressing high levels of telomerase or by inactivating downstream signaling events, for example by loss of p53 function. Some cells, including subsets of B cells, may avoid the telomere checkpoints altogether, and high levels of telomerase could make such B cells more vulnerable to tumor development. Loss of p53 function also inactivates the telomere checkpoint. This is expected to be a rare event, as both copies of the normal *p53* allele in a cell must typically be lost or mutated in order to continue proliferation in the presence of many short and dysfunctional telomeres.[3] Loss of p53 function results in chromosome fusions and breakage that drive genetic instability and facilitate malignant progression. This is illustrated in CML, where the onset of blast crisis and additional genetic changes is inversely correlated with the length of telomeres in Philadelphia-positive chronic-phase cells.[49]

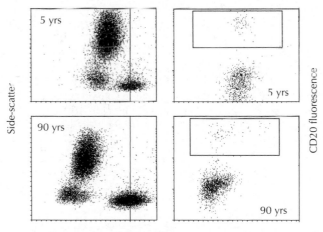

**Figure 13.4** Telomere length analysis in subpopulation of human nucleated blood cells using flow FISH (GM Baerlocher and PM Lansdorp, unpublished observations). For this type of analysis, nucleated blood cells following red cell lysis are hybridized with a fluorescently labeled telomere probe together with fixed cow thymocytes (with long telomeres: vertical bars, left panels) as internal controls. Following wash steps to remove unlabeled probe and incubation with labeled antibodies (e.g. phycoerythrin-labeled anti-CD20: right panels) the cells are analyzed by flow cytometry. Note the decline in telomere fluorescence (on a linear scale) with age in both granulocytes (with high side-scatter: left panels) and lymphocytes (low side-scatter, increased heterogeneity with age: left panels) and the presence of some CD20+ B cells with very long telomeres in the 90-year-old normal donor.

## Acknowledgments

Work in the author's laboratory is funded by NIH Grant AI29524 and by grants from the Canadian Institutes of Health Research and the National Cancer Institute of Canada with funds from the Terry Fox run. Part of this article was previously published in: Verfaillie CM, Pera MF, Lansdorp PM. *Hematology 2002, American Society of Hematology Education Program*. Stem cells: hype and reality. The American Society of Hematology, Blood, Washington, DC, pp 369–391, 2002. Copyright American Society of Hematology, used by permission.

## REFERENCES

1. Moyzis RK, Buckingham JM, Cram LS et al. A highly conserved repetitive DNA sequence, (TTAGGG)$_n$, present at the telomeres of human chromosomes. *Proc Natl Acad Sci USA* 1988; **85**: 6622–6.

2. Collins K, Mitchell JR. Telomerase in the human organism. *Oncogene* 2002; **21**: 564–79.

3. Martens UM, Zijlmans JMJM, Poon SSS et al. Short telomeres on human chromosome 17p. *Nat Genet* 1998; **18**: 76–80.

4. Blackburn EH. Telomere states and cell fates. *Nature* 2000; **408**: 53–6.

5. Smogorzewska A, van Steensel B, Bianchi A et al. Control of human telomere length by TRF1 and TRF2. *Mol Cell Biol* 2000; **20**: 1659–68.

6. Baumann P, Cech TR. Pot1, the putative telomere end-binding protein in fission yeast and humans. *Science* 2001; **292**: 1171–5.

7. Griffith JD, Comeau L, Rosenfield S et al. Mammalian telomeres end in a large duplex loop. *Cell* 1999; **97**: 503–14.

8. Karlseder J, Broccoli D, Dai Y et al. p53- and ATM-dependent apoptosis induced by telomeres lacking TRF2. *Science* 1999; **283**: 1321–5.

9. Zhu XD, Kuster B, Mann M et al. Cell-cycle-regulated association of RAD50/MRE11/NBS1 with TRF2 and human telomeres. *Nat Genet* 2000; **25**: 347–52.

10. Watson JD. Origin of concatameric T4 DNA. *Nat New Biol* 1972; **239**: 197–201.

11. Olovnikov AM. A theory of marginotomy. The incomplete copying of template margin in enzymic synthesis of polynucleotides and biological significance of the phenomenon. *J Theor Biol* 1973; **41**: 181–90.

12. Wellinger RJ, Ethier K, Labrecque P et al. Evidence for a new step in telomere maintenance. *Cell* 1996; **85**: 423–33.

13. Makarov VL, Hirose Y, Langmore JP. Long G tails at both ends of human chromosomes suggest a C strand degradation mechanism for telomere shortening. *Cell* 1997; **88**: 657–66.

14. Petersen S, Saretzki G, von Zglinicki T. Preferential accumulation of single-stranded regions in telomeres of human fibroblasts. *Exp Cell Res* 1998; **239**: 152–60.

15. Lansdorp PM. Repair of telomeric DNA prior to replicative senescence. *Mech Ageing Dev* 2000; **118**: 23–34.

16. Henle ES, Han Z, Tang N et al. Sequence-specific DNA cleavage by $Fe^{2+}$-mediated Fenton reactions has possible biological implications. *J Biol Chem* 1999; **274**: 962–71.

17. Oikawa S, Kawanishi S. Site-specific DNA damage at GGG sequence by oxidative stress may accelerate telomere shortening. *FEBS Lett* 1999; **453**: 365–8.

18. Hoeijmakers JHJ. Genome maintenance mechanisms for preventing cancer. *Nature* 2001; **411**: 366–74.

19. Hemann MT, Strong MA, Hao LY et al. The shortest telomere, not average telomere length, is critical for cell viability and chromosome stability. *Cell* 2001; **107**: 67–77.

20. Blackburn EH. Switching and signaling at the telomere. *Cell* 2001; **106**: 661–73.

21. Abraham RT. Cell cycle checkpoint signaling through the ATM and ATR kinases. *Genes Dev* 2001; **15**: 2177–96.

22. Hande MP, Balajee AS, Tchirkov A et al. Extra-chromosomal telomeric DNA in cells from $Atm^{-/-}$ mice and patients with ataxia-telangiectasia. *Hum Mol Genet* 2001; **10**: 519–28.

23. Serra V, von Zglinicki T. Human fibroblasts in vitro senesce with a donor-specific telomere length. *FEBS Lett* 2002; **516**: 71–4.

24. Frenck RW, Jr., Blackburn EH, Shannon KM. The rate of telomere sequence loss in human leukocytes varies with age. *Proc Natl Acad Sci USA* 1998; **95**: 5607–10.

25. Rufer N, Brummendorf TH, Kolvraa S et al. Telomere fluorescence measurements in granulocytes and T lymphocyte subsets point to a high turnover of hematopoietic stem cells and memory T cells in early childhood. *J Exp Med* 1999; **190**: 157–67.

26. Mitchell JR, Wood E, Collins K. A telomerase component is defective in the human disease dyskeratosis congenita. *Nature* 1999; **402**: 551–5.

27. Vulliamy T, Marrone A, Goldman F et al. The RNA component of telomerase is mutated in autosomal dominant dyskeratosis congenita. *Nature* 2001; **413**: 432–5.

28. Dokal I. Dyskeratosis congenita. A disease of premature ageing. *Lancet* 2001; **358**(Suppl): S27.

29. Blasco MA, Lee H-W, Hande MP et al. Telomere shortening and tumor formation by mouse cells lacking telomerase RNA. *Cell* 1997; **91**: 25–34.

30. Henson JD, Neumann AA, Yeager TR et al. Alternative lengthening of telomeres in mammalian cells. *Oncogene* 2002; **21**: 598–610.

31. Grompe M, D'Andrea A. Fanconi anemia and DNA repair. *Hum Mol Genet* 2001; **10**: 2253–9.

32. Kirkwood TB, Holliday R. The evolution of ageing and longevity. *Proc R Soc Lond B Biol Sci* 1979; **205**: 531–46.

33. Hayflick L, Moorhead PS. The serial cultivation of human diploid strains. *Exp Cell Res* 1961; **25**: 585–621.

34. Hastie ND, Dempster M, Dunlop MG et al. Telomere reduction in human colorectal carcinoma and with ageing. *Nature* 1990; **346**: 866–8.

35. Harley CB, Futcher AB, Greider CW. Telomeres shorten during ageing of human fibroblasts. *Nature* 1990; **345**: 458–60.

36. de Lange T, Shiue L, Myers R et al. Structure and variability of human chromosome ends. *Mol Cell Biol* 1990; **10**: 518–27.

37. Bodnar AG, Ouellette M, Frolkis M et al. Extension of lifespan by introduction of telomerase into normal human cells. *Science* 1998; **279**: 349–53.

38. Vaziri H, Benchimol S. Reconstitution of telomerase activity in normal human cells leads to elongation of telomeres and extended replicative life span. *Curr Biol* 1998; **8**: 279–82.

39. Mathon NF, Lloyd AC. Cell senescence and cancer. *Nat Rev Cancer* 2001; **1**: 203–13.

40. Cooke HJ, Smith BA. Variability at the telomeres of the human X/Y pseudoautosomal region. *Cold Spring Harb Symp Quant Biol* 1986; **51**: 213–19.

41. Allshire RC, Gosden JR, Cross SH et al. Telomeric repeat from *T. thermophila* cross-hybridizes with human telomeres. *Nature* 1988; **332**: 656–9.

42. Counter CM, Avilion AA, LeFeuvre CE et al. Telomere shortening associated with chromosome instability is arrested in immortal cells which express telomerase activity. *EMBO J* 1992; **11**: 1921–9.

43. Ohyashiki JH, Sashida G, Tauchi T et al. Telomeres and telomerase in hematologic neoplasia. *Oncogene* 2002; **21**: 680–7.

44. Rufer N, Dragowska W, Thornbury G et al. Telomere length dynamics in human lymphocyte subpopulations measured by flow cytometry. *Nat Biotechnol* 1998; **16**: 743–7.

45. Edelstein-Keshet L, Israel A, Lansdorp P. Modelling perspectives on aging: Can mathematics help us stay young? *J Theor Biol* 2001; **213**: 509–25.

46. Slagboom PE, Droog S, Boomsma DI. Genetic determination of telomere size in humans: a twin study of three age groups. *Am J Hum Genet* 1994; **55**: 876–82.

47. Rufer N, Brummendorf TH, Chapuis B et al. Accelerated telomere shortening in hematological lineages is limited to the first year following stem cell transplantation. *Blood* 2001; **97**: 575–7.

48. Antonchuk J, Sauvageau G, Humphries RK. *HoxB4*-induced expansion of adult hematopoietic stem cells ex vivo. *Cell* 2002; **109**: 39–45.

49. Brummendorf TH, Mak J, Baerlocher GM et al. Longitudinal studies of telomere length in feline blood cells point to a rapid turnover of stem cells in the first year of life. *Blood* 2000; **96**: 455a.

50. Bianchi A, Smith S, Chong L et al. TRF1 is a dimer and bends telomeric DNA. *EMBO J* 1997; **16**: 1785–94.

# 14 Angiogenesis and tumor development

**William T Bellamy**

## Introduction

Angiogenesis, the formation of new blood vessels from an existing vascular network, is distinguished from vasculogenesis, a process that occurs during the developmental period. Angiogenesis plays a central role in both physiologic processes and pathologic disorders. Under normal conditions, it is a complex process regulated through interactions between endothelial cells, growth factors and cytokines, and the extracellular matrix.[1-6] Physiologic angiogenesis is characterized by a very tightly controlled balance between angiogenic growth factors and inhibitors, and occurs during the monthly reproductive cycle to generate the endometrium, to form the corpus luteum, and during pregnancy to build the placenta.[1] Angiogenesis also occurs following tissue injury and is key to proper wound healing. In pathologic disorders such as diabetic retinopathies, rheumatoid arthritis, and cancer, there is an uncontrolled proliferation of vessels that subsequently develop in a disorganized manner.[1-6] Tumors produce large amounts of angiogenic growth factors that act to upset the normally well-controlled balance between pro- and anti-angiogenic factors, thus stimulating the proliferation of new vessels. It has now become well established that the viability and growth of tumors is dependent on this process. When solid tumors such as lung, breast, and colon cancers are less than 2 mm³ in size, all cells within the tumor mass can receive required nutrients and oxygen through diffusion; however, for these tumors to grow further, there is a strict requirement for a vascular supply, provided through the process of angiogenesis. Clinical studies have demonstrated that both the number and density of microvessels in several different human cancers directly correlate with invasion and metastasis and predict for an unfavorable prognosis.[7-11] Such findings are consistent with the belief that angiogenesis is both an independent prognostic marker of outcome and a mechanistic target for therapy. While it is well established that the growth of solid tumors is dependent upon neovascularization, the role of angiogenesis in hematopoietic malignancies has only recently been appreciated (see below).

## The angiogenic process

Both physiologic and pathologic angiogenesis, as mentioned above, are initiated by an imbalance between pro- and anti-angiogenic factors. The initiation of this process has been termed the 'angiogenic switch' and in tumors is associated with the activation of several proto-oncogenes, including *ras*, *src*, and others, as well as by inactivation of the tumor suppressor gene, *p53*.[12-14] Once the angiogenic process begins, a number of well-orchestrated events begin to occur. First, under the influence of pro-angiogenic growth factors such as vascular endothelial growth factor (VEGF) and basic fibroblast growth factor (bFGF, FGF-2), endothelial cells, which under normal circumstances are quiescent, begin to proliferate. There is an increase in vascular permeability, mediated by VEGF, allowing the release of fibrin into the interstitial space. The release of fibrin acts as a scaffolding for the growth of the newly forming vessels. Proteolytic enzymes such as the matrix metalloproteinases (MMP) are produced to dissolve the basement membrane, thus facilitating vascular growth. Following the binding of the growth factor to its receptor located on the surface of the endothelial cell, a series of signaling pathways are activated. The endothelial cells begin to proliferate and migrate into the interstitial space along a chemotactic gradient towards the source of the angiogenic factor(s). Specific integrins are expressed on the vascular endothelium ($\alpha_v\beta_3$, $\alpha_v\beta_5$) and help to guide the vessels. Ultimately, the newly formed vascular sprouts will begin to roll up and form a tube. These vascular tubes then anastomose to form patent vessels. Smooth muscle cells and pericytes then provide structural support to stabilize the vascular network. When comparing physiologic and pathologic angiogenesis, there are significant differences.

Physiologic angiogenesis is self-limited temporally; once the immediate need is met, the balance between stimulators and inhibitors is restored and the process terminates. Evidence now suggests that physiologic angiogenesis may be regulated in a tissue-specific manner, with specific tissues employing unique angiogenic regulators.[15] Frequently, tumor angiogenesis is uncontrolled and unlimited in time, and is characterized by a 30- to 40-fold increase in endothelial cell proliferation. In addition, there are morphologic differences in the vessels formed in tumor angiogenesis. Normal vasculature has a predominance of straight, non-branching microvessels, while in tumors, there is often a complex, tortuous architecture. Tumor vasculature has generally widened lumens, fewer associated smooth muscle cells and pericytes, irregular blood flow, regions of vascular stasis, and high permeability. Finally, in tumor-derived angiogenesis, there may be involvement of growth factors, such as placental growth factor (PlGF), that, while not critical for angiogenesis during development, clearly have the capacity to stimulate new vessel growth in the tumor.[16]

## Tumor angiogenesis

Angiogenesis is a key component of cancer progression and metastasis.[7–11] It was not until 1971, when Folkman[17] published his theory on tumor angiogenesis, that the concept of tumor-initiated angiogenesis was recognized. All tumors begin their existence as a small, avascular cluster of cells, growing above the basement membrane (carcinoma in situ). Tumors at this stage rely upon nearby blood vessels for oxygen and diffusion of nutrients. In the absence of angiogenesis, tumor growth would remain dormant at a size of only 2–3 mm$^3$, with the size being limited by the diffusion of oxygen and nutrients. Progression from in situ tumors to invasive and metastatic solid tumors requires, and is correlated with, the formation of new microvessels. As the tumor accumulates additional genetic changes, a small percentage of the tumor cells gain the ability to express genes encoding angiogenic growth factors. This theory was initially met with much skepticism, but has now been recognized as a cornerstone of tumor growth. It is now established that angiogenesis is not only essential for tumor growth but is also implicated in the initial progression from a premalignant tumor to a cancer,[3,13] invasion of the cancer cells into the circulation,[18] and growth of dormant micrometastases into frank metastatic lesions.[19] As a component of tumor growth, inflammatory cells that infiltrate the tumor also produce and release angiogenic growth factors and thus help stimulate the growth and spread of the tumor.[5,20]

## Angiogenic factors

Angiogenesis is influenced by a number of positive and negative regulatory factors. Soluble molecules (e.g. growth factors), non-cellular constituents of tissues (extracellular matrix), and peri-endothelial cellular elements (e.g. pericytes) contribute to the character and extent of vessel growth.[4–6]

The first recognized angiogenic growth factor, bFGF, was reported in 1984.[21] This was followed in 1989 by the discovery of VEGF.[22] It was soon realized that VEGF was identical to a molecule previously characterized as a mediator of vascular permeability, vascular permeability factor (VPF), discovered in 1979 by Dvorak.[23] Although angiogenesis is influenced by a number of regulatory factors, VEGF is a central player in this process. VEGF is a multifunctional cytokine commonly expressed by many tumors.[24–26] In support of its role in tumor growth, levels of VEGF mRNA and protein expression correlate positively with malignant progression and poor outcome in numerous human tumors.[27–29] Consistent with the notion of an angiogenic switch, VEGF expression is positively activated by both Ras- and Src-mediated oncogenic pathways.[30,31] While it is presently unclear what fraction of neovascular growth can be attributed to VEGF as opposed to other polypeptides with angiogenic activity, a critical role of VEGF in tumor growth in vivo was demonstrated by Kim et al,[32] who showed that the addition of neutralizing antibodies to VEGF resulted in a marked suppression of tumor growth in human tumor xenografts, thus providing the first direct evidence that tumor growth was VEGF-dependent.

In addition to its effects on vascular permeability, VEGF is a potent mitogen and survival factor for endothelial cells and promotes endothelial cell proliferation and survival. VEGF displays chemotactic effects on endothelial cells and increases the expression of proteolytic enzymes in endothelial cells involved in stromal degradation.[24] Its activity is mediated through interactions with high-affinity tyrosine kinase receptors. To date, three cell surface receptors have been identified that bind VEGF and its family members (reviewed in reference 4). All three consist of an extracellular domain with seven immunoglobulin-like loops, a transmembrane region, followed by a kinase domain that is divided into two parts by the insertion of a non-catalytic 100-amino-acid residue sequence. The first of these is known as VEGF receptor 1 (VEGFR1; also known as Flt1: Fms-like tyrosine kinase 1), and binds both VEGF-A, VEGF-B, and PlGF.[4] In addition to its expression on vascular endothelial cells, VEGFR1 is also present on smooth muscle and monocytes.[4] The role of VEGFR1 in pathologic angiogenesis is perplexing. In adult endothelial cells, VEGFR1 phosphorylation has been difficult to demonstrate, thus leading most investigators to the belief that VEGFR2 (see below) is playing a dominant role in this process. However, evidence is beginning to emerge suggesting that VEGFR1 may indeed be playing an important role. Ribozymes targeting VEGFR1 mRNA are effective in halting angiogenesis.[33] Conversely, overexpression of PlGF, a VEGFR1-selective ligand, has been shown to stimulate tumor progression.[34] The second receptor, VEGFR2 (also known as Flk1 (fetal liver kinase) or KDR (kinase domain receptor)) binds VEGF as well as VEGF-C through VEGF-E.[4] VEGFR3, the most recently described member of the VEGFR family, was previously designated Flt4. This receptor appears to be restricted predominantly to endothelial cells lining lymphatic channels, although it is functionally expressed in a certain subset of leukemic cells.[4,35] Ligands for VEGFR3 include VEGF-C and VEGF-D.[4] In addition to the three high-affinity VEGF receptors, an additional receptor that binds VEGF in an isoform-specific manner has been identified.[36] Neuropilin-1 (NP-1) belongs to the collapsing/semaphorin family of receptors that mediate neuronal cell guidance. In conjunction with VEGFR2, NP-1 binds specifically to sequences found in exon 7 and therefore binds $VEGF_{165}$ but not $VEGF_{121}$. Binding of $VEGF_{165}$ by NP-1 appears not to signal directly but rather acts to enhance VEGFR2-mediated chemotaxis,[36] as well as to enhance the survival of breast cancer cells.[37]

In addition to bFGF and VEGF, other pro-angiogenic growth factors include platelet-derived growth factor (PDGF), transforming growth factor β (TGF-β), interleukin-8 (IL-8), the angiopoietins, and many others (Table 14.1). Negative factors that act to suppress angiogenesis include platelet factor 4 (PF4), thrombospondin-1, tissue inhibitors of metalloproteinases (TIMP), prolactin, angiostatin, endostatin, and interferon-α (IFN-α) (Table 14.2). An interesting phenomenon that has been demonstrated is the production of endogenous angiogenic inhibitors by the primary tumor. These inhibitors are believed to suppress the angiogenic growth of distant metastases.[38] Surgical removal of experimental primary tumors lowers the level of these endogenous inhibitors and thereby promotes metastatic growth, a phenomenon that mirrors clinical experience.

There is growing evidence that the level of circulating angiogenic factors may have significant prognostic value and other clinical implications in various human cancers. Circulating VEGF expression has been the most widely studied of the angiogenic factors, and is generally believed to be a good reflection of tumor angiogenic activity in various cancers. Numerous studies have demonstrated a strong correlation between elevated tumor expression of VEGF and advanced disease or poor prognosis in various cancers.[39]

## Table 14.1 Pro-angiogenic growth factors

Acidic fibroblast growth factor (aFGF)
Angiogenin
Angiopoietin-1
Basic fibroblast growth factor (bFGF, FGF-2)
Hepatocyte growth factor (HGF)
Insulin-like growth factor (IGF)
Interleukin-6 (IL-6)
Interleukin-8 (IL-8)
Platelet-derived growth factor (PDGF)
Platelet endothelial cell adhesion molecule (CD-31, PECAM)
Placental growth factor (PlGF)
Transforming growth factor α and β (TGF-α and -β)
Tumor necrosis factor α (TNF-α)
Vascular endothelial growth factor (VEGF, VPF):
    VEGF-B
    VEGF-C
    VEGF-D

## Table 14.2 Endogenous angiogenic inhibitors

Angiopoietin-2 (in the absence of VEGF)
Angiostatin (fragment of plasminogen)
Endostatin (fragment of collagen XVIII)
Interferon-α, -β, and -γ (IFN-α, -β, and -γ)
Interleukin-10
Platelet factor 4 (PF4)
Prolactin (16 kDa fragment)
Thrombospondin-1
Tissue inhibitors of metalloproteinases (TIMP)
Soluble Flt1 receptor
Soluble bFGF receptor
Vasostatin (fragment of calreticulin)

# Angiogenesis and hematopoiesis

Human bone marrow is a heterogeneous mixture of various cell types, including hematopoietic stem cells, endothelial cells, osteoblasts, and other supporting elements. Cells within the marrow cavity form a continuous network in which stromal cells are interspersed with hematopoietic and endothelial progenitors. Hematopoiesis is regulated by several cytokines, including granulocyte and granulocyte – macrophage colony-stimulating factors (G-CSF and GM-CSF), IL-3, IL-4, IL-6, and IL-8.[40] Recent evidence suggests that the growth factors involved in angiogenesis also promote hematopoietic stem cell growth. bFGF has been shown to regulate hematopoiesis by acting on stromal cells, early and committed hematopoietic progenitors, and some mature blood cells.[41,42]

A role for VEGF in embryonic hematopoiesis was suggested by results from knockout mice. The loss of a single *VEGF* allele results in embryonic lethality.[43] *VEGF*[+/−] embryos were found to be devoid of most endothelial and hematopoietic cells in the blood island, the site of active hematopoiesis during early embryogenesis, and die around day 10 of embryonic development as a consequence of the absence of vascular structures. In the absence of VEGFR2, hemangioblasts fail to differentiate into endothelial cells,[44] while, in the absence of VEGFR1, the vascular defect is due to an increase in the number of hemangioblasts.[45] Such studies demonstrated the essential role of VEGF and its receptors during development.

With the discovery that, in the adult, VEGFR2 was expressed on a subset of multipotent human stem cells in the bone marrow and that VEGF was produced by hematopoietic stem cells in response to cytokine stimulation,[46–48] there was a realization that VEGF plays a key role not only in angiogenesis but also in normal hematopoiesis. CD34[+] VEGFR2[+] progenitor cells display pluripotent activity, whereas CD34[+] VEGFR2[−] cells are committed progenitors.[48] Stimulation with VEGF has been shown to mobilize both endothelial precursors as well as hematopoietic stem cells.[49] Studies have demonstrated that tumor angiogenesis is associated with the recruitment of both of these cell types and that this recruitment of VEGF-responsive bone marrow-derived precursors is both necessary and sufficient for tumor angiogenesis.[50]

# Angiogenesis in hematologic tumors

While it is well established that growth in solid tumors is dependent on angiogenesis, the role of this process in hematologic tumors is not fully appreciated. Increased microvessel density has now been described in several hematologic malignancies, including multiple myeloma, B-cell non-Hodgkin lymphoma (NHL), myelodysplastic syndromes (MDS), and acute and chronic leukemias representing both lymphocytic and myeloid lineages. As discussed below, hematologic tumor cells are capable of producing several angiogenic growth factors, including VEGF, VEGF-C, and bFGF, as well as expressing receptors for these molecules (Tables 14.3 and 14.4). Thus, different angio-regulatory molecules may be operating in a given hematopoietic tumor. Such findings suggest that the angiogenic process is commonly activated in these malignancies and is likely playing a functional role. While these findings suggest a role for angiogenesis, they do not prove that these tumors are dependent on this process; the elevated microvessel densities that are observed may reflect an epiphenomenon secondary to the elevation of a variety of cytokines, including VEGF. If one considers the pro-survival role of VEGF, however, the elevation of such factors begins to become more evident. That said, there is also evidence to support a direct role for angiogenesis in many of these tumors. Direct inhibitors of vascular endothelial cells such as endostatin have been shown to prolong survival in these

**Table 14.3 Angiogenic growth factor expression in human hematopoietic tumor cell lines**

| Cell line | Disease | Phenotype | bFGF | VEGF | Ang-1 |
|---|---|---|---|---|---|
| Jurkat | Acute T-cell leukemia | T-cell | Neg | Pos | Neg |
| Molt-4 | Acute lymphoblastic leukemia | T-cell | Neg | Pos | Neg |
| CCRF-CEM | Acute lymphoblastic leukemia | T-cell | Neg | Pos | Pos |
| Raji | Burkitt lymphoma (EBV-pos) | B-cell | Neg | Pos | Neg |
| Ramos | Burkitt lymphoma (EBV-neg) | B-cell | Pos | Pos | Neg |
| HUT 78 | Cutaneous T-cell lymphoma | T-cell | Pos | Pos | Neg |
| Granta | Mantle cell lymphoma | B-cell | NA | Pos | NA |
| Granta4 | Mantle cell lymphoma | B-cell | NA | Pos | NA |
| U-937 | Histiocytic lymphoma | Monocytic | Pos | Pos | Pos |
| HL-60 | Promyelocytic leukemia | Myeloid | Neg | Pos | Pos |
| KG-1 | Acute myeloid leukemia | Myeloid | NA | Pos | NA |
| K-562 | Chronic myelogenous leukemia | Myeloid | Pos | Pos | Pos |
| NALM 16 | Acute lymphocytic leukemia | Non-T, non-B | Neg | Pos | Neg |
| 8226 | Multiple myeloma | Plasma cell | Pos | Pos | Pos |
| U266 | Multiple myeloma | Plasma cell | NA | Pos | Neg |

Expression was established by immunohistochemistry, reverse transcriptase polymerase chain reaction (RT–PCR), and northern blot analysis.
bFGF, basic fibroblast growth factor; VEGF, vascular endothelial growth factor; Ang-1, angiopoietin-1; EBV, Epstein–Barr virus; Neg, negative; Pos, positive; NA, not assessed.

**Table 14.4 Vascular endothelial growth factor (VEGF) receptor expression in human hematopoietic tumor cell lines**

| Cell line | Disease | VEGFR1 | VEGFR2 | NP-1 |
|---|---|---|---|---|
| HL-60 | AML | Pos | Neg | Pos |
| KG-1 | AML | Neg | Pos | Pos |
| NALM | ALL | Pos | Neg | Pos |
| Jurkat | ALL | Pos | Neg | NA |
| CCRF-CEM | ALL | Pos | Neg | NA |
| Molt-4 | ALL | Pos | Neg | NA |
| 8226 | Multiple myeloma | Neg | Neg | Neg/Pos[a] |
| U-266 | Multiple myeloma | Pos | Neg | Neg |
| IM-9 | Multiple myeloma | Pos | Neg | Neg |
| U-937 | Histiocytic lymphoma | Pos | Neg | Neg |
| Raji | Burkitt lymphoma (EBV-pos) | Pos | Neg | Neg |
| Ramos | Burkitt lymphoma (EBV-neg) | Pos | Neg | Neg |
| Hut78 | T-cell lymphoma | Pos | Neg | Neg |
| Granta | Mantle cell lymphoma | Pos | Neg | Neg |
| Granta4 | Mantle cell lymphoma | Neg | Neg | Neg |

Expression was established by immunohistochemistry, reverse transcriptase polymerase chain reaction (RT–PCR), and northern blot analysis.
VEGFR1, VEGF receptor 1 (Flt1); VEGFR2, VEGF receptor 2 (KDR); NP-1, neuropilin-1; AML, acute myeloid leukemia; ALL, acute lymphoblastic leukemia; EBV, Epstein–Barr Virus; Pos, positive; Neg, negative; NA, not assessed.
[a] Positive in the presence of bone marrow stromal cells.

diseases.[51,52] The following is a brief overview of the involvement of angiogenesis in hematologic malignancies.

## Multiple myeloma

Multiple myeloma (also known as plasma cell myeloma or simply as myeloma) is a B-cell neoplasia in which there is an accumulation of terminally differentiated B cells (plasma cells), primarily in the bone marrow. In most patients, the disease follows a course in which the plasma cells are predominantly in a non-proliferative phase in the bone marrow. This may be followed by an active phase in which a small percentage of proliferating tumor cells (usually < 5%) may be detected among the predominantly non-proliferating plasma cells. Finally, there is a fulminant phase with an increase in the proliferating plasmablastic compartment and in which extramedullary disease may be observed.[53] The growth of myeloma cells in the bone marrow is subject to both autocrine and paracrine regulation, and malignant plasma cells secrete a number of cytokines that act on bone marrow stromal cells (Figure 14.1).

In myeloma patients, there is a strong correlation between increased angiogenesis, as measured by microvessel density and survival. The first report demonstrating a high correlation between increased bone marrow microvascular density, plasma cell label-

ing index (a measure of proliferative activity in myeloma), and disease activity in myeloma patients was published in 1994.[54] Subsequent studies have confirmed the prognostic value of bone marrow angiogenesis in myeloma.[55–61] (Table 14.5) The increased microvessel density in myeloma has been associated with elevated levels of angiogenic cytokines, such as bFGF and VEGF, as well as MMP-2, in addition to increased marrow levels of mast cells, which are known to secrete a variety of angiogenic factors.[54,56,57,62–64]

**Table 14.5 Bone marrow angiogenesis in plasma cell disorders[a]**

| Group | Median MVD (per 400× field) | Angiogenesis grade (%) |
|---|---|---|
| Normal marrow | 1.3 | 0 |
| MGUS | 3 | 1 |
| Smoldering myeloma | 4 | 3 |
| Newly diagnosed myeloma | 11 | 29 |
| Relapsed myeloma | 20 | 42 |

MVD, microvascular density; MGUS, monoclonal gammopathy of undetermined significance.
[a] Adapted from reference 61.

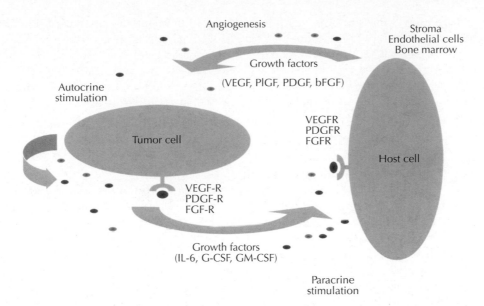

**Figure 14.1** Potential interaction in the bone marrow between tumor cells and bone marrow stromal cells. Tumor cells elaborate a variety of growth factors, including angiogenic cytokines that may act on the stromal cells to stimulate angiogenesis or the release of hematopoietic cytokines through a paracrine mechanism. In addition, subsets of tumor cells possess receptors for angiogenic growth factors such as vascular endothelial growth factor (VEGF) and basic fibroblast growth factor (bFGF), which may act on the cells in an autocrine manner to stimulate cell proliferation or mediate survival. PlGF, placental growth factor; PDGF, platelet-derived growth factor; IL-6, interleukin-6; G-CSF, granulocyte colony-stimulating factor; GM-CSF, granulocyte–macrophage CSF; . . . R, . . . receptor.

In addition to its potent angiogenic and pro-survival activities, VEGF has the potential to impact several key areas related to tumor growth and progression through autocrine- and paracrine-based mechanisms. Plasma cell expression of VEGF was observed in the bone marrow from 78% of myeloma patients,[62] and elevated levels of VEGF in the bone marrow correlate with the stage of the disease.[64] While neither the VEGFR1 nor the VEGFR2 receptors were found to be expressed by malignant plasma cells, both were markedly elevated in the normal marrow myeloid and monocytic cells surrounding the tumors in these patients. Such a pattern of expression is consistent with a paracrine role of VEGF in myeloma, although an autocrine mechanism cannot be ruled out at present. In support of a paracrine role for VEGF in myeloma, elevated levels of IL-6 induce VEGF expression in endothelial cells,[65] and elevated VEGF levels, in turn, stimulate IL-6.[62, 66]

Paracrine control mechanisms are increasingly recognized as being important for tumor growth. While the requirement of tumor–stromal interactions is well established in myeloma, the involvement of angiogenic factors, which act primarily on the stromal elements, is not fully appreciated. In myeloma, the stromal compartment is involved in interactions between the malignant plasma cells and the microenvironment of the bone marrow by means of cell–cell contact, adhesion molecules, and the release of cytokines.[53] Adhesion of myeloma cells to bone marrow stromal cells has been shown to upregulate VEGF

secretion, mediated through VEGFR1, by marrow stromal cells as well as malignant plasma cells.[67,68] In normal bone marrow as well as that of myeloma patients, endothelial cells are found in close contact with hematopoietic cells and have been demonstrated to produce IL-6, a key growth factor in myeloma.[66] Exposure of microvascular endothelial cells to VEGF results in increased expression of several growth factor cytokines, including IL-6.[62]

The potential effects of VEGF in myeloma are not limited to the neoplastic plasma cell alone. Bone disease in myeloma is the most common presenting clinical symptom, resulting in pathologic fractures and bone pain.[53] This serious complication is due in part to increased bone resorption secondary to the activation of osteoclasts.[69] Numerous osteoclast-activating factors, including tumor necrosis factor α (TNF-α), IL-1β, and IL-6, are released by myeloma cells directly or by the normal marrow cells in response to the myeloma cells.[69] Several studies have demonstrated that VEGF can directly or indirectly, through its stimulatory actions on TNF-α and IL-1β, stimulate the activation of osteoclasts, thus contributing to the lytic lesions in myeloma.[70,71]

Immunoassay of plasma cell extracts revealed significant higher levels of bFGF in patients with active myeloma than in those with smoldering myeloma or monoclonal gammopathy of undetermined significance (MGUS).[50] In vitro studies indicate that antibodies directed against bFGF inhibit the ability of conditioned media from myeloma patients to stimulate angiogenesis in a CAM assay.[59] The association of the bFGF receptor syndecan-1 (CD138) in the growth and progression of myeloma and the occurrence of the translocation involving the *FGFR3* gene in myeloma provide additional evidence for the role of angiogenesis in the pathogenesis of this disease.[72,73]

Considerable interest has been generated in targeting angiogenesis and angiogenic growth factors in myeloma and, by extension, other hematologic diseases. Thalidomide, an agent introduced to treat morning sickness in pregnant women, was marketed in Europe and Australia with disastrous consequences in the 1950s. The drug never completely disappeared, and its pariah status has recently begun to be lifted due to the recognition of its activity in several disease states, including cancer. Thalidomide undergoes rapid and spontaneous non-enzymatic hydrolytic cleavage at physiologic pH to generate up to 50 metabolites, some of which possess anti-angiogenic activity.[74] In experimental systems, thalidomide has been shown to inhibit angiogenesis induced by bFGF and VEGF.[75,76] Results of thalidomide use in myeloma are particularly promising, with thalidomide demonstrated to be beneficial in approximately one-third of patients with refractory disease, both as a single agent and in combination therapies.[58,77–82] Serial measurements of bone marrow microvessel density, however, have failed to reveal a consistent reduction among responders.[58] In addition, plasma levels of bFGF, VEGF, IL-6, and TNF-α do not appear to change appreciably in patients responding to thalidomide,[83] thus raising questions related to its mechanism of action in myeloma.

Although its anti-angiogenic effects are believed to contribute to its antimyeloma activity, thalidomide has additional effects on the cell, including inhibition of TNF-α, stimulating cytotoxic T-cell proliferation and increasing the secretion of IFN-γ and IL-2, induction of cytokine production by type 2 T helper cells, inhibition of cytokine production by type 1 T helper cells, and regulation of adhesion molecule expression. There also appears to be a direct effect on the myeloma cell and/or bone marrow stromal cell to inhibit tumor growth and survival (reviewed in reference 74).

Currently, thalidomide analogs are being examined for their efficacy and safety in myeloma patients. The first of these to reach clinical trials is CC-5013 (Revimid). As a class, these IMiDs are more potent than thalidomide at inhibiting TNF-α production and have been shown to induce apoptosis via a caspase-8-mediated mechanism in both myeloma cell lines and patient-derived material.[84] IMiDs have also been shown to target the bone marrow microenvironment by enhancing the production of IL-2 and IFN-γ relative to that achieved following treatment with thalidomide.[85]

Additional agents with anti-angiogenic properties are being assessed in myeloma, and include the proteasome inhibitor PS-341, the humanized anti-VEGF antibody bevacizumab, and several small-molecule receptor tyrosine kinase inhibitors of the VEGF pathway such as SU-5416 (Table 14.6).

### Acute myeloid leukemia

Acute myeloid leukemia (AML) is characterized by an accumulation of immature myeloid blasts in the bone marrow, finally resulting in disturbed production of normal hematopoietic cells. Different mechanisms have been recognized that contribute to the growth

---

**Table 14.6  Anti-angiogenic agents in clinical trials in hematologic malignancies**[a]

| Agent | Mechanism | Status |
|---|---|---|
| PTK787/ZK2284 | Small-molecule inhibitor of VEGF and PDGF receptors | Phase I |
| SU6668 | Small-molecule inhibitor of VEGF, FGF, and PDGF receptors | Phase I/II |
| 2-Methoxyestradiol | Inhibition of endothelial cells | Phase I/II |
| Prinomastat (AG3340) | Synthetic MMP inhibitor | Phase II |
| Neovastat | Natural MMP inhibitor | Phase II |
| Bevacizumab (Avastin) | Humanized anti-VEGF antibody | Phase II |
| PS-341 | Proteasome inhibitor | Phase II |
| CC-5013 (Revimid) | Immunomodulatory thalidomide analog | Phase II |
| Inteferon-α | Inhibition of bFGF and VEGF production | Phase II/III |
| Thalidomide | Unknown | Phase II/III |

VEGF, vascular endothelial growth factor; (b)FGF, (basic) fibroblast growth factor; PDGF, platelet-derived growth factor; MMP, matrix metalloproteinases.
[a] For a complete listing of angiogenesis inhibitors in clinical trials, the reader is referred to the website http://www.cancer.gov/clinical_trials/.

advantage of the leukemic progenitor cell. It has been demonstrated that AML cells can produce growth factors, including IL-1, IL-6, and GM-CSF, that act in an autocrine or paracrine manner, leading to spontaneous in vitro proliferation of AML cells and making them less susceptible to programmed cell death (apoptosis).

Microvessel density in AML was found to be significantly greater in leukemic bone marrow biopsy samples from untreated patients than in those from normal patient controls.[86] Following successful induction therapy, the microvessel density was shown to decrease by approximately 60% in one of these studies.[87] Additional studies have also demonstrated increased angiogenesis in AML.[88,89] Elevated VEGF levels displayed a positive correlation with both shorter overall and disease-free survival times, and proved to be an independent predictor of outcome in AML patients with high white blood cell and blast counts.[90] Interestingly, cellular VEGF levels were found to be significantly lower in one study of pediatric AML patients compared with adult AML patients, while there was no difference in VEGFR2 levels.[91] Similar to adult AML, higher VEGF and VEGFR2 levels in pediatric patients correlated with higher white blood cell counts, but, unlike the adult situation, VEGF and VEGFR-2 expression did not correlate with survival.[91] A more recent study produced contradictory results, demonstrating that VEGF expression was an independent prognostic variable in pediatric AML.[92] VEGF-stimulated endothelial cells secrete different growth factors, such as GM-CSF, G-CSF, IL-6, and macrophage colony-stimulating factor (M-CSF), that affect AML cell behavior.[62,93]

Overexpression and secretion of VEGF in approximately 70% of AML specimens has been reported in conjunction with a corresponding expression of the VEGFR1 and VEGFR2 receptors in AML blasts in approximately 50% and 20% of cases, respectively.[93] The presence of VEGFR1 and VEGFR2 on many of these cells raises the question whether VEGF acts to stimulate the cells in an autocrine manner. Using VEGFR+ cells derived from AML patients, a functional autocrine mechanism has been established.[94] With the identification of an autocrine mechanism operating in diseases such as AML, the possibility exists that overexpression of angiogenic factors in leukemias may serve two purposes. First, factors such as VEGF could promote the growth and proliferation of hematopoietic cells through direct effects. Second, they could activate pathways related to leukemic cell survival. The first suggestion that VEGF acted as a survival factor came from studies in which it was demonstrated that VEGF reduced apoptotic cell death in normal hematopoietic stem cells and tumor cell lines following exposure to ionizing radiation or chemotherapeutic agents,[95,96] in part by inducing the expression of the anti-apoptotic gene mcl-1. More

recently, it has been shown that VEGF promotes survival of endothelial cells by increasing Bcl-2 levels.[97] VEGF stimulation has also been demonstrated to increase levels of heat-shock protein 90 (Hsp90), a molecule observed to mediate anti-apoptotic and survival-promoting effects of VEGF via activation of the MAPK cascade. Elevated Hsp90 levels also serve to increase the expression of Bcl-2 and are thus likely contribute to the survival advantage of VEGFR+ leukemia subsets.[98] VEGF-C is secreted from endothelial cells in response to stimulation with bFGF or IL-1.[35] Expression of its specific receptor, VEGFR3, has been demonstrated in a subset of leukemic cells that, when stimulated by VEGF-C, promoted increased leukemia survival and proliferation.[35] The improvement in survival was apparently due to an increased Bcl-2/Bax ratio and served to protect the leukemic cells from the apoptotic effects of several cytotoxic chemotherapeutic agents.

Other angiogenic molecules reported in AML include the matrix metalloproteinases (MMP). These are a family of zinc- and calcium-dependent endopeptidases that are able to degrade extracellular matrix components. The action of MMP is counteracted by the interaction with tissue inhibitors of MMP (TIMP). Metalloproteinase-2 (MMP-2) and MMP-9 efficiently degrade native collagen types IV and V, fibronectin, and elastin to facilitate the invasion of interstitial stroma by endothelial cells.[99] MMP-2 secretion is frequently found in AML cells, but not in normal hematopoietic progenitor cells.[100] In contrast, MMP-9 is expressed in AML cells, normal mononuclear cells, and CD34+ cells.[100,101]

As in myeloma, there is an interest in targeting angiogenesis in AML. A phase I/II dose-escalating trial of thalidomide was performed to study its safety and efficacy in patients with AML.[102] A total of 20 patients, including 10 with secondary AML defined as a history of myelodysplasia, other antecedent hematologic disorders, or previous exposure to cytostatic drugs or radiotherapy, were entered into the study. Of 13 patients receiving thalidomide for longer than 4 weeks, 4 achieved a partial response. VEGF plasma levels decreased in 3 of the responders, whereas an increase was observed in 5 of 6 non-responders. In contrast to findings with thalidomide in myeloma, microvessel densities decreased significantly in the responding patients. More recently, several reports have documented inhibitory effects by small-molecule inhibitors targeting VEGFR1 and VEGFR2, such as SU5416, on the growth of a human myeloid leukemia cell line and in AML blasts, independently from their effects on angiogenesis.[103–105]

## Acute lymphoblastic leukemia

A correlation between angiogenesis and bFGF levels has been found in acute lymphoblastic leukemia

(ALL).[106] In this study of childhood ALL, there was a significant increase in the microvessel density as well as serum and urinary bFGF at diagnosis compared with a controlled group of non-leukemic patients without marrow involvement. Additional studies have demonstrated the expression of both VEGF and VEGFR1 in human ALL cell lines, thus raising the possibility that it may be playing a role in certain cases.[62]

## Chronic myelogenous leukemia

Chronic myelogenous leukemia (CML) is a clonal myeloproliferative disorder resulting from the BCR–ABL fusion oncogene.[107] As with the acute leukemias, increased angiogenesis, as evidenced by increased microvessel density, has been reported in the chronic leukemias. The bone marrow microvessel density in patients with CML is approximately twice that of controls and correlates with production of VEGF in these patients.[108,109] CML is among the diseases with the largest number of bone marrow vessels, and it came top of the list when the relative areas of vascular beds in the bone marrow of various diseases were calculated. While high VEGF levels have been demonstrated to correlate with shorter survival of patients in chronic CML, the impact of VEGF expression on the course of chronic CML is unknown and no significant differences have been observed in VEGF levels based on the phase of the disease.[110]

Murine cells transfected with BCR–ABL constructs have been shown to secrete a variety of angiogenic factors, including VEGF, bFGF, IL-8, and MMP-2 and -9 and to stimulate angiogenesis in in vitro models.[111] Myeloblasts from the bone marrow of Philadelphia-positive CML patients secreted up to 10 times more VEGF, bFGF, and IL-8 as compared with myeloblasts obtained from normal donors.[111] In addition, peripheral blood mononuclear cells isolated from CML patients expressed both MMP-2 and MMP-9.

## Chronic lymphocytic leukemia

Bone marrow MVD from patients with B-cell chronic lymphocytic leukemia (CLL) was significantly increased when compared with normal bone marrows,[112] and correlated with the clinical stage. Increased intracellular levels of VEGF and expression of VEGFR2 correlated with a poor prognosis in patients with CLL.[113–115]

In addition to VEGF, increased intracellular, urinary, and plasma levels of bFGF have been reported in CLL and have been shown to correlate with disease stage.[112,113,116,117] Mechanistically, increased intracellular bFGF levels have been demonstrated to increase the expression of Bcl-2, thereby augmenting apoptotic resistance.[118]

While it has now been well established that B-CLL cells produce several pro-angiogenic factors, it has also been demonstrated that they are capable of producing and secreting several anti-angiogenic molecules, including endostatin, IFN-α, and thrombospondin-1.[117] The significance of this finding is unclear, but it is interesting to speculate that it might be related to the angiogenic switch that occurs in hematologic tumors just as it does in solid tumors. Mutations in p53 are fairly common in advanced CLL and are known to downregulate thrombospondin-1.[119]

## Myelodysplasia

Myelodysplastic syndromes (MDS) are preleukemic disorders, particularly in patients who present with measurable leukemia burden or unfavorable karyotype. Ineffective hematopoiesis, the hallmark of MDS, arises from underlying genetic aberrations leading to alterations in cytokine regulation and response to cytokines, with a consequent increased apoptosis of hematopoietic progenitor cells and aberrant hematopoiesis.[120] Generally 35–40% of MDS cases transform to AML, and most patients die from infection or bleeding.[120]

The microvessel density has been found to be significantly greater in patients with advanced MDS, including those with refractory anemia with excess blasts in transformation (RAEB-t) or chronic myelomonocytic leukemia (CMML) compared with refractory anemia with excess blasts (RAEB), refractory anemia (RA), or refractory anemia with ring sideroblasts (RARS).[121] Following successful induction chemotherapy, the microvessel density has been demonstrated to decrease significantly.[87]

Cytologically, VEGF is expressed by immature myeloid elements, particularly leukemic monocytoid precursors, but not erythroid elements or lymphocytes (Figure 14.2).[94] Increased expression of VEGF in MDS appears to correlate with the high frequency of ras proto-oncogene activation found in these tumors, which is known to induce VEGF gene expression. Foci of abnormal localization of immature precursors (ALIP) often indicate transformation to a higher grade of MDS. These foci of myelomonocytic precursors coexpress VEGF and VEGFR1, suggesting the possibility of an autocrine mechanism. Support for this was derived from VEGF neutralization studies that were shown to suppress leukemia progenitor formation in a concentration-dependent manner, whereas recombinant human (rHu)VEGF promoted the growth of leukemia colonies.[94] rHuVEGF promoted in vitro expansion of myeloid progenitors while inhibiting the formation of erythroid bursts and multipotent progenitors; thus, excessive local elaboration of VEGF may accelerate apoptotic death of receptor-naive erythroid progenitors.[94] VEGF neutralization also suppressed the concentrations of TNF-α and IL-1β in

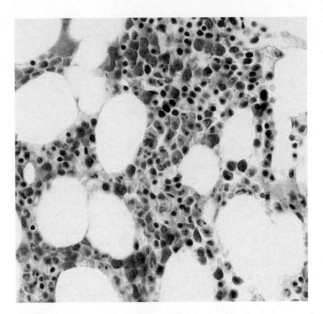

**Figure 14.2** Immunohistochemical staining for vascular endothelial factor (VEGF) in the bone marrow of a patient with MDS. VEGF was expressed in a diffuse cytoplasmic pattern predominantly in the myeloid and monocytic precursors. (400× magnification)

supernatants from control bone marrow mononuclear cultures, whereas the addition of rHuVEGF resulted in increased levels of these cytokines, thereby suggesting an additional mechanism where non-VEGFR-expressing cells may also be affected.

MDS have few therapeutic options, none of which is curative, particularly if hematopoietic stem cell transplantation is not an option.[122] As in other hematologic malignancies, there is an increased interest in therapies directed against angiogenesis in MDS. In several clinical trials examining the use of thalidomide in MDS patients, responses have been reported.[123–125] Although no complete responses have been described, there has been marked hematologic improvement, particularly in the erythroid series, with several previously transfusion-dependent patients becoming transfusion-independent. As in myeloma, it is unclear whether the reduction in blast cells that is observed in the bone marrow of high-risk MDS patients is attributable to a cytotoxic effect of thalidomide on the malignant cells or to a modulation of their interaction with the bone marrow microenvironment.

## Lymphomas

Elevated levels of angiogenesis and angiogenic growth factors are also associated with adverse prognosis in patients with non-Hodgkin lymphoma (NHL). Excessive angiogenesis has been shown in lymph nodes of patients with hyperplastic and dysplastic B-cell disorders, such as Castleman's disease.[126] In a study of 88 patients with B-cell NHL representing mixed subtypes, there was an increase in the microvessel density in lymph nodes that correlated with the severity of the disease, increasing from low-grade to high-grade subtypes (i.e. follicular versus diffuse large cell; Figure 14.3).[127] Increased angiogenesis, as reflected by microvessel density, has also been described in T-cell lymphomas such as mycosis fungoides.[128]

VEGF has been implicated in the overall course of this disease, however. Elevated levels of both VEGF and bFGF have been reported in NHL and are associated with an adverse prognosis, with those patients having elevated levels of both growth factors in the highest-risk group.[129] VEGF is expressed in the tumor vasculature as well as in the malignant cells in the majority of NHL patient samples studied to date. The expression of VEGF and its receptors was related to tumor grade, with a higher percentage of VEGF-positive cells in the intermediate/high-grade group than in low-grade lymphomas. These findings were in contrast to reactive lymphoid tissues, where there was an absence of VEGF expression in normal lymphocytes. In addition

**(a)**  **(b)**

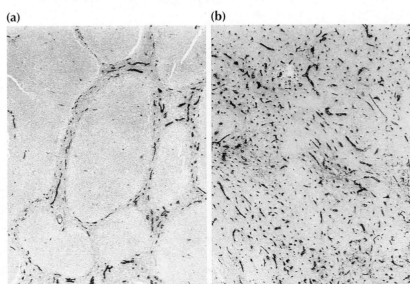

**Figure 14.3** CD31-related antigen staining of vasculature in non-Hodgkin lymphoma. (a) A case of follicular lymphoma demonstrating staining primarily limited to the perifollicular areas. (b) Large cell lymphoma demonstrating a diffuse pattern of vascular staining. (40× magnification)

to VEGF expression, the neoplastic lymphocytes from both low-grade and high-grade lymphomas were found to express VEGFR1 and VEGFR2, with VEGFR1 being observed more frequently but VEGFR2 being expressed solely in the higher-grade tumors. In another series of NHL patients, VEGF was expressed in 96% of cases.[130] Both hypoxia-inducible factors 1α and 2α were only weakly expressed in these cases, suggesting that VEGF expression may not be hypoxically driven in the setting of NHL. Expression of the anti-apoptotic factor MCL1 correlated with VEGF expression and was found to be elevated in patients with progressive NHL as compared with those achieving a complete remission.[131] VEGF expression has also been demonstrated in Hodgkin lymphoma, where it was found to be expressed in the Reed–Sternberg cells.[132] Although there was expression of VEGF in the tumor cells, there was no correlation between VEGF expression and the subtype of Hodgkin lymphoma or with microvessel density. Immunohistochemical detection of bFGF and its receptor FGFR1 has also been demonstrated in patients with NHL, but the expression did not correlate with either serum bFGF levels or microvascular densities.[133] Patients whose tumors expressed bFGF did, however, have a poor prognosis.

Serum levels of both VEGF and bFGF are elevated in NHL and correlate with high-grade disease and poor prognosis.[129,134] The highest prognostic power was observed when VEGF and serum bFGF levels were examined in combination. The risk of death in patients whose VEGF and bFGF levels were both within the highest quartiles was nearly three times greater than it was for other patients.[129]

Evidence for a functional role of VEGFR2 during lymphoma growth was provided by experiments studying the effects of a function-blocking antibody for VEGFR2 that has been demonstrated to inhibit proliferation in mice bearing human tumors.[135] Based on such findings, inhibition of VEGF or signaling by VEGFR1 and VEGFR2 may be effective in the treatment of hematologic malignancies, since it potentially interferes with both hallmarks of tumor growth – angiogenesis and tumor cell proliferation. Mantle cell lymphoma, an aggressive subtype of NHL, has been reported to respond to single-agent thalidomide.[136] Clinical trials are currently underway examining the efficacy of a humanized anti-VEGF antibody, bevacizumab, in refractory NHL.

## Conclusions

Numerous studies have now established the presence of elevated angiogenesis and the expression of a variety of angiogenic growth factors in hematopoietic malignancies, suggesting a role in the pathobiology of these diseases. There is increasing evidence that angiogenic growth factors play a role in hematologic malignancies. Production of these factors by malignant hematopoietic cells may serve as both an autocrine growth stimulus and a diffusible paracrine signal mediating the local generation of growth factors that foster tumor survival and self-renewal. Adding support to the hypothesis that angiogenic factors are playing a functional role in these tumors are the recent reports that thalidomide has been demonstrated to be effective in patients with refractory myeloma and other hematologic diseases. Although the mechanism responsible for such efficacy remains to be established, thalidomide has been demonstrated to possess anti-angiogenic activity. The presence of tumor angiogenesis and the elevated expression of angiogenic growth factors thus suggest new targets for therapeutic intervention in these disorders, and the initiation of clinical trials to assess anti-angiogenic therapies is well underway.

## Acknowledgment

This work was supported in part by funding from NIH Grant CA 90821, the Multiple Myeloma Research Foundation.

## REFERENCES

1. Folkman J, Clinical applications of research on angiogenesis. *N Engl J Med* 1995; **333**: 1757–63.
2. Folkman J. Angiogenesis in cancer, vascular, rheumatoid and other diseases. *Nat Med* 1995; **1**: 27–31.
3. Hanahan D, Weinberg RA. The hallmarks of cancer. *Cell* 2000; **100**: 57–70.
4. Veikkola T, Karkkainen M, Claesson-Welsh L et al. Regulation of angiogenesis via vascular endothelial growth factor receptors. *Cancer Res* 2000; **60**: 203–12.
5. Carmeliet P. Mechanisms of angiogenesis and arteriogenesis. *Nat Med* 2000; **3**: 389–95.
6. Folkman J. Angiogenesis. In: Braunwald E, Fauci AS, Kasper DL et al (eds) *Harrison's Textbook of Internal Medicine*, 15th edn. New York: McGraw-Hill, 2001: 517–30.
7. Weidner N, Semple JP, Welch WR et al. Tumor angiogenesis and metastasis – correlation in invasive breast carcinoma. *N Engl J Med* 1991; **324**: 1–8.
8. Weidner N, Carroll PR, Flax J et al. Tumor angiogenesis correlates with metastasis in invasive prostate carcinoma. *Am J Pathol* 1993; **143**: 401–9.
9. Fontanini G, Bigini D, Vignati S et al. Microvessel count predicts metastatic disease and survival in non-small cell lung cancer. *J Pathol* 1995; **177**: 57–63.
10. Meiter D, Crawford SE, Rademaker AW et al. Tumor angiogenesis correlates with metastatic disease, N-myc amplification, and poor outcome in human neuroblastoma. *J Clin Oncol* 1996; **14**: 405–14.
11. Gasparini G, Harris AL. Clinical importance of the

determination of tumor angiogenesis in breast carcinoma: much more than a new prognostic tool. *J Clin Oncol* 1995; **13**: 765–82.

12. Rak J, Filmus J, Finkenzeller G et al. Oncogenes as inducers of tumor angiogenesis. *Cancer Metastasis Rev* 1995; **14**: 263–77.

13. Hanahan D, Folkman J. Patterns and emerging mechanisms of the angiogenic switch during tumorigenesis. *Cell* 1996; **86**: 353–64.

14. Yu JL, Rak JW, Coomber BL et al. Effect of *p53* status on tumor response to antiangiogenic therapy. *Science* 2002; **295**: 1525–8.

15. Lecouter J, Kowalski J, Foster et al. Identification of an angiogenic mitogen selective for endocrine gland endothelium. *Nature* 2001; **412**: 877–84.

16. Carmeliet P, Moons L, Luttun A et al. Synergism between vascular endothelial growth factor and placental growth factor contributes to angiogenesis and plasma extravasation in pathological conditions. *Nat Med* 2001; **7**: 575–83.

17. Folkman J. Tumor angiogenesis: therapeutic implications. *N Engl J Med* 1971; **285**: 1182–6.

18. Liotta LA, Stracke ML. Tumor invasion and metastases: biochemical mechanisms. *Cancer Treat Res* 1998; **40**: 223–38.

19. Holmgren L, O'Reilly MS, Folkman J. Dormancy of micrometastases: balanced proliferation and apoptosis in the presence of angiogenesis suppression. *Nat Med* 1995; **1**: 149–53.

20. Sunderkotter C, Steinbrink K, Goebeler M et al. Macrophages and angiogenesis. *J Leukocyte Biol* 1994; **55**: 410–22.

21. Shing Y, Folkman J, Sullivan R et al. Heparin-affinity: purification of a tumor-derived capillary endothelial cell growth factor. *Science* 1984; **223**: 1296–9.

22. Leung DW, Cachianes G, Kuang W-J et al. Vascular endothelial growth factor is a secreted angiogenic mitogen. *Science* 1989; **246**: 1306–9.

23. Dvorak HF, Orenstein NS, Carvalho AC et al. Induction of a fibrin-gel investment: an early event in line 10 hepatocarcinoma growth mediated by tumor-secreted products. *J Immunol* 1979; **122**: 166–74.

24. Brown LF, Detmar M, Claffey K et al. Vascular permeability factor/vascular endothelial growth factor: a multifunctional angiogenic cytokine. In: Goldberg ID, Rosen EM (eds) *Regulation of Angiogenesis*. Basel: Birkhäuser, 1997: 233–69.

25. Bellamy WT. Expression of vascular endothelial growth factor and its receptors in multiple myeloma and other hematopoietic malignancies. *Semin Oncol* 2001; **28**: 551–9.

26. Ferrara N, Gerber HP. The role of vascular endothelial growth factor in angiogenesis. *Acta Haematol* 2001; **106**: 148–56.

27. Berger DP, Herbstritt L, Dengler WA et al. Vascular endothelial growth factor (VEGF) mRNA expression in human tumor models of different histologies. *Ann Oncol* 1995; **6**: 817–25.

28. Brown L, Berse B, Jackman R. Expression of vascular permeability factor (vascular endothelial growth factor) and its receptors in breast cancer. *Hum Pathol* 1995; **26**: 86–91.

29. Ohta Y, Endo Y, Tanaka M et al. Significance of vascular endothelial growth factor messenger RNA expression in primary lung cancer. *Clin Cancer Res* 1996; **2**: 1411–16.

30. Rak J, Mitsuhashi Y, Bayko L et al. Mutant *ras* oncogenes upregulate VEGF expression: implications for induction and inhibition of tumor angiogenesis. *Cancer Res* 1995; **55**: 4575–80.

31. Fleming RY, Ellis LM, Parikh NU et al. Regulation of vascular endothelial growth factor expression in human colon carcinoma cells by activity of src kinase. *Surgery* 1997; **122**: 501–7.

32. Kim JK, Li B, Winer J et al. Inhibition of vascular endothelial growth factor-induced angiogenesis suppresses tumor growth in vivo. *Nature* 1993; **362**: 841–4.

33. Weng DE, Usman N. Angiozyme: a novel angiogenesis inhibitor. *Curr Oncol Rep* 2001; **3**: 141–6.

34. Hiratsuka S, Maru Y, Okada A et al. Involvement of the Flt-1 tyrosine kinase (vascular endothelial growth factor receptor-1) in pathological angiogenesis. *Cancer Res* 2001; **61**: 1207–13.

35. Dias S, Choy M, Alitalo K et al. Vascular endothelial growth factor (VEGF)-C signaling through Flt-4 (VEGFR-3) mediates leukemic cell proliferation, survival, and resistance to chemotherapy. *Blood* 2002; **99**: 2179–84.

36. Soker S, Takashima S, Miao HQ et al. Neuropilin-1 is expressed by endothelial and tumor cells as an isoform-specific receptor for vascular endothelial growth factor. *Cell* 1998; **92**: 735–45.

37. Bachelder RE, Crago A, Chung C et al. Vascular endothelial growth factor is an autocrine survival factor for neuropilin-expressing breast carcinoma cells. *Cancer Res* 2001; **61**: 5736–40.

38. Cao Y, O'Reilly MS, Marshall B et al. Expression of angiostatin cDNA in a murine fibrosarcoma suppresses primary tumor growth and produces long-term dormancy of metastases. *J Clin Invest* 1998; **101**: 1055–63.

39. Poon RT, Fan ST, Wong J. Clinical implications of circulating angiogenic factors in cancer patients. *J Clin Oncol* 2001; **19**: 1207–25.

40. Zon LI. Developmental biology of hematopoiesis. *Blood* 1995; **86**: 2876–91.

41. Gabbianelli M, Sargiacomo M, Pelosi E et al. Pure human hematogenic progenitors: permissive action of basic fibroblast growth factor. *Science* 1990; **249**: 1561–4.

42. Wilson EL, Rifkin DB, Kelly F. Basic fibroblast growth factor stimulates myelopoiesis in long-term human bone marrow cultures. *Blood* 1994; **77**: 954–60.

43. Ferrara N, Carver Moore K et al. Heterozygous embryonic lethality induced by targeted inactivation of the *VEGF* gene. *Nature* 1996; **380**: 439–42.

44. Shalaby F, Rossant J, Yamaguchi TP et al. Failure of blood-island formation and vasculogenesis in Flk1-deficient mice. *Nature* 1995; **376**: 62–6.

45. Fong G-H, Rossant J, Gertsenstein M et al. Role of the Flt1 receptor tyrosine kinase in regulating the assembly of vascular endothelium. *Nature* 1995; **376**: 66–70.

46. Bautz F, Rafii S, Kanz L et al. Expression and secretion of vascular endothelial growth factor-A by cytokine-stimulated hematopoietic progenitor cells. Possible role in the hematopoietic microenvironment. *Exp Hematol* 2000; **28**: 700–6.

47. Kabrun N, Buhring HJ, Choi K et al. Flk-1 expression defines a population of early embryonic hematopoietic precursors. *Development* 1997; **124**: 2039–48.

48. Ziegler BL, Valtieri M, Porada GA et al. KDR receptor: a key marker defining hematopoietic stem cells. *Science* 1999; **285**: 1553–8.

49. Hattori K, Dias S, Heissig B et al. Vascular endothelial growth factor and angiopoietin-1 stimulate postnatal hematopoiesis by recruitment of vasculogenic and hematopoietic stem cells. *J Exp Med* 2001; **193**: 1005–14.

50. Lyden D, Hattori K, Dias S et al. Impaired recruitment of bone-marrow-derived endothelial and hematopoietic precursor cells blocks tumor angiogenesis and growth. *Nat Med* 2001; **7**: 1194–2020.

51. Folkman J. Angiogenesis-dependent diseases. *Semin Oncol* 2001; **28**: 536–42.

52. Scappaticci FA, Smith R, Pathat A et al. Combination angiostatin and endostatin gene transfer induces synergistic antiangiogenic activity in vitro and antitumor efficacy in leukemia and solid tumors in mice. *Mol Ther* 2001; **3**: 186–96.

53. Bataille R, Harousseau JL. Multiple myeloma. *N Engl J Med* 1997; **336**: 1657–64.

54. Vacca A, Ribatti D, Roneali L et al. Bone marrow angiogenesis and progression in multiple myeloma. *Br J Haematol* 1994; **87**: 503–8.

55. Vacca A, Di Loreto M, Ribatti D et al. Bone marrow of patients with active multiple myeloma: angiogenesis and plasma cell adhesion molecules LFA-1, VLA-4, LAM-1 and CD44. *Am J Hematol* 1995; **50**: 9–14.

56. Nguyen M, Tran C, Barsky S et al. Thalidomide and chemotherapy combination: preliminary results of preclinical studies. *Int J Oncol* 1997; **10**: 965–9.

57. Rajkumar SV, Fonseca R, Witzig TE et al. Bone marrow angiogenesis in patients achieving complete response after stem cell transplantation for multiple myeloma. *Leukemia* 1999; **13**: 469–72.

58. Singhal S, Mehta J, Desikan R et al. Antitumor activity of thalidomide in refractory multiple myeloma. *N Engl J Med* 1999; **341**: 1565–71.

59. Vacca A, Ribatti D, Presta M et al. Bone marrow neovascularization, plasma cell angiogenic potential, and matrix metalloproteinase-2 secretion parallel progression of human multiple myeloma. *Blood* 1999; **93**: 3064–73.

60. Rajkumar SV, Leong T, Roche PC et al. Prognostic value of bone marrow angiogenesis in multiple myeloma. *Clin Cancer Res* 2000; **6**: 3111–16.

61. Rajkumar SV, Measa R, Fonseca R et al. Bone marrow angiogenesis in 400 patients with monoclonal gammopathy of undetermined significance, multiple myeloma, and primary amyloidosis. *Clin Cancer Res* 2002; **8**: 2210–16.

62. Bellamy WT, Richter L, Frutiger Y et al. Expression of vascular endothelial growth factor (VEGF) and its receptors in hematopoietic malignancies. *Cancer Res* 1999; **59**: 728–33.

63. Ribatti D, Vacca A, Nico B et al. Bone marrow angiogenesis and mast cell density increase simultaneously with progression of human multiple myeloma. *Br J Cancer* 1999; **79**: 451–5.

64. Di Raimondo F, Azzaro MP, Palumbo G et al. Angiogenic factors in multiple myeloma: higher levels in bone marrow than in peripheral blood. *Haematologica* 2000; **85**: 800–5.

65. Cohen T, Nahari D, Cerem LW et al. Interleukin 6 induces the expression of vascular endothelial growth factor. *J Biol Chem* 1996; **271**: 736–41.

66. Dankhar B, Padro T, Leo R et al. Vascular endothelial growth factor and interleukin-6 in paracrine tumor-stromal cell interactions in multiple myeloma. *Blood* 2000; **95**: 2630–6.

67. Gupta D, Treon S, Shima Y et al. Adherence of multiple myeloma cells to bone marrow stromal cells upregulates vascular endothelial growth factor secretion: therapeutic applications. *Leukemia* 2001; **15**: 1950–61.

68. Podar K, Tai Y-T, Davies FE et al. Vascular endothelial growth factor triggers signaling cascades mediating multiple myeloma cell growth and migration. *Blood* 2001; **98**: 428–35.

69. Croucher PI, Apperley JF. Bone disease in myeloma. *Br J Haematol* 1998; **103**: 902–10.

70. Deckers MM, Karperien M, van der Bent C et al. Expression of vascular endothelial growth factors and their receptors during osteoblast differentiation. *Endocrinology* 2000; **141**: 1667–74.

71. Nakagawa M, Kaneda T, Arakawa T et al. Vascular endothelial growth factor (VEGF) directly enhances osteoclastic bone resorption and survival of mature osteoclasts. *FEBS Lett* 2000; **473**: 161–4.

72. Witzig TE, Kimlinger T, Stenson M et al. Syndecan-1 expression on malignant cells from the blood and marrow of patients with plasma cell proliferative disorders and B-cell chronic lymphocytic leukemia. *Leuk Lymphoria* 1998; **31**: 167–75.

73. Chesi M, Nardini E, Brents LA et al. Frequent translocation t(4;14)(p16.3;q32.3) in multiple myeloma is associated with increased expression and activating mutations of fibroblast growth factor receptor 3. *Nat Genet* 1997; **16**: 260–4.

74. Richardson P, Hideshima T, Anderson K. Thalidomide: emerging role in cancer medicine. *Annu Rev Med* 2002; **53**: 629–57.

75. D'Amato RJ, Loughnan MS, Flynn E et al. Thalidomide is an inhibitor of angiogenesis. *Proc Natl Acad Sci USA* 1994; **91**: 4082–5.

76. Kenyon BM, Browne F, D'Amato RJ. Effects of thalidomide and related metabolites in a mouse corneal model of neovascularization. *Exp Eye Res* 1997; **64**: 971–8.

77. Weber DM, Gavino M, Delasalle K et al. Thalidomide alone or with dexamethasone for multiple myeloma. *Blood* 1999; **94**: 604a.

78. Kneller A, Raanani P, Hardan I et al. Therapy with thalidomide in refractory multiple myeloma – the revival of an old drug. *Br J Haematol* 2000; **108**: 391–3.

79. Rajkumar SV, Fonseca R, Dispenzieri A et al. Thalidomide in the treatment of relapsed multiple myeloma. *Mayo Clin Proc* 2000; **75**: 897–901.

80. Barlogie B, Desikan R, Eddlemon P et al. Extended survival in advanced and refractory multiple myeloma after single-agent thalidomide: identification of prognostic factors in a phase 2 study of 169 patients. *Blood* 2001; **98**: 492–4.

81. Bertolini F, Mingrone W, Alietti A et al. Thalidomide in multiple myeloma, myelodysplastic syndromes and histiocytosis. Analysis of clinical results and of surrogate angiogenesis markers. *Ann Oncol* 2001; **12**: 987–90.

82. Kyle RA, Rajkumar SV. Therapeutic application of thalidomide in multiple myeloma. *Semin Oncol* 2001; **28**: 583–7.

83. Neben K, Moehler T, Kraemer A et al. Response to thalidomide in progressive multiple myeloma is not mediated by inhibition of angiogenic cytokine secretion. *Br J Haematol* 2001; **115**: 605–8.

84. Mitsiades N, Mitsiades CO, Poulaki V et al. Apoptotic signaling induced by immunomodulatory thalidomide

analogs in human multiple myeloma cells: therapeutic implications. *Blood* 2002; **99**: 4525–30.

85. Hideshima T, Chauhan D, Shima Y et al. Thalidomide and its analogs overcome drug resistance of human multiple myeloma cells to conventional chemotherapy. *Blood* 2000; **96**: 2943–50.

86. Hussong J, Rodgers GM, Shami PJ. Evidence of increased angiogenesis in patients with acute myeloid leukemia. *Blood* 2000; **95**: 309–13.

87. Pardo T, Ruiz S, Bieker R et al. Increased angiogenesis in the bone marrow of patients with acute myeloid leukemia. *Blood* 2000; **95**: 2637–44.

88. de Bont ES, Rosati S, Jacobs S et al. Increased bone marrow vascularization in patients with acute myeloid leukemia: a possible role for vascular endothelial growth factor. *Br J Haematol* 2001; **113**: 296–304.

89. Kini AR, Peterson LC, Tallman MS et al. Angiogenesis in acute promyelocytic leukemia: induction by vascular endothelial growth factor and inhibition by all-*trans* retinoic acid. *Blood* 2001; **97**: 3919–24.

90. Aguayo A, Estey E, Kantarjian H et al. Cellular vascular endothelial growth factor is a predictor of outcome in patients with acute myeloid leukemia. *Blood* 1999; **94**: 3717–21.

91. Jeha S, Smith FO, Estey E et al. Comparison between pediatric acute myeloid leukemia (AML) and adult AML in VEGF and KDR (VEGF-R2) protein levels. *Leuk Res* 2002; **26**: 399–402.

92. de Bont ESJM, Fidler V, Meeuwsen T et al. Vascular endothelial growth factor secretion is an independent prognostic factor for relapse-free survival in pediatric acute myeloid luekmeia patients. *Clin Cancer Res* 2002; **8**: 2856–61.

93. Fielder W, Graeven U, Ergun S et al. Vascular endothelial growth factor, a possible paracrine growth factor in human acute myeloid leukemia. *Blood* 1997; **89**: 1870–5.

94. Bellamy WT, Richter L, Sirjani D et al. Vascular endothelial cell growth factor (VEGF) is an autocrine promoter of abnormal localized immature myeloid precursors (ALIP) and leukemia progenitor formation in myelodysplastic syndromes. *Blood* 2001; **97**: 1427–34.

95. Katoh O, Tauchi H, Kawaishi K et al. Expression of the vascular endothelial growth factor (VEGF) receptor gene, *KDR*, in hematopoietic cells and inhibitory effect of VEGF on apoptotic cell death caused by ionizing radiation. *Cancer Res* 1995; **55**: 5687–92.

96. Katoh O, Takahashi T, Oguri T et al. Vascular endothelial growth factor inhibits apoptotic death in hematopoietic cells after exposure to chemotherapeutic drugs by inducing MCL-1 acting as an antiapoptotic factor. *Cancer Res* 1998; **58**: 5565–9.

97. Nor JE, Christensen J, Mooney DJ et al. Vascular endothelial growth factor (VEGF)-mediated angiogenesis is associated with enhanced endothelial cell survival and induction of Bcl-2 expression. *Am J Pathol* 1999; **154**: 375–84.

98. Dias S, Shmelkov S, Lam G et al. VEGF165 promotes survival of leukemic cells by Hsp-90-mediated induction of Bcl-2 expression and apoptosis inhibition. *Blood* 2002; **99**: 2532–40.

99. Mignatti P, Rifkin DB. Biology and biochemistry of proteinases in tumor invasion. *Physiol Rev* 1993; **73**: 161–95.

100. Janowska-Wieczorek A, Marquez LA, Matsuzaki A et al. Expression of matrix metalloproteinases (MMP-2 and -9)

and tissue inhibitors of metalloproteinases (TIMP-1 and -2) in acute myelogenous leukemia blasts: comparison with normal bone marrow cells. *Br J Haematol* 1999; **105**: 402–11.

101. Ries C, Loher F, Zang C et al. Matrix metalloproteinases production by bone marrow mononuclear cells from normal individuals and patients with acute and chronic myeloid leukemia or myelodysplastic syndromes. *Clin Cancer Res* 1999; **5**: 1115–24.

102. Steins MB, Padro T, Bieker R et al. Efficacy and safety of thalidomide in patients with acute myeloid leukemia. *Blood* 2002; **99**: 834–9.

103. Smolich BD, Yuen HA, West K et al. The antiangiogenic protein kinase inhibitors SU5416 and SU6668 inhibit the SCF receptor (c-kit) in a human myeloid leukemia cell line and in acute myeloid leukemia blasts. *Blood* 2001; **97**: 1413–21.

104. Lin B, Podar K, Gupta D et al. The vascular endothelial growth factor receptor tyrosine kinase inhibitor PTK787/ZK222584 inhibits growth and migration of multiple myeloma cells in the bone marrow microenvironment. *Cancer Res* 2002; **62**: 5019–26.

105. Mesters RM, Padro T, Bieker R et al. Stable remission after administration of the receptor tyrosine kinase inhibitor SU5416 in a patient with refractory acute myeloid leukemia. *Blood* 2001; **98**: 241–3.

106. Perez-Atayde AR, Sallan SE, Tedrow U et al. Spectrum of tumor angiogenesis in the bone marrow of children with acute lymphoblastic leukemia. *Am J Pathol* 1997; **150**: 815–21.

107. Deininger MWN, Goldman JM, Melo JV. The molecular biology of chronic myeloid leukemia. *Blood* 2000; **96**: 3343–57.

108. Aguayo A, Kantarjian H, Manshouri T et al. Angiogenesis in acute and chronic leukemias and myelodysplastic syndromes. *Blood* 2000; **96**: 2240–5.

109. Lundberg LG, Lerner R, Sundelin P et al. Bone marrow in polycythemia vera, chronic myelocytic leukemia, and myelofibrosis has an increased vascularity. *Am J Pathol* 2000; **157**: 15–19.

110. Verstovsek S, Kantarjian H, Manshouri T et al. Prognostic significance of cellular vascular endothelial growth factor expression in chronic phase chronic myeloid leukemia. *Blood* 2002; **99**: 2265–7.

111. Janowska-Wieczorek A, Majka M, Marquez-Curtis L et al. Bcr–abl-positive cells secrete angiogenic factors including matrix metalloproteinases and stimulate angiogenesis in vivo in Matrigel implants. *Leukemia* 2002; **16**: 1160–6.

112. Kini AR, Kay NE, Peterson LC. Increased bone marrow angiogenesis in B-cell chronic lymphocytic leukemia. *Leukemia* 2000; **14**: 1414–18.

113. Aguayo A, O'Brien S, Ketting M et al. Clinical relevance of intracellular vascular endothelial growth factor levels in B-cell chronic lymphocytic leukemia. *Blood* 2000; **96**: 768–70.

114. Molica S, Vitelli G, Levato D et al. Increased serum levels of vascular endothelial growth factor predict disk of progression in early B-cell chronic lymphocytic leukaemia. *Br J Haematol* 1999; **107**: 605–10.

115. Ferrajoli A, Manshouri T, Estrov Z et al. High levels of vascular endothelial growth factor receptor-2 correlate with shortened survival in chronic lymphocytic leukemia. *Clin Cancer Res* 2001; **7**: 795–9.

116. Duensing S, Atzpodien J. Increased intracellular and

plasma levels of basic fibroblast growth factor in B-cell chronic lymphocytic leukemia. *Blood* 1995; **85**: 1978–80.

117. Kay NE, Bone ND, Tschumper RC et al. B-CLL cells are capable of synthesis and secretion of both pro- and anti-angiogenic molecules. *Leukemia* 2002; **16**: 911–19.

118. Konig A, Menzel T, Lynen S et al. Basic fibroblast growth factor (bFGF) upregulates the expression of bcl-2 in B cell chronic lymphocytic leukemia cell lines resulting in delaying apoptosis. *Leukemia* 1997; **11**: 258–65.

119. Grant S, Kyshtoobayeva A, Kurosaki T et al. Mutant p53 correlates with reduced expression of thrombospondin-1, increased angiogenesism and metastatic progression in melanoma. *Cancer Detect Prevent* 1998; **22**: 185–94.

120. Silverman L, Holland JF, Frei E et al. The myelodysplastic syndrome. In: Holland JF, Frei E (eds) *Cancer Medicine*, 5th edn Hamilton, Ontario: Decker, 2000: 1931–46.

121. Pruneri G, Bertolini F, Soligo D et al. Angiogenesis in myelodysplastic syndromes. *Br J Cancer* 1999; **81**: 1398–401.

122. Preisler HD. The treatment of myelodysplastic syndromes. *Cancer* 1999; **86**: 1893–9.

123. Raza A, Meyer P, Dutt D et al. Thalidomide produces transfusion independence in long-standing refractory anemias of patients with myelodysplastic syndromes. *Blood* 2001; **98**: 958–65.

124. Zorat F, Shetty V, Dutt D et al. The clinical and biological effects of thalidomide in patients with myelodysplastic syndromes. *Br J Haematol* 2001; **115**: 881–94.

125. Strupp C, Germing U, Aivado M et al. Thalidomide for the treatment of patients with myelodysplastic syndromes. *Leukemia* 2002; **16**: 1–6.

126. Foss HD, Araujo I, Demel G et al. Expression of vascular endothelial growth factor in lymphomas and Castleman's disease. *J Pathol* 1997; **183**: 44–50.

127. Ribatti D, Vacca RD, Nico B et al. Angiogenesis spectrum in the stroma of B-cell non-Hodgkin's lymphomas. An immunohistochemical and ultrastructural study. *Eur J Haematol* 1996; **56**: 45–53.

128. Vacca A, Moretti S, Ribatti D et al. Progression of mycosis fungoides is associated with changes in angiogenesis and expression of the matrix metalloproteinases 2 and 9. *Eur J Cancer* 1997; **33**: 1685–92.

129. Salven P, Orpana A, Teerenhovi L et al. Simultaneous elevation in the serum concentrations of the angiogenic growth factors VEGF and bFGF is an independent predictor of poor prognosis in non-Hodgkin lymphoma: a single-institution study of 200 patients. *Blood* 2000; **96**: 3712–18.

130. Stewart M, Talks K, Leek R et al. Expression of angiogenic factors and hypoxia inducible factors HIF 1, HIF 2 and CA IX in non-Hodgkin's lymphoma. *Histopathology* 2002; **40**: 253–60.

131. Kuramoto K, Sakai A, Shigemasa K et al. High expression of *MCL1* gene related to vascular endothelial growth factor is associated with poor outcome in non-Hodgkin's lymphoma. *Br J Haematol* 2002; **116**: 158–61.

132. Doussis-Anagnostopoulou IA, Talks KL, Turley H et al. Vascular endothelial growth factor (VEGF) is expressed by neoplastic Hodgkin–Reed–Sternberg cells in Hodgkin's disease. *J Pathol* 2002; **197**: 677–83.

133. Pazgal I, Zimra Y, Tzabar C et al. Expression of basic fibroblast growth factor is associated with poor outcome in non-Hodgkin's lymphoma. *Br J Cancer* 2002; **86**: 1770–5.

134. Bertolini F, Paolucci M, Peccatori F et al. Angiogenic growth factors and endostatin in non-Hodgkin's lymphoma. *Br J Haematol* 1999; **106**: 504–9.

135. Dias S, Hattori K, Heissig B et al. Inhibition of both paracrine and autocrine VEGF/VEGFR-2 signaling pathways is essential to induce long-term remission of xeno-transplanted human leukemias. *Proc Natl Acad Sci USA* 2001; **98**: 10857–62.

136. Wilson EA, Jobanputra S, Jackson R et al. Response to thalidomide in chemotherapy-resistant mantle cell lymphoma: a case report. *Br J Haematol* 2002; **119**: 128–30.

# 15 Lymphoproliferations associated with human T-cell leukemia/lymphoma virus type 1 or 2 infection

Renaud Mahieux and Antoine Gessain

## Introduction

Since the early discovery of leukemia/sarcoma avian retroviruses by Ellerman and Bang in 1908, a long period had elapsed, covering most of the 20th century, with a succession of ups and downs for oncogenic viruses. In 1980, after 70 years of search, the first human oncoretrovirus (human T-cell leukemia/lymphoma type 1 or HTLV-1) was isolated by the group of Gallo,[1] and soon after independently, by Japanese researchers, in a sample of a rare and peculiar T-cell leukemia (named adult T-cell leukemia/lymphoma [ATLL]) that had been uncovered in Japan in 1977.[2,3]

Exogenous retroviruses (i.e. viruses that are transmitted horizontally) naturally cause leukemias in many animal out-bred species such as cats, cattle, gibbon, mice etc. These exogenous viruses do not contain an oncogene per se, i.e. a gene that encodes for a protein that is directly involved in cellular transformation. In humans, three families of exogenous retroviruses (i.e. oncoretroviruses, lentiviruses and spumaviruses) have been described. Of these, the spumaviruses have not yet been linked to any pathology. In contrast, oncoretroviruses (such as HTLV-1 and HTLV-2) and lentiviruses (human immunodeficiency virus [HIV]-1 and HIV-2) have been strongly associated with lymphoid malignancies. With respect to HIVs, there is no evidence that any of the proteins that are encoded by HIV-1 or HIV-2 can directly cause any human lymphoid neoplasia. The frequent B-cell lymphomas that are observed in acquired immune deficiency syndrome (AIDS) patients seem most likely, at least for a large part of them, to result from the reactivation of latent viruses such as Epstein–Barr virus. Similarly, a probable reactivation of human herpesvirus 8 is linked to the development of Kaposi sarcoma and primary effusion lymphomas in HIV-infected patients. In fact, HTLV-1 remains at this time the only human retrovirus that is the etiological agent of a human leukemia or of a lymphoma. However, even in that case, a number of other events have to occur, usually over a long latency period, before cancer will develop. By contrast, HTLV-2, the second human retrovirus to be isolated, has not yet been conclusively associated with any malignant lymphoproliferation.

In this chapter, after a review on the molecular and epidemiological aspects of HTLV-1 and HTVL-2, it will present the current knowledge of the clinical, epidemiological, viromolecular and therapeutic characteristics of ATLL that is associated with HTLV-1 infection. This chapter will also discuss the controversial association of HTLV-1 or of a related virus with some cutaneous T-cell lymphomas such as mycosis fungoides (MF) and Sézary syndrome. Finally, data regarding the possible association of HTLV-2 and rare CD8 lymphoproliferative disorders will be briefly presented.

## HTLV-1: A human oncogenic retrovirus

### Epidemiology and associated diseases

HTLV-1 infection was found to be endemic, in the south western islands of the Nippon Archipelago (Kyushu-Shikoku), then in large parts of the Caribbean area, in intertropical Africa, Central and South America, and in some restricted areas of the Middle East and Melanesia (reviewed in[4,5]). It is estimated that HTLV-1 infects 15–20 million individuals throughout the world. The HTLV-1 antibody prevalence rate varies from 0.2–10% among adults, depending on the geographical area. Furthermore, significant variations in prevalence exist in endemic areas, with a puzzling micro-epidemiology associated to foci of high prevalence. In Japan, where nationwide surveys were carried out in the early 1980s, the prevalence rate in blood donors varied initially from 0.1–1% in central Japan, to 2–10% in the Kyushu island.[6] Even there, foci of higher prevalence were observed. In this HTLV-1 endemic area, a female preponderance has been observed. The prevalence increases with age, reaching eventually 20–50% of the female population aged 60 and above.[4,5]

The two major diseases associated with HTLV-1 (ATLL and tropical spastic paraparesis/HTLV-1-associated myelopathy [TSP/HAM]) are present in all the endemic areas[1,7] (Table 15.1) with however significant differences in the incidence as well as prevalence. While the incidence of ATLL exhibits minor variations (1–5/100 000/year) in Japan, in the Caribbean area, and in South America,[8–11] the incidence of TSP/HAM seems to be higher in the Caribbean islands and in some countries of South America than in Japan.

Three modes of contamination are known for HTLV-1, and via any of these routes, infected cells are essential for transmission:

1. Mother-to-child transmission,[5,12,13] in which efficiency varies from 10–20% and which occurs after prolonged breast-feeding (with HTLV-1-infected milk lymphocytes), mainly after the baby is 6–9 months of age, i.e. when the protective IgG maternal antibodies decrease. In Japan, advice to HTLV-1-seropositive mothers not to breast-feed their babies led to a very significant decrease in mother-to-child transmission of the virus with however, for yet unknown reasons, inconsistent results according to areas. The excess of non-Hodgkin T-cell lymphomas (T-NHL – corresponding to the lymphoma type of ATLL), observed among adults in the Caribbean, especially in Jamaica, appears to be directly related to the HTLV-1 infection, and more specifically to an early infection.[9,14] Though, the prevention of HTLV-1 vertical transmission could result in a 70–80% reduction in such HTLV-1-associated T-NHL among infected adults in high HTLV-1 endemic areas.

2. HTLV-1 is also sexually transmitted.[9] Japanese studies clearly demonstrated higher transmission efficiency from male to female than from female to male. Such differences might account for the increase in the HTLV-1 seroprevalence with age that is observed in females.

3. The intravenous route of infection, mainly by blood transfusion, appears to be the most efficient mode for HTLV-1 transmission. This risk was estimated to reach 15–60% after the transfusion of a tainted lymphoid cellular blood product. Contamination through blood is associated with a

## Table 15.1 Diseases associated with HTLV-1 infection*

| Adult disease | Association |
| --- | --- |
| Adult T-cell leukemia/lymphoma | ++++ |
| Tropical spastic paraparesis/HTLV-I-associated myelopathy | ++++ |
| Intermediate uveitis (frequent in Japan) | +++ |
| Infective dermatitis (rare) | +++ |
| Polymyositis | +++ |
| HTLV-I-associated arthritis | ++ |
| Pulmonary infiltrative pneumonitis | ++ |
| Invasive cervical cancer | + |
| Small cell carcinoma of lung | + |
| Sjögren disease | + |

| Childhood | Association |
| --- | --- |
| Infective dermatitis (frequent in Jamaica) | ++++ |
| Tropical spastic paraparesis/HTLV-I-associated myelopathy (rare) | ++++ |
| Adult T-cell leukemia/lymphoma (very rare) | ++++ |
| Persistent lymphadenopathy | ++ |

*The strength of association is based on epidemiological studies as well as molecular data, animal models and intervention trials. ++++: proven association; +++: probable association; ++: likely association; +: possible association.

specific risk of developing TSP/HAM.[15] By contrast, the risk of developing ATLL after acquiring HTLV-1 through blood transfusion seems extremely rare. For these reasons, the screening of the blood donations was implemented in Japan, starting in 1986, in French Caribbean in 1989, in the USA in 1989, in Canada in 1990, in France in 1991, and in Denmark and the Netherlands in 1994.[16]

## Cellular tropism and viral receptor

While HTLV-1 can infect several different cell types of various origin in vitro, it has been thought for long to preferentially infect CD4+ lymphoid cells in vivo. However, some data also indicated that CD8+ cells constitute an additional in vivo reservoir for the virus.[17] Recent reports have brought new insights on the HTLV receptor.[18,19] These authors first reported that quiescent CD4 and CD8 T lymphocytes did not express the HTLV receptor and that the HTLV receptor was an early activation marker in neonatal and adult T lymphocytes, detected as early as 4 h following T-cell receptor (TCR) stimulation. Finally, after 20 years of intensive scrutiny, an HTLV-1 receptor was identified and reported to be the ubiquitous glucose transporter Glut-1.[20] Glut-1 is also a receptor for HTLV-2.

## Molecular biology

### Genetic organization

As members of the oncoviridae subfamily, the HTLVs (Figure 15.1), together with the BLV, and STLV represent a group (delta-type retroviruses) that is distinct from avian and murine oncoretroviruses. They do not harbor oncogene sequences of cellular origin, but rather specific genes encoding regulatory proteins (Tax and Rex), that regulate the viral replication and interact with the host cell machinery.[21,22]

The genetic organization of HTLV-1 is shown on Figure 15.2. The HTLV-1 genome encodes three major (structural/enzymatic) proteins, i.e. Gag, Pol and Env, whose genes are flanked by the long terminal repeat (LTR). The HTLV-1 LTR, which contains several regulatory elements, is divided into three regions: U3, R and U5. U3 contains the polyadenylation signal, the TATA box and the 3 Tax responsive elements (TREs). R contains the transcription initiation site and the Rex responsive element (RRE). In addition to these structural and enzymatic genes, a region referred to as the X region is present at the 3′ end of the genome.

Like other retroviruses, the *gag* gene is translated from the full length RNA to yield a precursor polyprotein (Pr53) that is subsequently cleaved by the viral protease to yield the matrix (p19), the capsid (p24) and the nucleocapsid (p15). The protease is in a frame distinct from *gag* and its synthesis is accomplished with a ribosomal frameshift. A second ribosomal

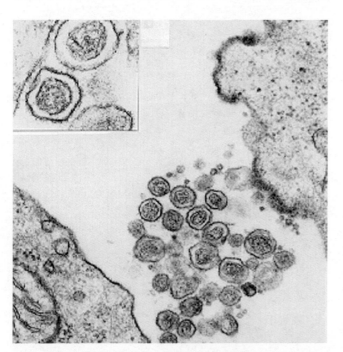

**Figure 15.1** Type C retroviral particles in the extracellular spaces of a CD4+ lymphoid cell line infected by HTLV-1. The cell line has been established from the long-term culture, in presence of interleukin 2, of the peripheral blood lymphocytes obtained from a patient with a TSP/HAM.

frameshift event is necessary to express the *pol* gene. The *env* gene encodes two envelope glycoproteins: the surface glycoprotein (gp46) and the transmembrane glycoprotein (gp21), which are themselves cleaved by cellular proteases from a larger precursor.[23] The X region located at the 3′ end of the genome contains at least four open reading frames (ORFs). The ORFs III and IV are transcribed through a single polycistronic doubly spliced mRNA. These ORFs encode two major regulatory proteins: Tax and Rex. The Rex protein acts at the post-transcriptional level to regulate viral gene expression. It increases the expression of viral structural and enzymatic protein by facilitating the shuttling from the nucleus to the cytoplasm of unspliced mRNAs coding for Gag, Pol and Env proteins.[24]

Using reverse transcriptase/polymerase chain reaction (PCR), alternatively spliced mRNAs coding for the ORF I and II of the pX region have also been discovered (for a review, see [25]). These mRNAs encode three proteins named p12[I], p13[II] and p30[II]. The p12[I] is a proline- and leucine-rich hydrophobic protein of 99 amino acids, which is localized in the cellular endomembranes and bears structural and functional analogies with the E5 oncoprotein of the bovine papilloma virus. p12[I] interacts specifically with the interleukine-2 receptor β and γ chains, but not with the α chain. It enhances STAT5 activation, suggesting its possible involvement in the mechanism of T-cell transformation. p12[I] also binds calcineurin and modulates NFAT activation to promote early virus infection of T lymphocytes.[26]

The functions of the p13[II] and p30[II] are also under intense examination. Recent reports suggest that p13[II] might alter mitochondrial permeability and morphology without however inducing apoptosis. p13[II] acts as a negative regulator of cell growth and underscores a link between mitochondria, Ca(2+) signaling, and tumorigenicity.[27]

The role of p30[II] is more controversial. Some authors reported that the protein can be viewed as a factor that activates transcriptions from the HTLV LTR when expressed at low levels, while it would repress the same promoter when highly expressed.[28] These results were not confirmed by others.[29] p30[II] also binds to, and retains in the nucleus, the doubly spliced mRNA encoding the Tax and Rex proteins. Because Tax and Rex are positive regulators of viral gene expression, their inhibition by p30[II] reduces virion production. p30(II) inhibits virus expression by reducing Tax and Rex protein expression.

### Tax protein and its role in leukemogenesis

Tax is a 40-kDa phosphoprotein that can be detected both in the cytoplasm and nucleus of the cells, depending on the cell line used for the transfection. Several lines of evidence have demonstrated a central

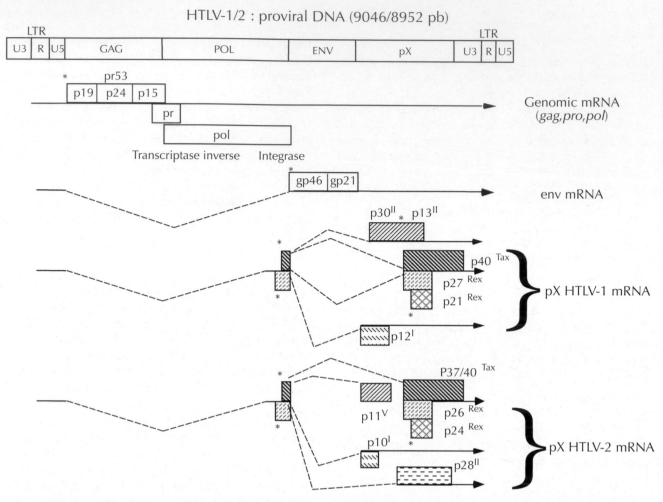

**Figure 15.2** Genomic structure of the HTLV-1/2 proviruses and of the different mRNAs with their corresponding encoded proteins.

role for the 40-kDa Tax protein in the immortalization or transformation of HTLV-1-infected cells (for a review see[30]):

1. The transduction of the *tax* gene into primary human T lymphocytes using a defective simian herpesvirus is sufficient to immortalize them.[31] Other experiments have further demonstrated that ablating Tax expression prevents the cell transformation as well as induces a G1 arrest. This suggests a role for Tax in the disregulation of the G1/S transition.[32]
2. Similarly, the expression of Tax or the co-trans-fection of Tax and Ras in rodent fibroblasts or T lymphocytes is sufficient to transform them.[33]
3. Wild-type Tax can also convert IL-2-dependent murine CTLL cells to an IL-2-independent stage.[34]
4. Tax transgenic animals expressing Tax under the control of the granzyme B promoter develop peripheral lymphomas consisting of CD8+ and natural killer cells.[35]

Tax does not bind directly to DNA, but rather interacts with several cellular proteins being either transcriptional factors or modulators of cellular function.

Therefore, the viral transactivator has the unique ability to activate 3 major cellular transduction pathways:

1. Tax binds to members of the activating transcription factor/cyclic AMP-responsive element-binding protein (ATF/CREB) family of transcription factors to stimulate their dimerization and their association onto the viral Tax TRE sequence to promote viral transcription.[36]
2. Tax also activates transcription from the serum response factor (SRF). Tax interactions with CREB-binding protein (CBP) and p300- and CBP-associated factor (p/CAF) were found to be essential for Tax activation of both the CREB/ATF and the SRF-mediated transcription.[37]
3. Finally another remarkable aspect of the Tax protein resides in its ability to activate permanently the NF-κB pathway (for a review, see [38]).

Through such pathways, Tax has pleiotropic effects: not only does it transactivate the viral promoter, but it is also able to activate or repress the expression or functions of a wide array of genes (see[21,30] for a review and Figure 15.3). Many of them are regulators of the

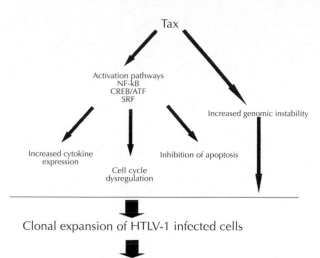

**Figure 15.3** Pleiotropic effects of Tax expression. Tax does not bind directly to DNA, but rather interacts with several cellular proteins being either transcriptional factors or modulators of cellular function. Therefore, the viral transactivator has the unique ability to activate three major cellular transduction pathways such as NF-κB, ATF/CREB (activating transcription factor/cyclic AMP-responsive element-binding protein) and SRF (serum response factor). Through such pathways, Tax not only transactivates the viral promoter, but it is also able to activate or repress the expression or functions of a wide array of genes including regulators of the cell cycle (p21, p53, p16$^{INKA}$), or of apoptosis (Bcl-2, Bcl-X$_L$, and caspases) or cytokines, or their receptor, as interleukin-2, IL-2 receptor α chain, IL-15, II -6. All these genes play a crucial role in T-lymphocyte growth and function. Their dysregulation could therefore be linked to tumorigenesis. Tax has also an important effect on the maintenance of the genomic stability. It inhibits DNA repair, (via DNA topoisomerase 1 and human telomerase reverse transcriptase (hTERT) transcription) and acts also as a transrepressor of the human β-polymerase gene.

cell cycle (p21, p53, p16$^{INKA}$), or of apoptosis (Bcl-2, Bcl-X$_L$, and caspases).[21,39,40] Tax also enhances the expression of interleukin-2 (IL-2), IL-2 receptor (IL-2R) α chain, IL-15, IL-6 and granulocyte–macrophage colony-stimulating factor (GM-CSF). It was also recently shown that Tax was a repressor of TGF-β1 signaling through JNK/c-Jun constitutive activation. All these genes play a crucial role in T-lymphocyte growth and function. Their dysregulation could therefore be linked to tumorigenesis.[41]

Tax may also have an effect on the maintenance of the genomic stability (for a review, see [30]). It is competent for inhibiting DNA repair via the suppression of the nucleotide-excision repair (NER) and the base excision repair (BER) pathways.[42] Tax acts also as a transrepressor of the human β-polymerase gene.[43] Lately,

Yoshida et al have proposed that Tax physically interacts both in vitro and in vivo with the DNA topoisomerase 1, which plays a role in DNA repair.[44] Consequently, the enzyme is partially inactivated. Finally, recent data showed that Tax can inhibit human telomerase reverse transcriptase (hTERT) transcription, which is the rate-limiting factor of telomerase activity.[45,46] hTERT repression by Tax at an early phase of carcinogenesis might contribute to the massive ploidy changes associated with the development of HTLV-1-associated malignancies.

# Hematological manifestations of HTLV-1 infection: ATLL

ATLL is a malignant lymphoproliferation of T cells, mostly CD4-activated T cells, characterized by the clonal integration of one or more HTLV-1 proviruses in the tumor cells.[11,47,48] Present in every HTLV-1 endemic area, ATLL presents a wide clinical diversity. This makes the diagnosis occasionally difficult at the onset of the disease.

## Epidemiology

ATLL was first discovered and reported by Takatsuki et al in the Southwestern regions of Japan, where it has a high incidence.[2,10,11,49,50] It was then described in Caribbean immigrants living in the UK by Catovsky et al.[51] Later, ATLL cases were reported in most of the HTLV-1 endemic areas, i.e. intertropical Africa, South and Central America and Iran.[52–55] Sporadic cases of ATLL have also been described in areas of low HTLV-1 endemicity such as Europe and the USA, often in immigrant patients originating from HTLV-1 endemic regions. Despite this wide geographical distribution, reliable data concerning the ATLL prevalence and incidence are available only for Japan, some Caribbean areas and Brazil.

A nationwide study in Japan revealed that 50% of ATLL patients were registered from Kyushu and 25% were from large metropolitan cities.[10,50] However, 80% of the latter patients were born in Kyushu. In Japan, the ATLL sex ratio (male/female) is roughly 1.4. Age- and sex-specific incidence rates of ATLL in Japan showed a steep increase with age after 40. These rates then reach a plateau at the age of 50 in males, but keep on increasing in females until 70 years of age. In Japan, the average age of those with ATLL is 57 years,[10,50] while it is roughly 40–45 years in the Caribbean and in South America (Brazil, Columbia, and French Guyana). This suggests the presence of yet unknown cofactors that are linked to the pathogenesis of ATLL. In Japan, the annual incidence of ATLL cases is estimated to be 700, while the number of HTLV-1 carriers is 1.2 million. This gives an estimated yearly incidence of ATLL in the range of 0.6–1.5 for 1000 adult HTLV-1 carriers older than 40.[10,50,56] In Jamaica, this rate is similar.[9,52] The additive lifetime risk for developing an ATLL among HTLV-1 carriers was estimated to be 1–5% for both sexes in Japan and Jamaica. Strikingly, a much higher incidence is observed in the Noir-Marrons population in French Guyana ([53] and Gessain et al, unpublished).

Studies performed in Brazil,[54,57] Gabon, and French Guyana[53] concluded that the ATLL prevalence is usually underestimated, until a specific disease research is performed. This is mostly due to the severity and rapid evolution of the disease and to confusion of ATLL with similar diseases, such as Sézary syndrome, MF or other types of T-cell non-Hodgkin lymphoma (NHL). In addition, HTLV-1 serological confirmatory tests such as western blot and/or molecular investigations are not easily available in most tropical countries.

## Diagnosis and classification of ATLL

### Diagnosis

The diagnostic criteria for ATLL have been defined by Takatsuki et al:[2,49,58]

1. Histologically and/or cytologically proven lymphoid malignancy with T-cell surface antigens (mostly CD2, CD3 and CD4 positive).
2. Abnormal T lymphocytes always present in the peripheral blood except in the lymphoma type of ATLL. These abnormal T lymphocytes include the typical ATLL flower cells, as well as some small and mature T lymphocytes with incised or lobulated nuclei that are characteristic of the chronic or smoldering type of ATLL.
3. Antibodies to HTLV-1 must be present in the patient's serum at diagnosis.

### Classification

The main clinical features of ATLL are summarized in Table 15.2.

### Table 15.2  Main clinical features of ATLL

| | Japan* | Caribbean† |
|---|---|---|
| Age at onset | 58 years (range 27–82) | 47 years |
| Sex ratio male/female | 1.4 | 0.6 |
| Lymphadenopathy | 60% | 70% |
| Hepatomegaly | 26% | 27% |
| Splenomegaly | 22% | 31% |
| Specific skin lesion | 39% | 41% |
| Hypercalcemia | 32% | 51% |

*From references[49,58] based on a series of 187 patients;
†From reference [159] based on a series of 57 patients seen in the UK, 46 of Caribbean origin.

Because of the diversity in the clinical presentation, and in the evolution, Shimoyama and the members of the lymphoma study group in Japan ([59,60] Table 15.3) have proposed a classification of ATLL into four major subtypes: a smoldering type,[61] a chronic type, a lymphoma type[62] and a leukemic/acute type. Both chronic and smoldering types can progress into an acute form of leukemia or lymphoma following a progressive aggravation of the clinical picture. This classification is very useful to discriminate ATLL from other types of leukemias or lymphomas, including cutaneous T-cell lymphomas. An accurate diagnosis is indeed critical for therapeutic decision since, based on Japanese studies, patients with smoldering type and about 30% of those with chronic ATLL have a somewhat 'good prognosis', even without being treated with chemotherapy.[59,60,63] A classification of the different clinical stages of ATLL has been proposed by Shirono et al[64] based on the expression of Ki 67 antigen in the peripheral blood T lymphocytes. Aggressive ATLL (death occurring within 1 year, mean survival: 105 days) is defined by a percentage of Ki 67+-positive cells greater than 18% in the peripheral blood T lymphocytes. Stable ATLL (mean survival of 750 days) are defined by a percentage of Ki 67+ cells lower than 18%. The criteria for determining the diagnosis of ATLL for epidemiological studies have also been proposed,[65] (Table 15.4). These could be used in order to compare the epidemiological characteristics of ATLL in areas such as the Caribbean, Central and South America and intertropical Africa. Interestingly, a recent report demonstrated that distinct sets of genes are up- or down-regulated during the transition from the chronic to acute phase of ATL.[66]

## Cytological, immunovirological and molecular features of ATLL

All ATLL cases are, by definition, associated with HTLV-1 infection. ATLL patients' sera contain specific antibodies directed against HTLV-1 antigens, as demonstrated by Western blot. Particle agglutination, enzyme-linked immunosorbent assay (ELISA) or immunofluorescence assays can also be used to titer these sera.

A high number of abnormal peripheral blood lymphocytes is commonly detected in acute and chronic ATLL patients, while anemia, neutropenia or thombocytopenia are rarely observed. ATLL cells are variable in size and characteristics according to the subtype: in the typical acute leukemia type, most of the lymphoid abnormal cells exhibit a multi-lobulated nuclei (flower cells) as seen in Figure 15.4. In terminal crisis, the cells often greatly vary in size (10–40 µ). They display a cytoplasmic basophilia and a marked nuclear lobulation. Some cells may resemble Sézary cells. In chronic ATLL, cells are generally small and of

## Table 15.3  Diagnosis criteria for clinical subtypes of HTLV-1-associated ATLL

|  | Smoldering | Chronic | Lymphoma | Acute |
|---|---|---|---|---|
| Anti-HTLV-I antibody | + | + | + | + |
| Lymphocyte (×10³/μl) | <4 | ≥4† | <4 | * |
| Abnormal T lymphocytes | ≥5%§ | +‡ | ≤1% | +‡ |
| Flower cells of T-cell marker | # | # | No | + |
| LDH | ≤1.5N | ≤2N | * | * |
| Corrected Ca (mEq/l) | <5.5 | <5.5 | * | * |
| Histology proven lymphadenopathy | No | * | + | * |
| Tumor lesion |  |  |  |  |
| Skin and/or lung | *§ | * | * | * |
| Lymph node | No | * | Yes | * |
| Liver | No | * | * | * |
| Spleen | No | * | * | * |
| Central nervous system | No | No | * | * |
| Bone | No | No | * | * |
| Ascites | No | No | * | * |
| Pleural effusion | No | No | * | * |
| Gastrointestinal tract | No | No | * | * |

N: normal upper limit;*no essential qualification except terms required for other subtype(s). ‡typical flower cells seen occasionally; †accompanied by T lymphocytosis (3.5×10³/μl or more); ‡if abnormal T lymphocytes are less than 5% in peripheral blood, histology-proven tumor lesion is required; §histology-proven skin and/or pulmonary lesion(s) is required if abnormal T lymphocytes are less than 5% in peripheral blood. Adapted from reference [59].

## Table 15.4  Registry criteria for definition of ATLL.

**Definition of ATL**

Clinical/routine laboratory criteria

| Hypercalcemia | 1 point |
|---|---|
| Skin lesions* | 1 point |
| Leukemic phase† | 1 point |

Research laboratory criteria

| T-cell lymphoma or leukemia | 2 points |
|---|---|
| HTLV-I antibody | 2 points |
| TAC-positive tumor cells | 1 point |
| HTLV-I-positive tumors‡ | 2 points |

**ATL classification**

| Classical | ≥7 points |
|---|---|
| Probable | 5 or 6 points |
| Possible | 3 or 4 points |
| Inconsistent with ATL | <3 points |

**Exclusion criteria**

B-cell positivity, nodular or follicular lymphoma, lymphoblastic lymphoma, small lymphocytic lymphoma

*Lymphomatous cells documented morphologically; †More than 2% abnormal lymphocytes. ‡Determined by PCR or Southern blot analysis of the DNA of tumoral cells and indicating a monoclonal integration of HTLV-I provirus(es). Adapted from reference [65].

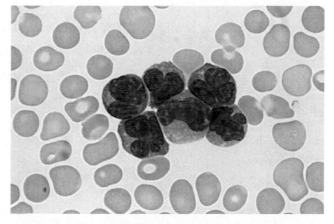

**Figure 15.4** Peripheral blood smear from a Caribbean ATLL leukemic patient showing a cluster of atypical lymphoid cells with multilobulated nuclei (May Grunwald Giemsa staining).

uniform shape; with minor nuclear abnormalities such as indentation or convolutions. In smoldering ATLL cases, cells are often relatively large with a bi- or trifoliate nucleus.[67]

ATLL cells are mature T cells of helper/inducer phenotype (CD2+, CD3+, CD4+, CD7−, CD8−) displaying activation markers (CD25+, HLA DP+, DQ+, DR+).[49,68,69] CD4−, CD8− ATLL cells are unusual, but a decrease of the CD3/T-cell receptor expression is common.[70]

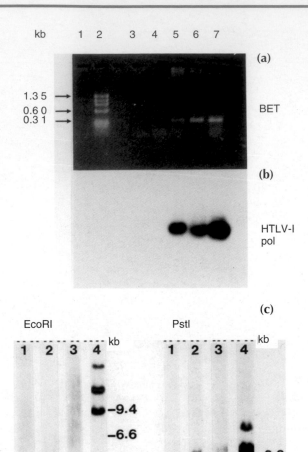

**Figure 15.5** (a) Ethidium-bromide-stained agarose gel analysis of PCR products generated with specific HTLV-1 *pol* primers. High molecular weight DNA were extracted from negative controls (lanes 1, 3 and 4), PBMCs and cutaneous tumor of a lymphoma type ATLL with skin lesions (lanes 5 and 6), and from an HTLV-1 infected cell line (lane 7). (b) Southern-blot analysis of the same gel after transfer of the PCR product to a nylon membrane and hybridization with a specific *pol* HTLV-1 oligomer of 30 base pairs. Positive specific amplification was observed in lanes 5, 6 and 7. (c) Southern blot analysis: control peripheral blood mononuclear cells (lane 1), PBMCs of an ATLL with a defective HTLV-1 provirus (lane 2), PBMCs of the patient with the skin tumors (lane 3) and cutaneous tumor biopsy of the same patient (lane 4). Because there is no known EcoRI site in the HTLV-1 provirus, the observation of three bands in lane 4 denotes a clonal integration of three proviral genomes in the DNA of the cutaneous lesions. Pst I digestion generates three internal bands, one of them of 2.4 Kb can be detected with the HTLV-1 probe. This observation indicates also a polyclonal integration of the HTLV-1 provirus in the PBMCs of this patient.

Phenotypic changes in ATLL have also been observed in some patients during the clinical course of the disease, i.e. typical CD4+CD8− ATLL cells changed into CD4+CD8+. A case of CD20-positive ATLL has also been described.

The lymph node histology often demonstrates infiltration by medium and large T cells with irregular nuclei effacing the nodal architecture, a pattern consistent with the diagnosis of pleiomorphic large T-cell lymphoma.[62] However there is no specific histological pattern for ATLL.[54,60,71]

The cytogenetic abnormalities found in ATLL are not specific but are more frequent in the acute and lymphoma type than in the chronic or the smoldering types.[72] They include various karyotypic abnormalities on chromosome 14: 14 q 32, 14 q 11 translocations and 6q deletions. There are also abnormalities such as trisomies 3,7 and 21 as well as X chromosome monosomy or loss of the Y chromosome.

Mutations on the p53 encoding tumor-suppressing gene are detected in 20–30% of ATLL patients, mostly in advanced cases, suggesting the involvement of the p53 mutation in a late stage of leukemogenesis, or as a consequence of the cancerous transformation.[73] However, several laboratories have also shown that wild type p53 was transcriptionally inactive in HTLV-1-infected cells and that the Tax protein alone could inactivate p53 function.[39]

HTLV-1 sequences can always be amplified from the DNA extracted from tumoral cells.[74] These PCR products can be cloned and sequenced, allowing the determination of the viral genotype (HTLV-1 molecular subtype). However, a positive PCR signal does not demonstrate the link between HTLV-1 and the tumoral status of the cells. In fact, proviral DNA can also be amplified from the PBMCs of any HTLV-1-seropositive individual (Figure 15.5). The demonstration by Southern blot analysis of the clonal integration of HTLV-1 provirus in the tumoral cells (leukemic, lymph nodes, skin infiltrate, pleural or ascitic fluid) represents the gold standard to define biologically ATLL ([47,48,75,76], Figure 15.5). Indeed, monoclonal integration of the HTLV-1 provirus is never detected in the malignant cells from patients with other T-cell malignancies, even if patients are HTLV-1 seropositive. In 5–20% of the cases, the integrated HTLV-1 proviruses are defective (Figure 15.5). The pX region is generally conserved, while deletions occur preferentially in *gag*, *pol*, and/or *env* sequences. Using Southern blot and long PCR, a Japanese study of 72 various ATLL subtypes, revealed two main types of defective viruses.[75] The first one retained both LTR and lacked internal sequences in the 5′ region of the provirus. The second one retained only one LTR, while the 5′ LTR was preferentially deleted. This second type was more frequently detected in the acute and lymphoma type samples than in the chronic type.

In most cases, only one copy of the provirus is integrated in the tumoral cells, while two or three copies are detected in 5–20% of ATLL cases. Some authors have suggested that the HTLV-1 integration pattern in the host DNA may be linked to the severity of the disease.[77,78] In a study conducted on 89 ATLL cases, a band whose size was greater than 9 kb was detected in 83 patients while an 'extraordinary' integration pattern of HTLV-1 proviral DNA was detected in six patients. Three showed two bands and three exhibited one band smaller than 9 kb. The patients with such 'extraordinary' integration pattern had clinical characteristics (including an extremely aggressive clinical course) different from those of the other 83 patients.[77,78] These data are however controversial since the genomic DNA extracted from some patients with chronic ATLL also contained two proviral copies, while some patients with aggressive ATLL had only one proviral copy.[79]

Numerous studies have demonstrated that the presence of HTLV-1 oligo or monoclonal populations was not characteristic of a malignant proliferation.[80–82] Indeed, some healthy carriers as well as 10–20% of all TSP/HAM exhibit a proviral clonal integration that can sometimes be detected by classical Southern blot analysis.[80] Furthermore, oligoclonal or polyclonal proliferation of HTLV-1-infected T cells can also be detected by inverse PCR in most TSP/HAM patients as well as in healthy HTLV-1-seropositive carriers.[83] Some clones were shown to persist in vivo several years in the same infected individual. The detection of a clonal proliferation of HTLV-1-infected cells that are not malignant could therefore be used as a molecular tool for monitoring groups at risk for the development of ATLL. It could also be instrumental for detecting residual ATLL cells after bone marrow transplantation.[81,84]

## Clinical features and complications

### Hypercalcemia

It is a very frequent and rather specific biological feature of ATLL. It is present in 20–30% of the patients at admission and in more than 50% of them during the entire clinical course with or without lytic bone lesions,[49,58,85] (Table 15.2). The degree of hypercalcemia might be linked to the expression of the parathyroid hormone (PTH)-related protein (PTHrP) gene in cooperation with IL-1 and TGF-β. Interestingly, the HTLV-1 Tax protein has been shown to transactivate the PTHrP promoter.[86] It has recently been suggested that ATLL cells induce the differentiation of hematopoietic precursor cells to osteoclasts via receptor activator nuclear factor κB ligand (RANKL), expressed on their surface, in cooperation with M-CSF (Macrophage colony stimulating factor). This may ultimately cause hypercalcemia.[41]

### Cutaneous lesions

Skin infiltration of a clonal population of HTLV-1 tumoral cells represents a frequent clinical feature of ATLL. It is found in 20–40% of all ATLL types and in more than 50% of smoldering ATLL patients ([61], Table 15.3). Various cutaneous lesions have been described. They include papules, nodules, erythroderma, plaques, tumors and ulcerative lesions. ATLL cells densely infiltrate both dermis and epidermis, forming Pautrier micro-abscesses (Figure 15.6).[87–89] When skin lesions dominate the clinical picture, the disease is often referred to as cutaneous ATLL.[87–89] In such cases, clinico-pathological differentiation of these lesions with other cutaneous T-cell lymphomas (CTCLs) might be difficult to establish and requests molecular studies. Interestingly, a recent study showed that HTLV-1-immortalized T cells and fresh ATLL cells frequently express CCR4.[90] Thus, the frequent involvement of skin in ATLL may be accounted for, in part, by the frequent expression of CCR4. However, only a fraction of patients have skin lesions. It is thus evident that CCR4 positivity of the leukemic cells per se is not sufficient for skin invasion. Other factors such as expression of cutaneous lymphocyte antigen (CLA) by leukemic cells and inflammatory responses in lesional skin leading to up-regulation of thymus and activation-regulated chemokine (TARC) and macrophage-derived chemokine (MDC) are also likely to contribute to skin involvement of ATLL. Fresh leukemic cells derived from patients with acute ATLL also produce vascular endothelial growth factor (VEGF) and basic fibroblast growth factor (bFGF) proteins. Angiogenesis, cell adhesion, and communication are likely to contribute to the development of ATLL.[91,92]

Infective dermatitis (ID), a rare dermatological condition originally described in Jamaica in 1966 was subsequently linked in 1990 to HTLV-1 infection.[93,94] ID is a relapsing skin disease with infectious and

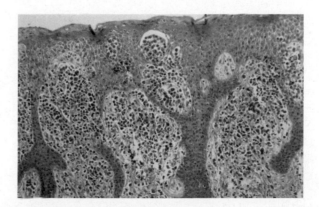

**Figure 15.6** Histology of skin invasion in a Caribbean patient with a cutaneous ATLL showing an infiltration of the dermis and epidermis with presence of Pautrier abscess. These tumoral cells were CD2+, CD3+, CD4+, CD8- and CD25+.

dermatitis-like features that is distinct from atopic dermatitis. So far, most cases of ID have been described in children living in Jamaica, however few cases have been reported in other HTLV-1 endemic areas including west Africa.[95] ID has been described in some patients with ATLL[94,96] and it has been suggested that ID defines a group of patients at increased risk for ATLL development.[93,96]

## Infectious complication

The frequency of opportunistic infections (*Pneumocystis carinii*, herpes viruses etc.), is quite high in patients with ATLL,[97] indicating that T-cell-mediated immunity is severely impaired in such patients. Furthermore, a mild T-cell immune deficiency state has been reported among HTLV-1 healthy carriers.[5] Infestation by *Strongyloides stercoralis* (*SS*) is quite frequent among HTLV-1-seropositive carriers and *SS*-infected individuals are often infected by HTLV-1 in highly endemic areas such as the Okinawa islands and Caribbean area. Numerous studies showed the presence of *SS* in acute or lymphoma ATLL, suggesting that infection by *SS* may play a significant role as a candidate cofactor for HTLV-1 induced leukemogenesis.[98] A study in Martinique, French West Indies, indicated that ATLL patients infected with *SS* were younger (39 vs. 70 years) and survived longer (median survival 167 d vs. 30 d) than uninfected patients.[99] A monoclonal integration of HTLV-1 proviral DNA has been detected by Southern blot in some patients infected with *SS* but who did not have overt ATLL.[100] In addition, Gabet et al demonstrated that the mean circulating HTLV-1 proviral load was more than five times higher in HTLV-1 carriers who were infected with strongyloidiasis than in those without *SS* infection. Such increased proviral load was found to result from the extensive proliferation of a restricted number of infected clones.[98] The positive effect of *SS* on clonal expansion was however reversible under effective treatment against strongyloidiasis in only one patient.

Pulmonary complications are also very frequent in ATLL patients. These are either leukemic infiltrate or infections. Gastrointestinal tract infiltration by ATLL cells is quite frequent while central nervous system localization rarely occurs in ATLL (10%).

## Differential diagnosis: other cutaneous T-cell lymphomas

The difference between smoldering or chronic forms of ATLL and other post-thymic T-cell malignancies, including cutaneous T-cell lymphoma may be difficult to establish. In cases of cutaneous lesions, only molecular studies can distinguish HTLV-1-related specific skin malignancies from cutaneous lesions of other etiology, which could also occur among HTLV-1 carriers.[61,76,87-89] Histopathologic data may also closely resemble cutaneous lesions that are present in other T-cell lymphomas that are not linked to HTLV-1 infection. Similarly, the presence of activated T-cell markers such as CD25, HLA-DR, HLA-DP, can also be found in some cases of CTCL. Therefore, an HTLV-1-positive serology combined to the presence of circulating ATLL-like cells, together with an HTLV-1 positive PCR signal on the DNA extracted from PBMCs and/or from tumor biopsy cells, are important clues in favor of an ATLL diagnosis. Nevertheless, they do not demonstrate a direct etiologic link between the presence of the virus and the cutaneous lesions since these features are also present among healthy HTLV-1-seropositive individuals. Therefore, the definitive evidence for a causal link between HTLV-1 and a cutaneous T-cell tumoral proliferation is the demonstration by Southern blot analysis of the monoclonal HTLV-1 proviral integration in the tumor cells of the skin infiltrate.[88]

In summary, according to Matutes et al,[54] the features that could be considered as specific of an ATLL are hypercalcemia, peripheral blood cell morphology and the presence of clonally integrated HTLV-1 in the neoplastic cells. Some features such as skin and lymph node histology, immunological markers and certain chromosome abnormalities can be found in other T-cell leukemias or lymphomas and thus do not distinguish them from ATLL.

## Therapeutic aspects of ATLL

The survival rate of ATLL patients, especially those who develop the acute leukemic or lymphomas forms, remains very poor and such tumor remains one of the most severe lymphoproliferations. Treatment of ATLL patients using conventional chemotherapy has indeed very limited benefit, since HTLV-1 cells are resistant to most apoptosis-inducing agents (for a review, see [101-103]). In a Japanese survey coordinated by Shimoyama based on 818 ATLL cases, the median survival time was 9 months, with a survival rate of only 27% and 10% at 2 and 4 years, respectively. The situation is very contrasted when subtypes are considered, with a 4-year survival rate of 66% for the smoldering type, of 27% for the chronic type and of 5–6% for the lymphoma and acute types.[59,63] Furthermore, spontaneous regression can also be observed in few cases of ATLL.[59,63]

The main prognostic factors associated with a poor response and a poor survival rate in ATLL patients are: a high lactic acid dehydrogenase (LDH) value, high leukemic counts (both reflecting a high tumor burden), hypercalcemia, and a poor clinical performance.[101] Furthermore, the main obstacles to an efficient response to treatment are: infectious complications (*Pneumocystis carinii, Cryptococcus meningitis*, disseminated herpes zoster), hypercalcemia, and liver or kidney dysfunction. Various strategies including classical combination chemotherapy, deoxycoformycin, leucocytopheresis, photochemotherapy, low-dose total-body irradiation, interferon, monoclonal antibodies directed against the IL-2 receptor, GM-CSF-supported combination chemotherapy and allogenic hematopoeitic stem cells transplant[104] have been used during clinical trials.[101,105] However these therapeutic regimens induce in very few long-term disease-free survival.

Zidovudine (AZT), which was originally synthesized as part of an anti-cancer drug discovery program, has been shown to inhibit HTLV-1 transmission in vitro.[106] Gill et al[107] initiated a clinical trial on 19 ATLL patients (including those with acute and lymphoma types) using interferon-α (INF-α) in combination with AZT. A major response was achieved in 58% of patients, including a remission in 26% (five out of 19). In France, Hermine et al[108] also reported the efficacy of such a therapeutic regimen in five ATLL patients (four acute and one smoldering cases). A more recent study confirms the efficacy and safety of AZT/INF-α in ATLL, with some high response and complete remission (CR). However, despite some with impressive prolonged CR of more than 3 years, most of the patients relapse, stressing the need for additional therapy after achieving CR with AZT/INF.[109,110] Initial treatment of ATL patients with CHOP therapy has also temporary beneficial effects.[110] Other studies performed in Jamaica and Great Britain found a response rate to be lower than in the two previous studies.[111]

In vitro, retinoic-acid[112,113] or arsenic trioxide (As$_2$O$_3$), in combination with INF-α can induce cell death in HTLV-1-transformed cells.[114,115] The mechanism involves the reversion of the NF-κB activation as well as the degradation of the Tax-1 protein.[116] The current authors also recently demonstrated that in vitro As$_2$O$_3$ treatment could induce apoptosis in all HTLV-1/2 cell lines tested, whether they were IL-2 dependent or independent, as well as in cells obtained from HTLV-1 ATLL patients. The apoptosis is correlated with caspase-3 activation, and caspase-3-dependent cleavage of Poly (ADP-ribose) polymerase (PARP), as well as of Bcl-2. The cleavage of Bcl-2 promotes the release of cytochrome c from the mitochondria.[117] The cell death might involve the down-regulation of NF-κB. Phase II clinical trials with As$_2$O$_3$ are ongoing.[118] The first results show that in vivo, arsenic/IFNα treatment is feasible and exhibits an anti-leukemia effect in ATL patients with a very poor prognosis despite a significant toxicity. More recently, NF-κB inhibitors were found to be efficient for preventing the tumor growth in NOD-SCID/gamma (null) animals previously inoculated with HTLV-1-infected cells.[119] Proteasome inhibitor PS-341 combined or not to anti-Tac therapy

was partially successful for treating NOD/SCID animals or Tax transgenic mice.[120,121]

# Risk factors for ATLL development and pathogenesis

Among HTLV-1 carriers, the risk factors for developing ATLL as well as the determinants of disease progression remain largely unknown. There could be viral factors, host genetic factors or environmental ones.[122]

## Viral factors

Soon after the discovery of TSP/HAM, a question arose as to whether the same virus could induce two different diseases (ATLL and TSP/HAM). In fact, it could be hypothesized that, as it is the case with murine leukemia viruses, specific mutations in structural and/or regulatory viral genes could direct HTLV-1 tissue tropism and pathogenesis. Such questions led numerous groups to study the sequence of the LTR and of the *env* gene of HTLV-1 in ATLL or TSP/HAM patients. These works demonstrated that the few nucleotide changes observed between isolates were specific of the geographical origin of the patients but not of the associated pathologies (ATLL, TSP/HAM).[123] However, Japanese researchers have proposed that one Tax-specific molecular subgroup (within the Cosmopolitan subtype) was more frequently found in TSP/HAM, as compared to ATLL and asymptomatic carriers.[124] Regarding molecular epidemiology, based on sequence and/or RFLP analysis of more than 500 HTLV-1 isolates originating from the main viral endemic areas, four major molecular geographical subtypes (or genotypes) emerged. Their existence is strongly supported by phylogenetic analysis (high bootstrap values). Each of these genotypes (Cosmopolitan [A], Central African [B], Melanesian [C] and Central-African-Pygmies [D]) appeared to arise from ancient interspecies transmission between monkeys infected by STLV-1 (the simian counterpart of HTLV-1) and humans. It is worthwhile to note that STLV-1, which infects several Old World monkey species, can also cause in some infected animals 'ATLL-like' diseases.[125]

Regarding *host genetic factors*, several arguments strongly suggest the existence of such factors involved in the HTLV-1 infection *per se* as well as in the development of ATLL or of TSP/HAM among HTLV-1-infected individuals. Ethnic and familial aggregations of ATLL have been reported in different HTLV-1 endemic areas.[53] Furthermore, numerous HLA studies performed in Japan and Jamaica have also suggested that some class I as well as class II HLA alleles may predispose to ATLL.[126] The authors suggest that

HLA-A\*26, B\*4002 and B\*4801 predispose to ATLL, because of the limited recognition of the HTLV-1 Tax peptide anchor motifs and epitope capable of generating anti-HTLV-1 Tax cytotoxic T cells (CTLs).[126] Consistent with these results, others have also suggested that at some stage of the ATLL development, HTLV-1-infected cells can escape the immune system (reviewed in [41]). This could in part be due to mutations in the Tax 11-19 epitope, which is the major target of the antiviral cellular response.[127] Some polymorphisms of the tumor necrosis factor alpha gene (TNF-α), have been shown to be associated with ATLL in comparison with asymptomatic carriers. Furthermore, among an endemic population of African origin, a major gene predisposing to HTLV-1 infection in children has also been detected.[128]

Regarding *environmental factors*, the mode of infection, the infectious dose and the age of infection seem decisive for developing ATLL or TSP/HAM.[122] Thus, early HTLV-1 infection of babies through infected breast-milk appears to be a major risk factor, especially for developing ATLL but not for TSP/HAM. Several studies conducted in Japan as well as in the Caribbean area and in Brazil have demonstrated that, most if not all the mothers of ATLL patients, were infected with HTLV-1.[129,130] Interestingly, the acquisition of HTLV-1 through blood transfusion represents an important risk factor for developing TSP/HAM but not for ATLL. Indeed, cases of post-transfusion ATLL are exceptional. It has been hypothesized that the route of infection and size of the initial inoculum allow HTLV-1 to infect different target cell populations (CD4, dendritic cells, etc.). Finally, as described earlier, the role of *SS* infection as a cofactor in ATLL among HTLV-1 carriers is obvious.

## Pathogenesis of ATLL

The fact that in man, oncogenesis proceeds, in most cases, from a multistage process is widely accepted.

For ATLL, the first step seems to be the primary infection through prolonged breast-feeding (>6 months) of a child born from an HTLV-1-infected mother (Figure 15.7). After few replication cycles using the viral reverse transcriptase, a clonal expansion of HTLV-1-infected cells arises progressively. The HTLV-1 provirus is integrated at random in the genome of the host. It is now hypothesized that HTLV-1 replicates and increases its copy number through the proliferation of infected cells, thus using the cellular DNA polymerase, which possesses a proof-reading activity and not the reverse transcriptase, an error prone DNA polymerase. Such a model could explain, in part, the very high genetic stability of HTLV-1, by contrast to other retroviruses.

The second step is thus the clonal proliferation of the infected CD4+ lymphocytes, which is linked to the pleiotropic effects of Tax (Figure 15.3). As seen earlier, this includes the activation of several cellular cytokines such as IL2, IL15, the dysregulation of the cell cycle, the inhibition of apoptosis and the promotion of genetic instability. The observation of an oligoclonal or a monoclonal integration of HTLV-1 in the PBMCs (Peripheral blood mononuclear cells) of TSP/HAM patients or of HTLV-1 healthy carriers suggests that neither the monoclonal integration of the virus nor the CD4+ cell proliferation per se is sufficient to cause the disease. The exact roles of cofactors, such as infection by *SS* are largely unknown. The level of Tax expression in vivo in HTLV-1-infected individuals, is still a matter of debate. Several

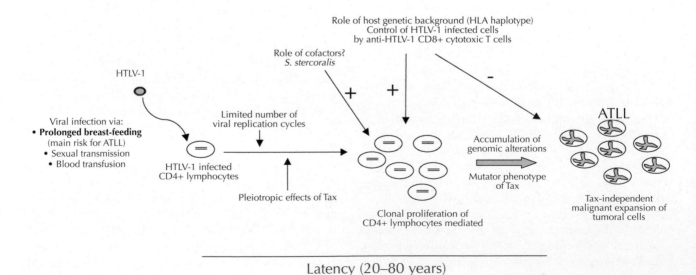

**Figure 15.7** Pathogenesis of ATLL. Natural course from HTLV-1 primary infection by prolonged breast-feeding to ATLL onset (adapted from [41]).

observations paradoxically suggest that HTLV-1 was transcriptionally silent in most infected cells. With the use of new procedures, Hannon et al[131] recently showed that a high proportion of naturally infected CD4[+] peripheral blood mononuclear cells (between 10% and 80%) isolated from TSP/HAM patients or HTLV-1 asymptomatic carriers were capable of expressing Tax. Furthermore, they provided direct evidence that autologous CD8[+] T cells rapidly kill CD4[+] cells that express Tax in vitro by a perforin-dependent mechanism. Those results suggested that virus-specific CTLs participate in a highly efficient immune surveillance mechanism that persistently destroys Tax-expressing HTLV-1-infected CD4[+] T cells in vivo. Such CTL control of the HTLV-1-infected cell proliferation may also result in the prevention of ATLL. The role of the genetic background, especially HLA haplotypes, in such CTL control could be crucial.

A third critical step toward ATLL leukemogenesis would be the accumulation of alteration of the host genome of ATLL cells mediated in part by the mutator phenotype of Tax linked to its action on the DNA damage repair machinery. Furthermore, at the ATLL stage, low levels of HTLV-1 tax mRNA are present in the ATLL cells.[132] Different hypotheses (deletion and/or methylation of the 5'LTR, nonsense or missense mutations of the tax gene) have been proposed to explain such phenomenon, which could facilitate the escape of the ATLL cells from the host immune system. This correlates to the fact that ATLL patients also appear to have an impaired CD8[+] T-cell response.[133]

Community-based prospective studies allowing the comparison of multiple characteristics between the ATLL cases and controls with minimal bias are ongoing in order to define precisely the risk factors associated to ATLL development.[41,134] However the rare occurrence and the long latency period of ATLL makes difficult such long-term prospective studies.

## IS HTLV-1 associated with cutaneous T-cell lymphomas other than ATLL?

As described earlier, there are some strong similarities between the clinical and histopatological features of some types of ATLL and other CTCLs including Sézary syndrome, MF and CD30 anaplastic large-cell CTCLs.[61,87–89] This led a number of investigators to determine whether HTLV-1 (including defective non-replicative forms) or a related virus might be present in such post-thymic mature T-lymphoproliferations.[135–138] This possibility was under active investigation in the 1990s, and a matter of controversy.[139] Several groups had thus demonstrated the presence of HTLV-1 proviral sequences in the DNA extracted from

the PBMCs and/or the cutaneous lesions of HTLV-1 seronegative Sézary syndrome as well as in MF patients originating from the USA, Sweden, UK and Italy.[135,137,138] In these studies, the amplified PCR product was either a part of the pX region (mostly tax and/or rex) or, in some cases, pol and other gene fragments. Sequencing revealed a complete identity with the HTLV-1 prototypic sequence. Other groups failed to detect HTLV-1 sequences in similar patients originating from France, Portugal, Spain or the USA.[140] The presence of defective HTLV-1 provirus was also detected in some patients suffering from CD30 anaplastic large-cell CTCLs.

It is therefore widely accepted that the only HTLV-1-associated lymphoproliferation is ATLL.

## Lymphoproliferative diseases associated with HTLV-2

HTLV-2, the second human oncoretrovirus to be discovered, was isolated in 1982 from a T-cell line established from the splenic cells of a patient suffering from a hairy T-cell leukemia.[141,142] A number of further isolates have been obtained from intravenous drug abusers, healthy HTLV-2-seropositive carriers and rare cases of CD8[+] lymphoproliferative diseases and chronic neuro-myelopathies. This virus is endemic in some Amerindian populations in which the HTLV-2 seroprevalence can reach up to 50%[142] as well as in some rare African Pygmie populations.[143] Furthermore HTLV-2 is also endemic/epidemic (1–30% of seroprevalence) in intravenous drug user (IVDU) population that is present in the large American cities.[142] It is also detected (0.5–10%) in some groups of IVDUs from European countries including the UK, Italy, Ireland and Spain.[144] From a molecular point of view, three main molecular subtypes have been discovered (A, B and D), with a nucleotidic divergence of 4–7% depending on the studied gene.[142,144]

While based on epidemiological and phylogenetic analyses, HTLV-1 and STLV-1 can be considered as 'Old World' viruses present in Africa and Asia, probably for millennia; HTLV-2, on the contrary, appears as a 'New World' virus brought from Asia into the Americas by migrations of population through the Bering strait, some 10 000 to 40 000 years ago. The presence of HTLV-2 in west and central Africa, especially in remote populations (Pygmies), raised however the possibility that HTLV-2 has also been present in Africa over a long period of time.[143,144]

Among HTLV-2-infected individuals, the virus is mainly present in the T CD8[+] lymphocyte subpopulation in vivo.[145] An overall increase of T CD8[+] cells is often detected in such individuals.[146] In vitro, the growth of PBMCs obtained from HTLV-2-seropositive individuals often leads to the establishment of mainly T CD8+ transformed cell lines. This preferential tropism is however not exclusive, and HTLV-2 can also infect the T CD4+ lymphocytes.[147]

The etiological role of HTLV-2 has been suggested in some rare cases of CTCL, or of T CD8 lymphoproliferative disorders.[142,148,149] A review of the literature on the possible involvement of HTLV-2 in such diseases revealed only six published cases where a clear evidence of HTLV-2 infection (by specific serological and/or molecular means) has been demonstrated in CD8+ lymphoproliferations (reviewed in [149,150], Table 15.5). These patients, originated from the USA. They include a case of T hairy cell leukemia,[151] cases of large granular leukemia (LGL) and of cutaneous T-cell lymphoma[149,151–153] and two cases of Sézary-like diseases.[154,155] However, in none of these cases could a clonal integration of HTLV-2 be demonstrated in the malignant tumoral cells. In the so-called 'hairy T-cell leukemia',[156] the virus was oligoclonally integrated in the CD8+ cells, while the clonal tumoral cells, which did not contain an integrated provirus (i.e. negative by Southern blot), were of B-cell type (as it is the case for most, if not all, hairy cell leukemias). In one LGL patient, the HTLV-2 provirus was detected in the normal CD3+, CD8+ cells, but not in tumoral large granular lymphocytes of NK phenotype (CD3+ and CD18+) that did not contain proviral sequences (PCR nega-

tive).[153] In the other case, HTLV-2 was only detected in the DNA of a cell lysate, from paraffin-embedded slides of a bone marrow biopsy. It was not possible to ascertain the role of HTLV-2 in the pathogenesis of this disease in this last patient, who had a clonal lymphoproliferation of CD3+, CD8+, CD57+ phenotype.[151] A large study involving 51 patients failed to demonstrate any association of LGL with HTLV-2 infection. In fact, only one patient with a NK (CD3−) phenotype LGL leukemia was HTLV-2 positive, but there was no evidence for a clonal proviral integration in the neoplastic cells.[152] In the two patients who developed MF or Sézary-like syndrome, in whom clonal proliferation was not demonstrated, the search for the presence of HTLV-2 in the tumoral cells was not performed.[154,155] The last case, is the best documented.[149] An HIV-1 and HTLV-2 co-infected IVDU developed a clonal CD3+, CD8+, CD4− CTCL. It was positive for HTLV-2 by immunostaining and PCR. The copy number of both HTLV-2 and a specific V β clonotype DNA was much higher in the patient's skin than in the peripheral blood. This finding further supports the hypothesis that HTLV-2 was directly involved in the pathogenesis of the lymphoma.

In contrast to HTLV-1, whose etiological role in ATLL is now well established, there is thus currently neither a serological association nor molecular evidence that would definitely suggest that HTLV-2 is etiologically associated to a malignant lympho-

**Table 15.5  T CD8+ lymphoproliferative disorders with clear evidence of HTLV-2 infection by serological and/or molecular means**

| Case (Ref.) | Age/sex | Diagnosis | Pathology | HTLV-2 serology | HTLV-2 molecular data | HTLV-2 isolation | HTLV-2 molecular subtype | HTLV-2 clonal integration |
|---|---|---|---|---|---|---|---|---|
| NRA[156] | 74/M | T-cell variant of hairy cell leukemia | Tumoral B clonal proliferation T CD8 lymphoid reactive proliferation | + WB | + (Southern blot sequence) | + (Transformed cell line) | 2-B | oligoclonal in CD8 cells |
| Patient 10[151] | 88/M | Large granular leukemia | Lymphoid clonal proliferation CD3+, CD8+, CD57+ | + ELISA-specific WB | + PCR, sequence | ND | 2-A | ND |
| Patient 2[154] | 40/M | Severe dermatitis Sézary-like/HIV-1+ | CD8 lymphoid cutaneous infiltrate | + WB | Southern blot | Transformed cell line: cocultivation with BJAB | 2-A | ND |
| [153] | 45/M | Large granular lymphocytosis | NK (CD3−, CD16−) cells proliferation not clonal | + WB | + by PCR in T CD8+ cells only | ND | ND | ND |
| EB[155] | 52/F | Mycosis fungoides | ND | + WB | + by PCR sequence | Cell line | 2-A | ND |
| [149] | 38/M | Cutaneous T-cell lymphoma / HIV-1+ | Clonal CD3+, CD8+, CD4− lymphoid proliferation | + WB | + by PCR sequence | Transformed cell line | 2-A | ND |

ND: not done; WB: Western blot; PCR: polymerase chain reaction. Adapted from reference[150].

proliferative disease. In order to gain new insight on such an issue, further studies are indeed needed in the HTLV-2 highly endemic population, including especially patients who are HTLV-2 and HIV-1 co-infected.

# Conclusion

Prospective studies on HTLV-1-infected individuals should therefore be developed. They shall put together molecular biologists, clinicians and epidemiologists. Among HTLV-1-infected individuals, they should allow the characterization of a high-risk biological profile for ATLL, so that preventive interventions or pre-clinical therapies could be envisaged.[134]

The vaccine approach[157,158] could also be pursued through the establishment of acceptable recombinant viral vaccines of proper experimental models, in which ATLL syndromes could be obtained. Furthermore, the characterization of 'disease susceptibility genes' is being actively pursued for HTLV-1-associated diseases.[128]

# Acknowledgments

This work was supported by grants from l'Association de Recherche sur le Cancer (ARC #4781), from ARECA and from la Fondation de France to RM. RM is supported by INSERM.

## REFERENCES

1. Poiesz BJ, Ruscetti FW, Gazdar AF et al. Detection and isolation of type C retrovirus particles from fresh and cultured lymphocytes of a patient with cutaneous T-cell lymphoma. *Proc Natl Acad Sci U S A* 1980; **77**: 7415–19.
2. Takatsuki T. Adult T-cell leukemia in Japan. In: Seno STS, Irino S, eds. *Topics in Hematology*. Amsterdam: Excerpta Medica 1977: 73–77.
3. Yoshida M, Miyoshi I, Hinuma Y. Isolation and characterization of retrovirus from cell lines of human adult T-cell leukemia and its implication in the disease. *Proc Natl Acad Sci U S A* 1982; **79**: 2031–5.
4. Gessain A. Epidemiology of HTLV-1. In: Holsberg PHD (eds) *Human T-cell lymphotropic virus type 1*. Chichester: Wiley 1996: 34–63.
5. Mueller N. The epidemiology of HTLV infection. *Cancer causes control* 1991; **2**: 37–52.
6. Hinuma Y, Komoda H, Chosa T et al. Antibodies to adult T-cell leukemia-virus-associated antigen (ATLA) in sera from patients with ATL and controls in Japan: a nation-wide sero-epidemiologic study. *Int J Cancer* 1982; **29**: 631–5.
7. Gessain A, Barin F, Vernant JC et al. Antibodies to human T-lymphotropic virus type-I in patients with tropical spastic paraparesis. *Lancet* 1985; **2**: 407–10.
8. Kondo T, Kono H, Miyamoto N et al. Age- and sex-specific cumulative rate and risk of ATLL for HTLV-I carriers. *Int J Cancer* 1989; **43**: 1061–4.
9. Murphy EL, Hanchard B, Figueroa JP et al. Modelling the risk of adult T-cell leukemia/lymphoma in persons infected with human T-lymphotropic virus type I. *Int J Cancer* 1989; **43**: 250–3.
10. Tajima K. The 4th nation-wide study of adult T-cell leukemia/lymphoma (ATL) in Japan: estimates of risk of ATL and its geographical and clinical features. The T- and B-cell Malignancy Study Group. *Int J Cancer* 1990; **45**: 237–43.
11. Yamaguchi K, Watanabe T. Human T lymphotropic virus type-I and adult T-cell leukemia in Japan. *Int J Hematol* 2002; **76** (Suppl)2: 240–5.
12. Takahashi K, Takezaki T, Oki T et al. Inhibitory effect of maternal antibody on mother-to-child transmission of human T-lymphotropic virus type I. The Mother-to-Child Transmission Study Group. *Int J Cancer* 1991; **49**: 673–7.
13. Ureta-Vidal A, Angelin-Duclos C, Tortevoye P et al. Mother-to-child transmission of human T-cell-leukemia/lymphoma virus type I: implication of high antiviral antibody titer and high proviral load in carrier mothers. *Int J Cancer* 1999; **82**: 832–6.
14. Manns A, Cleghorn FR, Falk RT et al. Role of HTLV-I in development of non-Hodgkin lymphoma in Jamaica and Trinidad and Tobago. The HTLV Lymphoma Study Group. *Lancet* 1993; **342**: 1447–50.
15. Gout O, Baulac M, Gessain A et al. Rapid development of myelopathy after HTLV-I infection acquired by transfusion during cardiac transplantation. *N Engl J Med* 1990; **322**: 383–8.
16. Taylor GP. The epidemiology of HTLV-I in Europe. *J Acquir Immune Defic Syndr Hum Retrovirol* 1996; **13**: S8–14.
17. Hanon E, Stinchcombe JC, Saito M et al. Fratricide among CD8(+) T lymphocytes naturally infected with human T cell lymphotropic virus type I. *Immunity* 2000; **13**: 657–64.
18. Nath MD, Ruscetti FW, Petrow-Sadowski C et al. Regulation of the cell-surface expression of an HTLV-I binding protein in human T cells during immune activation. *Blood* 2003; **101**: 3085–92.
19. Manel N, Kinet S, Battini JL et al. The HTLV receptor is an early T-cell activation marker whose expression requires de novo protein synthesis. *Blood* 2003; **101**: 1913–18.
20. Manel N, Kim FJ, Kinet S et al. The ubiquitous glucose transporter GLUT-1 is a receptor for HTLV. *Cell* 2003; **115**: 449–59.
21. Mesnard JM, Devaux C. Multiple control levels of cell proliferation by human T-cell leukemia virus type 1 Tax protein. *Virology* 1999; **257**: 277–84.
22. Johnson JM, Harrod R, Franchini G. Molecular biology and pathogenesis of the human T-cell leukaemia/lymphotropic virus Type-1 (HTLV-1). *Int J Exp Pathol* 2001; **82**: 135–47.
23. Delamarre L, Rosenberg AR, Pique C, Pham D, Callebaut I, Dokhelar MC. The HTLV-I envelope glycoproteins: structure and functions. *J Acquir Immune Defic Syndr Hum Retrovirol* 1996; **13**: S85–91.
24. Inoue J, Itoh M, Akizawa T, Toyoshima H, Yoshida M. HTLV-1 Rex protein accumulates unspliced RNA in the nucleus as well as in cytoplasm. *Oncogene* 1991; **6**: 1753–7.

25. Albrecht B, Lairmore MD. Critical role of human T-lymphotropic virus type 1 accessory proteins in viral replication and pathogenesis. *Microbiol Mol Biol Rev* 2002; **66**: 396–406.

26. Kim SJ, Ding W, Albrecht B, Green PL, Lairmore MD. A conserved calcineurin-binding motif in human T lymphotropic virus type 1 p12I functions to modulate nuclear factor of activated T cell activation. *J Biol Chem* 2003; **278**: 15550–7.

27. Silic-Benussi M, Cavallari I, Zorzan T et al. Suppression of tumor growth and cell proliferation by p13II, a mitochondrial protein of human T cell leukemia virus type 1. *Proc Natl Acad Sci U S A* 2004; **101**: 6629–34.

28. Zhang W, Nisbet JW, Bartoe JT, Ding W, Lairmore MD. Human T-lymphotropic virus type 1 p30(II) functions as a transcription factor and differentially modulates CREB-responsive promoters. *J Virol* 2000; **74**: 11270–7.

29. Nicot C, Dundr M, Johnson JM et al. HTLV-1-encoded p30II is a post-transcriptional negative regulator of viral replication. *Natl Med* 2004; **10**: 197–201.

30. Jeang KT, Giam CZ, Majone F, Aboud M. Life, death and Tax: role of HTLV-I oncoprotein in genetic instability and cellular transformation. *J Biol Chem* 2004; **279**: 31991–4.

31. Grassmann R, Fleckenstein B, Desrosiers RC. Viral transformation of human T lymphocytes. *Adv Cancer Res* 1994; **63**: 211–44.

32. Liang MH, Geisbert T, Yao Y, Hinrichs SH, Giam CZ. Human T-lymphotropic virus type 1 oncoprotein tax promotes S-phase entry but blocks mitosis. *J Virol* 2002; **76**: 4022–33.

33. Pozzatti R, Vogel J, Jay G. The human T-lymphotropic virus type I tax gene can cooperate with the ras oncogene to induce neoplastic transformation of cells. *Mol Cell Biol* 1990; **10**: 413–17.

34. Iwanaga Y, Tsukahara T, Ohashi T et al. Human T-cell leukemia virus type 1 tax protein abrogates interleukin-2 dependence in a mouse T-cell line. *J Virol* 1999; **73**: 1271–7.

35. Grossman WJ, Kimata JT, Wong FH, Zutter M, Ley TJ, Ratner L. Development of leukemia in mice transgenic for the tax gene of human T-cell leukemia virus type I. *Proc Natl Acad Sci U S A* 1995; **92**: 1057–61.

36. Yin MJ, Gaynor RB. HTLV-1 21 bp repeat sequences facilitate stable association between Tax and CREB to increase CREB binding affinity. *J Mol Biol* 1996; **264**: 20–31.

37. Jiang H, Lu H, Schiltz RL et al. PCAF interacts with tax and stimulates tax transactivation in a histone acetyltransferase-independent manner. *Mol Cell Biol* 1999; **19**: 8136–45.

38. Sun SC, Harhaj EW, Xiao G, Good L. Activation of I-kappaB kinase by the HTLV type 1 Tax protein: mechanistic insights into the adaptor function of IKKgamma. *AIDS Res Hum Retroviruses* 2000; **16**: 1591–6.

39. Pise-Masison CA, Mahieux R, Radonovich M et al. Insights into the molecular mechanism of p53 inhibition by HTLV type 1 Tax. *AIDS Res Hum Retroviruses* 2000; **16**: 1669–75.

40. Yoshida M. Multiple viral strategies of HTLV-1 for dysregulation of cell growth control. *Annu Rev Immunol* 2001; **19**: 475–96.

41. Matsuoka M. Human T-cell leukemia virus type I and adult T-cell leukemia. *Oncogene* 2003; **22**: 5131–40.

42. Gatza ML, Watt JC, Marriott SJ. Cellular transformation by the HTLV-I Tax protein, a jack-of-all-trades. *Oncogene* 2003; **22**: 5141–9.

43. Jeang KT, Widen SG, Semmes OJt, Wilson SH. HTLV-I trans-activator protein, tax, is a trans-repressor of the human beta-polymerase gene. *Science* 1990; **247**: 1082–4.

44. Suzuki T, Uchida-Toita M, Andoh T, Yoshida M. HTLV-1 tax oncoprotein binds to DNA topoisomerase I and inhibits its catalytic activity. *Virology* 2000; **270**: 291–8.

45. Gabet AS, Mortreux F, Charneau P et al. Inactivation of hTERT transcription by Tax. *Oncogene* 2003; **22**: 3734–41.

46. Sinha-Datta U, Horikawa I, Michishita E et al. Transcriptional activation of hTERT in HTLV-1 transformed cells through the NF-kB pathway. *Blood* 2004 (In Press).

47. Yamaguchi K, Sciki M, Yoshida M, Nishimura H, Kawano F, Takatsuki K. The detection of human T cell leukemia virus proviral DNA and its application for classification and diagnosis of T cell malignancy. *Blood* 1984; **63**: 1235–40.

48. Yoshida M, Seiki M, Yamaguchi K, Takatsuki K. Monoclonal integration of human T-cell leukemia provirus in all primary tumors of adult T-cell leukemia suggests causative role of human T-cell leukemia virus in the disease. *Proc Natl Acad Sci U S A* 1984; **81**: 2534–7.

49. Takatsuki K, Yamaguchi K, Matsuoka M. Adult T-cell leukemia. In: Holsberg PHD (ed.) *Human T Cell Lymphotropic Virus Type 1*. New York: Wiley 1996: 219–46.

50. Anonymous. The third nation-wide study on adult T-cell leukemia/lymphoma (ATL) in Japan: characteristic patterns of HLA antigen and HTLV-I infection in ATL patients and their relatives. The T- and B-cell Malignancy Study Group. *Int J Cancer* 1988; **41**: 505–12.

51. Catovsky D, Greaves MF, Rose M et al. Adult T-cell lymphoma-leukaemia in Blacks from the West Indies. *Lancet* 1982; **1**: 639–43.

52. Hanchard B. Adult T-cell leukemia/lymphoma in Jamaica: 1986–1995. *J Acquir Immune Defic Syndr Hum Retrovirol* 1996; **13**: S20–5.

53. Gerard Y, Lepere JF, Pradinaud R et al. Clustering and clinical diversity of adult T-cell leukemia/lymphoma associated with HTLV-I in a remote black population of French Guiana. *Int J Cancer* 1995; **60**: 773–6.

54. Matutes E, Schulz T, Serpa MJ, de Queiroz-Campos-Araujo A, de Oliveira MS. Report of the second international symposium on HTLV in Brazil. *Leukemia* 1994; **8**: 1092–4.

55. Fouchard N, Mahe A, Huerre M et al. Cutaneous T cell lymphomas: mycosis fungoides, Sezary syndrome and HTLV-I-associated adult T cell leukemia (ATL) in Mali, West Africa: a clinical, pathological and immunovirological study of 14 cases and a review of the African ATL cases. *Leukemia* 1998; **12**: 578–585.

56. Arisawa K, Soda M, Endo S et al. Evaluation of adult T-cell leukemia/lymphoma incidence and its impact on non-Hodgkin lymphoma incidence in southwestern Japan. *Int J Cancer* 2000; **85**: 319–24.

57. Pombo de Oliveira MS, Matutes E, Schulz T et al. T-cell malignancies in Brazil. Clinico-pathological and molecular studies of HTLV-I-positive and -negative cases. *Int J Cancer* 1995; **60**: 823–7.

58. Takatsuki. ATL and HTLV-1 related diseases. In: KT (ed.) *Adult T-cell Leukaemia*. Oxford: Oxford University Press 1994: 1–27.

59. Shimoyama M. treatment of patients with adult T-cell leukemia-lymphoma: an overview. In: Takatsuki K, Hinuma Y, Yoshida M (eds) *Advances in Adult T-cell Leukemia and HTLV-1 Research*. Tokyo: Japan Scientific Societies Press 1992: 43–6.

60. Shimoyama M. Diagnostic criteria and classification of clinical subtypes of adult T-cell leukaemia-lymphoma. A report from the Lymphoma Study Group (1984–87). *Br J Haematol* 1991; **79**: 428–37.

61. Yamaguchi K, Nishimura H, Kohrogi H, Jono M, Miyamoto Y, Takatsuki K. A proposal for smoldering adult T-cell leukemia: a clinicopathologic study of five cases. *Blood* 1983; **62**: 758–66.

62. Yamaguchi K, Yoshioka R, Kiyokawa T, Seiki M, Yoshida M, Takatsuki K. Lymphoma type adult T-cell leukemia – a clinicopathologic study of HTLV related T-cell type malignant lymphoma. *Hematol Oncol* 1986; **4**: 59–65.

63. Shimoyama M. Chemotherapy of ATL. In: Takatsuki K (ed.) *Adult T-cell Leukaemia*. Oxford University Press 1994: 221–36.

64. Shirono K, Hattori T, Takatsuki K. A new classification of clinical stages of adult T-cell leukemia based on prognosis of the disease. *Leukemia* 1994; **8**: 1834–7.

65. Levine PH, Cleghorn F, Manns A et al. Adult T-cell leukemia/lymphoma: a working point-score classification for epidemiological studies. *Int J Cancer* 1994; **59**: 491–3.

66. Tsukasaki K, Tanosaki S, DeVos S et al. Identifying progression-associated genes in adult T-cell leukemia/lymphoma by using oligonucleotide microarrays. *Int J Cancer* 2004; **109**: 875–81.

67. Kamihira S. Hemato-cytological aspects of adult T-cell leukemia. In: Takatsuki KHY, Yoshida M (ed.) *Advances in Adult T-cell Leukemia and HTLV-1 Research*. Tokyo: Scientific Societies Press 1992: 17–32.

68. Shirono K, Hattori T, Hata H, Nishimura H, Takatsuki K. Profiles of expression of activated cell antigens on peripheral blood and lymph node cells from different clinical stages of adult T-cell leukemia. *Blood* 1989; **73**: 1664–71.

69. Uchiyama T, Ishikawa T, Kondo A. Pathophysiology of ATL cells: cell growth characteristics. In: Takatsuki T (ed.) *Adult T-cell Leukemia*. Oxford University Press 1994: 181–203.

70. Suzushima H, Asou N, Nishimura S et al. Double-negative (CD4– CD8–) T cells from adult T-cell leukemia patients also have poor expression of the T-cell receptor alpha beta/CD3 complex. *Blood* 1993; **81**: 1032–9.

71. Ohshima K, Suzumiya J, Sato K et al. Survival of patients with HTLV-I-associated lymph node lesions. *J Pathol* 1999; **189**: 539–45.

72. Shimoyama M, Sakurai M, Kamada N. Chromosomal aberrations in adult T-cell leukemia-lymphoma: summary of a karyotype review committee report. In: Takatsuki K, Hinuma Y, Yoshida M (eds) *Advances in Adult T-cell Leukemia and HTLV-1 Research*. Tokyo: Scientific Societies Press 1992: 95–105.

73. Sakashita A, Hattori T, Miller CW et al. Mutations of the p53 gene in adult T-cell leukemia. *Blood* 1992; **79**: 477–80.

74. Chadburn A, Athan E, Wieczorek R, Knowles DM. Detection and characterization of human T-cell lymphotropic virus type I (HTLV-I) associated T-cell neoplasms in an HTLV-I nonendemic region by polymerase chain reaction. *Blood* 1991; **77**: 2419–30.

75. Tamiya S, Matsuoka M, Etoh K et al. Two types of defective human T-lymphotropic virus type I provirus in adult T-cell leukemia. *Blood* 1996; **88**: 3065–73.

76. Tanaka T, Takahashi K, Ideyama S, Imamura S, Noma T. Demonstration of clonal proliferation of T lymphocytes in early neoplastic disease. Studies with probes for the beta-chain of the T cell receptor and human T cell lymphotropic virus type I. *J Am Acad Dermatol* 1989; **21**: 218–23.

77. Shimamoto Y, Kobayashi M, Miyamoto Y. Clinical implication of the integration patterns of human T-cell lymphotropic virus type I proviral DNA in adult T-cell leukemia/lymphoma. *Leuk Lymphoma* 1996; **20**: 207–15.

78. Shimamoto Y, Suga K, Shibata K, Matsuzaki M, Yano H, Yamaguchi M. Clinical importance of extraordinary integration patterns of human T- cell lymphotropic virus type I proviral DNA in adult T-cell leukemia/lymphoma. *Blood* 1994; **84**: 853–8.

79. Kato N, Sugawara H, Aoyagi S, Mayuzumi M. Lymphoma-type adult T-cell leukaemia-lymphoma with a bulky cutaneous tumour showing multiple human T-lymphotropic virus-1 DNA integration. *Br J Dermatol* 2001; **144**: 1244–8.

80. Furukawa Y, Fujisawa J, Osame M et al. Frequent clonal proliferation of human T-cell leukemia virus type 1 (HTLV-1)-infected T cells in HTLV-1-associated myelopathy (HAM-TSP). *Blood* 1992; **80**: 1012–16.

81. Takemoto S, Matsuoka M, Yamaguchi K, Takatsuki K. A novel diagnostic method of adult T-cell leukemia: monoclonal integration of human T-cell lymphotropic virus type I provirus DNA detected by inverse polymerase chain reaction. *Blood* 1994; **84**: 3080–5.

82. Wattel E, Vartanian JP, Pannotier C, Wain-Hobson S. Clonal expansion of human T-cell leukemia virus type I-infected cells in asymptomatic and symptomatic carriers without malignancy. *J Virol* 1995; **69**: 2863–8.

83. Cavrois M, Leclercq I, Gout O, Gessain A, Wain-Hobson S, Wattel E. Persistent oligoclonal expansion of human T-cell leukemia virus type 1-infected circulating cells in patients with tropical spastic paraparesis/HTLV-1 associated myelopathy. *Oncogene* 1998; **17**: 77–82.

84. Leclercq I, Mortreux F, Morschhauser F et al. Semiquantitative analysis of residual disease in patients treated for adult T-cell leukaemia/lymphoma (ATLL). *Br J Haematol* 1999; **105**: 743–51.

85. Tannir N, Riggs S, Velasquez W, Samaan N, Manning J. Hypercalcemia, unusual bone lesions, and human T-cell leukemia-lymphoma virus in adult T-cell lymphoma. *Cancer* 1985; **55**: 615–19.

86. Ejima E, Rosenblatt JD, Massari M et al. Cell-type-specific transactivation of the parathyroid hormone-related protein gene promoter by the human T-cell leukemia virus type I (HTLV- I) tax and HTLV-II tax proteins. *Blood* 1993; **81**: 1017–24.

87. Takahashi K, Tanaka T, Fujita M, Horiguchi Y, Miyachi Y, Imamura S. Cutaneous-type adult T-cell leukemia/lymphoma. A unique clinical feature with monoclonal T-cell proliferation detected by Southern blot analysis. *Arch Dermatol* 1988; **124**: 399–404.

88. Gessain A, Moulonguet I, Flageul B et al. Cutaneous type of adult T cell leukemia/lymphoma in a French West Indian woman. Clonal rearrangement of T-cell receptor beta and gamma genes and monoclonal integration of HTLV-I proviral DNA in the skin infiltrate. *J Am Acad Dermatol* 1990; **23**: 994–1000.

89. Su IJ, Wu YC, Chen YC, Hsieh HC, Cheng AL, Wang CH,

Kadin ME. Cutaneous manifestations of postthymic T cell malignancies: description of five clinicopathologic subtypes. *J Am Acad Dermatol* 1990; **23**: 653–62.

90. Yoshie O, Fujisawa R, Nakayama T et al. Frequent expression of CCR4 in adult T-cell leukemia and human T-cell leukemia virus type 1-transformed T cells. *Blood* 2002; **99**: 1505–11.

91. El-Sabban ME, Merhi RA, Haidar HA et al. Human T-cell lymphotropic virus type 1-transformed cells induce angiogenesis and establish functional gap junctions with endothelial cells. *Blood* 2002; **99**: 3383–9.

92. Bazarbachi A, Abou Merhi R, Gessain A et al. Human T-cell lymphotropic virus type I-infected cells extravasate through the endothelial barrier by a local angiogenesis-like mechanism. *Cancer Res* 2004; **64**: 2039–46.

93. La Grenade L, Manns A, Fletcher V et al. Clinical, pathologic, and immunologic features of human T-lymphotrophic virus type I-associated infective dermatitis in children. *Arch Dermatol* 1998; **134**: 439–44.

94. Hanchard B, LaGrenade L, Carberry C et al. Childhood infective dermatitis evolving into adult T-cell leukaemia after 17 years. *Lancet* 1991; **338**: 1593–4.

95. Mahe A, Meertens L, Ly F et al. Human T-cell leukaemia/lymphoma virus type 1-associated infective dermatitis in Africa: a report of five cases from Senegal. *Br J Dermatol* 2004; **150**: 958–65.

96. Tsukasaki K, Yamada Y, Ikeda S, Tomonaga M. Infective dermatitis among patients with ATL in Japan. *Int J Cancer* 1994; **57**: 293.

97. White JD, Zaknoen SL, Kasten-Sportes C et al. Infectious complications and immunodeficiency in patients with human T-cell lymphotropic virus I-associated adult T-cell leukemia/lymphoma. *Cancer* 1995; **75**: 1598–607.

98. Gabet AS, Mortreux F, Talarmin A et al. High circulating proviral load with oligoclonal expansion of HTLV-1 bearing T cells in HTLV-1 carriers with strongyloidiasis. *Oncogene* 2000; **19**: 4954–60.

99. Plumelle Y, Gonin C, Edouard A et al. Effect of *Strongyloides stercoralis* infection and eosinophilia on age at onset and prognosis of adult T-cell leukemia. *Am J Clin Pathol* 1997; **107**: 81–87.

100. Nakada K, Yamaguchi K, Furugen S et al. Monoclonal integration of HTLV-I proviral DNA in patients with strongyloidiasis. *Int J Cancer* 1987; **40**: 145–8.

101. Hermine O, Wattel E, Gessain A, Bazarbachi A. Adult T cell leukemia, a review of established and new treatments. *BioDrugs* 1998; **10**: 447–62.

102. Hermine O, Arnulf B, Bazarbachi A. Treatment of adult-T cell leukemia/lymphoma: clinical results of new therapeutic approaches. *AIDS Res Hum Retroviruses* 2001; **17**: S–29.

103. Siegel RS, Gartenhaus RB, Kuzel TM. Human T-cell lymphotropic-I-associated leukemia/lymphoma. *Curr Treat Options Oncol* 2001; **2**: 291–300.

104. Kami M, Hamaki T, Miyakoshi S et al. Allogeneic haematopoietic stem cell transplantation for the treatment of adult T-cell leukaemia/lymphoma. *Br J Haematol* 2003; **120**: 304–9.

105. Yamada Y, Tomonaga M, Fukuda H et al. A new G-CSF-supported combination chemotherapy, LSG15, for adult T cell leukemia-lymphoma: Japan Clinical Oncology Group Study 9303. *Br J Haematol* 2001; **113**: 375–82.

106. Zhang J, Balestrieri E, Grelli S et al. Efficacy of 3′-azido 3′deoxythymidine (AZT) in preventing HTLV-1 transmis-

sion to human cord blood mononuclear cells. *Virus Res* 2001; **78**: 67–78.

107. Gill PS, Harrington W Jr., Kaplan MH et al. Treatment of adult T-cell leukemia-lymphoma with a combination of interferon alfa and zidovudine. *N Engl J Med* 1995; **332**: 1744–8.

108. Hermine O, Bouscary D, Gessain A et al. Brief report: treatment of adult T-cell leukemia-lymphoma with zidovudine and interferon alfa. *N Engl J Med* 1995; **332**: 1749–51.

109. Hermine O, Allard I, Levy V, Arnulf B, Gessain B, Bazarbachi A. A prospective phase II clinical trial with the use of zidovudine and interferon-alpha in the acute and lymphoma forms of adult T-cell leukemia/lymphoma. *Hematol J* 2002; **3**: 276–82.

110. Besson C, Panelatti G, Delaunay C et al. Treatment of adult T-cell leukemia-lymphoma by CHOP followed by therapy with antinucleosides, alpha interferon and oral etoposide. *Leuk Lymphoma* 2002; **43**: 2275–9.

111. White JD, Wharfe G, Stewart DM et al. The combination of zidovudine and interferon alpha-2B in the treatment of adult T-cell leukemia/lymphoma. *Leuk Lymphoma* 2001; **40**: 287–94.

112. Fujimura S, Suzumiya J, Anzai K et al. Retinoic acids induce growth inhibition and apoptosis in adult T-cell leukemia (ATL) cell lines. *Leuk Res* 1998; **22**: 611–18.

113. Darwiche N, El-Sabban M, Bazzi R et al. Retinoic acid dramatically enhances the arsenic trioxide-induced cell cycle arrest and apoptosis in retinoic acid receptor alpha-positive human T-cell lymphotropic virus type-I-transformed cells. 2001; **2**: 127–35.

114. Bazarbachi A, El-Sabban ME, Nasr R et al. Arsenic trioxide and interferon-alpha synergize to induce cell cycle arrest and apoptosis in human T-cell lymphotropic virus type I-transformed cells. *Blood* 1999; **93**: 278–83.

115. El-Sabban ME, Nasr R, Dbaibo G et al. Arsenic-interferon-alpha-triggered apoptosis in HTLV-I transformed cells is associated with tax down-regulation and reversal of NF-kappaB activation. *Blood* 2000; **96**: 2849–55.

116. Nasr R, Rosenwald A, El-Sabban ME et al. Arsenic/interferon specifically reverses 2 distinct gene networks critical for the survival of HTLV-1-infected leukemic cells. *Blood* 2003; **101**: 4576–82.

117. Mahieux R, Pise-Masison C, Gessain A et al. Arsenic trioxide induces apoptosis in HTLV-1 and HTLV-2 infected cells by a caspase-3 dependent mechanism involving Bcl-2 cleavage. *Blood* 2001; **98**: 3762–9.

118. Hermine O, Dombret H, Poupon J et al. Phase II trial of arsenic trioxide and alpha interferon in patients with relapsed/refractory adult T-cell leukemia/lymphoma. *Hematol J* 2004; **5**: 130–4.

119. Dewan MZ, Terashima K, Taruishi M et al. Rapid tumor formation of human T-cell leukemia virus type 1-infected cell lines in novel NOD-SCID/gammac(null) mice: suppression by an inhibitor against NF-kappaB. *J Virol* 2003; **77**: 5286–94.

120. Tan C, Waldmann TA. Proteasome inhibitor PS-341, a potential therapeutic agent for adult T-cell leukemia. *Cancer Res* 2002; **62**: 1083–6.

121. Mitra-Kaushik S, Harding JC, Hess J, Ratner L. Effects of the Proteasome inhibitor PS-341 on tumor growth in HTLV-1 Tax transgenic mice and Tax tumor transplants. *Blood* 2004 (In Press)

122. Barmak K, Harhaj E, Grant C, Alefantis T, Wigdahl B. Human T cell leukemia virus type I-induced disease:

pathways to cancer and neurodegeneration. *Virology* 2003; **308**: 1–12.

123. Slattery JP, Franchini G, Gessain A. Genomic evolution, patterns of global dissemination, and interspecies transmission of human and simian T-cell leukemia/lymphotropic viruses. *Genome Res* 1999; **9**: 525–40.

124. Furukawa Y, Yamashita M, Usuku K, Izumo S, Nakagawa M, Osame M. Phylogenetic subgroups of human T cell lymphotropic virus (HTLV) type I in the tax gene and their association with different risks for HTLV-I-associated myelopathy/tropical spastic paraparesis. *J Infect Dis* 2000; **182**: 1343–9.

125. Akari H, Ono F, Sakakibara I et al. Simian T cell leukemia virus type I-induced malignant adult T cell leukemia-like disease in a naturally infected African green monkey: implication of CD8+ T cell leukemia. *AIDS Res Hum Retroviruses* 1998; **14**: 367–71.

126. Yashiki S, Fujiyoshi T, Arima N et al. HLA-A*26, HLA-B*4002, HLA-B*4006, and HLA-B*4801 alleles predispose to adult T cell leukemia: the limited recognition of HTLV type 1 tax peptide anchor motifs and epitopes to generate anti-HTLV type 1 tax CD8(+) cytotoxic T lymphocytes. *AIDS Res Hum Retroviruses* 2001; **17**: 1047–61.

127. Furukawa Y, Kubota R, Tara M, Izumo S, Osame M. Existence of escape mutant in HTLV-I tax during the development of adult T-cell leukemia. *Blood* 2001; **97**: 987–93.

128. Plancoulaine S, Gessain A, Joubert M et al. Detection of a major gene predisposing to human T lymphotropic virus type I infection in children among an endemic population of African origin. *J Infect Dis* 2000; **182**: 405–12.

129. Bartholomew C, Jack N, Edwards J et al. HTLV-I serostatus of mothers of patients with adult T-cell leukemia and HTLV-I-associated myelopathy/tropical spastic paraparesis. *J Hum Virol* 1998; **1**: 302–5.

130. Pombo-de-Oliveira MS, Carvalho SM, Borducchi D et al. Adult T-cell leukemia/lymphoma and cluster of HTLV-I associated diseases in Brazilian settings. *Leuk Lymphoma* 2001; **42**: 135–44.

131. Hanon E, Hall S, Taylor GP et al. Abundant tax protein expression in CD4+ T cells infected with human T-cell lymphotropic virus type I (HTLV-I) is prevented by cytotoxic T lymphocytes. *Blood* 2000; **95**: 1386–92.

132. Kannagi M, Matsushita S, Harada S. Expression of the target antigen for cytotoxic T lymphocytes on adult T-cell leukemia cells. *Int J Cancer* 1993; **54**: 582–8.

133. Arnulf B, Thorel M, Poirot Y et al. Loss of the ex vivo but not the reinducible CD8+ T-cell response to Tax in human T-cell leukemia virus type 1-infected patients with adult T-cell leukemia/lymphoma. *Leukemia* 2004; **18**: 126–32.

134. Okayama A, Stuver S, Matsuoka M et al. Role of HTLV-1 proviral DNA load and clonality in the development of adult T-cell leukemia/lymphoma in asymptomatic carriers. *Int J Cancer* 2004; **110**: 621–5.

135. Hall WW. Human T cell lymphotropic virus type I and cutaneous T cell leukemia/lymphoma. *J Exp Med* 1994; **180**: 1581–5.

136. Capesius C, Saal F, Maero E et al. No evidence for HTLV-I infection in 24 cases of French and Portuguese mycosis fungoides and Sézary syndrome (as seen in France). *Leukemia* 1991; **5**: 416–19.

137. Ghosh SK, Abrams JT, Terunuma H, Vonderheid EC, DeFreitas E. Human T-cell leukemia virus type I tax/rex DNA and RNA in cutaneous T-cell lymphoma. *Blood* 1994; **84**: 2663–71.

138. Manca N, Piacentini E, Gelmi M et al. Persistence of human T cell lymphotropic virus type 1 (HTLV-1) sequences in peripheral blood mononuclear cells from patients with mycosis fungoides. *J Exp Med* 1994; **180**: 1973–8.

139. Zucker-Franklin D, Coutavas EE, Rush MG, Zouzias DC. Detection of human T-lymphotropic virus-like particles in cultures of peripheral blood lymphocytes from patients with mycosis fungoides. *Proc Natl Acad Sci U S A* 1991; **88**: 7630–4.

140. Bazarbachi A, Soriano V, Pawson R et al. Mycosis fungoides and Sézary syndrome are not associated with HTLV-I infection: an international study. *Br J Haematol* 1997; **98**: 927–33.

141. Kalyanaraman VS, Sarngadharan MG, Robert-Guroff M, Miyoshi I, Golde D, Gallo RC. A new subtype of human T-cell leukemia virus (HTLV-II) associated with a T-cell variant of hairy cell leukemia. *Science* 1982; **218**: 571–3.

142. Hall WW, Ishak R, Zhu SW et al. Human T lymphotropic virus type II (HTLV-II): epidemiology, molecular properties, and clinical features of infection. *J Acquir Immune Defic Syndr Hum Retrovirol* 1996; **13**: S204–14.

143. Gessain A, Mauclere P, Froment A et al. Isolation and molecular characterization of a human T-cell lymphotropic virus type II (HTLV-II), subtype B, from a healthy Pygmy living in a remote area of Cameroon: an ancient origin for HTLV-II in Africa. *Proc Natl Acad Sci U S A* 1995; **92**: 4041–5.

144. Vandamme AM, Bertazzoni U, Salemi M. Evolutionary strategies of human T-cell lymphotropic virus type II. *Gene* 2000; **261**: 171–80.

145. Ijichi S, Ramundo MB, Takahashi H, Hall WW. In vivo cellular tropism of human T cell leukemia virus type II (HTLV-II). *J Exp Med* 1992; **176**: 293–6.

146. Rosenblatt JD, Plaeger-Marshall S, Giorgi JV et al. A clinical, hematologic, and immunologic analysis of 21 HTLV-II-infected intravenous drug users. *Blood* 1990; **76**: 409–17.

147. Wang TG, Ye J, Lairmore MD, Green PL. In vitro cellular tropism of human T cell leukemia virus type 2. *AIDS Res Hum Retroviruses* 2000; **16**: 1661–8.

148. Perzova RN, Loughran TP, Dube S, Ferrer J, Esteban E, Poiesz BJ. Lack of BLV and PTLV DNA sequences in the majority of patients with large granular lymphocyte leukaemia. *Br J Haematol* 2000; **109**: 64–70.

149. Poiesz B, Dube D, Dube S et al. HTLV-II-associated cutaneous T-cell lymphoma in a patient with HIV-1 infection. *N Engl J Med* 2000; **342**: 930–6.

150. Fouchard N, Flageul B, Bagot M et al. Lack of evidence of HTLV-I/II infection in T CD8 malignant or reactive lymphoproliferative disorders in France: a serological and/or molecular study of 169 cases. *Leukemia* 1995; **9**: 2087–92.

151. Loughran TP Jr., Coyle T, Sherman MP, Starkebaum G, Ehrlich GD, Ruscetti FW, Poiesz BJ. Detection of human T-cell leukemia/lymphoma virus, type II, in a patient with large granular lymphocyte leukemia. *Blood* 1992; **80**: 1116–19.

152. Heneine W, Chan WC, Lust JA et al. HTLV-II infection is rare in patients with large granular lymphocyte leukemia. *J Acquir Immune Defic Syndr* 1994; **7**: 736–7.

153. Martin MP, Biggar RJ, Hamlin-Green G, Staal S, Mann D. Large granular lymphocytosis in a patient infected with HTLV-II. *AIDS Res Hum Retroviruses* 1993; **9**: 715–19.

154. Kaplan MH, Hall WW, Susin M et al. Syndrome of severe skin disease, eosinophilia, and dermatopathic lymphadenopathy in patients with HTLV-II complicating human immunodeficiency virus infection. *Am J Med* 1991; **91**: 300–9.

155. Zucker-Franklin D, Hooper WC, Evatt BL. Human lymphotropic retroviruses associated with mycosis fungoides: evidence that human T-cell lymphotropic virus type II (HTLV-II) as well as HTLV-I may play a role in the disease. *Blood* 1992; **80**: 1537–45.

156. Rosenblatt JD, Giorgi JV, Golde DW et al. Integrated human T-cell leukemia virus II genome in CD8+ T cells from a patient with 'atypical' hairy cell leukemia: evidence for distinct T and B cell lymphoproliferative disorders. *Blood* 1988; **71**: 363–9.

157. Kazanji M, Tartaglia J, Franchini G et al. Immunogenicity and protective efficacy of recombinant human T-cell leukemia/lymphoma virus type 1 NYVAC and naked DNA vaccine candidates in squirrel monkeys (Saimiri sciureus). *J Virol* 2001; **75**: 5939–48.

158. Bomford R, Kazanji M, De The G. Vaccine against human T cell leukemia-lymphoma virus type I: progress and prospects. *AIDS Res Hum Retroviruses* 1996; **12**: 403–5.

159. Matutes E, Catovsky D. ATL of Caribbean origin. In: Takatsuki K (ed.) *Adult T-cell Leukemia*. Oxford University Press 1994: 114–38.

# 16 Immunosuppression: Epstein–Barr virus and other herpesviruses in hematological malignancies

Martine Raphaël, Fanny Baran-Marszak, and Hélène A Poirel

## Introduction

Immunodeficiency, either primary or acquired, is associated with an increased incidence of lympho-proliferative disorders (LPD) and lymphoma. Among the pathogenic mechanisms underlying the primary immune disorders (PID), which are widely heterogeneous, defective immune surveillance of herpesviruses, particularly to Epstein–Barr virus (EBV), is involved in the majority of PID, leading to EBV-driven LPD. These EBV-driven LPD are observed in PID where the T-cell defect is partial or complete, as in severe combined immunodeficiency (SCID), Wiskott–Aldrich syndrome (WAS), combined variable immunodeficiency disorder (CVID), and X-linked lymphoproliferative syndrome (XLP, Duncan syndrome).[1,2] In acquired immunodeficiency, two main clinical settings are described: the post-transplant lymphoproliferative disorders (PTLD) occurring after transplantation and the lymphoid neoplasms developing in HIV-infected patients (AIDS-related lymphomas). In PTLD, the pathogenic mechanisms are mainly linked to the immune defect with respect to EBV, especially in early lesions.[3–5] In HIV infection, in addition to the immune defect with respect to the oncogenic viruses EBV and Kaposi sarcoma-associated herpesvirus (KSHV; also known as human herpesvirus 8, HHV8), antigenic stimulation and genomic abnormalities involving known oncogenes also play a role.[5,6]

## Epstein–Barr virus

EBV (HHV4), a γ-herpesvirus with double tropism for lymphoid and epithelial cells, shares the same biologic properties as the other viruses from this subfamily, such as latent infection in lymphocytes, cell proliferation, and an association with cancer.[7] EBV, the causal agent of infectious mononucleosis, is also an etiologic agent in nasopharyngeal carcinoma and in lymphoid proliferations, including Burkitt lymphoma, Hodgkin lymphoma, extranodal NK/T-cell lymphoma nasal type, and LPD and lymphomas in immunosuppressed patients.[8] Like other herpesviruses, EBV has a protein core wrapped with DNA, a nucleocapsid, a protein tegument, and an envelope with external glycoprotein spikes. The most abundant EBV outer envelope protein is gp350/220, which binds to CD21, the EBV receptor, on the surface of B lymphocytes.[9]

The EBV genome, which has been entirely sequenced, is linear, double-stranded 172 kbp DNA, and contains terminal repeats (TR), internal repeats (IR1–4), and unique sequence domains (U1–U5). EBV can manifest two different life cycles: latent and replicative, but in lymphoid cells, EBV is mostly latent. EBV exists in different forms: circular or episomal during latency, and linear in the replicative cycle.[8,9] Circularization of the EBV genome is obtained by the joining of 500 bp tandem-repeat DNA sequences at both ends of the linear molecule. Because different episomes can have different numbers of TR, the analysis of the structure of the termini can also be used to assess the clonality of the lymphoid proliferation.[10]

In lymphoblastoid cell lines (LCL) and in recently EBV-infected lymphocytes, six different nuclear proteins, EBNA (Epstein–Barr nuclear antigens) 1, 2, 3A, 3B, 3C, and LP, three different integral membrane proteins, LMP (latent membrane proteins) 1, 2A, and 2B, and two small non-polyadenylated RNAs (EBV-encoded RNAs, EBER) are expressed. Two types of EBV – EBV1/EBVA and EBV2/EBVB – are identified based on the genomic differences on genes encoding for EBNALP, 2, 3A, 3B, and 3C. EBV2 is more frequent in Africa where half of the Burkitt lymphoma (BL) are associated with EBV2.[9]

Recombinant EBV technologies developed in several laboratories have allowed identification of the proteins and their roles in continuously proliferating lymphoblastoid cell lines and in human malignancies. Recombinant EBV genetic analysis of transformation using specifically mutated cloned restriction fragments of viral DNA transfected into infected cells is one of the experimental strategies used to analyze viral genes essential for transformation. The P3HR1 strain of EBV, which is deleted for a DNA segment that contains all of the EBNA2 exons and the last two exons of EBNALP, is unable to immortalize B cells. Among other approaches to analyze EBV-transformed genes are marker rescue of a transformation-defective EBV genome, the mini-EBV genome, and recombinant cloning of EBV as a bacterial artificial chromosome (BAC).[11]

EBV may lead to B-cell immortalization by activating a set of host cellular genes. EBNALP and EBNA2 are the first viral proteins to be expressed after cellular infection. EBNA2, a specific transactivator of the BamHI C-promoter (Cp) and the promoters of LMP1 and LMP2, is a key viral protein in the immortalization of B cells. Thus, EBNA2 transactivates viral genes such as LMP1 and LMP2 and cellular genes, including CD21, CD23, and the fgr oncogene, as well as the c-myc oncogene,[9] and represses transcription of the immunoglobulin heavy-chain locus.[12] EBNA2 is tethered to cellular genes with the cellular repressor RBP-J involved in the Notch signaling pathway. In the latter, after activation by ligands belonging to the Delta, Serrate, Lag-2 (DSL) family of proteins, the extracellular part of the Notch receptor is cleaved, releasing the intracellular part of Notch (Notch-IC), which is translocated to the nucleus, where it interacts with RBP-J and modulates gene expression. In fact, EBNA2, resembling the physiologically switched-on form of this gene modulator, can be regarded as a viral functional equivalent to the activated Notch receptor, Notch-IC. However, Notch-IC cannot maintain B-cell proliferation in the absence of EBNA2.[13,14] Thus, EBNA2 should be able to transactivate genes that can lead to cellular transformation and neoplasms. Moreover, cooperation between EBNALP and EBNA2 may induce the cell cycle transition from $G_0$ to $G_1$ by inducing cyclin D2.[15]

EBNA3A, 3B, and 3C, encoded by three genes that are likely to have had a common origin, have structural similarities and probably similar roles in cell growth transformation. EBNA3A and 3C are essential for B-cell immortalization. It has been shown that EBNA3C upregulates LMP1 expression and CD21 mRNA, cooperates with RAS,[15] and downregulates p27, one of the proteins involved in cell cycle regulation.[16]

EBNA1 is the only EBNA protein that associates with chromosomes during mitosis and there are at least three independent domains mediating EBNA1 binding. EBNA1 activates the origin of replication OriP during S phase and may also contribute to the partition and/or retention of the viral genome during mitosis.[17]

The LMP1 protein, which is expressed in a wide variety of malignancies, may contribute to EBV-driven neoplasia.[18] Evidence of its oncogenic properties was demonstrated by the acquired malignant phenotype of rodent fibroblasts induced by LMP1.[19] The different functions of LMP1 that confer its oncogenic ability can be summarized as induction of DNA synthesis together with suppression of apoptosis by the induction of anti-apoptotic genes such as BCL2, MCL1, BFL1, A20, and c-IAP. The potential indirect role of LMP1 in angiogenesis and metastasis has also been involved.[20] LMP1 is regarded as a constitutively active receptor, mimicking the activation of B cells via the tumor necrosis factor receptor (TNFR) activation pathway Two regions of LMP1, CTAR1/TES1 and CTAR2/TES2, are critical for B-cell immortalization. The CTAR1 domain binds with TNFR-associated factors (TRAF) 1, 2, 3, and 5, which suggests a similarity between LMP1 and the superfamily of TNF receptors and a mimicry of the CD40/CD40-ligand activation pathway.[21] LMP1, as a key transforming viral protein, activates very complex signaling cascades, including the NF-κB, MAPK, JNK, p38, and JAK–STAT pathways through its C terminus, plays a leading role in most of the pleiotropic malignant effects.[9,20,21] Its involvement in the PI3K/Akt signaling pathway has also been identified.[20] Interferon regulatory factor 7 (IRF7), which was cloned and identified in the context of EBV infection, is regulated by LMP1, which induces its expression, activation by phosphorylation, and nuclear translocation. Thus, IRF7 appears to be a cellular mediator of LMP1 in EBV latency and transformation.[22]

Two small non-polyadenylated RNAs, EBER1 and EBER2, are the most abundant viral transcripts in latently EBV-infected cells. They are therefore used as targets for in situ hybridization to detect EBV in tissue; however, examples of EBER-negative latent infection do exist.[23] EBER, which are involved in the interferon response, may also have a role in oncogenesis. In fact, they are also implicated in the maintenance of the malignant phenotype in BL cells by conferring resistance to various stimuli that normally induce apoptosis.[24] They also induce transcription of IL-10 as an autocrine growth factor in BL[25] and contribute to the local immune deficiency.

EBV, using many different signaling pathways to induce lymphocyte proliferation and survival, generates a highly complex molecular crosstalk between signaling events inducing transcription of the genes encoding the cytokines interleukin-6 (IL-6) and IL-10, signaling molecules linked to the cell cycle and molecules implicated in the inhibition of apoptosis.[26,27] The use of gene array technology to analyze virally regulated cellular genes in EBV-transformed Burkitt cell lines have identified several functional groups of genes involved in the cell cycle, apoptosis, and signal transduction pathways, including the TNFR and interferon pathways. Moreover, this study has identified the involvement of three families of transcription factors: Rel/NF-κB, STAT1, and the Ets-related proteins spi-B, Elf-1, and Ets-1.[28]

Approximately 1 in $10^3$–$10^4$ peripheral blood B lymphocytes are latently infected. In the general healthy population, the persistence of EBV is related to its ability to use the cellular machinery of the normal B cell during immunopoiesis. Recent studies have identified the memory B cell as a reservoir of EBV,[29] and have demonstrated that these latently infected B cells express the same restricted pattern of latent genes previously found only in EBV-associated tumors.[30] EBV-infected B cells have to evade the germinal center reaction to gain access to the B-cell memory compartment, the reservoir of EBV. The latent gene expression of EBV depends on the location and differentiation state of the infected B cell. In newly infected B cells, all nine latent proteins and both EBER are expressed under the transactivation of EBNA2. Whereas in the germinal center, viral gene expression is restricted to LMP1, LMP2, the EBER, and EBNA1, in memory B cells in the tonsils and in peripheral blood, the latency is characterized as latency 0, with only the EBER and LMP2 transcripts being expressed.[31]

Thus, four types of latency (0, I, II, and III) have been described from analysis of EBV latent gene expression in LCL, primary infection and persistence of EBV, and tumors. They are characterized by differential expression of latent genes; the four types of EBV latency are summarized in Table 16.1.

The replicative life cycle of EBV appears when latently infected lymphocytes become permissive for virus replication.[32] BZLF1 and BRLF1 are the immediate early genes expressed at the induction of the lytic cycle. These genes are transactivators of early EBV lytic gene expression, such as that of BHLF1, BHRF1, BSMLF1, and BALF2. Several EBV early genes are linked to DNA replication, including those encoding DNA polymerase (BALF5), major DNA-binding protein (BALF2), ribonucleotide reductase (BORF2 and BaRF1), thymidine kinase (BXLF1), and endoalkaline exonuclease (BGLF5). The late genes are mostly involved in encoding structural viral proteins, the most abundant of which is gp350/220 (encoded by BLLF1), which is found on the virus and in the plasma membrane of lytically infected cells.[9]

Because some EBV sequences have homology to cellular genes, it appears that some lytic genes have been appropriated from the primate genome. These genes are the EBV immediate early gene BZLF1, which is closely related to the jun/fos family, the early gene BHRF1, with functional homology to the BCL2 gene, one of the most important anti-apoptotic genes, and the late gene BCRF1, which is close to the human IL-10 gene. IL-10, which is involved in proliferation and terminal B-cell differentiation, can induce local immunosuppression by blunting the initial interferon, natural killer (NK), and CD8+ T-cell response.[9]

## EBV and immunodeficiency

Identifying positive serology to EBV, epidemiological studies show that more than 95% of adults in all populations worldwide are infected with EBV.[8] In the general population, however, only a very few proportion of people develop LPD. In contrast, patients with immunodeficiencies have a 60–200 times greater risk of developing LPD. This observation reflects two fundamental features: (1) a tightly controlled and strong cellular immune response to EBV-infected cells, (2) the ability of the virus to establish interactions with cellular genes, leading to a breakdown of cellular homeostasis control, including both cell cycle and apoptosis.

**Table 16.1.  Types of EBV latency**

|  | Latency | | | | Functions |
| --- | --- | --- | --- | --- | --- |
|  | 0 | I | II | III |  |
| EBERS | +/– | + | + | + | Interferon response, resistance to apoptosis, transcription of IL-10 |
| EBNA1 | ARN | + | + | + | Partition/retention of viral genome |
| EBNA2 | – | – | – | + | Transcription, tethered to RBP-J |
| EBNA3A | – | – | – | + | Transcription |
| EBNA3B | – | – | – | + | Transcription |
| EBNA3C | – | – | – | + | Cell cycle interaction |
| EBNAl P | – | – | – | + | Cooperation with EBNA2 |
| LMP1 | – | – | + | + | Activation pathways: NF-κB, STAT1 |
| LMP2A | ARN | – | + | + | B-cell receptor interaction |
| LMP2B | – | – | + | + | ? |

ARN, acute retinal necrosis

Defective T-cell control in immunosuppressed patients is one of the key pathogenic mechanisms in EBV-related LPD. There is evidence of virus-specific T-cell mediated immunity, with restriction mainly through HLA class I but also through HLA class II (reviewed in reference 33). The specific response against different viral antigens determined by the HLA class I of the responder has been demonstrated using expansion and subsequent cloning of reactive T cells and a complex viral system with vaccinia recombinants expressing individual viral genes.[34,35] Immunological studies have been conducted using mapped antigenic peptide epitopes within the primary sequence of several of the viral proteins expressed in transformed cells,[36] the interferon-γ (IFN-γ) Elispot assay for quantitative detection of EBV-specific CD8+ cells,[37] together with the use of synthetic peptides and tetramer technology.[38] These studies have demonstrated the lack of a specific T-cell response and the long-term restoration of immunity against EBV infection by adoptive transfer of gene-modified virus-specific T lymphocytes.[39] Besides a quantitative defect, studies of the functional diversity of the CD8+ T-cell response to EBV have shown that EBV-specific CD8+ T cells that express type 2 cytokines (IL-4, IL-5, IL-6, IL-10, and IL-13) possess the ability to activate resting B cells.[40] This is in accordance with previous experiments in SCID mice engrafted with human peripheral blood lymphocytes, showing that the presence of T cells is required for the development of EBV-induced lymphoproliferative disorders.[41]

Targets of EBV CD8+ T cells are immunogenic latency proteins such as EBNA3C, EBNA2, and LMP1,[8,42] as well as immediate early and early lytic cycle proteins.[43] EBNA1, which is a major latent protein of EBV, does not generate a specific CD8+ T-cell response due to selective inhibition of processing by glycine–alanine repeats.[44] However, recent immunological data have shown that CD4+ cells are specific for EBNA1.[45]

Besides the defective T-cell response to a given antigen, the importance of the role of different processing of the epitope and its presentation has also been demonstrated.[46] Recent data show that the interaction of EBV with monocytes can prevent the development of dendritic cells, suggesting that interference with the dendritic cell functions plays a role in escaping the virus-specific immune response.[47] The secretion of IL-10 by EBV-infected B cells[48] and by a subset of CD8+ T cells leads to an enhancement of immunosuppression.[40,49]

As a consequence of the lack of the immune control, there is an increase in viral load. This increase has been demonstrated in immunodeficient patients by semiquantitative and quantitative polymerase chain reaction (PCR).[50] The relationship between the high viral load and the occurrence of LPD has been demonstrated in post-transplant patients,[50] although in HIV patients, the link between a high viral load and the occurrence of a lymphoma is less clearly demonstrated.[51]

The importance of these mechanisms of immune surveillance in limiting the growth advantage of EBV-infected cells is clearly illustrated in immunodeficient patients. Regressions of LPD have been reported after reduction of immunosuppression[4] and also after infusion of blood lymphocytes or in vivo activated EBV-specific cytotoxic T-lymphocyte cultures of donor origin in bone marrow recipients developing lymphomas.[52–54]

# KSHV/HHV8

In 1994, using a new technique of viral identification, representational difference analysis (RDA), a new human γ-herpesvirus was identified[55,56] in an AIDS-related Kaposi sarcoma (KS) biopsy. The same virus was identified in a peculiar lymphoma confined predominantly to the body cavities and persisting as effusion, now named primary effusion lymphoma (PEL), that had developed in AIDS patients.[57] This virus has also been identified in HIV-related multicentric Castleman disease (MCD),[58] which is frequently associated with secondary tumors such as KS and lymphomas. This virus was named Kaposi sarcoma-associated herpesvirus (KSHV) or human herpesvirus 8 (HHV8). KSHV/HHV8 has sequence similarity to the oncogenic herpesvirus saimiri (HVS), EBV, and murine herpesvirus 68 (MHV68), and leads, like these transforming viruses, to neoplasms. The complete genome of KSHV/HHV8 was sequenced from both KS biopsy and PEL cell lines (BC1).[59,60] The virus consists of a long unique coding region (LUR) flanked by 800 bp terminal repeat sequences. The LUR comprises 81 open reading frames (ORF). A large number of genes pirated from eukaryotic cellular DNA are recognized, mimicking cytokine and cytokine response pathways. Comparisons between KSHV/HHV8 and EBV have shown similarities in the use of cellular machinery by these two viruses, both virus employing the same signaling cascades to survive in their hosts.[61]

The cellular genes pirated by KSHV/HHV8 include those specifying functions associated with signal transduction, immune evasion, and cellular proliferation and survival. Thus, they can be categorized according to their function. Genes involved in cell proliferation are v-cyclin (ORF72),[62] v-GPCR (ORF74),[63] and v-IRF (K9).[64] The latter two have oncogenic potential and transform 3T3 cells.[63,64] Apoptosis inhibitors are encoded by v-BCL2 (ORF16),[65] v-FLIP (ORF71), and v-IL-6 (ORFK2).[66] Broad-spectrum chemokine antagonists are also encoded by the

KSHV/HHV8 genes v-*MIP-I* (ORFK4), v-*MIP-II* (ORFK6), and v-*MIPIII* (ORFK4-2). The virally encoded chemokines v-MIP-I and v-MIP-II bind to both CC and CXC receptors preferentially over cellular chemokines.[67] The protein encoded by v-*NCAM* (ORFK14) has an intercellular signaling function. The captured eukaryotic genes have acquired unique properties abrogating normal responses; for example, the D-type cyclin encoded by KSHV/HHV8 does not respond to the cell cycle inhibitors p16 and p21 after binding to CDK6.[68]

Like EBV, KSHV/HHV8 is latently present in B lymphocytes. A punctuate nuclear staining detected after immunofluorescence using KSHV/HHV8 immune sera as well as immunoblots detected a 222−234 kDa doublet, leading to the discovery of a latent antigen, latency-associated nuclear antigen (LANA, LNA, or LNA1), encoded by ORF73. Serological assays based on antibodies to LANA and to a recombinant structural (capsid-related) protein encoded by ORF65, and then polymerase chain reaction (PCR) detection on peripheral blood mononuclear cells, semen, and saliva, has allowed wide epidemiological studies.[69]

The gene expression of KSHV/HHV8 in PEL is important for understanding the pathogenetic role of this virus in this peculiar lymphoma. Three KSHV/HHV8 gene products, v-GPCR,[63] v-IRF,[64] and kaposin,[70] can induce transformation of rodent fibroblasts, and K1 can substitute for the transforming protein of HVS.[71] In PEL-derived cell lines, associated or not with EBV,[59] KSHV/HHV8 is latent, with only a minority being replicated. Exposure of these cells lines to 12-tetradecamoylphorbol 13-acetate (TPA) or butyrate can induce an increase in virus-producing cells. Based on the responsiveness of PEL cells lines to TPA-induction, three classes of transcription of KSHV/HHV8 genes have been identified: class I genes, which are constitutively transcribed; class II, which are transcribed in the absence of TPA with much higher expression after exposure to TPA; and class III, reflecting lytic viral replication transcribed only following TPA induction.[72] Studies on PEL, using reverse transcriptase (RT)–PCR, revealed the expression of v-*BCL2*, v-*IL-6*, v-*MIP-I*, v-*MIP-II*, v-*cyclin*, and v-*GPCR*.[73] High levels of KSHV/HHV8 viral load and human IL-6 and IL-10 correlate with exacerbation of MCD in HIV-infected patients.[74−76] Interaction between LANA and cellular IL-6 was demonstrated through the AP1 response element.[77] Moreover, LANA inhibits p53, leading to protection against apoptosis of KSHV/HHV8-infected cells. These pathogenic mechanisms can lead in MCD to a spectrum of LPD having the features of plasmablastic lymphoma. Thus, oncogenes encoded by KSHV/HHV8 can potentially induce cell transformation and suppress host defense mechanisms.

# EBV-associated hematological malignancies in immunosuppression

Whatever the immunodeficiency, it is now well established that the EBV-related LPD induced in the context of immunosuppression result from the cooperative action of several EBV genes, interactions between the virus and the cell in complex signaling pathways, and cooperation with genetic aberrations of the cellular genome.[26] However, besides the role of EBV, cellular genetic abnormalities are also present and may have synergy with the role of the viruses, leading to very aggressive LPD in the context of immunodeficiency.

## EBV-associated tumors in PID

In PID, the cause of the LPD is related to the underlying primary immune defect.[2] In the case of EBV-related LPD, the defective immune surveillance of EBV is the primary mechanism. This is present in XLP, WAS, SCID, and some CVID.[78] The absence of T-cell control may be complete, as in fatal infectious mononucleosis (FIM) due to mutations of the SAP/SLAM protein leading to a deficient immune response to EBV.[79,80] The defect can be partial, as in lymphomatoid granulomatosis, mostly linked to WAS, a complex PID where T cells, B cells, neutrophils, platelets, and macrophages are deficient.[81,82]

Most LPD in patients with PID are of B-cell lineage, displaying B-cell markers corresponding to their differentiation status. EBV infection of B cells often leads to downregulation of these B antigens, which may be negative or expressed in only some of the neoplastic cells. On the contrary, activation molecules such as CD30 often related to the presence of the expression of the EBV latent protein LMP1, which is expressed in most cases, is upregulated and present in a variable number of EBV-infected B cells.

FIM, primarily seen in patients with XLP, results from the proliferation of EBV-positive B cells in the absence of effective immune surveillance. This abnormal B-cell proliferation is systemic, involving both lymphoid and non-lymphoid organs, most commonly the terminal ileum. This EBV-related LPD is characterized by a highly polymorphous proliferation of lymphoid cells with plasmacytoid and immunoblastic differentiation, and some Reed–Sternberg-like cells may be seen. FIM may be polyclonal at the genetic level.[78,83]

Lymphomatoid granulomatosis is an EBV-driven proliferation of B cells associated with a marked T-cell infiltration, mostly located in extranodal sites: lung, skin, brain, and kidney. The lymphoid proliferation is characterized by an angiocentric and angiodestructive infiltrate, often with extensive necrosis. Variable numbers of atypical large EBV-infected B cells are described, and this lymphoproliferative disorder may progress to diffuse large cell lymphoma (DLBCL),[82] which can be observed de novo in PID.[84]

## EBV and post-transplant lymphoproliferative disorders (PTLD)

The overall incidence of PTLD for solid organ transplant recipients is 2%. However, the frequency of PTLD varies from less than 1% in renal allografts to 5% after heart–lung or liver–bowel allografts.[85,86] After bone marrow transplantation, the risk of PTLD is low (1%), except after mismatched bone marrow transplantation, T-cell-depleted bone marrow, or immunosuppressive therapy for graft-versus-host disease, where the occurrence rate of lymphoma can reach 20%.[87] In solid organ recipients, the majority of PTLD are of host origin, while in marrow allograft recipients, they are of donor origin.[87] EBV-related PTLD tend to occur earlier after transplantation, with a median interval of 6–10 months, than EBV-negative lymphomas, which tend to occur later than 5 years following the transplant.[5,88]

The majority of PTLD associated with EBV infection occurring in a setting of iatrogenic impaired T-cell immune surveillance are EBV-induced polyclonal, oligoclonal, or monoclonal B-cell proliferations.[85,86,89,90] A physical association of LMP1 with TRAF molecules was demonstrated in EBV-positive PTLD, showing that LMP1-mediated signaling through the TRAF system plays a role in the pathogenesis of PTLD.[91] PTLD comprise a spectrum ranging from early EBV-driven polyclonal proliferations resembling infectious mononucleosis to lymphomas of predominantly B-cell or less often T-cell type. Several categories have been identified according to clinical presentation, morphology, and phenotypic and molecular features[85,86,89,90] (Table 16.2).

Early lesions, often arising within the first 2 years, and seen more frequently in children or in adult solid organ recipients who have not had prior EBV infection, are characterized as plasmacytic hyperplasia (PH) and infectious mononucleosis-like (IM-like). The lymphoid proliferation involves lymph nodes or tonsils and adenoids and may regress spontaneously or after reduction in immunosuppression. Plasmacytic hyperplasia contain numerous plasma cells and rare immunoblasts, while the IM-like lesion in lymph nodes or tonsils has the typical morphologic features of IM, with paracortical expansion and numerous immunoblasts in a background of T cells and plasma cells. Immunoblasts are EBV-infected B cells expressing LMP1. Small monoclonal or oligoclonal bands on Southern blots probed for episomal EBV genomes may be detected in these lesions. Some cases may be followed by polymorphic or monomorphic PTLD.[92]

---

**Table 16.2  Histological categories of post-transplant lymphoproliferative disorders[90]**

- Early lesions
   - Reactive plasmacytic hyperplasia
   - Infectious mononucleosis-like
- Polymorphic PTLD
- Monomorphic PTLD (classified according to the WHO lymphoma classification)
   - B-cell neoplasms:
      - Diffuse large B-cell lymphoma
      - Burkitt lymphoma (classical or atypical)
      - Plasma cell myeloma
      - Plasmacytoma-like lesions
   - T-cell neoplasms
      - Peripheral T-cell lymphoma, not otherwise categorized
      - Other types
- Hodgkin lymphoma and Hodgkin lymphoma-like

---

Polymorphic PTLD, developing mostly in extranodal localizations in one or multiple sites (including the allograft), are destructive lesions effacing the architecture with some areas of necrosis. They are composed of a range of lymphoid cell types, including immunoblasts, plasma cells, and intermediate-sized lymphoid cells. Clonal rearrangements of immunoglobulin genes and/or EBV genomes are frequent, and the presence of distinct clones at different sites in the same patient has been demonstrated. There are no genetic abnormalities involving oncogenes such as c-MYC, RAS, and p53, but chromosomal abnormalities/imbalances may be detected by comparative genomic hybridization (CGH).[93] These lesions contain numerous EBV-infected cells detected by in situ hybridization using EBER probes. The EBV-infected lymphoid cells express EBV latent genes such as LMP1 and EBNA2, reflecting in the majority of cases a type III latency pattern of EBV.[94,95] The evolution of these lesions is variable; reduction of immunosuppression can lead to regression of the PTLD, while some cases can evolve to a monomorphic lymphoma.[85,86]

Monomorphic PTLD are mostly DLBCL with clonal immunoglobulin gene rearrangements in virtually all cases. These lymphomas satisfy the histological criteria according to the WHO classification. The majority are subclassified as immunoblastic with plasmacytic features.[89,90] Many cases are CD30+, containing EBV genomes that are in clonal episomal form, and the three types of EBV latency are also described in these tumors. Genetic abnormalities involving mutations of the BCL6 and RAS genes, c-MYC rearrangement and mutations, and numerous chromosomal imbalances such as in the region containing BCL2 are present in the great majority of cases.[92,93]

Monomorphic T-PTLD showing clonal T-cell receptor gene rearrangements occur after a longer interval from the graft than B-cell lymphoma. They are classified according to the categories of T-cell lymphomas recognized in the WHO classification and are variable with respect to EBV positivity, about 25% showing clonal episomal EBV genomes.[89,90]

Other PTLD where EBV is virtually always present are Hodgkin lymphoma and Hodgkin-like lesions showing infiltrates with morphologic and immunophenotypic features of classical Hodgkin lymphoma, including the expression of CD15 and CD30; some have B-cell antigen expression. Some cases have responded to therapy for Hodgkin lymphoma, while others have been clinically aggressive.[89,90]

Polymorphic and less often monomorphic PTLD may regress with reduction in immune suppression; a proportion of cases of both types fail to regress, and require cytotoxic chemotherapy.[4] Overall, the mortality rate of PTLD in solid organ allograft recipients is approximately 60%, while that of marrow allograft recipients with PTLD is 80%. Administration of antibody to CD20 antigen has been useful in abrogating PTLD development in some cases.[96] Monitoring for evidence of reactivation of EBV infection may provide an early warning of PTLD development,[50] leading to a better clinical management of PTLD.

## EBV and AIDS-related lymphomas

Lymphomas that develop in HIV-positive patients are predominantly aggressive B-cell lymphomas, and in a proportion of cases they are the initial manifestation of AIDS. The incidence of Hodgkin lymphoma may be increased up to eight-fold. These lymphomas are heterogeneous, and include lymphomas usually diagnosed in immunocompetent patients, as well as those seen much more often in the setting of HIV infection and some appearing in other immunodeficiencies.[97] AIDS-related lymphomas are heterogeneous, reflecting several pathogenic mechanisms. The herpesviruses EBV and KSHV/HHV8 play a major role in some categories of HIV-related lymphomas. Disruption of the cytokine network, with high serum levels of IL-6 and IL-10, is a feature of HIV-related lymphomas associated with EBV or KSHV/HHV8. Other pathogenetic aspects of lymphomas are also involved, such as chronic antigen stimulation, genetic abnormalities involving the c-MYC and BCL6 genes, as well as tumor suppressor genes.[6,98] EBV is identified in the neoplastic cells of approximately 60% of HIV-related lymphomas, but the detection of EBV varies considerably with localization and histological subtype.[99]

The most common HIV-associated lymphomas include BL, DLBCL, plasmablastic lymphomas of the oral cavity, Hodgkin lymphoma, lymphoproliferative disorders, and lymphomas associated with KSHV/HHV8, particularly PEL (Table 16.3).[97]

Besides classical BL, the morphological variant of BL with plasmacytoid differentiation is nearly confined to AIDS patients and represents about 20% of NHL cases in these patients. Those developing such tumors have more pronounced immunosuppression than in classical BL. Medium-sized cells with more abundant basophilic cytoplasm are characteristic, as is an eccentric nucleus, often with one centrally located prominent nucleolus. The cells often contain cytoplasmic immunoglobulin, and EBV is positive in about 50–70% of cases. At the molecular level, HIV-associated BL, like other BL, have genetic abnormalities affecting band 8q24, the location of the c-MYC locus.[100] Besides the truncation within or around the c-MYC locus, point mutations in the first intron–first exon regulatory regions and amino-acid substitutions in the second exon are also detected and contribute to the deregulation of c-MYC.[98]

DLBCL having centroblastic features are associated with EBV in 30% of cases and represent about 25% of HIV-related lymphomas. The immunoblastic variant, usually exhibiting plasmacytoid features as in

**Table 16.3 Categories of HIV-associated lymphomas and frequency of EBV[97]**

| Categories of HIV-associated lymphomas | EBV-positivity (%) |
|---|---|
| Lymphomas also occurring in immunocompetent patients | |
| Burkitt lymphoma | 30–70 |
| Classical | 30 |
| With plasmacytoid differentiation | 50–70 |
| Atypical | 30–50 |
| Diffuse large cell lymphoma | 20–100 |
| Centroblastic | 20–30 |
| Immunoblastic | 90–100[a] |
| Extranodal marginal zone B-cell lymphoma of MALT type (rare) | |
| Peripheral T-cell lymphoma (rare) | |
| Classical Hodgkin lymphoma | |
| Lymphomas occurring more specifically in HIV-positive patients | |
| Primary effusion lymphoma | 90 |
| Plasmablastic lymphoma of the oral cavity | 50 |
| Lymphomas also occurring in other immunodeficiency states | |
| Polymorphic B-cell lymphoma (PTLD-like) | 90 |

[a] In primary central nervous system lymphomas, almost all cases are associated with EBV.

primary central nervous system lymphoma, is associated with EBV in 90–100% of cases, and often occurs late in the course of HIV disease.[101] Phenotypic markers that allow distinction between mature B cells as virgin B-cell, germinal center B-cell, and post-germinal center, namely BCL6, MUM1/IRF4, and CD138, are differentially expressed in AIDS-related lymphomas according to their origin. Two main categories are identified: lymphomas reflecting the germinal center, which are $BCL_6^+$,$MUM_1$/$IRF_4^-$,$CD138^-$, and those belonging to the post-germinal center expression pattern $BCL_6^-$,$MUM_1$/$IRF_4^+$,$CD138^+$. In EBV-positive lymphomas expressing high amounts of LMP1, BCL6 may be downregulated.[102] Another interaction between EBV latent protein and the regulatory cell protein is abrogation of the inverse relationship between the p27$^{Kip}$ inhibitor of cell cycle expression and a high rate of proliferation in these tumors.[103]

Plasmablastic lymphoma of the oral cavity, a rare lymphoid neoplasm, localized in the oral cavity or the jaw, and having plasmablastic features is rapidly growing, with a high mitotic index. The large tumor cells display a diffuse pattern of growth interspersed by macrophages. Some cells display cytoplasmic immunoglobulins. EBV is present in more than 50% of cases, but no association with KSHV/HHV8 has been detected.[104]

Polymorphic lymphoid proliferations resembling polymorphic PTLD, mostly EBV-positive, may be seen in adults and also in children, but are much less common than in the post-transplant setting, comprising less than 5% of AIDS-related lymphomas.[105]

Most cases of Hodgkin lymphoma correspond to either the mixed cellularity or lymphocyte-depleted forms of classical Hodgkin lymphoma. Some cases of nodular sclerosis Hodgkin lymphoma are also seen. HIV-related Hodgkin lymphoma is associated with EBV in nearly all cases; the pattern of EBV latent gene expression is characteristic of latency II (EBER+ LMP1+EBNA2-).[106]

KSHV/HHV8-related LPD and lymphoma develop in HIV-infected patients because KSHV/HHV8 is highly pathogenic in the context of HIV infection and immunosuppression. The LPD, which are almost all of B-cell origin, include PEL (initially termed body cavity-based lymphomas) and MCD associated with micro or frank plasmablastic lymphoma.

PEL, a rare lymphoma with lymphomatous effusions, was not fully characterized until the discovery of KSHV/HHV8. It represents a distinct clinicopathological entity, based on morphological, immunophenotypic, molecular, and viral features. Typically presenting with either pleural or peritoneal effusion, it can present as a solid tumor mass, most commonly affecting the gastrointestinal tract or soft tissue. PEL is associated with both Kaposi sarcoma and MCD in HIV-positive patients. Tumor cells exhibit variable cell types, from large immunoblastic or plasmablastic cells to cells with more anaplastic morphology and plasmacytoid differentiation, or Reed–Sternberg cells may be seen. The tumor cells originate from post-germinal center B cells and express CD45, CD38, CD138, and also activation markers such as CD30. However, they are usually negative for B-cell markers such as CD19, CD20, and CD79a, as well as for surface and cytoplasmic immunoglobulins. At the molecular level, they are characterized as late differentiated B cells with rearranged and mutated immunoglogulin genes. No c-*MYC* abnormalities have been found. This rare lymphoma has a very aggressive clinical outlook, with a median survival of less than 6 months.[107,108]

Plasmablastic lymphoma in the context of MCD is a lymphoproliferative disorder that can lead to frank plasmablastic lymphoma, associated in all cases with KSHV/HHV8.[109] A variable number of KSHV/HHV8-positive scattered large lymphoid cells are detected in the mantle zone. These cells, having the morphology of plasmablasts, containing large amounts of IgM, and expressing exclusively λ light chain, are proliferating (Ki67+). These plasmablasts may coalesce to form confluent clusters with the constitution of micro-lymphomatous lesions and sometimes frank plasmablastic lymphomas. Although of monotype IgMλ, the KSHV/HHV8 microlymphomatous lesions are polyclonal, while frank plasmablastic lymphomas are monoclonal. This molecular spectrum is similar to those described in EBV-driven lymphoproliferative disorders. The characteristic of these KSHV/HHV8-associated plasmablastic lymphomas is the lack of somatic mutations in their rearranged heavy and light chains, suggesting their origin from a naive B cell. The plasmablastic features of these lymphomas without somatic Ig gene mutations are evidence in favor of the role of KSHV/HHV8 driving infected cells to differentiate into plasmablasts without going through the germinal center.[110]

## REFERENCES

1. Report of a WHO scientific group. Primary immunodeficiency diseases. *Clin Exp Immunol* 1997; **109**(suppl 1): 1–28.
2. Elenitoba-Johnson KS, Jaffe ES. Lymphoproliferative disorders associated with congenital immunodeficiencies. *Semin Diagn Pathol* 1997; **14**: 35–47.
3. Ferry JA, Jacobson JO, Conti D et al. Lymphoproliferative disorders and hematological malignancies following organ transplantation. *Mod Pathol* 1989; **16**: 252–8.
4. Leblond V, Sutton L, Doreen R et al. Post transplant lymphoproliferative disorders after organ transplantation: a report of 24 cases observed in a single center. *J Clin Oncol* 1995; **13**: 1131–8.

5. Swinnen LJ. Transplantation-related lymphoproliferative disorder: a model for human immunodeficiency virus-related lymphomas. *Semin Oncol* 2000; **27**: 402–8.

6. Carbone A. AIDS-related non Hodgkin's lymphomas: from pathology and molecular pathogenesis to treatment. *Hum Pathol* 2002; **90**: 235–43.

7. Epstein MA, Achong BG, Barr YM. Virus particles in cultured lymphoblasts from Burkitt's lymphoma. *Lancet* 1964; **i**: 702–4.

8. Rickinson AB, Kieff E. Epstein–Barr virus. In: Fields BN, Knipe DM, Howley PM et al (eds) *Fields Virology*, 3rd edn. Philadelphia: Lippincott–Raven, 1996: 2397–445.

9. Kieff E. Epstein–Barr virus and its replication. In: Fields BN, Knipe PM, Howley PM et al (eds) *Fields Virology*, 3rd edn. Philadelphia: Lippincott–Raven, 1996: 2343–95.

10. Kaplan MA, Ferry JA, Harris NL, Jacobson JO. Post-transplant lymphoproliferative disorders: episomal EBV is a more reliable marker of clonality than immunoglobulin gene rearrangement. *Am J Clin Pathol* 1994; **101**: 590–6.

11. Izumi KM. Identification of EBV transforming genes by recombinant EBV technology. *Semin Cancer Biol* 2001; **11**: 407–14.

12. Jochner N, Eick D, Zimber-Strobl U et al. Epstein–Barr virus nuclear antigen 2 is a transcriptional suppressor of the immunoglobulin μ gene: implications for the expression of the translocated c-*myc* gene in Burkitt's lymphoma cells. *EMBO J* 1996; **15**: 375–82.

13. Zimber-Strobl U, Strobl. EBNA2 and Notch signaling in Epstein–Barr virus mediated immortalization of B lymphocytes. *Semin Cancer Biol* 2001; **11**: 423–34

14. Fujiwara J. Epstein–Barr virus nuclear protein 2-induced activation of the EBV-replicating cycle in Akata cells: analysis by tetracycline-regulated expression. *Curr Top Microbiol* 2001; **258**: 35–47.

15. Manet E, Bourillot PY, Waltzer L et al. EBV genes and B cell proliferation. *Crit Rev Oncol Hematol* 1998; **28**: 129–37.

16. Parker GA, Touitou R, Allday MJ. Epstein–Barr virus EBNA3C can disrupt multiple cell cycle chekpoints and induce nuclear division divorced from cytokinesis. *Oncogene* 2000; **19**: 700–9.

17. Maréchal V, Dehee A, Chikhi-Brachet R et al. Mapping EBNA-1 domains involved in binding to metaphase chromosomes. *J Virol* 1999; **73**: 4385–92.

18. Rickinson AB. Epstein–Barr in action in vivo. *N Engl J Med* 1998; **338**: 1413–21.

19. Wang D, Leibowitz D, Kieff E. An EBV membrane protein expressed in immortalized lymphocytes transformed established rodent cells. *Cell* 1985; **43**: 831–40.

20. Eliopoulos A, Young LS. LMP1 structure and signal transduction. *Semin Cancer Biol* 2001; **11**: 435–44.

21. Mosialos G, Birkenbach M, Yalamanchite R et al. The Epstein–Barr virus transforming protein LMP1 engages signaling proteins for the TNF factor receptor family. *Cell* 1995; **80**: 389–99.

22. Zhang L, Pagano JS. Interferon regulatory factor 7: a key cellular mediator of LMP1 in EBV latency and transformation. *Semin Cancer Biol* 2001; **11**: 445–53.

23. Takada K, Nanbo A. The role of EBERs in oncogenesis. *Semin Cancer Biol* 2001; **11**: 461–7.

24. Komano J, Maruo S, Kurozumi K et al. Oncogenic role of Epstein–Barr virus-encoded RNAs in Burkitt's lymphoma cell line Akata. *J Virol* 1999; **73**: 9827–31.

25. Kitagawa N, Goto M, Kurozumi K et al. Epstein–Barr virus-encoded poly(A)⁻ RNA supports Burkitt's lymphoma growth through interleukin-10 induction. *EMBO J* 2000; **19**: 6742–50.

26. Rowe M. Cell transformation induced by Epstein–Barr virus – living dangerously. *Semin Cancer Biol* 2001; **11**: 403–5.

27. Brennan P. Signaling events regulating lymphoid growth and survival. *Semin Cancer Biol* 2001; **11**: 403–5.

28. Baran-Marszak F, Fagard R, Girard B et al. Gene array identification of Epstein–Barr virus-regulated cellular genes in EBV-converted Burkitt lymphoma cell lines. *Lab Invest* 2002; **82**: 1463–80.

29. Thorley-Lawson DA, Babcock GJ. A model for persistent infection with Epstein–Barr virus: the stealth virus of human B cells. *Life Sci* 1999; **65**: 1433–53.

30. Babcock GJ, Thorley-Lawson DA. Tonsillar memory B cell latently infected with Epstein–Barr virus express the restricted pattern of latent gene previously found only in Epstein–Barr virus associated tumors. *Proc Natl Acad Sci USA* 2000; **97**: 12250–5.

31. Thorley-Lawson DA. Epstein–Barr virus: exploiting the immune system. *Nat Rev Immunol* 2001; **1**: 75–82.

32. Rowe M, Lear AL, Croom-Carter D et al. Three pathways of Epstein–Barr virus gene activation from EBNA1-positive latency in B lymphocytes. *J Virol* 1992; **66**: 122–32.

33. Rickinson AB, Moss DJ. Human cytotoxic T lymphocyte responses to Epstein–Barr virus infection. *Annu Rev Immunol* 1997; **15**: 405–31.

34. Wallace LE, Rickinson AB, Rowe M. Epstein MA. Epstein–Barr virus-specific cytotoxic T-cell clones restricted through a single HLA antigen. *Nature* 1982; **207**: 413–15.

35. Murray R, Kurilla M, Brooks J et al. Identification of target antigens for the human cytotoxic response to Epstein–Barr virus (EBV): implication for the immune control of EBV-positive malignancies. *J Exp Med* 1992; **176**: 157–68.

36. Steven NM, Leese AM, Annels NE et al. Epitope focusing in the primary cytotoxic T cell response to Epstein–Barr virus and its relationship to T cell memory. *J Exp Med* 1996; **184**:1801–13.

37. Yang J, Lemas VM, Flinn IW et al. Application of the Elispot assay to the characterization of CD8⁺ response to Epstein–Barr virus antigens. *Blood* 2000; **95**: 241–8.

38. Altman JD, Moss PAH, Goulder PJR et al. Phenotypic analysis of antigen specific T-lymphocytes. *Science* 1996; **274**:94–6 [Erratum 1998; **280**: 1821].

39. Heslop HE, Ng CYG, Li C et al. Long term restoration of immunity against Epstein–Barr virus infection by adoptive transfer of gene-modified virus specific T lymphocytes. *Nat Med* 1996; **2**: 551–5.

40. Nazaruk RA, Rochford R, Hobbs MV et al. Functional diversity of the CD8⁺ T-cell response to Epstein–Barr virus (EBV): implications for the pathogenesis of EBV-associated lymphoproliferative disorders. *Blood* 1998; **91**: 3875–83.

41. Veronese ML, Veronesi A, d'Andrea E et al. Lymphoproliferative disease in human peripheral blood mononuclear cell-injected SCID mice. I. T lymphocytes requirement for B cell tumor generation. *J Exp Med* 1992; **176**: 1763–7.

42. Pai S, Khanna R. Role of LMP1 in immune control of EBV infection. *Semin Cancer Biol* 2001; **11**: 455–60.

43. Steven NM, Annels NE, Kumar A et al. Immediate early and early lytic cycle proteins are frequent targets of the Epstein–Barr virus-induced cytotoxic T cell response. *J Exp Med* 1997; **185**: 1605–17.

44. Levitskaya J, Coram M, Levitsky V et al. Inhibition of antigen processing by the internal repeat region of the

Epstein–Barr virus nuclear antigen-1. *Nature* 1995; **375**: 685–8.

45. Paludan C, Bickham K, Nikiforow S et al. Epstein–Barr nuclear antigen 1-specific CD4+ Th1 cell kill Burkitt's lymphoma cells. *J Immunol* 2002; **169**: 1593–603.

46. Gavioli R, Vertuani S, Masucci MG. Proteasome inhibitors reconstitute the presentation of cytotoxic T-cell epitopes in Epstein–Barr virus-associated tumors. *Int J Cancer* 2002; **101**: 532–8.

47. Li L, Liu D, Hutt-Fletcher L et al. Epstein–Barrr virus inhibits the development of dendritic cells by promoting apoptosis of their monocytes precursors in the presence of granulocyte–macrophage colony-stimulating factor and interleukin-4. *Blood* 2002; **99**: 3725–34.

48. Emilie D, Touitou R, Raphaël M et al. In vivo production of IL-10 by malignant cells in AIDS lymphomas. *Eur J Immunol* 1992; **22**: 2937–42.

49. Frisan T, Sjöberg J, Dolcetti R et al. Local suppression of Epstein–Barr virus (EBV) specific cytotoxicity in biopsies of EBV positive Hodgkin's disease. *Blood* 1995; **86**: 1493–501.

50. Wagner HJ, Fisher L, Jabs WJ et al. Longitudinal analysis of Epstein–Barr viral load in plasma and in peripheral blood mononuclear cells of transplanted patients by real-time polymerase chain reaction. *Transplantation* 2002; **74**: 656–64.

51. Dehée A, Asselot C, Piolot T et al. Quantification of Epstein–Barr virus load in peripheral blood of human immunodeficiency virus-infected patients using real-time PCR. *J Med Virol* 2001; **65**: 543–52.

52. Papadopulos AB, Landanyi M, Emmanuel D et al. Infusion of donor leukocytes to Epstein–Barr virus associated lymphoproliferative disorders after allogenic bone marrow transplantation. *N Engl J Med* 1994; **330**: 1185–91.

53. Rooney CM, Smith CA, Ng CY et al. Infusion of cytotoxic T cells for the prevention and treatment of Epstein–Barr virus-induced lymphoma in allogenic transplant recipients. *Blood* 1998; **92**: 1549–55.

54. Haque T, Amiot PL, Helling N et al. Reconstitution of EBV specific T cell immunity in solid organ transplant recipients. *J Immunol* 1998; **160**: 6204–9.

55. Chang Y, Cesarman E, Pessin MS et al. Identification of herpesvirus-like DNA sequences in AIDS-associated Kaposi's sarcoma. *Science* 1994; **266**: 1865–9.

56. Moore PS, Gao SJ, Dominguez et al. Primary characterization of a herpesvirus agent associated with Kaposi's sarcoma. *J Virol* 1996; **70**: 549–58.

57. Cesarman E, Chang Y, Moore PS et al. Kaposi's sarcoma-associated herpesvirus-like DNA sequences in AIDS-related body-cavity-based lymphomas. *N Engl J Med* 1995; **332**: 1186–91.

58. Soulier J, Grollet L, Oksenhendler E et al. Kaposis's sarcoma-associated herpesvirus-like DNA in multicentric Castleman disease. *Blood* 1995; **86**: 1276–80.

59. Cesarman E, Moore PS, Rao PH et al. In vitro establishment and characterization of two acquired immunodeficiency syndrome-related lymphoma cell lines (BC-1 and BC-2) containing Kaposis's sarcoma-associated herpesvirus-like (KSHV) DNA sequences. *Blood* 1995; **86**: 2708–14.

60. Russo JJ, Bohenzky RA, Chien MC et al. Nucleotide sequence of the Kaposi's sarcoma-associated herpesvirus (HHV8). *Proc Natl Acad Sci USA* 1996; **93**: 14862–7.

61. Moore PS, Boschoff C, Weiss RA et al. Molecular mimicry of human cytokine and cytokine response pathway gene by KSHV. *Science* 1996; **274**: 1739–44.

62. Chang Y, Moore PS, Talbot SJ et al. Cyclin encoded by KS herpes virus. *Nature* 1996; **382**: 410.

63. Bais C, Santomasso B, Coso O et al. Kaposi's sarcoma-associated herpesvirus (KSHV/HHV8) G protein-coupled receptor is a viral oncogene and angiogenesis activator. *Nature* 1998; **391**: 86–9.

64. Gao SJ, Boshoff C, Jayachandra S et al. KSHV ORF K9 (v-IRF) is an oncogene which inhibits the interferon signalling pathway. *Oncogene* 1997; **15**: 1979–85.

65. Sarid R, Sato T, Bohenzky RA et al. Kaposi's sarcoma-associated herpesvirus (KSHV) encodes a functional bcl-2 homologue. *Nat Med* 1997; **3**: 293–8.

66. Molden J, Chang Y, You Y et al. Kaposi's sarcoma-associated herpesvirus-encoded cytokine homologue (v-IL6) activates signaling through the shared gp130 receptor subunit. *J Biol Chem* 1997; **272**: 19625–31.

67. Kladal TN, Rosenkilde MM, Coulin F et al. A broad spectrum chemokine antagonist encoded by Kaposi's sarcoma-associated herpesvirus. *Science* 1997; **277**: 1656–9.

68. Swanton C, Mann DJ, Fleckenstein B et al. Herpesviral cyclin/Cdk6 complexes evade inhibition by Cdk inhibitor proteins. *Nature* 1997; **390**: 184–7.

69. Schulz TF. Kaposi's sarcoma-associated herpes virus (human herpesvirus 8). *J Gen Virol* 1998; **79**:1573–91.

70. Muralidhar S, Pumfery AM, Hassani M et al. Identification of kaposin (open reading frame K12) as a human herpesvirus 8 (Kaposi's sarcoma-associated herpesvirus) transforming gene. *J Virol* 1998; **72**: 4980–8.

71. Lee H, Veazey R, Williams et al. Deregulation of cell growth by the K1 gene of Kaposi's sarcoma-associated herpesvirus. *Nat Med* 1998; **4**: 435–40.

72. Sarid R, Flore O, Bohenzky RA et al. Transcription mapping of the Kaposi's sarcoma-associated herpesvirus (human herpesvirus 8) genome in a body cavity-based lymphoma cell line (BC-1). *J Virol* 1998; **72**: 1005–12.

73. Terruya-Feldstein J, Zauber P, Setsuda JE et al. Expression of human herpesvirus-8 oncogene and cytokine homologues in a HIV-seronegative patient with Castleman's disease and primary effusion lymphoma. *Lab Invest* 1998; **78**: 1637–42.

74. Oksenhendler E, Carcelain G, Aoki Y et al. High levels of human herpesvirus-8 viral load, human interleukin-6, interleukin-10 and C-reactive protein correlate with exacerbation of multicentric Castleman's disease in HIV-infected patients. *Blood* 2000; **96**: 2069–73.

75. Aoki Y, Tosato G, Fonville TW et al. Serum viral interleukin-6 in AIDS-related multicentric Castleman's disease. *Blood* 2001; **97**: 2526–7.

76. An J, Lichtenstein AK, Brent G et al. The Kaposi sarcoma-associated herpesvirus (KSHV) induces cellular interleukin 6 expression: role of the KSHV latency-associated nuclear antigen and the AP1 response element. HHV8 latent nuclear antigen upregulates cellular IL-6 expression through the AP1 response element. *Blood* 2002; **99**: 649–54.

77. Friborg JJ, Kong W, Hottiger MO et al. p53 inhibition by the LANA protein of KSHV protects against cell death. *Nature* 1999; **402**: 889–94.

78. Purtilo DT, Strobach RS, Okano M, Davis, J. Epstein–Barr virus-associated lymphoproliferative disorders. *Lab Invest* 1992; **67**: 5–23.

79. Gilmour KC, Cranston T, Jones A et al. Diagnosis of X-linked lymphoproliferative disease by analysis of SLAM-associated protein expression. *Eur J Immunol* 2000; **30**: 1691–7.

80. Tangye SG, Phillips JH, Lanier LL et al. Functional requirement for SAP in 2B4-mediated activation of human natural killer cells as revealed by the X-linked lymphoproliferative syndrome. *J Immunol* 2000; **165**: 2932–6.

81. Ilowite NT, Fligner CL, Ochs H et al. Pulmonary angiitis with atypical lymphoreticular infiltrates in Wiskott–Aldrich syndrome: possible relationship of lymphomatoid granulomatosis and EBV infection. *Clin Immunol Immunopathol* 1986; **41**: 479–84.

82. Jaffe ES, Wilson WH. Lymphomatoid granulomatosis: pathogenesis, pathology, and clinical implications. *Cancer Surv* 1997; **30**: 233–48.

83. Tinguely M, Vonlanthen R, Muller E et al. Hodgkin's disease-like lymphoproliferative disorders in patients with different underlying immunodeficiency states. *Mod Pathol* 1998; **11**: 307–12.

84. Canioni D, Jabado N, Macintyre E et al. Lymphoproliferative disorders in children with primary immunodeficiencies: immunological status may be more predictive of the outcome than the other criteria. *Histopathology* 2001; **38**: 146–59.

85. Nalesnik M, Jaffe R, Starzl T et al. The pathology of post-transplant lymphoproliferative disorders occurring in the setting of cyclosporine A–prednisone immunosuppression. *Am J Pathol* 1988; **133**: 173–92.

86. Ferry J, Jacobson J, Conti D et al. Lymphoproliferative disorders and hematologic malignancies following organ transplantation. *Mod Pathol* 1989; **2**: 583–92.

87. Curtis RE, Travis LB, Rowlings PA et al. Risk of lymphoproliferative disorders after bone marrow transplantation: a multiinstitutional study. *Blood* 1999; **94**: 2208–16.

88. Leblond V, Davi F, Charlotte F et al. Posttransplant lymphoproliferative disorders not associated with Epstein–Barr virus: a distinct entity? *J Clin Oncol* 1998; **16**: 2052–9.

89. Harris NL, Ferry JA, Swerdlow SH. Posttransplant lymphoproliferative disorders: summary of Society for Hematopathology Workshop. *Semin Diagn Pathol* 1997; **14**: 8–14.

90. Harris NL, Swerdlow SH, Frizzera G, Knowles DM. Posttransplant lymphoproliferative disorders. In: Jaffe ES, Harris NL, Stein H, Vardiman JW (eds) *World Health Organization Classification of Tumours. Pathology and Genetics of Tumours of Haematopoietic and Lymphoid Tissues.* Lyon: IARC Press, 2001: 264–9.

91. Leibowitz D. Epstein–Barr virus and a cellular signaling pathway in lymphomas from immunosuppressed patients. *N Engl J Med* 1998; **338**: 1413–21.

92. Knowles DM, Cesarman E, Chadburn A et al. Correlative morphologic and molecular genetic analysis demonstrates three distinct categories of posttransplantation lymphoproliferative disorders. *Blood* 1995; **85**: 552–65.

93. Poirel AH, Scneider A, Meddeb M et al. Characteristic pattern of chromosomal gains and losses in posttransplantation lymphoproliferative disorders (PTLDs): corelation with EBV and clinical status. In: *Proceedings of the American Society of Hematology, 2002* (abst).

94. Rowe M, Niedobitek G, Young LS. Epstein–Barr virus gene expression in post-transplant lymphoproliferative disorders. *Springer Semin Immunopathol* 1998; **20**: 389–403.

95. Rea D, Fourcade C, Leblond V et al. Patterns of EBV latent and replicative gene expression in EBV B-cell lymphoproliferative disorders after organ transplantation. *Transplantation* 1994; **58**: 317–24.

96. Milpied N, Vasseur B, Parquet N et al. Humanized anti-CD20 monoclonal antibody (rituximab) in posttransplant B-lymphoproliferative disorder: a retrospective analysis on 32 patients. *Ann Oncol* 2000; **11**(suppl 1): 113–16.

97. Raphaël M, Borisch B, Jaffe ES. Lymphomas associated with infection by the human immune deficiency virus (HIV). In: Jaffe ES, Harris NL, Stein H, Vardiman JW (eds) *World Health Organization Classification of Tumours. Pathology and Genetics of Tumours of Haematopoietic and Lymphoid Tissues.* Lyon: IARC Press, 2001: 260–3.

98. Carbone A. The spectrum of AIDS-related lymphoproliferative disorders. *Adv Clin Pathol* 1997; **1**: 13–19.

99. Hamilton-Dutoit SJ, Raphaël M, Audouin J et al. In situ demonstration of Epstein–Barr virus small RNAs (EBER 1) in acquired immunodeficiency syndrome-related lymphomas: correlation with tumor morphology and primary site. *Blood* 1993; **82**: 619–24.

100. Davi F, Delecluse HJ, Guiet P et al. Burkitt-like lymphomas in AIDS patients: characterization within a series of 103 human immunodeficiency virus-associated non-Hodgkin's lymphomas. Burkitt's Lymphoma Study Group. *J Clin Oncol* 1998; **16**: 3788–95.

101. Camilleri-Broët S, Davi F, Feuillard J et al. AIDS-related primary brain lymphomas: histopathological and immunohistochemical study of 51 cases. *Hum Pathol* 1997; **28**: 367–74.

102. Carbone A, Gaidano G, Gloghini A et al. Differential expression of BCL-6 CD138/syndecan-1 and Epstein–Barr virus-encoded latent membrane protein-1 identifies distinct histogenetic subsets of acquired immunodeficiency syndrome-related non Hodgkin's lymphoma. *Blood* 1998; **91**: 747–55.

103. Gloghini A, Gaidano G, Larocca LM et al. Expression of cyclin-dependent kinase inhibitor p27 (Kip1) in AIDS-related diffuse large cell lymphoma is associated with Epstein–Barr virus-encoded latent membrane protein 10. *Am J Pathol* 2002; **160**: 163–71.

104. Delecluse HJ, Anagnostopoulos I, Dallenbach F et al. Plasmablastic lymphomas of the oral cavity: a new entity associated with the human immunodeficiency virus infection. *Blood* 1997; **89**: 1413–20.

105. Martin A, Flaman JM, Frebourg T et al. Functional analysis of the p53 protein in AIDS-related non-Hodgkin's lymphomas and polymorphic lymphoproliferations. *Br J Haematol* 1998; **101**: 311–17.

106. Audouin J, Diebold J, Pallesen G. Frequent expression of Epstein–Barr virus latent membrane protein-1 in tumour cells of Hodgkin's disease in HIV-positive patients. *J Pathol* 1992; **167**: 381–4.

107. Carbone A, Gaidano G. HHV-8-positive body-cavity-based lymphoma: a novel lymphoma entity. *Br J Haematol* 1997; **97**: 515–22.

108. Nador RG, Cesarman E, Chadburn A et al. Primary effusion lymphoma: a distinct clinicopathologic entity associated with the Kaposi's sarcoma-associated herpes virus. *Blood* 1996; **88**: 645–56.

109. Dupin N, Diss TL, Kellam P et al. HHV-8 is associated with a plasmablastic variant of Castleman disease that is linked to HHV8-positive plasmablastic lymphoma. *Blood* 2000; **95**: 1406–12.

110. Du MQ, Liu H, Diss TC et al. Kaposi sarcoma-associated herpesvirus infects monotypic (IgMλ) but polyclonal naive B-cells in Castleman disease and associated lymphoproliferative disorders. *Blood* 2000; **97**: 2130–6.

# 17 Acquired genetic changes in myeloid malignancies

## Cristina Mecucci and Anne Hagemeijer

## Introduction

### Cytogenetic findings

Chromosomal changes can be detected in the majority of cases of acute myeloid leukemia (AML) or myelodysplastic syndromes (MDS). These abnormalities are an acquired and clonal intrinsic feature of leukemia. They are the visible indicator of malignant transformation: with response to treatment, the malignant clone may disappear, but in the case of relapse, the leukemic cells carry the same original aberration, sometimes with additional changes.

Recurrent patterns of numerical changes (gain and loss) or structural changes (translocation, inversion, deletion, and duplication) have been identified and found to be characteristic of specific subtypes of leukemia.

Several chromosomal rearrangements, and the molecular abnormalities that they produce, identify distinct clinical subgroups with predictable clinical features and therapeutic responses.

De novo AML and therapy-related AML (t-AML) may exhibit different karyotype changes. In AML in children and young adults, there is a predominance of balanced translocations; in the aged and in secondary leukemia, there is a predominance of numerical and unbalanced abnormalities. Complex karyotypes (more than three abnormalities) are particularly ominous in all age groups (Figure 17.1).

### Gene rearrangements

Molecular analyses of recurrent translocations have revealed how genes controlling cell proliferation, survival, or apoptosis are rearranged or modified and become oncogenic. As a consequence of translocation of chromosome segments, genes are recombined illegitimately (gene fusion) and give rise to a new hybrid gene encoding chimeric neoproteins. Many of these

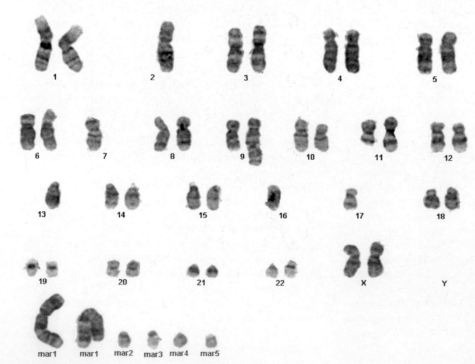

**Figure 17.1** G-banded abnormal complex karyotype from bone marrow cells of an aged patient with refractory anemia and very short survival (5 months from diagnosis).

oncoproteins are transcription factors. Master genes have been identified that may recombine with a variety of other genes; this gives rise to different translocations and to leukemia that can be of different phenotype. Examples of 'multipartner' genes are *MLL* on 11q23, *ETV6* on 12p13 and *RUNX1* (*AML1*) on 21q22.

Chromosomal translocations can also lead to altered transcription of intact genes through positioning them ectopically under the control of other constitutively active promoters or transcriptional enhancers. While this is more common in lymphoid malignancies, including acute lymphoblastic leukemia (ALL), chromosomal translocations involving the formation of chimeric fusion proteins are more frequently seen in myeloid malignancies.

Chromosome numerical changes and deletions result in gene imbalance. Deletions are suggestive of a mechanism of leukemogenesis by tumor suppression. Many studies are currently concentrating on the definition of tumor suppressor genes on 5q, 7q, and 20q, which are sites of recurrent deletions. Mutations resulting in transcriptional upregulation of a gene also occur.

In addition to numerical or structural chromosomal changes that can be detected with classical cytogenetics or fluorescence in situ hybridization (FISH), an increasing number of molecular changes are being identified with higher-resolution techniques, including gene amplification, deletions, internal domain duplications, and point mutations in growth factor receptors or signaling molecules. From the molecular identification of these changes, two general classes of leukemia-inducing changes are emerging: those conferring a proliferative and/or survival advantage, and those impairing hematopoietic differentiation. While the former class can be molecularly targeted by specific small-molecule inhibitors, the latter class might be targeted by compounds that restore or promote hematopoietic differentiation.

In summary, leukemia, like other malignancies, arises as a consequence of a major genetic insult and/or a cascade of more subtle mutations. Current molecular studies provide information on these mechanisms of leukemogenesis, and additional insight is gained into the genetic control of normal hematopoiesis.

## Methods of detection

Genetic abnormalities of leukemic cells are investigated using a number of different techniques: classical karyotype analysis using banding techniques, FISH, Southern blotting, reverse-transcriptase polymerase chain reaction (RT–PCR), and immunological detection of a specific oncoprotein.

### Classical cytogenetics

This provides a complete picture of genetic changes at the chromosomal level. It is performed on leukemic cells in metaphase, obtained after short-term culture with or without the use of growth factors or mitogens.

Cytogenetics provides information on specific changes, on the complexity of abnormalities, and on the presence of more than one leukemic clone. Apparently normal karyotype may harbor a genetic defect at submicroscopic level that can be detected using molecular methods.

### FISH

FISH makes use of specific DNA probes directly or indirectly labeled with fluorochromes and hybridized on cellular DNA in metaphase or interphase. The method is highly specific and the characteristics of the probes determine its sensitivity. Currently, the probes used are chromosome-specific (centromeric, subtelomeric, whole paint) or locus/gene-specific. For the detection of translocations, a double-color strategy (also applicable on interphase cells) is usually applied using gene-specific probes (Figure 17.2, see Plate 2).

Some probe combinations detect a 'fusion signal' in leukemic cells; other probes are designed as 'break apart', giving a split signal in rearranged genes such as *MLL* and *ETV6* (Figure 17.2, see Plate 2). FISH can be combined with other detection methods,

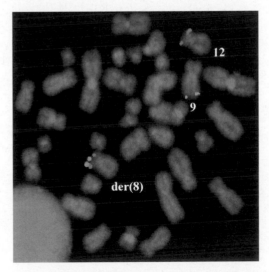

**Figure 17.2** Double-color metaphase FISH in a patient with a cryptic *ETV6–ABL1* fusion gene and only a t(8;12)(p12;p13) translocation on classical cytogenetics. Red signals mark the *ETV6* gene both in the abnormal 12p and in the abnormal 8 derived from the chromosomal translocation. Green signals label the *ABL1* gene in both the normal chromosome 9 and the abnormal 8. See Plate 2.

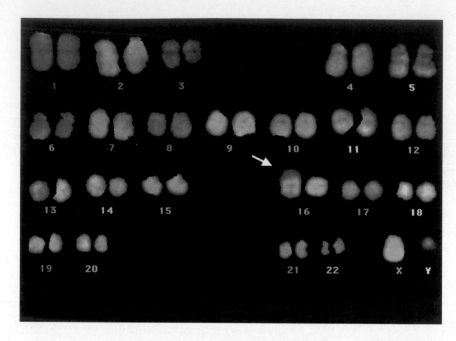

**Figure 17.3** AML with extra material in the short arm of chromosome 16 derived from chromosome 1 (arrow), as revealed by multicolor FISH karyotype. See Plate 2.

such as cytology, cytochemistry, and immunology, which allows the investigation of selected subsets of cells.

Complex painting probes allowing 24-color karyotyping are also available, and are useful in analysis of complex abnormalities, and sometimes the detection of cryptic changes (Figure 17.3, see Plate 2).

### RT–PCR

This technique amplifies the 'fusion transcript' characteristic of a given translocation. RT–PCR detects known fusion events with high sensitivity and is particularly useful for detecting residual disease. The new Taqman technology makes quantitative assessment of transcripts in real time, which allows the evaluation of therapeutic response, monitoring of remission, and prediction of relapse.

### cDNA microarray

Fluorescently labeled mRNA of leukemic cells can be hybridized to a high-density cDNA microarray. This provides a quantitative assessment of transcripts (genome-wide) and has proven very useful to determine the specific expression profile associated with specific cytogenetic subtypes of leukemia.[1]

## Fusion genes

Fusion genes are generated by chromosome translocations or inversions. A summary is given in Table 17.1. Most of them will be discussed separately.

Frequently occurring translocations in AML are t(15;17) in 7% (95% of acute promyelocytic leukemia (APL)); t(8;21) in 10%; inv(16) in 9%; t(11q23) in 5–7%, and t(3q) in 5%. All other translocations have

a frequency of 1% or less, with some age-related and geographical differences. Correlations between specific cytogenetic subgroups and prognosis are shown in Table 17.2.

### t(15;17)(q22;q21): PML/RARA

Acute promyelocytic leukemia (APL, AML-M3) is characterized by a specific reciprocal translocation that involves chromosome 17q21 in more than 95% of cases. The *RARA* (retinoic acid receptor α) gene at 17q21 recombines with the *PML* (promyelocytic leukemia) gene at 15q22.[2] Both fusion products, PML–RARα and RARα–PML may be present in leukemic cells. In transgenic mice, the PML/RARα fusion protein is expressed in the myeloid lineage. APL with t(15;17) is responsive to treatment with all-*trans*-retinoic acid (ATRA). Mice developed an abnormal hematopoiesis resembling a myeloproliferative disorder, but only 10% of them, after a latency of 12–14 months, developed an acute leukemia with clinical and hematological features mirroring human APL, including responsiveness to retinoic acid treatment.[3]

Molecular analysis of APL without the classical t(15;17) has documented the existence of complex or simple variant translocations, involving chromosomes 15 and/or 17 plus other chromosomes.[4] Moreover, masked translocations/insertions with apparently normal chromosomes 15 and 17 have been shown. Among simple variants, in a subgroup of AML with morphological features intermediate between M2 and M3 subtypes, a t(11;17)(q23;q22) results in fusion of the *RARA* gene with the *PLZF* (promyelocytic leukemia zinc finger) gene.[5] This t(11;17)/*PLZF–RARA* APL represents a distinct entity characterized by poor response to chemotherapy, little or no response to treatment with ATRA, and a bad prognosis, worse than t(15;17)/APL

**Table 17.1 Summary of specific translocations and inversions found in myeloid malignancies, the genes involved, and the main clinicopathological associations**

| Cytogenetic abnormality | Genes involved[a] | Fusion gene product | Main pathological association[b] |
|---|---|---|---|
| t(15;17)(q22;q21) | PML; RARA | PML–RARA | |
| t(5;17)(q35;q21) | NPM; RARA | NPM–RARA | |
| t(11;17)(q23;q21) | PLZF; RARA | PLZF–RARA | AML-M3 (APL) |
| t(11;17)(q13;q21) | NUMA; RARA | NUMA–RARA | |
| t(17;17)(q11;q21) | STAT5b; RARA | STAT5b–RARA | |
| t(8;21)(q22;q22) | ETO; RUNX1 | RUNX1–ETO | AML-M2 |
| t(3;21)(q26;q22) | EAP or MDS or EVI1; RUNX1 | RUNX1–EVI1 RUNX1–MDS1–EVI1 | t-AML, MDS, CML-BC |
| t(16;21)(q24;q22) | MTG16; RUNX1 | RUNX1–MTG16 | t-MDS/AML |
| inv(16)(p13q22)/t(16;16) | MYH11; CBFB | CBFB–MYH11 | AML-M4$_{Eo}$ |
| t(9;22)(q34;q11) | ABL; BCR | BCR–ABL | AML-M1, biphenotype |
| t(6;9)(p23;q34) | DEK; CAN | DEK–CAN | AML-M1, MDS |
| t(8;16)(p11;p13) | MOZ; CBP | MOZ–CBP | AML-M5B, erythrophagocytosis |
| inv(8)(p11;q13) | MOZ; TIF2 | MOZ–TIF2 | |
| t(8;22)(p11;q13) | MOZ; p300 | MOZ–P300 | t-AML |
| t(1;22)(p13;q13) | OTT; MAL | OTT–MAL | AML-M7, childhood |
| t(3;5)(q25;q35) | MLF1; NPM | NPM–MLF1 | MDS, AML (M6) |
| t(16;21)(p11;q22) | FUS; ERG | FUS–ERG | AML (M2, M7, M5) |
| t(9;11)(p22;q23) | AF9; MLL | MLL AF9 | AML-M5 |
| t(6;11)(p25;q23) | AF6; MLL | MLL–AF6 | |
| t(10;11)(p12;q23) | AF10; MLL | MLL–AF10 | AML-M4/M5/t-AML, |
| t(11;19)(q23;p13.1) | MLL; ELL | MLL–ELL | sometimes mixed-lineage |
| t(11q23) | MLL; other | MLL–other | |
| t(7;11)(p15;p15) | NUP98; HOXA9 | NUP98 HOXA9 | AML-M2 |
| t(2;11)(q31;p15) | HOXD11 or 13; NUP98 | NUP98–HOXD11/13 | MDS/AML |
| t(1;11)(q23;p15) | PMX1; NUP98 | NUP98–PMX1 | t-AML |
| t(11p15) | NUP98; other | NUP98–other | |
| t(5;12)(q33;p13) | PDGFBR; ETV6 | ETV6–PDGFβR | MDS |
| t(12;22)(p13;q11) | ETV6; MN1 | MN1–ETV6 | AML, MPD |
| t(12)(p13) | ETV6; other | ETV6–other | AML, MDS |
| t(3;3)/inv(3)(q21;q26) | EVI1; ribophorin | — | AML, MDS |
| t(1;3)(p36;q21) | MEL1; ribophorin | — | AML, MDS |
| t(2;3)(p25;q26) | ?; EVI1 | — | MDS, AML, CML-BC |

[a] RUNX1 was formerly termed AML1.

[b] AML, acute myeloid leukemia; APL, acute promyelocytic leukemia; MDS, myelodysplastic syndromes; t-, therapy-related; CML-BC, chronic myeloid leukemia in blast crisis; MPD, myeloproliferate disorders.

(Figure 17.4). In other rare cases, the RARA gene recombines with the NPM (nucleophosmin) gene in the presence of a t(5;17)(q35;q21). Similarly to t(11;17)/APL, this entity is refractory to ATRA treatment. Other partners of RARA are the NuMA (nuclear mitotic apparatus) gene in the t(11;17)(q13;q21), and the STAT5b gene in the t(17;17)(qll;q21).[6–8] In both translocations, the leukemia presents with morphological, immunophenotypic, and clinical features overlapping those of t(15;17)/APL.

Serial screenings of APL patients by RT–PCR assay for the PML/RARα fusion protein on bone marrow cells

is helpful to predict clinical course after treatment.[9] A negative result of RT–PCR at the end of therapy is strongly associated with long-term remission, whereas persistent positive tests are highly predictive of relapse.

In addition to t(15;17), secondary chromosomal changes have been reported in 25–40% of APL cases.[10] The most frequent additional change is trisomy 8. Other abnormalities may involve chromosomes 9, 17, 7, 21, 16, 6, and 12. The prognostic value of additional cytogenetic abnormalities in APL is controversial. However, in a large cohort of patients uniformly treated with ATRA in combination with chemotherapy, no differences were found in terms of clinical and biological features, event-free survival, risk of relapse, and overall survival.

**Table 17.2 Prognostic value of karyotype in acute myeloid leukemia**

**Good**
t(15;17)(q22;q21) in acute promyelocytic leukemia
t(8;21)(q22;q22)
inv(16)(p13q22)

**Intermediate**
Normal karyotype, –Y
Single translocation not in other categories

**Intermediate – Poor**
Trisomy 8
t(11q23)

**Poor**
t(6;9)(p21;q34)
t(9;22)(q34;q11)

**Very poor**
–5, –7, 7q–
t/inv(3)(q21–q26)
Complex (>3) abnormalities

## t(8;21)(q22;q22): *RUNX1–ETO*

The t(8;21)(q22;q22) translocation is found in around 10% of AML cases, predominantly those of M2 subtype, with a good response to chemotherapy, high remission rate, and long median survival. Immunophenotyping is particularly useful to identify this type of myeloid leukemia with significant high expression of the CD19 antigen.[11] Fusion occurs between the *RUNX1* gene (previously called *AML1*), a core binding factor (CBF) at chromosome 21q22, and the *ETO* gene, a transcription factor at chromosome 8q22. The RUNX1–ETO fusion protein acts as an inhibitor of transcription through heterodimerization with the CBFβ domain and subsequent interaction with CBF DNA-binding sites (Figure 17.5). CBF is a heterodimer consisting of a DNA binding α subunit (AML1, CBFα, RUNX1) and a β subunit (CBFβ), which enhances the DNA-binding affinity of the α subunit. CBF acts as a transcriptional organizer that, depending on the cellular context and the target gene, can recruit transcriptional activators and co-activators, or transcriptional repressors. The RUNX1–ETO fusion protein acts as a dominant-negative inhibitor of the native CBF complex through recruitment of the nuclear corepressor complex.[12]

FISH and PCR studies revealed the existence of RUNX1–ETO[+] leukemias in the absence of the

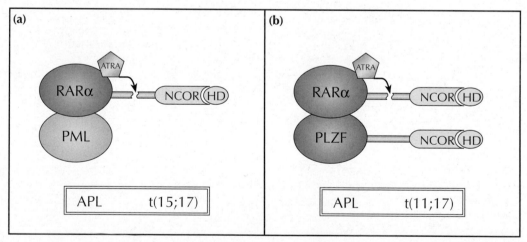

**Figure 17.4** Schematic representation of the mechanism of all-*trans*-retinoic acid (ATRA) responsiveness and refractoriness in APL associated with t(15;17) (a) and t(11;17) (b), respectively. The link between RARα and the nuclear corepressor–histone deacetylase (NCOR–HD) complex is broken by ATRA. The link between PLZF and NCOR–HD is not broken by ATRA.

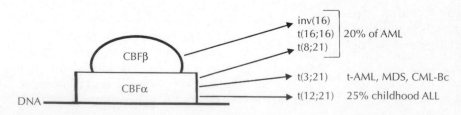

**Figure 17.5** Schematic representation of the core binding factor, CBF, which is composed of two subunits. Disruption and rearrangement of the genes encoding for RUNX1 (AML1, CBFα) and CBFβ are found as recurrent aberrations in AML and ALL.

classical t(8;21).[13] Cytogenetically, these cases are characterized by complex variant translocations involving 8q22, 21q22, or another chromosome, masked translocations, and insertions.[14] The RUNX1–ETO fusion protein, which consists of the N terminus of RUNX1 fused to nearly the full length of ETO, is not sufficient to drive the leukemogenic process, as demonstrated in transgenic mice.[15] The prognostic significance of RT–PCR for RUNXI–ETO has not been completely clarified, owing to the presence of the RUNX1–ETO fusion protein in case of long-term hematological remission.[16] A good correlation, however, was found between negative PCR results and the absence of relapse in a prospective study of patients with t(8;21).

Additional chromosome aberrations are estimated to occur in around 70–80% of AML cases with t(8;21). The most frequent additional abnormalities are represented by loss of a sex chromosome, partial deletion of the long arm of chromosome 9, and, less frequently, trisomy 8 and partial deletion of the long arm of chromosome 7. Whereas the loss of a sex chromosome does not influence the clinical outcome of the disease, a partial deletion of the long arm of chromosome 9 seems to be related to an unfavorable prognosis.[17]

### inv(16)(p13q22/t(16;16)(p13;q22): *CBFB–MYH11*

inv(16)(p13q22) and t(16;16)(p13;q22) are associated with the M4Eo subset of AML and, less frequently, with the M2 and M5 subtypes. Prognosis is relatively good. However, quantitative molecular monitoring may identify a group with low copy number at low or non-existing risk of relapse, and a group with higher numbers of transcripts at high risk for relapse.[18] The chimeric gene consists of the 5′ part of CBFβ, a transcription factor at 16q22 that interacts with the RUNX1 DNA-binding factor (Figure 17.5), and the 3′ coding sequence of *MYH11* at 16p13, encoding the smooth muscle myosin heavy chain (SMMHC). This results in a CBFβ–SMMHC fusion protein, which in a dominant-negative way inhibits CBF function through mobilization of the nuclear corepressor complex or through RUNX1 sequestration in the cytoplasm. By applying molecular investigations, masked inv(16) have been identified, including cases with an inverted 16 that is also involved in a translocation with another chromosome, as well as submicroscopic rearrangements in leukemias with normal karyotype or trisomy of chromosome 8 and/or 22.[19,20] Molecular studies using RT–PCR revealed that the frequency of this change is higher than reported using conventional cytogenetics. Molecular studies are also highly sensitive in monitoring the disease during and at the end of therapy. However, the value of molecular monitoring in inv(16) cases is limited, since *CBFB–MYH11* transcripts can be detected in long-term remission patients.

FISH with appropriate probes for the 16p13 region detects accompanying deletions in the p arm, including the *MPR* gene, in around 20% of patients.[21] No significant differences in the survival of patients with or without 16p deletions associated with inv(16)/t(16;16) were observed.[21]

Additional karyotypic abnormalities are present in about half of the patients with inv(16)/t(16;16). Trisomy 8, 21, and 22 are common. No prognostic differences were found on comparing patients with inv(16) alone versus patients with additional karyotypic abnormalities.[22]

### t(6;9) (p23;q34): DEK–CAN

The t(6;9)(p23;q34) fuses the 5′ part of *DEK*, coding for a nuclear DNA-binding protein, located on chromosome 6p23, to the 3′ part of the *CAN* (also known as *NUP214*) gene, located on chromosome 9q34, encoding for a nucleoporin. The *DEK–CAN* chimeric gene is transcribed into the DEK–CAN 165 kDa protein, whereas no transcription could be detected from the reciprocal *CAN–DEK* fusion.[23] This rare translocation may be found in both AML and MDS. It is frequently associated with bone marrow basophilia and predicts an unfavorable prognosis. The *CAN* gene has also been activated by fusion of its 3′ half to the *SET* gene, located at 9q34, in a case of acute undifferentiated leukemia.[24] The *SET–CAN* fusion gene contains a single open reading frame (ORF), coding for a 155 kDa chimeric SET–CAN protein. Since *CAN* recombines with either *DEK* or *SET*, its role as an oncogene, activated by fusion of its 3′ part to different genes, has been suggested.

### t(8;16)(p11;p13): MOZ–CBP

The t(8;16)(p11;p13) is a hallmark of AML, including both M4 and M5 subtypes.[25] Typical features are erythrophagocytosis from bone marrow blast cells, extramedullary infiltration, and disseminated intravascular coagulation (DIC). The malignant disorder affects both infants and adults, as a de novo or as a therapy-related or occupationally related AML. At chromosome 8p11, the breakpoint was identified within the *MOZ* (monocytic leukemia zinc finger protein) gene, a zinc finger protein with acetyltransferase activity. This gene is also rearranged in other 8p11 changes, involving *TIF2* in inv(8)(p11;q13)[26] and *p300* in t(8;22)(p11;q13).[27]

At chromosome 16p13, the gene implicated is *CBP* (CREB (cAMP response element binding)-binding protein), which codes for a transcriptional adaptor/coactivator protein, and which undergoes monoallelic mutations, with loss of one functional copy, in the Rubinstein–Taybi constitutional syndrome. The *CBP* gene has also been identified as the target of a t(11;16)(q23;p13) in therapy-related AML/MDS, in which it rearranges with *MLL*.[28]

### t(1;22)(p13;q13): *OTT–MAL*

The t(1;22)(p13;q13) is a specific cytogenetic marker of acute megakaryocytic leukemia (AML-M7 subtype) in infants, presenting with extensive infiltration of abdominal organs and rare response to therapy. This translocation is usually found as an isolated anomaly in infants younger than 6 months, while hyperdiploid or complex karyotypes are more often found in infants older than 6 months.[29] Duplication of the derivative chromosome 1, i.e. der(1)t(1;22), is one of the most frequent additional chromosomal changes. Recently, other genes involved in this translocation have been identified in two infants with AML-M7 carrying a classical and a variant t(1;22).[30] The gene on chromosome 22 was named *MAL* (megakaryocytic acute leukemia), and may be involved in chromatin organization, whereas the gene on chromosome 1 was named *OTT* (one twenty-two) and seems to be related to the *Drosophila* split-end (spen) family of proteins. The OTT–MAL fusion product, encoded by the der(22) and detectable by PCR assay, contains almost all of the identified domains of both the OTT and MAL proteins. Its role in the pathogenesis of leukemia has not yet been established. The reciprocal MAL–OTT fusion product has not been detected.

### t(3;5)(q25;q35): *NPM–MLF1*

The t(3;5)(q25;q35) is found in MDS and AML preceded by MDS, and predicts a bad prognosis. This translocation has been observed in all FAB subtypes except M3 (APL), with a higher incidence in AML-M6. Bone marrow specimens consistently show an increased number of megakaryocytes and trilineage dysplasia.

Both genes involved in this chromosomal change have been identified. At chromosome 5q35, the target gene is *NPM* (nucleophosmin, protein B23, NO38, numatrin) a nucleolar phosphoprotein, which is already known for its involvement in the t(2;5)/*NPM–ALK* in large cell lymphomas, and as a partner of the *RARA* gene in the t(5;17)/*NPM–RARA* variant translocation in APL. At chromosome 3q25, a novel gene named *MLF1* (myelodyspasia/myeloid leukemia factor 1) has been identified. The *MLF1* gene encodes a 31 kDa protein expressed in the cytoplasm.[31] The chimeric NPM–MLF1 protein is transported into the nucleus by NPM, and is expressed at high level in the nucleolus. In vitro studies showed that NPM–MLF1 induces apoptotic cell death of the expressing cells, which can be rescued by anti-apoptotic proteins such as BCL2. These findings suggest that the pro-apoptotic effect of the NPM–MLF1 fusion protein plays a role in causing ineffective hematopoiesis and MDS in the t(3;5) translocation, while the evolution to AML would imply an additional event with activation of anti-apoptotic proteins.[32]

# Promiscuous genes: *MLL, NUP98, ETV6*

A number of reciprocal translocations producing fusion genes in AML are promiscuous recombinations of one specific gene with multiple genomic partners. The paradigm for such phenomenon in AML is the *MLL* gene, which is known to recombine with more than 40 different genes. In this section, we also include a discussion of both *NUP98* and *ETV6* recombinations in AML.

### *MLL*/11q23

*MLL* (alternatively called *ALL1*, *HRX*, and *Htrx-1*) is the human homolog of the *Drosophila trithorax* gene, which encodes a putative DNA-binding protein involved in the control of embryonic development. It is a 90 kb gene with 36 exons, characterized by multiple zinc finger DNA-binding domains. Murine models suggest that MLL plays an important role in hematopoietic differentiation as regulator of transcription of other genes, namely the *HOX* genes.[33] *MLL* gene translocations involve different chromosomal partners, some of which have not been completely characterized at a molecular level. In AML, the t(9;11), t(10;11), t(6;11), and t(11;19) are most frequent (Table 17.1). Using standard cytogenetics, only some *MLL* translocations can be detected. Molecular analyses and FISH are necessary in cases negative for classical cytogenetics. These cases are represented by reciprocal translocations between chromosome bands sharing the same staining property, such as the t(6;11)(q27;q23), by complex translocations involving more than one chromosome in addition to 11q23, and by a cryptic insertion either of the 5′ end of *MLL* into a partner chromosome or of the 3′ end of a partner gene into the 11q23 band.[34,35] Accompanying deletions of the 3′ end of *MLL* have also been identified in a number of cases by applying FISH probes for the 3′ and 5′ ends of *MLL* in double-color experiments.

The *MLL* gene also rearranges by internal tandem duplication of the portion spanning exons 2–6 in AML cases with normal karyotype or in the presence of trisomy 11.[36] Rearrangement of *MLL* by self-fusion can be detected only by molecular studies, which have further demonstrated that the partially duplicated *MLL* is transcribed into mRNA capable of encoding a partially duplicated protein. These findings suggest that the *MLL* gene plays a critical role in leukemogenesis on its own, regardless of the partner genes involved in translocations.

The *MLL* breakpoints map in the same 8.3 kb breakpoint cluster region (bcr). Within the bcr, two different breakpoints have been identified. In infant leukemias and in leukemias induced by DNA topoisomerase II inhibitors, the breakpoints occur in the 3′

half of the bcr, so that a similar mechanism of DNA damage has been hypothesized.[37,38] In the majority of de novo leukemias, breakpoints map at the 5′ half of the bcr. In vivo experiments in knock-in models with the t(9;11) translocation evidenced a long period of latency before the onset of leukemia, suggesting that the *MLL* rearrangement per se is not sufficient for the expression of a full leukemic phenotype.[39] The disruption of normal Ikaros function in *MLL–AF4* in infants further supports this hypothesis.[40]

Rearrangements of *MLL* occur in about 80% of acute lymphoplastic leukemia (ALL) and AML of infants, in de novo AML, and therapy-related leukemias, mainly following treatment with anti-topoisomerase II or intercalating topoisomerase II inhibitors, but also after alkylating agents and/or radiotherapy. The prognostic significance of these rearrangements has not been definitively established, except for the t(4;11)(q21;q23), which is associated with a poor prognosis.[41]

Despite the distribution of *MLL* rearrangements between ALL and AML according to current morphological/immunological classifications, a unique expression profile is emerging for all the acute leukemias bearing an *MLL* translocation.[42]

## NUP98/11p15

The 98 kDa nucleoporin protein (NUP98) is a member of a nucleoporin family characterized by FXFG or FG repeats. It is located at the nucleoplasmic side of the nuclear pore complex and regulates nucleo-cytoplasmic transport of proteins and RNA by its docking function.

Rearrangement of the *NUP98* gene was first identified by cloning the t(7;11)(p15;p15) translocation in de novo and therapy-related AML/MDS and in chronic myeloid leukemia (CML). Since this translocation is most frequently observed in Oriental populations and found only sporadically in Caucasians, a racial or geographical predisposition has been hypothesized. In this translocation, the partner of *NUP98* is the homeobox gene *HOXA9*.[43,44]

The *HOX* genes are a superfamily of transcription factor genes organized in class I, corresponding to four clusters (A, B, C, and D) on chromosomes 7, 17, 12, and 2, respectively, and class II, with a divergent homeodomain, dispersed throughout the genome. The *HOXA9* gene consists of three exons, and the translocation breakpoint lies between exons 1A and 1B. The *NUP98* breakpoint is located on either intron 11 or 12. The *NUP98–HOXA9* chimeric transcript, originating from this translocation, contains the FG repeat docking site of *NUP98* and most of the coding region of *HOXA9*. The reciprocal *HOXA9–NUP98* has never been detected. The NUP98–HOXA9 fusion protein is predicted to function as an aberrant transcription factor deregulating *HOX*-responsive genes. The leuke-

### Table 17.3 Summary of *NUP98* fusions reported in acute myeloid leukemia/myelodysplastic syndromes

| | |
|---|---|
| t(7;11)(p15;p15) | *NUP98–HOXA9/A11/A13* |
| t(2;11)(q31;p15) | *NUP98–HOXD11/D13* |
| t(1;11)(q23;p15) | *NUP98–PMX1* |
| inv(11)(p15q22) | *NUP98–DDX10* |
| t(11;17)(p15;q21) | *NUP98–? HOXB[a]* |
| t(11;12)(p15;q13) | *NUP98–? HOXC[a]* |
| t(11;20)(p15;q11) | *NUP98–TOP1* |
| t(9;11)(p22;p15) | *NUP98–LEDGF* |
| t(5;11)(q35;p15) | *NUP98–NSD1* |
| t(8;11)(p12;p15) | *NUP98–NSD3* |

[a] Not yet molecularly demonstrated.

mogenic potential of the NUP98–HOXA9 protein has been tested in vitro by transformation of NIH3T3 fibroblasts, and in vivo on transplanted mice. Fusion partners of *NUP98* are summarized in Table 17.3.

In all of the *NUP98* rearrangements identified so far, a chimeric transcript from the 5′ portion of *NUP98* is fused in-frame to the 3′ portion of the partner gene, while the reciprocal fusion transcript has only been sporadically detected.[45,46] These findings suggest that the NUP98 N-terminal part, containing the FG repeats, may play an important role in leukemogenesis.

## ETV6/12p13

The human *ETV6* (ETS-variant gene 6) encodes a member of the ETS family of transcription factors. The gene spans 240 kb and consists of eight exons encoding a helix–loop–helix (HLH) domain (exons 3 and 4) and a DNA-binding domain (exons 6–8). The first chromosomal translocation affecting *ETV6* was a t(5;12)(q33;p13) found in a patient with chronic myelomonocytic leukemia (CMML). The molecular consequence of this translocation is fusion of the 5′ HLH domain of *ETV6* to the transmembrane and tyrosine kinase domains of the *PDGFBR* (platelet-derived growth factor β receptor) gene.[47] In addition to the t(5;12) translocation, involvement of *ETV6* has also been reported in number of translocations associated with myeloid (Figure 17.6) as well as lymphoid leukemias.[48]

*ETV6* displays different functions in the fusion transcripts derived from these rearrangements. The t(1;12) and the t(12;15)(p13;q25) are rare *ETV6* translocations in myeloid disorders, each having been described in only one case of AML. The t(1;12) results in the ETV6–ARNT chimeric protein, which contains the 5′ end of ETV6 and almost the entire ARNT (aryl hydrocarbon receptor nuclear translocator) component.[49] The t(12;15), which is also found in congenital fibrosarcoma, fuses the *ETV6* gene with the *NTRK3* (neurotropin-3 receptor) gene. The resulting

*ETV6–NTRK3* fusion transcript contains the HLH dimerization domain of *ETV6* and the protein tyrosine kinase domain of *NTRK3*, and may contribute to leukemogenesis by dysregulation of the NTRK3 signal transduction pathway.[50]

A particular type of fusion has been found in the t(3;12)(q26;p13) and in the t(12;13)(p13;q12), where *ETV6* drives the expression of the partner genes, namely of *MDS1/EVI1* in the t(3;12), and of *CDX2* in the t(12;13).[51,52]

The t(4;12)(q12;p13) translocation is typically associated with CD7+ AML in adults and with B-lymphoid leukemias in children. The involvement of *ETV6* in this rearrangement was first demonstrated by FISH in two AML cases. The partner gene at 4q12 was identified as *BTL* (Brx-like translocated in leukemia), now renamed *CHIC2*.[53] The *CHIC2–ETV6* transcript, but not the reciprocal *ETV6–CHIC2*, was detected by molecular studies in four AML-M0 patients. Of note is the ectopic expression of the *GSH2* gene, located upstream of *CHIC2* and most probably upregulated by *ETV6* regulator sequences.

Similarly to the t(4;12), in the t(7;12)(q36;p13) rearrangement, both the HLH and DNA-binding domains of ETV6 are present in the fusion protein. The t(7;12)(q36;p13), associated with myeloid malignancies of children characterized by poor prognosis, fuses the *ETV6* gene to the *HLXB9* homeobox gene, with the expression only of the *HLXB9–ETV6* fusion transcript.[54]

The t(9;12)(q34;p13) was found in ALL and in AML cases using molecular and FISH investigations, since it is rarely detectable by classical cytogenetics. This translocation results in the fusion of the 5′ part of *ETV6* to the 3′ part of *ABL1*, producing a chimeric ETV6–ABL1 protein with elevated tyrosine kinase activity.[55]

The t(12;22)(p13;q11), observed in different myeloid malignancies, including myeloproliferative disorders (MPD), MDS, and AML, fuses the *ETV6* gene to the *MN1* gene already known for its involvement in 22q rearrangements of meningioma. Both reciprocal chimeric transcripts, *ETV6–MN1* and *MN1–ETV6*, are expressed in tumor cells. The MN1–ETV6 chimeric protein, which contains the 3′ DNA-binding domain of ETV6, acts as a transcription factor, whose transforming potential has been shown in NIH3T3 cells.[56]

## Chromosomal changes resulting in altered gene expression: 3q21–q26

Recurrent structural changes of chromosome 3 in AML involve bands q21 and q26, and include an inv(3)(q21q26), a translocation, and an insertion between the long arms of both homologs broken at q21 and q26, and reciprocal translocations, namely t(3;21)(q26;q22), t(3;13)(q26;q14), t(3;7)(q26;q22), t(3;12)(q26;p13). Activation of *EVI1* at 3q26 has been identified as the common denominator of these cytogenetic changes.[57] The abnormal expression is due to the activity of the enhancer of the *ribophorin I* gene at 3q21 in the typical inversion, but also as result of translocations leading to a fusion gene, such as the t(3;12) translocation (Figure 17.6). Another gene that has been shown to be activated by a non-random reciprocal translocation in AML, namely the t(1;3)(p36;q21) translocation, is *MEL1* at 1p36, which belongs to the same family of *EVI1*.[58] Interestingly the gene involved at 3q21 is the *ribophorin I* gene, as in the inv(3).

The leukemias associated with these genetic lesions are disorders with a very poor prognosis. A specific hematological feature is the high number of platelets at presentation, even in the presence of massive blastic infiltration in the bone marrow. Cytogenetically, inv(3) is frequently associated with monosomy 7.

### t(2;3)(p23;q26)

The t(2;3)(p22–p23;q26–q28) is a rare non-random translocation observed in myeloid disorders such as MDS, AML, and blastic phases of Philadelphia (Ph)-positive and Ph-negative MPD. In the majority of cases, it is associated with other chromosomal aberrations, particularly –5/del(5)(q) and –7/del(7)(q), and it is also found in therapy-induced myeloid disorders. The molecular counterpart of this translocation is still unknown. Conventional cytogenetics shows heterogeneity for both 2p and 3q breakpoints. Overexpression of *EVI1*, possibly due to translocation, has been shown. However, RACE–PCR did not identify the translocation partner on chromosome 2p.[59]

## Gene amplification

Over-representation of a chromosomal region, from three to multiple copies, so-called 'gene amplification', is a recently discovered leukemogenetic event in which putative oncogene(s) within the over-represented region are thought to be involved. Some cases show an intrachromosomal amplification, as jumping translocation of the same DNA sequence to different partner chromosomes or as a marker chromosome/ring with contiguous amplified region and homogeneously staining region (hsr). Some cases have extrachromosomal amplification on double minutes (dmin).

In AML, two recurrent regions of amplification have been identified: 8q24 and 11q23.[60–62] Amplification of the 8q24 region has been found sporadically in AML.

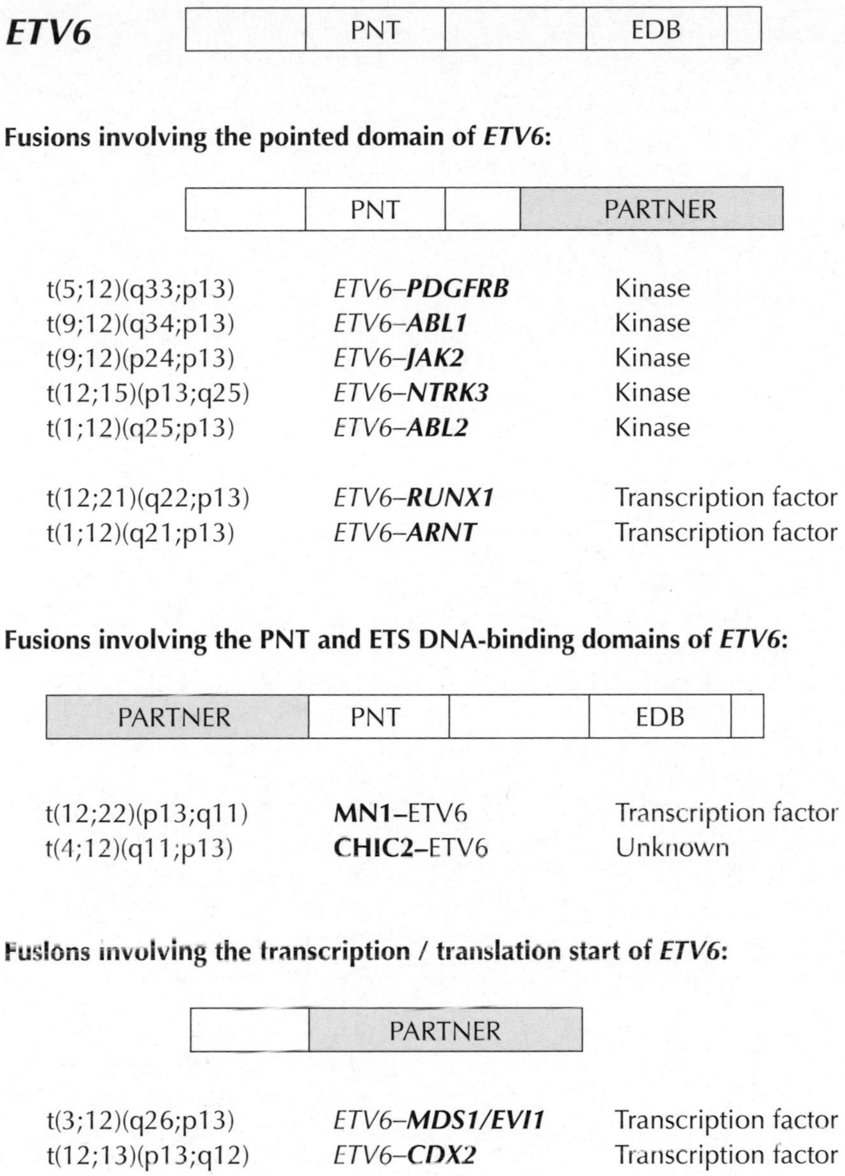

**ETV6**  | PNT | EDB |

**Fusions involving the pointed domain of ETV6:**

| PNT | | PARTNER |

| t(5;12)(q33;p13) | ETV6–**PDGFRB** | Kinase |
| t(9;12)(q34;p13) | ETV6–**ABL1** | Kinase |
| t(9;12)(p24;p13) | ETV6–**JAK2** | Kinase |
| t(12;15)(p13;q25) | ETV6–**NTRK3** | Kinase |
| t(1;12)(q25;p13) | ETV6–**ABL2** | Kinase |
| t(12;21)(q22;p13) | ETV6–**RUNX1** | Transcription factor |
| t(1;12)(q21;p13) | ETV6–**ARNT** | Transcription factor |

**Fusions involving the PNT and ETS DNA-binding domains of ETV6:**

| PARTNER | PNT | | EDB |

| t(12;22)(p13;q11) | **MN1**–ETV6 | Transcription factor |
| t(4;12)(q11;p13) | **CHIC2**–ETV6 | Unknown |

**Fusions involving the transcription / translation start of ETV6:**

| | PARTNER |

| t(3;12)(q26;p13) | ETV6–**MDS1/EVI1** | Transcription factor |
| t(12;13)(p13;q12) | ETV6–**CDX2** | Transcription factor |

**Figure 17.6** Schematic representation of the known *ETV6* fusion partners, illustrating the different mechanism involving *ETV6* in the production of oncogenic fusion proteins in myeloid disorders. Fusion partners of *ETV6* are shown in bold, their function is described in the last column. PNT, pointed domain (oligomerization domain); EDB, ETS DNA-binding domain.

Cytogenetically, all cases with dmin were shown to contain c-*MYC* amplicons.

*MLL* amplifications have been described in de novo AML/MDS and in therapy-related AML/MDS, especially if alkylating agents have been included in the treatment. Patients are in general old and have a bad prognosis.[62]

Besides c-*MYC* and *MLL*, other regions may contain the target genes of genomic amplification in myeloid disorders.[61] *RUNX1* amplifications have also been documented, but are more frequently associated with ALL.[63]

# Gene mutation

More recently, recurrent genetic mutations have been identified in leukemic cells. These mutations detectable by molecular techniques constitute an additional marker of the leukemic clone that can be used for diagnosis, prognosis, and follow-up of residual disease. The genes most often studied are summarized in Table 17.4.[64–73] Among these, the receptor tyrosine kinase as well as the *RAS* oncogene have gained in importance because selective inhibitors are being developed to treat AML by selective molecular targeting, with encouraging preliminary results.

**Table 17.4 Gene mutations in acute myeloid leukemia (AML)/myelodysplastic syndromes (MDS)**

| | |
|---|---|
| *FLT3* (13q12) | • Receptor tyrosine kinase class III |
| | • Expressed in hematopoietic lineage |
| | • ITD (internal tandem duplication) of juxtamembrane domain in 20% of AML, associated with poor prognosis |
| | • Mutation Asp 835 in 7% of AML. Prognostic implication uncertain |
| *c-KIT* (4q12) | • Receptor tyrosine kinase class III |
| | • Expressed in CD34+ cells, mast cells and melanocytes |
| | • Expressed in 65% of AML |
| | • Mutation in 8%, sometimes associated with inv(16) |
| *N-RAS* (1p22) | • GTP-binding protein |
| *K-RAS* (12p12) | • Major switch in signal transduction by activation of kinase cascade: MAPK, PI3K, and others |
| | • Ubiquitously expressed |
| | • Mutations at codon 12, 13, or 61 in 25% of MDS and AML |
| *WT1* (11p13) | • Zinc finger transcription factor |
| | • Tumor suppressor gene implicated in Wilms' tumor |
| | • Expressed in CD34+ cells, not in mature cells |
| | • Highly expressed in 75% of AML. Can be used for monitoring of residual disease |
| | • Mutation in 15% of AML |
| *CEBPA* (19q13) | • Transcription factor with tumor suppressor gene function expressed in myeloid/myelomonocytic cells |
| | • Mutated in 7% of AML |
| *RUNX1* (21q22) | • Core binding factor CBFA2 involved in t(8;21), t(3;21), etc. |
| | • Biallelic mutation in 5% of AML (FAB-M0), trisomy 21 with AML |
| | • Mutations reported in a familial platelet disorder with predisposition to AML (FPD/AML) |
| *TP53* (17p13) | • Nuclear phosphoprotein involved in control of cell cycle, proliferation, and apoptosis |
| | • Tumor suppressor gene implicated mainly in solid tumors |
| | • Deletion of one allele and mutation observed in 5% of AML and MDS |
| *MLL* (11q23) | • Internal tandem duplication (discussed under promisuous genes) |

## Trisomies

Among numerical chromosomal changes, trisomies are the most commonly occurring as isolated karyotypic aberrations in AML. Well-established trisomies in AML are listed in Table 17.5.

The most frequent change is trisomy 8, often as an additional change to more typical structural rearrangements. The incidence as a primary anomaly is higher in other myeloid disorders, such as MDS and MPD. A specific pathogenetic role of this trisomy in AML has been strongly supported by expression profiling showing a significant difference with leukemias with a normal karyotype due to a more pronounced downregulation of apoptosis-regulating genes.[74] These results have been related to a lack of response of trisomy 8-bearing leukemic cells to cytarabine,[75] a drug inducing apoptosis. Interestingly some authors have focused on the meiotic origin of this trisomy, which would be present as a part of constitutional mosaicism in the bone marrow of affected patients.[76] The trisomic clone would undergo preferential expansion in the proliferating malignant population. In a subgroup of cases, the trisomy may be the first step in the evolution of AML associated with a more advanced polysomy, such as tetrasomy 8.

**Table 17.5 Most frequent autosomal trisomies occurring as single anomalies in myeloid malignancies**

| Trisomy | Disease (frequency as % of all cases) |
|---|---|
| +4 | AML (<1%), MDS (rare) |
| +6 | AML (<1%), MDS (<1%), hypoplastic MDS (rare) |
| +8 | AML (3–4%), MDS (3–6%), CMPD (4–7%) |
| +9 | AML (<1%), MDS (<1%), CMPD[a] (21%) |
| +11 | AML (1%), MDS (1%) |
| +13 | AML (<1%), MDS (rare) |
| +14 | AML, MDS (rare) |
| +21 | AML (1–3%), MDS (<1%), CMPD (<1%) |

AML, acute myeloid leukemia; MDS, myelodysplastic syndromes; CMPD, chronic myeloproliferative disorders.
[a] Especially polycythemia vera, often associated with +9.

AML with trisomy 4 likely originates from an early myeloid precursor, as suggested by the occurrence of the lesion either in MDS with a high blast component or in AML. This trisomy is consistently found in cases with double minutes and *c-MYC* amplification.

Studies of the molecular counterpart have focused on the duplication of a mutated form of the c-*KIT* gene as well as on c-*KIT* overexpression in leukemic cells with trisomy 4.[77,78]

Other recurrent trisomies in AML involve chromosomes 13, 14, and 21.

# Myelodysplastic syndromes

The incidence of karyotypic abnormalities is less pronounced in the MDS group (50% of cases) than in AML (80%). Structural changes, such as complete or partial deletions, are found more typically in MDS than in AML (Table 17.6), where reciprocal translocations represent the most frequent primary aberration. Moreover, the incidence of MDS deletions has been increasing since the application of loss of heterozygosity (LOH) studies as well as FISH investigations on interphase nuclei. In cases with progression of MDS to overt AML, a clonal karyotypic evolution, i.e. the appearance of new chromosomal anomalies in addition to those present at diagnosis, may be observed. However, additional chromosomal changes with a predictive value for evolution to AML have not been definitively established.

The fact that the same change may occur in MDS as well as in de novo AML suggests that, at least in those cases, the malignant clone originates from a genetic insult at the level of a multipotent stem cell and that the clinico-hematological findings of the malignant disorder are related to additional factors influencing the balance between cell growth, survival, and differentiation of bone marrow populations.

Strong correlations between typical cytogenetic changes and prognosis of MDS have been well documented.[79]

## Table 17.6 Primary chromosome deletions in myelodysplastic syndromes

del(3)(p14–21)s
del(5)(q13q33)/–5s
del(6)(p21)
del(6)(q21)
del(7)(q22q32–35)/–7s
del(9)(q13q2?)
del(11)(q14q23)
del(12)(p13)
del(13)(q14q22)
del(17)(p13)
del(18)(p11)
del(20)(q11q13)
–Y

s, secondary disorder.

For a listing of critical genomic rearrangements in MDS the reviews in references 80 and 81 are recommended. Here some entities with specific cytogenetic–hematological correlations will be presented.

## Typical deletions in MDS

### del(7)/–7

Chromosome 7 is often involved, either as a partial deletion of the long arm (7q–) or as loss of one homolog (–7), in different types of MDS. Monosomy 7 is the most frequent aberration in myeloid proliferations in children.[82] Both the 7q– and the –7 changes are consistently associated with MDS or AML induced by radiotherapy and/or chemotherapy for a previous lymphoma or solid tumor. Alkylating agents have mostly been implicated. Interestingly, loss of 7q is also the result of a genomic imbalance due to the t(1;7)(q10;p10) translocation consistently found in secondary MDS.

Despite its frequency, the biological significance of monosomy 7 is still undefined. An intriguing observation is that a clone with monosomy 7 may emerge during the evolution of a number of genetic conditions predisposing to MDS/AML, such as Fanconi anemia, Shwachman syndrome, familial myelodysplasia, and Kostman syndrome. In the last syndrome, the emergence of a monosomy 7 is possibly favored by treatment with granulocyte colony-stimulating factor (G-CSF). In the multistep process of malignant transformation, monosomy 7 in children may be preceded by mutations of the *RAS* and/or *NF1* genes.[83]

Monosomy 7 is a marker of poor prognosis in both children and adults, and very serious infectious complications are related to a deep disturbance of chemotaxis.

### The 5q– syndrome

The WHO Classification keeps this syndrome separate from all other refractory anemias.[84] It is a distinct clinico-hematological disease characterized by macrocytic anemia, normal or elevated platelet count, and trilineage bone marrow dysplasia with typical monolobulated micromegakaryocytes. The disorder significantly affects aged women. The prognosis is relatively good, with a chronic course and very rare evolution to acute leukemia. However, the need for intensive support with red cell transfusions may lead to serious complications from hemosiderosis. Attempts of treatments with different growth factors, including erythropoietin, granulocyte–macrophage colony-stimulating factor (GM-CSF), and G-CSF, have been successful in controlling anemia only in sporadic cases of 5q– syndrome.

The chromosomal rearrangement is always an interstitial deletion, with loss of a variable extent of material. The minimal common deletion is located at band 5q31, in which a number of genes responsible for regulation of growth and/or differentiation of hematopoietic cells are located. The critical molecular event underlying the 5q– syndrome, however, is still unknown.[85]

Combined immunophenotypic and FISH studies have shown that the cell of origin of the 5q– change is an early progenitor such as a CD34+CD19+ lymphomyeloid stem cell.[86] Similarly to the Ph chromosome, T lymphocytes are not involved.

The occurrence of a 5q– chromosome is not limited to the 5q– syndrome,[87] since it can also be found in other MDS, such as refractory anemia with excess of blasts (RAEB), and secondary MDS, especially after radiotherapy or alkylating agents for a previous malignancy. In those cases the anomaly may result not only from simple deletions, but also from unbalanced translocations, such as t(5;17). In secondary MDS, loss of an entire homolog (monosomy 5) is also frequent. A 5q– in a complex karyotype is associated with bad prognosis.

### The 17p– syndrome

A deletion on the short arm of chromosome 17 may result from different types of chromosomal rearrangements, i.e. unbalanced translocations, isochromosome of the long arm, and simple deletions. The anomaly is usually associated with other rearrangements. A common molecular event is the involvement of the TP53 gene at 17p13: a TP53 mutation is found in around 70% of patients with 17p deletion and MDS, so that both TP53 alleles are abnormal, one being deleted and the second mutated. The typical hematological stigmata of the 17p– syndrome are represented by dysgranulopiesis, with pseudo Pelger–Hüet hypolobulated nuclei and small vacuoles in the cytoplasm of neutrophils. Prognosis is usually adverse.[88]

Chromosome 17p is also a hot site for rearrangements arising after radiochemotherapy or exposure to environmental toxics.

### 20q–

del(20)(q11q13) has been reported in a large spectrum of myeloid malignancies: in approximately 5% of MDS, in 10–15% of polycythemia vera (PV), and less frequently in AML. It is a primary change not associated with poor prognosis in PV. In MDS, the prognostic value of 20q– is more controversial, although as an isolated karyotypic anomaly it has been associated with relatively low-risk disorders.

Experimental data are in favor of 20q– occurring in a progenitor common to granulomonocytes and erythroid cells. A peculiar cellular kinetics of cells bearing a 20q– chromosome has been described, in that positive bone marrow granulocytes are not discharged into the peripheral blood.[89] Whether this phenomenon reflects a high level of apoptosis of granulocytes in leukemic bone marrow with 20q– remains to be determined.

The size of the deletion is heterogeneous. FISH studies have indicated an SRD (shortest region of deletion) of less than 1 Mb in MPD and a somewhat larger one (3 Mb) in MDS.[90] Putative candidate genes have been analyzed for deletion or mutations on the second allele.

## Myelodysplastic– myeloproliferative disorders

This category, which contains a subgroup of diseases with morphological signs of both MDS and chronic MPD, has recently been introduced in the WHO Classification.[84] Cytogenetically, changes common to MDS and Phi-negative CML as well as myelofibrosis have been described, including iso(14q), trisomy 14, monosomy 7, –Y, and t(5;12). The reciprocal translocation t(5;12), originally described in CMML and resulting in a fusion gene between PDGFBR on 5q33 and ETV6 on 12p13, is very interesting, as other changes involving the PDGFBR gene with alternative partners have also been found in hematological cases diagnosed as MDS or atypical CML.[91–93] Tyrosine kinase inhibitors, such as imatinib, are able to induce hematological remission in malignancies with PDGFBR gene rearrangements.

## t(8)(p11) Myeloproliferative syndrome

A new syndrome has recently been identified.[94] It presents as a CML-like myeloid hyperplasia, with marked eosinophilia, a high incidence (60%) of T-cell non-Hodgkin lymphoma, and rapid progression to AML. It results from various translocations, all involving the FGFR1 (fibroblast growth factor receptor 1) gene at 8p11.3. FGFR1 is a transmembrane tyrosine kinase receptor. Its tyrosine kinase domain is fused to other transcription factors as a consequence of chromosomal translocations: t(8;13) encodes ZnF198–FGFR1, t(6;8) FOP–FGFR1; t(8;9) CEP110–FGFR1, and t(8;22) BCR–FGFR1. This syndrome is associated with a very poor prognosis.

# REFERENCES

1.  Golub TR. Genomic approaches in the pathogenesis of hematologic malignancy. *Curr Opin Hematol* 2001; **8**: 252–61.

2.  de Thé H, Chomienne C, Lanotte M et al. The t(15;17) translocation of acute promyelocytic leukaemia fuses the retinoic acid receptor α gene to a novel transcribed locus. *Nature* 1990; **347**: 558–61.

3.  He L-Z, Tribioli C, Rivi R et al. Acute leukemia with promyelocytic features in *PML/RARα* transgenic mice. *Proc Natl Acad Sci USA* 1997; **94**: 5302–7.

4.  Brunei V, Lafage-Pochitaloff M et al. Variant and masked translocations in acute promyelocytic leukemia. *Leuk Lymphoma* 1996; **22**: 221–8.

5.  Licht JD, Chomienne C, Goy A et al. Clinical and molecular characterization of a rare syndrome of acute promyelocytic leukemia associated with translocation (11;17). *Blood* 1995; **85**: 1083–94.

6.  Pandolfi PP. In vivo analysis of the molecular genetics of acute promyelocytic leukemia. *Oncogene* 2001; **20**: 5726–35.

7.  Arnould C, Philippe C, Bourdon V et al. The signal transducer and activator of transcription *STAT5b* gene is a new partner of retinoic acid receptor α in acute promyelocytic-like leukemia. *Hum Mol Genet* 1999; **8**: 1741–9.

8.  Wells RA, Catzavolos C, Kamel-Reid S. Fusion of retinoic acid receptor α to NuMA, the nuclear mitotic apparatus protein, by a variant translocation in acute promyelocytic leukemia. *Nat Genet* 1997; **17**: 109–13.

9.  Jurcic JG, Nimer SD, Scheinberg DA et al. Prognostic significance of minimal residual disease detection and PML/RAR-α isoform type: long term follow-up in acute promyelocytic leukemia. *Blood* 2001; **98**: 2651–6.

10. De Botton S, Chevret S, Sanz M et al. Additional chromosomal abnormalities in patients with acute promyelocytic leukemia (APL) do not confer poor prognosis: results of APL 93 trial. *Br J Haematol* 2000; **111**: 801–6.

11. Ferrara F, Di Noto R, Annunziata M et al. Immunophenotypic analysis enables the correct prediction of t(8,21) in acute myeloid leukaemia. *Br J Haematol* 1998; **102**: 744–8.

12. Friedman AD. Leukemogenesis by CBF oncoproteins. *Leukemia* 1999; **13**: 1932–42.

13. Andrieu V, Radford-Weiss I, Troussard X et al. Molecular detection of t(8;21)/*AML1/ETO* in AML M1/M2: correlation with cytogenetics, morphology and immunophenotype. *Br J Haematol* 1996; **92**: 855–65.

14. Gallego M, Carroll AJ, Gad GS et al. Variant t(8;21) rearrangements in acute myeloblastic leukemia of childhood. *Cancer Genet Cytogenet* 1994; **75**: 139–44.

15. Yuan Y, Zhou L, Miyamoto T et al. *AML1–ETO* expression is directly involved in the development of acute myeloid leukemia in the presence of additional mutations. *Proc Natl Acad Sci USA* 2001; **98**: 10398–403.

16. Morschhauser F, Cayuela JM, Martini S et al. Evaluation of minimal residual disease using reverse-transcription polymerase chain reaction in t(8;21) acute myeloid leukemia: a multicenter study of 51 patient. *J Clin Oncol* 2000; **18**: 788–94.

17. Schoch C, Haase D, Haferlach T et al. Fifty-one patients with acute myeloid leukemia and translocation t(8;21)(q22;q22): an additional deletion in 9q is an adverse prognostic factor. *Leukemia* 1996; **10**: 1288–95.

18. Buonamici S, Ottaviani E, Testoni N et al. Real-time quantitation of minimal residual disease in inv(16)-positive acute myeloid leukemia may indicate risk for clinical relapse and may identify patients in a curable state. *Blood* 2002; **99**: 443–9.

19. Dierlamm J, Stul M, Vranckx H et al. FISH identifies inv(16)(p13q22) masked by translocations in three cases of acute myeloid leukemia. *Genes Chromosomes Cancer* 1998; **22**: 87–94.

20. Aventin A, La Starza R, Nomdedeu J et al. Typical *CBFβ/MYH11* fusion due to insertion of the 3′-*MYH11* gene into 16q22 in acute monocytic leukemia with normal chromosomes 16 and trisomies 8 and 22. *Cancer Genet Cytogenet* 2000; **123**: 137–39.

21. Martinet D, Muhlematter D, Leeman M et al. Detection of 16p deletions by FISH in patients with inv(16) or t(16;16) and acute myeloid leukemia (AML). *Leukemia* 1997; **11**: 964–70.

22. Marlton P, Keating M, Kantarjian H et al. Cytogenetic and clinical correlates in AML patients with abnormalities of chromosome 16. *Leukemia* 1995; **9**: 965–71.

23. Soekarman D, von Lindern M, Daenen S et al. The translocation (6;9)(p23;q34) shows consistent rearrangement of two genes and defines a myeloproliferative disorder with specific clinical features. *Blood* 1992; **79**: 2990–7.

24. Von Lindern M, van Baal S, Wiegant J et al. *Can*, a putative oncogene associated with myeloid leukemogenesis, may be activated by fusion of its 3′ half to different genes: characterization of the *set* gene. *Mol Cell Biol* 1992; **12**: 3346–55.

25. Velloso ER, Mecucci C, Michaux L et al. Translocation t(8;16)(p11;p13)in acute nonlymphocytic leukemia: report on two new cases and review of the literature. *Leuk Lymphoma* 1996; **21**: 137–42.

26. Carapetti M, Aguiar RCT, Goldman JM, Cross NCP. A novel fusion between *MOZ* and the nuclear receptor coactivator *TIF2* in acute myeloid leukemia. *Blood* 1998; **91**: 3127–33.

27. Chaffanet M, Gressin L, Preudhomme C et al. *MOZ* is fused to *p300* in acute monocytic leukemia with t(8;22). *Genes Chromosomes Cancer* 2000; **28**: 138–44.

28. Sobulo OM, Borrow J, Tomek R et al. *MLL* is fused to *CBP*, a historic acetyltransferase in therapy-related acute myeloid leukemia with a t(11;16)(q23;p13.3). *Proc Natl Acad Sci USA* 1997; **94**: 8732–7.

29. Carroll A, Civin C, Schneider N et al. The t(1;22)(p13;q13) is nonrandom and restricted to infants with acute megakaryoblastic leukemia: a Pediatric Oncology Group study. *Blood* 1991; **78**: 748–52.

30. Mercher T, Busson-Le Coniat M, Monni R et al. Involvement of a human gene related to the *Drosophila spen* gene in the recurrent t(1;22) translocation of acute megakaryocytic leukemia. *Proc Natl Acad Sci USA* 2001; **98**: 576–9.

31. Yoneda-Kato N, Look AT, Kirstein MN et al. The t(3;5)(q25.1;q34) of myelodysplastic syndrome and acute myeloid leukemia produces a novel fusion gene, *NPM–MLF1*. Oncogene 1996; **12**: 265–75.

32. Yoneda-Kato N, Fukuhara S, Kato J. Apoptosis induced by the myelodysplastic syndrome-associated NPM-MLF1 chimeric protein. *Oncogene* 1999; **18**: 3716–24.

33. Yu BD, Hess JL, Horning SE et al. Altered *Hox* expression and segmental identity in *MLL* mutant mice. *Nature* 1995; **378**: 505–8.

34. Angioni A, La Starza R, Mecucci C et al. Interstitial insertion of *AF10* into the *ALL1* gene in a case of infant acute lymphoblastic leukemia. *Cancer Genet Cytogenet* 1998; **107**: 107–10.

35. von Bergh A, Gargallo P, De Prijck B et al. Cryptic t(4;11) eoncoding *MLL–AF4* due to insertion of 5′ *MLL* sequences in chromosome 4. *Leukemia* 2001; **15**: 595–600.

36. Schichman SA, Caligiuri MA, Gu Y et al. *ALL–1* partial duplication in acute leukemia. *Proc Natl Acad Sci USA* 1994; **91**: 6236–9.

37. Felix CA, Lange BJ. Leukemia in infants. *Oncologist* 1999, **4**: 225–40.

38. Strick R, Strissel PL, Borgers S et al. Dietary bioflavonoids induce cleavege in the *MLL* gene and may contribute to infant leukemia. *Proc Natl Acad Sci USA* 2000; **97**: 4790–5.

39. Corral J, Lavenir I, Impery H et al. An *MLL/A9* fusion gene made by homologous recombination causea acute leukemia in chimeric mice: a method to create fusion oncogenes. *Cell* 1996; **85**: 853–61.

40. Sun L, Heerema N, Crotty L et al. Expression of dominant-negative and mutant isoforms of the antileukemic transcription factor Ikaros in infant acute lymphoblastic leukemia. *Proc Natl Acad Sci USA* 1999; **96**: 680–5.

41. Harrison CJ. The detection and significance of chromosomal abnormalities in childhood acute lymphoblastic leukemia. *Blood Rev* 2001; **15**: 19–59.

42. Armstrong S, Staunton JE, Silverman LB et al. *MLL* translocations specify a distinct gene expression profile that distinguishes a unique leukemia. *Nat Genet* 2002; **30**: 41–7.

43. Borrow J, Shearman AM, Stanton VP et al. The t(7;11)(p15;p15) translocation in acute myeloid leukemia fuses the genes for nucleoporin *NUP98* and class I homeoprotein *HOXA9*. *Nat Genet* 1996; **12**: 159–67.

44. Kroon E, Thorsteins U, Mayotte N et al. *NUP98/HOXA9* expression in hemopoietic stem cells induces chronic and acute myeloid leukemias in mice. *EMBOJ* 2001; **20**: 350–61.

45. Lam DH, Aplan PD. *NUP98* gene fusions in hematologic malignancies. *Leukemia* 2001; **15**: 1689–95.

46. Rosati R, La Starza R, Veronese A et al. *NUP98* is fused to the *NSD3* gene in acute myeloid leukemia associated with t(8;11)(p11.2;p15). *Blood* 2002; **99**: 3857–60.

47. Golub TR, Barker GF, Lovett M, Gilliland DG. Fusion of PDGF receptor β to a novel *ets*-like gene, *tel*, in chronic myelomonocytic leukemia with t(5;12) chromosome translocation. *Cell* 1994; **77**: 307–16.

48. Wlodarska I, Mecucci C, Baens M et al. *ETV6* gene rearrangements in hematopoietic malignant disorders. *Leuk Lymphoma* 1996; **23**: 287–95.

49. Salomon-Nguyen F, Della-Valle V, Mauchauffe M et al. The t(1;12)(q21;p13) translocation of human acute myeloblastic leukemia results in a *TEL–ARNT* fusion. *Proc Natl Acad Sci USA* 2000; **97**: 6757–62.

50. Eguchi M, Eguchi-Ishimae M, Tojo A et al. Fusion of *ETV6* to neurotrophin-3 receptor *TRKC* in acute myeloid leukemia with t(12;15)(p13;q25). *Blood* 1999; **93**: 1355–63.

51. Peeters P, Wlodaeska I, Baens M et al. Fusion of *ETV6* to *MDS/EVI1* as a result of t(3;12)(q26;p13) in myeloproliferative disorders. *Cancer Res* 1997; **15**: 564–9.

52. Chase A, Reiter A, Burci L et al. Fusion of *ETV6* to the caudal-related homeobox gene *CDX2* in acute myeloid leukemia with the t(12;13)(p13;q12). *Blood* 1999; **93**: 1025–31.

53. Cools J, Bilhou-Nabera C, Wlodarska I et al. Fusion of a novel gene, *BTL*, to *ETV6* in acute myeloid leukemias with a t(4;12)(q11–q12;p13). *Blood* 1999; **94**: 1820–4.

54. Beverloo HB, Panagopoulos I, Isaksson M et al. Fusion of the homeobox gene *HLXB9* and the *ETV6* gene in infant acute myeloid leukemias with the t(7;12)(q36;p13). *Cancer Res* 2001; **15**: 5374–7.

55. Papadopoulos P, Ridge SA, Boucher CA et al. The novel activation of *ABL* by fusion to an *ets*-related gene, *TEL*. Cancer Res 1995; **55**: 34–8.

56. Buijs A, van Rompaey L, Molijn AC et al. The MN1–TEL fusion protein, encoded by the translocation (12;22)(p13;q11) in myeloid leukemia, is a transcription factor with transforming activity. *Mol Cell Biol* 2000; **20**: 9281–93.

57. Nucifora G. The *EVI1* gene in myeloid leukemia. *Leukemia* 1997; **11**: 2022–31.

58. Mochizuki N, Shimizu S, Nagasawa T et al. A novel gene, *MEL1*, mapped to 1p36.3, is highly homologous to the *MDS1/EVI1* gene and is transcriptionally activated in t(1;3)(p36;q21)-positive leukemia cells. *Blood* 2000; **96**: 3209–14.

59. Poppe B, Yigit N, Marynen P et al. Molecular characterization of a t(2;3)(p23;p26). A recurrent translocation involving the *EVI1* gene. *Blood* 2001; **98**: 564a.

60. Falzetti D, Vermeesch JR, Matteucci C et al. Microdissection and FISH investigations in acute myeloid leukemia: a step forward to full identification of complex karyotypic changes. *Cancer Genet Cytogenet* 2000; **118**: 28–34.

61. Salt SN, Qadir MU, Conroy JM et al. Double minute chromosomes in acute myeloid leukemia and myelodysplastic syndrome: identification of new amplification regions by fluorescence in situ hybridization and spectral karyotyping. *Genes Chromosomes Cancer* 2002; **34**: 42–7.

62. Michaux L, Wlodarska I, Stul M et al. *MLL* amplification in myeloid leukemias: a study of 14 cases with multiple copies of 11q23. *Genes Chromosomes Cancer* 2000; **29**: 40–7.

63. Hilgenfeld E, Padilla-Nash H, McNeil N et al. Spectral karyotyping and fluorescence in situ hybridization detects novel chromosomal aberrations, a recurring involvement of chromosome 21 and amplification of the *MYC* oncogene in acute myeloid leukemia M2. *Br J Haematol* 2001; **113**: 305–17.

64. Schnittger S, Schoch C, Dugas M et al. Analysis of *FLT3* length mutations in 1003 patients with acute myeloid leukemia: correlation to cytogenetics, FAB subtype, and prognosis in the AMLCG study and usefulness as a marker for the detection of minimal residual disease. *Blood* 2002; **100**: 59–66.

65. Longley BJ, Reguera MJ, Ma Y. Classes of c-KIT activating mutations: proposed mechanisms of action and implications for disease classification and therapy. *Leuk Res* 2001; **25**: 571–6.

66. Reylly JT. Class III receptor tyrosine kinases: role in leukemogenesis. *Br J Haematol* 2002; **116**: 744–56.

67. Janssen J, Steenvorden A, Lyons J et al. *Ras* gene mutations in acute and chronic myelocytic leukemias, chronic myeloproliferative disorders, and myelodysplastic syndromes. *Proc Natl Acad Sci USA* 1987; **84**: 9228–32.

68. King-Underwood L, Pritchard-Jones K. Wilms' tumor (*WT1*) gene mutations occur mainly in acute myeloid leukemia and may confer drug resistance. *Blood* 1998; **91**: 2961–8.

69. Pabst T, Mueller BU, Zhang P et al. Dominant-negative mutations of *CEBPA*, encoding CCAAT/enhancer binding protein-α (C/EBPα), in acute myeloid leukemia. *Nat Genet* 2001; **27**: 263–70.

70. Song WJ, Sullivan MG, Legare RD et al. Haploinsufficiency of *CBFA2* causes familial thrombocytopenia with propensity to develop acute myelogenous leukaemia. *Nat Genet* 1999; **23**: 166–75.

71. Preudhomme C, Warot-Loze D, Roumier C et al. High incidence of biallelic mutations in the Runt domain of the *AML1* gene in M0 acute myeloid leukemia and in myeloid malignancies with acquired trisomy 21. *Blood* 2000; **96**: 2862–9.

72. Krug U, Ganser A, Koeffler HP. Tumor suppressor genes in normal and malignant hematopoiesis. *Oncogene* 2002; **21**: 3475–95.

73. Christiansen DH, Andersen MK, Pedersen-Bjergaard J. Mutations with loss of heterozygosity of *p53* are common in therapy-related myelodysplasia and acute myeloid leukemia after exposure to alkylating agents and significantly associated with deletion or loss of 5q, a complex karyotpye, and a poor prognosis. *J Clin Oncol* 2001; **19**: 1405–13.

74. Virtaneva K, Wright FA, Tanner SM et al. Expression profiling reveals fundamental biological differences in acute myeloid leukemia with isolated trisomy 8 and normal cytogenetics. *Proc Natl Acad Sci USA* 2001; **98**: 1124–9.

75. Byrd JC, Lawrence D, Arthur D et al. Patients with isolated trisomy 8 in acute myeloid leukemia are not cured with cytarabine-based chemotherapy: results from Cancer and Leukemia Group B 8461. *Clin Cancer Res* 1998; **4**: 1235–41.

76. Minelli A, Morerio C, Maserati E et al. Meiotic origin of trisomy in neoplasms: evidence in a case of erythroleukemia. *Leukemia* 2001; **15**: 971–5.

77. Ferrari S, Grande A, Zucchini P et al. Overexpression of c-*kit* in a leukemic cell population carrying a trisomy 4 and its relationship with the proliferative capacity. *Leuk Lymphoma* 1993; **9**: 495–501.

78. Beghini A, Ripamonti CB, Castorina P et al. Trisomy 4 leading to duplication of a mutated *KIT* allele in acute myeloid leukemia with mast cell involvement. *Cancer Genet Cytogenet* 2000; **119**: 26–31.

79. Greenberg P, Cox C, LeBeau MM et al. International scoring system for evaluating prognosis in myelodysplastic syndromes. *Blood* 1997; **89**: 2079–88.

80. Mecucci C, La Starza R. Cytogenetics of myelodysplastic syndromes. *FORUM Trends Exp Clin Med* 1999; **9**: 4–13.

81. Pedersen-Bjergaard J, Andersen MK, Christiansen DH, Nerlov C. Genetic pathways in therapy related myelodysplasia and acute myeloid leukemia. *Blood* 2001; **99**: 1909–12.

82. Hasle H, Arico M, Basso G et al. Myelodysplastic syndrome, juvenile myelomonocytic leukemia, and acute myeloid leukemia associated with complete or partial monosomy 7. European Working Group on MDS in childhood (EWOG-MDS). *Leukemia* 1999; **13**: 376–85.

83. Shannon KM, Watterson J, Johnson P et al. Monosomy 7 myeloproliferative disease in children with neurofibromatosis type 1: epidemiology and molecular analysis. *Blood* 1992; **9**: 1311–18.

84. Jaffe ES, Harris NL, Stein H, Vardiman JW (eds). *World Health Organization Classification of Tumours. Pathology and Genetics of Tumours of Hematopoietic and Lymphoid Tissues*. Lyon: IARC Press, 2001.

85. Lai F, Gogley LA, Joslin J et al. Transcript map and comparative analysis of the 1.5-Mb commonly deleted segment of human 5q31 in malignant myeloid diseases with a del(5q). *Genomics* 2001; **71**: 235–45.

86. Nilsson L, Astran-Grundstrom I, Arvidsson I et al. Isolation and characterization of hematopoietic progenitor/stem cells in 5q-deleted myelodysplastic syndromes: evidence for involvement at the hematopoietic stem cell level. *Blood* 2000; **96**: 2012–21.

87. Van den Berghe H, Michaux L. 5q–, twenty-five years later: a synopsis. *Cancer Genet Cytogenet* 1997; **94**: 1–7.

88. Lai JL, Preudhomme C, Zandecki M et al. Myelodysplastic syndromes and acute myeloid leukemia with 17p deletion. An entity characterized by specific dysgranulopoiesis and a high incidence of *p53* mutations. *Leukemia* 1995; **9**: 370–81.

89. Asimakopoulos FA, Holloway TL, Nacheva EP et al. Detection of chromosome 20q deletions in bone marrow metaphases but not peripheral blood granulocytes in patients with myeloproliferative disorders or myelodysplastic syndromes. *Blood* 1996; **87**: 1561–70.

90. Bench AJ, Nacheva EP, Hood TL et al. Chromosome 20 deletions in myeloid malignancies: reduction of the common deleted region, generation of a BAC/PAC contig and identification of candidate genes. UK Cancer Cytogenetics Group (UKCCG). *Oncogene* 2000; **19**: 3902–13.

91. Magnusson MK, Meade KE, Brown KE et al. Rapaptin-5 is a novel fusion partner to platelet-derived growth factor β receptor in chronic myelomonocytic leukemia. *Blood* 2001; **98**: 2518–25.

92. Ross TS, Bernard OA, Berger R, Gilliland DG. Fusion of huntingtin interacting protein 1 to platelet-derived growth factor β receptor (PDGFβR) in chronic myelomonocytic leukemia with t(5;7)(q33;q11.2). *Blood* 1998; **91**: 4419–26.

93. Schwaller J, Anastasiadou E, Cain D et al. H4 (*Dl0S170*), a gene frequently rearranged in papillary thyroid carcinoma, is fused to the platelet-derived growth factor receptor β gene in atypical chronic myeloid leukemia with t(5;10)(q33;q22). *Blood* 2001; **97**: 3910–18.

94. Macdonald D, Reiter A, Cross NC. The 8p11 myeloproliferative syndrome: a distinct clinical entity caused by constitutive activation of FGFR1. *Acta Haematol* 2002; **107**: 101–7.

# 18 Cytogenetic and molecular abnormalities in lymphoid malignancies

**William B Slayton and Stephen P Hunger**

## The nature of oncogenes and tumor suppressor genes

Remarkably, the basic tenets of molecular cytogenetics and molecular oncology were outlined in the early 1900s by Theodor Boveri.[1] He hypothesized that gain of 'growth-promoting' chromosomes or loss of 'growth-inhibitory' chromosomes might each cause unrestrained cell growth and cancer. We now know that Boveri's general concept was correct, and that alterations in chromosomes play a pivotal role in oncogenesis. The details are both more complicated and more elegant than Boveri imagined. The important functional unit is not the chromosome, but rather individual genes located on the chromosomes. Consistent with Boveri's original hypothesis, the genes responsible for oncogenesis fall into two broad classes: growth-promoting oncogenes and growth-inhibitory tumor suppressor genes (TSG).

Identification and characterization of genes involved in the pathogenesis of human cancer has been a major biomedical advancement of the past quarter century. Cytogenetic and molecular genetic characterization of recurrent changes observed in leukemias and lymphomas has played a crucial role in these advances and has revealed two fundamental axioms: first, that specific, cytogenetically-evident changes occur non-randomly, and are often tightly linked with distinct clinical subtypes of disease; second, that these cytogenetic changes are harbingers of alterations in oncogenes/TSG, and can facilitate identification of these genes.[2] We now know that cancer is the cumulative phenotypic manifestation of mutations in oncogenes and/or TSG. In most, and likely all, cases, full expression of the malignant phenotype requires that mutations occur in a number of different oncogenes/TSG.[3]

## Mechanisms of oncogene activation and TSG inactivation

Visible cytogenetic alterations occur in a substantial majority of lymphoid malignancies. Cytogenetic abnormalities are classified as structural or numerical.[4] Structural changes include translocations (rearrangements that involve two or more different chromosomes) and inversions (rearrangements within a single chromosome). Numerical changes include deletion or gain of all or a portion of individual chromosomes.

Chromosomal translocations are detected cytogenetically or molecularly in the majority of cases of acute lymphoblastic leukemia (ALL) and non-Hodgkin lymphoma (NHL). Translocations cause altered expression of, and/or structural changes in, cellular proto-oncogenes by one of two mechanisms. First, proto-oncogenes can be translocated into the vicinity of active regulatory elements of another gene, usually one of the immunoglobulin (*Ig*) or T-cell receptor (*TCR*) genes, causing dysregulated expression of a structurally intact (or occasionally truncated) protein. Translocations in B-lineage leukemias/lymphomas often involve chromosome bands 14q32 (heavy-chain gene, *IgH*), 2q12 (light-chain gene, *Igκ*), or 22q11 (light-chain gene, *Igλ*), while T-lineage malignancies involve 14q11 (*TCRδ* or *TCRα*) or 7q35 (*TCRβ*). The second class of translocations are those that create fusion genes encoding chimeric proteins that possess novel structural and functional properties not present in the constituent wild-type proteins. This type of translocation most commonly affects transcription factors, often fusing a DNA-binding and/or protein oligomerization domain from one protein with effector domains, such as a transcriptional activation domain (TAD), from another. These translocations typically occur in introns of each gene; exons of the two genes are then joined together during mRNA splicing. Creation of a functional chimera generally requires that the joined exons from each gene are in the same reading frame.[5]

Numerical changes are conceptually easy to envision, but their functional consequences have been difficult to elucidate. Cytogenetically visible deletions involve loss of millions of base pairs of DNA encoding many different genes. Smaller deletions also occur that are not cytogenetically evident, but can be detected by molecular techniques. Current evidence indicates that the important target of deletions is usually one specific TSG. Molecular analyses of solid tumors have shown that when deletions are observed, the other allele of the relevant TSG is usually mutated, leading to complete loss of protein function. It is also possible that the remaining allele may not be altered and that an alteration in dosage of one or more genes is the critical consequence of the deletion. Identification of the critical target gene(s) is a daunting challenge. The consequences of complete or partial chromosome gains are poorly defined. Chromosome gains may result in higher levels of expression of certain proteins by altering gene dosage. This hypothesis is difficult to test, and the critical genes affected by chromosome additions remain unknown.

Other types of mutations affect a small number of nucleotides, and can be detected only by targeted molecular techniques. Point mutations alter one nucleotide and can be grouped into neutral alterations/polymorphisms that do not alter protein coding, missense mutations that substitute one amino acid for another while maintaining an open reading frame, and nonsense mutations that create a stop codon. Frameshift mutations are insertions or deletions of a small number of nucleotides (not divisible by three) that alter the reading frame and generally lead to protein truncation.

Different types of mutations, with different functional consequences, occur in oncogenes and TSG. Missense mutations in oncogenes cause a gain of function, and are dominant, genetically and functionally, as they promote transformation even though the normal protein from the wild-type allele is still expressed. In contrast, missense mutations in TSG generally inactivate the protein product. For example, missense mutations in *TP53* generate mutant p53 proteins that are impaired in important transcriptional and cell cycle-regulatory functions.[6] Nonsense and frameshift mutations almost always inactivate the function of proteins encoded by TSG by eliminating essential functional domains or by creating unstable proteins that are degraded rapidly. These mutations are typically genetically and functionally recessive, because the remaining wild-type allele still produces a normal protein that can perform the necessary cellular functions. In general, both alleles of a TSG must be inactivated to significantly alter cell growth. Frequently, each allele is inactivated by different mechanisms – for example, point mutation of one allele and deletion of the other. In some instances, TSG mutations may act in a so-called dominant-negative manner and exert their phenotype even in the presence of a non-mutated wild-type allele.

# Methods used to detect genetic alterations

It is critical to karyotype leukemias and lymphomas at initial diagnosis and relapse, because specific cytogenetic abnormalities may clarify the diagnosis, provide important prognostic information, or identify patients who might benefit (or fail to benefit) from specific therapeutic interventions. A detailed discussion of the techniques of cytogenetic analysis is outside the scope of this text. However, it is critical to emphasize that cancer karyotypes are performed on cells derived from direct preparations or short-term (24−72 hours) unstimulated cultures of malignant cells, as contrasted with analyses performed to detect constitutional cytogenetic abnormalities, which use mitogens to stimulate T cells to divide. Chromosome abnormalities are classified by the well-accepted International System for Human Cytogenetic Nomenclature (ISCN) which is updated periodically.[7]

Molecular cytogenetics is now an important complement to conventional cytogenetics. Fluorescence in situ hybridization (FISH) uses DNA probes that are hybridized to metaphase or interphase chromosomes and visualized directly or indirectly with fluorescent dyes or fluorochromes. FISH can be used to determine gene copy number, to map the relation of genes to one another, and to detect translocations or inversions by using multiple probes labeled with different fluorochromes. Figure 18.1 (see Plate 3) shows how two color split-apart FISH probes can be used to detect *E2A* translocations in interphase cells.[8] Alternatively, differentially labeled probes can be used for two different genes that give separate signals normally and merge to create a fusion signal when a translocation has occurred.[9]

Multicolor FISH (m-FISH) and spectral karyotyping (SKY) use a larger number of probes and allow each chromosome to be visualized in a unique color.[2] SKY and m-FISH are not yet used for routine clinical analyses, but can help identify the consequences of complicated or cryptic abnormalities that might be missed by FISH or by standard cytogenetics. Comparative genomic hybridization (CGH) involves cohybridization of tumor and control DNA to normal chromosome spreads and can identify region of chromosomes that have been amplified or deleted, but does not detect structural rearrangements such as translocations.[10]

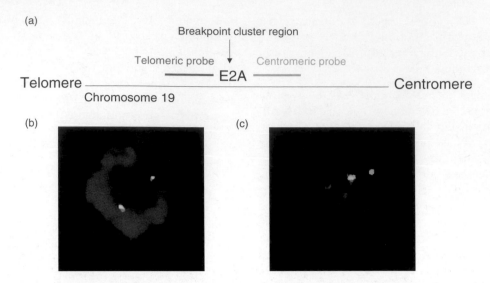

**Figure 18.1** Detection of *E2A* translocations in interphase cells via two-color 'split apart' FISH. (a) Schematic depiction of the *E2A* gene on chromosome 19 and location of probes centromeric (green) and telomeric (red) to *E2A*. (b) Interphase FISH of a normal cell shows two fused red/green or yellow signals from the adjacent signals on each chromosome 19 homologue. (c) Interphase FISH of a cell with a t(1;19)(q23;p13) shows one fused red/green signal from the normal chromosome 19, and single red and green signals from the der(1) and der(19) chromosomes, respectively. See Plate 3.

Other methods of detecting alterations in oncogenes and TSGs rely upon molecular techniques to analyze DNA, RNA, or proteins directly. This is feasible only for recurring abnormalities with previously defined molecular consequences. Important techniques include Southern blotting to detect gene rearrangement or gene copy number, polymerase chain reaction (PCR), which can be used to amplify diagnostic sequences or to produce sufficient material for other analyses, and methods to determine primary DNA sequence. As an understanding of these techniques is an important prerequisite for the discussions to follow, the underlying concepts will be reviewed briefly.

Southern blotting can be used to detect gene rearrangements that result from chromosomal translocations.[11] Technical considerations make this approach useful for detecting translocations that cluster within an area of less than approximately 20 kilobases (kb). Pulsed-field gel electrophoresis, which is generally available only in research laboratories, can be used to detect rearrangements that are spread out over a larger region of the genome. Figure 18.2 illustrates the use of Southern blot analysis to detect rearrangements within the 11q23 gene *MLL*, a frequent target of fusion gene-creating chromosomal translocations in acute leukemias.[12,13]

It is critical to determine the presence or absence of specific translocations that create fusion genes encoding chimeric mRNA and proteins in ALL and NHL. The DNA rearrangements that produce translocations almost always occur within introns of each gene. Because introns can range in size from less than one hundred to hundreds of thousands of nucleotides, the genomic breakpoints may vary widely in location from one patient to another, and fusion products often cannot be amplified reliably from DNA with a standard set of primers. For this reason, RNA is usually the preferred starting material for PCR (RNA–PCR or reverse transcriptase (RT)–PCR), as removal of introns during mRNA splicing fuses specific exons of each gene to one another, and fusion transcripts can be consistently amplified from almost all patients with a given translocation using a standard set of primers. Figure 18.3 demonstrates how RT–PCR can be used to amplify *E2A–PBX1* chimeric mRNAs produced by the t(1;19)(q23;p13).[14] Multiplex PCR uses a combination of primers that can detect a variety of fusion transcripts derived from chromosome translocations. One group has developed a set of multiplex PCR reagents capable of detecting any of 29 common translocations that occur in acute leukemia.[15]

Quantitative real-time PCR provides a way to quantify the number of copies of a particular RNA species in a given sample. This technique uses a fluorescent dye that is incorporated into the amplified DNA. Levels of fluorescence are measured with each PCR cycle and compared to calibrated standard controls. Real-time PCR can be used to quantitate minimal residual disease (MRD) by measuring levels of RNA transcripts derived from chromosome translocations or DNA copies of clonotypic *Ig/TCR* gene rearrangements during treatment of patients with leukemia or lymphoma.[16] This approach can stratify patients into groups with differential risks of relapse based on early response to therapy, and may become a major component of future systems for risk stratification.[17]

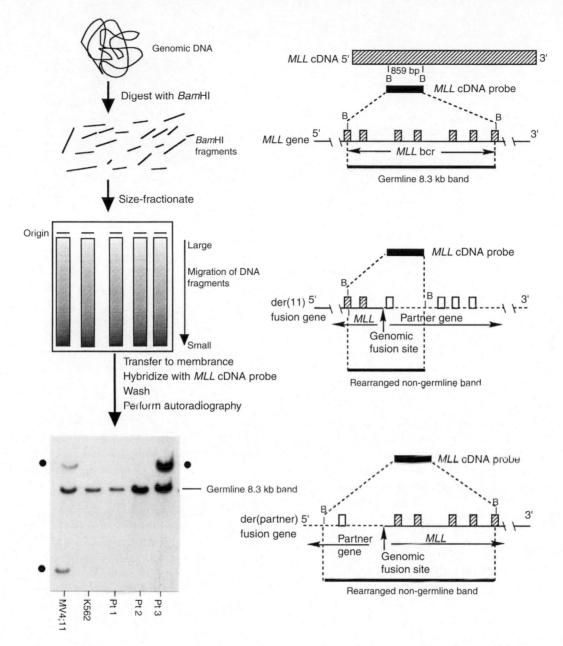

**Figure 18.2** Southern blot detection of *MLL* gene rearrangements. The structures of germline and fusion *MLL* genes are schematically depicted at right (exons are denoted by filled (*MLL*) or empty (partner gene) boxes). In the germline *MLL* gene, restriction enzyme *Bam*HI sites (B) flank the breakpoint cluster region (bcr) in which translocations occur, and the *MLL* cDNA probe will hybridize with an 8.3 kb germline band. Following translocation, two *MLL* fusion genes are potentially created, one on the der(11) chromosome and one on the der(partner chromosome), and the *MLL* cDNA probe will hybridize with one or two rearranged non-germline bands of unique size. The process of Southern blot analysis is shown at left. Genomic DNA is first digested with the restriction enzyme *Bam*HI, generating DNA fragments of various sizes that are size-fractionated by electrophoresis in agarose gel, generating a continuous smear of DNA fragments. The fragments are then denatured, transferred to a charged nylon membrane, and immobilized on the membrane. The membrane is then incubated with a radioactively labeled DNA probe, in this case the 859 bp *MLL Bam*HI cDNA fragment depicted at top right. To eliminate non-specific background hybridization, the blot is washed under stringent conditions. The hybridized blot is then exposed to X-ray film and developed. As can be seen in the autoradiograph at bottom left, a single 8.3 kb germline *MLL* band is seen in the cell line K562 and patients 1 and 2, each of which lacks *MLL* translocations. One *MLL*-rearranged band is present in patient 3, an infant with ALL and a t(11;19)(q23;p13.3). Two *MLL*-rearranged bands are present in MV4;11, a t(4;11)-ALL cell line.

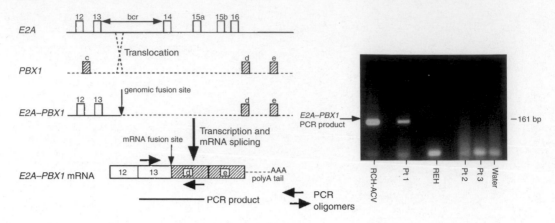

**Figure 18.3** RT–PCR analysis of *E2A–PBX1* fusion mRNAs produced by the t(1;19)(q23;p13). Portions of germline *E2A* and *PBX1* genes and the *E2A–PBX1* fusion gene produced by the t(1;19)(q23;p13) are depicted at the top left. To perform RT–PCR, RNA is isolated from the sample and a cDNA copy is made using reverse transcriptase and an oligodT primer that anneals to the polyA mRNA tail. PCR is then performed using oligomers complementary to *E2A* and *PBX1* sequences on opposite DNA strands. A specific product can only be amplified from cells containing a t(1;19) and *E2A–PBX1* fusion, as these genes are normally located on different chromosomes. At right are size-fractionated PCR products from RCH-ACV (a t(1;19)-ALL cell line), REH (an ALL cell line lacking a t(1;19)), three patients (one of whom (no. 1) had a t(1;19) and two (nos 2 and 3) who did not), and a negative control reaction containing no input DNA (water).

Advances in automated nucleotide sequencing have made it easier to directly analyze amplified DNA for mutations in specific genes. Microarray analysis has been a powerful tool to study the expression of a large number of genes in a single experiment (see Chapter 20).[18]

## Chromosome translocations: prototypic examples

Chromosome translocations comprise the largest group of well-characterized mutations in lymphoid malignancies. A comprehensive listing of the hundreds of translocations that have been characterized molecularly is impractical and rapidly outdated. Table 18.1 lists prototypical examples of the major types of proteins that are activated by chromosome translocations in lymphoid malignancies.

An increasing number of oncogenes are recurrent targets of chromosome translocations. In some cases, these translocations involve juxtaposition with more than one of the *Ig/TCR* loci. For example, c-*MYC* is involved in translocations with each of the three *Ig* loci, at least one of the *TCR* genes and at least one other gene.[19] In Burkitt lymphoma or leukemia, the t(8;14)(q24;q32) juxtaposes c-*MYC* with the *IgH* regulatory elements and results in dysregulated high-level expression of c-*MYC*. c-MYC is a transcription factor that turns on expression of target genes that result in entry into S phase, decreased growth factor requirements, and escape from normal regulation of cell cycle progression.[19] Other genes are fused to different partner genes by several different translocations. The extreme example is *MLL*, which is fused to a myriad of different partner genes by translocations in ALL and AML that involve more than 30 different partner loci.[20]

In T-ALL, chromosomal translocations juxtapose a wide variety of genes with one of the *TCR* loci, resulting in dysregulated expression of structurally intact proteins. The majority of these proteins possess structural features and functional properties of transcription factors, and are not expressed normally in T cells, underscoring the prominent role of aberrant transcription regulation in oncogenesis.[21] Transcription factors are grouped into functional classes or families on the basis of conserved protein motifs involved in DNA binding and protein oligomerization. Genes involved in T-ALL translocations encode members of the basic helix–loop–helix (bHLH) (TAL1, TAL2, and LYL1), bHLH-leucine zipper (ZIP) (c-MYC), LIM domain (LMO1 and LMO2), and homeodomain (HOX11) families.[22] The involvement of different members of protein subfamilies with highly similar DNA-binding properties (e.g. TAL1, TAL2, and LYL1, or LMO1 and LMO2) is particularly striking. Several of these transcription factors play important roles in the development of the hematopoietic system. HOX11 is required for formation of the spleen and TAL1/SCL is essential for development of all hematopoietic lineages.[23,24]

Some translocations observed in B-lineage ALL also cause dysregulated expression of structurally intact proteins, including transcription factors such as c-MYC and growth factors such as interleukin-3 (IL-

**Table 18.1 Major classes and examples of mutations leading to lymphoid malignancies**

| Class | Protein | Translocation | Function |
|---|---|---|---|
| Transcription factor | c-MYC | t(8;14)(q24;q32) | Regulates genes involved in cell cycle progression and apoptosis |
| | E2A–PBX1 | t(1;19)(q23;p13) | Heterodimerizes with Hox proteins, blocks differentiation, and transforms lymphoid cells |
| | TAL1/SCL | t(1;14)(p32;q11) | Required for definitive hematopoiesis; regulates genes involved in proliferation of myeloid progenitors |
| | HOX11 | t(7;10)(q35;q24) | Required for formation of the spleen. Immortalizes hematopoietic cells |
| | LMO2 | t(11;14)(p13;q11) | Complexes with other proteins that regulate definitive hematopoiesis (SCL/GATA-1/GATA-2) |
| Growth factor | IL-3 | t(5;14)(q31;q32) | Dysregulated cytokine production produces autocrine and paracrine effects on early hematopoietic progenitors |
| Kinase | BCR–ABL | t(9;22)(q34;q11) | Constitutive kinase action has proliferative and anti-apoptotic functions |
| | NPM–ALK | t(2;5)(p23;q35) | Constitutive ALK kinase activates pathways involved in cell proliferation, transformation, and survival |
| Cell cycle protein | CCND1 | t(11;14)(q13;q32) | Activates cell cycle progression of centrocytic cells |
| Apoptosis regulator | BCL 2 | t(14;18)(q32;q21) | Translocation dysregulates expression of this prototypical suppressor of apoptosis |

3). However, the majority create fusion genes that encode fusion proteins, many of which are chimeric transcription factors. Prominent examples include E2A–PBX1 and E2A–HLF, encoded by the t(1;19) and t(17;19), respectively.[25] In both cases, chimeras contain the N-terminal portion of E2A, including two experimentally defined TAD, fused to heterologous DNA-binding domains, a homeodomain in the case of E2A–PBX1 and a bZIP in the case of E2A–HLF. E2A–PBX1 and E2A–HLF bind to DNA sequences that are completely different from one another and from wild-type E2A, and activate target gene transcription. The E2A gene encodes at least two splice-variant proteins, E12 and E47, that contain bHLH elements involved in protein dimerization as well as DNA binding.[26] E2A is a transcriptional regulator of B-cell development, is involved in the initiation of immunoglobulin gene rearrangement, and is absolutely required for proper B-cell development.[27] E2A fusion proteins act as chimeric transcription factors in vitro and transform hematopoietic cells in a variety of experimental systems.[25] Despite recognition of completely different target DNA sequences, E2A–PBX1 and E2A–HLF transgenic mice develop T-cell malignancies with very similar features.[28–30] The E2A gene behaves as a TSG in mice. Almost all of the rare E2A-null mice that survive the immediate perinatal period later develop T-cell tumors that have a striking similar phenotype to those that develop in E2A–PBX1 and E2A–HLF transgenic mice.[31] These and other observations suggest that transformation mediated by E2A chimeras may involve mechanisms

other than direct transcriptional effects on target gene expression.[32] Complicating this picture further, recent data suggest that wild-type E2A can also function as an oncogene and can collaborate with c-MYC to induce tumors in a murine model system.[33]

Another major class of genes that are activated by a variety of mechanisms, including translocations, in lymphoid malignancies are those that encode tyrosine kinases. The prototype is BCR–ABL, the product of the t(9;22)(q34;q11), which occurs in chronic myeloid leukemia (CML), ALL, and acute myeloid leukemia (AML) (see Chapter 41).[34] The rational development of imatinib (STI571, (Gleevec/Glivec)) and its remarkable clinical efficacy in patients with CML[35] have prompted great scientific and clinical interest in small-molecule inhibitors of activated tyrosine kinases in cancer. One excellent candidate for such therapeutic strategies is anaplastic lymphoma kinase (ALK), which is fused to many other genes in anaplastic large cell lymphoma (ALCL) and inflammatory myofibroblastic tumors (IMT).[36] NPM–ALK, produced by the t(2;5)(p23;q35) in ALCL, is the founding member of this family. Experimental data indicate that the critical contribution of NPM and all other ALK fusion partners is an oligomerization domain that leads to constitutive activation of ALK tyrosine kinase activity.[36] General tyrosine kinase inhibitors can inhibit the activity of NPM-ALK in vitro and induce apoptosis of ALCL cell lines.[37] It can be anticipated that specific inhibitors of ALK will be developed and tested in patients with ALCL in the near future.

In NHL, specific translocations are frequently associated with distinct clinicopathologic subtypes of lymphoma. For example, the t(14;18)(q32;q21) or one of its variants are present in about 90% of follicular lymphomas (FL) and 20–30% of B-lineage diffuse large cell lymphomas (DLCL).[38] These translocations lead to dysregulated expression of BCL2, which inhibits programmed cell death.[39] A large body of evidence indicates that the clinically aggressive DLCL that contain a t(14;18) generally arise from more indolent t(14;18)-positive FL following acquisition of additional mutations in important growth-regulatory genes. Strikingly, a common second mutation in both *BCL2*-expressing animal models and human lymphomas is acquisition of translocations activating c-*MYC* expression.[38,40] Expression of c-*MYC* by itself promotes both proliferation and apoptosis; thus, the concomitant expression of *BCL2* and c-*MYC* has synergistic effects that allow cells to proliferate rapidly and survive.

Another important translocation in NHL is the t(11;14)(q13;q32), which is detected in 50–70% of mantle cell lymphomas (MCL), a recently delineated subtype of B-cell NHL.[41] This translocation juxtaposes *CCND1* with the *IgH* locus, causing dysregulated expression of cyclin D1. In contrast to other lymphoid malignancies, almost all MCL overexpress cyclin D1, making this a useful diagnostic feature. It is not clear what genetic alterations cause cyclin D1 overexpression in the 30–50% of MCL lacking detectable gene rearrangements. Possibilities include translocations outside the region detected by commonly utilized molecular probes and more subtle mutations in *CCND1* regulatory elements.

# Other recurrent mutations in lymphoid malignancies

Numerical alterations also play an important role in the pathogenesis of lymphoid malignancies. Additions of genetic material occur frequently, but the molecular consequences are not well-understood. For example, hyperdiploidy with a modal chromosomal number of more than 53 chromosomes is common in childhood ALL and is associated with an excellent prognosis.[4] Although certain chromosomes are duplicated more frequently than others, the specific consequences of duplication are unknown. It is possible that abnormalities of this type do not have specific consequences in the sense that translocations do, but rather are themselves phenotypic effects of other important genetic changes. Arguing against this possibility are the facts that duplications occur non-randomly, and are usually stable within a clone.[42] Single chromosome gains are also associated with specific subclasses of lymphoid malignanices, such as

the frequent occurrence of trisomy 12 in chronic lymphocytic leukemia (CLL).[43]

Chromosomal deletions are crucial harbingers of TSG in solid tumors, and are generally assumed to denote similar alterations in hematopoietic malignancies. Until recently, the target genes affected by deletions in leukemias have proved elusive. Two tightly linked and functionally related genes on chromosome 9, *INK4A* and *INK4B*, have been identified as the targets of deletions/mutations in a wide variety of malignancies, including ALL.[44,45] These genes encode proteins of approximately 16 kDa (p16$^{INK4a}$) and 15 kDa (p15$^{INK4b}$), members of a large family of cyclin-dependent kinase inhibitors (CDI or CKI), which interact with specific cyclin-dependent protein kinase (CDK)/cyclin complexes and negatively regulate cell cycle progression (see Chapter 4).

There are a number of other areas of recurrent deletion in lymphoid malignancies. In many solid tumors, detailed molecular analysis of recurrent deletions has led to identification of a critical single TSG within the common deleted segment.[3] In tumors such as colon cancer, one allele of the TSG is inactivated by deletion and one by point mutation. Identification of the point mutation allows one to focus on the critical gene from the region. To date, it has been very difficult to find such TSG within the areas of common deletion in lymphoid malignancies. This raises the possibility that different mechanisms may be operative in lymphoid malignancies. An example is provided by recent investigations of CLL. More than half of cases of CLL contain mono- or bi-allelic deletions of 13q14.[43] A common deleted segment of about 1 million base pairs has been identified and sequenced, but no single gene has been found that is consistently altered in CLL. A recent study identified micro-RNA genes *miR15* and *miR16* from the common deleted segment of 13q14 and demonstrated that both genes are deleted or downregulated in more than half of CLL cases.[46] These findings may facilitate identification of the target genes involved in other recurrent deletions in lymphoid malignancies.

Mutations in the *TP53* TSG are detected in a wide range of hematopoietic malignancies.[6] Their occurrence is not random, but rather is disease-specific and generally linked with advanced stage and poor prognosis. For example, mutations are rare in B-lineage ALL and T-ALL at the time of initial diagnosis. At relapse, *TP53* mutations are found in a significant minority of T-ALL, but are still uncommon in B-lineage ALL.[47,48] Similarly, approximately 15% of CLL contain *TP53* mutations at diagnosis versus 40–50% of transformed CLL (Richter syndrome).[49] A significant percentage (about 30%) of aggressive high-grade B-lineage NHL have *TP53* mutations, whereas they are rare in clinically indolent low-grade B-lineage NHL.[50]

# Chromosomal abnormalities, prognosis, and treatment decisions

Many cytogenetic and molecular abnormalities are tightly associated with distinct clinical subtypes of disease and have important prognostic or therapeutic implications. Perhaps the best example of this is the t(15;17) and *PML–RARA* fusion in acute promyelocytic leukemia (APL) (see Chapter 17). In childhood ALL, contemporary risk group stratification relies heavily on the presence or absence of specific cytogenetic abnormalities in the leukemic clone, including translocations and changes in ploidy. Patients with t(9;22) and *BCR–ABL* fusion and t(12;21) and *TEL–AML1* fusion or hyperdiploidy comprise two opposite ends of the spectrum. While there is no tight linkage of t(9;22)/*BCR–ABL* fusion with unique clinical features, the outcome of patients with this abnormality is extremely poor and few patients with *BCR–ABL1*⁺ ALL are cured with chemotherapy alone.[51] For this reason, many centers and cooperative groups now routinely perform RT–PCR for *BCR–ABL* fusion mRNA in patients with ALL. When it is detected, patients are offered alternative therapies. Until recently, this was usually early allogeneic bone marrow transplantation. New studies are also investigating the combination of intensive chemotherapy with imatinib. In contrast, about 40% of children less than 10 years of age with ALL will have either *TEL–AML1* fusion or a hyperdiploid DNA content.[52] Children with *TEL–AML1*⁺/hyperdiploid ALL have a particularly good prognosis with modern chemotherapy and may have cure rates as high as 90%. Many contemporary clinical trials use the presence of either of these features in treatment stratification algorithms. However, the *BCR–ABL*⁺ and the *TEL–AML1*⁺/hyperdiploid group are not completely homogeneous. Some *BCR–ABL*⁺ patients will be cured with combination chemotherapy alone, and some *TEL–AML1*⁺/hyperdiploid patients will relapse. An ongoing challenge is to dissect the heterogeneity that exists even within molecularly defined groups at the extremes of the prognostic spectrum. Measures of early treatment response and/or gene expression profiles may help refine these groups.

# Summary and perspectives

In this chapter, we have reviewed cytogenetic and molecular abnormalities in lymphoid malignancies. We have discussed different types of mutations that occur in proto-oncogenes and tumor suppressor genes, how they are detected, and how they contribute to malignant transformation. We have also highlighted the association between specific cytogenetic and molecular abnormalities and distinct clinical subtypes of disease or treatment outcomes. These associations are now recognized as important diagnostic criteria in leukemia and lymphoma classification systems, and are used to stratify therapy. It is anticipated that these trends will continue and that there will be further movement towards genetically based classification systems and the use of rationally designed therapies targeted at the fundamental molecular lesions that cause lymphoid malignancies.

# Acknowledgment

WBS is supported by NIH Grant HL03962.

## REFERENCES

1. Boveri T. *Zur Frage der Enstehung Maligner Tumoren.* Jena: Fischer, 1914.
2. Rowley JD. The role of chromosome translocations in leukemogenesis. *Semin Hematol* 1999; **36**(4 Suppl 7): 59–72.
3. Fearon ER, Vogelstein B. A genetic model for colorectal tumorigenesis. *Cell* 1990; **61**: 759–67.
4. Raimondi SC. Current status of cytogenetic research in childhood acute lymphoblastic leukemia. *Blood* 1993; **81**: 2237–51.
5. Hunger SP, Devaraj PE, Foroni L et al. Two types of genomic rearrangements create alternative E2A–HLF fusion proteins in t(17;19)-ALL. *Blood* 1994; **83**: 2970–7.
6. Imamura J, Miyoshi I, Koeffler HP. p53 in hematologic malignancies. *Blood* 1994; **84**: 2412–21.
7. Mitelman F (ed). *ISCN (1995): An International System for Human Cytogenetic Nomenclature.* Basel: S Karger, 1995.
8. Boomer T, Varella-Garcia M, McGavran L et al. Detection of *E2A* translocations in leukemias via fluorescence in situ hybridization. *Leukemia* 2001; **15**: 95–102.
9. Tkachuk DC, Westbrook CA, Andreeff M et al. Detection of *bcr–abl* fusion in chronic myelogeneous leukemia by in situ hybridization. *Science* 1990; **250**: 559–62.
10. Kallioniemi A, Kallioniemi OP, Sudar D et al. Comparative genomic hybridization for molecular cytogenetic analysis of solid tumors. *Science* 1992; **258**: 818–21.
11. Southern EM. Detection of specific sequences among DNA fragments separated by gel electrophoresis. *J Mol Biol* 1975; **98**: 503–17.
12. Hunger SP, Tkachuk DC, Amylon MD et al. *HRX* involvement in de novo and secondary leukemias with diverse chromosome 11q23 abnormalities. *Blood* 1993; **81**: 3197–203.
13. Thirman MJ, Gill HJ, Burnett RC et al. Rearrangement of the *MLL* gene in acute lymphoblastic and acute myeloid leukemias with 11q23 chromosomal translocations. *N Engl J Med* 1993; **322**: 909–14.

14. Hunger SP, Gallili N, Carroll AJ et al. The t(1;19)(q23;p13) results in consistent fusion of *E2A* and *PBX1* coding sequences in acute lymphoblastic leukemias. *Blood* 1991; **77**: 687–93.

15. Pallisgaard N, Hokland P, Riishoj DC et al. Multiplex reverse transcription–polymerase chain reaction for simultaneous screening of 29 translocations and chromosomal aberrations in acute leukemia. *Blood* 1998; **92**: 574–88.

16. Pongers-Willemse MJ, Verhagen OJ et al. Real-time quantitative PCR for the detection of minimal residual disease in acute lymphoblastic leukemia using junctional region specific TaqMan probes. *Leukemia* 1998; **12**: 2006–14.

17. Cave H, van der Werff ten Bosch J, Suciu S et al. Clinical significance of minimal residual disease in childhood acute lymphoblastic leukemia. European Organization for Research and Treatment of Cancer – Childhood Leukemia Cooperative Group. *N Engl J Med* 1998; **339**: 591–8.

18. Moos PJ, Raetz EA, Carlson MA et al. Identification of gene expression profiles that segregate patients with childhood leukemia. *Clin Cancer Res* 2002; **8**: 3118–30.

19. Kuppers R, Dalla-Favera R. Mechanisms of chromosomal translocations in B cell lymphomas. *Oncogene* 2001; **20**: 5580–94.

20. Ayton PM, Cleary ML. Molecular mechanisms of leukemogenesis mediated by MLL fusion proteins. *Oncogene* 2001; **20**: 5695–707.

21. Cleary ML. Oncogenic conversion of transcription factors by chromosomal translocations. *Cell* 1991; **66**: 619–22.

22. Rabbitts TH. Chromosomal translocations in human cancer. *Nature* 1994; **372**: 143–9.

23. Roberts CW, Shutter JR, Korsmeyer SJ. Hox11 controls the genesis of the spleen. *Nature* 1994; **368**: 747–9.

24. Porcher C, Swat W, Rockwell K et al. The T cell leukemia oncoprotein SCL/tal-1 is essential for development of all hematopoietic lineages. *Cell* 1996; **86**: 47–57.

25. Hunger SP. Chromosomal translocations involving the *E2A* gene in acute lymphoblastic leukemia: clinical features and molecular pathogenesis. *Blood* 1996; **87**: 1211–24.

26. Murre C, McCaw PS, Baltimore D. A new DNA binding and dimerization motif in immunoglobulin enhancer binding, daughterless, MyoD, and myc proteins. *Cell* 1989; **56**: 777–83.

27. Bain G, Maandag EC, Izon DJ et al. E2A proteins are required for proper B cell development and initiation of immunoglobulin gene rearrangements. *Cell* 1994; **79**: 885–92.

28. Dedera DA, Waller EK, LeBrun DP et al. Chimeric homeobox gene *E2A–PBX1* induces proliferation, apoptosis, and malignant lymphomas in transgenic mice. *Cell* 1993; **74**: 833–43.

29. Honda H, Inaba T, Suzuki T et al. Expression of E2A–HLF chimeric protein induced T-cell apoptosis, B-cell maturation arrest, and development of acute lymphoblastic leukemia. *Blood* 1999; **93**: 2780–90.

30. Smith KS, Rhee JW, Naumovski L et al. Disrupted differentiation and oncogenic transformation of lymphoid progenitors in *E2A–HLF* transgenic mice. *Mol Cell Biol* 1999; **19**: 4443–51.

31. Bain G, Engel I, Robanus Maandag EC et al. E2A deficiency leads to abnormalities in αβ T-cell development and to rapid development of T-cell lymphomas. *Mol Cell Biol* 1997; **17**: 4782–91.

32. Bayly R, LeBrun DP. Role for homodimerization in growth deregulation by E2a fusion proteins. *Mol Cell Biol* 2000; **20**: 5789–96.

33. Mikkers H, Allen J, Berns A. Proviral activation of the tumor suppressor *E2a* contributes to T cell lymphomagenesis in Eμ-*Myc* transgenic mice. *Oncogene* 2002; **21**: 6559–66.

34. Sawyers CL. Chronic myeloid leukemia. *N Engl J Med* 1999; **340**: 1330–40.

35. Kantarjian H, Sawyers C, Hochhaus A et al. Hematologic and cytogenetic responses to imatinib mesylate in chronic myelogenous leukemia. *N Engl J Med* 2002; **346**: 645–52.

36. Duyster J, Bai R-Y, Morris SW. Translocations involving anaplastic lymphoma kinase (ALK). *Oncogene* 2001; **20**: 5623–37.

37. Turturro F, Arnold MD, Pulforde K. Model of inhibition of the NPM–ALK kinase activity by herbimycin A. *Clin Cancer Res* 2002; **8**: 240–245.

38. Yunis JJ, Frizzera G, Oken MM et al. Multiple recurrent genomic defects in follicular lymphoma. A possible model for cancer. *N Engl J Med* 1987; **316**: 79–84.

39. Korsmeyer SJ. *Bcl-2* initiates a new category of oncogenes: regulators of cell death. *Blood* 1992; **80**: 879–86.

40. McDonnell TJ, Korsmeyer SJ. Progression from lymphoid hyperplasia to high-grade malignant lymphoma in mice transgenic for the t(14;18). *Nature* 1991; **349**: 254–6.

41. Weisenburger DD, Armitage JO. Mantle cell lymphoma – an entity comes of age. *Blood* 1996; **87**: 4483–94.

42. Moorman AV, Clark R, Farrell DM et al. Probes for hidden hyperdiploidy in acute lymphoblastic leukemia. *Genes Chromosomes Cancer* 1996; **16**: 40–5.

43. Navarro B, Garcia-Marco JA, Jones D et al. Association and cloncal distribution of trisomy 12 and 13q14 deletions in chronic lymphocytic leukemia. *Br J Haematol* 1998; **102**: 1330–4.

44. Kamb A, Gruis NA, Weaver-Feldhaus J et al. A cell cycle regulator potentially involved in genesis of many tumor types. *Science* 1994; **264**: 436–40.

45. Nobori T, Miura K, Wu DJ et al. Deletions of the cyclin-dependent kinase-4 inhibitor gene in multiple human cancers. *Nature* 1994; **368**: 753–6.

46. Calin GA, Dan Dumitru C, Shimizu M et al. Frequent deletions and downregulation of micro-RNA genes *miR15* and *miR16* at 13q14 in chronic lymphocytic leukemia. *Proc Natl Acad Sci USA* 2002; **99**: 15524–9.

47. Hsiao MH, Yu AL, Yeargin J et al. Nonhereditary *p53* mutations in T-cell acute lymphoblastic leukemia are associated with the relapse phase. *Blood* 1994; **83**: 2922–30.

48. Gump J, McGavran L, Wei Q et al. Analysis of *TP53* mutations in relapsed childhood acute lymphoblastic leukemia. *J Pediatr Hematol Oncol* 2001; **23**: 416–19.

49. Gaidano G, Ballerini P, Gong JZ et al. *p53* mutations in human lymphoid malignancies: association with Burkitt lymphoma and chronic lymphocytic leukemia. *Proc Nat Acad Sci USA* 1991; **88**: 5413–17.

50. Lo Coco F, Gaidano G, Louie DC et al. *p53* mutations are associated with histologic transformation of follicular lymphoma. *Blood* 1993; **82**: 2289–95.

51. Arico M, Valsecchi MG, Camitta B et al. Outcome of treatment in children with Philadelphia chromosome-positive acute lymphoblastic leukemia. *N Engl J Med* 2000; **342**: 998–1006.

52. Pui CH, Relling MV, Campana D et al. Childhood acute lymphoblastic leukemia. *Rev Clin Exp Hematol* 2002; **6**: 161–80.

# 19 Analysis of clonality using X-chromosome inactivation patterns

**Rosemary E Gale**

## Introduction

The vast majority of human malignancies are derived from a single cell and are thus clonal in origin. Assessment of clonality has therefore been used to assist in the diagnosis of hematological malignancies. However, the distinction between malignant and non-malignant proliferations is not always clear-cut, and the clonality results must always be interpreted in the context of the type of analysis performed and the clinical information available (Table 19.1). The finding of a nonconstitutive clonal chromosome abnormality in a cell population almost always represents a malignancy and will usually define a disease-specific abnormality. The same cannot always be assumed in situations where clonality has been demonstrated using a less specific marker, for example, clonal lymphoid populations determined by immunoglobulin or T-cell receptor gene rearrangements can be reactive. Conditions such as benign monoclonal gammopathy are caused by clonal B-cell proliferations and are apparently neoplastic (nonreactive) but are not considered to be malignant. In essential thrombocythemia, demonstration of a clonal population of cells using X-chromosome inactivation patterns (XCIPs) is thought to indicate a malignant disorder, but in the absence of strokes and coronary thromboses some patients can live for years, not unduly troubled by the cell proliferation per se.

Current understanding of the complex pathways leading to cellular transformation in vivo remains limited and clonal analysis of different cell populations can be helpful in determining the target cell of the malignant transformation. In chronic myeloid leukemia (CML), where the Philadelphia chromosome can be identified in neutrophils, monocytes, erythroid progenitors and some B lymphocytes, it can be concluded that the disease arose at the 'stem cell level'. The converse is not invariably the case, however. The finding that a specific clonal marker is restricted to the neutrophil lineage does not necessarily mean that the disease arose in a late neutrophil precursor. It could have arisen at the stem cell level but other molecular events involved in the transformation process might have restricted proliferation to the neutrophil lineage. Furthermore, an acquired hyperproliferative phase

---

**Table 19.1  Assessment of clonality in hematological malignancies**

Cytogenetic analysis
  (Chromosome loss, gain, partial deletion, inversion or translocation)
  Conventional karyotyping
  Karyotyping plus surface immuno-phenotyping
  Fluorescent in situ hybridization (FISH)
  FISH plus immunophenotyping
Molecular detection of somatic mutations
  (Detection of chromosome loss, translocations, inversions or point mutations)
  Restriction fragment length polymorphisms
  Microsatellite instability
  (RT)-PCR across breakpoint regions
  Single-stranded conformation polymorphism analysis
  Heteroduplex analysis
  Denaturing gradient gel electrophoresis
  Mismatch detection analysis
  Allele-specific oligonucleotide hybridization
Lymphocyte gene rearrangements
  Surface expression of κ and λ light chains on B cells
  Rearrangement of immunoglobulin heavy and light chain genes
  Rearrangement of T-cell receptor genes
X-chromosome inactivation patterns (see Table 19.2)
  Protein expression, e.g. G6PD
  DNA differential methylation, e.g. PGK, HUMARA
  mRNA expression, e.g. G6PD

may be polyclonal in nature, only becoming clonal with the acquisition of a further 'hit'.

This chapter will consider techniques and interpretation of clonality using XCIPs. Technical aspects of cytogenetic analysis, immunoglobulin and T-cell receptor gene rearrangement studies and molecular analysis of somatic mutations are dealt with elsewhere.

## X-chromosome inactivation patterns

Despite extensive progess in the identification of disease-specific molecular markers in hematological malignancies in recent years, clonal analysis using XCIPs in females remains a useful tool for the study of disorders because it does not require prior knowledge of a disease-specific abnormality. Instead it is based on the (pre-supposed) single-cell origin of a malignancy and determines the relative contribution of the two X chromosomes to the cell population under study. In mammalian female cells, one of the two X chromosomes is always inactivated at an early stage in embryogenesis, a process called Lyonization, after Mary Lyon, who first described it.[1] Which chromosome is inactivated is random and is stably inherited as such by all daughter cells,[2] so that a constitutional

mosaic pattern is thereby laid down in each female (Figure 19.1). In a normal or reactive population, the cells should all demonstrate the same active X chromosome. An XCIP therefore has two basic requirements: the ability to distinguish between the two X chromosomes, which is achieved using an X-linked polymorphic marker, and the ability to differentiate between the active and inactive X chromosomes, which depends on the type of analysis employed (Table 19.2).

With the first descriptions of this technique using glucose-6-phosphate dehydrogenase (G6PD) analysis,

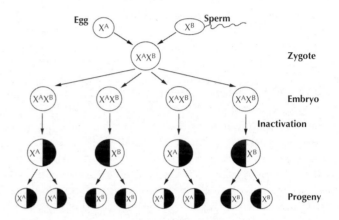

**Figure 19.1** X-chromosome inactivation.

**Table 19.2 Analysis of X-chromosome inactivation patterns**

| Sample | Gene/locus | Polymorphism | Technique | Heterozygosity* (%) | References |
|---|---|---|---|---|---|
| Protein | Glucose-6-phosphate dehydrogenase (G6PD) | Amino acid substitution | Gel electrophoresis | 30 (Negro) | 3, 5 |
| DNA | Phosphoglycerate kinase (PGK) | RFLP | Southern blotting<br>PCR | 32 | 6<br>9 |
| | Hypoxanthine phospho-ribosyl transferase (HPRT) | RFLP | Southern blotting | 17 | 6 |
| | DXS16 | RFLP | Southern blotting | 33 | 88 |
| | DXS255 (M27β) | VNTR | Southern blotting | 78 | 7, 89 |
| | Human androgen receptor (AR) | VNTR | PCR | 90 | 11,14 |
| | Monoamine oxidase A (MAOA) | VNTR | PCR | 75 | 10 |
| | Fragile X (FMR1) | VNTR | PCR | 45 | 12 |
| | DXS 15-134 | VNTR | PCR | 46 | 13 |
| RNA | G6PD | RFLP | RT-PCR + ASA<br>RT-PCR-LDR | 17 | 20, 21, 23<br>19 |
| | Iduronate-2-sulphatase (IDS) | RFLP | RT-PCR + ASA | 40 | 21, 22 |
| | Palmitoylated membrane protein, p55 | RFLP | RT-PCR + ASA | 40 | 19, 23 |
| | Bruton tyrosine kinase (BTK) | RFLP | RT-PCR + ASA | 39 | 90 |
| | Four-and-a-half LIM domain 1 (FHL1) | RFLP | RT-PCR + ASA | 48 | 90 |

*Figures are population-dependent. RFLP: restriction fragment length polymorphism; VNTR: variable number tandem repeat sequence; PCR: polymerase chain reaction; RT: reverse transcription; ASA: allele-specific analysis; LDR: ligase detection reaction.

both objectives could be achieved simultaneously as isoenzymes of the expressed protein product can be electrophoretically separated.[3,4] Furthermore, as a housekeeping gene the protein is detectable in all cell types, even enucleated red cells. However, despite the existence of more than 400 variant forms, the frequency of heterozygotes is low, reaching its highest (approximately 35%) in females of African origin who are of heterozygous for the common B type and either the A or A− isoenzyme.[5] To date no other X-linked genes with suitable polymorhic proteins have been described.

During the 1980s the search for polymorphic markers detectable using restriction enzymes revealed a number in X-lined genes that are present at sufficiently high frequency and can be analyzed using Southern blotting. They include base substitutions, as in the phosphoglycerate kinase (PGK) and hypoxanthine phosphoribosyl transferase (HPRT) genes,[6] and variable number tandem repeat (VNTR) sequences such as the DXS255 locus recognized by the M27β probe.[7] Discrimination between active and inactive X-chromosomes depends on differential methylation patterns at these loci and can be demonstrated using methylation-sensitive enzymes such as HpaII and HhaI.[8] DNA is first digested with the relevant restriction enzyme to enable separation of the two alleles, then divided into two aliquots, one of which is further digested with the appropriate methylation-sensitive enzyme. A relative ratio of expression of the two alleles can be obtained by comparison of the intensity of bands present after the first and second enzyme digestions (Figure 19.2) and results are usually reported either as the percentage expression of the two alleles (75%:25%, 50%:50%, 25%:75% etc.) or as a ratio of expression of the two alleles (3.0, 1.0, 0.25 etc.).

These loci have been used extensively in clonality assays, but Southern blotting analysis requires large amounts of DNA and there can be difficulties of interpretation due to the complexity of some methylation patterns.[8] Attention therefore has turned to genes that are amenable to polymerase chain reaction (PCR) analysis, i.e. where the polymorphism and differential methylation sites are situated close together, within approximately one kilobase of each other. Suitable loci include the BstXI restriction enzyme polymorphism in the PGK gene,[9] and VNTRs in the monoamine oxidase A gene,[10] the human androgen receptor (AR) gene,[11] the fragile X (FMR1) gene[12] and at locus DXS15-134.[13] To date, the human AR assay (HUMARA) is the most widely used due to the high level of heterozygosity of the AR gene in most populations, approximately 90%. PCR does not maintain methylation of the alleles so DNA is first digested with the methylation-sensitive enzyme, cutting only unmethylated (active) alleles and leaving uncut the methylated (inactive) alleles, which are thus available for PCR amplification. For quantitative purposes a

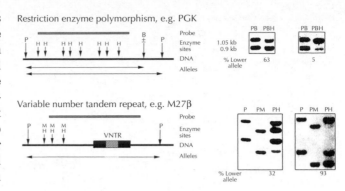

**Figure 19.2** Clonal analysis using Southern blotting. For a restriction enzyme polymorphism such as the polymorphic Bst XI site in the PGK gene, DNA is first digested with Pst I (P) and Bst XI (B) to distinguish the two alleles of 0.9 and 1.05kb (PB). Further digestion with the methylation-sensitive enzyme *Hpa II (H)* cuts the unmethylated alleles, which are then too small to be detected. The intensity of the remaining 0.9 and 1.05 kb, undigested by *Hpa II (H)* bands reflects the relative expression of the alleles (PBH). Alternatively, for a variable number tandem repeat sequence (VNTR) as identified by the M27 (β probe), DNA is first digested with Pst I to separate the two alleles of differing sizes (P). Digestion with Msp I (M), which is not affected by methylated cytosines, reduces each allele by approximately 500bp (PM). Digestion with its methylation-sensitive isoschizomer *Hpa II* (PH) demonstrates the proportion of each allele that is unmethylated and allows calculation of the relative expression of each allele.

radioactive or fluorescent-labeled primer is incorporated. PCR products of VNTR alleles can be directly separated electrophoretically on the basis of their size. Single nucleotide substitutions require prior digestion with the relevant restriction enzyme to allow separation of the alleles (Figure 19.3).

PCR-based clonal analysis has been successfully applied to small samples of DNA obtained from purified populations of cells or individual hemopoietic colonies grown in culture. Its speed and ease of analysis are obviously advantageous, and provided a number of technical considerations are carefully addressed such as extra bands due to Taq slippage, preferential amplification of shorter alleles, and heteroduplex formation that can interfere with restriction enzyme digestion, quantitative results comparable with Southern blotting can be obtained.[14]

An alternative DNA-based PCR method that uses chemical modification to differentiate between the active and inactive alleles has been recently described.[15,16] DNA is first treated with sodium bisulphite, which converts all unmethylated cytosines to uracil but does not alter the methylated cytosines. One or two separate PCRs are then performed using

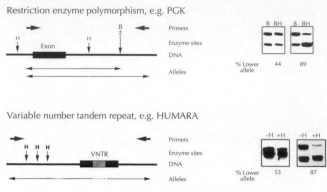

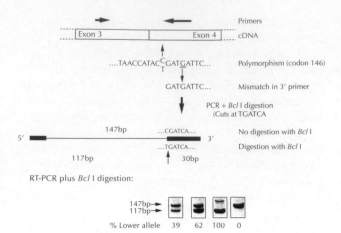

**Figure 19.3** Clonal analysis using DNA-based PCR. The polymorphism and differentially methylated cytosines must lie sufficiently close together to allow amplification across both sites. PCR is performed on aliquots of DNA either undigested or pre-digested with the methylation-sensitive enzyme *Hpa II (H)*, which cuts the unmethylated alleles, i.e. leaving intact the methylated alleles for amplification. The two alleles are then separated either by polymorphic enzyme digestion, as with the Bst XI site (B) in the PGK gene, or by different size alleles due to a VNTR sequence, as in the AR gene.

**Figure 19.4** Clonal analysis using the C/T polymorphic site at codon 146 in the iduronate-2-sulphatase mRNA. PCR is performed on cDNA using a 3′ primer, which introduces a G -> C mismatch to create a Bcl I enzyme restriction site in products from the T-containing alleles but not the C-containing alleles. After RT-PCR and Bcl I digestion, the relative proportion of the two bands reflects expression of the two alleles.

primers that are specific for methylated DNA in one reaction and/or unmethylated DNA in the other. Although only one PCR is necessary, the complementary results obtained from both reactions act as confirmation of the pattern obtained. This method circumvents false results arising from incomplete restriction enzyme digestion of unmethylated alleles, and although it has not yet been widely tested, it may be particularly useful for analysis of hematopoietic colonies where restriction enzyme digestion of small numbers of cells can be problematic.

A more direct approach to overcome the problem of complex DNA methylation patterns has been the introduction of methods using RNA, where relative expression of the two alleles can by analyzed directly at the transcript level. Genes suitable for this analysis must contain the polymorphism in their coding sequence, although it will not necessarily change the amino acid sequence, and be expressed in the cells of interest. Three single base substitutions have been used in a number of studies; all are house-keeping genes with widespread tissue expression: G6PD (different from the A/A− variants),[17] iduronate-2-sulphatase (IDS)[18] and the palmitoylated membrane protein p55.[19] Together they provide a reasonably high degree of heterozygosity in most population groups (Table 19.2). Several different methods have been reported after the reverse-transcription step: either (1) PCR followed by allele-specific oligonucleotide hybridization,[20] (2) PCR using a mismatch primer to introduce a suitable restriction site plus restriction enzyme digestion specific to one of the alleles (Figure 19.4),[21,22] (3) PCR with allele-specific

primers,[23] or (4) PCR plus the ligase detection reaction with specific primers to distinguish the two alleles.[19] Quantitative, reproducible results have been reported which correlate well with DNA-based assays.[19,22] The VNTRs in the AR[24] and FMR1[25] genes also occur within the coding sequence and mRNA expression of these genes may be studied in some tissues.

RNA-based assays have a number of advantages over those using DNA. Not only are they less likely to be affected by aberrant or complex methylation patterns, but there is no requirement for the polymorphic site to be in close proximity to a site demonstrating the differential expression. Primers can be designed across an exon/intron boundary to eliminate interference from contaminating DNA. Furthermore, where appropriate, enucleated cells such as reticulocytes and platelets can be studied. However, important factors that may influence RNA assays but not those based on DNA include variation between tissues in the level of transcript expression and degree of sample purity required. For example, platelet contamination of T lymphocytes may give a false pattern for the latter cell population. In view of all these considerations, wherever possible results should be confirmed using more than one assay.

The loci mentioned earlier have all been reported in studies using XCIPs for analysis of clonality. With the sequencing of the entire X-chromosome as part of the Human Genome Project and the creation of a database for single nucleotide polymorphisms (SNPs) in the human genome (http://www.ncbi.nlm.nih.gov/SNP/), it is likely that many other useful polymorphic X-linked loci will be identified in the next few years. Of

1844 X-linked SNPs in the database in March 2001, Vasques and Pereira reported that 141 were within expressed sequences corresponding to 99 different genes.[26] Thus it should soon be possible to find a suitable marker for XCIP analysis in any female. However, a number of nonpseudoautosomal genes have been found to either completely escape[27,28] or show variable X-inactivation[29] and gene expression may be tissue restricted.[26] Therefore any new marker should be carefully evaluated for its suitability before application to patient samples.

## Interpretation of results

Despite the widespread use of XCIPs to address questions of clonality and lineage involvement in hematological disorders, many of the studies appear to have contradictory results. Recent evidence suggests that much of this confusion has probably arisen from the definition of a clonal XCIP and the failure to take into account other mechanisms that can mimic this. Since Lyonization is a random process, it has been argued that a normal polyclonal pattern will show approximately 50% expression of each allele, and the patterns that diverge from this indicate the presence of monoclonal or oligoclonal hematopoiesis. A skewed or imbalanced XCIP indicative of the presence of a clonal population of cells has therefore arbitrarily been taken to mean >75% expression of one allele, i.e. an allele ration of >3 or <.25.[6] A number of studies have shown, however, that there is considerable variation in the XCIPs obtained from blood or bone marrow of hematologically normal females, with an imbalanced or skewed Lyonization pattern in approximately 20–25%.[30–32] This degree of skewing may relate to the size of the primordial stem cell pool committed to hematopoiesis at the time of X-inactivation, since the smaller the number of hematopoietic stem cells present at that time, the greater the number of individuals that will be observed with a skewed XCIP.[33] Consequently an apparently 'clonal' XCIP does not necessarily represent a clonal population of cells but may simply reflect the constitutive Lyonization pattern for that individual. Therefore, to interpret an XCIP in a tissue sample from an individual requires knowledge of their normal pattern.

Blood or bone marrow from a patient pre-dating the transforming event is rarely available for comparison to show that the pattern has altered and therefore alternative tissues such as skin, cultured fibroblasts and buccal mucosa have been used. However, these may not be appropriate controls as XCIPs appear to be tissue specific and can vary widely between tissues of the same individual, possibly because the progenitor cell pool size varies for different tissues.[34,35] For most myeloid disorders, T lymphocytes are a suitable comparative control as they are not generally involved in the clonal process but derive from the same pluripotent stem cell and therefore will have the same constitutional XCIP.[36] However, where there are doubts regarding possible T-cell involvement in the disorder, assessment of clonality in individuals may not be feasible and large-scale studies to determine the distribution patterns for a particular disorder relative to the normal population may be necessary.

Further complication has arisen with the recent observation that XCIPs can change with age; approximately 40% of hematologically normal females ≥75 years of age acquire a skewed XCIP in their myeloid cells.[37–39] These results are not necessarily indicative of a preleukemic phase or of stem cell depletion but may reflect random changes in stem cell usage, with fewer of the original stem cell pool actively contributing to the myeloid population. Longtitudinal studies in cats, analysis of XCIPs in elderly monozygotic twins, and the study of different tissues from elderly females have all suggested that there may be a genetic component to this shift and that it results from a selective advantage of cells expressing one particular X chromosome.[35,40–42] This proliferative or competitive advantage must, however, be small as it takes many years in humans before it is evident, and longtitudinal studies of up to 3 years have shown stable XCIPs.[43,44] Whatever the cause of this phenomenon, it has important implications for the use of these tests in the diagnosis of diseases of the elderly, which are arbitrarily defined as occurring in those >65 years of age. An imbalanced myeloid XCIP in the presence of a balanced T-cell XCIP cannot be interpreted in these patients as evidence of clonal hematopoiesis. Balanced myeloid XCIPs, however, can be used to indicate the presence of polyclonal hematopoiesis. Acquired skewing is also the probable cause of a number of cases of X-linked disorders that only present in the later years of life, such as late-onset X-linked sideroblastic anemia.[45]

Finally, in addition to the importance of evaluating an XCIP with respect to a relevant tissue control and the age of the individual, technical considerations must also be taken into account. Unlike direct analysis of a clonal marker such as demonstration of the presence of a fusion transcript by RT-PCR, this technique is not sufficiently sensitive for detection of a small population of clonal cells on a predominantly polyclonal background. Results are generally highly reproducible, but duplicate analysis of samples can give quite wide variations,[14] and only values differing by >20% are considered to be significantly different.

## Application of techniques

### Chronic myeloid leukemia

CML was the first hematological disorder shown to have a clonal origin when, in 1967, Fialkow and colleagues examined G6PD isoenzymes in the red cells and granulocytes of three female patients and demonstrated that they expressed only the A type, whereas fibroblasts had both A and B types.[46] Subsequent studies concluded that the disease arose in a stem cell common to myeloid, erythroid, and megakaryocytic cells, and (at least in some cases) B-lymphoid cells.[47,48] With the identification of the leukemia-specific t(9;22) translocation giving rise to the bcr/abl fusion transcript and protein, there has been little further diagnostic application of XCIPs in CML. A number of studies have, however, used this technique to demonstrate a return of polyclonal hematopoiesis after interferon- or high-dose chemotherapy-induced cytogenetic remission[49,50] and/or autografting with Philadelphia-negative, bcr/abl negative, peripheral blood stem cells.[51] It has shown that, whereas Philadelphia-negative, bcr/abl-negative, CD34+ progenitors obtained from early chronic phase CML were polyclonal, in late chronic phase and accelerated phase CML the progenitors were mainly Philadelphia-positive, bcr/abl positive and clonal, and a polyclonal state could not be induced by chemotherapy.[52]

# Chronic myeloproliferative disorders

XCIPs have a potentially useful role in the diagnosis of polycythemia vera (PV), essential thrombocythemia (ET) and agnogenic myeloid metaplasia. Although characterized by the excessive proliferation of one or more hematopoietic cell lineages, their diagnosis is often one of exclusion and they may be difficult to distinguish from reactive processes accompanying various infectious, inflammatory, or neoplastic disorders. Although a variable proportion transform to acute leukemia (3–20%), relatively few patients present with clonal chromosomal abnormalities. Early studies suggested that they are clonal disorders of stem cell origin, with single G6PD isoenzyme types only observed in granulocytes, red cells and platelets.[53,54] However, only small numbers of heterozygous patients were studied, results were compared with skin or cultured fibroblasts, not T lymphocytes, and age-related skewing was not taken into account. More recent studies have indicated that in ET and to a lesser extent PV, a significant proportion of patients may have polyclonal granulocyte and T-cell patterns.[9,21,39,55–58] This may reflect heterogeneity of lineage involvement in these disorders, with restriction of the clonal population to the dominant cell type in some patients. PCR analysis of individual colonies demonstrated that one out of three PV patients had evidence for a clonal population in erythroid progenitors, whereas neutrophils had a balanced XCIP despite an increased neutrophil count.[9] In ET, although mono-

clonal platelets with polyclonal neutrophils have been reported in a small number of patients; this lineage restriction is uncommon.[21,55,57] Of clinical significance, polyclonal myelopoiesis in ET patients correlates with a reduced susceptibility of thrombotic complications.[55,57]

These findings suggest that, unlike CML, where a specific marker is present in nearly all patients, the chronic myeloproliferative disorders may be genotypically heterogeneous despite many apparent phenotypic similarities. XCIPs may therefore be a useful tool to subclassify patients and to search for more specific molecular abnormalties that, to date, have proved remarkably elusive. Long-term follow-up studies are required to determine whether clonal myelopoiesis evolves from polyclonal disease through the acquisition of further pathogenic alterations, and whether myelofibrosis only develops in clonal patients or correlates with the development of clonal myelopoiesis. Since many patients have a relatively stable disease over long periods of time, such information may have particular relevance to the use of potentially leukemogenic therapy, especially in younger patients.

## Aplastic anemia and paroxysmal nocturnal hemoglobinuria

The defect in acquired aplastic anemia (AA) affects multiple cell lineages and patients have a high incidence of evolution to a clonal disease with increasing time from diagnosis. Current data suggests that immune destruction causes the pancytopenia, and there is little evidence to indicate a possible causal link between AA and clonal disease with, for example, clonal expansion of a defective stem cell or reduction of the stem cell pool to a clonal composition. Clonal cytogenetic abnormalities are rare and XCIPs suggest that most patients have polyclonal hematopoiesis.[59,60] Furthermore, XCIPs have not been useful in predicting development of a clonal disorder. In one study, three of four patients with clonal hematopoiesis showed no sign of clonal evolution after more than 1 year of follow-up; conversely six patients with polyclonal hematopoiesis developed paroxysmal nocturnal hemoglobinuria (PNH), acute myeloid leukemia (AML) or monosomy 7.[59] However, it must be noted that these techniques are relatively insensitive and will not detect minor clonal populations. This problem is particularly evident for PNH where the abnormal cells deficient in phosphatidylinositol glycan anchored proteins (PIG-AP) are known to be clonal,[60–62] but their presence may be obscured by normal cells, so that unsorted cells from AA or PNH patients harboring PIG-AP-deficient cells may have a polyclonal XCIP.[59] These PIG-AP-deficient cells appear to be unique in that, although they carry an acquired, specific clonal marker, they have no growth advantage and are not considered to be neoplastic.[63]

## Myelodysplastic syndromes and acute myeloid leukemia

The myelodysplastic syndromes (MDSs) and AML are clonal stem cell disorders frequently characterized by disease-specific karyotypic abnormalities. Monoclonal or skewed XCIPs can be demonstrated in myeloid cells, consistent with the presence of a predominant clone.[30,64] Nevertheless, polyclonal hematopoiesis has been reported in a number of patients with diagnostic features of MDS, who can remain stable over many years before transformation.[65,66] Nonclonal progenitor cells have been shown to persist in some MDS patients.[67]

Before the molecular identification of some of the commonest translocations and deletions, XCIPs were used to determine the extent of lineage involvement in these disorders.[64,68–70] Results were often contradictory, at least in some studies because suitable control tissues were not included. Most studies now indicate that a disease-specific defect can be identified in myeloid, erythroid and sometimes B-lymphoid cells, but the involvement of T-lymphoid cells in clonal development of MDS remains controversial.[71] Acute promyelocytic leukemia is unusual in that early progenitor cells (CD34+, CD38-) are not only PML/RARα negative by RT-PCR but also polyclonal by XCIP analysis.[72] Early studies indicated that there may be heterogeneity of lineage involvement in AML, with lineage restriction of clonal progenitor cells in some younger but not older patients.[73] These results led to the suggestion that AML in the elderly may represent evolution from a preleukemic, myelodysplastic state. However, with the recent knowledge of acquired skewing of XCIPs in myeloid cells of the elderly, this issue needs to be re-evaluated.

Clonal analysis has been used to demonstrate that restoration of polyclonal hematopoiesis in morphological remission can be achieved post high-dose chemotherapy in MDS,[74–76] and to confirm that nonclonal CD34+ progenitor cells can be harvested for autologous peripheral blood transplantation.[77] A recent study has also suggested that low-risk MDS patients with clonal and nonclonal patterns may have differing responses to antithymocyte or antilymphocyte globulin.[78] In AML, although some studies have suggested that remission may be clonal in approximately one-third of patients,[79] implying that this indicated the return to a pre-leukemic state, T cells were not included in these studies and at least some cases can probably be explained by a constitutionally imbalanced Lyonization pattern. Where T cells have been studied in parallel with remission granulocytes or bone marrow,[30] or where the disappearance of leukemia-specific products such as the PML/RARα fusion product in acute promyelocytic leukemia has been correlated with XCIPs,[50] the results suggest that clonal remission is infrequent, and when present is often associated with trilineage myelodysplasia.[80,81] An XCIP, however, will not distinguish between a truly clonal remission with repopulation by potentially leukemic cells, and an apparent clonal remission induced by regeneration from a small stem cell pool. In general, studies post allogeneic or autologous bone marrow transplantation have demonstrated that repopulation is polyclonal,[82,83] although monoclonal/oligoclonal hemopoiesis of donor origin has been reported in two patients.[84]

The risk of developing therapy-related myelodysplasia or AML after high-dose therapy and, in particular, autologous stem cell transplantation, is substantial and does not necessarily correlate with the presence of cytogenetic abnormalities.[85] Studies have therefore attempted to use analysis of XCIPs to follow disease progression. However, although clonal evolution can be detected in some patients through demonstration of progressively changing patterns,[86,87] such studies are limited by the frequency of constitutionally skewed XCIPs and require careful interpretation of the results obtained. Furthermore, this technology will not identify the presence of minor clonal populations on a polyclonal background, and polyclonal hematopoiesis can persist despite myelodysplastic features.[87]

In conclusion, clonal analysis with XCIPs can be used to provide information regarding clones of cells, both in disease entities as a whole and for selected patients, but the technology has a number of limitations and great care in the interpretation of data from individual patients is required.

## REFERENCES

1. Lyon MF. Gene action in the X-chromosome of the mouse (Mus musculus L.). Nature 1961; 190: 372–3.

2. Gartler SM, Riggs AD. Mammalian X-chromosome inactivation. Annu Rev Genet 1983; 17: 155–90.

3. Beutler E, Yeh M, Fairbanks VF. Normal human female as a mosaic of X-chromosome activity: studies using the gene for G6PD deficiency as a marker. Proc Natl Acad Sci U S A 1962; 48: 9–16.

4. Fialkow PJ. Use of genetic markers to study cellular origin of development of tumors in human females. Adv Can Res 1972; 15: 191–226.

5. Boyer SH, Porter IH, Weilbacher RG. Electrophoretic heterogeneity of glucose-6-phosphate dehydrogenase and its relationship to enzyme deficiency in man. Proc Natl Acad Sci U S A 1962; 48: 1868–76.

6. Vogelstein B, Fearon ER, Hamilton SR et al. Clonal analy-

sis using recombinant DNA probes from the X-chromosome. *Cancer Res* 1987; **47**: 4806–13.

7. Boyd Y, Fraser NJ. Methylation patterns at the hypervariable X-chromosome locus DXS255 (M27β): correlation with X-inactivation status. *Genomics* 1990; **7**: 182–7.

8. Gale RE, Wainscoat JS. Clonal analysis using X-linked DNA polymorphisms. *Br J Haematol* 1993; **85**: 2–8.

9. Gilliland DG, Blanchard KL, Levy J et al. Clonality in myeloproliferative disorders: Analysis by means of the polymerase chain reaction. *Proc Natl Acad Sci U S A* 1991; **88**: 6848–52.

10. Hendriks R, Chen Z-Y, Hinds H et al. An X chromosome inactivation assay based on differential methylation of a CpG island coupled to a VNTR polymorphism at the 5′ end of the monoamine oxidase A gene. *Hum Mol Genet* 1992; **1**: 187–94.

11. Allen RC, Zoghbi HY, Moseley AB et al. Methylation of *HpaII* and *HhaI* sites near the polymorphic CAG repeat in the human androgen-receptor gene correlates with X chromosome inactivation. *Am J Hum Genet* 1992; **51**: 1229–39.

12. Lee S-T, McGlennen RC, Litz CE. Clonal determination by the fragile X *(FMRI)* and phosphoglycerate kinase *(PGK)* genes in hematological malignancies. *Cancer Res* 1994; **54**: 5212–16.

13. Okamoto T, Okada M, Wada H et al. Clonal analysis of hematopoietic cells using a novel polymorphic site of the X chromosome. *Am J Hematol* 1998; **58**: 263–6.

14. Gale RE, Mein CA, Linch DC, Quantification of X-chromosome inactivation patterns in haematological samples using the DNA-based HUMARA assay. *Leukemia* 1996; **10**: 362–7.

15. Kubota T, Nonoyama S, Tonoki H et al. A new assay for the analysis of X-chromosome inactivation based on methylation-specific PCR. *Hum Genet* 1999; **104**: 49–55.

16. Uchida T, Ohashi H, Aoki E et al. Clonality analysis by methylation-specific PCR for the human androgen-receptor gene (HUMARA-MSP). *Leukemia* 2000; **14**: 207–12.

17. Beutler E, Kuhl W. The NT 1311 polymorphism of G6PD: G6PD Mediterranean mutation may have originated independently in Europe and Asia. *Am J Hum Genet* 1990; **47**: 1008–12.

18. Hopwood JJ, Bunge S, Morris CP et al. Molecular basis of mucopolysaccharidosis type II: mutations in the iduronate-2-sulphatase gene. *Hum Mutation* 1993; **2**: 435–42.

19. Luhovy M, Liu Y, Belickova M et al. A novel clonality assay based on transcriptional polymorphism of X chromosome gene p55. *Biol Blood Marrow Transplant* 1995; **1**: 81–7.

20. Curnutte JT, Hopkins PJ, Kuhl W, Beutler E. Studying X inactivation. *Lancet* 1992; **339**: 749.

21. El-Kassar N, Hetet G, Briere J, Grandchamp B. Clonality analysis of hematopoiesis in essential thrombocythaemia: Advantages of studying T lymphocytes and platelets. *Blood* 1997; **89**: 128–34.

22. Harrison CN, Gale RE, Linch DC. Quantification of X-chromosome inactivation patterns using RT-PCR of the polymorphic iduronate-2-sulphatase gene and correlation of the results obtained with DNA-based techniques. *Leukemia* 1998; **12**: 1834–9.

23. Liu Y, Phelan J, Go RCP et al. Rapid determination of clonality by detection of two closely-linked X chromosome exonic polymorphisms using allele-specific PCR. *J Clin Invest* 1997; **99**: 1984–90.

24. Busque L, Zhu J, DeHart D et al. An expression based clonality assay at the human androgen receptor locus (HUMARA) on chromosome X. *Nucleic Acids Res* 1994; **22**: 697–8.

25. Fu Y-H, Kuhl DPA, Pizzuti A et al. Variation of the CGG repeat at the fragile X site results in genetic instability: resolution of the Sharman paradox. *Cell* 1991; **67**: 1047–58.

26. Vasques LR, Pereira LV. Allele-specific X-linked gene activity in normal human cells assayed by expressed single nucleotide polymorphisms (cSNPs). *DNA Res* 2001; **8**: 173–7.

27. Miller AP, Willard HF. Chromosomal basis of X chromosome inactivation: identification of a multigene domain in Xp11.21-p11.22 that escapes X inactivation. *Proc Natl Acad Sci U S A* 1998; **95**: 8709–14.

28. Kutsche R, Brown CJ. Determination of X-chromosome inactivation status using X-linked expressed polymorphisms identified by database searching. *Genomics* 2000; **65**: 9–15.

29. Anderson CL, Brown CJ. Polymorphic X-chromosome inactivation of the human TIMP 1 gene. *Am J Hum Genet* 1999; **65**: 699–708.

30. Gale RE, Wheadon H, Goldstone AH et al. Frequency of clonal remission in acute myeloid leukaemia. *Lancet* 1993; **341**: 138–42.

31. Fey MF, Liechti-Gallati S, von Rohr A et al. Clonality and X-inactivation patterns in hematopoietic cell populations detected by the highly informative M27β DNA probe). *Blood* 1994; **83**: 931–8.

32. Puck JM, Stewart CC, Nussbaum RL. Maximum-likelihood analysis of human T-cell X-chromosome inactivation patterns: normal women versus carriers of X-linked severe combined immunodeficiency. *Am J Hum Genet* 1992; **50**: 742–8.

33. Gale RE, Linch DC. Interpretation of X-chromosome inactivation patterns. *Blood* 1994; **84**: 2376–7.

34. Gale RE, Wheadon H, Boulos P, Linch DC. Tissue specificity of X-chromosome inactivation patterns. *Blood* 1994; **83**: 2899–905.

35. Sharp A, Robinson D, Jacobs P. Age- and tissue-specific variation of X chromosome inactivation ratios in normal women. *Hum Genet* 2000; **107**: 343–9.

36. Keller G, Paige G, Gilboa E, Wagner EF. Expression of a foreign gene in myeloid and lymphoid cells derived from multipotent haematopoietic precursors. *Nature* 1985; **318**: 149–54.

37. Busque L, Mio R, Mattioli J et al. Nonrandom X-inactivation patterns in normal females: Lyonization ratios vary with age. *Blood* 1996; **88**: 59–65.

38. Gale RE, Fielding AK, Harrison CN, Linch DC. Acquired skewing of X-chromosome inactivation patterns in myeloid cells of the elderly suggests stochastic clonal loss with age. *Br J Haematol* 1997; **98**: 512–19.

39. Champion KM, Gilbert JGR, Asimakopoulos FA et al. Clonal haemopoiesis in normal elderly women: implications for the myeloproliferative disorders and myelodysplastic syndromes. *Br J Haematol* 1997; **97**: 920–6.

40. Abkowitz JL, Taboada M, Shelton GH et al. An X chromosome gene regulates hematopoietic stem cell kinetics. *Proc Natl Acad Sci U S A* 1998; **95**: 3862–6.

41. Christensen K, Kristiansen M, Hagen-Larsen H et al. X-linked genetic factors regulate hematopoietic stem-cell kinetics in females. *Blood* 2000; **95**: 2449–51.

42. Vickers MA, McLeod E, Spector TD, Wilson IJ. Assessment of mechanism of acquired skewed X inactivation by analysis of twins. *Blood* 2001; **97**: 1274–81.

43. Prchal JT, Prchal JF, Belickova M et al. Clonal stability of blood cell lineages indicated by X-chromosomal transcriptional polymorphism. *J Exp Med* 1996; **183**: 561–7.

44. van Dijk JP, Heuver L, Stevens-Linders E et al. Acquired skewing of Lyonization remains stable for a prolonged period in healthy blood donors. *Leukemia* 2002; **16**: 362–7.

45. Cazzola M, May A, Bergamaschi G et al. Familial-skewed X-chromosome inactivation as a predisposing factor for late-onset X-linked sideroblastic anemia in carrier females. *Blood* 2000; **96**: 4363–5.

46. Fialkow PJ, Gartler SM, Yoshida A. Clonal origin of chronic myelocytic leukemia in man. *Proc Natl Acad Sci U S A* 1967; **58**: 1468–71.

47. Fialkow PJ, Jacobson RJ, Papayannopoulou T. Chronic myelocytic leukemia: Clonal origin in a stem cell common to the granulocyte, erythrocyte, platelet and monocyte/macrophage. *Am J Med* 1977; **63**: 125–30.

48. Martin PJ, Najfeld V, Hansen JA et al. Involvement of the B-lymphoid system in chronic myelogenous leukemia. *Nature* 1980; **237**: 49–50.

49. Claxton D, Deisseroth A, Talpaz M et al. Polyclonal hematopoiesis in interferon-induced cytogenetic remissions of chronic myelogenous leukemia. *Blood* 1992; **79**: 997–1002.

50. Lo Coco F, Pelicci PG, D'Adamo F et al. Polyclonal hematopoietic reconstitution in leukemia patients at remission after suppression of specific gene rearrangements. *Blood* 1993; **82**: 606–12.

51. Bergamaschi G, Podesta M, Frassoni F et al. Restoration of normal polyclonal haemopoiesis in patients with chronic myeloid leukaemia autografted with Ph-negative peripheral stem cells. *Br J Haematol* 1994; **87**: 867–70.

52. Delforge M, Boogaerts MA, McGlave PB, Verfaillie CM. BCR/ABL–CD34+HLA-DR–progenitor cells in early chronic phase, but not in more advanced phases, of chronic myelogenous leukemia are polyclonal. *Blood* 1999; **93**: 284–92.

53. Adamson JW, Fialkow PJ, Murphy S et al. Polycythemia vera: Stem-cell and probable clonal origin of the disease. *N Engl J Med* 1976; **295**: 913–16.

54. Fialkow PJ, Faguet GB, Jacobson RJ et al. Evidence that essential thrombocythemia is a clonal disorder with origin in a multipotent stem cell. *Blood* 1981; **58**: 916–19.

55. Harrison CN, Gale RE, Machin SJ, Linch DC. A large proportion of patients with a diagnosis of essential thrombocythemia do not have a clonal disorder and may be at lower risk of thrombotic complications. *Blood* 1999; **93**: 417–24.

56. Ferraris AM, Mangerini R, Racchi O et al. Heterogeneity of clonal development in chronic myeloproliferative disorders. *Am J Hematol* 1999; **60**: 158–60.

57. Chiusolo P, La Barbera EO, Laurenti L et al. Clonal hemopoiesis and risk of thrombosis in young female patients with essential thrombocythemia. *Exp Hematol* 2001; **29**: 670–6.

58. Shih LY, Lin TL, Dunn P et al. Clonality analysis using X-chromosome inactivation patterns by HUMARA–PCR assay in female controls and patients with idiopathic thrombocytosis in Taiwan. *Exp Hematol* 2001; **29**: 202–8.

59. Raghavachar A, Janssen JWG, Schrezenmeier H et al. Clonal hematopoiesis as defined by polymorphic X-linked loci occurs infrequently in aplastic anemia. *Blood* 1995; **86**: 2938–47.

60. Mortazavi Y, Chopra R, Gordon-Smith EC, Rutherford TR. Clonal patterns of X-chromosome inactivation in female patients with aplastic anemia studies using a novel reverse transcription polymerase chain reaction method. *Eur J Haematol* 2000; **64**: 385–95.

61. Bessler M, Hillmen P, Luzzatto L. Clonal origin of abnormal granulocytes in paroxysmal nocturnal hemoglobinuria. *Blood* 1992; **80**: 844–5.

62. Ohashi H, Hotta T, Ichikawa A et al. Peripheral blood cells are predominantly chimeric of affected and normal cells in patients with paroxysmal nocturnal hemoglobinuria: Simultaneous investigation on clonality and expression of glycophosphatidylinositol-anchored proteins. *Blood* 1994; **83**: 853–9.

63. Araten DJ, Nafa K, Pakdeesuwan K, Luzzatto L. Clonal populations of hematopoietic cells with paroxysmal nocturnal hemoglobinuria genotype and phenotype are present in normal individuals. *Proc Natl Acad Sci U S A* 1999; **96**: 5209–14.

64. van Kamp H, Fibbe WE, Jansen RPM et al. Clonal involvement of granulocytes and monocytes, but not of T and B lymphocytes and natural killer cells in patients with myelodysplasia: Analysis by X-linked restriction fragment length polymorphisms and polymerase chain reaction of the phosphoglycerate kinase gene. *Blood* 1992; **80**: 1774–80.

65. Busque L, Kohler S, DeHart D et al. High incidence of polyclonal granulocytopoiesis in myelodysplastic syndromes (MDS). *Blood* 1993; **82**(Suppl 1): 196a.

66. Culligan DJ, Bowen DT, May A et al. Refractory anaemia with preleukaemic polyclonal haemopoiesis and the emergence of monoclonal erythropoiesis on disease progression. *Br J Haematol* 1995; **89**: 675–7.

67. Asano H, Ohashi H, Ichihara M et al. Evidence for non-clonal hematopoietic progenitor cell populations in bone marrow of patients with myelodysplastic syndromes. *Blood* 1994; **84**: 588–94.

68. Janssen JWG, Buschle M, Layton M et al. Clonal analysis of myelodysplastic syndromes: evidence of multipotent stem cell origin. *Blood* 1989; **73**: 248–54.

69. Tefferi A, Thibodeau SN, Solberg LA. Clonal studies in the myelodysplastic syndrome using X-linked restriction fragment length polymorphisms. *Blood* 1990; **75**: 1770–3.

70. Abrahamson G, Boultwood J, Madden J et al. Clonality of cell populations in refractory anaemia using combined approach of gene loss and X-linked restriction fragment length polymorphism-methylation analyses. *Br J Haematol* 1991; **79**: 550–5.

71. Boultwood J, Wainscoat JS. Clonality in the myelodysplastic syndromes. *Int J Hematol* 2001; **73**: 411–15.

72. Turhan AG, Lemoine FM, Debert C et al. Highly purified primitive hematopoietic stem cells are PML-RARA negative and generate nonclonal progenitors in acute promyelocytic leukemia. *Blood* 1995; **85**: 2154–61.

73. Fialkow PJ, Singer JW, Raskind WH et al. Clonal development, stem cell differentiation, and clinical remissions in acute nonlymphocytic leukemia. *N Engl J Med* 1987; **317**: 468–73.

74. Ito T, Ohashi H, Kagami Y et al. Recovery of polyclonal hematopoiesis in patients with myelodysplastic syndromes following successful chemotherapy. *Leukemia* 1994; **8**: 839–43.

75. Delforge M, Demuynck H, Verhoef G et al. Patients with high-risk myelodysplastic syndrome can have polyclonal or clonal haemopoiesis in complete haematological remission. *Br J Haematol* 1998; **102**: 486–94.

76. Aivado M, Rong A, Germing U et al. Long-term remission after intensive chemotherapy in advanced myelodysplastic syndromes is generally associated with restoration of polyclonal haemopoiesis. *Br J Haematol* 2000; **110**: 884–6.

77. Delforge M, Demuynek H, Vandenberghe P et al. Polyclonal primitive hematopoietic progenitors can be detected in mobilized peripheral blood from patients with high-risk myelodysplastic syndromes. *Blood* 1995; **86**: 3660–7.

78. Aivado M, Rong A, Stadler M et al. Favourable response to antithymocyte or antilymphocyte globulin in low-risk myelodysplastic syndrome patients with a 'non-clonal' pattern of X- chromosome inactivation in bone marrow cells. *Eur J Haematol* 2002; **68**: 210–16.

79. Fialkow PJ, Janssen JWG, Bartram CR. Clonal remissions in acute nonlymphocytic leukemia: Evidence for a multi-step pathogenesis of the malignancy. *Blood* 1991; **77**: 1415–17.

80. Jowitt SN, Liu Yin JA, Saunders MJ, Lucas GS. Clonal remissions in acute myeloid leukaemia are commonly associated with features of trilineage myelodysplasia during remission. *Br J Haematol* 1993; **85**: 698–705.

81. Jinnai I, Nagai K, Yoshida S et al. Incidence and characteristics of clonal hematopoiesis in remission of acute myeloid leukemia in relation to morphological dysplasia. *Leukemia* 1995; **9**: 1756–61.

82. Nash R, Storb R, Neiman P. Polyclonal reconstitution of human marrow after allogeneic bone marrow transplantation. *Blood* 1988; **72**: 2031–7.

83. Saunders MJ, Jowitt SN, Liu Yin JA. Clonality studies in patients undergoing allogeneic and autologous bone marrow transplantation for haematological malignancies. *Bone Marrow Transplant* 1995; **15**: 81–5.

84. Turhan AG, Humphries RK, Phillips GL et al. Clonal hematopoiesis demonstrated by X-linked DNA polymorphisms after allogeneic bone marrow transplantation. *N Engl J Med* 1989; **320**: 1655–61.

85. Gilliland DG, Gribben JG. Evaluation of the risk of therapy-related MDS/AML after autologous stem cell transplantation. *Biol Blood Marrow Transplant* 2002; **8**: 9–16.

86. Gale RE, Bunch C, Moir DJ et al. Demonstration of developing myelodysplasia/acute myeloid leukaemia in haematologically normal patients after high-dose chemotherapy and autologous bone marrow transplantation using X-chromosome inactivation patterns. *Br J Haematol* 1996; **93**: 53–8.

87. Mach-Pascual S, Legare RD, Lu D et al. Predictive value of clonality assays in patients with non-Hodgkin's lymphoma undergoing autologous bone marrow transplant: A single institution study. *Blood* 1998; **91**: 4496–503.

88. Khalifa MM, Struthers JL, Maurice S et al. Methylation of *HpaII* site at the human DXS 16 locus on Xp22 as an assay for abnormal patterns of X inactivation. *Am J Med Genet* 2001; **98**: 64–9.

89. Gale RE, Wheadon H, Linch DC. Assessment of X-chromosome inactivation patterns using the hypervariable probe M27β in normal hemopoietic cells and acute myeloid leukemic blasts. *Leukemia* 1992; **6**: 649–55.

90. Liu E, Guan Y, Pastore Y et al. Novel assay for clonality of hematopoiesis by detection of transcriptional polymorphisms of X chromosome genes BTK and FHL1 using SSCP analysis. *Blood* 2001; **98**(Suppl 1): 110a.

# 20 Gene expression profiling in leukemias using microarrays

Torsten Haferlach, Wolfgang Kern, Alexander Kohlmann,
Susanne Schnittger, and Claudia Schoch

## Introduction

The classical methods to diagnose leukemias are cyto-morphology and histology, which are both supplemented by cytochemistry and multiparameter immunophenotyping to refine classifications. Furthermore, insights into the genetic basis of the leukemia have substantially increased the diagnostic importance of cytogenetics, fluorescence in situ hybridization (FISH), and polymerase chain reaction (PCR). Besides the detailed classification of leukemias based on the knowledge provided by the different methods, the selection of disease-specific therapeutic approaches has become a reality, for example the use of all-trans-retinoic acid (ATRA) in acute promyelo-cytic leukemia (APL).[1] Also, the significant efficacy of imatinib (STI571), a specific tyrosine kinase inhibitor, in BCR–ABL-positive acute lymphoblastic leukemia (ALL) and chronic myeloid leukemia (CML) patients demonstrates the impressive advances in developing tailored disease-specific therapeutic approaches based on a molecular rationale.[2] As knowledge of disease-specifically altered pathways increases, microarray technology that can provide a vast amount of data on significantly altered gene expression may become an essential tool for optimization of leukemia classification. It also allows the detection of new biologically and clinically relevant subtypes in leukemia, and may guide therapeutic decisions in the near future. In addition, the development of new drugs may be within the focus of such functional genomic approaches in leukemia.

## Gene expression profiling using microarrays

### Technical aspects

Microarrays contain precisely positioned DNA probes designed to specifically monitor the expression levels of genes in a highly parallel manner. Common to all expression profiling approaches is the heteroduplex formation: structural features of nucleic acids enable every nucleic acid strand to recognize complementary sequences through base pairing. After the process of hybridization, complementary fluorescently tagged nucleotides can be detected.[3,4] A detailed overview of the various options available for array-based expression analyses can be found elsewhere.[5] Briefly, a number of basically different microarray platforms are available: filter arrays (formerly considered as macroarrays due to their lower probe density), in situ synthesized oligonucleotide arrays, and spotted glass slide arrays. The latter two vary according to the immobilized probe (i.e. cDNA, oligonucleotides, or genomic fragments) and according to the choice of substrate for surface modification.

In situ synthesized oligonucleotide arrays for expression monitoring contain hundreds of thousands of gene-specific polynucleotides fabricated at high spatial resolution at precise locations on a surface. Laser confocal fluorescence scanning enables the measurement of molecular hybridization events on the array (Figure 20.1, see Plate 3). On a current commercial chip design (e.g. HG-U133 plus 2.0 microarrays from Affymetrix), about 42 000 human genes are represented and thereby probably cover most human genes. Each sequence is represented by multiple oligonucleotides designed to hybridize to different regions of the same RNA. An additional level of redundancy comes from the use of mismatch control probes that are identical to their perfect match partners except for a single base difference in a central position. In contrast, spotted glass slide arrays are usually designed for two-color competitive hybridization. Co-hybridized preparations of both test RNA and reference RNA compete for the spotted DNA probe.[5] Compared with commercially available in situ synthesized arrays with a predetermined number and selection of genes, spotted glass slide arrays can be produced at low cost at core facilities and may only focus on particular genes of interest.

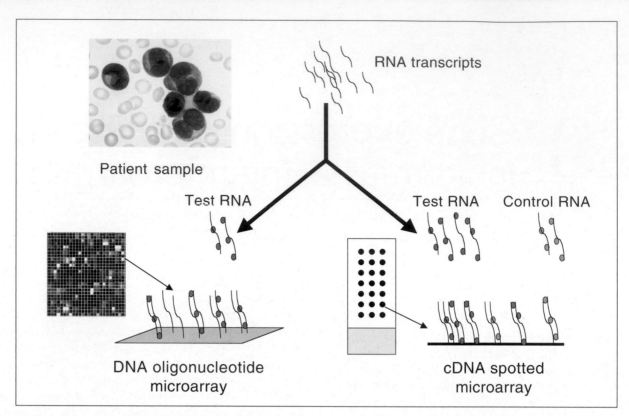

**Figure 20.1** Schematic illustration of microarray technology. For DNA oligonucleotide microarrays, one sample is hybridized per experiment. The detection is accomplished by a fluorescent dye, and results in an absolute expression level for each gene. The oligonucleotides are synthesized in situ onto the array surface. For spotted microarrays, the test RNA is co-hybridized with control RNA. Following detection of the signals, the ratio of differentially tagged test and control RNA is calculated. See Plate 3.

## Data mining, interpretation, and storage

Microarray studies generate vast quantities of data. After image processing, the first step of analysis is to produce a large number of quantified gene expression values. These values represent absolute fluorescence signal intensities as a direct result of hybdridization events on the array surface. It is also possible to qualitatively rate gene expression as absent/present detection call calculations.[6,7] Before analyzing the data, it is a routine procedure to normalize the data.[8]

Data mining, the discovery of non-obvious information, often uses mathematical techniques that have traditionally been used to identify patterns in complex data. There are two different approaches to analyze the data: the supervised approach and the unsupervised approach. Typically, it is of great interest to correlate array data directly to, for example, clinical, cytomorphological, or cytogenetic features. The application of a supervised analysis then requires the grouping of patients according to predefined characteristics. There are several statistical algorithms available that can identify statistically significant differentially expressed genes. A detailed overview can be found elsewhere.[9] After detecting differential gene expression, it is often necessary to accurately classify

samples into known groups. Again, a wealth of machine-learning literature can be found elsewhere.[10–13] Ideally, class prediction is done by dividing the gene expression data into training sets and test sets. First, a number of differentially expressed markers are selected to differentiate between groups that are already known (Figure 20.2). This list of genes is then used to predict independent samples in a test set, based on their discrete gene expression characteristics.

By contrast, clustering is an unsupervised method for organizing expression data into groups with similar signatures. It can be used both to reduce the complexity of the matrix-like data and to visualize it in a more understandable way, as well as predicting the categorization of unknown samples. Patterns in the data are discovered solely from the data itself, as there is no previous knowledge or grouping of the data. Two-dimensional hierarchical clustering[14] sorts both patients and genes according to similarities and leads to a tree-structured dendrogram, which can easily be viewed and explored (Figure 20.3a, Plate 2). It is clear that this hierarchical structure provides potentially useful information about the relationship between adjacent clusters. Common crossing points represent similar patient characteristics as well as similarities with regard to the coexpression of distinct genes. By

# Data  patient samples →

| | inv(16) | inv(16) | M3v | M3v | M3v | inv(3) | inv(3) | inv(3) |
|---|---|---|---|---|---|---|---|---|
| | Avg Diff | Avg Diff | Avg Diff | Avg Diff | Avg Diff | Avg Diff | Avg Diff | Avg Diff |
| 714_at | 11.3 | 4.4 | 5.3 | 12.4 | 5.1 | 5.9 | 5.2 | 24.2 |
| 41349_at | 20.2 | 27.1 | 14.6 | 14.4 | 3 | 12.4 | 1.9 | 15.2 |
| 36919_r_at | 35.5 | 37.8 | 26.4 | 33.1 | 44.5 | 26.2 | 36.6 | 26.6 |
| 40119_at | 19.2 | 58.3 | 24.4 | 12.1 | 9.6 | 12.1 | 14.2 | 23.4 |
| 36140_at | 721.2 | 442 | 365.9 | 683.7 | 787 | 616.4 | 335.1 | 758.2 |
| 31909_at | 19.4 | 19.9 | 9 | 1.3 | 4 | 8.3 | 52.3 | 3.4 |
| 35355_at | 44.1 | 66.2 | 45.5 | 78.1 | 94.4 | 11.3 | 9.6 | 61.8 |
| 35958_at | 9.3 | 8.6 | 7.3 | 2.8 | 18.5 | 3.2 | 54.7 | 12 |
| 36788_at | 1.7 | 6.8 | 1.4 | 7 | 3 | 9.5 | 1.4 | 8.6 |
| 1988_at | 105.2 | 59.9 | 3.7 | 2.2 | 7.9 | 6.9 | 196.1 | 197.6 |
| 40169_at | 98.5 | 115.1 | 161.6 | 148.9 | 269.9 | 220.2 | 143 | 182.1 |
| 180_at | 6.9 | 5.7 | 91.9 | 28.1 | 15.8 | 176.3 | 29.9 | 17 |
| 38947_at | 12.8 | 8 | 6 | 3.9 | 8.8 | 7.9 | 27.5 | 4.7 |
| 34698_at | 4 | 20.8 | 1.1 | 14 | 9.6 | 3 | 17.2 | 2 |
| 37705_at | 112.8 | 119 | 107.6 | 86.8 | 135 | 77.7 | 135.7 | 28.4 |
| 34724_at | 5 | 23.7 | 3 | 5.7 | 6.6 | 7.7 | 3 | 3 |
| 31683_at | 8.6 | 4.4 | 3.4 | 5.9 | 7.6 | 6.1 | 48.7 | 4.3 |
| 31838_at | 36.6 | 51.3 | 35.3 | 15.4 | 10.4 | 3.6 | 43.2 | 9 |
| ... | ... | ... | ... | ... | ... | ... | ... | ... |

*represented genes* ↓

**Figure 20.2** Schematic representation of a matrix-like gene expression raw data set. Individual patient samples are ordered in columns, while gene expression values are given in rows.

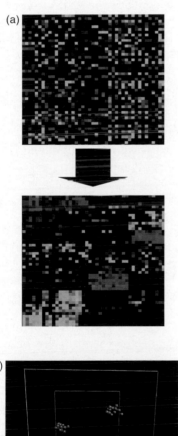

(a)

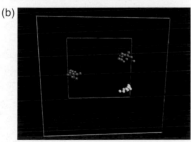

(b)

**Figure 20.3** Two-dimensional hierarchical clustering (a) orders primary expression data. Genes with similar expression patterns are grouped together. Displayed graphically, the relationship among genes can be explored intuitively. Principal component analysis (PCA) (b) is a classical analysis technique to reduce the dimensionality of the data set. New uncorrelated variables summarize characteristical features of the original data. See Plate 4.

use of a detailed gene annotation, it is possible to find functional groupings of genes based on their similarity among the gene expression profiles. This information can be used to gain new insights into physiological pathways (www.ingenuity.com), and may also help to characterize previously uncharacterized genes.[14] A structured and normalized annotation of the respective genes and gene products, essential for all evaluations, is provided by the Gene Ontology consortium.[15] Public available databases such as NetAffx provide regularly updated functional gene annotations.[16] Furthermore, relevant gene information is connected to other various databases such as OMIM (www.ncbi.nlm.nih.gov/omim/), SWISSPROT (http://us.expasy.org/sprot/).

Principal component analysis (PCA) is another technique that can be used to reduce the dimensionality of array data and visualize large data sets in an understandable way.[17] The multidimensional and matrix-like structured array data set (with patient samples in columns and gene expression intensities in rows) is reduced to a new set of variables (i.e. the principle components) by transformation (Figure 20.3, see Plate 4). Since the variation of the original data can be retained and explained by a smaller number of transformed variables, PCA projects the data into a new two- or three-dimensional space and may provide valuable insight into the data (Figure 20.3b, see Plate 4).

The effective annotation of microarray experiments is a major task, which has been approached by the Microarray Gene Expression Data (MGED) group (www.mged.org).[18] This consortium defines standards for the annotation of microarray experiments (MIAME: minimum information about a microarray experiment), as well as a standard data-exchange format (MAGE-ML: microarray gene expression markup language). Based on these standards, global expression databases have been established with the aim of giving access to, sharing, and comparing microarray data. In accordance with the MGED recommendations, ArrayExpress (www.ebi.ac.uk/arrayexpress) is such a public repository for microarray data. The NCBI has launched the Gene Expression Omnibus (GEO), a gene expression and hybridization array data repository, as well as an online resource for the retrieval of gene expression data from any organism or artificial source (www.ncbi.nlm.nih.gov/geo/).

# Acute myeloid leukemia (AML)

Following the pivotal work of Golub et al,[19] who provided data on the applicability of microarrays and new biostatistical analysis methods, several more detailed analyses have been performed over the last few years. These analyses have provided not only a 'class prediction' (prediction of a tumor entity based on specific gene expression profiles of selected informative genes),[19–21] but also a 'class discovery' (discovery of new subentities within groups formerly regarded as homogeneous entities).[22–25] This discovery is not limited to the pure identification of new biological entities of leukemia, but also includes the definition of prognostically different groups,[22,24] which is anticipated to influence therapeutic strategies. Thus, it seems a realistic goal to predict response to therapy, relapse risk, and even risk of developing a secondary AML as suggested in children treated for ALL.[24]

## Class prediction in AML

The first study applying the microarray technology to AML samples demonstrated that both ALL and AML are characterized by distinct and specific gene expression profiles.[19] The distinction between ALL and AML is routine daily practice and is necessary for therapeutic decisions. Today, it is based on cytomorphology, cytochemistry, and immunophenotyping. Golub et al[19] showed that this distinction is also possible solely on the basis of gene expression profiles. In bone marrow samples from 27 patients with ALL and 11 patients with AML, a total of only 50 discriminatory genes were demonstrated to allow the separation of these large and heterogeneous entities from each other. In 36 out of the 38 cases, the molecular diagnosis of leukemia was made correctly based on the gene expression profile as analyzed on the microarray. These analyses represented the first and a major step towards molecular diagnostics of acute leukemias.

Moos et al[26] confirmed this finding and were able to discriminate in 51 childhood leukemias between AML and ALL as well as to subdivide B-lineage from T-lineage ALL using their cDNA arrays representing 4608 genes.

## Class prediction on the basis of cytomorphology

Haferlach et al[27] addressed the question whether French–American–British (FAB) subtypes show distinct gene expression patterns allowing the prediction of subtype based solely on the expression status of a limited set of genes using microarrays (U133A, Affymetrix). All 130 analyzed cases were characterized by cytomorphology and cytogenetics. Reverse transcriptase (RT)–PCR was carried out in all cases with M2/t(8;21), M3(APL), and M4Eo.

Immunophenotyping was performed in all M0 cases. Based on the expression signature of only 1–3 genes, it was possible to separate M3, M3v, M4Eo, and M6 from all other subtypes with 100% accuracy. Comparison between M2 and M4 resulted in the lowest accuracy (85%), which demonstrates the arbitrariness of selecting a threshold of over 20% positivity for non-specific esterase in the FAB system. As shown in Figure 20.4, however, the percentage of myeloperoxidase (MPO)- or non-specific esterase (NSE)-positive cells as measured by cytochemistry correlates highly with microarray signal intensities across all different FAB subtypes.

## Correlation of gene and protein expression

To compare expression data obtained by microarray analyses with protein expression data determined by multiparameter flow cytometry, which is a standard method for diagnosing and subclassifying AML and ALL, Kern et al[28] analyzed 39 relevant markers in 113 patients with newly diagnosed AML and ALL and 4 normal bone marrow samples by both methods in parallel (Affymetrix U133A microarray). A high degree of correlation between protein expression and RNA abundance was observed with regard to both positivity/negativity and quantitative data. Thus, in 1512 of 2187 (69.1%) comparisons, congruent results were obtained with regard to positivity or negativity of expression, respectively. Moreover, among the genes most relevant for diagnosing and subclassifying AML and ALL, i.e. CD13 (Figure 20.5), CD33, MPO, CD22, CD79a, CD19, CD10, and terminal deoxyribonucleotidyl transferase (TdT), congruent results were obtained in 75–100%. These data are considered evidence that protein expression is highly correlated with mRNA abundance in AML and ALL. By taking advantage of these observations, new antigens may be identified that are expressed on the cell surface of AML and ALL cells and that may be promising targets to monitor minimal residual disease.

## Prediction of genetic abnormalities

Schoch et al[29] demonstrated that the cytogenetically defined subtypes – AML with t(8;21), AML with t(15;17), and AML with inv(16) – are characterized by different and specific gene expression profiles. The

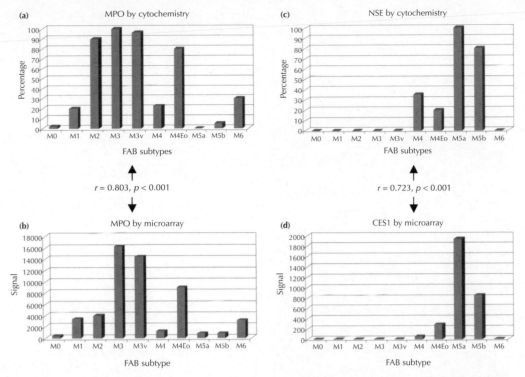

**Figure 20.4** Comparison between cytochemistry and gene expression in AML (*n* = 130). Percentage of myeloperoxidase (MPO)- or non-specific esterase (NSE)-positive cells as measured by cytochemistry on bone marrow smears in the different FAB subtypes in comparison with signal of MPO or CES1 (carboxylesterase 1) measured on the microarray in the same cases.

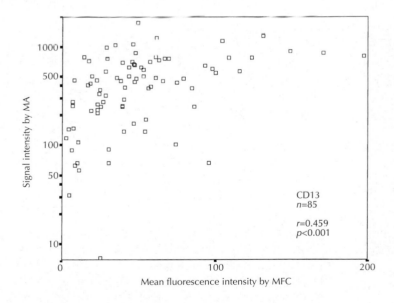

**Figure 20.5** Correlation of protein and mRNA levels in AML. Mean fluorescence intensities for CD13 obtained by multiparameter flow cytometry (MFC) are plotted against signal intensities for CD13 obtained by microarray analysis (MA) in 85 cases with AML (Spearman rank correlation).

underlying basic genetic alterations lead to patterns of gene expression that can be unequivocally detected by microarrays (Figure 20.6, see Plate 4). A minimum set of only 13 genes was sufficient to accurately predict the karyotypes in the respective AML samples.

A further step consisted in the addition of samples with AML carrying aberrations of chromosome 11q23, i.e. *MLL* rearrangements, representing an analysis of AML subtypes with recurring chromosomal aberrations as defined by the WHO.[30] Based on

the gene expression profiles, a minimum set of 39 genes was sufficient to classify samples as normal bone marrow or AML with one of the aberrations t(8;21), t(15;17), inv(16), or 11q23 rearrangements. A principal component analysis as calculated based on the expression intensities of these 39 genes visualizes this (Figure 20.7, see Plate 5).

The same approach was described by Debernardi et al,[31] when investigated 28 cases of AML with t(8;21), t(15;17), and inv(16), also including cases with dif-

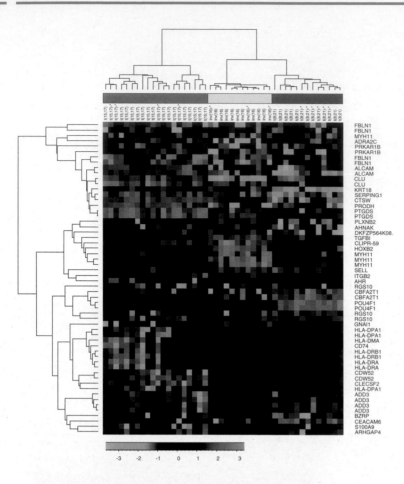

-3  -2  -1  0  1  2  3

**Figure 20.6** Hierarchical clustering based on U133A expression data of 45 AML samples (columns) comprising the subgroups t(15;17) (*n* = 20), t(8;21) (*n* = 13), and inv(16) (*n* = 12) versus 36 informative genes represented by 58 U133A chip design probesets (rows). New patient samples, which were not previously hybridized to U95Av2 microarrays are marked by asterisks. The normalized expression value for each gene is coded by color, with the scale shown at the lower left (standard deviation from mean). Red cells represent high expression and green cells low expression. The previously published set of diagnostic markers is given by respective gene symbols. See Plate 4.

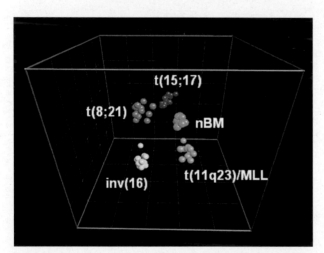

**Figure 20.7** Principal component analysis based on U133A expression data of WHO-classified AML subtypes with recurrent chromosome aberrations and normal bone marrow mononuclear cells from healthy volunteers. Sixty AML samples comprising the color-coded subgroups t(15;17) (*n* = 20), t(8;21) (*n* = 13), inv(16) (*n* = 12), and t(11q34)/*MLL* gene rearrangement-positive samples (*n* = 15) can be discriminated accurately, and are different from normal bone marrow nBM (*n* = 9). See Plate 5.

ferent 11q23 aberrations as well as 10 AML patients with a normal karyotype using U95A arrays (Affymetrix). In comparison with the data set described above, many discriminating genes were found in this independent cohort of AML cases. Furthermore, the expression status of specific genes correlated with 11q23 as well as with AML with normal karyotype. The latter group was characterized by a distinctive upregulation of members of the class I homeobox A and B gene families, implying a common underlying genetic lesion for AML with normal karyotype.

Virtaneva et al[32] focused on AML with trisomy 8 as the sole cytogenetic aberration and asked whether this subgroup could be separated from AML with a normal karyotype based on its gene expression profile. CD34+ cells were analyzed after Ficoll–Hypaque gradient centrifugation, labeled with a secondary antibody conjugated to magnetic beads, and purified over a magnetic column. However, in this analysis using HuGeneFL arrays (Affymetrix), full separation of both cytogenetically different AML subgroups was not possible. This may be due to trisomy 8 not being the disease-defining abnormality but rather a secondary aberration in addition to pathogenetically essential but not yet identified molecular events. Nonetheless, a gene dosage effect was clearly demonstrated, since many genes coded on chromosome 8 were expressed at higher levels in the group of AML with trisomy 8.

## AML subtypes characterized by molecular mutations

As 40–45% of AML cases show no chromosomal rearrangements in chromosome banding analysis, molecular studies are necessary to identify the underlying genetic defects. Several mutations have been found, the most frequent being length and point mutations within the *FLT3* gene and partial tandem duplications within the *MLL* gene (*MLL*-PTD).

In a cohort of 1992 unselected newly diagnosed AML cases, 125 (6.3%) had an *MLL*-PTD.[33] This mutation occurs mainly in cytogenetically normal AML, and like *MLL*-translocations (tMLL) is characterized by an unfavorable prognosis. Similar to translocations of 11q23 involving the *MLL* gene, *MLL*-PTD occur significantly more frequently in AML secondary to a previous cytotoxic therapy. Schnittger et al[33] asked whether it is possible to discriminate *MLL*-PTD cases from AML cases with normal karyotype without this aberration as well as from AML with tMLL based on different gene expression patterns using U133A microarrays (Affymetrix). By pairwise comparison, it was not possible to define a specific expression profile discriminating *MLL*-PTD-positive from negative cases. However, a specific expression profile was found for the various *MLL* translocations compared with the *MLL*-PTD group and normal karyotype group. Many of the discriminating genes encode for DNA-binding proteins involved in transcriptional regulation and developmental processes.

## Class discovery in AML

A main focus in gene expression profiling studies of leukemias will be to refine the subcategorization in subgroups with so-far identical patterns of diagnostic results but different clinical outcomes. This is urgently needed, especially in the two major groups of AML, i.e. AMC with normal karyotype (45% of patients) and AML with complex aberrant karyotype (15% of patients).

Qian et al[34] were able to identify distinct subtypes of therapy-related AML (t-AML) when analyzing CD34+ hematopoietic progenitor cells from 14 patients using U95A microarrays (Affymetrix). Gene expression patterns typical of arrested differentiation in early progenitor cells were commonly detected in all cases. Furthermore, two specific characteristics could be found. Cases with a −5/del(5q) had higher expression levels of genes involved in cell cycle control, checkpoints, or growth and a loss of expression of the gene encoding interferon consensus sequence-binding protein. Another subgroup was characterized by downregulation of transcription factors involved in early hematopoiesis and overexpression of proteins involved in signal transduction (e.g. FLT3) and cell survival (e.g. BCL2). Targeting these different pathways may lead to more specific treatment approaches in this very poor-prognosis group of AML.

## Estimation of prognosis in AML

Yagi et al[35] analyzed 54 pediatric AML cases using Affymetrix U95A arrays and focused on the reproducibility of some FAB subtypes and especially on gene patterns to predict outcome. After unsupervised clustering, they were able to differentiate patients with t(8;21) from those with inv(16) as well as from those demonstrating an AML M4/5 or AML M7 phenotype or immunophenotype by specific gene expression signatures. Within this unsupervised analysis, no specific profile was found that correlated with the prognosis of the patients. For further calculations, data were analyzed supervised with respect to outcome and prognosis. A subset of 35 genes was selected that was independent of the morphology or karyotype of the patients; some of these genes are associated with cell cycle regulation or apoptosis. By hierarchical cluster analysis, patients could be classified into high-risk and low-risk groups with respect to event-free survival ($p<0.001$).

# Myelodysplastic syndromes

Biologically, MDS is linked very closely to AML. Therefore, specific gene expression patterns discriminating MDS from AML and identifying cases with a high likelihood of progression to AML are of great interest. However, only a limited number of studies have focused on this topic.[36,37]

# Acute lymphoblastic leukemia (ALL)

As demonstrated by Golub et al,[19] ALL can be distinguished from AML based on the expression status of a small number of genes. In addition, Moos et al[26] could discriminate in 51 childhood leukemias between AML and ALL as well as between B- and T-lineage ALL using cDNA arrays with 4608 genes. Furthermore, they identified cases with low- and high-risk ALL, respectively, and predicted patients having a *TEL–RUNX1 (AML1)* fusion transcript.

Armstrong et al[23] were the first to demonstrate that childhood ALL with chromosomal aberrations involving the *MLL* gene can be regarded as a molecularly defined entity distinct from other ALL (U95A, Affymetrix). *MLL*-positive ALL had a distinct gene expression profile consistent with an early hematopoieteic progenitor expressing multilineage markers and specific *HOX* genes. Also comparison of these ALL cases with *MLL* aberrations with other ALL cases as well as with AML samples resulted in a clear separation between all three groups.

A milestone in microarray analysis with respect to class discovery, class prediction, and prediction of outcome was the report by Yeoh et al[24] on 327 childhood ALL cases analyzed by Affymetrix U95A arrays. Patients were discriminated according to their cytogenetic and immunological as well as their molecular subtype of ALL, i.e. T-ALL, *E2A–PBX1, BCR–ABL, TEL–RUNX1*, and *MLL* gene rearrangements, and hyperdiploid ALL. Yeoh et al[24] not only could predict the therapeutic outcome in most children with ALL, but also found specific genes in the ALL blasts at diagnosis that indicate an increased risk of developing therapy-induced AML after successful treatment of ALL.

### Prediction of response in ALL

Hofmann et al[38] analyzed 25 bone marrow samples from 19 patients with Philadelphia(Ph)-positive ALL all treated with the BCR–ABL tyrosine kinase inhibitor imatinib using HuGeneFL arrays (Affymetrix). Patients were selected according to their cytogenetic response to the drug, and 95 genes were identified to predict the treatment outcome in all cases. Another 56 genes were found to predict leukemia cells that had secondary resistance to the drug after remission had been achieved. Resistant cells expressed ATP synthetases such as ATP5A1 and ATP5C1 and had a significantly reduced expression of the pro-apoptotic gene *BAK1* and the cell cycle control gene *p15INK4B*.

Cheok et al[39] elucidated the genomics of cellular responses to treatment with methotrexate and mercaptopurine given alone or in combination before and after in vivo treatment in 60 childhood ALL cases (U95A, Affymetrix). A total of 124 differentially expressed genes were identified capable of accurately discriminating the four possible treatment groups. Genes included those involved in apoptosis, mismatch repair, cell cycle control, and stress response. These data indicate that leukemia cells in different patients react in a similar manner after specific treatments and therefore share common pathways of genomic responses to different drug schedules. This may also open the way to future trials to predict outcome of treatment protocols by gene expression profiling at diagnosis.

Ross et al[40] rehybridized 132 childhood ALL probes from their previous cohort to the Affymetrix U133 set and identified almost 60% of new discriminating genes in comparison with their previous analysis with U95A.[24] As a proportion of these new genes were highly ranked as class discriminators and led to an overall diagnostic accuracy of 97% in several analyses, the authors suggested that these gene expression profiles be assessed in a prospective clinical trial. The main clinical focus should be at diagnosis of ALL with respect to accuracy, practicality, and cost-effectiveness in comparison with standard diagnostic techniques.

# Summary of gene expression profiling of acute leukemias

An overview of important publications with respect to AML and ALL is given in Table 20.1.

# Chronic myeloid leukemia (CML)
## Class discovery

Ohmine et al[41] used DNA microarrays (HO-1–3, Mergen, San Leandro, CA, USA) and analyzed the expression profiles of 3456 genes in purified AC133+ hematopoietic stem cells in 13 CML patients and healthy volunteers. They were able to find the potential inhibitor of STAT proteins, *PIASy*, to be downregulated in association with stage progression of CML. Accordingly, the forced expression of *PIASy* induced apoptosis in a CML cell line. The authors conclude that microarray analysis may help to identify molecular events that underlie stage progression in CML.

## Prediction of response

Cohen et al[42] analyzed 94 patients with CML treated with interferon and in some cases with bone marrow transplantation. All were proven Philadelphia-positive, at least by FISH. Thirty-four patients were studied at diagnosis, 60 at different time points during therapy. In 14 of 96 patients major deletion of the region proximal to the rearranged *ABL* gene on 9q was found. These patients had a significantly shorter chronic phase of the disease as compared with the non-deletion 9q patients ($p=0.0144$). Using Human 1.2 Atlas Arrays (Clontech, Palo Alto, CA, USA), a number of genes were found to be differentially expressed between these two groups of patients. These genes were involved especially in cell adhesion and migration. The authors concluded that this finding may help to identify a subgroup of CML patients with a relatively poor prognosis and may lead to the adaptation of treatment strategies.

# Chronic lymphocytic leukemia (CLL)
## Class prediction

Aalto et al[43] analyzed 34 patients with CLL using Clontech microarrays and found significant expression differences in 78 genes compared with the reference, tonsillar B lymphocytes. Within these genes, a cluster of genes was associated ($p<0.05$) with 11q23 deletions detected by FISH and also with unfavorable Binet stages B or C. As most of these genes had not been discussed with respect to progression in CLL, the authors concluded that gene expression profiling

**Table 20.1  Summary of studies approaching the diagnosis and classification of acute leukemias based on gene expression profiling**

| Standard method | Results | Ref | Study population | Technology |
|---|---|---|---|---|
| Cytomorphology, cytochemistry | Differentiation between ALL and AML | 19 | Adult acute leukemias ($n = 72$) | Affymetrix Hu6800 |
| | | 26 | Pediatric acute leukemias ($n = 51$) | cDNA array, 4608 genes |
| | Subclassification of AML FAB subtypes | 51 | Adult AML ($n = 130$) | Affymetrix U133A |
| | | 35 | Pediatric AML ($n = 54$) | Affymetrix U95A |
| Immunophenotyping | Protein expression as measured by flow cytometry correlates with gene expression | 28 | Adult ALL ($n = 28$), adult AML ($n = 85$) | Affymetrix U133A |
| | Differentiation between ALL of B- and T-lineage | 19 | Adult ALL ($n = 27$) | Affymetrix Hu6800 |
| | | 24 | Pediatric ALL ($n = 360$) | Affymetrix U95A |
| | | 26 | Pediatric ALL ($n = 39$) | cDNA array, 4608 genes |
| | | 40 | Pediatric ALL ($n = 132$) | Affymetrix U133A+B |
| Cytogenetics | Identification of specific gene expression profiles of cytogenetic subgroups | 23 | ALL ($n = 47$), *MLL* rearrangement | Affymetrix U95A |
| | | 24 | Pediatric ALL ($n = 360$), hyperdiploid, t(12;21), t(9;22), t(1;19), *MLL* rearrangement | Affymetrix U95A |
| | | 40 | Pediatric ALL ($n = 132$), hyperdiploid, t(12;21), t(9;22), t(1;19), *MLL* rearrangement | Affymetrix U133A+B |
| | | 29 | Adult AML ($n = 37$), t(8;21), inv(16), t(15;17) | Affymetrix U95A |
| | | 31 | Adult AML ($n = 27$), pediatric AML ($n = 1$), t(8;21), inv(16), t(15;17), 11q23, normal | Affymetrix U95A |
| | | 52 | Adult AML ($n = 65$), t(8;21), inv(16), t(15;17), *MLL* rearrangement | Affymetrix U133A |
| | | 35 | Pediatric AML ($n = 54$), t(8;21), inv(16), t(9;11), *MLL* rearrangement | Affymetrix U95A |
| | Gene dose effect in trisomy 8 | 32 | Adult AML ($n = 20$), trisomy 8 sole, normal karyotype | Affymetrix HuGeneFL |
| Molecular genetics | Gene expression profile of AML *MLL*-PTD+ vs *MLL*-PTD– vs t(*MLL*) | 33 | Adult AML ($n = 55$) | Affymetrix U133A |
| Response to therapy | Prediction of response to imatinib in Ph+ ALL | 38 | Adult Ph+ ALL ($n = 19$) | Affymetrix HuGeneFL |
| | Prognosis in pediatric AML | 35 | Pediatric AML ($n = 54$) | Affymetrix U95A |

in CLL may provide important information about leukemogenesis and may help not only to define risk groups but also to design treatments aimed at specific molecular targets.

In their important analysis, Rosenwald et al[44] used the lymphochip, investigating 17 856 genes in 33 CLL patients, and were able to define a specific pattern of expression profile in all CLL. This was irrespective of rearranged immunoglobulins (Ig) being present or not in these patients. Nonetheless, the expression of hundreds of other genes correlated clearly with Ig mutational status. This latter group included many genes the expression of which is modulated during mitogenic B-cell receptor signaling. Genes identified were used to build a CLL subtype predictor that may help in the clinical subclassification of patients with CLL.

Another marker recently correlated with CLL prognosis is CD38 expression as measured by flow cytometry. CD38+ patients with B-CLL are characterized by advanced stage, an inferior responsiveness to chemotherapy, and a shorter survival. Dürig et al[45] used Hugen FL arrays with 5600 genes and analyzed 25 CD38+ CLL versus 45 CD38- patients. In concordance with others, they showed that B-CLL display a common gene expression profile that is, however, largely independent of CD38 positivity. Nonetheless, 14 genes differed significantly between the two groups, including genes involved in the regulation of cell survival. Using an unsupervised hierarchical cluster analysis in 76 CLL samples, two major subgoups of patients were identified comprising 20 versus 50 patients. Patients in the smaller group were characterized by a coordinate high expression of a large number of ribosomal and other translocation-associated genes and had a better clinical outcome. Thus, CD38 status may be measured by microarray platforms in comparison with flow cytometry or immunohistology, and gene expression profiling

may also define different prognostic subgroups in CLL.

Wiestner et al[46] focused on ZAP70 in 107 CLL patients using the lymphochip with 13 868 human cDNAs. The mRNA expression of ZAP70 was found to be an excellent surrogate marker for the distinction between Ig mutated and non-mutated CLL subtypes and was also able to identify patients with a divergent clinical course. In 93% of cases, ZAP70 expression correlated correctly with Ig mutation subtype. In comparison with all the other genes investigated, ZAP70 was the best to predict outcome in CLL: high expression levels identified a group of CLL patients with a progressive form of the disease, with a median time to treatment following diagnosis of 6.4 years in comparison with the other group, with an interval of more than 10 years.

Jelinek et al[47] used U95A arrays (Affymetrix) to analyze 38 cases of B-CLL in comparison with 10 age-matched healthy controls. They identified 70 genes that discriminate leukemic cells from normal B cells. These genes were able to create a diagnostic signature tested in an idependent cohort of 21 B-CLL and 20 normal subjects, leading to a perfect specificity and sensitivity of class prediction. Furthermore, a group of 31 genes was identified to distinguish between

**Table 20.2 Summary of studies approaching diagnosis, prognosis and classification of chronic leukemias based on gene expression profiling**

| Standard method | Results | Ref | Study population | Technology |
|---|---|---|---|---|
| Immunophenotyping | Global gene expression signature in CLL | 47 | Adult CLL (n = 35) | Affymetrix U95A |
| | Homogeneous phenotype in CLL versus memory B cells | 49 | Adult CLL (n = 34) | Affymetrix U95A |
| Cytogenetics | CML with additional deletion of 9q | 42 | Adult CML (n = 14/94) | Clontech |
| | Distinct expression profile in CLL with del(11)q23, or with Binet stages B and C | 43 | Adult CLL (n = 34); 9 with 11q23 | Clontech |
| Molecular genetics | ZAP70 demonstrates distinct gene expression profile in CLL | 46 | Adult CLL (n = 107) | Lymphochip |
| | Gene expression and immunoglobulin mutation genotype in CLL | 44 | Adult CLL (n = 33) | Lymphochip |
| Response to therapy; prognostic marker | Prognostic markers in CLL involved in lymphocyte trafficking | 48 | Adult CLL (n = 54) | Incyte Pharmaceuticals |
| | Progression of CML | 41 | Adult CML (n = 13) | ExpressCHIP, HO-1–3, Mergen |
| | Genes correlated with outcome in CLL | 45 | Adult CLL (n = 70) | Affymetrix HuGeneFL |

patients with Rai stage 0 and Rai stage 4, suggesting that the gene expression pattern may be associated with disease progression.

## Class discovery

Stratowa et al[48] analyzed 54 peripheral blood samples from B-CLL patients using the Clontech arrays with 1024 selected genes. Several genes were identified as correlating significantly with patient survival and/or with the clinical stage of the disease. Most of these genes coded either for cell adhesion molecules such as L-selectin and $\beta_2$ integrin or for factors that induce cell adhesion molecules. The authors therefore concluded that prognosis of CLL may also be related to a defect in lymphocyte trafficking.

Klein et al[49] analyzed 34 peripheral blood samples from CLL patients and enriched CLL cells by MACS (Miltenyi). Sequences of $IgV_H$ status were known in all patients. Using Affymetrix U95A microarrays, they compared leukemia cells with CD19+ enriched cord blood cells and found that CLL display a common and characteristic gene expression profile that is largely independent of their $IgV_H$ genotype. However, on the basis of a restricted number of less than 30 differentially expressed genes, they were able to predict IgV mutated and non-mutated samples. Further genes were identified in comparison with purified normal B cells that indicate that CLL profiles are more closely related to memory B cells than to those derived from naive B cells or CD5+ B cells, as well as from germinal center centroblasts or centrocytes.

## Summary of gene expression profiling of chronic leukemias

A short overview of important publications with respect to CML and CLL is given in Table 20.2.

# Conclusions

Microarray technology provides a means for comprehensive and simultaneous analysis of the expression status of thousands of genes. The resulting signature allows the identification of a distinct molecular leukemic genotype. It is anticipated that the application of microarrays will significantly improve molecular diagnostics in leukemia,[50] and will provide deep insights into the pathogenetic alterations of malignant and non-malignant haematopoietic cells, which will allow the discovery of new entities, new prognostic markers, and markers for follow-up monitoring of minimal residual disease. Furthermore, it is expected that the results of microarray experiments will allow the identification of disease-specific target structures and the design of novel and specific drugs. Several studies have already shown that a variety of different diagnostic and prognostic questions can already be answered by gene expression profiling (Tables 20.1 and 20.2). Gene expression analyses are limited, however, to the RNA level and thus cannot be used to analyze alterations at the protein level, for example the phosphorylation and dephosphorylation of proteins. These aspects will be covered by other novel techniques such as proteomics.

## REFERENCES

1. Fenaux P, Le Deley MC, Castaigne S et al. Effect of all trans retinoic acid in newly diagnosed acute promyelocytic leukemia. Results of a multicenter randomized trial. European APL 91 Group. Blood 1993; 82: 3241–9.
2. Kantarjian H, Sawyers C, Hochhaus A et al. Hematologic and cytogenetic responses to imatinib mesylate in chronic myelogenous leukemia. N Engl J Med 2002; 346: 645–52.
3. Southern E, Mir K, Shchepinov M. Molecular interactions on microarrays. Nat Genet 1999; 21: 5–9.
4. Lockhart DJ, Dong H, Byrne MC et al. Expression monitoring by hybridization to high-density oligonucleotide arrays. Nat Biotechnol 1996; 14: 1675–80.
5. Holloway AJ, van Laar RK, Tothill RW et al. Options available – from start to finish – for obtaining data from DNA microarrays II. Nat Genet 2002; 32(Suppl): 481–9.
6. Liu WM, Mei R, Di X et al. Analysis of high density expression microarrays with signed-rank call algorithms. Bioinformatics 2002; 18: 1593–9.
7. Lipshutz RJ, Fodor SP, Gingeras TR et al. High density synthetic oligonucleotide arrays. Nat Genet 1999; 21: 20–4.
8. Quackenbush J. Microarray data normalization and transformation. Nat Genet 2002; 32(Suppl): 496–501.
9. Slonim DK. From patterns to pathways: gene expression data analysis comes of age. Nat Genet 2002; 32(Suppl): 502–8.
10. Hastie T, Tibshirani R, Friedman J. The Elements of Statistical Learning. New York: Springer-Verlag, 2001.
11. Vapnik V. Statistical Learning Theory. New York: Wiley, 1998.
12. Furey TS, Cristianini N, Duffy N et al. Support vector machine classification and validation of cancer tissue samples using microarray expression data. Bioinformatics 2000; 16: 906–14.
13. Brown MP, Grundy WN, Lin D et al. Knowledge-based analysis of microarray gene expression data by using support vector machines. Proc Natl Acad Sci USA 2000; 97: 262–7.
14. Eisen MB, Spellman PT, Brown PO et al. Cluster analysis and display of genome-wide expression patterns. Proc Natl Acad Sci USA 1998; 95: 14863–8.
15. Ashburner M, Ball CA, Blake JA et al. Gene ontology: tool for the unification of biology. The Gene Ontology Consortium. Nat Genet 2000; 25: 25–9.
16. Liu G, Loraine AE, Shigeta R et al. NetAffx: Affymetrix probesets and annotations. Nucleic Acids Res 2003; 31: 82–6.

17. Yeung KY, Ruzzo WL. Principal component analysis for clustering gene expression data. *Bioinformatics* 2001; **17**: 763–74.

18. Brazma A, Hingamp P, Quackenbush J et al. Minimum information about a microarray experiment (MIAME) – toward standards for microarray data. *Nat Genet* 2001; **29**: 365–71.

19. Golub TR, Slonim DK, Tamayo P et al. Molecular classification of cancer: class discovery and class prediction by gene expression monitoring. *Science* 1999; **286**: 531–7.

20. Ramaswamy S, Tamayo P, Rifkin R et al. Multiclass cancer diagnosis using tumor gene expression signatures. *Proc Natl Acad Sci USA* 2001; **98**: 15149–54.

21. Ramaswamy S, Golub TR. DNA microarrays in clinical oncology. *J Clin Oncol* 2002; **20**: 1932–41.

22. Alizadeh AA, Eisen MB, Davis RE et al. Distinct types of diffuse large B-cell lymphoma identified by gene expression profiling. *Nature* 2000; **403**: 503–11.

23. Armstrong SA, Staunton JE, Silverman LB et al. *MLL* translocations specify a distinct gene expression profile that distinguishes a unique leukemia. *Nat Genet* 2002; **30**: 41–7.

24. Yeoh EJ, Ross ME, Shurtleff SA et al. Classification, subtype discovery, and prediction of outcome in pediatric acute lymphoblastic leukemia by gene expression profiling. *Cancer Cell* 2002; **1**: 133–43.

25. Zhan F, Hardin J, Kordsmeier B et al. Global gene expression profiling of multiple myeloma, monoclonal gammopathy of undetermined significance, and normal bone marrow plasma cells. *Blood* 2002; **99**: 1745–57.

26. Moos PJ, Raetz EA, Carlson MA et al. Identification of gene expression profiles that segregate patients with childhood leukemia. *Clin Cancer Res* 2002; **8**: 3118–30.

27. Haferlach T, Kohlmann A, Kern W et al. Gene expression profiling as a tool for the diagnosis of acute leukemias. *Semin Hematol* 2003; **40**: 281–95.

28. Kern W, Kohlmann A, Wuchter C et al. Correlation of protein expression and gene expression in acute leukemia. *Cytometry* 2003; **55B**: 29–36.

29. Schoch C, Kohlmann A, Schnittger S et al. Acute myeloid leukemias with reciprocal rearrangements can be distinguished by specific gene expression profiles. *Proc Natl Acad Sci USA* 2002; **99**: 10008–13.

30. Kohlmann A, Dugas M, Schoch C et al. Gene expression profiles of distinct cytogenetic AML subtypes as defined by the new WHO classification: a study of 45 patients. *Oncogenomics Conference 2002, Dublin, Ireland.*

31. Debernardi S, Lillington DM, Chaplin T et al. Genome-wide analysis of acute myeloid leukemia with normal karyotype reveals a unique pattern of homeobox gene expression distinct from those with translocation-mediated fusion events. *Genes Chromosomes Cancer* 2003; **37**: 149–58.

32. Virtaneva K, Wright FA, Tanner SM et al. Expression profiling reveals fundamental biological differences in acute myeloid leukemia with isolated trisomy 8 and normal cytogenetics. *Proc Natl Acad Sci USA* 2001; **98**: 1124–9.

33. Schnittger S, Kohlmann A, Haferlach T et al. Acute myeloid leukemia (AML) with partial tandem duplication of the *MLL*-gene (MLL-PTD) can be discriminated from *MLL*-translocations based on specific gene expression profiles. *Blood* 2002; **100**: 310a.

34. Qian Z, Fernald AA, Godley LA et al. Expression profiling of CD34+ hematopoietic stem/progenitor cells reveals distinct subtypes of therapy-related acute myeloid leukemia. *Proc Natl Acad Sci USA* 2002; **99**: 14925–30.

35. Yagi T, Morimoto A, Eguchi M et al. Identification of a gene expression signature associated with prognosis of pediatric AML. *Blood* 2003; **102**: 1849–56.

36. Miyazato A, Ueno S, Ohmine K et al. Identification of myelodysplastic syndrome-specific genes by DNA microarray analysis with purified hematopoietic stem cell fraction. *Blood* 2001; **98**: 422–7.

37. Hofmann WK, de Vos S, Komor M et al. Characterization of gene expression of CD34+ cells from normal and myelodysplastic bone marrow. *Blood* 2002; **100**: 3553–60.

38. Hofmann WK, de Vos S, Elashoff D et al. Relation between resistance of Philadelphia-chromosome-positive acute lymphoblastic leukaemia to the tyrosine kinase inhibitor STI571 and gene-expression profiles: a gene-expression study. *Lancet* 2002; **359**: 481–6.

39. Cheok MH, Yang W, Pui CH et al. Treatment-specific changes in gene expression discriminate in vivo drug response in human leukemia cells. *Nat Genet* 2003; **34**: 85–90.

40. Ross ME, Zhou X, Song G et al. Classification of pediatric acute lymphoblastic leukemia by gene expression profiling. *Blood* 2003; **102**: 2951–9.

41. Ohmine K, Ota J, Ueda M et al. Characterization of stage progression in chronic myeloid leukemia by DNA microarray with purified hematopoietic stem cells. *Oncogene* 2001; **20**: 8249–57.

42. Cohen N, Rozenfeld-Granot G, Hardan I et al. Subgroup of patients with Philadelphia-positive chronic myelogenous leukemia characterized by a deletion of 9q proximal to *ABL* gene: expression profiling, resistance to interferon therapy, and poor prognosis. *Cancer Genet Cytogenet* 2001; **128**: 114–19.

43. Aalto Y, El Rifa W, Vilpo L et al. Distinct gene expression profiling in chronic lymphocytic leukemia with 11q23 deletion. *Leukemia* 2001; **15**: 1721–8.

44. Rosenwald A, Alizadeh AA, Widhopf G et al. Relation of gene expression phenotype to immunoglobulin mutation genotype in B cell chronic lymphocytic leukemia. *J Exp Med* 2001; **194**: 1639–47.

45. Dürig J, Nuckel H, Huttmann A et al. Expression of ribosomal and translation-associated genes is correlated with a favorable clinical course in chronic lymphocytic leukemia. *Blood* 2003; **101**: 2748–55.

46. Wiestner A, Rosenwald A, Barry TS et al. *ZAP-70* expression identifies a chronic lymphocytic leukemia subtype with unmutated immunoglobulin genes, inferior clinical outcome, and distinct gene expression profile. *Blood* 2003; **101**: 4944–51.

47. Jelinek DF, Tschumper RC, Stolovitzky GA et al. Identification of a global gene expression signature of B-chronic lymphocytic leukemia. *Mol Cancer Res* 2003; **1**: 346–61.

48. Stratowa C, Loffler G, Lichter P et al. cDNA microarray gene expression analysis of B-cell chronic lymphocytic leukemia proposes potential new prognostic markers involved in lymphocyte trafficking. *Int J Cancer* 2001; **91**: 474–80.

49. Klein U, Tu Y, Stolovitzky GA et al. Gene expression profiling of B cell chronic lymphocytic leukemia reveals a homogeneous phenotype related to memory B cells. *J Exp Med* 2001; **194**: 1625–38.

50. Staudt LM. Molecular diagnosis of the hematologic cancers. *N Engl J Med* 2003; **348**: 1777–85.

51. Haferlach T, Kohlmann A, Dugas M et al. Gene expression profiling is able to reproduce different phenotypes in AML as defined by the FAB classification. *Blood* 2002; **100**: 195a.

52. Kohlmann A, Schoch C, Schnittger S et al. Molecular characterization of acute leukemias by use of microarray technology. *Genes Chromosomes Cancer* 2003; **37**: 396–405.

# 21 Detection of minimal residual disease in lymphoid malignancies

JJM van Dongen, T Szczepański, VHJ van der Velden, and AW Langerak

## Introduction

### Lymphoid malignancies

Lymphoid malignancies are categorized into four main groups: acute lymphoblastic leukemias (ALL), chronic lymphocytic leukemias (CLL), non-Hodgkin lymphomas (NHL), and multiple myelomas (MM). Together they represent about 76% of all hematopoietic malignancies and affect about 75 000 patients per year in the European Union (with some 375 million inhabitants). Figure 21.1 shows the age-related incidence of the four categories of lymphoid malignancies in the Netherlands.[1] Although the incidence of most malignancies increases with age, the highest incidence of ALL is seen in early childhood. This is in contrast to CLL and MM, which do not occur in children, are rare in young adults, but have progressively increasing incidence rates from the age of 50–60 years onwards. NHL represent the largest category (about 60%) of lymphoid malignancies and are found at all ages, with increasing incidence in older age groups (Figure 21.1).[1]

ALL are generally regarded as malignant counterparts of immature lymphoid cells, such as precursor B cells in the bone marrow (BM) and immature T cells in the cortical thymus.[2–4] The maturation arrest of CLL generally occurs in more mature differentiation stages. Most cells in NHL are also arrested in more mature differentiation stages, whereas MM are regarded as malignant counterparts of plasma cells.[2–4] However, it should be noted that malignant transformation probably occurs in earlier differentiation stages and that the offspring of the malignant clonogenic cells can further mature to form the dominant malignant cell population. This implies that reliable techniques for detection of malignant cells should also be able to detect malignant precursor cells.

Cytomorphological and histomorphological techniques generally form the basis for diagnosis and classification of lymphoid malignancies.[5] However, additional diagnostic techniques are frequently needed for reliable and reproducible diagnosis and classification. This includes immunophenotyping, analysis of immunoglobulin (Ig) and T-cell receptor (TCR) genes, and detection of chromosome aberrations with molecular techniques or via classical cytogenetics.[2–8]

Immunophenotyping appears to be useful for diagnosis and detailed classification of lymphoid malignancies as well as for detection of immunophenotypic aberrances and the recognition of subpopulations in the malignancy. Most lymphoid malignancies (93–95%) appear to belong to the B-cell lineage (Table 21.1).[2–4]

Virtually all lymphoid malignancies (>98%) have rearranged Ig and/or TCR genes. This is probably related to the fact that Ig and TCR gene rearrangements start early during lymphoid differentiation.

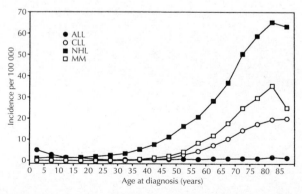

**Figure 21.1** Age-related incidence of the four types of lymphoid malignancies in the Netherlands in 1989–1991: acute lymphoblastic leukemia (ALL), chronic lymphocytic leukemia (CLL), non-Hodgkin lymphoma (NHL), and multiple myeloma (MM). Data are derived from The Netherlands Cancer Registry.[1]

**Table 21.1  B-lineage and T-lineage origin of lymphoid malignancies**

|  | ALL | | CLL | NHL | MM |
|---|---|---|---|---|---|
|  | Childhood | Adult |  |  |  |
| B-lineage | 80–85% | 75–80% | 95% (B-CLL, B-PLL, HCL) | 90–95% | 100% |
| T-lineage | 15–20% | 20–25% | 5% (LGL, T-PLL, CTLL, ATLL[a]) | 5–10% | 0% |

ALL, acute lymphoblastic leukemia; CLL, chronic lymphocytic leukemia; PLL, prolymphocytic leukemia; HCL, hairy cell leukemia; LGL, large granular lymphocyte leukemia; CTLL, cutaneous T-cell leukemia/lymphoma; ATLL, adult T-cell leukemia/lymphoma; NHL, non-Hodgkin lymphoma; MM, multiple myeloma.
[a] In Japan and Caribbean regions, ATLL occurs in essentially higher frequencies than in Europe and other Western countries.

Lymphoid malignancies are regarded as being derived from a single malignantly transformed cell, i.e. they are clonal diseases. Therefore, cells of a lymphoid malignancy in principle have identically rearranged Ig and TCR genes. This feature can be used as unique marker for identification of malignant (clonal) lymphoid cells between normal reactive (polyclonal) lymphoid cells.[6,7]

Chromosome aberrations are found in 25–40% of lymphoid malignancies, depending on the type of malignancy and on the applied technique, such as classical cytogenetics, fluorescence in situ hybridization (FISH), Southern blotting, or polymerase chain reaction (PCR).[8,8a,9] Chromosome aberrations are important genetic markers for classification of lymphoid malignancies, because they are directly related to the malignant transformation process.

## Detection of minimal residual disease

Current cytotoxic treatment protocols induce complete remission in most ALL patients, in some patients with CLL, in most NHL patients, and in a proportion of patients with MM.[10–12] The introduction of allogeneic and autologous stem cell transplantation (SCT) in treatment protocols has further increased the remission rates in ALL, NHL, and MM.[10–12] Nevertheless, many of these patients ultimately relapse. Apparently, the treatment protocols are not capable of killing all clonogenic malignant cells in these patients, even though they reached complete remission according to cytomorphological criteria. The detection limit of cytomorphological techniques is not lower than 1–5% of malignant cells, implying that these techniques can provide only superficial information about the effectiveness of the treatment. More sensitive techniques are needed for detection of lower frequencies of malignant cells during and after treatment, i.e. detection of minimal residual disease (MRD).[13] MRD techniques should reach sensitivities

of at least $10^{-3}$ (one malignant cell within thousand normal cells), but sensitivities of $10^{-4}$ to $10^{-6}$ are preferred. Such sensitivities allow 'true' MRD detection and thereby evaluation of the effectiveness of the total treatment and assessment of the contribution of each treatment phase (Figure 21.2).[13–15]

The application of MRD techniques is especially valuable in malignancies that potentially can be cured by use of cytotoxic therapy and/or SCT. This concerns ALL, several types of NHL, and possibly also MM. In these disease categories, MRD information either is already used or might be employed in the near future for adaptation of treatment.

During the last 20 years, several methods for MRD detection have been developed and evaluated. Most of these techniques appeared to have a limited sensitivity and/or applicability:

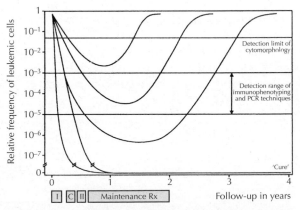

**Figure 21.2** Diagram of the putative relative frequencies of leukemic cells in peripheral blood or bone marrow of acute leukemia patients during and after chemotherapy and during development of relapse. The detection limit of cytomorphological techniques as well as the detection range of immunophenotyping and PCR techniques are indicated. I, induction treatment; C, consolidation treatment; II, re-induction treatment.

- *Cytogenetics*: sensitivity of $10^{-2}$. Applicability is limited to microscopically detectable chromosome aberrations and is dependent on the possibility to obtain cells in metaphase.
- *Cell culture systems*: sensitivity is variable, and standardized application on a routine basis is difficult.[16]
- *FISH techniques*: sensitivity of $10^{-2}$ to $10^{-3}$. Application is restricted to malignancies with a well-defined chromosome aberration for which suitable DNA probes are available.[17,18] The sensitivity of interphase FISH for translocations, inversions, and deletions is limited to 1–5%. The limited sensitivity of the classical fusion signal FISH is caused by artefactual colocalization of two independent (unlinked) breakpoint probe signals in normal cells, which might cause false positivity.[18] The sensitivity can be slightly increased by the application of metaphase FISH, which does not cause false-positive results but like conventional cytogenetics is dependent on the availability of cells in metaphase.[19] A better possibility to increase the sensitivity of FISH techniques is the application of 'split-signal' FISH, implying that the two differently labeled FISH probes are positioned at opposite sides of the breakpoint area, but sufficiently close to give a fusion signal in normal cells, whereas the signal is split in the case of a chromosome aberration.[20,21,21a] In principle, the split signal FISH will not result in false-positive results and thus has an essentially higher sensitivity ($10^{-2}$ to $10^{-3}$) than the fusion-signal FISH.
- *Southern blotting*: sensitivity of only $10^{-1}$ to $10^{-2}$, but application in virtually all lymphoid malignancies with rearranged Ig or TCR genes as well as in malignancies with well-defined chromosome aberrations for which suitable DNA probes are available.[22]

So far only two techniques are sufficiently sensitive, specific, and have a relatively broad applicability: immunophenotyping techniques and PCR techniques (Figure 21.2). The application of immunophenotyping techniques is based on the occurrence of aberrant or unusual immunophenotypes, whereas PCR techniques can be used for the detection of tumor-specific sequences, such as junctional regions of rearranged Ig and TCR genes or breakpoint fusion regions of chromosome aberrations.[14,15] Immunophenotyping and PCR techniques can reach sensitivities of $10^{-3}$ to $10^{-6}$, depending on the immunophenotype and genotype of the lymphoid malignancy. In ALL and MM, both immunophenotyping and PCR techniques can be used for MRD detection. However in CLL and NHL, immunophenotyping techniques are generally not sufficiently sensitive to reach levels of $10^{-3}$. Nevertheless, PCR analysis of Ig and TCR genes can be applied for MRD detection in the majority of these disease categories.

In this chapter, we shall discuss the technical aspects of immunophenotyping and PCR analysis for MRD detection. Subsequently, we shall summarize the clinical applications of these MRD techniques and discuss their clinical relevance in the four categories of lymphoid malignancies.

# MRD detection by immunophenotyping

## Aberrant immunophenotypes as targets for MRD detection

The resemblance of malignant lymphoid cells to cells of normal hematopoietic differentiation stages implies that the detectability of malignant cells is hampered by the presence of normal lymphoid cells within the cell sample.[14,15,23–26] Despite this inherent limitation on the detection of malignant cells, MRD detection is still possible because lymphoid malignancies might display unusual or aberrant antigen expression (Figure 21.3) or clonal patterns of Ig or TCR chain expression.[27–29]

Unusual or aberrant immunophenotypes are the result of cross-lineage antigen expression, asynchronous expression of antigens, antigen overexpression, absence of antigen expression, and/or ectopic antigen

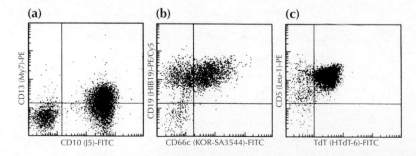

**Figure 21.3** Examples of uncommon and ectopic antigen expression in acute lymphoblastic leukemia (ALL). (a) Weak CD13 expression on CD10+ precursor B-ALL cells. (b) Cross-lineage expression of CD66c (KOR-SA3544) antigen on CD19+ precursor B-ALL cells. (c) Combined expression of the CD5 antigen and TdT constitutes a typical characteristic of T-ALL and is normally only found in cortical thymocytes but not in extrathymic locations such as bone marrow or peripheral blood.

expression.[14,15,25] The latter refers to the expression of particular antigens on cells outside their normal breeding sites or homing areas or to the expression of antigens that are normally only expressed on non-hematopoietic cells. Cross-lineage antigen expression represents the expression of typical B-lineage antigens on T-lineage cells or vice versa, or even of myeloid or other non-lymphoid antigens on cells of either B or T lineages.[14,15] Asynchronous antigen expression refers to the simultaneous expression of antigens that are normally not expressed during the same maturational stage.[14,15]

Clonal Ig molecules can be found in most chronic B-cell leukemias, B-cell NHL (B-NHL), and MM; they are detectable as single Ig light-chain expression, i.e. Igκ or Igλ.[27,28] In chronic T-cell leukemias and in T-NHL, expression of most clonal TCRαβ molecules is detectable with antibodies against the variable (V) domains of TCRβ chains; virtually no antibodies against variable domains of TCRα chains are available.[29-31] Antibodies against the various V domains of TCRγ and TCRδ chains might contribute to clonality assessment of suspect TCRγδ+ T-cell proliferations.[32]

Previously, immunophenotyping of hematopoietic malignancies was performed with fluorescence microscopy using single- and double-immunofluorescence (IF) stainings.[27] However, flow cytometry is superior in analyzing unusual and aberrant antigen expression, because it enables routinely multiparameter analysis with two scatter parameters and at least four fluorochrome (antigen) parameters.[33] This multiparameter analysis can involve both surface membrane and intracellular antigens.[34]

## Precursor B-cell ALL

Several categories of aberrant antigen expression in precursor B-cell ALL (precursor B-ALL) might be used for MRD detection in multiparameter flow cytometry (Table 21.2 and Figure 21.3). This concerns cross-lineage expression of T-lineage antigens (e.g. CD5 and CD7) or myeloid antigens (CD13, CD15, CD33, and CD66c), asynchronous expression of antigens (e.g. CD20 on CD45- cells), lack of CD45 expression (particularly the isoform CD45RA), and antigen overexpression (e.g. CD10 overexpression).[23-26,35-39,39a,39b] The finding of NG2 expression on the surface membrane of precursor B-ALL carrying the t(4;11) or t(11;19) represents an example of a true ectopic antigen expression.[40,41] The studies with cDNA microarrays, analyzing expression levels of thousands of genes, might further aid the discovery of new leukemia-specific markers.[42] Flow-cytometric investigations based on double/triple antigen stainings showed the presence of leukemia-associated phenotypes in 60–95% of precursor B-ALL patients.[38,43-45] Investigation of normal BM precursor B cells has enabled the establishment of multiparameter templates for normal B-cell development, whereas malignant precursor B lymphoblasts frequently display aberrant immunophenotypic features and thereby fall into so-called 'empty spaces' outside the normal B-lineage pathways.[46-48] Preliminary data indicate that the 'empty spaces' approach with triple or preferably quadruple antigen stainings identifies leukemia-associated immunophenotypes in virtually all patients.[47,49] The availability of specific antibodies to fusion proteins or ectopic antigens that are observed in precursor B-ALL with translocations, such as t(1;19) or t(12;21), might further facilitate the specific detection of malignant cells.[50]

It should be emphasized that combinations of typical B-cell precursor markers, such as CD10 antigen and terminal deoxynucleotidyl transferase (TdT), are not suitable for MRD detection in precursor B-ALL. This is owing to the background of normal TdT+ precursor B cells in BM (generally <10% of mononuclear cells) and peripheral blood (PB) (generally <0.4%).[23,51,52] Moreover, the levels of TdT+ (and TdT-) precursor B cells can be as high as 50% in regenerating BM after chemotherapy or after SCT.[23,53] Substantial expansions of normal precursor B cells in regenerating BM take place not only after maintenance therapy, but also during treatment.[54,55] At the end of short intervals after intensive induction and consolidation blocks, regeneration of B-cell development occurs in BM with large fractions of immature CD34+/TdT+ B cells. In contrast, in regenerating BM after cessation of maintenance treatment, the more mature TdT-/CD19+/CD10+ B cells are significantly increased, whereas the fraction of immature CD34+/TdT+ B cells is essentially smaller.[54,55] The extent of B-lineage regeneration in BM also differs per treatment protocol and seems to be dependent on the intensity of the preceding treatment.[54] Interestingly, after maintenance treatment, a substantial proportion (10–30%) of PB B cells express CD10, indicating that CD10+ B cells are easily released from regenerating BM after cessation of therapy.[55] The discrimination between normal and malignant precursor B cells can only be made on the basis of atypical features such as CD10 overexpression on precursor B-ALL cells or molecular clonality analysis. On one hand, moderately increased frequencies of CD19+/CD10+/TdT+ BM cells should never directly be interpreted as relapse of ALL, particularly during the high-dose cytotoxic treatment phases. On the other hand, substantial increase in B-cell precursors after chemotherapy, particularly with a homogeneous immunophenotype, may herald a relapse of the disease.

## T-cell ALL and T-lymphoblastic lymphoma

Nearly all T-cell ALL (T-ALL) express TdT as well as the pan-T-cell antigens CD2, cytoplasmic CD3 (CyCD3), CD5, and CD7. Additional T-cell antigens

## Table 21.2  Detection of MRD in cell samples from patients with a lymphoid malignancy

| Technique | Detection limit | Applicability | Requirements, limitations, and pitfalls |
|---|---|---|---|
| **Immunological marker analysis** | | | |
| • Multiparameter flow cytometry (scatter pattern and four membrane or intracellular antigens) | $10^{-2}$ to $10^{-4}$ | • 60–95% of childhood precursor B-ALL<br>• 80–90% of adult precursor B-ALL<br>• >95% of T-ALL and T-LBL<br>• >90% of MM | • Only applicable in cases with unusual or aberrant immunophenotype (including ectopic and tumor-specific antigen expression)<br>• Normal cell populations (especially in bone marrow) will influence the detection limit |
| • Single Ig light-chain expression: Igκ/Igλ ratio | $10^{-1}$ to $10^{-3}$ | • All Ig light-chain⁺ B-cell malignancies | • Weak SmIg light-chain expression on leukemic cells (e.g. in B-CLL) may hamper their detectability<br>• Occurrence of normal SmIg light-chain⁺ B cells will influence the detection limit |
| • Vβ-Vγ, and Vδ expression: increased TCR V-gene expression | $10^{-1}$ to $10^{-3}$ | • Virtually all TCR⁺ T-cell malignancies | • Occurrence of normal T cells will influence the detection limit<br>• Oligoclonal T-cell subsets might occur in the elderly |
| **PCR techniques** | | | |
| • Junctional regions of rearranged Ig and TCR genes (DNA level) | $10^{-3}$ to $10^{-5}$ | • >90% of precursor B-ALL<br>• >95% of T-ALL<br>• >93% of CLL<br>• >90% of B-NHL and MM<br>• >95% of T-NHL | • Rearrangements have to be detected and identified precisely by use of well-designed PCR primers<br>• The occurrence of somatic hypermutation of Ig genes in B-NHL and MM might prevent proper primer annealing and thereby inhibit detection and identification of Ig gene rearrangements at diagnosis and during follow-up<br>• Junctional regions have to be sequenced in order to design junctional region-specific probes for each individual patient<br>• Oligoclonality and clonal evolution at Ig or TCR gene level may cause false-negative results<br>• Occurrence of normal cells with rearrangements of the same gene segments as the malignant cells influence the detection limit |
| • Chromosome aberrations with well-defined breakpoints at DNA level | $10^{-4}$ to $10^{-6}$ | • 20–25% of T-ALL<br>• 30–35% of precursor B-ALL<br>• 25–40% of B-NHL | • Availability of well-designed PCR primers and/or (inverse) long-distance PCR approaches<br>• Fusion region oligonucleotide probes are useful for identification of PCR products from different patients |
| • Chromosome aberrations resulting in leukemia-specific fusion genes and fusion mRNA (PCR analysis after reverse transcription into cDNA: RT–PCR analysis) | $10^{-4}$ to $10^{-5}$ | • 40–45% of childhood precursor B-ALL<br>• 40–45% of adult precursor B-ALL<br>• 15–20% of T-ALL<br>• 20–25% of childhood NHL<br>• <5% of adult NHL | • Availability of well-designed RT–PCR primers<br>• Cross-contamination of RT–PCR products is the main pitfall (even cross-contamination between samples from different patients appears to occur; this cross-contamination is an underestimated problem)<br>• Detection limit is dependent on the expression level of the fusion gene transcript and the efficiency of the reverse transcriptase step |

ALL, acute lymphoblastic leukemia; LBL, lymphoblastic lymphoma; NHL, non-Hodgkin lymphoma; MM, multiple myeloma; CLL, chronic lymphocytic leukemia.

such as CD1, surface membrane CD3, CD4, and/or CD8 are also often expressed. T-lymphoblastic lymphomas (T-LBL) are lymphomatous counterparts of T-ALL and they also express TdT in combination with one or more T-cell antigens. In healthy individuals, the combination of T-cell marker and TdT expression is found in the cortical thymus, but is absent or rare in extrathymic locations such as BM or PB (<0.3% and <0.02%, respectively). Moreover, if T-cell marker+TdT+ cells are found in BM or PB, they only express CD2 and/or CD7 and no other T-cell antigens such as CD3, CD4, or CD8. Early microscopic dilution experiments have demonstrated that the T-cell antigen/TdT double IF staining technique (Figure 21.4)

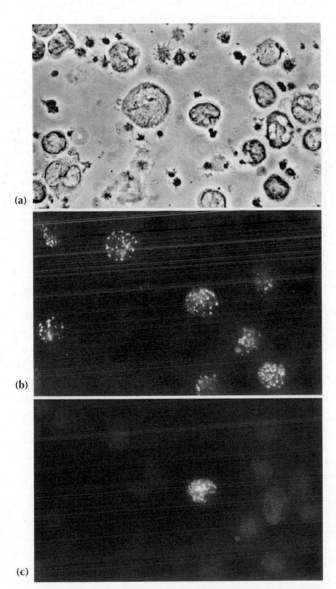

(a)

(b)

(c)

**Figure 21.4** Double-IF staining for a T-cell antigen and TdT on peripheral blood (PB) mononuclear cells of a T-cell acute lymphoblastic leukemia (T-ALL) patient at 20 weeks after diagnosis. (a) Phase-contrast morphology. (b) T-cell antigen-positive cells. (c) TdT+ cell. One cell expresses both the T-cell antigen and TdT, and is probably a T-ALL cell, whereas the other T-cell antigen-positive cells probably represent normal PB T lymphocytes.

has a detection limit of $10^{-4}$ to $10^{-5}$ and that detection of such ectopic double-positive cells via this technique can be used for evaluating the effectiveness of the applied cytotoxic treatment.[14,23] Currently, such analysis is routinely performed via flow-cytometric T-cell marker/TdT stainings, which allows MRD detection in 90% of T-ALL (Table 21.2 and Figure 21.3). Flow-cytometric analysis based on cross-lineage myeloid antigen expression, asynchronous antigen expression (e.g. CD34+/CD3+), and antigen overexpression (e.g. CD7++), can also be used for MRD detection in T-ALL.[56,57] Similarly to precursor B-ALL, multiparameter flow cytometry in T-ALL reveals 'empty spaces' outside the templates for normal T-cell development in BM and PB.[57] Together, the various leukemia-associated immunophenotypes can be employed for MRD detection in all T-ALL and T-LBL.[56,57] The presence of tumor-specific antigens resulting from chromosome aberrations may further increase the number of immunophenotypic MRD targets per T-ALL patient. One important candidate is the TAL1 protein, which is ectopically expressed in T-ALL with the *SIL–TAL1* fusion gene or *TAL1* gene translocations.[58,59]

## CLL and NHL

The relatively high frequencies of mature lymphoid cells in BM and PB hampers immunophenotypic MRD detection in patients with CLL of B or T lineage. In an analogous way, immunophenotypic MRD detection in B-cell or T-cell NHL (B-NHL or T-NHL) can also be hampered by the presence of mature lymphoid cells in lymph nodes and in potentially involved BM or PB compartments. Due to the normal background of lymphoid cells, low levels of MRD (<$10^{-3}$) will only be detectable if antibodies against tumor-associated antigens are used, e.g. antibodies directed against fusion proteins derived from chromosome aberrations that are specific for a particular type of CLL or NHL or antibodies directed against particular antigens that are normally not expressed on normal counterparts of CLL and NHL.

### Chronic B-cell leukemias and B-cell NHL

Single Ig light-chain (Igκ or Igλ) expression can be employed for the detection of Ig+ B-cell leukemias and Ig+ B-NHL, since normal and malignant B lymphocytes express only one type of Ig light chain.[27,28] The distribution of Igκ+ versus Igλ+ cells (the Igκ/Igλ ratio) can accurately be determined by analysis of Igκ and Igλ expression within the B-cell population in multicolor stainings, using CD19, CD20, and/or CD37 as pan-B-cell antigens. In normal B-cell populations, the Igκ/Igλ ratio ranges from 0.8 to 2.5. The size of the normal B-cell population in BM, PB, and lymph nodes obviously influences the detectability of leukemic B cells via analysis of the Igκ/Igλ ratio. Due to this normal background, the detection limit of routinely performed Ig light-chain/B-cell marker stainings in BM and PB is only $10^{-1}$ to $10^{-2}$ (Table 21.2 and Figure 21.5).[27,28]

The use of additional antigens in multicolor stainings may allow MRD detection with levels around $10^{-3}$

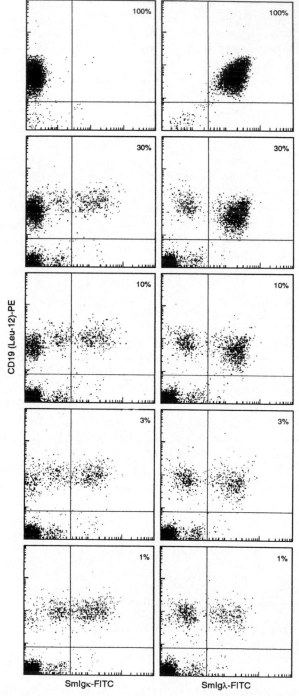

**Figure 21.5** SmIgκ/CD19 and SmIgλ/CD19 double-IF stainings on serial dilutions of SmIgλ+ B-cell non-Hodgkin lymphoma (B-NHL) cells in peripheral blood mononuclear cells of a healthy individual. The percentages of B-NHL cells that are present in each dilution step are indicated. The detection limit of SmIg/CD19 double-IF stainings is clearly influenced by the frequency of normal polyclonal B lymphocytes.

(Table 21.2). Such additional markers may involve antigens that are normally only expressed on a sub-population of B cells. Examples include the CD103 antigen on hairy cell leukemia (HCL) and the CD5 antigen on B-CLL and mantle cell lymphoma (MCL) cells.[60–62] Furthermore, protein products from particular chromosome aberrations may also be used as additional markers in IF stainings. Triple IF staining for $BCL_2$, a B-cell antigen and Ig light chain may be employed for MRD detection in patients with follicular lymphomas (FL), since BCL2 overexpression is observed in this type of B-NHL with t(14;18).[63] Similarly, the overexpression of cyclin D1 in MCL with t(11;14) or of MYC in Burkitt lymphomas with t(2;8), t(8;14), or t(8;22) may be employed for MRD detection of these types of B-NHL.[64]

With the advent of multiparameter flow cytometry, particularly with quadruple stainings, it now seems to be possible to identify quantitative differences in the levels of antigen expression in B-CLL as compared with normal B cells. This approach, analogous to the detection of 'empty spaces' outside the normal B-lineage development in ALL, can potentially reach sensitivities of $10^{-4}$.[65,66] In a report by Rawstron et al,[65] the combination of CD19/CD5/CD20/CD79b antibodies was claimed to be informative for MRD detection in PB in all tested B-CLL patients. For MRD monitoring in BM, at least one of the combinations CD19/CD5/CD20/CD79b, CD19/CD5/CD38/CD79b, and CD19/CD5/CD38/CD20 was found to be sufficiently sensitive and specific.[65]

### Chronic T-cell leukemias and T-NHL

The relatively high frequencies of T lymphocytes and natural killer (NK) cells in normal BM and PB samples and lymph nodes have their impact on the immunophenotypic detectability of leukemic T cells and T-NHL cells. Even the expression of the less common CD3+CD4−CD8−, CD3+CD4+CD8+ or TCRγδ+ phenotypes as well as antigen loss (absence of particular T-cell antigens) will generally result in detection limits of only $10^{-1}$ to $10^{-2}$.

The vast majority of chronic T-cell leukemias and T-NHL belong to the TCRαβ lineage, whereas only a minor fraction express TCRγδ. During the last decade or so, a large series of antibodies against the protein products of $V$ gene segments of most *TCRBV* gene families have been produced. Together, these Vβ antibodies recognize 60–70% of normal and malignant T cells with TCRβ chain expression.[29–31] Also, antibodies against most Vγ and Vδ domains of TCRγδ molecules have become available. These Vγ and Vδ antibodies might be useful for the detection and monitoring of malignant (clonal) TCRγδ+ T cells,[32] although the presence of normal TCRγδ+ T lymphocytes will interfere with these applications. This especially concerns Vγ9/V$_{\delta_2}$ phenotypes, because

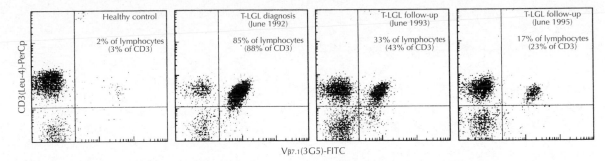

**Figure 21.6** Double-IF staining for CD3 and Vβ7.1. In a healthy individual, only a minor subpopulation of CD3+ T cells express Vβ7.1, whereas in a T-lineage large granular lymphocyte leukemia (T-LGL) patient at diagnosis (June 1992), virtually all CD3+ T lymphocytes expressed Vβ7.1. This single Vβ gene expression was in line with the clonally rearranged *TCRB* genes. Vβ7.1/CD3 double-IF stainings during follow-up allowed rapid and precise monitoring of the Vβ7.1+ T-LGL cells, which decreased to 43% and 23% of CD3+ T lymphocytes during follow-up.

most normal TCRγδ+ T lymphocytes have this TCR phenotype.[67] The application of Vβ, Vγ, and Vδ antibodies in well-chosen multicolor stainings can result in sensitivity levels of approximately $10^{-2}$ (Table 21.2). Such sensitivities do not allow true MRD detection, but may enable monitoring of T-cell leukemia patients during treatment (Figure 21.6) or predicting the possible outgrowth of a dominant subclone in the case of oligoclonal T-cell proliferations.

Detection of lower MRD levels (of about $10^{-3}$) in chronic T-cell leukemia or T-NHL is only possible upon analysis of tumor-associated antigens or translocation-specific fusion gene proteins. The availability of antibodies against the *NPM–ALK* fusion gene protein that is produced in anaplastic large cell lymphomas with t(2;5) can become important in this respect.[68]

## MM

Immunophenotypic MRD detection in MM patients suffers from the presence of normal plasma cells in BM. Analogously to normal B cells, the distribution of Igκ+ and Igλ+ producing cells (Igκ/Igλ ratio) can be determined within the plasma cell population via immunological marker analysis. Flow-cytometric detection of cytoplasmic single Ig light-chain production in combination with the plasma cell antigen CD138 may enable detection of MM cells, resulting in detection limits of $10^{-1}$ to $10^{-2}$ (Figure 21.7). Recent studies applying multiparameter flow cytometry have characterized phenotypic differences between normal and malignant plasma cells. While normal plasma cells are usually CD38+++, CD56–, CD45+, CD20–, CD28–, CD33–, and CD117–, their malignant counterparts typically show aberrant expression patterns of one or more of these antigens. Quadruple flow-cytometric stainings are now claimed to reach sensitivities of $10^{-4}$.[69]

# MRD detection by PCR analysis of rearranged Ig and TCR genes

## Rearrangement of Ig and TCR genes and formation of antigen receptor diversity

The variable domains of the Ig and TCR molecules are involved in antigen recognition and constitute the enormous antigen-specific receptor diversity of the immune system. Each variable domain is encoded by two or more gene segments, which were joined to each other via gene rearrangement processes during early lymphoid differentiation. The variable domains of IgH, TCRβ, and TCRδ chains are encoded by combinations of variable (*V*), diversity (*D*), and joining (*J*) gene segments, whereas variable domains of Igκ, Igλ, TCRα, and TCRγ chains are encoded by *V* and *J* gene segments. Based on the homology of their sequences, the *V*, *D*, and *J* gene segments are grouped in families. The rearrangement processes generally start with *D*-to-*J* joining, followed by *V*-to-*DJ* joining, as illustrated in Figure 21.8 for an Ig heavy-chain (*IGH*) gene rearrangement.[22]

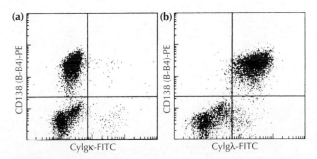

**Figure 21.7** Double-IF staining for the plasma cell antigen CD138 (B-B4) in combination with CyIgκ (a) and CD138 in combination with CyIgλ (b) on bone marrow cells from a multiple myeloma patient.

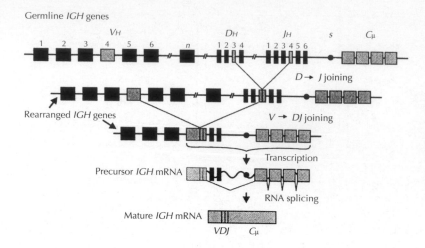

Germline *IGH* genes

**Figure 21.8** Schematic diagram of human *IGH* gene rearrangement. In this example, *D<sub>H3</sub>* is first joined to *J<sub>H4</sub>*, followed by *V<sub>H4</sub>*-to-*D<sub>H3</sub>*-*J<sub>H4</sub>* joining; as a result of the gene segment couplings, all intervening DNA sequences are deleted. The rearranged gene complex can be transcribed into precursor mRNA, which is further processed into mature mRNA by splicing out all non-coding intervening sequences.

Due to the multiple *V*, *D*, and *J* gene segments per Ig and TCR gene locus, many different *V(D)J* combinations can be made via the rearrangement process (Table 21.3). The *V(D)J* combinations and the combination of two protein chains with different variable domains per antigen receptor molecule (IgH and Igκ or Igλ, TCRα and TCRβ, TCRγ and TCRδ) determines the so-called combinatorial repertoire (Table 21.3). The combinatorial repertoire for Ig molecules and TCRαβ molecules (encoded by *TCRA* and *TCRB* genes) is at least $2 \times 10^6$. For TCRγδ molecules, the combinatorial repertoire is smaller (about 5000) due to the limited number of *V*, (*D*), and *J* gene segments in the TCRγ- and TCRδ-encoding genes, i.e. *TCRG* and *TCRD*, respectively (Table 21.3).[22]

The repertoire of Ig and TCR molecules is further extended by so-called junctional diversity, which is based on deletion of germline nucleotides by trimming the ends of the rearranging gene segments and by random insertion of nucleotides between the joined gene segments.[70,71] The insertion of nucleotides at the junction sites is mediated by the nuclear enzyme TdT, which adds nucleotides to 3′ ends of DNA breakpoints without the need for a template. The junctional diversity varies per Ig and TCR gene, depending on the number of junction sites per junctional region (*VJ*, or *VDJ*, or *VDDJ*, etc.) and upon the activity of TdT during the rearrangement process. For instance, junctional regions of *IGH* gene rearrangements are generally extensive (Figure 21.9) as compared with the relatively small junctional regions of the Igκ- and Igλ-encoding genes, i.e. *IGK* and *IGL*, respectively (Table 21.3).[72]

## Secondary rearrangements in Ig and TCR genes

Secondary rearrangements can replace or adapt preexisting rearrangements, depending on the involved Ig or TCR gene and the type of pre-existing rearrangement. *DJ* replacements concern the deletion of pre-existing *DJ* complexes by the joining of an upstream *D* gene segment to a downstream *J* gene segment. In a comparable way, *VJ* replacements can delete a pre-

**Table 21.3 Estimation of potential primary repertoire of human Ig and TCR molecules[a]**

| | Ig molecules | | | TCRαβ molecules | | TCRγδ molecules | |
|---|---|---|---|---|---|---|---|
| | IgH | Igκ | Igλ | TCRα | TCRβ | TCRγ | TCRδ |
| **Number of functional gene segments:** | | | | | | | |
| V gene segments | 40–46 | 34–37 | 30–33 | 45 | 44–47 | 6 | 6 |
| D gene segments | 25[b] | — | — | — | 2[b] | — | 3[b] |
| J gene segments | 6 | 5 | 4 | 50 | 13 | 5 | 4 |
| Combinatorial diversity | | >2 × 10⁶ | | | >2 × 10⁶ | | >5000 |
| Junctional diversity | ++ | ± | ± | + | ++ | ++ | ++++ |
| Estimation of total repertoire | | >10¹² | | | >10¹² | | >10¹² |

[a] Numbers are based on the IMGT (ImMunoGeneTics) database.[300,300a]

[b] In *TCRD* gene rearrangements, multiple *D* segments might be used; this implies that the number of junctions can vary from one to four. In *IGH* and *TCRB* gene rearrangements, generally only one *D* gene segment is used.

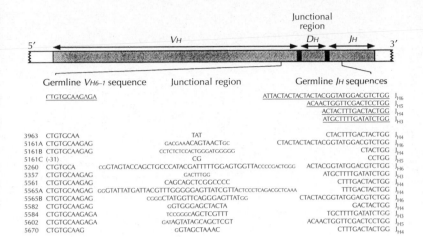

Germline *V*<sub>H6–1</sub> sequence    Junctional region    Germline *J*<sub>H</sub> sequences

| | | | | |
|---|---|---|---|---|
| | CTGTGCAAGAGA | | ATTACTACTACTACTACGGTATGGACGTCTGG | J<sub>H6</sub> |
| | | | ACAACTGGTTCGACTCCTGG | J<sub>H5</sub> |
| | | | ACTACTTTGACTACTGG | J<sub>H4</sub> |
| | | | ATGCTTTTGATATCTGG | J<sub>H3</sub> |
| 3963 | CTGTGCAA | TAT | CTACTTTGACTACTGG | J<sub>H4</sub> |
| 5161A | CTGTGCAAGAG | GACGAAACAGTAACTGC | CTACTACTACTACGGTATGGACGTCTGG | J<sub>H6</sub> |
| 5161B | CTGTGCAAGAG | CCTCTCTCCACTGGGATGGGGG | CTACTGG | J<sub>H4</sub> |
| 5161C (-31) | | CG | CCTGG | J<sub>H5</sub> |
| 5260 | CTGTGCA | CGGTAGTACCAGCTGCCCATACGATTTTTGGAGTGGTTAccccgactggg | ACTACGGTATGGACGTCTGG | J<sub>H6</sub> |
| 5357 | CTGTGCAAGAG | GACTTTGG | ATGCTTTTGATATCTGG | J<sub>H3</sub> |
| 5561 | CTGTGCAAGAG | CAGCAGCTCGGCCCC | CTTTGACTACTGG | J<sub>H4</sub> |
| 5565A | CTGTGCAAGAG | GGGTATTATGATTACGTTTGGGGGAGTTATCGTTActccctcagacgctcaaa | TTTGACTACTGG | J<sub>H4</sub> |
| 5565B | CTGTGCAAGAG | CGGGCTATGGTTCAGGGAGTTATGG | CTACTACGGTATGGACGTCTGG | J<sub>H6</sub> |
| 5582 | CTGTGCAAGAG | GGTGGGAGCTACTA | GACTACTGG | J<sub>H4</sub> |
| 5584 | CTGTGCAAGAGA | TCCCGGGCAGCTCGTTT | TGCTTTTGATATCTGG | J<sub>H3</sub> |
| 5602 | CTGTGCAAGAGA | GATAGTATAGCAGCTCGT | ACAACTGGTTCGACTCCTGG | J<sub>H5</sub> |
| 5670 | CTGTGCAAG | GGTAGCTAAAC | CTTTGACTACTGG | J<sub>H4</sub> |

**Figure 21.9** Schematic diagram of a *V*<sub>H</sub> gene segment joined to one of the *J*<sub>H</sub> gene segments via a junctional region. *IGH* junctional regions may contain one, or rarely two, *D*<sub>H</sub> gene segments. The presented *IGH* junctional region sequences are derived from precursor B-cell acute lymphoblastic leukemia (precursor B-ALL) patients and illustrate the deletion of nucleotides from the germline sequences as well as the size and composition of the junctional regions. *D*<sub>H</sub> gene segments and inserted nucleotides are indicated by capital letters and small capital letters, respectively.

existing *VJ* complex in the *IGK*, *IGL*, *TCRA*, and *TCRG* genes (Table 21.4).[73,74]

Another type of secondary rearrangements concerns *V* replacement in complete *V(D)J* complexes. The *V* gene segment of the *V(D)J* complex is replaced by a new upstream *V* gene segment. This process is mediated via a recombination signal sequence in the downstream part of the *V* gene segments of the *IGH*, *TCRB*, and *TCRG* genes.[75] Such signal sequences are not found within the *V* gene segments of the *IGK*, *IGL*, *TCRA*, and *TCRD* genes (Table 21.4).

Secondary rearrangements occur in immature B and T cells and have been found to replace pre-existing non-productive (out of-frame) rearrangements as well as productive (in-frame) rearrangements. Therefore, it is assumed that secondary rearrangements are not only involved in rescuing precursor B cells and T cells from non-productive rearrangements, but are also involved in receptor editing during selection processes of immature B cells in the BM and immature T cells in the thymus.[76] This implies that such secondary rearrangements can also occur in the malignant counterparts of immature lymphoid cells, i.e. precursor B-ALL and T-ALL.[76–85]

### Somatic mutations in Ig genes

The repertoire of Ig molecules can be further increased and adapted via antigen-induced somatic mutations in the *V(D)J* exon of rearranged Ig genes.[86] These point mutations occur in follicular center B lymphocytes and are not found in virgin B lymphocytes. They are assumed to serve affinity maturation and clonal selection, and precede or coincide with IgH class switching.

Consequently, also malignant counterparts of follicular center B lymphocytes and 'post-follicular' B-cell malignancies have somatically mutated *IGH*, *IGK*, and *IGL* genes.[87] In particular, B cell malignancies with Ig molecules of non-IgM class (IgG, IgA, etc.) show mutated Ig genes. In follicular B-cell lymphomas, the somatic mutation process can still be active, resulting in the formation of subclones with different specificities of the Ig molecules.[88] However, in post-follicular B-cell malignancies (e.g. MM), the somatically mutated *IGH*, *IGK*, and *IGL* genes remain stable.[89]

### Junctional regions as PCR targets for MRD detection

The junctional regions of rearranged Ig and TCR genes are unique 'fingerprint-like' sequences, which are assumed to be different in each lymphoid cell and thus also in each lymphoid malignancy.[14,22] Therefore, junctional regions can be used as tumor-specific targets for MRD–PCR analysis (Table 21.2).[90–93] The PCR primers for amplification of junctional regions are designed at opposite sides, generally within a distance of less than 500 bp. The size limitation of PCR products is an advantage for PCR analysis of junctional regions of rearranged Ig and TCR genes, because the distance between the vast majority of

### Table 21.4 Occurrence of secondary rearrangements in Ig and TCR genes

| | Ig genes | | | TCR genes | | | |
|---|---|---|---|---|---|---|---|
| | **IGH** | **IGK** | **IGL** | **TCRA** | **TCRB** | **TCRG** | **TCRD** |
| *DJ* replacement | I | – | – | – | (+) | – | (+) |
| *VJ* replacement | – | + | (+) | + | – | + | – |
| *V* replacement | + | – | – | – | + | (+) | – |

+, replacement reported to occur; (+), replacement can potentially occur, but is not (yet) reported; –, replacement not likely or impossible to occur.

germline gene segments is far too large to be covered by PCR amplification, whereas juxtaposed rearranged gene segments are easily amplified. For almost every possible gene rearrangement, a primer pair can be made. However, to reduce the number of PCR primers and PCR tests for detection of all possible rearrangements within a particular Ig or TCR locus, generally $V$ and $J$ consensus primers are designed that recognize (virtually) all $V$ and $J$ gene segments of the involved Ig or TCR locus, or $V$ family and $J$ family primers are designed that recognize (virtually) all $V$ and $J$ gene segments of one family.[90–93] The BLOMEO-2 Concerted Action '*PCR-based clonality studies for early diagnosis in lymphoproliferation disorders*'

(BMH4-CTgδ-3g3b) has developed 14 PCR multiplex tubes which can detect the majority of *IGH, IGK, IGL, TCRB, TCRG* and *TCRD* gene rearrangements.[93a]

For MRD–PCR studies, the various Ig and/or TCR gene rearrangements have to be identified in each lymphoid malignancy at diagnosis by using the various PCR primer sets (Table 21.2). It should be assessed whether the obtained PCR products are derived from the malignant cells and not from normal polyclonal cells with comparable Ig or TCR gene rearrangements. For this purpose, the PCR products are analyzed for their clonal origin, for example by heteroduplex analysis or by GeneScan analysis (Figure 21.10).[94,95] Subsequently, the

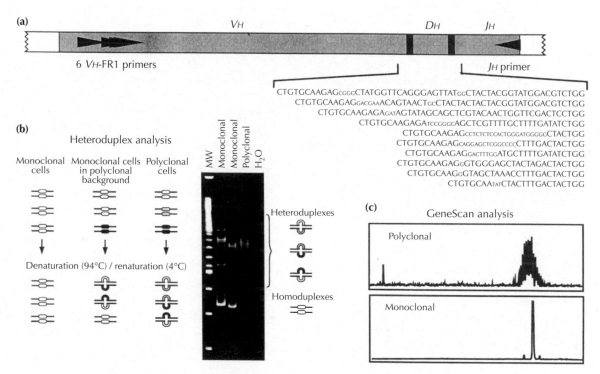

**Figure 21.10**  (a) Schematic diagram of $V_H$-$D_H$-$J_H$ junctional regions with primers for PCR analysis. The approximate positions of the $V_H$-family-specific framework 1 ($V_H$-FR1) primers as well as of a $J_H$ consensus primer are indicated. The presented junctional region sequences are derived from precursor B-ALL patients and illustrate the deletion of nucleotides from the germline sequences as well as the size and composition of the junctional regions. Nucleotides of $V_H$-$D_H$, and $J_H$ gene segments are indicated by capital letters, whereas small capital letters represent inserted nucleotides. (b) Schematic diagram of heteroduplex PCR analysis, in which the junctional region heterogeneity of PCR products of rearranged Ig or TCR genes is employed to discriminate between PCR products derived from monoclonal and polyclonal lymphoid cell populations. In heteroduplex analysis, PCR products are heat-denatured and subsequently rapidly cooled to induce duplex (homo- or heteroduplex) formation. In cell samples consisting of clonal lymphoid cells, the PCR products of rearranged Ig or TCR genes give rise to homoduplexes after denaturation and renaturation, whereas in samples that contain polyclonal lymphoid cell populations, the single-strand PCR fragments will mainly form heteroduplexes upon renaturation. In the case of an admixture of monoclonal cells in a polyclonal background, both homo- and heteroduplexes are formed. Because of differences in conformation, homo- and heteroduplexes can be separated from each other by electrophoresis in non-denaturing polyacrylamide gels. Homoduplexes with perfectly matching junctional regions migrate more rapidly through the gel than heteroduplex molecules with less perfectly matching junctional regions. The latter form a background smear of slower-migrating fragments. (c) Automated high-resolution fluorescence-based PCR fragment analysis for identification of clonally rearranged *IGH* genes (fluorescent GeneScan analysis). Polyclonal $V_H$-$J_H$ PCR products form a cluster of peaks reflecting a Gaussian distribution of average junctional region sizes in normal B cells. Monoclonal gene rearrangements form single high-fluorescence peaks, representing products of identical size.

precise nucleotide sequence of the junctional regions should be determined. This sequence information allows the design of junctional region-specific oligonucleotides (Table 21.2). These oligonucleotides can be used to detect malignant cells among normal lymphoid cells during follow-up of patients in two different ways. One possibility is the use of the oligonucleotides as patient-specific junctional region probes in hybridization experiments to detect PCR products derived from the malignant cells (Figures 21.11 and 21.12). The other possibility is to use the junctional region-specific oligonucleotides as PCR primers to amplify the rearrangements of the malignant clone specifically.

## Sensitivity of PCR analysis of junctional regions

Theoretically the detection limit of MRD–PCR analyses of junctional regions is maximally of order $10^{-6}$.

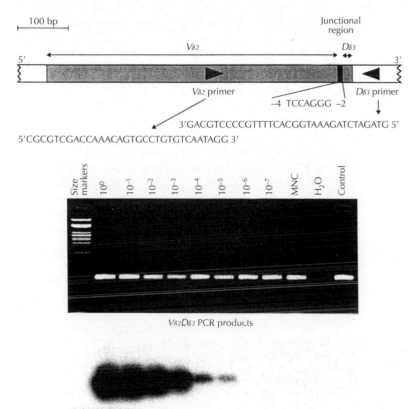

Hybridization with junctional region probe (CTGTGA<u>TCCAGGG</u>TGGGGGA)

**Figure 21.11** Precursor B-cell acute lymphoblastic leukemia (precursor B-ALL) patient with a $V\delta2$-$D\delta3$ rearrangement as a PCR target for MRD detection. The specificity of the junctional region is based on the deletion of six nucleotides and the random insertion of seven nucleotides. This sequence information was used for the design of a patient-specific junctional region probe. DNA from the ALL cells was diluted into DNA from normal mononuclear blood cells (MNC) and subjected to PCR analysis with $V\delta2$ and $D\delta3$ primers. PCR products were size-separated in an agarose gel, blotted onto a nylon membrane, and hybridized with the junctional region probe. In all dilution steps and in the MNC, $V\delta2$-$D\delta3$ PCR products were found, but only the first five dilution steps appeared to contain leukemia-derived PCR products, i.e. a sensitivity of $10^{-5}$ was reached.

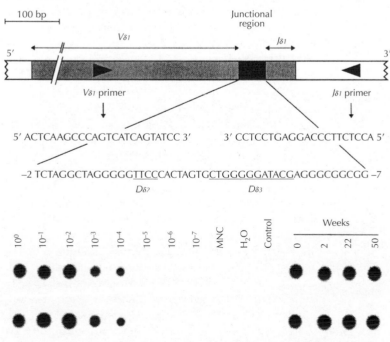

Dot blot hybirdization with junctional region probe (GGATACG<u>AGGGCGGCGG</u>TAA)

**Figure 21.12** A complete *TCRD* rearrangement was used to monitor a T-cell acute lymphoblastic leukemia (T-ALL) patient. The large junctional region of the $V\delta1$-$J\delta1$ rearrangement contained $D\delta2$ and $D\delta3$ sequences. The size of the junctional region was 48 nucleotides, the $D\delta2$ and $D\delta3$ sequences inclusive. PCR amplification was performed using $V\delta1$ and $J\delta1$ primers on DNA from the diagnosis dilution series and from bone marrow follow-up samples (in weeks). Hybridization of the spotted PCR products with the junctional region probe resulted in a sensitivity of $10^{-4}$. All follow-up time points tested gave a signal representative of a high tumor load of $\geq 10^{-2}$, based on comparison with the signals from the diagnosis dilution series. This patient had a clinical relapse 50 weeks after diagnosis. According to molecular MRD detection, this patient was persistently positive and never reached remission.

This is based on the assumption that one million cells, equivalent to about 6.5 μg of DNA, can be tested in one reaction tube, although generally only 1 μg of DNA is used per tube.[14] However, the sensitivity of MRD–PCR analysis of junctional regions is also dependent on the type of rearrangement, on the size of the junctional region, and on the 'background' of normal lymphoid cells with comparable Ig or TCR gene rearrangements. Junctional regions of complete $VDJ$ rearrangements are extensive, whereas junctional regions of $VJ$ rearrangements are 3–4 times smaller. Normal cells can contain the same rearranged gene segments as the leukemic cells. For instance, $V_{\delta 1}\text{-}J_{\delta 1}$ rearrangements frequently occur in T-ALL, but also in a small fraction (0.1–2%) of normal blood T cells; $V_{\gamma 1}\text{-}J_{\gamma 1.3}$ and $V_{\gamma 1}\text{-}J_{\gamma 2.3}$ rearrangements occur in many T-cell malignancies, but are also found in a large fraction (70–90%) of normal blood T cells. This might significantly influence sensitivity levels, particularly taking into account the abundance of polyclonal $V_{\gamma}\text{-}J_{\gamma}$ joinings in normal T cells in postinduction follow-up samples.[96] Therefore, MRD–PCR analysis of long $V_{\delta 1}$-$J_{\delta 1}$ junctional regions in PB samples is generally more sensitive ($10^{-4}$ to $10^{-5}$) than MRD–PCR analysis of short $V_{\gamma}\text{-}J_{\gamma}$ junctional regions ($10^{-3}$ to $10^{-4}$).[97,98] Similarly, substantial expansions of normal precursor B cells with polyclonal $IGH$ gene rearrangements in regenerating BM during and after therapy might affect the sensitivity of MRD detection using Ig gene rearrangements as PCR targets.[54,55]

## MRD–PCR analysis of junctional regions in ALL

### Ig and TCR gene rearrangements in precursor B-ALL

Virtually all precursor B-ALL (96%) have rearranged $IGH$ genes.[99,100] In most cases (80–90%), this concerns complete $V_H\text{-}D_H\text{-}J_H$ rearrangements on at least one allele. Incomplete $D_H\text{-}J_H$ rearrangements can be identified in 22% of patients, being the sole $IGH$ gene rearrangements in only 5% of patients.[100] The usage of $V_H$ gene segments in complete $V_H\text{-}D_H\text{-}J_H$ rearrangements seems to reflect the proximity to $J_H$ gene segments, with the preferential utilization of the most downstream $V_{H6}$ segment.[100,101] Most precursor B-ALL contain $IGK$ gene rearrangements (30%) or deletions (50%); even 20% of precursor B-ALL cases have $IGL$ gene rearrangements.[99,102–104,104a] Deletions in the $IGK$ genes are predominantly mediated via the $IGK$ deleting element ($Kde$) sequence, which implies that $IGK$ gene deletions can be identified as $Kde$ rearrangements. Such rearrangements occur in 50% of cases, whereas in 20% even biallelic $Kde$ rearrangements are found.[103] Interestingly, the size of the junctional regions in $Kde$ rearrangements is relatively extensive in precursor B-ALL as compared with similar rearrangements in mature B-cell malignancies.[105]

Cross-lineage TCR gene rearrangements occur at high frequency in childhood precursor B-ALL: $TCRB$, $TCRG$, and $TCRD$ gene rearrangements and/or deletions are found in 35%, 60%, and 90% of cases, respectively.[106,107,107a] However, the spectrum of cross-lineage TCR gene rearrangements in precursor B-ALL is very limited. $TCRB$ gene rearrangements are restricted to the $J_{\beta 2}$ region.[107] This is in contrast to normal T cells and T-ALL, which employ both $J_{\beta 1}$ and $J_{\beta 2}$ gene regions.[108] $TCRG$ gene rearrangements in childhood precursor B-ALL are most frequently (about 70%) rearrangements to $J_{\gamma 1}$ region gene segments.[107] Remarkably, 80% of $TCRD$ gene rearrangements represent incomplete $V_{\delta 2}\text{-}D_{\delta 3}$ or $D_{\delta 2}\text{-}D_{\delta 3}$ joinings,[107,109] whereas complete rearrangements to the $J_{\delta 1}$ gene segment, characteristic of normal T cells and T-ALL blasts (particularly TCRγδ+ [32,110]), have been reported in precursor B-ALL only anecdotally.[111] Furthermore, $V_{\delta 2}\text{-}D_{\delta 3}$ rearrangements are prone to continuing rearrangements, particularly to $J_{\alpha}$ gene segments with concomitant deletion of the $C_{\delta}$ exons and subsequent $V_{\alpha}\text{-}J_{\alpha}$ recombination.[85,112] In fact, about 40% of $TCRD$ gene deletions in childhood precursor B-ALL probably result from a $V_{\delta 2}\text{-}J_{\alpha}$ recombination, while the remaining approximately 60% of $C_{\delta}$ deletions most probably are caused by $V_{\alpha}\text{-}J_{\alpha}$ rearrangements.[107] Interestingly, the occurrence of cross-lineage TCR gene rearrangements seems to be age-dependent.[113,114] For example, the incidence of incomplete $V_{\delta 2}\text{-}D_{\delta 3}$ gene rearrangements significantly decreases with patient age, while $TCRG$ gene rearrangements are rarely found in patients below 2 years of age.[113–115,115a]

### TCR and Ig gene rearrangements in T-ALL

Subclassification of T-ALL into CD3−, TCRγδ+, and TCRαβ+ subgroups reveals major differences in TCR gene rearrangement patterns.[102,116] Although the frequency of TCR gene rearrangements in the total group of T-ALL is very high, approximately 10% of CD3− T-ALL still have all TCR genes in germline configuration;[102,116] this mainly concerns immature CD1−CD3− T-ALL of the prothymocytic/pre-T-ALL subgroup. The $TCRD$ genes in CD3− T-ALL are rearranged in most cases (approximately 80%) and contain biallelic deletions in approximately 10% of cases.[116,117] As expected, all TCRγδ+ T-ALL have $TCRG$ and $TCRD$ gene rearrangements and the vast majority (approximately 95%) also contain $TCRB$ gene rearrangements.[32,117] All TCRαβ+ T-ALL contain $TCRB$ and $TCRG$ gene rearrangements and have at least one deleted $TCRD$ allele (= $TCRA$ rearrangement); the second $TCRD$ allele is also deleted in two-thirds of cases.[102,117] Analysis of the $TCRG$ gene configuration in T-ALL showed that TCRγδ+ T-ALL display a less mature $TCRG$ immunogenotype as compared with TCRαβ+ and most CD3− cases.[118] This is reflected by significantly higher usage of the more downstream $V_{\gamma}$ genes and the more upstream $J_{\gamma 1}$ segments in TCRγδ+ T-ALL.[32,118] Despite the described immunobiological differences between the T-ALL subsets, in virtually all childhood T-ALL (>95%), *TCRG* and/or *TCRD* junctional regions are potentially suitable targets for MRD monitoring.[98,117,118]

Cross-lineage Ig gene rearrangements occur at a relatively low frequency in T-ALL (approximately 20%) and almost exclusively involve *IGH* genes.[102] Interestingly, cross-lineage *IGH* gene rearrangements occur more frequently in CD3⁻ T-ALL (approximately 20%) and TCRγδ⁺ T-ALL (approximately 50%) than in TCRαβ⁺ T-ALL (less than 5%).[119] Heteroduplex PCR analysis showed a high frequency (approximately 80%) of incomplete $D_H$-$J_H$ rearrangements, as well as preferential usage of $D_{H6-19}$ and the most downstream $D_{H7-27}$ gene segment together with the most upstream $J_{H1}$ and $J_{H2}$ gene segments. Complete $V_H$-$J_H$ recombinations comprised only 18% of cross-lineage *IGH* gene rearrangements in T-ALL patients.[119]

## Ig/TCR gene rearrangements as MRD–PCR targets in ALL

Junctional regions of *IGH*, *IGK* (especially *Kde*), *TCRG*, and *TCRD* gene rearrangements are convenient MRD–PCR targets, because they require only a limited number of PCR primer sets. Furthermore, the vast majority (over 90%) of precursor B-ALL patients can be monitored by application of junctional regions of *IGH*, *IGK*, *TCRG*, and/or *TCRD* gene rearrangements (Table 21.5). In virtually all T-ALL (over 95%) *TCRG* and/or *TCRD* junctional regions are suitable targets for MRD monitoring (Table 21.5).

## Oligoclonality and clonal evolution of Ig and TCR gene rearrangements

Ig and TCR gene rearrangements in precursor B-ALL and T-ALL might be prone to subclone formation due to continuing rearrangements or secondary rearrangements mediated via the active recombinase enzyme system in these immature lymphoid malignancies (reviewed in reference 120). The *IGH* gene rearrangements in particular are known to change in the time period between diagnosis and relapse. In fact, at diagnosis, multiple *IGH* gene rearrangements are already found in 30–40% of precursor B-ALL, indicating the presence of biclonality or oligoclonality.[99] The problem of oligoclonality at diagnosis is the uncertainty as to which clone is going to emerge at relapse, and should be monitored with MRD–PCR analysis. Most continuing or secondary *IGH* gene rearrangements represent $V_H$ to $D_H$-$J_H$ rearrangements or $V_H$ replacements, respectively.[80,81] During these rearrangements the $D_H$-$J_H$ junctional region remains unaffected, leading to the concept of designing the primers around the relatively stable $D_H$-$J_H$ region in order to prevent false-negative PCR results.[80,81,121]

TCR gene oligoclonality is rarely seen at diagnosis in T-ALL.[77,102,118] In contrast, combined Southern blot and PCR data show that the frequency of oligoclonality in the cross-lineage TCR gene rearrangements of precursor B-ALL is approximately 20%, which is slightly less than in the *IGH* gene.[107] Initially, subclone formation at diagnosis was thought to be less

---

**Table 21.5 Frequencies of identifiable Ig and TCR gene rearrangements as MRD–PCR targets in acute lymphoblastic leukemia (ALL)[a]**

| Gene | Rearrangement type | Precursor B-ALL | T-ALL |
|------|-------------------|-----------------|-------|
| *IGH* | $V_H$-$J_H$ | 93% | 5% |
| | $D_H$-$J_H$ | 20% | 23% |
| | Total *IGH* | 98% | 23% |
| *IGK* | $V_\kappa$-*Kde* | 45% | 0% |
| | Intron RSS–*Kde* | 25% | 0% |
| | total *IGK*–*Kde* | 50% | 0% |
| *TCRG* | $V_\gamma$-$J_\gamma$ | 55% | 95% |
| *TCRD* | $V_\delta$-$J_{\delta 1}$ or $D_\delta$-$J_{\delta 1}$ | <1% | 50% |
| | $V_{\delta 2}$-$D_{\delta 3}$ or $D_{\delta 2}$-$D_{\delta 3}$ | 40% | 5% |
| | Total *TCRD* | 40% | 55% |
| At least one PCR target | | >95%[b] | >95%[b] |
| At least two PCR targets | | 90%[b] | 90%[b] |
| At least three PCR targets | | ~65% | ~50% |

[a] The indicated frequencies solely refer to the presence of PCR-detectable rearrangements.
[b] When a high sensitivity of ≤10⁻⁴ is included as an extra criterion, the frequency of at least one sensitive PCR target drops to 85–90% and the frequency of at least two sensitive PCR targets drops to approximately 80%.

frequent for the *TCRD* gene complex, as suggested by Southern blotting.[117] However, PCR heteroduplex analysis and sequencing have shown that $V_{\delta 2} D_{\delta 3}$ and $D_{\delta 2} D_{\delta 3}$ rearrangements in newly diagnosed precursor B-ALL are oligoclonal in 30–40% of cases.[82,107,113] $V_{\delta 2}$ $D_{\delta 3}$ rearrangements are also prone to continuing rearrangements, particularly to $J_\alpha$ gene segments with concomitant deletion of the $C_\delta$ exons.[82,85]

False-negative results due to clonal evolution are a major drawback of using Ig/TCR gene rearrangements as PCR targets for MRD detection. Changes in Ig/TCR gene rearrangement patterns at relapse occur at high frequency in childhood precursor B-ALL, particularly when subclone formation is already present at diagnosis.[77,83,84,122] Monoclonal MRD–PCR targets in childhood precursor B-ALL are characterized by high stability, with approximately 90% of all targets detectable at relapse. In contrast, only 40% of the oligoclonal MRD–PCR targets are preserved at relapse.[122] Therefore, it is probably important to discriminate between monoclonal and oligoclonal Ig/TCR rearrangements, which requires a combined Southern blot and PCR approach. Southern blotting is particularly informative for detection of oligoclonality in *IGH* and *IGK* gene rearrangements,[99,102] whereas heteroduplex PCR analysis in combination with Southern blotting is informative for detection of oligoclonal *TCRD* gene rearrangements.[82,107] At present, the *IGK-Kde* gene rearrangements are considered to be the most stable MRD–PCR targets, probably because they are rarely oligoclonal and represent end-stage rearrangements, which do not allow continuing or secondary rearrangements.[122,123]

Despite the high frequency of immunogenotypic changes in childhood ALL at relapse, at least one rearranged *IGH*, *TCRG*, and/or *TCRD* allele remains stable in 75–90% of precursor B-ALL and in 90% of T-ALL.[77,83,84,122,124,124a,b,c] More importantly, in most ALL patients, at least two suitable PCR targets are available (Table 21.5). Therefore, it is now generally accepted that MRD–PCR studies should preferably employ at least two Ig/TCR targets per patient. Such approach should result in a major reduction of false-negative MRD results.

## PCR analysis of Ig genes in mature B-cell malignancies

All mature Ig+ B-cell malignancies contain *IGH* gene rearrangements, most of them on both alleles. Igκ+ B-cell malignancies contain one rearranged *IGK* allele (about 80% of cases) or two rearranged alleles (about 20% of cases).[102,103] *IGL* gene rearrangements are rare in Igκ+ B-cell malignancies (Table 21.6). Igλ+ B-cell malignancies contain *IGL* gene rearrangements on one allele (about 75%) or both alleles (about 25%) and also have at least one deleted *IGK* allele, but generally biallelic *IGK* gene deletions are found (Table 21.6).[125]

The Ig gene rearrangements in mature B-cell malignancies provide several PCR targets for MRD studies (Table 21.2). Indeed, in most chronic B-cell leukemias, the Ig gene rearrangements can easily be detected and used as MRD–PCR targets, because they generally do not contain somatic mutations.[126] However in many B-NHL, especially follicular and

### Table 21.6 Frequencies (%) of detectable Ig and TCR gene rearrangements and deletions in mature lymphoid malignancies

| | IGH | IGK | | IGL | TCRB | TCRG | TCRD | |
| | R | R | D | R | R | R | R | D |
|---|---|---|---|---|---|---|---|---|
| **B-lineage** | | | | | | | | |
| Smκ+ B-CLL, B-PLL, HCL, and MM | 100 | 100 | 0 | 5 | <5 | <5 | 0 | 0 |
| Smλ+ B-CLL, B-PLL, HCL, and MM | 100 | 25 | 75 | >98 | <5 | <5 | 0 | 0 |
| **T-lineage** | | | | | | | | |
| ATLL, MF/SS, and T-PLL[a] | <5 | 0 | | 0 | 100 | 100 | 10–25 | 75–90 |
| **LGL**[b] | | | | | | | | |
| TCRαβ+ LGL | <5 | 0 | | 0 | 100 | 100 | <25 | >75 |
| TCRγδ+ LGL | 0 | 0 | | 0 | ~50 | 100 | 100 | 0 |
| NK-LGL | 0 | 0 | | 0 | 0 | 0 | 0 | 0 |

R, at least one rearranged allele; D, both alleles deleted; CLL, chronic lymphocytic leukemia; PLL, prolymphocytic leukemia; HCL, hairy cell leukemia; MM, multiple myeloma; ATLL, adult T-cell leukemia/lymphoma; MF/SS, mycosis fungoides/Sézary syndrome; LGL, large granular lymphocyte leukemia.
[a] The vast majority of ATLL, MF/SS, and T-PLL probably belong to the TCRαβ lineage.
[b] Most LGL leukemias express TCRαβ (70–80%), some express TCRγδ (10–15%), and some belong to the NK lineage (10–15%).

post-follicular B-NHL, as well as in MM, somatic mutations in the Ig genes may lead to false-negative results, because of the inability of proper PCR primer annealing.[86,89] This problem can partly be overcome by use of multiple V and J consensus primer sets in the hope that at least one primer set is not hampered by the somatic mutations. Such an approach is successful in 70–90% of cases.[127] In addition, $D_H$-$J_H$ rearrangements as well as recombinations involving the Kde might provide extra MRD–PCR targets. Such a complementary approach involving all possible rearrangements in Ig loci will provide optimal targets in MRD–PCR studies in over 90% of cases.

The somatic mutation process tends to focus on the V(D)J exon of the rearranged IGH, IGK, and IGL genes, whereas further upstream and downstream sequences are progressively less affected. Consequently, the leader sequences upstream of the V(D)J exon and the constant (C) gene segments at the downstream side are probably much less affected by somatic mutations. Therefore, it would be worthwhile to use V leader primers and C primers for RT–PCR analysis of Ig gene transcripts. At the DNA level, this approach will not work easily because of the large intervening distance between the V leader primer and the C primer: 8–10 kb for rearranged IGH genes, 3.5–5 kb for rearranged IGK genes, and 2–2.5 kb for rearranged IGL genes. Sequencing of the V(D)J exons in the obtained RT–PCR products should allow the design of patient-specific V and J primers and junctional region probes for MRD–PCR studies at the DNA level. Nevertheless, it should be noted that false-negative results can still be obtained in follicular B-NHL, which may have an active somatic mutation machinery, leading to subclones that are no longer recognized by the patient-specific primers and/or probes. However, in post-follicular B-NHL and MM, the described approach should work smoothly, because their V(D)J exons are assumed to remain stable throughout the disease course.[89]

### PCR analysis of TCR genes in mature T-cell malignancies

The mature T-cell malignancies should be discriminated from T-ALL and lymphoblastic T-NHL, which are regarded as thymus-derived malignancies based on their positivity for TdT. Mature (post-thymic) T-cell malignancies do not have TdT expression and frequently express TCR molecules. Most chronic T-cell leukemias, such as adult T-cell leukemia/lymphoma (ATLL), mycosis fungoides/Sézary syndrome (MF/SS), and T-cell prolymphocytic leukemia (T-PLL), express TCRαβ molecules, whereas small subsets of large granular lymphocytic leukemias (T-LGL) belong to the TCRγδ lineage or natural killer (NK)-cell lineage (Table 21.6). Also, most T-NHL belong to the TCRαβ lineage, although small categories of TCRγδ+ T-

NHL have been identified (e.g. hepatosplenic T-cell lymphoma).[5]

TCRG gene rearrangements are found in virtually all mature T-lineage malignancies, except for NK-LGL leukemias.[102] In fact, all Ig and TCR genes are in germline configuration in NK-LGL leukemias. Southern blot analysis also showed that all malignancies belonging to the TCRαβ lineage have TCRB gene rearrangements and most of them biallelic TCRD gene deletions (Table 21.6).[108] Thus, MRD studies in mature T-cell malignancies can generally use junctional regions of rearranged TCRG genes as PCR targets (Table 21.2). TCRB genes might also be used as MRD–PCR targets, although the currently available Vβ and Jβ consensus primers are less suitable for reliable detection of all Vβ and Jβ gene segments.[128] With the newly developed BIOMED-2 multiplex PCR strategy for TCRB detection, it is possible to precisely and relatively easy identify most Vβ-Jβ and Dβ-Jβ joinings, which are detectable by Southern blot analysis of TCRB gene rearrangements.[93a,128a,b] Alternatively, It is possible to determine the precise TCRB gene rearrangement via RT–PCR analysis of TCRB gene transcripts using multiple Vβ family primers in combination with a single Cβ primer.[31] As soon as the involved Vβ and Jβ gene segments as well as the junctional region are identified via sequencing, suitable primers and patient-specific junctional region probes can be used for MRD–PCR studies at the DNA level.

In contrast to mature B-cell malignancies, TCR genes are not affected by somatic mutations. For this reason, it should be relatively easy to monitor mature T-cell malignancies during and after treatment.

## MRD detection by PCR analysis of chromosome aberrations

### Chromosome aberrations as PCR targets for MRD detection

Breakpoint fusion regions of chromosome aberrations can be employed as tumor-specific PCR targets for MRD detection in which the PCR primers are chosen at opposite sides of the breakpoint fusion region. Amplification of breakpoint fusion sequences at the DNA level with standard PCR techniques can only be used for chromosome aberrations in which the breakpoints of different patients cluster in a relatively small breakpoint area of preferably less than 2 kb, as PCR products should not exceed about 2 kb in routine MRD–PCR analysis. This is the case in t(14;18), where the BCL2 gene is juxtaposed to one of the J gene segments of the IGH locus. Other examples include T-ALL-associated aberrations such as t(11;14)(p13;q11), t(1;14)(p34;q11), t(10;14)(q24;q11), and the TAL1 deletions. Despite the clustering of the breakpoints, the nucleotide sequences of the breakpoint fusion regions of the above chromosome aberrations differ per patient. Therefore, these breakpoint fusion regions represent unique patient-specific and sensitive PCR targets for MRD detection.[58,129,130]

In most translocations, however, breakpoints of different patients are more widespread, resulting in breakpoint regions of over 2 kb. This implies that in each individual patient, the exact breakpoint has to be determined for PCR primer design, which is more laborious and time-consuming. Recently, simplified strategies have been developed to determine precise DNA breakpoint sequences in ALL patients with t(4;11) and t(12;21) based on multiple long-distance PCR and long-distance inverse PCR, respectively, followed by cloning and sequencing.[131,132] Alternatively, several malignancies with chromosome aberrations have tumor-specific fusion genes that are transcribed into fusion-gene mRNA molecules that are similar in individual patients despite distinct breakpoints at the DNA level. After reverse transcription into cDNA, these fusion-gene mRNA molecules can therefore be used as appropriate targets for MRD–PCR analysis. Examples include *BCR–ABL* transcripts in the case of precursor B-ALL with t(9;22), *E2A–PBX1* mRNA in most pre-B-ALL with t(1;19), *MLL–AF4* transcripts in pro-B-ALL with t(4;11), and *NPM-ALK* mRNA in large cell anaplastic lymphoma with t(2;5).[8,133–136]

An advantage of using chromosome aberrations as tumor-specific PCR targets for MRD detection is their stability during the disease course. However, MRD detection of chromosome aberrations by PCR is not always applicable, because in many lymphoid malignancies, no PCR-detectable chromosome aberrations have yet been found. Depending on the type of tumor-specific PCR target, detection limits of $10^{-4}$ to $10^{-6}$ can be reached by using chromosome aberrations as MRD–PCR targets (Table 21.2). However, because of the high sensitivity of PCR techniques, cross-contamination of RT–PCR products between patient samples is a major pitfall in PCR-mediated MRD studies, resulting in up to 20% of false-positive results.[136] Such cross-contamination is difficult to recognize, since leukemia-specific fusion-gene mRNA PCR products are not patient-specific. This is in contrast to PCR products obtained from breakpoint fusion regions at the DNA level, such as in t(14;18) and *TAL1* deletions, which can be identified by the use of patient-specific oligonucleotide probes.

## ALL

MRD detection is possible in several types of childhood and adult precursor B-ALL because of the presence of particular leukemia-specific fusion gene transcripts, which can be used as MRD–PCR targets. Examples are *BCR–ABL* fusion transcripts, which are especially observed in adult ALL cases with t(9;22), *E2A–PBX1* mRNA in most pre-B-ALL with t(1;19), *MLL–AF4* transcripts that are found at high frequencies in infant pro-B-ALL with t(4;11), and *TEL–AML1* fusion mRNA in childhood precursor B-ALL with t(12;21).[134] In this way, RT–PCR analysis of leukemia-specific fusion gene mRNA for detection of low levels of MRD ($<10^{-4}$) can be applied in 40–45% of precursor-B-ALL (Table 21.7).

**Table 21.7 Chromosome aberrations in ALL as (RT–)PCR targets for MRD detection[a]**

| Aberration | Target (mRNA or DNA) | Frequency of applicability (%)[b] | | |
|---|---|---|---|---|
| | | | Children | Adults |
| **Precursor B-ALL** | | | | |
| t(9;22)(q34;q11) | *BCR–ABL* (mRNA) | | 5–8 | 30–35 |
| t(1;19)(q23;p13) | *E2A–PBX1* (mRNA) | | 5–8 | 3–4 |
| t(4;11)(q21;q23) | *MLL–AF4* (mRNA) | | 3–5[c] | 3–4 |
| 11q23 aberrations | Aberrant *MLL* (mRNA) | | 5–6 | <5 |
| t(12;21)(p13;q22) | *TEL–AML1* (mRNA) | | ~30 | 1–3 |
| | | Total: | 40–45 | 40–45 |
| **T-ALL** | | | | |
| *TAL1* deletion | *SIL–TAL1* (DNA/mRNA) | | 10–25 | 5–10 |
| t(8;14)(q24;q11) | *MYC–TCRA/D* (DNA) | | | |
| t(11;14)(p15;q11) | *LMO1–TCRD* (DNA) | | | |
| t(11;14)(p13;q11) | *LMO2–TCRD* (DNA) | | 5–10 | 5–10 |
| t(1;14)(p34;q11) | *TAL1–TCRD* (DNA) | | | |
| t(10;14)(q24;q11) | *HOX11–TCRD* (DNA) | | | |
| | | Total: | 25–30 | 10–15 |

[a] The detection limit of PCR analysis of chromosome aberrations is $10^{-4}$ to $10^{-6}$.
[b] The indicated percentages represent frequencies within the precursor B-ALL and T-ALL groups.
[c] In infant ALL, the frequency of t(4;11) can be as high as 50%.

In contrast, MRD–PCR analysis of chromosome aberrations is only possible in 15–25% of T-ALL cases and mainly concerns *TAL1* deletions and to some extent t(1;14), t(10;14), and t(11;14) (Table 21.7). Similarly to chromosome aberrations in precursor B-ALL, *TAL1* deletions can be detected at the mRNA level via of *SIL–TAL1* fusion gene transcripts. However, the T-ALL-associated chromosome aberrations can also be analyzed at the DNA level. This latter approach has the advantage that the breakpoint fusion regions can be employed for sensitive patient-specific MRD detection by use of patient-specific oligonucleotides.[58,130]

## CLL

In CLL, MRD detection by (RT–)PCR analysis of chromosome aberrations is hardly possible, because of lack of frequently occurring well-defined chromosome aberrations that can be used as PCR targets. Once particular aberrations are identified that turn out to be common and specific for any of the CLL,

these may be employed for future MRD–PCR studies in these leukemias, either at the DNA level or at the mRNA level, depending on whether breakpoints cluster in small DNA regions or whether fusion genes are formed, respectively.

## NHL

In B-NHL, chromosomal aberrations frequently involve Ig genes. For example, in FL with t(14;18), the *BCL2* gene is joined to $J_H$ gene segments,[137] while in MCL with t(11;14), the *BCL1* gene is joined to $J_H$ gene segments.[138] Furthermore, in Burkitt lymphoma with t(8;14), t(2;8), and t(8;22), one of the Ig loci (*IGH*, *IGK*, and *IGL*, respectively) is coupled to the *MYC* gene.[139] In all of these B-NHL types, the breakpoints generally occur outside coding regions, implying that these translocations are not amenable to RT–PCR analysis for MRD detection, but should be studied at the DNA level. Therefore, the detectability of these chromosome aberrations is dependent on the clustering of the breakpoints of different patients in rela-

**Table 21.8 Frequent chromosome aberrations in NHL and their detectability by Southern blotting (SB) and PCR techniques**

| NHL type | Relative frequency (%) | | Chromosome aberrations | | Detectability per NHL type (%) | | Per total group of NHL (%) | |
|---|---|---|---|---|---|---|---|---|
| | Children | Adults | Type | Involved genes | SB | PCR (DNA/mRNA) | SB | PCR |
| FL | 5 | 20–30 | t(14;18) | *IGH–BCL2* | 80 | 65 (DNA) | 15–20 | 15–20 |
| | | | 3q27[a] | *BCL6* | 5–10 | 5 (DNA) | 1–3 | 1–2 |
| DLBCL | 10 | 25–35 | t(14;18) | *IGH–BCL2* | 20–30 | 15 (DNA) | 4–6 | 4–5 |
| | | | 3q27[a] | *BCL6* | 30–40 | 15 (DNA) | 5–9 | 5–10 |
| MCL | <1 | 5–10 | t(11;14) | *BCL1–IGH* | 70 | 25 (DNA) | 2–5 | 1–2 |
| BL | 35 | 2–3 | t(8;14) | *MYC–IGH* | 75–90 | <50 (DNA) | 1–2 | <1 |
| | | | t(2;8) | *IGK–MYC* | | | | |
| | | | t(8;22) | *IGL–MYC* | | | | |
| SLL | <1 | 15–20 | — | — | — | — | — | — |
| LPL | <1 | 2–3 | t(9;14)[b] | *PAX5–IGH* | ? | ? | ? | ? |
| MALT lymphoma | <1 | 15–20 | t(11;18) | *API2–MALT1* | ? | 20 (mRNA) | ? | 3–5 |
| PTCL | <1 | 7–10 | — | — | — | — | — | — |
| ALCL | 15 | 3–5 | t(2;5) | *NPM–ALK* | ? | 70–80 (mRNA) | ? | 2–4 |
| | — | | t(1;2) | *TPM3–ALK* | ? | 10–20 (mRNA) | ? | <1 |
| Precursor T-LBL | 30 | <1 | *TAL1* deletion | *SIL–TAL1* | 20 | 15–20 (DNA) | <1 | <1 |
| | | | t(1;14) | *TAL1–TCRD* | | | | |
| | | | t(10;14) | *HOX11–TCRD* | | | | |
| | | | t(11;14) | *RHOM1–TCRD* | | | | |
| | | | | | | Total: | 30–40 | 35–45 |

FL, follicular lymphoma; DLBCL, diffuse large B-cell lymphoma; MCL, mantle cell lymphoma; BL, Burkitt lymphoma; SLL, small lymphocytic lymphoma; LPL, lymphoplasmacytic lymphoma; MALT, mucosa-associated lymphoid tissue; PTCL, peripheral T-cell lymphoma; ALCL, anaplastic large cell lymphoma; T-LBL, T-lymphoblastic lymphoma.

?, unknown.

[a] Rearrangements to 3q27 (*BCL6* locus) involve Ig genes in at least 50% of cases, i.e. t(3;14); t(2;3), and t(3;22).

[b] Based on FISH experiments, the frequency of t(9;14) in LPL is at least 50%.

tively small DNA regions. Southern blotting can scan essentially larger DNA regions (10–15 kb) than PCR analysis (1–2 kb) and therefore detects higher frequencies of particular chromosome aberrations in B-NHL (Table 21.8). Nevertheless, in about 30% of B-NHL patients, chromosome aberrations can potentially be used for MRD–PCR studies at the DNA level. The t(14;18) has already proven to be an important and sensitive PCR target for MRD studies in FL due to the presence of a patient-specific breakpoint fusion region by coupling of the *BCL2* and *IGH* genes.[140]

In T-NHL, only a few well-defined translocations are known so far. This concerns the *NPM–ALK* fusion gene that is observed in large cell anaplastic lymphoma with t(2;5) and that can be used for RT–PCR analysis and potentially in some cases for PCR analysis at the DNA level as well.[135] Furthermore, T-LBL in childhood might have the same chromosome aberrations as found in T-ALL, such as *TAL1* deletions (Table 21.8).

## MM

In most MM, chromosome translocations involving *IGH* genes can be found, and several recurrent partner loci have been identified.[141,142] In contrast to the chromosome aberrations in B-NHL, in which breakpoints within the Ig loci are frequently targeted to $J_H$ gene segments, the translocations in MM often appear to involve the switch regions (*S*) of the *IGH* locus.[141] Such illegitimate *IGH* class switch rearrangements or illegitimate deletion of the functional $V_H$-($D_H$)-$J_H$ allele might result in the lack of IgH protein production and IgH⁻ MM phenotype.[143] Future application of these translocations as PCR targets for MRD detection awaits detailed study of the gene fusions in these chromosome aberrations.

# Quantification of MRD levels via PCR analysis of junctional regions and chromosome aberrations

MRD quantification by PCR analysis of Ig/TCR gene rearrangements and chromosome aberrations is a complex process, which is essential for reliable disease monitoring. First, the quantity and 'amplifiability' of isolated DNA/RNA should be ensured. In RT–PCR-based MRD monitoring, the number of fusion mRNA transcripts should be normalized to the number of transcripts of a housekeeping gene. Second minor variations in (RT-) PCR efficiency, primer annealing, and primer extension may lead to major variations after 30–35 PCR cycles. The disadvantages of such PCR endpoint quantification might

(partly) be overcome by using serial dilutions of DNA/RNA isolated from the leukemic cell sample at diagnosis into DNA/RNA of normal mononuclear cells (Figures 21.11 and 21.12).[97] The same dilution series of diagnosis DNA/RNA is generally used to determine the tumor load in a follow-up sample in a semiquantitative manner by comparison of the hybridization signals. This approach gives an indication of the tumor burden in the follow-up sample. More accurate methods are needed to define the tumor load in remission samples, since it is clear for several malignancies that the level of MRD (not simply its presence) provides important prognostic information. A more precise but also more laborious quantification method is based on limiting dilution of MRD-positive remission samples.[144,145] To make this assay reliable, it is necessary to perform replicate experiments to determine the level of MRD positivity. Another less tedious strategy for quantitative PCR uses an internal standard that is coamplified with the target of interest.[146] The internal standard is added in a limited but constant number of copies in each reaction. Quantification by competitive PCR is performed by comparing the PCR signal of the specific target DNA with that of known concentrations of an internal standard, the competitor.[146]

Finally, if the main purpose of the MRD detection is only the recognition of high-risk ALL patients, the sensitivities for detection of clonal Ig/TCR gene rearrangements of $10^{-2}$ to $10^{-3}$ might be sufficient. Such detection levels might be achieved with high-resolution electrophoresis systems such as radioactive fingerprinting or fluorescent gene scanning, without the need for application of patient-specific oligonucleotides.[147,148,148a]

## Real-time quantitative PCR

Within the last few years, a novel technology has become available – 'real-time' quantitative PCR (RQ–PCR).[149,150,150a,b] In contrast to the PCR endpoint quantification techniques decribed above, RQ–PCR permits accurate quantification during the exponential PCR amplification phase. The first available RQ–PCR technique was based on TaqMan technology (Figure 21.13). This assay exploits the $5' \rightarrow 3'$ nuclease activity of the *Taq* polymerase to detect and quantify specific PCR products as the reaction proceeds.[151] Upon amplification, an internal target-specific TaqMan probe (hydrolysis probe) conjugated with a reporter and a quencher dye is degraded, resulting in emission of a fluorescent signal by the reporter dye that accumulates during the consecutive PCR cycles. Because of the real-time detection, the method has a very large dynamic detection range over five orders of magnitude, thereby eliminating the need for performing serial dilutions of follow-up samples (Figure 21.13). Quantitative data can be obtained in a short

**(a)**

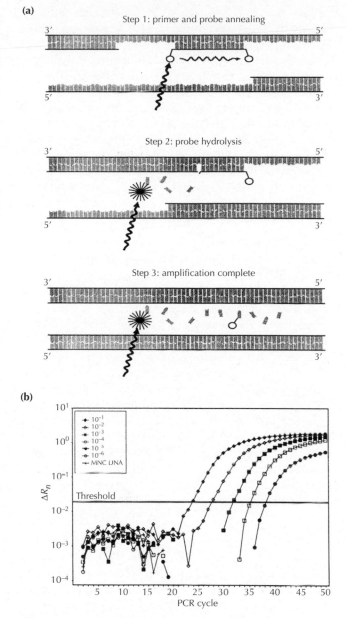

**(b)**

**Figure 21.13** Real-time quantitative (RQ)–PCR analysis by use of the TaqMan technique. (a) The TaqMan probe contains a reporter dye and a quencher dye, which prevents emission of the reporter dye as long as the reporter dye and the quencher dye are closely linked. During the extension phase of each PCR cycle, the annealed TaqMan probe is hydrolyzed by the $5' \rightarrow 3'$ exonuclease activity of the *Taq* polymerase, thereby separating the reporter dye from the quencher dye. This results in a fluorescent signal ($\Delta R_n$), which further increases during each subsequent PCR cycle. (b) Example of an RQ–PCR analysis using the TaqMan approach. Tenfold dilutions of a diagnostic sample in normal mononuclear cell (MNC) DNA were analyzed using an *IGH* rearrangement and an ASO primer.

**(a)**

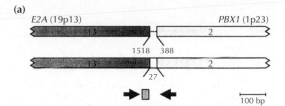

**(b)**

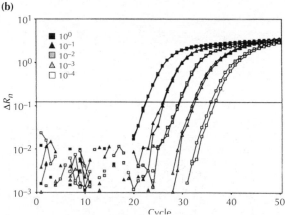

**Figure 21.14** RQ–RT–PCR analysis of *E2A–PBX1* fusion gene transcripts for MRD detection. (a) Schematic diagram of the classical *E2A–PBX1* fusion transcript (upper) and the variant transcript (lower) with an insertion of 27 nucleotides. The arrows and the bar indicate the relative position of the primers and the TaqMan probe, respectively. (b) Example of an RQ–PCR analysis using the TaqMan approach. Tenfold dilutions of a diagnostic sample in normal mononuclear cell cDNA were analyzed using the forward primer and probe positioned in the *E2A* gene and the reverse primer located in the *PBX1* gene. RQ–PCR analysis of the *E2A–PBX1* fusion gene transcript resulted in a sensitivity of $10^{-4}$.

period of time, since post-PCR processing is not necessary. Several groups have shown that RQ–PCR via the TaqMan technology can be used for the quantitative detection of MRD using leukemia-specific chromosome aberrations as PCR targets as well as junctional regions of Ig and TCR gene rearrangements (Figures 21.14 and 21.15).[152–158,158a]

Another type of RQ–PCR technology exploits hybridization probes via the so-called fluorescence resonance energy transfer (FRET) technique, which is usually performed using rapid-cycle RQ–PCR (LightCycler) technology. This method requires two hybridization probes complementary to neighboring sequences – one labeled with a fluorochrome at the 3' end and the other carrying a fluorochrome at the 5' end. One fluorochrome is a donor fluorochrome, whereas the other (the acceptor) emits fluorescent light if it is positioned close to the donor dye. Fluorescence is measured during each annealing step, when both probes hybridize to adjacent target sequences on the same strand.[149,159] Also, in this hybridization probe-based RQ–PCR analysis, the fluorescent signal increases exponentially during the consecutive cycles, in line with the amount of PCR product formed.

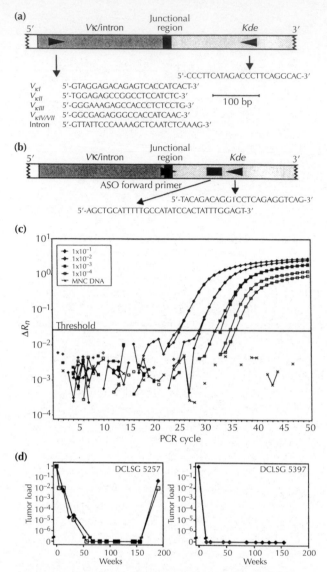

**Figure 21.15** (a) Schematic representation of an *IGK Kde* rearrangement. The position and sequences of the primers used for target identification at diagnosis are indicated.[105] (b) Position of the patient-specific junctional region primer and the position and sequences of the TaqMan probe and the *Kde* reverse primer used for MRD detection via RQ–PCR analysis during follow-up of patients.[123] (c) RQ–PCR amplification plot of a $V_{\kappa II}$ *Kde* rearrangement in a precursor B-ALL patient using a junctional region-specific primer in combination with the *Kde* TaqMan probe and primer. Tenfold dilutions of the diagnostic sample in normal mononuclear cell (MNC) DNA were analyzed at an annealing temperature of 60°C; a reproducible sensitivity of $10^{-4}$ was reached. Normal MNC DNA did not show amplification in any of the four wells tested. (d) Two examples of MRD kinetics during the follow-up as measured with *IGK-Kde* gene rearrangements as RQ–PCR targets. Patient 5257 had high MRD levels at the end of induction treatment and during early consolidation, and consequently was assigned to the MRD-based high-risk group. Patient 5397 was assigned to MRD-based low-risk group, because of the rapid MRD clearance, which was followed by long-term complete remission.[123]

A third possibility for RQ–PCR is detection of SYBR Green I (DNA intercalating dye) fluorescence during PCR, employing patient-specific primers.[149,160] The SYBR Green I dye binds to the minor groove of double-stranded DNA, which greatly enhances its fluorescence. During the consecutive PCR cycles, the amount of double-stranded PCR product will increase, and therefore more SYBR Green I dye can bind to DNA and emit its fluorescence. Maximal SYBR Green I dye binding will occur at the end of each elongation phase. This approach is most cost-effective and is sufficiently sensitive for MRD detection.[160] Future studies should assess whether SYBR Green I-based detection of PCR products also ensures satisfactory specificity.

For each of the above-mentioned RQ–PCR methods, a real-time amplification plot is generated (Figures 21.14 and 21.15). The cycle at which the fluorescence signal exceeds a certain background fluorescence level, referred to as the threshold cycle ($C_T$), is directly proportional to the amount of target DNA present in the sample. Using these approaches, a dilution series of the diagnostic sample can be made, and the amount of residual leukemic cells in follow-up samples obtained during or after treatment can be calculated by using the standard curve of the diagnostic sample. If fusion gene transcripts from chromosome aberrations are used as PCR target for the detection of MRD, copy numbers of fusion gene transcripts can be calculated by referring to a dilution curve of known amounts of plasmids containing (part of) the fusion gene transcript.

With current RQ–PCR methodology, a reproducible sensitivity of $10^{-4}$ can be reached for the majority of currently used MRD–PCR targets. The reproducible sensitivity of a TaqMan primer/probe combination is usually defined as the dilution step with a maximal difference in $C_T$ value of 1.5 between the duplicate dilution samples. Furthermore, the $C_T$ values of the reproducible sensitivity have to be at least three cycles lower than the $C_T$ values found with any non-specific amplification in normal mononuclear cell DNA. In addition to the reproducible sensitivity, the maximal sensitivity can be defined as the maximal 10-fold dilution of the diagnostic sample giving specific but non-reproducible amplification ($\Delta C_T > 1.5$) or giving specific amplification[150a] in one out of the two duplicate wells only.

## Specific clinical applications of MRD detection

### Detection of CNS involvement in ALL patients

The incidence of central nervous system (CNS) involvement in ALL patients at diagnosis is relatively low according to classical morphological criteria for the presence of distinct blasts and/or increased cerebrospinal fluid (CSF) pleocytosis (>5 cells/μl). However, prior to the use of CNS prophylaxis, up to 50% of ALL patients suffered from meningeal relapse, indicating the high frequency of asymptomatic CNS involvement in ALL patients.[161] Therefore, the introduction of preventive therapy for meningeal leukemia is regarded to be a milestone in the progress of leukemia treatment.[162,163]

Normal CSF does not contain TdT[+] or CD34[+] progenitor cells, which implies that their presence provides evidence for meningeal leukemic infiltration. Microscopic immunophenotyping of CSF samples at diagnosis showed the presence of TdT[+] cells in about 25% (11 of 43) of children with ALL, whereas only 1 of the 11 positive cases had overt CNS leukemia according to cytomorphological criteria.[164] During follow-up, 6 children developed CNS leukemia, all belonging to the group with TdT[+] CSF at diagnosis. This implies that TdT staining of CSF samples has high prognostic value and should supplement classical cytomorphology.[164] Monitoring of MRD in CSF samples of more than 100 patients with a TdT[+] malignancy during a 5-year follow-up period showed the development of overt CNS involvement in 70% of the patients with repeated finding of TdT[+] cells in CSF, despite normal cell morphology.[104] On the other hand, patients with increased CSF pleocytosis and/or CSF cells with 'suspicious' morphology but TdT negativity (probably indicative of activated lymphocytes) had no evidence of subsequent CNS disease.[164,165]

Knowledge of the ALL-specific immunophenotypes allows CSF investigation with multiparameter flow-cytometry. The finding of cells with such aberrant immunophenotype is almost always associated with CNS involvement or impending CNS relapse.[166] In contrast, the absence of cells with the ALL-specific immunophenotype in CSF samples suspected of CNS leukemia was reflecting CNS infection or toxicity.[166]

Patient-specific *TCRD* rearrangements have been used as an MRD–PCR target for the detection of CNS involvement in childhood precursor B-ALL.[167] Identical rearrangements were found in both BM and CSF in 43% of the analyzed patients, which confirms the clinical assumption that asymptomatic CNS involvement occurs much more frequently than diagnosed on the basis of classical cytomorphological criteria.[167] Moreover, preliminary data indicate that the molecular finding of MRD in CSF during ALL treatment as assessed via patient-specific Ig/TCR gene rearrangements is inevitably associated with subsequent CNS relapse.[168]

### Early diagnosis of ALL in cases of 'smoldering leukemia'

Hypoplastic bone marrow in ALL patients at presentation is a rare phenomenon, which occurs with a frequency of about 2% in childhood ALL and is rarely seen in cases of adult ALL.[169,170] In contrast to aplastic anemia, the presence of relatively high frequencies of CD10[+]TdT[+] cells in BM and PB is a distinct feature in hypoplastic bone marrow with smoldering leukemia.[51] A few case reports have been published demonstrating the presence of identical clonal cell populations during the hypoplastic phase, the subsequent recovery phase, and the phase characterized by overt leukemia, using patient-specific Ig/TCR gene rearrangements as PCR targets.[171,172] In contrast, monoclonal gene rearrangements could not be detected in patients with idiopathic hypoplastic anemia.[172]

### Diagnosis of leukemia/lymphoma in patients with unexplained cytopenias

In a proportion of patients, unexplained cytopenias might mask underlying malignancies. In a comprehensive multiparameter flow-cytometric study of 121 patients with pancytopenias and/or refractory anemias, Wells et al[173] showed the presence of an abnormal cell population in 17 cases. Further immunophenotyping confirmed the diagnosis of HCL in 8 patients, NHL in 2 patients, and acute myeloid leukemia (AML)/myelodysplastic syndrome (MDS) in the remaining 7 patients. Importantly, the diagnosis of a lymphoid malignancy in 6 patients, which were previously diagnosed as MDS, resulted in a major treatment modification and deferral of SCT is already introduced.[173]

### Detection of bone marrow involvement during 'isolated' extramedullary relapse of ALL

'Isolated' extramedullary relapse (e.g. in CNS or testis) is usually associated with detectable MRD levels in BM. This is in concordance with the clinical observation that full systemic reinduction therapy is required in these patients to prevent impending hematological relapse.[23,174–176] Nevertheless, some ALL patients with isolated CNS relapse were reported without detectable MRD levels in BM.[146,174,177] MRD positivity of histologically normal end-of-treatment testicular biopsies was shown to be followed by overt testicular relapse.[178] Nevertheless, in some patients, testicular relapse did occur despite MRD negativity in testicular biopsies. Moreover, PCR-based MRD assays at the time of a unilateral testicular relapse allow reliable exclusion of occult leukemic blasts in the histologically normal contralateral testis.[178]

### Detection of bone marrow involvement during initial staging of NHL

Immunophenotypic and molecular detection of BM involvement has not yet been implemented into clinical staging of NHL. Initial evaluation of the tumor burden is based on cytomorphological findings, with requirement for bilateral BM aspirations and biopsies in high-grade lymphoma.[179] Several studies demonstrated the presence of aberrant CD5+TdT+ cells in BM of children with T-LBL.[23,180] Similarly, BM involvement detected by *BCL2–IGH* PCR analysis is a constant feature not only of advanced-stage FL with t(14;18) but also of localized stages I and II.[181,182] Preliminary results of a PCR-based MRD study of *IGH* genes in B-NHL demonstrated a higher incidence of BM involvement than suggested by cytomorphological findings.[183] Further prospective studies should reveal whether detection of submicroscopic BM involvement with sensitivities of $10^{-3}$ to $10^{-5}$ would improve prediction of clinical outcome in lymphoma patients. If so, MRD-positive patients might receive more intensive treatment, including SCT.

## MRD detection in autologous bone marrow grafts

### Detection of MRD in autologous grafts in ALL patients

Autologous purged bone marrow transplantation (BMT) and autologous peripheral blood stem cell transplantation (PBSCT) following intensified chemotherapy are currently being evaluated as new treatment modalities in aggressive lymphoproliferative diseases. These treatment strategies are used in high-risk ALL patients in second complete remission who do not have a matched related donor. PCR studies showed that MRD positivity of the autologous BM graft before purging is the most predictive factor of treatment failure in ALL, regardless of a successful purging procedure (MRD-negative graft).[184] In fact, the remission duration after autologous SCT significantly correlates with MRD levels before the purging procedure. On the other hand, infusion of MRD-negative purged grafts in patients with MRD-negative pretransplantation BM is associated with durable clinical remission.[185] The study of *BCR-ABL*+ ALL patients revealed that autologous BM grafts are more heavily contaminated with leukemic cells as compared with autologous PBSC grafts.[186] Although the purging procedure might be more effective for autologous BM grafts, the chance of obtaining an MRD-negative autologous BM graft after purging is significantly lower than that of achieving an MRD-negative PBSC graft.[186] Detection of MRD in autologous BM or PBSC grafts is associated with an increased risk of relapse in ALL patients after transplantation.[187] In addition, ex vivo gene marking of autologous BM grafts suggest that residual malignant clonogenic cells in the autologous grafts are responsible for relapse after transplantation.[188]

### Detection of MRD in autologous grafts in B-NHL patients

Several studies have focused on autologous SCT in B-NHL with t(14;18), where BM infiltration is common at the time of diagnosis.[181] Also, PBSC harvests are frequently contaminated by lymphoma cells, with MRD levels comparable to those in BM.[189,190] Even CD34+CD19+ progenitors with t(14;18) could be identified in BM and PB.[191,192] In fact, mobilization regimens before PBSCT might result in increased PB contamination with tumor cells, which was clearly shown for MCL.[193] With the currently available techniques, it is possible to effectively purge autologous grafts of FL cells, as assessed by the disappearance of clonal *BCL2–IGH* PCR products.[194–196] In contrast, the purging procedure in MCL is generally unsuccessful.[193,196,197] Also, PCR analysis of *IGH* gene junctional regions showed that purging in autologous BM harvests can be successful in 50% of FL cases, but is generally ineffective in patients with DLBCL.[198] Preliminary RQ–PCR data indicate that successful purging of t(14;18)-positive cells is only possible in patients with a low tumor burden in stem cell harvests.[199] It is virtually impossible to achieve MRD negativity after purging when PBSC aphereses contain more than 1% CD19+ B cells.[200] Initial data suggested that patients transplanted with MRD–PCR-negative autologous grafts showed significantly longer disease-free survival in comparison with those whose marrow contained residual clonal lymphoma cells after purging.[201] Subsequent studies did not show a significant correlation between the PCR status of the reinfused bone marrow and FL outcome.[202,203]

### Detection of MRD in autologous grafts in MM patients

High-dose chemotherapy followed by autologous SCT is also becoming a treatment of choice for MM patients. Positive selection of CD34+ PBSC results in the reduction of contaminating tumor cells by at least two orders of magnitude, but residual MM-specific *IGH* gene rearrangements are frequently detectable.[204–206] Only highly purified (over 99.9%) CD34+ PBSC of MM patients are MRD-negative.[206,207] Preliminary observations indicate that transplantation of MM patients with purged PBSC seems to be associated with better event-free survival as compared with SCT with unmanipulated grafts.[208]

# Clinical value of MRD detection during and after treatment

Clinical MRD studies have mainly been performed in lymphoid malignancies of B lineage, such as precursor B-ALL, chronic B-cell leukemia, B-NHL, and MM. A few studies have also included T-ALL, but virtually no studies on MRD monitoring in chronic T-cell leukemias or peripheral (post-thymic) T-NHL have been reported.

## ALL

Most MRD studies in ALL have concerned childhood patients. The initial retrospective and small prospective studies with relatively short follow-up indicated that detection of MRD in childhood ALL has potent clinical value, although the results of these clinical studies were not fully concordant (summarized in references 72 and 209). This could be attributed to differences in sensitivities of MRD monitoring as well as to differences in the intensity of the cytotoxic treatment protocols. Several recent large prospective studies have confirmed the clinical value of MRD monitoring, justifying incorporation of the MRD information to refine risk-group assignment in current childhood ALL treatment protocols.[43,124,210–215]

### Clinical value of MRD detection for assessment of early response to first-line cytotoxic treatment in childhood ALL

The most significant application of MRD monitoring in childhood ALL is the assessment of the initial response to chemotherapy.[216] For example, a blast count in PB of less than 1000/μl after 1 week of prednisone therapy within BFM treatment protocols was found to be an important prognostic factor.[217] As a logical continuation of these clinical findings, low levels or absence of MRD after completion of induction therapy predicts good outcome, as found by PCR-based MRD studies.[124,144,210,211,214,218,218a,b] Meta-analysis of published MRD studies showed that approximately 50% of children with ALL are MRD-positive at the end of induction treatment and approximately 45% of these MRD-positive patients will ultimately relapse.[209] The risk of relapse has been found to be proportional to the detected MRD levels.[124,144,210,219] The level of MRD–PCR positivity after induction therapy is the most powerful prognostic factor. Multivariate analyses showed that this prognostic value is independent of other clinically relevant risk factors, including age, blast count at diagnosis, immunophenotype at diagnosis, presence of chromosome aberrations, response to prednisone, and classical clinical risk group assignment, provided that sensitive and accurate MRD quantification on adequate BM samples is performed.[124,210,211] Such sensitive and accurate MRD detection can be achieved via RQ–PCR analysis of junctional regions of Ig and TCR gene rearrangements (Figure 21.15).[98,123,158,220]

The meaning of MRD positivity differs according to the cytogenetic subgroup of ALL. Philadelphia chromosome-positive (Ph+) ALL with t(9;22) is characterized by high drug resistance and a very poor prognosis.[221] This leukemia subtype is also associated with an increased percentage of MRD-positive patients and increased MRD levels at the end of induction treatment.[222] Chemotherapy can lower the degree of MRD by only 2–3 logs in most Ph+ ALL patients, which is not enough for prolonged hematological remission. Nevertheless, in some patients with favorable prognostic features (e.g. low initial leukocyte count or good prednisone response), the disease can be

controlled with intensive chemotherapy.[221] MRD monitoring might identify this small drug-sensitive subgroup of Ph+ patients.[223] However, due to the poor prognosis of ALL with t(9;22) and the very low frequency of complete cure in this patient group, this preliminary observation should be confirmed by large multicenter studies. The same holds true for other cytogenetic ALL subgroups with increased risk of relapse, such as precursor B-ALL with t(4;11). It is possible to identify a small subgroup of t(4;11)-positive patients with rapid achievement of molecular remission after intensive chemotherapy and/or allogeneic SCT and persistent PCR negativity in long-term complete remission.[224] Therefore, prospective MRD monitoring can be used for assessment of treatment response and can be applied for individualization of therapy in order to further improve the outcome of high-risk t(4;11) positive leukemia, including infant ALL patients.[225] MRD studies in patients with the prognostically favorable *TEL–AML1* aberration suggest that the MRD levels at the end of induction therapy are generally below the threshold associated with bad outcome.[226] Nevertheless, using quantitative MRD analysis of early treatment response, it is possible to identify the subgroup of *TEL–AML1+* patients with slower kinetics of tumor reduction being at higher risk of leukemia relapse.[226,227]

The results from the large prospective study of the International BFM Study Group (I-BFM-SG) utilizing Ig and TCR gene rearrangements as MRD–PCR targets indicated that MRD analysis at a single time point is not sufficient for recognition of patients with poor prognosis as well as patients with good prognosis.[124] In contrast, combined information on the kinetics of tumor load decrease at the end of induction treatment and before consolidation treatment appeared to be highly informative. This combined MRD information distinguishes patients at low risk with MRD negativity at both time points (5-year relapse rate of 2%); patients at high risk with an intermediate ($10^{-3}$) or high ($\geq 10^{-2}$) degree of MRD at both time points (5-year relapse rate of 80%); and the remaining patients at intermediate risk (5-year relapse rate of 22%) (Figure 21.16).[124] The group of patients at MRD-based high risk is larger than any previously identified high-risk group (approximately 15%) and has an unprecedented high 5-year relapse rate of 80%. This group might benefit from further intensification of treatment protocols, including SCT during first remission or novel treatment modalities, such as including antibodies conjugated with immunotoxins or tyrosine kinase inhibitors. On the other hand, the MRD-based low-risk patients make up a group of a substantial size (approximately 45%), comparable to the frequency of survivors of childhood ALL before treatment intensification was introduced.[163] Within the MRD-based low-risk group, half of the patients have already low ($\leq 10^{-4}$) or undetectable MRD levels after 2 weeks of

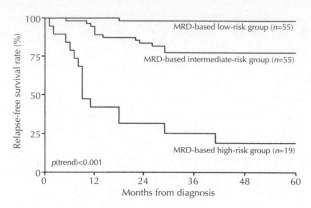

**Figure 21.16** Relapse-free survival rates of the three MRD-based risk groups of children treated for ALL according to protocols of the International BFM Study Group. The three risk groups were defined by combined MRD information at the end of induction treatment (time point 1) and before consolidation treatment (time point 2).[124] Patients in the low-risk group have MRD negativity at both time points (43% of patients), patients in the high-risk group have MRD degrees of $\geq 10^{-3}$ at both time points (15% of patients), and the remaining patients form the MRD-based intermediate-risk group (43% of patients). The numbers of patients at risk are given in parentheses for each group at 24 months and 48 months after time point 2.

treatment.[212] This group in particular might profit from treatment reduction.

The reported clinical MRD studies all show the prognostic value of MRD information, but the definition of MRD-based risk groups, the relative distribution of patients over these groups, and the corresponding relapse rates are different between the studies. Most probably, these differences are related to the treatment protocol, the sensitivity of the MRD technique, and the timing of the follow-up BM samples. Therefore, it is important to realize that for each ALL treatment protocol, optimal time points and sensitivities for determination of early treatment response ('MRD window') should be determined. Modifications of chemotherapy regimens and the corresponding BM sampling time points might result in loss of clinical significance of MRD information if the MRD window is not adjusted appropriately.[228,228a]

### Clinical value of MRD detection for assessment of response to reinduction treatment after relapse of ALL

The predictive value of MRD monitoring is particularly clear after first relapse.[229,230] This can be perceived as assessment of early treatment response after second induction treatment. The BFM group demonstrated the high prognostic value of MRD detection at day 36 of the ALL-REZ treatment protocol. Patients with MRD levels below $10^{-3}$ ($n = 16$) had a probability of relapse-free survival rate of 86%, whereas MRD

levels equal or more to $10^{-3}$ ($n = 10$) were uniformly predictive of dismal outcome (with zero probability of relapse-free survival).[230] These first MRD results in relapsed childhood ALL look very promising, but need further confirmation because of the limited number of studies patients.

### Differences in MRD kinetics between precursor B-ALL and T-ALL of childhood

The MRD data suggest slower kinetics of leukemia clearance in T-ALL as compared with precursor B-ALL patients.[214,231,232] In a study by Dibenedetto et al,[231] nearly all T-ALL patients (16 of 17) were found to be MRD-positive at the end of induction treatment, while a later time point at the beginning of maintenance treatment carried the most significant prognostic information. All but one (7 of 8) MRD-positive patients at this *late* time point subsequently relapsed, while all 8 MRD-negative patients remained in continuous complete remission.[231] This is in contrast to the MRD study of the I-BFM-SG, which showed that PCR-based measurement of *early* treatment response at two consecutive time points after induction treatment and before consolidation treatment results in highly prognostic MRD information: approximately 25% low-risk patients with 0% relapses, 50% intermediate-risk patients with 25% relapses, and 25% high-risk patients with 100% relapses.[232]

### Clinical value of continuous MRD monitoring in childhood ALL

Continuous MRD monitoring in childhood ALL has shown that a steady decrease of MRD levels to negative PCR results during treatment is associated with favorable prognosis,[233] whereas persistence of high MRD levels or steady increase of MRD levels generally leads to clinical relapse (Figure 21.17).[124,234–236] Therefore, persisting MRD levels during treatment can be regarded as a good indicator of in vivo resistance to treatment. PCR-based MRD monitoring was shown to be able to select the group of 'poor responders' with early relapse during maintenance treatment.[124,210,211] Sequential sampling generally shows positive MRD–PCR results prior to clinical relapse. However, the time span between the reappearance of MRD positivity and overt hematological relapse might be too short for earlier implementation of reinduction treatment.[237]

Low levels of MRD after therapy might be associated with late development of relapse, but absence of MRD at the end of treatment is not sufficient to assure that the patient is cured.[124,236] Despite the high sensitivity of most MRD techniques, it should be noted that MRD negativity does not exclude the presence of leukemic cells in the patient, because each MRD test only screens a minor fraction of all BM and PB leukocytes. Curiously, one report claims that multiple PCR analy-

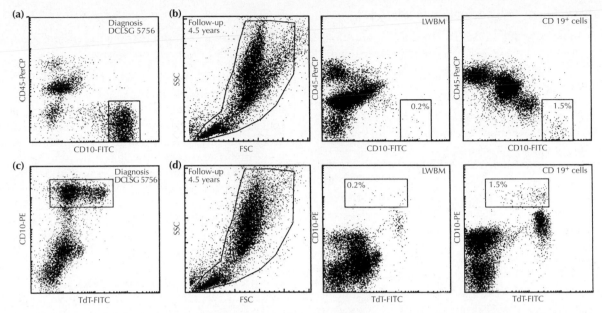

**Figure 21.17** Flow-cytometric detection of MRD in a precursor B-cell acute lymphoblastic leukemia (precursor B-ALL) patient by use of CD45/CD10/CD19 (a, b) and TdT/CD10/CD19 (c,d) triple labelings. The leukemia-specific immunophenotypic detection was based on CD10 overexpression and CD45 negativity. In the follow-up bone marrow (BM) sample, taken 4.5 years from the diagnosis of ALL, the population of cells with leukemia-specific immunophenotype comprised 0.2% of BM cells, i.e. 1.5% of CD19+ cells. At that time, the patient was in complete clinical remission of the leukemia. However, he underwent the overt hematological relapse of precursor B-ALL, 9 months after this positive MRD test. (Courtesy of Dr EG van Lochem)

ses (testing a higher cell number) gave evidence for residual leukemia at very low levels in about 90% (15 of 17) of patients remaining in long-term clinical remission.[238] In 7 out of these 15 patients, this PCR result was confirmed in a blast colony assay. So far, these data have not been confirmed by other investigators, even not by using extremely sensitive 10-fold PCR analyses (sensitivities $10^{-6}$ to $10^{-7}$).[124] In contrast, large prospective studies showed 0–10% of patients being positive at the end of treatment; the majority of the MRD-positive patients relapsed later on.[124,236]

These combined data suggest that continuous MRD monitoring in childhood ALL has limited value and might only be useful for a subgroup of patients with a relatively slow early response to treatment, i.e. patients at high risk of relapse and for patients at intermediate risk of relapse.

### Clinical value of MRD detection before and/or after stem cell transplantation in childhood ALL

MRD monitoring is particularly informative for ALL patients undergoing BMT. In the extensive study of Knechtli et al,[147] high levels of MRD–PCR positivity ($10^{-2}$ to $10^{-3}$) before allogeneic BMT were invariably associated with relapse after transplantation, while the 2-year event-free survival rate in patients with a low level of MRD positivity ($10^{-3}$ to $10^{-5}$) approximated 36%. This study involved patients receiving T-cell-depleted grafts, while two other studies showed

that the strong graft-versus-leukemia (GVL) effect associated with non-depleted grafts might overcome high levels of MRD positivity in selected cases.[239–241]

In contrast, MRD negativity before allogeneic transplantation significantly correlated with better outcome and a 2-year event-free survival rate greater than 70%.[147,240–242] Similar results were obtained in the study of pre-BMT samples with multiparameter flow cytometry, with disease-free-survival rates of 33% and 74% for MRD-positive and MRD-negative patients, respectively.[243] Therefore, patients with a high MRD burden prior to BMT might be offered alternative treatment (e.g. further cytoreduction before BMT, intensified conditioning, and/or early post-BMT immunotherapy) in order to improve their generally poor outcome.[147,240–242]

MRD–PCR positivity in ALL patients after BMT is suggestive of impending relapse.[244,244a] This is true both for high-risk patients transplanted in first remission and for patients subjected to BMT in second remission after leukemia relapse. MRD was shown to occur in post-BMT samples in 88% of patients who subsequently relapsed, while only 22% of patients in long-term complete remission showed MRD at any time after BMT, mostly at low levels.[244] The patients with persistent MRD positivity after BMT might be candidates for early treatment with immunotherapy, including donor lymphocyte infusions to increase the GVL effect.[243,244,244a]

### Clinical value of MRD detection in adult ALL

Preliminary results of MRD studies in adult ALL using junctional regions of Ig/TCR genes as MRD–PCR targets showed molecular responses to chemotherapy similar to those in childhood ALL, but with higher frequencies of persistent MRD positivity in adults.[245,246] Not only the frequencies of MRD positivity but also the MRD levels in adult patients were significantly higher than in comparably treated children; this points towards a higher frequency of in vivo drug resistance in adult ALL.[246,247,247a] A single prospective MRD study in t(9;22)-negative adult precursor B-ALL patients demonstrated the strong predictive value of MRD information at all investigated time points within 2 years of treatment.[248] The prognostic value of semiquantitative MRD data was most significant 3–5 months after remission induction and beyond. In contrast to childhood ALL, the prognostic value of pre-BMT MRD levels was inferior to MRD information after allogeneic BMT.[248]

### Comparison of MRD monitoring between bone marrow and peripheral blood in ALL

One of the serious limitations of continuous MRD monitoring is the need for multiple traumatic BM aspirations. Replacement of BM sampling by PB sampling has been a topic of debate in MRD studies for the last 15 years or so. Both early immunophenotypic data[14,23] and a RQ–PCR study[249] showed a very good concordance between MRD levels in BM and PB in T-ALL patients. This strong correlation was independent of the follow-up time point, underlining the disseminated character of T-ALL. Therefore, BM sampling might be replaced by PB sampling in T-ALL.[249] In contrast, MRD levels in precursor B-ALL differed significantly between BM and PB.[249,250,250a] The data from a single PCR study showed an 11.7-fold difference between BM and PB during induction treatment of precursor B-ALL patients.[250,250a] Recent RQ–PCR-based results show a highly variable ratio between MRD levels in BM and PB, ranging from 1 to more than 1000.[249] This implies that no simple straightforward relationship exists between MRD levels in paired BM and PB samples of precursor B-ALL patients – particularly not at later time points (>3 months). The difference between BM and PB might be less pronounced in Ph+ precursor B-ALL, most probably because of a generally higher degree of MRD as compared with other ALL subtypes. Nevertheless, PB sampling cannot easily replace BM sampling for MRD detection in precursor B-ALL patients. Moreover, the differences in MRD levels between BM and PB are additionally influenced by the degree of dilution of BM aspirates with PB. This is suggested by the finding of a 4.1-fold greater mean MRD level in trephine BM biopsies as compared with BM aspirates.[251]

### B-CLL

### Persistence of residual disease in patients treated with conventional chemotherapy

B-CLL typically occurs at an advanced age, is characterized by an indolent course, and frequently requires no specific treatment.[252] Immunophenotypic monitoring of residual disease in B-CLL was traditionally based on overexpression of the CD5 antigen on CD20+ cells or an abnormal Igκ/Igλ ratio within a B-cell-enriched population or on CD37+-gated B cells.[28,253,254] With such an approach, characterized by a limited sensitivity of about $10^{-2}$, residual leukemic cells were detected in the majority of B-CLL patients in cytomorphological remission after conventional chemotherapy. This finding was confirmed by the persistence of clonal *IGH* gene rearrangements as detected by Southern blotting.[255] Immunophenotypic remission after chemotherapy was associated with significantly longer relapse-free survival of patients, but this remission was not related to prolonged overall survival.[255] Immunophenotypic MRD analysis after treatment of B-CLL with fludarabine plus prednisone showed that the vast majority of patients in complete clinical remission had no detectable immunophenotypically aberrant cells.[256] Relapse-free survival in this group was significantly longer compared with patients with MRD positivity by flow cytometry. Reappearance of cells with the B-CLL immunophenotype preceded overt clinical relapse by 3–14 months.[256] Similarly, in the study by Brugiatelli et al,[256] immunophenotypically defined remission after chemotherapy was associated with a significantly longer relapse-free survival of patients, but this remission was not related to prolonged overall survival. Persistence of immunophenotypically defined MRD was associated with a more rapid progression of B-CLL.[257] During disease progression, there was no evidence for clonal evolution, which is in line with the absence of secondary rearrangements in B-CLL.[258]

### Value of MRD monitoring in B-CLL patients treated with SCT

In a subgroup of patients with high-risk B-CLL, particularly those under the age of 60 years, intensive treatment (including autologous or allogeneic SCT) is being increasingly used (reviewed in reference 259). For patients in advanced-stage B-CLL referred for SCT, more sensitive PCR analyses of *IGH* junctional regions with sensitivities of $10^{-3}$ to $10^{-5}$ would be preferred. With such sensitive MRD detection, none of the patients reach molecular remission after conventional or salvage chemotherapy.[258] Following allogeneic or autologous B-cell-purged SCT, a subset of disease-free patients could be identified without detectable MRD.[258,260–262] In contrast, persistence of MRD–PCR positivity after SCT might be associated with impending relapse.[258] Esteve et al[66,263] analyzed patients in complete remission after SCT with combined flow-cytometric and molecular analyses, reaching sensitivities of $\leq 10^{-4}$. Six out of seven patients who were MRD-positive at the first evaluation 3 months after autologous SCT experienced disease relapse, while only 1 of 11 MRD-negative patients at the same time point subsequently relapsed.[66,263] This implies a high prognostic value of MRD after autologous SCT. Concerning MRD monitoring at later time points, some investigators have reported MRD positivity for several months or even several years in B-CLL patients in complete clinical remission after SCT.[261,264,265] In this aspect, quantitative MRD data might be particularly informative for discrimination between patients with persistently low MRD levels in stable clinical remission and those with increasing MRD levels at high risk of relapse. Rawstron et al[65] used multiparameter flow cytometry and quantitatively assessed MRD in patients treated with PBSCT and/or humanized anti-CD52 antibody (CAMPATH-1H). All patients with MRD levels above $5 \times 10^{-4}$ at the end of treatment experienced rapid B-CLL progression. Virtually all patients with MRD levels below $5 \times 10^{-4}$ remained progression-free, although in half of these patients MRD levels subsequently increased.[65]

In conclusion, MRD data in B-CLL are preliminary, mostly retrospective, and largely qualitative, and the clinical value of MRD in this leukemia type should be fully established. It is clear that MRD kinetics in B-CLL differ according to the treatment protocol. Nevertheless, patients with high-risk B-CLL in particular should definitely profit from more precise, quantitative treatment monitoring. Assessment of MRD after autologous SCT especially might reveal prognostically significant information.

## B-NHL

### Limited value of MRD monitoring in PB in FL patients treated with conventional chemotherapy

MRD detection might be particularly important in the subgroup of high- and intermediate-grade lymphomas, where circulating lymphoma cells are frequently found in BM and PB. The vast majority of clinical studies have concentrated on FL with t(14;18) using the BCL2–IGH fusion gene as a DNA target for PCR-based MRD analysis.[181,182,192,266–274] Most of the patients suffering from this disease harbor lymphoma cells in BM or PB at diagnosis, with BM being more informative than PB for MRD monitoring.[181,182,267] More than half of the patients convert to MRD negativity during the first year of cytotoxic treatment, which is associated with a longer relapse-free survival.[268] In patients with advanced t(14;18)-positive NHL (stage III/IV) treated with conventional induction therapy, no obvious correlation was found between the presence or absence of t(14;18)-positive cells in circulation and relapse-free survival.[269] Using

RQ–PCR, Mandigers et al[275] prospectively assessed the response to induction chemotherapy in PB of FL patients. Half of the patients converted to PCR negativity, while another one-third had very low levels of MRD as measured in a BCL2–IGH RQ–PCR assay. However, this molecular response in PB was not associated with a better progression-free survival.[275]

Apparently, MRD monitoring in PB has limited value in FL patients, but MRD monitoring in BM might be more valuable.

### MRD kinetics in FL patients treated with chimeric CD20 antibody

A combination of chemotherapy and chimeric (mouse–human) anti-CD20 antibody (rituximab) treatment has been shown to produce durable clinical remission in a subgroup of FL patients accompanied by PCR negativity.[270,276] Patients who achieved sustained molecular remission had significantly better clinical outcome at 3-year follow-up as compared with persistently MRD-positive patients or those who converted to MRD–PCR positivity.[276]

t(14;18)-positive B cells can even be effectively cleared from PB and/or BM in a subset of patients treated with rituximab as *single* first-line treatment.[277] PCR negativity in PB 1 month after treatment completion can identify patients with a significantly lower rate of disease progression during the first year of follow-up.[277] Although a significant subset of patients remained MRD-negative 1 year after completion of rituximab treatment, the prognostic significance of such molecular remission should be established after longer follow-up.

### Negativity or persistence of low MRD levels in FL patients in complete remission after SCT

MRD studies for the presence of BCL2–IGH transcripts in patients treated with purged autologous SCT showed that the patients in continuous molecular remission after SCT had significantly higher relapse-free survival as compared with patients with persistent PCR positivity.[203,271] In another group of patients treated with autologous PBSCT, reappearance of PCR positivity at any time post transplantation was associated with an increased relapse risk.[192] Diametrically different conclusions were drawn from another study, in which the majority of patients after purged autologous SCT remained MRD–PCR-positive and no correlation was found between MRD–PCR status and relapse-free survival.[273]

Furthermore, circulating t(14;18)-positive cells were detected in patients in long-term clinical remission after radiation therapy for localized FL.[274] RQ–PCR data indicate that patients in continuous clinical remission after high-dose chemotherapy supported by autologous BMT might become transiently MRD-negative.[202] More frequently *BCL2–IGH* fusion genes are persistently found with stable levels within one order of magnitude.[202] Further investigations and standardization on multicenter level are required to establish the quantitative criteria for molecular remission in FL and the potential applicability of MRD information for clinical decision-making.

### BCL2–IGH fusions in normal individuals – reality or contamination?

It should be noted that positive results in sensitive *BCL2–IGH* PCR studies should be interpreted with caution, because the presence of t(14;18)-positive B cells has also been reported in healthy individuals.[278,278a] Also an international multicenter study revealed a high variability of *BCL2–IGH* PCR results between different laboratories, with an unexpectedly high frequency of false-positive results.[279] Such false-positive results, due to normal t(14;18)-positive cells or intralaboratory contamination, can be prevented by routine design of patient-specific oligonucleotides directed against the fusion-region sequence of the *BCL2–IGH* junction.[280]

### Persistent MRD positivity in MCL patients

Using *IGH* gene rearrangements and *BCL1–IGH* fusion genes as DNA targets, MCL patients were found to be continuously MRD-positive in BM and/or PB during chemotherapy.[193,197] In the majority of MCL patients, MRD levels in BM and PB vary between $10^{-2}$ and $10^{-3}$, indicating extensive dissemination of MCL cells and significant resistance to conventional chemotherapy schemes.[193] With more intensive treatment, including a combination of rituximab and conventional chemotherapy, approximately one-third of MCL patients can reach a MRD–PCR-negative status.[281] However, in the majority of cases, this conversion to PCR negativity is transient and molecular remission is not associated with better progression-free-survival.

### Value of MRD monitoring in B-NHL after autologous or allogeneic SCT

Persistence of MRD–PCR positivity in BM after autologous SCT was shown to be associated with impending clinical relapse, whereas all patients with eradication of PCR-detectable lymphoma cells remained in continuous clinical remission.[198] Nevertheless, persistence of patient-specific *IGH* gene rearrangements during long-term complete remission has also been reported.[282] MRD was investigated with patient-specific PCR techniques in a group of patients with advanced-stage FL or MCL.[283] After high-dose sequential chemotherapy, it was possible to harvest MRD–PCR-negative autologous BM grafts in most FL patients. None of the patients who received an MRD–PCR-negative BM graft relapsed at a median follow-up of 24 months.[283] These combined MRD studies indicate that transplantation with MRD-negative

autologous BM or PBSC grafts is a promising treatment modality in patients with FL.

In contrast, it is virtually impossible to harvest autologous MRD-negative BM or PBSC grafts in MCL.[193,197,283] Reinfusion of MRD-positive grafts is uniformly associated with the relapse of MCL.[197] Preliminary data suggest that high-dose chemoradiotherapy followed by autologous PBSCT might result in molecular remission in a subset of MCL patients.[284,284a] MRD–PCR-negativity after PBSCT is strongly predictive of progression-free survival.[284,284a] These promising data should be confirmed for larger groups of patients. Currently, for patients with advanced MCL allogeneic SCT remains the only effective treatment regimen, and preliminary data show conversion to MRD negativity after SCT, which is related to long-term hematological remission.[197,285]

### MM

Detection of MRD in MM is a quite recent issue because of progress in the treatment of this formerly incurable disease. In particular, the application of high-dose chemotherapy in combination with allogeneic or autologous SCT has increased the overall survival and possibly leads to ultimate cure of MM.[11,286] This treatment eradicates not only malignant plasma cells but also putative malignant B lymphocytes, which are found to be clonally related to the MM cells.[12] The malignant event apparently affects B lymphocytes with somatically mutated *IGH* genes before IgH class switching occurs; they are characterized by CD45RO, high-density CD38 expression, and CD56 expression.[287] Rearranged *IGH* genes of MM cells contain somatic mutations, but show no further intraclonal variation.[89]

Some studies have shown that after high-dose sequential chemoradiotherapy, malignant plasma cells might still be detectable by MRD–PCR analyses in PB and BM harvests as well as in BM after autologous transplantation, whereas clonally related B lymphocytes (before IgH class switching) were not detectable in the cell harvests.[288] Persistent MRD positivity is a frequent finding in MM patients in complete remission after conventional chemotherapy or after high-dose chemotherapy followed by single or tandem autologous SCT (with MRD levels ranging from $10^{-4}$ to $10^{-2}$).[208,289] This combination of chemotherapy and autologous SCT results in a more significant reduction of residual malignant plasma cell levels as compared with conventional chemotherapy.[290] However, only a small subset (5–15%) of MM patients in long-term complete remission after autologous SCT ultimately reach an MRD–PCR-negative status (sensitivity $10^{-3}$ to $10^{-4}$).[289,291,292] Nevertheless, even patients in transient molecular remission have a significantly lower relapse rate and a significantly longer relapse-free survival.[292]

In contrast, up to 70% of MM patients in long-term complete remission after high-dose chemotherapy and allogeneic SCT remain persistently MRD-negative, indicating that complete eradication of the malignant clone and real 'cure' of MM become realistic goals.[286,289,292,293]

# Conclusions

Several immunophenotyping and PCR techniques are available for MRD detection in patients with a lymphoid malignancy, as summarized in Table 21.9. Especially in precursor B-ALL and T-ALL, multiple sensitive MRD techniques can be used, showing a high correlation of the obtained results between different methodologies.[294–296] Each MRD technique has its advantages and disadvantages, which have to be weighed carefully to make an appropriate choice (see Table 21.2). On the one hand, false-positive and false-negative results should be prevented, but, on the other hand, the MRD techniques should be sufficiently sensitive and quantitative. These requirements can generally be met with RQ–PCR analysis of chromosome aberrations, if adequate precautionary measures are taken to prevent cross-contamination of PCR products. Speed and relatively low costs will also play a role in the choice of MRD techniques, and can be achieved with multiparameter flow-cytometric MRD analysis, which is also inherently quantitative. RQ–PCR analysis of junctional regions of Ig/TCR gene rearrangements is time-consuming and expensive, but has the advantage of broad applicability in all categories of lymphoid malignancies, as well as the advantage of high sensitivity levels (Table 21.9).

Although most MRD techniques are relatively sensitive, one should realize that MRD negativity does not exclude the presence of malignant cells.[297] Generally each MRD test only screens $10^5$–$10^6$ cells, which represent a minor fraction of the total amount of lymphoid cells. In addition, it might well be that the distribution of low numbers of malignant lymphoid cells throughout the body is not homogeneous and that the investigated cell sample is therefore not fully representative.[298,299]

Finally, the clinical impact of MRD detection in the various categories of lymphoid malignancies is not yet established (Table 21.10). In ALL, the main application of MRD information was shown to be the evaluation of early treatment response, with precise measurement of tumor load reduction during remis-

## Table 21.9  Applicability of MRD techniques in lymphoid malignancies[a]

| | Flow-cytometric immunophenotyping | | PCR analysis | |
| --- | --- | --- | --- | --- |
| | Aberrant immunophenotypes ($10^{-3}$ to $10^{-4}$) | Igκ/Igλ distribution or TCR-V analysis ($10^{-1}$ to $10^{-2}$)[b] | Junctional regions of Ig/TCR genes ($10^{-4}$ to $10^{-5}$) | Chromosome aberrations ($10^{-4}$ to $10^{-6}$) |
| Precursor B-ALL: | | | | |
|    Children | 70–90% | — | ~95% | 40–45% |
|    Adults | 70–80% | — | ~95% | 35–40% |
| T-ALL: | | | | |
|    Children | | | >95% | 25–30% |
|    Adults | ~95% | 30–35%[c] | | 10–15% |
| Chronic B-cell leukemias | — | >95% | >95% | — |
| Chronic T-cell leukemias | — | 60–65%[d] | ~95% | — |
| B-NHL | — | >95% | 70–80%[e] | 25–30% |
| T-NHL | 20–25%[f] | 50–60%[d] | ~95% | 10–15% |
| MM | — | >95% | 60–70%[e] | — |

ALL, acute lymphoblastic leukemia; NHL, non-Hodgkin lymphoma. MM, multiple myeloma.
[a] The percentages indicate the applicability of the MRD techniques to the category of lymphoid malignancies.
[b] The sensitivity of flow-cytometric detection of Igκ/Igλ distribution or TCR-V gene usage can be improved to about $10^{-3}$ in triple labelings with specific markers such as BCL2, cytoplasmic CD3, and ALK proteins.
[c] Based on the expression of TCRαβ molecules (20% of cases) and TCRγδ molecules (about 10% of cases).
[d] TCR-V antibodies recognize TCR chains in 65–70% of TCRαβ molecules and in most TCRγδ molecules.
[e] Somatic mutations hamper primer annealing in some of the patients with B-NHL, B-CLL, or multiple myeloma.
[f] Based on T-ALL-like immunophenotype in T-lymphoblastic lymphoma and NPM–ALK expression in about 50% of large cell anaplastic lymphomas of T-cell lineage.

**Table 21.10 Prognostic value and clinical applicability of MRD detection in different lymphoid malignancies**

| Disease category | Type of MRD application | | | |
| --- | --- | --- | --- | --- |
| | Early response to front-line treatment | Continuous monitoring for therapy titration | MRD assessment before SCT | MRD assessment after SCT |
| ALL | ++ | + | ++ | + |
| B-CLL | – | +?* | +? | + |
| B-NHL | – | +?* | +? | + |
| MM | – | +?* | +? | + |

ALL, acute lymphoblastic leukemia; CLL, chronic lymphocytic leukemia; NHL, non-Hodgkin lymphoma; MM, multiple myeloma.
++ value of MRD detection proven by prospective studies;
+ potentially clinically relevant (e.g. in a subset of patients) but not yet proven by large prospective studies;
+? MRD results are statistically significant but their clinical implication is not yet established;
* only relevant for patients treated with more aggressive protocols and/or including anti-CD20 antibody;
– MRD detection has no additional value as compared with conventional cytomorphological techniques.

sion induction therapy. In mature lymphoid malignancies, the value of MRD information might probably rely on monitoring over a clinically relevant disease-specific time span, with the possibility of attuning the treatment based on MRD results. Further studies are required to fully define the disease-specific 'MRD windows' for clinically reliable MRD monitoring in CLL, NHL, and MM. Current prospective studies have to demonstrate whether MRD information can be used for adaptation of treatment protocols and how the persistence of MRD positivity during long-term complete remission should be interpreted.

## REFERENCES

1. Visser O, Coebergh JWW, Schouten LJ, Dijck JAAM (eds). *Incidence of cancer in the Netherlands 1995*. Utrecht: Vereniging van Integrale Kankercentra, 1998.
2. Foon KA, Todd RF. Immunologic classification of leukemia and lymphoma. *Blood* 1986; **68**: 1–31.
3. Greaves MF. Differentiation-linked leukemogenesis in lymphocytes. *Science* 1986; **234**: 697–704.
4. Van Dongen JJM, Adriaansen HJ, Hooijkaas H. Immunophenotyping of leukaemias and non-Hodgkin's lymphomas. Immunological markers and their CD codes. *Neth J Med* 1988; **33**: 298–314.
5. Jaffe ES, Harris NL, Stein H, Vardiman JW (eds). *World Health Organization Classification of Tumours. Pathology and Genetics of Tumours of Haematopoietic and Lymphoid Tissues*. Lyon: IARC Press, 2001.
6. O'Connor N, Gatter KC, Wainscoat JS et al. Practical value of genotypic analysis for diagnosing lymphoproliferative disorders. *J Clin Pathol* 1987; **40**: 147–50.
7. Korsmeyer SJ. Antigen receptor genes as molecular markers of lymphoid neoplasms. *J Clin Invest* 1987; **79**: 1291–5.
8. Rabbitts TH. Chromosomal translocations in human cancer. *Nature* 1994; **372**: 143–9.
8a. Szczepanski T, Van der Velden VHJ, Van Dongen JJM. Classification systems for acute and chronic leukaemias. *Best Pract Res Clin Haematol* 2003; **16**: 561–82.
9. Look AT. Oncogenic transcription factors in the human acute leukemias. *Science* 1997; **278**: 1059–64.
10. Schrappe M, Camitta B, Pui CH et al. Long-term results of large prospective trials in childhood acute lymphoblastic leukemia. *Leukemia* 2000; **14**: 2193–4.
11. Vesole DH, Barlogie B, Jagannath S et al. High-dose therapy for refractory multiple myeloma: improved prognosis with better supportive care and double transplants. *Blood* 1994; **84**: 950–6.
12. Billadeau D, Ahmann G, Greipp P, Van Ness B. The bone marrow of multiple myeloma patients contains B cell populations at different stages of differentiation that are clonally related to the malignant plasma cell. *J Exp Med* 1993; **178**: 1023–31.
13. Szczepański T, Orfao A, van der Velden VHJ et al. Minimal residual disease in leukaemia patients. *Lancet Oncol* 2001; **2**: 409–17.
14. Van Dongen JJM, Breit TM, Adriaansen HJ et al. Detection of minimal residual disease in acute leukemia by immunological marker analysis and polymerase chain reaction. *Leukemia* 1992; **6**: 47–59.
15. Campana D, Pui CH. Detection of minimal residual disease in acute leukemia: methodologic advances and clinical significance. *Blood* 1995; **85**: 1416–34.
16. Estrov Z, Grunberger T, Dube ID et al. Detection of residual acute lymphoblastic leukemia cells in cultures of bone marrow obtained during remission. *N Engl J Med* 1986; **315**: 538–42.
17. Anastasi J, Thangavelu M, Vardiman JW et al. Interphase cytogenetic analysis detects minimal residual disease in a case of acute lymphoblastic leukemia and resolves the question of origin of relapse after allogeneic bone marrow transplantation. *Blood* 1991; **77**: 1087–91.
18. Nylund SJ, Ruutu T, Saarinen U et al. Detection of minimal residual disease using fluorescence DNA in situ

hybridization: a follow-up study in leukemia and lymphoma patients. *Leukemia* 1994; **8**: 587–94.

19. El-Rifai W, Ruutu T, Vettenranta K et al. Follow-up of residual disease using metaphase-FISH in patients with acute lymphoblastic leukemia in remission. *Leukemia* 1997; **11**: 633–8.

20. Van der Burg M, Beverloo HB, Langerak AW et al. Rapid and sensitive detection of all types of MLL gene translocations with a single FISH probe set. *Leukemia* 1999; **13**: 2107–13.

21. Van der Burg M, Smit B, Brinkhof B et al. A single split-signal FISH probe set allows detection of *TAL1* translocations as well as *SIL–TAL1* fusion genes in a single test. *Leukemia* 2002; **16**: 755–61.

21a. Van der Burg M, Poulsen TS, Hunger SP, Beverloo HB, Smit EM, Vang-Nielsen K, Langerak AW, Van Dongen JJM. Split-signal FISH for detection of chromosome aberrations in acute lymphoblastic leukemia. *Leukemia* 2004; **18**: 895–908.

22. Van Dongen JJM, Wolvers-Tettero ILM. Analysis of immunoglobulin and T cell receptor genes. Part I: Basic and technical aspects. *Clin Chim Acta* 1991; **198**: 1–91.

23. Van Dongen JJM, Hooijkaas H, Adriaansen HJ et al. Detection of minimal residual acute lymphoblastic leukemia by immunological marker analysis: possibilities and limitations. In: Hagenbeek A, Löwenberg B (eds) *Minimal Residual Disease in Acute Leukemia* Dordrecht: Martinus Nijhoff, 1986: 113–33.

24. Smith RG, Kitchens RL. Phenotypic heterogeneity of TDT+ cells in the blood and bone marrow: implications for surveillance of residual leukemia. *Blood* 1989; **74**: 312–19.

25. Campana D, Coustan-Smith E, Janossy G. The immunologic detection of minimal residual disease in acute leukemia. *Blood* 1990; **76**: 163–71.

26. Macedo A, Orfao A, Ciudad J et al. Phenotypic analysis of CD34 subpopulations in normal human bone marrow and its application for the detection of minimal residual disease. *Leukemia* 1995; **9**: 1896–901.

27. Van Dongen JJM, Adriaansen HJ, Hooijkaas H. Immunological marker analysis of cells in the various hematopoietic differentiation stages and their malignant counterparts. In: Ruiter DJ, Fleuren GJ, Warnaar SO (eds) *Application of Monoclonal Antibodies in Tumor Pathology*. Dordrecht: Martinus Nijhoff, 1987: 87–116.

28. Peters RE, Janossy G, Ivory K et al. Leukemia-associated changes identified by quantitative flow cytometry. III. B-cell gating in CD37/κ/λ clonality test. *Leukemia* 1994; **8**: 1864–70.

29. Van Dongen JJM, van den Beemd MWM, Schellekens M et al. Analysis of malignant T cells with the Vβ antibody panel. *Immunologist* 1996; **4**: 37–40.

30. Van den Beemd MWM, Boor PPC, Van Lochem EG et al. Flow cytometric analysis of the Vβ repertoire in healthy controls. *Cytometry* 2000; **40**: 336–45.

31. Langerak AW, van Den Beemd R, Wolvers-Tettero ILM et al. Molecular and flow cytometric analysis of the Vβ repertoire for clonality assessment in mature TCRαβ T-cell proliferations. *Blood* 2001; **98**: 165–73.

32. Langerak AW, Wolvers-Tettero ILM, van den Beemd MWM et al. Immunophenotypic and immunogenotypic characteristics of TCRγδ+ T cell acute lymphoblastic leukemia. *Leukemia* 1999; **13**: 206–14.

33. Terstappen LW, Loken MR. Five-dimensional flow cytometry as a new approach for blood and bone marrow differentials. *Cytometry* 1988; **9**: 548–56.

34. Groeneveld K, te Marvelde JG, van den Beemd MW et al. Flow cytometric detection of intracellular antigens for immunophenotyping of normal and malignant leukocytes. *Leukemia* 1996; **10**: 1383–9.

35. Drach J, Drach D, Glassl H et al. Flow cytometric determination of atypical antigen expression in acute leukemia for the study of minimal residual disease. *Cytometry* 1992; **13**: 893–901.

36. Hurwitz CA, Gore SD, Stone KD, Civin CI. Flow cytometric detection of rare normal human marrow cells with immunophenotypes characteristic of acute lymphoblastic leukemia cells. *Leukemia* 1992; **6**: 233–9.

37. Mori T, Sugita K, Suzuki T et al. A novel monoclonal antibody, KOR-SA3544 which reacts to Philadelphia chromosome-positive acute lymphoblastic leukemia cells with high sensitivity. *Leukemia* 1995; **9**: 1233–9.

38. Dworzak MN, Fritsch G, Fleischer C et al. Comparative phenotype mapping of normal vs. malignant pediatric B-lymphopoiesis unveils leukemia-associated aberrations. *Exp Hematol* 1998; **26**: 305–13.

39. Campana D, CoustanSmith E. Detection of minimal residual disease in acute leukemia by flow cytometry. *Cytometry* 1999; **38**: 139–52.

39a. Campana D, Coustan-Smith E. Advances in the immunological monitoring of childhood acute lymphoblastic leukaemia. *Best Pract Res Clin Haematol* 2002; **15**: 1–19.

39b. Hrusak O, Porwit-MacDonald A. Antigen expression patterns reflecting genotype of acute leukemias. *Leukemia* 2002; **16**: 1233–50.

40. Behm FG, Smith FO, Raimondi SC et al. Human homologue of the rat chondroitin sulfate proteoglycan, NG2, detected by monoclonal antibody 7.1, identifies childhood acute lymphoblastic leukemias with t(4;11)(q21;q23) or t(11;19)(q23;p13) and *MLL* gene rearrangements. *Blood* 1996; **87**: 1134–9.

41. Smith FO, Rauch C, Williams DE et al. The human homologue of rat NG2, a chondroitin sulfate proteoglycan, is not expressed on the cell surface of normal hematopoietic cells but is expressed by acute myeloid leukemia blasts from poor-prognosis patients with abnormalities of chromosome band 11q23. *Blood* 1996; **87**: 1123–33.

42. Chen JS, Coustan-Smith E, Suzuki T et al. Identification of novel markers for monitoring minimal residual disease in acute lymphoblastic leukemia. *Blood* 2001; **97**: 2115–20.

43. Coustan-Smith E, Behm FG, Sanchez J et al. Immunological detection of minimal residual disease in children with acute lymphoblastic leukaemia. *Lancet* 1998; **351**: 550–4.

44. Ciudad J, San Miguel JF, Lopez-Berges MC et al. Prognostic value of immunophenotypic detection of minimal residual disease in acute lymphoblastic leukemia. *J Clin Oncol* 1998; **16**: 3774–81.

45. Griesinger F, Piró-Noack M, Kaib N et al. Leukaemia-associated immunophenotypes (LIAP) are observed on 90% of adult and childhood acute lymphoblastic leukaemia: detection in remission marrow predicts outcome. *Br J Haematol* 1999; **105**: 241–55.

46. Lucio P, Parreira A, van den Beemd MW et al. Flow cytometric analysis of normal B cell differentiation: a frame of reference for the detection of minimal residual disease in precursor-B-ALL. *Leukemia* 1999; **13**: 419–27.

47. Weir EG, Cowan K, LeBeau P, Borowitz MJ. A limited antibody panel can distinguish B-precursor acute

lymphoblastic leukemia from normal B precursors with four color flow cytometry: implications for residual disease detection. *Leukemia* 1999; **13**: 558–67.

48. Ciudad J, San Miguel JF, Lopez-Berges MC et al. Detection of abnormalities in B-cell differentiation pattern is a useful tool to predict relapse in precursor-B-ALL. *Br J Haematol* 1999; **104**: 695–705.

49. Lucio P, Gaipa G, van Lochem EG et al. BIOMED-1 concerted action report: flow cytometric immunophenotyping of precursor B-ALL with standardized triple-stainings. BIOMED-1 Concerted Action Investigation of Minimal Residual Disease in Acute Leukemia: International Standardization and Clinical Evaluation. *Leukemia* 2001; **15**: 1185–92.

50. Sang BC, Shi L, Dias P et al. Monoclonal antibodies specific to the acute lymphoblastic leukemia t(1;19)-associated E2A/PBX1 chimeric protein: characterization and diagnostic utility. *Blood* 1997; **89**: 2909–14.

51. Knulst AC, Adriaansen HJ, Hählen K et al. Early diagnosis of smoldering acute lymphoblastic leukemia using immunological marker analysis. *Leukemia* 1993; **7**: 532–6.

52. Farahat N, Lens D, Zomas A et al. Quantitative flow cytometry can distinguish between normal and leukaemic B-cell precursors. *Br J Haematol* 1995; **91**: 640–6.

53. Smedmyr B, Bengtsson M, Jakobsson A et al. Regeneration of CALLA (CD10$^+$), TdT$^+$ and double-positive cells in the bone marrow and blood after autologous bone marrow transplantation. *Eur J Haematol* 1991; **46**: 146–51.

54. Van Lochem EG, Wiegers YM, van den Beemd R et al. Regeneration pattern of precursor-B-cells in bone marrow of acute lymphoblastic leukemia patients depends on the type of preceding chemotherapy. *Leukemia* 2000; **14**: 688–95.

55. Van Wering ER, van der Linden-Schrever BE, Szczepański T et al. Regenerating normal B-cell precursors during and after treatment of acute lymphoblastic leukaemia: implications for monitoring of minimal residual disease. *Br J Haematol* 2000; **110**: 139–46.

56. Van Dongen JJM, Szczepański T, de Bruijn MAC et al. Detection of minimal residual disease in acute leukemia patients. *Cytokines Mol Ther* 1996; **2**: 121–33.

57. Porwit-MacDonald A, Bjorklund E, Lucio P et al. BIOMED-1 concerted action report: flow cytometric characterization of CD7$^+$ cell subsets in normal bone marrow as a basis for the diagnosis and follow-up of T cell acute lymphoblastic leukemia (T-ALL). *Leukemia* 2000; **14**: 816–25.

58. Breit TM, Mol EJ, Wolvers-Tettero ILM et al. Site-specific deletions involving the *tal-1* and *sil* genes are restricted to cells of the T cell receptor α/β lineage: T cell receptor δ gene deletion mechanism affects multiple genes. *J Exp Med* 1993; **177**: 965–77.

59. Delabesse E, Bernard M, Meyer V et al. *TAL1* expression does not occur in the majority of T-ALL blasts. *Br J Haematol* 1998; **102**: 449–57.

60. Geisler CH, Larsen JK, Hansen NE et al. Prognostic importance of flow cytometric immunophenotyping of 540 consecutive patients with B-cell chronic lymphocytic leukemia. *Blood* 1991; **78**: 1795–802.

61. Robbins BA, Ellison DJ, Spinosa JC et al. Diagnostic application of two-color flow cytometry in 161 cases of hairy cell leukemia. *Blood* 1993; **82**: 1277–87.

62. Molot RJ, Meeker TC, Wittwer CT et al. Antigen expression and polymerase chain reaction amplification of mantle cell lymphomas. *Blood* 1994; **83**: 1626–31.

63. Hermine O, Haioun C, Lepage E et al. Prognostic significance of bcl-2 protein expression in aggressive non-Hodgkin's lymphoma. *Blood* 1996; **87**: 265–72.

64. De Boer CJ, Schuuring E, Dreef E et al. Cyclin D1 protein analysis in the diagnosis of mantle cell lymphoma. *Blood* 1995; **86**: 2715–23.

65. Rawstron AC, Kennedy B, Evans PA et al. Quantitation of minimal disease levels in chronic lymphocytic leukemia using a sensitive flow cytometric assay improves the prediction of outcome and can be used to optimize therapy. *Blood* 2001; **98**: 29–35.

66. Esteve J, Villamor N, Colomer D et al. Stem cell transplantation for chronic lymphocytic leukemia: different outcome after autologous and allogeneic transplantation and correlation with minimal residual disease status. *Leukemia* 2001; **15**: 445–51.

67. Borst J, Wicherink A, Van Dongen JJM et al. Non-random expression of T cell receptor γ and δ variable gene segments in functional T lymphocyte clones from human peripheral blood. *Eur J Immunol* 1989; **19**: 1559–68.

68. Pulford K, Lamant L, Morris SW et al. Detection of anaplastic lymphoma kinase (ALK) and nucleolar protein nucleophosmin (NPM)–ALK proteins in normal and neoplastic cells with the monoclonal antibody ALK1. *Blood* 1997; **89**: 1394–404.

69. Almeida J, Orfao A, Ocqueteau M et al. High-sensitive immunophenotyping and DNA ploidy studies for the investigation of minimal residual disease in multiple myeloma. *Br J Haematol* 1999; **107**: 121–31.

70. Tonegawa S. Somatic generation of antibody diversity. *Nature* 1983; **302**: 575–81.

71. Davis MM, Björkman PJ. T-cell antigen receptor genes and T-cell recognition. *Nature* 1988; **334**: 395–402.

72. Szczepański T, Flohr T, van der Velden VHJ et al. Molecular monitoring of residual disease using antigen receptor genes in childhood acute lymphoblastic leukaemia. *Best Pract Res Clin Haematol* 2002; **15**: 37–57.

73. Reth MG, Jackson S, Alt FW. *VHDJH* formation and *DJH* replacement during pre-B differentiation: non-random usage of gene segments. *EMBO J* 1986; **5**: 2131–8.

74. Marolleau JP, Fondell JD, Malissen M et al. The joining of germ-line *Vα* to *Jα* genes replaces the preexisting *Vα–Jα* complexes in a T cell receptor αβ positive T cell line. *Cell* 1988; **55**: 291–300.

75. Reth M, Gehrmann P, Petrac E, Wiese P. A novel *VH* to *VHDJH* joining mechanism in heavy-chain-negative (null) pre-B cells results in heavy-chain production. *Nature* 1986; **322**: 840–2.

76. Alt FW, Blackwell TK, Yancopoulos GD. Development of the primary antibody repertoire. *Science* 1987; **238**: 1079–87.

77. Beishuizen A, Verhoeven MA, van Wering ER et al. Analysis of Ig and T-cell receptor genes in 40 childhood acute lymphoblastic leukemias at diagnosis and subsequent relapse: implications for the detection of minimal residual disease by polymerase chain reaction analysis. *Blood* 1994; **83**: 2238–47.

78. Bird J, Galili N, Link M et al. Continuing rearrangement but absence of somatic hypermutation in immunoglobulin genes of human B cell precursor leukemia. *J Exp Med* 1988; **168**: 229–45.

79. Wasserman R, Yamada M, Ito Y et al. *VH* gene rearrangement events can modify the immunoglobulin heavy chain

during progression of B-lineage acute lymphoblastic leukemia. *Blood* 1992; **79**: 223–8.

80. Kitchingman GR. Immunoglobulin heavy chain gene *VH–D* junctional diversity at diagnosis in patients with acute lymphoblastic leukemia. *Blood* 1993; **81**: 775–82.

81. Steenbergen EJ, Verhagen OJ, van Leeuwen EF et al. Distinct ongoing Ig heavy chain rearrangement processes in childhood B-precursor acute lymphoblastic leukemia. *Blood* 1993; **82**: 581–9.

82. Ghali DW, Panzer S, Fischer S et al. Heterogeneity of the T-cell receptor δ gene indicating subclone formation in acute precursor B-cell leukemias. *Blood* 1995; **85**: 2795–801.

83. Steward CG, Goulden NJ, Katz F et al. A polymerase chain reaction study of the stability of Ig heavy-chain and T-cell receptor δ gene rearrangements between presentation and relapse of childhood B-lineage acute lymphoblastic leukemia. *Blood* 1994; **83**: 1355–62.

84. Taylor JJ, Rowe D, Kylefjord H et al. Characterisation of non-concordance in the T-cell receptor γ chain genes at presentation and clinical relapse in acute lymphoblastic leukemia. *Leukemia* 1994; **8**: 60–6.

85. Steenbergen EJ, Verhagen OJ, van Leeuwen EF et al. Frequent ongoing T-cell receptor rearrangements in childhood B-precursor acute lymphoblastic leukemia: implications for monitoring minimal residual disease. *Blood* 1995; **86**: 692–702.

86. Rajewsky K, Forster I, Cumano A. Evolutionary and somatic selection of the antibody repertoire in the mouse. *Science* 1987; **238**: 1088–94.

87. Cleary ML, Galili N, Trela M et al. Single cell origin of bigenotypic and biphenotypic B cell proliferations in human follicular lymphomas. *J Exp Med* 1988; **167**: 582–97.

88. Cleary ML, Meeker TC, Levy S et al. Clustering of extensive somatic mutations in the variable region of an immunoglobulin heavy chain gene from a human B cell lymphoma. *Cell* 1986; **44**: 97–106.

89. Bakkus MH, Heirman C, Van Riet I et al. Evidence that multiple myeloma Ig heavy chain VDJ genes contain somatic mutations but show no intraclonal variation. *Blood* 1992; **80**: 2326–35.

90. Breit TM, Wolvers-Tettero ILM, Hählen K et al. Extensive junctional diversity of γδ T-cell receptors expressed by T-cell acute lymphoblastic leukemias: implications for the detection of minimal residual disease. *Leukemia* 1991; **5**: 1076–86.

91. Yamada M, Hudson S, Tournay O et al. Detection of minimal disease in hematopoietic malignancies of the B-cell lineage by using third-complementarity-determining region (CDR-III)-specific probes. *Proc Natl Acad Sci USA* 1989; **86**: 5123–7.

92. d'Auriol L, Macintyre E, Galibert F, Sigaux F. In vitro amplification of T cell γ gene rearrangements: a new tool for the assessment of minimal residual disease in acute lymphoblastic leukemias. *Leukemia* 1989; **3**: 155–8.

93. Hansen-Hagge TE, Yokota S, Bartram CR. Detection of minimal residual disease in acute lymphoblastic leukemia by in vitro amplification of rearranged T-cell receptor δ chain sequences. *Blood* 1989; **74**: 1762–7.

93a. Van Dongen JJM, Langerak AW, Bruggemann M, Evans PAS, Hummel M, Lavender FL, Delabesse E, Davi F, Schuuring E, Garcia-Sanz R, van Krieken JHJM, Droese J, Gonzalez D, Bastard C, White HE, Spaargaren M, Gonzalez M, Parreira A, Smith JL, Morgan GJ, Kneba M, Macintyre EA. Design and standardization of PCR primers and protocols for detection of clonal immunoglobulin and T-cell receptor gene recombinations in suspect lymphoproliferations: Report of the BIOMED-2 Concerted Action BMH4-CT98-3936. *Leukemia* 2003; **17**: 2257–317.

94. Langerak AW, Szczepański T, van der Burg M et al. Heteroduplex PCR analysis of rearranged T cell receptor genes for clonality assessment in suspect T cell proliferations. *Leukemia* 1997; **11**: 2192–9.

95. Linke B, Bolz I, Fayyazi A et al. Automated high resolution PCR fragment analysis for identification of clonally rearranged immunoglobulin heavy chain genes. *Leukemia* 1997; **11**: 1055–62.

96. Van Wering ER, van der Linden-Schrever BEM, van der Velden VHJ et al. T lymphocytes in bone marrow samples of children with acute lymphoblastic leukemia during and after chemotherapy might hamper PCR-based minimal residual disease studies. *Leukemia* 2001; **15**: 1031–3.

97. Pongers-Willemse MJ, Seriu T, Stolz F et al. Primers and protocols for standardized MRD detection in ALL using immunoglobulin and T cell receptor gene rearrangements and *TAL1* deletions as PCR targets. Report of the BIOMED-1 Concerted Action: Investigation of Minimal Residual Disease in Acute Leukemia. *Leukemia* 1999; **13**: 110–18.

98. Van der Velden VHJ, Wijkhuijs JM, Jacobs DCH et al. T cell receptor γ gene rearrangements as targets for detection of minimal residual disease in acute lymphoblastic leukemia by real-time quantitative PCR analysis. *Leukemia* 2002; **16**: 1372–80.

99. Beishuizen A, Hählen K, Hagemeijer A et al. Multiple rearranged immunoglobulin genes in childhood acute lymphoblastic leukemia of precursor B-cell origin. *Leukemia* 1991; **5**: 657–67.

100. Szczepański T, Willemse MJ, van Wering ER et al. Precursor-B-ALL with *DH–JH* gene rearrangements have an immature immunogenotype with a high frequency of oligoclonality and hyperdiploidy of chromosome 14. *Leukemia* 2001; **15**: 1415–23.

101. Mortuza FY, Moreira IM, Papaioannou M et al. Immunoglobulin heavy-chain gene rearrangement in adult acute lymphoblastic leukemia reveals preferential usage of *J(H)*-proximal variable gene segments. *Blood* 2001; **97**: 2716–26.

102. Van Dongen JJM, Wolvers-Tettero ILM. Analysis of immunoglobulin and T cell receptor genes. Part II: Possibilities and limitations in the diagnosis and management of lymphoproliferative diseases and related disorders. *Clin Chim Acta* 1991; **198**: 93–174.

103. Beishuizen A, Verhoeven MA, Mol EJ, van Dongen JJM. Detection of immunoglobulin kappa light-chain gene rearrangement patterns by Southern blot analysis. *Leukemia* 1994; **8**: 2228–36.

104. Tümkaya T, van der Burg M, Garcia Sanz R et al. Immunoglobulin lambda isotype gene rearrangements in B-cell malignancies. *Leukemia* 2001; **15**: 121–7.

104a. Van Der Burg M, Barendregt BH, Szczepanski T, Van Wering ER, Langerak AW, Van Dongen JJM. Immunoglobulin light chain gene rearrangements display hierarchy in absence of selection for functionality in precursor-B-ALL. *Leukemia* 2002; **16**: 1448–53.

105. Beishuizen A, de Bruijn MAC, Pongers-Willemse MJ et al. Heterogeneity in junctional regions of immunoglobulin κ deleting element rearrangements in B cell leukemias: a

new molecular target for detection of minimal residual disease. *Leukemia* 1997; **11**: 2200–7.

106. Felix CA, Wright JJ, Poplack DG et al. T cell receptor α-, β-, and γ-genes in T cell and pre-B cell acute lymphoblastic leukemia. *J Clin Invest* 1987; **80**: 545–56.

107. Szczepański T, Beishuizen A, Pongers-Willemse MJ et al. Cross-lineage T-cell receptor gene rearrangements occur in more than ninety percent of childhood precursor-B-acute lymphoblastic leukemias: alternative PCR targets for detection of minimal residual disease. *Leukemia* 1999; **13**: 196–205.

107a. Szczepański T, Van der Velden VH, Hoogeveen PG, De Bie M, Jacobs DC, Van Wering ER, Van Dongen JJM. Vd2-Ja rearrangements are frequent in precursor-B-acute lymphoblastic leukemia but rare in normal lymphoid cells. *Blood* 2004; **103**: 3798–804.

108. Langerak AW, Wolvers-Tettero ILM, van Dongen JJM. Detection of T cell receptor β (*TCRB*) gene rearrangement patterns in T cell malignancies by Southern blot analysis. *Leukemia* 1999; **13**: 965–74.

109. Biondi A, Francia di Celle P, Rossi V et al. High prevalence of T-cell receptor Vδ2–(D)–Dδ3 or Dδ1/2–Dδ3 rearrangements in B-precursor acute lymphoblastic leukemias. *Blood* 1990; **75**: 1834–40.

110. Breit TM, Wolvers-Tettero ILM, Hählen K et al. Limited combinatorial repertoire of γδ T-cell receptors expressed by T-cell acute lymphoblastic leukemias. *Leukemia* 1991; **5**: 116–24.

111. Bierings M, Szczepański T, van Wering ER et al. Two consecutive immunophenotypic switches in a child with immunogenotypically stable acute leukaemia. *Br J Haematol* 2001; **113**: 757–62.

112. Yokota S, Hansen-Hagge TE, Bartram CR. T-cell receptor δ gene recombination in common acute lymphoblastic leukemia: preferential usage of Vδ2 and frequent involvement of the Jα cluster. *Blood* 1991; **77**: 141–8.

113. Szczepański T, Langerak AW, Wolvers-Tettero ILM et al. Immunoglobulin and T cell receptor gene rearrangement patterns in acute lymphoblastic leukemia are less mature in adults than in children: implications for selection of PCR targets for detection of minimal residual disease. *Leukemia* 1998; **12**: 1081–8.

114. Brumpt C, Delabesse E, Beldjord K et al. The incidence of clonal T-cell receptor rearrangements in B-cell precursor acute lymphoblastic leukemia varies with age and genotype. *Blood* 2000; **96**: 2254–61.

115. Peham M, Panzer S, Fasching K et al. Low frequency of clonotypic Ig and T-cell receptor gene rearrangements in t(4;11) infant acute lymphoblastic leukaemia and its implication for the detection of minimal residual disease. *Br J Haematol* 2002; **117**: 315–21.

115a. Van der Velden VHJ, Szczepanski T, Wijkhuijs JM, Hart PG, Hoogeveen PG, Hop WC, Van Wering ER, Van Dongen JJM. Age-related patterns of immunoglobulin and T-cell receptor gene rearrangements in precursor-B-ALL: implications for detection of minimal residual disease. *Leukemia* 2003;**17**:1834–44.

116. Van Dongen JJM, Comans-Bitter WM, Wolvers-Tettero ILM, Borst J. Development of human T lymphocytes and their thymus-dependency. *Thymus* 1990; **16**: 207–34.

117. Breit TM, Wolvers-Tettero ILM, Beishuizen A et al. Southern blot patterns, frequencies and junctional diversity of T-cell receptor δ gene rearrangements in acute lymphoblastic leukemia. *Blood* 1993; **82**: 3063–74.

118. Szczepański T, Langerak AW, Willemse MJ et al. T cell receptor γ (*TCRG*) gene rearrangements in T cell acute lymphoblastic leukemia reflect 'end-stage' recombinations: implications for minimal residual disease monitoring. *Leukemia* 2000; **14**: 1208–14.

119. Szczepański T, Pongers-Willemse MJ, Langerak AW et al. Ig heavy chain gene rearrangements in T-cell acute lymphoblastic leukemia exhibit predominant *DH6-19* and *DH7-27* gene usage, can result in complete *V–D–J* rearrangements, and are rare in T-cell receptor αβ lineage. *Blood* 1999; **93**: 4079–85.

120. Szczepański T, Pongers-Willemse MJ, Langerak AW, van Dongen JJM. Unusual immunoglobulin and T-cell receptor gene rearrangement patterns in acute lymphoblastic leukemias. *Curr Top Microbiol Immunol* 1999; **246**: 205–15.

121. Szczepański T, Willemse MJ, Kamps WA et al. Molecular discrimination between relapsed and secondary acute lymphoblastic leukemia – proposal for an easy strategy. *Med Pediatr Oncol* 2001; **36**: 352–8.

122. Szczepański T, Willemse MJ, Brinkhof B et al. Comparative analysis of Ig and TCR gene rearrangements at diagnosis and at relapse of childhood precursor-B-ALL provides improved strategies for selection of stable PCR targets for monitoring of minimal residual disease. *Blood* 2002; **99**: 2315–23.

123. Van der Velden VHJ, Willemse MJ, van der Schoot CE et al. Immunoglobulin κ deleting element rearrangements in precursor-B acute lymphoblastic leukemia are stable targets for detection of minimal residual disease by real-time quantitative PCR. *Leukemia* 2002; **16**: 928–36.

124. Van Dongen JJM, Seriu T, Panzer-Grumayer ER et al. Prognostic value of minimal residual disease in acute lymphoblastic leukaemia in childhood. *Lancet* 1998; **352**: 1731–8.

124a. Szczepański T, Van der Velden VHJ, Raff T, Jacobs DC, van Wering ER, Bruggemann M, Kneba M, van Dongen JJM. Comparative analysis of T-cell receptor gene rearrangements at diagnosis and relapse of T-cell acute lymphoblastic leukemia (T-ALL) shows high stability of clonal markers for monitoring of minimal residual disease and reveals the occurrence of second T-ALL. *Leukemia* 2003; **17**: 2149–56.

124b. Li A, Zhou J, Zuckerman D, Rue M, Dalton V, Lyons C, Silverman LB, Sallan SE, Gribben JG. Sequence analysis of clonal immunoglobulin and T-cell receptor gene rearrangements in children with acute lymphoblastic leukemia at diagnosis and at relapse: implications for pathogenesis and for the clinical utility of PCR-based methods of minimal residual disease detection. *Blood* 2003; **102**: 4520–26.

124c. Germano G, del Giudice L, Palatron S, Giarin E, Cazzaniga G, Biondi A, Basso G. Clonality profile in relapsed precursor-B-ALL children by GeneScan and sequencing analyses. Consequences on minimal residual disease monitoring. *Leukemia* 2003; **17**: 1573–82.

125. van der Burg M, Tumkaya T, Boerma M et al. Ordered recombination of immunoglobulin light chain genes occurs at the *IGK* locus but seems less strict at the *IGL* locus. *Blood* 2001; **97**: 1001–8.

126. Wagner SD, Martinelli V, Luzzatto L. Similar patterns of Vκ gene usage but different degrees of somatic mutation in hairy cell leukemia, prolymphocytic leukemia, Waldenström's macroglobulinemia, and myeloma. *Blood* 1994; **83**: 3647–53.

127. Derksen PW, Langerak AW, Kerkhof E et al. Comparison of different polymerase chain reaction-based approaches for clonality assessment of immunoglobulin heavy-chain gene rearrangements in B-cell neoplasia. *Mod Pathol* 1999; **12**: 794–805.

128. Kneba M, Bolz I, Linke B, Hiddemann W. Analysis of rearranged T-cell receptor β-chain genes by polymerase chain reaction (PCR) DNA sequencing and automated high resolution PCR fragment analysis. *Blood* 1995; **86**: 3930–7.

128a. Droese J, Langerak AW, Groenen PJTA, Bruggemann M, Neumann P, Wolvers-Tettero ILM, Van Altena MC, Kneba M, Van Dongen JJM. Validation of BIOMED-2 multiplex PCR tubes for detection of *TCRB* gene rearrangements in T-cell malignancies. *Leukemia* 2004; **18**: in press.

128b. Sandberg Y, Heule F, Lam K, Lugtenburg PJ, Wolvers-Tettero ILM, Van Dongen JJM, Langerak AW. Molecular immunoglobulin/T- cell receptor clonality analysis in cutaneous lymphoproliferations. Experience with the BIOMED-2 standardized polymerase chain reaction protocol. *Haematologica* 2003; **88**: 659–70.

129. Van Dongen JJM, Szczepański T, Adriaansen HJ. Immunobiology of leukemia. In: Henderson ES, Lister TA, Greaves MF (eds) *Leukemia*. Philadelphia: WB Saunders Company, 2002.

130. Breit TM, Beishuizen A, Ludwig WD et al. *tal-1* deletions in T-cell acute lymphoblastic leukemia as PCR target for detection of minimal residual disease. *Leukemia* 1993; **7**: 2004–11.

131. Wiemels JL, Cazzaniga G, Daniotti M et al. Prenatal origin of acute lymphoblastic leukaemia in children. *Lancet* 1999; **354**: 1499–503.

132. Reichel M, Gillert E, Breitenlohner I et al. Rapid isolation of chromosomal breakpoints from patients with t(4;11) acute lymphoblastic leukemia: implications for basic and clinical research. *Cancer Res* 1999; **59**: 3357–62.

133. Privitera E, Rivolta A, Ronchetti D et al. Reverse transcriptase/polymerase chain reaction follow-up and minimal residual disease detection in t(1;19)-positive acute lymphoblastic leukaemia. *Br J Haematol* 1996; **92**: 653–8.

134. Nakao M, Yokota S, Horiike S et al. Detection and quantification of *TEL/AML1* fusion transcripts by polymerase chain reaction in childhood acute lymphoblastic leukemia. *Leukemia* 1996; **10**: 1463–70.

135. Morris SW, Kirstein MN, Valentine MB et al. Fusion of a kinase gene, *ALK*, to a nucleolar protein gene, *NPM*, in non-Hodgkin's lymphoma. *Science* 1994; **263**: 1281–4.

136. Gleissner B, Rieder H, Thiel E et al. Prospective *BCR–ABL* analysis by polymerase chain reaction (RT–PCR) in adult acute B-lineage lymphoblastic leukemia: reliability of RT–nested-PCR and comparison to cytogenetic data. *Leukemia* 2001; **15**: 1834–40.

137. Cleary ML, Sklar J. Nucleotide sequence of a t(14;18) chromosomal breakpoint in follicular lymphoma and demonstration of a breakpoint-cluster region near a transcriptionally active locus on chromosome 18. *Proc Natl Acad Sci USA* 1985; **82**: 7439–43.

138. Williams ME, Meeker TC, Swerdlow SH. Rearrangement of the chromosome 11 *bcl-1* locus in centrocytic lymphoma: analysis with multiple breakpoint probes. *Blood* 1991; **78**: 493–8.

139. Leder P, Battey J, Lenoir G et al. Translocations among antibody genes in human cancer. *Science* 1983; **222**: 765–71.

140. Lee MS, Chang KS, Cabanillas F et al. Detection of minimal residual cells carrying the t(14;18) by DNA sequence amplification. *Science* 1987; **237**: 175–8.

141. Bergsagel PL, Chesi M, Nardini E et al. Promiscuous translocations into immunoglobulin heavy chain switch regions in multiple myeloma. *Proc Natl Acad Sci USA* 1996; **93**: 13931–6.

142. Nishida K, Tamura A, Nakazawa N et al. The Ig heavy chain gene is frequently involved in chromosomal translocations in multiple myeloma and plasma cell leukemia as detected by in situ hybridization. *Blood* 1997; **90**: 526–34.

143. Szczepański T, van 't Veer MB, Wolvers-Tettero ILM et al. Molecular features responsible for the absence of immunoglobulin heavy chain protein synthesis in an IgH⁻ subgroup of multiple myeloma. *Blood* 2000; **96**: 1087–93.

144. Brisco MJ, Condon J, Hughes E et al. Outcome prediction in childhood acute lymphoblastic leukaemia by molecular quantification of residual disease at the end of induction. *Lancet* 1994; **343**: 196–200.

145. Ouspenskaia MV, Johnston DA, Roberts WM et al. Accurate quantitation of residual B-precursor acute lymphoblastic leukemia by limiting dilution and a PCR-based detection system: a description of the method and the principles involved. *Leukemia* 1995; **9**: 321–8.

146. Cave H, Guidal C, Rohrlich P et al. Prospective monitoring and quantitation of residual blasts in childhood acute lymphoblastic leukemia by polymerase chain reaction study of δ and γ T-cell receptor genes. *Blood* 1994; **83**: 1892–902.

147. Knechtli CJ, Goulden NJ, Hancock JP et al. Minimal residual disease status before allogeneic bone marrow transplantation is an important determinant of successful outcome for children and adolescents with acute lymphoblastic leukemia. *Blood* 1998; **92**: 4072–9.

148. Delabesse E, Burtin ML, Millien C et al. Rapid, multifluorescent TCRG *Vγ* and *Jγ* typing: application to T cell acute lymphoblastic leukemia and to the detection of minor clonal populations. *Leukemia* 2000; **14**: 1143–52.

148a. Guidal C, Vilmer E, Grandchamp B, Cave H. A competitive PCR-based method using *TCRD*, *TCRG* and *IGH* rearrangements for rapid detection of patients with high levels of minimal residual disease in acute lymphoblastic leukemia. *Leukemia* 2002; **16**: 762–4.

149. Van der Velden VHJ, Szczepański T, van Dongen JJM. Polymerase chain reaction, real-time quantitative. In: Brenner S, Miller JH (eds) *Encyclopedia of Genetics*. London: Academic Press, 2001: 1503–6.

150. Heid CA, Stevens J, Livak KJ, Williams PM. Real time quantitative PCR. *Genome Res* 1996; **6**: 986–94.

150a. Van der Velden VHJ, Hochhaus A, Cazzaniga G, Szczepanski T, Gabert J, Van Dongen JJM. Detection of minimal residual disease in hematologic malignancies by real-time quantitative PCR: principles, approaches, and laboratory aspects. *Leukemia* 2003; **17**: 1013–34.

150b. Szczepanski T, van der Velden VHJ, van Dongen JJM. Real-time quantitative (RQ)-PCR for the detection of minimal residual disease in childhood acute lymphoblastic leukemia. *Haematologica* 2002; **87 Suppl. 1**: 183–91.

151. Holland PM, Abramson RD, Watson R, Gelfand DH. Detection of specific polymerase chain reaction product by utilizing the 5′→3′ exonuclease activity of *Thermus aquaticus* DNA polymerase. *Proc Natl Acad Sci USA* 1991; **88**: 7276–80.

152. Kreuzer KA, Lass U, Bohn A et al. LightCycler technology for the quantitation of *bcr/abl* fusion transcripts. *Cancer Res* 1999; **59**: 3171–4.

153. Luthra R, McBride JA, Cabanillas F, Sarris A. Novel 5′ exonuclease-based real-time PCR assay for the detection of t(14;18)(q32;q21) in patients with follicular lymphoma. *Am J Pathol* 1998; **153**: 63–8.

154. Marcucci G, Livak KJ, Bi W et al. Detection of minimal residual disease in patients with *AML1/ETO*-associated acute myeloid leukemia using a novel quantitative reverse transcription polymerase chain reaction assay. *Leukemia* 1998; **12**: 1482–9.

155. Mensink E, van de Locht A, Schattenberg A et al. Quantitation of minimal residual disease in Philadelphia chromosome positive chronic myeloid leukaemia patients using real-time quantitative RT–PCR. *Br J Haematol* 1998; **102**: 768–74.

156. Pallisgaard N, Clausen N, Schroder H, Hokland P. Rapid and sensitive minimal residual disease detection in acute leukemia by quantitative real-time RT–PCR exemplified by t(12;21) *TEL–AML1* fusion transcript. *Genes Chromosomes Cancer* 1999; **26**: 355–65.

157. Pongers-Willemse MJ, Verhagen OJHM, Tibbe GJM et al. Real-time quantitative PCR for the detection of minimal residual disease in acute lymphoblastic leukemia using junctional regions specific TaqMan probes. *Leukemia* 1998; **12**: 2006–14.

158. Verhagen OJHM, Willemse MJ, Breunis WB et al. Application of germline *IGH* probes in real-time quantitative PCR for the detection of minimal residual disease in acute lymphoblastic leukemia. *Leukemia* 2000; **14**: 1426–35.

158a. Gabert J, Beillard E, Van der Velden VH, Bi W, Grimwade D, Pallisgaard N, Barbany G, Cazzaniga G, Cayuela JM, Cave H, Pane F, Aerts JL, De Micheli D, Thirion X, Pradel V, Gonzalez M, Viehmann S, Malec M, Saglio G, Van Dongen JJM .Standardization and quality control studies of 'real-time' quantitative reverse transcriptase polymerase chain reaction of fusion gene transcripts for residual disease detection in leukemia - a Europe Against Cancer program. *Leukemia* 2003; **17**: 2318–57.

159. Eckert C, Landt O, Taube T et al. Potential of LightCycler technology for quantification of minimal residual disease in childhood acute lymphoblastic leukemia. *Leukemia* 2000; **14**: 316–23.

160. Nakao M, Janssen JW, Flohr T, Bartram CR. Rapid and reliable quantification of minimal residual disease in acute lymphoblastic leukemia using rearranged immunoglobulin and T-cell receptor loci by LightCycler technology. *Cancer Res* 2000; **60**: 3281–9.

161. Pinkel D, Woo S. Prevention and treatment of meningeal leukemia in children. *Blood* 1994; **84**: 355–66.

162. Mahmoud HH, Rivera GK, Hancock ML et al. Low leukocyte counts with blast cells in cerebrospinal fluid of children with newly diagnosed acute lymphoblastic leukemia. *N Engl J Med* 1993; **329**: 314–19.

163. Rivera GK, Pinkel D, Simone JV et al. Treatment of acute lymphoblastic leukemia. 30 years' experience at St. Jude Children's Research Hospital. *N Engl J Med* 1993; **329**: 1289–95.

164. Hooijkaas H, Hählen K, Adriaansen HJ et al. Terminal deoxynucleotidyl transferase (TdT)-positive cells in cerebrospinal fluid and development of overt CNS leukemia: a 5-year follow-up study in 113 children with a TdT-positive leukemia or non-Hodgkin's lymphoma. *Blood* 1989; **74**: 416–22.

165. Campana D. Applications of cytometry to study acute leukemia: in vitro determination of drug sensitivity and detection of minimal residual disease. *Cytometry (Commun Clin Cytometry)* 1994; **18**: 68–74.

166. Subira D, Castanon S, Roman A et al. Flow cytometry and the study of central nervous disease in patients with acute leukaemia. *Br J Haematol* 2001; **112**: 381–4.

167. Januszkiewicz DA, Nowak JS. Molecular evidence for central nervous system involvement in children with newly diagnosed acute lymphoblastic leukemia. *Hematol Oncol* 1995; **13**: 201–6.

168. De Haas V, Vet M, Verhagen M et al. Early detection of central nervous system relapse by polymerase chain reaction in children with B-precursor acute lymphoblastic leukemia. *Ann Hematol* 2002; **81**: 59–61.

169. Sills RH, Stockman JA. Preleukemic states in children with acute lymphoblastic leukemia. *Cancer* 1981; **48**: 110–12.

170. Escudier SM, Albitar M, Robertson LE et al. Acute lymphoblastic leukemia following preleukemic syndromes in adults. *Leukemia* 1996; **10**: 473–7.

171. Ishikawa K, Seriu T, Watanabe A et al. Detection of neoplastic clone in the hypoplastic and recovery phases preceding acute lymphoblastic leukemia by in vitro amplification of rearranged T-cell receptor δ chain gene. *J Pediatr Hematol Oncol* 1995; **17**: 270–5.

172. Morley AA, Brisco MJ, Rice M et al. Leukaemia presenting as marrow hypoplasia: molecular detection of the leukaemic clone at the time of initial presentation. *Br J Haematol* 1997; **98**: 940–4.

173. Wells DA, Hall MC, Shulman HM, Loken MR. Occult B cell malignancies can be detected by three-color flow cytometry in patients with cytopenias. *Leukemia* 1998; **12**: 2015–23.

174. Goulden N, Langlands K, Steward C et al. PCR assessment of bone marrow status in 'isolated' extramedullary relapse of childhood B-precursor acute lymphoblastic leukaemia. *Br J Haematol* 1994; **87**: 282–5.

175. Neale GA, Pui CH, Mahmoud HH et al. Molecular evidence for minimal residual bone marrow disease in children with 'isolated' extra-medullary relapse of T-cell acute lymphoblastic leukemia. *Leukemia* 1994; **8**: 768–75.

176. O'Reilly J, Meyer B, Baker D et al. Correlation of bone marrow minimal residual disease and apparent isolated extramedullary relapse in childhood acute lymphoblastic leukaemia. *Leukemia* 1995; **9**: 624–7.

177. Yamada M, Wasserman R, Lange B et al. Minimal residual disease in childhood B-lineage lymphoblastic leukemia. Persistence of leukemic cells during the first 18 months of treatment. *N Engl J Med* 1990; **323**: 448–55.

178. Lal A, Kwan E, al Mahr M et al. Molecular detection of acute lymphoblastic leukaemia in boys with testicular relapse. *Mol Pathol* 1998; **51**: 277–81.

179. Sandlund JT, Downing JR, Crist WM. Non-Hodgkin's lymphoma in childhood. *N Engl J Med* 1996; **334**: 1238–48.

180. Bradstock KF, Kerr A. Immunological detection of covert leukaemic spread in mediastinal T-cell lymphoblastic lymphoma. *Leuk Res* 1985; **9**: 905–11.

181. Gribben JG, Freedman A, Woo SD et al. All advanced stage non-Hodgkin's lymphomas with a polymerase chain reaction amplifiable breakpoint of *bcl-2* have residual cells containing the *bcl-2* rearrangement at evaluation and after treatment. *Blood* 1991; **78**: 3275–80.

182. Lambrechts AC, Hupkes PE, Dorssers LC, van't Veer MB.

Translocation (14;18)-positive cells are present in the circulation of the majority of patients with localized (stage I and II) follicular non-Hodgkin's lymphoma. *Blood* 1993; **82**: 2510–16.

183. Kurokawa T, Kinoshita T, Ito T et al. Detection of minimal residual disease B cell lymphoma by a PCR-mediated RNase protection assay. *Leukemia* 1996; **10**: 1222–31.

184. Vervoordeldonk SF, Merle PA, Behrendt H et al. PCR-positivity in harvested bone marrow predicts relapse after transplantation with autologous purged bone marrow in children in second remission of precursor B-cell acute leukaemia. *Br J Haematol* 1997; **96**: 395–402.

185. Balduzzi A, Gaipa G, Bonanomi S et al. Purified autologous grafting in childhood acute lymphoblastic leukemia in second remission: evidence for long-term clinical and molecular remissions. *Leukemia* 2001; **15**: 50–6.

186. Atta J, Fauth F, Keyser M et al. Purging in BCR–ABL-positive acute lymphoblastic leukemia using immunomagnetic beads: comparison of residual leukemia and purging efficiency in bone marrow vs peripheral blood stem cells by semiquantitative polymerase chain reaction. *Bone Marrow Transplant* 2000; **25**: 97–104.

187. Seriu T, Yokota S, Nakao M et al. Prospective monitoring of minimal residual disease during the course of chemotherapy in patients with acute lymphoblastic leukemia, and detection of contaminating tumor cells in peripheral blood stem cells for autotransplantation. *Leukemia* 1995; **9**: 615–23.

188. Brenner MK, Rill DR, Holladay MS et al. Gene marking to determine whether autologous marrow infusion restores long-term haemopoiesis in cancer patients. *Lancet* 1993; **342**: 1134–7.

189. Hardingham JE, Kotasek D, Sage RE et al. Molecular detection of residual lymphoma cells in peripheral blood stem cell harvests and following autologous transplantation. *Bone Marrow Transplant* 1993; **11**: 15–20.

190. Leonard BM, Hetu F, Busque L et al. Lymphoma cell burden in progenitor cell grafts measured by competitive polymerase chain reaction: less than one log difference between bone marrow and peripheral blood sources. *Blood* 1998; **91**: 331–9.

191. Macintyre EA, Belanger C, Debert C et al. Detection of clonal CD34+19+ progenitors in bone marrow of BCL2–IgH-positive follicular lymphoma patients. *Blood* 1995; **86**: 4691–8.

192. Moos M, Schulz R, Martin S et al. The remission status before and the PCR status after high-dose therapy with peripheral blood stem cell support are prognostic factors for relapse-free survival in patients with follicular non-Hodgkin's lymphoma. *Leukemia* 1998; **12**: 1971–6.

193. Jacquy C, Lambert F, Soree A et al. Peripheral blood stem cell contamination in mantle cell non-Hodgkin lymphoma: the case for purging? *Bone Marrow Transplant* 1999; **23**: 681–6.

194. Gribben JG, Saporito L, Barber M et al. Bone marrows of non-Hodgkin's lymphoma patients with a bcl-2 translocation can be purged of polymerase chain reaction-detectable lymphoma cells using monoclonal antibodies and immunomagnetic bead depletion. *Blood* 1992; **80**: 1083–9.

195. Di Nicola M, Siena S, Corradini P et al. Elimination of bcl-2–IgH-positive follicular lymphoma cells from blood transplants with high recovery of hematopoietic progenitors by the Miltenyi CD34+ cell sorting system. *Bone Marrow Transplant* 1996; **18**: 1117–21.

196. Tarella C, Corradini P, Astolfi M et al. Negative immunomagnetic ex vivo purging combined with high-dose chemotherapy with peripheral blood progenitor cell autograft in follicular lymphoma patients: evidence for long-term clinical and molecular remissions. *Leukemia* 1999; **13**: 1456–62.

197. Andersen NS, Donovan JW, Borus JS et al. Failure of immunologic purging in mantle cell lymphoma assessed by polymerase chain reaction detection of minimal residual disease. *Blood* 1997; **90**: 4212–21.

198. Zwicky CS, Maddocks AB, Andersen N, Gribben JG. Eradication of polymerase chain reaction detectable immunoglobulin gene rearrangement in non-Hodgkin's lymphoma is associated with decreased relapse after autologous bone marrow transplantation. *Blood* 1996; **88**: 3314–22.

199. Ladetto M, Sametti S, Donovan JW et al. A validated real-time quantitative PCR approach shows a correlation between tumor burden and successful ex vivo purging in follicular lymphoma patients. *Exp Hematol* 2001; **29**: 183–93.

200. Straka C, Oduncu F, Drexler E et al. The CD19+ B-cell counts at peripheral blood stem cell mobilization determine different levels of tumour contamination and autograft purgability in low-grade lymphoma. *Br J Haematol* 2002; **116**: 695–701.

201. Gribben JG, Freedman AS, Neuberg D et al. Immunologic purging of marrow assessed by PCR before autologous bone marrow transplantation for B-cell lymphoma. *N Engl J Med* 1991; **325**: 1525–33.

202. Hirt C, Dölken G. Quantitative detection of t(14;18)-positive cells in patients with follicular lymphoma before and after autologous bone marrow transplantation. *Bone Marrow Transplant* 2000; **25**: 419–26.

203. Apostolidis J, Gupta RK, Grenzelias D et al. High-dose therapy with autologous bone marrow support as consolidation of remission in follicular lymphoma: long-term clinical and molecular follow-up. *J Clin Oncol* 2000; **18**: 527–36.

204. Lemoli RM, Fortuna A, Motta MR et al. Concomitant mobilization of plasma cells and hematopoietic progenitors into peripheral blood of multiple myeloma patients: positive selection and transplantation of enriched CD34+ cells to remove circulating tumor cells. *Blood* 1996; **87**: 1625–34.

205. Schiller G, Vescio R, Freytes C et al. Transplantation of CD34+ peripheral blood progenitor cells after high-dose chemotherapy for patients with advanced multiple myeloma. *Blood* 1995; **86**: 390–7.

206. Willems P, Croockewit A, Raymakers R et al. CD34 selections from myeloma peripheral blood cell autografts contain residual tumour cells due to impurity, not to CD34+ myeloma cells. *Br J Haematol* 1996; **93**: 613–22.

207. Vescio RA, Hong CH, Cao J et al. The hematopoietic stem cell antigen, CD34, is not expressed on the malignant cells in multiple myeloma. *Blood* 1994; **84**: 3283–90.

208. Barbui AM, Galli M, Dotti G et al. Negative selection of peripheral blood stem cells to support a tandem autologous transplantation programme in multiple myeloma. *Br J Haematol* 2002; **116**: 202–10.

209. Foroni L, Harrison CJ, Hoffbrand AV, Potter MN. Investigation of minimal residual disease in childhood and adult acute lymphoblastic leukaemia by molecular analysis. *Br J Haematol* 1999; **105**: 7–24.

210. Cave H, van der Werff ten Bosch J, Suciu S et al. Clinical significance of minimal residual disease in childhood acute lymphoblastic leukemia. *N Engl J Med* 1998; **339**: 591–8.

211. Jacquy C, Delepaut B, Van Daele S et al. A prospective study of minimal residual disease in childhood B-lineage acute lymphoblastic leukaemia: MRD level at the end of induction is a strong predictive factor of relapse. *Br J Haematol* 1997; **98**: 140–6.

212. Panzer-Grumayer ER, Schneider M, Panzer S et al. Rapid molecular response during early induction chemotherapy predicts a good outcome in childhood acute lymphoblastic leukemia. *Blood* 2000; **95**: 790–4.

213. Biondi A, Valsecchi MG, Seriu T et al. Molecular detection of minimal residual disease is a strong predictive factor of relapse in childhood B-lineage acute lymphoblastic leukemia with medium risk features. A case control study of the International BFM Study Group. *Leukemia* 2000; **14**: 1939–343.

214. Nyvold C, Madsen HO, Ryder LP et al. Precise quantification of minimal residual disease at day 29 allows identification of children with acute lymphoblastic leukemia and an excellent outcome. *Blood* 2002; **99**: 1253–8.

215. Dworzak MN, Froschl G, Printz D et al. Prognostic significance and modalities of flow cytometric minimal residual disease detection in childhood acute lymphoblastic leukemia. *Blood* 2002; **99**: 1952–8.

216. Donadieu J, Hill C. Early response to chemotherapy as a prognostic factor in childhood acute lymphoblastic leukaemia: a methodological review. *Br J Haematol* 2001; **115**: 34–45.

217. Riehm H, Reiter A, Schrappe M et al. Corticosteroid-dependent reduction of leukocyte count in blood as a prognostic factor in acute lymphoblastic leukemia in childhood (therapy study ALL-BFM 83). *Klin Padiatr* 1987; **199**: 151–60.

218. Wasserman R, Galili N, Ito Y et al. Residual disease at the end of induction therapy as a predictor of relapse during therapy in childhood B-lineage acute lymphoblastic leukemia. *J Clin Oncol* 1992; **10**: 1879–88.

218a. Coustan-Smith E, Sancho J, Behm FG, Hancock ML, Razzouk BI, Ribeiro RC, Rivera GK, Rubnitz JE, Sandlund JT, Pui CH, Campana D. Prognostic importance of measuring early clearance of leukemic cells by flow cytometry in childhood acute lymphoblastic leukemia. *Blood* 2002; **100**: 52–8.

218b. Marshall GM, Haber M, Kwan E, Zhu L, Ferrara D, Xue C, Brisco MJ, Sykes PJ, Morley A, Webster B, Dalla Pozza L, Waters K, Norris MD. Importance of minimal residual disease testing during the second year of therapy for children with acute lymphoblastic leukemia. *J Clin Oncol* 2003; **21**: 704–9.

219. Gruhn B, Hongeng S, Yi H et al. Minimal residual disease after intensive induction therapy in childhood acute lymphoblastic leukemia predicts outcome. *Leukemia* 1998; **12**: 675–81.

220. Brüggemann M, Droese J, Bolz I et al. Improved assessment of minimal residual disease in B cell malignancies using fluorogenic consensus probes for real-time quantitative PCR. *Leukemia* 2000; **14**: 1419–25.

221. Arico M, Valsecchi MG, Camitta B et al. Outcome of treatment in children with Philadelphia chromosome-positive acute lymphoblastic leukemia. *N Engl J Med* 2000; **342**: 998–1006.

222. Brisco MJ, Sykes PJ, Dolman G et al. Effect of the Philadelphia chromosome on minimal residual disease in acute lymphoblastic leukemia. *Leukemia* 1997; **11**: 1497–500.

223. Cazzaniga G, Rossi V, Biondi A. Monitoring minimal residual disease using chromosomal translocations in childhood ALL. *Best Pract Res Clin Haematol* 2002; **15**: 21–35.

224. Cimino G, Elia L, Rapanotti MC et al. A prospective study of residual-disease monitoring of the *ALL1/AF4* transcript in patients with t(4;11) acute lymphoblastic leukemia. *Blood* 2000; **95**: 96–101.

225. Szczepański T, Pongers-Willemse MJ, Hählen K, van Dongen JJM. Intensified therapy for infants with acute lymphoblastic leukemia: results from the Dana-Farber Cancer Institute Consortium. *Cancer* 1998; **83**: 1055–7.

226. De Haas V, Oosten L, Dee R et al. Minimal residual disease studies are beneficial in the follow-up of *TEL/AML1* patients with B-precursor acute lymphoblastic leukaemia. *Br J Haematol* 2000; **111**: 1080–6.

227. Seeger K, Kreuzer KA, Lass U et al. Molecular quantification of response to therapy and remission status in *TEL-AML1*-positive childhood ALL by real-time reverse transcription polymerase chain reaction. *Cancer Res* 2001; **61**: 2517–22.

228. Zur Stadt U, Harms DO, Schluter S et al. MRD at the end of induction therapy in childhood acute lymphoblastic leukemia: outcome prediction strongly depends on the therapeutic regimen. *Leukemia* 2001; **15**: 283–5.

228a. Hoelzer D, Gokbuget N, Ottmann O, Pui CH, Relling MV, Appelbaum FR, Van Dongen JJM, Szczepanski T. Acute lymphoblastic leukemia. *Hematology (Am Soc Hematol Educ Program)* 2002; 162–92.

229. Steenbergen EJ, Verhagen OJ, van Leeuwen EF et al. Prolonged persistence of PCR-detectable minimal residual disease after diagnosis or first relapse predicts poor outcome in childhood B-precursor acute lymphoblastic leukemia. *Leukemia* 1995; **9**: 1726–34.

230. Eckert C, Biondi A, Seeger K et al. Prognostic value of minimal residual disease in relapsed childhood acute lymphoblastic leukaemia. *Lancet* 2001; **358**: 1239–41.

231. Dibenedetto SP, Lo Nigro L, Mayer SP et al. Detectable molecular residual disease at the beginning of maintenance therapy indicates poor outcome in children with T-cell acute lymphoblastic leukemia. *Blood* 1997; **90**: 1226–32.

232. Willemse MJ, Seriu T, Hettinger K et al. Detection of minimal residual disease identifies differences in treatment response between T-ALL and precursor-B-ALL. *Blood* 2002; **99**: 4386–93.

233. Nizet Y, Van Daele S, Lewalle P et al. Long-term follow-up of residual disease in acute lymphoblastic leukemia patients in complete remission using clonogeneic IgH probes and the polymerase chain reaction. *Blood* 1993; **82**: 1618–25.

234. Neale GA, Menarguez J, Kitchingman GR et al. Detection of minimal residual disease in T-cell acute lymphoblastic leukemia using polymerase chain reaction predicts impending relapse. *Blood* 1991; **78**: 739–47.

235. Yokota S, Hansen-Hagge TE, Ludwig WD et al. Use of polymerase chain reactions to monitor minimal residual disease in acute lymphoblastic leukemia patients. *Blood* 1991; **77**: 331–9.

236. Goulden NJ, Knechtli CJ, Garland RJ et al. Minimal resid-

ual disease analysis for the prediction of relapse in children with standard-risk acute lymphoblastic leukaemia. *Br J Haematol* 1998; **100**: 235–44.

237. Biondi A, Yokota S, Hansen-Hagge TE et al. Minimal residual disease in childhood acute lymphoblastic leukemia: analysis of patients in continuous complete remission or with consecutive relapse. *Leukemia* 1992; **6**: 282–8.

238. Roberts WM, Estrov Z, Ouspenskaia MV et al. Measurement of residual leukemia during remission in childhood acute lymphoblastic leukemia. *N Engl J Med* 1997; **336**: 317–23.

239. Schneider M, Hettinger K, Matthes-Martin S et al. Influence of transplantation regimen on prognostic significance of high-level minimal residual disease before allogeneic stem cell transplantation in children with ALL. *Bone Marrow Transplant* 2001; **28**: 1087–9.

240. Bader P, Hancock J, Kreyenberg H et al. Minimal residual disease (MRD) status prior to allogeneic stem cell transplantation is a powerful predictor for post transplant outcome in children with ALL. *Leukemia* 2002; **16**: 1668–72.

241. Uzunel M, Mattsson J, Jaksch M et al. The significance of graft-versus-host disease and pretransplantation minimal residual disease status to outcome after allogeneic stem cell transplantation in patients with acute lymphoblastic leukemia. *Blood* 2001; **98**: 1982–4.

242. Van der Velden VHJ, Joosten SA, Willemse MJ et al. Real-time quantitative PCR for detection of minimal residual disease before allogeneic stem cell transplantation predicts outcome in children with acute lymphoblastic leukemia. *Leukemia* 2001; **15**: 1485–7.

243. Sanchez J, Serrano J, Gomez P et al. Clinical value of immunological monitoring of minimal residual disease in acute lymphoblastic leukaemia after allogeneic transplantation. *Br J Haematol* 2002; **116**: 686–94.

244. Knechtli CJ, Goulden NJ, Hancock JP et al. Minimal residual disease status as a predictor of relapse after allogeneic bone marrow transplantation for children with acute lymphoblastic leukaemia. *Br J Haematol* 1998; **102**: 860–71.

244a. Uzunel M, Jaksch M, Mattsson J, Ringden O. Minimal residual disease detection after allogeneic stem cell transplantation is correlated to relapse in patients with acute lymphoblastic leukaemia. *Br J Haematol* 2003; **122**: 788–94.

245. Scholten C, Fodinger M, Mitterbauer M et al. Kinetics of minimal residual disease during induction/consolidation therapy in standard-risk adult B-lineage acute lymphoblastic leukemia. *Ann Hematol* 1995; **71**: 155–60.

246. Foroni L, Coyle LA, Papaioannou M et al. Molecular detection of minimal residual disease in adult and childhood acute lymphoblastic leukaemia reveals differences in treatment response. *Leukemia* 1997; **11**: 1732–41.

247. Brisco MJ, Hughes E, Neoh SH et al. Relationship between minimal residual disease and outcome in adult acute lymphoblastic leukemia. *Blood* 1996; **87**: 5251–6.

247a. Vidriales MB, Perez JJ, Lopez-Berges MC, Gutierrez N, Ciudad J, Lucio P, Vazquez L, Garcia-Sanz R, del Canizo MC, Fernandez-Calvo J, Ramos F, Rodriguez MJ, Calmuntia MJ, Porwith A, Orfao A, San-Miguel JF. Minimal residual disease in adolescent (older than 14 years) and adult acute lymphoblastic leukemias: early immunophenotypic evaluation has high clinical value. *Blood* 2003; **101**: 4695–700.

248. Mortuza FY, Papaioannou M, Moreira IM et al. Minimal residual disease tests provide an independent predictor of clinical outcome in adult acute lymphoblastic leukemia. *J Clin Oncol* 2002; **20**: 1094–104.

249. Van der Velden VHJ, Jacobs DCH, Wijkhuijs AJM et al. Minimal residual disease levels in bone marrow and peripheral blood are comparable in children with T cell acute lymphoblastic leukemia (ALL), but not in precursor-B-ALL. *Leukemia* 2002; **16**: 1432–36.

250. Brisco MJ, Sykes PJ, Hughes E et al. Monitoring minimal residual disease in peripheral blood in B-lineage acute lymphoblastic leukaemia. *Br J Haematol* 1997; **99**: 314–19.

250a. Coustan-Smith E, Sancho J, Hancock ML, Razzouk BI, Ribeiro RC, Rivera GK, Rubnitz JE, Sandlund JT, Pui CH, Campana D. Use of peripheral blood instead of bone marrow to monitor residual disease in children with acute lymphoblastic leukemia. *Blood* 2002; **100**: 2399–402.

251. Sykes PJ, Brisco MJ, Hughes E et al. Minimal residual disease in childhood acute lymphoblastic leukaemia quantified by aspirate and trephine: is the disease multifocal? *Br J Haematol* 1998; **103**: 60–5.

252. Rozman C, Montserrat E. Chronic lymphocytic leukemia. *N Engl J Med* 1995; **333**: 1052–7.

253. Brugiatelli M, Callea V, Morabito F et al. Immunologic and molecular evaluation of residual disease in B-cell chronic lymphocytic leukemia patients in clinical remission phase. *Cancer* 1989; **63**: 1979–84.

254. Lavabre-Bertrand T, Janossy G, Exbrayat C et al. Leukemia-associated changes identified by quantitative flow cytometry. II. CD5 over-expression and monitoring in B-CLL. *Leukemia* 1994; **8**: 1557–63.

255. Robertson LE, Huh YO, Butler JJ et al. Response assessment in chronic lymphocytic leukemia after fludarabine plus prednisone: clinical, pathologic, immunophenotypic, and molecular analysis. *Blood* 1992; **80**: 29–36.

256. Brugiatelli M, Claisse JF, Lenormand B et al. Long-term clinical outcome of B-cell chronic lymphocytic leukemia patients in clinical remission phase evaluated at phenotypic level. *Br J Haematol* 1997; **97**: 113–18.

257. Cabezudo E, Matutes E, Ramrattan M et al. Analysis of residual disease in chronic lymphocytic leukemia by flow cytometry. *Leukemia* 1997; **11**: 1909–14.

258. Provan D, Bartlett-Pandite L, Zwicky C et al. Eradication of polymerase chain reaction-detectable chronic lymphocytic leukemia cells is associated with improved outcome after bone marrow transplantation. *Blood* 1996; **88**: 2228–35.

259. Van Besien K, Keralavarma B, Devine S, Stock W. Allogeneic and autologous transplantation for chronic lymphocytic leukemia. *Leukemia* 2001; **15**: 1317–25.

260. Rabinowe SN, Soiffer RJ, Gribben JG et al. Autologous and allogeneic bone marrow transplantation for poor prognosis patients with B-cell chronic lymphocytic leukemia. *Blood* 1993; **82**: 1366–76.

261. Dreger P, von Neuhoff N, Kuse R et al. Early stem cell transplantation for chronic lymphocytic leukaemia: a chance for cure? *Br J Cancer* 1998; **77**: 2291–7.

262. Esteve J, Villamor N, Colomer D et al. Hematopoietic stem cell transplantation in chronic lymphocytic leukemia: a report of 12 patients from a single institution. *Ann Oncol* 1998; **9**: 167–72.

263. Esteve J, Villamor N, Colomer D, Montserrat E. Different clinical value of minimal residual disease after autologous and allogenic stem cell transplantation for chronic lymphocytic leukemia. *Blood* 2002; **99**: 1873–4.

264. Magnac C, Sutton L, Cazin B et al. Detection of minimal residual disease in B chronic lymphocytic leukemia (CLL). *Hematol Cell Ther* 1999; **41**: 13–18.

265. Mattsson J, Uzunel M, Remberger M et al. Minimal residual disease is common after allogeneic stem cell transplantation in patients with B cell chronic lymphocytic leukemia and may be controlled by graft-versus-host disease. *Leukemia* 2000; **14**: 247–54.

266. Corradini P, Ladetto M, Pileri A, Tarella C. Clinical relevance of minimal residual disease monitoring in non-Hodgkin's lymphomas: a critical reappraisal of molecular strategies. *Leukemia* 1999; **13**: 1691–5.

267. Gribben JG, Neuberg D, Barber M et al. Detection of residual lymphoma cells by polymerase chain reaction in peripheral blood is significantly less predictive for relapse than detection in bone marrow. *Blood* 1994; **83**: 3800–7.

268. Lopez-Guillermo A, Cabanillas F, McLaughlin P et al. The clinical significance of molecular response in indolent follicular lymphomas. *Blood* 1998; **91**: 2955–60.

269. Lambrechts AC, Hupkes PE, Dorssers LC, van't Veer MB. Clinical significance of t(14;18)-positive cells in the circulation of patients with stage III or IV follicular non-Hodgkin's lymphoma during first remission. *J Clin Oncol* 1994; **12**: 1541–6.

270. Czuczman MS, Grillo-Lopez AJ, White CA et al. Treatment of patients with low-grade B-cell lymphoma with the combination of chimeric anti-CD20 monoclonal antibody and CHOP chemotherapy. *J Clin Oncol* 1999; **17**: 268–76.

271. Gribben JG, Neuberg D, Freedman AS et al. Detection by polymerase chain reaction of residual cells with the *bcl-2* translocation is associated with increased risk of relapse after autologous bone marrow transplantation for B-cell lymphoma. *Blood* 1993; **81**: 3449–57.

272. Von Neuhoff N, Dreger P, Suttorp M et al. Comparison of different strategies of molecular genetic monitoring following autologous stem cell transplantation in patients with follicular lymphoma. *Bone Marrow Transplant* 1998; **22**: 161–6.

273. Johnson PW, Price CG, Smith T et al. Detection of cells bearing the t(14;18) translocation following myeloablative treatment and autologous bone marrow transplantation for follicular lymphoma. *J Clin Oncol* 1994; **12**: 798–805.

274. Finke J, Slanina J, Lange W, Dolken G. Persistence of circulating t(14;18)-positive cells in long-term remission after radiation therapy for localized-stage follicular lymphoma. *J Clin Oncol* 1993; **11**: 1668–73.

275. Mandigers CM, Meijerink JP, Mensink EJ et al. Lack of correlation between numbers of circulating t(14;18)-positive cells and response to first-line treatment in follicular lymphoma. *Blood* 2001; **98**: 940–4.

276. Rambaldi A, Lazzari M, Manzoni C et al. Monitoring of minimal residual disease after CHOP and rituximab in previously untreated patients with follicular lymphoma. *Blood* 2002; **99**: 856–62.

277. Colombat P, Salles G, Brousse N et al. Rituximab (anti-CD20 monoclonal antibody) as single first-line therapy for patients with follicular lymphoma with a low tumor burden: clinical and molecular evaluation. *Blood* 2001; **97**: 101–6.

278. Limpens J, Stad R, Vos C et al. Lymphoma-associated translocation t(14;18) in blood B cells of normal individuals. *Blood* 1995; **85**: 2528–36.

278a. Ladetto M, Drandi D, Compagno M, Astolfi M, Volpato F, Voena C, Novarino A, Pollio B, Addeo A, Ricca I, Falco P, Cavallo F, Vallet S, Corradini P, Pileri A, Tamponi G,

Palumbo A, Bertetto O, Boccadoro M, Tarella C. PCR-detectable nonneoplastic Bcl-2/IgH rearrangements are common in normal subjects and cancer patients at diagnosis but rare in subjects treated with chemotherapy. *J Clin Oncol* 2003; **21**: 1398–403.

279. Johnson PW, Swinbank K, MacLennan S et al. Variability of polymerase chain reaction detection of the *bcl-2–IgH* translocation in an international multicentre study. *Ann Oncol* 1999; **10**: 1349–54.

280. Galoin S, al Saati T, Schlaifer D et al. Oligonucleotide clonospecific probes directed against the junctional sequence of t(14;18): a new tool for the assessment of minimal residual disease in follicular lymphomas. *Br J Haematol* 1996; **94**: 676–84.

281. Howard OM, Gribben JG, Neuberg DS et al. Rituximab and CHOP induction therapy for newly diagnosed mantle-cell lymphoma: molecular complete responses are not predictive of progression-free survival. *J Clin Oncol* 2002; **20**: 1288–94.

282. Scholten C, Hilgarth B, Hilgarth M et al. Predictive value of clone-specific CDR3 PCR in high-grade non-Hodgkin's lymphoma: long-term persistence of a clone-specific rearrangement in a patient with secondary high-grade NHL in remission after high-dose therapy. *Br J Haematol* 1997; **97**: 246–7.

283. Corradini P, Astolfi M, Cherasco C et al. Molecular monitoring of minimal residual disease in follicular and mantle cell non-Hodgkin's lymphomas treated with high-dose chemotherapy and peripheral blood progenitor cell autografting. *Blood* 1997; **89**: 724–31.

284. Pott C, Schrader C, Derner N et al. Molecular remission predicts progression-free survival in mantle cell lymphoma after peripheral blood stem cell transplantation. *Ann Oncol* 2002; **13**: 69a.

284a. Gianni AM, Magni M, Martelli M, Di Nicola M, Carlo-Stella C, Pilotti S, Rambaldi A, Cortelazzo S, Patti C, Parvis G, Benedetti F, Capria S, Corradini P, Tarella C, Barbui T. Long-term remission in mantle cell lymphoma following high-dose sequential chemotherapy and in vivo rituximab-purged stem cell autografting (R-HDS regimen). *Blood* 2003; **102**: 749–55.

285. Corradini P, Ladetto M, Astolfi M et al. Clinical and molecular remission after allogeneic blood cell transplantation in a patient with mantle-cell lymphoma. *Br J Haematol* 1996; **94**: 376–8.

286. Bird JM, Russell NH, Samson D. Minimal residual disease after bone marrow transplantation for multiple myeloma: evidence for cure in long-term survivors. *Bone Marrow Transplant* 1993; **12**: 651–4.

287. Bergsagel PL, Smith AM, Szczepek A et al. In multiple myeloma, clonotypic B lymphocytes are detectable among CD19+ peripheral blood cells expressing CD38, CD56, and monotypic Ig light chain. *Blood* 1995; **85**: 436–47.

288. Corradini P, Voena C, Astolfi M et al. High-dose sequential chemoradiotherapy in multiple myeloma: residual tumor cells are detectable in bone marrow and peripheral blood cell harvests and after autografting. *Blood* 1995; **85**: 1596–602.

289. Corradini P, Voena C, Tarella C et al. Molecular and clinical remissions in multiple myeloma: role of autologous and allogeneic transplantation of hematopoietic cells. *J Clin Oncol* 1999; **17**: 208–15.

290. San Miguel JF, Almeida J, Mateo G et al. Immunophenotypic evaluation of the plasma cell compartment in multiple myeloma: a tool for comparing the

efficacy of different treatment strategies and predicting outcome. *Blood* 2002; **99**: 1853–6.

291. Bjorkstrand B, Ljungman P, Bird JM et al. Double high-dose chemoradiotherapy with autologous stem cell transplantation can induce molecular remissions in multiple myeloma. *Bone Marrow Transplant* 1995; **15**: 367–71.

292. Martinelli G, Terragna C, Zamagni E et al. Molecular remission after allogeneic or autologous transplantation of hematopoietic stem cells for multiple myeloma. *J Clin Oncol* 2000; **18**: 2273–81.

293. Cavo M, Terragna C, Martinelli G et al. Molecular monitoring of minimal residual disease in patients in long-term complete remission after allogeneic stem cell transplantation for multiple myeloma. *Blood* 2000; **96**: 355–7.

294. Neale GAM, CoustanSmith E, Pan Q et al. Tandem application of flow cytometry and polymerase chain reaction for comprehensive detection of minimal residual disease in childhood acute lymphoblastic leukemia. *Leukemia* 1999; **13**: 1221–6.

295. Malec M, Bjorklund E, Soderhall S et al. Flow cytometry and allele-specific oligonucleotide PCR are equally effective in detection of minimal residual disease in ALL. *Leukemia* 2001; **15**: 716–27.

296. De Haas V, Breunis WB, Dee R et al. The *TEL–AML1* real-time quantitative polymerase chain reaction (PCR) might replace the antigen receptor-based genomic PCR in clinical minimal residual disease studies in children with acute lymphoblastic leukaemia. *Br J Haematol* 2002; **116**: 87–93.

297. Morley A. Quantifying leukemia. *N Engl J Med* 1998; **339**: 627–9.

298. Beishuizen A, Verhoeven MA, Hählen K et al. Differences in immunoglobulin heavy chain gene rearrangement patterns between bone marrow and blood samples in childhood precursor B-acute lymphoblastic leukemia at diagnosis. *Leukemia* 1993; **7**: 60–3.

299. Martens AC, Schultz FW, Hagenbeek A. Non-homogeneous distribution of leukemia in the bone marrow during minimal residual disease. *Blood* 1987; **70**: 1073–8.

300. Lefranc MP, Giudicelli V, Ginestoux C et al. IMGT, the international ImMunoGeneTics database. *Nucleic Acids Res* 1999; **27**: 209–12.

300a. Lefranc MP. IMGT databases, web resources and tools for immunoglobulin and T cell receptor sequence analysis, http://imgt.cines.fr. *Leukemia* 2003; **17**: 260–6.

# 22 Detection of minimal residual disease in myeloid malignancies

Jesús F San Miguel, Marcos González, and Alberto Orfao

## Introduction

Some myeloid malignances could be considered potentially curable with the treatment strategies currently available. In fact, around one-third of patients with acute myeloid leukemia (AML) are leukemia-free at 5 years. In addition, the use of AML-oriented therapy, including stem cell transplantation (SCT), in young patients with high-risk myelodysplastic syndromes (MDS) results in an actuarial 2-year survival rate of 20–30%. Finally, 30–50% of patients with chronic myeloid leukemia (CML) are theoretically cured following allogeneic SCT. However, relapses due to the persistence of low numbers of residual neoplastic cells that are undetectable by conventional morphological techniques – minimal residual disease (MRD) – still represent a major challenge.[1–7] Owing to this, patients are indiscriminately subjected to consolidation treatments, including SCT, in order to eradicate MRD, with the risk of certain cases being either over- or undertreated. Therefore, more sensitive techniques are needed to evaluate the effectiveness of different treatment protocols and to lay the foundations for the design of patient-adapted consolidation therapies that would reduce the risk of both relapse and overtreatment. In addition, sensitive methods for detecting MRD could be also used to assess the efficacy of ex vivo purging protocols for autologous stem cells prior to reinfusion.

The efficacy and applicability of the different methodological approaches that are available for the detection of MRD depend on three main features:[8]

- *Specificity:* discrimination between malignant and normal cells, without false-negative and false-positive results.
- *Sensitivity:* Leukemic cells are undetectable by morphology when their number falls below 1–5% of total bone marrow (BM) nucleated cells, and consequently the detection limit of a MRD technique must be at least $10^{-3}$, i.e. discrimination of 1 leukemic cell among 1000 normal cells.

- *Reproducibility:* The technique should allow for easy standardization and rapid collection of results for their clinical application.[7,8]

In addition, the possibility of predicting whether or not the residual leukemic cells are really the clonogenic cells responsible for an impending relapse would be of great clinical benefit.

At present, the strategies used in MRD detection are usually based on the identification at diagnosis of singular characteristics of the leukemic cells that allow us to distinguish them from residual normal cells in complete remission samples. Based on these leukemia-associated characteristics, a patient's probe can be 'custom-built' at diagnosis for the identification of possible residual leukemic cells during follow-up. Accordingly, techniques for MRD detection can be classified based on the type of cell marker used to identify the malignant cell clone, as follows:[8,9]

- morphology;
- cell culture techniques that evaluate the pattern of in vitro colony growth;
- cytogenetic characteristics of blast cells evaluated either by conventional chromosome analysis or by fluorescence in situ hybridization (FISH);
- the analysis of total cell DNA contents detected by flow cytometry;
- the immunophenotypic profile of blast cells assessed by multiparametric flow cytometry;
- DNA sequences analyzed by polymerase chain reaction (PCR).

It should be noted that these techniques cannot be used indiscriminately for all types of leukemias, but they should be adapted depending on the markers (cytogenetic, immunological, molecular, etc.) that characterize the malignant clone. Thus, immunophenotyping is ideal for T-cell acute lymphoblastic leukemia, while PCR analysis is the method of choice for CML. Ideally, two or more techniques should be simultaneously explored in each patient, in order to define the best approach for investigation of MRD (Figure 22.1).

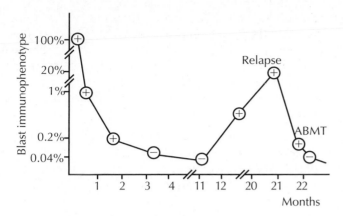

**Figure 22.1** Simultaneous monitoring of MRD in an acute promyelocytic leukemia by immunophenotyping (results on the vertical axis are expressed as the number of residual blast cells) and by RT–PCR (results are expressed in circles as + or –).

In this chapter, we shall first review the pros and cons of the different techniques for investigation of MRD, and then we shall focus on the detection of MRD in myeloid malignancies, including AML, MDS, and CML. As we have already mentioned, the utility of the MRD techniques varies depending on the type of disorder, and therefore AML, MDS, and CML will be discussed separately. Table 22.1 illustrates the applicability and sensitivity of the different methods in these myeloid disorders. In Table 22.2 we have summarized some of the most relevant general conclusions on MRD detection in myeloid malignancies. More specific conclusions for each type of leukemia and individual technique are specified in the corresponding sections of the text.

## Table 22.1 Applicability[a] and sensitivity of MRD techniques in myeloid malignancies

|  | Morphology | Cell cultures | Cytogenetics/FISH | DNA ploidy by flow cytometry | Phenotype | PCR |
|---|---|---|---|---|---|---|
| **AML** |  |  |  |  |  |  |
| Applicability | 100% | 100%[b] | 40–70% | <5% | 70–80% | 40% |
| Sensitivity | $10^{-2}$ | $10^{-2}$ | $10^{-2}$–$10^{-3}$ | $10^{-4}$–$10^{-5}$ | $10^{-4}$–$10^{-5}$ | $10^{-4}$–$10^{-6}$ |
| **MDS** |  |  |  |  |  |  |
| Applicability | NA | NSE | 40–70% | <5% | NSE | NSE |
| Sensitivity |  |  | $10^{-2}$ | $10^{-4}$–$10^{-5}$ |  |  |
| **CML** |  |  |  |  |  |  |
| Applicability | NA | NSE | 90–95% | <5% | NSE | 95–100% |
| Sensitivity |  |  | $10^{-3}$ | $10^{-4}$–$10^{-5}$ |  | $10^{-5}$–$10^{-6}$ |

AML, acute myeloid leukemia; MDS, myelodysplastic syndromes; CML, chronic myeloid leukemia; FISH, fluorescence in situ hybridization; PCR, polymerase chain reaction; NA, not applicable; NSE, not sufficiently explained.
[a] Applicability is defined to as the proportion of cases in which the technique is applicable.
[b] By either CFU-L or CFU-GM assays.

## Table 22.2 General conclusions on MRD detection in myeloid malignancies

- Prospective studies to evaluate the utility and specificity of the techniques used for MRD detection are still needed in some myeloid malignancies (e.g. myelodysplastic syndromes)
- The applicability of MRD techniques varies depending on the type of leukemia
- Assessment of the quality of the response to induction treatment by immunological or molecular methods is of prognostic value
- The terms 'immunological/molecular response' provide complementary information to morphological complete remission
- Evaluation of residual cells should be performed in the stem cell harvest to be used for autologous transplantation and to assess the efficacy of purging methods
- It is important to define relevant clinical time points to measure MRD, since sequential studies are laborious and expensive
- Switches from negative to positive results are highly predictive of impending relapse
- MRD negativity does not exclude the existence of minimal numbers of residual leukemic cells, since only $10^6$ cells are usually screened.

# Methodological considerations concerning MRD techniques

## Morphology

Morphology is not a real MRD technique but the current gold standard for the definition of complete remission (CR). As mentioned above, the sensitivity of morphological analysis for the detection of leukemic cells is low ($10^{-2}$, which represents a possible residual tumor burden of up to $10^{11}$ cells). Moreover, special difficulties emerge in regenerating bone marrow samples, and the need for routine bone marrow examination to detect relapse in acute leukemia has been questioned.[10,11]

## Cell cultures

The investigation of the persistence of leukemic cell colonies (colony-forming units leukemic, CFU-L) or the existence of an abnormal growth pattern of colony-forming units granulocyte–macrophage (CFU-GM) can represent a useful approach for MRD detection in myeloid leukemias.[12,13] A major concern with CFU-L assays is the discrimination between leukemic colonies and normal CFU-GM, which may be difficult to establish, especially if we consider that we are not dealing with diagnostic samples but with specimens from patients in morphological CR. However, the leukemic colonies grow faster than normal CFU-GM, so the former should be scored by days 3–6 and the latter by day +14. The characterization of each individual colony by means of tumor-specific markers such as cytogenetics, immunophenotype, or molecular markers will contribute to the unequivocal assessment of the leukemic origin of cells grown in vitro. Interestingly, the investigation of tumor markers (i.e. chromosomal aberrations or junctional regions of rearranged immunoglobulins) in the cells of the CFU-L has shown that these cells may be more sensitive than the uncultured BM cells for showing up residual disease, since the tumor marker has been detected in the colony but not on the fresh cells.[12,14] However, a major problem with this approach is that CFU-L may persist in patients who remain in continuous CR for many years and who are therefore cured,[15] suggesting that in these cases, CFU-L are not really the clonogenic cells responsible for disease progression. Another possible pitfall of this approach for MRD detection is the presence of suboptimal culture conditions for leukemic cell growth, which would generate false-negative results.

## Cytogenetics and FISH

Chromosomal abnormalities, both numerical and structural, are specific leukemic markers. However, the sensitivity of conventional cytogenetics for their detection is low ($10^{-2}$). Thus, although it is a most valuable technique for diagnostic purposes, it is not very useful for residual disease.[16] Two additional limitations of cytogenetics are related to the fact that (i) analysis is restricted to metaphases, which are difficult to obtain in several types of leukemias, and (ii) when cells are cultured to obtain metaphases, a clonal selection can be induced.

FISH can be considered as cytogenetic studies at a molecular level, since it allows the identification of specific DNA sequences, both in chromosome metaphases and interphase nuclei using either chromosome-specific and/or gene-specific DNA probes. The possibility of studying interphase nuclei is particularly useful for the analysis of malignant disorders with low proliferative index. A limiting factor on the level of detection of chromosome changes with FISH is the efficiency of the hybridization process. The sensitivity of FISH when using centromeric probes for detection of trisomies is relatively low (around 1%), and even lower (10%) for monosomies. These figures are based on the false-positive (0.2–1%) and false-negative (0.5–5%) rates obtained upon analyzing normal diploid cells.[17,18] Nevertheless, when two or more numerical chromosome aberrations coexist, the possibility of false-positive and/or false-negative signals decreases, leading to an increased sensitivity of up to $10^{-3}$ to $10^{-5}$.[18] The detection of chromosomal translocations (e.g. BCR–ABL) by FISH, using probes that either flank or span a translocation breakpoint, can be used to identify the presence of such marker chromosomes in interphase and metaphase cells through the identification of one fused signal.[19] However, its sensitivity for MRD detection is again low ($10^{-2}$), due to the possibility of artifactual colocalization of the two fluorochrome signals.[19] An increase in sensitivity of up to one logarithmic decade is achieved for those probes that split into two signals once a translocation occurs, such as for t(16;16) or inv(16) and 11q23 abnormalities. An attractive possibility is the combination of FISH and immunophenotypical analysis, either simultaneously or after cell sorting on the basis of leukemic-associated immunophenotypic characteristics, which would notably increase the sensitivity since it would identify individual tumor cells with a double marker: chromosome/antigen.[9,10]

## Measurement of DNA ploidy by flow cytometry

The analysis of cell DNA contents by flow cytometry allows the identification of clonal abnormalities – DNA aneuploidy – present in leukemic cells through comparison of the DNA contents of the tumor cells with that of normal diploid cells in the same cell cycle phase. In cases with an aneuploid cell population, this could be easily monitored during follow-up. For the identification of an aneuploid peak, a gain or loss of total DNA greater than 5% is usually required.

Therefore, the sensitivity of this technique is similar to that of morphology when used alone. Nevertheless, we have shown that with simultaneous staining for DNA content and leukemic-associated antigens that identify the cells from the malignant clone, the sensitivity increases to between $10^{-4}$ and $10^{-5}$, allowing a specific and sensitive detection of aneuploid cell populations during follow-up.[2]

## Immunophenotype

Immune marker analysis and PCR studies are the two most commonly employed methods for the detection of MRD.[2,4-8] Immunophenotypic analysis is theoretically an optimum method because of its relative speed and simplicity. In addition, it provides a quantitative evaluation of the number of cells present in the sample. However, it has two potential major pitfalls that could limit its specificity: (i) the lack of leukemia-specific antigens in most cases – with the exception of some proteins resulting from fusion genes such as BCR–ABL or PML–RARα, although reliable monoclonal antibodies (MoAbs) for their detection are not yet available – and (ii) the occurrence of phenotypic changes at relapse. Regarding the first problem, our group[20,21] as well as several others[5,6,22-24] using large panels of MoAbs in three- and four-color combinations analyzed by flow cytometry, have shown that leukemic cells frequently display uncommon or aberrant phenotypic features that allow us to distinguish them from normal cells. These phenotypic aberrations generally concern cross-lineage antigen expression, maturational asynchronic antigen expression, abnormal differentiation pathways, antigen overexpression, altered light scatter patterns, and/or ectopic antigen expression.[5,8,9,25,26] Such aberrations constitute unique phenotypic patterns that can be used as 'leukemia-associated' markers that will contribute to the specific identification of residual malignant cells during follow-up. In spite of initial concerns about the sensitivity of immunophenotyping for the detection of low numbers of leukemic cells, both in vitro dilutional experiments mixing-up leukemic and normal cells[1,4-6] and in vivo studies[2,21,22,24-26] point to a sensitivity ranging between $10^{-4}$ and $10^{-5}$, depending on the type of leukemia and the combination of monoclonal antibodies used for monitoring residual neoplastic cells.

An additional advantage of immunophenotypical studies is that they provide dynamic information concerning the differentiation of leukemic cells as regards their maturational blockade.

## Molecular biology

Leukemic cells may display two types of tumor-specific markers that can be used for MRD detection at a molecular level: breakpoint fusion regions of chromosome abnormalities and junctional regions of rearranged immunoglobulin (Ig) and T-cell receptor (TCR) genes.[6,7,27] These targets can be analyzed by Southern blot or PCR techniques. The first method has a low sensitivity ($10^{-2}$), and thus is not really an MRD detection technique. By contrast, PCR is one of the best tools for the investigation of residual leukemia, with a potential detection limit of up to $10^{-6}$, depending on the type of leukemia-specific PCR target. The junctional regions of rearranged Ig and TCR genes are 'fingerprint-like' sequences, which differ from one lymphocyte to the other and thus also within each lymphoid leukemia.[7,8] The strategy for MRD detection using this target implies the identification at diagnosis of the various possible patterns of Ig and/or TCR gene rearrangements and then determination of the precise nucleotide sequence of the junctional region in order to design a patient-specific probe or primer for the detection of residual leukemic cells during follow-up. MRD via chromosomal abnormalities is simpler and can be analyzed either at the DNA level – so long as that the breakpoint occurs at a constant region of small size (<2 kb) – or at the RNA level. For this second choice (the most common one), the translocation should produce a leukemia-specific fusion mRNA that can be used as PCR target after reverse transcription into cDNA (RT–PCR).[27] In contrast to Ig/TCR gene rearrangements, translocations are not patient-specific but rather tumor-specific markers. Although PCR techniques are potentially very powerful for MRD detection, they have several limitations (including subclone formation and clonal evolution, cross-contamination of PCR products between patient samples, amplification of sequences of normal cells, and poor quality of DNA or RNA samples) – all of these problems may lead to either false-positive or false-negative results in MRD investigations.[6,7,28] Moreover, quality control studies have shown a great variability in both intra- and inter-laboratory results. Therefore, improvement in the standardization of this methodology is still required. In this context, a collaborative program carried out through a BIOMED-1 concerted action led to the development of standardized nested RT–PCR assays, suitable for the detection of MRD as well as for diagnostic screening.[27] MRD studies by qualitative or semiquantitative PCR analysis have been shown to be clinically relevant in some particular situations (childhood ALL, BCR–ABL in CML patients following allogeneic transplant and PML–RARα in acute promyelocytic leukemia (APL) patients after consolidation therapy).[27] However, these methods fail to demonstrate clinical impact in leukemias associated with other chromosome aberrations (e.g. AML–ETO). This is probably due to the fact that this 'endpoint' PCR analysis does not allow a precise quantitative evaluation of the number of residual tumor cells in the sample. Thus, a quantitative PCR assay (e.g. competitive PCR) could improve the predictive capacity of RT–PCR in some chromosome aberrations (e.g. *M-BCR* in CML, *CBFβ–MYH11*, *AML1–ETO*). However, competitive PCR techniques are labor-intensive, prone to cross-contamination, and time-consuming, which precludes their use in both standardization protocols and large prospective therapeutic trials. More recently, automated real-time quantitative PCR (RQ–PCR) technology has demonstrated its reliability and potential utility for MRD studies on different fusion transcripts (e.g. *M-BCR, PML–RARα, and AML1–ETO*) and for the detection of clonal rearrangements of Ig and TCR genes.[29,30] The results of a Europe Against Cancer program of standardization and quality control studies of RQ–PCR for MRD detection of fusion-gene transcripts in leukemia have been published.[29]

# Detection of MRD in AML: clinical studies

Although experience in MRD detection is more limited in AML than it is in ALL, several clinical studies including small series of patients have been reported, based mainly on either molecular or immunophenotypical methods for the assessment of residual neoplastic cells.[1,31–35] In this review, we shall comment on clinical results reported for the different techniques available for MRD detection in AML and discuss possible pitfalls of these techniques.

## Morphology in AML

Relapse of AML patients is classically defined by the presence of 5% or more myeloblasts, morphologically identified in BM samples. As we have already mentioned, this is not a sensitive assay, particularly in those patients receiving chemotherapy, due to the difficulty in making a morphological distinction between leukemic blast cells and normal regenerating myeloid precursor cells. In fact, although the morphological assessment of BM is a very specific outcome-predictor assay for patients displaying over 5% blast cells following AML induction therapy – refractory disease with very poor prognosis – in the remaining patients (<5% blast cells, 'morphological CR'), its predictive value is uncertain since some of these patients will remain in continuous CR while many others will relapse. Moreover, there is some controversy surrounding the value of routine morphological BM examinations to detect recurrence of AML. Accordingly, several cooperative groups such as Cancer and Leukemia Group B (CALGB), the Eastern Cooperative Oncology Group (ECOG), and the Southwestern Oncology Group (SWOG) have called for serial marrow aspirations every 2–3 months for the first year and every 3–5 months for the following 2 years. However, two reports including 69[36] and 444[11]

relapsed AML patients showed that an abnormality in peripheral blood cell counts preceded or coexisted with BM relapse in 97% and 84% of cases, respectively. According to these results, BM aspirations for morphological examinations would be superfluous in over 80% of AML patients, providing that peripheral blood counts are frequently obtained (i.e. weekly). However, this would depend on the age of the patient and the planned therapy, since patients who are candidates for an allogeneic transplant may benefit from an earlier detection of relapse. In addition, as we shall discuss below, the situation may be completely different if the BM sample is going to be examined for residual cells using other MRD techniques.

## Cell cultures in AML

Few studies have been performed to evaluate the clinical value of investigating the growth of leukemic colonies (CFU-L) for MRD detection in AML. In a series of 43 AML patients in remission before autologous transplantation, Miller et al[12] found that the assay was not predictive of relapse, since CR samples from 80% of the patients showed CFU-L growth. However, they observed that the sensitivity of the clonogenic cells to 4-hydroperoxycyclophosphamide (4-HC) used to purge the autografts correlated with outcome; of the 23 patients in which the CFU-L were sensitive to 4-HC treatment, only 18% relapsed, while of the 22 resistant AML patients, 77% had relapsed. Gerhartz and Schmetzer[14] combined immunophenotyping with CFU-L analysis, demonstrating growth of colonies with abnormal antigen coexpression in 17 out of 19 AML patients in morphological CR. Although this pattern was associated with relapse, frequent false-positive results occurred in sustained remission.

A different approach to the exploitation of cell cultures for investigation of MRD is based on the hypothesis that the persistence of residual leukemic hemopoiesis will alter the growth pattern of normal granulomonocytic progenitors (CFU-GM) in AML patients. For this reason, we explored the utility of the CFU-GM assay in predicting relapse in 36 de novo AML patients in morphological CR.[13] Our results showed that all patients who achieved a normal CFU-GM growth pattern remained in CR, but that a median of 6 months after chemotherapy is necessary before a stable growth pattern is achieved. Leukemic relapse was always preceded by an abnormal CFU-GM pattern, although there were cases with anomalous growth who remained in CR.

## Cytogenetics and FISH in AML

In spite of its low sensitivity, conventional cytogenetics has proved to be a reliable marker for monitoring response to therapy in AML patients due to its high specificity. The persistence of cells in CR samples that show the same karyotypic abnormality found at diagnosis has traditionally been considered a high-risk prognostic factor for impending relapse. Accordingly, Freireich et al[16] studied 71 AML patients in morphological CR who had specific karyotypic abnormalities at diagnosis (inv (16), t(15;17), trisomy 8, etc.). In 20 patients, the cytogenetic aberration persisted in CR samples and all of them relapsed within the next 78 weeks. Nevertheless, from the remaining 51 patients with normal cytogenetics at CR, 25 have also relapsed. Therefore, although false-positive results are unlikely to occur, false negatives are relatively frequent. A possible explanation for these latter cases is the technical inability to obtain metaphases from the leukemic cell clone when the number of these cells is very low.

Preliminary reports suggest that due to its high specificity and the possibility of analyzing both metaphase chromosomes and interphase nuclei, FISH is a promising approach to detect low numbers of residual leukemic cells. At present, the reported experience of the detection of MRD in AML is still scanty and, as mentioned above, the sensitivity usually found to be low ($10^{-2}$) unless combined with other methods. Nylund et al[17] analyzed the predictive value of the investigation of trisomy 8 and t(15;17) in both metaphase and interphase nuclei obtained from BM samples in morphological CR from 11 AML patients. Eight patients had trisomy 8 at diagnosis, and this alteration was detected during follow-up in either metaphase or interphase cells from 3 and 2 patients respectively, who subsequently relapsed. In addition, in one patient, the use of appropriate probes showed persistence of residual cells with t(15;17) prior to relapse. By contrast, two M3 leukemias that became FISH-negative remained in clinical remission. Zhao et al[37] analyzed residual leukemic cells in 10 APL patients in clinical remission. In 6 of them, no cells with t(15;17) were found, and all these cases remained in CR for 25–33 months after the first FISH study. In 4 patients who had a relapse, FISH evaluation showed low numbers (2–4%) of residual cells with t(15;17) before relapse (1–14 months' interval between FISH detection and clinical relapse). Interestingly, these 4 cases were negative by conventional cytogenetics for t(15;17).

In an attempt to increase the sensitivity of FISH techniques, Varella-Garcia et al[38] sorted CD34+ cells from CR AML patients and analyzed by FISH the genetic aberrations detected at diagnosis, reaching a sensitivity of detection of 1 leukemic cell in $10^4$ normal cells. They have used this approach to study 20 AML patients in morphological CR. Residual disease was observed prior to relapse in 5 of 7 evaluable patients. In contrast, out of the 12 AML patients in whom residual disease was undetectable, 11 remained in continuous CR for a median period of 38 weeks.

## DNA aneuploidy in AML

The reported incidence of DNA aneuploidy detected by flow cytometry in AML ranges between 5% and 35%. In our experience, only 10 out of 205 de novo AML patients (4.9%) had DNA aneuploidy, many of these cases corresponding to tetraploid AML patients.[39] Therefore, this approach would only be applicable to a minority of AML patients, which, as previously discussed, together with its low sensitivity, indicate that it is useless for MRD investigation in AML.

## Immunophenotyping in AML

### Basis of MRD detection in AML

A precise identification of leukemic cells is essentially based on the ability to clearly distinguish them from the normal cells present in the specimen. Accordingly, phenotypic patterns of normal cells present in all types of samples used for the diagnosis of hematological malignancies must be well established. It has traditionally been considered that leukemic cells reflect the immunophenotypic characteristics of normal cells blocked at a certain differentiation stage. However, as we have previously mentioned, the use of multiparametric flow-cytometric analyses and large panels of MoAb combinations has shown that leukemic cells frequently display aberrant or uncommon phenotypic features that allow their distinction from normal cells.[21,22,24,26,40–42] Table 22.3 shows several phenotypic patterns based on the assessment of myeloid antigens

**Table 22.3  Acute myeloid leukemia: incidence of the most frequent phenotypic patterns that are absent or present at very low frequencies ($<10^{-4}$) in normal bone marrow**

| Phenotypic pattern | Incidence (%) |
|---|---|
| **Asynchronous antigen expression** | |
| CD33++ HLA-DR- CD34- CD15- CD14- | 17 |
| CD33- CD13+ | 14 |
| CD117+ CD33+ HLA-DR- | 11 |
| CD34+ HLADR- CD33+ | 9 |
| CD34+ CD56+ | 8 |
| CD33+ CD13- | 7 |
| CD117+ CD11b+ | 6 |
| CD117+dim CD34- CD15- | 6 |
| CD34+ CD11b+ | 5 |
| **Cross-lineage antigen expression** | |
| CD2+ | 21 |
| CD7+ | 9 |
| **Antigen overexpression** | |
| CD33+++ | 11 |
| CD34+++ | 9 |

that are undetectable ($<10^{-4}$) or present at very low frequencies ($<10^{-3}$ cells) in normal adult BM and therefore suitable for MRD investigation in those AML cases in which blast cells display such phenotypes. Although preliminary studies reported a variable incidence of aberrant or 'leukemia-associated' phenotypes in AML, ranging from 30% to 85% depending on the criteria used for their definition and the panel of monoclonal antibodies employed,[5,7,21,22,24,26,31,41,43–45] more recent reports[21,22,24] consistently find aberrant phenotypes in 70–80% of patients (Table 22.4). In our experience, 75% of AML patients display aberrant phenotypes, two or more aberrations coexisting in most of them (56%).[21,41] Therefore, according to these results, immunophenotypical detection of MRD is feasible in three-quarters of AML patients. The most common type of leukemia-associated phenotype found is the presence of asynchronous antigen expression (in 78% of aberrant cases), caused by the coexistence of two antigens that are not simultaneously expressed in normal differentiation or by the lack of reactivity for the panmyeloid antigens CD13 and CD33. Examples of these phenotypic aberrations are CD34+CD56+, CD34+CD11b+, CD34+CD14+, CD117+HLA-DR+CD15+, and CD33+CD13-CD15+, CD33-CD13+CD15+. Cross-lineage expression of lymphoid-associated markers (e.g. CD2, CD7, and CD19) in myeloid blast cells is observed in around one-third of cases.[40,41] Finally, abnormal light scatter patterns and overexpression of the myeloid cell-related markers (CD34, CD13, CD33, CD15, and CD14) contribute to the definition of around 15% and 20% of leukemia-associated phenotypes, respectively.[21,40,41] The sensitivity of this approach for the identification of residual AML blast cells ranges between $10^{-4}$ and $10^{-5}$, depending on the type of aberration explored and the normal background. Since the strategy for MRD detection using immunological methods has up till now relied mainly on the identification of residual cells with the same phenotypic aberration detected at diagnosis, a possible major limitation on this type of study is the existence of phenotypic switches during the evolution of the disease. In this sense, several groups, including our own,[1,6,21,22,25,40,44,46] have observed that at relapse, changes in the expression of individual markers

(CD15, CD14, CD11b, and HLA-DR) are relatively common in AML, involving between 63% and 90% of cases, depending on the number of antigens tested. Such changes are usually maturation-associated, more immature blast cell populations being present at relapse.[22,41] Despite this instability, such phenotypic modifications do not usually affect antigens that define the 'leukemia-associated phenotypes',[25] and, in our experience, only occur in 16% of all AML patients.[46] Accordingly, in cases with more than one 'leukemic phenotype', simultaneous investigation of all of them will reduce the possibility of false-negative results due to the occurrence of a phenotypic switch. Moreover, the systematic use of multiple antibody panels analyzed by multiparameter flow cytometry would have the potential to identify different aberrant phenotypic patterns from residual leukemic cells during follow-up, but at the expense of increased cost.

Until recently, the immunophenotypic detection of MRD was based on the antigenic characteristics of the predominant blast cell population at diagnosis.[5,31,44] However, it is well known that several leukemic subpopulations with different phenotypic characteristics may be present at diagnosis,[5,20,22,43] and perhaps a minor one may be the resistant clone responsible for relapse. In our experience, 80% of AML patients have two or more cell populations, often small in size, containing less than 10% blast cells.[20] These subpopulations frequently correspond to different stages of maturation of the neoplastic clone. According to this observation, the investigation of MRD should be based on the phenotypic characteristics of each subpopulation. An additional conclusion from the study of cell subsets in AML is that some of the reported phenotypic switches are not real, but correspond to an expansion, during disease evolution, of a very small cell subpopulation that went undetected at diagnosis. Figure 22.2 illustrates an APL that relapsed with an immature CD34+ phenotype (100% of cells), while at diagnosis most leukemic cells were more mature and only 10% of the blast cells expressed this specific CD34+ phenotype.

### Clinical results

Although the number of reports on the clinical value of immunophenotypic detection of MRD in AML has increased in recent years, the information so far available is still scanty, and sometimes not based on five or six parameter flow cytometry studies but simply on double marker combinations. Early studies by Adriaansen et al[31] and Campana et al,[1] based on the aberrant coexpression of terminal deoxynucleotidyl transferase (TdT) and myeloid markers (CD13/CD33) (cross-lineage marker expression), showed the value of this phenotypic combination to detect MRD in AML patients. The criteria used to define TdT positivity at diagnosis were different in the two studies, since Adriaansen et al[31] included all cases that displayed

---

**Table 22.4  Incidence of leukemia-associated immunophenotypes in acute myeloid leukemia**

| Leukemic phenotype | Incidence (%) |
|---|---|
| Asynchronous antigen expression | 60–70 |
| Cross-lineage antigen expression | 30–40 |
| Antigen overexpression | 20–30 |
| Abnormal light scatter | 15–20 |
| Overall | 70–80 |

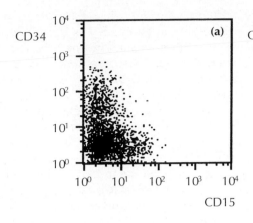 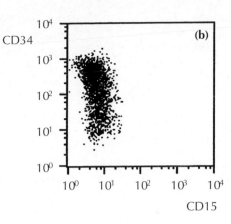

**Figure 22.2** Acute promyelocytic leukemia: at diagnosis (a), only 10% of blast cells expressed CD34 antigen, while at relapse (b), most leukemic cells (90%) expressed it.

over 1% TdT+ myeloid leukemic cells, while for Campana et al,[1] the cut-off value was much higher. In this latter series, from the seven patients included, residual disease persisted during follow-up in four patients, all of whom subsequently relapsed, by contrast, only one of the three negative cases relapsed. In the series by Adriaansen et al,[31] 9 of the 10 relapses observed were preceded, over a period of 14–38 weeks, by a gradual increase of TdT+CD13+ cells. In five additional patients who remained in continuous CR, TdT+ CD13+ blast cells were detected, but their number did not increase during follow-up. It should be noted that later studies showed that early lymphoid progenitors may coexpress the myeloid-related CD13 and CD33 markers, which could at least partially explain these findings.[47] Drach et al[44] followed three patients who also displayed a lineage infidelity (CD13+CD7+) and in whom the persistence of these cells was predictive of relapse. Campana and Pui[25] studied by multiparameter flow cytometry 13 children in CR after BMT. In 4 patients, residual leukemic cells were observed, and all relapsed within 2 months after the phenotypical detection. In the remaining 9 patients, leukemic cells were not detected, and 7 of them remain in CR with a median follow-up of more than 1 year after transplant. The other two patients relapsed and, according to the authors, should be considered false-negative cases. Reading et al[43] studied 16 AML patients in morphological CR using three-color stainings analyzed at flow cytometry: 6 had over 0.2% phenotypically aberrant cells in the first-remission BM aspirate, and all relapsed between 1 and 7 months later. Conversely, of the 10 patients with less than 0.2% aberrant cells, only 1 relapsed during the follow-up period. These findings are consistent with those of Wörman et al,[32] who also quantitated the number of residual cells in a series of 45 adult patients. In two-thirds of cases over 0.5% phenotypically aberrant cells were detected in the first-CR bone marrow samples, and half of these patients relapsed within 1 year. As far as our own experience is concerned,[21] in a series of 126 AML patients followed for a median period of 2 years, we have observed that the immunophenotypic enumeration of residual cells with leukemia-associated phenotypes on the first-remission BM sample, obtained at the end of induction therapy, correlates with both disease-free and overall survival. Accordingly, four different risk group categories could be established based on the MRD levels: (1) very low-risk ($<10^{-4}$ residual leukemic cells); (2) low-risk (between $10^{-3}$ and $10^{-4}$ residual tumor cells); (3) intermediate-risk (between $10^{-2}$ and $10^{-3}$ residual neoplastic cells); and (4) high-risk ($>10^{-2}$ residual leukemic cells); the relapse-free survival rates at 3 years for these risk groups were 100%, 85%, 55%, and 25%, respectively. An adverse prognostic impact of MRD levels was also observed once APL and non-APL AML cases were analyzed separately; multivariate analysis of prognostic factors showed that the MRD level together with cytogenetics were the most powerful independent prognostic factors for predicting disease-free survival.[21]

Reports by other groups have confirmed our observations. Accordingly, Vendetti et al[24] and Lahuerta et al[48] have found that the persistence of $3.5\times10^{-4}$ or more and over $8\times10^{-3}$ immunophenotypically aberrant cells either at the end of consolidation or prior to transplantation, respectively, strongly predict relapse.

Taking all this data together we can state that:

- The persistence or the increase in the number of phenotypically abnormal cells during follow-up of AML patients is usually associated with relapse.
- The number of aberrant cells in the remission BM aspirate correlates with relapse. This indicates that for predicting outcome in AML patients achieving CR, immunological evaluation of residual disease is more accurate than morphological examination. Therefore, the term 'immunological remission' is complementary to 'morphological CR'.
- The enumeration during follow-up of residual leukemic cells by immunophenotyping may also help to individualize the therapeutic approaches in AML patients in order to reduce both over- and undertreatment during the consolidation and intensification phases.

## Molecular biology in AML

Chromosomal translocations, including t(15;17), t(8;21), inv(16), 11q23 aberrations, t(6;9), and t(9;22), which together account for 30–40% of AML cases (Table 22.5), are the most efficient tumor-specific PCR targets in AML patients.[27] However, in order to cover a larger number of patients, other potential MRD–PCR targets (e.g. *WT1* and *FLT3*) have been developed. Moreover, other strategies could be used for MRD monitoring in patients without cytogenetic abnormalities in the allograft setting, such as detection of the Y chromosome or chimerism studies on FACS-sorted material (e.g. cells with the immunophenotypic characteristics of the original leukemic clone).[49] In addition, approximately 10–15% of AML patients have cross-lineage Ig or TCR gene rearrangements[50] with identifiable junctional regions, but clinical MRD–PCR studies using this approach have not been reported.

In this section, we shall comment on the clinical applications of MRD–PCR studies, concentrating on those for which clinical information is currently available.

### Molecular monitoring of PML–RARα transcripts in AML with t(15;17)(q22;q21)

This reciprocal chromosomal translocation is a specific characteristic associated with APL, including both the hypergranular (French–American–British (FAB) AML-M3) and microgranular (FAB AML-M3v) variants, secondary APL, and the promyelocytic blast crisis of CML leukemia.[51] As a consequence of the translocation, two chimeric genes, *PML–RARα*

(detected in 100% of cases) and *RARα–PML* (detected in 70% of AML patients) are formed. The *PML* breakpoints cluster within three regions (intron 6 bcr-1 or L-long-form, exon 6 bcr-2 or V-variable-form, and intron 3 bcr-3 or S-short-form) that fuse with the 3′ portion of *RARα* intron 2.[51] Using appropriate primers, it is possible to amplify the different *PML/RARα* mRNA isoforms by RT–PCR in all APL cases, even if cytogenetic analysis has failed to identify t(15;17). The detection of *PML/RARα* has therapeutic implications, since the rare APL cases with the variant t(11;17) failed to respond to all-*trans*-retinoic acid (ATRA).[51] Moreover, a reduced sensitivity to ATRA has also been described in patients with the bcr-2 (or V) isoform. However, the number of cases is limited and most of these patients display additional cytogenetic abnormalities, so that no clear conclusions can be drawn.[52,53]

Several groups using conventional nested RT–PCR have reported that molecular monitoring of *PML–RARα* is clinically relevant in APL.[33,51,54,55] These studies revealed that qualitative RT–PCR positivity after consolidation treatment was highly predictive of clinical relapse, whereas a PCR-negative result was associated with prolonged disease-free survival. On the other hand, studies performed within the first months after induction revealed PCR-positive results in nearly 50% of the cases, but this early positivity does not correlate with response to treatment.[51,55] However, a study from the UK Medical Research Council (MRC) has shown that analysis of the kinetics of *PML–RARα* transcript reduction could be a useful parameter to identify subgroups of patients with a different risk of relapse.[56] These

### Table 22.5 Detection of chromosome translocations by RT–PCR

| Cytogenetic abnormality | Individual genes | AML subtype | Frequency of applicability (%) |
|---|---|---|---|
| t(15;17)(q22;q21) | PML/RARα | AML-M3 (APL) | 10–30[a] |
| Variants: | | | |
| t(11;17)(q23;q21) | PLZF/RARα | AML-M3-like | – |
| t(5;17)(q35;q21) | NPM/RARα | AML-M3-like | – |
| t(8;21)(q22;q22) | AML1/ETO | AML-M2,-M1,-M4 | 8–10 |
| inv(16)(p13;q22) | CBFβ/MYH11 | AML-M4Eo,-M4 | 3–5 |
| t(16;16)(p13;q22) | | | |
| 11q23 aberrations | | | |
| Translocations | MLL | | |
| der(11)(q23) | | | |
| t(9;11)(p22;q23) | MLL/AF9 | AML-M4-,M5 | 8–10 |
| t(11;19)(p23;p13) | MLL/ENL or ELL | | |
| t(6;9)(q21;q26) | DEK/CAN | AML | 2 |
| t(9;22)(q34;q11) | BCR/ABL | AML | 1–2 |
| inv(3)(q21;q26) | EVI1 | AML-M1 | <1 |
| t(3;3)(q21;q26) | | | |

[a] The incidence of t(15;17) in some areas of Europe (Italy) and some US and South American Latino populations is higher (30%).

studies[33,51,54-56] indicate that patients in whom *PML-RARα* transcripts persist at the end of consolidation therapy or patients who convert to RT–PCR positivity after a negative result are at great risk of relapse. Indeed, preliminary data suggest that early treatment at the stage of molecular relapse leads to improved survival in comparison with patients who were retreated in overt hematological relapse.[57] Moreover, MRD studies are of value to predict outcome following autologous SCT in APL patients in second CR.[51,55]

At present, the availability of modern protocols containing concomitant ATRA plus quemotherapy had produced a remarkable improvement in the outcome of APL patients, associated with a relapse risk of only 10–20%.[51,53] Thus, the major limitation of qualitative RT–PCR assays is their failure to identify these small subgroup of patients who ultimately relapse, which may be a reflection of RNA quality and/or assay sensitivity.[58] Previous European quality control programs show that the number of unsuitable samples for MRD studies ranged from 20% to 50% due to poor quality samples that could potentially give rise to 'false-negative' results.[51,55] The sensitivity of conventional nested RT–PCR for detection of *PML-RARα* transcripts is lower than in other translocations, such as *AML1-ETO*, which could explain also the existence of false-negative results.[27] Interestingly, the detection of *RARα-PML* is more sensitive than that of *PML-RARα*, since in 8 out of 30 CR samples in which both chimeric genes were simultaneously analyzed, *RARα-PML* transcripts were detected while *PML-RARα* was negative.[58,59] However, study of this transcript can produce both false-negative results (*RARα-PML* negative in patients who ultimately relapse) and false-positive results (persistence of *RARα-PML* fusion mRNA in patients in long-term remission).[58,59] Taking all this data together, we can see that there is still room for improvement in MRD detection in APL, and RQ–PCR could provide additional information to overcome these limitations (quantitation of *PML-RARα* and control gene transcripts to determine the exact level of MRD and identification of poor quality samples).[29] Preliminary studies using RQ–PCR are encouraging, and a retrospective analysis found that RQ–PCR increased rates of MRD detection in comparison with the qualitative assay and was an independent predictor of relapse risk and overall survival. However, it is clear that this new approach needs to be evaluated in the context of large-scale multicenter clinical trials to establish guidelines to use RQ–PCR data for clinical decision-making.[29]

### Molecular monitoring of AML1–ETO transcripts in AML with t(8;21) (q22;q22)

The t(8;21) is one of the most frequent chromosomal abnormalities in AML (7–20%), especially in the FAB M2 subtype (20–40%), with a higher incidence in younger patients.[60,61] Although most t(8;21) (90%) have been described in AML-M2, it has also been reported in about 3–6% of AML-M1 and, less frequently, in AML-M4 and other myeloproliferative syndromes.[60,61] Myeloid leukemias with t(8;21) show common features, both morphological (blasts with abundant cytoplasm with large vacuoles, numerous granules, and prominent Auer rods) and immunological (CD19, CD56, and CD34 expression, with absence or dim reactivity for CD33).[61]

Molecular characterization of t(8;21) has shown that it involves the *AML1 (RUNX1)* gene on chromosome 21 and the *ETO* gene on chromosome 8, which fuse to form a new hybrid gene on the der(8) chromosome.[60] In contrast to t(15;17) and inv(16), the breakpoints within the *AML1* gene and the *ETO* gene occur in an area highly conserved within a single intron of both genes; therefore, an identically sized band is detected by RT–PCR in nearly all patients.[60,61]

From a clinical point of view, this translocation has been associated with good response to chemotherapy (cytarabine), a high remission rate, and prolonged disease-free survival. For these reasons, and because *AML1-ETO* has also been described in AML patients negative by conventional cytogenetics,[61] molecular screening for *AML1-ETO* would be advisable for all AML patients where morphology and/or immunophenotyping suggest the presence of t(8;21). This should avoid overtreatment strategies such as allogenic SCT in patients who can be cured with standard chemotherapy.

Studies of MRD in patients with t(8;21) suggest that conventional nested RT–PCR may have limited value. Accordingly, *AML1-ETO* fusion transcripts have been found in patients in long-term remission after chemotherapy or autologous SCT and even allogeneic SCT.[60,62,63] These data suggest that patients who are considered to be clinically cured may still have molecular evidence of MRD, suggesting that t(8;21) may represent only one of the necessary steps for the development of leukemia and that additional genetic abnormalities may be required for the overt clinical expression of the acute leukemia. Thus, the finding that in AML patients with t(8;21), the *AML1-ETO* fusion can also be expressed in non-leukemic stem cells, monocytes, and B cells is concordant with this hypothesis.[63] Moreover, these data are probably a reflection of the higher levels of the sensitivity achieved with qualitative RT–PCR for *AML1-ETO* ($10^{-5}$ to $10^{-6}$) as compared with those achieved for other AML fusion genes, such as *PML-RARα* ($10^{-4}$). In line with this hypothesis, a study has shown that conventional *AML1-ETO* RT–PCR is predictive of outcome when a single-step PCR (sensitivity of $10^{-4}$) instead of nested PCR (sensitivity of $10^{-6}$) is carried out.[64]

In order to improve the predictive value of qualitative RT–PCR studies, a quantitative analysis of *AML1-ETO* transcripts has been developed.

Miyamoto et al,[65] by studying peripheral blood stem cell (PBSC) harvest samples from 15 patients collected after both the first and the second consolidation cycles, have found that in all patients the number of *AML1–ETO* transcripts was lower in the second PBSC harvest than in the first. However, no correlation was found between the number of *AML1–ETO* transcripts in the infused PBSC harvest and the clinical outcome after autologous blood SCT (ABSCT). Other competitive RT–PCR studies performed by the Manchester group[66] have shown that this method could help to predict relapse for up 6 months before the onset of overt relapse and, furthermore, it is able to identify MRD threshold levels above which patients would relapse within 3–6 months. On the other hand, patients with low or undetectable levels of *AML1–ETO* transcripts were associated with maintenance of continuous CR. Data produced to date, from RQ–PCR have essentially confirmed results obtained by competitive RT–PCR, but experience is limited to small numbers of patients. These encouraging results suggest that RQ–PCR assay could be applied in large-scale clinical trials.

### Molecular monitoring of CBFβ–MYH11 transcripts in AML with inv(16) and t(16;16) (p13;q22)

The pericentric inversion of chromosome 16 – inv(16)(p13;q22) – and the less common but molecularly similar t(16;16)(p13;q22) are closely associated with the M4Eo AML subtype (in nearly 100% of cases), although they may also be detected in AML cases with FAB M2, M4, and M5 morphology and in MDS.[35,67] This chromosomal abnormality involves the *CBFβ* gene on 16q22 and the *MYH11* gene on 16p13, which produce the *CBFβ–MYH11* fusion gene. RT–PCR assays have been developed to detect *CBFβ–MYH11* fusion transcripts, showing that this assay can detect chimeric mRNA in over 90% of cases with inv(16) or t(16;16). These studies have demonstrated the existence of a marked molecular heterogeneity, and at least seven types of fusion transcripts (A–H) have been reported, type A being the predominant (80% of AML patients with inv(16) or t(16;16)).

The value of molecular monitoring of MRD in AML patients with *CBFβ–MYH11* by qualitative RT–PCR still needs to be determined; preliminary results are limited and contradictory.[27,35,67,68] In most reports, the large majority of patients in continuous CR were found to be qualitative RT–PCR-negative, but some long-term survivors remained PCR-positive. Moreover, about 10–20% of PCR-negative patients eventually relapsed, suggesting that the achievement of PCR negativity is not predictive of cure. Studies using both competitive and real-time quantitative assays suggest that MRD monitoring can provide prognostic information on the response to treatment and can identify patients at high risk of relapse.[29] Moreover, Marcucci et al[69] reported that a cut-off level

of 10 *CBFβ–MYH11* transcripts during remission can discriminate patients at different risks of relapse. However, due to the limited numbers of patients so far analyzed by RQ-PCR, longitudinal studies in large series of patients are still necessary in order to confirm these preliminary data.

### Other chromosomal translocations: 11q23 aberrations, t(6;9)(p23;q34), and t(9;22)(q34;q11)

Molecular cloning of genes involved in additional chromosomal translocations in AML – 11q23 rearrangements, t(6;9), and t(9;22) – have made it possible to design sensitive RT–PCR assays for MRD monitoring.[27] However, the incidence of these chromosomal translocations is low (<5%) and up to now there have been no reports of any clear correlation with specific morphological or immunological features of AML that would orientate the investigation of these translocations to restricted subgroups of patients.

Translocations involving chromosome 11, band q23, have been detected in a variety of hematopoietic malignancies, occurring in 7–10% of ALL, 5–6% of AML, and 85% of secondary leukemias following treatment with topoisomerase II inhibitors.[70] Although over 20 partner loci have been shown to be involved in balanced 11q23 translocations, the most common translocations in AML are t(9;11)(p22;q23), t(11;19)(q23;p13.1), and t(11;19)(q23;p13.3). In de novo AML, the 11q23 translocations have typically been associated with monocytic differentiation, as defined by FAB M4 and M5. In infant AML, 11q23 rearrangements are associated with hyperleukocytosis and a poor prognosis. In contrast, in adult cases, no association with specific clinical or prognostic features has been found. The gene on chromosome 11 interrupted by the 11q23 translocations is referred to as the *MLL* gene (mixed-lineage leukemia), and fuses with the *AF9* gene in t(9;11) and with *ENL* or *ELL* in t(11;19).[70] The cloning of these partner genes has led to the development of an RT–PCR assay for the detection of the der(11)-derived chimeric mRNA in diagnostic leukemic samples. Molecular monitoring of MRD in leukemia with 11q23 rearrangement has so far been restricted to the analysis of t(4;11) in infant ALL, showing that remission samples lacked evidence of *MLL–AF4* fusion transcripts.

The t(6;9)(p23;q34) can be found in 2–4% of all AML patients (subtypes FAB M1, M2, and M4) and in some cases of refractory anemia with excess blasts (RAEB).[27] This translocation is associated with a subtype of AML with a bad prognosis that occurs in young people. Although, initially, t(6;9)(p23;q34) was also related with increase of basophils, myelodysplastic features, and immature phenotype (TdT+), these associations have not been confirmed in recent studies. The two genes involved in this translocation, *DEK* on 6q23 and *CAN* on 9q34, produce a chimeric fusion mRNA that is expressed and detected by RT–PCR. The genomic breakpoints within both genes are restricted to a precise site, a uniform *DEK–CAN* fusion transcript being observed in all cases. A study by Nakano et al[71] reported that in a young patient who relapsed after PBSC transplantation, RT–PCR assay was able to detect the fusion transcript in the harvested stem cell sample. Further studies are necessary to confirm its clinical value for MRD monitoring.

Approximately 1–2% of de novo AML display the reciprocal translocation t(9;22)(q34;q11). Although no MRD studies of Philadelphia-positive AML have been reported, a strategy similar to that for CML or Ph+ ALL could be used as discussed below.

### Genetic markers for MRD study other than chromosome aberrations

Since at least half of AML patients do not have a suitable fusion gene target for MRD detection, there is a need to identify alternative molecular markers for MRD monitoring. Such potential targets include *FLT3* and WT1.

The *FLT3* (Fms-like tyrosine kinase) gene encode a receptor tyrosine kinase that is closely related to two well-known receptors, Kit and Fms, and is expressed predominantly in primitive hematopoitic CD34+.[72] Studies have shown that an internal tandem duplication (ITD) in the *FLT3* gene is a somatic mutation detected almost exclusively in AML, occurring in 20–30% of AML patients.[72] Controversy exists regarding the prognostic significance of these mutations, but in the largest study (854 patients) reported to date,[73] an *FLT3* IDT was associated with increased risk of relapse and with adverse disease-free survival, event-free survival, and overall survival, suggesting that detection of *FLT3* ITD should be included as a routine test at diagnosis. An RQ–PCR assay for *FLT3* ITD with high sensitivity and specificity has been reported, detecting between 0.01% and 0.001% of *FLT3* ITD-positive ADN in a background of 1 μg of normal bone marrow DNA.[74] However, these assays are labor-intensive, requiring the development of patient-specific primers (the size and location of the somatic mutations is different in each patient) as well as optimization procedures similar to those carried out for MRD assays based on IgH *VDJ* rearrangements in ALL. Moreover, these assays require that relapsed patients must have the same *FLT3* ITD as that observed at diagnosis, but a recent study has shown that one of 12 patients did not have an *FLT3* ITD at relapse. Thus, further studies to explore the stability of *FLT3* at relapse are needed.

The Wilms' tumor gene 1 (*WT1*) is a tumor suppressor gene that plays a key role in the carcinogenesis of Wilms' tumor. Several studies have shown that *WT1* is expressed in all AML, ALL, and CML, and that the expression levels correlate inversely with prognosis.[75] Moreover, monitoring of *WT1* expression by quantitative RT–PCR in patients with acute leukemia in remission can contribute to the prediction of impending hematological relapses. Moreover, quantification of *WT1* transcripts at specific time points (post induction and post consolidation) is prognostically valuable.[76] However, these results have not been reproduced by other groups, and the prognostic relevance in de novo AML of *WT1* transcript detection by RT–PCR in CR has not been demonstrated.[77] Data from RQ–PCR assay have been reported and appear to be encouraging, providing a basis for the evaluation of these targets by RQ–PCR in a large number of patients.[78]

## Myelodysplastic syndromes

Patients with poor-prognosis MDS under the age of 60 years are increasingly being treated with intensive chemotherapy, including SCT. Although the efficacy and effectiveness of these treatment modalities are inferior to those obtained in primary AML, CR rates varying from 20% to 60% have been reported.[79] In this latter subset of patients, the investigation of the quality of remission and the monitoring of residual disease will contribute to a better assessment of the efficacy of these new treatment strategies. Although theoretically most of the techniques used for MRD in AML could be applied to MDS, the information available so far is almost restricted to cytogenetic evaluation, including FISH analysis. Regarding the use of molecular techniques for MRD detection in female patients, PCR analysis of X-chromosome inactivation patterns may contribute to the assessment of clonal remission. Although chromosomal translocations are rare in MDS, if present they could be exploited as previously described for AML. In secondary MDS, the existence of balanced translocations involving chromosome ends 11q23 and 21q12 are increasingly being reported, and could also constitute a useful target for PCR analysis. However, in MDS, the most common cytogenetic abnormalities are numeric chromosomal changes or deletions such as 5q–/–5 7q–/–7, +8, 12p–, and 20q–.[79] In this context, large numbers of nondividing cells can be analyzed using interphase FISH and appropriate probes that would allow the demonstration of a small population of residual cells following therapy. Nylund et al[80] analyzed, by FISH, metaphase cells from two MDS patients with trisomy 8: following BMT, only normal cells were detected, and both patients remained in CR 9 and 24 months later. Flactif et al[81] re-examined three patients with clonal –7 after CR was achieved following intensive chemotherapy: interphase FISH showed normal cells in all three cases.

Few studies have been devoted to the investigation of the immunophenotypic characteristics of MDS.[82–85]

Although some of these studies[83,85-87] were based on a comparative analysis with normal cell differentiation for the definition of phenotypic profiles present in MDS, which would allow the identification of the myelodysplastic clone during follow-up, with a few exceptions,[83,86] they were restricted to the analysis of only a subset of bone marrow cells corresponding to either the erythroid,[85] neutrophil,[87] or CD34+ compartments.[86] In our experience, MDS frequently display aberrant phenotypic features such as the existence of asynchronous antigen expression, antigen overexpression, and differentiation blockade at early stages of maturation for the different myeloid cell lineages present in bone marrow, although these abnormalities may only involve a subset of all clonal cells.[88] In this sense, it has been pointed out that the ratio between immature/mature myeloid cells and the number of CD34+ cells may have prognostic implications, and consequently may represent valuable parameters for monitoring treatment.[82] More recently, Stetler-Stevenson et al[83] showed that multiparameter flow cytometry detected immunophenotypic abnormalities in virtually all of the 45 well-established MDS patients they analyzed. Such abnormalities included aberrations involving the maturing neutrophil-lineage cells – i.e. decreased granularity (84%), absence of CD64 (66%) and CD10 (11%) expression, reactivity for CD56 (21%), and abnormal CD11b/CD16 (70%) and CD13/CD16 (78%) differentiation patterns – as well as in the monocytic lineage CD56+ (33%), together with increased numbers of CD45+dim precursor cells (53%), and coexpression of CD2 (27%) and other lymphoid-associated markers (38%) on myeloid cells. Nevertheless, unlike AML, MDS still lacks a precise definition for the patterns of phenotypic aberrations that would allow a sensitive detection of the clonal dysplastic cells, which is a prerequisite for a correct inmmunophenotypic investigation of MRD in MDS patients.

## Chronic myeloid leukemia

CML has been one of the first malignancies to benefit from MRD studies. Two types of techniques have been used in these patients: molecular cytogenetics (FISH) and PCR. In fact, the terms 'cytogenetic and molecular remission' have already been included in the medical decision process concerning treatment strategies in CML.

### FISH

One of the major goals in the therapeutic control of CML patients who achieve CR is the early detection of MRD and relapse, especially following allogeneic transplantation, in order to use new treatment rescue strategies such as donor lymphocyte infusion (DLI).

FISH permits the identification of the BCR–ABL fusion gene in metaphase and interphase cells, which is particularly attractive for monitoring response to therapy in CML patients. The use of a yeast artificial chromosome (YAC) probe spanning the breakpoint region within the BCR gene and a cosmid probe flanking the breakpoint within the ABL gene, in a dual-color hybridization assay, provides a relatively high specificity with a decrease in the incidence of false-positive results to less than 0.5%.[19] Although this sensitivity is still lower than that of PCR, one of the advantages of FISH is that it is based on hybridization between the DNA of BCR–ABL probes and the genomic DNA, while the PCR technique explore the production of transcript RNA. Therefore, with FISH, it is feasible to detect the two types of BCR–ABL translocations (p210 and p190) in a single test. In addition, contamination is much less frequent in FISH than it is in PCR.

Amiel el al,[89] in five CML patients post BMT, have compared the sensitivity and specificity of FISH with cytogenetics and PCR with regards in the ability to detect the Philadelphia chromosome (Ph). The BCR–ABL translocation was detected in four of the five patients during the first 3 months following transplant. The proportion of residual positive cells ranged between 1% and 3%. A good correlation between FISH and PCR was observed. Knuutila's group[90] have used metaphase FISH for the detection of residual leukemic cells in 25 patients with CML following allogeneic BMT. According to their experience, three main conclusions can be drawn:

- The absence of residual leukemic cells is highly predictive of continuing remission (16 out of the 17 patients with no residual Ph+ cells remained in complete cytogenetic response (CCR).
- During the first 6 months, residual leukemic cells can be detected in about 25% of cases, but if the number of residual cells remains stable, it is not predictive of relapse, although careful follow-up is indicated.
- An increase in the amount of residual leukemic cells in subsequent samples is highly predictive of relapse (as observed in two of the three patients in whom relapse occurred).

Zhao et al[37] applied FISH to examine 10 CML patients who achieved complete cytogenetic remission following interferon-α (IFN-α) treatment. In six patients, residual BCR–ABL+ cells were observed, indicating that FISH is more sensitive than conventional cytogenetics for the detection of MRD in CML. This has also been confirmed by Cox-Froncillo et al.[91]

### RT–PCR

The Philadelphia chromosome, resulting from the reciprocal t(9 : 22) translocation, occurs in more than

95% of patients with CML, in about 30% (20–55%) of adult and 2–10% of childhood ALL, and in less than 2% of AML. At the molecular level, part of the *ABL* proto-oncogene is translocated from chromosome 9 into the *BCR* gene on chromosome 22, which results in the formation of a *BCR–ABL* chimeric gene. In the majority of CML cases and 30% of adult ALL, the *BCR* breakpoint is located at M-bcr. In contrast, in 50–70% of adult ALL cases, the majority of pediatric ALL and rare cases of AML the m-bcr region is involved.[92]

RT–PCR detection of BCR/ABL transcripts is possible in virtually all CML (>95%), even in those cases missed by standard cytogenetics (up to 10% of CML). However, a 3–5% of Ph+ CML escape molecular detection by conventionally used primer combinations.[93] The sensitivity of RT–PCR is usually down to $10^{-5}$ to $10^{-6}$. Therefore, RT–PCR is particularly useful in patients undergoing allogenic or autologous SCT as well as in those who achieve a cytogenetic complete response following IFN-α treatment. Several MRD–PCR studies have been performed in patients in clinical and cytogenetic remission after allogenic SCT in order to evaluate the incidence and significance of PCR-positive cells. The results reported so far have been conflicting, although a consensus appears to exist on the fact that most patients (>75%) are PCR-positive in the first 6 months after BMT and this positivity does not correlate with outcome.[93] After 1 year post BMT, the number of PCR-positive patients decrease to 20–40%, negativity being associated with withdrawal of immunosuppressive treatment and with both acute and chronic graft-versus-host disease (GVHD). However, 44% of patients without GVHD also have PCR-negative assays, suggesting the presence of mechanisms capable of suppression or eradication of CML independently of GVHD.[94] The existence of PCR-positive cells in a late post-transplant period again does not correlate with relapse, since such cells have been observed even several years after BMT without any signs of disease progression. Of greater value are sequential follow-up studies that allow patients to be divided into three main groups: persistently positive, intermittently negative, and persistently negative. These three groups have, respectively, a low, intermediate and high probability of maintaining remission.[94,95] Several MRD studies have also been carried out on patients in cytogenetic response after IFN-α. The majority of these studies found that IFN-α does not eradicate the disease. Consequently, a large proportion of the patients who achieve CCR are PCR-positive, their incidence being 90% or more within the first year and slightly less (60–80%) in long-term cytogenetic remission patients. However, the existence of PCR-positive cells

can be detected for a long period of time without relapse, suggesting that in these cases, the clonogenic potential of the residual leukemic clone is low. Moreover, patients taken off IFN-α therapy after CCR do not relapse in a short period of time, indicating that IFN-α may have a particular remnant effect.[96]

The limitations of qualitative PCR for predicting relapse in individual patients has led to the development of quantitative techniques based on competitive RT–PCR. Competitive RT–PCR techniques have been successfully used in the monitoring of MRD in CML patients both after allogenic SCT and during treatment with IFN-α.[93] This is particularly important in patients who are candidates for donor lymphocyte infusion (DLI), since response apparently correlates with residual tumor burden. Olavarria et al[97] showed that the probability of relapse correlates with the number of *BCR–ABL* transcripts found 3–5 months after SCT. Thus, they defined three levels of *BCR–ABL* transcripts – negative, positive at low level (<100 copies per µg RNA), and positive at high level – which correlate with the cumulative incidence of relapse (16.7%, 42.9%, and 86.4%, at 3 years after SCT, respectively; $p=0.0001$). However, some authors consider the use of competitive RT–PCR for clinical decision-making to be premature, since this technique is difficult to standardize. Several groups have reported that real-time quantitative (RQ–PCR) could be an alternative, and have applied it successfully to monitor MRD in CML patients.[29] A study from Radich et al[98] on 379 CML patients explored the significance of *BCR–ABL* molecular quantification by RQ–PCR at 18 months onwards after SCT. Quantification was performed on 344 samples from 85 qualitative RT–PCR-positive patients, and showed that the slope of the *BCR–ABL* change was significantly steeper in those patients destined to relapse compared with those who did not ($p=0.002$). Moreover, quantitative values for these patients who did not relapse tended to be quite low, with a median *BCR–ABL* level of 24 copies per µg RNA (62% of samples had fewer than 100 copies of *BCR–ABL* per µg RNA). These data suggest that the prognostic significance of a qualitative *BCR–ABL* can be refined using an RQ–PCR assay. However, this latter technique is associated with some caveats that may affect its use for monitoring and guiding therapy; for example, *BCR–ABL* can be detected in normal individuals (although at levels not detectable by standard RT–PCR assay), and some patients display high levels of transcripts without relapse (15% of patients in the study by Radich et al[98] had more than 1000 copies). Thus, early therapeutic interventions based on *BCR–ABL* quantification should only be offered within a research setting.

322 Detection of minimal residual disease in myeloid malignancies

## REFERENCES

1. Campana D, Coustan-Smith E, Janossy G. The immuno-logic detection of minimal residual disease in acute leukemia. *Blood* 1990; **76**: 163–71.
2. Orfao A, Ciudad J, Lopez-Berges MC et al. Acute lymphoblastic leukemia (ALL): detection of minimal residual disease (MRD) at flow cytometry. *Leuk Lymphoma* 1994; **13** (Suppl 1): 87–90.
3. San Miguel JF, Bartram C, Campana D, Andreeff M. Minimal residual disease in hematologic malignancies. *Rev Invest Clin* 1994; Suppl: 147–52.
4. Sievers EL, Loken MR. Detection of minimal residual disease in acute myelogenous leukemia. *J Pediatr Hematol Oncol* 1995; **17**: 123–33.
5. Terstappen LW, Konemann S, Safford M et al. Flow cytometric characterization of acute myeloid leukemia. Part 1. Significance of light scattering properties. *Leukemia* 1991; **5**: 315–21.
6. van Dongen JJ, Breit TM, Adriaansen HJ et al. Detection of minimal residual disease in acute leukemia by immunological marker analysis and polymerase chain reaction. *Leukemia* 1992; **6**(Suppl 1): 47–59.
7. van Dongen JJ, San Miguel J. Techniques for detection of minimal residual disease in leukemia patients. In: *Meet the Expert Sessions of the Second EHA*. Oxford: Blackwell Science, 1996: 39–46.
8. San Miguel J, Bartram C, Campana D, Andreeff M. Minimal residual disease in haematological malignancies. *XXV Congress of the International Society of Hematology. Education Program (Rev Invest Clin Suplemento)*, 1994: 147–52.
9. San Miguel JF, van Dongen JJ. Methods for detection of minimal residual disease. In: Buchner T, Hiddeman B, Wormann G (eds) *Acute Leukemias. VI. Prognostic Factors and Treatment Strategies*. Berlin: Springer-Verlag, 1997: 307–12.
10. Campana D. Determination of minimal residual disease in leukemia patients. *Br. J. Haematol* 2003; **121**: 823–38.
11. Estey E, Pierce S. Routine bone marrow exam during first remission of acute myeloid leukemia. *Blood* 1996; **87**: 3899–902.
12. Miller CB, Zehnbauer BA, Piantadosi S et al. Correlation of occult clonogenic leukemia drug sensitivity with relapse after autologous bone marrow transplantation. *Blood* 1991; **78**: 1125–31.
13. del Canizo MC, Mota A, Orfao A et al. Value of colony forming unit–granulocyte macrophage assay in predicting relapse in acute myeloid leukaemia. *J Clin Pathol* 1996; **49**: 450–2.
14. Gerhartz HH, Schmetzer H. Detection of minimal residual disease in acute myeloid leukemia. *Leukemia* 1990; **4**: 508–16.
15. Estrov Z, Grunberger T, Dube ID et al. Detection of residual acute lymphoblastic leukemia cells in cultures of bone marrow obtained during remission. *N Engl J Med* 1986; **315**: 538–42.
16. Freireich EJ, Cork A, Stass SA et al. Cytogenetics for detection of minimal residual disease in acute myeloblastic leukemia. *Leukemia* 1992; **6**: 500–6.
17. Nylund SJ, Ruutu T, Saarinen U et al. Detection of minimal residual disease using fluorescence DNA in situ hybridization: a follow-up study in leukemia and lymphoma patients. *Leukemia* 1994; **8**: 587–94.
18. Tabernero D, San Miguel JF, Garcia-Sanz M et al. Incidence of chromosome numerical changes in multiple myeloma: fluorescence in situ hybridization analysis using 15 chromosome-specific probes. *Am J Pathol* 1996; **149**: 153–61.
19. Bentz M, Cabot G, Moos M et al. Detection of chimeric *BCR–ABL* genes on bone marrow samples and blood smears in chronic myeloid and acute lymphoblastic leukemia by in situ hybridization. *Blood* 1994; **83**: 1922–8.
20. Macedo A, Orfao A, Gonzalez M et al. Immunological detection of blast cell subpopulations in acute myeloblastic leukemia at diagnosis: implications for minimal residual disease studies. *Leukemia* 1995; **9**:993–8.
21. San Miguel JF, Vidriales B, Lopez-Berges C et al. Early immunophenotypical evaluation of minimal residual disease in acute myeloid leukemia identifies different patients risk groups and may contribute to postinduction treatment stratification. *Blood* 2001; **98**: 1746–51.
22. Baer MR, Stewart CC, Dodge RK et al. High frequency of immunophenotype changes in acute myeloid leukemia at relapse: implications for residual disease detection (Cancer and Leukemia Group B Study 8361). *Blood* 2001; **97**: 3574–80.
23. Terstappen LW. Identification and characterization of plasma cells in normal human bone marrow by high-resolution flow cytometry. *Blood* 1990; **76**: 1739–47.
24. Venditti A, Buccisano F, Del Poeta G, Maurillo L et al. Level of minimal residual disease after consolidation therapy predicts outcome in acute myeloid leukemia. *Blood* 2000; **96**: 3948–52.
25. Campana D, Pui CH. Detection of minimal residual disease in acute leukemia: methodologic advances and clinical significance. *Blood* 1995; **85**: 1416–34.
26. Macedo A, Orfao A, Vidriales MB et al. Characterization of aberrant phenotypes in acute myeloblastic leukemia. *Ann Hematol* 1995; **70**: 189–94.
27. van Dongen JJ, Macintyre EA, Gabert JA et al. Standardized RT–PCR analysis of fusion gene transcripts from chromosome aberrations in acute leukemia for detection of minimal residual disease. Report of the BIOMED-1 Concerted Action: Investigation of Minimal Residual Disease in Acute Leukemia. *Leukemia* 1999; **13**: 1901–28.
28. Yin JA, Tobal K. Detection of minimal residual disease in acute myeloid leukaemia: methodologies, clinical and biological significance. *Br J Haematol* 1999; **106**: 578–90.
29. Gabert J, Beillard E, van der Velden VHJ et al. Standardization and quality control studies of 'real-time' quantitative reverse transcriptase polymerase chain reaction (RQ–PCR) of fusion gene transcripts for residual disease detection in leukemia (A Europe Against Cancer Program). *Leukemia* 2003; **17**: 2318–57.
30. Verhagen O, Willemse MJ, Breunis WB et al. Application of germline IgH probes in real-time quantitative PCR for the detection of minimal residual disease in acute lymphoblastic leukemia. *Leukemia* 2000; **14**: 1426–35.
31. Adriaansen HJ, Jacobs BC, Kappers-Klunne MC et al. Detection of residual disease in AML patients by use of double immunological marker analysis for terminal deoxynucleotidyl transferase and myeloid markers. *Leukemia* 1993; **7**: 472–81.

32. Wörman B, Griesinger F, Innig G. Detection of residual leukemic cells in patients with acute myeloid leukemia based on cell surface antigen expression. *Sangre (Barc)* 1992; **37**: 133–5.

33. Lo CF, Diverio D, Pandolfi PP et al. Molecular evaluation of residual disease as a predictor of relapse in acute promyelocytic leukaemia. *Lancet* 1992; **340**: 1437–8.

34. Miyamoto T, Nagafuji K, Akashi K et al. Persistence of multipotent progenitors expressing *AML1/ETO* transcripts in long-term remission patients with t(8;21) acute myelogenous leukemia. *Blood* 1996; **87**: 4789–96.

35. Tobal K, Johnson PR, Saunders MJ et al. Detection of *CBFB/MYH11* transcripts in patients with inversion and other abnormalities of chromosome 16 at presentation and remission. *Br J Haematol* 1995; **91**: 104–8.

36. Muller E, Sauter C. Routine bone marrow punctures during remission of acute myelogenous leukemia. *Leukemia* 1992; **6**: 419.

37. Zhao L, Chang KS, Estey EH et al. Detection of residual leukemic cells in patients with acute promyelocytic leukemia by the fluorescence in situ hybridization method: potential for predicting relapse. *Blood* 1995; **85**: 495–9.

38. Varella-Garcia M, Hogan CJ, Odom LF et al. Minimal residual disease (MRD) in remission t(8;21) AML and in vivo differentiation detected by FISH and CD34+ cell sorting. *Leukemia* 2001; **15**: 1408–14.

39. Vidriales MB, Orfao A, Lopez-Berges MC et al. DNA aneuploidy in acute myeloblastic leukemia is associated with a high expression of lymphoid markers. *Cytometry* 1995; **22**: 22–5.

40. San Miguel JF, Martinez A, Macedo A et al. Immunophenotyping investigation of minimal residual disease is a useful approach for predicting relapse in acute leukemia patients. *Blood* 1997; **90**: 2465–70.

41. Macedo A, Orfao A, Ciudad J et al. Phenotypic analysis of CD34 subpopulations in normal human bone marrow and its application for the detection of minimal residual disease. *Leukemia* 1995; **9**: 1896–901.

42. Coustan-Smith E, Behm FG, Hurwitz CA et al. N-CAM (CD56) expression by CD34+ malignant myeloblasts has implications for minimal residual disease detection in acute myeloid leukemia. *Leukemia* 1993; **7**: 853–8.

43. Reading CL, Estey EH, Huh YO et al. Expression of unusual immunophenotype combinations in acute myelogenous leukemia. *Blood* 1993; **81**: 3083–90.

44. Drach J, Drach D, Glassl H et al. Flow cytometric determination of atypical antigen expression in acute leukemia for the study of minimal residual disease. *Cytometry* 1992; **13**: 893–901.

45. Thomas X, Campos L, Archimbaud E et al. Surface marker expression in acute myeloid leukaemia at first relapse. *Br J Haematol* 1992; **81**: 40–4.

46. Macedo A, San Miguel JF, Vidriales MB et al. Phenotypic changes in acute myeloid leukaemia: implications in the detection of minimal residual disease. *J Clin Pathol* 1996; **49**: 15–18.

47. Olweus J, Lund-Johansen F, Terstappen LW. CD64/Fc γRI is a granulo-monocytic lineage marker on CD34+ hematopoietic progenitor cells. *Blood* 1995; **85**: 2402–13.

48. Lahuerta JJ, Montalban MA, de la Serna J et al. Minimal residual disease by flow cytometry immediatelly before autologous stem cell transplantation in acute myeloid leukemia: a critical factor in outcome? Blood 1999; **94**(Suppl 1): 979–87.

49. Thiede C, Bornhauser M, Oelschlagel U et al. Sequential monitoring of chimerism and detection of minimal residual disease after allogeneic blood stem cell transplantation (BSCT) using multiplex PCR amplification of short tandem repeat-markers. *Leukemia* 2001; **15**: 293–302.

50. Sanchez-Garcia I, San Miguel JF, Gonzalez-Sarmiento R. Immunoglobulin lambda chain gene rearrangement in a case of acute nonlymphoblastic leukemia. *Leukemia* 1999; **13**: 485–7.

51. Grimwade D. The pathogenesis of acute promyelocytic leukaemia: evaluation of the role of molecular diagnosis and monitoring in the management of the disease. *Br J Haematol* 1999; **106**: 591–613.

52. Slack JL, Willman CL, Andersen JW et al. Molecular analysis and clinical outcome of adult APL patients with the type V PML–RARα isoform: results from Intergroup Protocol 0129. *Blood* 2000; **95**: 398–403.

53. Gonzalez M, Barragan E, Bolufer P et al. Pretreatment characteristics and clinical outcome of acute promyelocytic leukaemia patients according to the PML–RARα isoforms: a study of the PETHEMA group. *Br J Haematol* 2001; **114**: 99–103.

54. Diverio D, Rossi V, Avvisati G et al. Early detection of relapse by prospective reverse transcriptase- polymerase chain reaction analysis of the *PML/RARα* fusion gene in patients with acute promyelocytic leukemia enrolled in the GIMEMA–AIEOP multicenter 'AIDA' trial. GIMEMA–AIEOP multicenter 'AIDA' Trial. *Blood* 1998; **92**: 784–9.

55. Lo CF, Diverio D, Falini B et al. Genetic diagnosis and molecular monitoring in the management of acute promyelocytic leukemia. *Blood* 1999; **94**: 12–22.

56. Burnett AK, Grimwade D, Solomon E et al. Presenting white blood cell count and kinetics of molecular remission predict prognosis in acute promyelocytic leukemia treated with all-*trans* retinoic acid: result of the randomized MRC trial. *Blood* 1999; **93**: 4131–43.

57. Lo CF, Diverio D, Avvisati G, Petti MC et al. Therapy of molecular relapse in acute promyelocytic leukemia. *Blood* 1999; **94**: 2225–9.

58. Grimwade D, Howe K, Langabeer S et al. Minimal residual disease detection in acute promyelocytic leukemia by reverse-transcriptase PCR: evaluation of PML–RARα and RARα–PML assessment in patients who ultimately relapse. *Leukemia* 1996; **10**: 61–6.

59. Tobal K, Saunders MJ, Grey MR, Yin JA. Persistence of RARα–PML fusion mRNA detected by reverse transcriptase polymerase chain reaction in patients in long-term remission of acute promyelocytic leukaemia. *Br J Haematol* 1995; **90**: 615–18.

60. Nucifora G, Rowley JD. *AML1* and the 8;21 and 3;21 translocations in acute and chronic myeloid leukemia. *Blood* 1995; **86**: 1–14.

61. Porwit-MacDonald A, Janossy G, Ivory K et al. Leukemia-associated changes identified by quantitative flow cytometry. IV. CD34 overexpression in acute myelogenous leukemia M2 with t(8;21). *Blood* 1996; **87**: 1162–9.

62. Guerrasio A, Russo C, Martinelli G et al. Polyclonal haemopoieses associated with long-term persistence of the *AML1-ETO* transcript in patients with FAB M2 acute myeloid leukaemia in continous clinical remission. *Br J Haematol* 1995; **90**: 364–8.

63. Miyamoto T, Weissman IL, Akashi K. *AML1/ETO*-expressing nonleukemic stem cells in acute myelogenous

leukemia with 8;21 chromosomal translocation. *Proc Natl Acad Sci USA* 2000; **97**: 7521–6.

64. Morschhauser F, Cayuela JM, Martini S et al. Evaluation of minimal residual disease using reverse-transcription polymerase chain reaction in t(8;21) acute myeloid leukemia: a multicenter study of 51 patients. *J Clin Oncol* 2000; **18**: 788–94.

65. Miyamoto T, Nagafuji K, Harada M et al. Quantitative analysis of *AML1/ETO* transcripts in peripheral blood stem cell harvests from patients with t(8;21) acute myelogenous leukaemia. *Br J Haematol* 1995; **91**: 132–8.

66. Tobal K, Newton J, Macheta M et al. Molecular quantitation of minimal residual disease in acute myeloid leukemia with t(8;21) can identify patients in durable remission and predict clinical relapse. *Blood* 2000; **95**: 815–19.

67. Liu PP, Hajra A, Wijmenga C, Collins FS. Molecular pathogenesis of the chromosome 16 inversion in the M4Eo subtype of acute myeloid leukemia. *Blood* 1995; **85**: 2289–302.

68. Costello R, Sainty D, Blaise D et al. Prognosis value of residual disease monitoring by polymerase chain reaction in patients with *CBFβ/MYH11*-positive acute myeloblastic leukemia. *Blood* 1997; **89**: 2222–3.

69. Marcucci G, Caligiuri MA, Dohner H et al. Quantification of *CBFβ/MYH11* fusion transcript by real time RT–PCR in patients with INV(16) acute myeloid leukemia. *Leukemia* 2001; **15**: 1072–80.

70. Rubnitz JE, Behm FG, Downing JR. 11q23 rearrangements in acute leukemia. *Leukemia* 1996; **10**: 74–82.

71. Nakano H, Shimamoto Y, Suga K, Kobayashi M. Detection of minimal residual disease in a patient with acute myeloid leukemia and t(6;9) at the time of peripheral blood stem cell transplantation. *Acta Haematol* 1995; **94**: 139–41.

72. Yokota S, Kiyoi H, Nakao M et al. Internal tandem duplication of the *FLT3* gene is preferentially seen in acute myeloid leukemia and myelodysplastic syndrome among various hematological malignancies. A study on a large series of patients and cell lines. *Leukemia* 1997; **11**: 1605–9.

73. Kottaridis PD, Gale RE, Frew ME et al. The presence of a *FLT3* internal tandem duplication in patients with acute myeloid leukemia (AML) adds important prognostic information to cytogenetic risk group and response to the first cycle of chemotherapy: analysis of 854 patients from the United Kingdom Medical Research Council AML 10 and 12 trials. *Blood* 2001; **98**: 1752–9.

74. Stirewalt DL, Willman CL, Radich JP. Quantitative, real-time polymerase chain reactions for *FLT3* internal tandem duplications are highly sensitive and specific. *Leuk Res* 2001; **25**: 1085–8.

75. Inoue K, Ogawa H, Yamagami T et al. Long-term follow-up of minimal residual disease in leukemia patients by monitoring *WT1* (Wilms tumor gene) expression levels. *Blood* 1996; **88**: 2267–8.

76. Garg M, Moore H, Tobal K, Liu Yin JA. Predictive and prognosis significance of quantitative analysis of *WT1* gene transcripts by competitve RT–PCR in acute leukemia. *Br J Haematol* 2001; **113**(Suppl 1): 28.

77. Gaiger A, Schmid D, Heinze G et al. Detection of the *WT1* transcript by RT–PCR in complete remission has no prognostic relevance in de novo acute myeloid leukemia. *Leukemia* 1998; **12**: 1886–94.

78. Kreuzer KA, Saborowski A, Lupberger J et al. Fluorescent 5'-exonuclease assay for the absolute quantification of Wilms' tumour gene (*WT1*) mRNA: implications for monitoring human leukaemias. *Br J Haematol* 2001; **114**: 313–18.

79. San Miguel JF, Sanz GF, Vallespi T et al. Myelodysplastic syndromes. *Crit Rev Oncol Hematol* 1996; **23**: 57–93.

80. Nylund SJ, Ruutu T, Saarinen U, Knuutila S. Metaphase fluorescence in situ hybridization (FISH) in the follow-up of 60 patients with haemopoietic malignancies. *Br J Haematol* 1994; **88**: 778–83.

81. Flactif M, Lai JL, Preudhomme C, Fenaux P. Fluorescence in situ hybridization improves the detection of monosomy 7 in myelodysplastic syndromes. *Leukemia* 1994; **8**: 1012–18.

82. Oertel J, Huhn D. CD34 immunophenotyping of blasts in myelodysplasia. *Leuk Lymphoma* 1994; **15**: 65–9.

83. Stetler-Stevenson M, Arthur DC, Jabbour N et al. Diagnostic utility of flow cytometric immunophenotyping in myelodysplastic syndrome. *Blood* 2001; **98**: 979–87.

84. Woodlock TJ, Seshi B, Sham RL et al. Use of cell surface antigen phenotype in guiding therapeutic decisions in chronic myelomonocytic leukemia. *Leuk Res* 1994; **18**: 173–81.

85. Kuiper-Kramer PA, Huisman CM, Molen-Sinke J et al. The expression of transferrin receptors on erythroblasts in anaemia of chronic disease, myelodysplastic syndromes and iron deficiency. *Acta Haematol* 1997; **97**: 127–31.

86. Kanter-Lewensohn L, Hellstrom-Lindberg E, Kock Y et al. Analysis of CD34-positive cells in bone marrow from patients with myelodysplastic syndromes and acute myeloid leukemia and in normal individuals: a comparison between FACS analysis and immunohistochemistry. *Eur J Haematol* 1996; **56**: 124–9.

87. Bowen KL, Davis BH. Abnormal patterns of expression of CD16 (FcR-III) and CD11b (CRIII) antigens by developing neutrophils in the bone marrow of patients with myelodisplastic syndrome. *Lab Hematol* 1997; **3**: 292–8.

88. del Canizo C, Fernandez ME, Lopez A et al. Immunophenotypic analysis of myelodysplastic syndromes. Its prognostic significance. *Blood* 2002 (in press).

89. Amiel A, Yarkoni S, Slavin S et al. Detection of minimal residual disease state in chronic myelogenous leukemia patients using fluorescence in situ hybridization. *Cancer Genet Cytogenet* 1994; **76**: 59–64.

90. el Rifai W, Ruutu T, Vettenranta K et al. Minimal residual disease after allogeneic bone marrow transplantation for chronic myeloid leukaemia: a metaphase-FISH study. *Br J Haematol* 1996; **92**: 365–9.

91. Cox-Froncillo MC, Cantonetti M, Masi M et al. Cytogenetic analysis is non-informative for assessing the remission rate in chronic myeloid leukemia (CML) patients on interferon-α (IFN-α) therapy. *Cancer Genet Cytogenet* 1995; **84**: 15–18.

92. Deininger MW, Goldman JM, Melo JV. The molecular biology of chronic myeloid leukemia. *Blood* 2000; **96**: 3343–56.

93. Lion T. Monitoring of residual disease in chronic myelogenous leukemia: methodological approaches and clinical aspects. *Leukemia* 1996; **10**: 896–900.

94. Pichert G, Roy DC, Gonin R et al. Distinct patterns of minimal residual disease associated with graft-versus-host disease after allogeneic bone marrow transplantation for chronic myelogenous leukemia. *J Clin Oncol* 1995; **13**: 1704–13.

95. Radich JP, Gehly G, Gooley T et al. Polymerase chain reaction detection of the *BCR–ABL* fusion transcript after allogeneic marrow transplantation for chronic myeloid leukemia: results and implications in 346 patients. *Blood* 1995; **85**: 2632–8.

96. Bilhou-Nabera C, Marit G, Gharbi MJ et al. Chronic myelocytic leukemia patients achieving complete cytogenetic conversion under interferon alpha therapy: minimal residual disease follow-up. *Leukemia* 1995; **9**: 2067–70.

97. Olavarria E, Kanfer E, Szydlo R et al. Early detection of *BCR–ABL* transcripts by quantitative reverse transcriptase–polymerase chain reaction predicts outcome after allogeneic stem cell transplantation for chronic myeloid leukemia. *Blood* 2001; **97**: 1560–5.

98. Radich JP, Gooley T, Bryant E et al. The significance of bcr-abl molecular detection in chronic myeloid leukemia patients 'late', 18 months or more after transplantation. *Blood* 2001; **98**: 1701–7.

# 23 Drug resistance and its modification in hematological malignancies

**Jean-Pierre Marie**

## Introduction

Hematological neoplasms are usually primarily sensitive to chemotherapy, but the relapse rate is still high, except for Hodgkin lymphoma and childhood acute lymphoblastic leukemia (ALL). Drug resistance is therefore a major cause of chemotherapeutic failure and patient death in hemato-oncology.

A mathematical model for the development of drug resistance in tumors was proposed in 1979 by Goldie and Coldman.[1] This model was based on the postulate that cancer cells have a high spontaneous mutation rate, leading, over time, to the emergence of cells resistant to chemotherapeutic drugs. In accordance with this hypothesis, it was suggested that a reduction in the rate of emergence of resistant cells could be achieved by simultaneous administration of multiple drugs with different targets. However, despite combination chemotherapies, treatment failures were observed in lymphoid and myeloid malignancies, and relapses occurred in more than half of the cases in acute myeloid leukemia (AML) and adult ALL.

It is therefore clear that a better understanding of the mechanisms involved in drug resistance is still warranted for the development of new therapeutic strategies.

## Measurement of drug resistance in clinical samples

In vitro assays have been developed to test the drug resistance of clinical samples (mainly acute leukemia).[2] Clonogenic assays offer the advantage of testing the drug sensitivity of progenitor cells, and have been successfully correlated with clinical outcome in AML: resistance to both anthracyclines and cytarabine (cytosine arabinoside, Ara-C) was highly correlated with clinical failure in adult AML, and was one of the best predictive variables in a multivariate analysis.[3] Unfortunately, these clonogenic assays are time-consuming and cannot be automated. For these reasons, other viability tests have been developed. The most commonly used assay is the MTT assay, which relies on the ability of the mitochondria of living cells to convert a soluble tetrazolium salt (MTT) into an insoluble formazan. The formazan precipitate is purple, it can be dissolved, and its extinction can be read on a 96-well plaque reader. The extinction is linearly correlated with the number of viable cells in suspension. The 4-day MTT assay is an efficient tool for large-scale drug-resistance testing, and results have shown good correlation with prognosis in childhood ALL.[4]

## Classification of drug resistance (Table 23.1)

The efficacy of cytostatic antineoplastic therapy is determined by a sequential cascade of events, including drug delivery, drug–target interaction, and the induction of cellular damage. The first part of this cascade corresponds to the 'pharmacological' resistance, and up to now has been the most widely studied mechanism of resistance.

Classically, resistance is divided into extrinsic and intrinsic causes.

### Extrinsic resistance

This corresponds to an inability of the drug to reach the tumor cell. This is the case when the bioavailability of the oral form varies greatly from patient to patient, as with 6-mercaptopurine in ALL.[5] Defects in tumor vascularization, frequently observed in solid tumors, are also probably relevant for hematological malignancies.[6]

## Table 23.1  Drug-resistance classification

| Proximal | Distal |
|---|---|
| Low uptake (nucleoside receptors for cytarabine) | No DNA synthesis (low S phase) |
| Efflux: ABC proteins (P-gp, MRPs, BCRP, . . .) | Target mutations (topoisomerases) |
| Cellular traffic (LRP) | Increased DNA repair (increased DNA-PK) |
| Chelation (GSTs) Activation/catabolism (cytarabine/ deoxycytidine enzymes) | Delay to chemo/ radiotherapy-induced apoptosis (*bcl-2* family, *p53* mutations, Cdk inhibitors) |

### Intrinsic resistance

This is directly due to the properties of the tumor cell. This phenomenon can be observed in vitro, and can be classified as *simple resistance*, when the cells are resistant to only one drug, or as *multidrug resistance* (MDR), when a cross resistance is observed for chemostatic drugs with different biochemical targets. This latter type of resistance is mainly observed in patients, and can be due to several mechanisms. The underlying pharmacological mechanism corresponds mainly to active efflux of drugs out of the tumor cells. Molecular profiles giving rise to broader forms of resistance are now under investigation, and it is believed that a defect in drug-induced apoptosis is at least partly responsible.

### Proximal and distal resistance

Another approach is to consider the resistance mechanisms as *proximal resistance*, when the events occur before the drug reaches the target (decreased influx,

increased efflux or catabolism, reduced synthesis of active form, and compartmentalization), and *distal resistance*, when the mechanisms are not linked to the intracellular pharmacokinetics: decreased cell division, increased DNA repair, and increased anti-apoptosis proteins (or decreased pro-apoptosis proteins) (Figure 23.1).

## Proximal (pharmacological) drug resistance

### ABC proteins

MDR cells are resistant to several naturally occurring plant or microbial products, but are not resistant to synthetic compounds such as cisplatin, or to nucleotide analog such as cytarabine (Table 23.2). The resistant tumor cells maintain lower intracellular drug concentrations than their sensitive counterparts,[7] and in the large majority of cases express transport proteins that are responsible for active efflux of the drugs.

The first – and probably most important – protein described in cellular models of MDR is P-glycoprotein (P-gp), encoded by the *ABCB1* (*MDR1*) gene. This transmembrane protein belongs to a superfamily of ABC (ATP-binding cassette) proteins, specialized for energy-dependent cellular transport.[8] The genes coding for these proteins are highly conserved between species, from bacteria to humans. Besides P-gp other members of the ABCC family (MRP1–6, multidrug resistance-associated proteins), with low homology with P-gp, have been described (for a review, see reference 9).

A small ABC protein, ABCG2 (or BCRP), was described simultaneously by three different groups. It was described as a 'specific' ABC protein of the placenta (ABCP), as a new ABC protein expressed in a *MDR1⁻ MRP1⁻* breast cell line resistant to anthracy-

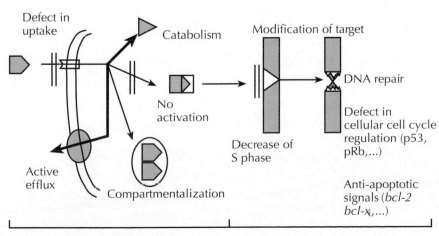

'Pharmalogical' or 'proximal' resistance mechanisms    'Distal' resistance mechanisms

**Figure 23.1** Drug-resistance mechanisms.

## Table 23.2  Drugs and P-glycoprotein (P-gp)

| Expelled by P-gp | Not expelled by P-gp |
|---|---|
| Anthracyclines | Alkylating agents: |
|    Daunorubicin |    Chlorambucil |
|    Doxorubicin |    Cyclophosphamide |
|    THP-Adriamycin | |
|    Idarubicin | |
| Mitoxantrone | |
| Amsacrine | |
| Vinca alkaloids: | Purine and pyrimidine |
| | analogs: |
|    Vinblastine |    6-Mercaptopurine |
|    Vincristine |    6-Thioguanine |
|    Vinorelbine |    Cytarabine |
| Taxanes | |
| Epipodophyllotoxins: | Bleomycin |
|    Etoposide | Carmustine, lomustine |
|    Teniposide) | Glucocorticoids |
| Dactinomycin | |
| Mitomycin C | |
| Topotecan | |
| Homoharringtonine | |

cline (BCRP), and in a colon carcinoma cell line resistant to mitoxantrone (MXR1).[8]

The expression of these genes is believed to confer resistance – the evidence for this being that the transfection of their cDNA in sensitive cell lines gives rise to the MDR phenotype (Table 23.3).[10–12]

P-gp, the MRPs, and BCRP are not unique to drug-resistant cells, and are expressed by tissues with excretory–secretory functions. In hematopoietic cells, progenitor cells express P-gp and BCRP, but not MRP. These localizations suggest that these proteins are involved in the protection of organisms (and cells of vital importance) against natural xenobiotics.[13]

A few years ago, several workshops[14,15] proposed a consensus on technical recommendations for measuring P-gp. Protein detection and, more importantly, functional test by flow cytometry are recommended for leukemic samples. Several monoclonal antibodies,

recognizing an external epitope, are available for protein expression, and several fluorescent probes can be used, with and without specific inhibitors, for measuring the drug efflux.

## ABC proteins in hematological malignancies

The MDR phenotype conferred by expression of the *MDR1* gene can be 'disease-related', as in AML and probably in adult T-cell leukemia/lymphoma (ATLL), or 'treatment-related', as in ALL, non-Hodgkin lymphoma (NHL), and multiple myeloma (MM).

### Acute myetoid leukemia

Several studies have reported a high frequency of *MDR1* gene expression in AML. Large multicentric studies (for a review, see 16) showed between one-third and one-half of 'positive' cases at diagnosis, whatever the technique used, and usually a higher proportion of positive cases were described in elderly patients.[17] The MDR phenotype is associated with markers of bad prognosis, such as CD34 and CD7.

Except for the promyelocytic subtype (FAB M3), which is devoid of P-gp expression,[18] all the other AML subtypes are able to express the MDR phenotype. In the majority of cases, the functional tests (dye efflux) were correlated with P-gp expression, except in CD34- cells, like myelomonocytic and monoblastic leukemias. For that reason, dye efflux appears to be more informative than quantification of P-gp itself in AML.

The MDR phenotype is also frequent in the myelodysplastic syndromes (MPS)[19] and the blast crisis of chronic myeloid leukemia (CML) – both of which are known to be diseases with particularly bad prognosis.

The correlation between *MDR1* gene expression and treatment outcome is well documented in AML (for a review, see reference 16): many studies have reported a relationship between either the absence of remission (refractory disease and death during aplasia) and the overexpression of P-gp, or the overexpression of P-gp and refractory disease.

More discordant results have been published concerning the incidence of MRP expression in AML:[20] the range of MRP expression is narrow compared with

## Table 23.3  Resistance spectrum of *MDR1*, *MRP*, and *LRP* genes

| | Anthracyclines | Vincristine | Paclitaxel | Melphalan | Cisplatin |
|---|---|---|---|---|---|
| *MDR1* | ++ | ++ | ++ | – | – |
| *MRP* | ++ | ++ | – | – | – |
| *LRP* | ++ | ++ | ? | + | + |

++/+, confers resistance; –, does not confer resistance; ?, not described.

that of P-gp, and a basal expression is found in all cases. One-third of patients present with high expression. The prognostic value of MRP itself has not yet been clearly determined, but a functional test measuring efflux due to P-gp and MRP1 (using calcein AM and modulators) has clearly shown that both P-gp and MRP1 functions are of prognostic importance in adult AML.[21] The roles of other MRPs are still under investigation.[22]

Discordant results have been published concerning the incidence of expression and the prognostic value of BCRP in leukemia. The frequency of expression ranges from 5%[23] to 30%[24,25] in adult AML, and, so far, no large series have been published concerning functional assay and prognostic value of this protein in adult acute leukemia. In pediatric AML, BCRP has been linked to a worse prognosis.[26]

### Acute lymphoblastic leukemia

Except for a few studies, the incidence of *MDR1* overexpression in untreated patients with ALL has generally been found to be low (<10%) at diagnosis and even at relapse, except during the latest stage of the disease, when clinical drug resistance is usually observed (for a review, see reference 16).

The MDR phenotype in ALL is found only in ALL subgroups with a bad prognosis: adult ALL (often Philadelphia chromosome-positive) and a subtype of CD7'CD4-CD8 ALL, which is thought to originate from a hematopoietic stem cell.

P-gp expression was not found to be predictive for induction treatment failure in childhood ALL. This could be explained by the predominant role of corticosteroids – which are not expelled by P-gp – as the major drugs in ALL. In adult ALL, a recent study showed that protein expression, but not function (?), predicted the achievement of complete remission in patients treated according to the GIMEMA ALL0496 protocol.[27]

Few publications have concerned MRP in ALL,[20] but all have shown a measurable level of MRP at diagnosis – comparatively higher than in AML cells – and some cases showed an increase after treatment. The prognostic value of MRP expression is at present not clearly demonstrated.

Until now, only one publication has described a low incidence of BCRP expression in pediatric ALL, with no prognostic significance.[28]

### Multiple myeloma

The limited bone marrow infiltration by plasma cells (15–60%) in MM argues for the use of immunocytochemistry as the method of choice for determining the MDR phenotype in this disease. An alternative technique is double labeling with anti-CD56 or anti-CD38 antibodies, together with another antibody against P-gp. A low incidence of P-gp in malignant plasma cells has been observed at diagnosis.[29] This incidence increased during progression, depending on the dose of anthracyclines and vinca alkaloids received, and reached 85% in patients refractory to VAD (vincristine, doxorubicin, and dexamethasone). This positivity is a factor of clinical resistance to VAD,[30] and even to melphalan. MRP expression is detectable in the majority of myeloma cells, but does not increase dramatically after treatment – the significance of this expression is not known.

### Chronic lymphocytic leukemia

In chronic lymphocytic leukaemia (CLL), several authors have described a large majority of patients expressing P-gp, either before or after chemotherapy (for a review, see reference 19). Semiquantitative studies have shown that expression is moderate, and does not change after chemotherapy. The MDR phenotype is also detected in normal B lymphocytes, and therefore is probably constitutive in CLL, but expressed at a low level, and seems not to be implicated in clinical drug resistance.[31]

CLL cells express variable levels of MRP at diagnosis and after treatment, but the amount of MRP does not influence the course of the disease.[31]

### Non-Hodgkin lymphoma

The majority of the cases published in the literature have been from retrospective studies, using immunohistochemical detection of P-gp on frozen lymph node sections (for a review, see reference 32).

In no report could any difference be observed between high- and low-grade lymphoma, or between B and T subtypes, except for adult T-cell leukemia/lymphoma (ATLL), which frequently expressed the MDR phenotype at presentation.

Several studies have addressed the question of the clinical significance of the MDR phenotype in NHL (for reviews, see references 16 and 32). In short series, the absence of P-gp was associated with a better response, but in the larger series of high-risk lymphoma, no correlation with treatment result was noted.

The *MRP* gene is expressed at a low level in all cases of lymphoma (low- or high-grade), and the level does not differ before and after chemotherapy, except in a very few patients.[33]

### Lung resistance protein/major vault protein

An additional protein has been described in a wide variety of P-gp-negative MDR cancer cell lines and in clinical samples. This protein is a non-ABC, MDR-associated protein originally termed lung resistance-related protein (LRP), and now idenified as the major vault protein (MVP) (for a review, see reference 34). Vaults are highly conserved among species, supporting the notion that their function is essential to eukaryotic cells. It was hypothesized that vaults mediate the bidirectional transport of a variety of substrates between the nucleus and the cytoplasm. So far, the cDNA of LRP/MVP has been unable to confer the MDR phenotype; therefore, a proof of the involvement of LRP/MVP in the MDR phenotype has not been demonstrated.

In the majority of cases of AML, LRP/MVP expression is low,[35] but detectable by RT–PCR.

The clinical significance of LRP expression is still controversial,[35,36] and functional tests specific for LRP need to be developed.

## Pharmacological resistance to cytarabine

Cytarabine plays a key role in the achievement and consolidation of complete remission in AML, and is also widely used at high dose as rescue treatment in refractory ALL and AML. This nucleotide analog is not expelled by ABC proteins, and is of particular interest in patients expressing P-gp or MRP. In vitro resistance to cytarabine has been given as a main parameter for predicting treatment failure[37,38] or relapse[39] after conventional doses of cytarabine and anthracyclines in AML.

After transport into the cell, cytarabine must be phosphorylated to its active triphosphate form (arabinosylcytosine triphosphate, Ara-CTP) by a series of kinase enzymes (Figure 23.2). The ability of fresh human leukemic cells to retain the cellular concentration of Ara-CTP has been correlated with the duration of remission in patients treated with cytarabine and

anthracyclines.[40] Although Ara-CTP is an inhibitor of DNA polymerase α, it is also a substrate, and is in competition with deoxycytidine triphosphate (dCTP, the natural compound) for DNA incorporation. It is thought that the incorporation of Ara-CTP into DNA is responsible for the lethal effect of this drug. Factors that reduce the intracellular concentration of Ara-CTP may induce chemoresistance in AML patients. These factors include reduced influx of cytarabine by the hENT1 transporter, reduced phosphorylation by deoxycytidine kinase (dCK), and increased degradation by high-$K_m$ cytoplasmic 5′-nucleotidase (5NT) and/or cytidine deaminase (CDD). It has been suggested that expression of DNA Pol, 5NT, and hENT1 at diagnosis may be resistance mechanisms to cytarabine in AML patients.[41–43]

# Distal drug resistance

Alkylation of DNA, and more specifically the formation of DNA interstrand crosslinks, has been considered to be responsible for the cytotoxicity of alkylating agents. Resistance to these agents has been reported to be secondary to (i) alterations in the kinetics of the DNA crosslinks formed by these agents, (ii) overexpression of metallothionein, (iii) changes in apoptosis, and (iv) altered DNA repair activity (for a review, see reference 44).

## p53 and proteins regulating the cell cycle

The ultimate success of genotoxic anticancer agents is determined by the ability of malignant cells to initiate an apoptotic response to induced DNA damage.[45] Among the numerous factors known to modulate can-

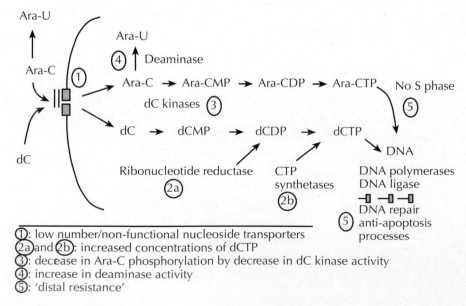

**Figure 23.2** Resistance to cytarabine (cytosine arabinoside; i.e. arabinosylcytosine, Ara-C). Ara-CM/D/TP, arabinosylcytosine mono/di/triphosphate; dC, deoxycytidine; dCM/D/TP, deoxycytidine mono/di/triphosphate.

cer-related apoptosis, p53 and the Bcl-2 family are the most extensively characterized proteins. p53 is activated in response to DNA damage (Figure 23.3), and stops the cell in $G_1$ phase (via p21), permitting DNA repair, whereas apoptosis can be considered to be a failsafe mechanism to rid the organism of cells with severely damaged DNA. In cases of non-functional p53, the threshold of DNA damage leading to apoptosis increases, and this could contribute to drug resistance.[46] In hematological malignancies, p53 is usually functional at diagnosis, but mutations have been described during progression of the disease in both lymphoid and myeloid leukemias as well as in lymphomas,[47] and this progression corresponds mainly to highly resistant tumors.

Genetic alterations affecting the p16[INK4A] and cyclin D1 (Figure 23.3) proteins, which govern phosphorylation of the retinoblastoma protein (pRb) and control exit from $G_1$ phase of the cell cycle,[48] are frequent in cancer, including ALL and mantle cell lymphoma, and are associated with an aggressive course of the disease. The first evidence of in vitro correlation between pRb pathway alterations and drug sensitivity has been described (for a review, see reference 49), opening a new field of investigation for a better understanding of drug resistance.

In chronic lymphocytic leukemia (CLL), a high cell content of p27, a universal cyclin–cyclin-dependent kinase (cdk) inhibitor, is correlated with poor survival but increased survival in the presence of drugs such as fludarabine.[50]

## Anti-apoptosis proteins and signals

Analysis of the t(14;18) translocation in follicular lymphoma has permitted the description of the *bcl-2* (B-cell lymphoma 2) oncogene. The anti-apoptotic properties of Bcl-2 and Bcl-$x_L$, another member of the same family, are now well documented, and their overexpression has been shown to protect tumor cell lines from the toxicity of several chemotherapeutic agents (for a review, see reference 51). The clinical impact of Bcl-2/Bcl-$x_L$ overexpression on drug resistance has not been demonstrated, but correlations have been described between high Bcl-2 cell content and clinical drug resistance in NHL[52] and AML,[53] but not in ALL.[54] On the other hand, Bax expression correlates with drug sensitivity to doxorubicin, cyclophosphamide, and chlorambucil in CLL,[55] and relapse in childhood ALL is associated with a decrease of the Bax/Bcl-2 ratio.[56]

The chimeric protein BCR–ABL, specific to chronic myeloid leukemia (CML) and frequent in adult ALL, has been shown to confer resistance to genotoxic agent-induced apoptosis (by cytarabine, daunorubicin, etoposide, etc.) in vitro, via prolongation of cell cycle arrest at the $G_2$/M restriction point, without altering either the p53 pathway or DNA repair.[57] Imatinib (STI571, Gleevec/Glivec), a specific anti-tyrosine kinase drug, is a very potent inhibitor of BCR–ABL effects, but resistance to this drug has been described in patients, as a result of amplification or mutations in the chimeric BCR–ABL protein (for a review, see reference 58).

Signals from the microenvironment could be strong stimulators for tumor cell survival and resistance to chemotherapy. In AML, the role of bone marrow endothelial cells has begun to be explored, and has revealed paracrine loops, involving vascular endothelial growth factor (VEGF) and its receptors.[59]

In CLL, tumor cells express and are receptive to BlyS/BAFF, a signal of survival for normal B lymphocytes. An autocrine loop responsible for tumor cell survival has been described.[60]

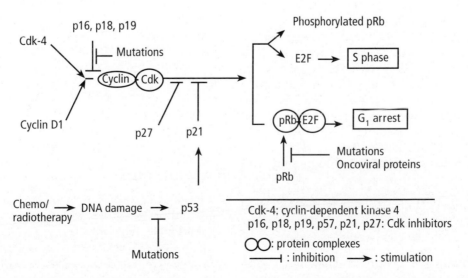

**Figure 23.3** Cell cycle control.

# Reversal of the MDR phenotype

## P-gp inhibition

Numerous compounds have been identified that inhibit the efflux activity of P-gp and reverse cellular resistance in experimental systems (for a review, see reference 61). This has led to the strategy of concomitant administration of chemotherapy and an 'MDR modulator' to reverse clinical drug resistance. These compounds act mainly as competitive or non-competitive inhibitors, by binding to similar drug substrate-binding sites, or to other P-gp sites that cause allosteric changes of the molecule, resulting in a decrease in cytotoxic drug binding.

The most widely used modulators in randomized phases III in leukemia are quinine and cyclosporins (cyclosporin A (cyclosporine, CsA) and PSC833, an analog of cyclosporin D). More recently, other compounds, specially designed and developed for modulation of drug resistance, have entered phase I trials, namely VX710, LY335979, and XR9576.

The first large randomized study of an MDR modulator in hemato-oncology tested the usefulness of the addition of quinine to a combination of mitoxantrone and high-dose cytarabine in 315 bad-prognosis adult leukemia cases (relapsing/refractory/secondary).[62] Global results showed no difference between the groups with or without quinine, but it was noted that (i) clinical drug resistance was higher in the control group and (ii) the toxic death rate was higher in the quinine group. The clinical toxicity of quinine could have masked the clinical benefit of MDR reversal.

The same kind of results were observed with PSC833 (10-fold more potent than CsA and without any renal or immunosuppressive toxicity) in elderly untreated patients:[63] the Cancer and Leukemia Group B (CALGB) phase III trial consisted of standard doses of cytarabine, with daunorubicin 60 mg/m² (40 with PSC833) and etoposide 100 mg/m² (60 with PSC833) daily for 3 days without (ADE) or with (ADEP) PSC833 (10 mg/kg/day by 3-day infusion). The ADEP arm was closed after randomization of 120 patients because of excessive early mortality. Nevertheless, disease-free survival (median 7 months verses 8 months; $p = 0.38$) and overall survival (approximately 33% alive at 1 year) did not differ and were similar to historical results. For patients with PSC833-modulated efflux, the median disease-free survival was 5 months with ADE and 14 months with ADEP ($p = 0.07$).

Several other phase III clinical trials in relapsed myeloid leukemia and multiple myeloma with PSC833 have now been completed, with globally negative results.[64]

On the other hand, the Southwest Oncology Group (SWOG) conducted a randomized phase III study on 226 patients, randomly assigned to sequential treatment with cytarabine 3 g/m² daily for 5 days, followed by daunorubicin 45 mg/m²/day (continuous infusion) on days 6–8, with or without intravenous CsA (16 mg/kg/day).[65] Addition of CsA significantly reduced the frequency of resistance and increased the relapse-free and overall survival. The effect of CsA on survival was greatest in patients with P-gp⁺ leukemic cells. The same cooperative group performed another randomized trial with the same arms in blast crisis of CML, but in this disease CsA was unable to improve the complete response or survival rates.[66]

Other P-gp inhibitors are now in phase II trials – mainly in solid tumors. LY335979 is a quinoline derivative, specific to P-gp, and delivered orally, with a weak effect on pharmacokinetics of co-administered drugs.[67] Phase II is now completed in AML, and a phase III trial is now beginning in the USA. XR9576, an anthranilic acid derivative, delivered orally or intravenously, is now in a phase I/II trial.[68]

## Reversion of other ABC pumps

GG120918, a derivative of acridonecarboxamide, was developed as an inhibitor of P-gp, but has also been described as a potent inhibitor of BCRP.[69] VX-710 (Biricodar), a pipecolinate derivative, is a modulator of P-gp and MRP1. It has no effect on doxorubicin pharmacokinetics, although an increase in bilirubin was noted in a phase II trial.[70]

# Reversal of other kinds of resistance

## Resistance to cytarabine

High-dose (1–3 g/m²/12 h × 8–12) infusion (2–3 h) of cytarabine is a very potent treatment in secondary/relapsing/refractory AML and in ALL. Resistance to standard doses of cytarabine (100–200 mg/m²/day × 7 days) is usually overcome by increasing the dose, because of the competition between this nucleoside and natural deoxycytidine (dC): more cytarabine will enter the cell, more will be phosphorylated, and more will be incorporated into DNA. The cellular concentration of Ara-CTP in circulating leukemic cells during high-dose infusion of this drug is strongly correlated with clinical outcome,[71] confirming the importance of cytarabine uptake and of cytarabine phosphorylation.

It has also been proposed to prime leukemic myeloid progenitors with growth factors granulocyte and granulocyte–macrophage colony-stimulating factors (G-CSF and GM-CSF) before cytarabine treatment. After several large trials, the value of this approach is inconclusive (for a review, see reference 72).

## Inhibitors of farnesyl transferase

The membrane-associated G proteins encoded by the *ras* family of proto-oncogenes are potential target for new therapeutic agents. The Ras proteins are activated downstream of protein tyrosine kinases, and in turn trigger a cascade of phosphorylation events through sequential activation of Raf, MEK1, and ERK1 and 2. To be active, the Ras proteins have to be farnesyled. Therefore, several inhibitors of farnesyl transferase have recently been developed. A phase I trial in refractory/relapsing acute leukemia with R115777 (Janssen) demonstrated a significant inhibition of ERK phosphorylation in bone marrow after treatment, and clinical response occurred in 29% of the patients (including 2 complete responses in 34 evaluable patients).[73] In *BCR–ABL*[+] cells resistant to imatinib, another farnesyl transferase inhibitor, SCH66336 (Schering-Plough) was able to restore apoptosis usually induced by imatinib alone.[74]

## Restoring apoptosis: *bcl-2* antisense therapy

Restoration of drug-induced apoptosis could be obtained in vitro with *bcl-2* antisense oligonucleotides. A phase I study of *bcl-2* antisense therapy was performed in relapsed *bcl-2*[+] NHL, using 14 days of subcutaneous infusion of G3139, an 18-mer oligonucleotide complementary to the first codons of *bcl-2*.[75] A steady-state concentration of the antisense oligonucleotide was achieved without major toxicity, although few responses were observed. Another phase I trial was performed in refractory/relapsed acute leukemia, treated with 10 days of G3139 (continuous infusion) together with fludarabine, cytarabine, and G-CSF. A steady-state concentration of G3139 was achieved after 24 hours without major toxicity, and 6 of 20 patients achieved CR.[76] A randomized phase III trial is now running in untreated elderly patients with AML.

## REFERENCES

1. Goldie J, Coldman A. A mathematical model for relating the drug sensitivity of tumors to their spontaneous mutation rate. *Cancer Treat Res* 1979; **63**: 1727–31.

2. Veerman A, Pieters R. Drug sensitivity assays in leukemia and lymphoma. *Br J Haematol* 1990; **74**: 381–4.

3. Delmer A, Marie J, Thevenin D et al. Multivariate analysis of prognostic factors in acute myeloid leukemia: value of clonogenic leukemic cell properties. *J Clin Oncol* 1989; **7**: 738–46.

4. Pieters R, Huismans D, Loonen A et al. Relation of cellular drug resistance to long term clinical outcome in childhood acute lymphoblastic leukemia. *Lancet* 1991; **338**: 399–403.

5. Zimm S, Collins J, Riccarrdi R et al. Variable bioavailability of oral mercaptopurine: Is maintenance chemotherapy in acute lymphoblastic leukemia being optimally delivered? *N Engl J Med* 1983; **308**: 1005–9.

6. Padro T, Ruiz S, Bieker R et al. Increased angiogenesis in the bone marrow of patients with acute myeloid leukemia. *Blood* 2000; **95**: 2637–44.

7. Biedler J, Riehm H. Cellular resistance to actinomycin D in Chinese hamster in vitro: cross resistance, radioautographic and cytogenetic studies. *Cancer Res* 1970; **30**: 1174–80.

8. Klein I, Sarkadi B, Varadi A. An inventory of the human ABC proteins. *Biochim Biophys Acta* 1999, **1461**: 237–62.

9. Borst P, Evers R, Kool M et al. A family of drug transporters: the multidrug resistance-associated proteins. *J Natl Cancer Inst* 2000; **92**: 1295–302.

10. Gros P, Fallows D, Croop J, Housman D. Chromosome-mediated gene transfer of multidrug resistance. *Mol Cell Biol* 1986; **6**: 3785–90.

11. Grant C, Valdimarsson G, Hipfner D et al. Overexpression of multidrug resistance-associated protein (MRP) increases resistance to natural product drugs. *Cancer Res* 1994; **54**: 357–61.

12. Litman T, Brangi M, Hudson E et al. The multidrug-resistant phenotype associated with overexpression of the new ABC half-transporter, MXR (ABCG2). *J Cell Sci* 2000; **113**: 2011–21.

13. Litman T, Druley TE, Stein WD, Bates SE. From MDR to MXR: new understanding of multidrug resistance systems, their properties and clinical significance. *Cell Mol Life Sci* 2001; **58**: 931–59.

14. Beck W, Grogan T, Willman C et al. Methods to detect P-glycoprotein-associated multidrug resistance in patients' tumors: consensus recommendations. *Cancer Res* 1996; **56**: 3010–20.

15. Marie P, Huet S, Faussat A et al. Multicentric evaluation of the MDR phenotype in leukemia. *Leukemia* 1997; **11**: 1086–94.

16. Marie P, Zhou D, Gurbuxani S et al. MDR1/P-glycoprotein in haematological neoplasms. *Eur J Cancer* 1996; **32A**: 1034–8.

17. Leith CP, Kopecky KJ, Chen IM et al. Frequency and clinical significance of the expression of the multidrug resistance proteins MDR1/P-glycoprotein, MRP1, and LRP in acute myeloid leukemia: a Southwest Oncology Group study. *Blood* 1999; **94**: 1086–99.

18. Paietta E, Andersen J, Racevskis J et al. Significantly lower P-glycoprotein expression in acute promyelocytic leukemia than in other types of acute myeloid leukemia: immunological, molecular and functional analyses. *Leukemia* 1994; **8**: 968–73.

19. Sonneveld P, Van Dongen J, Hagemeijer A et al. High expression of multidrug resistance P-glycoprotein in high-risk myelodysplasia is associated with immature phenotype. *Leukemia* 1993; **7**: 963–9.

20. Broxterman H, Giaccone G, Lankelma J et al. Multidrug resistance proteins and other drug transport-related resistance to natural product agents. *Curr Opin Oncol* 1995; **7**: 532–40.

21. Legrand O, Simonin G, Beauchamp-Nicoud A et al. Simultaneous activity of MRP1 and Pgp is correlated with in vitro resistance to daunorubicin and with in vivo resistance in adult acute myeloid leukemia. *Blood* 1999; **94**: 1046–56.

22. van der Kolk DM, de Vries EG, Noordhoek L et al. Activity and expression of the multidrug resistance proteins P-gly-

coprotein, MRP1, MRP2, MRP3 and MRP5 in de novo and relapsed acute myeloid leukemia. *Leukemia* 2001; **15**: 1544−53.

23. Abbott BL, Colapietro AM, Barnes Y et al. Low levels of ABCG2 expression in adult AML blast samples. *Blood* 2002; **100**: 4594−601.

24. Ross DD, Karp JE, Chen TT, Doyle LA. Expression of breast cancer resistance protein in blast cells from patients with acute leukemia. *Blood* 2000; **96**: 365−8.

25. van der Kolk DM, Vellenga E, Scheffer GL et al. Expression and activity of breast cancer resistance protein (BCRP) in de novo and relapsed acute myeloid leukemia. *Blood* 2002; **99**: 3763−70.

26. Steinbach D, Sell W, Voigt A et al. *BCRP* gene expression is associated with a poor response to remission induction therapy in childhood acute myeloid leukemia. *Leukemia* 2002; **16**: 1443−7.

27. Tafuri A, Gregorj C, Petrucci MT et al. MDR1 protein expression is an independent predictor of complete remission in newly diagnosed adult acute lymphoblastic leukaemia. *Blood* 2002; **100**: 974−81.

28. Sauerbrey A, Sell W, Steinbach D et al. Expression of the BCRP gene (*ABCG2/MXR/ABCP*) in childhood acute lymphoblastic leukaemia. *Br J Haematol* 2002; **118**: 147−50.

29. Grogan T, Spiers C, Salmon S et al. P-glycoprotein expression in human plasma cell myeloma: correlation with prior chemotherapy. *Blood* 1993; **81**: 490−5.

30. Epstein J, Xiao H, Oba B. P-glycoprotein expression in plasma cell myeloma is associated with resistance to VAD. *Blood* 1989; **74**: 913−17.

31. Marie P, Simonin G, Legrand O et al. Glutathione-S-transferases p, a, m mRNA expression in normal lymphocytes and chronic lymphocytic leukemia. *Leukemia* 1995; **9**: 1742−7.

32. Yuen A, Sikic B. Multidrug resistance in lymphomas. *J Clin Oncol* 1994; **12**: 2453−9.

33. Zhan Z, Sandor V, Gamelin E et al. Expression of the multidrug resistance-associated protein gene in refractory lymphoma: quantitation by a validated polymerase chain reaction assay. *Blood* 1997; **89**: 3795−800.

34. Izquierdo M, Scheffer G, Flens M et al. Major vault protein LRP-related multidrug resistance. *Eur J Cancer* 1996; **32A**: 979−84.

35. List A, Spiers C, Grogan T et al. Overexpression of the major vault transporter protein lung-resistance protein predicts treatment outcome in acute myeloid leukemia. *Blood* 1996; **87**: 2464−9.

36. Legrand O, Simonin G, Zittoun R, Marie JP. Lung resistance protein (LRP) gene expression in adult acute myeloid leukemia: a critical evaluation by three techniques. *Leukemia* 1998; **12**: 1367−74.

37. Lacombe F, Belloc F, Dumain P et al. Detection of cytarabine resistance in patients with acute myelogenous leukemia using flow cytometry. *Blood* 1994; **84**: 716−23.

38. Schuurhuis G, Broxterman H, Ossenkoppele G et al. Functional multidrug resistance phenotype associated with combined overexpression of Pgp/MDR1 and MRP together with 1-β-D-arabinosylcytosine sensitivity may predict clinical response in acute myeloid leukemia. *Clin Cancer Res* 1995; **1**: 81−93.

39. Klumper E, Ossenkoppele G, Pieters R et al. In vitro resistance to cytosine arabinoside, not to daunorubicin, is associated with the risk of relapse in de novo acute myeloid leukaemia. *Br J Haematol* 1996; **93**: 903−10.

40. Rustum Y, Preisler H. Correlation between leukemic cell retention of cytosine arabinoside and response to therapy. *Cancer Res* 1979; **39**: 42−9.

41. Gati W, Paterson A, Larratt L et al. Sensitivity of acute leukemia cells to cytarabine is a correlate of cellular *es* nucleoside transporter site content measured by flow cytometry with SAENTA fluorescein. *Blood* 1997; **90**: 346−53.

42. Galmarini CM, Graham K, Thomas X et al. Expression of high $K_m$ 5′-nucleotidase in leukemic blasts is an independent prognostic factor in adults with acute myeloid leukemia. *Blood* 2001; **98**: 1922−6.

43. Galmarini CM, Thomas X, Calvo F et al. In vivo mechanisms of resistance to cytarabine in acute myeloid leukaemia. *Br J Haematol* 2002; **117**: 860−8.

44. Panasci L, Xu ZY, Bello V, Aloyz R. The role of DNA repair in nitrogen mustard drug resistance. *Anticancer Drugs* 2002; **13**: 211−20.

45. Fisher D. Apoptosis in cancer therapy: crossing the threshold. *Cell* 1994; **78**: 539−42.

46. Harris C. Structure and function of the *p53* tumor suppressor gene: clues for rational cancer therapeutic strategies. *J Natl Cancer Inst* 1996; **88**: 1442−55.

47. Imamura J, Miyishi I, Koeffler H. *p53* in hematologic malignancies. *Blood* 1994; **84**: 2412−21.

48. Sherr C. Cancer cell cycles. *Science* 1996; **274**: 1672−7.

49. Kohn K. Regulatory genes and drug sensitivity. *J Natl Cancer Inst* 1996; **88**: 1255−6.

50. Vrhovac R, Delmer A, Tang R et al. Prognostic significance of the cell cycle inhibitor p27$^{Kip1}$ in chronic B-cell lymphocytic leukemia. *Blood* 1998; **91**: 4694−700.

51. Reed J. Bcl-2: prevention of apoptosis as a mechanism of drug resistance. *Hematol Oncol Clin North Am* 1995; **9**: 451−73.

52. Hermine O, Haioun C, Lepage E et al. Prognostic significance of bcl-2 protein expression in aggressive non-Hodgkin's lymphoma. Groupe d'Etude des Lymphomes de l'Adulte (GELA). *Blood* 1996; **87**: 265−72.

53. Campos L, Rouault J, Sabido O et al. High expression of bcl-2 protein in acute myeloid leukemia cells is associated with poor response to chemotherapy. *Blood* 1993; **81**: 3091−6.

54. Campos L, Sabido O, Sebban C et al. Expression of *BCL-2* proto-oncogene in adult acute lymphoblastic leukemia. *Leukemia* 1996; **10**: 434−8.

55. Bosanquet AG, Sturm I, Wieder T et al. Bax expression correlates with cellular drug sensitivity to doxorubicin, cyclophosphamide and chlorambucil but not fludarabine, cladribine or corticosteroids in B cell chronic lymphocytic leukemia. *Leukemia* 2002; **16**: 1035−44.

56. Prokop A, Wieder T, Sturm I et al. Relapse in childhood acute lymphoblastic leukemia is associated with a decrease of the Bax/Bcl-2 ratio and loss of spontaneous caspase-3 processing in vivo. *Leukemia* 2000; **14**: 1606−13.

57. Bedi A, Barber J, Bedi G et al. Bcr−abl-mediated inhibition of apoptosis with delay of G$_2$/M transition after DNA damage: a mechanism of resistance to multiple anticancer drugs. *Blood* 1995; **86**: 1148−58.

58. Nimmanapalli R, Bhalla K. Mechanisms of resistance to imatinib mesylate in Bcr−Abl-positive leukemias. *Curr Opin Oncol* 2002; **14**: 616−20.

59. Dias S, Choy M, Alitalo K, Rafii S. Vascular endothelial growth factor (VEGF)-C signaling through FLT-4 (VEGFR-

3) mediates leukemic cell proliferation, survival, and resistance to chemotherapy. *Blood* 2002; **99**: 2179–84.

60. Novak AJ, Bram RJ, Kay NE, Jelinek DF. Aberrant expression of B-lymphocyte stimulator by B chronic lymphocytic leukemia cells: a mechanism for survival. *Blood* 2002; **100**: 2973–9.

61. Robert J. Multidrug resistance in oncology: diagnostic and therapeutic approaches. *Eur J Clin Invest* 1999; **29**: 536–45.

62. Solary E, Witz B, Caillot D et al. Combination of quinine as a potential reversing agent with mitoxantrone and cytarabine for the treatment of acute leukemias: a randomized multicentric study. *Blood* 1996; **88**: 1198–205.

63. Baer MR, George SL, Dodge RK et al. Phase 3 study of the multidrug resistance modulator PSC-833 in previously untreated patients 60 years of age and older with acute myeloid leukemia: Cancer and Leukemia Group B study 9720. *Blood* 2002; **100**: 1224–32.

64. Bates SF, Chen C, Robey R et al. Reversal of multidrug resistance: lessons from clinical oncology. *Novartis Found Symp* 2002; **243**: 83–96.

65. List AF, Kopecky KJ, Willman CL et al. Benefit of cyclosporine modulation of drug resistance in patients with poor-risk acute myeloid leukemia: a Southwest Oncology Group study. *Blood* 2001; **98**: 3212–20.

66. List AF, Kopecky KJ, Willman CL et al. Cyclosporine inhibition of P-glycoprotein in chronic myeloid leukemia blast phase. *Blood* 2002; **100**: 1910–12.

67. Dantzig AH, Law KL, Cao J, Starling JJ. Reversal of multidrug resistance by the P-glycoprotein modulator, LY335979, from the bench to the clinic. *Curr Med Chem* 2001; **8**: 39–50.

68. Mistry P, Stewart AJ, Dangerfield W et al. In vitro and in vivo reversal of P-glycoprotein-mediated multidrug resistance by a novel potent modulator, XR9576. *Cancer Res* 2001; **61**: 749–58.

69. Maliepaard M, van Gastelen MA, Tohdo A et al. Circumvention of breast cancer resitance protein (BCRP)-mediated resistance to camptothecins in vitro using non-substrate drugs or the BCRP inhibitor GF120918. *Clin Cancer Res* 2001, 7: 935–41.

70. Peck RA, Hewett J, Harding MW et al. Phase I and pharmacokinetic study of the novel MDR1 and MRP1 inhibitor Biricodar administered alone and in combination with doxorubicin. *J Clin Oncol* 2001; **19**: 3130–41.

71. Plunkett W, Gandhi V, Grunewald R et al. Pharmacologically directed design of AML therapy. In: Gale RP (ed) *Acute Myelogenous Leukemia: Progress and Controversies*. New York: Wiley-Liss, 1990: 481–92.

72. Terpstra W, Löwenberg B. Application of myeloid growth factors in the treatment of acute myeloid leukemia. *Leukemia* 1997; **11**: 315–27.

73. Karp JE, Lancet JE, Kaukmann SH et al. Clinical and biologic activity of the farnesyltransferase inhibitor R115777 in adults with refractory and relapsed acute leukemias: a phase 1 clinical–laboratory correlative trial. *Blood* 2001; **97**: 3361–3369.

74. Hoover RR, Mahon FX, Melo JV, Daley GQ. Overcoming STI571 resistance with the farnesyl transferase inhibitor SCH66336. *Blood* 2002; **100**: 1068–71.

75. Waters JS, Webb A, Cunningham D et al. Phase I clinical and pharmacokinetic study of bcl-2 antisense oligonucleotide therapy in patients with non-Hodgkin's lymphoma. *J Clin Oncol* 2000; **18**: 1812–23.

76. Marcucci C, Byrd JC, Dai G et al. Phase 1 and pharmacodynamic studies of G3139, a Bcl-2 antisense oligonucleotide, in combination with chemotherapy in refractory or relapsed acute leukemia. *Blood* 2003; **101**: 425–32.

# 24 The theoretical basis of chemotherapy for hematological malignancy

**AK McMillan and DC Linch**

## Introduction

In situations where chemotherapy is given with curative intent, multiple agents are usually used in combination. These are administered in pulses, with the non-treatment intervals being required for recovery from the drug-induced toxicities. The drug components of a regimen typically have different modes of action, so that the antitumor effects will be additive at least and the limiting side-effects will hopefully be non-overlapping. In hemato-oncology practice, there have been continual attempts to improve patient outcomes by increasing the doses of the chemotherapy agents employed, and the theoretical basis of dose escalation is discussed below.

## The Skipper experiments

Skipper and co-workers published a series of fundamental papers in the early 1960s that have impacted greatly on subsequent clinical practice. The most important of these was entitled 'On the criteria and kinetics associated with curability of experimental leukaemia'.[1] These experiments reported studies using the intraperitoneal injection of L1210 leukemic cells in a mouse model. The underlying assumption was that small numbers of viable leukemia cells are ultimately lethal and, therefore, if a cure is to be achieved, the aim must be to eradicate each last tumor cell from the experimental animal. In the experiments reported in this paper, a logarithmic relationship was demonstrated between the size of tumor cell inoculum and the duration of survival of an animal without treatment. At a level of intensity of therapy where some animals might have either zero or one cell remaining, the Poisson distribution equation becomes applicable and a cure rate of around 40% would be expected. The antileukemic agent amethopterin was administered every other day after varying sizes of leukemia cell aliquot ranging over five logs of cell dose. The results showed an increase in the percentage of animals who survived 100 days from 0% through 8%, 82%, 96%, to 100% survival with each log decrease in the size of the inoculum. These experiments led to the concept of log-kill, which states that the relationship between the number of surviving tumor cells and chemotherapy dose is logarithmic rather than linear. The important corollary of this is that, with the decrease in the numbers of residual cells remaining after dose escalation, it becomes progressively harder to eradicate any further cells as the tumor burden decreases.

To translate these data to the clinical arena involves not only an understanding of the increase in complexity of factors in clinical practice, but also an understanding of the role of the immune system. 'Immune surveillance' may mean that it is not essential to eradicate every last cell, as it was in the above experiments when injections of syngeneic tumor cells were given in an experimental mouse model. Nevertheless, the principles operating are probably similar, so that, for a given patient, the threshold number of surviving cells below which patients may be cured is likely to be constant. The rules governing whether a reduction to below this threshold can be achieved are likely to adhere to the principles of log-kill outlined above. Therefore, the same log increase in chemotherapy dose will progressively eradicate fewer and fewer cells as the possibility of cure is approached. A further useful concept articulated by Skipper and colleagues is the observation that clinical remission may be achieved when large numbers of tumor cells remain. In this situation, some animals may have no detectable leukemic cells, but because they have received a dose of chemotherapy insufficient to eradicate every last cell, these mice are destined to relapse. In the same way, patients treated with inadequate doses of chemotherapy may achieve remission but will inevitably relapse due to occult tumor cells remaining. The mathematical equivalent of this, as described in the seminal paper, is that after a single dose of a chemotherapy agent that will reduce a $10^4$ cell population by 4 logs to an average of 1 leukemia cell per animal (99.99% cell kill), there will be an anticipated 40% cure rate. However, the same dose administered to animals bearing $10^6$ leukemia cells would be expected to result in an average of $10^2$ leukemia cells surviving, with virtually no cures.

Chemotherapy scheduling was also considered by Skipper, so for a tumor with a very high growth rate, such as the leukemia model used in these experiments, there is a high likelihood of regrowth of tumor between doses, which can make repeated intermittent dose scheduling ineffective. If a single large dose of treatment is used, as long as toxicity to the host is sustainable, it could be shown to be more effective. Again, when consideration is given to actual clinical practice, it can be seen that tumor growth fraction and toxicity to the patient's vital organs will modify the optimum schedule. The idea of using large doses of single-agent therapy has been encompassed into the high-dose sequential therapy developed by Gianni and colleagues.[2] Their results are very encouraging, but confirmation in other trials of the efficacy of this strategy is required

Lastly, as a result of these experiments, Skipper commented on the existence of anatomical compartments that can be readily invaded by leukemia cells but not as readily penetrated by most chemotherapy agents – this for instance being in accord with the concept of the blood–brain barrier.

# The Goldie–Coldman hypothesis

The experiments of Skipper suggest how a single chemotherapy agent can be used optimally, but as most chemotherapy regimens contain multiple agents, it is important to also consider the work of Goldie and Coldman.[3] The hypothesis of Goldie and Coldman was based solely on theoretical mathematical modeling and not on laboratory or clinical data. The hypothesis related the drug sensitivity of a tumor to the rate of spontaneous mutation towards phenotypic drug resistance. In their summary, they state that 'the proportion, as well as the absolute numbers of resistant cells, will therefore increase with time and the fraction of resistant cells within tumour colonies of the same size will vary depending on whether the mutation occurs as an early or late event.' They go on to state that, from their mathematical model, 'the probability of the appearance of a resistant phenotype increases with the mutation rate and furthermore, for any population of tumours with a non-zero mutation rate, the likelihood of there being at least one resistant cell may go from a condition of low to high probability over a very short interval in the tumour's biologic

history.' From these theoretical assumptions, it can be concluded that the probability of the number of resistant cells in a tumor is not linearly related to the size of the tumor, but increases rapidly as the number of cells increases. This means that at certain times in certain tumors there is a period when the tumor's susceptibility to chemotherapy is changing rapidly. This, in turn, leads to the conclusion that tumors early in their growth history can be expected to have a much better likelihood of cure than tumors that have reached an advanced stage, and it supports the concept of early dose intensification. It is clearly not possible to alter the rate of mutation, but the use of effective and independently acting agents in combination will have the effect of reducing the value for the effective spontaneous mutation rate. This is because it is then a requirement for the cell to spontaneously become resistant to two mechanisms of drug action simultaneously – and this is a less likely event. An analogy for this observation is the combination of antimicrobial chemotherapy agents used in the treatment of mycobacterial infection.

# Relative dose intensity (RDI)

Models of dose intensity were further refined with the concept of relative dose intensity (RDI). This suggests that the efficacy of a chemotherapy regimen is not just due to the total drug dose administered, but is more closely related to the dose delivered over unit time. To quantify and allow comparison of protocols, Hryniuk et al[4] defined RDI as the amount of drug delivered per unit time expressed as milligrams per square meter per week relative to an arbitrarily chosen standard single drug for the tumor being studied. In the case of a combination regimen, RDI is the decimal fraction of the ratio of the test regimen compared with the standard regimen. A major limitation, however, in the determination of the RDI is the lack of single-agent trials that allow the accurate assignment of the relative efficacies of the different components of a combination chemotherapy regimen for a specific tumor type. Using the Hryniuk model, for instance, regimens such as MACOP-B (used in non-Hodgkin lymphoma, NHL) have considerably higher RDIs than standard CHOP therapy, and yet the clinical results with these regimens are similar.[5] With different assumptions about the relative efficacies of the individual drugs, it is possible to derive broadly similar RDIs more closely in accord with the clinical data, although the relationship between RDI and tumor response does not appear to be as clear as in Hodgkin lymphoma.[6] A further limitation of the RDI, and other mathematical models relating administered chemotherapy dose to tumor control, is that it fails to take into account the marked interindividual variation in drug absorption and metabolism that have been well documented. In many situations, the extent of hematological toxicity may more closely reflect the true drug exposure (TDE) rather than the amount of drugs administered over unit time or the individual's intrinsic marrow sensitivity. A recent analysis of patients with advanced Hodgkin lymphoma treated in Germany with the COPP/ABVD regimen indicated that those patients with relatively marked hematological toxicity received lower drug doses with reduced dose intensity, as a result of the toxicity, and yet achieved better disease control.[7] This has important clinical implications, as, in some circumstances, the philosophy of using growth factors to achieve 'full dose on time' may merely increase the drug delivery to those patients who have already received the highest TDE.

Toxicity may also be dependent on dose intensity, and this is normally the case with hematopoietic toxicity. In some cases, toxicity may be related to the 'area under the curve', as has been demonstrated for carboplatin-induced hematopoietic toxicity,[8] whereas with other toxicities, such as anthracycline cardiac toxicity, peak drug levels may also be relevant. These issues must be considered carefully in the scheduling of any intensive drug regimen.

## Summation dose intensity (SDI)

In contrast to RDI, summation dose intensity (SDI)[9] is an attempt to measure to what extent giving drugs in combination impairs giving the maximum total dose of an individual drug. If drugs are given in combination and there is no toxicity created by their use together then the summation dose intensity of a three-drug protocol will be 3. In reality, the use of drugs in combination almost always means that some reduction in dose will be required, so, for example, Frei[10] uses the example of the MOPP protocol, where the summation dose intensity for the four drugs is 3.2 out of a possible 4, and contrasts this with the CMF protocol (used for breast cancer), where the summation dose intensity is only 1.2 out of a possible 3. In a third example, this time with respect to high-dose therapy and stem cell transplantation, the transplant conditioning schedule of three breast cancer protocols varied between 2.0 and 2.7, illustrating good additive dose escalation.

## The effective dose approach

Hasenclever and colleagues[6] have revisited the Skipper model in the setting of malignant lymphomas and have defined a 'generalized Skipper model' (GSM) by combining the Skipper concepts with a representation of the tumor heterogeneity with respect to the growth characteristics and chemosensitivity of that tumor type. Each tumor is assumed to have a specific chemosensitivity status and a characteristic latency time, which is derived from the time to disease progression after an initial response observed in clinical trials. The effective dose is then defined as

$$\frac{\text{total dose}}{1 + \text{treatment duration/average latency time}}.$$

Using such models, the authors went on to propose that in Hodgkin lymphoma, where there is a long latency time (estimated to be 490 days), increasing the total dose is most likely to improve results and there is relatively little concern about tumor regrowth between treatment cycles. In histologically aggressive NHL, by contrast, the estimated latency time is 132 days and the tumor regrowth between cycles is a major concern, implying that the way forward is to shorten the intervals between therapy. Furthermore, they have suggested that a raised lactate dehydrogenase (LDH) is a surrogate measure of proliferation rate and thus latency time, and a more time-intense schedule is particularly important in those patients with a raised LDH at presentation. These concepts have formed the basis for the recent lymphoma trials in Germany,[11–13] and the results of these trials can be further used to modify and enhance the model.

## Examples of dose intensification not requiring stem cell transplantation

A good illustration of an improvement in outcome with increased dose intensity is Burkitt lymphoma in adults. Historically, the survival rate was between 50% and 60%, but regimens such as CODOX-M/IVAC, which utilize a marked increase in dose intensity, as well as multiple chemotherapy agents, have produced survival rates in excess of 70%.[14,15] It is interesting to note that this intensification of therapy has been achieved without the use of high-dose therapy and stem cell rescue but rather by changes in schedule and the addition of the hematopoietic growth factors. The use of growth factors to enable dose escalation should, therefore, be distinguished from the use of growth factors to maintain dose intensity with conventional-dose regimens (see above). The improvement attributable to CODOX-M/IVAC and a number of other modern Burkitt lymphoma regimens can be seen as a combination of the application of dose intensity (as per the Skipper log-kill hypothesis) and also the application of non-cross-resistant combination therapy (as per the Goldie and Colman hypothesis). Two further examples of increasing dose intensity, but this time without changing the drug combination, come from the German Hodgkin's Disease Study Group (BEACOPP versus escalated BEACOPP)[11] and also from the German Non-Hodgkin Lymphoma Study Group trial, where a comparision was made between identical doses of CHOP or CHOP plus etoposide chemotherapy given over the standard 3 weeks or in the same dosage with a 2-week cycle accelerated by the use of hematopoietic growth factors.[12] In both of these cases, since exactly the same drugs are used, the improvement is only attributable to the increase in dose intensity achieved by the change in scheduling. The improvement in outcome with the escalated BEACOPP (freedom from treatment failure at 5 years 87%, versus 76% with standard BEACOPP) and time-accelerated CHOP in elderly patients (event-free survival at 5 years 44% with CHOP-14, versus 33% with CHOP-21) reflects the value of designing protocols from first principles and supports the concept of the GSM and effective dose model. Prior to these trials, the justification of various dose-intensity models has largely been derived from retrospective analysis of trial populations, where it has been shown that the worst outcome is achieved in patients where the relative dose intensity is poor. However, this can be a self-fulfilling prophecy, since the patients with a poor performance status at the outset (who are known to do badly) will also be the same patients in whom it is difficult to achieve the planned degree of dose intensity during treatment.

# Drug selection in high-dose therapy and stem cell transplantation strategies

Special consideration needs to be given to drug selection in high-dose chemotherapy given with rescue by the infusion of hematopoietic stem cells. In this circumstance, where hematopoietic toxicity is effectively bypassed by the reinfusion of stem cells, close consideration has to be given to the toxicity profile of the agents in use. A good example of this is the anthracycline class of cytotoxics, whose dose-limiting toxicity is cardiac, and even though a drug such as doxorubicin is one of the most effective drugs in first-line lymphoma therapy, it is of little value in high-dose chemotherapy. By contrast, alkylating agents such as melphalan are the most frequently used class of drugs, since doses can be escalated markedly over conventional dose levels, once hematopoietic toxicity has been excluded, before other critical organ toxicity (pulmonary, renal, or hepatic) becomes a consideration. The potential utility of drug classes in high-dose therapy can be assessed by their 'dose escalation index', which is the ratio of their maximum tolerated dose in conventional therapy and the increased dose achieved after stem cell rescue. The potential value of escalated therapy with stem cell rescue with respect to a particular tumor is also a property of the shape of the dose–response curve for the particular combination of a tumor/drug pair. Tumors where there is phase

III evidence for the efficacy of high-dose chemotherapy, such as relapsed high-grade NHL,[16] tend to be those illustrating a steep dose–response relationship, so that the higher doses of drugs delivered generate significantly higher tumor cell kill. Tumors where there is no evidence for the efficacy of high-dose therapy, such as breast cancer,[17] tend to be those where the dose–response relationship is less steep.

# Use of biological agents

In recent years, a number of biological agents have been introduced into the treatment of hematological malignancies, one of the most striking examples of which is the use of rituximab in combination with CHOP in the treatment of histologically aggressive NHL.[18] Whether this can just be considered as another chemotherapeutic agent in the chemotherapy dose models is not clear. Thus, the addition of rituximab to CHOP-14 could further improve the results, but it is equally possible that when rituximab is used, there is no benefit in any further escalation over standard CHOP.

# Maintenance therapy

Maintenance therapy comprising relatively low-dose therapy given over a long period of time has now been largely abandoned, except in acute lymphoblastic leukemia, as a result of clinical experience. The aim is to continue tumor reduction after the patient has achieved remission so as to bring about a cure. The drugs are often given on a semicontinuous schedule, and this type of scheduling has the theoretical advantage of being more active against any tumor cells that are in deep $G_0$ and only infrequently enter the cell cycle (when they become more accessible to chemotherapy attack).

# Chemotherapy infusion and 'third spacing'

In tumors where the growth fraction is low (e.g. myeloma), alternative strategies for delivering the most effective use of chemotherapy may become applicable. One of the current standard treatments for myeloma is the VAD chemotherapy regimen,[19] where the total dose and dose intensity are low but because the drugs are infused over a 4-day period, the area under the curve (AUC) in pharmacological terms is probably the key to the observed efficacy. The AUC has also proved a useful concept in dosing drugs where the toxicity threshold is close to the therapeutic level – for example carboplatin, where renal and hepatic handling are of particular importance. A further example of the importance of the AUC is the observed toxicity noted with the phenomenon known as 'third spacing', which is where a drug is able to partition into extravascular fluid spaces such as pleural effusions or ascites, from where it is slowly returned to the intravascular space. This results in the prolonged presence of low drug concentrations and in turn increases the AUC and the risk of toxicity. This phenomenon has been well described for methotrexate[20] and cytarabine and more recently fludarabine.[21] There had been an expectation that infusional therapy might be a means of either increasing efficacy or decreasing toxicity in other tumors, but there are few clinical data to support this.[22]

## Rescue strategies

It is not necessarily the case that theoretical principles can always be used to explain the value of clinipcal strategies. An example of where a frequently used strategy is not fully understood is the use of folinic acid (leucovorin) to rescue patients after very high doses of intravenous methotrexate. The true mechanism is probably unknown,[23] although the rationale for this is often said to be that the folinic acid

allows normal tissues to recover without also 'rescuing' the tumor cells. The strategy has been used in a wide range of tumors, including head and neck cancer and NHL, and it is also said to allow the delivery of high doses of drug to protected compartments such as the central nervous system. The stated rationale is dependent upon alterations in the enzyme pathway of DNA synthesis (e.g. dihydrofolate reductase), but the experimental evidence for this is inconclusive.[24] To complicate the situation, the start of rescue protocols after less than 36–42 hours is probably too early to allow a genuine rescue phenomenon to occur with the administration of the folinic acid.[25]

## Conclusions

A sound knowledge of the principles underlying the practice of chemotherapy is fundamental to good clinical practice. The work of Skipper and of Goldie and Coldman indicates that dose intensity and scheduling may explain different outcomes between different regimens and should help in the design of future protocols. An understanding of the interaction between biological agents and chemotherapy should emerge from the results of ongoing trials.

## REFERENCES

1. Skipper HE, Schabel FM Jr, Wilcox WS. Experimental evaluation of potential anticancer agents XII. On the criteria and kinetics associated with 'curability' of experimental leukaemia. *Cancer Chemother Rep* 1964; **35**: 1–111.
2. Gianni AM. High-dose chemotherapy and autologous bone marrow transplantation compared with MACOP-B in aggressive B-cell lymphoma. *N Engl J Med* 1997; **336**: 1290–7.
3. Goldie JH, Coldman AJ. A mathematic model for relating the drug sensitivity of tumors to their spontaneous mutation rate. *Cancer Treat Rep* 1979; **63**: 1727–33.
4. Hryniuk W, Levine MN. Analysis of dose intensity for adjuvant chemotherapy trials in stage II breast cancer. *J Clin Oncol* 1986; **4**: 1162–70.
5. Fisher RI, Gaynor ER, Dahlberg S. Comparison of a standard regimen (CHOP) with three intensive chemotherapy regimens for advanced non-Hodgkin's lymphoma. *N Engl J Med* 1993.
6. Hasenclever DBO, Gerike T, Loeffler M. Modelling of chemotherapy: the effective dose approach. *Ann Haematol* 2001; **80**: B89–94.
7. Brosteanu O, Hasenclever D, Loeffler M, Diehl V. Low acute hematological toxicity during chemotherapy predicts reduced disease control in advanced Hodgkin's disease. *Ann Haematol* 2004; **83**: 176–82.
8. Calvert AH, Newell DR, Gumbrell LA et al. Carboplatin dosage: prospective evaluation of a simple formula based on renal function. *J Clin Oncol* 1989; **7**: 1748–56.
9. Frei E 3rd, Elias A, Wheeler C et al. The relationship between high-dose treatment and combination chemotherapy: the concept of summation dose intensity. *Clin Cancer Res* 1998; **4**: 2027–37.
10. Frei E. Pharmacologic strategies for high dose therapy. In: Armitage J (ed) *High Dose Cancer Therapy*. Baltimore: Williams and Wilkins, 1995: 3–17.
11. Diehl V, Franklin J, Pfreundshah M et al. Standard and increased dose BEACOPP chemotherapy compared with COPP-ABVD for advanced Hodgkin's disease. *N Engl J Med* 2003; **348**: 2386–95.
12. Pfreundschuh M, Trumper L, Kloess M et al. 2-weekly or 3-weekly CHOP chemotherapy with or without etoposide for the treatment of elderly patients with aggressive lymphomas: results of the NHL-B2 trial of the DSHNHL. *Blood* 2004; **104**: 634–41.
13. Pfreundschuh M, Trumper L, Kloess M et al. 2-weekly or 3-weekly CHOP chemotherapy with or without etoposide for the treatment of young patients with good prognosis (normal LDH) aggressive lymphomas: results of the NHL-B1 trial of the DSHNHL. *Blood* 2004; **104**: 626–33.
14. Magrath I, Adde M, Shad A et al. Adults and children with small non-cleaved-cell lymphoma have a similar excellent outcome when treated with the same chemotherapy regimen. *J Clin Oncol* 1996; **14**: 925–34.
15. Mead GM, Sydes MR, Walewski J et al. An international evaluation of CODOX-M and CODOX-M alternating with IVAC in adult Burkitt's lymphoma: results of United Kingdom Lymphoma Group LY06 study. *Ann Oncol* 2002; **13**: 1264–72.
16. Philip T, Guglielmi C, Hagenbeek A et al. Autologous bone marrow transplantation as compared with salvage chemotherapy in relapses of chemotherapy-sensitive non-Hodgkin's lymphoma. *N Engl J Med* 1995; **333**: 1540–5.

17. Dicato M. High-dose chemotherapy in breast cancer: Where are we now? *Semin Oncol* 2002; **29**(3 Suppl 8): 16–20.

18. Coiffier B, Lepage E, Briere J et al. CHOP chemotherapy plus rituximab compared with CHOP alone in elderly patients with diffuse large B-cell lymphoma. *N Engl J Med* 2002; **346**: 235–42.

19. Barlogie B, Smith L, Alexanian R. Effective treatment of advanced multiple myeloma refractory to alkylating agents. *N Engl J Med* 1984; **310**: 1353–6.

20. Evans W, Pratt C. Effect of pleural effusion on high-dose methotrexate kinetics. *Clin Pharmacol Ther* 1978; **23**: 68–72.

21. Mahadevan A, Kanegaonkar R, Hoskin PJ. Third space sequestration increases toxicity of fludarabine – a case report. *Acta Oncol* 1997; **36**: 441.

22. Boyd DB et al. COPBLAM III: infusional combination chemotherapy for diffuse large-cell lymphoma. *J Clin Oncol* 1988; **6**: 425–33.

23. Ackland SP, Schilsky RL. High-dose methotrexate: a critical reappraisal. *J Clin Oncol* 1987; **5**: 2017–31.

24. Jolivet J. Biochemical and pharmacologic rationale for high-dose methotrexate. *NCI Monogr* 1987; **5**: 61–5.

25. Borsi JD, Sagen E, Romslo I et al. Rescue after intermediate and high-dose methotrexate: background, rationale, and current practice. *Pediatr Hematol Oncol* 1990; **7**: 347–63.

# 25 Humoral immunotherapy and the use of monoclonal antibodies

Peter T Daniel

## Introduction

Significant advances have been achieved in the therapy of hematopoeitic malignancies. Polychemotherapy regimens in combination with radiotherapy, or bone marrow or stem cell transplantation yield high rates of complete remission. Nevertheless, a significant percentage of these remissions is not durable and therapy only prolongs survival. Primary or acquired resistance to DNA-damaging agents is the major problem of these conventional therapeutic strategies. In addition, the gains achieved by high-dose chemotherapy have been paralleled by an increase in drug-related multiorgan toxic side-effects, thereby limiting further dose escalation.

Recent developments in antibody technology have provided novel approaches to further improve the treatment of leukemia and lymphoma. In fact, the introduction of monoclonal antibodies in the treatment of different types of B-cell lymphoma has already shown impressive clinical efficacy. This has opened up the field, and antibodies targeted against a broad range of surface markers are now being successfully advertised as 'magic bullets' not only in the treatment of lymphoproliferative diseases but also in solid tumors and for immunosuppression in the control of autoimmune and graft-versus-host disease.

## The history of antibody therapy

It was in the year 1897 when Paul Ehrlich developed the concept of immune bodies as the correlate for specific immunity and protection from infectious diseases. The basis for this concept was created only a few years earlier, in 1890, by Emil von Behring and Shibasaburo Kitasato, the founders of serotherapy, in their work on the transfer of specific immunity and protection from tetanus and diphtheria in experimen-tal animals. Despite the interest in immune mechanisms and serotherapy in cancer starting as early as the start of the 20th century, the bulk of the work in this field has been done since the 1950s. Early investigations of serotherapy in malignant disease have been reviewed elsewhere.[1-3] The discovery of the molecular basis for antibody diversity by Susumu Tonegawa[4] and the development of novel techniques for the immortalization of B cells and the production of monoclonal antibodies (mAbs) by Milstein and Köhler[5] finally enabled the field for the use of specifically defined mAbs in diagnosis and therapy.

The generation of mAbs against tumor cells led rapidly to the discovery of novel tumor-associated markers that allowed new classifications and refined the diagnosis of lymphoid and myeloid malignancies. Ideally, the antibody should specifically target the tumor cell, and have no cross-reactivity with normal cells, since binding to non-malignant tissues will reduce effective tumor targeting. Moreover, the recognition of normal tissue by antibodies might cause severe damage to the patient. The majority of these tumor antigens are, however, not tumor-specific but only tumor-associated and therefore can also be found on the corresponding non-malignant counterparts. These antigens, which are often lineage-specific, can still serve as a target for tumor eradication provided that stem cells in the lineage of the normal cell are antigen-negative and hence able to reconstitute the cellular compartment or the tissue involved. A large number of tumor-associated antigens that may serve as putative targets for therapy have been identified by techniques such as Serex or more straightforward methods that measure genome-wide differential expression of gene products on the RNA or protein level, such as cDNA or oligonucleotide microarrays, differential display polymerase chain reaction (PCR), or proteome analyses. Truly tumor-specific antigens, in contrast, can be created by chromosomal translocations or point mutations leading to the formation of neo-antigens such as the BCR–ABL fusion protein in chronic myeloid leukemia (CML). Such neo-antigens may also be found by the use of Serex, which employs low-titer antibodies found in patients' sera in an expression cloning strategy that yields the tumor antigen from a corresponding cDNA library.[6] Nevertheless, the vast majority of these antigens represent embryofetal genes that are turned on in consequence of deregulated gene expression in tumor cells such as the cancer–testis antigens, i.e. tumor-associated antigens.[7] Additional tumor-specific antigens being exploited in sero- and immunotherapy are the individual antigen receptors (idiotypes) found on the malignant lymphoid T or B cells (see below).

Due to the increasing number of monoclonal antibodies in the literature, which often reacted with the same molecule expressed during a distinct cellular differentiation stage, a unifying nomenclature was introduced. Based on the structures recognized by the antibodies, so-called clusters of differentiation (CD) were defined. Table 25.1 shows the expression pattern and lineage restriction of a few selected CD molecules identified as useful targets for antibody-based immunotherapy. These target structures were selected according to their biological properties, for example lineage restriction, expression levels, and signaling properties, or simply for historical reasons. Today, the vast majority of antibodies employed in anticancer therapy have been genetically engineered, in most instances, to replace antigenic murine structures by corresponding human framework sequences.

## Recombinant antibodies

Classical mAbs are almost exclusively of murine origin. These antibodies were generated by immuniza-tion of mice and fusion of spleen cells from immunized animals containing a few antigen-specific cells with a murine plasmacytoma cell line followed to obtain immortalized hybridoma cells that secrete antibodies against the specific antigen employed for immunization.[5] Such mAbs are xenogeneic proteins and therefore highly immunogenic. Individuals receiving murine monoclonals have been found to produce high titers of human anti-mouse antibodies (HAMA) within a few weeks after the first dose.[8,9] These HAMA can neutralize the murine mAbs. This can reduce the efficacy of such antibody applications in vivo to the short time period before the neutralizing antibodies are detectable. Thus, efforts were undertaken to reduce the immunogenicity of the foreign proteins. One such approach was the generation of human mAbs by hybridoma technology, which, however, was not successful since the human hybridomas proved to be unstable and therefore not suitable for mass production. This, together with the need to facilitate the production of mAbs, which are still mainly produced in eukaryotic cells, led to the establishment of recombinant DNA technologies.[10,11] The murine variable regions that contain the antibody recognition sites – the complementarity-defining regions (CDRs) – can now be cloned using PCR strategies. The structure of an IgG molecule is depicted in Figure 25.1. The cDNAs coding for the variable regions of the heavy and light chains of the murine immunoglobulins can be cloned and fused to the constant regions of human antibody cDNAs to produce human-like, chimeric monoclonal antibodies.[12] Apart from the murine variable regions, these chimeric antibodies resemble human self-structures, which largely reduces immunogenicity. Unfortunately, the few remaining amino acids of the murine variable regions can still be recognized as non-self and elicit neutralizing HAMA.

| | **Stage of maturation** | | | |
|---|---|---|---|---|
| **Lineage** | **Early immature** | **Late immature and mature** | **Late, activated** | **Broad expression** |
| T lymphocyte | CD1, CD7 | CD3, CD4, CD8 | CD25, CD30, CD95 | CD2, CD5, CD7, CD45, CD52 |
| B lymphocyte | CD10, CD38 | sIgM, CD21, CD22, CD37, CD79 | CD5, CD23, CD30, CD38, CD79, CD95 | CD19, CD20, CD45, CD52, Idiotype |
| Myelomonocytic | CD33 | – | CD16 | CD13, CD14, CD15, CD45, CD52 |
| Stem cells | CD34, HLA-DR | – | – | – |
| Carcinoma | | | | EpCAM, HER2/neu, EGFR |

Table 25.1 Surface markers targeted in antibody therapy

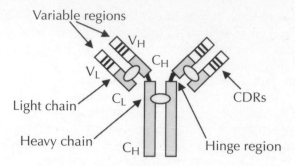

**Figure 25.1** Domain structure of IgG antibodies. C, constant region; V, variable region; H, heavy chain; L, light chain; CDRs, complementarity-defining regions, i.e. the three regions defining specificity of the antigen-binding region. They are located in the variable regions of the heavy and light chains ($V_H$ and $V_L$).

Thus, efforts have been made to further decrease immunogenicity by grafting the regions responsible for antigen binding, i.e. the CDRs, to the constant parts of human heavy and light chains. This results in fully humanized antibodies. Nevertheless, due to the unique structure of their antigen-binding groove, these humanized antibodies still retain immunogenicity, and a humoral HAMA response has been observed against their foreign regions.

It should be noted, moreover, that a HAMA immune response can interfere with antibody-based detection systems in clinical chemistry and lead to falsely elevated assay results. Examples are sandwich enzyme-linked immunosorbent assay (ELISA) systems for the detection of hormones or tumor markers. Such falsely elevated markers may misguide clinical decisions, and therefore caution should be exercised when such assays are performed on the sera of patients receiving antibody therapy.

Another promising development is the generation of recombinant single-chain antibodies. These consist of the variable region of the PCR-cloned antibody light chain fused to the variable region of the PCR-cloned heavy chain by means of an artificial linker peptide (Figure 25.2). Such single-chain variable region fragments (scFvs) can be easily produced in bacteria on a large scale as compared with eukaryotic cell-produced mAbs.[13] In addition, the scFvs are much smaller than the original intact antibodies and therefore have different pharmacodynamic properties, such as improved tissue penetration (Table 25.2). In a similar approach, natural or genetically engineered ligands for surface receptors are employed to target receptor-bearing cells (see the discussion of immunotoxins later in this chapter).

To allow recognition of the antibody type employed, e.g. human, humanized or of murine origin, a nomen-

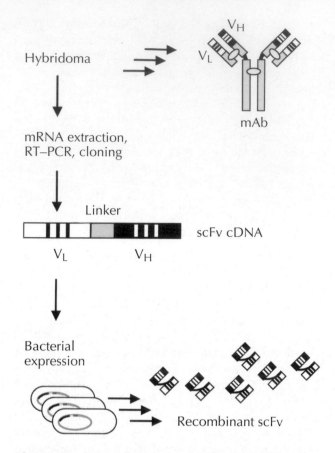

**Figure 25.2** Recombinant DNA technologies for the production of monoclonal antibodies (mAbs). The variable regions of the heavy and light chain of a mAb can be cloned from the mRNA of a mAb-producing hybridoma using reverse transcriptase polymerase chain reaction (RT–PCR). Fusion of the cDNAs via a bridging linker yields the cDNA for the expression of a single-chain Fv fragment (scFv). The expression of such a scFv in bacteria allows the mass production of mAbs without the need for sophisticated eukaryotic cell culture techniques as in the case of the original hybridoma. Similar cloning techniques may be employed to humanize mAbs from mAbs of animal origin, i.e. to replace animal mAb framework sequences by the corresponding human sequences, mostly derived from human IgG1, while retaining the complementarity-defining regions.

clature has been introduced in which the generic name of the antibody has a suffix indicating its origin (Table 25.3). Thus, rituximab (IDEC-C2B8, i.e. chimeric 2B8) is a chimeric antibody (against human CD20) where the constant regions are derived from human IgG1 and the variable regions of the heavy and light chains are derived from the original IDEC-2B8 murine mAb.

## Table 25.2 Targeting properties of different forms of antibodies

|  | IgG | bsAb | F(ab')$_2$ | Fab' | scFv | Diabody |
|---|---|---|---|---|---|---|
| Molecular weight (kDa) | 150 | 300 | 100 | 50 | 20 | 40 |
| Complement activation | Yes | Yes | No | No | No | No |
| ADCC | Yes | Yes | No | No | No | No |
| Blood half-life | 1–3 d | 1–3 d | ~ 1 d | ~ 3 h | ~ 1 h | ~ 1 h |
| Accumulation in | Liver | Liver | Liver | Kidney | Kidney | Kidney |
| Tumor penetration | Low | Low | Better | Good | Best | Good |

bsAb, bispecific antibody; scFv, single-chain antibody; diabody, bispecific scFv; ADCC, antibody-dependent cell-mediated cytotoxicity

## Table 25.3 Nomenclature for therapeutic monoclonal antibodies

| Suffix to generic name | Origin |
|---|---|
| -umab | Human |
| -zumab | Humanized |
| -ximab | Chimeric |
| -omab | Murine |
| -amab | Rat |
| -emab | Hamster |
| -imab | Primate |

# Serotherapy with unconjugated monoclonal antibodies

Despite their intellectual appeal, the initial therapeutic efficiency of unmodified tumor-reactive mAbs has been disappointing. In particular, the results of clinical studies in patients with solid tumors have shown little efficacy. In contrast to the disappointing results in carcinomas, however, some limited success had been reported with tumor-reactive antibodies in non-Hodgkin lymphoma (NHL), acute myeloid leukemia (AML), and T-cell leukemias. The first lymphoma patient was treated in 1979 by the group of Nadler and Schlossman.[14] Despite the presence of soluble, blocking antigen in the circulation, a transient decrease in the numbers of circulating tumor cells was observed during and shortly after three infusions of the mAb. No side-effects were encountered on infusing doses up to 150 mg, and this study, despite the rather limited clinical success, pioneered the use of mAbs in the serotherapy of cancer. It is now clear that in many cases, the antibody doses employed might have been too low. Modern biotechnology and bioreactors were required to permit the gram-wise application of engineered antibodies in today's clinical studies.

Many of the early mAb trials focused on lymphoid neoplasms. mAbs capable of inducing tumor regression include mAbs to CD5, CD25, and CD52 (Campath-1) on T-cell leukemias and lymphomas, and mAbs to CD5, CD19, CD20, CD21, CD22, CD37, CD52, HLA-DR, and the surface antigen receptor (idiotype) in B-cell neoplasms (Table 25.1). CD30 is restricted to a small subset of activated T and B cells, and may serve as a target structure for the treatment of Hodgkin and anaplastic large cell or other CD30/Ki-1$^+$ lymphomas. Typical AML blasts may express the following surface markers: HLA-DR, CD45, CD33, CD34, CD13, CD15, and CD14, which can serve as targets for mAb therapy (Table 25.1). Efforts have therefore been made to also treat myeloid leukemias through this approach. The remarkable potency of these agents to kill leukemia and lymphoma cells has been demonstrated in trials of conjugated and unconjugated mAbs (see below).

## Effector functions of mAbs

Unless the targeted structure is critical for the survival of the cell or for its proliferation, such as a growth factor or cell death receptor, binding of the antibody alone is not cytotoxic. There is considerable experimental and some clinical evidence that the nature of the antitumor response thereby largely depends on the ability of the mAb to activate immunological mechanisms (Figure 25.3). These are mainly complement-mediated cell lysis and antibody-dependent cell-mediated cytotoxicity (ADCC). They are determined by the antibody isotype: human or humanized IgM, IgG1, IgG2, and IgG3 can efficiently activate the complement cascade, leading to pore formation in the mAb-coated cell. Complement is a central component of the innate immune system involved in protection against pathogens. It induces death of targets either indirectly by attracting and activating phagocytes or directly by formation of a membrane pore, the membrane attack complex (MAC). Antibody-targeted cells may escape, however, from complement lysis through upregulation of the CD55 and CD59 receptors that play a role in inactivation of complement on antibody-targeted cells.[15] Thus, induction of CD55 and CD59 has recently been

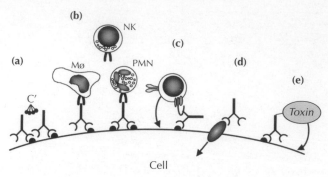

**Figure 25.3** Effector mechanisms of mAbs. (a) Activation of the complement cascade (C′), which leads to the insertion of pore-forming channels in the cell membrane and lysis of the target cell. (b) Antibody-dependent cell-mediated cytotoxicity (ADCC): granulocytes (polymorphonuclear cells, PMN), monocytes/macrophages (Mø), and natural killer cells (NK) can bind to mAb-coated tumor cells via Fc receptors and kill them. (c) Targeting of T cells by bispecific mAbs leads to polyclonal, T-cell receptor-independent T-cell activation and target cell lysis. (d) Direct negative signaling by mAbs via activation of a signaling cascade upon binding to a surface receptor (growth arrest, apoptosis). (e) Killing of the target cell by toxins or radionuclides bound to the mAb, which is only used as a carrier to specifically target the cytotoxic compound to the tumor cell.

observed to correlate with failure of the anti-CD20 mAb rituximab to clear chronic lymphocytic leukemia (CLL) cells from the circulation.[16]

Binding of IgG isotypes, especially IgG1, IgG2, and IgG3, can attract Fc-receptor-bearing cells such as natural killer (NK) cells, granulocytes, and macrophages, which can then lyse the target cell (Figure 25.4). Differences, however, exist with regard to the species origin of the mAbs (e.g. murine, rat, or human). In

particular, murine IgG1 mAbs bind little, if at all, to Fc receptors and do not activate complement (Figure 25.5).

More recently, it has been recognized that complement may cause other 'non-classical' effects that may not be aimed directly at the killing of pathogens. Products of complement activation collaborate with the adaptive immune system to enhance responses to antigens. The MAC of complement, apart from lysing cells, can also trigger diverse events in target cells, including cell activation, proliferation, resistance to subsequent complement attack, and either resistance to or induction of apoptosis.[17] Moreover, attraction of phagocytes for ADCC either by bound antibodies or complement products results in induction of apoptosis in the affected target cell.[18] This is mediated either through direct triggering of apoptosis by death-inducing ligands on the surface of the immune effector cell or by releasing apoptosis-promoting enzymes such as granzyme B into the target cell through channels formed by perforins. This indicates that antibody effector functions are more complex than previously believed.

## Signaling functions of antibodies

Some tumor cells can produce growth factors that can bind to the corresponding receptors on the same or neighboring cells. The blocking of such autocrine or paracrine loops leads to cell cycle arrest or apoptosis (programmed cell death: Figure 25.6). Targeting the low-affinity interleukin-2 receptor (IL-2R) α chain (CD25) in T-cell malignancies or the IL-6 in multiple myeloma can disrupt autocrine or paracrine tumor cell stimulation both in vitro and in animal models. In adult T-cell leukemia (ATL) the infusion of anti-CD25 mAbs results in a significant rate of complete responses (CR) or partial responses (PR).[19] In multiple myeloma, recent evidence suggests that an IL-6-like

| Humanized mAbs: | IgG1 | IgG2 | IgG3 | IgG4 | IgM (pentameric) |
|---|---|---|---|---|---|
| Complement fixation | +++ | + | ++ | − | ++++ |
| Fc-receptor binding (ADCC) | ++ | (+) | ++ | (+) | − |

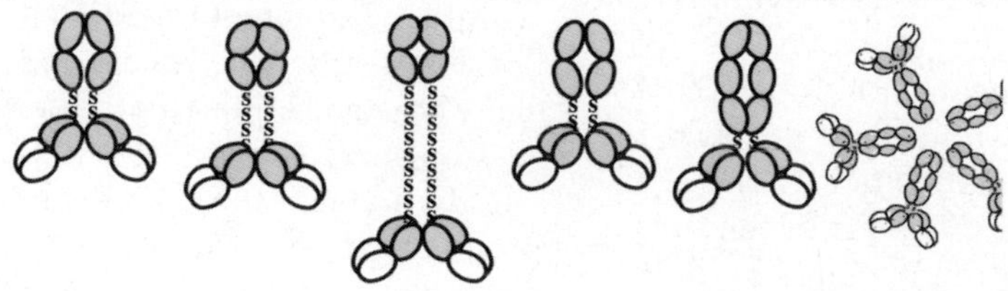

| Murine mAbs | IgG1 | IgG2a | IgG2b | IgG3 | IgM |
|---|---|---|---|---|---|
| Complement fixation | − | + | ++ | (+) | +++ |
| Fc-receptor binding (ADCC) | − | + | − | + | − |

**Figure 25.4** Activation of complement and ADCC by human or murine mAb isotypes.

| | Human Ab | | | | Murine Ab | | | |
|---|---|---|---|---|---|---|---|---|
| | IgG1 | IgG2 | IgG3 | IgG4 | IgG1 | IgG2a | IgG3b | IgG3 |
| CD64 (high-affinity RI) | + | − | + | (+) | − | + | − | + |
| CD32 (medium-affinity RII) | + | (+) | + | (+) | − | − | + | − |
| CD16 (low-affinity RIII) | + | − | + | − | (+) | + | − | + |

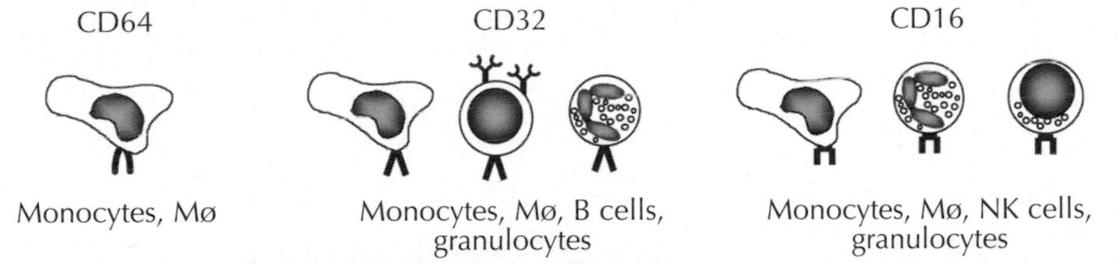

**Figure 25.5** Affinity of human and murine Abs for different Fc receptor (FcR) classes. Expression of CD16 (FcRIII), CD32 (FcRII), and CD64 (FcRI) by cells that can mediate (ADCC) is indicated.

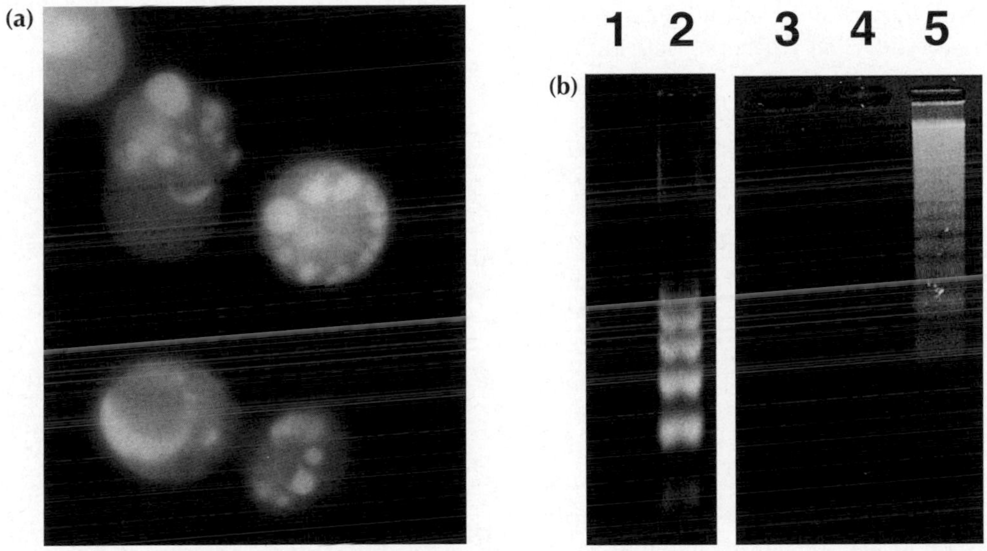

CD64 — Monocytes, Mø

CD32 — Monocytes, Mø, B cells, granulocytes

CD16 — Monocytes, Mø, NK cells, granulocytes

**Figure 25.6** Induction of apoptosis (programmed cell death) by antibodies against surface receptors. Apoptosis-inducing antibodies often mimick natural ligands, and mAbs against some surface receptors can trigger a death signaling cascade. Examples of this phenomenon are mAbs against the antigen receptors of B (or T) cells and the CD95 (APO-1/Fas) receptor. Apoptosis leads to destruction of the cell and is accompanied by chromatin condensation and DNA fragmentation to oligonucleosomal fragments. (a) Apoptosis of BL41 Burkitt lymphoma cells 16 hours after triggering with an anti-IgM mAb. DNA was visualized by ultraviolet light after acridine orange staining. Instead of a homogeneous staining, the nuclei show a patchy texture due to chromatin condensation and nuclear fragmentation. (b) Oligonucleosomal fragmentation of the genomic DNA (so-called DNA ladder). Low-molecular-weight (fragmented) DNA was prepared after hypotonic lysis of apoptotic cells and was separated by agarose gel electrophoresis. BL41 cells were triggered for apoptosis by antigen receptor (surface IgM) crosslinking for 24 hours (lane 1, medium control; lane 2, anti-IgM Ab). Jurkat T cells were triggered for apoptosis by anti-CD95 mAb for 16 hours (lane 3, medium control; lane 4, IgG3 control mAb; lane 5, anti-CD95 (clone anti-APO-1 IgG3κ).

cytokine is produced by virally infected bone marrow stroma cells and stimulates plasma cell growth and survival. Stimulation via the IL-6R could thus be the causative agent for the disease as previously suggested.[20] Disappointingly, the use of an anti-IL-6R mAb in a phase I study in seven patients with multiple myeloma did not lead to a significant clinical response.[21] Interestingly, myeloma cell proliferation was clearly decreased, indicating that IL-6 inhibition eventually might show efficacy in the future. Notably, the dose of the mAb was low in this study and only 20 mg per day were applied over a 12-day period. In another study, 11 myeloma patients were injected with 10–40 mg anti-IL-6 mAb: 1 had a PR and 7 showed stable disease.[22] In both studies, low-grade fever resolved and C-reactive protein (CRP) levels decreased, showing that the mAb was able to specifically block some IL-6-mediated effects. Clinical studies are underway to determine the clinical efficacy of IL-6 inhibition either by antibodies or pharmacological inhibitors of IL-6R signal transduction.

Antibody binding can also lead to direct negative signaling. This has been investigated in great detail with antibodies directed against the antigen receptors of normal and malignant T or B cells. Thus, anti-idiotypic but also plain anti-IgM or anti-IgD antibodies can mimic the natural ligand of the surface immunoglobulins, i.e. the antigen, and lead to cell cycle arrest in $G_1$ phase. Negative signaling for growth of B-NHL cells also can be exerted through antibodies against CD19, CD20, and the TAPA antigen. These molecules associate with the antigen receptor (e.g. surface IgM or IgD), and crosslinking them by mAbs mediates signal transduction events such as calcium fluxes, activation of receptor-associated kinases (Fyn, Lyn, and Blk), and activation of the mitogen-associated protein kinase (MAPK) cascade. Both animal experiments and clinical data show that antibodies directed against surface immunoglobulin, CD19, or CD20 can lead to tumor regression, and experimental evidence suggests that this is due to negative signaling (e.g. cell cycle arrest). Most likely, however, the immunological mechanisms described above contribute to the growth inhibition in vivo, and careful selection of the antibody isotype might increase the therapeutic effect.[23]

In this vein, the direct induction of apoptosis by a tumor cell-reactive mAb is one of the most interesting developments and is a result of signal transduction events delivered by mimicking physiological ligands by the mAb. This has been demonstrated for mAbs directed against the antigen receptors of malignant T- or B-lymphoid cells, including anti-idiotypic mAbs[24–26] (Figure 25.6 – compare Figure 25.11). Other apoptosis-promoting molecules include the T-cell receptor-associated CD3-antigen ε-chain, the MHC class II molecules, CD20, CD30, CD52, and the CD95 (APO-1/Fas) molecule[12,23,25,27–29] (Figure 25.6).

## Obstacles in antibody therapy

Further issues for mAb therapy are mainly of pharmakokinetic and pharmakodynamic nature. Early studies indicated that neutralization of therapeutic antibodies may occur by HAMA/HACA (human anti-chimera antibody) humoral immune responses. Interestingly, the broad clinical use of chimeric antibodies such as the anti-CD20 chimeric antibody rituximab clearly demonstrated that HACA responses are limited in lymphoma patients and do not affect the clinical efficacy of rituximab.[30] Likewise, the occurrence of HAMA responses in up to 60% of patients treated with the entirely murine antibodies [131]I-tositumomab or [90]Y-ibritumomab tiuxetan or other radiolabeled murine antibodies does not appear to affect clinical efficacy or result in high percentages of hypersensitivity reactions.[31] This may be due to the high doses of the foreign protein and the fact that lymphoma patients are often immunocompromised. One of the major obstacles is, however, the insufficient tumor penetration of the large mAbs (150 kDa), particularly into bulky tumors. This furthermore depends on the mAb isotype, affinity, and epitope density on the target cell.[23] In addition, a pressure gradient from the core to the periphery of tumors and insufficient tumor vascularization makes it difficult for drugs and mAbs to reach the cells in the tumor core (Table 25.4). Thus, in high-affinity mAbs, the majority of the mAb may be absorbed around the initial tumor cell layers surrounding the supplying blood vessels.[32] This insufficient tumor tissue penetration may severely affect the clinical efficacy, as observed in the case of the anti-CD19 antibody anti-B4 coupled to a ricin toxin.[33] Tumor cell heterogeneity is another problem, and selection of clones that express low antigen density or even of antigen-negative clones can occur. Furthermore, tumor cells can evade the mAb by shedding the antigen, as in the case of the CD25 and CD30 antigens. This has been observed in ATL cells, where the CD25 antigen can be found in large quantities in the circulation.[19,34] In contrast, the CD19 antigen, a pan-B-cell marker, is not released from the cell surface.[32] Resistance to host

---

**Table 25.4 Difficulties encountered in serotherapy with monoclonal antibodies (mAbs)**

**Delivery**
- Non-specific binding of the mAb to normal tissue
- Absorbance of the mAb by shedded antigen
- Downmodulation of the tumor antigen by mAb binding
- Inactivation by neutralizing antibodies (HAMA)
- Inefficient penetration of the mAb macromolecules into bulky tumors
- Absorption of the mAb in the first tumor cell layers surrounding the blood vessels
- Short half-life of some antibodies

**Tumor cell evasion**
- Inefficient host cytotoxic mechanisms (complement, ADCC)
- Tumor cell resistance to host cytotoxic mechanisms
- Lack or heterogeneity of tumor antigen expression
- Selection of tumor cell clones with mutated epitopes

**Toxicity**
- Allergic reactions, serum sickness
- Targeting of host cytotoxicity towards non-malignant tissue
- Direct toxicity to normal cells

immune mechanisms such as complement lysis has been described in vitro, e.g. as a consequence of upregulation of endogenous complement-inhibitory receptors such as CD55 and CD59.[16]

# Clinical use of unlabeled antibodies

In clinical studies, a humanized chimeric anti-CD20 antibody (rituximab) has now been established as a complement to classical chemotherapy in low- and high-grade B-NHL.[35] Notably, the vast majority of the more or less positive data on the clinical efficacy of rituximab are derived from phase I/II trials. Evidence from prospective phase III trials where rituximab alone or rituximab plus chemotherapy were compared with standard regimens is unfortunately still scarce despite the fact that an estimated over 50 000 patients worldwide have been treated with rituximab.

The human CD20 antigen shows lineage-specific expression on all B lymphocytes except plasma cells, pro-B precursor B cells, and hematopoetic stem cells. It is found in high density on the surface of most NHL and does not shed into the serum. CD20 is a non-glycosylated phosphoprotein that is essential for regulation of growth and differentiation of activated B cells. Crosslinking of CD20 by rituximab triggers calcium fluxes that result in growth arrest in $G_1$ phase of the

cell cycle and trigger apoptosis in targeted B cells (Figure 25.7). In addition, ADCC and complement lysis have been described as effector mechanisms (reviewed in reference 36). There is an ongoing discussion as to which of these mechanisms is the major one determining the clinical efficacy of rituximab (or that of other mAbs).

A phase I/II study in 166 patients (median age 58 years, 151 patients evaluable) with low-grade B-NHL in relapse after prior polychemotherapy showed an overall response of 48%, including 10 patients (6%) with a CR, with a median time to progression of 13 months in responders. Patients received 375 mg rituximab as a single agent weekly for 4 weeks. The mAb infusion led to a rapid B-cell depletion, which recovered 9–12 months after therapy and did not result in a major decrease in IgM/IgG levels or increased susceptibility to infection. No neutralizing HAMAs were observed and only 3 patients developed HACA. The majority of adverse events occurred during the first infusion and were grade 1 or 2; fever and chills were the most common events. Only 12% of patients had grade 3 and 3% grade 4 toxicities.[37] These results are comparable to those obtained in historic controls with the use of the nucleoside analogs fludarabine and cladribine.

High-grade B-NHL shows a similar density of the CD20 antigen as compared with follicular lymphoma. Rituximab as a single agent was employed in first-line

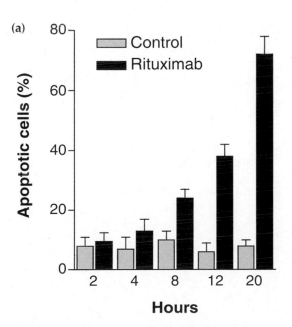
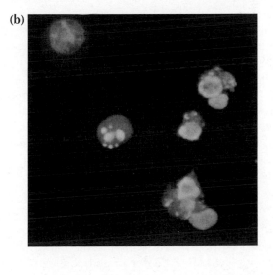

**Figure 25.7** Induction of apoptosis by the anti-CD20 mAb rituximab. BL41 Burkitt lymphoma cells were incubated in the presence of rituximab or an isotype-matched control antibody immobilized by coating of the mAbs to the plastic of the culture dish. Rituximab, but not the control antibody, induced apoptosis, as determined by flow-cytometric measurement of genomic DNA fragmentation. (a) Percentages of cells with a hypodiploid DNA content are shown. Apoptosis started to be detectable at 8 hours and reached a maximum at 20-hour culture with rituximab. (b) Apoptotic morphology of rituximab-treated BL41 cells was visualized by staining of cellular DNA with acridine orange under ultraviolet light. The upper left of the photograph shows a non-apoptotic cell with intact nucleus and homogeneously distributed chromatin.

therapy in elderly patients above 60 years of age or as second- or third-line therapy in younger patients in first or second relapse. This randomized multicenter phase I/II trial compared eight cycles of weekly rituximab at 375 mg/m² with one cycle at 375 mg/m² followed by seven weekly cycles at 500 mg/m². There was a slight tendency for more pronounced adverse reactions in the higher-dose arm and, as expectable, no difference regarding the therapeutic efficacy.[38] Of the 54 patients, 9% achieved a CR and 31% a PR. These response rates are concordant with those observed in the plethora of additional, more or less uninformative, phase I/II trials that can be found in the literature.

Interestingly, there is evidence that lymphoma subtypes may respond differently to such anti-CD20 treatment. In low-grade lymphoma, good overall response rates of approximately 50% were seen in follicular lymphoma, whereas immunocytoma with lymphoplasmacytoid differentiation showed a far worse response. This may be due to differences in the level of CD20 expression. Notably, another phase I/II study in 70 patients with therapy-refractory follicular lymphoma demonstrated that pretreatment status matters, as the highest number of responders (80%) was found in patients who had received only one prior course of chemotherapy.[39] This indicates that chemotherapy utilizes similar effector mechanisms as rituximab and that prior chemotherapies may select for resistance to antibody therapy. In line with other studies and in contrast to other NHL subtypes, immunocytoma showed an overall response rate of 28% among 28 patients, and in B-CLL a rate of only 14% among 29 patients.[39] A rather interesting phase II trial investigated the efficacy of retreatment with rituximab in patients with low-grade or follicular NHL who relapsed after a response to rituximab therapy. The overall response rate in 57 assessable patients was 40% (11% CR and 30% PR). The median time to progression (TTP) in responders and the median duration of response (DR) as estimated by Kaplan–Meier analyses were 17.8 months and 16.3 months (range 3.7+ to 25.1 months), respectively.[40]

Better results as compared with rituximab monotherapy can be obtained when rituximab is combined with conventional chemotherapy.[41] In fact, in vitro studies demonstrated that rituximab sensitizes B-lymphoma cells to drug-induced apoptosis.[42] This is very similar to the anti-HER2/*neu* antibody trastuzumab (Herceptin), which sensitizes breast carcinoma cells to anthracycline-induced cell death.[43] Upon ligation of CD20, rituximab activates the mitochondrial pathway of apoptosis,[44] which mediates the final demise of the targeted cell through a caspase-3-dependent pathway.[45] Anticancer drugs depend critically on the same mitochondrial cell death pathway. Thus, the molecular basis for the synergism between rituximab and anti-

cancer drugs appears to be lowering of the threshold for mitochondrial activation in apoptosis.

A phase II trial in newly diagnosed or relapsed low-grade lymphoma yielded a CR in 58% and a PR in 42% of the patients when CHOP (cyclophosphamide, doxorubicin, vincristine, and prednisone) was combined with rituximab for six cycles every 3 weeks. Rituximab was administered prior to CHOP and did not increase toxicity when compared to historic controls. Remissions were sustained, with 74% of the patients remaining in remission at 29 months.[46] This favorable effect of combined rituximab/CHOP was also established by a large randomized multicenter trial by the Groupe d'Etude des Lymphomes de l'Adult (GELA) in elderly patients with high-grade B-NHL (Figure 25.8). Previously untreated patients with diffuse large B-cell lymphoma, 60–80 years old, were randomized to receive either an optimal 'standard' regimen of eight cycles of CHOP every 3 weeks (197 patients) or eight cycles of CHOP plus rituximab given on day 1 of each cycle (202 patients). This trial clearly established a significantly higher rate of CR of

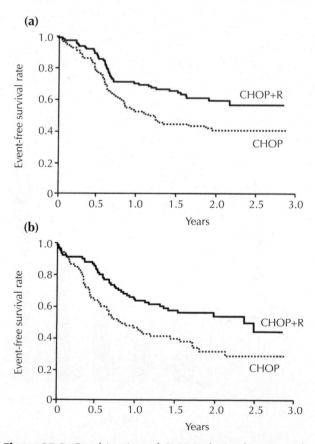

**Figure 25.8** Combination of CHOP chemotherapy with rituximab in first-line therapy of high-grade B-NHL. Patients received either eight cycles of CHOP or eight cycles of CHOP plus rituximab (CHOP+R). CHOP+R-treated patients showed a significantly better event-free survival. This was apparent in patients younger or older than 70 years (a and b, respectively). Adapted from reference 47.

76% in the group that received CHOP plus rituximab as compared with the group that received CHOP alone (63% CR). Both event-free and overall survival times were significantly higher in the CHOP-plus-rituximab group during a median 2-year follow-up. Notably, clinically relevant toxicities were not significantly greater with CHOP plus rituximab. This indicates that the addition of rituximab to the CHOP regimen increases CR rates and prolongs event-free and overall survival in elderly patients with diffuse large B-cell lymphoma, without a clinically significant increase in toxicity.[47] Nevertheless, it remains to be established whether these remissions are durable and really result in sustained prolongation of event-free survival. In this context, a promising finding is the propensity of this immunochemotherapy regimen to overcome resistance as a consequence of *bcl-2* overexpression in this patient cohort.[48]

In contrast, rituximab does not improve response rates and duration of remission in low-grade B-NHL patients treated with interferon-α2a (IFN-α2a).[49] Nevertheless, promising data were generated in low-grade B-NHL in a randomized phase III study by the German Low-Grade Lymphoma Study Group. This trial evaluated rituximab in combination with FCM (fludarabine, cyclophosphamide, and mitoxantrone) in a randomized setting versus FCM alone in patients with relapsed or refractory follicular, mantle cell, or lymphoplasmacytic lymphoma. An interim analysis of 94 evaluable patients demonstrated a significantly higher response rate for rituximab plus FCM (overall response rate, ORR 83%; CR rate 35%) as compared with FCM alone (ORR 58%; CR rate 13%), with no increase in toxicity. Superiority of rituximab plus FCM was seen both in follicular lymphoma (*n*=53; ORR 92% versus 75%; CR rate 40% versus 21%) and, most strikingly, in mantle cell lymphoma (*n*=38; ORR 65% versus 33; CR rate 35% versus 0%). Moreover, a trend towards longer overall and disease-free survival for rituximab plus FCM was reported.[50]

In contrast, the efficacy of rituximab is low in immunocytoma and quite limited in B-CLL.[39,51] Of 28 patients treated with four intravenous infusions of rituximab 375 mg/m$^2$ over 4 weeks, only 7 responded with a PR.[52] This may very well be due to the generally lower expression of CD20 in B-CLL as compared with follicular and high-grade lymphomas such as diffuse large B-cell lymphoma. Moreover, toxicities are in general more pronounced in B-CLL, probably as a consequence of the large number of circulating malignant B cells. Thus, in particular, CLL patients with high peripheral blood B-cell counts are prone to potentially lethal tumor lysis syndrome accompanied by fever, chills, nausea, seizure and thrombocytopenia. Such syndromes may arise following the secretion of tumor necrosis factor α (TNF-α), IFN-γ and IL-6 upon the first infusion of rituximab.[53] It remains to be established whether the addition of conventional

chemotherapy such as nucleoside analogs may improve these so-far unsatisfactory results. A recent phase II study indicates in fact that such a combination with fludarabine shows increased efficacy in B-CLL. The overall response rate (CR + PR) was 87% (27 of 31 evaluable patients). Of 20 previously untreated patients, 17 (85%) responded. Of 31 patients, 10 achieved a CR (5 of 20 untreated, 5 of 11 pretreated, 9 of 21 Binet stage B, and 1 of 10 Binet stage C). The median duration of response was 75 weeks. Given this so-far limited success, a recent trial employed repetitive courses of four cycles of weekly rituximab at 375 mg/m$^2$ that were given in 6-month intervals in responding patients. By using this maintenance treatment approach in 44 patients, an overall response rate of 58% with 9% CR was obtained (28 patients received one or more additional courses).[54] There is, however, no evidence from randomized trials available that would support the usefulness of such a maintenance therapy.

A reason for concern regarding the clinical use of rituximab is the prolonged impairment of antibody production, leading to an increased risk of viral and bacterial infections. Pure red blood cell aplasia due to parvovirus B19 infection has been reported after administration of rituximab,[55] as have acute viral hepatitis B[56] and bacterial pneumonia.[57] Nevertheless, this profound suppression of humoral immune responses has recently been recognized as a therapeutic feature that is now successfully exploited in immunosuppressive regimens in autoimmune diseases (see below).

An antibody approach more suitable to B-CLL may come from the revival of the anti-CD52 mAb alemtuzumab (Campath-1H, humanized rat IgG1). CD52 is highly expressed on over 95% of peripheral blood lymphocytes and monocytes and in the majority of T- and B-cell neoplasias. Low-level expression is found on granulocytes, and hematopoeitic stem cells are void of CD52. The physiological function of CD52 on these cell types remains so far enigmatic. The mechanism of action of Campath-1 is based on complement activation and ADCC.

Studies performed in the late 1980s showed a rather limited effect of Campath-1 in various B-cell malignancies, depending on the isotype (IgG2a or IgM).[58] The first two patients with advanced NHL treated with humanized alemtuzumab both showed a PR.[59] Likewise, 11 of 15 T-prolymphocytic lymphoma (T-PLL) patients treated with alemtuzumab achieved a PR.[60] In low-grade NHL, a multicenter phase II trial applied alemtuzumab in 50 patients at 30 mg intravenously three times per week over 12 weeks, and showed a CR in only 4% and a PR in 16% of the patients. It became apparent, however, that, apart from fever and chills in 80% of the patients, alemtuzumab therapy is associated with a very significant risk of hematologic toxicities: 28% of patients showed grade 3–4 neutropenia and 22% grade 3–4 thrombocytopenia. In addition, a long-lasting lymphopenia was induced by alemtuzumab treatment. The latter is the underlying reason for the high rate of severe infectious complications, including viral and fungal infections, with 28% of the patients developing pneumonitis. As in the case of rituximab, this feature is now used in immunosuppressive therapies, and in the control of graft-versus-host disease (GVHD: see below).

Other phase II studies with alemtuzumab showed similar response rates and spectra of severe complications. Especially in B-CLL, higher response rates were observed: 29 patients who had relapsed after an initial response ($n = 8$) or were refractory to chemotherapy ($n = 21$) were treated with alemtuzumab administered intravenously 30 mg three times a week for a maximum period of 12 weeks. Eleven patients (38%) achieved a PR and one (4%) a CR. Three of 8 patients (38%) with a relapse and 9 of 21 refractory patients (43%) responded to alemtuzumab therapy. CLL cells were rapidly eliminated from blood in 28 of 29 patients (97%). CR in the bone marrow was obtained in 36% and splenomegaly resolved completely in 32%.[61] These results are supported by a more recent phase II trial in CLL first-line therapy.[62] This phase II study determined the efficacy and safety of alemtuzumab over a prolonged treatment period of 18 weeks in 41 patients with symptomatic B-CLL. Injections were administered subcutaneously three times a week. An overall response rate of 87% (with a CR in 19% and a PR in 68%) was achieved in 38 evaluable patients. CLL cells were cleared from the blood in 95% of patients in a median time of 21 days. CR or nodular PR in the bone marrow was observed in 66% of the patients and most patients achieved this after 18 weeks of treatment. Notably, a 87% overall response rate (with a CR in 29%) was established in the lymph nodes. Transient injection site skin reactions were seen in 90% of patients. Rigor, rash, nausea, dyspnea, and hypotension were, however, rare or absent. Transient grade 4 neutropenia developed in 21% of the patients. Infections were rare, mainly due to cotrimoxazole prophylaxis, but 10% of patients developed cytomegalovirus (CMV) reactivation. Thus, alemtuzumab is highly effective as first-line treatment in patients with B-CLL, but requires caution in view of the impressive immunosupression by this compound.

### More antibodies to come . . .

In addition to antibodies against CD20 and CD52, a variety of antibodies are currently being developed for the treatment of T- and B-NHL and lymphoid and myeloid leukemias. CD22 is a 135 kDa B-cell-restricted sialoglycoprotein present in the cytoplasm of virtually all B-lineage cells but expressed on the B-cell surface only at mature stages of differentiation. CD22 expression is high in follicular mantle and marginal zone B cells and weak in germinal center B cells. In B-cell malignancies, CD22 expression ranges from 60% to 80%, depending on the histological type and on the assays used. The function of the CD22 molecule is uncertain, although recent studies have suggested roles for the molecule both as a component of the B-cell activation complex and as an adhesion molecule. After binding to antibodies, CD22 is rapidly internalized. This provides a potent costimulatory signal in primary B-cells and proapoptotic signals in neoplastic B cells. In preclinical studies, CD22 has been shown to be an effective target for immunotherapy of B-cell malignancies using either naked, unconjugated or toxin-labeled or radiolabeled mAbs.[63] Clinical trials in patients with low- and high-grade NHL are now ongoing with a humanized unconjugated anti-CD22 antibody (epratuzumab) used as single agent or in combination with other mAbs (e.g. rituximab) and/or chemotherapy. Preliminary data from these studies has shown that such approaches are effective and well-tolerated.

Newer antibodies in development as single agents and in combinations include apolizumab (Hu1D10), a humanized antibody against an epitope of HLA-DR, and IDEC-152, a primatized anti-CD23 antibody. BL22, anti-CD22 immunotoxin with impressive activity in hairy cell leukemia, is in phase II trials in CLL as well. Antibodies employed in the treatment of solid tumors are discussed separately (see below).

## Immunotoxins

Because of the low intrinsic cytotoxicity of most mAbs, antibody–toxin conjugates (immunotoxins) have been constructed (reviewed in reference 64). Conventional immunotoxins are capable of inducing responses in patients with hematological malignancies, with dose-limiting toxicities being thrombocytopenia, hepatic damage, and especially vascular leak syndrome.[65] The latter is characterized by an increase in vascular permeability accompanied by extravasation of fluids and proteins and resulting in interstitial edema and organ failure. Manifestations include fluid retention, increase in body weight, peripheral edema, pleural and pericardial effusions, ascites, anasarca, and, in severe forms, signs of pulmonary and cardiovascular failure. Symptoms are highly variable among patients. The pathogenesis of vascular leak syndrome is poorly understood, but involves both direct damage to endothelial cells by the toxin and release of cytokines and of inflammatory mediators by targeted leukocytes that lead to alterations in cell–cell and cell–matrix adhesion and cytoskeletal function of vascular endothelial cells. Vascular leakage is the major dose-limiting toxicity in immunotoxin therapy and, in some cases, necessitates the cessation of therapy.

Newer immunotoxins contain a recombinant ligand, either the variable domains (Fv) of a mAb or a growth factor, fused to a truncated bacterial toxin. The antibody portion of the immunotoxin is used to focus the toxin specifically to the targeted cell population. The cytotoxic effect of the immunotoxin therefore does not rely on the activation of immune helper mechanisms or of growth-inhibitory or apoptosis-inducing signaling. The mAb is only used as a vehicle to target the toxin to the tumor cell. Conjugates with potent toxins have been produced either by chemical crosslinking or, more recently, by genetically engineered recombinant fusion proteins with scFvs. Genetically engineered immunotoxins have been proven to be more potent as compared with the chemical production procedure. Using a similar approach, toxins have been fused to non-antibody-derived ligands such as cytokines that may be employed to target the toxin to cytokine receptor-expressing tumor cells (e.g. the IL-2R). Recombinant fusion toxins have several potential advantages over conventional immunotoxin chemical conjugates, including (1) a defined toxin–ligand junction; (2) efficient and relatively inexpensive production on a large scale from bacteria; (3) shorter plasma half-lives, which might avoid the diffuse endothelial damage that leads to vascular leak syndrome; and (4) the ability to genetically engineer mutations in the recombinant toxin to increase its potency or lower its non-specific toxicity.

The two major varieties of recombinant fusion toxins are growth factor fusion toxins, containing a growth factor fused to a truncated toxin, and recombinant immunotoxins, containing the Fv domains of an antibody fused to a truncated toxin. In either case, the ligand is used to bind selectively to tumor cells while the toxin kills the target cell following internalization.[66]

The toxins employed in most conjugates are Diphtheria toxin, Pseudomonas exotoxin, the plant-derived ricin, and, more recently, the bacterial toxin calicheamicin. Most toxins possess domains specific for cell binding (B chain), toxin translocation (B chain), and toxic activity (A chain). Ricin tends to bind via its B chain to galactose carbohydrate moieties expressed on most cell types.[67] Therefore, to prevent non-specific binding to untargeted tissue, so-called 'blocked' ricin is produced in which blocking affinity ligands are attached to the ricin B chain. This has been proven advantageous over the removal of the B chain from the toxin, since the translocation-mediating B-chain moieties and consequently higher biological activity are retained in the complex.

Nanogram quantities of the pure toxin would be lethal to the patient if not bound to a targeting moiety, for example an antibody, an scFv fragment, or a growth factor, to target it directly to a specific tumor cell. This also implies that only mAbs with low cross-reactivity with normal tissues are selected for the generation of immunotoxins.

In contrast to antibody therapy with unconjugated mAbs, it is advantageous in the case of immunotoxins that the target antigen be internalized together with the bound immunotoxin. This allows the toxin component to exert action. In the case of Diphtheria toxin and Pseudomonas exotoxin, the mode of action is based on inhibition of protein synthesis and ATP depletion through ADP ribosylation, which inactivates elongation factor 2 (EF2) and turns off the transcriptional machinery of the cell. Similarly, ricin inactivates protein synthesis by disrupting N-terminal glycosidation of 28S-rRNA via the catalytically active A chain. Like Diphtheria toxin and Pseudomonas exotoxin, ricin thereby inactivates ribosomes by rendering their 60S subunit unable to bind EF2. In contrast, calicheamicin is a member of the enediyne class of antitumor antibiotics, i.e. a 'small molecule' and not a protein like the toxins described above. This toxin is therefore discussed below, in the context of drug–antibody conjugates.

Using such compounds in vitro, up to a $5 \log_{10}$ reduction of tumor cells has been reported. These immunotoxins are efficient at nanomolar concentrations in vitro and in vivo to eliminate malignant cells. In fact, while gram quantities of unlabeled mAbs have often been administered to demonstrate clinical efficacy, milligram quantities of immunotoxins can suffice to eliminate an established tumor in vivo in animal models. A major disadvantage of immunotoxins as compared with unconjugated mAbs or radiolabeled mAbs (see below) is, however, their increased immunogenicity. The macromolecular toxins are of mostly bacterial origin and therefore lead rapidly to the production of neutralizing antibodies, which may also be present prior to therapy due to vaccination (Diphtheria toxin) or natural exposure (Pseudomonas exotoxin).

Immunotoxins against CD5, CD19, CD22, and CD38 (B-NHL), against CD3, CD5, CD7, and CD25 (T-NHL), and against CD30 (anaplastic large cell NHL and Hodgkin's disease) have been successfully employed in vitro and in experimental animals in vivo to eliminate malignant cells.[64] A phase I study of a murine anti-CD22 mAb (RFB4) coupled with deglycosylated ricin A chain (dgA) in 26 patients with relapsed B-NHL showed short-term responses of 30–78 days with 1 CR and 5 PR.[68] Patients were treated for up to 24 days; vascular leak syndrome was dose-limiting and in 1 patient rhabdomyolysis was encountered. A high percentage (37%) of patients developed antibodies against the murine Ig or the dgA. Animal experiments show that the efficiency of this toxin can be increased by combination with an anti-CD19 antibody as carrier (HD37-dgA[69]). An anti-CD19-blocked ricin (anti-B4-blocked ricin) immunotoxin was administered in 12 patients as a 7-day continuous infusion during complete remission after autologous bone marrow transplantation (ABMT) for relapsed B-NHL.[70] Again, vascular leakage was dose-limiting. Anti-immunotoxin responses developed in 7 patients, but 11 of the 12 patients remained in CR 13–26 months after ABMT. Another phase I trial was conducted with daily bolus injections of the anti-B4-blocked ricin immunotoxin.[71] In this trial, 25 patients were treated with increasing immunotoxin doses for 5 days; the main toxicities were reversible elevation of aminotransferases, thrombocytopenia, and fever. One CR and two PR were observed. Nine patients developed a humoral immune response against the immunotoxin that may be directed against either the antibody component or the toxin itself. Additional adverse side-effects reported in other phase I trials with anti-B4-blocked ricin are fatigue, nausea, hypoalbuminemia, myalgia, dyspnea, and capillary leak syndrome. A later phase II trial in 16 patients with relapsed CD19+ NHL, conducted to evaluate the efficacy of anti-B4-blocked ricin when administered at the previously established maximum tolerated dose using a daily bolus for 5 consecutive days, failed to establish the clinical efficacy of this compound. Immunohistochemical analysis of tissue samples provided some insight into the low efficacy and showed poor penetration into lymphoid tissue.[33] To this end, phase II trials were undertaken in which anti-B4-blocked ricin was either combined with aggressive polychemotherapy in 25 patients with low-grade NHL[72] or as adjuvant therapy to patients in CR after ABMT for B-NHL.[73] These trials yielded interesting data regarding the efficacy of such combination regimens, but so far they have not allowed determination of the contribution of the immunotoxin. Nevertheless, such an adjuvant approach might overcome the limitations imposed by the poor tissue penetration. Apart from problems arising from pharmakokinetics, toxic side-effects of the toxins might be the limiting factor in future developments in immunotoxin-based therapeutic strategies. In the case of the dgA-conjugated anti-CD19 antibody HD37, such adverse effects that may be dose-limiting are vascular leak syndrome, aphasia, rhabdomyolysis, and acrocyanosis with reversible superficial distal digital skin necrosis in the absence of overt evidence of systemic vasculitis.[74] In fact, a phase I study in 22 patients that employed a combination regimen of dgA conjugated to mAbs directed against CD22 (RFB4-dgA) and CD19 (HD37-dgA) reported two therapy-related fatal complications.[75] So far, apart from these toxicity profiles no trial data have been published for RFB4-dgA and HD37-dgA that would allow assessment of the clinical efficacy of these interesting compounds in the therapy of B-NHL. Finally, the toxicity of dgA chain-containing immunotoxins in patients with NHL is exacerbated by prior radiotherapy, and this may affect the clinical applicability of dgA immunotoxins in pretreated patients.[76]

In contrast, denileukin diftitox (DAB389IL2, Ontak) is a recently US Food and Drug Administration (FDA)-approved growth factor fusion toxin containing human IL-2 and *Diphtheria* toxin and is effective in chemotherapy-resistant cutaneous T-cell lymphoma (CTCL). Denileukin diftitox is an IL-2R-specific ligand fusion protein that may potentially be selective for IL-2R-expressing malignancies. Its activity in the treatment of cutaneous T-cell lymphoma has established the feasibility of utilizing such a targeted therapeutic in disseminated disease with acceptable toxicity. Data from a phase I trial suggest that the definition of activity in other cancer types, including other NHL, is warranted. Denileukin diftitox and its predecessor, DAB(486)IL-2, have shown clinical activity in a variety of diseases, including B-NHL, CTCL, Hodgkin lymphoma, psoriasis, rheumatoid arthritis, and HIV infection. The highest response rates were observed in CTCL, and this became the focus of clinical trials leading to its subsequent approval by the FDA for this disease.[77] In a recent clinical trial, patients with biopsy-proven CTCL that expressed CD25 were treated with denileukin diftitox administered on 5 consecutive days every 3 weeks for up to eight cycles. Overall, 30% of the 71 patients with CTCL treated with denileukin diftitox had an objective response (20% PR; 10% CR). Adverse events consisted of flu-like symptoms (fever, chills, nausea, and myalgias/arthralgias), acute infusion-related events (hypotension, dyspnea, chest pain, and back pain), and a vascular leak syndrome with hypotension, hypoalbuminemia, and edema. In addition, 61% of the patients experienced transient elevations of hepatic aminotransferase levels, with grade 3–4 in 17%. Hypoalbuminemia occurred in 79%, including 15% with grade 3–4 toxicity.[78]

Anti-Tac(Fv)-PE38 (LMB-2) and RFB4(dsFv)-PE38 (BL22) are two recombinant immunotoxins, targeting the CD25 low-affinity IL-2R and CD22, respectively, in which Fvs of mAbs targeting these antigens are fused to truncated *Pseudomonas* exotoxin. BL22 is a recombinant *Pseudomonas* exotoxin-based immunotoxin under development by the US National Cancer Institute (NCI) for the treatment of B-cell malignancies. It is composed of the disulfide-stabilized Fv portion of the anti-CD22 antibody RFB4 genetically fused to a truncated form of *Pseudomonas* exotoxin A. It has entered phase I trials for the treatment of B-NHL.[79] Both LMB-2 and BL22 have exhibited clinical activity in patients with hematological malignancies, with less vascular leak syndrome and probably less immunogenicity than the larger conventional immunotoxin conjugates. In a phase I trial of LMB-2 in 35 patients with various hematological malignacies, one hairy cell leukemia (HCL) patient achieved a CR, which was ongoing at 20 months. Seven PR were observed in patients with CTCL, HCL, B-CLL, Hodgkin lymphoma, and ATL. Responding patients had 2–5 $\log_{10}$ reductions of circulating malignant cells, improvement in skin lesions, and regression of lymphomatous masses and splenomegaly. All four patients with HCL responded to treatment. Thus, LMB-2 has clinical activity in CD25+ hematological malignancies.[80]

Two other immunotoxins, RFT5.dgA (anti-CD25) and Ki-4.dgA (anti-CD30) were assessed in Hodgkin lymphoma regarding their toxicity and clinical efficacy in phase I/II trials. The immunotoxins were constructed by linking the mAbs RFT5 or Ki-4 to dgA. Both immunotoxins showed potent specific activity against Hodgkin lymphoma cells in vitro and in vivo in animal xenotransplant models, and were subsequently evaluated in phase I/II clinical trials in humans. Of the 18 patients treated at the maximum tolerable dose of RFT5.dgA, 17 were evaluable for clinical response and showed 2 PR, 1 minor response (MR), and stable disease (SD) in 5 patients. Of 17 patients treated with Ki-4.dgA, 15 were evaluable for clinical response, and responses included 1 PR, 1 MR, and 2 SD. Toxicities were comparable to those observed in other trials with dgA immunotoxins.[81] It remains, however, to be established whether these compounds overcome the limitations observed with similar dgA immunotoxin constructs directed against CD19 in B-NHL immunotherapy.

Apart from these hallmark examples, a plethora of new recombinant immunotoxins are currently being engineered and developed to target a variety of hematological and solid tumor antigens. The impression is, however, that the efficacy of immunotoxin constructs is overall lower as compared with that of radiolabeled immunoconjugates. The reasons for this phenomenon may reside in poor tumor penetration, humoral immune responses against the toxin component, and the toxicity profiles of the employed toxins. Exceptions to this rule are, however, conjugates with calicheamicin, as evidenced by the clinical efficacy of gemtuzumab ozogamicin, an anti-CD33–calicheamicin conjugate (see below).

# Targeting of anticancer drugs by the use of antibodies

A special form of immunotoxin can be produced by linking cytostatic drugs to mAbs. Since a major advantage of the immunotoxin approach consists, however, in circumventing primary or acquired resistance mechanisms to conventional cytostatic drugs, the clinical efficacy of such a targeting of the classical anticancer compounds remains to be elucidated,

especially in view of the well-known resistance mechanisms. In contrast to drug conjugates employing conventional anticancer drugs, gemtuzumab ozogamicin, a conjugate of the bacterial toxin calicheamicin, has been successfully employed in the treatment of myeloid leukemias. Calicheamicin is a naturally occurring hydrophobic enediyne antibiotic that was isolated from *Micromonospora echinospora calichensis*.[82] It exerts potent antitumor activity and has been shown to induce apoptotic cell death in the picomolar range (Figure 25.9). Calicheamicin binds to the minor groove of the DNA helix, preferentially to the 3′ ends of oligopurine tracts, and causes sequence-selective oxidation of deoxyribose and bending of the DNA helix by an induced-fit mechanism of DNA target recognition.[83] In addition, calicheamicin and other naturally occurring enediyne antibiotics, including esperamicin, neocarcinostatin, kedarcidin, and dynemicin, constitute a unique class of reactive compounds that can undergo aromatization to produce biradicals. Phosphodiester-bond breakage of DNA was shown, however, to be dispensable for the apoptosis-inducing activity. Furthermore, prevention of apoptosis was observed in analogs that were electronically stabilized to impair aromatic rearrangements and generation of biradicals.[84] Thus, apart from enforcing a conformational change in DNA structure and the induction of DNA strand breaks, additional signaling events appear to be critically involved in the activation of apoptosis by calicheamicin and its analogs. Notably, calicheamicin induces apoptosis through a p53-independent mechanism, and this may explain part of its impressive clinical activity. Execution of apoptosis then proceeds via the mitochondrial pathway through an entirely Bax-dependent manner that is susceptible to suppression by the anti-apoptotic Bcl-2 and Bcl-x$_L$.[85] Conjugates to CD33, which is expressed on more than 90% of myeloid leukemic blasts, are currently being evaluated in the therapy of AML (reviewed in reference 86). In this line, treatment of a patient with the anti-CD33–calicheamicin immunoconjugate gemtuzumab ozogamicin (CDR-grafted humanized P67.6, CMA-676, Mylotarg) led to molecular remission of Philadelphia/*BCR–ABL*+ AML.[87] In vitro data obtained in 122 patients with relapsed AML indicate that gemtuzumab ozogamicin is rapidly and specifically targeted to CD33+ cells, followed by internalization and subsequent induction of apoptosis.[88] After evaluating a series of phase II studies, the US FDA approved gemtuzumab ozogamicin for the treatment of patients with CD33+ AML in first relapse who are 60 years of age or older and who are not considered candidates for other types of cytotoxic chemotherapy. Among 277 adult patients with CD33+ AML in first relapse, 26% experienced an overall response after gemtuzumab ozogamicin monotherapy.[89] Despite the fact that myelosuppression, hyperbilirubinemia, and elevated hepatic transaminases were commonly

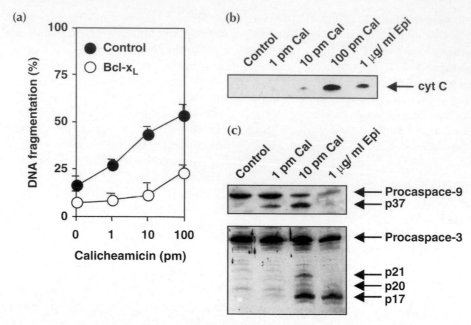

**Figure 25.9** Calicheamicin induces apoptosis via the mitochondrial pathway of apoptosis. BJAB Burkitt-like lymphoma cells (mock or Bcl-x$_L$ transfectants) were incubated in the presence or absence of calicheamicin. (a) Calicheamicin induced apoptosis readily at picomolar concentrations. Apoptosis was determined by flow-cytometric measurement of genomic DNA fragmentation. Percentages of cells with a hypodiploid DNA content are shown. Apoptosis could be inhibited by overexpression of Bcl-x$_L$, an inhibitor of mitochondrial activation and cytochrome c release during apoptosis. (b) Western blot analysis of cytosolic extracts showed that calicheamicin (Cal) induces cytochrome c (cyt c) release from mitochondria. Induction of cytochrome c release by the anthracycline epirubicin (Epi) served as a positive control. Notably, calicheamicin-induced cytochrome c release at 100 pM was more pronounced as compared with the conventional anticancer drug epirubicin at 1 $\mu$g/ml (1.72 $\mu$M). (c) Western blot analysis for caspase cleavage. Calicheamicin induces processing of the initiator caspase-9 and the executioner caspase-3, which are downstream effectors of the mitochondrial death pathway.

observed, the incidences of severe infections and mucositis were relatively low in comparison with conventional chemotherapy. Preliminary reports in pediatric patients also report gemtuzumab ozogamicin to be reasonably well tolerated and to show clinical efficacy.[90] Data from study regimens combining gemtuzumab ozogamicin and conventional chemotherapy suggest an unusually high remission induction rate in de novo AML patients.[91] More recent data indicate, however, that prior gemtuzumab ozogamicin exposure significantly increases the risk of potentially fatal hepatic veno-occlusive disease in patients who undergo myeloablative allogeneic stem cell transplantation[92] or additional chemotherapy.[93] The underlying pathological mechanism is so far unknown, but appears to be a feature of calicheamicin acting on vascular endothelial cells.

A prodrug approach in order to reach higher local anticancer drug concentrations is the mAb-mediated targeting of enzyme–mAb conjugates to tumor cells. These enzymes can produce high local cytotoxic concentrations of otherwise non-toxic compounds. An example of this is the use of horseradish peroxidase to produce high local concentrations of reactive oxygen compounds or the targeting of a prodrug-converting enzyme such as carboxypeptidase G2 or cytosine deaminase.

# Radioimmunotherapy

Radiolabeling of mAbs was an early development in immunoassay techniques. Later, it was found that mAbs also allow the specific delivery of high doses of a radiolabel to tumor cells. This can be exploited both for diagnostic immune scintigraphy and for the delivery of therapeutic radiation doses to tumor cells, i.e. radioimmunotherapy (reviewed in reference 94). Thus, radionuclides are an appropriate alternative for targeting cytotoxicity to tumor cells. In contrast to drug or toxin immunoconjugates, radiolabeled mAbs can kill cells that are not in direct contact with the mAb target and there is no need for the labeled mAb to be internalized, as in the case of immunotoxins. The killing of neighboring cells depends largely on the choice of radionuclide, for example the type of emission ($\alpha$, $\beta$, or $\gamma$), the isotope half-life, and the energy transfer. The attractive feature of radioimmunotherapy is the prospect that most normal tissues can be spared from intensive radiation. Therefore, as in the case of other mAb conjugates, the radionuclide should be linked tightly to the mAb without affecting targeting. Considerable progress has been made in the chemistry of mAb radiolabeling. Some radionuclides (e.g. iodine) can be conjugated directly to the mAb, while others are linked by an intermediary group, such as chelators for radiometals.

Each radionuclide decays at a specific rate and releases particular radioactive emissions. The β decay from iodine-131 ($^{131}$I) travels a relatively short distance of less than 1 mm. Other β-emitting isotopes, such as yttrium-90 ($^{90}$Y), have a higher maximum energy and diffuse their radiation effect over a larger distance within tissues, showing path lengths of several millimeters. Moreover, $^{90}$Y offers several advantages over $^{131}$I, since radiometals such as $^{90}$Y are better retained within target cells after cellular internalization of antigen–antibody complexes. Because $^{90}$Y is a pure β emitter, large doses can be given safely in an outpatient setting with fewer consequences for medical personnel or patients' families. In contrast, α particles traverse much shorter distances of only 30–90 $\mu$m. They nonetheless possess an approximately ten fold higher energy and are often several thousandfold more efficient at a short range than β emitters. A single hit by an α particle to the nucleus is sufficient to kill a cell. This is also true for low-energy electrons such as those emitted by $^{125}$I, which deposit their energy over very short distances in the nanometer range (Table 25.5).

Phase I trials in B-NHL demonstrated that conjugates such as $^{131}$I-labeled anti-CD20, anti-CD22, anti-CD37, and anti-HLA-DR can induce tumor regression for several months. Toxicities include mainly suppression of hematopoiesis, which can last for several months.[95–98] The doses of radioactivity that can be delivered to the tumor by 'high-dose' radiolabeled mAbs are in the range of 40–50 Gy, with limited toxicity to bone marrow and other organs. Similar data were obtained with a $^{90}$Y-labeled anti-idiotype mAb in relapsed B-NHL.[99]

Significant PR and CR rates of 50–70% can be achieved by the use of radiolabeled antibodies in relapsed and even chemoresistant NHL patients. Nevertheless, early studies showed that only a few patients receiving such radioimmunotherapeutics as single agents had a disease-free survival longer than 5 years. It was therefore postulated that higher, potentially myeloablative, doses combined with bone marrow or stem cell transplantation might yield a higher rate of CR and longer disease-free survival.[100] It was suggested that such high-dose radioimmunotherapy be applied only in patients with a 'favorable'

**Table 25.5  Radionuclides employed for antibody labeling in radioimmunotherapy**

| Nuclide | Decay | Emission | Half-life | Energy (keV) | Range (mm) |
|---|---|---|---|---|---|
| Iodine-131 ($^{131}$I) | β | β | 8.02 d | 971 | 0.8 |
|  |  | γ |  | 364 |  |
| Yttrium-90 ($^{90}$Y) | β | β | 64.1 h | 2280 | 2.7 |
| Copper-67 ($^{67}$Cu) | β | β | 61.8 h | 577 | 0.4 |
|  |  | γ |  | 300 |  |
| Lutetium-177 ($^{177}$Lu) | β | β | 6.7 d | 498 | 0.3 |
|  |  | γ |  | 321 |  |
| Rhenium-186 ($^{186}$Re) | β | β | 3.7 d | 1072 | 1.1 |
|  |  | γ |  | 143 |  |
| Rhenium-188 ($^{188}$Re) | β | β | 17 h | 2120 | 2.4 |
|  |  | γ |  | 155 |  |
| Bismuth-212 ($^{212}$Bi) | α | α | 60.6 min | 6090 | ≤ 0.1 |
|  |  | γ |  | 328 |  |
|  | β | β |  | 2248 |  |
|  |  | γ |  | 727 |  |
| Bismuth-213 ($^{213}$Bi) | α | α | 45.6 min | 5869 | ≤ 0.1 |
|  |  | γ |  | 324 |  |
|  | β | β |  | 1420 |  |
|  |  | γ |  | 807 |  |
| Polonium-213 ($^{213}$Po) | α | α | 4.2 $\mu$s | 8537 | ≤ 0.1 |
|  |  | γ |  | 779 |  |

*Source:* Nuclide table at: Nuclear Data Evaluation Laboratory, Korea Atomic Energy Research Institute: http://www.kaeri.re.kr

biodistribution. Notably, the majority of patients without bulky disease, small spleen and tumor load below 500 g should show such a favorable distribution in almost all instances. This possible bias in selecting patients with a more favorable prognosis must be considered when interpreting clinical data obtained from patients treated with account taken of favorable/unfavorable biodistribution. Often, such high-dose radioimmunotherapy results in severe, long-lasting myelosuppression and should therefore be combined with (autologous) stem cell support.[101–103] Depending on the dose, onset of leuko- and thrombocytopenia occurs on day 7–10, with complete aplasia around week 2–3. At this time, remaining radioactivity has dropped to a level that permits reinfusion of bone marrow stem cells (15–20 mCi in the case of [131]I). Using such a protocol, neutrophils recover after 7–10 days, whereas thrombopenia (mostly grade 3) may persist far longer – in some cases for more than 100 days after stem cell transplantation.

The murine [90]Y-labeled IDEC-Y2B8 anti-CD20 antibody ([90]Y-ibritumomab tiuxetan, Zevalin) was the first radiolabeled antibody to obtain approval from the FDA for non-myeloablative therapy of relapsed or refractory low-grade, follicular, or transformed B-cell lymphoma, including rituximab-refractory transformed NHL.[104] Like ibritumomab tiuxetan, [131]I-tositumomab (B1, Bexxar) is a murine antibody directed against the CD20 antigen expressed on the surface of normal and malignant B lymphocytes. Recently, the FDA has approved [131]I-tositumomab for the treatment of patients with CD20+ follicular NHL whose disease is refractory to rituximab and has relapsed following chemotherapy. [131]I-Tositumomab is given according to a patient-specific dosimetric pretherapeutic study, whereas [90]Y-ibritumomab tiuxetan has been developed in such a manner that this pretherapy dosimetry is not needed, and is administered on a body-weight basis.[105] As with most drugs, there is considerable interpatient variability in the clearance rate (or total body residence time) of radioimmunoconjugates. The clearance rate of [131]I-tositumomab in clinical trials has varied by as much as fivefold. The advantage of radioimmunotherapy with [131]I, which emits both γ rays and β particles, is that by scanning it allows for the determination of the patient-specific total body residence time by the administration of a trace-labeled dose of the radionuclide (i.e. dosimetric dose). By administration of the dosimetric dose, and determination of the patient's residence time (a measure of how long the radionuclide is retained in the body), the patient-specific maximally tolerated therapeutic radiation dose is determined in order to maximize efficacy while minimizing organ and bone marrow toxicity. Both [131]I-tositumomab and [90]Y-ibritumomab tiuxetan require, however, a pretherapy cold antibody dosing in order to clear peripheral B cells and improve biodistribution of the radiolabeled antibody, i.e. to improve tumor targeting. This is achieved by infusion of unlabeled tositumomab with [131]I-tositumomab and of unlabeled rituximab prior to [90]Y-ibritumomab tiuxetan. The current [90]Y-ibritumomab tiuxetan regimen consists of pretreatment with rituximab (250 mg/m[2] intravenously) on days 1 and 8, then [90]Y-ibritumomab tiuxetan (0.4 mCi/kg intravenously, with a maximum of 32 mCi) on day 8. An imaging/dosimetry dose of indium-111 ([111]In)-labelled ibritumomab tiuxetan (5 mCi) may be injected after rituximab (day 1) for dosimetry and imaging purposes.[106]

Interestingly, both [90]Y-ibritumomab tiuxetan and [131]I-tositumomab have shown higher and more durable responses than the 'naked' antibodies, but they also have dose-limiting toxicities, predominantly myelotoxicity. Infusional adverse reactions are minimal for [131]I-tositumomab, as compared with [90]Y-ibritumomab tiuxetan, and both show minimal non-hematological toxicities, with absence of hair loss or mucositis and generally mild nausea.[107] Because of the usually high release of [131]I from [131]I-tositumomab, thyroid blockage is required. This does not, however, preclude a complication of hypothyroidism even with such blockage. Some patients have shown myelodysplasia after long-term follow-up following [131]I-tositumomab, but they were also heavily pretreated with chemotherapy, which could have contributed to this complication.[108]

In the USA, [131]I-tositumomab can now be given in most (but not all) states on an outpatient basis providing that the total effective dose equivalent to another individual from exposure to a treated patient is below 500 mrem.[109,110] [90]Y-Ibritumomab tiuxetan and other products using pure β emitters such as [90]Y can be used throughout the USA on an outpatient basis. Because [90]Y is a pure β emitter, the [90]Y-ibritumomab tiuxetan regimen is routinely administered as an outpatient procedure by using plastic shielding during the procedure. Once the radioimmunoconjugate has been administered, the risk of radiation exposure to healthcare workers and family members is minimal. The primary route of biological elimination of [90]Y-ibritumomab tiuxetan is through the urinary system, with approximately 7% of the total being activity administered being eliminated over the course of 1 week. Standard universal precautions, which should already be in place in healthcare facilities, should be sufficient to prevent radiation exposure to personnel working with patients who have been treated with [90]Y-ibritumomab tiuxetan. Written radiation safety instructions for patients are not required, but basic instructions to the patient and his or her family may help further minimize the risk of radiation exposure and help alleviate patient and family concerns.[111]

Both products have been studied predominantly as single-cycle therapy. A recent phase II trial in 30 patients with relapsed or refractory NHL yielded an overall response rate of 83% (37% CR, 6.7% CR unconfirmed, and 40% PR). Of these patients, 83% had a follicular lymphoma and 67% showed bone marrow involvement. Patients had a median of two prior therapies. The Kaplan–Meier estimated median time to progression (TTP) was 9.4 months. In responders, the Kaplan–Meier estimated median TTP was 12.6 months, with 35% of data censored. Toxicity was primarily hematological, transient, and reversible. The incidences of grade 4 neutropenia, thrombocytopenia, and anemia over 33%, 13%, and 3%, respectively. Notably, this regimen was evaluated in patients with mild thrombocytopenia (100–149 × 10$^9$ platelets.[112] A phase II trial with [131]I-tositumomab in 60 patients with chemotherapy-refractory low-grade or transformed low-grade B-NHL demonstrated an overall response in 39 patients (65% CR + PR) after [131]I-tositumomab, as compared with 17 patients (28%) achieving a PR or CR after their last chemotherapy. The median duration of response was 6.5 months after [131]I-tositumomab, as compared with 3.4 months after the last chemotherapy.[108] A multicenter single-arm study in 40 patients with follicular lymphoma showed efficacy of [131]I-tositumomab in patients who were either resistant to or relapsed after rituximab treatment. A total of 29% of the patients had a CR and the median duration of response had not been reached after a follow-up of 25 months. The results of this study were supported by demonstration of durable responses in four other single-arm studies enrolling 190 patients in rituximab-naive follicular lymphoma, where the overall response rates ranged between 47% and 64% and the median duration of response from 12 to 18 months.[113]

Phase II trials have been performed to determine the efficacy of combinations of [131]I-tositumomab and CHOP (cyclophosphamide, doxorubicin, vincristine, and prednisone) chemotherapy in follicular lymphoma: 90 patients with previously untreated, advanced-stage follicular lymphoma underwent six cycles of CHOP followed 4–8 weeks later by [131]I-tositumomab. Treatment was well tolerated; reversible myelosuppression was the main adverse event, and was more severe during CHOP chemotherapy than following radioimmunotherapy. The overall response rate to the entire treatment regimen was 90%, including 67% CR (plus unconfirmed CR) and 23% PR. Interestingly, 27 (57%) of those patients who achieved less than a CR following CHOP improved their remission status after [131]I-tositumomab. After a median follow-up of 2.3 years, the 2-year progression-free survival rate was estimated at 81%, with a 2-year overall survival rate of 97%.[114]

There is now evidence that high-dose radioimmunotherapy may be superior to 'conventional' high-dose chemotherapy, both followed by autologous peripheral blood stem cell transplantation (PBSCT). A comparison of 125 high-dose radioimmunotherapy plus PBSCT patients treated with [131]I-tositumomab (n=27) or conventional high-dose therapy (n=98) showed an improved overall and progression free survival for the high-dose radioimmunotherapy group. The estimated 5-year overall and progression-free survival rates were 67% and 48%, respectively, for high-dose radioimmunotherapy and 53% and 29%, respectively, for conventional high-dose therapy. Notably, the 100-day treatment-related mortality rate was 3.7% in the high-dose radioimmunotherapy group and 11% in the conventional high-dose therapy group.[102] Similar data are now available for relapsed mantle zone lymphoma: 16 patients received a median of three prior treatments, and 7 had chemotherapy-resistant disease. Among 11 patients with measurable disease, the CR and overall response rates were 91% and 100%, respectively. The overall survival rate at 3 years from transplantation was estimated at 93%, with a progression-free survival rate of 61%.[101]

A recent phase III randomized study compared radioimmunotherapy with [90]Y-ibritumomab tiuxetan with a control immunotherapy, rituximab, in 143 patients with relapsed or refractory low-grade, follicular, or transformed CD20+ NHL. The overall response rate was 80% for the [90]Y-ibritumomab tiuxetan group versus 56% for the rituximab group. CR rates were significantly better in the [90]Y-ibritumomab tiuxetan, at 30%, as compared with 16% in the rituximab group. An additional 4% achieved an unconfirmed CR in each group. The Kaplan–Meier estimated median duration of response was 14.2 months in the [90]Y-ibritumomab tiuxetan group versus 12.1 months in the control group, and the time to progression was 11.2 months versus 10.1 months in all patients. Durable responses of more than 6 months were significantly more frequent for [90]Y-ibritumomab tiuxetan radioimmunotherapy, versus 64%, 47% for rituximab. As expected, reversible myelosuppression was the primary toxicity noted with radioimmunotherapy.[115]

A further study evaluated the response to [90]Y-ibritumomab tiuxetan radioimmunotherapy in 54 patients with rituximab-refractory follicular lymphoma. The overall response rate for the 54 patients was 74% (15% CR and 59% PR). The Kaplan–Meier estimated time to progression was 6.8 months (range 1.1–25.9+ months) for all patients and 8.7 months for responders. Adverse events were primarily hematological, with grade 4 neutropenia in 35%, thrombocytopenia in 9%, and anemia in 4% of the patients.[115]

Finally, radioimmunotherapy with the anti-CD20 [131]I-tositumomab in patients with low-grade NHL does not induce loss of acquired humoral immunity against common antigens. Despite a temporary depletion of peripheral blood B cells and a decline in T-cell subpopulations, no reduction in serum immunoglobulin levels was observed. Almost all patients remained seropositive against rubella, mumps, varicella zoster, measles, and tetanus antigens during a 1 to 2-year follow-up, and no significant reductions in antibody concentrations to tetanus or measles were detected. Thus, acquired humoral immunity against common antigens appears to be preserved despite a temporary depletion of immune cells.[116]

In analogy to the data obtained with the use of radio-labeled anti-CD20 antibodies, patients with relapsed and chemoresistant Hodgkin lymphoma may benefit from radioimmunotherapy with [131]I- or [90]Y-labeled antibodies against ferritin.[117] Overall, 134 patients with recurrent Hodgkin lymphoma were treated in five different studies with intravenous antiferritin, labeled with [131]I or [111]In for diagnostic purposes and with [90]Y for therapeutic purposes. Patients with recurrent, end-stage Hodgkin lymphoma obtained a 60% response rate following [90]Y-labeled antiferritin. One-half of the therapy responses were complete.[118] Complete responders survived significantly longer than partial responders (2 years versus 1 year), and patients with a PR survived longer than patients with progressive disease (1 year versus 4 months). The underlying principle is, however, not tumor cell targeting and tumor-targeted irradiation but rather seems to be related to a sort of unspecific 'internal' total body irradiation. It remains to be established whether better results can be obtained with the use of radiolabeled anti-CD30 monoclonals that are currently in preclinical development.

For diagnosis and treatment of T-cell neoplasias, mainly three target structures are currently being evaluated: CD5, CD7, and CD25. Radiolabeling of the anti-CD25 mAb anti-Tac with the β emitter [90]Y increases efficiency as compared with the unlabeled mAb. In a phase I/II trial, 18 patients received up to eight treatment cycles with 5–15 mCi per infusion.[119] Two patients had a CR and 7 a PR. The duration of the responses was 1–33+ months and freedom from progression ranged from 2 to 45+ months, as compared with a median survival time of 9 months in a historical control group of untreated patients. A phase I study in patients with CTLC and B-CLL using a [131]I-labeled T101 anti-CD5 antibody showed a PR in 5 of the 10 treated patients. The median response duration was 23 weeks. One CTCL patient who subsequently received electron-beam irradiation to a residual lesion was disease-free after 6 years.[120] Notably, rapid antigenic modulation of CD5 on circulating T and B cells was observed and recovery of non-malignant T-cell populations occurred within 2–3 weeks. Interestingly, suppression of normal B-cell populations persisted after 5+ weeks. Anti-CD7 antibodies are still in preclinical development, but show interesting activities both as unlabeled or radiolabeled therapeutics.

Although radioimmunotherapy with radiolabeled intact mAbs has demonstrated efficacy in the treatment of lymphoma, it provides low tumor-to-normal-tissue radionuclide target ratios and unwanted prolonged radiation exposure to the bone marrow. To overcome these obstacles, the administration of the radionuclide was separated from that of the antibody by using an anti-IL-2 Rα antibody scFv–streptavidin fusion protein, followed by radiolabeled biotin to treat lymphoma or leukemia xenografted mice. This pretargeting approach provided extremely rapid and effective tumor targeting and cure of xenotransplanted mice when combined with the β emitter [90]Y or the α emitter bismuth-213 ([213]Bi) as radionuclides.[121] The use of such genetically engineered fusion proteins should allow better tumor penetration as compared with conventional anti-CD25 antibodies such as anti-Tac–[213]Bi conjugates.[122] Nevertheless, the clinical efficacy of this approach remains to be established.

Like other radiolabeled antibodies against tumor-associated antigens, radiolabeled anti-CD33 antibodies are capable of reducing large tumor burdens. CD33 is a 67 kDa cell surface glycoprotein found on most myeloid leukemia cells and on committed myelo-monocytic and erythroid progenitor cells. It is not found on lymphoid or non-hematopoietic cells. So far, three anti-CD33 antibodies have been evaluated in clinical radioimmunotherapy of myeloid leukemias: M195, HuM195, and p67. M195 is a murine monoclonal IgG2a antibody, HuM195 is a humanized antibody constructed by grafting the complementarity determining region of M195 onto the constant region and variable framework of human IgG1. Notably, and in contrast to the murine H195, the humanized HuM195 can mediate the killing of leukemia cells by ADCC. p67 is an anti-CD33 antibody that was tested in the past for efficacy in the radiotherapy of myeloid leukemias. To determine the intrinsic clinical efficacy of such unlabeled antibodies, 50 adult patients with relapsed or refractory AML were randomized to receive HuM195 at a dose of 12 or 36 mg/m² by intravenous infusion over 4 hours on days 1–4 and 15–18. No hepatic, renal, or cardiac toxicities were observed, and other adverse events such as nausea, vomiting, mucositis, and diarrhea were uncommon. In addition, anti-HuM195 responses were not detected. Of 49 evaluable patients, two CR and one PR were observed. Decreases in blast counts ranging from 30% to 74% were seen in nine additional patients. This indicates that HuM195 as a single agent has minimal antileukemic activity in patients with relapsed or refractory AML, with activity being confined to patients with a low burden of disease.[123] Such antibodies against CD33, however, target not only the AML blasts but also the normal bone marrow. This explains the extensive myelotoxicity of anti-CD33 radioimmunotherapies and is why these mAbs may be employed for myeloablative therapeutic schedules (reviewed in reference 124).

A [131]I-p67 anti-CD33 conjugate was studied in nine patients with advanced AML. Of these patients, only four had a 'favorable biodistribution', defined as a higher dose of radiation delivered to the marrow and spleen than to other organs. These four patients then received therapeutic doses of [131]I-p67 (110–330 mCi) together with cyclophosphamide (120 mg/kg) and total body irradiation (12 Gy) as a conditioning regimen for allogeneic BMT. Although the therapy was well tolerated, three of the four patients relapsed.[125] In view of the short half-life of [131]I-p67 in the bone marrow (9–41 hours) and the unfavorable biodistribution in many patients, the further focus of this study group was on the use of an [131]I-anti-CD45 radioimmunoconjugate as reviewed elsewhere.[126] The anti-CD33 murine antibody P67.6 was, however, developed successfully as an immunoconjugate with calicheamicin: gemtuzumab ozogamicin[127] (see above). Similar problems regarding the half-life of radiolabeled constructs in targeting CD33+ blasts in bone marrow were encountered when [131]I conjugates of M195 and HuM195 were employed. Moreover, [131]I labeling of tyrosine residues in the hypervariable region partially affects antigen binding by M195 and HuM195 anti-CD33 antibodies.[128] Therefore, and in view of the unfavorably long half-life of [131]I, and the need for isolation, current trials employ a [90]Y conjugate of HuM195. An early phase I study with a [131]I–H195 conjugate in acute promyelocytic leukemia (APL) in relapse showed promising results when combined with differentiation therapy using all-*trans*-retinoic acid (ATRA).[129] The median disease-free survival of the 7 patients was 8 months (range 5.5–33 months). The results of this trial compare favorably with those of other regimens for APL in relapse. In a more recent phase I trial, [90]Y-HuM195 was studied in patients with relapsed or refractory AML. Nineteen patients were treated with escalating doses of [90]Y-HuM195 (0.1–0.3 mCi/kg). Apart from myelosuppression lasting 9–62 days, adverse side-effects were limited to transient low-grade liver function abnormalities, which occurred in 11 of the 19 patients. Up to 56 and 75 Gy were delivered to the marrow and spleen, respectively. Thirteen patients had reductions in bone marrow blasts, and one patient achieved a CR lasting 5 months. All patients treated with 0.3 mCi/kg had hypocellular bone marrow biopsies performed 2 or 4 weeks after treatment, without evidence of leukemia.[124] These results compare well with those of a phase I/II study where [131]I-M195 or [131]I-HuM195 were given in combination with busulfan and cyclophosphamide as conditioning for allogeneic BMT in 31 patients with relapsed/refractory AML (*n*=16), accelerated/myeloblastic CML (*n*=14), or advanced myelodysplastic syndrome (MDS) (*n*=1).[130] At 59+, 87+, and 90+ months following BMT, three patients with relapsed AML remained in complete remission. This indicates that [90]Y-HuM195 might be useful as conditioning before stem cell transplantation, and

clinical studies are currently being undertaken to determine the value of such preparative regimens for autologous and non-myeloablative allogeneic stem cell transplantation.

In addition, radiolabeling with [213]Bi, an α emitter, can be used in such an adjuvant setting to eliminate minimal residual disease. The advantages of the short-range α emitters versus other radiolabels are shown in Table 25.5. As low as 1 particle per cell may suffice to kill a targeted cell. The combination of this regimen with a consolidation therapy with conventional AML chemotherapy appears promising. To enhance the potency of native HuM195 while avoiding the non-specific cytotoxicity of β-emitting constructs, the α-emitting isotope [213]Bi was conjugated with HuM195. Eighteen patients with relapsed and refractory AML leukemia or chronic myelomonocytic leukemia (CMML) were treated with 10–37 MBq/kg [213]Bi-HuM195. No significant extramedullary toxicity was seen. All 17 evaluable patients developed myelosuppression, with a median time to recovery of 22 days. Nearly all the [213]Bi-HuM195 rapidly localized to and was retained in areas of leukemic involvement, including the bone marrow, liver, and spleen. Absorbed dose ratios between these sites and the whole body were 1000-fold greater than those seen with β-emitting constructs in this antigen system and patient population.[131] Of 15 evaluable patients, 14 (93%) had reductions in circulating blasts, and 14 (78%) of 18 patients had reductions in the percentage of bone marrow blasts.[132]

# Purging strategies

High-dose chemoradiotherapy followed by ABMT or PBSCT has been shown to result in long-term disease-free survival of selected patients with malignant B-NHL. A problem that may affect the clinical outcome of ABMT or PBSCT in NHL is tumor infiltration of the marrow and, as a consequence, contamination of the graft. To prevent reinfusion of residual tumor cells in the transplant, a number of in vitro techniques have been developed for 'purging' autografts. These include chemoseparation with cytotoxic drugs, use of mAbs in conjunction with complement-mediated lysis, toxin-conjugated mAbs, or immunoconjugates with magnetic particles (Figure 25.10).[133,134] In B-NHL, murine mAbs against the CD19, CD22, and CD37 antigens have been employed for immunomagnetic purging of B-NHL cells from human bone marrow.[135] Using a cocktail of these antibodies in combination with indirect labeling via sheep anti-mouse-coated immunomagnetic beads, a more than 5 $\log_{10}$ reduction of malignant B cells from bone marrow can be achieved. The concomitant reduction of colony-forming units (CFU) is low, in the range of 20%. In 21 patients with B-NHL (18 low-grade and

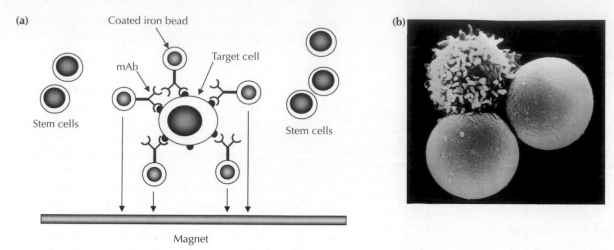

**Figure 25.10** Immunomagnetic purging of transplants with mAbs. Stem cell preparations can be contaminated with tumor cells. To eliminate the tumor cells from the transplant, these cells can be depleted by staining with mAbs against tumor-associated antigens. (a) Stained cells can be depleted with coated iron beads and are removed from the transplant by magnetic separation. (b) Raster scanning electron microscopy of two antibody-coated magnetic beads bound to a tumor cell.

3 high-grade) treated with high-dose chemotherapy followed by ABMT with purging, CR was achieved in 8 and PR in 6.[136] A cocktail of anti-CD19, CD20, CD22, CD23, and CD37 was used for purging. After myeloablative treatment with total body irradiation and cyclophosphamide at 200 mg/kg body weight hematopoietic reconstitution was observed after a median of 21.5 days (white cell count $> 10^9/l$), 27.5 days (neutrophils $0.5 \times 10^9/l$), and 27 days (platelets $> 20 \times 10^9/l$). Using marker genes, a sensitive PCR-based detection of contaminating tumor cells is possible. One of these tumor-specific markers is generated by t(14;18) translocations in B-NHL, leading to fusion of the *bcl-2* gene with the IgH enhancer. Thus, it has been shown that purging can remove virtually all tumor cells down to PCR-negativity of the purged transplant.[137] The use of magnetic beads proves to be advantageous if compared with the previously employed complement lysis-mediated purging. The latter requires antibody isotypes capable of activating complement, and does not reach the high log rates in purging achieved with immunobeads.

Additional purging efforts have focused on the CD14, CD15, and the CD33 antigens in AML. Anti-CD33 mAbs bind to normal myeloid cells in the marrow and to monocytes in the periphery. In the bone marrow, 20–30% of cells express CD33, including a fraction of metamyelocytes, most myelocytes and promyelocytes, and virtually all myeloblasts. Among the progenitor cells approximately 50% of CFU granulocyte–erythrocyte–macrophage–megakaryocyte (CFU-GEMM), more than 95% of CFU granulocyte–macrophage (CFU-GM), and a variable fraction of burst-forming units erythroid (BFU-E), CFU-E, and CFU megakaryocyte (CFU-Mk) are CD33+. The earlier hematopoietic stem cells express CD34 but not CD33, suggesting that CD33 can be used as a target for depletion of CD33+

AML cells. Purging of bone marrow for ABMT with anti-CD33 mAbs in AML significantly delays engraftment of the transplant,[138] as compared with purging allografts with anti-CD10 mAbs in ALL,[139,140] indicating that CD33+ marrow cells are important in the early phase of hematopoietic reconstitution after ABMT. In analogy, a cocktail of CD14 and CD15 mAbs, which do not bind to multilineage progenitor cells, has been used for complement-dependent purging of AML cells in ABMT in a multicenter phase II trial.[141] As in anti-CD33 studies, engraftment of purged bone marrow was strongly delayed. This approach can lead to long-term disease-free-survival in about 50% of patients with relapsed AML.

The need for graft purging is nevertheless still controversial. A beneficial effect for marrow purging in ABMT for B-NHL was suggested by Gribben et al[142] in 1991. However, none of the clinical trials performed so far has demonstrated in a controlled way that transplant purging has an effect on relapse rates. The largest patient numbers have been investigated in AML.[138,141] Nevertheless, most of these strategies failed to significantly improve the outcome of patients in controlled studies. This, together with the purging-related costs, has so far prevented the clinical introduction of purging of bone marrow or stem cell preparations.

# Anti-idiotypes and idiotype vaccination

The idiotypic determinants of surface immunoglobulin (Ig) on B-lymphoma cells were the first tumor-specific antigens to be discovered.[143] Malignant B cells express an individual B-cell receptor (Ig) with a unique antigen recognition site (idiotype). Immunization of mice with B-NHL cells led to the generation of anti-idiotypic antibodies (anti-Id) that recognized only the idiotype of the malignant B cell but not the majority of non-malignant B cells of the patient (Figure 25.11). These anti-Ids are to a large extent truly tumor-specific. It was therefore tempting to use these anti-Id mAbs for the therapy of B-cell lymphoma.[144,145] In contrast to a tumor-associated mAb, e.g. anti-CD20,[146] the normal B-cell pool remains untouched and no immune suppression is to be feared. The disadvantage of this strategy is that an idiotype-specific antibody has to be produced against every individual idiotype. Fortunately, the existence of 'shared idiotypes' was discovered by Levy and co-workers. These are idiotypic determinants on B-lymphoma cells shared by different patients, which can be recognized by one anti-idiotypic mAb. This facilitated the production of anti-idiotypic antibodies, since appropriate anti-idiotypic mAbs for an individual patient could be identified by screening a library of existing anti-idiotypes.

So far, only a few patients have been treated using anti-idiotypic antibodies, although the principle was introduced in the early 1980s. A compilation of data from phase I trials shows that anti-idiotypic antibodies alone or in combination with IFN-α induced a CR or PR in 68% of 34 treated patients.[143,145,147,148] A more favorable response was seen in those patients in whom the anti-Id mAbs induce signal transduction (tyrosine phosphorylation) in malignant B cells.[149] It is conceivable that some anti-Id mAbs bind to the B-cell antigen receptor but do not deliver an activating signal. There are therefore several possible mechanisms for the antitumor effect of these anti-idiotypes. Opsonization of the tumor cell, ADCC, and destruction by complement activation do not appear to be the major mechanisms of tumor cell elimination. In other models, the activation of the antigen receptor of malignant B cells was shown to lead to cell cycle arrest and apoptosis. Figure 25.6 shows the induction of apoptosis in human BL41 Burkitt lymphoma cells by anti-IgM antibodies.[26,27] Direct signaling for cell cycle arrest or apoptosis is therefore the most probable mechanism of anti-Id action.

In experimental animals or patients treated with anti-Ids, selection of tumor cell subclones with mutated idiotypic determinants has been observed during anti-idiotypic therapy.[150] This may lead to escape from immune recognition. An alternative approach to the direct infusion of anti-idiotypic Ig is to induce a broad antitumor response by active immunization with tumor-derived idiotype vaccines. Vaccination with tumor-derived immunoglobulins leads to polyclonal antibody and T-cell responses. These responses are capable of recognizing multiple antigenic determinants on the individual idiotype, and may thus may prevent the escape of tumor cells by idiotype mutations. These anti-idiotype vaccinations can protect experimental animals from tumor cell challenge and can cure animals – even those with established lymphomas. In a long-term follow-up of a phase I study, it was shown that 20 of 41 patients with low-grade B-NHL developed specific anti-idiotypic immunity upon immunization with a tumor-Ig – KLH conjugate.[151] The clinical outcome for those patients who mounted a specific immune response was a freedom from progression of 7.9 years, as compared with 1.3 years for those who did not. This suggests that idiotypic vaccination might be a potent tool to improve the treatment of B-NHL. A promising new approach might be the use of idiotypic DNA vaccines. These are simple plasmids containing the variable region sequences of the malignant B-cell Ig. These have been used successfully for vaccination in NHL patients to generate an anti-idiotypic humoral and T-cell response.[152] Nevertheless, no clinical data are yet available regarding the efficacy of this type of

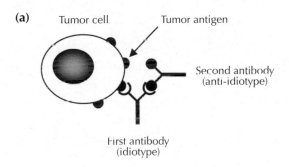

**(a)**

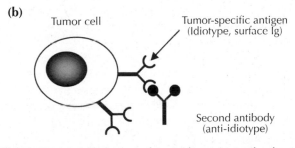

**(b)**

**Figure 25.11** Idiotypic and anti-idiotypic antibody response against a tumor cell. (a) The individual antigen-binding region of a mAb (idiotype) against a (tumor) antigen (idiotope) can be recognized by the immune system and lead to the formation of anti-idiotypic antibodies. These can mimic the antigen and form a so-called 'internal' image of the idiotope (i.e. a structure derived from the self immune system). Such anti-idiotypic antibodies are currently being investigated in tumor vaccination studies with the aim of raising a protective immune response against the tumor antigen. (b) In the case of malignant B lymphocytes, anti-idiotypic antibodies can be raised by immunizing mice with tumor cells. These anti-idiotypic mAbs can then be used to induce tumor regression upon injection of a tumor cell-carrying host.

tumor-specific DNA vaccination. A more feasible approach might be the use of dendritic cell (DC) vaccination in which the DC are loaded with tumor-derived Id proteins. The results of two phase I studies in 35 patients have been published.[153] Among 10 patients with measurable lymphoma, 8 mounted T-cell proliferative anti-Id responses, and 4 had clinical responses (2 CR, 1 PR, and 1 molecular response). Twenty-five additional patients were vaccinated after first chemotherapy, and 15 of 23 (65%) who completed the vaccination schedule mounted T-cell or humoral anti-Id responses. Notably, six patients with disease progression after primary DC vaccination received booster injections of Id–KLH protein, and tumor regression was observed in three of them (two CR and one PR). This suggests clinical efficacy, validation of which in a controlled trial is desirable.

## Targeting T cells to tumor cells by using bifunctional antibodies

It is generally accepted that tumor cells can carry tumor-specific antigens. Chromosomal translocations lead to the formation of novel non-self determinants such as the BCR–ABL fusion protein, and point mutations (e.g. in CDK4 as in malignant melanoma) create altered self structures that can be recognized by specific T cells. Theoretically, these tumor-specific antigens can be exploited by tumor vaccination strategies to elicit a tumor-specific T-cell response leading to tumor cell elimination in a fashion comparable to transplant rejection. Nevertheless, T-cell targeting to tumor cells can also be achieved by so-called bispecific antibodies (bsAbs), which form a bridge between the tumor cell and T cells, or other immunological effector cells such as NK cells or monocytes (Figure 25.12). One arm of these bsAbs reacts with the tumor-specific or tumor-associated antigen, while the other arm reacts with a structure on the immune effector cell, mediating both bridging and activation of the cytotoxic machinery. These antibodies can be produced by (1) chemical crosslinking of intact antibodies or F(ab)′ fragments, (2) by fusion of two antibody producing hybridomas to 'quadromas' (Figure 25.13), or (3) by recombinant DNA technologies. One strategy to achieve this is to fuse two single-chain antibodies (scFv) to a recombinant bsAb (scFv$_2$), also termed a 'diabody', by the introduction of an additional linker peptide. Effector cells that may be targeted by bispecific antibodies include T and NK cells and phagocytes such as neutrophils or monocytes/macrophages (Table 25.6). Apart from these cytotoxic effector cells, death receptors such as CD95/Fas have been targeted by bispecific antibodies to allow for specific activation of these killer receptors on the cancer cell without harming non-malignant tissues such as the liver (reviewed in reference 29).

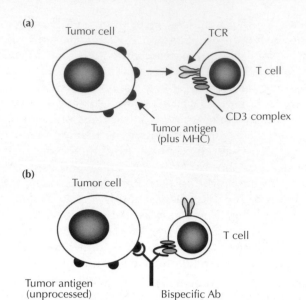

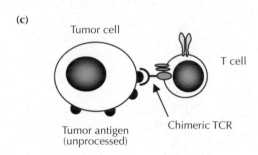

**Figure 25.12** Targeting of cytotoxic T lymphocytes (CTL) to tumor cells by bispecific antibodies or chimeric T-cell receptors. (a) CTL capable of recognizing tumor cells have been found in 'immunogenic' cancers such as malignant melanoma and renal cell carcinoma. The CTL recognize the tumor cell through tumor antigens presented in the groove of mainly MHC class I molecules. This leads to activation of the T-cell receptor (TCR) and signal transduction via the TCR-associated CD3 complex. (b) Monoclonal antibodies against tumor antigens and antibodies against the CD3 complex (in most cases against the CD3 ε chain, such as the OKT3 mAb) can be combined to produce a bispecific antibody. Commonly used tumor-associated antigens for bsAbs are CD19, CD20, or CD22 in B-NHL. The bsAb binds with one arm to the tumor-associated antigen and to the CD3 complex with the second arm. This activates the CD3 signaling cascade and T-cell activation independently of the TCR. (c) A novel recombinant DNA technology is under current development, and may lead to rapid progress in tumor immunology: Artificial chimeric TCRs can be produced by fusion of a recombinant single-chain antibody (scFv) to the ζ or γ chain of the CD3 complex. Such cDNAs for chimeric TCR can be introduced into T-cells via retroviral expression vectors. These fusion proteins can lead to efficient signal transduction, T-cell activation, and generation of CTL. The T cells then express the artificial TCR, and have been shown to specifically kill tumor cells.

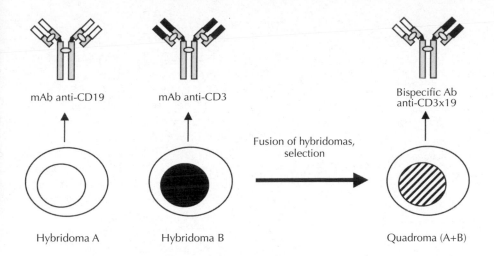

mAb anti-CD19

mAb anti-CD3

Hybridoma A

Hybridoma B

Fusion of hybridomas, selection

Bispecific Ab
anti-CD3x19

Quadroma (A+B)

**Figure 25.13** Generation of bispecific Abs (bsAbs). Individual mAb-producing hybridoma cells can be fused to quadromas, which then produce bsAbs. After selection of bsAb-producing clones, the bsAbs can be purified, for example by high-performance liquid chromatography (HPLC).

| **Table 25.6 Effector cells and molecules for bispecific antibodies** | |
| --- | --- |
| **Effector** | **Trigger molecule** |
| T cells | CD3 ε chain |
| NK cells | Fcγ RIII (CD16) |
| Monocytes/macrophages | Fcγ RI (CD64) |
| | Fcα RI (CD89) |
| | Fcγ RIIIa (CD16) |
| Granulocytes | Fcγ RI (CD64) |
| | Fcα RI (CD89) |
| Death receptors | CD95/Fas |
| | TRAIL receptors DR4, DR5 |

The bridging mediated by such bsAbs mimics specific activation of the immune effector cell. Thus, a bsAb consisting of an anti-CD3ε mAb and an anti-CD19 mAb moiety (CD3×CD19) can polyclonally activate T cells in the presence of CD19+ B-lymphoma cells by crosslinking of the T-cell receptor (TCR)/CD3 complex.[154] This bypasses the need for specific TCR/MHC/peptide interaction, leading to proliferation of the T cell (which would normally be unreactive against the lymphoma cells) and to the generation of cytotoxic T lymphocytes (CTL). In the presence of the bridging bsAb, these CTL can specifically lyse the B-lymphoma cells (Figure 25.14a). Costimulation via agonistic anti-CD28 mAbs increased the efficiency of CTL generation by mimicking the binding of its physiological ligand, B7.1 (CD80) or B7.2 (CD86).[155] It is generally accepted that this costimulation (signal 2) complements the CD3/TCR-mediated activation signals (signal 1), to allow the induction of a productive immune response. Otherwise, the stimulation by the bsAb alone could lead to induction of T-cell unresponsiveness (anergy) or to an abortive immune response due to deletion of inadequately activated T cells.[155] In an animal model, SCID mice carrying xeno-transplanted human Burkitt lymphoma cells could be cured by injection of CD3×CD19 bsAb in combination with an anti-CD28 mAb (Figure 25.14). This adequate costimulation was a prerequisite for efficient lymphoma cell elimination and therapeutic efficacy of the CD3×CD19 bsAb.[156] Likewise, a study using a CD3×CD30 mAb in combination showed that costimulation via CD28 is a prerequisite for efficient bsAb therapy of lymphoma.[157] The use of CD3×CD19 bsAbs in phase 1 studies in patients with low-grade B-NHL such as CLL leads to T-cell activation in vivo and a strong reduction in the number of the malignant cells. Unfortunately, CLL cell elimination is so far incomplete and, upon cessation of bsAb antibody infusions, the malignant cell pool is rapidly replenished. Additional studies are therefore required to clarify whether higher bsAb doses, repeated injections, and additional costimulation are required to increase the therapeutic efficiency of bsAbs. In this vein, recombinant diabodies generated by genetic fusion of two scFv antibody fragments may circumvent such problems: extremely low doses of the recombinant bsAb were sufficient to efficiently generate a cytolytic T-cell response against lymphoma cells in vitro, even in the absence of a second, costimulatory signal (Figure 25.15, see Plate 5).[158] While this propensity to trigger and mediate cytolytic T-cell responses is impressive, it remains to be clarified whether treatment by the use of these recombinant bs scFv is restricted to high efficacy against the malignant B-cell population without concomittant toxicities such as massive polyclonal T- and B-cell activation leading to cytokine secretion, shock, and vascular leakage syndrome.

Recombinant DNA techniques may also overcome some of the drawbacks of T-cell targeting with bsAbs. Chimeric TCR have been created by fusing scFv molecules recognizing tumor-related antigens to the signal-transducing molecules of the TCR/CD3 complex, for example the γ or ζ chains.[159] These chimeric molecules function as 'surrogate' T-cell receptors and mediate antigen recognition, and are therefore termed T bodies. The intracellular part of the molecule (CD3 γ or ζ chain) then triggers signal transduction cascades, T-cell activation and generation of cytotoxic

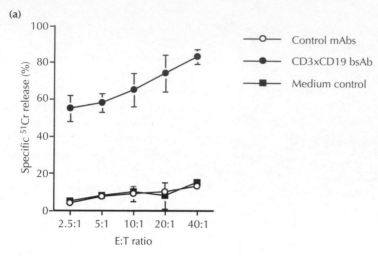

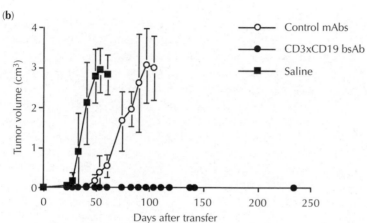

**Figure 25.14** Bispecific antibodies can bridge between tumor cells and lead to specific lysis by T cells that are otherwise unspecific for the tumor cell. (a) T cells were polyclonally activated by a CD3×CD19 bsAb that links CD19 on the surface of a malignant B cell to the CD3 ε chain on a T cell for a 4-day period. T cells received a second, costimulatory signal via an agonistic antibody against CD28. The activated T cells were then incubated with chromium-51 ($^{51}$Cr)-labeled Raji Burkitt lymphoma cells. Only low alloreactive lysis is observed in the absence of bsAb. Addition of CD3×CD19 bsAbs induces tumor cell lysis, even at low effector-to-target (E:T) cell ratios as measured by specific $^{51}$Cr release. (b) A CD3×CD19 bsAb was employed to inhibit tumor growth of Raji Burkitt lymphoma cells that were xenotransplanted into SCID mice. Subcutaneous injection of tumor cells alone led to rapid tumor growth. Co-injection of polyclonally activated human T cells at an E:T ratio of 1 : 1 slows down but does not prevent tumor growth. Animals that received the human T cells, CD3×CD19 bsAb, and costimulatory anti-CD28 mAb were saved from tumor growth.[156]

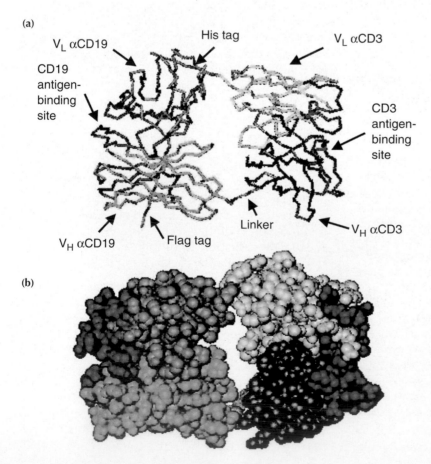

**Figure 25.15** Three-dimensional (3D) structure of a recombinant bispecific single-chain antibody (diabody). An scFv antibody against CD19 was fused by a linker to an scFv against CD3. This diabody construct is highly efficient in activating resting T cells and inducing a CTL response and target cell lysis of CD19+ malignant B cells.[158] (a) Backbone of the peptide chain. (b) Rendering of the 3D surface structure. Green, $V_H$ of the anti-CD19 scFv; purple, $V_L$ of the anti-CD19 scFv; gray, $V_H$ of the anti-CD3 scFv; light blue, $V_L$ of the anti-CD3 scFv; yellow, linker peptide; orange, His tag; darker blue, Flag tag (employed for detection and purification of the recombinant protein) (see Plate 5).

T cells (Figure 25.12). In vitro experiments are promising, but the clinical relevance remains to be elucidated. Nevertheless, a gene therapy approach to deliver and express these chimeric T-cell receptors in patients' T cells might finally exploit the power of the immune system to eliminate tumors.

## Targeting solid tumors

To date, there have been few successful attempts to treat solid tumors with antibodies or immunotoxins. The treatment of solid tumors is more difficult owing to the tight junctions between tumor cells, the high interstitial pressure, and the heterogeneous blood supply. Moreover, a higher rate of HAMA or HACA responses is observed in patients with solid tumors receiving mAb therapy. This may be due to the higher grade of immunocompetence as compared with often-immunocompromised lymphoma and leukemia patients.

The most promising data so far come from the use of antibodies to block growth factor signaling. Therapeutic targets for this approach are the epider-

mal growth factor (EGF) receptors, i.e. EGFR itself and homologs such as the HER2/*neu* receptor (Figure 25.16). The concept of using a mAb directed against EGFR was first proposed in the 1980s as a means to block the receptor from its activating ligands, transforming growth factor α (TGF-α) and EGF, thereby preventing the cascade of tyrosine kinase activation and mitogenic signal transduction in tumor cells. This led to the development of a human–murine chimeric antibody, cetuximab (C225, IMC-225), which binds with a 10-fold higher affinity than the natural ligands without delivering an activating signal and induces downregulation of the inactivated receptor.[160] Cetuximab thereby induces cell cycle arrest in $G_1$, presumably through induction of the cyclin-dependent kinase inhibitor p27, which inhibits the cyclin-dependent kinase cdk2. Moreover, expression of apoptosis-inducing proteins is induced, and inhibitors of angiogenesis and metastasis-associated metalloproteinases are downregulated.[161] Finally, ADCC and complement lysis add to the inhibitory effects of cetuximab. Several phase I and phase I/II trials showed good tolerability and only a low rate of adverse reactions, with 4% of the patients developing detectable HACA, an acneiform rash in

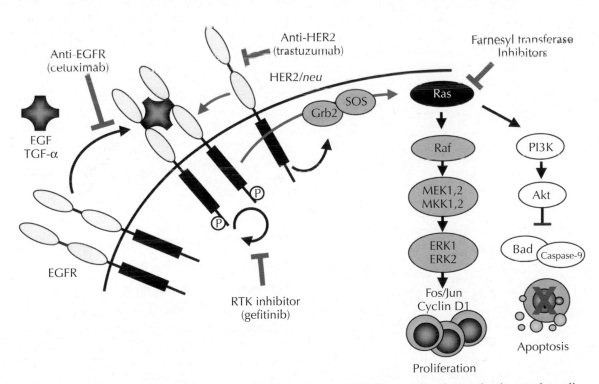

**Figure 25.16** Targeting of epidermal growth factor (EGF) receptor (EGFR) signaling by antibodies and small molecules. Ligand binding of EGF or transforming growth factor α (TGF-α) to the EGFR triggers activation of the receptor tyrosine kinase (RTK) activity of the EGFR, leading to recruitment of adapter molecules (Grb2 and SOS) that mediate activation of the p21[Ras] pathway. This results in activation of MAPK and PI3/Akt kinase signaling, which turn on proliferation and inhibit apoptosis. Blocking of ligand binding to the EGFR by the anti-EGFR mAb cetuximab blocks ligand binding and abrogates ligand-induced EGFR signaling. Similarly, the anti-HER2/*neu* antibody trastuzumab interferes with HER2/*neu* signaling and crosstalk with the EGFR. These antibodies therefore inhibit proliferation of EGFR+ or HER2/*neu*+ tumor cells and sensitize these cells for apoptosis. Similarly, small-molecule kinase inhibitors may interfere with signaling, inhibit proliferation, and abrogate survival signals. Examples are gefitinib (ZD1983, Iressa), an EGFR RTK inhibitor, and the various inhibitors of p21[Ras] farnesylation.

9%, and anaphylactic reactions in 2%, managed successfully by standard therapies. Notably, other trials reported severe skin toxicities when combining cetuximab with paclitaxel. In combination with radiotherapy in 15 patients with head and neck cancer, a 100% overall response was found: 13 patients had a CR and 2 a PR. Even though radiochemotherapy already yields a high rate of CR in head and neck cancer, these results for cetuximab are better than those for historic controls of a 50–60% CR rate.[162] Another trial in head and neck cancer showed a 67% CR rate when cetuximab was combined with cisplatin.[163] Phase III trials are now underway to validate the efficacy of radiation or cisplatin in combination with cetuximab. Trials in other carcinomas, including colorectal and pancreatic carcinoma, showed activity in advanced and chemorefractory patients when cetuximab was combined with irinotecan/5-fluorouracil or gemcitabine. Trials are currently being performed to evaluate the efficacy in first-line therapy. Additional antibodies against EGFR – ICR62, EMD55900, and ABX-EGF, a fully humanized antibody – are now in preclinical and clinical development. Moreover, MDX-447, a bsAb against EGFR and FcRγ1 (CD64), has entered clinical trials. From 36 evalubale patients with various clinically advanced carcinomas, 9 showed stabilization of the disease for 3–6 months upon therapy with MDX-447.[164] Other constructs currently being evaluated in phase I trials aim at targeting of cytotoxic T lymphocytes by anti-EGFR×CD3 bsAbs in combination with costimulation by a second bsAb against CD28. It remains to be established if these antibodies compare favorably against the novel small-molecule EGFR kinase inhibitors such as gefitinib (ZD1839, Iressa) and erlotinib (OSI-774, Tarceva).

HER2/neu, also known as c-ErbB2, is expressed by breast, ovarian, gastric, and prostate tumors of subsets of patients with these disorders. HER2/neu, the product of the proto-oncogene c-erbB2, is a 185 kDa transmembrane receptor with protein tyrosine kinase activity that is a member of the EGFR family. This receptor is modestly expressed in normal adult tissues; however, it is strongly associated with epithelial solid malignancies and is overexpressed in approximately 25–35% of human gastric, lung, prostate, and breast carcinomas. HER2/neu overexpression is found in approximately 10% of breast carcinomas and is inversely related to estrogen receptor expression; it is correlated with poor prognosis. Antibodies directed against HER2/neu were developed in the mid to late 1980s.[165,166] Trastuzumab (Herceptin), a humanized IgG1 mAb that contains human framework constant immunoglobulin regions associated with the complementarity-determining regions of the murine antibody 4D5, is now employed clinically. Trastuzumab was shown to be effective when administered as a single agent in HER2/neu-overexpressing breast cancer when administered weekly in a phase II trial.[167] Moreover, it was shown to enhance the antitumor activity of paclitaxel and doxorubicin when studied in mice bearing HER2/neu-overexpressing human breast cancer xenografts.[168] In fact, trastuzumab shows clinical synergy when combined with anthracyclines such as doxorubicin in patients with metastatic breast cancer.[169]

In another approach, attempts were made to treat micrometastasis in a neoadjuvant setting with the mAb edrecolomab (17-1A, Panorex) directed against the EpCAM antigen, a pan-epithelial cell marker. Initial reports from a phase II trial showed impressive improvement of overall survival when edrecolomab was given in an adjuvant setting.[170] The mode of action depends on ADCC and complement lysis as an immune effector mechanism. Nevertheless, these data could not be confirmed in a large phase III trial, and this led to the discontinuation of this compound. Interestingly, edrecolomab was shown to sensitize carcinoma cells for chemotherapy, much like trastuzumab. In the adjuvant therapy of breast cancer, a reduction of EpCAM+ disseminated tumor cells was achieved by sequential immunochemotherapy plus edrecolomab.[171] A phase I study showed moderate toxicity of combined edrecolomab and capecitabine in 27 patients with advanced or metastatic adenocarcinoma. Of the 18 patients evaluable for response, 1 had a CR and 2 a PR. Nine patients had disease stabilization lasting a median of 17.5 weeks (range 14.5–28+).[172] A fully humanized IgG1 antibody against EpCAM, MT201, is now under preclinical development and shows improved immune effector mechanisms.[173] It remains to be seen whether, in view of the data obtained with edrecolomab, any therapeutic benefit may derive from such novel anti-EpCAM antibodies or even edrecolomab alone or in combination with other cancer treatment modalities.

# Immune suppression by antibody therapy

## Suppression of B-cellular immune responses

The potency of antibodies to suppress humoral immune responses became evident when rituximab entered clinical use. Patients receiving this or other antibodies that eliminate neoplastic B cells show a profound and long-lasting depletion of non-malignant B cells from peripheral and lymphoid tissues. The good therapeutic efficacy, coupled with limited toxicity (consisting primarily of infusion-related events), has led to the recent use of this agent for the treatment of autoimmune disorders, with the aim of interfering with or, at best, abolishing autoantibody production. In fact, several case reports and phase I studies indicate that rituximab can be applied successfully for the therapy of autoimmune hemolytic anemia (AIHA) and mixed cryoglobulinemia (MC). Nevertheless, considering the type of autoantibody responsible for hemolysis, it appears that a better response can be achieved in patients with cold-agglutinin disease, as compared with warm-autoantibody AIHA.[174,175]

A combination of rituximab, cyclophosphamide, and dexamethasone was applied in eight CLL patients with steroid-refractory AIHA. All eight achieved a remission of their AIHA. The median pretreatment hemoglobin level was 8.3 g/dl, and this increased post treatment to 14.3 g/dl. Five of the eight patients converted to Coombs negativity with this treatment regimen. The median duration of response was 13 months (range 7–23 months), and retreatment was also effective in achieving a response on relapse of AIHA.[176] In pediatric AIHA, 15 children were given rituximab. All patients had previously received two or more courses of immunosuppressive therapy; two patients had undergone splenectomy. After completing treatment, all children received intravenous immunoglobulin for 6 months. Treatment was well tolerated. With a median follow-up of 13 months, 13 patients (87%) responded, whereas 2 showed no improvement. Median hemoglobin levels increased significantly from 7.7 g/dl to a 2-month post-treatment level of 11.8 g/dl, with a concomittant decrease in reticulocyte count. An increase in platelet count was observed in patients with concomitant thrombocytopenia (Evans syndrome). Three responder patients relapsed 7, 8, and 10 months after rituximab infusion, respectively. Notably, all three again achieved disease remission upon a second course of rituximab. These results indicate that rituximab alone or rituximab-based combination regimens are highly effective treatment modalities for steroid-refractory AIHA.[177]

Likewise, 20 patients with MC and hepatitis C virus (HCV)-positive chronic active liver disease, resistant to IFN-$\alpha$ therapy received a 'standard' regimen of 375 mg/m$^2$ rituximab intravenously once a week for 4 consecutive weeks. Of the 20 patients, 16 (80%) showed a CR, characterized by a rapid improvement of clinical signs (disappearance of purpura and weakness arthralgia and improvement of peripheral neuropathy) and a decline in cryocrit. CR was associated with a significant reduction of rheumatoid factor (RF) activity and anti-HCV antibody titers. Decline of IgG anti-HCV titers in the cryoprecipitates was usually associated with a favorable response, and no differences in the dynamics of B-cell depletion and recovery were found between responders and non-responders. No severe side-effects were reported. Molecular monitoring of the B-cell response revealed disappearance, i.e. deletion of peripheral clones, in the responders. Nevertheless, rituximab had a clearly negative impact on hepatitis C viremia; HCV RNA increased approximately twice the baseline levels in the responders, whereas it remained much the same in the non-responders. Of 16 responders, 12 (75%)

remained in remission throughout the follow-up. These results indicate that rituximab has clinical and biological activity in patients with HCV-associated MC. The long-term consequences of the increased viremia in the responders must, however, be clarified before this treatment modality may enter clinical routine.[178] Similar data were reported in a parallel study in 15 patients with HCV-associated MC.[179]

Additional disorders where rituximab has shown activity in suppression of disease activity are autoimmune thrombocytopenias, some patients with rheumatoid arthritis,[180] and other autoimmune disorders (reviewed in reference 181). Compared with the other immunosuppressive agents used for the treatment of antibody-mediated autoimmune disorders, rituximab presents the advantage of inducing selective B-cell immunosuppression, sparing cellular immunity mediated by T cells and NK cells. Moreover, the specific impairment of antibody production can be easily corrected by prophylactic intravenous immunoglobulin administration, which allows maintenance of normal IgG levels for the whole period of B-cell depletion.

## Suppression of T-cell responses

Acute and chronic graft-versus-host disease (GVHD) remain major obstacles to successful allogeneic hematopoietic stem cell transplantation, contributing substantially to morbidity and non-relapse mortality. Better understanding of the immunopathophysiology of GVHD has identified a number of targets for intervention that provide a more rational and probably also more effective approach as compared with antithymocyte immunoglobulin. Among newly developed agents suitable for the prevention and treatment of GVHD, several mAbs have shown promising results. Those currently available, such as infliximab against TNF-$\alpha$ and anti-IFN-$\gamma$, are capable of blocking the action of these effector cytokines. Antibodies directed against activated T cells, including anti-CD25 (daclizumab), humanized engineered non-FcR-binding anti-CD3 IgG2 (visilizumab[182]), and ABX-CBL, an IgM murine mAb binding to CD147/basigin, a signaling receptor for cyclophilin B,[183] may offer more specificity than the more broadly acting pan-T-cell-depleting agents, and show promising results in the treatment of steroid-resistant acute GVHD.[184] Antibody targeting of the T-cell activation-associated antigen CD147 prevents TCR stimulation-dependent reorganization and clustering of membrane microdomains. Triggering CD147 induces a displacement of the GPI-anchored coreceptors CD48 and CD59 from such microdomains in human T lymphocytes. This perturbation of microdomains is accompanied by a selective inhibition of TCR-mediated T-cell proliferation.[185] Daclizumab binds to the IL-2R $\alpha$ chain (see below) and interferes with IL-2 signaling, which is critically involved in the maintenance of T-cell responses. In contrast, antibodies against the CD3 signaling complex such as visilizumab or muronomab activate signaling functions of the TCR signal transduction machinery that, in the absence of adequate costimulatory signals, lead to apoptosis and T-cell deletion or T-cell anergy.[155,156] In addition, these antibodies exert immune effector functions such as ADCC and complement lysis.

Notably, such T-cell depletion approaches carry the risk of reducing graft-versus-tumor effects and of increasing susceptibility to virus reactivation, but offer significant benefits in terms of reduced mortality and morbidity from GVHD. Finally, the clinical investigation of antibodies to adhesion molecules (such as LFA-1) or distal effector mechanisms (such as CD95/FasL or TNF-α) may offer another level of specificity. Alemtuzumab (Campath-1H) has been used successfully for the prevention of acute GVHD. Two protocols are currently favored: (1) simple addition of alemtuzumab to the stem cell infusion[187] and (2) administration in vivo prior to the transplant – especially in the context of non-myeloablative conditioning regimens.[188] Both of these give excellent control of GVHD with minimal graft rejection (reviewed in references 189 and 190).

Apart from their application in the prevention or treatment of GVHD, these antibodies have been employed successfully in the treatment of allograft rejection in organ transplantation.[191] Additional applications include the treatment of autoimmune diseases. T-cell activation and cellular immune responses in these disease conditions are modulated by IL-2 through binding to IL-2R. Three forms of the receptor are recognized based on IL-2 binding affinity. The high-affinity receptor is heterotrimer composed of α, β, and γ polypeptide chains. The α chain – also known as the TAC (T-cell activation) antigen or CD25 – is a unique subunit of the IL-2R (IL-2α). Together with the β-chain it forms the high affinity IL-2R (IL-2R). Resting T cells express few IL-2Rα; however, when activated, the expression of IL-R2α rapidly increases. Humanized anti-TAC (daclizumab) has been shown to reduce the incidence of renal and cardiac allograft rejection,[191] as well as decreasing the severity of GVHD in patients undergoing HLA-matched allogeneic BMT.[184,189] In addition, anti-CD25 IL-2R antibody therapy with daclizumab, given intravenously with intervals of up to 4 weeks, instead of standard immunosuppressive therapy, appeared to prevent the expression of severe sight-threatening autoimmune uveitis in 8 of 10 patients treated over a 12-month period, with noted improvements in visual acuity.[192] Notably, antibodies against the IL-2R β chain, which is shared between the high-affinity IL-2R and IL-15R, have yielded similarly potent

immunosuppressive activities in preclinical models in vitro and in vivo.

The Anti-CD3 ε-chain murine mAb muronomab (OKT3) has been employed in the past to deplete T cells from allogeneic grafts and to suppress T-cell responses in vivo both in GVHD and in organ transplant rejection. Nevertheless, the reports on its clinical efficacy are mixed, which may be due to the intrinsic T-cell stimulatory property of this antibody. Early data seem to indicate that these limitations do not apply in the case of HuM291, a humanized murine IgG2 mAb against the human CD3 complex. This antibody has undergone preclinical and clinical testing for various indications, where it was noted to profoundly deplete normal circulating T cells. It is now under consideration for clinical testing against CD3+ T-NHL. In chimpanzee studies, HuM291 induced virtually complete peripheral blood T-cell depletion as early as 6 hours after administration. T-cell counts increased as the HuM291 concentration in the circulation declined, indicating that the T-cell depletion in these animals was reversible. A multiple dose-escalation study of HuM291 given intravenously to renal transplant patients experiencing acute rejection was performed in 14 patients. Profound T-cell depletion was achieved, and its extent and duration appeared to be dose-dependent, with the highest dose leading to T-cell counts below 100 cells/mm³ for 14 to 28 days. A multicenter study evaluating the safety and pharmacology of HuM291 administered as a single subcutaneous injection to patients with mild or moderate psoriasis has now begun.

Like 'naked' antibodies, immunotoxins and radioimmunotherapeutics have entered clinical trials aiming at immune suppression. With regard to the immunotoxin denileukin diftitox (DAB(389)IL-2 Ontak), the potential to target the high-affinity IL-2R supports the development of this agent in transplantation and in autoimmune diseases. Denileukin diftitox has so far been examined in clinical trials of psoriasis and rheumatoid arthritis and has shown promising results.

Additional promising target structures include the CD40 ligand (CD154) or other costimulatory ligands and the inhibitory ligand CTLA4. In preclinical models, the administration of a fusion protein genetically engineered by linking CTLA4 and the Fc part of IgG (CTLA4–Ig) can prolong the survival of allogeneic BMT recipient mice, although this effect was not complete. CTLA4–Ig blocks the interaction of CD28 on T cells and B7 molecules on antigen-presenting cells (APC) in this setting. In addition, an anti-CD154 mAb, which can interfere with the interaction of CD154 on T cells and CD40 on APC, can induce long-term graft survival in such a murine model.[193,194] It is noteworthy that the combined administration of CTLA4–Ig and an anti-CD40L mAb can prevent allograft rejection in primates. Moreover, clinical data indicate that blockade of the CD40/CD154 pathway enhances T-cell-depleted allogeneic bone marrow engraftment under non-myeloablative and irradiation-free conditioning therapy.[195]

# Side-effects and nursing techniques

The most distressing problem of intravenous mAb therapy is the possibility of severe allergic reactions. These include fever, chills, and rigors, and usually occur during the first 30 minutes of the mAb infusion. This acute risk increases with repeated injections. In contrast to these early reactions, fever that develops late in therapy (hours to days after injection) may be due to the development of HAMA. Continuation of infusion in the latter case can lead to symptoms such as facial palsy, hypotension, and acute renal tubular necrosis. The rapidity of dose administration appears to relate to the severity of symptoms. Thus, an infusion for 4–6 hours both decreases the severity of the reaction and allows discontinuation of the infusion rapidly enough in the case of hypersensitivity as compared with bolus intravenous injection. Prolonged infusion may also be associated with a decrease in pulmonary problems such as dyspnea and respiratory obstruction. Throat tightness, cough, dyspnea, stridor, or chest pain are early indicators of hypersensitivity, and should always lead to immediate discontinuation of the infusion. Tumor lysis and the formation of circulating immune complexes due to HAMA or shedded tumor antigens may lead to immune deposits, complement activation, and, in most cases, transient renal damage and elevation of serum creatinine. Premedication with antipyretics may help prevent fever, while chills and rigor usually respond well to low-dose opiates. Medications to be administered in case of more severe hypersensitivity include intravenous $H_1$ and $H_2$ histamine receptor antagonists, high-dose intravenous steroids, and hydration. It has been reported that, upon rapid relief of symptoms, the infusion may be continued slowly without the occurrence of additional hypersensitivity reactions.

In the case of immunotoxins, in contrast, the side-effects can be severe, and their systemic toxicity is a dose-limiting factor in clinical use. Unfortunately, despite the use of different toxins, there is substantial overlap with regard to toxicity profiles. The most commonly observed side-effect is capillary leak syndrome, most probably due to non-specific endothelial damage. As in cytokine therapy with IL-2, this can range from simple weight gain and moderate peripheral edema to severe hypotension, pleural effusion, and lung edema. Fever, myalgia, and anorexia are frequently observed. Neurological disorders such as aphasia have been described, as have liver toxicity and severe rhabdomyolysis.

# Conclusions and future directions

Despite the scarcity of cancer-specific antigens, mAbs have been demonstrated to be more or less selective anticancer agents. Nevertheless, the complexity and variety of human cancers dictate so far that no single agent or approach is sufficient to cure the disease. Each cancer type and stage may require a different agent or a combination of modalities. Several unlabeled mAbs and, recently, radiolabeled antibodies have shown promising results in clinical phase II and III studies. It is now mandatory to evaluate whether the increases in complete remissions and the so-far observed prolongation of disease-free survival are sustained and move forward cancer therapy. Disappointing results in the past are in part due to an excess of tumor burden: minimal residual disease appears therefore to be a most promising target for mAb therapy in the near future. A list of ongoing clinical trials for monoclonal antibody serotherapy in cancer can be accessed at the cancer.gov server of the US National Cancer Institute (http://cancer.gov/cancerinformation).

In conclusion, it is clear that mAbs are still far from being the 'magic bullet' that Paul Ehrlich dreamed of. They nonetheless provide novel therapeutic approaches that contribute to the steady – if slow – improvement in the treatment of leukemias, lymphomas, and an array of other malignancies.

## REFERENCES

1. Bodey B, Siegel SE, Kaiser HE. Human cancer detection and immunotherapy with conjugated and non-conjugated monoclonal antibodies. *Anticancer Res* 1996; **16**: 661–74.
2. Bruland OS. Cancer therapy with radiolabeled antibodies. An overview. *Acta Oncol* 1995; **34**: 1085–94.
3. Huang YW, Vitetta ES. Immunotherapy of multiple myeloma. *Stem Cells Dayt* 1995; **13**: 123–34.
4. Tonegawa S, Somatic generation of antibody diversity. *Nature* 1983; **302**: 575–81.
5. Köhler G, Milstein C. Continuous cultures of fused cells secreting antibody of predefined specificity. *Nature* 1975; **256**: 495–7.
6. Tureci O, Sahin U, Pfreundschuh M. Serological analysis of human tumor antigens: molecular definition and implications. *Mol Med Today* 1997; **3**: 342–9.

7. Chen YT, Scanlan MJ, Sahin U et al. A testicular antigen aberrantly expressed in human cancers detected by autologous antibody screening. *Proc Natl Acad Sci USA* 1997; **94**: 1914–18.

8. Goldman-Leikin R, Kaplan E, Zimmer A, Kazikiewicz J. Long-term persistence of human anti-murine antibody responses following radioimmunodetection and radioimmunotherapy of cutaneous T cell lymphoma patients using [131]I-T101. *Exp Hematol* 1988; **16**: 861–4.

9. Shawler D, Bartholomew R, Smith L, Dillman R. Human immune response to multiple injections of murine monoclonal Ig. *J Immunol* 1985; **135**: 1530–5.

10. Riechmann L, Clark M, Waldmann H, Winter G. Reshaping human antibodies for therapy. *Nature* 1988; **332**: 323–7.

11. Orlandi R, Gussow DH, Jones PT, Winter G. Cloning immunoglobulin variable domains for expression by the polymerase chain reaction. *Proc Natl Acad Sci USA* 1989; **86**: 3833–7.

12. Coney LR, Daniel PT, Sanborn D, Dhein J et al. Apoptotic cell death induced by a mouse–human anti-APO-1 chimeric antibody leads to tumor regression. *Int J Cancer* 1994; **58**: 562–7.

13. Skerra A. Bacterial expression of immunoglobulin fragments. *Curr Opin Immunol* 1993; **5**: 256–62.

14. Nadler LM, Stashenko P, Hardy R et al. Serotherapy of a patient with a monoclonal antibody directed against a human lymphoma-associated antigen. *Cancer Res* 1980; **40(9)**: 3147–54.

15. Golay J, Zaffaroni L, Vaccari T et al. Biologic response of B lymphoma cells to anti-CD20 monoclonal antibody rituximab in vitro: CD55 and CD59 regulate complement-mediated cell lysis. *Blood* 2000; **95**: 3900–8.

16. Bannerji R, Kitada S, Flinn IW et al. Apoptotic-regulatory and complement-protecting protein expression in chronic lymphocytic leukemia: relationship to in vivo rituximab resistance. *J Clin Oncol* 2003; **21**: 1466–71.

17. Cole DS, Morgan BP. Beyond lysis: how complement influences cell fate. *Clin Sci (Lond)* 2003; **104**: 455–66.

18. Stacey NH, Bishop CJ, Halliday JW et al. Apoptosis as the mode of cell death in antibody-dependent lymphocytotoxicity. *J Cell Sci* 1985; **74**: 169–79.

19. Waldmann TA, White JD, Goldman CK et al. The interleukin-2 receptor: a target for monoclonal antibody treatment of human T cell lymphotrophic virus-I induced adult T cell leukemia. *Blood* 1993; **82**: 1701–12.

20. Hilbert DM, Kopf M, Mock BA et al. Interleukin 6 is essential for in vivo development of B lineage neoplasms. *J Exp Med* 1995; **182**: 243–8.

21. Bataille R, Barlogie B, Lu Z et al. Biologic effects of anti-interleukin-6 murine monoclonal antibody in advanced multiple myeloma. *Blood* 1995; **86**: 685–91.

22. Emilie D, Wijdenes J, Gisslebrecht C et al. Administration of anti-interleukin-6 monoclonal antibody to patients with acquired immunodeficiency syndrome and lymphoma: effect on lymphoma growth and on B clinical symptoms. *Blood* 1994; **84**: 2472–9.

23. Dhein J, Daniel PT, Trauth BC et al. Induction of apoptosis by monoclonal antibody anti-APO-1 class switch variants is dependent on cross-linking of APO-1 cell surface antigens. *J Immunol* 1992; **149**: 3166–73.

24. Bargou RC, Bommert K, Weinmann P et al. Induction of Bax-α precedes apoptosis in a human B lymphoma cell line: potential role of the *bcl-2* gene family in surface IgM-mediated apoptosis. *Eur J Immunol* 1995; **25**: 770–5.

25. Daniel PT, Krammer PH. Activation induces sensitivity towards APO-1 (CD95) mediated apoptosis in human B cells. *J Immunol* 1994; **153**: 5624–32.

26. Mapara MY, Weinmann P, Bommert K et al. Involvement of NAK-1, the human nur77 homologue, in surface IgM-mediated apoptosis in Burkitt lymphoma cell line BL41. *Eur J Immunol* 1995; **25**: 2506–10.

27. Daniel PT, Oettinger U, Bargou R et al. Activation-induced cell death in human B cells: lack of CD95 (APO-1/Fas) ligand expression and function. *Eur J Immunol* 1997; **27**: 1029–34.

28. Lücking-Famira KM, Daniel PT, Möller P et al. APO-1 (CD95) mediated apoptosis in human T-ALL engrafted in SCID mice. *Leukemia* 1994; **8**: 1825–33.

29. Daniel PT, Sturm I, Wieder T, Schulze-Osthoff K. The kiss of death: promises and failures of death receptors and ligands in cancer therapy. *Leukemia* 2001; **15**: 1022–32.

30. Piro LD, White CA, Grillo-Lopez AJ et al. Extended rituximab (anti-CD20 monoclonal antibody) therapy for relapsed or refractory low-grade or follicular non-Hodgkin's lymphoma. *Ann Oncol* 1999; **10**: 655–61.

31. Goldenberg DM. The role of radiolabeled antibodies in the treatment of non-Hodgkin's lymphoma: the coming of age of radioimmunotherapy. *Crit Rev Oncol Hematol* 2001; **39**: 195–201.

32. Schmid J, Moller P, Moldenhauer G et al. Monoclonal antibody uptake in B-cell lymphomas: experimental studies in nude mouse xenografts. *Cancer Immunol Immunother* 1993; **36**: 274–80.

33. Multani PS, O'Day S, Nadler LM, Grossbard ML. Phase II clinical trial of bolus infusion anti-B4 blocked ricin immunoconjugate in patients with relapsed B-cell non-Hodgkin's lymphoma. *Clin Cancer Res* 1998; **4**: 2599–604.

34. Waldman TA. Immune receptors: targets for therapy of leukemia/lymphoma, autoimmune diseases and for the prevention of allograft rejection. *Annu Rev Immunol* 1992; **10**: 675–704.

35. Maloney DG, Liles TM, Czerwinski DK et al. Phase I clinical trial using escalating single-dose infusion of chimeric anti-CD20 monoclonal antibody (IDEC-C2B8) in patients with recurrent B-cell lymphoma. *Blood* 1994; **84**: 2457–66.

36. Plosker GL, Figgitt DP. Rituximab: a review of its use in non-Hodgkin's lymphoma and chronic lymphocytic leukaemia. *Drugs* 2003; **63**: 803–43.

37. McLaughlin P, Grillo-Lopez AJ, Link BK et al. Rituximab chimeric anti-CD20 monoclonal antibody therapy for relapsed indolent lymphoma: half of patients respond to a four-dose treatment program. *J Clin Oncol* 1998; **16**: 2825–33.

38. Coiffier B, Haioun C, Ketterer N et al. Rituximab (anti-CD20 monoclonal antibody) for the treatment of patients with relapsing or refractory aggressive lymphoma: a multicenter phase II study. *Blood* 1998; **92**: 1927–32.

39. Foran JM, Rohatiner AZ, Cunningham D et al. European phase II study of rituximab (chimeric anti-CD20 monoclonal antibody) for patients with newly diagnosed mantle-cell lymphoma and previously treated mantle-cell lymphoma, immunocytoma, and small B-cell lymphocytic lymphoma. *J Clin Oncol* 2000; **18**: 317–24.

40. Davis TA, Grillo-Lopez AJ, White CA et al. Rituximab anti-CD20 monoclonal antibody therapy in non-Hodgkin's lymphoma: safety and efficacy of retreatment. *J Clin Oncol* 2000; **18**: 3135–43.

41. Czuczman MS, Fallon A, Mohr A et al. Rituximab in combination with CHOP or fludarabine in low-grade lymphoma. *Semin Oncol* 2002; **29**(1 Suppl 2): 36–40.

42. Demidem A, Lam T, Alas S et al. Chimeric anti-CD20 (IDEC-C2B8) monoclonal antibody sensitizes a B cell lymphoma cell line to cell killing by cytotoxic drugs. *Cancer Biother Radiopharm* 1997; **12**: 177–86.

43. Lee S, Yang W, Lan KH et al. Enhanced sensitization to Taxol-induced apoptosis by herceptin pretreatment in ErbB2-overexpressing breast cancer cells. *Cancer Res* 2002; **62**: 5703–10.

44. Ghetie MA, Bright H, Vitetta ES. Homodimers but not monomers of Rituxan (chimeric anti-CD20) induce apoptosis in human B-lymphoma cells and synergize with a chemotherapeutic agent and an immunotoxin. *Blood* 2001; **97**: 1392–8.

45. Mathas S, Rickers A, Bommert K et al. Anti-CD20- and B-cell receptor-mediated apoptosis: evidence for shared intracellular signaling pathways. *Cancer Res* 2000; **60**: 7170–6.

46. Czuczman MS, Grillo-Lopez AJ, White CA et al. Treatment of patients with low-grade B-cell lymphoma with the combination of chimeric anti-CD20 monoclonal antibody and CHOP chemotherapy. *J Clin Oncol* 1999; **17**: 268–76.

47. Coiffier B, Lepage E, Briere J et al. CHOP chemotherapy plus rituximab compared with CHOP alone in elderly patients with diffuse large-B-cell lymphoma. *N Engl J Med* 2002; **346**: 235–42.

48. Mounier N, Briere J, Gisselbrecht C et al. Rituximab plus CHOP (R-CHOP) overcomes bcl-2-associated resistance to chemotherapy in elderly patients with diffuse large B-cell lymphoma (DLBCL). *Blood* 2003; **101**: 4279–84.

49. Davis TA, Maloney DG, Grillo-Lopez AJ et al. Combination immunotherapy of relapsed or refractory low-grade or follicular non-Hodgkin's lymphoma with rituximab and interferon-α-2a. *Clin Cancer Res* 2000; **6**: 2644–52.

50. Hiddemann W, Dreyling M, Unterhalt M. Rituximab plus chemotherapy in follicular and mantle cell lymphomas. *Semin Oncol* 2003; **30**(1 Suppl 2): 16–20.

51. Byrd JC, Waselenko JK, Maneatis TJ et al. Rituximab therapy in hematologic malignancy patients with circulating blood tumor cells: association with increased infusion-related side effects and rapid blood tumor clearance. *J Clin Oncol* 1999; **17**: 791–5.

52. Huhn D, von Schilling C, Wilhelm M et al. Rituximab therapy of patients with B-cell chronic lymphocytic leukemia. *Blood* 2001; **98**: 1326–31.

53. Winkler U, Jensen M, Manzke O et al. Cytokine-release syndrome in patients with B-cell chronic lymphocytic leukemia and high lymphocyte counts after treatment with an anti-CD20 monoclonal antibody (rituximab, IDEC-C2B8). *Blood* 1999; **94**: 2217–24.

54. Hainsworth JD, Litchy S, Barton JH et al. Single-agent rituximab as first-line and maintenance treatment for patients with chronic lymphocytic leukemia or small lymphocytic lymphoma: a phase II trial of the Minnie Pearl Cancer Research Network. *J Clin Oncol* 2003; **21**: 1746–51.

55. Song KW, Mollee P, Patterson B et al. Pure red cell aplasia due to parvovirus following treatment with CHOP and rituximab for B-cell lymphoma. *Br J Haematol* 2002; **119**: 125–7.

56. Dervite I, Hober D, Morel P. Acute hepatitis B in a patient with antibodies to hepatitis B surface antigen who was receiving rituximab. *N Engl J Med* 2001; **344**: 68–9.

57. Ghielmini M, Schmitz SF, Burki K et al. The effect of rituximab on patients with follicular and mantle-cell lymphoma. Swiss Group for Clinical Cancer Research (SAKK). *Ann Oncol* 2000; **11**(Suppl 1): 123–6.

58. Dyer MJ, Hale G, Hayhoe FG, Waldmann H. Effects of CAMPATH-1 antibodies in vivo in patients with lymphoid malignancies: influence of antibody isotype. *Blood* 1989; **73**: 1431–9.

59. Hale G, Dyer MJ, Clark MR et al. Remission induction in non-Hodgkin lymphoma with reshaped human monoclonal antibody CAMPATH-1H. *Lancet* 1988; **ii**: 1394–9.

60. Pawson R, Dyer MJ, Barge R et al. Treatment of T-cell prolymphocytic leukemia with human CD52 antibody. *J Clin Oncol* 1997; **15**: 2667–72.

61. Osterborg A, Dyer MJ, Bunjes D et al. Phase II multicenter study of human CD52 antibody in previously treated chronic lymphocytic leukemia. European Study Group of CAMPATH-1H Treatment in Chronic Lymphocytic Leukemia. *J Clin Oncol* 1997; **15**: 1567–74.

62. Lundin J, Kimby E, Bjorkholm M et al. Phase II trial of subcutaneous anti-CD52 monoclonal antibody alemtuzumab (Campath-1H) as first-line treatment for patients with B-cell chronic lymphocytic leukemia (B-CLL). *Blood* 2002; **100**: 768–73.

63. Cesano A, Gayko U. CD22 as a target of passive immunotherapy. *Semin Oncol* 2003; **30**: 253–7.

64. Kreitman RJ. Toxin-labeled monoclonal antibodies. *Curr Pharm Biotechnol* 2001; **2**: 313–25.

65. Baluna R, Vitetta ES. Vascular leak syndrome: a side effect of immunotherapy. *Immunopharmacology* 1997; **37**: 117–32.

66. Kreitman RJ. Chimeric fusion proteins – *Pseudomonas* exotoxin-based. *Curr Opin Invest Drugs* 2001; **2**: 1282–93.

67. Grossbard M, Nadler L. Monoclonal antibody therapy for indolent lymphomas. *Semin Oncol* 1993; **20**: 118–35.

68. Amlot PL, Stone MJ, Cunningham D et al. A phase I study of an anti-CD22-deglycosylated ricin A chain immunotoxin in the treatment of B-cell lymphomas resistant to conventional therapy. *Blood* 1993; **82**: 2624–33.

69. Ghetie MA, Tucker K, Richardson J et al. The antitumor activity of an anti-CD22 immunotoxin in SCID mice with disseminated Daudi lymphoma is enhanced by either an anti-CD19 antibody or an anti-CD19 immunotoxin. *Blood* 1992; **80**: 2315–20.

70. Grossbard ML, Gribben JG, Freedman AS et al. Adjuvant immunotoxin therapy with anti-B4-blocked ricin after autologous bone marrow transplantation for patients with B cell non-Hodgkin's lymphoma. *Blood* 1993; **81**: 2263–71.

71. Grossbard ML, Freedman AS, Ritz J et al. Serotherapy of B-cell neoplasms with anti-B4-blocked ricin: a phase I trial of daily bolus infusion. *Blood* 1992; **79**: 576–85.

72. Longo DL, Duffey PL, Gribben JG et al. Combination chemotherapy followed by an immunotoxin (anti-B4-blocked ricin) in patients with indolent lymphoma: results of a phase II study. *Cancer J* 2000; **6**: 146–50.

73. Grossbard ML, Multani PS, Freedman AS et al. A phase II study of adjuvant therapy with anti-B4-blocked ricin after autologous bone marrow transplantation for patients with relapsed B-cell non-Hodgkin's lymphoma. *Clin Cancer Res* 1999; **5**: 2392–8.

74. Stone MJ, Sausville EA, Fay JW et al. A phase I study of bolus versus continuous infusion of the anti-CD19

immunotoxin, IgG-HD37-dgA, in patients with B-cell lymphoma. *Blood* 1996; **88**: 1188–97.

75. Messmann RA, Vitetta ES, Headlee D et al. A phase I study of combination therapy with immunotoxins IgG-HD37–deglycosylated ricin A chain (dgA) and IgG-RFB4–dgA (Combotox) in patients with refractory CD19+, CD22+ B cell lymphoma. *Clin Cancer Res* 2000; **6**: 1302–13.

76. Schindler J, Sausville E, Messmann R et al. The toxicity of deglycosylated ricin A chain-containing immunotoxins in patients with non-Hodgkin's lymphoma is exacerbated by prior radiotherapy: a retrospective analysis of patients in five clinical trials. *Clin Cancer Res* 2001; **7**: 255–8.

77. Foss FM. DAB(389)IL-2 (ONTAK): a novel fusion toxin therapy for lymphoma. *Clin Lymphoma* 2000; **1**:110–16; discussion 7.

78. Olsen E, Duvic M, Frankel A et al. Pivotal phase III trial of two dose levels of denileukin diftitox for the treatment of cutaneous T-cell lymphoma. *J Clin Oncol* 2001; **19**: 376–88.

79. Barth S. Technology evaluation: BL22, NCI. *Curr Opin Mol Ther* 2002; **4**: 72–5.

80. Kreitman RJ, Wilson WH, White JD et al. Phase I trial of recombinant immunotoxin anti-Tac(Fv)-PE38 (LMB-2) in patients with hematologic malignancies. *J Clin Oncol* 2000; **18**: 1622–36.

81. Schnell R, Borchmann P, Staak JO et al. Clinical evaluation of ricin A-chain immunotoxins in patients with Hodgkin's lymphoma. *Ann Oncol* 2003; **14**: 729–36.

82. Maiese WM, Lechevalier MP, Lechevalier HA et al. Calicheamicins, a novel family of antitumor antibiotics: taxonomy, fermentation and biological properties. *J Antibiot* 1989; **42**: 558–63.

83. Salzberg AA, Dedon PC. DNA bending is a determinant of calicheamicin target recognition. *Biochemistry* 2000; **39**: 7605–12.

84. Hiatt A, Merlock R, Mauch S, Wrasidlo W. Regulation of apoptosis in leukemic cells by analogs of dynemicin A. *Bioorg Med Chem* 1994; **2**: 315–22.

85. Prokop A, Wrasidlo W, Lode H et al. Induction of apoptosis by enediyne antibiotic calicheamicin theta II proceeds through a caspase-mediated mitochondrial amplification loop in an entirely Bax-dependent manner. *Oncogene* 2003; **22**: 9107–20.

86. Nabhan C, Tallman MS. Early phase I/II trials with gemtuzumab ozogamicin (Mylotarg^R) in acute myeloid leukemia. *Clin Lymphoma* 2002; **2**(Suppl 1): S19–23.

87. de Vetten MP, Jansen JH, van der Reijden BA et al. Molecular remission of Philadelphia/*bcr–abl*-positive acute myeloid leukaemia after treatment with anti-CD33 calicheamicin conjugate (gemtuzumab ozogamicin, CMA-676). *Br J Haematol* 2000; **111**: 277–9.

88. van der Velden VH, te Marvelde JG, Hoogeveen PG et al. Targeting of the CD33–calicheamicin immunoconjugate Mylotarg (CMA-676) in acute myeloid leukemia: in vivo and in vitro saturation and internalization by leukemic and normal myeloid cells. *Blood* 2001; **97**: 3197–204.

89. Sievers EL. Antibody-targeted chemotherapy of acute myeloid leukemia using gemtuzumab ozogamicin (Mylotarg). *Blood Cells Mol Dis* 2003; **31**: 7–10.

90. Zwaan CM, Reinhardt D, Corbacioglu S et al. Gemtuzumab ozogamicin: first clinical experiences in children with relapsed/refractory acute myeloid leukemia treated on compassionate-use basis. *Blood* 2003; **101**: 3868–71.

91. Voutsadakis IA. Gemtuzumab ozogamicin (CMA-676, Mylotarg) for the treatment of CD33+ acute myeloid leukemia. *Anticancer Drugs* 2002; **13**: 685–92.

92. Wadleigh M, Richardson PG, Zahrieh D et al. Prior gemtuzumab ozogamicin exposure significantly increases the risk of veno-occlusive disease in patients who undergo myeloablative allogeneic stem cell transplantation. *Blood* 2003; **102**: 1578–82.

93. Stadtmauer EA. Trials with gemtuzumab ozogamicin (Mylotarg^R) combined with chemotherapy regimens in acute myeloid leukemia. *Clin Lymphoma* 2002; **2**(Suppl 1): S24–8.

94. Goldenberg DM. Advancing role of radiolabeled antibodies in the therapy of cancer. *Cancer Immunol Immunother* 2003; **52**: 281–96.

95. Juweid M, Sharkey RM, Markowitz A et al. Treatment of non-Hodgkin's lymphoma with radiolabeled murine, chimeric, or humanized LL2, an anti-CD22 monoclonal antibody. *Cancer Res* 1995; **55**(Suppl): 5899s–907s.

96. Bernstein ID, Eary JF, Badger CC et al. High dose radiolabeled antibody therapy of lymphoma. *Cancer Res* 1990; **50**(Suppl): 1017s–21s.

97. Press OW, Eary JF, Badger CC et al. Treatment of refractory non-Hodgkin's lymphoma with radiolabeled MB-1 (anti-CD37) antibody. *J Clin Oncol* 1989; **7**: 1027–38.

98. Kaminski MS, Zasadny KR, Francis IR et al. Radioimmunotherapy of B cell lymphoma with 131J anti-B1 (anti-CD20) antibody. *N Engl J Med* 1993; **329**: 459–65.

99. White CA, Halpern SE, Parker BA et al. Radioimmunotherapy of relapsed B cell lymphoma with yttrium 90 anti-idiotype monoclonal antibodies. *Blood* 1996; **87**: 3640–9.

100. Press OW, Eary J, Badger CC et al. High-dose radioimmunotherapy of lymphomas. *Cancer Treat Res* 1993; **68**: 13–22.

101. Gopal AK, Rajendran JG, Petersdorf SH et al. High-dose chemoradioimmunotherapy with autologous stem cell support for relapsed mantle cell lymphoma. *Blood* 2002; **99**: 3158–62.

102. Gopal AK, Gooley TA, Maloney DG et al. High-dose radioimmunotherapy versus conventional high-dose therapy and autologous hematopoietic stem cell transplantation for relapsed follicular non-Hodgkin's lymphoma: a multivariable cohort analysis. *Blood* 2003 **102**: 2351–7.

103. Press OW, Eary JF, Appelbaum FR et al. Radiolabeled-antibody therapy of B-cell lymphoma with autologous bone marrow support. *N Engl J Med* 1993; **329**: 1219–24.

104. Grillo-Lopez AJ. Zevalin: the first radioimmunotherapy approved for the treatment of lymphoma. *Expert Rev Anticancer Ther* 2002; **2**: 485–93.

105. Wahl RL. The clinical importance of dosimetry in radioimmunotherapy with tositumomab and iodine I 131 tositumomab. *Semin Oncol* 2003; **30**(2 Suppl 4): 31–8.

106. Witzig TE, Flinn IW, Gordon LI et al. Treatment with ibritumomab tiuxetan radioimmunotherapy in patients with rituximab-refractory follicular non-Hodgkin's lymphoma. *J Clin Oncol* 2002; **20**: 3262–9.

107. Witzig TE, White CA, Gordon LI et al. Safety of yttrium-90 ibritumomab tiuxetan radioimmunotherapy for relapsed low-grade, follicular, or transformed non-Hodgkin's lymphoma. *J Clin Oncol* 2003; **21**: 1263–70.

108. Kaminski MS, Zelenetz AD, Press OW et al. Pivotal study of iodine I 131 tositumomab for chemotherapy-refractory low-grade or transformed low-grade B-cell non-Hodgkin's lymphomas. *J Clin Oncol* 2001; **19**: 3918–28.

109. Rutar FJ, Augustine SC, Kaminski MS et al. Feasibility and safety of outpatient Bexxar therapy (tositumomab and iodine I 131 tositumomab) for non-Hodgkin's lymphoma based on radiation doses to family members. *Clin Lymphoma* 2001; **2**: 164–72.

110. Siegel JA, Kroll S, Regan D et al. A practical methodology for patient release after tositumomab and [131]I-tositumomab therapy. *J Nucl Med* 2002; **43**: 354–63.

111. Zhu X. Radiation safety considerations with therapeutic [90]Y Zevalin. *Health Phys* 2003; **85**(2 Suppl): S31–5.

112. Wiseman GA, Gordon LI, Multani PS et al. Ibritumomab tiuxetan radioimmunotherapy for patients with relapsed or refractory non-Hodgkin lymphoma and mild thrombocytopenia: a phase II multicenter trial. *Blood* 2002; **99**: 4336–42.

113. Espicom Research. Hematological cancer. *Cancer Drug News* 2003; **83**: 5–11.

114. Press OW, Unger JM, Braziel RM et al. A phase 2 trial of CHOP chemotherapy followed by tositumomab/iodine I 131 tositumomab for previously untreated follicular non-Hodgkin lymphoma: Southwest Oncology Group Protocol S9911. *Blood* 2003; **102**: 1606–12.

115. Witzig TE, Gordon LI, Cabanillas F et al. Randomized controlled trial of yttrium-90-labeled ibritumomab tiuxetan radioimmunotherapy versus rituximab immunotherapy for patients with relapsed or refractory low-grade, follicular, or transformed B-cell non-Hodgkin's lymphoma. *J Clin Oncol* 2002; **20**: 2453–63.

116. Nordoy T, Kolstad A, Tuck MK et al. Radioimmunotherapy with iodine-131 tositumomab in patients with low-grade non-Hodgkin's B-cell lymphoma does not induce loss of acquired humoral immunity against common antigens. *Clin Immunol* 2001; **100**: 40–8.

117. Vriesendorp HM, Quadri SM, Wyllie CT et al. Fractionated radiolabeled antiferritin therapy for patients with recurrent Hodgkin's disease. *Clin Cancer Res* 1999; **5**(10 Suppl): 3324s–9s.

118. Vriesendorp HM, Morton JD, Quadri SM. Review of five consecutive studies of radiolabeled immunoglobulin therapy in Hodgkin's disease. *Cancer Res* 1995 **55**: 5888s–92s.

119. Waldmann TA, White JD, Carrasquillo JA et al. Radioimmunotherapy of interleukin-2Rα-expressing adult T cell leukemia with yttrium-90-labeled anti-Tac. *Blood* 1995; **86**: 4063–75.

120. Foss FM, Raubitscheck A, Mulshine JL et al. Phase I study of the pharmacokinetics of a radioimmunoconjugate, [90]Y-T101, in patients with CD5-expressing leukemia and lymphoma. *Clin Cancer Res* 1998; **4**: 2691–700.

121. Zhang M, Zhang Z, Garmestani K et al. Pretarget radiotherapy with an anti-CD25 antibody–streptavidin fusion protein was effective in therapy of leukemia/lymphoma xenografts. *Proc Natl Acad Sci USA* 2003; **100**: 1891–5.

122. Zhang M, Yao Z, Garmestani K et al. Pretargeting radioimmunotherapy of a murine model of adult T-cell leukemia with the alpha-emitting radionuclide, bismuth 213. *Blood* 2002; **100**: 208–16.

123. Feldman E, Kalaycio M, Weiner G et al. Treatment of relapsed or refractory acute myeloid leukemia with humanized anti-CD33 monoclonal antibody HuM195. *Leukemia* 2003; **17**: 314–18.

124. Burke JM, Jurcic JG, Scheinberg DA. Radioimmunotherapy for acute leukemia. *Cancer Control* 2002; **9**: 106–13.

125. Appelbaum FR, Matthews DC, Eary JF et al. The use of radiolabeled anti-CD33 antibody to augment marrow irradiation prior to marrow transplantation for acute myelogenous leukemia. *Transplantation* 1992; **54**: 829–33.

126. Feldman EJ. Monoclonal antibody therapy in acute myeloid leukemia. *Curr Hematol Rep* 2003; **2**: 73–7.

127. Hamann PR, Hinman LM, Hollander I et al. Gemtuzumab ozogamicin, a potent and selective anti-CD33 antibody–calicheamicin conjugate for treatment of acute myeloid leukemia. *Bioconjug Chem* 2002; **13**: 47–58.

128. Nikula TK, Bocchia M, Curcio MJ et al. Impact of the high tyrosine fraction in complementarity determining regions: measured and predicted effects of radioiodination on IgG immunoreactivity. *Mol Immunol* 1995; **32**: 865–72.

129. Jurcic JG, Caron PC, Miller WJ et al. Sequential targeted therapy for relapsed acute promyelocytic leukemia with all-*trans* retinoic acid and anti-CD33 monoclonal antibody M195. *Leukemia* 1995; **9**: 244–8.

130. Burke JM, Caron PC, Papadopoulos EB et al. Cytoreduction with iodine-131-anti-CD33 antibodies before bone marrow transplantation for advanced myeloid leukemias. *Bone Marrow Transplant* 2003; **32**: 549–56.

131. Sgouros G, Ballangrud AM, Jurcic JG et al. Pharmacokinetics and dosimetry of an alpha-particle emitter labeled antibody: [213]Bi-HuM195 (anti-CD33) in patients with leukemia. *J Nucl Med* 1999; **40**: 1935–46.

132. Jurcic JG, Larson SM, Sgouros G et al. Targeted alpha particle immunotherapy for myeloid leukemia. *Blood* 2002; **100**: 1233–9.

133. Kiesel S, Haas R, Moldenhauer G et al. Removal of cells from a malignant B-cell line from bone marrow with immunomagnetic beads and with complement and immunoglobulin switch variant mediated cytolysis. *Leukemia Res* 1987; **11**: 1119–25.

134. Freedman AS, Nadler LM. Developments in purging in autotransplantation. *Hematol Oncol Clin North Am* 1993; **7**: 687–715.

135. Kvalheim G, Sorensen O, Fodstad O et al. Immunomagnetic removal of B lymphoma cells from human bone marrow: a procedure for clinical use. *Bone Marrow Transplant* 1988; **3**: 31–41.

136. Ogniben E, Hohaus S, Kvalheim G et al. Successful autologous transplantation of immuno-magnetic bead purged bone marrow in Non-Hodgkin's lymphoma. *Adv Bone Marrow Purging Process* 1992 : 189–95.

137. Gribben JG, Saporito L, Barber M et al. Bone marrows of non-Hodgkin's lymphoma patients with a *bcl-2* translocation can be purged of polymerase chain reaction-detectable lymphoma cells using monoclonal antibodies and immunomagnetic bead depletion. *Blood* 1992; **80**: 1083–9.

138. Robertson MJ, Soiffer RJ, Freedman AS et al. Human bone marrow depleted of CD33-positive cells mediates delayed but durable reconstitution of hematopoiesis: clinical trial of MY9 monoclonal antibody-purged autografts for the treatment of acute myeloid leukemia. *Blood* 1992; **79**: 2229–36.

139. Billet AL, Sallan SE. Autologous bone marrow transplantation in childhood acute lymphoblastic leukemia with use of purging. *Am J Pediatr Hematol Oncol* 1993; **15**: 162–8.

140. Simonsson B, Burnett AK, Prentice HG et al. Autologous bone marrow transplantation with monoclonal antibody purged marrow for high risk acute lymphoblastic leukemia. *Leukemia* 1989; **3**: 631–6.

141. Selvaggi KJ, Wilson JW, Mills LE et al. Improved outcome for high-risk acute myeloid leukemia patients using autologous bone marrow transplantation and monoclonal antibody-purged bone marrow. *Blood* 1994; **83**: 1698–705.

142. Gribben JG, Freedman AS, Neuberg D et al. Immunologic purging of marrow assessed by PCR before autologous bone marrow transplantation for B cell lymphoma. *N Engl J Med* 1991; **325**: 1525–33.

143. Levy R, Miller RA. Therapy of lymphoma directed at idiotypes. *J Natl Cancer Inst* 1990; **10**: 61–8.

144. Rankin EM, Hekman A, Somers R, ten Bokkel Huinink W. Treatment of two patients with monoclonal anti-idiotype antibodies. *Blood* 1985; **65**: 1373–81.

145. Meeker TC, Lowder JL, Maloney DG et al. A clinical trial of anti-idiotype therapy for B cell malignancy. *Blood* 1985; **65**: 1349–63.

146. Reff ME, Carner K, Chambers KS et al. Depletion of B cells in vivo by a chimeric mouse human monoclonal antibody to CD20. *Blood* 1994; **83**: 435–45.

147. Brown SL, Miller RA, Horning SJ et al. Treatment of B-cell lymphomas with anti-idiotype antibodies alone and in combination with α interferon. *Blood* 1989; **73**: 651–61.

148. Lowder JN, Meeker TC, Campbell M et al. Studies on B lymphoid tumors treated with monoclonal anti-idiotype antibodies: correlation with clinical responses. *Blood* 1987; **69**: 199–210.

149. Vuist WMJ, Levy R, Maloney DG. Lymphoma regression induced by monoclonal anti-idiotypic antibodies correlates with their ability to induce Ig signal transduction and is not prevented by tumor expression of high levels of bcl-2 protein. *Blood* 1994; **83**: 899–906.

150. Meeker T, Lowder J, Stewart S et al. Emergence of idiotype variants during treatment of B cell lymphoma with anti-diotype antibodies. *N Engl J Med* 1985; **312**: 1658–65.

151. Hsu FJ, Caspar C, Czwerinski D et al. Tumor-specific idiotype vaccines in the treatment of patients with B cell lymphoma – long term results of a clinical trial. *Blood* 1997; **89**: 3129–35.

152. Timmerman JM, Singh G, Hermanson G et al. Immunogenicity of a plasmid DNA vaccine encoding chimeric idiotype in patients with B-cell lymphoma. *Cancer Res* 2002; **62**: 5845–52.

153. Timmerman JM, Czerwinski DK, Davis TA et al. Idiotype-pulsed dendritic cell vaccination for B-cell lymphoma: clinical and immune responses in 35 patients. *Blood* 2002; **99**: 1517–26.

154. Bohlen H, Manzke O, Patel B et al. Cytolysis of leukemic B cells by T cells activated via two bispecific antibodies. *Cancer Res* 1993; **53**: 4310–14.

155. Daniel P, Kroidl A, Cayeux S et al. Co-stimulatory signals through B7.1/CD28 prevent T-cell apoptosis during target cell lysis. *J Immunol* 1997; **159**: 3808–15.

156. Daniel PT, Kroidl A, Kopp J et al. Immunotherapy of B-cell lymphoma with CD3×19 bispecific antibodies: costimulation via CD28 prevents 'veto' apoptosis of antibody-targeted cytotoxic T cells. *Blood* 1998; **92**: 4750–7.

157. Renner C, Jung W, Sahin U et al. Cure of xenografted human tumors by bispecific monoclonal antibodies and human T cells. *Science* 1994; **264**: 833–5.

158. Loffler A, Kufer P, Lutterbuse R et al. A recombinant bispecific single-chain antibody, CD19 × CD3, induces rapid and high lymphoma-directed cytotoxicity by unstimulated T lymphocytes. *Blood* 2000; **95**: 2098–103.

159. Hwu P, Shafer GE, Treisman J et al. Lysis of ovarian cancer cells by human lymphocytes redirected with a chimeric gene composed of an antibody variable region and the Fc receptor γ chain. *J Exp Med* 1993; **178**: 361–6.

160. Goldstein NI, Prewett M, Zuklys K et al. Biological efficacy of a chimeric antibody to the epidermal growth factor receptor in a human tumor xenograft model. *Clin Cancer Res* 1995; **1**: 1311–18.

161. Mendelsohn J, Dinney CP. The Willet F. Whitmore, Jr., Lectureship: blockade of epidermal growth factor receptors as anticancer therapy. *J Urol* 2001; **165**: 1152–7.

162. Robert F, Ezekiel MP, Spencer SA et al. Phase I study of anti-epidermal growth factor receptor antibody cetuximab in combination with radiation therapy in patients with advanced head and neck cancer. *J Clin Oncol* 2001; **19**: 3234–43.

163. Shin DM, Donato NJ, Perez-Soler R et al. Epidermal growth factor receptor-targeted therapy with C225 and cisplatin in patients with head and neck cancer. *Clin Cancer Res* 2001; **7**: 1204–13.

164. Curnow RT. Clinical experience with CD64-directed immunotherapy. An overview. *Cancer Immunol Immunother* 1997; **45**: 210–15.

165. Hudziak RM, Lewis GD, Winget M et al. p185HER2 monoclonal antibody has antiproliferative effects in vitro and sensitizes human breast tumor cells to tumor necrosis factor. *Mol Cell Biol* 1989; **9**: 1165–72.

166. Drebin JA, Link VC, Weinberg RA, Greene MI. Inhibition of tumor growth by a monoclonal antibody reactive with an oncogene-encoded tumor antigen. *Proc Natl Acad Sci USA* 1986; **83**: 9129–33.

167. Baselga J, Tripathy D, Mendelsohn J et al. Phase II study of weekly intravenous recombinant humanized anti-p185HER2 monoclonal antibody in patients with HER2/neu-overexpressing metastatic breast cancer. *J Clin Oncol* 1996; **14**: 737–44.

168. Baselga J, Norton L, Albanell J et al. Recombinant humanized anti-HER2 antibody (Herceptin) enhances the antitumor activity of paclitaxel and doxorubicin against HER2/neu overexpressing human breast cancer xenografts. *Cancer Res* 1998; **58**: 2825–31.

169. Slamon DJ, Leyland-Jones B, Shak S et al. Use of chemotherapy plus a monoclonal antibody against HER2 for metastatic breast cancer that overexpresses HER2. *N Engl J Med* 2001; **344**: 783–92.

170. Riethmüller G, Schneider-Gadicke E, Schlimok G et al. Randomised trial of monoclonal antibody for adjuvant therapy of resected Dukes' C colorectal carcinoma. German Cancer Aid 17-1A Study Group. *Lancet* 1994; **343**: 1177–83.

171. Kirchner EM, Gerhards R, Voigtmann R. Sequential immunochemotherapy and edrecolomab in the adjuvant therapy of breast cancer: reduction of 17-1A-positive disseminated tumour cells. *Ann Oncol* 2002; **13**: 1044–8.

172. Makower D, Sparano JA, Wadler S et al. A pilot study of edrecolomab (Panorex, 17-1A antibody) and capecitabine in patients with advanced or metastatic adenocarcinoma. *Cancer Invest* 2003; **21**: 177–84.

173. Naundorf S, Preithner S, Mayer P et al. In vitro and in vivo activity of MT201, a fully human monoclonal antibody for pancarcinoma treatment. *Int J Cancer* 2002; **100**: 101–10.

174. Finazzi G. Rituximab in autoimmune cytopenias: for which patients? *Haematologica* 2002; **87**: 113–14.

175. Saito K, Sakurai J, Ohata J et al. Involvement of CD40 ligand–CD40 and CTLA4–B7 pathways in murine acute

graft-versus-host disease induced by allogeneic T cells lacking CD28. *J Immunol* 1998; **160**: 4225–31.

176. Gupta N, Kavuru S, Patel D et al. Rituximab-based chemotherapy for steroid-refractory autoimmune hemolytic anemia of chronic lymphocytic leukemia. *Leukemia* 2002; **16**: 2092–5.

177. Zecca M, Nobili B, Ramenghi U et al. Rituximab for the treatment of refractory autoimmune hemolytic anemia in children. *Blood* 2003; **101**: 3857–61.

178. Sansonno D, De Re V, Lauletta G et al. Monoclonal antibody treatment of mixed cryoglobulinemia resistant to interferon alpha with an anti-CD20. *Blood* 2003; **101**: 3818–26.

179. Zaja F, De Vita S, Mazzaro C et al. Efficacy and safety of rituximab in type II mixed cryoglobulinemia. *Blood* 2003; **101**: 3827–34.

180. De Vita S, Zaja F, Sacco S et al. Efficacy of selective B cell blockade in the treatment of rheumatoid arthritis: evidence for a pathogenetic role of B cells. *Arthritis Rheum* 2002; **46**: 2029–33.

181. Silverman GJ, Weisman S. Rituximab therapy and autoimmune disorders: prospects for anti-B cell therapy. *Arthritis Rheum* 2003; **48**: 1484–92.

182. Carpenter PA, Appelbaum FR, Corey L et al. A humanized non-FcR-binding anti-CD3 antibody, visilizumab, for treatment of steroid-refractory acute graft-versus-host disease. *Blood* 2002; **99**: 2712–19.

183. Deeg HJ, Blazar BR, Bolwell BJ et al. Treatment of steroid-refractory acute graft-versus-host disease with anti-CD147 monoclonal antibody ABX-CBL. *Blood* 2001; **98**: 2052–8.

184. Jacobsohn DA, Vogelsang GB. Novel pharmacotherapeutic approaches to prevention and treatment of GVHD. *Drugs* 2002; **62**: 879–89.

185. Staffler G, Szekeres A, Schutz CJ et al. Selective inhibition of T cell activation via CD147 through novel modulation of lipid rafts. *J Immunol* 2003; **171**: 1707–14.

186. Daniel PT, Kroidl A, Cayeux S et al. Costimulatory signals through B7.1/CD28 prevent T cell apoptosis during target cell lysis. *J Immunol* 1997; **159**: 3808–15.

187. Chakrabarti S, MacDonald D, Hale G et al. T-cell depletion with Campath-1H 'in the bag' for matched related allogeneic peripheral blood stem cell transplantation is associated with reduced graft-versus-host disease, rapid immune constitution and improved survival. *Br J Haematol* 2003; **121**: 109–18.

188. Kottaridis PD, Milligan DW, Chopra R et al. In vivo CAMPATH-1H prevents GvHD following nonmyeloablative stem-cell transplantation. *Cytotherapy* 2001; **3**: 197–201.

189. Bruner RJ, Farag SS. Monoclonal antibodies for the prevention and treatment of graft-versus-host disease. *Semin Oncol* 2003; **30**: 509–19.

190. Hale G. Alemtuzumab in stem cell transplantation. *Med Oncol* 2002; **19**(Suppl): S33–47.

191. Carswell CI, Plosker GL, Wagstaff AJ. Daclizumab: a review of its use in the management of organ transplantation. *BioDrugs* 2001; **15**: 745–73.

192. Nussenblatt RB, Fortin E, Schiffman R et al. Treatment of noninfectious intermediate and posterior uveitis with the humanized anti-Tac mAb: a phase I/II clinical trial. *Proc Natl Acad Sci USA* 1999; **96**: 7462–6.

193. Blazar BR, Taylor PA, Panoskaltsis-Mortari A et al. Blockade of CD40 ligand–CD40 interaction impairs CD4+ T cell-mediated alloreactivity by inhibiting mature donor T cell expansion and function after bone marrow transplantation. *J Immunol* 1997; **158**: 29–39.

194. Pan Y, Luo B, Sozen H et al. Blockade of the CD40/CD154 pathway enhances T-cell-depleted allogeneic bone marrow engraftment under nonmyeloablative and irradiation-free conditioning therapy. *Transplantation* 2003; **76**: 216–24.

# 26 T-cell-mediated immunotherapy of cancer

**Rienk Offringa, Rene EM Toes, Maaike E Ressing, Marloes LH de Bruijn, and Cornelis JM Melief**

## Immunotherapy of cancer

The mere fact that tumors can develop and progress in cancer patients indicates that the tumor cells have apparently escaped the attention of – or at least destruction by – the patients' immune systems. In the past, this notion has led to the suggestion that tumor cells may lack antigenic structures. At present, as a result of extensive experimental research using both murine tumor models and material from human cancer patients, it has become clear that many tumors do express an aberrant repertoire of antigenic determinants that can, in principle, be recognized by the immune system.[1,2] Furthermore, work, especially with murine tumor models, has indicated several ways in which the immune system can be stimulated or redirected to destroy tumor cells.[3,4]

Attempts to develop immunotherapeutic approaches for the treatment of cancer have mainly focused on three arms of the immune system:[5]

- natural killer (NK) cells and lymphokine-activated killer (LAK) cells;
- T cells;
- antibodies.

Of these effector mechanisms, NK and LAK cells are relatively easily induced, stimulation with lymphokines (especially interleukin (IL)-2) usually sufficing. The other side of the coin is the poor specificity of the immune effector cells obtained, as well as the severe side-effects elicited by most lymphokines when administered systemically to patients.[6,7] The induction of antigen-specific immunity requires more detailed knowledge of the target molecules exhibited by the tumor cells and of the methods by which immunity against these targets can be induced. Although these factors make the induction of antigen-specific antitumor immunity far more challenging, the superior selectivity of such effector mechanisms makes it worth the trouble. Both antibodies and T lymphocytes have been found to be capable of specif-

ically recognizing and eliminating tumor cells.[3,4,8–11] The spread of antibodies, however, depends strongly on the vascularization of the tumor tissue,[12] whereas T lymphocytes have the capacity to migrate through tissues and in this manner to track down their targets, even if these targets are located outside the bloodstream or in multiple sites of the body. This property makes T lymphocytes especially valuable in the fight against solid tumors and metastasizing tumors. In fact, T cells possess most of the desirable properties of a 'magic bullet', the highly effective and specific antitumor agent that represents the ultimate goal of cancer research. In this chapter, we shall therefore focus on the antitumor T-cell response and on various approaches that can be employed to activate or redirect this immune response.

The approaches used to activate and/or redirect the T-cell immune response can be subdivided into two categories:

- *adoptive immunotherapy*, involving the generation of the desired tumor-reactive T cells outside the patient (usually in vitro), followed by transfer of the resulting effector cells to the patient;
- *active immunotherapy*, involving the administration of vaccines and/or lymphokines to the tumor-bearing host with the objective of reprogramming the host's immune system.

Active immunotherapy has the obvious advantage that no manipulation of immune effector cells of the patient outside the body is required. Although in vitro culture conditions can be easily created for the growth and expansion of human lymphocytes, it is far more complicated to create a setting in which T cells are obtained that exhibit the desired antigen-specificity and reactivity. On the other hand, the feasibility of active immunotherapy depends strongly on the state of the patient's immune system. As a result of poor general health status, tumor-mediated immunosuppression, and/or the immunosuppressive effects of conventional chemo- or radiotherapy, the condition of a patient's immune system may not be sufficient for the induction of an immune response against even the most optimal vaccine.

## Cytokines; genetically engineered tumor cells

Selective induction of antitumor T-cell immunity is supported by knowledge of the repertoire of tumor-associated peptides that are presented to the T-cell immune system in the context of major histocompatibility complex (MHC) molecules. Unfortunately, identification of tumor-associated antigens, both in general and in the case of a given patient, is very time-consuming. Using basically two approaches, this laborious process can be circumvented:

(i)   by cytokine treatment;
(ii)  by vaccination with genetically engineered tumor cells.

Cancer patients can be treated by systemic or, in the case of certain solid tumors, local administration of lymphokines that are known to stimulate the T-cell immune response in a non-specific fashion. The lymphokines that have been used most frequently, in both experimental and clinical settings, are IL-2 and interferons.[6,13,14] The major action of IL-2 is to strongly enhance the activity and proliferation of T cells, whereas interferons act through elevation of the antigen processing and MHC expression on (amongst others) tumor cells and through T-cell activation. As already implied by the mode of action of these lymphokines, the effects of lymphokine therapy are non-specific, causing activation of the immune system in general rather than of the antitumor immune response. Furthermore, systemically administered lymphokines cause pleiotropic effects such as severe toxicity.[13]

Following these considerations, vaccination protocols were developed involving genetically engineered tumor cells that produce lymphokines. This approach in principle combines three desired features:

(i)   the presence of an antigenic stimulus without the need to know the identity of the relevant tumor-associated antigens;
(ii)  the local and temporary presence of T-cell stimulatory lymphokines;
(iii) especially in the case of interferon-producing tumor vaccines, the increased antigen-presenting capacity of the tumor cells.

One of the first examples of successful vaccination with modified tumor cells involved IL-2 gene-modified tumor cells. This approach, when tested in murine tumor models, did not involve toxicity and induced strong protective antitumor immunity, which in some cases not only prevented tumor growth but could also lead to destruction of existing tumors.[15,16]

A wide variety of cytokines have been tested similarly, including interferon (IFN)-γ, IL-4, and granulocyte–macrophage colony-stimulating factor (GM-CSF).[17] Although for most lymphokines cases have been described where lymphokine gene-transduced tumor cells could be used as an effective antitumor vaccine, the efficacy of a given lymphokine appears to depend strongly on the experimental setting. An important parameter in this setting is the antigenicity of the tumor that is to be genetically modified. Tumor cells that present sufficient levels of immunogenic, MHC-bound peptides at their surface are more likely to constitute an effective vaccine after, for instance, IL-2 gene transduction, whereas tumor cells exhibiting very low MHC expression may especially benefit from IFN-γ gene transduction, which in an autocrine fashion promotes antigen presentation by the tumor cells. Tumor cells genetically engineered to secrete GM-CSF have the advantage of promoting induction of antitumor immunity through cross-priming, involving the recruitment of professional antigen-presenting cells (APC) of host origin.[17] Professional APC such as dendritic cells (DC) express high levels of class I and II MHC antigens.[18,19] Consequently, also in the case of class II-negative tumors, the involvement of professional APC will result in the presentation of tumor-derived antigenic peptides in the context of both class I and class II MHC, causing the concerted activation of both cytotoxic T lymphocyte (CTL)-mediated and T-helper cell (Th)-mediated immunity. Moreover, professional APC express on their surfaces various molecules that can provide costimulatory signals to T cells when bound by their corresponding receptors on the T-cell surface. The most prominent costimulatory molecules are B7.1 and B7.2, which, through interaction with the CD28 molecules on T cells, can provide a strong costimulatory impulse to antigen-triggered T cells.[20–22] The importance of B7-mediated costimulation has been well illustrated by the observation that B7 gene transduction can significantly increase the immunogenicity of tumor cells.[23–25] The first interpretation of such experiments was that coexpression on the tumor cell surface of MHC-bound antigen and B7 led to direct priming of T cells without the intervention of professional APC. More recent data, however, have indicated that, also in the case of vaccination with gene-transduced cells, cross-priming by host APC constitutes a major mechanism of immune activation.[26–29] The important role of host APC-mediated cross-priming points to a clear advantage of vaccination with (genetically engineered) tumor cells: there is no absolute need for the tumor cell vaccine to be autologous. Partly MHC-matched and completely allogenic tumors as well as tumors that fail to express MHC, can be used as an effective antitumor vaccine, provided that the non-autologous tumor and the tumor in the patient share the relevant tumor-associated antigens.[30–32] Especially in the case of tumor types that are known to express a tumor-related repertoire of antigens (e.g. melanomas),[2] this advantage may allow the development of 'off-the-shelf' tumor cell vaccines that can be applied to a significant fraction of patients suffering from these types of cancer.

# Peptide-based vaccines for the induction of antitumor T-cell immunity

The promising results obtained with different vaccines consisting of genetically engineered tumor cells indicate that this approach will be valuable for the induction of antitumor T-cell immunity against at least certain types of tumors. However, naturally arising tumors are rarely good APC. Although certain tumors arise preferentially in immunosuppressed individuals, most types of cancer develop in immunocompetent hosts and therefore in the face of a functional immune system. In cases where insufficient antigen processing, MHC expression, or costimulation are the limiting factors, genetic modification through transduction of the appropriate gene can be employed to provide the cells with sufficient antigen-presenting capacity to induce an effective antitumor response. However, when the level of tumor-associated antigens is the limiting factor, genetic engineering as described above is not likely to result in an effective vaccine.[33] In that case, a vaccine is required that harbors increased doses of the relevant tumor antigens. This can be valid for vaccination against virus-induced tumors, which, owing to immunoselection, may express only modest levels of the viral oncogene products and may even have switched off the expression of viral genes not required for transformation, but is especially relevant with respect to the induction of T-cell immunity against tumor-associated self-antigens. As many of the latter antigens are also expressed by certain normal somatic cells, the T-cell immune system is likely to exhibit at least partial tolerance against such antigens.[34] Vaccination with sufficient amounts of the appropriate antigens may in such cases be required to alleviate the absence of antitumor T-cell reactivity.

Elucidation of the three-dimensional structure of the MHC–antigen complex[35] pointed towards new directions for the development of vaccines for the induction of specific T-cell immunity. Since the antigens presented in the context of the MHC molecules are peptides of limited length, this opens the possibility of developing vaccines composed of selected synthetic peptides. The development of such molecularly defined vaccines is further supported by the rapidly increasing knowledge of the repertoire of proteins that are aberrantly expressed by certain types of tumors.[1,2] Moreover, peptide-binding motifs are available for many MHC molecules, and can be used to predict the peptides within the primary sequence of a tumor-associated antigen that are most likely to bind to the MHC molecules concerned.[36,37] The actual binding of selected peptides to the MHC can subsequently be measured by means of several different peptide-binding assays.[38-41] Based on these binding assays, a new assay was developed that measures the stability of the MHC–peptide complexes.[42] Since the stability of these complexes was shown to correlate more accurately with the immunogenicity of peptides than binding affinity as measured by other assays, the stability assay constitutes a valuable new step in the selection of immunogenic peptides.[43]

Further improvement in epitope prediction comes from in vitro proteasomal cleavage analysis of long peptides containing high-affinity MHC class I-binding sequences.[44] It was found that for proper MHC class I processing and cell surface presentation of antigen sequences, precise proteasomal cleavage of the C termini of the epitopes is required. Because of this requirement, approximately 70% of all high-affinity MHC class I-binding sequences never make it to the cell surface, because of the lack of such a cleavage site.

The efficacy of peptide-based vaccines for the induction of protective T-cell responses was first demonstrated in virus-infected mice. Vaccination with selected class I MHC-binding peptides from lymphocytic choriomeningitis virus (LCMV) and Sendai virus, emulsified in incomplete Freund's adjuvant (IFA) and injected subcutaneously, was shown to induce a vigorous peptide-specific CTL response that protected the mice against a lethal challenge with the virus concerned.[45,46] Similarly, the peptide vaccination approach was applied in a murine tumor model featuring human papillomavirus 16 (HPV16)-transformed cells. To identify the CTL epitopes presented by these tumor cells, the HPV16 E6 and E7 oncoproteins were screened for peptides that bound with high affinity to the relevant class I MHC molecules. The peptides selected were subsequently tested for their capacity to induce protective immunity against a tumorigenic dose of the HPV16-transformed cells. One of the HPV16 E7-derived peptides was shown to elicit strong peptide- and tumor-specific T-cell immunity, preventing the outgrowth of HPV16-induced tumors.[47] Encouraged by the efficacy of peptide vaccination in this murine tumor model, an HPV16 peptide epitope vaccine was developed for use in patients suffering from HLA-A*0201+ HPV16+ cervical carcinomas. The combination of HLA-A*0201 and HPV16 was chosen because of the frequent occurrence of HLA-A*0201 in the human population (40%) and of HPV16 DNA in cervical carcinomas (60%). Peptides derived from HPV16 E6 and E7 were selected for their capacity to bind to HLA-A*0201 and to reproducibly induce peptide-specific T-cell immunity in both HLA-A*0201-transgenic mice and human HLA-A*0201+ peripheral blood mononuclear cell (PBMC) cultures.[39,48,49] A vaccine consisting of the two most immunogenic HPV16 E7-derived peptides in combination with a pan-HLA-DR-binding T-helper peptide (PADRE), emulsified in an IFA-like adjuvant, was subsequently tested in HLA-A*201+, HPV16+ cervical carcinoma patients in a phase I/II clinical trial. None of the patients suffered from serious side-effects following repeated injection of the peptide vaccine, whereas several patients, who were selected on the basis of recurrent or residual cervical carcinoma unresponsive to conventional treatment, have displayed stable disease for over 1 year. Although the effects of vaccination on HPV16-specific T-cell immunity await further evaluation, measurement of the pre-existing CTL immunity against one of the selected HPV16 E7-derived peptides in HLA-A*0201+ HPV16+ cervical cancer patients has shown that such CTL memory can be observed in a minority of these patients, whereas the majority showed influenza-specific CTL memory.[49] These data suggest that natural CTL responses against HPV16 can occur in patients, but are apparently insufficient in these cases (since these patients suffer from cervical carcinoma) and even absent from the majority of such patients. These findings support the notion that the induction of HPV16-specific T-cell immunity in these patients constitutes a valuable strategy for the immunotherapy of cervical cancer. Similarly, several melanoma patients have been vaccinated with an HLA-A1-binding peptide that is derived from the MAGE-3 melanoma-associated antigen. Although also in these patients clear-cut effects of vaccination on the antigen-specific T-cell response have not yet been documented, striking tumor regression in a small number of patients indicates that peptide-based antitumor vaccines may indeed be effective in inducing antitumor T-cell immunity in certain cases.[50]

In another report, melanoma patients were vaccinated with a gp100 melanocyte differentiation antigenic peptide, modified at one amino-acid position for enhanced HLA-A2 binding. Again the results were promising in a proportion of patients, with 13 out of 41 patients achieving objective anti-cancer responses.[51]

Various other groups have reported beneficial effects of vaccination with MHC class I-binding peptides in patients with metastatic melanoma.[52–54] The problem with this approach is that, clinically, most patients, even those with ostensibly complete remissions, eventually relapse. Moreover, as argued below, vaccination with exact MHC class I-binding peptides is far from optimal.

## Optimal antigen presentation; dendritic cells

Although murine models have shown the potency of peptide-based vaccines, experiments with these models have also revealed alarming limitations. For instance, repetitive and systemic intraperitoneal injections of mice with high doses of an immunogenic exact MHC class I-binding LCMV peptide in IFA, which at low doses induced protective immunity, caused suppression rather than induction of peptide-specific CTL immunity.[55] Furthermore, in a murine tumor model featuring adenovirus type 5 (Ad5)-transformed cells, vaccination with exact MHC class I-binding Ad5-derived tumor-specific peptides was shown to abrogate the peptide-specific CTL response, leading to enhanced tumor growth in the vaccinated mice.[56,57] Importantly, in contrast to the LCMV model, the adverse effect of Ad5 peptide vaccination on T-cell immunity was observed at peptide doses and with a mode of antigen delivery that in the case of other peptides (LCMV, Sendai, and HPV16 E7) was shown to induce protective CTL immunity. To explain what might go wrong in the case of vaccination with the Ad5 peptides, it is important to consider the mechanism by which soluble exact MHC class I-binding peptides, when injected into mice, modulate the T-cell immune response. The subcutaneously injected peptides in IFA form a depot from which the peptides diffuse throughout the body. Here, they bind to available MHC molecules on the surfaces of somatic cells. Most of these cells, although expressing the appropriate MHC molecules, lack the rich repertoire of costimulatory molecules present on professional APC. At moderate levels of peptide presentation, antigenic trigger and costimulation are still in balance, causing appropriate activation of the relevant T cells. However, at excessive peptide doses, as for instance in the case of the LCMV model,[55] the antigenic stimulus may greatly exceed the costimulatory capacity of the peptide-presenting somatic cells. As a result, the T cells become inappropriately stimulated, causing them to undergo programmed, activation-induced cell death (apoptosis) or to enter a state of unresponsiveness (anergy). In accordance with this notion, evidence was found that especially the Ad5 peptides, when injected subcutaneously in IFA, spread rapidly throughout the body.[56,57] In this setting, even modest doses of such peptides are likely to cause excessive peptide presentation and therefore inactivation of the peptide-specific T cells. The relevance of the context of antigen presentation, rather than the peptide itself, to the outcome of peptide vaccination is further supported by the observation that the same Ad5 peptides, when loaded ex vivo onto autologous dendritic cells (DC), did serve as an effective vaccine for the induction of protective antitumor immunity.[58]

The inadequacy of exact MHC class I-binding peptides as vaccines was recently also demonstrated in a murine study in which the vaccine potency of exact MHC class I-binding peptides was compared with that of long peptides incorporating both MHC class I and class II epitopes in therapy of established

HPV16-induced murine tumors. Only a long peptide containing an immunodominant HPV16 E7 MHC class I epitope in addition to a class II epitope coadministered with CpG, a powerful Toll-like receptor 9 (TLR9) agonist, was capable of tumor eradication in 80% of mice with established palpable tumors, whereas the exact MHC class I-binding peptide alone admixed with CpG was completely ineffective.[59] These results correlated with CTL response inductions by these vaccine formulations, a markedly stronger CTL response being observed with the long peptide vaccine. The CpG interacts with TLR9 on DC, causing activation of the DC to robust and powerful APC. Even in the absence of CpG, long peptides (32–35 amino acids long), containing both MHC class I and class II epitopes, induce a powerful CTL response after only two vaccinations.[59] In this case, DC become activated due to CD40L upregulation on activated CD4+ T cells interacting with CD40 on DC, causing DC activation.[60]

The formidable antigen-presenting capacity of DC has also been illustrated by experiments in various murine vaccination models. DC loaded ex vivo either with synthetic peptides or with unfractionated acid-eluted tumor peptides were shown to elicit protective antitumor T-cell immunity that not only prevented development of tumors but in some cases also resulted in the regression of pre-existing tumors.[61–64] Consequently, the efficacy of DC in the induction of T-cell immunity both in vitro and in vivo against human tumors is the subject of intensive studies. Peptide-loaded autologous DC were shown to serve as effective stimulator cells for the induction of peptide-specific CTL responses in human PMBC cultures.[60,65] Four patients suffering from B-cell lymphoma were vaccinated with autologous DC that had been pulsed ex vivo with tumor-specific idiotype immunoglobulin protein, followed by booster immunizations with these proteins in the absence of DC. All patients developed cellular antitumor responses, whereas tumor regressions were observed in three of the patients.[66] Taken together, there is no doubt that DC will serve as a valuable component in vaccines. A major point that needs further study, however, concerns the source of DC that is to be used and the protocols that are to be employed for isolation and expansion. DC can be isolated from a limited quantity of peripheral blood, or from the CD34+ fraction of human bone marrow, and expanded in vitro with a culture protocol involving stimulation with GM-CSF and IL-4.[67–70] However, the yield of DC and their phenotype and antigen-presenting capacity, as well as the stability of this phenotype, are still not well controlled, calling for better-defined culture conditions.[71,72] For proper evaluation of the value of DC vaccination in cancer patients, both clinical and immunological criteria should be defined. Examples of rigorously controlled studies are to be found in references 73–75. A recent discussion of the future of cancer vaccination with ex vivo activated DC can be found in reference 76. Proper DC activation and quality control of DC preparations administered to patients is of the utmost importance. Improperly activated DC are more likely to tolerize than to vaccinate.[77]

# Genetically engineered, molecularly defined vaccines

Notwithstanding the increased immunostimulatory capacity of peptide-loaded DC in comparison with free peptide in adjuvant, peptide-based vaccines are intrinsically limited by the fact that they will comprise only a select set of peptides that bind to certain MHC molecules, although part of this disadvantage can be circumvented by the use of long peptides. Clearly, vaccines that harbor or encode entire tumor-associated antigens can, in principle, be the source of a greater variety of immunogenic peptides. When designing a vaccine covering an entire antigen, one is left basically with two options: a recombinant protein encoded by a dedicated gene construct in, for instance, *Escherichia coli* or baculovirus expression systems, or a gene construct that, when introduced into the recipient, can encode the proteins of choice at the site of injection.

Experience is accumulating with both types of vaccines. Injection of various recombinant proteins was shown to induce specific T-cell immunity that protected against virus infection or tumor growth.[78–80] Furthermore, vaccination of mice with purified HPV16 E7 protein, synthesized in *E. coli*, has been shown to protect mice against a subsequent challenge with a tumorigenic dose of HPV16-transformed cells, and this protection was accompanied by the presence of HPV16 E7-specific CTL immunity.[81,82] Like peptide-based vaccines, whole protein-based vaccines can probably be improved through modifications that promote presentation of the resulting immunogenic peptides by professional APC such as DC. This goal can be reached by in vitro incubation of DC preparations with the protein(s) of choice, followed by injection of the protein-pulsed DC. A vaccination trial involving injection of B-cell lymphoma patients with autologous DC that have been pulsed with lymphoma-specific immunoglobulin preparations is in fact based on this principle.[66] Alternatively, proteins can be targeted for uptake by DC in vitro (and probably in vivo) by attaching mannose groups to these proteins. Mannosylated proteins are taken up not only through macropinocytosis, but also through endocytosis via the mannose receptor that is expressed at high levels on DC.[83]

Over the past few years, an enormous body of work has been done with respect to the efficacy of vaccines comprising genes. As a DNA construct is the starting point of virtually all recombinant vaccines, the simplest method of vaccination involves injection of the DNA construct itself. In fact, DNA vaccination using gene constructs encoding tumor antigens and/or lymphokines has been shown to elicit strong T-cell responses against tumor-associated antigens in several model systems.[84-87] In most cases, DNA vaccination involves intramuscular or intradermal injection of DNA. The intradermal route was generally found to be more efficient – most likely as a result of the higher numbers of professional APC in the skin.[87-89] DNA vaccination requires uptake of naked DNA by somatic cells, and can therefore be regarded as in vivo DNA transfection. Conceivably, the efficiency with which these cells take up DNA is limited, since most somatic cells are highly differentiated and non-proliferative. Attempts to increase DNA uptake have involved the injection of muscle regeneration drugs, which have been reported to facilitate the uptake and transcription of the DNA.[90] Alternatively, DNA constructs can be transferred (mostly intradermally) using the gene-gun technology, which utilizes an adjustable shock wave that accelerates DNA-coated gold particles into target cells or tissues. Compared with other gene-delivery methods, the gene-gun technique can achieve up to 100-fold higher gene expression levels, conceivably as a result of the fact that this technology leads to delivery of the DNA at the intracellular level.[91,92] This may overcome a potential problem with DNA vaccination, namely the fact that naked DNA is highly sensitive to degradation by ubiquitous nucleases. This problem is even more pronounced with respect to vaccination protocols employing extremely nuclease-sensitive RNA molecules. Packaging of these nucleic acids into liposomes constitutes an alternative way to shield these molecules from destruction by nuclease activity.

Instead of such 'artificial wrappings', recombinant viruses can be used to transfer the gene(s) of interest. Many viruses are capable of eliciting powerful and lifelong immunity. Moreover, viruses can be regarded as nature's own gene-transduction tool; the capsid shields the nucleic acids from nucleases and functions as an efficient carrier for gene transduction, sometimes even in a cell-specific manner. Finally, a wealth of information is available about the topography of the genomes of various viruses and about sites into which foreign sequences of considerable length can be introduced. Most research on experimental virus-based antitumor vaccines has been performed with recombinant vaccinia virus (rVac).[93-95] For example, rVac encoding HPV16 E7 were shown to elicit strong E7-specific T-cell immunity in vaccinated rodents.[81,96,97] An rVac vaccine encoding the E6 and E7 proteins of HPV16 and HPV18 has been used to vaccinate cervical carcinoma patients in a phase I/II clinical trial.[98] Other viruses that have received much

attention as potential tools for vaccination are recombinant human adenoviruses (rAd) and recombinant canarypox and fowlpox viruses.[99,100] A recombinant fowlpox virus encoding the model tumor antigen b-gal was shown to inhibit tumor development when injected into mice bearing b-gal-expressing tumors.[101] A recombinant canarypox vaccine (ALVAC) expressing the tumor-associated antigen p53 has been shown to protect mice from a challenge with highly tumorigenic mutant-p53-overexpressing tumor cells.[102] Interestingly, the tumor protection was equally effective regardless of whether the virus encoded mutant or wild-type p53, indicating that the protective immune response was apparently directed against wild-type p53-derived epitopes and that immunization with such virus-based vaccines apparently works well in inducing immunity against self-proteins. Indeed, in a phase I study of tumor vaccination in patients with colorectal cancer, ALVAC-p53, containing the entire human wild-type p53 sequence, was capable of inducing T-helper 1 type T-cell responses characterized by IFN-γ production.[103,104] Similar canarypox vector constructs encoding the tumor-associated antigens epithelial cellular adhesion molecule (Ep-CAM) or MAGE-3 were also shown to induce specific T-cell responses to these antigens.[105,106] Similarly, rAd encoding tumor-associated antigens were shown to induce protective antitumor immunity in murine tumor models.[107,108]

The first promising results obtained with recombinant virus vaccines have boosted the development of a great variety of these vaccines. Optimization of the processing and presentation of the virus-encoded immunogens to T cells has received considerable attention. To optimize presentation of peptide antigens for recognition by class II-restricted T cells, viruses have been made that encode the HPV16 E7 protein fused to a lysosomal-associated membrane protein, LAMP-1, which reroutes the antigens to the MHC class II pathway.[97,109] Indeed, LAMP-1 targeting of the E7 protein increases the efficiency with which the vaccine induces T-helper as well as CTL responses. As a role for the ubiquitin-mediated proteolytic pathway has been postulated in the proteasome-mediated degradation of proteins into antigenic peptide fragments, modifications of the gene product that promote ubiquitinylation may also constitute a way to increase processing and presentation of the relevant peptide epitopes. For instance, the rate of MHC class I presentation of b-gal was found to be enhanced when this antigenic protein contained an acidic or basic N terminus that was conjugated to a ubiquitin subunit.[110] Alternatively, recombinant viruses have been made that contain minigenes encoding antigenic peptides preceded by an N-terminal ER-insertion sequence, bypassing the requirements for both proteolysis and transport of the antigenic peptides.[93,94] Finally, rAd have been made carrying synthetic genes that encode polypeptides consisting of antigenic peptides alternated by short spacer sequences to allow processing of the polypeptide into the proper peptides. A single rAd vaccine encoding a 'string-of-beads' arrangement of immunogenic peptides derived from the HPV16 E7 as well as the Ad5 E1A and E1B oncoproteins was shown to elicit strong, REM-protective T-cell immunity against both HPV16- and Ad5-induced tumors in mice.[111] The ability to induce T-cell responses against oncoprotein-derived peptides through immunization with such poly-epitope rAd offers a clear advantage over immunization strategies in which the vaccine carries functional oncogenes, in that it largely eliminates the risk of introduction of functional oncogenes into infected cells and thereby of transformation of these cells. Note that oncoproteins especially are attractive targets for immunotherapy of cancer, since their expression is generally required for tumor growth, making the development of tumor variants lacking these antigens unlikely.

In addition to the design of the antigen-encoding gene, the presence of additional genes encoding immunostimulatory lymphokines or costimulatory molecules is likely to improve the efficacy of the vaccine. This is illustrated by the enhanced immunogenicity of rVAC-based vaccines that, in addition to the antigen, encoded either IL-2 or B7-1.[112,113]

## Transfer of in vitro expanded tumor-reactive T lymphocytes

Active immunotherapy relies on triggering the host immune response in vivo. Although appropriate vaccine formulations are likely to elicit the desired immune responses in healthy individuals and in cancer patients at an early stage of the disease, this approach may come too late for patients who have advanced stages of cancer and/or have already undergone conventional cytostatic treatment. In the latter cases, the poor state of the patient's immune system requires adoptive immunotherapy – the transfer of ready-made effector mechanisms to the patient. In murine tumor models, this approach has been shown to cause regression of large established tumors. For instance, large established Ad5-induced tumors can be eradicated by adoptive transfer of in vitro expanded Ad5-specific CTL.[114,115] Since the CTL were administered intravenously, whereas the tumors were located at a subcutaneous site, these results indicate that the CTL are apparently capable of tracking down the tumor cells and that in vitro culture did not affect this homing capacity. Importantly, however, the CTL only succeed in eradicating the tumors when IL-2 is given simultaneously, as a subcutaneous depot in IFA. Although this does not cause major side-effects in mice, systemic administration of IL-2 in humans is

very troublesome. Adoptive immunotherapy in humans will therefore benefit greatly from approaches to provide the CTL more physiologically with a mitogenic stimulus. In fact, the most physiological solution is represented by Th cells. The therapeutic efficacies of Th and CTL against viruses and tumors have been investigated in different murine models. For instance, in mice suffering from Rauscher murine leukemia virus-induced disease, it was shown that Rauscher-specific CD4+ and CD8+ cells only gave partial resistance, whereas a combined transfer resulted in complete protection against these tumors.[116]

Although in the human situation highly defined and purified Th and CTL populations against tumors are not yet available, adoptive transfer of less well-characterized effector populations is being tested in a clinical setting. For instance, the only curative treatment for chronic myeloid leukemia (CML) is currently allogeneic bone marrow transplantation (BMT). Of the patients treated by BMT, approximately 20% show leukemia recurrence. Full remission in such patients can subsequently be achieved by adoptive immunotherapy involving the infusion of viable buffy coat cells from the marrow donor. The beneficial effect of both BMT and buffy coat transfusion is intimately connected with the antileukemic activity of transplanted T cells.[117–125] Unfortunately, the effectiveness of this treatment is compromised by the fact that in many cases the donor-type T cells, in addition to the graft-versus-leukemia (GVL) response, exhibit graft-versus-host (GVH) activity. Increased knowledge of the identity of the leukemia-associated antigens, in combination with culture techniques that can be used to selectively expand the GVL-reactive T-cell population, are needed for improvement of the specificity of this antileukemic treatment. In vitro restimulation of donor-derived lymphocytes with DC generated from peripheral blood cells of patients with CML was shown to result in T-cell populations that exhibited vigorous cytotoxic activity against CML cells while showing low reactivity against MHC-matched normal bone marrow cells.[126] The bone marrow can serve as an alternative source for such DC. Culturing of CD34+ cells purified from the bone marrow of CML patients in the presence of GM-CSF, IL-4, and tumor necrosis factor (TNF)-α was shown to result in DC-enriched cell suspensions in which the DC expressed the BCR–ABL gene.[127] This implies that such DC should be capable of presenting peptides derived from the BRC–ABL fusion region in their class I and/or class II MHC molecules, and could be used for the induction of T-cell responses against this tumor-associated junctional amino-acid sequence.[128] Similarly, immunotherapeutic protocols for the treatment of Epstein–Barr virus (EBV)-induced B-cell lymphoma have been developed, involving the adoptive transfer of donor-derived, EBV-specific CTL.[129,130]

Another source of tumor-specific T cells in humans is constituted by patient-derived lymphocytes.

Melanoma-reactive CTL have been isolated and expanded in vitro from PBMC, draining lymph nodes, and tumor-infiltrating lymphocytes (TIL). In selected cases, adoptive transfer of TIL cultures together with IL-2 resulted in the regression of metastatic melanoma.[131]

Recently, partial tumor regressions were seen in 6 out of 13 patients with metastatic melanoma who were treated with a non-myeloablative conditioning regimen, causing lymphodepletion, in combination with ex vivo expanded tumor-reactive T cells containing mainly T cells directed against melanocyte differentiation antigens. Many of these patients also developed autoimmune vitiligo. The lymphodepletion may have deleted suppressor T-cell populations, as well have allowed better expansion of tumorreactive T cells.[132]

A third source of tumor-reactive T cells is the blood of HLA-typed healthy donors. Through stimulation of human PBMC cultures with selected tumor-associated peptide epitopes, CTL cultures have been obtained that exhibit peptide-specific reactivity as well as reactivity against tumor cells presenting the relevant MHC–peptide complex. As with induction of T-cell immunity in vivo (see above), induction of bona fide T-cell immunity in vitro depends strongly on proper antigen presentation, sufficient costimulation, and the appropriate cytokines. At present, DC appear to provide the best context for antigenic stimulation of T cells in vitro.[64,65,76]

# Conclusions

Clearly, modulation of the tumor-reactive T-cell response constitutes a highly promising approach for the immunotherapy of cancer. Depending on the tumor type and the clinical situation, the desired T-cell response can be elicited either through vaccination of the patient or through stimulation and expansion of patient- or donor-derived T-cell populations in vitro, followed by adoptive transfer of these T cells into the patient. In both cases, the successful induction of effective, tumor-reactive T-cell immunity will depend on accurate knowledge of the relevant tumor-associated T-cell epitopes and of the costimulatory signals required for appropriate T-cell activation. Considering the rate at which our insight into these aspects of the T-cell immune response is increasing, it is conceivable that within the foreseeable future effective immunotherapeutic modalities will indeed become available against at least certain types of cancer.

## REFERENCES

1. Melief CJM, Kast WM. Potential immunogenicity of oncogene and tumor suppressor gene products. *Curr Opin Immunol* 1993; **5**: 709–13.

2. Boon T, Van der Bruggen P. Human tumor antigens recognized by T lymphocytes. *J Exp Med* 1996; **183**: 725–9.

3. Melief CJM, Kast WM. T-cell immunotherapy of tumors by adoptive transfer of cytotoxic T lymphocytes and by vaccination with minimal essential epitopes. *Immunol Rev* 1995; **146**: 167–77.

4. Melief CJM, Offringa R, Toes REM, Kast WM. Peptide-based cancer vaccines. *Curr Opin Immunol* 1996; **8**: 651–7.

5. Melief CJM, Toes REM, Medema JP et al. Strategies for immunotherapy of cancer. *Adv Immunol* 2000; **75**: 235–82.

6. Rosenberg SA. Immunotherapy of cancer using interleukin 2: current status and future prospects. *Immunol Today* 1988; **9**: 58–62.

7. Rosenberg SA, Yannelli JR, Yang JC et al. Treatment of patients with metastatic melanoma with autologous tumor-infiltrating lymphocytes and interleukin 2. *J Natl Cancer Inst* 1994; **15**: 1159–66.

8. Waldmann TA. Monoclonal antibodies in diagnosis and therapy. *Science* 1991; **252**: 1652–62.

9. Grossbard ML, Press OW, Appelbaum FR et al. Monoclonal antibody-based therapies of leukemia and lymphoma. *Blood* 1992; **80**: 863–78.

10. Vitetta ES, Thorpe PE, Uhr JW. Immunotoxins: magic bullets or misguided missiles? *Immunol Today* 1993; **14**: 252–9.

11. Dillman RO. Antibodies as cytotoxic therapy. *J Clin Oncol* 1994; **12**: 1497–515.

12. Shockley TR, Lin K, Sung C et al. A quantitative analysis of tumor specific monoclonal antibody uptake by human melanoma xenografts: effects of antibody immunological properties and tumor antigen expression levels. *Cancer Res* 1992; **52**: 357–66.

13. Rosenberg SA, Lotze MT, Yang CJ et al. Experience with the use of high-dose interleukin-2 in the treatment of 652 cancer patients. *Ann Surg* 1989; **210**: 474–85.

14. Rosenberg SA, Lotze MT, Yan JC. Combination therapy with interleukin-2 and α-interferon for the treatment of patients with advanced cancer. *J Clin Oncol* 1989; **7**: 1863–74.

15. Gansbacher B, Zier K, Daniels B et al. Interleukin-2 gene transfer into tumors abrogates tumorigenicity and induces protective immunity. *J Exp Med* 1990; **172**: 1217–24.

16. Connor J, Bannerji R, Saito S et al. Regression of bladder tumors in mice treated with interleukin-2 gene-modified tumor cells. *J Exp Med* 1993; **177**: 1127–34.

17. Pardoll DM. Paracrine cytokine adjuvants in cancer immunotherapy. *Annu Rev Immunol* 1995; **13**: 399–415.

18. Melief CJM. Dendritic cells as specialized antigen presenting cells. *Res Immunol* 1989; **140**: 902–21.

19. Steinman RM. The dendritic cell system and its role in immunogenicity. *Annu Rev Immunol* 1991; **9**: 271–89.

20. Schwartz RH. Costimulation of T lymphocytes: the role of CD28, CTLA-4 and B7/BB1 in interleukin-2 production and immunotherapy. *Cell* 1992; **71**: 1065–8.

21. Freeman GJ, Gribben JG, Boussiotis VA et al. Cloning of

B7-2: a CTLA-4 counter-receptor that stimulates human T cell proliferation. *Science* 1993; **262**: 909–11.

22. Jenkins MK, Johnson JG. Molecules involved in T cell costimulation. *Curr Opin Immunol* 1993; **5**: 361–7.

23. Townsend SE, Allison JP. Tumor rejection after direct costimulation of CD8+ T cells by B7-transfected melanoma cells. *Science* 1993; **259**: 368–70.

24. Yang G, Hellstrom KE, Hellstrom I, Chen L. Antitumor immunity elicited by tumor cells transfected with B7-2, a second ligand for CD28/CTLA-4 costimulatory molecules. *J Immunol* 1995; **154**: 2794–800.

25. Johnston JV, Malacko AR, Minuzo MT et al. B7–CD28 costimulation unveils the hierarchy of tumor epitopes recognized by major histocompatibility complex class I-restricted cytolytic T lymphocytes. *J Exp Med* 1996; **183**: 791–800.

26. Huang L, Soldevilla G, Leeker M et al. The liver eliminates T cells undergoing antigen-triggered apoptosis. *Immunity* 1994; **1**: 741–9.

27. Wu T-C, Huang AYC, Jaffee EM et al. A reassessment of the role of B7-1 expression in tumor rejection. *J Exp Med* 1995; **182**: 1415–21.

28. Bevan MJ. Antigen presentation to cytotoxic T lymphocytes in vivo. *J Exp Med* 1995; **182**: 639–41.

29. Huang AYC, Bruce AT, Pardoll DM, Levitsky HI. Does B7.1 expression confer antigen-presenting capacity to tumors in vivo? *J Exp Med* 1996; **183**: 769–76.

30. Gooding LR, Edwards CB. H-2 antigen requirements in the in vitro induction of SV-40-specific cytotoxic T lymphocytes. *J Immunol* 1980; **124**: 1258–62.

31. Huang AYC, Golumbek P, Ahmadzadeh M et al. Role of bone marrow-derived cells in presenting MHC class I-restricted tumor antigens. *Science* 1994; **264**: 961–5.

32. Osanto S, Brouwenstijn N, Vaessen N et al. Immunization with interleukin-2 transfected melanoma cells. *Hum Gene Ther* 1993; **4**: 323–30.

33. Chen L, McGowan P, Ashe S et al. Tumor immunogenicity determines the effect of B7 costimulation on T cell-mediated tumor immunity. *J Exp Med* 1995; **179**: 523–32.

34. Schoenberger SP, Sercarz EE. Harnessing self-reactivity in cancer immunotherapy. *Semin Immunol* 1996; **8**: 303–9.

35. Bjorkman PJ, Parham P. Structure, function, and diversity of class I major histocompatibility complex molecules. *Annu Rev Biochem* 1990; **59**: 253–88.

36. Rammensee HG, Friede T, Stevanovic S. MHC ligands and peptide motifs: first listing. *Immunogenetics* 1995; **41**: 178–228.

37. D'Amaro J, Houbiers JGA, Drijfhout JWD et al. A computer program for predicting possible cytotoxic T lymphocyte epitopes based on HLA class I peptide-binding motifs. *Hum Immunol* 1995; **43**: 13–18.

38. Nijman HW, Houbiers JGA, Vierboom MPM et al. Identification of peptide sequences that potentially trigger HLA-A2.1-restricted cytotoxic T lymphocytes. *Eur J Immunol* 1993; **23**: 1215–19.

39. Kast WM, Brandt RMP, Sidney J et al. Role of HLA-A motifs in identification of potential CTL epitopes in human papillomavirus type 16 E6 and E7 proteins. *J Immunol* 1994; **152**: 3904–12.

40. Feltkamp MCW, Vierboom MPM, Toes REM et al. Competition inhibition of cytotoxic T lymphocyte (CTL) lysis, a more sensitive method to identify candidate CTL epitopes that antibody-detected MHC class I stabilization. *Immunol Lett* 1995; **47**: 1–8.

41. Van der Burg SH, Ras E, Drijfhout JWD et al. An HLA class I peptide binding assay based on competition for binding to class I molecules on intact human B cells: identification of conserved HIV-1 polymerase peptides binding to HLA-A0301. *Hum Immunol* 1995; **44**: 189–98.

42. Van der Burg SH, Visseren MJW, Brandt RMP et al. Immunogenicity of peptides bound to MHC class I molecules depends on the MHC–peptide complex stability. *J Immunol* 1996; **156**: 3308–14.

43. Van der Burg SH, Visseren MJW, Offringa R, Melief CJM. Do epitopes derived from autoantigens display low affinity for MHC class I? *Immunol Today* 1997; **18**: 97–8.

44. Kessler JH, Beekman NJ, Bres-Vloemans SA et al. Efficient identification of novel HLA-A*0201-presented cytotoxic T lymphocyte epitopes in the widely expressed tumor antigen PRAME by proteasome-mediated digestion analysis. *J Exp Med* 2001; **193**: 73–88.

45. Schulz M, Zinkernagel RM, Hengartner H. Peptide-induced antiviral protection by cytotoxic T cells. *Proc Natl Acad Sci USA* 1991; **88**: 991–3.

46. Kast WM, Roux L, Curren J et al. Protection against lethal Sendai virus infection by in vivo priming of virus-specific cytotoxic T lymphocytes with an unbound peptide. *Proc Natl Acad Sci USA* 1991; **88**: 2283–7.

47. Feltkamp MCW, Smits HL, Vierboom MPM et al. Vaccination with a cytotoxic T lymphocyte epitope-containing peptide protects against a tumor induced by human papillomavirus type 16-transformed cells. *Eur J Immunol* 1993; **23**: 2242–9.

48. Ressing ME, Sette A, Brandt RMP et al. Human CTL epitopes encoded by human papillomavirus type 16 E6 and E7 identified through in vivo and in vitro immunogenicity studies of HLA-A*0201-binding peptides. *J Immunol* 1995; **154**: 5934–43.

49. Ressing ME, van Driel WJ, Celis E et al. Occasional memory cytotoxic T-cell responses of patients with human papillomavirus type 16-positive cervical lesions against a human leukocyte antigen-A *0201-restricted E7-encoded epitope. *Cancer Res* 1996; **56**: 582–8.

50. Marchand M, Weynants P, Rankin E et al. Tumor regression responses in melanoma patients treated with a peptide encoded by gene *MAGE-3*. *Int J Cancer* 1995; **63**: 883–5.

51. Rosenberg SA, Yang JC, Schartzentruber DJ et al. Immunologic and therapeutic evaluation of a synthetic peptide vaccine for the treatment of patients with metastatic melanoma. *Nat Med* 1998; **4**: 321–7.

52. Jager E, Hohn H, Necker A et al. Peptide-specific CD8+ T-cell evolution in vivo: response to peptide vaccination with Melan-A/MART-1. *Int J Cancer* 2002; **98**: 376–88.

53. Speiser DE, Lienard D, Pittet MJ et al. In vivo activation of melanoma-specific CD8+ T cells by endogenous tumor antigen and peptide vaccines. A comparison to virus-specific T-cells. *Eur J Immunol* 2002; **32**: 731–41.

54. Valmori D, Dutoit V, Ayyoub M et al. Simultaneous CD8+ T cell responses to multiple tumor antigen epitopes in a multipeptide melanoma vaccine. *Cancer Immun* 2003; **28**: 3–15.

55. Aichele P, Brduscha-Riem K, Zinkernagel RM et al. T cell priming versus T cell tolerance induced by synthetic peptides. *J Exp Med* 1995; **182**: 261–6.

56. Toes REM, Offringa R, Blom RJJ et al. Peptide vaccination can lead to enhanced tumor growth through specific T-cell tolerance induction. *Proc Natl Acad Sci USA* 1996; **93**: 7855–60.

57. Toes REM, Blom RJJ, Offringa R et al. Functional deletion of tumor-specific cytotoxic T lymphocytes induced by peptide immunization can lead to the inability to reject tumors. *J Immunol* 1996; **156**: 3911–18.

58. Toes RE, Schoenberger SP, van der Voort EI et al. Activation or frustration of anti-tumor responses by T-cell-based immune modulation. *Semin Immunol* 1997; **9**: 323–7.

59. Zwaveling S, Ferreira Mota SC, Nouta J et al. Established human papillomavirus type 16-expressing tumors are effectively eraducated following vaccination with long peptides. *J Immunol* 2002; **169**: 350–8.

60. Bakker ABH, Van der Burg SH, Huijbens RJF et al. Analogues of CTL epitopes with improved MHC class I binding capacity elicit anti-melanoma CTL recognizing the wild type epitope. *Int J Cancer* 1997; **70**: 302–9.

61. Mayordomo JI, Zorina T, Storkus WJ et al. Bone marrow-derived dendritic cells pulsed with synthetic tumour peptides elicit protective and therapeutic antitumour immunity. *Nat Med* 1995; **1**: 1297–302.

62. Mayordomo JI, Loftus DJ, Sakamoto H et al. Therapy of murine tumors with p53 wild-type and mutant sequence peptide-based vaccines. *J Exp Med* 1996; **183**: 1357–65.

63. Zitvogel L, Mayordomo JI, Tjandrawan T et al. Therapy of murine tumors with tumor peptide-pulsed dendritic cells: dependence of T cells, B7 costimulation, and T helper cell 1-associated cytokines. *J Exp Med* 1996; **183**: 87–97.

64. Porgador A, Snyder D, Gilboa E. Induction of antitumor immunity using bone marrow-generated dendritic cells. *J Immunol* 1996; **156**: 2918–26.

65. Van Elsas A, Van der Burg SH, Van der Minne CE et al. Peptide-pulsed dendritic cells induce tumoricidal cytotoxic T lymphocytes from healthy donors against stably HLA-A*0201-binding peptides from Melan-A/MART-1 self antigen. *Eur J Immunol* 1996; **26**: 1683–9.

66. Hsu FJ, Benkie C, Fagnoni F et al. Vaccination of patients with B-cell lymphoma using autologous antigen-pulsed dendritic cells. *Nat Med* 1996; **2**: 52–8.

67. Romani N, Gruner S, Brang D et al. Proliferating dendritic cell progenitors in human blood. *J Exp Med* 1994; **180**: 83–5.

68. Sallusto F, Lanzavecchia A. Efficient presentation of soluble antigen by cultured human dendritic cells is maintained by granulocyte/macrophage colony-stimulating factor plus interleukin 4 and downregulated by tumor necrosis factor. *J Exp Med* 1994; **179**: 1109–21.

69. Reid CDL, Stackpoole A, Meager A, Tikerpea J. Interactions of tumor necrosis factor with granulocyte macrophage colony-stimulating factor and other cytokines in the regulation of dendritic cell growth in vitro from early bipotent CD341 progenitors in human bone marrow. *J Immunol* 1992; **149**: 2681–702.

70. Egner W, Hart DNJ. The phenotype of freshly isolated and cultured human bone marrow allostimulatory cells: possible heterogeneity in bone marrow dendritic cell populations. *Immunology* 1995; **85**: 611–28.

71. Romani N, Reider D, Heuer M et al. Generation of mature dendritic cells from human blood. An improved method with special regard to clinical applicability. *J Immunol Meth* 1996; **196**: 137–51.

72. Bender A, Sapp M, Schuler G et al. Improved methods for the generation of dendritic cells from nonproliferating progenitors in human blood. *J Immunol Meth* 1996; **196**: 121–35.

73. Schuler-Thurner B, Schultz ES, Berger TG et al. Rapid induction of tumor-specific type 1 T helper cells in metastatic melanoma patients by vaccination with mature, cryopreserved, peptide-loaded monocyte-derived dendritic cells. *J Exp Med* 2002; **195**: 1279–88.

74. Banchereau J, Palucka AK, Dhodapkar M et al. Immune and clinical responses in patients with metastatic melanoma to CD34+ progenitor-derived dendritic cell vaccine. *Cancer Res* 2001; **61**: 6451–8.

75. Geiger JD, Hutchinson RJ, Hohenkirk LF et al. Vaccination of pediatric solid tumor patients with tumor lys pulsed dendritic cells can expand specific T cells and mediated tumor regression. *Cancer Res* 2001; **61**: 8513–19.

76. Figdor CG, De Vries IJM, Lesterhuis WJ, et al. Dendritic cell immunotherapy: Mapping the way. *Nat Med* 2004; **10**: 475–80.

77. Steinman RM, Hawiger D, Nussenzweig MC. Tolerogenic dendritic cells. *Annu Rev Immunol* 2003; **21**: 685–711.

78. Schirmbeck R, Zerrahn J, Kuhrober A et al. Immunization with soluble simian virus 40 large T antigen induces a specific response of CD31 CD42 CD81 cytotoxic T lymphocytes in mice. *Eur J Immunol* 1992; **22**: 759–66.

79. Bachmann MF, Kündig TM, Freer G et al. Induction of protective cytotoxic T cells with viral proteins. *Eur J Immunol* 1994; **24**: 2128–36.

80. Hariharan K, Braslawski G, Black A et al. The induction of cytotoxic T cells and tumor regression by soluble antigen formulation. *Cancer Res* 1995; **55**: 3486–9.

81. Zhu X, Tommasino M, Vousden K et al. Both immunization with protein and recombinant vaccinia virus can stimulate CTL specific for the E7 protein of human papilloma virus 16 in H-2d mice. *Scand J Immunol* 1995; **42**: 557–63.

82. De Bruijn ML, Schuurhuis DH, Vierboom MP et al. Immunization with human papillomavirus type 16 (HPV16) oncoprotein-loaded dendritic cells as well as protein in adjuvant induces MHC class I-restricted protection to HPV16-induced tumor cells. *Cancer Res* 1998; **58**: 724–31.

83. Sallusto F, Cella M, Danieli C, Lanzavecchia A. Dendritic cells use macropinocytosis and the mannose receptor to concentrate macromolecules in the major histocompatibility complex II compartment: downregulation by cytokines and bacterial products. *J Exp Med* 1995; **182**: 389–400.

84. Schirmbeck R, Böhm W, Reimann J. DNA vaccination primes MHC class I restricted, simian virus 40 large tumor antigen specific CTL in H-2d mice that reject syngeneic tumors. *J Immunol* 1996; **157**: 3550–8.

85. Bright RK, Beames B, Shearer MH, Kennedy R. Protection against a lethal tumor challenge with SV40-transformed cells by the direct injection of DNA encoding SV40 large tumor antigen. *Cancer Res* 1996; **56**: 1126–30.

86. Irvine KR, Rao JB, Rosenberg SA, Restifo NP. Cytokine enhancement of DNA immunization leads to effective treatment of established pulmonary metastases. *J Immunol* 1996; **156**: 238–45.

87. Rakhmilevich AL, Turner J, Ford MJ et al. Gene gun-mediated skin transfection with interleukin 12 gene results in regression of established primary and metastatic murine tumors. *Proc Natl Acad Sci USA* 1996; **93**: 6291–6.

88. Corr M, Lee DJ, Carson DA, Tighe H. Gene vaccination with naked plasmid DNA: mechanism of CTL priming. *J Exp Med* 1996; **184**: 1555–60.

89. Kumar V, Sercarz E. Genetic vaccination: the advantages of going naked. *Nat Med* 1996; **2**: 857–9.

90. Wang B, Ugen EU, Srikantan V et al. Gene inoculation generates immune responses against human immunodeficiency virus type 1. *Proc Natl Acad Sci USA* 1993; **90**: 4156–63.

91. Pertmer TM, Eisenbraun MD, McCabe D et al. Gene gun-based nucleid acid immunization: elicitation of humoral and cytotoxic T lymphocyte responses following epidermal delivery of nanogram quantities of DNA. *Vaccine* 1995; **13**: 1427–30.

92. Yang N-S, Sun WH. Gene gun and other non-viral approaches for cancer gene therapy. *Nat Med* 1995; **1**: 481–3.

93. Restifo NP, Bacik I, Irvine KR et al. Antigen processing in vivo and the elicitation of primary CTL responses. *J Immunol* 1995; **154**: 4414–22.

94. McCabe BJ, Irvine KR, Nishimura MI et al. Minimal determinant expressed by a recombinant vaccinia virus elicits therapeutic antitumor cytolytic T cell response. *Cancer Res* 1995; **55**: 1741–7.

95. Hodge JW, Schlom J, Donohue SJ et al. A recombinant vaccinia virus expressing human prostate specific antigen (PSA): safety and immunogenicity in a nonhuman primate. *Int J Cancer* 1995; **63**: 231–7.

96. Meneguzzi G, Cerni C, Kieny MP, Lathe R. Immunization against human papillomavirus type 16 tumor cells with recombinant vaccinia viruses expressing E6 and E7. *Virology* 1991; **181**: 62–9.

97. Wu T-Z, Guarnieri FG, Stavely-O'Carroll KF et al. Engineering an intracellular pathway for major histocompatibility complex class II presentation of antigens. *Proc Natl Acad Sci USA* 1995; **92**: 11671–5.

98. Borysiewicz LK, Fiander A, Nimako M et al. A recombinant vaccinia virus encoding human papillomavirus types 16 and 18, E6 and E7 proteins as immunotherapy for cervical cancer. *Lancet* 1996; **347**: 1523–7.

99. Randrianarison-Jewtoukoff V, Perricaudet M. Recombinant adenoviruses as vaccines. *Biologicals* 1995; **23**: 145–57.

100. Plotkin SA, Cadoz M, Meignier B et al. Safety and use of canarypox vectored vaccines. *Dev Biol Stand* 1995; **84**: 165–70.

101. Wang N, Bronte V, Chen PW et al. Active immunotherapy of cancer with a nonreplicating recombinant fowlpox virus encoding a model tumor-associated antigen. *J Immunol* 1995; **154**: 4685–92.

102. Roth J, Dittmer D, Rea D et al. p53 as a target for cancer vaccines: recombinant canarypox virus vectors expressing p53 protect mice against lethal tumor cell challenge. *Proc Natl Acad Sci USA* 1996; **93**: 4781–6.

103. Van der Burg SH, Menon AG, Redeker A et al. Induction of p53-specific immune responses in colorectal cancer patients receiving a recombinant ALVAC-p53 candidate vaccine. *Clin Cancer Res* 2002; **8**: 1019–27.

104. Menon AG, Kuppen PJ, Van der Burg SH et al. Safety of intravenous administration of a canarypox virus encoding the human wild-type *p53* gene in colorectal cancer patients. *Cancer Gene Ther* 2003; **10**: 509–517.

105. Ullenhag GJ, Frodin JE, Mosolits S et al. Immunization of colorectal carcinoma patients with a recombinant canarypox virus expressing the tumor antigen CAM-KSA (ALVAC-KSA) and granulocyte macrophage colony-stimulating factor induced a tumor-specific cellular response. *Clin Cancer Res* 2003; **9**: 2447–56.

106. Karanikas V, Lurquin C, Colau D et al. Monoclonal anti-MAGE-3 CTL responses in melanoma patients displaying tumor regression after vaccination with a recombinant canarypox virus. *J Immunol* 2003; **171**: 4898–904.

107. Chen PW, Wang M, Bronte V et al. Therapeutic antitumor response after immunization with a recombinant adenovirus encoding a model tumor-associated antigen. *J Immunol* 1996; **156**: 224–31.

108. Zhai Y, Yang JC, Kawakami Y et al. Antigen-specific tumor vaccines. Development and characterization of recombinant adenoviruses encoding MART1 and gp100 for cancer therapy. *J Immunol* 1996; **156**: 700–10.

109. Lin KY, Guarnieri FG, Stavely-O'Carroll KF et al. Treatment of established tumors with a novel vaccine that enhances major histocompatibility class II presentation of tumor antigen. *Cancer Res* 1996; **56**: 21–6.

110. Grant EP, Michalek MT, Goldberg AL, Rock KL. Rate of antigen degradation by the ubiquitin–proteasome pathway influences MHC class I presentation. *J Immunol* 1995; **155**: 3750–8.

111 Toes RE, Hoeben RC, van der Voort EI et al. Protective anti-tumor immunity induced by vaccination with recombinant adenoviruses encoding multiple tumor-associated cytotoxic T lymphocyte epitopes in a string-of-beads fashion. *Proc Natl Acad Sci USA* 1997; **94**: 14 660–5.

112. Bronte V, Tsung K, Rao JB et al. IL-2 enhances the function of recombinant poxvirus-based vaccines in the treatment of established pulmonary metastasis. *J Immunol* 1995; **154**: 5282–92.

113. Hodge JW, McLaughlin JP, Abrams SI et al. Admixture of a recombinant vaccinia virus containing the gene for the costimulatory molecule B7 and a recombinant vaccinia virus containing a tumor-associated antigen gene results in enhanced specific T-cell responses and antitumor immunity. *Cancer Res* 1995; **55**: 3598–603.

114. Kast WM, Offringa R, Peters PJ et al. Eradication of adenovirus E1-induced tumors by E1a-specific cytotoxic T lymphocytes. *Cell* 1989; **59**: 603–15.

115. Toes REM, Offringa R, Blom HJJ et al. An adenovirus type 5 early region 1B-encoded CTL epitope-mediating tumor eradication by CTL clones is down-modulated by an activated ras oncogene. *J Immunol* 1995; **154**: 3396–405.

116. Hom RC, Finberg RW, Mullaney S, Ruprecht RM. Protective cellular retroviral immunity requires both CD41 and CD81 immune T cells. *J Virol* 1991; **65**: 220–4.

117. Kolb HJ, Mittelmüller J, Clemm C et al. Donor leukocyte transfusions for treatment of recurrent chronic myelogenous leukemia in marrow transplanted patients. *Blood* 1990; **76**: 2462–5.

118. Cullis JO, Jiang YZ, Schwarer AP. Donor leukocyte infusions for chronic myelogenous leukemia in relapse after allogeneic bone marrow transplantation. *Blood* 1992; **79**: 1379–81.

119. Bär BMAM, Schattenberg A, Mensink EJBM et al. Donor leukocyte infusions for chronic myeloid leukemia relapsed after allogeneic bone marrow transplantation. *J Clin Oncol* 1993; **11**: 513–19.

120. Helg C, Roux E, Beris P. Adoptive immunotherapy for recurrent CML after BMT. *Bone Marrow Transplant* 1993; **12**: 125–9.

121. Johnson BD, Weiler MB, Truitt RL. Adoptive immunotherapy with normal donor cells after allogeneic bone marrow transplantation provides an antileukemia

response without grafts-versus-host disease. *J Cell Biochem* 1993; **17**: 133–41.

122. Szer J, Grigg AP, Phillips GL. Donor leukocyte infusions after chemotherapy for patients relapsing with acute leukemia following allogeneic BMT. *Bone Marrow Transplant* 1993; **11**: 109–11.

123. Marmont AM. The graft versus leukemia (GVL) effect after allogeneic bone marrow transplantation for chronic myelogenous leukemia (CML). *Leuk Lymphoma* 1993; **11**(Suppl 1): 221–6.

124. Porter DL, Roth MS, McGarigle C et al. Induction of graft-versus-host disease as immunotherapy for relapsed chronic myeloid leukemia. *N Engl J Med* 1994; **330**: 1185–91.

125. Van Rhee F, Feng L, Cullis JO. Relapse of chronic myelogeneous leukemia after allogeneic bone marrow transplantation: the case for giving donor leukocyte transfusions before the onset of hematological relapse. *Blood* 1994; **83**: 3377–83.

126. Choudhury A, Gajewski JL, Liang JC et al. Use of leukemic dendritic cells for the generation of antileukemic cellular cytotoxicity against Philadelphia chromosome-positive myelogenous leukemia. *Blood* 1996; **89**: 1133–42.

127. Smit WM, Rijnbeek M, van Bergen CA et al. Generation of dendritic cells expressing *bcr–abl* from CD34-positive chronic myeloid leukemia precursor cells. *Hum Immunol* 1997; **53**: 216–23.

128. Mannering SI, McKenzie JL, Fearnley DB, Hart DN. HLA-DR1-restricted bcr–abl (b3a2)-specific CD41 T lymphocytes respond to dendritic cells pulsed with b3a2 peptide and antigen-presenting cells exposed to b3a2 containing cell lysates. *Blood* 1997; **90**: 290–7.

129. Smith CA, Ng CY, Loftin SK et al. Adoptive immunotherapy for Epstein–Barr virus-related lymphoma. *Leuk Lymphoma* 1996; **23**: 213–20.

130. Bollard CM, Savoldo B, Rooney CM, Heslop HE. Adoptive T-cell therapy for EBV-associated post-transplant lymphoproliferative disease. *Acta Haematol* 2003; **110**: 139–48.

131. Rosenberg SA, Packard BS, Aebersold PM et al. Use of tumor-infiltrating lymphocytes and interleukin-2 in the immunotherapy of patients with metastatic melanoma. *N Engl J Med* 1988; **319**: 1676–80.

132. Dudley ME, Wunderlich JR, Robbins PF et al. Cancer regression and autoimmunity in patients after clonal repopulation with antitumor lymphocytes. *Science* 2002; **298**: 850–4.

# 27 Interference with signaling pathways in malignant disease

**Asim Khwaja**

## Introduction

All normal cells are influenced by changes in their environment. The decision to move, to die, or to divide depends on extracellular factors, including a variety of cytokines and matrix proteins. Although some hormones may pass through the plasma membrane and interact directly with nuclear receptors, the majority of these factors affect the cell by interacting with external surface receptors that span the membrane – following ligand binding, a message is transmitted via dedicated signaling molecules inside the cell to the appropriate components of the cellular machinery. The molecules involved in transducing these messages form signaling modules, which often have complex relationships with each other.

The formation of cancer in humans is thought to involve a process whereby the sequential acquisition of genetic change in a number of key cellular pathways results in malignancy. Thus, many cancers share a number of attributes that set them apart from their normal counterparts: they may be independent of the normal requirement for external growth factors and less sensitive to signals that normally inhibit growth; they are often less susceptible to apoptosis and can proliferate without limits; in many instances, tumors stimulate the formation of new blood vessels and are also able to spread to sites distant from their origin.[1,2] Many of these changes in cellular behavior can be attributed to abnormalities in the biochemical pathways that are normally involved in signal transduction. An increasing number of abnormalities in signaling components have been identified, and these may either be relatively tumor-specific, for example mutations in the Flt3 tyrosine kinase receptor in AML,[3] or they may be found in a variety of malignancies, such as activating mutations in Ras proteins. Normal mechanisms of signal transduction are discussed in Chapter 3. This chapter will outline some of the abnormalities in signaling pathways that are found in hematological malignancies (Table 27.1) and will focus on approaches in the development of therapies that are targeted to these abnormalities.

## Abnormal tyrosine kinase signaling

Tyrosine kinases are normally activated in response to growth factor signaling, and this is often the earliest biochemical event that follows cytokine–receptor binding.[4] As discussed in Chapter 3, a number of growth factor receptors have intrinsic tyrosine kinase activity, for example c-Kit (the stem cell factor receptor) and Flt3, whereas other receptors utilize cytoplasmic tyrosine kinases, in particular of the Janus (JAK) and Src families. Tyrosine kinases are involved in the development of hematological malignancies in several ways: first, by mutation of receptor tyrosine kinases resulting in their constitutive activation, for example c-Kit in mast cell disorders[5] and Flt3 in acute myeloid leukemia (AML);[6] second, as components of fusion genes resulting from chromosomal translocation, for example BCR–ABL in chronic myeloid leukemia (CML) and acute lymphoblastic leukemia (ALL) and TEL–PDGFR in chronic myelomonocytic leukemia (CMML);[7] third, tyrosine kinases may be activated by overexpression or by the, inappropriate, autocrine or paracrine production of growth factors. In addition, tumor cells may secrete factors such as vascular endothelid growth factor (VEGF) that stimulate tyrosine kinase activity in normal host cells resulting in new blood vessel formation.

### Mutations in receptor tyrosine kinases

There are approximately 90 known protein tyrosine kinases (TK) in the human genome, of which two-thirds are receptor TK (RTK).[4] Signaling via RTK is normally a result of ligand-induced dimerization –

**Table 27.1 Constitutive activation of signaling pathways in hematological malignancies; inhibitors that have in vitro and/or clinical inhibitory activity are listed**

| Abnormal pathway | Genetic alteration | Disease | Inhibitor(s) |
|---|---|---|---|
| **Receptor tyrosine kinases** | | | |
| c-Kit | Point mutations (eg D816) | AML, mastocytosis | SU6577 |
| Flt3 | Point mutations (eg D835) | AML | PKC412, SU11248, CT53518, |
| | Internal tandem duplication | AML | CEP701 |
| PDGFRα | Fusion with *FIP1L1* interstitial deletion 4q12 | Hypereosinophilic syndrome | Imatinib, PKC412 |
| PDGFRβ | Fusion with *ETV6* (*TEL*) t(5;12) | CMML | Imatinib |
| FGFR1 | Fusion with *ZNF198* t(8;13) | Stem cell MPD | SU6668, SU5402 |
| | Fusion with *BCR* t(8;22) | CML | |
| FGFR3 | Overexpression t(4;14) | Myeloma | |
| ALK | Fusion with *NPM* t(2;5) | Anaplastic NHL | |
| TRK | Fusion of *TRKC* with *ETV6* t(12;15) | AML | CEP751 |
| | Activating deletion of *TRKA* 1q21 | AML | |
| **Cytoplasmic tyrosine kinases** | | | |
| ABL | Fusion with *BCR* t(9;22) | CML, ALL | Imatinib |
| | Fusion with *ETV6* t(9;12) | CML, AML | |
| ARG | Fusion with *ETV6* t(1;12) | AML | Imatinib |
| JAK2 | Fusion with *ETV6* t(9;12) | ALL, atypical CML | AG490 |
| Syk | Fusion with *FTV6* t(9;12) | MDS | BAY61-3606, piceatannol |
| **Ras pathway** | | | |
| Ras | Point mutations N- and Ki-*ras* | AML, CMML, JMML | Farnesyltransferase inhibitors |
| NF1 | Loss, point mutation | JMML | Farnesyltransferase inhibitors |
| **NF κB pathway** | Activated by Tax (HTLV-I) | ATLL | Proteasomal inhibitor |
| | Activated by EBV | Hodgkin lymphoma, Burkitt lymphoma | PS341/bortezomib, SPC839 |
| | c-*REL* amplification 2p14 | DLBCL | (IKK-2 inhibitor), aspirin |
| | *BCL10* amplification t(1;14) | MALT lymphoma | |
| **PI3K pathway** | Loss/mutation of *PTEN* | Lymphoma, myeloma | LY294002, wortmannin (PI3K inhibitors) |
| | Activated tyrosine kinases, Ras | Various | RAD001, CCI779 (mTOR inhibitors) |

PDGFR, platelet-derived growth factor receptor; FGFR, fibroblast growth factor receptor; ALK, anaplastic lymphoma kinase; PI3K, phosphatidylinositol 3'-kinase; AML, acute myeloid leukemia; CMML, chronic myelomonocytic leukemia; MPD, myeloproliferative disorder; CML, chronic myeloid leukemia; NHL, non-Hodgkin lymphoma; ALL, acute lymphoblastic leukemia; MDS, myelodysplastic syndrome; JMML, juvenile myelomonocytic leukemia; ATLL, adult T-cell leukemia/lymphoma; DLBCL, diffuse large B-cell lymphoma.

this results in phosphorylation in *trans* by the dimeric partner in a region known as the activation loop, which in the resting state occludes the active site of the kinase in *cis* and prevents substrate and/or ATP access. This phosphorylation leads to repositioning of the activation loop away from the active site and allows substrate to gain access.[4] The importance of this mechanism in preventing unwarranted activation of RTK is underscored by the fact that point mutations in the activation loop result in constitutive kinase activation and are found in a variety of hematological tumors, such as c-Kit in AML and mast cell disorders and Flt3 in AML (see below). In addition to the role of the activation loop in regulating kinase activity, the juxtamembrane region has also been implicated in autoinhibition. Crystal structural studies of the EphB2 TK suggest that the unphosphorylated juxtamembrane domain can interact with part of the kinase domain, resulting in catalytic repression.[4] This inhibition is relieved by phosphorylation of the juxtamembrane region after initial kinase activation following ligand binding. Oncogenic mutations can also affect this region, most notably in AML by internal tandem duplications of the *flt3* gene, and this is thought to relieve the normal constraints imposed by the juxtamembrane domain on catalytic activity.

### c-Kit

The c-Kit protein (CD117) is the receptor for stem cell factor (SCF, Steel factor), and is normally expressed on hematopoietic stem and progenitor cells (Figure 27.1). Expression is usually downregulated with maturation and differentiation, except in mast cell

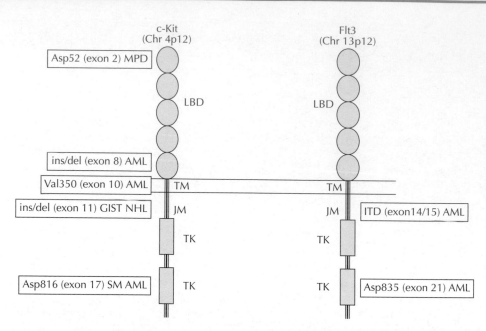

**Figure 27.1** Schematic representation of the c-Kit and Flt3 receptor tyrosine kinases. Sites of described mutations are shown. LBD, ligand-binding domain; TM, transmembrane domain; JM, juxtamembrane domain; TK, tyrosine kinase domain; MPD, myeloproliferative disorder; AML, acute myeloid leukemia; GIST, gastrointestinal stromal tumor; NHL, non-Hodgkin lymphoma; SM, systemic mastocytosis; ITD, internal tandem duplication.

development. Mutations in c-*kit* have been described in a number of hematological and related disorders. These are predominantly of three types: point mutations in the activation loop (exon 17) found in mast cell disorders, AML, and sinonasal lymphomas; mutations and in-frame insertions/deletions in the regulatory juxtamembrane region (exon 11), which are typically found in gastrointestinal stromal tumors (GIST); and mutations in the extracellular ligand-binding domain (exon 8), found in AML (reviewed in reference 8).

In systemic mastocytosis, virtually all adult patients are reported to have point mutations in the activation loop, mainly at asparate 816.[9] Systemic mastocytosis is associated with myeloid malignancies, in particular with AML and advanced myelodysplastic syndrome (MDS), classified as systemic mastocytosis with associated clonal hematological non-mast-cell lineage disease (SM-AHNMD).[10] The underlying mechanism of this association is not clear: it has been reported that the D816 mutation was present in the abnormal mast cells but not the leukemia cells in a patient with AML[11] but also that the mutation was present in both mast cells and myelomonocytic cells in a patient with associated CMML.[12] Studies in patients with indolent mastocytosis (without an associated hematological disorder) and the c-*kit* D816V mutation have utilized immunophenotype-based separation of mast cells, T and B lymphocytes, and monocytes to address which cell types were derived from the same clone. In the majority of cases, significant numbers of B lymphocytes and monocytes also have the D816V mutation, but T lymphocytes are usually not involved.[13,14] This is reminiscent of results obtained in recognized myeloproliferative stem cell disorders such as CML, and suggests that mastocytosis could be considered as part of this spectrum of disorders. Presumably, further genetic abnormalities are acquired in the stem/progenitor cells of some individuals, resulting in the development of more aggressive myeloid malignancy. A recent report of seven patients with SM-AHNMD showed two patients to have AML with t(8;21), two to have AML/refractory anemia with excess blasts 1 (RAEB-1) with chromosome 5 deletions, and one AML patient with an 11q23 abnormality.[15] t(8;21) in association with systemic mastocytosis has also been reported by others, and although numbers are small outcome does not appear to be favorable as in standard t(8;21)-positive AML.

In AML, c-*kit* mutations are found most frequently in patients with associated inv(16) and t(8;21) abnormalities.[8] These translocations result in the expression of the fusion genes *CBFβ–MYH11* and *AML1–ETO* respectively – CBFβ and AML1 both belong to the core binding factor (CBF) family, and this group of leukemias, which carries a relatively good prognosis, is known as CBF-AML.[16] Beghini and colleagues[17] showed in a small study that a high proportion of CBF-AML patients had a c-*kit* D816 mutation, and have also suggested that this may be associated with mast cell differentiation and high presenting white count. Reilly's group[18] has shown in a study of 110 patients with CBF-AML that 9% have a D816 mutation but that an additional 19% (predominantly those with inv(16)) have a D419 mutation. Overall, nearly 32% of patients with inv(16) had a c-*kit* mutation, compared with 13% with t(8;21). Although the D816 mutations have been shown to be constitutively active, this has not been demonstrated for the extracellular domain D419 abnormality.

### Flt3

The Flt3 receptor is expressed on hematopoietic stem and progenitor cells and is an important regulator of hematopoiesis (Figure 27.1). Mutations of *flt3* are largely restricted to patients with AML and comprise two main types: the internal tandem duplication

(ITD) and the D835 point mutation.[19] The more common abnormality results from in-frame duplication of 12–204 DNA base pairs of the intracellular juxtamembrane region of the receptor. This ITD is found in about 25% of adult AML cases (under the age of 60 years),[20] with a lower incidence (about 12%) in children.[21] Mutation detection is relatively simple, requiring a single polymerase chain reaction (PCR) step. The presence of an flt3 ITD is associated with a high white count and, in most series, with a higher relapse rate. ITD are more common in patients with promyelocytic leukemia, especially the variant kind, and less common in those with CBF abnormalities or complex karyotypes.[19] The mutant receptor is constitutively active, resulting in ligand-independent stimulation of the phosphatidylinositol 3′-kinase (PI3K), MAPK, and STAT5 pathways.[22,23] Expression of flt3-ITD can transform factor-dependent hematopoietic cell lines to growth factor independence.[23] When flt3-ITD is expressed in a murine progenitor transplant model, it induces an aggressive myeloproliferative disorder (rather than AML).[24] Expression of flt3-ITD into stem cells from a PML–RARα transgenic mouse leads to the accelerated development of promyelocytic AML, which is still all trans-retinoic acid (ATRA)-sensitive.[25] This suggests that flt3-ITD, which is commonly found in AML M3, can cooperate with PML–RARα in the development of overt leukemia. In about 10% of patients who present with flt3-ITD, and in whom the mutation is undetectable in remission, the mutation is not present at clinical relapse.[26] This indicates, at least in a subset of cases, that the flt3-ITD is a secondary phenomenon that is not required for maintenance of the leukemic phenotype. In addition to flt3-ITD, about 8% of AML cases have a D835 mutation.[19] This residue in the activation loop is at a homologous site to c-kit D816, and its point mutation results in constitutive activation of flt3. Therefore, in adult AML, about a third of all patients have an activating mutation in flt3, making this the single most frequently mutated known gene in this disease.

## Chromosomal translocations resulting in constitutive tyrosine kinase activation

A number of translocations known to generate constitutively active tyrosine kinases are found in hematological malignancies, of which the most intensely studied is the t(9;22) resulting in the generation of BCR–ABL in CML and ALL.

### BCR–ABL

The t(9;22) translocation fuses BCR genetic sequences upstream to those encoding c-ABL, resulting in a sequence that encodes for one of three BCR–ABL fusion proteins: p185 associated with ALL, p210 associated with CML, and p230 associated with a more indolent chronic neutrophilic leukemia.[27,28] ABL is a tyrosine kinase with important functions in regulation of the cell cycle and apoptosis, in particular in response to DNA damage and in interactions with the actin cytoskeleton. The BCR–ABL fusion proteins have markedly increased tyrosine kinase activity compared with ABL and lead to inappropriate autophosphorylation and phosphorylation of many substrates.[29] There is constitutive activation of several signaling pathways, with activation of the Ras and PI3K pathways believed to be critical in maintaining the abnormal phenotype.[30,31] The adapter proteins Grb2 and Crkl probably play an important role in maintaining prolonged activation of signaling pathways that are normally only transiently activated in cells following growth factor stimulation.[32,33] In addition, activation of the transcription factors NF-κB, c-Jun, and c-Myc have all been implicated in BCR–ABL-mediated transformation.[7] There is some debate as to whether BCR–ABL has a significant anti-apoptotic effect. Cell lines overexpressing the fusion protein are usually factor-independent, but some groups have not detected such an effect in cells taken from patients with CML.[34–36] In addition, evidence from patients treated with the ABL kinase inhibitor imatinib suggests that total eradication of BCR–ABL progenitors does not occur[37] – this may be because inhibition of ABL kinase activity does not trigger apoptosis of leukemia progenitors but results in negation of their proliferative advantage over normal cells, allowing non-CML cells to repopulate the blood and marrow.[38]

Transgenic mice expressing p210[BCR–ABL] usually develop lymphoid malignancies, but the expression of BCR–ABL by retroviral transduction in a murine bone marrow transplantation model can lead to the generation of a CML-like disorder.[39,40] Tenen's group[41] has generated a conditional transgenic mouse model expressing p210 regulated by tetracycline administration. These animals rapidly develop a precursor B-cell leukemia akin to Ph-positive human ALL that regresses on readministration of tetracycline (which turns off BCR–ABL expression). ABL is also involved in fusion with TEL (ETV6) in the t(9;12), which is an uncommon translocation but has been reported in CML, AML, and ALL.[42]

### PDGFRβ

Platelet-derived growth factor receptor β (PDGFRβ) is a receptor tyrosine kinase normally expressed on mesenchymal cells and involved in proliferation and migration. It is located on chromosome 5q33, and in hematological malignancies is predominantly involved in the pathophysiology of CMML. A number of fusion partners have been described, the most common being TEL (ETV6). The TEL–PDGFRβ fusion protein is the product of the t(5;12) translocation and fuses TEL to the intracytoplasmic domain of PDGFRβ.[43,44] TEL is able to dimerize via its helix–loop–helix domain, and this leads to constitutive activation of the intrinsic tyrosine kinase activity of the cytoplasmic portion of PDGFRβ. The other reported partners also have dimerization capability, and all result in constitutive kinase activity. TEL–PDGFRβ has been shown to be capable of transforming interleukin-3 (IL-3)-dependent cell lines to factor independence. The intracytoplasmic domain of PDGFRβ is known to transduce a variety of signals, including activation of Src, Ras, PI3K, and phospholipase C(PLC).[45] A myeloproliferative disease can be induced in a *TEL–PDGFβR* transgenic model.[46]

### PDGFRα

Gilliland and colleagues[47] have recently described a recurring translocation involving PDGFRα found in a high proportion of patients with hypereosinophilic syndrome (HES). This condition, which is typified by eosinophilia of unknown cause with associated tissue damage, has been ill-understood up to now. It has been suggested that patients with clonal eosinophilia should be classified as having a chronic eosinophilic leukemia.[48] The presence of an interstitial deletion on chromosome 4q12 in one patient with HES resulted in the identification of the fusion of a novel gene *Fip-1-like 1* (*FIP1L1*) to the intracytoplasmic portion of PDGFRα. The *FIP1L1–PDGFRα* fusion (which is usually undetectable by conventional cytogenetic analysis) was subsequently found in 9 of 16 patients with HES – the protein has constitutive activation of tyrosine kinase activity and can render hematopoietic cells factor-independent.[47] PDGFRα kinase activity is exquisitely sensitive to the ABL inhibitor imatinib, which has been used to successfully manage HES (see below). The presence of a clonal abnormality in patients previously thought to have non-clonal disease indicates that we need to rethink our view of HES as a clinical entity.

### FGFR1

The gene for fibroblast growth factor receptor 1 (*FGFR1*) is located on chromosome 8p11 and is fused to a number of partners, most commonly *ZNF198*, in a myeloproliferative disorder (MPD) known as the 8p11 myeloproliferative syndrome (EMS).[49] Patients with this sydrome present with a Ph-negative MPD with marked bone marrow and blood eosinophilia. In addition, the majority of patients have an associated non-Hodgkin lymphoma, which is usually of T-cell origin. The same cytogenetic abnormality is found in the MPD cells as in the lymphoma, suggesting that the initial genetic change takes place in a pluripotent stem cell. The disease usually rapidly evolves to a blastic acute leukemia phase, which is commonly of myeloid phenotype[49] although cases transforming to B-ALL have also been reported.[50] *FGFR1* is also involved in the variant t(8;22), which results in a fusion with the *BCR* gene and presents as CML.[51] FGFR inhibitors

have been described, but there are no clinical reports of their use in hematological disorders with specific translocations.[52]

### ALK

Anaplastic lymphoma kinase (ALK) is a tyrosine kinase receptor that is normally expressed in a developmentally restricted way in the central nervous system.[53] The ligand for ALK is pleiotropin,[54] and ALK was originally identified in the t(2;5) translocation in anaplastic large cell lymphoma.[55] In this translocation, the N-terminal 117 amino acid residues of the nucleolar protein nucleophosmin (NPM) are joined to the entire intracytoplasmic domain of ALK. This fusion is sufficient to transform fibroblasts, and retrovirally mediated transduction of *NPM–ALK* into mouse bone marrow leads to B-lineage large cell lymphoma.[56] The NPM segment is required for oligomerization of the fusion protein, which leads to activation of ALK kinase activity.[57,58] Other partners for ALK have also been described, all of which contain multimerization domains in what is a recurring theme in RTK fusion proteins.[59] NPM–ALK expression results in the activation of multiple signaling pathways, of which PI3K and STAT5 have been postulated as being critical for malignant transformation.[60–62]

### JAK2

The JAK family of cytosolic tyrosine kinases are critical for hematopoiesis but are rare partners in translocation events in hematopoietic malignancies. Fusion of *TEL* (*ETV6*) to *JAK2* has been reported in ALL and a case of atypical CML in transformation.[63,64] In many cases of AML and ALL, constitutive activation of JAKs and various STAT proteins (signal transducers and activators of transcription) has been reported.[65–67] The mechanism by which this activation takes place is unclear, but could involve autocrine production of stimulatory cytokines such as granulocyte–macrophage colony-stimulating factor (GM-CSF)[68,69] and IL-6.[70]

# Inappropriate activation of downstream signaling proteins

A number of signaling modules are activated by cytokines following initial stimulation of tyrosine kinase activity. These pathways can also be activated by activating mutations of positive regulators or deletion of negative regulators, and may be useful targets for therapeutic intervention.

## Ras

Many different physiological processes are regulated by guanine nucleotide-binding proteins that act as molecular switches. Conformational changes as a result of binding GTP enable these proteins to interact with target enzymes (also known as effectors). The interaction is limited by the intrinsic GTPase activity of the protein (converting bound GTP to GDP), which may be enhanced by catalytic mechanisms involving GTPase activating proteins (GAPs). There are two broad classes of such proteins: heterotrimeric G-proteins, which are classically associated with hormone receptors, and members of the Ras superfamily (also known as small GTPases), which are monomeric proteins of about 20–25 kDa in size.[71] The Ras superfamily includes subfamilies that are involved in related processes. The Ras subfamily is mainly involved in cell survival, growth, and differentiation; the Rho subfamily in cytoskeletal organization; the Rab subfamily in vesicular transport; the Ran subfamily in nuclear protein and RNA transport; and the Arf subfamily predominantly in membrane trafficking.[72]

Four alleles of *ras* have been described: Harvey (H), Kirsten (Ki) A and B, and neuroblastoma (N). Knockout studies have shown that H-Ras and N-Ras, either alone or in combination, are not required for normal mouse development whereas loss of Ki-Ras results in embryonic death (reviewed in reference 73). The reasons for this difference are not fully understood, but are most likely due to the ubiquitous expression of Ki-Ras. Ras is activated in response to a large number of stimuli, including growth factors and extracellular matrix–integrin interactions. Ras proteins are switched to the 'on' GTP-bound state by the positive action of guanine nucleotide exchange factors,[74] of which the best characterized is the son-of-sevenless (SOS) protein, or, less frequently, by the inhibition of GAPs such as p120[Ras-GAP] [75] and neurofibromin (NF1) (Figure 27.2). Point mutations at conserved residues in Ras that lead to constitutive activation by maintaining it in the GTP-bound state are found at a high frequency in human malignancies.[73] In hematopoietic tumors, mutations are found mainly in N-*ras* and Ki-*ras*.

For full biological activity, H-Ras must undergo post-translational modification by prenylation, resulting in its association with cellular membranes (reviewed in reference 76). The critical first step in this process is the covalent attachment of a farnesyl (15-carbon chain) group to cysteine 186 at the C-terminal end of the protein. The terminal three amino acids are then cleaved by a specific protease and the C terminus is methylated. The final modification step required for effective membrane localization is palmitoylation (covalent attachment of a 16-carbon moiety) at the C-terminal region. H-, Ki-, and N-Ras all undergo farnesylation, but only Ki-Ras is not additionally palmitoylated. Rather it relies on a cluster of C-terminal basic residues that interact with acidic phospholipids on the inner leaflet of the plasma membrane. Other members of the Ras superfamily, such as Rho, are not farnesylated but undergo geranylgeranylation (addition of a 20-carbon chain). These processes are catalyzed by specific enzymes: farnesyltransferase, geranylgeranyltransferases, prenyl protein-specific proteases, etc.

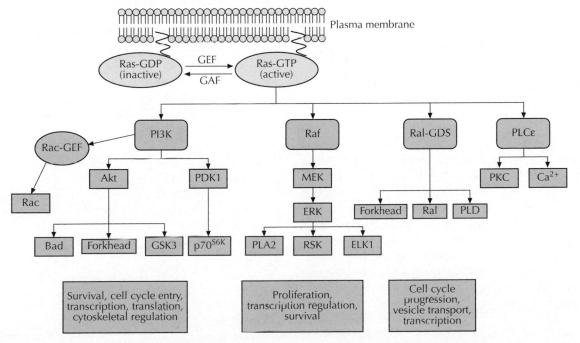

**Figure 27.2** Activation of the Ras signaling pathway regulates a number of cellular functions. Ras at the plasma membrane is activated in response to a GEF (guanine nucleotide exchange factor) and is inactivated by a GAP (GTPase-activating protein). GTP-bound Ras interacts with a number of effectors, including phosphatidylinositol 3′-kinase (PI3K), Raf, Ral–guanine nucleotide dissociation stimulator (Ral-GDS) and phospholipase Cε (PLCε).

## Ras targets

Activation of Ras proteins has been shown to be involved in the control of cell proliferation, survival, differentiation and movement (Figure 27.2). The first Ras target or effector to be described was the serine/threonine kinase Raf-1.[77] Raf-1 and the related B-Raf and A-Raf proteins sit at the head of a signaling pathway that results in the activation of the ERK type of MAPK (mitogen-activated protein kinases) and subsequently in transcriptional activation.[78] Activation of ERKs can also regulate non-nuclear substrates such as phospholipase A2 (PLA2) and myosin light-chain kinase (MLCK).[79,80] The duration of activation of the ERK pathway can play an important part in dictating the cellular response. Prolonged ERK activation was shown originally to result in neuronal cell differentiation rather than proliferation,[81] and thrombopoietin (TPO) may function in a similar way to regulate megakaryocyte maturation.[82] Although many of the biological effects of Ras were initially attributed to the activation of Raf, it has since become clear that other important effectors exist, including PI3K, Ral-GDS and phospholipase Cε (PLCε). The best characterized of these is the catalytic subunit of the PI3K,[83] and it is clear that, at least in some cell types, this activity is important for the anti-apoptotic[84] and cytoskeletal effects of Ras.[85] Importantly, the full effects of oncogenic Ras in promoting malignant transformation are probably reliant on cooperation between the various effectors.

## Ras mutations

Point mutations at codons 12, 13, and 61 are commonly found in AML and in MDS, most often in CMML. Interestingly, Ras mutations rarely coexist with oncogenic tyrosine kinase mutations such as Flt3, TEL–PDGFRβ and BCR–ABL. Constitutively active tyrosine kinases result in the activation of normal cellular Ras, and the rarity of coexisting mutations suggest that the Ras pathway is sufficient in many malignancies to provide similar transforming signals as active tyrosine kinases. In AML and other hematological malignancies, mutations are usually found in N-*ras* and less commonly in Ki-*ras*. These mutations result in a greatly reduced ability to hydrolyze GTP, resulting in a molecule that is always in the 'on' position. Although the incidence of *ras* mutations varies greatly between published series, overall it is approximately 20% in AML.[86–89] The presence of activating *ras* mutations in myeloid leukemia has been known of for some time, but the biological significance of this feature is not clear. In one study, AML colonies taken from cases with N-*ras* mutations grown in vitro were examined and it was shown that the proportion of colonies containing no mutant allele ranged from 5% to 57%.[90] This suggests that *ras* mutations are post-initiation events in AML

and may contribute to the outgrowth of more malignant subclones. In hematopoietic cell lines, the expression of activated Ras usually confers growth factor independence, but data from primary AML samples are lacking. Published data are not clear on whether the presence of an activating *ras* mutation is associated with an adverse outcome.

*ras* mutations are frequently found in myeloma, but there is some dispute about the true rate of abnormality.[91] One large series found activating mutations in 39% of samples examined.[92] In some reports, this has coincided with more advanced disease, *ras* mutations being found at very high frequency in plasma cell leukemias.[93] Although the introduction of oncogenic *ras* into myeloma cell lines can lead to a reduction in factor dependence and inhibition of apoptosis,[94] whether this is true in cases with ('natural') *ras* mutations is unclear.

Recently, activating mutations in the B-*raf* gene have been found at high frequency in human tumors, in particular in melanomas and colon carcinoma.[95] Although comprehensive large-scale screens of primary tissue in hematological malignancies have not been reported, no mutations have been found in myeloma/plasma cell lines or in selected cases of AML.[96,97]

## JMML and NF1

Neurofibromin, the product of the *NF1* gene, is a GAP for Ras and is important in some cell types for converting Ras to the inactive GDP-bound state. Infants and children with neurofibromatosis type I (NF1) have a markedly increased risk of developing myeloid malignancies such as juvenile myelomonocytic leukemia (JMML), monosomy 7 syndrome/MDS, and AML.[98] *ras* point mutations are often found in JMML patients without NF1 syndrome, but not in JMML patients with NF1 syndrome.[99,100] In NF1 patients with leukemia, there is frequent loss of heterozygosity of *NF1*, with retention of the mutant allele.[101] Loss of NF1 GAP activity is responsible for increased levels of Ras-GTP, with a hypersensitive response to GM-CSF.[102,103] Hematopoietic reconstitution of mice with *NF1*-deficient stem cells results in a myeloproliferative syndrome akin to JMML. Therefore, it appears that overactivation of the Ras signaling pathway is important in the development of myeloid malignancy in individuals with NF1.

## PI3K

Phosphoinositides phosphorylated on the 3'-hydroxyl group of the inositol ring are transiently found in many cell types stimulated with growth factors and in cells transformed by a variety of oncogenes. The enzymatic activity responsible for this is termed PI3K, and was originally purified as a heterodimer composed of an 85 kDa regulatory and a 110 kDa catalytic subunit.[104] Subsequent investigation has shown that there is a family of such kinases, but for the purposes of this chapter we will focus on the canonical pathway. The major lipid products of growth factor-stimulated PI3K are derived from the phosphorylation of phosphatidylinositol 4,5-bisphosphate – this yields first phosphatidylinositol 3,4,5-trisphosphate ($PIP_3$) and then, by the action of inositol 5′-phosphatases, phosphatidylinositol 3,4,-bisphosphate.[105] $PIP_3$ has been implicated in the subsequent activation of several targets, including the Rho family GTP-binding protein Rac, the serine kinase Akt/PKB, and certain atypical members of the PKC family (reviewed in reference 106). The active lipid products are downregulated predominantly by the action of the PTEN (phosphatase and tensin homolog) phosphatase, which acts to remove the 3′-phosphate from the inositol phospholipids. In addition, Src homology 2 domain-containing inositol 5′-phosphatase (SHIP), which removes the 5′-phosphate from $PIP_3$, is also involved in the control of PI3K signaling.[107] PI3K activity has been shown to be involved in many diverse physiological processes, including cell proliferation, cytoskeletal rearrangements and chemotaxis, the oxidative burst of phagocytic cells, cell survival, and glucose transport.[106]

PI3K is involved in malignant change in a variety of tumors, as is most clearly shown by the loss of the *PTEN* gene, which acts as a tumor suppressor.[108,109] This is fairly common in tumors such as prostate and pancreatic cancers and in glioblastomas. Loss of *PTEN* is, however, uncommon in lymphomas and myeloid leukemias.[110–112] Activation of the PI3K targets Akt and p70$^{S6K}$ is commonly seen in leukemia and myeloma – as this pathway can be activated by tyrosine kinases and by Ras, it is possible that in the majority of cases there is no evolutionary pressure within the tumor cells for the loss of *PTEN*, but further studies would be needed to confirm this.

### NFκB

Nuclear factor κB refers to a group of closely related protein dimers that bind to a common DNA sequence motif (reviewed in reference 113). There are five family members, which fall into two classes: those that do not require proteolytic processing (RELA/p65, c-REL, and RELB) and those that are processed to generate p50 and p52 proteins (NFκB1/p105 and NFκB2/p100). These two groups form dimers, of which the most common is p50$^{RELA}$. In the canonical NFκB pathway, dimers composed of RELA, c-REL, and p50 are restrained in the cytoplasm by association with an inhibitor of κB proteins (IκB). Triggering of the pathway, commonly by cytokines and in response to infection, results in phosphorylation of IκB, which targets this protein for ubiquitination and subsequent degradation by the proteasome. The liberated NFκB dimers can now translocate to the nucleus, where they induce the transcription of a number of targets – these include genes that regulate the immune system, inflammation, apoptosis, and proliferation. It is thought that NFκB may be one of the links between chronic inflammation and the development of malignant change, such as is seen in infections with *Helicobacter pylori*.

NFκB has been shown to be activated in a variety of hematological malignancies, in particular those affecting lymphoid tissues. As its targets include apoptosis regulators such as the BCL2 family members BFL1/A1 and BCL-X$_L$ and cellular inhibitors of apoptosis (IAP) as well as D- and G-type cyclins, it is an attractive candidate for mediating many of the key features of malignancy.[114] NFκB is directly activated by the Tax oncoprotein of HTLV-I, which is implicated in the development of T-cell leukemia.[115] The c-REL locus at 2p14 is frequently amplified in diffuse large B-cell lymphomas.[116] Epstein–Barr virus (EBV), which is implicated in the development of Burkitt lymphoma, some cases of Hodgkin lymphoma, and lymphoproliferative disorders in immunocompromised patients, can activate NFκB via latent membrane protein 1 (LMP1) and EBV nuclear antigen 2 (EBNA2).[113] In MALT lymphomas associated with t(1;14), a truncated BCL10 is amplified by translocation and leads to activation of NFκB.[117] In addition, the t(11;18) translocation associated with MALT lymphomas that are less sensitive to H. *pylori* eradication results in the formation of a fusion protein AP12–MALT1 that activates NFκB.[118] The NFκB pathway may be important in the pathophysiology of *BCR–ABL*-induced disease,[119] and has been found to be constitutively active in a high proportion of AML cells, including the most primitive CD34$^+$CD38$^-$ fraction believed to include leukemia-initiating cells.[120]

## Signaling components as therapeutic targets

Hematologists have been used to using signal transduction-directed therapy for some years. Cyclosporin A suppresses the immune system by inhibiting a key Ca$^{2+}$/calmodulin-dependent protein phosphatase known as PP2B or calcineurin. In addition, rapamycin, which is also used as an immunosuppressant, inhibits the protein kinase mTOR (target of rapamycin), which plays a crucial role in T-cell proliferation signaling. The identification of aberrant or overactive signaling pathways in hematopoietic malignancies has raised the possibility of interfering with these pathways in a targeted manner for therapeutic purposes.

For many years, it was felt that blocking signal transduction pathways for treating malignancy would be ineffective for a number of reasons. As human tumor development is thought to be the result of multiple genetic changes within a cell, targetting a single signaling pathway was predicted to be futile. However, it appears that tumors may become 'addicted' to certain oncogenic pathways and that the inactivation, even transiently, of these pathways can trigger cell death or differentiation.[121] The evidence for this largely comes from transgenic murine models of tumor development using regulatable oncogenes. Most frequently, these are controlled by tetracycline, which can be added or withdrawn from the mouse diet to assess the effects of turning on and then switching off an oncogene. For example, Felsher and Bishop showed that transgenic mice expressing *myc* developed T-cell and myeloid leukemias and that these regressed on switching off *myc* due to the induction of cell cycle arrest, differentiation, and apoptosis (reviewed in reference 122). Similar results have been obtained with *BCR–ABL* transgenic mice,[41] and it appears that even brief inactivation of the oncogene may be sufficient to trigger tumor regression. Clearly, these tumor models do not accurately reproduce the development of tumors in humans, but they do suggest that inactivation of signaling pathways may be beneficial in some malignancies. In addition, it appears that some hematological disorders, in particular chronic myeloproliferative disorders such as CML, may not be the result of multiple genetic changes but develop as a consequence of activating mutations or translocations of tyrosine kinases. As is shown in more detail below, such malignancies appear to respond to blockade of the single dysregulated signaling pathway.

Another theoretical worry with signal transduction inhibitors has been that many of the pathways involved, such as Ras and PI3K, are critical for the function of normal cells. Downward[73] has postulated that as tumor cells often have high levels of anti-apoptotic signaling activity, this may allow the cell to accumulate and tolerate other genetic changes that would normally be deleterious (such as DNA damage due to loss of cell cycle control). Therefore, inhibition of the dysregulated survival pathway, on which the tumor cell is now reliant, could lead to cell death due to the accumulated active death signals that the cell has previously been able to withstand. Normal cell counterparts in this model would be more able to tolerate blockade of the pathway as they have lower intrinsic levels of death signals. However, the issue of the extent to which a therapeutic window is present and if toxicity to normal tissues is acceptable may have to be empirically assessed for each pathway.

Finally with signaling inhibitors, the issue of specificity has also been raised. In particular, many agents that block kinase activity do so by competing for ATP binding – this region of kinases is highly conserved and it had been felt by many that specific inhibitors would be near impossible to develop. However, we now know that a number of ATP-competitive inhibitors also make contacts with regions of the kinase that are not directly involved in ATP binding and that this can confer some specificity as these areas are less conserved. In addition, as is illustrated by the use of imatinib in the treatment of CML, inhibitors that are not completely specific for their target may still be extremely valuable drugs. This realization, and the clinical success of imatinib, has resulted in virtually all large pharmaceutical and biotechnology companies having major programs in the area of signal transduction inhibition.

## Tyrosine kinase inhibitors

### BCR–ABL-positive leukemias

The results of clinical studies with the ABL inhibitor imatinib (CGP57148, STI571, Gleevec/Glivec) is considered in detail in Chapters 32 and 41. This section will review the mechanism by which imatinib acts, briefly consider the results obtained in CML and ALL, and discuss problems of resistance.

Druker and colleagues[123] were the first to show in the mid 1990s that the ATP-competitive compound STI571 (later named imatinib) could inhibit ABL kinases at low micromolar concentrations. It inhibited the growth of cell lines expressing BCR–ABL in vitro and inhibited tumor formation using similar cells in syngeneic mice. At low concentrations, it inhibited CML colony growth in semisolid assays with much less of an effect on progenitors from normal individuals. Extensive profiling has shown that imatinib is relatively selective for ABL – additional kinases that are inhibited are ARG (a close relative of ABL), c-Kit, and both PDGFRα and β.[124] Crystal structure analysis of the ABL–imatinib complex has shown that imatinib binds to ABL when it is in an inactive conformation and presumably locks it in this state, preventing it from becoming activated and then transferring phosphates to target proteins.[125,126] This may partly explain some of the selectivity of imatinib, as inactive kinase conformations are thought to be structurally more varied than active ones.

The clinical results with imatinib in chronic phase CML have been dramatic from the outset, and the drug is now licensed for use in this disease. Doses of 400 mg/day and above have been associated with very high hematological and cytogenetic response rates.[127] It is not clear if imatinib exerts its effects by selectively inducing apoptosis in BCR–ABL-positive cells or by decreasing the proliferative advantage of the malignant clone (or indeed both). There is a large body of in vitro data showing that BCR–ABL-positive cells undergo apoptosis in response to imatinib, but these experiments mostly involve cells that have been engineered to be dependent on the fusion protein for survival and proliferation. It is possible to isolate quiescent phenotypically primitive (CD34+)

BCR–ABL-positive cells from patients with CML in chronic phase that are resistant to the effects of imatinib[38] – this suggests that ABL inhibitors may not be able to induce apoptosis of all leukemic progenitors. The clinical responses to imatinib in chronic phase CML have been durable and contrast with results seen in patients with blast crisis of CML or with relapsed Ph-positive ALL.[128] Although there is a significant response to single-agent imatinib in these patients, this is typically of short duration but may be useful as preparation for more aggressive therapy or as part of a combination with cytotoxic drugs.

Soon after the trials with imatinib were initiated, it became apparent that clinical resistance was a problem in advanced disease (reviewed in reference 129). There are a number of potential mechanisms by which this could occur. First, there may be binding proteins in the plasma that become upregulated and reduce the amount of available intracellular imatinib. It has been suggested that increased levels of $\alpha_1$ acid glycoprotein may mediate this,[130] but the evidence is not conclusive.[131] Second, further genetic abnormalities could develop within the leukemia cells that render them resistant to the effects of imatinib (clonal evolution). Additional chromosomal aberrations have been described in a significant proportion of patients with imatinib resistance by Hochaus et al,[132] but it is not clear if these render the cells less sensitive to the effects of the drug. Third, gene amplification of BCR–ABL could result in cells that are resistant to the effects of imatinib if there is a threshold level of kinase activity that is sufficient to confer a biological advantage to the leukemia clone. Amplification was initially shown to be a factor in imatinib resistance of leukemia cell lines and has been detected in a proportion of patients.[132–134] In some instances, the clone with amplified BCR–ABL has been shown to decline if drug is temporarily withdrawn. Finally, resistance could develop as a result of mutations within BCR–ABL that lead to decreased binding of imatinib. The first report of such a mutation indicated a high frequency of C-to-T change at nucleotide 1091 resulting in the alteration of a threonine at position 315 to isoleucine (T315I).[134] This mutation retains kinase activity and is resistant to imatinib in vitro. Analysis of the crystal structure complex of ABL and imatinib shows that position 315 is a key residue for imatinib binding. A number of further mutations have now been described and it has been shown that in some patients these are already present at low levels prior to the initiation of imatinib therapy.[129,135–137]

The problems with resistance to imatinib monotherapy are likely to become increasingly significant as more patients are treated for longer periods. One approach to circumvent resistance would be to use structurally unrelated ABL kinase inhibitors either to treat patients who are resistant to imatinib or in combination at the initiation of therapy. For example, the drug PD166326 will inhibit the imatinib-resistant E255K BCR–ABL mutant.[138] However, neither PD166236 nor another inhibitor PD180970 effectively inhibit the common T315I mutant.[139] Alternative approaches may be to target BCR–ABL using other drugs such as geldanamycin, which reduces BCR–ABL protein levels by inhibiting the function of the molecular chaperone and heat-shock protein Hsp90.[140] Other avenues that are being tested are to combine imatinib with drugs that work in a non-ABL-targeted fashion such as cytotoxic agents (e.g. cytarabine), interferon-$\alpha$, and farnesyltransferase inhibitors (see below).

### Hypereosinophilic syndrome and mast cell disease

The effectiveness of imatinib in HES was first described in a case report in 2001[141] and this has been followed by further reports showing high response rates at low doses (100–200 mg/day).[142–145] In a number of patients, this is due to dysregulation of the PDGFR$\alpha$ receptor as a result of fusion to the FIP1L1 gene[47] (see above), but a significant number of responders do not have this or any other detectable molecular abnormalities. Gilliland and colleagues[47,146] reported the development of imatinib resistance in one of their cohort of patients due to a point mutation, echoing the problems seen in BCR–ABL-mediated disease. This mutant was still sensitive to an alternative kinase inhibitor, PKC412.[47,146]

The common c-Kit mutation found in mast cell disease (D816V) is insensitive to imatinib.[147] However, there may be patients with systemic mast cell disease who respond to this drug,[148] and it has been postulated that this could be due to the inhibition of wild-type c-Kit or of another unidentifed kinase.

### Flt3 mutant leukemia

There are a number of compounds that are in early clinical trials for mutant Flt3-positive AML, including PKC412 (Novartis), SU11248 (Sugen), CEP701 (Cephalon) and CT53518 (Millenium).[149] They all inhibit other kinases in addition to Flt3 and have demonstrable activity against flt3-ITD-positive cell lines in vitro and in animal models.[150–152] So far, results from clinical studies have only been presented orally and in abstract form and show a modest response rate in AML with single-agent therapy. It is possible that significant beneficial effects of Flt3 inhibitors would be seen in combination with conventional cytotoxic agents.

### Inhibitors of Ras

Several compounds have been identified that effectively inhibit Ras farnesylation.[153] The rationale for their development was to inhibit Ras targeting to the plasma membrane and thereby suppress oncogenic Ras-mediated tumor growth. This would have to be achieved without toxicity to cells expressing normal Ras and without adversely affecting the function of other farnesylated proteins such as nuclear lamins and rhodopsin. Considering the importance of Ras to myriad normal cell functions, this approach required that cells expressing activated Ras would be more sensitive to Ras inhibition, a view supported by some experimental data. In tumor models, a CAAX peptidomimetic was shown to cause regression of tumors generated in MMTV–v-H-*ras* transgenic mice.[154] However, the majority of human malignancies bear Ki- or N-*ras* mutations. It has been shown that Ki-Ras is much less sensitive to FTase inhibitors (FTI) than is H-Ras;[73] in addition in cells treated with FTI, both Ki- and N-Ras (but not H-Ras) can undergo alternative modification by geranylgeranylation and thereby remain associated with the membrane fraction.[155] This may help to explain the relative lack of toxicity of these compounds on normal cells, but also raises questions about their use in human cancer. Furthermore, data derived from a Ras-transformed fibroblast experimental system suggests that the effects of FTI is dependent on inhibition of RhoB function, which presumably acts downstream of Ras.[156,157] FTI have also been shown to inhibit growth of tumor cells that do not express mutant Ras.[158]

The most extensive clinical experience of Ras inhibition in hematological malignancies is with the oral agent R115777 (Tipifarnib, Janssen),[159] which is a non-peptidomimetic FTI.[160,161] Treatment of 35 adults with poor-risk acute leukemia showed only two complete remissions but some clinical response in 29% of patients.[162] None of the patients had *ras* mutations, emphasizing the fact that FTI, although designed with a rational target, may be exerting their effects in ways that were not previously predicted. Activity in pancreatic cancer, where *ras* mutations are virtually universal, emphasizes this point, as no responses were seen to single-agent therapy.[163] A further study with R115777 has shown activity in CML, albeit transient, a low response rate in myeloma, and modest activity in myelofibrosis.[164] The number of patients who have been treated with R115777 are still small, and further studies, utilizing combinations with conventional cytotoxics in AML and perhaps with ABL kinase inhibitors in CML, are awaited.

## Proteasomal inhibitors

The proteasome is a multicomponent complex found in all cell types that is involved in protein degradation, in particular of proteins that have been modified by ubiquitination.[165] These include cell cycle-regulatory components, p53, cytokine receptors, and the NFκB inhibitor IκB. In vitro studies show that tumor cells in general have high proteasomal activity and have a greater propensity to undergo cell cycle arrest or apoptosis in response to inhibitors compared with

normal counterparts.[166] This is likely to be multifactorial due to the reduced breakdown of a variety of proteins. The boronic acid dipeptide bortezomib (PS-341)[167] is a proteasomal inhibitor that is most advanced in its clinical evaluation in hematological malignancies and solid tumors.[168,169] A phase I study[170] showed significant activity in patients with plasma cell dyscrasias where significant in vitro effects had previously been found.[171] A subsequent phase II trial in nearly 200 patients with relapsed, refractory myeloma showed a response rate of 35%, with 10% having a complete or near-complete response.[172] Two-thirds of the patients had previously had a stem cell transplant and 83% had received thalidomide. Bortezomib has to be given intravenously, but was well tolerated in this group of patients with advanced disease and will be evaluated as antimyeloma therapy earlier in the course of the disease. Further studies in Waldenström's macroglobuliemia and non-Hodgkin lymphomas are also under way.

## Raf/MEK, PI3K and mTOR inhibitors

A number of tumors show increased MAPK activity. In some malignancies, for example melanoma, this is a consequence of activating mutations in Raf itself (B-Raf),[95] but more frequently increased activity is probably due to activation of upstream regulators such as tyrosine kinases and Ras. Two compounds targeting this pathway are in clinical development – the Raf inhibitor BAY 43–9006[173] and the MEK (MAPK/ERK kinase, MAPKK) inhibitor CI-1040[174] – but there are no results as yet in hematological malignancies.

A number of in vitro studies using the PI3K inhibitors LY294002 and wortmannin have shown that blockade of this pathway may have activity in a wide variety of tumors.[175] However, there have been concerns that the involvement of PI3K in the survival and proliferation of normal cells would result in excessive toxicity. Attention has now switched to developing isoform-specific PI3K inhibitors – there may be differential activation of α, β, γ, and δ isoforms in abnormal cells compared with normal tissues, and inhibitors that selectively target each isoform may be valuable. In addition, there is evidence that inhibiting one of the downstream targets of the PI3K pathway known as mTOR (mamalian target of rapamycin) may inhibit tumor cell proliferation.[176] There are a number of trials with inhibitors related to rapamycin (CCI-779 and RAD001)[177,178] currently running, but detailed results are not as yet available.

# Conclusions

Enormous advances have been made, and are continuing to be made, in understanding signal transduction pathways in normal and malignant cells. It is likely that in the next decade an increasing number of compounds targeted to specific abnormalities in signaling pathways in malignant cells will be identified. A coordinated combination of laboratory and clinical research will be needed to evaluate whether this approach of rational drug development will result in clinically useful agents.

## REFERENCES

1. Hanahan D, Weinberg RA. The hallmarks of cancer. *Cell* 2000; **100**: 57–70.
2. Hahn WC, Weinberg RA. Rules for making human tumor cells. *N Engl J Med* 2002; **347**: 1593–603.
3. Nakao M, Yokota S, Iwai T et al. Internal tandem duplication of the *flt3* gene found in acute myeloid leukemia. *Leukemia* 1996; **10**: 1911–18.
4. Blume-Jensen P, Hunter T. Oncogenic kinase signalling. *Nature* 2001; **411**: 355–65.
5. Metcalfe DD, Akin C. Mastocytosis: molecular mechanisms and clinical disease heterogeneity. *Leuk Res* 2001; **25**: 577–82.
6. Kiyoi H, Towatari M, Yokota S et al. Internal tandem duplication of the *FLT3* gene is a novel modality of elongation mutation which causes constitutive activation of the product. *Leukemia* 1998; **12**: 1333–7.
7. Scheijen B, Griffin JD. Tyrosine kinase oncogenes in normal hematopoiesis and hematological disease. *Oncogene* 2002; **21**: 3314–33.
8. Reilly JT. Class III receptor tyrosine kinases: role in leukaemogenesis. *Br J Haematol* 2003; **116**: 744–57.
9. Valent P, Akin C, Sperr WR et al. Diagnosis and treatment of systemic mastocytosis: state of the art. *Br J Haematol* 2003; **122**: 695–717.
10. Valent P, Horny HP, Escribano L et al. Diagnostic criteria and classification of mastocytosis: a consensus proposal. *Leuk Res* 2001; **25**: 603–25.
11. Sperr WR, Walchshofer S, Horny HP et al. Systemic mastocytosis associated with acute myeloid leukaemia: report of two cases and detection of the c-kit mutation Asp-816 to Val. *Br J Haematol* 1998; **103**: 740–9.
12. Sotlar K, Fridrich C, Mall A et al. Detection of c-kit point mutation Asp-816→ Val in microdissected pooled single mast cells and leukemic cells in a patient with systemic mastocytosis and concomitant chronic myelomonocytic leukemia. *Leuk Res* 2002; **26**: 979–84.
13. Akin C, Kirshenbaum AS, Semere T et al. Analysis of the surface expression of c-kit and occurrence of the c-kit Asp816Val activating mutation in T cells, B cells, and myelomonocytic cells in patients with mastocytosis. *Exp Hematol* 2000; **28**: 140–7.
14. Yavuz AS, Lipsky PE, Yavuz S et al. Evidence for the involvement of a hematopoietic progenitor cell in systemic mastocytosis from single-cell analysis of mutations in the c-kit gene. *Blood* 2002; **100**: 661–5.
15. Pullarkat VA, Bueso-Ramos C, Lai R et al. Systemic mastocytosis with associated clonal hematological non-mast-cell lineage disease: analysis of clinicopathologic features and activating c-kit mutations. *Am J Hematol* 2003; **73**: 12–17.
16. Dash A, Gilliland DG. Molecular genetics of acute myeloid leukaemia. *Best Pract Res Clin Haematol* 2001; **14**: 49–64.
17. Beghini A, Peterlongo P, Ripamonti CB et al. c-kit mutations in core binding factor leukemias. *Blood* 2000; **95**: 726–7.

18. Care RS, Valk PJ, Goodeve AC et al. Incidence and prognosis of c-*KIT* and *FLT3* mutations in core binding factor (CBF) acute myeloid leukaemias. *Br J Haematol* 2003; **121**: 775–7.
19. Kottaridis PD, Gale RE, Linch DC. *Flt3* mutations and leukaemia. *Br J Haematol* 2003; **122**: 523–38.
20. Kottaridis PD, Gale RE, Frew ME et al. The presence of a *FLT3* internal tandem duplication in patients with acute myeloid leukemia (AML) adds important prognostic information to cytogenetic risk group and response to the first cycle of chemotherapy: analysis of 854 patients from the United Kingdom Medical Research Council AML 10 and 12 trials. *Blood* 2001; **98**: 1752–9.
21. Zwaan CM, Meshinchi S, Radich JP et al. *FLT3* internal tandem duplication in 234 children with acute myeloid leukemia (AML): prognostic significance and relation to cellular drug resistance. *Blood* 2003; **102**: 2387–94.
22. Hayakawa F, Towatari M, Kiyoi H et al. Tandem-duplicated *Flt3* constitutively activates STAT5 and MAP kinase and introduces autonomous cell growth in IL-3-dependent cell lines. *Oncogene* 2000; **19**: 624–31.
23. Mizuki M, Fenski R, Halfter H et al. *Flt3* mutations from patients with acute myeloid leukemia induce transformation of 32D cells mediated by the Ras and STAT5 pathways. *Blood* 2000; **96**: 3907–14.
24. Kelly LM, Liu Q, Kutok JL et al. *FLT3* internal tandem duplication mutations associated with human acute myeloid leukemias induce myeloproliferative disease in a murine bone marrow transplant model. *Blood* 2002; **99**: 310–18.
25. Kelly LM, Kutok JL, Williams IR et al. PML/RARα and FLT3–ITD induce an APL-like disease in a mouse model. *Proc Natl Acad Sci USA* 2002; **99**: 8283–8.
26. Kottaridis PD, Gale RE, Langabeer SE et al. Studies of *FLT3* mutations in paired presentation and relapse samples from patients with acute myeloid leukemia: implications for the role of *FLT3* mutations in leukemogenesis, minimal residual disease detection, and possible therapy with FLT3 inhibitors. *Blood* 2002; **100**: 2393–8.
27. Shtivelman E, Lifshitz B, Gale RP, Canaani E. Fused transcript of *abl* and *bcr* genes in chronic myelogenous leukaemia. *Nature* 1985; **315**: 550–4.
28. Clark SS, McLaughlin J, Timmons M et al. Expression of a distinctive *BCR–ABL* oncogene in Ph1-positive acute lymphocytic leukemia (ALL). *Science* 1988; **239**: 775–7.
29. Deininger MW, Goldman JM, Melo JV. The molecular biology of chronic myeloid leukemia. *Blood* 2000; **96**: 3343–56.
30. Cortez D, Kadlec L, Pendergast AM. Structural and signaling requirements for BCR–ABL-mediated transformation and inhibition of apoptosis. *Mol Cell Biol* 1995; **15**: 5531–41.
31. Skorski T, Bellacosa A, Nieborowska-Skorska M et al. Transformation of hematopoietic cells by BCR/ABL requires activation of a PI-3K/Akt-dependent pathway. *EMBO J* 1997; **16**: 6151–61.

32. Tari AM, Arlinghaus R, Lopez-Berestein G. Inhibition of Grb2 and Crkl proteins results in growth inhibition of Philadelphia chromosome positive leukemic cells. *Biochem Biophys Res Commun* 1997; **235**: 383–8.

33. Senechal K, Halpern J, Sawyers CL. The CRKL adaptor protein transforms fibroblasts and functions in transformation by the *BCR–ABL* oncogene. *J Biol Chem* 1996; **271**: 23255–61.

34. Albrecht T, Schwab R, Henkes M et al. Primary proliferating immature myeloid cells from CML patients are not resistant to induction of apoptosis by DNA damage and growth factor withdrawal. *Br J Haematol* 1996; **95**: 501–7.

35. Amos TA, Lewis JL, Grand FH et al. Apoptosis in chronic myeloid leukaemia: normal responses by progenitor cells to growth factor deprivation, X-irradiation and glucocorticoids. *Br J Haematol* 1995; **91**: 387–93.

36. Bedi A, Zehnbauer BA, Barber JP et al. Inhibition of apoptosis by BCR–ABL in chronic myeloid leukemia. *Blood* 1994; **83**: 2038–44.

37. Bhatia R, Holtz M, Niu N et al. Persistence of malignant hematopoietic progenitors in chronic myelogenous leukemia patients in complete cytogenetic remission following imatinib mesylate treatment. *Blood* 2003; **101**: 4701–7.

38. Graham SM, Jorgensen HG, Allan E et al. Primitive, quiescent, Philadelphia-positive stem cells from patients with chronic myeloid leukemia are insensitive to STI571 in vitro. *Blood* 2002; **99**: 319–25.

39. Daley GQ, Van Etten RA, Baltimore D. Induction of chronic myelogenous leukemia in mice by the *p210^{bcr/abl}* gene of the Philadelphia chromosome. *Science* 1990; **247**: 824–30.

40. Daley GQ. Animal models of *BCR/ABL*-induced leukemias. *Leuk Lymphoma* 1993; **11**(Suppl 1): 57–60.

41. Huettner CS, Zhang P, Van Etten RA, Tenen DG. Reversibility of acute B-cell leukaemia induced by *BCR–ABL1*. *Nat Genet* 2000; **24**: 57–60.

42. Cross NC, Reiter A. Tyrosine kinase fusion genes in chronic myeloproliferative diseases. *Leukemia* 2002; **16**: 1207–12.

43. Golub TR, Barker GF, Stegmaier K, Gilliland DG. The *TEL* gene contributes to the pathogenesis of myeloid and lymphoid leukemias by diverse molecular genetic mechanisms. *Curr Top Microbiol Immunol* 1997; **220**: 67–79.

44. Carroll M, Tomasson MH, Barker GF et al. The TEL/platelet-derived growth factor β receptor (PDGFβR) fusion in chronic myelomonocytic leukemia is a transforming protein that self-associates and activates PDGFβR kinase-dependent signaling pathways. *Proc Natl Acad Sci USA* 1996; **93**: 14845–50.

45. Heldin CH, Ostman A, Ronnstrand L. Signal transduction via platelet-derived growth factor receptors. *Biochim Biophys Acta* 1998; **1378**: F79–113.

46. Ritchie KA, Aprikyan AA, Bowen-Pope DF et al. The *Tel–PDGFRβ* fusion gene produces a chronic myeloproliferative syndrome in transgenic mice. *Leukemia* 1999; **13**: 1790–803.

47. Cools J, DeAngelo DJ, Gotlib J et al. A tyrosine kinase created by fusion of the *PDGFRA* and *FIP1L1* genes as a therapeutic target of imatinib in idiopathic hypereosinophilic syndrome. *N Engl J Med* 2003; **348**: 1201–14.

48. Vardiman JW, Harris NL, Brunning RD. The World Health Organization (WHO) classification of the myeloid neoplasms. *Blood* 2002; **100**: 2292–302.

49. Macdonald D, Reiter A, Cross NC. The 8p11 myeloproliferative syndrome: a distinct clinical entity caused by constitutive activation of *FGFR1*. *Acta Haematol* 2002; **107**: 101–7.

50. JabbarAl-Obaidi M, Rymes N, White P et al. A fourth case of 8p11 myeloproliferative disorder transforming to B-lineage acute lymphoblastic leukaemia. A case report. *Acta Haematol* 2002; **107**: 98–100.

51. Demiroglu A, Steer EJ, Heath C et al. The t(8;22) in chronic myeloid leukemia fuses *BCR* to *FGFR1*: transforming activity and specific inhibition of FGFR1 fusion proteins. *Blood* 2001; **98**: 3778–83.

52. Mohammadi M, McMahon G, Sun L et al. Structures of the tyrosine kinase domain of fibroblast growth factor receptor in complex with inhibitors. *Science* 1997; **276**: 955–60.

53. Iwahara T, Fujimoto J, Wen D et al. Molecular characterization of ALK, a receptor tyrosine kinase expressed specifically in the nervous system. *Oncogene* 1997; **14**: 439–49.

54. Stoica GE, Kuo A, Aigner A et al. Identification of anaplastic lymphoma kinase as a receptor for the growth factor pleiotrophin. *J Biol Chem* 2001; **276**: 16772–9.

55. Morris SW, Kirstein MN, Valentine MB et al. Fusion of a kinase gene, *ALK*, to a nucleolar protein gene, *NPM*, in non-Hodgkin's lymphoma. *Science* 1994; **263**: 1281–4.

56. Kuefer MU, Look AT, Pulford K et al. Retrovirus-mediated gene transfer of *NPM–ALK* causes lymphoid malignancy in mice. *Blood* 1997; **90**: 2901–10.

57. Fujimoto J, Shiota M, Iwahara T et al. Characterization of the transforming activity of p80, a hyperphosphorylated protein in a Ki-1 lymphoma cell line with chromosomal translocation t(2;5). *Proc Natl Acad Sci USA* 1996; **93**: 4181–6.

58. Bischof D, Pulford K, Mason DY, Morris SW. Role of the nucleophosmin (NPM) portion of the non-Hodgkin's lymphoma-associated NPM–anaplastic lymphoma kinase fusion protein in oncogenesis. *Mol Cell Biol* 1997; **17**: 2312–25.

59. Drexler HG, Gignac SM, von Wasielewski R et al. Pathobiology of *NPM–ALK* and variant fusion genes in anaplastic large cell lymphoma and other lymphomas. *Leukemia* 2000; **14**: 1533–59.

60. Bai RY, Ouyang T, Miething C et al. Nucleophosmin–anaplastic lymphoma kinase associated with anaplastic large-cell lymphoma activates the phosphatidylinositol 3-kinase/Akt antiapoptotic signaling pathway. *Blood* 2000; **96**: 4319–27.

61. Nieborowska-Skorska M, Slupianek A, Xue L et al. Role of signal transducer and activator of transcription 5 in nucleophosmin/anaplastic lymphoma kinase-mediated malignant transformation of lymphoid cells. *Cancer Res* 2001; **61**: 6517–23.

62. Slupianek A, Nieborowska-Skorska M, Hoser G et al. Role of phosphatidylinositol 3-kinase–Akt pathway in nucleophosmin/anaplastic lymphoma kinase-mediated lymphomagenesis. *Cancer Res* 2001; **61**: 2194–9.

63. Peeters P, Raynaud SD, Cools J et al. Fusion of *TEL*, the ETS-variant gene 6 (*ETV6*), to the receptor-associated kinase *JAK2* as a result of t(9;12) in a lymphoid and t(9;15) in a myeloid leukemia. *Blood* 1997; **90**: 2535–40.

64. Lacronique V, Boureux A, Valle VD et al. A TEL–JAK2 fusion protein with constitutive kinase activity in human leukemia. *Science* 1997; **278**: 1309–12.

65. Gouilleux-Gruart V, Gouilleux F, Desaint C et al. STAT-

related transcription factors are constitutively activated in peripheral blood cells from acute leukemia patients. *Blood* 1996; **87**: 1692–7.

66. Weber-Nordt RM, Egen C, Wehinger J et al. Constitutive activation of STAT proteins in primary lymphoid and myeloid leukemia cells and in Epstein–Barr virus (EBV)-related lymphoma cell lines. *Blood* 1996; **88**: 809–16.

67. Xia Z, Baer MR, Block AW et al. Expression of signal transducers and activators of transcription proteins in acute myeloid leukemia blasts. *Cancer Res* 1998; **58**: 3173–80.

68. Young DC, Griffin JD. Autocrine secretion of GM-CSF in acute myeloblastic leukemia. *Blood* 1986; **68**: 1178–81.

69. Bradbury D, Rogers S, Reilly IA et al. Role of autocrine and paracrine production of granulocyte–macrophage colony-stimulating factor and interleukin-1β in the autonomous growth of acute myeloblastic leukaemia cells – studies using purified CD34-positive cells. *Leukemia* 1992; **6**: 562–6.

70. Schuringa JJ, Wierenga AT, Kruijer W, Vellenga E. Constitutive Stat3, Tyr705, and Ser727 phosphorylation in acute myeloid leukemia cells caused by the autocrine secretion of interleukin-6. *Blood* 2000; **95**: 3765–70.

71. Kjeldgaard M, Nyborg J, Clark BF. The GTP binding motif: variations on a theme. *FASEB J* 1996; **10**: 1347–68.

72. Manser E. Small GTPases take the stage. *Dev Cell* 2002; **3**: 323–8.

73. Downward J. Targeting RAS signalling pathways in cancer therapy. *Nat Rev Cancer* 2003; **3**: 11–22.

74. Quilliam LA, Khosravi-Far R, Huff SY, Der CJ Guanine nucleotide exchange factors: activators of the Ras superfamily of proteins. *Bioessays* 1995; **17**: 395–404.

75. Downward J, Graves JD, Warne PH et al. Stimulation of p21Ras upon T-cell activation. *Nature* 1990; **346**: 719–23.

76. Gelb MH. Protein prenylation, et cetera: signal transduction in two dimensions. *Science* 1997; **275**: 1750–1.

77. Marshall CJ. Ras effectors. *Curr Opin Cell Biol* 1996; **8**: 197–204.

78. Treisman R. Regulation of transcription by MAP kinase cascades. *Curr Opin Cell Biol* 1996; **8**: 205–15.

79. Klemke RL, Cai S, Giannini AL et al. Regulation of cell motility by mitogen-activated protein kinase. *J Cell Biol* 1997; **137**: 481–92.

80. Leslie CC. Properties and regulation of cytosolic phospholipase A2. *J Biol Chem* 1997; **272**: 16709–12.

81. Marshall CJ. Specificity of receptor tyrosine kinase signaling: transient versus sustained extracellular signal-regulated kinase activation. *Cell* 1995; **80**: 179–85.

82. Rouyez MC, Boucheron C, Gisselbrecht S et al. Control of thrombopoietin-induced megakaryocytic differentiation by the mitogen-activated protein kinase pathway. *Mol Cell Biol* 1997; **17**: 4991–5000.

83. Rodriguez-Viciana P, Warne PH, Dhand R et al. Phosphatidylinositol-3-OH kinase as a direct target of Ras. *Nature* 1994; **370**: 527–32.

84. Khwaja A, Rodriguez-Viciana P, Wennstrom S et al. Matrix adhesion and Ras transformation both activate a phosphoinositide 3-OH kinase and protein kinase B/Akt cellular survival pathway. *EMBO J* 1997; **16**: 2783–93.

85. Rodriguez-Viciana P, Warne PH, Khwaja A et al. Role of phosphoinositide 3-OH kinase in cell transformation and control of the actin cytoskeleton by Ras. *Cell* 1997; **89**: 457–67.

86. Vogelstein B, Civin CI, Preisinger AC et al. RAS gene mutations in childhood acute myeloid leukemia: a

Pediatric Oncology Group study. *Genes Chromosomes Cancer* 1990; **2**: 159–62.

87. Ahuja HG, Foti A, Bar-Eli M, Cline MJ. The pattern of mutational involvement of *RAS* genes in human hematologic malignancies determined by DNA amplification and direct sequencing. *Blood* 1990; **75**: 1684–90.

88. Nakagawa T, Saitoh S, Imoto S et al. Multiple point mutation of N-*ras* and K-*ras* oncogenes in myelodysplastic syndrome and acute myelogenous leukemia. *Oncology* 1992; **49**: 114–22.

89. Neubauer A, Dodge RK, George SL et al. Prognostic importance of mutations in the ras proto-oncogenes in de novo acute myeloid leukemia. *Blood* 1994; **83**: 1603–11.

90. Bashey A, Gill R, Levi S et al. Mutational activation of the N-*ras* oncogene assessed in primary clonogenic culture of acute myeloid leukemia (AML): implications for the role of N-*ras* mutation in AML pathogenesis. *Blood* 1992; **79**: 981–9.

91. Bezieau S, Avet-Loiseau H, Moisan JP, Bataille R. Activating *Ras* mutations in patients with plasma-cell disorders: a reappraisal. *Blood* 2002; **100**: 1101–2; author reply 1103.

92. Liu P, Leong T, Quam L et al. Activating mutations of N- and K-*ras* in multiple myeloma show different clinical associations: analysis of the Eastern Cooperative Oncology Group phase III trial. *Blood* 1996; **88**: 2699–706.

93. Corradini P, Ladetto M, Voena C et al. Mutational activation of N- and K-*ras* oncogenes in plasma cell dyscrasias. *Blood* 1993; **81**: 2708–13.

94. Billadeau D, Liu P, Jelinek D et al. Activating mutations in the N and K-*ras* oncogenes differentially affect the growth properties of the IL-6-dependent myeloma cell line ANBL6. *Cancer Res* 1997; **57**: 2268–75.

95. Davies H, Bignell GR, Cox C et al. Mutations of the *BRAF* gene in human cancer. *Nature* 2002; **417**: 949–54.

96. Smith ML, Snaddon J, Neat M et al. Mutation of *BRAF* is uncommon in AML FAB type M1 and M2. *Leukemia* 2003; **17**: 274–5.

97. Bonello L, Voena C, Ladetto M et al. *BRAF* gene is not mutated in plasma cell leukemia and multiple myeloma. *Leukemia* 2003; **17**: 2238–40.

98. Miles DK, Freedman MH, Stephens K et al. Patterns of hematopoietic lineage involvement in children with neurofibromatosis type 1 and malignant myeloid disorders. *Blood* 1996; **88**: 4314–20.

99. Miyauchi J, Asada M, Sasaki M et al. Mutations of the N-ras gene in juvenile chronic myelogenous leukemia. *Blood* 1994; **83**: 2248–54.

100. Kalra R, Paderanga DC, Olson K, Shannon KM. Genetic analysis is consistent with the hypothesis that NF1 limits myeloid cell growth through p21Ras. *Blood* 1994; **84**: 3435–9.

101. Side L, Taylor B, Cayouette M et al. Homozygous inactivation of the *NF1* gene in bone marrow cells from children with neurofibromatosis type 1 and malignant myeloid disorders. *N Engl J Med* 1997; **336**: 1713–20.

102. Largaespada DA, Brannan CI, Jenkins NA, Copeland NG. Nf1 deficiency causes Ras-mediated granulocyte/macrophage colony stimulating factor hypersensitivity and chronic myeloid leukaemia. *Nat Genet* 1996; **12**: 137–43.

103. Bollag G, Clapp DW, Shih S et al. Loss of NF1 results in activation of the Ras signaling pathway and leads to aberrant growth in haematopoietic cells. *Nat Genet* 1996; **12**: 144–8.

104. Carpenter CL, Cantley LC. Phosphoinositide 3-kinase and the regulation of cell growth. *Biochim Biophys Acta* 1996; **1288**: M11–16.

105. Divecha N, Irvine RF. Phospholipid signaling. *Cell* 1995; **80**: 269–78.

106. Vanhaesebroeck B, Leevers SJ, Ahmadi K et al. Synthesis and function of 3-phosphorylated inositol lipids. *Annu Rev Biochem* 2001; **70**: 535–602.

107. Liu Q, Oliveira-Dos-Santos AJ, Mariathasan S et al. The inositol polyphosphate 5-phosphatase ship is a crucial negative regulator of B cell antigen receptor signaling. *J Exp Med* 1998; **188**: 1333–42.

108. Paez J, Sellers WR. PI3K/PTEN/AKT pathway. A critical mediator of oncogenic signaling. *Cancer Treat Res* 2003; **115**: 145–67.

109. Pendaries C, Tronchere H, Plantavid M, Payrastre B. Phosphoinositide signaling disorders in human diseases. *FEBS Lett* 2003; **546**: 25–31.

110. Aggerholm A, Gronbaek K, Guldberg P, Hokland P. Mutational analysis of the tumour suppressor gene *MMAC1/PTEN* in malignant myeloid disorders. *Eur J Haematol* 2000; **65**: 109–13.

111. Liu TC, Lin PM, Chang JG et al. Mutation analysis of *PTEN/MMAC1* in acute myeloid leukemia. *Am J Hematol* 2000; **63**: 170–5.

112. Sakai A, Thieblemont C, Wellmann A et al. *PTEN* gene alterations in lymphoid neoplasms. *Blood* 1998; **92**: 3410–15.

113. Karin M, Cao Y, Greten FR, Li ZW. NF-κB in cancer: from innocent bystander to major culprit. *Nat Rev Cancer* 2002; **2**: 301–10.

114. Karin M, Lin A. NF-κB at the crossroads of life and death. *Nat Immunol* 2002; **3**: 221–7.

115. Xiao G, Cvijic ME, Fong A et al. Retroviral oncoprotein Tax induces processing of NF-κB2/p100 in T cells: evidence for the involvement of IKKα. *EMBO J* 2001; **20**: 6805–15.

116. Rao PH, Houldsworth J, Dyomina K et al. Chromosomal and gene amplification in diffuse large B-cell lymphoma. *Blood* 1998; **92**: 234–40.

117. Willis TG, Jadayel DM, Du MQ et al. *Bcl10* is involved in t(1;14)(p22;q32) of MALT B cell lymphoma and mutated in multiple tumor types. *Cell* 1999; **96**: 35–45.

118. Akagi T, Motegi M, Tamura A et al. A novel gene, *MALT1* at 18q21, is involved in t(11;18) (q21;q21) found in low-grade B-cell lymphoma of mucosa-associated lymphoid tissue. *Oncogene* 1999; **18**: 5785–94.

119. Reuther JY, Reuther GW, Cortez D et al. A requirement for NF-κB activation in Bcr–Abl-mediated transformation. *Genes Dev* 1998; **12**: 968–81.

120. Guzman ML, Neering SJ, Upchurch D et al. Nuclear factor-κB is constitutively activated in primitive human acute myelogenous leukemia cells. *Blood* 2001; **98**: 2301–7.

121. Weinstein IB. Cancer. Addiction to oncogenes – the Achilles heal of cancer. *Science* 2002; **297**: 63–4.

122. Pelengaris S, Khan M, Evan G. c-*MYC*: more than just a matter of life and death. *Nat Rev Cancer* 2002; **2**: 764–76.

123. Druker BJ, Tamura S, Buchdunger E et al. Effects of a selective inhibitor of the Abl tyrosine kinase on the growth of Bcr–Abl positive cells. *Nat Med* 1996; **2**: 561–6.

124. Kurzrock R, Kantarjian HM, Druker BJ, Talpaz M. Philadelphia chromosome-positive leukemias: from basic mechanisms to molecular therapeutics. *Ann Intern Med* 2003; **138**: 819–30.

125. Schindler T, Bornmann W, Pellicena P et al. Structural mechanism for STI-571 inhibition of Abelson tyrosine kinase. *Science* 2000; **289**: 1938–42.

126. Nagar B, Bornmann WG, Pellicena P et al. Crystal structures of the kinase domain of c-Abl in complex with the small molecule inhibitors PD173955 and imatinib (STI-571). *Cancer Res* 2002; **62**: 4236–43.

127. Deininger MW, O'Brien SG, Ford JM, Druker BJ. Practical management of patients with chronic myeloid leukemia receiving imatinib. *J Clin Oncol* 2003; **21**: 1637–47.

128. Druker BJ. Perspectives on the development of a molecularly targeted agent. *Cancer Cell* 2002; **1**: 31–6.

129. von Bubnoff N, Peschel C, Duyster J. Resistance of Philadelphia-chromosome positive leukemia towards the kinase inhibitor imatinib (STI571, Glivec): a targeted oncoprotein strikes back. *Leukemia* 2003; **17**: 829–38.

130. Gambacorti-Passerini C, Barni R, le Coutre P et al. Role of α₁ acid glycoprotein in the in vivo resistance of human *BCR–ABL*⁺ leukemic cells to the ABL inhibitor STI571. *J Natl Cancer Inst* 2000; **92**: 1641–50.

131. Jorgensen HG, Elliott MA, Allan EK et al. α₁-acid glycoprotein expressed in the plasma of chronic myeloid leukemia patients does not mediate significant in vitro resistance to STI571. *Blood* 2002; **99**: 713–15.

132. Hochhaus A, Kreil S, Corbin AS et al. Molecular and chromosomal mechanisms of resistance to imatinib (STI571) therapy. *Leukemia* 2002; **16**: 2190–6.

133. Mahon FX, Deininger MW, Schultheis B et al. Selection and characterization of *BCR–ABL* positive cell lines with differential sensitivity to the tyrosine kinase inhibitor STI571: diverse mechanisms of resistance. *Blood* 2000; **96**: 1070–9.

134. Gorre ME, Mohammed M, Ellwood K et al. Clinical resistance to STI-571 cancer therapy caused by *BCR–ABL* gene mutation or amplification. *Science* 2001; **293**: 876–80.

135. Hochhaus A. Cytogenetic and molecular mechanisms of resistance to imatinib. *Semin Hematol* 2003; **40**: 69–79.

136. Roche-Lestienne C, Lai JL, Darre S et al. A mutation conferring resistance to imatinib at the time of diagnosis of chronic myelogenous leukemia. *N Engl J Med* 2003; **348**: 2265–6.

137. Hofmann WK, Komor M, Wassmann B et al. Presence of the BCR–ABL mutation Glu255Lys prior to STI571 (imatinib) treatment in patients with Ph⁺ acute lymphoblastic leukemia. *Blood* 2003; **102**: 659–61.

138. Huron DR, Gorre ME, Kraker AJ et al. A novel pyridopyrimidine inhibitor of Abl kinase is a picomolar inhibitor of Bcr–Abl-driven K562 cells and is effective against STI571-resistant Bcr–Abl mutants. *Clin Cancer Res* 2003; **9**: 1267–73.

139. La Rosee P, Corbin AS, Stoffregen EP et al. Activity of the Bcr–Abl kinase inhibitor PD180970 against clinically relevant Bcr–Abl isoforms that cause resistance to imatinib mesylate (Gleevec, STI571). *Cancer Res* 2002; **62**: 7149–53.

140. Neckers L. Hsp90 inhibitors as novel cancer chemotherapeutic agents. *Trends Mol Med* 2002; **8**: S55–61.

141. Schaller JL, Burkland GA. Case report: rapid and complete control of idiopathic hypereosinophilia with imatinib mesylate. *Med Gen Med* 2001; **3**: 9.

142. Gleich GJ, Leiferman KM, Pardanani A et al. Treatment of hypereosinophilic syndrome with imatinib mesilate. *Lancet* 2002; **359**: 1577–8.

143. Ault P, Cortes J, Koller C et al. Response of idiopathic

hypereosinophilic syndrome to treatment with imatinib mesylate. *Leuk Res* 2002; **26:** 881−4.

144. Pardanani A, Reeder T, Porrata LF et al. Imatinib therapy for hypereosinophilic syndrome and other eosinophilic disorders. *Blood* 2003; **101:** 3391−7.

145. Cortes J, Ault P, Koller C et al. Efficacy of imatinib mesylate in the treatment of idiopathic hypereosinophilic syndrome. *Blood* 2003; **101:** 4714−16.

146. Cools J, Stover EH, Boulton CL et al. PKC412 overcomes resistance to imatinib in a murine model of FIP1L1−PDGFRα-induced myeloproliferative disease. *Cancer Cell* 2003; **3:** 459−69.

147. Frost MJ, Ferrao PT, Hughes TP, Ashman LK. Juxtamembrane mutant V560GKit is more sensitive to imatinib (STI571) compared with wild-type c-kit whereas the kinase domain mutant D816VKit is resistant. *Mol Cancer Ther* 2002; **1:** 1115−24.

148. Pardanani A, Elliott M, Reeder T et al. Imatinib for systemic mast-cell disease. *Lancet* 2003; **362:** 535−6.

149. Sawyers CL. Finding the next Gleevec: FLT3 targeted kinase inhibitor therapy for acute myeloid leukemia. *Cancer Cell* 2002; **1:** 413−15.

150. Levis M, Allebach J, Tse KF et al. A FLT3-targeted tyrosine kinase inhibitor is cytotoxic to leukemia cells in vitro and in vivo. *Blood* 2002; **99:** 3885−91.

151. Weisberg E, Boulton C, Kelly LM et al. Inhibition of mutant FLT3 receptors in leukemia cells by the small molecule tyrosine kinase inhibitor PKC412. *Cancer Cell* 2002; **1:** 433−43.

152. Kelly LM, Yu JC, Boulton CL et al. CT53518, a novel selective FLT3 antagonist for the treatment of acute myelogenous leukemia (AML). *Cancer Cell* 2002; **1:** 421−32.

153. Gibbs JB, Oliff A, Kohl NE. Farnesyltransferase inhibitors: Ras research yields a potential cancer therapeutic. *Cell* 1994; **77:** 175−8.

154. Omer CA, Kohl NE. CA1A2X-competitive inhibitors of farnesyltransferase as anti-cancer agents. *Trends Pharmacol Sci* 1997; **18:** 437−44.

155. Whyte DB, Kirschmeier P, Hockenberry TN et al. K- and N-Ras are geranylgeranylated in cells treated with farnesyl protein transferase inhibitors. *J Biol Chem* 1997; **272:** 14459−64.

156. Zeng PY, Rane N, Du W et al. Role for RhoB and PRK in the suppression of epithelial cell transformation by farnesyltransferase inhibitors. *Oncogene* 2003; **22:** 1124−34.

157. Cox AD, Der CJ. Farnesyltransferase inhibitors: promises and realities. *Curr Opin Pharmacol* 2002; **2:** 388−93.

158. Sepp-Lorenzino L, Ma Z, Rands E et al. A peptidomimetic inhibitor of farnesyl:protein transferase blocks the anchorage-dependent and -independent growth of human tumor cell lines. *Cancer Res* 1995; **55:** 5302−9.

159. Norman P. Tipifarnib (Janssen Pharmaceutica). *Curr Opin Invest Drugs* 2002; **3:** 313−19.

160. Hahn SM, Bernhard E, McKenna WG. Farnesyltransferase inhibitors. *Semin Oncol* 2001; **28:** 86−93.

161. End DW, Smets G, Todd AV et al. Characterization of the antitumor effects of the selective farnesyl protein transferase inhibitor R115777 in vivo and in vitro. *Cancer Res* 2001; **61:** 131−7.

162. Karp JE, Lancet JE, Kaufmann SH et al. Clinical and biologic activity of the farnesyltransferase inhibitor R115777 in adults with refractory and relapsed acute leukemias: a phase 1 clinical–laboratory correlative trial. *Blood* 2001; **97:** 3361−9.

163. Cohen SJ, Ho L, Ranganathan S et al. Phase II and pharmacodynamic study of the farnesyltransferase inhibitor R115777 as initial therapy in patients with metastatic pancreatic adenocarcinoma. *J Clin Oncol* 2003; **21:** 1301−6.

164. Cortes J, Albitar M, Thomas D et al. Efficacy of the farnesyl transferase inhibitor R115777 in chronic myeloid leukemia and other hematologic malignancies. *Blood* 2003; **101:** 1692−7.

165. Adams J. The proteasome: structure, function, and role in the cell. *Cancer Treat Rev* 2003; **29**(Suppl 1): 3−9.

166. Mitchell BS. The proteasome – an emerging therapeutic target in cancer. *N Engl J Med* 2003; **348:** 2597−8.

167. Paramore A, Frantz S. Bortezomib. *Nat Rev Drug Discov* 2003; **2:** 611−12.

168. Adams J, Palombella VJ, Sausville EA et al. Proteasome inhibitors: a novel class of potent and effective antitumor agents. *Cancer Res* 1999; **59:** 2615−22.

169. Aghajanian C, Soignet S, Dizon DS et al. A phase I trial of the novel proteasome inhibitor PS341 in advanced solid tumor malignancies. *Clin Cancer Res* 2002; **8:** 2505−11.

170. Orlowski RZ, Stinchcombe TE, Mitchell BS et al. Phase I trial of the proteasome inhibitor PS-341 in patients with refractory hematologic malignancies. *J Clin Oncol* 2002; **20:** 4420−7.

171. Hideshima T, Richardson P, Chauhan D et al. The proteasome inhibitor PS-341 inhibits growth, induces apoptosis, and overcomes drug resistance in human multiple myeloma cells. *Cancer Res* 2001; **61:** 3071−6.

172. Richardson PG, Barlogie B, Berenson J et al. A phase 2 study of bortezomib in relapsed, refractory myeloma. *N Engl J Med* 2003; **348:** 2609−17.

173. Activity of the Raf kinase inhibitor BAY 43-9006 in patients with advanced solid tumors. *Clin Colorectal Cancer* 2003; **3:** 16−18.

174. Dancey JE. Agents targeting ras signaling pathway. *Curr Pharm Des* 2002; **8:** 2259−67.

175. Stein RC. Prospects for phosphoinositide 3-kinase inhibition as a cancer treatment. *Endocr Rel Cancer* 2001; **8:** 237−48.

176. Huang S, Houghton PJ. Inhibitors of mammalian target of rapamycin as novel antitumor agents: from bench to clinic. *Curr Opin Invest Drugs* 2002; **3:** 295−304.

177. Dancey JE. Clinical development of mammalian target of rapamycin inhibitors. *Hematol Oncol Clin North Am* 2002; **16:** 1101−14.

178. Huang S, Bjornsti MA, Houghton PJ. Rapamycins: mechanism of action and cellular resistance. *Cancer Biol Ther* 2003; **2:** 222−32.

# 28 Gene transfer in leukemia and related disorders

**Martin Pulè and Malcolm Brenner**

## Introduction

Two broad strategies of gene transfer are used in the treatment of leukemia and lymphoma. First, the tumor itself can be genetically modified. That is, tumor cells can be transduced with genes that 'repair' major functional defects, with a toxic gene that destroys the tumor cell, or with genes that express molecules that trigger an immune response against the tumor cell. Second, the host can be modified, so that T cells are redirected and their antitumor activity augmented, with suicide genes introduced to terminate potentially harmful immune reactions. Moreover, the drug sensitivity of normal host tissues can be decreased by delivering cytotoxic drug-resistance genes to sensitive tissues, thereby increasing the therapeutic index of chemotherapy. Host cells may also be transduced with marker genes, not for a direct therapeutic benefit, but merely as a means to follow their behavior and persistence.

Clinical studies of gene therapy must show that the potential benefits outweigh the potential risks; hence, most protocols for the treatment of malignant diseases are open only to patients with a poor prognosis, in whom the risk-to-benefit ratio is most likely to be favorable. It must be emphasized that these patients are ultimately not likely to prove the most suitable group for gene therapy. Instead, many of the approaches to be described in this chapter will probably be most valuable for the eradication of minimal residual disease remaining after conventional therapies.

## Methods for gene delivery

Table 28.1 summarizes the properties of the common types of virus-based gene-therapy vector.

### Retroviral vectors

In a typical retroviral vector,[1] the structural and replicative genes (*gag, pol,* and *env*) are replaced by one or more genes of interest, driven either by the retroviral promoter in the 5′ long-terminal repeat (LTR) or by an internal promoter. Currently, only oncoretrovirus-based vectors have clinical applications in cancer. The retroviral constructs are made in cell lines in which the missing retroviral genes are present in *trans* and thus reproduce and package a vector that is not replication-competent (illustrated in Figure 28.1, see Plate 6). Retroviral vectors have a wide target cell range, and the genetic information they convey is integrated into the host cell DNA. Because the transferred gene not only survives for the entire lifespan of the transduced cell, but is also present in that cell's progeny, these vectors are ideal for transferring genes into rapidly dividing cell populations, such as leukemic or normal lymphocytes or for gene therapy targeting hematopoietic stem cells (HSC). Provided that replication-competent virus is absent, the vector preparations appear to be non-toxic. Oncoretroviral vectors have several disadvantages. Expression of the transferred gene requires genomic integration by the virus (hence a population of dividing cells) so that the efficiency of transfer to many cell types may be low.[2] Such vectors are not well suited for in vivo use because they are generally unstable in complement and cannot be targeted to specific cell types. More recently, murine retroviruses were linked to leukemia induction in two children receiving corrective therapy for X-linked severe combined immunodeficiency (X-SCID) caused by defects in the common γ chain for lymphoid cytokine receptors. The leukemia appears to have been generated by insertional mutagenesis due to retroviral integration. While these events have clearly dampened enthusiasm for the use of murine retroviruses to correct immunodeficiency states, many hundreds of patients have received retrovirally transduced normal or malignant hematopoietic cells without any ill effects similar to those in the two SCID patients. This issue is discussed further in the section below on gene therapy as a cause of leukemia.

## Table 28.1  Main gene-therapy vectors in clinical use

| Vector | Vector genome | Packaging limit (kb) | Tropism | Immune response | Genome in transduced cells | Advantages | Disadvantages |
|---|---|---|---|---|---|---|---|
| Retrovirus | RNA | 8 | Only dividing cells | Weak | Integrated | Integrating, hence results in persisting gene transfer in daughter cells | Integration may cause oncogenesis |
| Lentivirus | RNA | 8 | Wide | Weak | Integrated | As retrovirus but can transduce non-dividing cells also | More complex to generate than retrovirus; integration may cause oncogenesis |
| HSV1 | dsDNA | 40–150 | Strong for neurons | Strong | Episomal | Large packaging capacity | Inflammatory response; only transient transgene expression in most cell types |
| AAV | ssDNA | <5 | Serotype dependent | Weak | Episomal and integrated | Simple and have capacity to integrate. Multiple serotypes | Small packaging limit |
| Adenovirus | dsDNA | 8–30 | Wide | Strong | Episomal | Very efficient transduction of nearly all cell types | Only transient expression, potent immune response to capsid |

HSV1, herpes simplex virus 1; AAV, adeno-associated virus; dsDNA, double-stranded DNA; ssDNA, single-stranded DNA.

## Lentiviruses

Lentiviral vectors, which also have been evaluated for their clinical utility,[3] can transduce hematopoietic progenitors[4] and primary acute lymphoblastic leukemia (ALL) cells,[5] and may be more effective than murine retroviruses in targeting primitive HSC such as those with a CD34+CD38- phenotype.[6] Despite their ability to infect and replicate in non-mitotic cells, lentiviruses pose several technical problems that must be overcome before clinical applications are feasible. For example, the toxicity of some HIV proteins has made the generation of stable packaging cells difficult.[7] There are also safety concerns with these vectors. In particular, the use of HIV-derived vector systems raises the possibility that wild-type HIV may be generated during vector production. Newer (third-generation) lentiviruses have self-inactivating features, and are likely to become the first vector of this type to be used clinically. As of mid 2004, the first protocols specifying lentiviral vectors have been approved.

## Adenoviruses

Adenoviruses infect a wide range of cell types and, unlike retroviruses, can transfer genes into non-dividing cells. Most adenoviral vectors are E1 (early protein) deletion mutants and therefore are not replication-competent.[8,9] Early genes in the E3 region can also be deleted to increase the 'space' for insertion of new genes.[8] These vectors are reasonably stable in vivo and can be used to infect cells in situ. Examples include gene transfer into respiratory epithelium (the cystic fibrosis transmembrane conductance regulator (*CFTR*) gene in cystic fibrosis[8]) or liver (genes encoding factor VIII and factor IX in hemophilia A or B[10]). However, adenoviral vectors are generally non-integrating, so that the gene products are expressed from episomal DNA. Since the episome is often lost after cell division and can be inactivated or lost even in a non-dividing cell, adenoviral vectors are unsuited for any application that requires long-term expression in a rapidly turning-over cell population or transfer into a stem cell and expression in that cell's progeny. Another limitation is that most adenoviral vectors elicit immune responses against the viral proteins themselves, which often prevents readministration of the vector. More significantly, cellular and humoral immune responses may be generated against low levels of adenoviral proteins, expressed even when cells are transduced by defective viruses. These responses

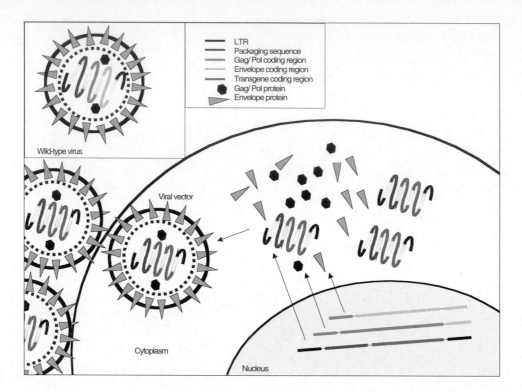

**Figure 28.1** Creation of a replication incompetent retroviral vector with a split packaging cell line. Wild-type retrovirus is shown in inset upper-left corner. Virus is composed of gag/pol and env proteins and a RNA genome. This genome codes for gag/pol and env proteins, hence upon infecting a host cell, all retroviral elements can be generated and virus can replicate. Split packaging line provides coding regions for gag/pol and env elements in trans. Coding region for our transgene (red) is preceded by a packaging signal (blue). Packaging signal has been removed from gag/pol and envelope coding regions. Hence virus is assembled as normal but our transgene replaces usual genome. Upon infecting a cell, our transgene is expressed but no gag/pol or env can be generated, and virus cannot replicate. For replication competent virus to be generated, packaging sequence, gag/pol and env elements would have to coincidentally recombine. (See Plate 6)

may destroy the target cell or simply downregulate expression of the transgene along with other virus-associated proteins. In addition, the entry of adenoviruses into many cell types will trigger innate immunity, with the release of cytokines, such as interleukin-8 (IL-8), which induce a non-specific but potentially highly destructive local inflammatory response.[11] Although these immunostimulatory attributes may render adenoviruses inherently unsuited for chronic application in diseases such as hemophilia A or B, they may be an asset when one intends to prepare a tumor vaccine (see below), emphasizing the importance of matching a vector's characteristics to its intended use. Aside from issues of immunostimulation, there are also concerns about recombination with endogenous adenoviruses, potentially leading to the release of novel variants into the environment. Finally, the wide host cell range of adenoviral vectors could hinder in vivo targeting to a specific cell type.

### Adeno-associated viruses (AAV)

As members of the *Parvoviridae* genus *Dependovirus*,[12] AAV typically depend upon coinfection with a helper virus, such as adenovirus, for efficient replication in the productive phase. The most unique feature of an AAV, however, is the latent phase of its life cycle. When the virus infects a permissive cell in the absence of helper virus, it achieves stable latency without obvious consequences for the host cell. In this phase, the viral genome can assume a number of integrated and episomal forms, but the predominant form in AAV2 latency in human cells appears to be a tandem head-to-tail integration within a region of chromosome 19 that has been termed the AAVS1 site.

In their native form, AAV consist of only 145 nucleotides at each end of the genome and two internal genes: *rep* and *cap*. Recombinant AAV vectors are generated by replacing *rep* and *cap* with the transgene of interest and retaining the ITR sequences. Providing permissive cells with *rep, cap*, and adenovirus helper functions ensures replication and packaging of these vectors. Plasmids can now be used to supply the genes needed for helper functions, enabling difficulties in generating a packaging line with stably integrated *cap* and *rep* to be overcome.[13] A recombinant herpesvirus that supplies *rep, cap*, and helper genes has also been generated.[14] In parallel with methods for producing AAV, purification techniques have also improved.[15]

The first rAAV2 vector developed for clinical studies was *CFTR*. In several phase I and phase II studies of cystic fibrosis patients,[15-18] safe, long-term, dose-dependent gene transfer was achieved with this vector, although lung inflammation continues to be an intrinsic barrier to successful gene therapy in this disease.

AAV vectors may also be useful in cancer gene therapy, for example, to transduce myeloma cells to express *B7.1* and *B7.2*[19] genes to generate a tumor vaccine. Selective killing of hepatocellular carcinoma cells by transfer of the herpes simplex virus 1 thymidine kinase gene (*HSV-tk*) by AAV has been reported in a mouse model.[20]

Whereas some of the major advantages of AAV vectors include stable integration, long-term expression, and ability to infect dividing and non-dividing cells, the major limitations include variations in AAV infectivity among different cell types and the small size of the recombinant genome that can be packaged. Future improvements are likely to include methods to retarget these vectors and increase the packaging size. The availability of multiple AAV serotypes with different tropisms may also increase their value.

### Liposomes/other physical methods

Among physical methods of gene transfer, cationic liposome/DNA complexes[21,22] have been tested most often in patients. These complexes fuse with the cell membrane and enter the endosomal uptake pathway; DNA released from the endosomes may then pass through the nuclear membrane and be expressed. The main advantage of liposomes is that they are non-toxic and can be given repeatedly. In some cell types, high levels of gene transfer have been obtained by this method,[22] and successful systemic administration has also been reported in large animal models.[23] However, the DNA transferred by liposomes does not integrate the genome, and despite the incorporation of a variety of ligands into the liposome–DNA complex,[24] the ability to target these vectors is still quite limited. More recently, successful gene transfer in vivo has been reported with use of a bio-ballistic ('gene gun') technique in which DNA coated onto colloidal gold particles is driven at high velocity by gas pressure into the cell.[25] Improved methods of electroporation may also be valuable for transducing normal and malignant hematopoietic progenitor cells with sufficient efficiency to allow therapeutic application.[26]

### Other vectors

Other vectors, including herpesviruses, have been proposed as high-efficiency transducers of normal and malignant hematopoietic cells, and are entering clinical trials. However, although these viruses may become future substitutes for currently available vector systems, most investigators now accept that no naturally occurring virus and no simple physical vector will ever prove suitable for all gene therapy purposes. Ultimately, therefore, entirely new synthetic or semisynthetic vectors will have to be developed. Possibilities include the generation of hybrid viral vectors, which may combine, for example, the in vivo stability of adenoviruses and the integrating capacity of retroviruses.[27] Alternative, fully synthetic vectors will be developed by combining components from multiple different vectors, allowing safe, efficient, and specific gene transfer and regulation. In the meantime, however, gene therapy protocols for leukemia will require investigators to circumvent the limitations of current vectors and to choose their agents on the basis of the most important feature required.

# Tumor cell modification

## Correction or deletion of underlying defects

The strategy of introducing genetic material into a hematologic malignancy to correct the genetic defect causing the neoplastic phenotype or to directly kill the malignant cell is seductively elegant. This approach would be highly relevant to the leukemias and lymphomas, which harbor a number of oncogenes and fusion transcripts that are specific to the malignant clone and frequently form a critical component of the malignant process. For example, efforts are being made to neutralize fusion transcripts such as *BCR–ABL* or activated oncogenes such as *MYB* (in chronic myeloid leukemia, CML), using ribozymes, antisense RNA, or wild-type genes.[28,29] Similarly, non-functional anti-oncogenes (tumor suppressor genes) such as *p53* may be replaced by wild-type genes in patients with acute myeloid leukemia (AML) or myelodysplasia (MDS).[13] Interest is also increasing in targeting the gene pathways involved in regulating apoptosis. Experimental models suggest that even minor perturbations in these pathways can greatly modify the sensitivity of cancer cells to chemotherapy.

Numerous obstacles must be overcome before the corrective approach is successful. The first set deal with the genetic change itself. Unless correction of a single defect is subsequently lethal to the malignant cell, the transfer of an individual corrective gene to a patient with $10^{11}$ or $10^{12}$ leukemic or lymphomatous cells will leave many cells that are effectively premalignant, with a high risk of later transformation. Moreover, many relevant gene defects produce molecules with 'transdominant' effects that will continue to produce a malignant phenotype, even if a wild-type gene is introduced. Hence, most approaches to correction attempt to silence transdominant malignant genes.

This can be achieved with ribozymes, antisense oligonucleotides, or double-stranded RNA or RNA interference, or by homologous recombination with a wild-type gene.[30,31] These 'subtractive' approaches to gene transfer are designed to destroy the function of an expressed gene rather than to add a new activity.

Ribozymes cleave specific sequences in targeted mRNA molecules. For clinical use, ribozymes that form hairpin or hammerhead structures are preferred because of their stability even in the absence of substrate and their activity under physiologic conditions. In viruses and other microorganisms, ribozymes function probably to autocatalyze their own cleavage into functional RNA, and perhaps also to destroy the RNA of invading organisms. For applications in gene transfer, ribozymes may be used to destroy transcripts originating from the unwanted host cell DNA sequence while leaving intact the mRNA originating from the transgene. Some ribozymes are currently under clinical investigation. The vascular endothelial growth factor (VEG-F)-targeted ribozyme, for example, is currently being investigated for a possible role in breast, lung, and colon cancer.

Antisense oligonucleotides are short synthetic stretches of DNA that hybridize with specific mRNA and can prevent translation of the target gene by inducing RNaseH digestion of target mRNA. In every in vivo experiment, oligonucleotides were found to be susceptible to natural phosphodiester backbone degradation by cellular nucleases. Several sugar, base, and backbone modifications have been investigated to improve stability. Replacement of the phosphate moiety by phosphorothioates results in compounds with serum stability and high RNA-binding affinity. Toxic effects are apparent at higher dose levels, including complement activation, thrombocytopenia, and heptotoxicity. Toxicity may be reduced by delivery in liposomes. Further modifications have concentrated on substitutions at the 2′ position with electronegative substituents, such as a 2-O-C-methylene bridge,[32] which enhance RNA binding. The sequence has to be carefully chosen to avoid hybridization of full-length oligonucleotides to unrelated targets. Preclinical studies and initial clinical results, however, did not substantiate concerns that toxicity would reflect non-specific inhibition of RNA. Normal healthy cells tolerate the transient loss of function better than cancer cells, which carry the pro-apoptotic burden of multiple genetic alterations and genomic instability. Several clinical studies have been reported using antisense oligonucleotides to target the c-*MYB* or *p53* genes, either as marrow-purging agents for the chronic or accelerated phase of CML or intravenously for refractory AML or CML in blast crisis, without significant clinical responses or associated toxicities.[33,34] An antisense *BCL2* oligonucleotide has also been administered to patients with refractory non-Hodgkin lymphoma (NHL), with objective clinical and biologic responses.[35] Several clinical studies of antisense oligonucleotide are underway.

RNA interference is an ancient mechanism of post-transcriptional gene silencing[36] in which short segments of double-stranded RNA direct RNases to digest specific sequences of mRNA. Initial attempts to harness this phenomenon for experimental manipulation of mammalian cells were foiled by non-specific antiviral defense mechanisms. The field advanced when synthetic duplexes of short RNAs were found to mediate specific and potent gene silencing.[37] Delivery of such molecules (e.g. in a lipid envelope) may facilitate application of this form of gene targeting to cancer therapy. Since RNA itself is fragile and costly, expression systems that allow the generation of siRNA inside the cell may be preferable alternatives,[38] and could be made part of a vector.

Introduction of a gene that directly kills tumor cells has frequently been used in gene therapy.[39] For example, a gene encoding an enzyme that metabolizes a drug to an active moiety, which then kills the tumor cell, can be expressed in cancer cells. The active molecule may also diffuse either through intercellular gap junctions or in the extracellular space and destroy adjacent tumor cells. In this way, transduction of even a small proportion of tumor cells can produce a large 'bystander' effect on adjacent tumor tissue. Unlike the corrective approach, the transgene is not specifically toxic to the tumor, and any normal cells that are transduced may be affected. For this reason, the main success has been in treating localized disease such as brain tumors. More recently, Hurwitz and colleagues[40–42] have injected bilateral retinoblastomas with adenovirus type 5 encoding the thymidine kinase gene, followed by administration of ganciclovir. Several patients showed a complete response of vitreal tumor deposits.

Bystander effects notwithstanding, a high proportion of tumor cells must be transduced if tumor modification is to be useful. Since current vectors cannot be targeted to tumor tissue and are relatively inefficient, most of the gene therapeutic approaches described so far are limited to the treatment of accessible local disease – rarely an option in hematologic cancers. Several developments may ultimately overcome this obstacle. Extensive efforts have been made to alter the envelope proteins of vectors to ablate their natural cell tropisms and replace them with new tumor-associated binding specificities.[43–47] It is also possible to make promoters that are active only in specific cell or tissue types. An example of this 'transcriptional targeting' is use of the carcinoembryonic antigen (*CEA*) promoter to drive a prodrug gene. This mediates selective gene expression in CEA-producing tumors. A combination of specific envelope (transductional targeting) and specific promoter (transcriptional targeting) may provide optimal specificity for tumor cells.

One can increase the efficiency of gene transfer to tumors by using conditionally replication-competent viruses. Viruses have been developed that will replicate in malignant but not in normal cells,[48] thereby providing multiple rounds of infection within tumor targets. Alternatively, normal cells could serve as vector carriers if they track to sites of tumor. The most obvious choice among cell carriers would be T cells or natural killer (NK) cells. Promoters that activate upon T-cell receptor (TCR) binding or after encounter with certain angiogenic factors could be used to trigger virus production and release. Systemic administration of vectors, particularly those derived from viruses, is also hampered by innate and adaptive immune responses. Inflammatory responses, specific antibodies, and cellular immune responses rapidly diminish the activity of even the largest doses of vector.[49] Efforts to induce selective and transient immunosuppression are only in their infancy.

## Tumor vaccines

One of the most commonly used strategies of cancer gene therapy is to enhance the immunogenicity of weak tumor antigens by transducing tumor cells to express immune-activating molecules. In murine model systems, tumor cells expressing such molecules have augmented immunogenicity. Injection of neoplastic cells (including those derived from lymphoid and myeloid malignancies) in doses that would normally establish a tumor instead recruits immune system effector cells and eradicates injected tumor cells.[50–53] Often, the animal is then resistant to challenges by further local injections of non-transduced parental tumor. The transduced tumor has therefore acted as a vaccine. In some models, established, non-transduced, parental malignant cells are also eradicated.[51] A number of different molecules have been successfully exploited in animal models. These include chemokines, such as lymphotactin;[54] agents that enhance antigen presentation, such as granulocyte–macrophage colony-stimulating factor (GM-CSF);[55–57] cytokines that enhance CD4+ cell activity, such as tumor necrosis factor α (TNF-α) and IL-7,[58,59] or that increase expression of class I MHC antigens, such as interferon-γ (IFN-γ),[60] or that amplify T-cell responses, such as IL-2.[61] Additionally, efforts have been made to express costimulatory molecules on tumor cells, including CD40 ligand (CD40L)[62–66] and B7.1,[67] or intercellular adhesion molecules such as ICAM-1 and ICAM-3.[68]

Translating this approach to human hematologic cancers is not straightforward. Although human leukemic cells are often readily available, they are difficult to grow in vitro (making murine retroviral transduction difficult), and they resist transduction with most currently available vectors. Leukemic cells may be heterogeneous, so that the population used to vaccinate may not express critical target antigens.[69] The use of an allogeneic cell line simplifies the logistics, but may result in the patient receiving a vaccine that does not express the appropriate target antigens. A phase I study of autologous AML cells engineered to secrete GM-CSF has recently commenced and is now extended to pediatric AML.[55] It has also proved feasible to express costimulator molecules such as CD40, CD40L, or B7.1 on primary tumor cells surfaces. We are using a combination of *CD40L* and *IL-2* gene transfer into pediatric ALL cells to generate an antitumor immune response in patients with high-risk disease who have entered remission. To date, this study has proved to be safe and has generated both cellular and humoral antileukemic immune responses in six out of eight patients treated.[70] Because these patients are treated in remission, it may be difficult to confirm whether there is any antileukemic activity. A similar study has begun for adults with chronic lymphocytic leukemia.[71] As an alternative to inducing expression in tumor cells directly, and as a throwback to the vaccine adjuvant days, some groups are testing vaccines composed of autologous tumor cells mixed with GM-CSF-producing bystander cells.[72]

In conclusion, genetic modification of tumor cells appears safe and is capable of generating specific humoral and cellular antitumor cytotoxic responses. There have been at least some reports of tumor regressions, and the approach is being evaluated in a wider range of tumors and in a larger number of patients, including those with leukemia.

## DNA vaccines

Nucleic acid vaccines induce an immune response against a protein expressed in vivo from a naked encoding gene. Nucleotide-based vaccines have a number of appealing features. They provide prolonged antigen expression that can continuously stimulate the immune system, probably through an intracellular antigenic reservoir resistant to antibody-mediated clearance. This may favor induction of immune memory even in the absence of booster immunization.[73] Codelivery with plasmids encoding cytokines or costimulatory molecules can further enhance the immune response.[74] Moreover, nucleotide vaccination leads to antigen presentation to both specific cytoxic T lymphocytes (CTL) and helper T cells. Preclinical experiments conducted in a mouse model of adult T-cell leukemia induced by the human T-cell leukemia virus I (HTLV-I) indicated a promising effect for a Tax-coding DNA vaccine against HTLV-I-induced tumors in vivo.[75] Immunization with DNA constructs encoding the idiotype (ld) of a murine B-cell lymphoma induced specific anti-ld antibody responses and protected mice against tumor challenge. Furthermore, use of DNA encoding an ld/GM-CSF fusion protein improved vaccine efficacy.[76] By introducing unmethylated CpG motifs into the transferred genes, one can achieve further enhancement of the host immune response, as these motifs are one of the most immunogenic components of bacterial DNA recognized by the vertebrate immune system.[77] Clinical trials of DNA vaccines are ongoing in patients with cutaneous T-cell lymphoma and melanoma.

# Host cell modification

## Immune system

In contrast to the meager clinical responses produced by tumor vaccines, the effects of adoptive transfer of T cells are quite dramatic. Recent studies of SV40 large T-antigen-dependent mouse tumor models of hepatocellular carcinoma and prostate cancer have shown that adoptive transfer of T cells from nontransgenic mice for which SV40 is non-self results in clear benefit.[78,79] In humans, allogeneic donor leukocyte infusion can render remissions in relapsed CML after bone marrow transplantation by rejection of minor histocompatability antigens that are foreign to the donor T cell.[80] Other human studies by Rooney et al[81] have shown that adoptive therapy with virus-specific T cells is safe, feasible, and active as prophylaxis and treatment for post-transplant Epstein–Barr virus (EBV) lymphoproliferative disorder.

Human malignant cells harbor other potential targets for the immune system, including mutated oncogenes or fusion proteins generated by chromosomal translocations.[82,83] Some lymphomas may express immunogenic virally encoded proteins.[84] Even normal proteins may be suitable targets if they are expressed in higher-than-usual quantities; tyrosinase and the MAGE series of proteins in melanoma cells are two good examples.[85] If tumor cells either express or are able to process and present these tumor-specific peptides, then malignancy-specific T cells administered in large enough doses should be effective treatment. However, generation of therapeutic doses of specific T cells is difficult, except in special cases where the tumors express viral proteins.

## Artificial T-cell receptors

One way of circumventing the lack of tumor antigen-specific T cells is to transduce T cells with chimeric surface proteins that transmit TCR signals in response to target cells. Such proteins have an extracellular domain (ectodomain), usually derived from immunoglobulin variable chains, that recognizes and binds target antigen. This domain is attached via a spacer to an intracytoplasmic signaling domain (endodomain), usually the cytoplasmic segment of the TCR ζ chain, which transmits an activation signal

to the T cell.[86] A wide variety of domains have been combined,[87] and the generation of these chimeras seems generally robust. This probably reflects the isolating effects of the lipid bilayer, which forces the extracellular and intracellular domains to remain structurally independent from each other. The structure of an artificial TCR is contrasted with that of a native TCR in Figure 28.2 (see Plate 7).

Immunoglobulin T-cell receptors (also called as IgTCR or T bodies) are the most commonly described constructs. They are created by joining the variable domain of an immunoglobulin with an intracytoplasmic signaling molecule. They unite the specificities of antibodies with the potency of cellular killing by transposing antibody recognition to T cells. T cells expressing these chimeric TCR are redirected to kill tumor cells that express antigen on their surface. The generation of T lymphocytes with an antibody-dictated specificity allows targeting toward any tumor-associated antigen for which a monoclonal antibody exists. In contrast to the lengthy process of selection and expansion of lymphocytes with native specificity for target antigens, large populations of antigen-redirected T lymphocytes can be obtained by simple retroviral transduction. Since chimeric TCR based on immunoglobulin provide T-cell activation in an MHC-unrestricted manner, mechanisms of tumor escape from T-cell recognition, such as downregulation of HLA class I molecules and defects in antigen processing, are bypassed. T-cell-mediated effector functions are much more likely to result in tumor cell lysis than humoral immune responses alone. Cytokine secretion upon T-cell activation by tumor antigen will result in the recruitment of additional components of the immune system, amplifying the antitumor immune response. Furthermore, unlike many intact antibodies, T cells can migrate through microvascular walls, extravasate, and penetrate the cores of solid tumors to exert their cytolytic activity.

These predictions have been tested in vivo. In a mouse model of ErbB2-expressing ovarian carcinoma, for example, autologous lymphocytes expressing scFv-ζ TCR directed against ErbB2 were infused into tumor-xenografted mice, resulting in total regression of the tumors.[88] Similarly, lymphocytes expressing scFv against CEA fused with FcεIg were effective at rejecting colon carcinomas in a mouse model of this tumor.[89] Chimeric receptors can also activate homing – ErbB2-targeted T cells labeled with fluorescent dye were specifically detected in the tumor tissue of SCID mice bearing ErbB2+ tumors.[90]

The first clinical trials of a chimeric TCR was performed with an HIV-Env-specific CD4ζ construct expressed in either autologous or syngeneic T cells.[91] No specific effect on HIV viral load could be demonstrated, and transduced T cells persisted only at very low levels. The outcome of this study is representa-

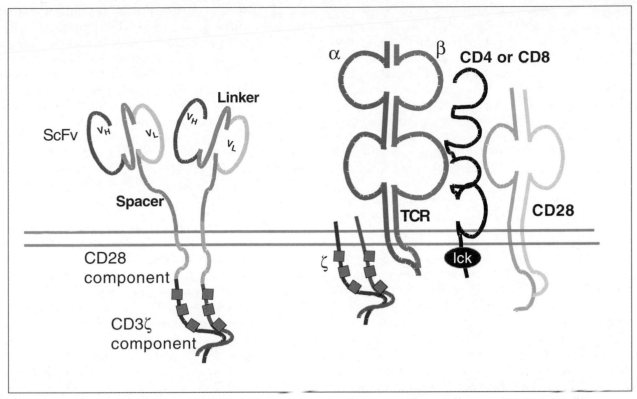

**Figure 28.2** Artificial TCR (dimer) and native TCR. Artificial receptor components can be divided into two groups. External section is involved with antigen recognition. This is usually composed of a Single Chain Variable Fragment (ScFv) derived from a monoclonal antibody. This is connected to the internal section of the receptor via a flexible spacer which allows the receptor multiple orientations. The internal section transmits signal. In this figure we show a signaling domain composed of a fusion of signaling portions of CD28 and CD3ζ. This receptor is capable of transmitting a CD3ζ signal and CD28 co-stimulatory signal upon antigen recognition. Simplicity of artificial receptor is contrasted to the complexity of the native TCR which requires an aggregate of multiple proteins to transmit a similar signal. See Plate 7.

tive of many others, and demonstrates the limitation of chimeric TCR. The signaling function of engineered chimeric proteins is much less effective than that of the native TCR, during which CD4 or CD8 coreceptors are recruited to the signaling complex via their interaction with class I and II MHC molecules. These coreceptors bring Src kinases to the TCR, promoting phosphorylation of TCR immunoreceptor tyrosine-based activation motifs (ITAM) and enhancing signaling severalfold.[92] Furthermore, the engagement of just the TCR is not sufficient to achieve full T-cell activation. A costimulatory signal from CD28 is required to cause clonal expansion and full activation of T cells. Chimeric receptors with just a TCR ζ-chain intracellular sequence do not fully activate naive T cells in transgenic mice.[93] In essence, chimeric TCR act as crude triggers of cell killing but lack the signaling components to fully activate and induce proliferation of T cells.

Deficient signaling may be overcome in a number of ways. The endodomains can be modified to transmit a more complete signal. For example, constructs containing endodomains composed of the intracellular segment of CD28 joined to that of CD3ζ were able to activate T cells and trigger killing of targets and pro-

liferation.[94,95] More complex endodomains involving portions of different costimulatory molecules have also been described.[96] Alternatively, investigators have generated 'bi-specific' T cells. Autologous T cells that recognize a powerful antigen unrelated to the tumor (e.g. allo or viral antigens) are expanded by repeated stimulation and subsequently transduced with a chimeric receptor before being returned to the patient. Activation via their native TCR leads to their persistence and activation. Recognition of tumor by their chimeric TCR triggers killing of targets. In other words, tumor killing is 'piggy-backed' onto a more potent antigen response.[97,98]

## T-cell modification to improve survival or overcome tumor evasion mechanisms

Adoptively transferred T cells must still face tumor evasion strategies, and hence frequently persist and function poorly in vivo.[99,100] Genetic modification may circumvent this obstacle. For example, IL-2 administration improves the survival of infused lymphocytes but is toxic at the required doses.[101] Genetically modified lymphocytes producing IL-2 should result in high local concentration and could improve their persistence without systemic toxicity. Liu and Rosenberg[102] transduced melanoma-reactive human T cells to secrete IL-2, and after stimulation these cells proliferated without addition of exogenous IL-2. Furthermore, transduction did not alter their specificity or ability to recognize tumor cells. An alternative strategy to promote survival is to transduce T cells with an anti-apoptotic gene. Transduction of T cells with a *BCLX*-expressing retroviral vector results in partial resistance to Fas antibody-induced apoptosis.[103] Unfortunately, concerns over oncogenesis (see below on gene therapy as a cause of leukemia) render these types of growth-promoting activities unlikely to be evaluated clinically in the near future.

The immunosuppressive cytokine transforming growth factor β (TGF-β) is secreted by many tumors. In murine models of both thymoma and malignant melanoma, transgenic mice genetically engineered so that all of their T cells are insensitive to TGF-β signaling were able to eradicate tumors.[104] In a preclinical human study, EBV-specific CTL were transduced with a retroviral vector expressing a mutant dominant-negative TGF-β type II receptor (DNR) that prevents the formation of the functional tetrameric receptor. Cytotoxicity, proliferation, and cytokine release assays showed that levels of exogenous TGF-β inhibitory to wild-type CTL had minimal inhibitory effects on DNR-transduced CTL.[105] If long-term murine toxicity studies continue to confirm that DNR-transduced CTL are not tumorigenic, this approach may be useful not only for Hodgkin lymphoma but also for other lymphomas and solid tumors that secrete TGF-β.

### Suicide genes

Suicide genes make transduced cells susceptible to an agent that is not ordinarily toxic. More than a dozen examples of these systems exist, but the most widely used clinically is the thymidine kinase gene from herpes simplex virus 1 (*HSV-tk*). This enzyme phosphorylates the prodrug ganciclovir, which results in the death of dividing cells when subsequently incorporated into DNA.

These genes have been used to treat relapsed leukemia after allogeneic stem cell transplantation. After this procedure, donor T cells contribute to a graft-versus-leukemia effect to reduce relapse, facilitate engraftment, and reduce opportunistic infections. Nevertheless, in a subset of patients, donor T cells can cause potentially lethal graft-versus-host disease (GVHD). The introduction of a 'suicide gene' in donor T cells that can be activated in vivo allows for their positive effects to be manifest, with the option of their possible subsequent deletion should GVHD ensue. Donor T lymphocytes transduced with *HSV-tk* have been administered to patients after T-cell depletion.[106,107] In these studies, administration of ganci-

clovir alone resulted in resolution of GVHD in five out of seven patients. Although these studies demonstrated proof of principle, *HSV-tk* therapy has several limitations. Ganciclovir must often be administered to treat cytomegalovirus (CMV) infection or reactivation after bone marrow transplantation, resulting in deletion of the needed donor T cells. HSV-tk is a virus-derived protein and is strongly immunogenic. Hence, cells expressing the protein are likely to survive only in immunosuppressed patients. Even then, an immune response may be detected.[106] In more immunocompetent patient groups, *HSV-tk*-transduced cells are rapidly deleted.[108]

More useful suicide genes encoding for non-immunogenic proteins with low basal toxicity but high efficacy after triggering are under development. For example, a suicide system has been developed that is based on endogenous pro-apoptotic molecules linked to modified FK506-binding proteins (FKBP). These molecules contain a binding site for a lipid-permeable chemical inducer of dimerization.[109] Administration of this dimerizing drug results in the aggregation of two or more chimeric pro-apoptotic molecules, leading to their activation and thus apoptosis. Similarly, inducible Fas is based on a self-protein and should be non-immunogenic.[110] Its inducer, AP1903, seems to lack toxicity.[111] Another possibility is to use inducible caspase molecules. These constructs may improve function, since caspases are downstream of Fas in the apoptosis-signaling cascade, distal to many anti-apoptotic molecules, such as c-FLIP and BCL2. Human *CD20* has also been proposed as a non-immunogenic suicide gene. Exposure to a monoclonal chimeric anti-CD20 antibody (rituximab), in the presence of complement, results in rapid killing of transduced cells.[112] This strategy precludes the need for coexpression of a surface marker for sorting. However, rituximab will result in the unwanted loss of B cells as well as donor T cells. Since transduction can never be 100% efficient in any of these systems, coexpression of a non-immunogenic selectable marker together with the suicide gene is required to allow for selection of suicide gene-expressing cells. An internal ribosomal entry site (IRES) or a linker sequence containing a cleavage site that will be cut by endogenous proteases post protein translation (e.g. FMDV 2A peptide) may be useful in obtaining reliable coexpression of both genes.[113]

### Sensitivity of host cells to cytotoxic drugs

If HSC could be rendered resistant to one or more cytotoxic drugs, they might be able to resist the myelosuppressive effects of cytotoxic drugs during leukemia therapy, allowing longer or more intensive therapy that could cure additional patients.[114–116]

The *MDR1* gene has been the most widely considered for human therapy. Its product, P-glycoprotein, functions as a drug efflux pump and confers resistance to many chemotherapeutic agents.[117] The feasibility of using *MDR1* to protect hemopoietic cells has been demonstrated by transgenic mouse experiments,[118,119] and retroviral transfer of *MDR1* to murine clonogenic progenitors conferred drug resistance both in vitro and in vivo.[119] These experiments with *MDR1*-containing vectors prove the principle that drug-resistance genes can be used to attenuate drug induced myelosuppression. It is likely that other drug resistance genes could function analogously. DNA methylguanine methyltransferases (MGMT) are enzymes that repair DNA damage induced by the nitrosoureas, a class of alkylating agents used widely in cancer chemotherapy. Preliminary data suggest that retrovirally mediated gene transfer of the human *MGMT* gene to mouse bone marrow cells results in protection of murine progenitors from toxicity produced by carmustine (BCNU).[120] Other drug resistance genes, including those for dihydrofolate reductase and topoisomerase II, are also under consideration for clinical testing. In a human breast cancer study, a significant proportion of hematopoietic cells were protected when expression levels of drug-resistance genes were adequate to reduce the sensitivity of stem cells to chemotherapeutic agents.[121]

The clinical application of drug-resistance gene transfer has several potential pitfalls. The low efficiency of stem cell transduction observed with current clinical protocols predicts that drug-induced myelosuppression cannot be ameliorated unless there is dramatic progress in vector targeting. There is also the risk of transferring the genes to neoplastic cells that contaminate the hematopoietic stem cell graft and produce drug-resistant relapse. Finally, toxicity to non-protected organs – including gut, heart, and lungs – may rapidly supervene when marrow resistance allows intensification of cytotoxic drug dosages.

# Gene marking

The underlying principle of gene marking is that the transfer of a unique DNA sequence into a host cell will allow its easy subsequent detection, thereby serving as a marker of these labeled cells. Gene marking is not intended for any direct therapeutic benefit, but rather to obtain information regarding the biology and function of adoptively transferred cells.

## In autologous stem cell transplantation

Autologous HSC rescue has shown promise as effective treatment for leukemias and lymphomas,[122–125] although disease recurrence continues to be the major cause of failure. Whether recurrence originates from stem cell harvest or residual disease is unclear.[122–127] Concern that the HSC may contain residual malignant cells has led to extensive evaluation of purging tech-

niques.[128–131] However, no method has been unequivocally shown to reduce the risk of relapse in naturally occurring disease,[127–132] and purging techniques usually slow engraftment due to damage to normal progenitor cells.

By marking stem cells prior to their infusion, we can determine if contaminating malignant cells in the stem cell harvest contribute to relapse following autologous stem cell transplantation.[133] The HSC product is marked at the time of harvest with retroviral vectors encoding the neomycin resistance gene (*neo*). Then, at relapse, it is possible to detect whether the marker gene is present in the malignant cells. Since 1991, this strategy had been studied in a variety of malignancies treated by autologous HSC transplantation,[133–137] including AML, CML, ALL, neuroblastoma, and lymphoma. In pediatric patients receiving autologous bone marrow transplantation as part of therapy for AML, 4 of 12 patients who received marked marrow relapsed. In 3 of the patients, detection of both the transferred marker and of a tumor-specific marker in the same cells at the time of relapse provided unequivocal evidence that the residual malignant cells in the marrow were a source of leukemic recurrence.

More difficult questions can be answered by simultaneously marking cells with different vectors. For instance, what are the effects of purging on relapse and engraftment? Comparison of two purging methods, 4-hydroperoxycyclophosphamide (4-HC) and culture with IL-2, by differential marking revealed greater contribution to hematopoietic reconstitution by 4-HC-purged marrow.[138] Notably, in these studies, marker gene levels were lower than in studies using unpurged marrow.

No in vitro assay can yet assess the capacity to repopulate the hematopoietic compartment. Differential marking in single patients allows comparison of these properties between different sources of stem cells (e.g. peripheral blood versus marrow), the function of different subpopulations, and the consequences of ex vivo manipulation, such as stromal support or cytokines. For instance, it is possible to use growth factors such as IL-1, IL-3, and stem cell factor to increase by 10- to 50-fold the numbers of hematopoietic progenitor cells.[139] It is not certain that such ex vivo data will be reflected by results in vivo. In primate and human studies, transplantation of marrow treated ex vivo with growth factor combinations that greatly augment both progenitor numbers and gene transfer rates yielded disconcertingly low levels of long-term gene expression in vivo.[139] The likeliest explanation for this seeming paradox is that many of the growth factors intended only to induce cycling in marrow stem cells also induce their differentiation and the loss of their self-renewal capacity. Another useful comparison is the repopulating capabilities of autologous bone marrow CD34+ cells and peripheral blood stream cells.[140] Judging by differential marking, the latter cells contributed to hematopoietic earlier and for longer times.

These marking studies also provided information on the transfer of marker genes to normal hematopoietic cells and showed that marrow autografts contribute to long-term hematopoietic reconstitution after transplantation.[141] Long-term transfer for more than 10 years has been seen in the mature progeny of marrow precursor cells, including peripheral blood T and B cells and neutrophils.[138]

### T-cell marking

Several studies have also shown the feasibility of gene-marking CTL to track their expansion, persistence and homing to sites of disease.[81,142,143] For example, gene marking of EBV-specific CTL for the prophylaxis and treatment of lymphoproliferative disorders post HSC transplantation has demonstrated the persistence of gene-marked CTL for 78 months post infusion. In addition, gene-marked EBV-CTL given as treatment for relapsed Hodgkin lymphoma have been shown to traffic to tumor sites.[143]

### New methodologies

Two new techniques will allow even more informative marking trials. Quantitative real-time polymerase chain reaction (PCR) enables simple, highly accurate quantification of integrant copy number that can easily be standardized against an internal control. This is a significant improvement over the semiquantitative PCR techniques used previously. In addition, every retroviral integration event results in a unique integration site in genomic DNA. The progeny of a transduced cell will bear the same integration site, and cutting of PCR-amplified flanking DNA with a restriction endonuclease yields multiple fragments whose lengths are unique to the integration site. The number of fragments from a given sample indicates 'clonality'. Individual fragments can be sequenced and the precise location of integration elucidated.[144] Detection systems specific to a particular provirus-flanking region can be developed and will allow precise tracking of an individual clone. This approach allows the evolution of clones and the true pluripotency of transduced cells to follow over time. We can even begin to hypothesize about such things as the number of true stem cells in harvested marrow or blood. Importantly, a reduction in the number of clones with a rise in marker levels may herald the emergence of integration-induced leukemogenesis, as described below.

## Gene therapy as a cause of leukemia

Any vector that randomly inserts its genetic information into the genome of target cells is, by definition,

causing insertional mutagenesis. Hence, the risk of insertional mutagenesis disrupting normal gene function, inactivating tumor suppressor genes, or activating oncogenes should be directly proportional to the number of insertion/integration events. However, the activation of a single proto-oncogene by itself should not be sufficient to convert a normal cell into a tumor cell – rather multiple gene disruptions would be required. Since current integrating vectors are inefficient, transducing a small proportion of cells with a low retroviral copy number, the risk of inducing a malignant change has always been considered to be small. Until recently, the only description of retroviral vector-related tumorigenesis in humans or non-human primates was in a monkey who developed T-cell lymphoma following transduction with a replication-competent retroviral vector. Analysis of the tumor revealed multiple integration sites caused by chronic productive retroviral infections,[145] further supporting the belief that the replication-incompetent retroviruses used clinically would not share this predisposition.

Unfortunately, this confidence was shattered by reports of two cases of T-ALL in 11 patients with common γ-chain deficiency (X-SCID) who received retrovirally corrected autologous stem cells.[146] Subsequent integration analysis revealed single integrations in each T-ALL line, both of which were proximate to *LMO2*, a locus known to be involved in T-cell growth and differentiation. Why was this single integration event sufficient to trigger leukemia? The common γ chain is involved in transmitting potent proliferative signals. In the construct used, expression was controlled by the retroviral long terminal repeat (LTR) rather than by the gene's native promoter system. Overexpression of the common γ chain together with activation of LMO2 at some stage of T-cell development may be sufficient for leukemogenesis. A similar observation was made when mice transplanted with stem cells transduced with truncated nerve growth factor receptor (dLNGFR) developed AML with a single integration involving the *Evi1* gene.[147] Like *LMO2*, disruption of *Evi1* was not felt to be sufficient on its own to cause AML. In other words, the transgene itself represents the 'second hit'. If this hypothesis is correct, the approaches that we have outlined for the gene therapy of leukemia are unlikely to prove problematic, since few involve the introduction of unregulated T-cell growth factors. While continued caution is essential, it is also important to remember that many hundreds of cancer patients have received retrovirally transduced cells without developing leukemia.

## Summing up

Figure 28.3 shows the distribution of attempts at cancer gene therapy thus far, and Table 28.2 lists some current studies of interest. Many obstacles must be

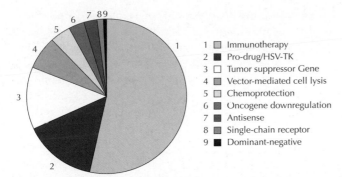

1 ☐ Immunotherapy
2 ■ Pro-drug/HSV-TK
3 ☐ Tumor suppressor Gene
4 ■ Vector-mediated cell lysis
5 ☐ Chemoprotection
6 ■ Oncogene downregulation
7 ■ Antisense
8 ■ Single-chain receptor
9 ■ Dominant-negative

**Figure 28.3** Distribution of cancer-gene therapy protocols in North America to date.

## Table 28.2 Some examples of current cancer gene-therapy protocols

| Study | Title, institution, and comments |
|---|---|
| 9803-242 | A phase I study of CD40L gene-transduced leukemia cells in patients with chronic lymphocytic leukemia<br><br>University of California, San Diego<br><br>Investigators here modified autologous CLL cells by transducing them with an adenovirus containing a coding sequence for CD40L. These CD40L-expressing autologous CLL cells are then administered to the patient as a tumor vaccine. This phase I study has now closed and demonstrated some clinical benefit. This approach is being pursued in a phase II study |
| 9705-188 | Autologous transplantation for chronic myelogenous leukemia with stem cells transduced with a methotrexate resistant DHFR and Anti-BCR/ABL containing vector and post transplant methotrexate administration<br><br>University of Minnesota, Minneapolis<br><br>This is an example of a study where the retroviral vector provides antisense sequences that directly target the genetic cause of the malignancy – in this case bcr/abl. Transduced marrow is also rendered resistant to methotrexate |
| 0310-608 | Administration of LMP2a specific cytotoxic T lymphocytes to patients with relapsed EBV-positive Hodgkin's disease<br><br>Baylor College of Medicine, Houston, Texas<br><br>In this study, gene-transfer technology is used to facilitate ex vivo selection and expansion of tumor-specific T cells. Dendritic cells are transduced with an adenovirus coding for a tumor antigen, LMP2. These transduced dendritic cells are used to selectively stimulate LMP2-specific T cells from peripheral blood mononuclear cells. Neither transduced cells nor vector are directly administered to the patient |
| 0005-400 | Transfer of the multidrug resistance gene, *MDR-1*, to hematopoietic progenitors from patients with high-risk lymphoma<br><br>University of Massachusetts Medical School Cancer Center, Worcester<br><br>This is an example of a chemoprotection study. Transduced, readministered marrow should be resistant to subsequent chemotherapy |
| 9907-330 | Autologous CD8+ T-lymphocyte clones transfected to express CD20-specific scFvFc-ζ as therapy for recurrent/refractory CD20+ lymphoma<br><br>City of Hope National Medical Center, Duarte, California<br><br>Investigators retarget T cells to recognize CD20 with an artificial T-cell receptor. This study will have the potential side-effect of depleting normal B cells as well as tumor cells |
| 0205-535 | Phase I study to evaluate the safety of cellular immunotherapy for high-risk CD19+ acute lymphoblastic leukemia after autologous hematopoietic stem cell transplantation using genetically modified CD19-redirected autologous cytolytic T-cell clones<br><br>City of Hope National Medical Center, Duarte, California<br><br>This study is similar to 9907-330, except here CD19 is targeted by an artificial receptor instead of CD20. As well as an artificial receptor, cells are engineered to express a suicide gene, *HSV-tk*. This renders T cells susceptible to ganciclovir. If unacceptable side-effects occur, the investigators have the option of administering ganciclovir, which will delete transduced T cells |
| 0301-564 | Autologous T cells retrovirally transduced to express anti-CEA-scFv-CD28ζ as therapy for adenocarcinoma<br><br>Beth Israel Deaconess Medical Center, Harvard Medical School, Boston, Massachusetts<br><br>The first proposed clinical study of second-generation artificial TCR that incorporate a CD28 signal as well as a ζ signal |

removed before the extraordinary potential of gene transfer can be fully exploited in therapy for hematologic malignancies. However, most advances in medicine proceed incrementally. Gene transfer is already being used successfully to complement conventional therapies for malignant hematologic disorders, it is facilitating the development of cytotoxic T-cell therapies for leukemia and lymphoma, and it is being explored as a means of generating leukemia vaccines. The benefits of this new technology can only increase as current limitations are progressively – albeit slowly – surmounted.

## REFERENCES

1. Bender MA, Palmer TD, Gelinas RE, Miller AD. Evidence that the packaging signal of Moloney murine leukemia virus extends into the *gag* region. *J Virol* 1987; **61**: 1639–46.

2. Brenner MK, Rill DR, Holladay MS et al. Gene marking to determine whether autologous marrow infusion restores long-term haemopoiesis in cancer patients. *Lancet* 1993; **342**: 1134–7.

3. Amado RG, Chen IS. Lentiviral vectors – the promise of gene therapy within reach? *Science* 1999; **285**: 674–6.

4. Sutton RE, Wu HT, Rigg R et al. Human immunodeficiency virus type 1 vectors efficiently transduce human hematopoietic stem cells. *J Virol* 1998; **72**: 5781–8.

5. Mascarenhas L, Stripecke R, Case SS et al. Gene delivery to human B-precursor acute lymphoblastic leukemia cells. *Blood* 1998; **92**: 3537–45.

6. Case SS, Price MA, Jordan CT et al. Stable transduction of quiescent CD34+CD38- human hematopoietic cells by HIV-1-based lentiviral vectors. *Proc Natl Acad Sci, USA* 1999; **96**: 2988–93.

7. Buchschacher GL Jr, Wong-Staal F. Development of lentiviral vectors for gene therapy for human diseases. *Blood* 2000; **95**: 2499–504.

8. Engelhardt JF, Yang Y, Stratford-Perricaudet LD et al. Direct gene transfer of human CFTR into human bronchial epithelia of xenografts with E1-deleted adenoviruses. *Nat Genet* 1993; **4**: 27–34.

9. Le Gal LS, Robert JJ, Berrard S et al. An adenovirus vector for gene transfer into neurons and glia in the brain. *Science* 1993; **259**: 988–90.

10. Smith TA, Mehaffey MG, Kayda DB et al. Adenovirus mediated expression of therapeutic plasma levels of human factor IX in mice. *Nat Genet* 1993; **5**: 397–402.

11. Amin R, Wilmott R, Schwarz Y, Trapnell B, Stark J. Replication-deficient adenovirus induces expression of interleukin-8 by airway epithelial cells in vitro. *Hum Gene Ther* 1995; **6**: 145–53.

12. Muzyczka N. Use of adeno-associated virus as a general transduction vector for mammalian cells. *Curr Top Microbiol Immunol* 1992; **158**: 97–129.

13. Clark KR, Voulgaropoulou F, Johnson PR. A stable cell line carrying adenovirus-inducible rep and cap genes allows for infectivity titration of adeno-associated virus vectors. *Gene Ther* 1996; **3**: 1124–32.

14. Conway JE, Rhys CM, Zolotukhin I et al. High-titer recombinant adeno-associated virus production utilizing a recombinant herpes simplex virus type I vector expressing AAV-2 Rep and Cap. *Gene Ther* 1999; **6**: 986–93.

15. Flotte T, Carter B, Conrad C et al. A phase I study of an adeno-associated virus-CFTR gene vector in adult CF patients with mild lung disease. *Hum Gene Ther* 1996; **7**: 1145–59.

16. Wagner JA, Moran ML, Messner AH et al. A phase I/II study of tgAAV-CF for the treatment of chronic sinusitis in patients with cystic fibrosis. *Hum Gene Ther* 1998; **9**: 889–909.

17. Wagner JA, Nepomuceno IB, Messner AH et al. A phase II, double-blind, randomized, placebo-controlled clinical trial of tgAAVCF using maxillary sinus delivery in patients with cystic fibrosis with antrostomies. *Hum Gene Ther* 2002; **13**: 1349–59.

18. Wagner JA, Reynolds T, Moran ML et al. Efficient and persistent gene transfer of AAV-CFTR in maxillary sinus. *Lancet* 1998; **351**: 1702–3.

19. van Gool SW, Barcy S, Devos S et al. CD80 (B7-1) and CD86 (B7-2): potential targets for immunotherapy? *Res Immunol* 1995; **146**: 183–96.

20. Su H, Chang JC, Xu SM, Kan YW. Selective killing of AFP-positive hepatocellular carcinoma cells by adeno-associated virus transfer of the herpes simplex virus thymidine kinase gene. *Hum Gene Ther* 1996; **7**: 463–70.

21. Gao X, Huang L. A novel cationic liposome reagent for efficient transfection of mammalian cells. *Biochem Biophys Res Commun* 1991; **179**: 280–5.

22. Nabel GJ, Nabel EG, Yang ZY et al. Direct gene transfer with DNA–liposome complexes in melanoma: expression, biologic activity, and lack of toxicity in humans. *Proc Natl Acad Sci, USA* 1993; **90**: 11307–11.

23. Templeton NS. Cationic liposome-mediated gene delivery in vivo. *Biosci Rep* 2002; **22**: 283–95.

24. Trubetskoy VS, Torchilin VP, Kennel S, Huang L. Cationic liposomes enhance targeted delivery and expression of exogenous DNA mediated by N-terminal modified poly(L-lysine)–antibody conjugate in mouse lung endothelial cells. *Biochim Biophys Acta* 1992; **1131**: 311–13.

25. Ito K, Shinohara N, Kato S. DNA immunization via intramuscular and intradermal routes using a gene gun provides different magnitudes and durations on immune response. *Biochim Biophys Acta* 2003; **39**: 847–54.

26. Lin-Hong L, Biagi E, Brenner M, Fratantoni J. Electroporation-mediated efficient non-viral gene delivery to CLL-B cells and application in immunotherapy. *Proc Am Soc Hematol* 2002: Abst 5538.

27. Yotnda P, Chen DH, Chiu W et al. Bilamellar cationic liposomes protect adenovectors from preexisting humoral immune responses. *Mol Ther* 2002; **5**: 233–41.

28. Rossi JJ. Therapeutic antisense and ribozymes. *Br Med Bull* 1995; **51**: 217–25.

29. Zhang Y, Mukhopadhyay T, Donehower LA et al. Retroviral vector-mediated transduction of K-ras antisense RNA into human lung cancer cells inhibits expression of the malignant phenotype. *Hum Gene Ther* 1993; **4**: 451–60.

30. Heise C, Sampson-Johannes A, Williams A et al. ONYX-015, an E1B gene-attenuated adenovirus, causes tumor-specific cytolysis and antitumoral efficacy that can be

augmented by standard chemotherapeutic agents. 1997; **3**: 639–45.

31. Parr MJ, Manome Y, Tanaka T et al. Tumor-selective transgene expression in vivo mediated by an E2F-responsive adenoviral vector. *Nat Med* 1997; **3**: 1145–9.

32. Wang H, Cai Q, Zeng X et al. Antitumor activity and pharmacokinetics of a mixed-backbone antisense oligonucleotide targeted to the RIα subunit of protein kinase A after oral administration. *Proct Natl Acad Sci, USA* 1999; **96**: 13989–94.

33. Bayever E, Iversen PL, Bishop MR et al. Systemic administration of a phosphorothioate oligonucleotide with a sequence complementary to *p53* for acute myelogenous leukemia and myelodysplastic syndrome: initial results of a phase I trial. *Antisense Res Dev* 1993; **3**: 383–90.

34. Gewirtz AM. Myb targeted therapeutics for the treatment of human malignancies. *Oncogene* 1999; **18**: 3056–62.

35. Waters JS, Webb A, Cunningham D et al. Phase I clinical and pharmacokinetic study of *bcl-2* antisense oligonucleotide therapy in patients with non-Hodgkin's lymphoma. *J Clin Oncol* 2000; **18**: 1812–23.

36. Fire A, Xu S, Montgomery MK et al. Potent and specific genetic interference by double-stranded RNA in *Caenorhabditis elegans*. *Nature* 1998; **391**: 806–11.

37. Elbashir SM, Harborth J, Lendeckel W et al. Duplexes of 21-nucleotide RNAs mediate RNA interference in cultured mammalian cells. *Nature* 2001; **411**: 494–8.

38. Brummelkamp TR, Bornards R, Agami R. A system for stable expression of short interfering RNAs in mammalian cells. *Science* 2002; **296**: 550–3.

39. Beltinger C, Fulda S, Kammertoens T et al. Herpes simplex virus thymidine kinase/ganciclovir-induced apoptosis involves ligand-independent death receptor aggregation and activation of caspases. *Proc Natl Acad Sci, USA* 1999; **96**: 8699–704.

40. Hurwitz A, Finci-Yeheskel Z, Milwidsky A, Mayer M. Regulation of cyclooxygenase activity and progesterone production in the rat corpus luteum by inducible nitric oxide synthase. *Reproduction* 2002; **123**: 663–9.

41. Hurwitz MY, Marcus KT, Chevez-Barrios P et al. Suicide gene therapy for treatment of retinoblastoma in a murine model. *Hum Gene Ther* 1999; **10**: 441–8.

42. Hurwitz RL, Brenner MK, Poplack DG, Horowitz MC. Retinoblastoma treatment. *Science* 1999; **285**: 663–4.

43. Bartlett JS, Kleinschmidt J, Boucher RC, Samulski RJ. Targeted adeno-associated virus vector transduction of nonpermissive cells mediated by a bispecific F(ab′γ)2 antibody. *Nat Biotechnol* 1999; **17**: 181–6.

44. Girod A, Ried M, Wobus C et al. Genetic capsid modifications allow efficient re-targeting of adeno-associated virus type 2. *Nat Med* 1999; **5**: 1438.

45. Grill J, Van Beusechem VW, Van D et al. Combined targeting of adenoviruses to integrins and epidermal growth factor receptors increases gene transfer into primary glioma cells and spheroids. *Clin Cancer Res* 2001; **7**: 641–50.

46. Krasnykh V, Belousova N, Korokhov N et al. Genetic targeting of an adenovirus vector via replacement of the fiber protein with the phage T4 fibritin. *J Viro* 2001; **75**: 4176–83.

47. Russell SJ, Cosset FL. Modifying the host range properties of retroviral vectors. *J Gene Med* 1999; **1**: 300–11.

48. Curiel DT. The development of conditionally replicative adenoviruses for cancer therapy. *Clin Cancer Res* 2000; **6**: 3395–9.

49. Pizzato M, Marlow SA, Blair ED, Takeuchi Y. Initial binding of murine leukemia virus particles to cells does not require specific Env–receptor interaction. *J Virol* 1999; **73**: 8599–11.

50. Colombo MP, Ferrari G, Stoppacciaro A et al. Granulocyte colony-stimulating factor gene transfer suppresses tumorigenicity of a murine adenocarcinoma in vivo. *J Ex Med* 1991; **173**: 889–97.

51. Fearon ER, Pardoll DM, Itaya T et al. Interleukin–2 production by tumor cells bypasses T helper function in the generation of an antitumor response. *Cell* 1990; **60**: 397–403.

52. Golumbek PT, Lazenby AJ, Levitsky HI et al. Treatment of established renal cancer by tumor cells engineered to secrete interleukin–4. *Science* 1991; **254**: 713–16.

53. Tepper RI, Pattengale PK, Leder P. Murine interleukin–4 displays potent anti-tumor activity in vivo. *Cell* 1989; **57**: 503–12.

54. Dilloo D, Bacon K, Holden W et al. Combined chemokine and cytokine gene transfer enhances antitumor immunity. *Nat Med* 1996; **2**: 1090–5.

55. DeAngelo DJ, Dranoff G, Galinsky I et al. A phase I study of vaccination with lethally irradiated, autologous myeloblasts engineered by adenoviral-mediated gene transfer to secrete granulocyte–macrophage colony-stimulating factor. *Blood* 2001; **98**: 463a.

56. Nelson WG, Simons JW, Mikhak B et al. Cancer cells engineered to secrete granulocyte–macrophage colony-stimulating factor using ex vivo gene transfer as vaccines for the treatment of genitourinary malignancies. *Cancer Chemother Pharmacol* 2000; **46**(Suppl): S07–72.

57. Soiffer R, Lynch T, Mihm M et al. Vaccination with irradiated autologous melanoma cells engineered to secrete human granulocyte–macrophage colony-stimulating factor generates potent antitumor immunity in patients with metastatic melanoma. *Proc Natl Acad Sci, USA* 1998; **95**: 13141–6.

58. Asher AL, Mule JJ, Kasid A, Restifo NP et al. Murine tumor cells transduced with the gene for tumor necrosis factor-α. Evidence for paracrine immune effects of tumor necrosis factor against tumors. *J Immunol* 1991; **146**: 3227–34.

59. Hock H, Dorsch M, Diamantstein T, Blankenstein T. Interleukin 7 induces CD4+ T cell-dependent tumor rejection. *J Exp Med* 1991; **174**: 1291–8.

60. Watanabe Y, Kuribayashi K, Miyatake S et al. Exogenous expression of mouse interferon gamma cDNA in mouse neuroblastoma C1300 cells results in reduced tumorigenicity by augmented anti-tumor immunity. *Pro Natl Acad Sci, USA* 1989; **86**: 9456–60.

61. Leimig T, Foreman N, Rill D et al. Immunomodulatory effects of human neuroblastoma cells transduced with a retroviral vector encoding interleukin-2. *Cancer Gene Ther* 1994; **1**: 253–8.

62. Banchereau J, Steinman RM. Dendritic cells and the control of immunity. *Nature* 1998; **392**: 245–53.

63. Dilloo D, Brown M, Roskrow M et al. CD40 ligand induces an antileukemia immune response in vivo. *Blood* 1997; **90**: 1927–33.

64. Fujita N, Kagamu H, Yoshizawa H et al. CD40 ligand promotes priming of fully potent antitumor CD4+ T cells in draining lymph nodes in the presence of apoptotic tumor cells. *J Immunol* 2001; **167**: 5678–88.

65. Kato K, Cantwell MJ, Sharma S, Kipps TJ. Gene transfer of

CD40-ligand induces autologous immune recognition of chronic lymphocytic leukemia B cells. *J Clin Invest* 1998; **101**: 1133–41.

66. Van Kooten C, Banchereau J. CD40–CD40 ligand: a multifunctional receptor–ligand pair. *Adv Immunol* 1996; **61**: 1–77.

67. Guinan EC, Gribben JG, Boussiotis VA et al. Pivotal role of the B7:CD28 pathway in transplantation tolerance and tumor immunity. *Blood* 1994; **84**: 3261–82.

68. Ranheim EA, Kipps TJ. Activated T cells induce expression of B7/BB1 on normal or leukemic B cells through a CD40-dependent signal. *J Exp Med* 1993; **177**: 925–35.

69. Wulf GG, Wang RY, Kuehnle I et al. A leukemic stem cell with intrinsic drug efflux capacity in acute myeloid leukemia. *Blood* 2001; **98**: 1166–73.

70. Rousseau RF, Biagi E, Yvon ES et al. Treatment of high-risk acute leukemia with an autologous vaccine expressing transgenic IL-2 and CD40L. *Blood* 2003; **44**: 1919.

71. Biagi E, Yvon E, Dotti G et al. Bystander transfer of functional human CD40 ligand from gene-modified fibroblasts to B-chronic lymphocytic leukemia cells. *Hum Gene Ther* 2003; **14**: 545–59.

72. Luznik L, Slansky JE, Jalla S et al. Successful therapy of metastatic cancer using tumor vaccines in mixed allogeneic bone marrow chimeras. *Blood* 2003; **101**: 1645–52.

73. Raz E, Carson DA, Parker SE et al. Intradermal gene immunization: the possible role of DNA uptake in the induction of cellular immunity to viruses. *Proc Natl Acad Sci, USA* 1994; **91**: 9519–23.

74. Kim JJ, Yang JS, Lee DJ et al. Macrophage colony-stimulating factor can modulate immune responses and attract dendritic cells in vivo. *Hum Gene Ther* 2000; **11**: 305–21.

75. Ohashi T, Hanabuchi S, Kato H et al. Prevention of adult T-cell leukemia-like lymphoproliferative disease in rats by adoptively transferred T cells from a donor immunized with human T-cell leukemia virus type 1 Tax-coding DNA vaccine. *J Virol* 2000; **74**: 9610–16.

76. Syrengelas AD, Chen TT, Levy R. DNA immunization induces protective immunity against B-cell lymphoma. *Nat Med* 1996; **2**: 1038–41.

77. Krieg AM, Wagner H. Causing a commotion in the blood: immunotherapy progresses from bacteria to bacterial DNA. *Immunol Today* 2000; **21**: 521–6.

78. Granziero L, Krajewski S, Farness P et al. Adoptive immunotherapy prevents prostate cancer in a transgenic animal model. *Eur J Immunol* 1999; **29**: 1127–38.

79. Romieu R, Baratin M, Kayibanda M et al. Passive but not active CD8+ T cell-based immunotherapy interferes with liver tumor progression in a transgenic mouse model. *J Immunol* 1998; **161**: 5133–7.

80. Drobyski WR, Roth MS, Thibodeau SN, Gottschall JL. Molecular remission occurring after donor leukocyte infusions for the treatment of relapsed chronic myelogenous leukemia after allogeneic bone marrow transplantation. *Bone Marrow Transplant* 1992; **10**: 301–4.

81. Rooney CM, Smith CA, Ng CY et al. Use of gene-modified virus-specific T lymphocytes to control Epstein–Barr-virus-related lymphoproliferation. *Lancet* 1995; **345**: 9–13.

82. Brenner MK, Heslop HE. Graft-versus-host reactions and bone-marrow transplantation. *Curr Opin Immunol* 1991; **3**: 752–7.

83. Melief CJ, Kast WM. Potential immunogenicity of oncogene and tumor suppressor gene products. *Curr Opin Immunol* 1993; **5**: 709–13.

84. Heslop HE, Rooney CM. Adoptive cellular immunotherapy for EBV lymphoproliferative disease. *Immunol Rev* 1997; **157**: 217–22.

85. van der BP, Traversari C, Chomez P et al. A gene encoding an antigen recognized by cytolytic T lymphocytes on a human melanoma. *Science* 1991; **254**: 1643–7.

86. Gross G, Gorochov G, Waks T, Eshhar Z. Generation of effector T cells expressing chimeric T cell receptor with antibody type-specificity. *Transplant Proc* 1989; **21**: 127–30.

87. Irving BA, Weiss A. The cytoplasmic domain of the T cell receptor ζ chain is sufficient to couple to receptor-associated signal transduction pathways. *Cell* 1991; **64**: 891–901.

88. Altenschmidt U, Klundt E, Groner B. Adoptive transfer of in vitro-targeted, activated T lymphocytes results in total tumor regression. *Proc Natl Acad Sci, USA* 1997; **159**: 5509–15.

89. Kershaw MH, Darcy PK, Trapani JA, Smyth MJ. The use of chimeric human Fcε receptor I to redirect cytotoxic T lymphocytes to tumors. *J Leukoc Biol* 1996; **60**: 721–8.

90. Moritz D, Wels W, Mattern J, Groner B. Cytotoxic T lymphocytes with a grafted recognition specificity for ERBB2-expressing tumor cells. *Proc Natl Acad Sci, USA* 1994; **91**: 4318–22.

91. Walker RE, Bechtel CM, Natarajan V et al. Long-term in vivo survival of receptor-modified syngeneic T cells in patients with human immunodeficiency virus infection. *Blood* 2000; **96**: 467–74.

92. Anderson SJ, Levin SD, Perlmutter RM. Involvement of the protein tyrosine kinase p56lck in T cell signaling and thymocyte development. *Adv Immunol* 1994; **56**: 151–78.

93. Brocker T, Karjalainen K. Signals through T cell receptor-ζ chain alone are insufficient to prime resting T lymphocytes. *J Exp Med* 1995; **181**: 1653–9.

94. Finney HM, Lawson AD, Bebbington CR, Weir AN. Chimeric receptors providing both primary and costimulatory signaling in T cells from a single gene product. *J Immunol* 1998; **161**: 2791–7.

95. Maher J, Brentjens RJ, Gunset G et al. Human T-lymphocyte cytotoxicity and proliferation directed by a single chimeric TCR-ζ/CD28 receptor. *Nat Biotechnol* 2002; **20**: 70–5.

96. Geiger TL, Nguyen P, Leitenberg D, Flavell RA. Integrated src kinase and costimulatory activity enhances signal transduction through single-chain chimeric receptors in T lymphocytes. *Blood* 2001; **98**: 2364–71.

97. Kershaw MH, Westwood JA, Hwu P. Dual-specific T cells combine proliferation and antitumor activity. *Nat Biotechnol* 2002; **20**: 1221–7.

98. Rossig C, Bollard CM, Nuchtern JG et al. Epstein–Barr virus-specific human T lymphocytes expressing antitumor chimeric T-cell receptors: potential for improved immunotherapy. *Blood* 2002; **99**: 2009–16.

99. Brodie SJ, Patterson BK, Lewinsohn DA et al. HIV-specific cytotoxic T lymphocytes traffic to lymph nodes and localize at sites of HIV replication and cell death. *J Clin Invest* 2000; **105**: 1407–17.

100. Rosenberg SA, Aebersold P, Cornetta K et al. Gene transfer into humans – immunotherapy of patients with advanced melanoma, using tumor-infiltrating lymphocytes modified by retroviral gene transduction. *N Engl J Med* 1990; **323**: 570–8.

101. Rosenberg SA, Lotze MT, Yang JC et al. Experience with

the use of high-dose interleukin-2 in the treatment of 652 cancer patients. *Ann Surg* 1989; **210**: 474–84.

102. Liu K, Rosenberg SA. Transduction of an *IL-2* gene into human melanoma-reactive lymphocytes results in their continued growth in the absence of exogenous IL-2 and maintenance of specific antitumor activity. *J Immunol* 2001; **167**: 6356–65.

103. Eaton D, Gilham DE, O'Neill A, Hawkins RE. Retroviral transduction of human peripheral blood lymphocytes with Bcl-X$_L$ promotes in vitro lymphocyte survival in pro-apoptotic conditions. *Gene Ther* 2002; **9**: 527–35.

104. Gorelik L, Flavell RA. Immune-mediated eradication of tumors through the blockade of transforming growth factor-beta signaling in T cells. *Nat Med* 2001; **7**: 1118–22.

105. Bollard CM, Rossig C, Calonge MJ et al. Adapting a transforming growth factor beta-related tumor protection strategy to enhance antitumor immunity. *Blood* 2002; **99**: 3179–87.

106. Bonini C, Ferrari G, Verzeletti S et al. *HSV-TK* gene transfer into donor lymphocytes for control of allogeneic graft-versus-leukemia. *Science* 1997; **276**: 1719–24.

107. Tiberghien P, Ferrand C, Lioure B et al. Administration of herpes simplex-thymidine kinase-expressing donor T cells with a T-cell-depleted allogeneic marrow graft. *Blood* 2001; **97**: 63–72.

108. Riddell SR, Elliott M, Lewinsohn DA et al. T-cell mediated rejection of gene-modified HIV-specific cytotoxic T lymphocytes in HIV-infected patients. *Nat Med* 1996; **2**: 216–23.

109. Clackson T, Yang W, Rozamus LW et al. Redesigning an FKBP-ligand interface to generate chemical dimerizers with novel specificity. *Proc Natl Acad Sci, USA* 1998; **95**: 10437–42.

110. Thomis DC, Marktel S, Bonini C et al. A Fas-based suicide switch in human T cells for the treatment of graft-versus-host disease. *Blood* 2001; **97**: 1249–57.

111. Iuliucci JD, Oliver SD, Morley S et al. Intravenous safety and pharmacokinetics of a novel dimerizer drug, AP1903, in healthy volunteers. *J Clin Pharmacol* 2001; **41**: 870–9.

112. Introna M, Barbui AM, Bambacioni F et al. Genetic modification of human T cells with CD20: a strategy to purify and lyse transduced cells with anti-CD20 antibodies. *Hum Gene Ther* 2000; **11**: 611–20.

113. Klump H, Schiedlmeier B, Vogt B et al. Retroviral vector-mediated expression of HoxB4 in hematopoietic cells using a novel coexpression strategy. *Gene Ther* 2001; **8**: 811–17.

114. Levin L, Hryniuk WM. Dose intensity analysis of chemotherapy regimens in ovarian carcinoma. *J Clin Oncol* 1987; **5**: 756–67.

115. Levin L, Simon R, Hryniuk W. Importance of multiagent chemotherapy regimens in ovarian carcinoma: dose intensity analysis. *J Natl Cancer Inst* 1993; **85**: 1732–42.

116. Murphy D, Crowther D, Renninson J et al. A randomised dose intensity study in ovarian carcinoma comparing chemotherapy given at four week intervals for six cycles with half dose chemotherapy given for twelve cycles. *Ann Oncol* 1993; **4**: 377–83.

117. Pastan I, Gottesman MM. Multidrug resistance. *Annu Rev Med* 1991; **42**: 277–86.

118. Mickisch GH, Licht T, Merlino GT et al. Chemotherapy and chemosensitization of transgenic mice which express the human multidrug resistance gene in bone marrow: efficacy, potency, and toxicity. *Cancer Res* 1991; **51**: 5417–24.

119. Mickisch GH, Merlino GT, Galski H et al. Transgenic mice that express the human multidrug-resistance gene in bone marrow enable a rapid identification of agents that reverse drug resistance. *Proc Natl Acad Sci, USA* 1991; **88**: 547–51.

120. Moritz T, Mackay W, Feng IJ. Gene transfer of O-6-methylguanine methyltransferase (MGMT) protects hematopoietic cells from nitrosourea (NU) induced toxicity in vitro and in vivo. *Blood* 1993; **81**(Suppl): 18a.

121. Moscow JA, Huang H, Carter C et al. Engraftment of MDR1 and NeoR gene-transduced hematopoietic cells after breast cancer chemotherapy. *Blood* 1999; **94**: 52–61.

122. Appelbaum FR, Buckner CD. Overview of the clinical relevance of autologous bone marrow transplantation. *Clin Haematol* 1986; **15**: 1–18.

123. Burnett AK, Tansey P, Watkins R et al. Transplantation of unpurged autologous bone-marrow in acute myeloid leukaemia in first remission. *Lancet* 1984; **2**: 1068–70.

124. Goldstone AH, Anderson CC, Linch DC et al. Autologous bone marrow transplantation following high dose chemotherapy for the treatment of adult patients with acute myeloid leukaemia. *Br J Haematol* 1986; **64**: 529–37.

125. Shpall EJ, Jones RB. Release of tumor cells from bone marrow. *Blood* 1994; **83**: 623–5.

126. Brugger W, Bross KJ, Glatt M et al. Mobilization of tumor cells and hematopoietic progenitor cells into peripheral blood of patients with solid tumors. *Blood* 1994; **83**: 636–40.

127. Rill DR, Santana VM, Roberts WM et al. Direct demonstration that autologous bone marrow transplantation for solid tumors can return a multiplicity of tumorigenic cells. *Blood* 1994; **84**: 380–3.

128. De Fabritiis P, Ferrero D, Sandrelli A et al. Monoclonal antibody purging and autologous bone marrow transplantation in acute myelogenous leukemia in complete remission. *Bone Marrow Transplant* 1989; **4**: 669–74.

129. Gambacorti-Passerini C, Rivoltini L, Fizzotti M et al. Selective purging by human interleukin-2 activated lymphocytes of bone marrows contaminated with a lymphoma line or autologous leukaemic cells. *Br J Haematol* 1991; **78**: 197–205.

130. Gorin NC, Aegerter P, Auvert B et al. Autologous bone marrow transplantation for acute myelocytic leukemia in first remission: a European survey of the role of marrow purging. *Blood* 1990; **75**: 1606–14.

131. Santos GW, Yeager AM, Jones RJ. Autologous bone marrow transplantation. *Annu Rev Med* 1989; **40**: 99–112.

132. Gribben JG, Freedman AS, Neuberg D et al. Immunologic purging of marrow assessed by PCR before autologous bone marrow transplantation for B-cell lymphoma. *N Engl J Med* 1991; **325**: 1525–33.

133. Brenner M, Krance R, Heslop HE et al. Assessment of the efficacy of purging by using gene marked autologous marrow transplantation for children with AML in first complete remission. *Hum Gene Ther* 1994; **5**: 481–99.

134. Cai Q, Rubin JT, Lotze MT. Genetically marking human cells – results of the first clinical gene transfer studies. *Cancer Gene Ther* 1995; **2**: 125–36.

135. Cornetta K, Tricot G, Broun ER et al. Retroviral-mediated gene transfer of bone marrow cells during autologous bone marrow transplantation for acute leukemia. *Hum Gene Ther* 1992; **3**: 305–18.

136. Deisseroth AB, Kantarjian H, Talpaz M et al. Autologous bone marrow transplantation for CML in which retroviral

markers are used to discriminate between relapse which arises from systemic disease remaining after preparative therapy versus relapse due to residual leukemia cells in autologous marrow: a pilot trial. *Br J Haematol* 1991; **2**: 359–76.

137. Santana VM, Brenner MK, Ihle J et al. A phase I trial of high-dose carboplatin and etoposide with autologous marrow support for treatment of stage D neuroblastoma in first remission: use of marker genes to investigate the biology of marrow reconstitution and the mechanism of relapse. *Cancer* 1991; **3**: 257–72.

138. Rill DR, Smith SS. Long-term in vivo fate of human hemopoietic cells transduced by Moloney-based retroviral vectors. *Blood* 2002; **84**: 96.

139. Dunbar CE, Bodine DM, Sorrentino B et al. Gene transfer into hematopoietic cells. Implications for cancer therapy. *Ann N Y Acad Sci* 1994; **716**: 216–24.

140. Dunbar CE, Cottler-Fox M, O'Shaughnessy JA et al. Retrovirally marked CD34-enriched peripheral blood and bone marrow cells contribute to long-term engraftment after autologous transplantation. *Blood* 1995; **85**: 3048–57.

141. Brenner MK, Rill DR, Heslop HE et al. Gene marking after bone marrow transplantation. *Eur J Cancer* 1994; **30A**: 1171–6.

142. Rooney CM, Smith CA, Ng CYC et al. Infusion of cytotoxic T cells for the prevention and treatment of Epstein–Barr virus-induced lymphoma in allogeneic transplant recipients. *Blood* 1998; **92**: 1549–55.

143. Roskrow MA, Rooney CM, Heslop HE et al. Administration of neomycin resistance gene marked EBV specific cytotoxic T-lymphocytes to patients with relapsed EBV-positive Hodgkin disease. *Hum Gene Ther* 1998; **9**: 1237–50.

144. Schmidt M, Hoffmann G, Wissler M et al. Detection and direct genomic sequencing of multiple rare unknown flanking DNA in highly complex samples. *Hum Gene Ther* 2001; **12**: 743–9.

145. Vanin EF, Kaloss M, Broscius C, Nienhuis AW. Characterization of replication-competent retroviruses from nonhuman primates with virus-induced T-cell lymphomas and observations regarding the mechanism of oncogenesis. *J Virol* 1994; **68**: 4241–50.

146. Hacein-Bey-Abina S, Le Deist F, Carlier F et al. Sustained correction of X-linked severe combined immunodeficiency by ex vivo gene therapy. *N Engl J Med* 2002; **346**: 1185–93.

147. Li Z, Dullmann J, Schiedlmeier B et al. Murine leukemia induced by retroviral gene marking. *Science* 2002; **296**: 497.

# 29 Allogeneic stem cell transplantation

Richard J O'Reilly, Esperanza B Papadopoulos, Trudy N Small, and
Stephen Mackinnon

## Introduction

Bone marrow transplantation (BMT) from a human leukocyte antigen (HLA)-matched sibling is considered the treatment of choice for patients with acute myeloid leukemia (AML)[1] or acute lymphoblastic leukemia (ALL)[2] at high risk for relapse in first remission and for all patients with acute leukemia in second or greater remission, aplastic anemia,[3] myelodysplastic syndromes (MDS; reviewed in reference 4), and several lethal forms of immunodeficiency, such as Wiskott–Aldrich syndrome and severe combined immunodeficiency (SCID; reviewed in reference 5). For selected patients with chronic myeloid leukemia (CML),[6] non-Hodgkin lymphoma (NHL),[7] or Hodgkin's disease,[8] as well as those with hemoglobinopathies, particularly β-thalassemia (reviewed in reference 9), allogeneic BMT may offer a considerable advantage over other forms of treatment.

Over the last 20 years, tremendous progress has been made in our understanding of the human histocompatibility gene complex and the cellular mechanisms giving rise to graft rejection and graft-versus-host (GVH) disease (GVHD). This has resulted in more precise HLA typing that has improved selection of potential unrelated donors, and has led to the emergence of more effective strategies to ensure engraftment and to prevent or ameliorate GVHD. Marked progress has also been made in supportive care measures and in the treatment and prevention of opportunistic infections following BMT. In this chapter, we shall describe the clinical features of allogeneic marrow grafts, focusing on the biologic and therapeutic determinants of a successful transplant at each of the different stages of its development. We shall also delineate the genetic and cellular characteristics of the graft and host that affect outcome. We shall then review recent advances in transplantation medicine and their impact on the results of allogeneic hematopoietic stem cell transplants applied to the treatment of hematopoietic malignancies.

## Clinical and biological characteristics of allogeneic BMT applied to the treatment of hematological neoplasia

### Identification of donors suitable for allogeneic BMT – the HLA gene complex: the major determinant of histocompatibility in human BMT

Experimental murine models demonstrating the relevance of matching for the major histocompatibility complex (MHC) to the prevention of lethal GVHD[10] paved the way for the initial successful applications of HLA-matched marrow grafts in humans.[11,12] The major histocompatibility region in humans, located on the short arm of chromosome 6, encodes a series of genes, each exhibiting an extensive degree of allelic polymorphism (Figure 29.1).[13] This complex is divided into:[13,14]

- class I genes (HLA-A, -B, and -C), encoding proteins expressed on the surface of all nucleated cells;
- class II genes (HLA-DR, -DQ, and -DP), encoding surface proteins on a more limited number of cell types, such as early hematopoietic cells, tissue macrophages, circulating monocytes, dendritic cells, endothelial cells, B cells, and activated T cells;
- class III genes, encoding other functional proteins, such as the complement proteins C2 and C4.

The HLA genes are codominantly expressed. Within a family, identification of parental haplotypes inherited by each sibling can usually be ascertained by serologic typing of HLA-A, -B, -C, and -DR determinants of a patient, siblings, and parents. Classically, histocompatibility within the HLA-D region can be defined by mutual unresponsiveness in mixed lymphocyte culture (MLC).[15] Parental HLA haplotypes are usually inherited en bloc, giving rise to a 1-in-4 likelihood

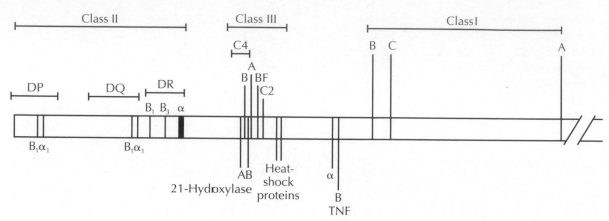

**Figure 29.1** Map of expressed genes of the HLA region on the short arm of chromosome 6.

that any two siblings will be genotypically HLA-matched. Because there are often more than two children in a sibship, HLA-identical siblings can usually be identified for 35–40% of individuals. For an additional 5% of patients, a phenotypic match or a partially HLA-mismatched family donor can be found.

An HLA-compatible unrelated donor can also be identified for a proportion of patients by searching among HLA-typed volunteer marrow donors participating in large registries. The combined pool of these registries now includes over 8 million volunteer donors. Currently, these registries can identify HLA-compatible unrelated donors for the majority of patients of European Caucasian ancestry, particularly patients inheriting common HLA-A, -B, and -DR haplotypes.[16,17] Unfortunately, because the number of volunteers derived from ethnic minorities is still limited, the proportion of successful searches for patients in these minority groups is much lower.

Despite serologic matching for HLA-A, -B, and -DR, the incidence of graft rejection and severe GVHD following a serologically matched unrelated BMT is significantly higher than that observed following an HLA-matched sibling BMT.[17,18] Based on these findings, several groups have been examining whether and to what degree unrelated serologically HLA-matched donor–recipient pairs are actually matched at the molecular level. More recently, molecular tissue typing of donor and recipient DNA by PCR-based techniques has generally been adopted. These sequence-based typing methods include single-strand conformational polymorphisms (SSCP) and sequence-specific oligonucleotide probes (SSOP).[19] These methodologies have allowed us to distinguish multiple molecular variants of many serologically defined alleles within of both HLA class I and class II. Reference strand-mediated conformation analysis (RSCA) is a novel conformational method that offers high resolution and high sample throughput for typing the HLA class I and class II genes. This technique differs from conventional sequence based typing methodologies in that the HLA type is assigned on the

basis of accurate measurement of conformation-dependent DNA mobility in polyacrylamide gel electrophoresis (PAGE). RSCA has been successfully applied in blind studies of HLA typing, demonstrating that it is reproducible, able to identify new alleles, and able to resolve ambiguous heterozygous combinations.[20] Several of these microvariants can also be distinguished in vitro by cloned alloreactive T cells. T cells reactive against certain microvariants, such as microvariants of HLA-B44, have been implicated as effectors of marrow allograft rejection[21] and GVHD.[22] One or more microvariant disparities between patients and potential unrelated donors serologically matched for HLA class I alleles have been detected in 30–48% of cases in different series.[23,24] Studies of the clinical relevance of these disparities to graft rejection and GVHD are now being conducted,[16,21] and will be discussed later in this chapter.

## Minor alloantigen systems contributing to graft rejection and GVHD following BMT in humans

Although the proteins encoded by the HLA gene complex are the major determinants of histocompatibility in humans, other alloantigens affect the engraftment of a hematopoietic stem cell graft in non-syngeneic hosts and the reactivity of donor lymphoid cells against the transplant recipient. Despite the use of aggressive pretransplant immunosuppression and post-transplant GVHD prophylaxis, marrow transplants from HLA genotypically identical siblings are still associated with a significant risk of graft rejection and GVHD (see below). These clinical manifestations of alloreactivity have been ascribed to the ability of host or donor T cells to react against minor alloantigens unique to the hematopoietic cells of the donor graft or host tissues, respectively. Several polymorphic minor alloantigenic systems, such as the MLS, H-Y, and QA-1 alloantigens, have been identified as potential targets of allointeractions in murine models.[25,26]

Although there have been reports linking the emergence of host-type minor alloantigen-reactive,

HLA-restricted T cells capable of inhibiting clonigenic donor hematopoietic cell growth with graft rejection and GVHD,[27,28] the minor alloantigens actually targeted during human marrow allograft rejections or GVHD remain poorly defined. One minor alloantigen, H-Y, which is encoded by the human Y chromosome, is expressed on male hematopoietic cells, and can be a target for cytotoxic T cells.[29–31] The increased risk of graft rejection in women transplanted with marrow from male donors and the increased likelihood of GVHD following transplantation of males with bone marrow derived from females have been hypothesized to be due to in vivo responses to the H-Y alloantigen.[32–35] An H-Y peptide epitope presented by HLA-A2, -A1, -B7, and -B60 has been isolated and sequenced. This nonameric peptide, FIDSYICQV, is encoded by a gene that maps to the centromeric portion of the Y chromosome.[36,37] HLA-A2-restricted H-Y-specific T cells have been implicated in the pathogenesis of marrow graft rejection.[38] Intriguingly, however, one large series has failed to implicate H-Y-specific responses in GVHD developing in HLA-matched male recipients of female sibling marrow bearing the appropriate HLA-restricting elements HLA-A2 or HLA-A1.[39]

Other human minor alloantigens encoded by autosomal genes have also been identified. Goulmy and coworkers[29,40] have generated T-cell clones from marrow allograft recipients that are HLA-restricted and recognize at least five antigens on hematopoietic cells (HA-1 to HA-5). These antigens appear to be the products of non-allelic genes that segregate in a Mendelian mode of inheritance. HA-1, HA-2, and HA-5 are expressed only by cells derived from the hematopoietic system, while HA-3 and HA-4 are expressed on a wider array of cell types.[40,41] Differences within HA-1 have been implicated in GVHD.[39]

The nature of the minor HA alloantigens targeted was completely unknown until 1995, when den Haan et al[42] succeeded in acid-eluting and isolating the HA-2 peptide antigen from its HLA-restricting element by reverse-phase high-performance liquid chromatography (HPLC). To distinguish the relevant peptide antigen, target cells with the same HLA-restricting element were pulsed with isolated peptides and exposed to HA-2 minor alloantigen-specific cytolytic T cells. Thereafter, the peptide was sequenced. The amino acid sequence of HA-2 revealed that this antigen belongs to the non-filamentous class I myosin family of proteins, which contribute to cell locomotion. Studies are currently underway to determine whether this protein displays allelic polymorphisms. More recently, the HA-1 minor alloantigen has also been isolated and sequenced. Interestingly, this antigen appears to have two different alleles that can be distinguished by HLA-restricted T cells.[43] Ultimately, typing for these alleles may improve the selection of donors comparably matched for their HLA determinants.

## Biologic and therapeutic determinants of engraftment

### Pretransplant immunosuppression and myeloablation

Allogeneic hematopoietic and lymphoid cell grafts are more susceptible to growth inhibition or rejection by host resistance systems than grafts of solid organs such as the kidney. As a consequence, durable engraftment and expansion of allogeneic marrow cells can only be achieved if the host's immune system is ablated. Only patients with SCID are sufficiently immunocompromised to permit consistent engraftment of unmanipulated HLA-matched marrow grafts without preparative treatment with immunosuppressive drugs. Although the preparative regimens utilized for patients with leukemia are largely designed to eliminate leukemic clones, they must also be sufficiently immunosuppressive and myeloablative to ensure engraftment of transplanted allogeneic hematopoietic cells. Initially, total-body irradiation (TBI) administered in a single dose of 10 Gy combined with cyclophosphamide was used for this purpose.[44] However, in the last 15 years, other cytoreduction regimens have been introduced that incorporate larger doses of fractionated TBI[45] and other chemotherapeutic agents such as etoposide,[46,47] cytarabine,[48,49] melphalan,[50] thiotepa[51–53] and fludarabine.[54] High-dose busulfan combined with cyclophosphamide has also been utilized to avoid the use of TBI.[55]

The concept that engraftment of hematopoietic cells can only be achieved if ablative doses of drugs are administered prior to transplant has been effectively challenged by durable engraftment with persistent mixed or full donor chimerism after less intensive, non-myelablative chemotherapeutic regimens. Such sublethal, non-ablative regimens may ultimately significantly extend the application of allogeneic stem cell transplants, permitting the transplantation of older patients, patients with more chronically debilitating hematopoietic malignancies such as myeloma, and patients with genetic disorders such as Fanconi anemia,[56] who tolerate current high-dose alkylating agent-based preparative regimens poorly. However, clinical trials with longer follow-up are still needed to adequately assess the potential of these promising approaches to induce durable engraftment and long-term eradications of the patient's underlying malignancy.

### Sources of allogeneic hematopoietic cells for transplantation

Until relatively recently, allogeneic transplants have almost exclusively used the donor's marrow as the source of hematopoietic stem cells. In the last 5–10 years, granulocyte colony-stimulating factor (G-CSF)-mobilized peripheral blood stem cells

(PBSC), which have been shown to be enriched for CD34+ primitive progenitors,[57–59] and umbilical cord blood cells derived from normal HLA-matched related or unrelated donors have been increasingly used as sources of hematopoietic progenitors for transplantation. Experience with allogeneic cord blood transplants will be summarized in a later section of this chapter. However, since many centers are now beginning to use donor PBSC instead of bone marrow, current estimates of the advantages and potential disadvantages of PBSC transplants (PBSCT) in comparison with BMT need to be briefly summarized. The potential advantages of G-CSF-stimulated PBSC are several. First, they can provide doses of CD34+ progenitors that are four- to fivefold higher than those contained in a marrow allograft.[58,59] This increased dose of progenitor cells facilitates engraftment. Furthermore, as noted above, PBSCT may contain tenfold more T cells than a marrow graft. These additional donor T cells may be associated with potentially good and harmful effects, namely ehhanced antileukemic effect and an increased incidence of GVHD. Lastly, at any given dose of progenitor cells, G-CSF-stimulated PBSC induce a somewhat more rapid reconstitution of platelet counts, and a comparably rapid recovery of neutrophil counts in the post-transplant period.[58–61]

The results of several randomized trials addressing the issues of acute and chronic GVHD, relapse, and survival have now been reported.[62–68] With the exception of the European Group for Blood and Marrow Transplantation (EBMT) trial,[63] among the studies listed, the cumulative incidence of acute GVHD was found to be statistically no different whether using PBSC or bone marrow stem cells. Interestingly, the EBMT study (the largest prospective trial) is also the only study using three doses of post-transplant methotrexate as opposed to the customary four doses given for acute GVHD prophylaxis. The probability of chronic GVHD developing has varied by report; four studies showed a significantly higher probability of chronic GVHD after allogeneic PBSCT than after allogeneic BMT. This includes a retrospective registry analysis of 824 patients who underwent allotransplantation.[69] In contrast, the other studies do not show a statistically significant difference. These studies showed, with one exception,[66] no obvious difference in the relapse rates between allogeneic PBSCT and BMT. Patients with low-risk disease had similar rates of disease-free survival irrespective of the stem cell source. On the other hand, two of the larger randomized trials[64,67] show a significant difference in overall survival favoring PBSCT, largely because of lower transplant-related mortality in patients with advanced-stage disease. There are also data indicating that recipients of allogeneic PBSCT have faster immune reconstitution than recipients of BMT.[70]

In summary, PBSC grafts may improve disease free survival in patients with advanced disease but may only lead to more chronic GVHD in patients with standard-risk disease without improving survival.

## The pre-engraftment period

Following infusion of the stem cell allograft, the hematopoietic progenitor cells migrate to the bone marrow and spleen. Marrow cellularity begins to recover 10–14 days following a transplant, and, by 10–21 days post grafting, neutrophils of donor origin can be detected in the circulation. Prior to this time, patients are profoundly pancytopenic and require intensive support with platelet and red cell transfusions as well as broad-spectrum antimicrobial therapy for presumed or documented infections. All blood products, including fresh frozen plasma (FFP), infused to support transplant recipients must be irradiated, since they contain allogeneic lymphocytes capable of inducing lethal third-party GVHD.[71]

Prior to neutrophil engraftment, patients are susceptible to both bacterial and fungal infections. The risk of neutropenic sepsis is increased by the toxicity of the conditioning regimen, which may be further exacerbated by methotrexate given to prevent GVHD. This can cause breakdown of the normal epithelial barriers to infection in the mouth and gut. Additionally, the use of tunneled central intravenous lines often leads to infections with gram-positive bacteria from the skin. Viral infections common during this period of neutropenia and lymphopenia principally include recurrences of herpes simplex virus (HSV) types 1 and 2.[72] These infections may cause significant morbidity. Herpes zoster infections may occur at any time in the post-transplant period, resulting in a cumulative risk of reactivation of herpes zoster in the first 2–3 years post transplant that can be as high as 50%.[73] Human herpes virus 6 (HHV6) may also be activated in this period, and has been implicated as a cause of marrow suppression, graft failure, pneumonitis and encephalitis.[74–76] The BK papovavirus is another virus that commonly reactivates during the post-transplant period. It has been implicated in the pathogenesis of encephalitis/encephalopathy, hepatitis, and, more commonly, hemorrhagic cystitis.[77–79] Severe enteritis in the early transplant period may be caused by rotavirus and adenovirus.[80,81] Adenovirus may also cause severe pneumonia, hepatitis, and hemorrhagic cystitis.[82,83]

Multiple strategies have been developed to decrease the incidence, morbidity, and mortality of these post-transplant infections. Prophylaxis with fluconazole or itraconazole has also been associated with reduced systemic fungal infections.[84–86] Lipid-based formulations of amphotericin have been used in the treatment of systemic fungal infections, with less renal toxicity.[87,88] Acyclovir prophylaxis reduces the incidence of genital and labial herpes simplex infections as well as herpes zoster infections.[89,90]

Some patients may develop clinical signs and symptoms of hepatic veno-occlusive disease (VOD). These include hepatomegaly, massive ascites, and jaundice.[91–93] This disorder is caused by damage to the endothelial lining of the hepatic sinusoids, which induces edema and obstruction to the flow of blood through hepatic capillaries and venules. This process may be mild, moderate, or severe.

Certain chemotherapeutic agents also have unique early side-effects requiring careful monitoring and prophylaxis. Cyclophosphamide can cause a cardiomyopathy resulting in decreased cardiac output, particularly in patients who have previously received high doses of anthracyclines or other cardiotoxic agents.[94,95] Cyclophosphamide can also induce mild to severe hemorrhagic cystitis, a complication that may be prevented by hydration sufficient to sustain a brisk diuresis or continuous direct bladder irrigation for patients who cannot tolerate high doses of parenteral fluids. Mesna may also be used to prevent this complication.[96–99] High-dose busulfan has been associated with neurotoxicity, including seizures, which can generally be prevented with phenytoin. Busulfan, melphalan, thiotepa, and TBI can cause injury to the pulmonary microvasculature, resulting in interstitial infiltrates and/or diffuse hemorrhages.[100] High-dose cytarabine can cause severe conjunctivitis, which is generally preventable with topical steroids.[101] Less frequently, this agent can cause cerebellar toxicity.

### Factors affecting engraftment and reconstitution of hematopoietic function

Engraftment post transplant is heralded by the development of donor-derived myeloid and erythroid progenitors in the marrow and the emergence of neutrophils in the blood, generally 10–21 days post transplant. Engraftment of donor hematopoietic and lymphoid cells can be ascertained by several techniques, including conventional cytogenetics,[102] detection of donor-specific restriction fragment length polymorphisms (RFLP),[103] or minisatellite allelic polymorphisms or, in sex-mismatched pairs, detection of X and Y probes using fluorescence in situ hybridization (FISH) techniques.[104] Persistent thrombocytopenia and leukopenia often complicate intercurrent infections due to viruses, such as cytomegalovirus (CMV)[105] and HHV6, as well as GVHD.[106]

Graft failure following allogeneic BMT is empirically defined either as a failure to develop donor marrow function or as marrow aplasia that occurs following initial hematologic reconstitution. Graft failure associated with immune rejection is also documented by the loss of donor lymphoid and hematopoietic cells in the bone marrow and circulation. Most graft failures occur within the first 2 months post transplant, but graft failures as late as 4–5 months post transplant have been reported.

The pre-BMT cytoreductive regimen utilized, the type of transplant administered, and the degree of HLA disparity between donor and host each contribute to the incidence of graft failure. For example, the incidence of graft failure following a transplant of unmodified marrow for aplastic anemia varies from 5% to 30%, depending on the patient's prior transfusion history, if conditioning with cyclophosphamide alone is utilized.[34,107,108] If, however, antithymocyte globulin (ATG) or total lymphoid irradiation are added to the conditioning regimen, consistent engraftment is observed.[3,109,110] Similarly, while unmodified marrow grafts from HLA-matched siblings administered to patients with leukemia cytoreduced with TBI and cyclophosphamide[17,111] are rarely associated with graft failure, unmodified grafts from HLA-disparate donors may fail as a result of graft rejection in a significant proportion of cases. Rates of 6–28% have been reported in similarly treated patients when HLA-disparate donors have been used. The risk of graft failure is increased in proportion to the number and type of HLA allodisparities unique to the donor.[112,113] Depletion of T cells from a marrow allograft renders the graft more susceptible to graft failure and rejection, even if the donor is an HLA-matched sibling.[40,148,149] Graft failure rates as high as 10–30% and 40–50% have been reported in leukemic recipients of T-cell-depleted HLA-matched[33,114–116] or two- to three-antigen-mismatched grafts[171], respectively.

Identification of the processes contributing to graft rejection and failure has spawned the development of increasingly effective strategies for their reversal or prevention. Principal among these has been the development of tolerable yet more immunosuppressive preparative regimens to eliminate residual host T cells. Examples are intensifications of standard preparative protocols to include additional immunosuppressive drugs such as cytarabine,[118] thiotepa,[49] and fludarabine,[56] and treatment of the host (either prior to or following the transplant) with T-cell-depleting monoclonal or hetero antibodies such as OKT3, Campath-1, and ATG.[33]

### Acute and chronic GVHD

GVHD is a pathologic process induced by engrafted immunocompetent donor T cells reacting against alloantigens expressed on host cells. The main targets of this reaction are cells originating from the host's lymphohematopoietic system.[119] Host dendritic cells appear to be the most potent stimulants of this reaction.[120] Indeed, recent studies in murine models suggest that functional host dendritic cells are essential for the stimulation and initiation of GVHD by alloreactive donor T cells in vivo.[121] In response to host alloantigens, donor T cells divide and mature into cytotoxic and helper T cells, which can either directly injure targeted host cells or recruit other cells, such as natural killer (NK) cells and monocytes, to kill host cells.[122,123] Indeed, such donor T cells specifically reactive against host unique HLA microvariant alleles or against host minor alloantigens have been isolated from the blood and affected tissues of patients suffering from acute GVHD.[22,39] These activated donor T cells also produce cytokines such as tumor necrosis factor α (TNF-α), which may further contribute to the observed pathology.[124,125]

Over the past 15 years, the specific types of T cells capable of initiating potentially lethal acute GVH reactions have been extensively characterized. In lethally irradiated mice transplanted with marrow and spleen cells from MHC-disparate donors, either CD8+ or CD4+ T cells may induce lethal GVHD, depending on whether the MHC disparity unique to the host is an MHC class I or class II determinant.[126,127] In mice bearing multiple MHC disparities and in outbred species, such as humans, however, depletion of all T-cell subsets is required to prevent GVHD. Selective depletion of CD4+ or CD8+ T cells alone is ineffective.[127,128] On the other hand, in murine models, when donor and recipient are H-2-matched but differ for one or more minor alloantigens, depletion of CD8+ T cells from the marrow and spleen cell graft may prevent GVHD.[129] In clinical trials, the incidence and severity of GVHD have also been reduced, but not eliminated, in HLA-matched sibling recipients of CD8+ T-cell-depleted marrow grafts administered with cyclosporine and methotrexate prophylaxis post transplant.[130]

The main manifestations of acute GVHD are an erythematous maculopapular skin rash, which may be focal or diffuse, hepatitis, enteritis, and delayed hematopoietic and lymphoid reconstitution.[131–133] The incidence and severity of acute GVHD are principally related to the type and the degree of allodisparity existing between donor and host.[5] GVHD is also strongly influenced by host factors such as patient age and sex, intensity of the preparative cytoreduction, presence or absence of concurrent infection, and type of resident microflora, as well as donor features such as gender, previous sensitization to host minor alloantigens by pregnancy, and the number of T cells contained in the marrow allograft.[32,134,135]

Chronic GVHD is a complex disorder, pathologically distinct from acute GVHD. Although chronic GVHD often develops in patients with antecedent acute GVHD, it may occur de novo late (conventionally defined as later than 100 days) after transplantation, particularly in association with tapering or discontinuation of immunosuppressive drug therapy. Chronic GVHD presents with localized or diffuse sclerotic changes of the skin, with hypo- and hyperpigmentation, focal lichen planus lesions, and, in severe cases, recurrent, superficial skin ulcerations, debilitating scars, and joint contractures. Systemic manifestations may include xerostomia, xerophthalmia, biliary cirrhosis, malabsorption, and failure to gain weight.[136] A minority of patients with chronic GVHD develop an obliterative bronchiolitis, which may result in chronic obstructive pulmonary disease and death due to respiratory failure or intercurrent pneumonia.[137]

Chronic GVHD also results in impaired hematopoiesis and delayed immune reconstitution. Persistent thrombocytopenia in patients with GVHD is associated with a very poor prognosis.[138] Prolonged humoral immunodeficiencies, including IgA, IgG2, and IgG4 subtype deficiencies, render these patients highly susceptible to recurrent pyogenic infections caused by *Streptococcus pneumoniae, Haemophilus influenzae* and other encapsulated organisms, similar to those observed in individuals with congenital agammaglobulinemia.[139,140]

Experimental findings suggest that chronic GVHD may be due to ineffectively controlled immunosuppressive and potentially autoreactive T-cell clones, potentially generated in response to populations of host-reactive donor T cells participating in acute GVHD reactions.

As will be discussed subsequently, multiple strategies have been utilized to prevent acute GVHD. However, even when drug prophylaxis with low-dose methotrexate and cyclosporine has been used, 30–50% of patients transplanted with unmodified HLA-identical sibling BMT have developed grade II–IV acute GVHD, requiring systemic immunosuppression with high doses of glucocorticoids.[141,142] Responses to steroid treatment, including stabilization and improvement of the skin rash and the hepatic and gastrointestinal abnormalities, are usually detected within 5–7 days of starting treatment. However, for patients with severe (grade III–IV) GVHD or moderate (grade II) GVHD that is refractory to steroid treatment,[142] prognosis is poor. Additional treatment with ATG, CD3-specific immunotoxins, or other T-cell-specific monoclonal antibodies can often result in complete or partial resolution of the skin manifestations of GVHD, but these agents are less effective in abrogating GVH-induced hepatic and gastrointestinal dysfunction.[143–145] These secondary therapies for steroid-refractory GVHD may also be relatively toxic, and commonly intensify the host's susceptibility to secondary infection.[143,144] Unfortunately, the majority of patients with steroid-refractory GVHD, unresponsive to these second-line therapies, will ultimately succumb to sequelae of GVHD or associated infections, particularly CMV-induced interstitial pneumonia, aspergillosis, and bacterial sepsis.[142,146,147]

Although chronic GVHD is reversible in a significant proportion of patients, responses must be measured over months to years. Without systemic immunosuppression, less than 25% of patients have survived over 18 months.[146,147] Prolonged treatment with prednisone coupled with azathioprine or cyclosporine can induce slow reversal in up to 76% of cases.[146,147] In addition, treatment with methoxypsoralen and ultraviolet irradiation may reverse the skin changes associated with chronic GVHD.[148] In steroid-refractory cases, treatments with other immunosuppressive agents, including clofazimine,[149] low-dose total lymphoid irradiation,[150] mycophenolic acid,[151] and thalidomide,[152] have been proposed, based on promising results in small reported series. Rates of responses described for these agents range from 10% to 55%. Other strategies, including the use of extracorporeal photopheresis, are also being explored.[153] The ultimate effectiveness of any or all of these second-line therapies is still in question. Indeed, in one prospective randomized trial, patients with acute GVHD treated with thalidomide to prevent chronic GVHD actually fared less well than those treated with a placebo.[154]

### Prevention of GVHD by prophylactic use of drugs or antibodies post transplantation

The excessive morbidity and mortality associated with severe GVHD, particularly in recipients of unrelated or HLA-non-identical related marrow transplants, as well as older adults even after HLA-matched sibling transplants, continuously underscore the need for more effective methods for preventing GVHD or abrogating its severity. In view of the essential role of donor T cells in the initiation of GVHD,[119] prevention and treatment have focused on two principal approaches:

- administration of combinations of immunosuppressive drugs immediately prior to and following unmodified BMT, in an effect to prevent or inhibit the proliferation and function of donor T cells that are host-reactive;
- manipulation of the marrow graft to remove alloreactive donor T cells capable of inducing GVHD.

Early studies in a dog model first demonstrated that low-dose methotrexate could significantly decrease the incidence and severity of acute GVHD following DLA-identical marrow grafts. Based on these studies, methotrexate prophylaxis was introduced in clinical trials in the 1970s. Unfortunately, despite such prophylaxis, 50–70% of individuals receiving HLA-identical sibling grafts still developed acute GVHD and 30% developed chronic GVHD. In subsequent randomized trials, cyclosporine alone was found to be equivalent to methotrexate in preventing GVHD.[155] However, the combination of cyclosporine and methotrexate reduced the incidence of acute grade II–IV GVHD following HLA-matched related BMT to 33%, compared with 54% with methotrexate alone (p=0.014), resulting in a significantly improved survival in prospective trials.[156,157] Unfortunately, this combination has had little effect on the incidence or severity of chronic GVHD.

Randomized phase III trials in both the related and unrelated setting comparing tacrolimus (FK506) with cyclosporine in combination with methotrexate for the prevention of GVHD following HLA-matched sibling transplants have demonstrated a significant reduction in the incidence of acute grade II–IV GVHD in those given tacrolimus versus cyclosporine.[158,159] In the sibling trial,[159] the incidence of grade III–IV acute GVHD was similar in both arms. There was no difference in the incidence of chronic GVHD between the tacrolimus and the cyclosporine. The relapse rates of the two groups were similar. The patients in the cyclosporine arm had a significantly better 2-year disease-free and overall survival than patients in the tacrolimus arm. There was a higher frequency of deaths from regimen-related toxicity in patients with advanced disease who received tacrolimus. There was no difference in the disease-free and overall survival in patients with non-advanced disease. The survival disadvantage in advanced-disease patients receiving tacrolimus warrants further investigation. In the unrelated donor trial,[160] there was a significant trend toward decreased severity of acute GVHD across all grades. The probability of grade II–IV acute GVHD in the tacrolimus group (56%) was significantly lower than in the cyclosporine group (74%; p=0.0002). Overall and relapse-free survival rates for the tacrolimus and cyclosporine arms at 2 years were 54% versus 50% (p=0.46) and 47% versus 42% (p=0.58), respectively.

In summary, both these trials showed a significant reduction in grade II–IV acute GVHD in the patients receiving tacrolimus and methotrexate. However, this reduction in acute GVHD did not result in improved survival or relapse-free survival, and was (at least in siblings) associated with an unexplained survival disadvantage in patients with advanced disease.

Other immunosuppressive agents, such as rapamicin,[160] mycophenolic acid,[161] and thalidomide,[162] are currently under investigation in BMT.

### T-cell-depleted marrow transplants for prevention of GVHD

GVHD can be effectively prevented in both HLA-matched and HLA-disparate recipients through the use of marrow grafts rigorously depleted of T lymphocytes prior to infusion. The most extensively evaluated techniques for T-cell depletion include:

- agglutination with soybean lectin followed by rosetting with sheep red blood cells (SBA-E⁻) as described by Reisner and co-workers;[163,164]

- depletion with Campath-1, a monoclonal antibody against CDw52 that binds human complement derived from the donor's own plasma;[165]
- T-cell depletion with one or more T-cell-specific mouse monoclonal antibodies and rabbit complement;[166-168]
- treatment with T-cell-specific immunotoxins;[169]
- immunoadsorption of T cells via monoclonal antibodies bound to immunomagnetic beads or polystyrene membranes;[170,171]
- positive selection of CD34+ stem cells by immunoadsorption.[172]

Less-selective techniques capable of reducing T cells by 1–1.5 $\log_{10}$, such as elutriation, are also being explored.[173] These techniques may differ by 1–2 $\log_{10}$-fold in the degree of T-cell depletion achieved.[174] The threshold dose of clonable T cells administered in a marrow allograft associated with a significant risk of GVHD following HLA-matched sibling BMT[175] has been established at $10^5$ clonable T cells/kg recipient weight. For this reason, grade II–IV acute GVHD and chronic GVHD are still reported from large series using techniques achieving less than a 2.5–3.0 $\log_{10}$ depletion of T cells, even when cyclosporine is given as additional prophylaxis against GVHD. This trend is even more evident following transplantation of HLA-disparate marrow grafts. For such patients, only methods that can reduce the dose of clonable T cells to less than $0.5 \times 10^5$/kg can prevent the development of severe acute GVHD in all but a small proportion (<15%) of cases.[5]

Although several series have shown that T-cell depletion of a marrow allograft may reduce the incidence and severity of acute GVHD and, with certain methods, chronic GVHD, a clear advantage of T-cell-depleted transplants over unmodified marrow grafts reflected in long-term disease-free survival has thus far been clearly documented only in patients with SCID transplanted from HLA-non-identical donors.[5] In such cases, T-cell-depleted BMT from HLA-A, -B, -D haplotype-disparate parental donors has been associated with rates of long-term disease-free survival with immunologic reconstitution comparable to those achieved with T-cell-replete HLA-identical sibling marrow grafts. However, for patients with leukemia and aplastic anemia, reductions in GVHD and GVH-associated mortality accrued by the use of T-cell-depleted BMT have, until recently, been largely counterbalanced by an increased incidence of graft failure or rejection. This situation has been changing rapidly. The use of tolerable, more effective immunosuppressive preparatory regimens has dramatically reduced the risk of graft failure following T-cell-depleted BMT,[176] resulting in a significant improvement in long-term and disease-free survival rates, particularly among older recipients of matched sibling grafts and recipients of marrow derived from unrelated donors. As T-cell-depleted marrow grafts

have become more widely utilized, it has also become clear that the increased risk of leukemic relapse ascribed to T-cell-depleted transplants is not observed in all leukemic groups. Although patients transplanted for CML are clearly at increased risk,[177,178] those transplanted for AML are not.[163,179-182] These observations, coupled with the finding that leukocyte infusions administered to patients relapsing post transplant induce durable remissions in a high proportion of patients relapsing with CML, but are usually ineffective when used to treat relapses of ALL or AML, have led to a re-examination of the basis of the enhanced resistance to leukemia conferred by a marrow graft – the so-called 'graft-versus-leukemia' (GVL) effect.

## GVL: enhanced resistance to leukemia conferred by marrow allograft and augmentation by post-transplant adoptive cell transfer

An enhanced resistance to leukemia conferred by a marrow allograft was first suggested by comparisons of unmodified marrow grafts derived from identical twins versus HLA-matched siblings applied to the treatment of AML in first remission.[183] Weiden et al[184] subsequently analyzed a large series of patients with leukemia, transplanted with marrow from HLA-matched siblings, and found that leukemic relapse was lower among patients developing moderate to severe acute GVHD and/or chronic GVHD. These data led investigators to speculate that the antileukemic effect of a marrow allograft is largely based on the activity of alloreactive T cells responsible for GVHD.

Early results of T-cell-depleted marrow grafts for the treatment of leukemia tended to support this general hypothesis, since the incidence of relapse following T-cell-depleted BMT was higher than that reported for unmodified grafts.[185] However, subsequent analyses demonstrated that the risk of relapse for patients transplanted for leukemias[44,186,187] is consistently increased only for patients transplanted for CML,[163,186,187] and is not significantly increased among patients transplanted for acute leukemias. Nevertheless, these findings have suggested that T cells exert a crucial role in transplants for CML – not only in facilitating engraftment of donor marrow but also in eradicating residual leukemic cells resistant to the myeloablative cytoreduction administered prior to transplant.

Strong evidence that donor lymphoid cells contribute directly to resistance against CML was first provided by Kolb et al,[188] who reported that infusions of donor-derived peripheral blood mononuclear cells could induce durable remissions in patients with CML who relapsed following an allogeneic BMT. This finding has since been confirmed by many centers.[188-198] Overall, approximately 75% of patients who relapse with CML post transplant can be induced into durable molecular remissions by this approach (Figure 29.2). The doses of T cells administered in the mononuclear cell fractions have generally been in the range $(1-10)\times10^8$/kg. Infusions of such large T-cell numbers, have, as expected, been associated with a significant incidence of acute GVHD, although approximately one-quarter of the patients treated have achieved remission without exhibiting signs of GVHD.[195,196] Stepwise T-cell dose-escalation studies administered to patients relapsing with CML in chronic phase more than 9 months post T-cell-depleted BMT have also shown that remissions can be regularly achieved with T-cell doses as low as $10^7$/kg,[195,196] without concomitant GVHD. Such T-cell doses, if given at the time of BMT, would be expected to induce GVHD in 60–70% of cases. However, when these doses are given later than 12 months post BMT, they have induced mild GVHD in less than 10% of HLA-matched recipients.[175,196]

The specific donor-derived effector cells that selectively induce regressions of CML post transplant are currently unknown. However, CD4+ T cells probably play a significant role in that the emergency of CD4+ donor T cells capable of differentially inhibiting the growth of host clonogenic CD34+ Philadelphia-chromosome (Ph)-positive CML progenitors has been a consistent correlate of remission induction.[199] Furthermore, adoptive transfer of CD8+ T-cell depleted mononuclear cells from the original HLA-matched marrow donor has been reported to induce remissions of CML without inducing GVHD.[200] The observation that when Ph+ host cells are eliminated following donor leukocyte infusions, residual Ph− presumptively non-leukemic host T cells are also eradicated[196,197] gives additional support to the hypothesis that the effectors are not leukemia-specific but are reacting against minor alloantigens expressed both on leukemic cells and on normal cells of the lymphohematopoietic system.

The role of alloreactive T cells as effectors of resistance against acute leukemias is less clear. In several series, including an analysis of the International Bone Marrow Transplant Registry (IBMTR) transplant compendium, recipients of T-cell-depleted marrow for the treatment of AML in early remission have not shown any increase in the risk of relapse post transplant.[193,194] In ALL, the GVL effect associated with a marrow allograft remains controversial. On the one hand, in the IBMTR compendium of transplant results, recipients of a T-cell-depleted HLA-matched transplant for the treatment of ALL have been found to experience a modest but significant increase in the rate of relapse over that observed in recipients of unmodified transplants. This finding has suggested that, in the majority of patients transplanted for ALL, GVL effects could not be distinguished from GVHD.[201] On the other hand, the use of donor leukocytes to promote GVHD in patients with ALL in relapse or secondary or greater remission at the time of transplant have not reduced the risk of relapse rate, although the donor leukocyte infusions did induce an increased incidence and severity of GVHD.[202] Similarly, donor leukocyte infusions have been largely ineffective in eradicating relapse of ALL occurring post transplant. Indeed, in recent compendia of the European and American experiences with donor leukocyte infusions to treat disease recurrence following allogeneic BMT, Kolb et al[194] and Collins et al[203] found respectively that whereas donor leukocyte infusions induced remissions in the majority of patients treated for cytogenetic (80–100%) or hematologic (70–80%) relapse of CML, only a small fraction of patients with relapsed AML or ALL achieved durable remissions. These latter findings suggest that the enhanced leukemia resistance conferred by a marrow allograft for AML or ALL may not be as dependent upon alloreactive T cells for its expression as for CML, or, conversely, that clonogenic AML and ALL cells may be less sensitive to the cytolytic and/or cytoinhibitory activity of alloreactive T cells than clonogenic CML progenitors – either because they are too numerous and are so rapidly replicating as to outstrip alloreactive T-cell populations emerging from the donor leukocyte infusions or because these leukemic cells do not express target or accessory structures needed for recognition and killing by such alloreactive T cells.[204] To address the former possibility, several groups are now evaluating the activity of donor leukocyte infusions administered after a course of induction chemotherapy designed to reduce leukemic populations as treatment for patients relapsing with AML or ALL post transplant.[205]

The facts that T-cell-depleted marrow grafts that effectively prevent GVHD are not associated with an increased rate of relapse when applied to patients

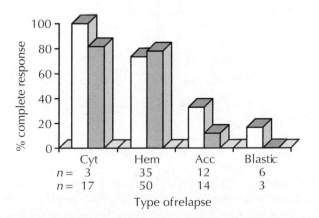

**Figure 29.2** Results of donor leukocyte infusions for treatment of relapsed chronic myeloid leukemia post bone marrow transplantation. White bars represent the results of Collins et al[203] and shaded bars those of Kolb et al.[194] Cyt, cytogenetic; Hem, hematologic; Acc, accelerated; n, number of patients in each study.

with AML and that alloreactive T cells may be only marginally active against ALL have fostered consideration of alternative cellular bases for the enhanced resistance to these leukemias conquered by a marrow allograft. Investigators exploring such mechanisms have focused on the detection, identification, and characterization of donor-derived cell populations developing after an unmodified or T-cell-depleted marrow allograft that are capable of discriminating between leukemic and non-leukemic host hematopoietic cells as measured by cytolysis or colony inhibition in vitro.

To date, three types of effector cells exhibiting this characteristic have been distinguished:

- donor-type NK cells;[206]
- donor T cells exhibiting broad, HLA-nonrestricted NK-like leukemocidal activity;[207]
- at low frequency, HLA-restricted donor T cells that can differentially inhibit the growth of clonogenic host leukemic cell populations.[199,208,209]

Of the non-T-cell populations that might contribute to an antileukemic effect, NK cells may be of particular importance. Two recently published studies have highlighted the GVL effect of HLA-C mismatching. The Japan Marrow Donor Program reported that in unrelated donor transplantation, matching at HLA-C was associated with a significantly higher relapse rate.[210] The Perugia group have reported that in the haploidentical setting, mismatching at HLA-C, as determined by killer inhibitory receptor (KIR) groupings, significantly reduced the incidence of relapse in patients with AML.[211]

Another strategy being evaluated in an effort to detect or generate leukemia-reactive T cells has been to establish mixed leukocyte cultures between HLA-matched or partially matched normal donor T lymphocytes and isolated host leukemic cells. T-cell lines and clones derived from such cultures have been assessed for their capacity to distinguish between leukemic and non-leukemic targets such as phytohemagglutinin (PHA)-stimulated T lymphoblasts and Epstein–Barr virus (EBV)-transformed normal B cells obtained from the host during remission. Using this approach, Sossman et al[208,209] generated CD3+CD4+ T-cell lines and HLA-DR, -DP-restricted CD4+ T-cell clones exhibiting selective, proliferative and cytotoxic responses against ALL cells derived from an HLA-A, -B, -D-mismatched patient. Faber et al[212] similarly generated HLA-restricted CD8+ leukemia-specific cytotoxic T cells from the peripheral blood lymphocytes of an HLA-matched sibling of a patient with AML. Although the frequency of such clones has been low when compared with the frequency of clones exhibiting reactivity against both normal and leukemic cells of the host, this latter study indicates the possibility of generating leukemia-selective cytotoxic T cells potentially lacking the potential

to induce GVHD, even from HLA-matched normal donors.

Taken together, the studies cited above have clearly shown that several effector systems may contribute to the antileukemic effect of an allogeneic BMT, including alloreactive potentially GVH-inducing T cells reactive against major and minor alloantigens expressed on both normal and leukemic cells, T cells reactive against differentiation antigens preferentially expressed on leukemic cells, and NK cells.

## Infections in the early stages of immune reconstitution

Interstitial pneumonias (IP) still constitute the major cause of death in the first 3 months post transplant. Between 25% and 35% of patients transplanted for leukemia develop this complication. Historically, over 50% of these cases were caused by CMV.[213] Other viruses, such as adenovirus,[83] respiratory syncytial virus (RSV),[214] influenza, and parainfluenza,[215] have gained prominence as methodologies to detect these viruses have improved, and more widespread use of prophylactic or pre-emptive therapy of CMV infections has reduced the incidence of CMV IP.[216–219] Pneumocystis carinii IP is much less common owing to the widespread use of cotrimoxazole[220] or pentamidine prophylaxis before and after marrow transplantation. However, the more intensive and prolonged administration of steroids, used either to prevent or to treat GVHD, has led to a significant increase in the incidence of Aspergillus pneumonia.[221–223]

CMV remains the most common cause of life-threatening infections in the post-transplant period. Approximately 70–90% of transplant recipients who are CMV-seropositive, or who receive grafts from seropositive donors, will become viremic post transplant during the first 3–6 months following engraftment.[224,225] In the absence of pre-emptive or prophylactic antiviral therapy, 30–40% of CMV-viremic patients will develop IP. In contrast, this complication is low among seronegative patients with seronegative donors who receive blood-product support from CMV-negative donors.[224] This finding, coupled with molecular analyses of CMV isolates from CMV-positive individuals, suggests that CMV disease post BMT usually results from reactivation of latent virus from the host or the graft.[226] Alloreactions between donor and host augment the risk of CMV disease. Thus recipients of HLA-matched related marrow grafts who develop moderate to severe GVHD have a higher incidence of CMV IP[227–229] when compared with allograft recipients without GVHD. Furthermore, CMV IP is a rare complication in recipients of syngeneic or autologous BMT.[230] More intensive cytoreductive regimens are also associated with an increased incidence of CMV disease.[229,231]

Over the last 15 years, a number of effective strategies have been developed to reduce the incidence of CMV IP and improve treatment outcome. The risk of developing CMV disease may be reduced to less than 2% by the exclusive use of either CMV-negative or filtered leukocyte-reduced blood products in CMV-negative donor–recipient pairs.[232,233]

In the late 1980s, several studies demonstrated that CMV IP could be effectively treated in 50–70% of affected marrow allograft recipients using combined therapy with ganciclovir and intravenous gammaglobulin.[234–237] Neither agent alone had a significant effect on the course of CMV IP. For patients unable to tolerate ganciclovir, primarily because of myelosuppression, foscarnet used in combination with gammaglobulin has also been reported as being effective.[238] Unfortunately, these antiviral combinations have often been ineffective in reversing overt CMV disease in recipients of unrelated BMT, prompting the evaluation of these agents in prophylactic strategies. Several groups have reported their experience either with pre-emptive antiviral therapy, i.e. therapy initiated at the time of CMV viremia, or with prophylactic therapy, initiated in all seropositive patients or recipients of marrow allografts from seropositive donors at the time of engraftment. Two randomized trials have demonstrated that early treatment of patients with detectable virus in body fluids (blood or broncheoalveolar lavage) significantly reduced the frequency of CMV IP, thereby reducing transplant-associated mortality.[216,217] Two other prospective randomized trials have demonstrated the effectiveness of prophylactic ganciclovir in reducing early CMV disease.[218,219] However, effective prophylaxis has ultimately not led to a reduction in transplant-associated mortality. The most recent study by Boeckh et al[219] revealed that although prophylactic ganciclovir was more effective than pre-emptive treatment in preventing early (<100 days) CMV disease, recipients of prophylactic ganciclovir had a higher incidence of late (>100 days) CMV disease, which was generally fatal. Furthermore, this prophylactic use of ganciclovir has been associated with neutropenia, which was severe enough in up to 30% of patients to warrant discontinuation of treatment. In such patients, the incidence of other infections was increased.[219,238] Given these results, the pre-emptive treatment of CML viremia appears to be the better approach. However, this strategy depends critically on access to viral detection methods that detect virus before the onset of overt disease. Although rapid viral detection methods, such as shell vial cultures, polymerase chain reaction (PCR) analysis and assays for the CMV pp65 early antigen, have markedly improved the ability to detect clinically occult viremia,[238–241] the impact of these tests depends on the type and vigilance of the surveillance schedules employed.

Currently, adoptive immunotherapy with donor-derived, in vitro selected and expanded, CMV-specific T-cell clones is being evaluated for the prevention of CMV disease. The preliminary results in clinical trials have been highly promising.[242] The adoptive transfer of $(3-10)\times10^7$ CMV-specific T cells/ml has induced significant levels of circulating CD8+ cells exhibiting CMV-specific cytotoxicity, which have been sustained for at least 8 weeks post infusion. Repeated doses have been infused without toxicity or GVHD. None of the first five patients who received these cloned cells developed CMV disease.[242] Larger trials of this approach have confirmed these results,[243] and have demonstrated the potential of adoptive cell transfer to restore specific antiviral immunity, thereby reducing post-transplant morbidity and mortality. In addition, the successful use of donor-derived interleukin-2 (IL-2)-activated T cells into which a suicide vector has been inserted to allow for elimination of infused cells in the event of GVHD has been reported.[244]

## Infections in the later stages of immune reconstitution

Immune reconstitution following a marrow allograft can be a protracted process, and is adversely affected by advanced patient age, post-transplant prophylaxis and treatment of GVHD, and transplants of HLA non-identical related or 'matched' unrelated donors.[245] Although T-cell populations (primarily CD8+ T cells) begin to redevelop within the first 2 months post transplant, CD4+ cell recovery may not occur for 6–18 months post BMT, and responses to mitogens and specific antigens may be severely depressed for 6–24 months.[133,245,246]

During the periods of profound T-cell deficiency between engraftment and 6–8 months post transplant, BMT patients are also at risk for polyclonal or oligoclonal B-cell lymphoproliferative disorders (LPD) and monoclonal lymphomas induced by EBV.[247,248] The risk of EBV-LPD following lectin-separated T-cell-depleted grafts has been reported to be as high as 6% for HLA-matched related and 12% for unrelated transplants when equine antithymocyte has been administered to the patients to prevent immune rejection.[248] Rates of EBV-LPD of approximately 6% have been recorded following HLA-matched transplants depleted with T-cell-specific mouse monoclonals,[249] and as high as 8–24% in recipients of HLA-non-identical grafts depleted of T cells with T-cell-specific monoclonal antibodies.[249,250] Similarly, Martin et al[251] have reported a 16% incidence of EBV-LPD in patients given infusions of certain T-cell-specific monoclonal antibodies for treatment of GVHD following unmodified marrow transplants. The EBV-LPD that arise post transplant are usually of donor rather than host origin.[249,251] The basis for these B-cell transformations remains unclear, but may in part reflect an inability of patients early post transplant to generate T cells capable of suppressing donor B-cell expansions.[252]

Prior to the 1990s, the majority of patients who developed an EBV-LPD died from these disorders. Specifically, monoclonal proliferations were refractory to classical chemotherapy, radiation and/or antiviral therapy. In 1993, Papadopoulos et al[253] first demonstrated that adoptive transfer of EBV-specific immunity by infusion of small doses of peripheral mononuclear cells derived from a patient's EBV-seropositive donor could induce complete and durable remissions of EBV-LPD in the majority of patients, including those with monoclonal EBV-associated lymphomas. These infusions were calculated to deliver in the range of $(0.5-1.0)\times10^6$ CD3+ T cells/kg. This finding has now been confirmed by several other groups.[254,255] The efficacy of this approach probably reflects the expansion of circulating EBV-specific cytotoxic T-cell precursors found in high frequency in the leukocytes of normal seropositive marrow donors.[256] Indeed, within 2 weeks following infusions of as few as $10^3$ EBV cytotoxic T-lymphocyte (CTL) precursors, frequencies of EBV-reactive CTL regularly increase from undetectable levels to frequencies as high as $1/10^4$ T cells in the blood.[252] Further substantiation of this hypothesis comes from the studies by Rooney et al,[255] which demonstrated sustained remissions following infusions of small numbers of genetically marked EBV-specific T cells derived from T-cell lines generated in vitro. Not all patients, especially children, have EBV-cytotoxic T cells available or even an EBV-seropositive donor. Recent reports have shown that rituximab, a humanized anti-CD20 monoclonal antibody, has been effective as both treatment and prophylaxis of EBV lymphoma.[257,258]

## Late complications of marrow transplants

The late sequelae of the TBI and chemotherapy used for cytoreduction prior to transplant may be mild to severe, depending on the type of agents used and their dose intensity. The toxicity of the transplant cytoreduction is also affected by the patient's age at transplant, as well as by the regimens used prior to referral for transplant to induce, consolidate, and maintain remissions of the primary disease. For example, toxicity induced by regimens incorporating myeloablative doses of TBI tends to be more profound and enduring than those induced by regimens that include myeloablative combinations of chemotherapeutic agents alone, and is more damaging when the radiation is given in a single large dose rather than in multiple fractions.[259,260]

One of the most devastating late complications resulting from damage induced by TBI and chemotherapy is leukoencephalopathy.[261] This complication occurs almost exclusively in patients transplanted for leukemia who have received cranial radiation and/or extended courses of intrathecal methotrexate as treatment or prophylaxis for central nervous system (CNS) leukemia prior to referral for transplantation. In such patients, the risk of leukoencephalopathy has been reported to be as high as 7%.[261] This complication usually induces severe symptoms, including slurred speech, confusion, ataxia, seizures, and spasticity, which may progress to coma and death. Less severe CNS toxicities may also be observed, in the form of neuropsychological dysfunctions and varying degrees of retardation.[262] However, the incidence of the latter complications has not been established. Transient neurologic toxicities, including tremors, seizures, and paresis, may also complicate the use of cyclosporine and tacrolimus for prophylaxis of GVHD.[263–265]

Endocrine abnormalities involving the thyroid, pituitary gland, and gonads are common late sequelae of BMT. Hypothyroidism, requiring hormone replacement, has been reported in 10%[266,267] and compensated hypothyroidism in an additional 34–36% of patients transplanted for leukemia. Analysis of gonadal function post BMT has revealed that the age and the type and intensity of the cytoreductive regimen utilized are important factors in determining whether ovarian function will recover in females. In one study, women younger than 27 years cytoreduced with cyclophosphamide alone regularly recovered ovarian function within the first year post transplant (median 6 months); however, more than 35% women older than 27 years had sustained ovarian failure.[268] Young women who received TBI and cyclophosphamide in preparation for BMT for leukemia have experienced a 55% incidence of permanent ovarian failure, compared with a 74% incidence in older women.[268] In a single-institution study of prepubescent females undergoing BMT following cytoreduction with hyperfractionated TBI and chemotherapy, at least 50% were able to enter puberty and sustain menarche.

A proportion of women who recover ovarian function post transplant may achieve successful pregnancies. Thus, in a long-term study by Sanders et al,[269] 110 of 708 women (15%) who were postpubescent at the time of BMT recovered normal ovarian function. Of these, 32 became pregnant. The proportion of pregnancies resulting in live births was 79%. There was a statistically higher incidence of spontaneous abortions ($p=0.02$) and preterm births ($p=0.01$) complicating the pregnancies of women who received TBI as part of their conditioning regimen as compared with those prepared with cyclophosphamide alone. Despite these complications, the children born were normal and had no higher an incidence of birth defects than that associated with pregnancies in the general population.

Deficiencies of Leydig cell function are rare in boys and men transplanted after preparation with cyclophosphamide with or without TBI.[270] Indeed, we have found that most prepubertal boys undergoing BMT following cytoreduction with hyperfractionated TBI and chemotherapy undergo a normal transition to puberty.[271] However, despite normal testosterone levels, many will have compensatory elevations of follicle-stimulating hormone (FSH). Unfortunately, spermatogenesis is eliminated or severely impaired, resulting in infertility in the majority of patients with leukemia who received TBI and up to one-third of patients given cyclophosphamide alone.[271] Of 618 postpubertal men evaluated by Sanders et al,[269] 157 had some level of spermatogenesis, including 66% of those treated with TBI. The partners of 35 of these men had one or more pregnancies, which were not associated with increased rates of spontaneous abortion, preterm delivery, or congenital abnormalities.[269]

The degree of growth retardation following transplantation is influenced by age at transplant, radiation schema (single dose versus fractionated or hyperfractionated), as well as prior CNS radiation. The effects of radiation on linear growth are complex and multifactorial, involving not only hypothalamic production of growth hormone-releasing factor (GHRF) but also the intrinsic growth potential of long bones. The use of hyperfractionated regimens of TBI has been associated with less impaired growth potential than standard-dose regimens.[272] Whether and to what degree treatment with growth hormone or GHRF can partially correct short stature in these cases is now under study.

TBI may induce cataracts in the late post-transplant period. Recipients of single-fraction high-dose TBI have the highest incidence – reported to be as high as 50%. For patients given fractionated TBI, the incidence is approximately 10–20%.[273]

Cytoreduction with alkylating agents has been associated with secondary malignancies post BMT – although, to date, the incidence of such neoplasms have been relatively limited[274,275] and lower than the incidence of secondary tumors recorded in patients given comparable or lower localized doses of radiation and chemotherapy for other neoplasms such as Hodgkin's disease. In a large study of 19 229 recipients of an allogeneic BMT at 235 centers,[275] the overall risk of solid tumors was 2.7 times that expected in the general population (8.3 times if the patient survived for more than 10 years post allogeneic BMT). The cumulative risk of a solid tumor developing post BMT was 2.2% at 10 years, increasing to 6.7% at 15 years. The most common solid tumors arising post BMT included malignant melanoma, squamous cell carcinomas of the buccal mucosa (particularly in patients with prior chronic GVHD), and cancers of the liver, CNS, thyroid, bone, and connective tissue. More prolonged follow-up is still needed before a full assessment of the risk of secondary neoplasms can be made.

# HLA-matched marrow transplants for leukemia

In the 1970s, BMT was utilized predominantly in patients with end-stage disease, whose leukemias were probably refractory to chemotherapy. In this poor-risk group of patients, a 13–18% disease-free survival (DFS) was observed, which increased to 25% in a subgroup of patients transplanted in good physical condition.[276] These results paved the way for exploration of the use of marrow transplantation in patients in better clinical condition, earlier in the course of their disease, when the leukemic cell burden was low and residual leukemic cells were still likely to be sensitive to the cytoreduction employed.[277] In 1979, the Seattle group[277] reported a series of patients with AML transplanted in first complete remission (CR) who achieved a 63% long-term DFS associated with only a 12% incidence of relapse. Subsequently, similar results were achieved in several other transplant centers, heralding the widespread use of HLA-matched marrow grafts to treat patients with acute leukemias in first or second remission and CML in first chronic phase. Approximately 25 years of this experience can now be evaluated. Furthermore, the results of allogeneic BMT can be compared with those achieved with chemotherapy as well as autologous transplants at different stages in the course of these leukemias.

# Acute myeloid leukemia

For patients with AML in second or later remission or relapse, an allogeneic HLA-matched marrow graft is generally regarded as the treatment of choice, since few of these patients have survived disease-free if treated with chemotherapy alone[278] (see Chapters 37 and 38). Marrow transplants from HLA-matched siblings following cytoreduction with cyclophosphamide coupled with TBI or busulfan have provided extended DFS for 20–40% in adults and 30–50% in children grafted in second CR.[279–282] Alternatively, some centers have proceeded directly to allogeneic transplant in first relapse, and report a 23% DFS.[283] The use of similar cytoreduction followed by an autologous, purged marrow graft obtained during second remission may also lead to long-term (5-year) DFS in up to one-third of cases.[284,285] Although autologous transplants are associated with a higher risk of relapse than HLA-matched marrow grafts (>50% versus 20–25%) and a lower probability of long-term DFS, in some centers they are considered the treatment of choice for patients in second remission who lack an HLA-matched donor, being somewhat superior to chemotherapy alone. A retrospective analysis performed by Busca et al[286] reported a similar DFS in 24 patients with AML in second or third CR given an unrelated (30%, *n*=9) or autologous (25%, *n*=12) BMT.

In the 1980s, four prospective randomized trials tried to address whether allogeneic BMT from an HLA-matched sibling or chemotherapy was the best postremission therapy for adults (<45 years) with AML in first CR.[279,287–289] In all four trials, relapse was significantly lower among transplanted patients (for BMT, the relapse rate was 9–40%; for chemotherapy, it was 71–88%). However, the lower relapse rate following transplant was counterbalanced by a higher rate of non-relapse mortality. Despite this, the 3- to 5-year DFS rates were superior in the transplant arms of each study, although these differences were statistically significant in only two.[279,288] Concerns regarding the results of these studies included the possibility of patient selection bias as well as the adequacy of treatment and supportive care administered to the chemotherapy control arms.[290] Although the postinduction therapy varied in each of the four chemotherapy arms, the drugs administered were representative of 'standard' consolidation or intensification regimens at the time.

To address concerns raised by the earlier trials, two large multicenter randomized studies were subsequently undertaken. These trials compared outcomes in recipients of chemotherapy alone with those of allogeneic or autologous marrow transplantation. In the first study, the UK Medical Research Council (MRC) AML-10 trial,[291] patients received two identical induction and consolidation courses, followed by allocations to the allogeneic transplantation arm if an HLA-matched donor was available or, if not, randomization to either the autologous transplantation or the observation-alone arm. Data were analyzed on an intention-to-treat basis. The 1063 patients under 55 years who entered complete remission were tissue-typed. Of these patients, 419 had a matched sibling donor and 644 had no match. When compared on a donor versus no donor basis, the risk of relapse was reduced in the donor arm (36% versus 52%; *p*=0.001) and the DFS rate improved (50% versus 42%; *p*=0.01), but the overall survival (OS) rate was not different (55% versus 50%; *p*=0.1). However, only 61% of patients with a donor underwent transplantation. When patients were subdivided into risk groups based on cytogenetics alone or with the addition of blast response to the first course, a reduction in relapse risk was seen in all risk groups and in three age cohorts (0–14, 15–34, and 35+ years). Significant benefit in DFS was only seen in the intermediate-risk cytogenetic group (50% versus 39%; *p*=0.004). The OS benefit was only seen in intermediate-risk patients (55% versus 44%; *p*=0.02). The reduction in risk of relapse in good-risk patients was attributable to patients with t(15;17) but not to patients with t(8;21) or inv(16). Allogeneic transplantation given after intensive chemotherapy was able to reduce relapse in all risk and age groups. However, owing to the competing effects of procedural mortality and an inferior response to chemotherapy if relapse does occur, there was a survival advantage only in patients at intermediate risk. This trial found no survival advantage in children, patients over 35 years, or good-risk disease. Criticisms of this trial have included the fact that almost 40% of those allocated to the allogeneic transplantation arm did not receive a transplant and that the allograft was performed only after four intensive courses of chemotherapy, which potentially could have adversely affected transplant-related mortality.

In a second trial, Zittoun and colleagues[292] compared patient outcome following intensive chemotherapy versus allogeneic or autologous transplantation. In this study, patients who achieved a complete remission after standard induction therapy (daunorubicin and cytarabine) and one course of intensive consolidation therapy (intermediate-dose cytarabine, 500–1000 mg/m$^2$ every 12 hours × 12 doses, and amsacrine, 120 mg/m$^2$/day × 3 doses) were allocated to an allogeneic transplant if an HLA-matched sibling was available or were randomized to an autologous transplant versus a second course of intensive chemotherapy with high-dose cytarabine (2 g/m$^2$ every 12 hours × 8 doses) and daunorubicin (45 mg/m$^2$/day × 3 doses) if the patient lacked a sibling donor. Patients over 45 years of age were excluded from the allogeneic transplant arm. The projected DFS rate at 4 years was 55% for the allogeneic arm, 48% for the autologous arm, and 30% for the intensive chemotherapy arm. The difference in outcome between the autologous transplant arm and intensive chemotherapy was statistically significant (*p*=0.05). The difference between the allogeneic arm and the chemotherapy arm was also statistically significant (*p*=0.04). Relapse in the allogeneic arm was 25%, versus 41% and 57% in the autologous and chemotherapy arms, respectively. In an intention-to-treat analysis, no significant differences in outcome were revealed between the two transplant groups.

In earlier trials comparing transplantation and chemotherapy, benefits from lower relapse rates in the allogeneic arm were offset by higher non-relapse mortality rates. In addition, questions have been raised as to whether the chemotherapy control arm in the study by Zittoun et al[292] contained 'optimal' therapy.[293] Thus, when the Cancer and Leukemia Group B (CALGB) examined the efficacy of sequential low-, intermediate-, or high-dose cytarabine as postremission intensification therapy in patients with AML under the age of 60, patients receiving the high-dose cytarabine regimen (3 g/m$^2$ every 12 hours × 6 doses) had a 44% probability of remaining in continuous remission at 4 years.[294] These results are similar to those achieved in the autologous arm of the Zittoun study. A follow-up study from the CALGB demonstrated that certain 'good'-risk cytogenetic abnormalities, such as t(8;21)(q22;q22) and inv(16)(p13q22), predict responsiveness to intensive chemotherapy with high-dose cytarabine. Patients in this study who had these 'good-risk' cytogenetic abnormalities achieved a 51% DFS rate when given high-dose cytarabine as postremission consolidation.[294] This result has prompted questions as to whether or not such good-risk patients should be considered candidates for any transplant approach.

To address these concerns, several multicenter analyses reanalyzed the results of transplantation to assess the impact of cytogenetic abnormalities on outcome following allogeneic or autologous BMT in patients with AML in first CR.[295,296] In a retrospective analysis of the IBMTR data, Gale et al[295] found that the DFS rate for patients with cytogenetic abnormalities associated with 'good-risk' AML was 56% (46–66%). A subsequent analysis of outcome following allogeneic BMT for AML in first CR conducted by the EBMT[296] demonstrated 5-year leukemia-free survival rates of 67%, 57%, and 29% for patients with favorable (abn(16) and t(8;21)), standard intermediate (t(15;17), pseudodiploid, hyperdiploid, and diploid) and poor-prognosis (abn(5) and/or (7), abn(11q) and hypodiploid) cytogenetic abnormalities, respectively. For patients with favorable or standard cytogenetic abnormalities, allogeneic BMT achieved remission duration and DFS rates that were significantly better than those recorded for autologous marrow grafts. However, for those with unfavorable karyotype, there was no difference in outcome following allogeneic or autologous BMT. Multivariate analysis of these data demonstrated that cytogenetics at diagnosis was the most important prognostic indicator of DFS and relapse.

While the results of more intensive chemotherapeutic regimens over the last 15 years have improved the outcomes for patients with AML, novel approaches to allogeneic transplantation using T-cell-depleted techniques have also been developed that result in a lower non-relapse mortality and diminish the incidence and severity of GVHD.[53,297,298] For example, a report from the Memorial Sloan–Kettering group[182] demonstrated a 77% DFS rate at 2 years in adult patients with AML transplanted in first CR (n=31), following cytoreduction with TBI, thiotepa, and cyclophosphamide. Bone marrows were T-cell-depleted with soybean lectin agglutination followed by rosetting with sheep red blood cells, resulting in a 2.5–3.0 $\log_{10}$ depletion of T cells. No patient experienced graft failure or grade II–IV acute GVHD. In this report, the relapse rate was 3.4% and the rate of non-leukemic mortality was 19.4%. Transplant teams from the Dana-Farber Cancer Center[181] and Ulm University Hospital[298] reported similar findings, with 63% and

80% DFS rates, respectively, for patients with AML transplanted in first remission. In these studies, the bone marrow grafts were T-cell-depleted utilizing the anti-CD6 monoclonal antibody or Campath-1G/1M, respectively. These studies demonstrate that advances in allogeneic transplantation techniques have led to a reduction in regimen-related mortality and to improved DFS rates. However, the long-term DFS rates recorded in these studies have so far only been reported for intensive chemotherapy or autologous BMT in adults. Given these developments, the selection of an 'optimal approach' for the treatment of adults with AML – particularly those older than 45 years – must await the results of planned or active protocols comparing these second-generation chemotherapy and transplantation regimens.

While current chemotherapy regimens for the treatment of AML in children have resulted in 3- to 5-year DFS rates ranging from 40% to 55%,[299–301] HLA-matched marrow grafts administered to children with AML in first remission have also achieved impressive results, with 49–80% of such patients surviving disease-free at 3–5 years post transplant.[280,302,303] For patients treated with allogeneic BMT for AML in first CR, pretransplant cytoreduction with cyclophosphamide coupled with TBI has yielded better results than preparative regimens combining busulfan and cyclophosphamide.[209,303,304] In an initial prospective trial conducted by the Children's Cancer Study Group (CCSG),[304] the DFS rate was superior for children who received an allogeneic HLA-matched BMT when compared with those randomized to non-ablative chemotherapy (p<0.05). A subsequent CCSG study[301] has compared chemotherapy versus an autologous transplant purged with 4-hydroperoxycyclophosphamide (4-HC) versus an allogeneic HLA-matched transplant administered after a standard or more intensively timed intensive course of DCTER induction chemotherapy. This study demonstrated an overall improvement in DFS in each post-remission treatment group when the more intensive DCTER regimen was used to induce remission. Again, however, the DFS rates for patients treated with allogeneic marrow grafts were significantly superior to those recorded for the postremission groups treated with either chemotherapy or a purged autologous marrow graft, irrespective of the induction treatment administered. Indeed, for those patients induced into remission with the more dose-intensive DCTER regimen, the DFS rate at 5 years for the allogeneic arm was 72%, which is significantly better than the 52% and 55% DFS rates achieved respectively with an autologous marrow graft or chemotherapy alone.[305]

In summary, HLA-identical sibling allogeneic stem cell transplantation is generally accepted as the therapy of choice for patients with AML in first remission who do not have favorable cytogenetics.

# Acute lymphoblastic leukemia

## Transplantation for ALL in first remission

Current treatment of ALL in childhood will result in long-term survival in more than 70% of patients[306–310] (see Chapter 31). For those children considered at an increased risk of relapse, more-intensive regimens have resulted in sustained DFS rates of 60–70%.[309,310] Because of these excellent results, it has been difficult to identify children with ALL who will clearly benefit from an allogeneic transplant in first remission. Indeed, allogeneic BMT in pediatric patients with high-risk ALL has led to long-term DFS rates of 56–84%, which are no superior to those that can currently be achieved with chemotherapy alone.[311–315]

The place of allogeneic marrow grafts in the treatment of adults with ALL who have achieved an initial remission is only slightly less controversial.[316] Current chemotherapeutic regimens induce remissions in 70–85% of adults, but only 20–51% of these patients will achieve long-term DFS, depending upon the characteristics of the ALL under treatment[317–319] (see also Chapter 32). In particular, for patients who, at initial diagnosis, present with disease features associated with a high risk of relapse, such as white cell count above 20 000/mm³, age over 60 years, CNS involvement, chromosomal translocations t(4;11), t(8;14), or t(9;22), null or B-cell phenotype, or failure to achieve remission within 5 weeks of induction therapy, the proportion who will survive in sustained remission is small. In contrast, in several series, HLA-matched marrow transplants have resulted in 3- to 5-year DFS rates of 30–71% in high-risk young adults (younger than 40 years) with ALL in first remission, with relapse rates post transplant of 9–35%. While DFS rates vary significantly, depending upon the type of cytoreduction[317–326] and the method of GVHD prophylaxis utilized,[311] the promising results achieved have suggested that allogeneic BMT may offer a significant advantage to adults with ALL with high-risk features in first CR.

Three prospective randomized trials have attempted to further define the optimal postremission therapy in adult patients with ALL. In the first of these, patients under the age of 40 years were allocated to an allogeneic BMT arm if they had an HLA-identical sibling. Patients younger than 40 years without a donor and those aged between 40 and 50 years were randomized to chemotherapy versus autologous BMT.[327] In this trial, which used an intention-to-treat analysis, the 5-year survival rates were similar in patients randomized to the allogeneic BMT arm and those randomized to the autologous BMT or chemotherapy arms. However, although there was no benefit from allogeneic BMT in adults with 'standard-risk' ALL, for those with high-risk features, there was a significant difference in overall and disease-free survival, favor-

ing the allogeneic BMT arm: 44% versus 20%, respectively. In the second prospective study, patients younger than 55 years who achieved a complete remission following induction were allocated to receive an allogeneic BMT if an HLA-identical sibling was available or were randomized to an autologous BMT with or without interleukin-2 (IL-2).[328] In this study, the 3-year probability of DFS was significantly higher in recipients of an HLA-identical sibling transplant than in the autologous transplant groups: 68% versus 26%. Post-transplant IL-2 had no effect on the DFS of patients in the autologous transplant group, whose main cause of failure was relapse. The third trial is the MRC UKALL XII/Eastern Cooperative Oncology Group (ECOG) E2993 to prospectively define the benefit of allogeneic and autologous BMT in adult Philadelphia chromosome-negative (Ph⁻) ALL in first CR.[329] All patients received two phases of standard induction and, if in CR, were assigned to allogeneic BMT if they had an HLA-matched sibling donor. Other patients were randomized to either standard consolidation/maintenance therapy or autologous BMT. The data were analyzed on an intent-to-treat basis. Standard risk was defined as Ph⁻, age 35 years or less, time to CR 4 weeks or less, and white cell count less than 30 000/mm³ for B-lineage and less than 100 000/mm³ for T-lineage. The actuarial 5-year event-free survival (EFS) rates for these 434 Ph⁻ patients, who had intended to undergo an allogeneic BMT ($n$=170) or were randomized ($n$=264), were 54% and 34%, respectively ($p < 0.04$). The study showed that allogeneic BMT conferred the most potent antileukemic effect for all adult patients with ALL in first CR and, despite increased early toxicity, appears to provide favorable long-term results.

In summary, these studies demonstrate that allogeneic BMT may be a preferred option for certain subsets of patients with adult ALL in first remission.

## Transplantation for ALL in second or greater remission or relapse

The results reported for HLA-matched sibling BMT applied to the treatment of children with ALL in second CR vary considerably both in DFS rates and in the incidence of relapse. Regimens utilizing single-dose TBI and cyclophosphamide have been associated with relapse rates ranging from 30% to 57% at 2 years, and DFS rates of 33–50%.[330,331] In contrast, regimens incorporating higher doses of hyperfractionated TBI followed by cyclophosphamide[280] or fractionated TBI administered with high-dose cytarabine,[332] etoposide,[322] or altered doses of cyclophosphamide[325] have resulted in long-term DFS rates of 59–64% at 5 years and relapse rates of 9–16%.

Meaningful comparisons between transplant results and those achieved with chemotherapy alone must take into consideration the characteristics of the patients treated – particularly the duration of first remission and the chemotherapy that they have previously received. Although children with ALL who relapse early in the course of their initial chemotherapy (e.g. in the first 18 months) may be induced into a second remission, they are unlikely to survive disease-free for more than 6–12 months. This contrasts with the results of chemotherapy alone in patients with ALL who relapse after completing 18–24 months of chemotherapy,[333] 40–81% of whom may survive disease-free. Given these results, it has been argued that a transplant is indicated for children who relapse early in the course of their disease, but not necessarily in those relapsing after a prolonged initial remission.

To address this issue, we and others have conducted retrospective analyses of single-center and multicenter experiences from this point of view.[334] In these studies, children with ALL in second remission whose initial relapse occurred while still on chemotherapy fared significantly better if they received an allogeneic BMT than if they were treated with chemotherapy alone. The five-year DFS rates for children transplanted ranged from 30% to 56%. For those patients treated with chemotherapy alone, the 5-year DFS rates reported since 1986 varied from 17% to 31%. These results indicate that allogeneic BMT is superior to chemotherapy for children with ALL who relapse within 1–2 years of achieving first remission. In our own series reported by Boulad et al,[334] and in those reported by Chessels et al[335] and Barrett et al,[336] transplants may also be superior to chemotherapy in children with ALL who relapse later in first remission. In our own single-center series, for those patients whose first remissions were later than 24 months, the 10-year DFS rate is 81% following allogeneic BMT, compared with 31% with chemotherapy alone.[334] In the multicenter analysis conducted by Chessels et al[335] and the large matched-pair study of children reported to the IBMTR and the Pediatric Oncology Group by Barrett et al,[336] the 5-year leukemia-free survival rates for children who received transplants were 55% and 53%, respectively, versus 18% and 32% for children treated with chemotherapy. Because of continuing concerns regarding treatment-allocation biases, however, prospective trials comparing allogeneic BMT versus aggressive chemotherapy are still needed to resolve this issue.

For adults with ALL who have failed to sustain an initial remission, an HLA-matched marrow graft is the treatment of choice. For adults transplanted in second remission, the reported extended DFS rates for transplant recipients range from 22% to 43%, with relapse, post transplant, representing the cause of failure in 26–56% of cases.[45,308,323,335] For children and adults transplanted in later remissions or relapse, the extended DFS is only 8–25% at 3–5 years post grafting.[45,311,337]

# Chronic myeloid leukemia

Until recently, allogeneic BMT was the treatment of choice for patients under the age of 60 with CML who have an HLA-compatible donor,[338] cure being achieved in 50–90% of patients transplanted in first chronic phase in reported series.[6,338–340] In the past, single-agent chemotherapy for CML has been found to be only palliative; it does not significantly prolong survival[341] (see also Chapter 41). Although certain multidrug chemotherapy regimens can transiently eradicate the Ph+ clone, re-emergence of Ph+ cells has ultimately occurred in almost all cases. As a result, these regimens have not resulted in a significant improvement in median survival.[342] Interferon-α (IFN-α), used as first-line therapy in CML, has induced hematologic remissions in as many as 70% of patients. However, complete cytogenetic remissions have been less common, occurring in fewer than 20% of patients.[343] Nevertheless, several randomized trials have shown a survival advantage in patients who receive IFN-α for the treatment of CML, compared with chemotherapy. For example, a large multi-institutional study from the Italian Cooperative Study Group published in 1994[344] demonstrated a statistically significant improvement in overall survival for patients treated with IFN-α compared with conventional therapy with hydroxyurea or busulfan, with median survival times of 72 months versus 52 months, respectively. Other investigators have demonstrated a similarly significant improvement in overall survival for those patients achieving a complete, major, or minor cytogenetic response versus those not achieving a cytogenetic response or historical controls treated with standard chemotherapy.[345,346] The French Chronic Myeloid Leukemia Study Group reported that treatment with IFN-α together with cytarabine conferred a significant improvement in survival (a 3-year survival rate of 85.7% versus 79.1%; $p=0.02$) as well as a higher hematologic response rate ($p=0.003$) when compared with treatment with IFN-α alone.[347] Major cytogenetic responses were observed 12 months after randomization in 126 of 311 patients treated with combination therapy (41%) compared with 75 of 314 patients with IFN-α alone (24%; $p<0.001$).

The recent introduction of imatinib (STI571, Gleevec/Glivec) has transformed the results of non-transplant therapy for CML. In newly diagnosed patients with CML, imatinib has been reported to induce complete cytogenetic remissions in 68% of patients.[348] Most patients who achieve complete cytogenetic remission remain PCR-positive for the BCR–ABL transcript, which suggests that imatinib is probably not curative. However, the reported incidence of progression to accelerated or blastic phase in these imatinib-treated patients was only 1.5% at 1 year. These exciting results have made the decision on which patients should proceed to allogeneic BMT more difficult. The lack of long-term follow-up in imatinib-treated patients at present only makes this decision more problematic.

Although imatinib has dramatically improved the response rates in patients with CML, at present, only allogeneic BMT has induced extended *disease-free* survival or cure for a significant proportion of patients, dependent on the phase of disease at BMT. Long-term survival rates ranging from 50% to 60% in multicenter studies and from 70% to 90% in single-institution trials have been achieved in patients transplanted in first chronic phase.[6,338–340] A retrospective study by the IBMTR, evaluating survival in patients given an HLA-matched sibling BMT versus hydrox-yurea or IFN-α therapy, has demonstrated at least a 7-year survival advantage in recipients of BMT.[349] In patients transplanted in later stages of CML, eradication of disease with BMT has been less successful. Long-term DFS has been achieved in 10–40% of patients transplanted in accelerated phase and 10–20% of those transplanted in blast crisis.[350,351]

Multiple factors have been analyzed to determine their effect on disease recurrence and non-leukemic mortality following a transplant for CML. Disease status at the time of transplant and time from diagnosis to transplant are viewed as significant predictors of subsequent relapse and survival.[352–354] In the three largest series reported to date,[178,354,355] patients transplanted in first chronic phase had a 5–30% probability of relapse, while those transplanted in accelerated phase had a 40% probability and patients transplanted while in blast crisis had a 60–80% probability.[356] The type and intensity of cytoreduction used to prepare patients may also affect post-transplant relapse rates. While the overall results of transplants administered after TBI and cyclophosphamide or conventionally dosed busulfan and cyclophosphamide are not significantly different,[6] a study from the Fred Hutchinson Cancer Research Center[357] demonstrated that higher steady-state plasma busulfan levels were associated with a statistically significant reduction in the cumulative incidence of relapse. Non-relapse mortality appears to be influenced by various other factors. Timing between diagnosis and transplant appears to have a significant impact on non-relapse mortality. An early study from the Fred Hutchinson Cancer Research Center[354] demonstrated a statistically significant advantage in actuarial survival for patients transplanted within the first 17 months from diagnosis compared with those transplanted beyond 17 months: 73% versus 54%, respectively. Their more recent results suggest that this difference is significant only when the transplant is delayed beyond 2 years from diagnosis.[338] A report from the IBMTR[340] demonstrated that chronic phase patients transplanted 1 year or less from diagnosis have significantly lower regimen-related mortality

and relapse rates, resulting in a significantly higher overall DFS compared with patients transplanted later than 1 year from diagnosis. These analyses are important for assessing the optimal timing for transplant in view of recent data regarding the efficacy of imatinib in the treatment of patients with CML. Identification of variables such as Sokal score that predict response to imatinib would greatly facilitate the selection of treatment options. At this time, many oncologists are questioning the role of allogeneic BMT as the first-line treatment of patients with newly diagnosed CML. Randomized trials comparing results of transplants administered early after diagnosis versus imatinib treatment will be required in these patient populations to resolve this issue.

The type of chemotherapy used prior to transplant also affects transplant results. The IBMTR found significantly lower disease-free and overall survival rates in the group of patients who had been treated with busulfan compared with hydroxyurea,[355] which was directly related to a significantly higher non-leukemic mortality in the busulfan-treated group. In a multivariate analysis of these results, both pre-transplant treatment and time to treatment were found to be independent predictors of outcome. On the other hand, T-cell-depleted marrow transplants that are effective in reducing or eliminating acute and chronic forms of GVHD are associated with a marked increase in the incidence of post-transplant relapse.[163,186,187] Indeed, relapse rates of 50–60% have been recorded among recipients of T-cell-depleted grafts,[163,186,187] compared with rates of 5–30% in recipients of unmodified marrow grafts.[6,358] Prior treatment with busulfan had a negative impact on transplant outcome, regardless of the time to transplant – presumably owing to the additional host toxicity induced by cumulative exposure to this drug. This study suggests that treatment with busulfan should be avoided in patients who are likely to undergo allogeneic BMT.

The presence or absence of acute and/or chronic GVHD can also impact significantly on the outcome of transplants for patients with CML. Although moderate to severe forms of acute GVHD can have a negative impact on overall survival (35% at 4 years in patients with moderate to severe acute GVHD, versus 74% in those with no or mild acute GVHD),[170] the development of GVHD is associated with a lower relapse rate – the so-called 'graft-versus-leukemia' (GVL) phenomenon. Indeed, an inverse correlation exists between the severity of acute GVHD and the incidence of relapse.[359] There is also a lower risk of relapse in patients who develop do novo chronic GVHD.[185]

As previously discussed, direct evidence of a GVL effect has been provided by numerous studies demonstrating the efficacy of donor leukocyte infusions for the induction of complete hematologic, cytogenetic, and molecular remissions in patients with CML relapsing post BMT.[188–198,360] The probability of attaining a molecular remission has been reported to be as high as 90% in patients who have received donor leukocyte infusions in cytogenetic or molecular relapse, compared with 70% for patients treated in hematologic chronic phase and 40% (n=20) for patients relapsing in accelerated phase (p=0.009).

Because of the striking results achieved with donor leukocyte infusions, several transplant groups have begun to re-evaluate T-cell-depleted transplants used in combination with post-transplant donor leukocytes to prevent and/or treat disease recurrence post allogeneic BMT as an approach for reducing non-leukemic mortality in older patients and patients who have received prolonged therapy prior to referral for transplant. Although several early studies demonstrated that T-cell-depleted transplants for CML are associated with high relapse rates, T-cell depletion reduces both the incidence and severity of acute and, in some cases, chronic GVHD, leading to decreased peritransplant morbidity and mortality, particularly in older patients.[178,339] A strategy currently under investigation in these 'older' patients is T-cell-depleted BMT followed by prophylactic or therapeutic donor leukocyte infusions 9–12 months post transplant, when the dose of T cells required to induce GVHD is higher. This strategy is particularly practical in patients with CML, because most relapses occur later than 6 months post transplant, and can be detected early by molecular techniques.[361,362] Studies have shown that repeated tests detecting BCR–ABL mRNA transcripts by PCR-amplified assays in the blood or marrow of patients post transplant is highly predictive of subsequent clinical relapse.[362] Ongoing studies are currently examining this approach for the treatment of CML.

# Myelodysplastic syndromes

The myelodysplastic syndromes (MDS; see Chapter 40) are a heterogeneous group of clonal hematologic disorders characterized by peripheral cytopenias and normal to increased marrow cellularity. In over 70% of cases, clonal cytogenetic abnormalities are observed, particularly single deletions of 5q, monosomy 7, and trisomy 8. According to the French–American–British (FAB) classification, five categories of MDS have been described, based on the percentage of blast cells in the marrow or blood, the presence of Auer rods in myelogenous precursors, and the presence of ringed sideroblasts (see Chapter 40): these include refractory anemia (RA), refractory anemia with ringed sideroblasts (RARS), refractory anemia with excess blasts (RAEB), refractory anemia with excess blasts in transformation (RAEB-t) and chronic myelomonocytic leukemia (CMML).[363] A sub-

group of patients exhibiting 'hypoplastic MDS' characterized by a hypocellular bone marrow with dysplastic features has been described.[364] Hypoplastic MDS is often confused with aplastic anemia (AA), particularly when there are no cytogenetic abnormalities or overt dysplastic features. As idiopathic myelofibrosis is often included in studies evaluating transplantation in patients with MDS, despite it being a myeloproliferative disorder, this discussion will include patients with this disorder (see also Chapter 42).

For patients lacking an HLA-matched donor, particularly older adults, treatment is primarily supportive. Intensive chemotherapeutic regimens have yielded only short-term remissions, and have been associated with significant morbidity and mortality.[365] Although certain subgroups of patients may respond to treatment with danazol, oxymethalone,[366] low-dose cytarabine,[367] azacytidine,[368] and supportive measures, such as the use of G-CSF or granulocyte–macrophage colony-stimulating factor (GM-CSF) to induce production of mature neutrophils[369,370] and/or erythropoietin to stimulate red cell production, these strategies have failed to produce sustained complete remissions in the majority of patients.

In contrast to these results, allogeneic BMT administered to patients prepared with TBI or busulfan and cyclophosphamide have led to sustained remissions of disease in approximately 30–73% of cases, depending on the disease status at the time of transplant.[371–375] Accumulated experience suggests that patients transplanted for RA or RARS enjoy better prospects for DFS (53–73%) than patients with RAEB (20–38%) or RAEB-t (14–27%). This difference reflects the extremely low incidence of disease relapse among patients transplanted for RA or RARS (0–6%), which contrasts with the high relapse rates (45–61%) associated with transplants for RAEB or RAEB-t.[371,372] A 10-year retrospective analysis of factors influencing the outcome of 71 consecutive recipients of an allogeneic transplant for the treatment of MDS demonstrated that younger age (less than 37 years), favorable FAB classification (i.e. RA), lack of prior chemotherapy before BMT, and cytoreduction with TBI and cyclophosphamide were significantly associated with better outcome.[376] Because of the improved outcome of transplantation for RA, new strategies are now being explored for the treatment of patients with RAEB and RAEB-t that either intensify the pretransplant cytoreductive regimen[377] or attempt to induce less than 5% blasts with intensive chemotherapy prior to proceeding to transplant.[372] These strategies are based on the hypothesis that reduction or elimination of blasts or cytogenetic evidence of disease prior to transplant may reduce the incidence of post-transplant relapse. However, these strategies will be successful only if peritransplant mortality is not increased by the more intensive therapy.

Cumulative evidence derived from single-patient reports indicates that patients treated with HLA-matched BMT for severe myelofibrosis and malignant myelosclerosis, once engrafted, may recover normal hematopoiesis and achieve complete resolution of fibrosis with sustained DFS.[378,379] However, the presence of marrow fibrosis may be associated with a delay in engraftment and with graft rejection.[371] Experience with BMT for this group of patients remains too limited to provide a meaningful probability of DFS.

## Lymphomas

Approximately 50% of adults and over 70% of children with intermediate and high-grade NHL will be cured by current dose-intensive multi-agent chemotherapy (see Chapter 36). Similarly, primary treatment of Hodgkin's disease is now curative for over 70% of cases (see Chapter 35). In view of these results, BMT has largely been reserved for patients who fail to attain or sustain a primary remission.

Although experience with allogeneic BMT for the treatment of NHL is fairly limited,[380] studies indicate that disease status at transplant as well as sensitivity to prior chemotherapy are the most important prognostic indicators of long-term DFS. Whereas patients with chemotherapy-refractory disease have only a 10–23% probability of extended DFS when treated with chemotherapy,[381–383] 25–44% of those transplanted in second remission and 88% of those transplanted in first remission have experienced long-term DFS.[384,385] To date, four published studies (three retrospective and one prospective) have comparatively addressed the relative merits of allogeneic BMT versus autologous BMT for adults with NHL, and have yielded conflicting results. In retrospective analyses, the probabilities of disease progression were not different for the allograft and autograft recipients in the Seattle series,[386] they were lower in allograft recipients in the Johns Hopkins series,[8] and they were lower only in allograft recipients with lymphoblastic lymphoma in the EBMT Registry series.[7] In the one study that demonstrated a lower rate of disease progression in allograft recipients, the overall progression-free survival was not significantly different in the allogeneic versus autologous BMT recipients – primarily because of GVHD complications in the allograft recipients.[7]

Evidence of an allogeneic graft-versus-lymphoma effect has been provided by a prospective comparative trial of allogeneic versus autologous BMT.[384] The progression-free survival rate was 24% in the autologous transplant group and 46% in the allogeneic transplant cohort at 2 years – a difference that was not statistically significant. However, the differing probabilities of disease progression (69% in the autologous group and 20% in the allogeneic group) were statistically significant. This distinction was seen both in patients with chemosensitive disease (60% versus 18%) and in those with chemoresistant disease (87% versus 18%). Disease progression was the cause of death in 82% of the autograft recipients but in only 25% of the allograft recipients. The allograft arm, however, had a significantly higher rate of non-relapse deaths – most commonly attributable to infection in the context of GVHD. Of the allograft recipients, 52% developed acute and 35% chronic GVHD respectively. Multivariate analysis revealed that the probability of relapse was lower in patients with chemosensitive disease and in patients receiving an allograft. While this study supports the notion that allogeneic BMT may contribute to a reduced risk of post-transplant relapse, this study and the Johns Hopkins trial[8] have also documented high allotransplant-related mortality rates, which have essentially eliminated any improvement in survival or DFS rates in the allogeneic BMT recipients.

Stem cell transplantation has been applied to children with NHL only after they have failed chemotherapy alone. For these patients, the use of allogeneic versus autologous transplantation depends on the quality of autologous marrow or PBSC that can be collected and the availability of a donor. Results accrued from the most recently published series of transplants for childhood NHL have documented results similar to those recorded in adults.[8,386–388]

These data indicate that if the allogeneic graft-versus-lymphoma effect could be harnessed without a prohibitive transplant-related mortality, this might result in improved DFS for patients with lymphoma. Recent studies using non-myeloablative or reduced-intensity conditioning regimens have demonstrated a marked reduction in mortality rates; however; longer follow-up will be needed to assess the ultimate relapse rates and DSF.

## Multiple myeloma

Until recently, therapy for multiple myeloma (see Chapter 34) has been limited to combination chemotherapy with or without IFN-α.[389–391] Although response rates of 40–70% have been achieved with a variety of different regimens, the median event-free survival is still only 3 years.[391,392] In view of the results of conventional chemotherapy and IFN-α, the use of more intensive, myeloablative chemotherapy regimens followed by allogeneic or autologous hematopoietic stem cell grafts is being explored.[393–395] Although several hundred patients have been treated with such transplants, relapse following autologous stem cell transplantation and transplant-related mortality following allogeneic BMT have remained major obstacles.[396,397]

Overall success rates with either approach have been modest. The 3-year survival rates at different stages of disease currently range from 30% to 60%.[398,399] The EBMT revealed overall survival rates of 32% at 4 years and 28% at 7 years for allograft recipients following TBI and intensive chemotherapy or high-dose chemotherapy alone.[399] The relapse-free survival rate for those patients rendered disease-free post BMT was 34% at 6 years. Favorable pretransplant prognostic factors that predicted a better outcome post transplant included female sex, stage I disease at diagnosis, one course of previous treatment, and the achievement of a complete remission before pretransplant conditioning. In addition, low levels of $\beta_2$-microglobulin and the diagnosis of IgA myeloma predicted a better outcome. Following transplant, only the attainment of a complete remission predicted improved transplant outcome. A comparison between 24 patients with myeloma treated with allogeneic BMT and a similarly treated group of patients treated with an autologous PBSCT[400] revealed no significant differences in event-free survival (median 16.7 for autologous PBSCT versus 31 months for allogeneic BMT; $p=0.8$). Transplant-related mortality was 12.5% in the autologous PBSCT recipients versus 25% for the allogeneic BMT group.

Cumulative results derived from single case reports and small published series have suggested that an allogeneic graft-versus-myeloma effect exists similar to that seen in CML. Vesole et al[401] were the first to report a marked tumor reduction after donor leukocyte infusions in patients with relapsed or persistent multiple myeloma following a marrow allograft. In a retrospective study by Lokhurst et al[402] of 13 consecutive recipients of donor leukocyte infusions administered for relapsed multiple myeloma post transplant, 4 achieved a partial remission and 4 a complete remission. Responses were observed at a median of 6 weeks (range 4–10 weeks). In this retrospective study, the only predictors of response were infusion of at least $10^8$cells/kg, and induction of overt GVHD.[401] Using a different approach, Kwak et al[403] succeeded in transferring myeloma idiotype-specific immunity from an actively immunized marrow donor, and hypothesized that this myeloma-specific form of adoptive cell therapy may also be used to enhance the antimyeloma effect of the allogeneic graft.

These developments in the treatment of multiple myeloma are promising. Translation to improved DFS will depend upon better selection of patients likely to benefit from this intensive approach, introduction of transplant earlier in the disease, and the development of better-tolerated transplant regimens. As in the case of lymphoma, one option is to employ the well-tolerated, less-intensive, non-myeloablative preparative regimen that can now be used with allogeneic PBSCT to secure durable engraftment.

# BMT for patients lacking an HLA-identical sibling donor

Over the last 15 years, there has been an enormous expansion in the use of allogeneic stem cell transplants from HLA partially mismatched related donors as well as from HLA-matched unrelated marrow or cord blood donors for the treatment of patients lacking an HLA-matched sibling. Experience with these transplants has also engendered several improvements in tissue typing and donor selection as well as new approaches to infection prophylaxis and supportive care, which have resulted in a limited but encouraging improvement in overall results. Thus, while the DFS rate for good-risk patients reported by the National Marrow Donor Program in 1993 was only 43%, several centers have recently reported 50–70% event-free survival rates for young adults and children with acute leukemias transplanted from early remission and first-chronic-phase CML. Similarly, unrelated cord blood transplants have been associated with a 40–50% DFS rate in good-risk patients.[404–406] In this section, we shall briefly review the current status of these different transplant approaches in the treatment of patients lacking a matched sibling donor.

## Unmodified marrow grafts from partially matched related donors

Ever since the first recognition of the importance of the HLA system in the definition of histocompatibility for BMT, multiple groups have explored the use of HLA partially matched related donors in an attempt to identify tolerable histoincompatibilities within the HLA region. The early studies focused on the use of HLA-haplotype-identical but MLC-compatible related donors because of murine models that had indicated that transplantation from MHC class II disparate donors were most likely to result in lethal GVHD.[407] Initial studies, conducted in children with SCID, supported this approach to donor selection, since allodisparities for HLA-A and/or -B on one haplotype were tolerated without lethal GVHD.[408,409] In a review of 10 such transplants,[410] 8 patients developed GVHD, which was severe in only 2. Five of these patients, however, died of infection less than 100 days post BMT, precluding an assessment of the incidence or severity of chronic GVHD. Of three patients who received HLA-D-incompatible marrow, none survived long enough to assess GVH reactions. Patients with SCID transplanted from donors HLA-disparate for both class I and class II determinants had a poor outcome. Of 19 evaluable patients, 3 had graft failure and 10 developed severe, fatal GVHD – none survived.

Experience with partially matched related donor marrow grafts in patients with aplastic anemia underscores the incremental risk of graft rejection when HLA-disparate grafts are administered to immunocompetent hosts, even after intensive treatment with immunosuppressive agents. In one large series of patients cytoreduced with cyclophosphamide alone, HLA-phenotypically matched non-sibling donor transplants were associated with consistent engraftment, while 7 or 11 grafts from one-HLA-locus-disparate donors and 3 of 3 transplants from two-locus-disparate donors were rejected.[411] Of the 13 patients who achieved sustained engraftment, grade II–IV GVHD was observed in 5 of 8 phenotypically matched and all 4 single-HLA-allele-disparate recipients.

In 1985, Beatty et al[412] reported that 75% of leukemic patients who received a one-antigen-mismatched related transplant following preparation with TBI and cyclophosphamide developed grade II–IV GVHD. However, the long-term DFS was similar to that observed following HLA-matched sibling BMT. In this series, no single allelic disparity (i.e. HLA-A, or -B, or -D) could be identified that resulted in a greater risk of severe GVHD. Subsequent studies on an expanded patient population from the same group, however, have modified this definition of tolerable incompatibilities in that donor–recipient pairs differing for HLA class II alleles on one haplotype have experienced a higher incidence of severe GVHD.[413] Graft rejections were observed in up to 9% of these single-HLA-allele-disparate transplants – an incidence higher than the less than 1% incidence of graft failure following an HLA-matched sibling graft. Transplants for leukemia from related donors differing at more than one HLA allele on the unshared haplotype had a 21% incidence of graft rejection and an 80–85% incidence of severe acute and chronic GVHD. In this latter group of patients, the overall survival rate was markedly inferior (<15%) to that observed following HLA-phenotypically matched or single-HLA-allele-disparate marrow transplants (40–45%). These data indicated that engraftment of unmodified bone marrow from a donor exhibiting unique HLA disparities requires a higher degree of pretransplant immunosuppression than that provided by TBI and cyclophosphamide in order to ensure consistent engraftment. In addition, such transplants were associated with a significantly higher incidence of severe acute and chronic GVHD. The complications of HLA-A or HLA-B single-allele-disparate marrow grafts – at least in patients transplanted for leukemia – are tolerable and may be associated with long-term DFS rates comparable to those achieved following HLA-matched sibling grafts.

## Transplants of unmodified marrow from unrelated donors

In 1977, the successful reconstitution of immunologic function in a child with SCID transplanted with marrow from an HLA-compatible unrelated donor was reported by our group.[414] Subsequent reports demonstrated that transplants from unrelated donors could restore hematopoiesis in patients with leukemia and aplastic anemia.[415,416] In 1988, the results of 40 patients with refractory forms of leukemia and aplastic anemia who received marrow grafts from unrelated, HLA-matched or partially mismatched donors obtained from a statewide registry developed in Iowa were reported.[416] Of these patients, 15% survived disease-free for longer than 1 year post transplant, albeit with severe acute GVHD in 67% of patients and chronic GVHD in all but one case. Although consistent engraftment was observed in leukemic patients prepared with TBI and cyclophosphamide, two out of four patients with aplastic anemia experienced graft failures despite cytoreduction with total lymphoid irradiation and cyclophosphamide.[416] Of five patients with aplastic anemia reported by Gajewski et al,[417] one suffered graft failure after preparation with total lymphoid irradiation and cyclophosphamide. These early experiences indicated an increased risk of both GVHD and graft failure following unrelated BMT.

Early results of unrelated BMT for the treatment of CML were more encouraging. In one study, 102 patients with CML received an unrelated transplant at one of four centers, 29% of whom experienced extended DFS.[418] In this series, those patients who received serologically matched unrelated transplants achieved a somewhat better long-term DFS (39%) than those transplanted from single-antigen-disparate unrelated donors (27%). Eighty percent of recipients of an unmodified unrelated graft in this series developed severe GVHD. In this series, although T-cell-depleted marrow transplantation was associated with less severe GVHD, long-term DFS was comparable to that observed following unmodified marrow transplants. In a subsequent report from Seattle of 52 patients with leukemia who received serologically matched unrelated marrow,[419] the incidence of grade II–IV acute GVHD was 79%, compared with 36% for patients transplanted from HLA-matched siblings. This incidence of grade II–IV GVHD is comparable to that seen following transplants of marrow from one- or two-HLA-allele-disparate related donors.[420]

Kernan et al[421] analyzed the initial 462 recipients of an unrelated BMT reported by the National Marrow Donor Program. Of these patients, 352 were transplants for leukemia, 38 for MDS or lymphomas, and 72 for non-malignant disorders, such as aplastic anemia and congenital disorders of immunity or metabolism. In this series, early or late graft failures were observed in 14% of cases, grade II–IV acute GVHD in

64% of cases, and grade III–IV acute GVHD in 47% of cases.[421] The incidence of severe grade III–IV acute GVHD was significantly increased among recipients of non-T-cell-depleted marrow grafts (60%) when compared with recipients of T-cell-depleted marrow (30%). Limited or extensive chronic GVHD was observed in 55% of patients – particularly among recipients of unmodified, marrow grafts. Despite the increased incidence of graft failure and severe acute and chronic GVHD, the DFS rate in good-risk patients was approximately 40%. However, for patients with advanced leukemias, the DFS rate was 20% or less. Similarly, patients with MDS or aplastic anemia had 18% and 29% DFS rates, respectively. A detailed analysis of the 196 patients with CML transplanted in this series[421] was subsequently reported,[422] demonstrating a two-year DFS rate of 45% for patients in first chronic phase transplanted within 1 year of diagnosis. For patients transplanted later than 1 year from diagnosis, a 36% DFS rate was observed.

As experience with matched unrelated BMT has increased, the results of these transplants have continued to improve. This progress probably reflects, in part, the introduction of molecular typing for HLA class II determinants, which has improved the selection of histocompatible donors. Recognition of the more profound and prolonged states of immunodeficiencies experienced by recipients of unrelated grafts[423,424] has also led to more aggressive and more extended use of antiviral and antifungal agents for prophylaxis against infections – particularly those due to CMV. In addition, as the follow-up of unrelated marrow grafts has lengthened, a strikingly reduced risk of relapse associated with unrelated donor-derived transplants when used in the treatment of several forms of leukemia, including CML and Ph+ ALL, has become apparent. As a result, DFS rates for adults younger than 50 years transplanted for CML in the first year after diagnosis have improved to up to 74% in the Seattle series.[425] In one series of patients who received an unrelated marrow graft for Ph+ ALL, the 2-year leukemia-free survival rate was 49%[426] – a result that is comparable to or better than results achieved with HLA-matched sibling transplants.[427]

The marked increase in severe acute and chronic GVHD in recipients of HLA-phenotypically matched unrelated marrow probably reflects alloreactions generated against molecular differences in class I and II alleles that can only be detected by more discriminatory molecular tissue typing approaches. Molecular differences at HLA-A, -B, -C as well as class II alleles undoubtedly also contribute to the increased frequency of allocytotoxic T cells generated in mixed lymphocyte cultures between HLA-phenotypically matched unrelated donor–recipient pairs when compared with mixed lymphocyte cultures between HLA-matched siblings.[428] Early studies using molecular typing techniques demonstrated that up to 30% of

HLA serologically matched unrelated donors will differ from their intended recipient by one or two alleles when analyzed by isoelectric focusing.[429,430] Subsequent reports demonstrated that microvariant disparities for class II determinants also occur at significantly increased frequency among HLA serologically matched unrelated donor–recipient pairs and that these disparities have major clinical significance.[144,307] More recent studies have also demonstrated that among HLA-A, -B serologically matched, DRB1 molecularly matched unrelated donor–recipient pairs, 48% will demonstrate at least one microvariant disparity at HLA-A or -B by molecular typing.[431] Differences among HLA-C typing have also been uncovered among HLA-A, -B serologically matched unrelated donor–recipient pairs.[432]

The clinical significance of these molecular disparities is currently under study. In one published report,[433] HLA-C disparities were found to be associated with an increased risk of graft rejection. However, this has not been confirmed in other studies. An increase in severe GVHD has also been reported following BMT from HLA-A or HLA-B singly mismatched unrelated donors.[434,435] Although overall survival was not significantly affected by single HLA-A or HLA-B disparities in young patients, it was markedly reduced among adult single-allele-disparate patients (19–40 years).[435] In addition, Petersdorf et al[436] had reported severe GVHD in 48% of recipients of unmodified HLA-A, -B serologically matched, DRB1-matched unrelated marrow transplants versus 70% among recipients with DRB1 mismatches. Recent reports from the NMDP have suggested that HLA DQ mismatching was the more important than mismatching at other loci in determining the outcome of unrelated transplantation in CML.[437] Other studies have found that mismatching for HLA-A or -C significantly increases the incidence of GVHD, while mismatching at class II was not linked to GVHD.[210] Similarly, there are conflicting reports on the significance of HLA-DP mismatching in the unrelated donor setting.[438–440] In summary, mismatch at the molecular level leads to an increased incidence of GVHD that usually, but not always, impacts adversely on survival. However, which of the HLA alleles are most important for this effect remains controversial and will require further study.

## Allogeneic cord blood transplants from related and unrelated donors

In 1984, Broxmeyer and co-workers first presented data from murine models supporting the possibility that umbilical cord blood might contain sufficient hematopoietic progenitors to reconstitute lethally irradiated allogeneic recipients.[441] This hypothesis was tested clinically in 1989 by Gluckman et al,[442] who reported a successful transplant of a patient with

Fanconi anemia using cord blood derived from an HLA-identical sibling. Subsequently, the number and characteristics of hematopoietic progenitor cells and lymphocytes in human umbilical cord blood have been extensively analyzed.[441,443] These studies have shown that the concentrations of colony-forming units granulocyte–macrophage (CFU-GM) and of colony-forming units granulocyte–erythroid– macrophage–megakaryocyte (CFU-GEMM) are 17- to 28-fold greater in umbilical cord blood than in adult blood,[444–446] and that early CD34+CD38− progenitors in umbilical cord blood have a much greater proliferative potential[447,448] and capacity for self-renewal.[448,449]

Based on these studies, several centers have initiated programs exploring the application of umbilical cord blood transplants derived from either HLA-matched or partially matched related or unrelated donors for the treatment of leukemias, aplastic anemia, and congenital disorders of hematopoiesis and metabolism.[404,450] Furthermore, cord blood banks have now been established at several centers, modelled on the cord blood program established at the New York Blood Center,[451] to provide a source of typed cryopreserved unrelated cord blood grafts for transplant purposes. Certain of these banks now include over 20 000 HLA-typed cord blood specimens, prescreened to exclude the possibility of transmission of congenitally acquired infections. The HLA typings of the cord bloods stored at these banks are now computer-linked with the major marrow donor registries, including the National Marrow Donor Program.

To date, cord blood transplants have been predominantly applied to the treatment of children and adolescents with leukemia, acquired aplastic anemia, or severe congenital cytopenias. This relatively restricted approach has been governed by concerns regarding the capacity of limited numbers of umbilical cord mononuclear cells to engraft in fully grown adults. Many adults have now been successfully engrafted with HLA-matched umbilical cord blood[406] – a fact that has kindled greater interest in the potential of such grafts in older patients. On the other hand,[452] retrospective analyses have supported concerns that low doses of cells place the patient at risk of graft failure. By 1995, it was estimated that over 450 unrelated cord blood transplants had been performed worldwide.[452] Two recent retrospective analyses of centers reporting to the International Cord Blood Registry[452,453] and to EuroCord,[406] coupled with two of the larger single-institution experiences,[405,454] have reported, and can be briefly summarized.

Umbilical cord blood transplants derived from sibling donors have enjoyed considerable success in the treatment of young patients with leukemia and other hematologic diseases. In an analysis of 62 patients transplanted between 1988 and 1995 who were reported to the International Cord Blood Registry and

78 patients (many or most of whom were also reported to the Registry) reported to the EuroCord Registry, cord blood grafts induced durable engraftment and hematopoietic reconstitution in 91% of the patients transplanted. Doses of nucleated cells varied, but median dose estimates in the two series were $3.7 \times 10^7$ and $4.7 \times 10^7$ nucleated cells/kg recipient weight, respectively. In the EuroCord Registry analysis, transplant doses providing less than $3.7 \times 10^6$ nucleated cells/kg were associated with a significantly increased risk of graft failure. Among those engrafted, low cell dose delayed recovery of platelets and, to a varying but lesser degree, neutrophils. The incidence of acute GVHD of grade II–IV severity was only 2% and 9% in the two series for patients receiving HLA-matched or one-HLA-allele-disparate grafts; and only 40–50% in two- or three-HLA-allele-disparate recipients. Survival at 1 year post transplant for the patients reported to the EuroCord Registry was 63% – a result similar to that which might be achieved in a comparable group of young patients transplanted with unmodified marrow.

The results of unrelated HLA-matched or partially compatible cord blood grafts in the two registry series and the single-institution experiences are inferior to those recorded for related cord blood grafts, but they are quite encouraging. The overall incidence of graft failure in recipients of unrelated cord blood grafts is strikingly similar to that recorded for related cord blood grafts (6–7% versus 9%). The risk of graft failure in each series is inversely proportional to cell dose, and increases with greater degrees of HLA disparity. On the other hand, the overall incidence of grade II–IV acute GVHD is much higher (57%), ranging from 33% in HLA-matched hosts to 73% in two- or three-HLA-allele-disparate hosts. Overall, however, the results from each series suggest a lower incidence of severe GVHD following a cord blood graft than a marrow graft for a given level of HLA disparity.

The basis for the apparent reduction in the capacity of a cord blood graft to induce GVHD is still unclear. The proportion of naive T cells is increased in umbilical cord blood relative to adult marrow, but the capacity of these cells to proliferate in response to an allogeneic stimulus is similar.[455,456] However, the effector functions of these T cells may differ in that activated umbilical cord blood T cells produce less inflammatory cytokines such as IL-2 and IL-12, and have less cytolytic activity than their adult T-cell counterparts in marrow allografts.[452,456–458] The NK cells in umbilical cord blood are comparable in number and general function to those detected in adult marrow.[459] Whether the antigen-presenting accessory cells, such as dendritic cells, are comparable in their function is still under study.

The overall results of unrelated cord blood grafts are strikingly inferior to those achieved with matched related cord blood or marrow allografts. In the European Registry,[406] survival at 12 months was 29% versus 63% in recipients of related cord blood grafts. This difference may, in part, reflect the consequences of the higher incidence of severe GVHD in unrelated cord blood transplant recipients. However, a major difference lies in the incidence of lethal infections – particularly infections due to CMV. Such infections may be particularly difficult to reverse when an immunologically naive, CMV-seronegative cord blood graft is transplanted into an unrelated adolescent or adult already harboring a latent infection.

Taken together, the results of unrelated cord blood transplants accrued thus far suggest that such transplants may be comparable to unrelated BMT when applied to children and young adults with leukemia or other lethal hematologic disorders. Such transplants appear to have certain unique advantages over unrelated BMT, including their immediate and enduring availability, their low risk of infection transmission, and their reduced potential to induce severe GVHD. Furthermore, pools of potential cord blood grafts can also be recruited from selected ethnic groups under-represented in existing marrow donor registries. Accurate assignments of donor HLA haplotypes can also be ascertained, since the maternal donors are usually also HLA-typed. On the other hand, these transplants also have several potential limitations in that the doses of progenitor cells and adequately competent alloreactive T cells are limited, which may limit the capacity of umbilical cord blood transplants to achieve engraftment in larger adults – particularly those presensitized to alloantigens by prior transfusion or pregnancy. The recovery of platelets in recipients of such grafts is also often delayed. Furthermore, the immunologic naivete of umbilical cord lymphocytes may preclude a sufficiently rapid and effective response to infection in adolescents and adults harboring latent herpesvirus infections such as CMV. Whether cord blood grafts will be comparable to adult marrow grafts in their capacity to confer enhanced leukemia resistance to the allogeneic host remains to be determined.

## T-cell-depleted HLA non-identical related and HLA-compatible unrelated marrow grafts

The principal limitation to the use of transplants from suitable matched unrelated donors is that such donors are not available for 30–50% of the patients lacking an HLA-matched sibling. Development of more sensitive techniques for the selection of unrelated donors, while important to our understanding of incompatibilities contributing to graft rejection, GVHD, and immunodeficiency, will nevertheless only serve to further restrict the number of patients for whom an 'adequately compatible' donor will be identified. There remains a continuing need to develop

transplant approaches that will result in consistent hematologic and immunologic reconstitution without severe or lethal GVHD when patient and donor are disparate at one more HLA alleles.

The potential of T-cell-depleted transplants from HLA-non-identical donors, including donors who are haplotype-disparate, has been clearly demonstrated when applied to BMT for the correction of SCID. In 1981, our group[460] reported that transplants of HLA-A, -B, -DR haplotype-disparate parental marrow depleted of T cells by agglutination with a soybean lectin followed by rosetting with sheep red blood cells could reconstitute hematopoietic and lymphoid function in children with leukemia or SCID without GVHD. Over the last 20 years, of our series of 55 children with SCID transplanted with HLA-haplotype-disparate parental marrow depleted of T cells by this technique, 74% currently survive with reconstitution of immunity and stable donor T-cell chimerism. In this series, fewer than 10% developed grade I acute GVHD. The actuarial DFS for this group is not different from that observed following unmodified HLA-matched grafts for SCID. Other centers incorporating this and other approaches to T-cell depletion have reported similar results.

Unfortunately, until recently, T-cell-depleted HLA-non-identical BMT for the treatment of leukemia and other acquired and genetic diseases of hematopoiesis was considerably less successful owing to the associated increased risk of graft failure. However, the introduction of more intensive cytoreductive and immunosuppressive regimens and alternative, less-extensive T-cell depletion techniques achieving only a 2.0–2.5 $\log_{10}$ depletion of T cells has reduced the frequency of rejection following transplants of T-cell-depleted marrow from HLA-matched unrelated or HLA-mismatched related donors without unduly increasing the incidence of severe GVHD. For example, in one series of patients transplanted with unrelated donor marrow depleted of T cells with the T10B9 monoclonal antibody plus complement, patients with acute leukemia in early remission or chronic phase CML achieved a 48% extended DFS.[461] In this series, in which a 2 $\log_{10}$ level of T-cell depletion was achieved, HLA-matched unrelated marrow grafts were associated with only a 20% incidence in grade II–IV GVHD. Similarly, in a compendium of unrelated marrow transplant results from four centers in the UK by Howard et al,[462] the incidence of engraftment was comparable to that observed following unmodified BMT. T-cell-depleted grafts in this series, which were associated with a markedly reduced incidence of acute GVHD, were also associated with a significantly improved DFS rate (60% versus 29% at 3 months) – a difference not observed among HLA-matched sibling transplant recipients. In a review of results of marrow grafts from donors identified by the National Marrow Donor Program for the treatment of

CML, McGlave et al[463] found that durable engraftment following T-cell-depleted grafts did not differ from that following unmodified grafts (94% versus 88%), reflecting the use of more effective immunosuppressive cytoreductive regimens for the T-cell-depleted grafts. In addition, the incidence of relapse following a T-cell-depleted unrelated graft (16% at 2 years) did not differ significantly from that observed following an unmodified graft (10% at 2 years). The finding of a low relapse rate following unrelated T-cell-depleted grafts applied to patients with CML stands in striking contrast with the markedly increased incidence of relapse of CML observed following T-cell-depleted grafts derived from matched siblings.[463,464] As a result, T-cell-depleted grafts were associated with a significant improvement in long-term DFS.

Over the last 10 years, the results of T-cell-depleted partially matched related and HLA-compatible unrelated marrow transplants in children have yielded particularly promising results. In 1989, Camitta et al[465] reported that 5 of 10 children with aplastic anemia achieved long-term reconstitution following transplantation of T10B9+C′ T-cell-depleted marrow derived from partially matched related or unrelated matched donors. A subsequent report published by this group in 1996 demonstrated that 15 of 28 (54%) children with aplastic anemia were alive, transfusion-independent, with a median follow-up of 2.75 years (range 1.1–8 years) following a T10B9 T-cell-depleted unrelated BMT. Casper et al[466] reported a 44% extended DFS rate in 50 children with leukemia who received T-cell-depleted (T10B9) unrelated transplants from serologically matched ($n=13$) or mismatched ($n=37$) donors. Similar DFS rates in children following unrelated transplants were reported utilizing both T-cell-depleted and T-cell-replete marrows for the treatment of first chronic phase CML and acute leukemia in early remission.[467,468]

Although HLA-A, -B, -DR haplotype-disparate BMT from related donors, if suitably depleted of T cells, can induce full hematologic and immune reconstitution without GVHD, the high risk of graft rejection in patients other than children with SCID has, until recently, limited its use in patients with leukemia. Over the last 15 years, however, more tolerable, intensive immunosuppressive cytoreductive regimens have been designed, often combining high-dose thiotepa or cytarabine with TBI and cyclophosphamide or fludarabine. In addition, supplementary immunosuppression with ATG, T-cell-specific monoclonal antibodies, and/or high-dose steroids has been employed to eliminate residual host T cells that could mediate immune rejection. These regimens have almost eliminated the risk of graft failure following T-cell-depleted grafts from matched related donors, and have markedly reduced graft rejection following transplants of T-cell-depleted mismatched related and unrelated donors.[469,470] The groups of Reisner et al

and Weissman et al introduced another approach to overcome host resistance, demonstrating[471–474] in murine models that the incidence and quality of engraftment of T-cell-depleted MHC-disparate grafts could be strikingly enhanced by increasing the stem cell dose. Based on these findings, Aversa et al[475] investigated the use of haplo-identical T-cell-depleted bone marrow plus G-CSF-stimulated peripheral blood progenitor cells depleted of T cells by lectin agglutination and rosetting with sheep red blood cells.[476,477] Combining T-cell-depleted bone marrow with G-CSF-stimulated PBSC resulted in a 5- to 10-fold increase in the number of CD34+ progenitor cells transplanted. Patients did not receive any post-transplant GVHD prophylaxis. Of the initial 17 patients transplanted with this technique (most with advanced or refractory leukemia), 16 achieved durable, full hematopoietic reconstitution, with grade III–IV GVHD developing in only one patient.[475] In an effort to reduce peritransplant mortality, this group subsequently substituted fludarabine for cyclophosphamide, in a cytoreductive regimen also including 8 Gy single-fraction TBI, thiotepa, and ATG. In a later series of patients, 54 of 60 patients transplanted achieved sustained engraftment and hematopoietic reconstitution. Twenty-six patients (43%) were alive disease-free 2–22 months (median 8 months) post transplant. Grade II or more GVHD was observed in fewer than 5% of patients, and chronic GVHD in none.

The group of Henslee-Downey et al[478] also reported promising results following partially T-cell-depleted mismatched related donors given cytarabine post transplant for the prevention of GVHD. Using T10B9-depleted bone marrow and cytoreduction with fractionated TBI, cytarabine, and cyclophosphamide, 72 patients received a one- ($n=13$), two- ($n=35$), or three- ($n=24$) HLA-allele mismatched transplant for good-risk ($n=20$) or high-risk ($n=52$) leukemia ($n=66$) or aplastic anemia/MDS ($n=6$). Of the 72 patients, 62 (87%) ultimately achieved durable engraftment and hematopoietic reconstitution. The risk of graft failure for transplants expressing one or two donor-unique HLA alleles was less than 5%; however, it was over 30% for HLA-A, -B, -DR-disparate grafts. The incidence of grade II–IV acute GVHD was low (16%), irrespective of the degree of HLA disparity. Chronic GVHD developed in 17–40 (35%) patients evaluable. The probability of DFS for the whole group was 30%, and was 53% for patients transplanted for acute leukemia in first or second remission or for chronic phase CML (good risk), and 23% for patients with more advanced or refractory disease. As in the Perugia series, infections, and, in the high-risk group, leukemic relapses, constituted the principal causes of death.

Taken together, these studies suggest that T-cell-depleted HLA-haplotype-disparate transplants, which have long been established as an efficacious treatment for SCID, are now becoming increasingly effective for the treatment of patients with leukemia. If these trends continue, this transplant approach should secure the possibility of an allogeneic transplant for almost all patients for whom a transplant is currently recognized as a treatment of choice. In the future, the choice between an unrelated bone marrow or cord blood donor or an HLA-mismatched related T-cell-depleted graft may increasingly be based on the relative ability of each type of stem cell graft to induce durable and complete hematopoietic and immunologic reconstitution as well as resistance to recurrent leukemia.

## Non-myeloablative/reduced-Intensity conditioning regimens for allogeneic transplantation

Conventional allogeneic transplantation for patients with hematological malignancies involve conditioning with high-dose chemotherapy with or without TBI to both eradicate the underlying malignancy and suppress the patient's immune system to prevent graft rejection. The bone marrow or PBSC serve to rescue patients from the lethal stem cell toxicity of the conditioning regimens. Consequently, the conditioning therapy's intensity would be limited only by toxicities to non-marrow organs, such as gut, lung, kidney, heart, and liver. These toxicities have generally restricted allogeneic transplantation to younger, medically fit patients. As the median age at diagnoses of patients with most hematologic malignancies range from 65–70 years, it follows that conventional allogeneic transplantaion benefits only a minority of patients with candidate diseases.

Many hematologic malignancies are not always eradicated by high doses of chemoradiotherapy, and some of the observed cures after allogeneic stem cell transplantation are likely due to immunologic graft-versus-tumor reactions. These observations, together with a better understanding of how to control both host and donor immune cell functions, resulted in a re-evaluation of how to perform allogeneic transplantation. Specifically, instead of relying on tumor eradication through intensive and toxic chemoradiation, the donor's immune cells might be used for that purpose, invoking graft-versus-tumor effects. Removing the high-dose cytotoxic therapy would allow treatment of those patients who are too old or medically infirm to qualify for conventional allogeneic transplantation. Therefore, in general, these regimens are most appropriate for these hematologic malignancies that are susceptible to the GVL effect of donor T cells. The best examples of these are CML, chronic lymphocytic leukemia (CLL), and follicular lymphoma; however, GVL effects have been documented to a lesser extent in myeloma and acute leukemia.[479]

In general, two different types of regimen have emerged. The first is based upon immunosuppressive chemotherapeutic drugs – usually fludarabine in combination with an alkylating agent.[480–484] The other approach is based upon low-dose (2 Gy) TBI with or without fludarabine.[485] A number of regimens have been proposed to reduce the toxicity associated with allogeneic transplantation. As a working definition, a truly non-myeloablative regimen should not eradicate host hematopoiesis and should allow relatively prompt hematopoietic recovery without a transplant. Many of the reduced-toxicity regimens referred to as non-myeloablative that include busufan or melphalan may require a transplant for hematologic recovery, and if the graft is rejected, prolonged aplasia typically occurs. These should be referred to as reduced-intensity regimens.

The major advantage of these regimens is a substantial reduction in transplant-related mortality. This has been achieved by a reduction in regimen-related toxicity, a short duration of neutropenia, and a reduced incidence of acute GVHD in the first few weeks after transplantation. There are also potential disadvantages of using these less intensive regimens. The major disadvantages are relapse of the underlying malignancy and consequent extensive chronic GVHD caused by early discontinuation of immunosuppression or donor leukocyte infusions to promote GVL effects. Inclusion of in vivo Campath-1H as part of the conditioning regimen has been reported to produce a low rate of both acute and chronic GVHD in both sibling and unrelated donor transplantation.

Most studies of non-myeloablative hematopoietic transplantation have been performed in elderly or medically debilitated patients unable to tolerate an ablative preparative regimen. Some studies have included younger patients with standard eligibility criteria; differences in patient selection generally preclude meaningful comparisons among regimens. The MD Anderson group initially evaluated the use of standard-dose purine analog-based chemotherapy as a non-ablative preparative regimen in patients with advanced myeloid leukemias.[486] Giralt et al[487] subsequently reported a study combining melphalan and fludarabine for the treatment of advanced acute leukemia; this is a more myelosuppressive regimen that should be considered a reduced-intensity regimen. It was sufficiently immunosuppressive to allow for engraftment from unrelated donors as well as matched siblings. The additional cytoreduction resulted in improved disease-free survival in AML patients, and suggests that cytoreduction of the malignancy by the preparative regimen has value. Slavin et al[484] reported the use of a reduced-toxicity preparative regimen consisting of busulfan (8 mg/kg), fludarabine, and ATG. Although less toxic than the commonly used ablative preparative regimens, this regimen has been particularly encouraging in CML.

Khouri et al[482,488] reported the use of fludarabine plus cyclophosphamide in 20 patients with indolent lymphoma; 9 patients received rituximab in addition to the chemotherapy. All patients achieved engraftment of donor cells. The cumulative incidence of acute grade II–IV GVHD was 20%. All patients achieved complete remission. None has had a relapse of disease at a median follow-up period of 21 months. The actuarial probability of being alive and in remission at 2 years was 84%. This regimen has been effective in achieving engraftment and its use has been extended to a range of malignancies by a number of investigators. The Seattle group has used minimally toxic conditioning with low-dose (2 Gy) TBI, with postgraft mycophenolate mofetil and cyclosporine to facilitate stable allogeneic engraftment.[485] Forty-five patients with hematologic malignancies, HLA-identical sibling donors, and relative contraindications to conventional stem cell transplantation were reported. Regimen toxicities and myelosuppression were mild, allowing 53% of eligible patients to have entirely outpatient transplantations. Non-fatal graft rejection occurred in 20% of patients. Grade II–III acute GVHD occurred in 47% of patients with sustained engraftment. With a median follow-up of 417 days, the survival rate was 66.7%, the non-relapse mortality rate 6.7%, and the relapse mortality rate 26.7%. Of the patients with sustained engraftment, 53% were in complete remission. Fludarabine has recently been given to some patients receiving this regimen as additional immunosuppression to reduce the incidence of graft rejection.

Allogeneic bone BMT is associated with a high risk of treatment-related mortality in multiple myeloma. Use of a non-ablative preparative regimen may reduce this morbidity while still inducing a graft-versus-myeloma effect. Giralt et al[489] reported results in 22 patients with myeloma who received a reduced-intensity conditioning regimen with fludarabine and melphalan. All patients received unmanipulated grafts from either HLA-matched sibling donors ($n=13$) or matched unrelated donors ($n=9$). Seven patients achieved complete remission. Six patients were alive with a median follow-up of 15 months. The actuarial survival and progression-free survival rates were 30% and 19% at 2 years. Others have reported similar results. This promising approach requires further study. A novel strategy under study in myeloma is the use of tandem autologous and allogeneic transplantation. High-dose therapy with autologous transplantation is initially performed to cytoreduce the malignancy, followed by a non-ablative allogeneic transplant with the goal of eradicating minimal residual disease. The preliminary results of this strategy were recently reported, with a low transplant-related mortality and a high complete remission rate, although follow-up is still limited.[490]

In summary, non-myeloablative or reduced-intensity conditioning regimens allow engraftment and generation of GVL effects. This approach is potentially curative for susceptible malignancies and reduces the risks of treatment-related mortality. This strategy can extend the use of allogeneic transplantation to older patients and those with comorbidities that preclude high-dose chemoradiotherapy. The indications for a non-myeloablative allogeneic transplant versus conventional transplant and non-transplant strategies need to be defined for each target malignancy in controlled clinical trials.

## REFERENCES

1. Nesbit ME, Buckley JD, Feig SA et al. Chemotherapy for induction of remission of childhood acute myeloid leukemia followed by marrow transplantation or multiagent chemotherapy: a report from the Children's Cancer Group. *J Clin Oncol* 1994; **12**: 127.

2. Kersey JH. Fifty years of studies of the biology and therapy of childhood leukemia. *Blood* 1997; **90**: 4243.

3. Storb R, Leisenring W, Anasetti C et al. Long-term follow-up of allogeneic marrow transplants in patients with aplastic anemia conditioned by cyclophosphamide combined with antithymocyte globulin. *Blood* 1997; **89**: 3890.

4. Anderson JE, Appelbaum FR, Storb R. An update on allogeneic marrow transplantation for myelodysplastic syndrome. *Leuk Lymphoma* 1995; **17**: 95–9.

5. O'Reilly RJ, Friedrich W, Small TN. Transplantation approaches for severe combined immunodeficiency disease, Wiskott–Aldrich syndrome, and other lethal genetic disorders. In: Foreman S, Blume K, Thomas ED (eds) *Bone Marrow Transplantation*. Cambridge, MA: Blackwell Scientific, 1994: 849–72.

6. Clift RA, Buckner CD, Thomas ED et al. Marrow transplantation for chronic myeloid leukemia: a randomized study comparing cyclophosphamide and total body irradiation with busulfan and total body irradiation with busulfan and cyclosphosphamide. *Blood* 1994; **84**: 2036–43.

7. Jones RJ, Ambinder RF, Piantadosi S, Santos GW. Evidence of a graft-versus-lymphoma effect associated with allogeneic bone marrow transplantation. *Blood* 1991; **77**: 649–53.

8. Verdonck LF, Dekker AW, Lokhorst HM et al. Allogeneic versus autologous bone marrow transplantation for refractory and recurrent low-grade non-Hodgkin's lymphoma. *Blood* 1997; **90**: 4201–5.

9. Lucarelli G, Giardini C, Angelucci E. Bone marrow transplantation in thalassemia. *Cancer Treat Res* 1997; **77**: 305–15.

10. Billingham RE. The biology of graft-versus-host reactions. *Harvey Lect* 1966–67; **62**: 22.

11. Bach FH, Albertini RJ, Joo P et al. Bone marrow transplantation in a patient with the Wiskott–Aldrich syndrome. *Lancet* 1968; **ii**: 1364–6.

12. Gatti RA, Meuwiissen HJ, Allen HD et al. Immunological reconstitution of sex-linked lymphopenic immunological deficiency. *Lancet* 1968; **ii**: 1366–9.

13. Bodmer WF. HLA 1987. In: Dupont B (ed) *Immunobiology of HLA*, Volume II: *Immunogenetics and Histocompatibility*. New York: Springer-Verlag, 1989: 1–9.

14. White PC. Molecular genetics of the class III region of the HLA complex in immunobiology of HLA. In: Dupont B (ed) *Immunobiology of HLA*, Volume II: *Immunogenetics and Histocompatibility*. New York: Springer-Verlag, 1989: 62–9.

15. Yunis EJ, Amos DB. Three closely linked genetic systems relevant to transplantation. *Proc Natl Acad Sci USA* 1971; **68**: 3031.

16. Sonnenberg FA, Eckman MH, Pauker SG. Bone marrow donor registries: the relation between registry size and probability of finding complete and partial matches. *Blood* 1989; **74**: 2569–78.

17. Anasetti C, Amos D, Beatty PG et al. Effect of HLA compatibility on engraftment of bone marrow transplants in patients with leukaemia or lymphoma. *N Engl J Med* 1989; **320**: 197–204.

18. Beatty PG, Dahlberg S, Mickelson EM et al. Probability of finding HLA-matched unrelated marrow donors. *Transplant Proc* 1988; **45**: 714–18.

19. Cereb N, May P, Lee S et al. Locus-specific amplification of HLA class I genes from genomic DNA: locus-specific sequences in the first and third introns of HLA-A, -B, and -C alleles. *Tissue Antigens* 1995; **45**: 1.

20. Arguello R, Pay AL, McDermott A et al. Complementary strand analysis: a new approach for allelic separation in complex polyallelic genetic systems. *Nucleic Acids Res* 1997; **25**: 2236–8.

21. Fleischhauer K, Kernan NA, O'Reilly RJ et al. Bone marrow allograft rejection by T lymphocytes recognizing a single amino acid difference in HLA-B44. *N Engl J Med* 1990; **323**: 1818–22.

22. Keever CA, Leong N, Cunningham I et al. HLA-B44-directed cytotoxic T cells associated with acute graft-versus-host disease following unrelated bone marrow transplantation. *Bone Marrow Transplant* 1994; **14**: 137–45.

23. Prasad VK, Kernan NA, Heller G et al. DNA typing for HLA-A and -B identifies disparities between patients and unrelated donors matched by HLA-A and -B serology and DRB1. *Blood* 1997; **90**: 562a.

24. Madrigal JH, Scott I, Arguello R et al. Factors influencing the outcome of bone marrow transplants using unrelated donors. *Immunol Rev* 1997; **157**: 153–66.

25. Davis AP, Roopenian DC. Complexity at the mouse minor histocompatibility locus H-4. *Immunogenetics* 1990; **31**: 7.

26. Korngold R, Sprent J. Lethal GVHD across minor H barriers. Nature of the effector cells and of the role of the H-2. *Immunology* 1983; **71**: 5.

27. Marijt WAF, Kernan NA, Diaz-Barrientos T et al. Multiple minor histocompatibility antigen-specific cytotoxic T lymphocyte clones can be generated during graft rejection after HLA-identical bone marrow transplantation. *Bone Marrow Transplant* 1995; **16**: 125–32.

28. Voogt PJ, Fibbe WE, Marijt WAF et al. Rejection of bone marrow graft by recipient-derived cytotoxic T lymphocytes against minor histocompatibility antigens. *Lancet* 1990; **335**: 131–4.

29. Goulmy E. Minor histocompatibility antigens in man and their role in transplantation. *Transplant Rev* 1988; **2**: 29.

30. Goulmy E, Termijtzlen A, Bradley BA, van Rood JJ. Y-antigen killing by T-cells of woman restricted by HLA. *Nature* 1977; **226**: 544–5.

31. Voogt PJ, Goulmy WE, Fibbe WE et al. Minor histocompatibility antigen H-Y is expressed on human hematopoietic progenitor cells. *J Clin Invest* 1988; **82**: 906–12.

32. Flowers MED, Pepe MS, Longton G et al. Previous donor pregnancy as a risk factor for acute graft-versus-host disease in patients with aplastic anaemia treated by allogeneic marrow transplantation. *Br J Haematol* 1990; **74**: 492–6.

33. Kernan NA, Bordignon C, Heller G et al. Graft failure after T-cell-depleted human leukocyte antigen identical marrow transplants for leukemia: I. Analysis of risk factors and results of secondary transplants. *Blood* 1989; **74**: 2227–36.

34. Storb R, Prentice RL, Thomas ED. Treatment of aplastic anemia by marrow transplantation from HLA identical siblings. *J Clin Invest* 1977; **59**: 625–32.

35. Gale RP, Bortin MM, van Bekkum DW et al. Risk factors for acute graft-versus-host disease. *Br J Haematol* 1987; **67**: 397–406.

36. O'Reilly AJ, Affara NA, Simpson E et al. A molecular deletion map of the Y chromosome long arm defining X and autosomal homologous regions and the localisation of the HYA locus to the proximal region of the Yq euchromatin. *Hum Mol Genet* 1992; **1**: 379.

37. Meadows L, Wang W, den Haan JM et al. The HLA-A*0201-restricted H-Y antigen contains a posttranslationally modified cysteine that significantly affects T cell recognition. *Immunity* 1997; **6**: 273–81.

38. Goulmy E. Human minor histocompatibility antigens: new concepts for marrow transplantation and adoptive immunotherapy. *Immunol Rev* 1997; **157**: 125.

39. Goulmy E, Schipper R, Pool JE et al. Mismatches of minor histocompatibility antigens between HLA-identical donors and recipients and the development of graft-versus-host disease after bone marrow transplantation. *N Engl J Med* 1996; **334**: 281.

40. Schreuder GM, Pool J, Blokland E et al. A genetic analysis of human minor histocompatibility antigens demonstrates Mendelian segregation independent of HLA. *Immunogenetics* 1993; **38**: 98–105.

41. deBueger M, Bakker A, van Rood JJ et al. Tissue distribution of human minor histocompatibility antigens: ubiquitous versus restricted tissue distribution indicates heterogeneity among human cytotoxic T lymphocyte-defined non-MHC antigens. *J Immunol* 1992; **149**: 1788–94.

42. den Haan, JMM, Sherman NE, Blokland E et al. Identification of a graft versus host disease-associated human minor histocompatibility antigen. *Science* 1995; **268**: 1476–80.

43. den Haan JM, Meadows LM, Wang W et al. The minor histocompatibility antigen HA-1: a diallelic gene with a single amino acid polymorphism. *Science* 1998; **279**: 1054.

44. Thomas ED, Buckner CD, Rudolph RII et al. Allogeneic marrow grafting for hematologic malignancy using HLA matched donor recipient sibling pairs. *Blood* 1971; **38**: 267–87.

45. Dinsmore R, Kirkpatrick D, Flomenberg N et al. Allogeneic bone marrow transplantation for patients with acute lymphoblastic leukemia. *Blood* 1983; **62**: 381–8.

46. Blume KG, Forman SJ, O'Donnell MR et al. Total body

irradiation and high-dose etoposide: a new preparatory regimen for bone marrow transplantation in patients with advanced hematologic malignancies. *Blood* 1987; **69**: 1015–20.

47. Schmitz N, Gassmann W, Rister M et al. Fractionated total body irradiation and high-dose VP 16-213 followed by allogeneic bone marrow transplantation in advanced leukemias. *Blood* 1988; **72**: 1567–73.

48. Champlin R, Jacobs A, Gale RP et al. High-dose cytarabine in consolidation chemotherapy or with bone marrow transplantation for patients with acute leukemia: preliminary results. *Semin Oncol* 1985; **12**(Suppl 3): 190–5.

49. Gordon BG, Warkentin PI, Strandjord SE et al. Allogeneic bone marrow transplantation for children with acute leukemia: long-term follow-up of patients prepared with high dose cytosine arabinoside and fractionated total body irradiation. *Bone Marrow Transplant* 1997; **20**: 5.

50. Helenglass G, Powles RL, McElwain TJ et al. Melphalan and total body irradiation (TBI) versus cyclophosphamide and TBI as conditioning for allogeneic matched sibling bone marrow transplants for acute myeloblastic leukemia in first remission. *Bone Marrow Transplant* 1988; **3**: 21–9.

51. Aversa F, Terenzi A, Carrotti A et al. Addition of thiotepa improves results in T-cell depleted bone marrow transplant for advanced leukemia. *Blood* 1993; **82**(Suppl 1): 81a.

52. Papadopoulos E, Carabasi M, Young JW et al. Results of T-cell depleted (TCD) allogeneic BMT after TBI, thiotepa and cyclosphosphamide in patients with leukemia. *Blood* 1992; **80**: 170a.

53. Papadopoulos EB, Boulad F, Carabasi MH et al. Improved disease-free survival in recipients of T cell depleted bone marrow allografts for acute non-lymphocytic leukemia in first remission. *Blood* 1994; **84**(Suppl 1): 331a.

54. Estey E, Plunkett W, Gandhi V et al. Fludarabine and ara-binosylcytosine therapy of refractory and relapsed acute myelogenous leukemia. *Leuk Lymphoma* 1993; **9**: 43.

55. Tutschka PJ, Copelan EA, Klein JP. Bone marrow transplantation for leukemia following a new busulfan and cyclophosphamide regimen. *Blood* 1987; **70**: 1382–9.

56. Kapelushnik J, Or R, Slavin S, Nagler A. A fludarabine-based protocol for bone marrow transplantation in Fanconi's anemia. *Bone Marrow Transplant* 1997; **20**: 1109–10.

57. Sheridan WP, Begley CG, Juttner CA et al. Effect of peripheral-blood progenitor cells mobilised by filgrastim (G-CSF) on platelet recovery after high-dose chemotherapy. *Lancet* 1992; **339**: 640–4.

58. Korbling M, Przepiorka D, Huh YO et al. Allogeneic blood stem cell transplantation for refractory leukemia and lymphoma: potential advantage of blood over marrow allografts. *Blood* 1995; **85**: 1659–65.

59. Urbano-Ispizua A, Solano C, Brunet S et al. Allogeneic peripheral blood progenitor cell transplantation: analysis of short-term engraftment and acute GVHD incidence in 33 cases. allo-PBPCT Spanish Group. *Bone Marrow Transplant* 1996; **18**: 35–40.

60. Russell JA, Brown C, Bowen T et al. Allogeneic blood cell transplants for haematological malignancy: preliminary comparison of outcomes with bone marrow transplantation. *Bone Marrow Transplant* 1996; **17**: 703–8.

61. Finke J, Brugger W, Bertz H et al. Allogeneic transplantation of positively selected peripheral blood CD34+ progenitor cells from matched related donors. *Bone Marrow Transplant* 1996; **18**: 1081–6.

62. Ringden O, Remberger M, Runde V et al. Peripheral blood stem cell transplantation from unrelated donors: a comparison with marrow transplantation. *Blood* 1999; **94**: 455–64.

63. Schmitz N, Beksac M, Hasenclever D et al. Transplantation of mobilized peripheral blood cells to HLA-identical siblings with standard-risk leukemia. *Blood* 2002; **100**: 761–7.

64. Bensinger WI, Martin PJ, Storer B et al. Transplantation of bone marrow as compared with peripheral-blood cells from HLA-identical relatives in patients with hematologic cancers. *N Engl J Med* 2001; **344**: 175–81.

65. Heldal D, Tjonnfjord G, Brinch L et al. A randomised study of allogeneic transplantation with stem cells from blood or bone marrow. *Bone Marrow Transplant* 2000; **25**: 1129–36.

66. Powles R, Mehta J, Kulkarni S et al. Allogeneic blood and bone-marrow stem-cell transplantation in haematological malignant diseases: a randomised trial. *Lancet* 2000; **355**: 1231–7.

67. Couban S, Simpson DR, Barnett MJ et al. A randomized multicenter comparison of bone marrow and peripheral blood in recipients of matched sibling allogeneic transplants for myeloid malignancies. *Blood* 2002; **100**: 1525–31.

68. Blaise D, Kuentz M, Fortanier C et al. Randomized trial of bone marrow versus lenograstim-primed blood cell allogeneic transplantation in patients with early-stage leukemia: a report from the Société Française de Greffe de Moelle. *J Clin Oncol* 2000; **18**: 537–46.

69. Champlin RE, Schmitz N, Horowitz MM et al. Blood stem cells compared with bone marrow as a source of hematopoietic cells for allogeneic transplantation. IBMTR Histocompatibility and Stem Cell Sources Working Committee and the European Group for Blood and Marrow Transplantation (EBMT). *Blood* 2000; **95**: 3702–9.

70. Ottinger HD, Beelen DW, Scheulen B et al. Improved immune reconstitution after allotransplantation of peripheral blood stem cells instead of bone marrow. *Blood* 1996; **88**: 2775–9.

71. Anderson KC, Weinstein HJ. Transfusion-associated graft-versus-host disease. *N Engl J Med* 1990; **323**: 315–21.

72. Zaia JA. Viral infections associated with bone marrow transplantation. *Hematol Oncol Clin North Am* 1990; **4**: 603.

73. Locksley RM, Flournoy N, Sullivan KM, Meyers JD. Infection with varicella-zoster virus after marrow transplantation. *J Infect Dis* 1985; **152**: 1172–8.

74. Knox K, Carrigan DR. In vitro suppression of bone marrow progenitor cell differentiation by human herpesvirus 6 infection. *J Infect Dis* 1992; **165**: 925–9.

75. Carrigan DR, Drobyski WR, Russler SK et al. Interstitial pneumonia associated with human herpesvirus 6 after marrow transplantation. *Lancet* 1991; **ii**: 147.

76. Singh N, Carrigan DR. Human herpesvirus-6 in transplantation: an emerging pathogen. *Ann Intern Med* 1996; **124**: 1065.

77. Arthur RR, Shah KV, Baust SJ et al. Association of BK viruria with hemorrhagic cystitis in recipients of bone marrow transplants. *N Engl J Med* 1986; **315**: 230–4.

78. Bedi A, Miller CB, Hanson JL et al. Association of BK virus with failure of prophylaxis against hemorrhagic cystitis. *J Clin Oncol* 1995; **13**: 1103.

79. O'Reilly RJ, Lee FK, Grossbard E et al. Papovavirus excretion following marrow transplantation: incidence and association with hepatic dysfunction. *Transplant Proc* 1981; **13**: 262–6.

80. Yolken RH, Bishop CA, Townsend TR et al. Infectious gastroenteritis in bone-marrow-transplant recipients. *N Engl J Med* 1982; **306**: 1010–12.

81. Troussard X, Bauduer F, Galler E et al. Virus recovery from stools of patients undergoing bone marrow transplantation. *Bone Marrow Transplant* 1993; **12**: 573–6.

82. Ambinder RF, Burns W, Forman M et al. Hermorrhagic cystitis associated with adenovirus infection in bone marrow transplantation. *Arch Intern Med* 1986; **146**: 1400–1.

83. Bruno B, Boeckh M, Davis C et al. Adenovirus infections in patients undergoing bone marrow transplantation. *Blood* 1997; **90**: 420a.

84. Goodman JL, Drew MD, Winston MD et al. A controlled trial of fluconazole to prevent fungal infections in patients undergoing bone marrow transplantation. *N Engl J Med* 1992; **326**: 845–51.

85. Slavin MA, Osborne B, Adams R et al. Efficacy and safety of fluconazole prophylaxis for fungal infections after marrow transplantation – a prospective, randomized, double-blind study. *J Infect Dis* 1995; **171**: 1545–52.

86. Prentice AG, Morgenstern GR, Prentice HG. Fluconazole v itraconazole prophylaxis in neutropenia following therapy for haematological malignancy. *Blood* 1997; **90**: 420a.

87. Wingard JR. Efficiacy of amphotericin B lipid complex injection (ABLC) in bone marrow transplant recipients with life-threatening systemic mycoses. *Bone Marrow Transplant* 1997; **19**: 343–7.

88. Uzun O, Anaissie EJ. Antifungal prophylaxis in patients with hematologic malignancies: a reappraisal. *Blood* 1995; **86**: 2063–72.

89. Saral R, Burns WH, Laskin OL et al. Acyclovir prophylaxis of herpes-simplex-virus infections. A randomized, double-blind, controlled trial in bone marrow transplant recipients. *N Engl J Med* 1981; **305**: 63–7.

90. Selby P, Jameson B, Watson J et al. Parenteral acyclovir for herpes virus infections of man. *Lancet* 1979; **ii**: 1267–70.

91. Ganem G, Giarardin M, Kuentz M et al. Veno-occlusive disease of the liver after allogeneic bone marrow transplantation in man. *Int J Radiat Oncol Biol Phys* 1988; **14**: 879–84.

92. Jones RJ, Lee KS, Beschorner WE et al. Veno-occlusive disease of the liver following bone marrow transplantation. *Transplantation* 1987; **44**: 778–83.

93. McDonald GB, Sharma P, Matthews DE et al. Veno-occlusive disease of the liver after bone marrow transplantation: diagnosis, incidence and predisposing factors. *Hepatology* 1984; **4**: 116–22.

94. Appelbaum FR, Strauchen JA, Graw RG. Acute lethal carditis caused by high-dose combination chemotherapy: a unique clinical and pathological entity. *Lancet* 1976; **i**: 58–65.

95. Gottdiener JS, Appelbaum FR, Ferrans VJ et al. Cardiotoxicity associated with high-dose cyclophosphamide therapy. *Arch Intern Med* 1981; **141**: 758–63.

96. Brugieres L, Hartmann O, Travagli et al. Hemmorrhagic cystitis following high-dose chemotherapy and bone marrow transplantation in children with malignancies: incidence, clinical course and outcome. *J Clin Oncol* 1989; **7**: 194–9.

97. Blacklock H, Ball L, Knight C et al. Experience with mesna in patients receiving allogeneic bone marrow transplants for poor prognostic leukaemia. *Cancer Treat Rev* 1983; **10**(Suppl A): 45–52.

98. Hows JM, Mehta A, Ward L et al. Comparison of mesna with forced diuresis to prevent cyclophosphamide induced haemorrhagic cystitis in marrow transplantation: a prospective randomized study. *Br J Cancer* 1984; **50**: 753–6.

99. Russell SJ, Vowels MR, Vale T. Haemorrhagic cystitis in paediatric bone marrow transplant patients: an association with infective agents, GVHD, and prior cyclophosphamide. *Bone Marrow Transplant* 1994; **13**: 533.

100. Crawford SW, Hackman RC, Clark JG. Open lung biopsy diagnosis of diffuse pulmonary infiltrates after marrow transplantation. *Chest* 1988; **94**: 949–53.

101. Vogler WR, Winton EF, Heffner LT et al. Opthalmological and other toxicities related to cytosine arabinoside and total body irradiation as preparatory regimen for bone marrow transplantation. *Bone Marrow Transplant* 1990; **6**: 405–9.

102. Sparks RS. Cytogenetic analysis in human bone marrow transplantation. *Cancer Genet Cytogenet* 1981; **4**: 345–52.

103. Blazar BR, Orr HT, Arthur DC et al. Restriction fragment length polymorphisms as markers of engraftment in allogeneic marrow transplantation. *Blood* 1985; **66**: 1436–44.

104. Hutchinson RM, Pringle JH, Potter L et al. Rapid identification of donor and recipient cells after allogeneic bone marrow transplantation using specific genetic markers. *Br J Haematol* 1989; **72**: 133–40.

105. Torok-Storb B, Boeckh M, Hoy C et al. Association of specific cytomegalovirus genotypes with death from myelosuppression after marrow transplantation. *Blood* 1997; **90**: 2097–102.

106. Baughan AS, Worsley AM, McCarthy DM et al. Haematological reconstitution and severity of graft-versus-host disease after bone marrow transplantation for chronic granulocytic leukaemia: the influence of previous splenectomy. *Br J Haematol* 1984; **56**: 445–54.

107. Champlin RE, Horowitz MM, van Bekkum DW et al. Graft failure following bone marrow transplantation for severe aplastic anemia: risk factors and treatment results. *Blood* 1989; **73**: 606–13.

108. Storb R, Epstein RB, Rudolph RH, Thomas ED. The effect of prior transfusion on marrow grafts between histocompatible canine siblings. *J Immunol* 1970; **107**: 409–13.

109. Castro-Malaspina H, Childs B, Laver J et al. Hyperfractionated total lymphoid irradiation and cyclophosphamide for preparation of previously transfused patients undergoing HLA-identical marrow transplantation for severe aplastic anemia. *Int J Radiat Oncol Biol Phys* 1994; **29**: 847–54.

110. Storb R, Etzioni R, Anasetti C et al. Cyclophosphamide combined with antithymocyte globulin in preparation for allogeneic marrow transplants in patients with aplastic anemia. *Blood* 1994; **84**: 841–9.

111. Dinsmore R, Kirkpatrick D, Flomenberg N et al. Allogeneic bone marrow transplantation for patients with acute nonlymphocytic leukemia. *Blood* 1984; **63**: 649–56.

112. Reisner Y, Martelli MF. Bone marrow transplantation across HLA barriers by increasing the number of transplanted cells. *Immunol Today* 1995; **16**: 437–40.

113. Donahue J, Homge M, Kernan NA. Characterization of cells emerging at the time of graft failure following bone marrow transplantation from an unrelated marrow donor. *Blood* 1993; **82**: 1023–9.

114. Hale G, Cobbold S, Waldmann H. T-cell depletion with Campath-1 in allogeneic bone marrow transplantation. *Transplantation* 1988; **45**: 753–9.

115. Martin PJ, Hansen JA, Torok-Storb B et al. Graft failure in patients receiving T-cell depleted HLA-identical allogeneic marrow transplants. *Bone Marrow Transplant* 1988; **3**: 345–56.

116. Martin PJ, Hansen JA, Buckner CD et al. Effects of in vitro depletion of T-cells in HLA-identical allogeneic marrow grafts. *Blood* 1985; **66**: 664–72.

117. O'Reilly RJ, Collins NH, Kernan NA et al. Transplantation of marrow depleted of T-cells by soybean lectin agglutination and E-rosette depletion: major histocompatibility complex-related graft resistance in leukemia transplant patients. *Transplant Proc* 1985; **17**: 455–9.

118. Bozdech MJ, Sondel PM, Trigg ME et al. Transplantation of HLA-haploidentical T-cell depleted marrow for leukemia: addition of cytosine arabinoside to the pretransplant conditioning prevents rejection. *Exp Hematol* 1985; **13**: 1201–10.

119. Steilein WJ, Billingham RE. An analysis of graft-versus-host-disease in syrian hamsters. *J Exp Med* 1970; **132**: 163–80.

120. Steinman RM. The dendritic cell system and its role in immunogenicity. *Annu Rev Immunol* 1991; **9**: 271–96.

121. Shlomchik DWD, Couzens MS, Tang CB, Emerson SG. Radioresistant host antigen presenting cells are required for acute graft-vs-host disease induction. *Blood* 1997; **90**(Suppl 1): 396a.

122. Ferrara JL, Guillen FJ, Dijken PJ et al. Evidence that large granular lymphocytes of donor origin mediate acute graft-versus-host disease. *Transplantation* 1989; **47**: 50–4.

123. Xun C, Brown SA, Jennings CD et al. Acute graft-versus-host-like disease induced by transplantation of human activated natural killer cells into SCID mice. *Transplantation* 1993; **56**: 409–17.

124. Piguet PF, Grau GE, Allet B, Vassali P. Tumor necrosis factor/cachectin is an effector of skin and gut lesions of the acute phase of graft-versus-host disease. *J Exp Med* 1987; **166**: 1280–9.

125. Ferrara JL. Cytokine dysregulation as a mechanism of graft versus host disease. *Curr Opin Immunol* 1993; **5**: 794–9.

126. Korngold R, Sprent J. Surface markers of T cells causing lethal graft-vs-host disease to class I vs class II H-2 differences. *J Immunol* 1985; **135**: 3004–10.

127. Sprent J, Schaefer M, Lo D, Korngold R. Properties of purified T cell subsets. II. In vivo responses to class I vs. class II H-2 differences. *J Exp Med* 1986; **163**: 998–1011.

128. Moser M, Sharrow SO, Shearer GM. Role of L3T4⁺ and Lyt-2⁺ donor cells in graft-versus-host immune deficiency induced across a class I, class II, or whole H-2 difference. *J Immunol* 1988; **140**: 2600–8.

129. Korngold R, Sprent J. Variable capacity of L3T4⁺ T cells to cause lethal graft-versus-host disease across minor histocompatibility barriers in mice. *J Exp Med* 1987; **165**: 1552–64.

130. Nimer SD, Giorgi J, Gajewski JL et al. Selective depletion of CD8⁺ cells for prevention of graft-versus-host disease after bone marrow transplantation. A randomized controlled trial. *Transplantation* 1994; **57**: 82–7.

131. Glucksberg H, Storb R, Fefer A et al. Clinical manifestations of GVHD in human recipients of marrow from HLA-matched sibling donors. *Transplantation* 1974; **18**: 295–304.

132. Vogelsang GB, Hess AD, Santos GW. Acute graft-versus-host disease: clinical characteristics in the cyclosporine era. *Medicine* 1988; **67**: 163–74.

133. Witherspoon RP, Lum LG, Storb R. Immunologic reconstitution after human marrow grafting. *Semin Hematol* 1984; **21**: 2–10.

134. Gale RP, Bortin MM, van Bekkum DW et al. Risk factors for acute graft-versus-host disease. *Br J Haematol* 1987; **67**: 397–406.

135. Hill GR, Crawford JM, Cooke KR et al. Total body irradiation and acute graft-versus-host disease: the role of gastrointestinal damage and inflammatory cytokines. *Blood* 1997; **90**: 3204–13.

136. Sullivan KM, Shulman HM, Storb R et al. Chronic graft-versus-host disease in 52 patients: adverse natural course and successful treatment with combination immunosuppression. *Blood* 1981; **57**: 267–76.

137. Holland K, Wingard JR, Beschorner WE et al. Bronchiolitis obliterans after bone marrow transplantation: relationship to chronic graft-versus-host disease and serum IgG. *Blood* 1988; **72**: 621–7.

138. Sullivan KM, Mori M, Witherspoon R et al. Alternating-day cyclosporine and prednisone (CSP/PRED) treatment of chronic graft-vs-host disease (GVHD): predictors of survival. *Blood* 1990; **76**(Suppl 1): 568a.

139. Sheridan JF, Tutschka PJ, Sedmak DD, Copelan EA. Immunoglobulin subclass deficiency and pneumococcal infection after bone marrow transplantation. *Blood* 1990; **75**: 1583–6.

140. Storek J, Saxon A. Reconstitution of B cell immunity following bone marrow transplantation. *Bone Marrow Transplant* 1992; **9**: 395–408.

141. Kennedy MS, Deeg HJ, Storb R et al. Treatment of acute graft-versus-host disease after allogeneic marrow transplantation: randomized study comparing corticosteroids and cyclosporine. *Am J Med* 1985; **78**: 978–83.

142. Martin PJ, Schoch G, Fisher DR et al. A retrospective analysis of therapy for acute graft-versus-host disease: initial treatment. *Blood* 1990; **76**: 1464–72.

143. Anasetti A, Martin PJ, Storb R et al. Treatment of acute graft-versus-host disease with a non-mitogenic anti-CD3 monoclonal antibody. *Transplantation* 1992; **54**: 844–51.

144. Byers VS, Henslee PJ, Kernan NA et al. Use of an anti-pan T-lymphocyte ricin A chain immunotoxin in steroid-resistant acute graft-versus-host disease. *Blood* 1990; **75**: 1426–32.

145. Herbelin C, Stephan J-L, Donadieu J et al. Treatment of steroid-resistant acute graft-versus-host disease with an anti-IL-2 receptor monoclonal antibody (BT 563) in children who received T cell-depleted, partially matched, related bone marrow transplants. *Bone Marrow Transplant* 1994; **13**: 563–9.

146. Sullivan KM, Witherspoon RP, Storb R et al. Alternating day cyclosporine and prednisone for treatment for high risk chronic graft-versus-host disease. *Blood* 1988; **72**: 555–61.

147. Sullivan KM, Witherspoon RP, Storb R et al. Prednisone and azathioprine compared with prednisone and placebo for treatment of chronic graft-versus-host disease: prognostic influence of prolonged thrombocytopenia after allogenic marrow. *Blood* 1988; **72**: 546–54.

148. Eppinger T, Ehninger G, Steinhart M et al. 8-Methoxypsoralen and ultraviolet: a therapy for cutaneous manifestations of graft-versus-host disease. *Transplantation* 1990; **50**: 807–11.

149. Lee SJ, Wegner SA, McGarigle CJ et al. Treatment of chronic graft-versus-host disease with clofazimine. *Blood* 1997; **89**: 2298–302.

150. Socie G, Devergie A, Cosset JM et al. Low-dose (one gray) total-lymphoid irradiation for extensive, drug-resistant chronic graft-versus-host disease. *Transplantation* 1990; **49**: 657–8.

151. Nash RA, Furlong T, Storb R et al. Mycophenolate mofetil (MMF) as salvage treatment for graft-versus-host disease (GVHD) after allogeneic hematopoetic stem cell transplantation. *Blood* 1997; **90**: 105a.

152. Vogelsang GV, Farmer EB, Hess AD et al. Thalidomide for the treatment of chronic graft versus host disease. *N Engl J Med* 1992; **326**: 1055–8.

153. Rabitsch W, Reiter E, Keil F et al. Extracorporeal photopheresis (ECP) in extensive chronic graft versus host disease (GVHD). *Blood* 1997; **90**: 376a.

154. Chao NJ, Parker PM, Niland JC et al. Paradoxical effect of thalidomide prophylaxis on chronic graft-vs.-host disease. *Biol Blood Marrow Transplant* 1996; **2**: 86–92.

155. Storb R, Deeg HJ, Thomas ED et al. Marrow transplantation for chronic myelocytic leukemia: a controlled trial of cyclosporine versus methotrexate for prophylaxis of graft-versus-host disease. *Blood* 1985; **66**: 698–702.

156. Storb R, Deeg HJ, Whitehead J et al. Methotrexate and cyclosporine compared with cyclosporine alone for prophylaxis of acute graft versus host disease after marrow transplantation for leukemia. *N Engl J Med* 1986; **314**: 729–35.

157. Storb R, Pepe M, Deeg HG et al. Long-term follow-up of a controlled trial comparing a combination of methotrexate plus cyclosporine with cyclosporine alone for prophylaxis of graft versus host disease in patients administered HLA-identical marrow grafts for leukemia. *Blood* 1992; **79**: 3091.

158. Nash RA, Antin JH, Karanes C et al. Phase 3 study comparing methotrexate and tacrolimus with methotrexate and cyclosporine for prophylaxis of acute graft-versus-host disease after marrow transplantation from unrelated donors. *Blood* 2000; **96**: 2062–8.

159. Ratanatharathorn V, Nash RA, Przepiorka D et al. Phase III study comparing methotrexate and tacrolimus (Prograf, FK506) with methotrexate and cyclosporine for graft-versus-host disease prophylaxis after HLA-identical sibling bone marrow transplantation. *Blood* 1998; **92**: 2303–14.

160. Granger DK, Cromwell JW, Chen SC et al. Prolongation of renal allograft survival in a large animal model by oral rapamycin monotherapy. *Transplantation* 1995; **59**: 183.

161. Basara N, Blau WI, Römer E et al. Mycophenolate mofetil for the treatment of acute and chronic GVHD in bone marrow transplant patients. *Bone Marrow Transplant* 1998; **22**: 61.

162. Chao NJ, Parker PM, Niland JC et al. Paradoxical effect of thalidomide prophylaxis on chronic graft vs.-host disease. *Biol Blood Marrow Transplant* 1996; **2**: 86–92.

163. O'Reilly RJ, Kernan NA, Cunningham I et al. Allogeneic transplants depleted of T-cells by soybean lectin agglutination and E-rosette depletion. *Bone Marrow Transplant* 1988; **3**: 3–6.

164. Reisner Y, Kapoor N, Kirkpatrick D et al. Transplantation for severe combined immunodeficiency with HLA-A,B,DR incompatible parental marrow fractionated by soybean agglutin and sheep red blood cells. *Blood* 1983; **61**: 341–8.

165. Hale G, Cobbold S, Waldmann H. T-cell depletion with Campath-1 in allogeneic bone marrow transplantation. *Transplant* 1988; **45**: 753–9.

166. Ash RC, Casper JT, Chitambar CR et al. Successful allogeneic transplantation of T-cell depleted bone marrow from closely HLA-matched unrelated donors. *N Engl J Med* 1990; **322**: 485–94.

167. Martin PJ, Hansen JA, Buckner CD et al. Effects of in vitro depletion of T cells in HLA-identical allogeneic marrow grafts. *Blood* 1985; **66**: 664–72.

168. Racadot E, Herve P, Beaujean F et al. Prevention of graft-versus-host disease in HLA-matched bone marrow transplantation for malignant disease: a multicentric study of 62 patients using 3 pan-T monoclonal antibodies and rabbit complement. *J Clin Oncol* 1987; **5**: 426–35.

169. Filipovich AH, Vallera DA, Youle RJ et al. Graft-versus-host disease prevention in allogeneic bone marrow transplantation from histocompatible siblings. *Transplantation* 1987; **44**: 62–9.

170. O'Reilly RJ, Carabasi MH, Collins NH et al. T-cell depletion and allogeneic bone marrow transplantation. *Semin Hematol* 1992; **29**: 20–6.

171. Vartdal F, Albrechtsen D, Ringden O et al. Immunomagnetic treatment of bone marrow allografts. *Bone Marrow Transplant* 1987; **2**(Suppl 2): 94.

172. DiPersio J, Martin B, Abboud C et al. Allogeneic BMT using bone marrow and CD34-selected mobilized PBSC; comparison to BM alone and mobilized PBSC alone. *Blood* 1994; **84**(Suppl 1): 91a.

173. Wagner JE, Santos GW, Noga SJ. Bone marrow graft engineering by counterflow contrifugal elutriation: results of a phase I–II clinical trial. *Blood* 1990; **75**: 1370–7.

174. Frame J, Collins NH, Cartagena T et al. T-cell depletion of human bone marrow: comparison of Campath-1 plus complement, anti-T-cell ricin A chain immunotoxin and soybean agglutin alone or in combination with sheep erythrocytes or immunomagnetic beads. *Transplantation* 1989; **47**: 984–8.

175. Kernan NA, Collins NH, Juliano I et al. Clonable T-lymphocytes in T-cell depleted bone marrow transplants correlate with development of graft-versus-host disease. *Blood* 1986; **68**: 770–3.

176. Soiffer RJ, Mauch P, Fairclough D et al. CD6+ T cell depleted allogeneic bone marrow transplantation from genotypically HLA nonindientical related donors. *Biol Blood Marrow Transplant* 1997; **3**: 11–17.

177. Gratwohl A, Hermans J, Niederwieser D et al. Bone marrow transplantation for chronic myeloid leukemia: long term results. *Bone Marrow Transplant* 1993; **12**: 509–16.

178. Goldman JM, Gale RP, Horowitz MM et al. Bone marrow transplantation for chronic myelogenous leukemia in chronic phase: increased risk for relapse associated with T-cell depletion. *Ann Intern Med* 1988; **108**: 806–14.

179. Hale G, Waldmann H. Campath-1 for prevention of graft-versus-host disease and graft rejection. Summary of results from a multi-centre study. *Bone Marrow Transplant* 1988; **3**: 11–14.

180. Antin JH, Bierer BE, Smith BR et al. Selective depletion of bone marrow T-lymphocytes with anti-CD5 monoclonal antibodies: effective prophylaxis for graft-versus-host disease in patients with hematologic malignancies. *Blood* 1991; **78**: 2139–49.

181. Soiffer RJ, Fairclough D, Robertson M et al. CD6-depleted allogeneic bone marrow transplantation for acute

leukemia in first complete remission. *Blood* 1997; **89:** 3039–47.

182. Papadopoulos EB, Carabasi MH, Castro-Malaspina H et al. T-cell-depleted allogeneic bone marrow transplantation as postremission therapy for acute myelogenous leukemia: freedom from relapse in the absence of graft-versus-host disease. *Blood* 1998; **91:** 1083.

183. Gale R, Champlin R. How does bone marrow transplantation cure leukaemia? *Lancet* 1984; **ii:** 28–30.

184. Weiden PL, Flournoy N, Thomas ED et al. Antileukemic effects of graft versus host disease in human recipients of allogeneic marrow grafts. *N Engl J Med* 1979; **300:** 1068–73.

185. Horowitz MM, Gale RP, Sondel PM et al. Graft versus leukemia reactions after bone marrow transplantation. *Blood* 1990; **75:** 555–62.

186. Marmont AM, Gale RP, Butturini A et al. T-cell depletion in allogeneic bone marrow transplantation: progress and problems. *Haematologica* 1989; **74:** 235–48.

187. Falkenburg JHF, Goselink HM, Van der Harst D et al. Growth inhibition of clonogenic leukemic precursor cells by minor histocompatability antigen-specific cytotoxic T-lymphocytes. *J Exp Med* 1991; **174:** 27–33.

188. Kolb HJ, Mittermuller J, Clemm CH et al. Donor leukocyte transfusions for treatment of recurrent chronic myelogenous leukemia in marrow transplant patients. *Blood* 1990; **76:** 2462–5.

189. Bar B, Schattenberg A, Mensink EJBM et al. Donor leukocyte infusions for chronic myeloid leukemia relapsed after allogeneic bone marrow transplantation. *J Clin Oncol* 1993; **11:** 513–19.

190. Drobyski WR, Keever CA, Roth MS et al. Salvage immunotherapy using donor leukocyte infusions as treatment for relapsed chronic myelogenous leukemia after allogeneic bone marrow transplantation: efficacy and toxicity of a defined T-cell dose. *Blood* 1993; **82:** 2310–18.

191. Helg C, Roux E, Beris P et al. Adoptive immunotherapy for recurrent CML after BMT. *Bone Marrow Transplant* 1993; **12:** 125–9.

192. Hertenstein B, Wiesneth M, Novotny J et al. Interferon-α and donor buffy coat transfusions for treatment of relapsed chronic myeloid leukemia after allogeneic bone marrow transplantation. *Transplantation* 1993; **56:** 1114–18.

193. Giralt SA, Hester J, Hugh Y et al. CD8+ depleted donor lymphocyte infusion as treatment for relapsed chronic myelogenous leukemia after allogeneic bone marrow transplantation: graft vs leukemia without graft vs host disease. *Blood* 1994; **84**(Suppl 1): 538.

194. Kolb HJ, Schattenberg A, Goldman JM et al. Graft-versus-leukemia effect of donor lymphocyte transfusions in marrow grafted patients. *Blood* 1995; **86:** 2041–50.

195. Mackinnon S, Hows JM, Goldman JM. Induction of in vitro graft-versus-leukemia activity following bone marrow transplantation for chronic myeloid leukemia. *Blood* 1990; **76:** 2037–45.

196. Mackinnon S, Papadoupoulos EB, Carabasi MH et al. Adoptive immunotherapy evaluating escalating doses of donor leukocytes for relapse of chronic myeloid leukemia following bone marrow transplantation: separation of graft-versus-host leukemia responses from graft-versus-host disease. *Blood* 1995; **86:** 1261–8.

197. Porter DL, Roth MS, McGarigle C et al. Induction of graft-versus-host disease as imunotherapy for relapsed chronic myeloid leukemia. *N Engl J Med* 1994; **330:** 100.

198. van Rhee F, Lin F, Cullis JO et al. Relapse of chronic myeloid leukemia after allogeneic bone marrow transplant: the case for giving donor leukocyte transfusions before the onset of hematologic relapse. *Blood* 1994; **83:** 3377.

199. Falkenburg JH, Smit WM, Willemze R. Cytotoxic T-lymphocyte (CTL) responses against acute or chronic myeloid leukemia. *Immunol Rev* 1997; **157:** 223–30.

200. Giralt S, Hester J, Huh Y et al. CD8+ depleted donor lymphocyte infusion as treatment for relapsed chronic myelogenous leukemia after allogeneic bone marrow transplantation: graft vs. leukemia without graft vs. host disease. *Blood* 1994; **84**(Suppl 1): 538a.

201. Barrett AJ, Horowitz MM. Transplants in ALL. *Bone Marrow Transplant* 1992; **10**(Suppl 1): 30–6.

202. Sullivan KM, Storb R, Buckner CD et al. Graft-versus-host disease as adoptive immunotherapy in patients with advanced hematologic neoplasms. *N Engl J Med* 1989; **320:** 828–34.

203. Collins RH Jr, Shpolberg O, Drobyski WR et al. Donor leukocyte infusions in 140 patients with relapsed malignancy after allogeneic bone marrow transplantation. *J Clin Oncol* 1997; **15:** 433.

204. Cardoso AA, Seamon MJ, Afonso HM et al. Ex vivo generation of human anti-pre-B leukemia-specific autologous cytolytic T cells. *Blood* 1997; **90:** 549–61.

205. Lewis S, Halvorson R, Thompson J et al. Novel approach to relapsed acute myelogenous leukemia (AML) following bone marrow transplantation (BMT). *Blood* 1995; **86**(Suppl 10): 565a.

206. Hercend T, Takvorian T, Nowill A et al. Characterization of natural killer cells with antileukemia activity following allogeneic bone marrow transplantation. *Blood* 1986; **67:** 722–8.

207. Albi N, Ruggeri L, Aversa F et al. Natural killer (NK)-cell function and antileukemic activity of a large population of CD3+/CD8+ T cells expressing NK receptors for histocompatibility complex class I after 'three-loci' HLA-incompatible bone marrow transplantation. *Blood* 1996; **87:** 3993–4000.

208. Sossman JA, Oettel KR, Smith SD et al. Specific recognition of human leukemic cells by allogeneic T-cells: II. Evidence for HIA-D restricted determinants on leukemic cells that are crossreactive with determinants present on unrelated nonleukemic cells. *Blood* 1990; **75:** 2005–16.

209. Sossman JA, Oettel KR, Hank JA et al. Specific recognition of human leukemic cells by allogeneic T-cell lines. *Transplantation* 1989; **48:** 486–95.

210. Sasazuki T, Juji T, Morishima Y et al. Effect of matching of class I HLA alleles on clinical outcome after transplantation of hematopoietic stem cells from an unrelated donor. Japan Marrow Donor Program. *N Engl J Med* 1998; **339:** 1177–85.

211. Ruggeri L, Capanni M, Urbani E et al. Effectiveness of donor natural killer cell alloreactivity in mismatched hematopoietic transplants. *Science* 2002; **295:** 2097–100.

212. Faber LM, Luxemburg-Heijs SAB, Willemze R, Falkenburg JHF. Generation of leukemia-reactive cytotoxic T lymphocyte clones from the HLA-identical bone marrow of a patient with leukemia. *J Exp Med* **176:** 1283–9.

213. Wingard J, Mellitis MB, Sostrin DY-H et al. Interstitial pneumonitis after allogeneic bone marrow transplanta-

tion. Nine-year experience at a single institution. *Medicine* 1988; **67**: 175–86.

214. Hertz MI, Englund JA, Snover D et al. Respiratory syncytial virus-induced acute lung injury in adult patients with bone marrow transplants: a clinical approach and review of the literature. *Medicine* 1989; **68**: 269–81.

215. Whimbey E, Champlin RE, Couch RB. Community respiratory virus infections among hospitalized adult bone marrow transplant recipients. *Clin Infect Dis* 1996; **22**: 778.

216. Goodrich JM, Mori M, Gleaves CA et al. Early treatment with ganciclovir to prevent cytomegalovirus disease after allogeneic bone marrow transplantation. *N Engl J Med* 1991; **325**: 1601.

217. Schmidt GM, Horak DA, Niland JC et al. The City of Hope–Stanford–Syntex CMV Study Group. A randomized controlled trial of prophylactic ganciclovir for cytomegalovirus pulmonary infection in recipients of allogenic bone marrow transplants. *N Engl J Med* 1991; **324**: 1005–11.

218. Winston DJ, Ho WG, Bartoni K et al. Ganciclovir prophylaxis of cytomegalovirus infection and disease in allogeneic bone marrow transplant recipients. *Ann Intern Med* 1993; **118**: 179.

219. Boeckh M, Gooley TA, Myerson D et al. Cytomegalovirus pp65 antigenemia-guided early treatment with ganciclovir versus ganciclovir at engraftment after allogeneic marrow transplantation: a randomized double-blind study. *Blood* 1996; **88**: 4063.

220. Hughes W, Kuhn S, Chaudhary J et al. Successful chemoprophylaxis for *Pneumocystis carinii* pneumonitis. *N Engl J Med* 1977; **297**: 1410–20.

221. O'Donnell MR, Schmidt GM, Tegtmeier B et al. Prophylactic low dose amphotericin B (AM-B) decreases systemic fungal infection (SFI) in allogeneic bone marrow transplant (BMT) recipients. *Blood* 1990; **76**(Suppl 1): 558a.

222. O'Donnell MR, Schmidt GM, Tegtmeier BR et al. Prediction of systemic fungal infection in allogeneic marrow recipients: impact of amphotericin prophylaxis in high-risk patients. *J Clin Oncol* 1994; **12**: 827–34.

223. Sayer HG, Longton G, Bowden R et al. Increased risk of infection in marrow transplant patients receiving methylprednisolone for graft-versus-host-disease prevention. *Blood* 1994; **84**: 1328.

224. Apperley JF, Goldman JM. Cytomegalovirus: biology, clinical features and methods for diagnosis. *Bone Marrow Transplant* 1988; **3**: 253–64.

225. Meyers JD, Fluornoy N, Thomas ED. Risk factors for cytomegalovirus infection after human marrow transplantation. *J Infect Dis* 1986; **153**: 478–88.

226. Winston DJ, Huang E, Miller MJ et al. Molecular epidemiology of cytomegalovirus infections associated with bone marrow transplantation. *Ann Intern Med* 1985: **102**: 16–20.

227. Churchill MA, Zaia JA, Forman SJ et al. Quantitation of human cytomegalovirus DNA in lungs from bone marrow transplant recipients with interstitial pneumonia. *J Infect Dis* 1987; **155**: 501–9.

228. Neiman PE, Reeves W, Ray G et al. A prospective analysis of interstitial pneumonia and opportunistic viral infection among recipients of allogeneic bone marrow grafts. *J Infect Dis* 1977; **136**: 754–67.

229. Weiner RS, Bortin MB, Gale RP et al. Interstitial pneu-

monitis after bone marrow transplantation: assessment of risk factors. *Ann Intern Med* 1986; **104**: 168–75.

230. Wingard JR, Chen DY, Burns WH et al. Cytomegalovirus infection after autologous bone marrow transplantation with comparison to infection after allogeneic bone marrow transplantation. *Blood* 1988; **71**: 1432.

231. Meyers JD, Fluornoy N, Thomas ED. Nonbacterial pneumonia after allogeneic marrow transplantation. A review of ten year's experience. *Rev Infect Dis* 1982; **4**: 1119–32.

232. Mackinnon S, Burnett AK, Crawford RJ et al. Seronegative blood products prevent primary cytomegalovirus infection after bone marrow transplantation. *J Clin Pathol* 1988; **41**: 948.

233. Bowden RA, Slichter SJ, Sayers M et al. A comparison of filtered leukocyte-reduced and cytomegalovirus (CMV) seronegative blood products for the prevention of transfusion-associated CMV infection after marrow transplant. *Blood* 1995; **86**: 3598–603.

234. Bratanow NC, Ash RC, Turner PA et al. Successful treatment of serious cytomegalovirus disease with 9-(1,3-dihydroxy-2-propoxymethyl)guanine and intravenous immunoglobulin in bone marrow transplant patients. *Exp Hematol* 1987; **15**: 541.

235. Emanuel D, Cunningham I, Jules-Elysee K et al. Cytomegalovirus pneumonia after bone marrow transplantation successfully treated with the combination of ganciclovir and high-dose intravenous immune globulin. *Ann Intern Med* 1988; **100**. 777–82.

236. Reed EC, Bowden RA, Dandiliker PS et al. Treatment of cytomegalovirus pneumonia with ganciclovir and intravenous cytomegalovirus immunoglobulin in patients with bone marrow transplants. *Ann Intern Med* 1988; **109**: 783–8.

237. Apperley JF, Marcus RE, Goldman JM et al. Foscarnet for cytomegalovirus pneumonitis. *Lancet* 1985; **i**: 1151.

238. Saltzberger B, Bowden RA, Hackman RC et al. Neutropenia in allogeneic marrow transplant recipients receiving ganciclovir for prevention of cytomegalovirus disease: risk factors and outcome. *Blood* 1997; **90**: 2502.

239. Boeckh M, Bowden RA, Goodrich JM et al. Cytomegalovirus antigen detection in peripheral blood leukocytes after allogeneic marrow transplantation. *Blood* 1992; **80**: 1358.

240. Einsele H, Steidle M, Vallbracht A et al. Early occurrence of human cytomegalovirus infection after bone marrow transplantation as demonstrated by the polymerase chain reaction technique. *Blood* 1991; **77**: 1104.

241. Gleaves CA, Smith TF, Shuster EA, Pearson GR. Rapid detection of cytomegalovirus in MRC–5 cells inoculated with urine specimens by using low-speed centrifugation and monoclonal antibody to an early antigen. *J Clin Microbiol* 1984; **19**: 917.

242. Riddell SR, Watanabe KS, Goodrich JM et al. Restoration of viral immunity in immunodeficient humans by the adoptive transfer of T cell clones. *Science* 1992; **257**: 238.

243. Walter EA, Greenberg PD, Gilbert MJ et al. Reconstitution of cellular immunity against cytomegalovirus in recipients of allogeneic bone marrow by transfer of T-cell clones from the donor. *N Engl J Med* 1995; **333**: 1038–44.

244. Bonini C, Ferrari G, Verzeletti S et al. *HSV-TK* gene transfer into donor lymphocytes for control of allogeneic graft versus leukemia. *Science* 1997; **276**: 1719.

245. Small TN, Avigan D, Dupont B et al. Immune reconstitu-

tion following T-cell depleted bone marrow transplantation: effect of age and post-transplant graft rejection prophylaxis. *Biol Blood Marrow Transplant* 1997; **3**: 65.

246. Keever CA, Small TN, Flomenberg N et al. Comparison of recipients of T-cell depleted marrow with recipients of conventional marrow grafts. *Blood* 1989; **73**: 1340–50.

247. Witherspoon RP, Fisher LD, Schoch G et al. Secondary cancers after bone marrow transplantation for leukemia or aplastic anemia. *N Engl J Med* 1989; **321**: 784–9.

248. O'Reilly RJ, Small TN, Papadopoulos E et al. Biology and adoptive cell therapy of Epstein–Barr virus-associated lymphoproliferative disorders in recipients of marrow allografts. *Immunol Rev* 1997; **157**: 195.

249. Zutter MM, Martin PJ, Sale GE et al. Epstein–Barr virus lymphoproliferation after bone marrow transplantation. *Blood* 1988; **72**: 520–9.

250. Fischer A. Bone marrow transplantation in immunodeficiency and osteoporosis. *Bone Marrow Transplant* 1989; **4**(Suppl 14): 12–14.

251. Martin PJ, Shulman HM, Schubach WH et al. Fatal Epstein–Barr-virus-associated proliferation of donor B-cells after treatment of acute graft-versus-host disease with a murine anti-T-cell antibody. *Ann Intern Med* 1984; **101**: 310–15.

252. Lucas K, Small T, O'Reilly RJ, Dupont B. The development of Epstein–Barr virus specific cellular immunity following allogeneic marrow transplantation. *Blood* 1994; **84**: 98.

253. Papadopoulos E, Ladanyi M, Emanuel D et al. Infusions of donor leukocytes as treatment of Epstein–Barr virus associated lymphoproliferative disorders complicating allogeneic marrow transplantation. *N Engl J Med* 1993; **330**: 1185–91.

254. Servida P, Rossini S, Traversari C et al. Gene transfer into peripheral blood lymphocytes for in vivo immunomodulation of donor anti-tumor immunity in a patient affected by EBV-induced lymphoma. *Blood* 1993; **82**: 214a.

255. Rooney CM, Smith CA, Ng CYC et al. Use of gene-modified virus-specific T lymphocytes to control Epstein–Barr-virus-related lymphoproliferation. *Lancet* 1995; **345**: 9.

256. Bourgault I, Gomez A, Gomard E, Levy JP. Limiting dilution analysis of the HLA-restriction of anti-Epstein–Barr virus specific cytolytic T lymphocytes. *Clin Exp Immunol* 1991; **84**: 501–7.

257. van Esser JW, Niesters HG, van der HB et al. Prevention of Epstein–Barr virus-lymphoproliferative disease by molecular monitoring and preemptive rituximab in high-risk patients after allogeneic stem cell transplantation. *Blood* 2002; **99**: 4364–9.

258. Kuehnle I, Huls MH, Liu Z et al. CD20 monoclonal antibody (rituximab) for therapy of Epstein–Barr virus lymphoma after hemopoietic stem-cell transplantation. *Blood* 2000; **95**: 1502–5.

259. Deeg HJ, Flournoy N, Sullivan KM et al. Cataracts after total body irradiation and marrow transplantation: a sparing effect of dose fractionation. *Int J Radiat Oncol Biol Phys* 1984; **10**: 957–64.

260. Sanders JE, Pritchard S, Mahoney P et al. Growth and development following marrow transplantation for leukemia. *Blood* 1986; **68**: 1129–35.

261. Thompson CB, Sanders JE, Flournoy N et al. The risks of central nervous system relapse and leukoencephalopathy in patients receiving marrow transplants for acute leukemia. *Blood* 1986; **67**: 195–9.

262. Wiznitzer M, Packer RJ, August CS, Burkey PA. Neurological complications of bone marrow transplantation in childhood. *Ann Neurol* 1984; **15**: 569–76.

263. Walker RW, Brochstein JA. Neurologic complications of immunosuppressive agents. *Neurol Clin* 1988; **6**: 261–78.

264. Ghany AM, Tutschka PJ, McGhee RB et al. Cyclosporine-associated seizures in bone marrow transplant recipients given busulfan and cyclophosphamide preparative therapy. *Transplantation* 1991; **52**: 310–15.

265. Woo M, Przepiorka D, Ippoliti C et al. Toxicities of tacrolimus and cyclosporin A after allogeneic blood cell transplantation. *Bone Marrow Transplant* 1997; **20**: 1095–8.

266. Leiper AD, Stanhope R, Lau T et al. The effect of total body irradiation and bone marrow transplantation during childhood and adolescence on growth and endocrine function. *Br J Haematol* 1987; **67**: 419–26.

267. Sklar CA, Kim TH, Ramsay NK. Thyroid dysfunction among long-term survivors of bone marrow transplantation. *Am J Med* 1982; **73**: 688–94.

268. Sanders JE, Buckner CD, Amos D et al. Ovarian function following marrow transplantation for aplastic anemia or leukemia. *J Clin Oncol* 1988; **6**: 813–18.

269. Sanders JE, Hawley J, Levy W et al. Pregnancies following high-dose cyclophosphamide with or without high-dose busulfan or total-body irradiation and bone marrow transplantation. *Blood* 1996; **87**: 3045–52.

270. Sklar CA, Kim TH, Ramsay NK. Testicular function following bone marrow transplantation performed during or after puberty. *Cancer* 1984; **53**: 1498–501.

271. Sarafoglou K, Boulad F, Gillio A, Sklar C. Gonadal function after bone marrow transplantation for acute leukemia during childhood. *J Pediatr* 1997; **130**: 210–16.

272. Huma Z, Boulad F, Black P et al. Growth in children after bone marrow transplantation for acute leukemia. *Blood* 1995; **86**: 819–24.

273. Tichelli A, Gratwohl A, Egger T et al. Cataract formation after bone marrow transplantation. *Ann Intern Med* 1993; **119**: 1175–80.

274. Deeg HJ, Sanders JE, Martin P et al. Secondary malignancies after marrow transplantation. *Exp Hematol* 1984; **12**: 660–6.

275. Curtis RE, Rowlings PA, Deeg HJ et al. Solid cancers after bone marrow transplantation. *N Engl J Med* 1997; **336**: 897–904.

276. Thomas ED, Buckner CD, Banaji M et al. One hundred patients with acute leukemia treated by chemotherapy, total body irradiation and allogeneic marrow transplantation. *Blood* 1977; **49**: 511–33.

277. Thomas ED, Buckner CD, Clift RA et al. Marrow transplantation for acute nonlymphoblastic leukemia in first remission. *N Engl J Med* 1979; **301**: 597–9.

278. Champlin RE, Gale RP. Acute myelogenous leukemia: recent advances in therapy. *Blood* 1987; **69**: 1551–62.

279. Appelbaum FR, Dahlberg S, Thomas ED et al. Bone marrow transplantation or chemotherapy after remission induction for adults with acute nonlymphoblastic leukemia: a prospective comparison. *Ann Intern Med* 1984; **101**: 581–8.

280. Brochstein JA, Kernan NA, Groshen S et al. Allogeneic bone marrow transplantation after hyperfractionated total-body irradiation and cyclophosphamide in children with acute leukemia. *N Engl J Med* 1987; **317**: 1618–24.

281. Clift RA, Buckner CD, Thomas ED et al. The treatment of

acute non-lymphoblastic leukemia by allogeneic marrow transplantation. *Bone Marrow Transplant* 1987; **2**: 243–58.

282. Dinsmore R, Kirkpatrick D, Flomenberg N et al. Allogeneic bone marrow transplantation for patients with acute nonlymphocytic leukemia. *Blood* 1984; **63**: 649–56.

283. Clift RA, Buckner CD, Appelbaum FR et al. Allogeneic marrow transplantation during untreated first relapse of acute myeloid leukemia. *J Clin Oncol* 1992; **10**: 1723–9.

284. Gorin NC, Aegerter P, Auvert B. Autologous bone marrow transplantation (ABMT) for acute leukemia in remission: Fifth European Survey. Evidence in favour of marrow purging. *Bone Marrow Transplant* 1989; **4**(Suppl 1): 206.

285. Yeager A, Kaizer H, Santos GW et al. Autologous bone marrow transplantation in patients with acute nonlymphocytic leukemia, using ex-vivo marrow treatment with 4-hydroperoxycyclophosphamide. *N Engl J Med* 1986; **315**: 141–7.

286. Busca A, Anasetti C, Anderson G et al. Unrelated donor or autologous marrow transplantation for treatment of acute leukemia. *Blood* 1994; **83**: 3077–84.

287. Champlin RE, Ho WG, Gale RP et al. Treatment of acute myelogenous leukemia: a prospective controlled trial of bone marrow transplantation versus consolidation chemotherapy. *Ann Intern Med* 1985; **102**: 285–91.

288. Conde E, Iriondo A, Rayon C et al. Allogeneic bone marrow transplantation versus intensification chemotherapy for acute myelogenous leukaemia in first remission: a prospective controlled trial. *Br J Haematol* 1988; **68**: 219–26.

289. Zander AR, Keating M, Dicke K et al. A comparison of marrow transplantation with chemotherapy for adults with acute leukemia of poor prognosis in first complete remission. *J Clin Oncol* 1988; **6**: 1548–57.

290. Mayer RJ. Current chemotherapeutic treatment approaches to the management of previously untreated adults with de novo acute myelogenous leukemia. *Semin Oncol* 1987; **14**: 385–96.

291. Burnett AK, Wheatley K, Goldstone AH et al. The value of allogeneic bone marrow transplant in patients with acute myeloid leukaemia at differing risk of relapse: results of the UK MRC AML 10 trial. *Br J Haematol* 2002; **118**: 385–400.

292. Zittoun RA, Mandelli F, Willemze R et al. Autologous or allogeneic bone marrow transplantation compared with intensive chemotherapy in acute myelogenous leukemia. *N Engl J Med* 1995; **332**: 217–23.

293. Mayer RJ, Davis RB, Schiffer CA et al. Intensive postremission chemotherapy in adults with acute myeloid leukemia. *N Engl J Med* 1994; **331**: 896–903.

294. Bloomfield CD, Lawrence D, Arthur CD et al. Cancer and Leukemia Group B. Curative impact of intensification with high-dose cytarabine (HiDAC) in acute myeloid leukemia varies by cytogenetic group. *Blood* 1994; **84**(Suppl 1): 111a.

295. Gale RP, Horowitz MM, Weiner RS et al. Impact of cytogenetic abnormalities on outcome of bone marrow transplantation in acute myelogenous leukemia in first remission. *Bone Marrow Transplant* 1995; **16**: 203–8.

296. Ferrant A, Labopin M, Frassoni F et al. Karyotype in acute myeloblastic leukemia: prognostic significance for bone marrow transplantation in first remission: a European Group for Blood and Marrow Transplantation study. Acute Leukemia Working Party of the European Group for Blood and Marrow Transplantation (EBMT). *Blood* 1997; **90**: 2931–8.

297. Bunjes D, Hertenstein B, Wiesneth M et al. In vivo/ex vivo T cell depletion reduces the morbidity of allogeneic bone marrow transplantation in patients with acute leukemias in first remission without increasing the risk of treatment failure: comparison with cyclosporin/methotrexate. *Bone Marrow Transplant* 1995; **15**: 563–8.

298. Soiffer R, Murray C, Fairclough D et al. CD6-depleted allogeneic BMT for adults with acute leukemia. *Blood* 1994; **84**(Suppl 1): 332a.

299. Creutzig V, Ritter J, Riehm H et al. Improved treatment results in childhood acute myelogenous leukemia: a report of the German Cooperative Study AML-BFM 78. *Blood* 1985; **65**: 298–304.

300. Weinstein HJ, Mayer RL, Rosenthal DS et al. Chemotherapy for acute myelogenous leukemia in children and adults: VAPA update. *Blood* 1983; **62**: 315.

301. Woods WG, Kobrinsky N, Buckley JD et al. Timed-sequential induction therapy improves postremission outcome in acute myeloid leukemia: a report from the Children's Cancer Group. *Blood* 1996; **87**: 4979–89.

302. Sanders JE, Thomas ED, Buckner CD et al. Marrow transplantation for children in first remission of acute nonlymphoblastic leukemia: an update. *Blood* 1985; **66**: 460.

303. Michel G, Gluckman E, Esperou-Bourdeau H et al. Allogeneic bone marrow transplantation for children with acute myeloblastic leukemia in first complete remission: impact of conditioning regimen without total-body irradiation – a report from the Société Française de Greffe de Moelle. *J Clin Oncol* 1994; **12**: 1217–22.

304. Nesbitt ME, Bukley JD, Feig SA et al. Chemotherapy for induction or remission of childhood acute myelogenous leukemia followed by marrow transplantation or multi-agent chemotherapy: a report from the Children's Cancer Group. *J Clin Oncol* 1994; **12**: 127–35.

305. Woods WG, Neudorf S, Gold S et al. Aggressive postremission (REM) chemotherapy is better than autologous bone marrow transplantation and allogeneic BMT is superior to both in children with acute myeloid leukemia (AML). *Proc Am Soc Clin Oncol* 1996; **15**: 368a (Abst 1091).

306. Tubergen D, Gilchest G, Coccia P et al. The role of intensified chemotherapy in intermediate risk acute lymphoblastic leukemia (ALL) of childhood. *Proc Am Soc Clin Oncol* 1990; **9**: 216.

307. Kersey JH. Fifty years of studies of the biology and therapy of childhood leukemia. *Blood* 1997; **90**: 4243–51.

308. Clavell LA, Gelber RD, Cohen JH et al. Four-agent induction and intensive asparaginase therapy for treatment of childhood acute lymphoblastic leukemia. *N Engl J Med* 1986; **315**: 657.

309. Steinherz PG, Gaynon P, Miller DR et al. Improved disease free survival of children with acute lymphoblastic leukemia at high risk for early relapse with the 'New York' regimen – a new intensive therapy protocol: a report from the Children's Cancer Study Group. *J Clin Oncol* 1986; **4**: 744–52.

310. Chessells JM, Bailey C, Richards SM. Intensification of treatment and survival in all children with lymphoblastic leukaemia: results of UK Medical Research Council trial UKALL X. Medical Research Council Working Party on Childhood Leukaemia. *Lancet* 1995; **345**: 653.

311. Barrett AJ, Horowitz MM, Gale RP et al. Marrow

transplantation for acute lymphoblastic leukemia: factors affecting relapse and survival. *Blood* 1989; **74**: 862–71.

312. Barrett AJ, Joshi R, Kendra JR et al. Prediction and prevention of relapse of acute lymphoblastic leukaemia after bone marrow transplantation. *Br J Haematol* 1986; **64**: 179–86.

313. Bordigoni P, Vernant JP, Souillet G et al. Allogeneic bone marrow transplantation for children with acute lymphoblastic leukemia in first remission: a cooperative study of the Groupe d'Etude de la Greffe de Moelle Osseuse. *J Clin Oncol* 1989; **7**: 747–53.

314. Chessells JM, Bailey C, Wheeler K, Richards SM. Bone marrow transplantation for high-risk childhood lymphoblastic leukaemia in first remission: experience in MRC UKALL X. *Lancet* 1992; **340**: 565–8.

315. Uderzo C, Valsecchi MG, Balduzzi A et al. Allogeneic bone marrow transplantation versus chemotherapy in high-risk childhood acute lymphoblastic leukaemia in first remission. Associazione Italiana di Ematologia ed Oncologia Pediatrica (AIEOP) and the Gruppo Italiano Trapianto di Midollo Osseo (GITMO). *Br J Haematol* 1997; **96**: 387–94.

316. Champlin RE, Gale RP. Acute lymphoblastic leukemia: recent advances in biology and therapy. *Blood* 1989; **73**: 2051–66.

317. Gaynor J, Chapmann D, Little C et al. A cause-specific hazard rate analysis of prognostic factors among 199 adults with acute lymphoblastic leukemia: the Memorial Hospital Experience since 1969. *J Clin Oncol* 1988; **6**: 1014–30.

318. Hoelzer D, Gale RP. Acute lymphoblastic leukemia in adults: recent progress, future directions. *Semin Hematol* 1987; **24**: 27–39.

319. Preti A, Kantarjian HM. Management of adult acute lymphocytic leukemia: present issues and key challenges. *J Clin Oncol* 1994; **12**: 1312–22.

320. Hoelzer D, Ludwig WD, Thiel E et al. Improved outcome in adult B-cell acute lymphoblastic leukemia. *Blood* 1996; **87**: 495–508.

321. Blaise D, Gaspard MH, Stoppa AM et al. Allogeneic or autologous bone marrow transplantation for acute lymphoblastic leukemia in first complete remission. *Bone Marrow Transplant* 1990; **5**: 7–12.

322. Blume KG, Forman SJ, Snyder DS et al. Allogeneic bone marrow transplantation for acute lymphoblastic leukemia during first complete remission. *Transplant Proc* 1987; **43**: 389–92.

323. Doney KC, Buckner CD, Kopecky KJ et al. Marrow transplantation for patients with acute lymphoblastic leukemia in first marrow remission. *Bone Marrow Transplant* 1987; **2**: 355–63.

324. Doney K, Fisher LD, Appelbaum FR et al. Treatment of adult acute lymphoblastic leukemia with allogeneic bone marrow transplantation. Multivariate analysis of factors affecting acute graft-versus-host disease, relapse, and relapse-free survival. *Bone Marrow Transplant* 1991; **7**: 453–9.

325. Hertzig RH, Bortin MM, Barrett AJ et al. Bone marrow transplantation in high-risk acute lymphoblastic leukaemia in first and second remission. *Lancet* 1987; **i**: 786–9.

326. Wingard JR, Piantadosi S, Santos GW et al. Allogeneic bone marrow transplantation for patients with high-risk acute lymphoblastic leukemia. *J Clin Oncol* 1990; **8**: 820–30.

327. Sebban C, Lepage E, Vernan J et al. Allogeneic bone marrow transplantation in adult acute lymphoblastic leukemia in first complete remission: a comparative study. *J Clin Oncol* 1994; **12**: 2580–7.

328. Attal M, Blasie D, Marit G et al. Consolidation treatment of adult acute lymphoblastic leukemia: a prospective, randomized trial comparing allogeneic versus autologous bone marrow transplantation and testing the impact of recombinant interleukin-2 after autologous bone marrow transplantation. *Blood* 1995; **86**: 1619–28.

329. Rowe JM, Richards SM, Burnett AK et al. Favorable results of allogeneic bone marrow transplantation (BMT) for adults with Philadelphia (Ph)-chromosome-negative acute lymphoblastic leukaemia (ALL) in first complete remission (CR): Results from the International ALL Trial. *Blood* 2001; **98** (Suppl 1): 481a.

330. Sanders JE, Thomas ED, Buckner CD, Doney K. Marrow transplantation for children with acute lymphoblastic leukemia in second remission. *Blood* 1987; **70**: 324.

331. Woods WG, Nesbit ME, Ransay NKC et al. Intensive therapy followed by bone marrow transplantation for patients with acute lymphocytic leukemia in second or subsequent remission: determination of prognostic factors (a report from the University of Minnesota Bone Marrow Transplantation Team). *Blood* 1983; **61**: 1182–9.

332. Coccia PF, Strandjord SE, Warkentin PI et al. High-dose cytosine arabinoside and fractionated total-body irradiation: an improved preparative regimen for bone marrow transplantation of children with acute lymphoblastic leukemia in remission. *Blood* 1988; **71**: 888–93.

333. Rivera GK, Buchanan G, Boyett JM et al. Intensive retreatment of childhood acute lymphoblastic leukemia in first bone marrow relapse: a Pediatric Oncology Group study. *N Engl J Med* 1986; **315**: 273.

334. Boulad F, Steinherz P, Reyes B et al. Allogeneic bone marrow transplantation (BMT) versus chemotherapy for the treatment of childhood acute lymphoblastic leukemia (ALL) in second remission (CR2): the MSKCC experience. *Blood* 1994; **84**(Suppl 1): 251a.

335. Chessels JM, Leiper AD, Richards SM et al. A second course of treatment for childhood acute lymphoblastic leukemia: long-term followup is needed to assess results. *Br J Haematol* 1994; **86**: 48–54.

336. Barrett AJ, Horowitz MM, Pollock BH et al. Bone marrow transplants from HLA identical siblings as compared with chemotherapy for children with acute lymphoblastic leukemia in a second remission. *N Engl J Med* 1994; **331**: 1253–8.

337. Sanders JE, Fluornoy N, Thomas ED et al. Marrow transplant experience in children with acute lymphoblastic leukemia: an analysis of factors associated with survival, relapse and graft-versus-host disease. *Med Pediatr Oncol* 1985; **13**: 165.

338. Clift RA, Appelbaum FR, Thomas ED. Treatment of chronic myeloid leukemia by marrow transplantation. *Blood* 1993; **82**: 1954–6.

339. Apperley JF, Jones L, Hale G et al. Bone marrow transplantation for patients with chronic myeloid leukaemia: T-cell depletion with Campath-1 reduces the incidence of graft-versus-host disease but may increase the risk of leukaemic relapse. *Bone Marrow Transplant* 1986; **1**: 53–60.

340. Goldman JM, Szydlo R, Horowitz MM et al. Choice of pre-transplant treatment and timing of transplants for chronic

myelogenous leukemia in chronic phase. *Blood* 1993; **82:** 2235–8.

341. Sokal JE, Baccarani M, Russo D, Tura S. Staging and prognosis in chronic myelogenous leukemia. *Semin Hematol* 1988; **25:** 49–61.

342. Talpaz M, Kantarjian H, Kurzrock R, Gutterman J. Therapy of chronic myelogenous leukemia: chemotherapy and interferons. *Semin Hematol* 1988; **25:** 62.

343. Talpaz M, Kantarjian H, Kurzrock R et al. Interferon-α produces sustained cytogenetic responses in chronic myelogenous leukemia. *Ann Intern Med* 1991; **114:** 532–8.

344. The Italian Cooperative Study Group on Chronic Myeloid Leukemia. Interferon alfa-a as compared with conventional chemotherapy for the treatment of chronic myeloid leukemia. *N Engl J Med* 1994; **330:** 820–5.

345. Kantarjian HM, Smith TL, O'Brien S et al. Prolonged survival in chronic myelogenous leukemia after cytogenetic response to interferon-α therapy. *Ann Intern Med* 1995; **122:** 254–61.

346. Schofield JR, Robinson WA, Murphy JR, Rovira DK. Low doses of interferon-α are as effective as higher doses in inducing remissions and prolonging survival in chronic myeloid leukemia. *Ann Intern Med* 1994; **121:** 736–44.

347. Guilhot F, Chastang C, Michallet M et al. Interferon alfa versus chemotherapy for chronic myeloid leukemia: a meta-analysis of seven randomized trials: Chronic Myeloid Trialists' Collaborative Group. *J Natl Cancer Inst* 1997; **89:** 1616–20.

348. Druker BJ. STI571 (Gleevec/Glivec, imatinib) versus interferon (IFN) + cytarabine as initial therapy for patients with CML: results of a randomized study. *Proc Am Soc Clin Oncol* 2002; **21:** 1a

349. Gale RP, Hehlmann R, Zhang MJ et al. Survival with bone marrow transplantation versus hydroxyurea or interferon for chronic myelogenous leukemia. The German CML Study Group. *Blood* 1998; **91:** 1810–19.

350. Champlin RE, Goldman JM, Gale RP. Bone marrow transplantation in chronic myelogenous leukemia. *Semin Hematol* 1988; **25:** 74–80.

351. Copelan EA, Grever MR, Kapoor N, Tutschka PJ. Marrow transplantation following busulfan and cyclophosphamide for chronic myelogenous leukaemia in accelerated or blastic phase. *Br J Haematol* 1989; **71:** 487–91.

352. Devergie A, Reiffers J, Vernant JP et al. Long-term follow-up after bone marrow transplantation for chronic myelogenous leukemia: factors associated with relapse. *Bone Marrow Transplant* 1990; **5:** 379–86.

353. McGlave PB, Arthur DC, Kim TH et al. Successful allogeneic bone marrow transplantation for patients in the accelerated phase of chronic granulocytic leukaemia. *Lancet* 1982; **ii:** 625–7.

354. Thomas ED, Clift RA. Indications for marrow transplantation in chronic myelogenous leukemia. *Blood* 1989; **73:** 861–4.

355. Goldman JM, Szydlo R, Horowitz MM et al. Choice of pre-transplant treatment and timing of transplants for chronic myelogenous leukemia in chronic phase. *Blood* 1993; **82:** 2235–8.

356. McGlave P, Arthur D, Haake R et al. Therapy of chronic myelogenous leukemia with allogeneic bone marrow transplantation. *J Clin Oncol* 1987; **5:** 1033–40.

357. Slattery JT, Clift RA, Buckner CD et al. Marrow transplantation for chronic myeloid leukemia: the influence of plasma busulfan levels on the outcome of transplantation. *Blood* 1997; **89:** 3055–60.

358. McGlave PB, Arthur DC, Kim TH et al. Successful allogeneic bone marrow transplantation for patients in the accelerated phase of chronic granulocytic leukaemia. *Lancet* 1982; **ii:** 625.

359. Gratwohl A, Hermans J, Apperley J. Acute graft-versus-host disease: grade and outcome in patients with chronic myelogenous leukemia. *Blood* 1995; **86:** 813–18.

360. Raanani P, Dazzi F, Sohal J et al. The rate and kinetics of molecular response to donor leucocyte transfusions in chronic myeloid leukaemia patients treated for relapse after allogeneic bone marrow transplantation. *Br J Haematol* 1997; **99:** 945–50.

361. Arcese W, Goldman JM, D'arcangelo E et al. Outcome for patients who relapse after allogeneic bone marrow transplantation for chronic myeloid leukemia. *Blood* 1993; **82:** 3211–19.

362. Roth MS, Antin JH, Ash R et al. Prognostic significance of Philadelphia chromosome-positive cells detected by the polymerase chain reaction after allogeneic bone marrow transplant for chronic myelogenous leukemia. *Blood* 1992; **79:** 276–82.

363. Bennett JM, Catovsky D, Daniel MT et al (FAB Cooperative Group). Proposals for the classification of the myelodysplastic syndromes. *Br J Haematol* 1982; **51:** 189–99.

364. Maschek H, Kaloutsi V, Rodriguez-Kaiser M et al. Hypoplastic myelodysplastic syndrome: incidence, morphology, cytogenetics and prognosis. *Ann Hematol* 1993; **66:** 117–22.

365. Kantarjian HM, Keating MJ, Walters RS et al. Therapy-related leukemia and myelodysplastic syndrome: clinical, cytogenetic and prognostic features. *J Clin Oncol* 1986; **4:** 1748–57.

366. Hurtado RM, Sosa RC, Majjuf AC et al. Refractory anaemia type I FAB treated with oxymetholone: long-term results. *Br J Haematol* 1993; **85:** 235–6.

367. Hellstrom-Lindberg E, Rober K-H, Gahrton G et al. Predictive model for the clinical response to low dose ara-C: a study of 102 patients with myelodysplastic syndromes or acute leukaemia. *Br J Haematol* 1992; **81:** 503–11.

368. Silverman LR, Holland JF, Nelson D et al. Trilineage response of myelodysplastic syndromes to subcutaneous azacytidine. *Proc Am Soc Clin Oncol* 1991; **10:** 747.

369. Antin JH, Smith BR, Holmes W, Rosenthal DS. Phase I/II study of recombinant human granulocyte macrophage colony-stimulating factor in aplastic anemia and myelodysplastic syndrome. *Blood* 1988; **72:** 705–13.

370. Negrin RS, Haeuber DH, Nagler A et al. Maintenance treatment of patients with myelodysplastic syndromes using recombinant human granulocyte colony-stimulating factor. *Blood* 1990; **76:** 36–43.

371. Appelbaum FR, Barrall J, Storb R et al. Bone marrow transplantation for patients with myelodysplasia: pre-treatment variables and outcome. *Ann Intern Med* 1990; **112:** 590–7.

372. DeWitte T, Hermans J et al. Prognostic variables in bone marrow transplantation for secondary leukaemia and myelodysplastic syndromes: a survey of the Working Party on Leukaemia. *Bone Marrow Transplant* 1991; **8**(Suppl 1): 40.

373. Arnold R, Heimpel H. Allogeneic bone marrow transplantation for myelodysplastic syndromes (MDS). *Bone Marrow Transplant* 1989; **4**(Suppl 4): 101–3.

374. Guinan EC, Tarbell NJ, Tantravahi R, Weinstein HJ. Bone marrow transplantation for children with myelodysplastic syndromes. *Blood* 1989; **73:** 619–22.

375. O'Donnell MR, Nademanee AP, Snyder DS et al. Bone marrow transplantation for myelodysplastic and myeloproliferative syndromes. *J Clin Oncol* 1987; **5:** 1822–6.

376. Sutton L, Chastang C, Ribaud P et al. Factors influencing outcome in de novo myelodysplastic syndromes treated by allogeneic bone marrow transplantation: a long-term study of 71 patients. Société Française de Greffe de Moelle. *Blood* 1996; **88:** 358–65.

377. Ratanatharathorn V, Karanes C, Uberti J et al. Busulfan-based regimens and allogeneic bone marrow transplantation in patients with myelodysplastic syndromes. *Blood* 1993; **81:** 2194–9.

378. Rappeport J, Parkman R, Belli J et al. Reversibility of myelofibrosis (MF) after bone marrow transplantation. *Blood* 1978; **52:** 589a.

379. Wolf JL, Spruce WE, Bearman RM et al. Reversal of acute ('malignant') myelosclerosis by allogeneic bone marrow transplantation. *Blood* 1982; **59:** 191–3.

380. Armitage JO. Bone marrow transplantation in the treatment of patients with lymphoma. *Blood* 1989; **73:** 1749.

381. Copelan EA, Kapoor N, Gibbons B, Tutschka PJ. Allogeneic marrow transplantation in non-Hodgkin's lymphoma. *Bone Marrow Transplant* 1990; **5:** 47.

382. Phillips GL, Herzig RH, Lazarus HM et al. High-dose chemotherapy, fractionated total-body irradiation, and allogeneic marrow transplantation for malignant lymphoma. *J Clin Oncol* 1986; **4:** 480.

383. Ernst P, Maraninchi D, Jacobsen N et al. Marrow transplantation for non-Hodgkin's lymphoma: a multicentre study from the European Co-operative Bone Marrow Transplant Group. *Bone Marrow Transplant* 1986; **1:** 81.

384. Ratanatharon V, Uberti J, Karanes C et al. Prospective comparative trial of autologous versus allogeneic bone marrow transplantation in patients with non-Hodgkin's lymphoma. *Blood* 1994; **84:** 1050–5.

385. Chopra R, Goldstone AH, Pearce R et al. Autologous versus allogeneic bone marrow transplantation for non-Hodgkin's lymphoma: a case-controlled analysis of the European Bone Marrow Transplant Group Registry data. *J Cin Oncol* 1992; **10:** 1690–5.

386. Appelbaum FR, Sullivan KM, Buckner CD et al. Treatment of malignant lymphoma in 100 patients with chemotherapy, total body irradiation, and marrow transplantation. *J Clin Oncol* 1987; **5:** 1340–7.

387. Vose JM, Anderson JR, Kessinger A et al. High dose chemotherapy and autologous hematopoietic stem cell transplantation for aggressive non-Hodgkin's lymphoma. *J Clin Oncol* 1993; **11:** 1846–51.

388. Bureo E, Ortega JJ, Munoz A et al. Bone marrow transplantation in 46 pediatric patients with non-Hodgkin's lymphoma. Spanish Working Party for Bone Marrow Transplantation in Children. *Bone Marrow Transplant* 1995; **15:** 353–9.

389. Gregory WM, Richards MA, Malpas JS. Combination chemotherapy versus melphalan and prednisone in the treatment of multiple myeloma: an overview of published trials. *J Clin Oncol* 1992; **10:** 334–42.

390. Mandelli F, Avvisati G, Amadori S et al. Maintenance treatment with recombinant interferon alfa-2b in patients with multiple myeloma responding to conventional induction chemotherapy. *N Engl J Med* 1990; **322:** 1430–4.

391. Barlogie B, Jagannath S, Epstein J et al. Biology and therapy of multiple myeloma in 1996. *Semin Hematol* 1997; **34**(Suppl 1): 67–72.

392. Barlogie B, Epstein J, Selvanayagam P, Alexanian R. Plasma cell myeloma: new biological insights and advances in therapy. *Blood* 1989; **73:** 865–79.

393. Anderson KC, Anderson J, Soiffer R et al. Monoclonal antibody purged bone marrow transplantation therapy for multiple myeloma. *Blood* 1993; **82:** 2568–76.

394. Barlogie B, Alexanian, Dicke KA et al. High-dose chemoradiotherapy and autologous bone marrow transplantation for resistant myeloma. *Blood* 1987; **70:** 869–72.

395. Schiller G, Vescio R, Freytes C et al. Transplantation of CD34+ peripheral blood progenitor cells after high-dose chemotherapy for patients with advanced multiple myeloma. *Blood* 1995; **86:** 390–7.

396. Billadeau D, Quam L, Thomas W et al. Detection and quantitation of malignant cells in the peripheral blood of multiple myeloma patients. *Blood* 1992; **80:** 1818–24.

397. Tricot G, Jagannath S, Vesole DH et al. Relapse of multiple myeloma after autologous transplantation: survival after salvage therapy. *Bone Marrow Transplant* 1995; **16:** 7–11.

398. Barlogie B, Gahrton G. Bone marrow transplantation in multiple myeloma. *Bone Marrow Transplant* 1991; **7:** 71–9.

399. Gahrton G, Tura S, Ljungman P et al. Prognostic factors in allogeneic bone marrow transplantation for multiple myeloma. *J Clin Oncol* 1995; **13:** 1312–22.

400. Varterasian M, Janakiraman N, Karanes C et al. Transplantation in patients with multiple myeloma: a multicenter comparative analysis of peripheral blood stem cell and allogeneic transplant. *Am J Clin Oncol* 1997; **20:** 462–6.

401. Vesole D, Tricot G, Jagannath S. Induction of graft-versus myeloma effect following allogeneic bone marrow transplantation. *Blood* 1994; **84:** 331a.

402. Lokhorst HM, Schattenberg A, Cornelissen JJ et al. Donor leukocyte infusions are effective in relapsed multiple myeloma after allogeneic bone marrow transplantation. *Blood* 1997; **90:** 4206–11.

403. Kwak LW, Taub DD, Duffey PL et al. Transfer of myeloma idiotype-specific immunity from an actively immunized marrow donor. *Lancet* 1995; **345:** 1016–20.

404. Wagner JE, Kernan NA, Steinbuch M et al. Allogeneic sibling umbilical-cord-blood transplantation in children with malignant and non-malignant disease. *Lancet* 1995; **346:** 214–19.

405. Gluckman E, Rocha V, Boyer-Chammard A et al. Outcome of cord-blood transplantation from related and unrelated donors. *N Engl J Med* 1997; **337:** 373–81.

406. Kurtzberg J, Laughlin M, Graham ML et al. Placental blood as a source of hematopoietic stem cells for transplantation into unrelated recipients. *N Engl J Med* 1996; **335:** 157–66.

407. Klein J, Park JM. Graft-versus-host reaction across different regions of the H-2 complex of the mouse. *J Exp Med* 1973; **137:** 1213–25.

408. Gatti RA, Meuwiissen JH, Allen HD et al. Immunological reconstitution of sex-linked lymphopenia immunological deficiency. *Lancet* 1968; **ii:** 1366–9.

409. Dupont B, O'Reilly RJ, Pollack MS, Good RA. Use of genotypically different donors in bone marrow transplantation. *Transplant Proc* 1979; **11:** 219–24.

410. Kenny AB, Hitzig WH. Bone marrow transplantation for severe combined immunodeficiency. Reported from 1968 to 1977. *Eur J Pediatr* 1979; **131**: 155–77.

411. Beatty PG, Bartolomeo P, Storb R et al. Treatment of aplastic anemia with marrow grafts from related donors other than HLA genotypically-matched siblings. *Clin Transplant* 1987; **1**: 117–24.

412. Beatty PG, Clift RA, Michelson EM et al. Marrow transplantation from related donors other than HLA-identical siblings. *N Engl J Med* 1985; **313**: 765–71.

413. Servida P, Gooley T, Hansen JA et al. Improved survival of haploidentical related donor marrow transplants mismatched for HLA-A or B versus HLA-DR. *Blood* 1996; **88**(Suppl 1): 484a.

414. O'Reilly RJ, Dupont B, Pahwa S et al. Reconstitution in severe combined immunodeficiency by transplantation of marrow from an unrelated donor. *N Engl J Med* 1977; **297**: 1311–18.

415. Hansen JA, Clift RA, Thomas ED et al. Transplantation of marrow from an unrelated donor to a patient with acute leukemia. *N Engl J Med* 1980; **303**: 565–7.

416. Gingrich RD, Ginder GD, Goeken D et al. Allogeneic marrow grafting with partially mismatched, unrelated donors. *Blood* 1988; **71**: 1375–81.

417. Gajewski J, Ho WG, Feig SA et al. Bone marrow transplantation using unrelated donors for patients with advanced leukemia or bone marrow failure. *Transplantation* 1990; **50**: 244–0.

418. McGlave PB, Beatty P, Ash R, Hows JM. Therapy for chronic myelogenous leukemia with unrelated donor bone marrow transplantation: results in 102 cases. *Blood* 1990; **75**: 1728–32. [Erratum: 1990; **76**: 654].

419. Beatty PG, Hansen JA, Longton GM et al. Marrow transplantation from HLA-matched unrelated donors for treatment of hematologic malignancies. *Transplantation* 1991; **51**: 443–7.

420. Beatty PG. Marrow transplantation using volunteer unrelated donors in a comparison of mismatched family donor transplants: a Seattle perspective. *Bone Marrow Transplant* 1994; **14**(Suppl 4): S39–41.

421. Kernan NA, Barsch G, Ash RC et al. Analysis of 462 transplantations from unrelated donors facilitated by the National Marrow Donor Program. *N Engl J Med* 1993; **328**: 593–602.

422. McGlave P, Bartsch G, Anasetti C et al. Unrelated donor marrow transplantation therapy for chronic myelogenous leukemia: initial experience of the National Marrow Donor Program. *Blood* 1993; **81**: 543–50.

423. Small TN, Flomenberg N, Black P et al. Comparison of immune reconstitution following T-cell depleted bone marrow transplantation from related versus unrelated donors. *Blood* 1991; **78**: 226a.

424. Marks DI, Cullis JO, Ward KN et al. Allogeneic bone marrow transplantation for chronic myeloid leukemia using sibling and volunteer unrelated donors: a comparison of complications in the first 2 years. *Ann Intern Med* 1993; **119**: 207–14.

425. Hansen JA, Gooley TA, Martin PJ et al. Bone marrow transplants from unrelated donors for patients with chronic myeloid leukemia. *N Engl J Med* 1998; **338**: 962–8.

426. Sierra J, Radich J, Hansen JA et al. Marrow transplants from unrelated donors for treatment of Philadelphia chromosome-positive acute lymphoblastic leukemia. *Blood* 1997; **90**: 1410–14.

427. Barrett AJ, Horowitz MM, Ash RC et al. Bone marrow transplantation for Philadelphia chromosome-positive acute lymphoblastic leukemia. *Blood* 1992; **79**: 3067–70.

428. Beatty PG, Hansen JA, Anasetti C et al. Significance of different levels of hisocompatibility in patients receiving marrow grafts from unrelated donors. *Exp Hematol* 1990; **15**: 509a.

429. Kernan NA, Khan R, Landrey C et al. Identification of unrelated bone marrow donors based on matching for class I IEF subtypes. *Blood* 1990; **76**: 548a.

430. Santamaria P, Reinsmoen NL, Lindstrom AL et al. Frequent HLA class I and DP sequence mismatches in serologically (HLA-A, HLA-B, HLA-DR) and molecularly (HLA-DRB1, HLA-DQA1, HLA-DQB1) HLA-identical unrelated bone marrow transplant pairs. *Blood* 1994; **83**: 280–7.

431. Prasad VK, Kernan NA, Heller G et al. DNA typing for HLA-A and -B identifies disparities between patients and unrelated donors matched by HLA-A and -B serology and DRB1. *Blood* 1997; **90**: 562a.

432. Prasad VK, Kernan NA, Heller G et al. HLA-C disparity between patients and unrelated donors matched by HLA-A and -B serology and DRB1. *Blood* 1997; **90**: 562a.

433. Petersdorf EW, Longton GM, Anasetti C et al. Association of HLA-C disparity with graft failure after marrow transplantation from unrelated donors. *Blood* 1997; **89**: 1818–23.

434. Beatty PG, Anasetti C, Hansen JA et al. Marrow transplantation from unrelated donors for treatment of hematologic malignancies: effect of mismatching for one HLA locus. *Blood* 1993; **81**: 249–53.

435. Davies SM, Shu XO, Blazar BR et al. Unrelated donor bone marrow transplantation: influence of HLA A and B incompatibility on outcome. *Blood* 1995; **86**: 1636–42.

436. Petersdorf EW, Longton GM, Anasetti C et al. The significance of HLA-DRB1 matching on clinical outcome after HLA-A, B, DR identical unrelated donor marrow transplantation. *Blood* 1995; **86**: 1606–13.

437. Petersdorf EW, Kollman C, Hurley CK et al. Effect of HLA class II gene disparity on clinical outcome in unrelated donor hematopoietic cell transplantation for chronic myeloid leukemia: the US National Marrow Donor Program Experience. *Blood* 2001; **98**: 2922–9.

438. Petersdorf EW, Gooley T, Malkki M et al. The biological significance of HLA-DP gene variation in haematopoietic cell transplantation. *Br J Haematol* 2001; **112**: 988–94.

439. Varney MD, Lester S, McCluskey J et al. Matching for HLA DPA1 and DPB1 alleles in unrelated bone marrow transplantation. *Hum Immunol* 1999; **60**: 532–8.

440. Shaw BE, Pay AL, Potter MN et al. HLA-DPB1 plays a role in the outcome of unrelated stem cell transplants in pairs completely matched at the other five transplantation loci. *Bone Marrow Transplant* 2002; **29**: 25.

441. Broxmeyer HE, Douglas GW, Hangoc G et al. Human umbilical cord blood as a potential source of transplantable hematopoietic stem/progenitor cells. *Proc Natl Acad Sci USA* 1989; **86**: 3828–32.

442. Gluckman E, Broxmeyer HA, Auerbach AD et al. Hematopoietic reconstitution in a patient with Fanconi's anemia by means of umbilical-cord blood from an HLA-identical sibling. *N Engl J Med* 1989; **321**: 1174–8.

443. Christensen RD, Harper TE, Rothstein G. Granulocyte–macrophage progenitor cells in term and preterm neonates. *J Pediatr* 1986; **109**: 1047–51.

444. Broxmeyer HE, Gluckman E, Auerbach A et al. Human umbilical cord blood: a clinically useful source of transplantable hematopoetic stem/progenitor cells. *Int J Cell Cloning* 1990; **8**(Suppl 1): 76–89.

445. Emerson SG, Sieff CA, Wang EA et al. Purification of fetal hematopoietic progenitors and demonstration of recombinant multipotential colony-stimulating activity. *J Clin Invest* 1985; **76**: 1286–90.

446. Haneline LS, Marshall KP, Clapp DW. The highest concentration of primitive hematopoietic progenitor cells in cord blood is found in extremely premature infants. *Pediatr Res* 1996; **39**: 820–5.

447. van den Ven C, Ishizawa L, Law P, Cairo MS. IL-11 in combination with SLF and G-CSF or GM-CSF significantly increases expansion of isolated CD34⁺ cell population from cord blood vs. adult bone marrow. *Exp Hematol* 1995; **23**: 1289–95.

448. Lu L, Xiao M, Shen RN et al. Enrichment, characterization, and responsiveness of single primitive CD34 human umbilical cord blood hematopoietic progenitors with high proliferative and replating potential. *Blood* 1993; **81**: 41–8.

449. Hao QL, Shah AJ, Thiemann FT et al. A functional comparison of CD34⁺CD38⁻ cells in cord blood and bone marrow. *Blood* 1995; **86**: 3745–53.

450. Kurtzberg J, Graham M, Casey J et al. The use of umbilical cord blood in mismatched related and unrelated hemapoietic stem cell transplantation. *Blood Cells* 1994; **20**: 275–83.

451. Rubinstein P, Dobrila L, Rosenfield RE et al. Processing and cryopreservation of placental/umbilical cord blood for unrelated bone marrow reconstitution. *Proc Natl Acad Sci USA* 1995; **92**: 10119–22.

452. Wagner JE, Kernan NA, Steinbuch M et al. Allogeneic sibling umbilical-cord-blood transplantation in children with malignant and non-malignant disease. *Lancet* 1995; **346**: 214–19.

453. Cairo MS, Wagner JE. Placental and/or umbilical cord blood: an alternative source of hematopoietic stem cells for transplantation. *Blood* 1997; **90**: 4665–78.

454. Wagner JW, Rosenthal J, Sweetman R et al. Successful transplantation of HLA-matched and HLA-mismatched umbilical cord blood from unrelated donors: analysis of engraftment and acute graft-versus-host disease. *Blood* 1996; **88**: 795–802.

455. Harris DT, Schumacher MJ, Locascio J et al. Phenotypic and functional immaturity of human umbilical cord blood T lymphocytes. *Proc Natl Acad Sci USA* 1992; **89**: 10006–10.

456. Risdon G, Gaddy J, Horie M, Broxmeyer HE. Alloantigen priming induces a state of unresponsiveness in human umbilical cord blood T cells. *Proc Natl Acad Sci USA* 1995; **92**: 2413–17.

457. Lee SM, Suen Y, Chang L et al. Decreased interleukin-12 (IL-12) from activated cord versus adult peripheral blood mononuclear cells and upregulation of interferon-γ, natural killer, and lymphokine-activated killer activity by IL-12 in cord blood mononuclear cells. *Blood* 1996; **88**: 945–54.

458. Bertotto A, Gerli R, Lanfrancone L et al. Activation of cord T lymphocytes. II. Cellular and molecular analysis of the defective response induced by anti-CD3 monoclonal antibody. *Cell Immunol* 1990; **127**: 247–59.

459. Chin TW, Ank BJ, Murakami D et al. Cytotoxic studies in human newborns: lessened allogeneic cell-induced (aug-

460. mented) cytotoxity but strong lymphokine-activated cytotoxicity of cord mononuclear cells. *Cell Immunol* 1986; **103**: 241–51.

460. Reisner Y, Kapoor N, Kirkpatrick D et al. Transplantation for acute leukemia with HLA-A and B non-identical parental marrow cells fractionated with soybean agglutinin and sheep blood cells. *Lancet* 1981; **ii**: 327–31.

461. Ash RC, Casper JT, Chitambar CR et al. Successful allogeneic transplantation of T-cell depleted bone marrow from closely HLA-matched unrelated donors. *N Engl J Med* 1990; **322**: 485–94.

462. Howard MR, Hows JM, Gore SM et al. Unrelated donor marrow transplantation between 1977 and 1987 at four centers in the United Kingdom. *Transplantation* 1990; **49**: 547–53.

463. McGlave P, Bartsch G, Anasetti C et al. Unrelated donor marrow transplantation therapy for chronic myelogenous leukemia: initial experience of the National Marrow Donor Program. *Blood* 1993; **81**: 543–50.

464. Hessner MJ, Endean DJ, Casper JT et al. Use of unrelated marrow grafts compensates for reduced graft versus leukemia reactivity after T-cell depleted allogeneic marrow transplantation for chronic myelogenous leukemia. *Blood* 1995; **86**: 3987–96.

465. Camitta B, Ash R, Menitove J et al. Bone marrow transplantation for children with severe aplastic anemia: use of donors other than HLA-identical siblings. *Blood* 1989; **74**: 1852–7.

466. Casper J, Camitta B, Truitt R et al. Unrelated bone marrow donor transplants for children with leukemia or myelodysplasia. *Blood* 1995; **85**: 2354–63.

467. Hongeng S, Krance RA, Bowman LC et al. Outcomes of transplantation with matched-sibling and unrelated donor marrow in children with leukaemia. *Lancet* 1997; **350**: 767–71.

468. Balduzzi A, Gooley T, Anasetti C et al. Unrelated donor marrow transplantation in children. *Blood* 1995; **86**: 3247–56.

469. Bozdech MJ, Sondel PM, Trigg ME et al. Transplantation of HLA-haploidentical T-cell depleted marrow for leukemia: addition of cytosine arabinoside to the pretransplant conditioning prevents rejection. *Exp Hematol* 1985; **13**: 1201–10.

470. Terenzi A, Lubin I, Lapidot T et al. Enhancement of T-cell depleted bone marrow allografts in mice by thiotepa. *Transplantation* 1990; **50**: 717.

471. Drizlikh G, Schmidt-Sole J, Yankelevich B. Involvement of the K and I regions of the H-2 complex in resistance to hemopoietic allografts. *J Exp Med* 1984; **159**: 1070.

472. Ferrara J, Lipton J, Hellman S et al. Engraftment following T-cell-depleted marrow transplantaion. I. The role of major and minor histocompatibility barriers. *Transplantation* 1987; **43**: 461.

473. Reisner Y, Itzicovitch L, Meshorer A, Sharon N. Hematopoietic stem cell transplantation using mouse bone-marrow and spleen cell fractionated by lectins. *Proc Natl Acad Sci USA* 1978; **75**: 2933.

474. van Bekkum DW, Löwenberg B. *Bone Marrow Transplantation: Biological Mechanisms and Clinical Practice.* New York: Marcel Dekker, 1985.

475. Aversa F, Tabilio A, Terenzi A et al. Successful engraftment of T-cell-depleted haploidentical 'three-loci, incompatible transplants in leukemia patients by addition of recombinant human granulocyte colony-stimulating

factor-mobilized peripheral blood progenitor cells to bone marrow inoculum. *Blood* 1994; **84**: 3948–55.

476. O'Reilly RJ, Kernan NA, Cunningham I et al. Allogeneic transplants depleted of T-cells by soybean lectin agglutination and E-rosette depletion. *Bone Marrow Transplant* 1988; **3**: 3 6.

477. Reisner Y, Kapoor N, Kirkpatrick D et al. Transplantation for severe combined immunodeficiency with HLA-A,B,DR incompatible parental marrow fractionated by soybean agglutin and sheep red blood cells. *Blood* 1983; **61**: 341–8.

478. Henlee-Downey PJ, Abhyankar SH, Parrish RS et al. Use of partially mismatched related donors extends access to allogeneic marrow transplant. *Blood* 1997; **89**: 3864–72.

479. Mackinnon S. Who may benefit from donor leucocyte infusions after allogeneic stem cell transplantation? *Br J Haematol* 2000; **110**: 12–17.

480. Giralt S, Cohen A, Mehra R et al. Preliminary results of fludarabine/melphalan or 2CDA/melphalan as preparative regimens for allogeneic progenitor cell transplantation in poor candidates for conventional myeloablative conditioning. *Blood* 1997; **90**(Suppl 1): 417.

481. Giralt S, Weber D, Aleman A et al. Non myeloablative conditioning with fludarabine/melphalan (FM) for patients with multiple myeloma (MM). *Blood* 1999; **94**(Suppl 1): 347.

482. Khouri IF, Keating M, Korbling M et al. Transplant-lite: induction of graft-versus-malignancy using fludarabine-based nonablative chemotherapy and allogeneic blood progenitor-cell transplantation as treatment for lymphoid malignancies. *J Clin Oncol.* 1998; **16**: 2817 24.

483. Kottaridis P, Milligan DW, Chopra R et al. In vivo CAMPATH 1H prevents graft-versus-host disease following nonmyeloablative stem cell transplantation. *Blood* 2000; **96**: 2419–25.

484. Slavin S, Nagler A, Naparstek E et al. Nonmyeloablative stem cell transplantation and cell therapy as an alternative to conventional bone marrow transplantation with lethal cytoreduction for the treatment of malignant and nonmalignant hematologic diseases. *Blood* 1998; **91**: 756–63.

485. McSweeney PA, Niederwieser D, Shizuru JA et al. Hematopoietic cell transplantation in older patients with hematologic malignancies: replacing high-dose cytotoxic therapy with graft-versus-tumor effects. *Blood* 2001; **97**: 3390–400.

486. Giralt S, Estey E, Albitar M et al. Engraftment of allogeneic hematopoietic progenitor cells with purine analog-containing chemotherapy: harnessing graft-versus-leukemia without myeloablative therapy. *Blood* 1997; **89**: 4531–6.

487. Giralt S, Thall PF, Khouri I et al. Melphalan and purine analog-containing preparative regimens: reduced-intensity conditioning for patients with hematologic malignancies undergoing allogeneic progenitor cell transplantation. *Blood* 2001; **97**: 631–7.

488. Khouri IF, Saliba RM, Giralt SA et al. Nonablative allogeneic hematopoietic transplantation as adoptive immunotherapy for indolent lymphoma: low incidence of toxicity, acute graft-versus-host disease, and treatment-related mortality. *Blood* 2001; **98**: 3595–9.

489. Giralt S, Aleman A, Anagnostopoulos A et al. Fludarabine/melphalan conditioning for allogeneic transplantation in patients with multiple myeloma. *Bone Marrow Transplant* 2002; **30**: 367–73.

490. Maloney D, Sahebi F, Stockerl-Goldstein KE et al. Combining an allogeneic graft-versus-myeloma effect with high-dose autologous stem cell rescue in the treatment of multiple myeloma. *Blood* 2001; **16**: 434a.

# 30 Epidemiology

### Jørgen H Olsen

## Introduction

Hematopoietic tissue is a prevalent site of cancer in large parts of the world. The number of new cases in 1990 was estimated at 570 000 (7% of all new cancers), which is only surpassed by cancers of the lung (1 040 000), breast (800 000), stomach (800 000), and colon/rectum (780 000).[1] In this chapter, the term 'hematological malignancies' includes the leukemias, Hodgkin's disease, the many forms of non-Hodgkin lymphoma (NHL), and multiple myeloma. The descriptive epidemiology of this heterogeneous group of cancers has been hampered by the many changes in disease classification that have been introduced over time; furthermore, different classification schemes have been used simultaneously in different countries and even in different regions of the same country. This chapter on the epidemiology of hematological malignancies emphasizes only the major diagnostic groups of leukemias, Hodgkin's disease, NHL, and multiple myeloma, although some aspects of the leukemias and NHL are discussed in further subgroupings.

## Incidence and mortality

Research into the causation and prevention of cancer has traditionally been based on descriptive statistics. A prominent example of such basic work is the series *Cancer Incidence in Five Continents*, published by the International Agency for Research on Cancer (IARC).[2] These publications describe the burden and patterns of hematological and other cancers in diverse populations, and can thus give rise to hypotheses that might explain the observed differences in risk.

The commonest measures used in descriptive statistics are incidence and mortality rates. The incidence rate is the number of new cases of a certain disease that develop in a population at risk, normally expressed as a number per 100 000 persons during 1 year. The incidence rate is widely used in epidemiology because it indicates disease frequency – or risk. The incidence rate directly reflects the burden of disease-causing agents, taking into account the latency of the disease measured. If exposure of a population to, for example, leukemogenic agents becomes more prevalent, the incidence of leukemia will eventually rise to a level that is determined simply by specific interactions between the target cells and the carcinogens. The rate of mortality from the disease is a more complex measure of disease burden, as the number of patients who are cured of the disease or who survive long enough to die from another cause influences it. With high cure rates and advantageous 5-year survival rates, as seen for many types of hematological cancers, the mortality rate typically underestimates the size of the cancer problem in a given population. However, often the mortality rate is used in epidemiology and clinical research when a proper instrument for population-based case finding – such as a cancer registry – is absent.

In Europe, nationwide incidence rates of hematological malignancies and other cancers are known only for the Nordic countries, Scotland, Estonia, Latvia, the Czech Republic, Slovakia, and Slovenia. England and Wales are covered by regional cancer registries with substantial variations in registration and completeness. Nationwide cancer registration either is in progress or has been initiated recently in the Netherlands, Belgium, Portugal, Greece, Austria, Cyprus, and Belarus. Well-functioning regional cancer registration exists to a greater or lesser extent in other European countries, including Ireland, Germany, France, Spain, Italy, Romania, Hungary, Poland, and Russia, but in general with a coverage of less than 10% of the national population.[2]

Outside Europe, all of Canada, New Zealand, and a major part of Australia are covered by cancer registration. About 10% of the population in the USA located in nine selected areas of the country is covered by population-based cancer incidence registries; these latter registries are coordinated by the Surveillance, Epidemiology, and End Results (SEER) program under the responsibility of the National Cancer Institute.[3] Few areas of the rest of the world are covered by routine cancer registration.

## Standardization of rates

With the striking exception of Hodgkin's disease, age is a major determinant of risk for hematological malignancies; for example, in the Nordic countries, the risk of NHL increases by 30-fold for men as well as women between the ages of 20 and 75 years (Table 30.1). This dependence on age means that it is important to adjust for differences in age composition when comparing the occurrence of hematological malignancies in two or more populations. Comparisons are usually made in one of two ways:

- by calculating age-adjusted (age-standardized) rates, which are averages of age-specific incidence rates weighted against a standard population;
- by calculating the cumulative incidence rate between age 0 and, for example, 74 years, which gives a number (lifetime risk) that indicates the probability that a person will develop the disease within the age range if still alive.

Examples of both measures are given in Table 30.2 for the commonest cancers and for all cancers combined for men and women in England and Wales and for similar sites in Japan (Hiroshima City). The incidence of hematological malignancies in England and Wales is believed to be representative of that of a large part of the European population. Grouped together, these malignancies rank fourth among men in England and Wales, with 24 new cases per 100 000 per year (only surpassed by cancers of the lung, colon/rectum, and prostate), and fourth among women, with 16 new cases per 100 000 per year (only surpassed by cancers of the breast, colon/rectum, and lung). These numbers are equivalent to lifetime risks (age 0–74 year) of 2.5% and 1.6%, respectively. Hematological cancers occur more rarely in Japan, where cancer of the stomach is by far the commonest type of cancer among both men and women (83 and 36 per 100 000 per year, respectively) (Table 30.2).

## Geographical variation

For most types of cancers, striking differences in frequency exist between countries. This is less true for hematological malignancies, but some international

### Table 30.1 Annual age-specific incidence of non-Hodgkin lymphoma in men and women in the five Nordic countries (Denmark, Finland, Iceland, Norway, and Sweden): 1993–97[4]

| Age (years) | Rate per 100 000 | |
|---|---|---|
| | Men | Women |
| 0–5 | 1.2 | 0.7 |
| 5–9 | 1.9 | 0.6 |
| 10–14 | 1.6 | 0.8 |
| 15–19 | 2.1 | 1.2 |
| 20–24 | 2.2 | 1.4 |
| 25–29 | 3.0 | 1.6 |
| 30–34 | 4.0 | 3.0 |
| 35–39 | 6.5 | 3.4 |
| 40–44 | 8.8 | 5.8 |
| 45–49 | 13.6 | 10.4 |
| 50–54 | 20.4 | 14.9 |
| 55–59 | 24.6 | 19.8 |
| 60–64 | 33.8 | 25.6 |
| 65–69 | 44.9 | 35.1 |
| 70–74 | 61.4 | 45.1 |
| 75–79 | 74.7 | 51.3 |
| 80–84 | 92.8 | 61.1 |
| 85+ | 84.8 | 54.4 |

### Table 30.2 Annual age-adjusted (World Standard Population) rates and cumulative incidence rates to age 74 years for all types of cancer combined for the five most frequent cancers among men and women in the UK and for similar sites in Japan[2]

| Cancer site | Age-adjusted rate per 100 000 | | Cumulative rate, age 0–74 years (%) | |
|---|---|---|---|---|
| | UK[a] | Japan[b] | UK[a] | Japan[b] |
| **Men** | | | | |
| All sites[c] | 261.1 | 322.3 | 29.9 | 38.6 |
| Lung | 62.4 | 39.6 | 7.8 | 4.7 |
| Colon/rectum | 33.9 | 51.0 | 3.9 | 6.3 |
| Prostate | 28.0 | 10.9 | 3.0 | 1.2 |
| *Hematological cancer* | *23.9* | *16.6* | *2.5* | *1.8* |
| Urinary bladder | 20.3 | 12.9 | 2.4 | 1.5 |
| Stomach | 16.1 | 83.1 | 1.9 | 10.1 |
| **Women** | | | | |
| All sites | 225.5 | 195.0 | 25.5 | 22.0 |
| Breast | 68.8 | 33.7 | 7.7 | 3.6 |
| Colon/rectum | 23.7 | 27.9 | 2.7 | 3.2 |
| Lung | 22.8 | 11.7 | 3.0 | 1.7 |
| *Hematological cancer* | *15.7* | *9.2* | *1.6* | *1.0* |
| Cervix uteri | 12.5 | 12.6 | 1.3 | 1.4 |
| Ovary | 12.4 | 6.6 | 1.4 | 0.7 |

[a]England and Wales, 1988–90. [b]Hiroshima City, 1986–90. [c]All sites but non-melanoma skin.

variation is seen for each of the main diagnostic groups of leukemia, Hodgkin's disease, NHL, and multiple myeloma. This is illustrated in Figures 30.1–30.4, which show the incidence of the hematological malignancies in selected countries around the world during the early 1990s. Some of the data were derived from particular areas within the countries, and do not necessarily represent national rates. In view of the variations in diagnostic practices and tumor classifications mentioned above, international comparisons should be interpreted with caution.

The leukemias (Figure 30.1) seem to occur at the highest rates in certain areas of Canada (Quebec, Ontario, Saskatchewan, and Yukon), among both men and women. Rates are also high among Whites in the USA, Australia, and Denmark. Leukemias are also relatively more common in other Western countries than registered in most parts of the world. There is little variation worldwide among women.

The highest rates for Hodgkin's disease (Figure 30.2) are reported in several areas of Europe and among Whites of each sex in many parts of the USA – Connecticut in particular (4.1 and 3.6 per 100 000 men and women, respectively). The lowest incidence rates are seen in Polynesia and in Asian populations.

In comparison with the incidence rates of Hodgkin's disease, relatively more international variation is seen for the combined group of NHL (Figure 30.3), with the absolutely highest rates in men and women observed in North America and Australia. An excep-

tionally high rate is seen among White males in San Francisco, with 25 new cases annually per 100 000 (lifetime risk 2.6%). For the group of NHL, the lowest rates are reported from Asia and Africa. However, Burkitt lymphoma, which is grouped with the NHL,

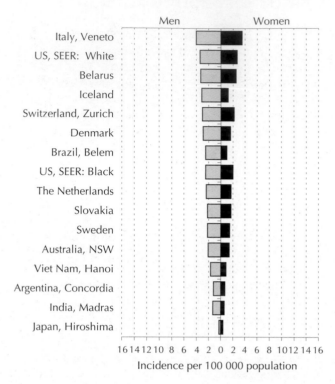

**Figure 30.2** Annual incidence of Hodgkin's disease per 100 000 men and women (World Standard Population) in selected countries during the early 1990s.[2]

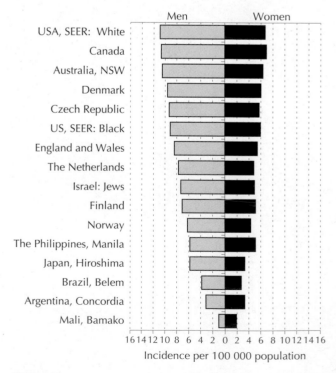

**Figure 30.1** Annual incidence of leukemia per 100 000 men and women (World Standard Population) is selected countries during the early 1990s.[2]

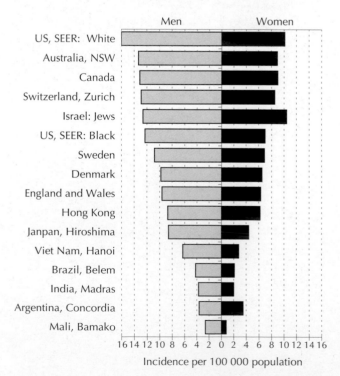

**Figure 30.3** Annual incidence of non-Hodgkin lymphoma per 100 000 men and women (World Standard Population) in selected countries during the early 1990s.[2]

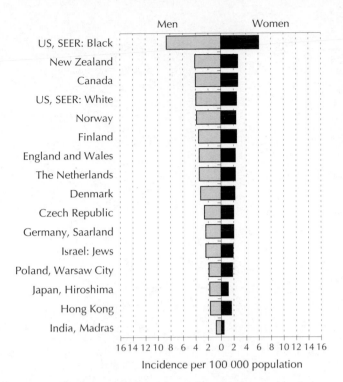

**Figure 30.4** Annual incidence of multiple myeloma per 100 000 men and women (World Standard Population) in selected countries during the early 1990s.[2]

**Table 30.3** Incidence rates of hematological cancers and their proportion relative to all cancers in major areas of the world served by reliable cancer registries[2,5,6]

| Major geographical areas | Period | Rate per 100 000[a] | Percentage of all cancers[b] |
|---|---|---|---|
| **Men** | | | |
| European Union[c] | 1997 | 25.4 | 7.7 |
| Australia[c] | 2000 | 30.8 | 8.2 |
| USA: White | 1992–99 | 35.5 | 9.5 |
| USA: Black | 1992–99 | 33.9 | 7.8 |
| Canada[c] | 2000 | 32.0 | 9.2 |
| **Women** | | | |
| European Union | 1997 | 16.8 | 7.4 |
| Australia | 2000 | 22.4 | 7.9 |
| USA: White | 1992–99 | 22.9 | 7.8 |
| USA: Black | 1992–99 | 21.7 | 7.8 |
| Canada | 2000 | 22.5 | 8.3 |

[a]World Standard Population. [b]All sites but non melanoma skin. [c]Estimates.

occurs endemically among children in tropical Africa and lowland New Guinea. In such high-risk areas, the rate is 5–8 cases per 100 000 children per year, which is double the rate of leukemia seen in children of Caucasian origin.

The highest incidence rates of multiple myeloma in the world (Figure 30.4) are found almost consistently among American Blacks. The lowest rates are seen in areas outside the Western world.

Table 30.3 lists the registered or estimated incidence rates of all hematological malignancies combined for those areas of the world with some reliable population-based cancer registries. The group of hematological malignancies represents approximately 8–9% of all cancers in men and around 8% of all cancers in women in Australia, the USA, and Canada. The proportion appears to be slightly lower in the European Union.

The proportion also varies by age (Figure 30.5). In England and Wales, the combined group of hematological malignancies accounts for up to 40% of all cancers during the first decade of life, but the proportion reveals a steep decline in subsequent age groups, reaching minimum of 5% around age 50 years.

Table 30.4 gives the incidence rates of each of the main diagnostic groups of hematological malignancies. Although the rates are higher among men than women, the relative distribution of hematological cancers into the different diagnostic groups is almost

the same for each sex. Some variation exists, however, between areas and between ethnic groups (Figure 30.6). Leukemia represents almost 35% of all hematological malignancies in Europe, a little more than 30% in the USA (Whites) and Canada, and some 25% among Black Americans. NHL is relatively more frequent in Canada and among Whites in the USA than in other populations, while multiple myeloma is a major hematological diagnosis among Black Americans.

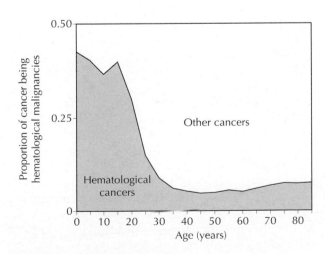

**Figure 30.5** Age-specific proportion of hematological malignancies out of all malignancies except non-melanoma skin cancer in England and Wales, both sexes combined, 1997.[6]

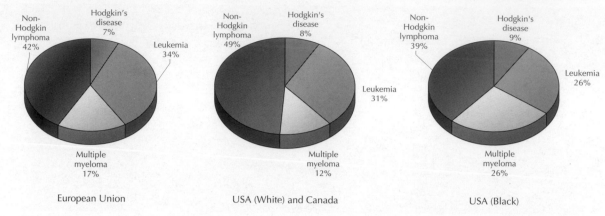

**Figure 30.6** Relative importance of hematological malignancies in some major populations of the world.[2,5,6]

**Table 30.4 Incidence rates of each of the main diagnostic groups of hematological malignancies in major areas of the world served by reliable cancer registries[2,5,6]**

| Major geographical area | Period | Rate per 100 000 population[a] | | | |
|---|---|---|---|---|---|
| | | Leukemia | Hodgkin's disease | Non-Hodgkin lymphoma | Multiple myeloma |
| **Men** | | | | | |
| European Union[b] | 1997 | 9.1 | 2.5 | 10.3 | 3.4 |
| Australia[b] | 2000 | 10.3 | 2.1 | 14.4 | 4.0 |
| USA: White | 1992–99 | 11.7 | 3.0 | 16.8 | 4.0 |
| USA: Black | 1992–99 | 8.9 | 2.5 | 14.1 | 8.4 |
| Canada[b] | 2000 | 10.4 | 2.7 | 14.6 | 4.3 |
| **Women** | | | | | |
| European Union | 1997 | 5.9 | 1.9 | 6.7 | 2.4 |
| Australia | 2000 | 6.9 | 1.9 | 10.8 | 2.8 |
| USA: White | 1992–99 | 7.2 | 2.5 | 10.6 | 2.6 |
| USA: Black | 1992–99 | 5.6 | 2.0 | 7.5 | 6.6 |
| Canada | 2000 | 6.8 | 2.2 | 10.5 | 3.0 |

[a]World Standard Population. [b]Estimates.

# Time trends and age curves

In Denmark, where cancer registration has been maintained on a nationwide scale for more than 50 years, the incidence of hematological malignancies has evolved as shown in Figures 30.7. Registration was also established relatively early in Norway (1953), Finland (1953), Iceland (1955), and Sweden (1958), which together with Denmark covered a population of 24 million in the 1990s. The evolving incidences in those countries are similar to those among men and women in Denmark. Although the rates differ between the sexes, the trends in rates are similar for men and women: there was a marked and relatively uniform increase for the group of NHL, which today is slightly more frequent than the combined group of leukemias; and a moderate increase was observed for the group of leukemias up to the mid-1980s, followed by a stable incidence. A slight but continuous increase was seen for the group of multiple myelomas, while the rate of Hodgkin's disease hardly changed.

## Epidemic of NHL

A steep increase over time in the incidence of NHL has been observed in many places other than the Nordic countries. Incidence data from the SEER program[7,8] and the IARC indicate that both mortality and incidence rates have been increasing for many years.[9] Greater increases among older persons, however, suggest a role for improvements in diagnosis, particularly during the 1950s and 1960s, but overall it is judged unlikely that the marked increase in time trends seen across country borders can be attributed entirely to data artifacts.[10] Accordingly, careful analyses of incidence data on NHL from Connecticut, USA show that there has been a 10.3% increase in risk every 5 years

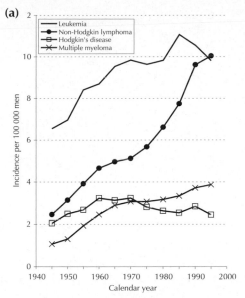
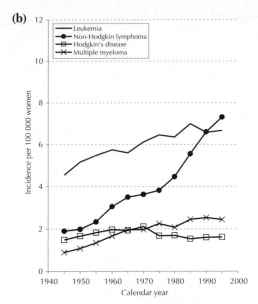

**Figure 30.7** Time trends in incidence rates of hematological malignancies among (a) men and (b) women in Denmark, 1943–98 (World Standard Population). *Source:* The Danish Cancer Registry (unpublished data).s

since 1965 for women and a 9.2% increase for men.[10] On the basis of SEER data, Groves et al[8] found age adjusted total NHL incidence rates that during the periods 1978–83 to 1990–95 increased by 77% and 53% in Black and White men, respectively, and 39% and 33% among Black and White women, respectively

### Age curves and cohort of birth

Figure 30.8 gives the age-specific incidence rates over time (age curves) for each of the major diagnostic group of hematological diseases in the population of Denmark. The incidence rate per 100 000 is plotted on a logarithmic scale. The distribution of each malignancy by age at diagnosis is somewhat different.

While some 25% of cases of multiple myeloma are diagnosed in people under the age of 60 years, 75% of cases of Hodgkin's disease are diagnosed in people under that age and 25% under the age of 30. Leukemias and NHL have an intermediate age distribution, with 40% of cases diagnosed in people under the age of 60.

Age-specific curves give a summary measure of the level of risk in each of a number of defined age groups; however, it must be kept in mind that each of the age groups are composed of individuals belonging to different generations. This will strongly influence the shape of the age-specific curve if the risk of cancer increases or decreases with time. To better evaluate the importance of changing exposure to carcinogens over generations, age-specific incidence curves are

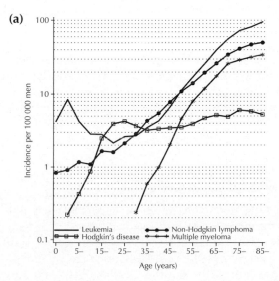
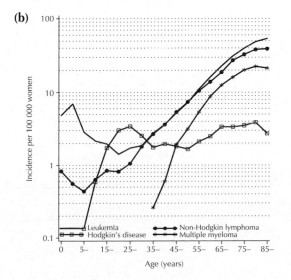

**Figure 30.8** Age-specific incidence rates of hematogical malignancies, among (a) men and (b) women, 1943–98. *Source:* The Danish Cancer Registry (unpublished data).

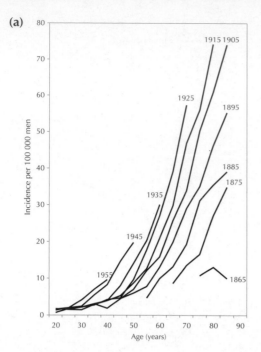
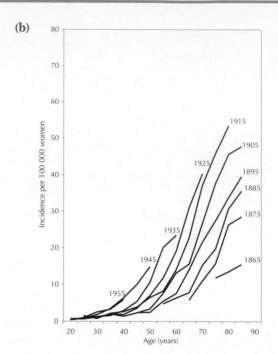

**Figure 30.9** Age-specific incidence rates of non-Hodgkin lymphoma among (a) men and (b) women, in Denmark, 1943–98, in selected 10-year birth cohorts. One point is shown for each mid-cohort. *Source:* The Danish Cancer Registry (unpublished data).

sometimes drawn for year-of-birth cohorts, as shown in Figure 30.9 for NHL in Denmark. The presentation of incidence data in this way shows clearly that the age-specific rates of NHL for both men and women are consistently higher in younger generations than in older generations, which also indicates that the over-all incidence of NHL in Denmark – and in other Western countries – will continue to increase, at least in the forthcoming two to three decades. This is so because the incidence rates of NHL in young adults may be used to make a prediction of the future lymphoma burden of the entire population, since the shape of the incidence curve in young adults indicates the magnitude of the NHL problem that will eventually be carried over to people of older ages.

## The leukemias

The leukemias are a group of malignancies of precursor cells of blood and tissue lymphocytes. For general purposes, they are distinguished by their cell type of origin (mainly lymphocytes, myelocytes, and monocytes) and by their clinicopathological behavior (acute, subacute, and chronic). Comparisons of the different subtypes are difficult because diagnostic methods and the accuracy of diagnosis vary, with different proportions remaining unspecified. Table 30.5 gives data on the frequencies of the subtypes of leukemia in general use in 18 selected populations.

A more detailed picture of the distribution of leukemias by subtype is given in Tables 30.6 and 30.7, which are based on approximately 13 700 notified

cases of leukemia in Denmark during the period 1978–98. The two commonest diagnosis used by oncologists during that period were 'lymphatic' (50%) and 'myeloid' (43%) leukemia, followed by 'leukemia not otherwise specified' (3%), 'hairy cell leukemia' (1%), and 'monocytic leukaemia' (1%) (Table 30.6). While some 80% of lymphatic leukemias are chronic and some 20% acute, the clinical pattern of the group of myeloid leukemias is almost the reverse, with some 30% of cases regarded as chronic and 70% as acute (Table 30.7). The picture may, however, be imprecise, since it reflects routine diagnosis in the healthcare system applied to a European national population over a 20-year period.

### Childhood leukemia

Although rare, leukemia is the most frequent cancer in children, accounting for one-third of all new cases. Unlike most other malignancies, it shows a distinct peak in childhood, rising to about 9–11 cases per 100 000 in children aged about 3 years, and decreasing in later childhood to around 2 cases per 100 000 per year (Figure 30.10). About 30% more cases are seen in boys than in girls, and some 80% are acute lymphoblastic leukemia (ALL).

During the last 50 years, when cancer registration has been in operation in the Nordic countries, the rate of childhood leukemia has remained stable. Interestingly, over this relatively long period, the peak of leukemia in childhood has also remained unchanged, with respect to both its extent and the age group most clearly affected. The incidence of

**Table 30.5  Age-standardized incidences of leukemias of different subtypes in selected areas of the world in the early 1990s (per 100 000 population)[2]**

| Area of registration | Leukemia subtype | | | |
| --- | --- | --- | --- | --- |
| | Lymphatic | Myeloid | Monocytic | Other leukemias |
| Canada | 4.6 | 3.1 | 0.2 | 0.2 |
| Belarus | 4.5 | 2.1 | 0.1 | 0.2 |
| US, SEER: White | 4.4 | 3.4 | 0.2 | 0.1 |
| Australia, NSW | 4.0 | 3.8 | 0.1 | 0.1 |
| Sweden | 3.5 | 2.7 | 0.1 | 0.7 |
| England and Wales | 3.3 | 3.0 | 0.1 | 0.1 |
| US, SEER: Black | 3.3 | 3.3 | 0.2 | 0.1 |
| The Netherlands | 3.1 | 2.7 | 0.2 | 0.2 |
| Algeria, Setif | 2.1 | 1.9 | — | — |
| Japan, Hiroshima | 1.9 | 2.8 | 0.1 | — |
| Argentina, Concordia | 1.8 | 0.3 | — | — |
| The Philippines, Manila | 1.7 | 1.9 | 0.1 | — |
| China, Shanghai | 1.3 | 1.5 | 0.5 | 0.1 |
| India, Madras | 1.1 | 1.2 | 0.1 | — |
| Brazil, Belem | 1.0 | 1.5 | — | — |
| Vietnam, Hanoi | 0.6 | 1.4 | 0.1 | 0.1 |

**Table 30.6  Distribution of notified leukemia subtypes in Denmark 1978–98[a]**

| Leukemia subtype | Number | % |
| --- | --- | --- |
| Lymphatic | 7 046 | 50 |
| Myeloid | 5 760 | 43 |
| Leukemia, NOS[b] | 435 | 3 |
| Hairy cell | 232 | 1 |
| Monocytic | 155 | 1 |
| Erythroleukemia | 63 | <1 |
| Acute myelofibrosis | 22 | <<1 |
| Megakaryocytic | 17 | <<1 |
| Myeloid sarcoma | 17 | <<1 |
| Eosinophilic | 6 | <<1 |
| Compound leukemia | 2 | <<1 |
| Lymphosarcoma cell leukemia | 2 | <<1 |
| All leukemias | 13 757 | 100 |

[a]Source: The Danish Cancer Registry (unpublished data).
[b]NOS, not otherwise specified.

**Table 30.7  Population-based distribution of lymphatic and myeloid leukemias in Denmark, 1978–92, by clinical behavior[a]**

| Leukemia subtype | Lymphatic | | Myeloid | |
| --- | --- | --- | --- | --- |
| | No. | % | No. | % |
| Acute/subacute | 1275 | 18 | 4105 | 71 |
| Chronic | 5633 | 80 | 1492 | 26 |
| Aleukemic | 10 | <1 | 9 | <1 |
| NOS[b] | 128 | 2 | 154 | 3 |
| All types | 7046 | 100 | 5760 | 100 |

[a]Source: The Danish Cancer Registry (unpublished data).
[b]NOS, not otherwise specified.

childhood leukemia seems to be lower in most non-Caucasian populations, and the peak at the age of 3 years is less marked. In Africa, there seems to be no childhood peak at all.[12]

## The lymphomas

Lymphoma is a malignancy of lymphocytes, the primary effector cells of the immune system. While Hodgkin's disease constitutes a rather uniform subgroup of lymphomas, distinguished by its histological appearance (the presence of Reed–Sternberg giant cells) and its clinical features, the remaining, largest group of lymphomas, namely NHL, is heterogeneous. The various subclassifications that have been proposed over the years are probably of little relevance to the etiology of these tumors.

On the basis of data from Europe and the USA, we know that extranodal NHL comprise approximately 30% of cases in adulthood. Of these, some 50% arise in the gastrointestinal organs (the stomach in particular) and some 10% each in the respiratory system, the central nervous system, and the uroginital organs. The remaining 20% of extranodal lymphomas can affect almost any other organ of the body.

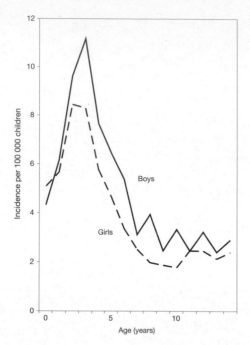

**Figure 30.10** Age-specific incidence rates of childhood leukemia, 1943–98.[11]

An analysis of the NHL reported to the SEER registries in the USA showed the following distribution according to the Working Formulation subtypes: diffuse subtypes (43%); follicular subtypes (18%); high-grade subtypes (12%); small lymhocytic lymphomas (9%); peripheral T-cell lymphomas (4%); and lymphomas not otherwise specified (NOS) (14%).[8] The analysis also showed that the follicular histological subtypes were two or three times more frequent among Blacks than among Whites, and that high-grade lymphomas were two to three times more frequent in men than in women.

### Burkitt lymphoma

Burkitt lymphoma is a distinct pathological entity arising from B lymphocytes. The classifical picture of the malignancy is that of a rapidly growing tumor of the jaws or abdominal viscera in a child aged 5–8 years. In most series, twice as many boys as girls develop the disease. In the endemic form, which is seen in tropical Africa and lowland New Guinea, evidence of the Epstein–Barr virus (EBV) is seen consistently in tumor tissue. The areas of high risk for Burkitt lymphoma coincide with those regions affected endemically by malaria; this environmental link with malaria is supported by studies of migrants.[13]

Awareness of the characteristics of Burkitt lymphoma has led to the observation that it seemingly constitutes a significant percentage (20–30%) of childhood NHL in most countries,[14] although the incidence rates are much higher in Africa (8 per 100 000 children, compared with 0.2 per 100 000 in Whites in the USA).

# Etiology

During the last five decades, a variety of risk factors for hematological malignancies have been suggested, many of which, however, have been based on unconfirmed data and inconsistent findings across studies. Taken together, verified risk factors explain only a minor proportion of these cancer types.

### The leukemias

Genetic factors seem to be involved in some cases of leukemia, childhood leukemia in particular. A well-known example is that persons with Down syndrome (trisomy 21) have an estimated 20- to 30-fold increased risk of developing acute leukemia of various cell types.[15] Although most common during childhood, all ages are apparently affected.[16] Other congenital disorders with extra chromosomes associated with leukemia are Kleinefelter syndrome and D-trisomy. Children with certain hereditary or congenital conditions accompanied by a tendency to chromosomal abnormalities or breaks have an elevated risk of acute leukemia. These disorders include Bloom syndrome, Fanconi anemia, and ataxia telangiectasia.[17] Von Recklinghausen's disease (neurofibromatosis type 1) is yet another congenital disorder that in some cases is linked with leukemia, particularly the rare juvenile chronic lymphocytic leukemia (CLL). The Li–Fraumeni cancer family syndrome, which is likely caused by germline mutations in the *p53* gene, and possibly other more or less well-characterized family syndromes and congenital disorders, have likewise been associated with increased risk of leukemia.[17] However, with the exception of the trisomies, these genetic and congenital abnormalities occur extremely rarely in the population and account for only a small proportion of leukemias.

There is overwhelming evidence that ionizing radiation is a risk factor for leukemia. The tumors induced are either acute forms or chronic myeloid leukemia (CML), with a mean latency of approximately 10 years.[18] The atomic bomb survivor studies carried out in Hiroshima and Nagasaki in Japan provide an important human experience from which estimates have been derived. The population is large and not selected because of disease or occupation. Studies of atomic bomb survivors, patients irradiated for benign diseases (ankylosing spondylitis, tinea capitis, or gynecological diseases), or given fluoroscopy for tuberculosis, and patients treated by ionizing radiation for malignant diseases show a dose–effect relationship measurable in absorbed doses over 0.1 Gy (10 rad).[18,19] The dose–response curve for doses below this level remains uncertain.

However, authoritative estimates predict that continuous lifetime exposure of 100 000 persons to an equivalent dose of 1 mSv of ionizing radiation per year will induce about 65 leukemias.[20] The greatest population exposure to ionizing radiation stems from natural background sources, which are about 2.9 mSv/year.[21] These sources include cosmic rays (0.27 mSv/year) and terrestrial radiation (0.28 mSv/year), internally deposited radionuclides (0.39 mSv/year), and radon (2.0 mSv/year), the last of which seems to be of relevance for lung cancer only. The greatest source of man-made radiation is from medical uses – therapeutic as well as diagnostic (0.53 mSv/year). Occupation, nuclear power, fallout from nuclear testing, and consumer products make only a minor contribution (0.11 mSv/year).[21] On the basis of these exposure assesments, it has been estimated that approximately 14% of all acute leukemias arising in a typical Western population are due to ionizing radiation from background sources.[19]

The excess risk, if any, of leukemia following low-dose radiation exposure of workers in nuclear installations in the UK and North America has been difficult to assess. Even the largest studies have had difficulties in providing risk estimates of useful precision, because the ranges of exposures were very small.[22–24] However, in a combined analysis of mortality data on approximately 96 000 workers employed for 6 months or longer in the nuclear industry in the USA, the UK, and Canada, the authors found that mortality from leukemia, excluding CLL, was significantly associated with cumulative external radiation dose. The analysis, which was based on 119 non-CLL leukemia deaths, suggested that the risk for these types of leukemias was increased by 22% for a cumulative protracted dose of 100 mSv compared with the no-exposure situation (0 mSv).[25]

A case–control study conducted in Denver, Colorado, USA first linked childhood cancer mortality with residential proximity to electric power lines, noting correlations between the current flow of the lines, their wiring configurations, and the estimated magnetic field exposures within residences.[26] Concurrently, in death certificate studies, positive associations were observed between adult leukemia and employment in an 'electrical occupation', suggesting a carcinogenic effect of electromagnetic fields from the electric power system.[27,28] Since then, numerous studies have investigated the relationship between extremely low-frequency (ELF) magnetic fields (in the 50–60 Hz frequency range) and cancer – leukemia in particular. The scientific evidence for an association has been assessed by an IARC working group.[29] The working group found that pooled analyses of data from a number of well-conducted studies showed a fairly consistent statistical association between a doubling of risk of childhood leukemia and ELF residential magnetic field strengths above 0.4 µT. The group concluded that there is limited evidence in humans for the carcinogenicity of ELF magnetic fields in relation to

childhood leukemia, and inadequate evidence in relation to all other cancers.

There is sufficient evidence that benzene causes acute myeloid leukemia (AML) in humans.[30] Since 1928, there have been many reports of leukemia in benzene-exposed shoe and leather workers. Benzene exposures are probably also the reason for the increased leukemia rates observed among rubber manufacturing workers, petroleum refinery workers, painters, pressmen, and printers. Table 30.8 lists the chemicals and industries that have been associated most consistently with an increased risk of leukemia. Most of the evaluations were made by working groups convened by the IARC on the basis of available scientific literature.

### Table 30.8 Drugs, chemicals, and industries recognized as presenting a leukemogenic risk

| Type of exposure | IARC group[a] |
| --- | --- |
| **Drugs** | |
| Melphalan | 1 |
| Cyclophosphamide | 1 |
| Busulfan | 1 |
| Chlorambucil | 1 |
| Semustine (methyl-CCNU) | 1 |
| MOPP and other combined chemotherapy regimens including alkylating agents Semustine (methyl-CCNU) | 1 |
| Epipodophyllotoxins | 2A/2B |
| Carmustine (BCNU) and related drugs other than semustine | —[b] |
| Treosulfane | 1 |
| Thiotepa | 2A |
| Chloramphenicol | 2A |
| **Other chemicals** | |
| Benzene | 1 |
| 1,3-Butadiene | 2A |
| Ethylene oxide | 2A |
| **Industries** | |
| Boot and shoe manufacture and repair | 1 |
| Rubber industry (certain occupations) | 1 |
| Petroleum refining | 2A |
| Paint manufacture and painting | 1 |
| Printing industry | 3 |
| Radiologists and X-ray technicians | —[b] |
| Nuclear industry workers | —[b] |

[a]IARC, International Agency for Research on Cancer. Group 1, The agent is carcinogenic to humans. Group 2A, the agent is probably carcinogenic to humans. Group 2B, the agent is possibly cinogenic to humans. Group 3, the agent is not classifiable as to its carcinogenicity to humans.
[b]Not evaluated by the IARC.

Several alkylating drugs and other chemotherapy agents are linked with highly increased risks of secondary AML among patients treated for various hematopoietic malignancies, and patients treated for some types of solid tumors, including ovarian cancer, small cell lung cancer, gastrointestinal malignancies, male germ cell tumors, and female breast cancer. Table 30.8 also lists these and other drugs associated with leukemia.

Leukemia has been linked with viral diseases in experimental settings; however, no conclusive epidemiologic evidence exists that confirm an association (but see ATLL under the discussion of NHL in the next subsection).

### Hodgkin's disease

Little is known about the etiology of Hodgkin's disease. There have been numerous reports of multiple occurrence of Hodgkin's disease within families, but such aggregations have not clearly been confirmed in population-based studies. No mutations that predispose to Hodgkin's disease have been identified to date.

There have been reports of unusual clusters of the disease in time and space (e.g. in high schools), which suggest that Hodgkin's disease might be contagious. Large, well-designed studies, however, have failed to confirm the initial reports,[31] although the potentially infectious nature of Hodgkin's disease is still debated. The candidate as an etiological infectious agent is the ubiquitous herpesvirus, the Epstein–Barr virus (EBV). Thus, in several case–control studies of patients with Hodgkin's disease, a moderate association was found with previous infections mononucleosis, a disease caused by EBV, and in support of such an association, molecular studies of tumor tissue from Hodgkin's disease patients have shown that 30–50% of cases in general are EBV-genome-positive.[31]

Overall, there is some evidence that occupational groups such as carpenters, joiners, and other woodworkers have a slightly increased risk of Hodgkin's disease, but the relevant exposures have not been identified.[32]

### NHL, other than Burkitt lymphoma

An increased risk of NHL has been clearly associated with immunodeficiency. Highly increased rates during childhood and early adulthood have been reported among patients with primary immunodeficiency disorders such as ataxia telangiectasia, common variable immunodeficiency, X-linked lymphoproliferative syndrome, or Wiskott–Aldrich syndrome, all of which are rare disorders. A much lower, but clearly excessive, risk of NHL is seen among patients with secondary, or acquired, immunodeficiency, such as that following immunosuppressive therapy in conjunction with organ or bone marrow transplantation, or human immunodeficiency viral (HIV) infection.[13,33] There is some evidence that several chronic connective tissue disorders, such as rheumatoid arthritis, systemic lupus erythematosus, and Sjögren syndrome, increase the risk of subsequent NHL.

Adult T-cell leukemia/lymphoma (ATLL), which constitutes only a small proportion of NHL in Western countries, but occur in clusters in, for example, Japan, is most likely caused by the human T-cell lymphotropic virus type I (HTLV-I). The presence of HTLV-I in endemic areas is thought to be the chief cause of lymphomas in persons under 60 years of age;[13] however, in general, this is a relatively rare infection and contributes little to the overall NHL incidence.

Not only viral infections seem to be related to NHL – an increasing body of evidence links chronic gastric infections with *Helicobacter pylori* to the development of malignant gastric neoplasia, including low-grade lymphomas arising from mucosa-associated lymphoid tissue (MALT).[34] In developing countries, the prevalence of infection with *H. pylori* increases rapidly during childhood, and continues to increase gradually throughout adult life, to reach a level of 80–90%. In most developed countries, the prevalence of infection is below 50%, with markedly decreasing trends over time. A low level of education and poor housing conditions have been associated with infection. Both oral–oral and oral–fecal routes of transmission of the bacteria have been postulated.[34]

Several studies have shown that blood transfusion recipients are at an increased risk of developing NHL, which suggests that a bloodborne agent may be responsible for this disease.[35–37]

A number of occupational exposures have been considered causes of NHL. Farming and herbicide application seem to be associated with increased rates of this malignancy, although the association is not definitively proven,[38,39] since specific exposures that may account for the increased risk have not been identified. Exposures to pesticides, including phenoxyacetic acid herbicides, have regularly been implicated. Besides farming, employment in rubber manufacture and in styrene–butadiene rubber production have been linked with increased risks of NHL.[30] Industrial exposures to ethylene oxide, chlorinated solvents (such as perchloro- and trichloroethylene), inks in the printing industry,[40,41] and of hairdressers and barbers to chemicals,[42] have been associated with this disease in some but not all studies. The general importance of these occupational exposures, some of which (pesticides and hair colorants) also affect the general population, is at present unknown. Exposure to radiation probably has little effect on the risk of NHL.

Left column, top heading "Multiple myeloma":

Individuals with monoclonal gammopathy of unknown significance (MGUS) are predisposed to developing multiple myeloma.[43] MGUS is an asymptomatic, non-malignant disorder involving proliferation of plasma cells and production of M-components. However, the cause of MGUS is unknown, and other causes of multiple myeloma are largely unrecognized. The increased incidence of the disease among US Blacks, however, indicates that genetic factors may be involved, although the higher rate could also be explained by race-specific environmental differences. In some but not all studies of occupation and industrial activities, farming was associated with multiple myeloma. Positive associations have also been reported for a history of occupational exposure to petroleum products. There is no convincing evidence of an association between exposure to ionizing radiation in therapeutic doses and multiple myeloma.

Heading "Survival":

Many reports are available on the prognosis of patients with hematological malignancies involved in clinical trials the main purpose of which was to test the efficacy of new treatments. The outcome, therefore, does not usually reflect the survival experience of patients with these malignancies in general, nor is it possible on the basis of trials to evaluate trends in survival over time. In contrast, population-based cancer registries continuously collect information on the incidence of and survival from malignant diseases over time in a defined population, i.e. on all individuals included in the population, regardless of prognostic factors.

Survival can be recorded as crude or relative. Crude survival rates represent the observed numbers of patients in a given population who survive a given length of time relative to the size of the initially diagnosed study population. Relative survival rates are adjusted for deaths due to causes that are not related to the disease under study and are computed by dividing the observed proportion or rate of patients who survive by the equivalent proportion of the background population of the same age and sex composition. If this survival ratio is 1.0, then the chance of the patients surviving is similar to that of the general population; if the ratio is below 1.0, then the patient group has less chance of surviving than the general population.

Recently, efforts have been made to collect data on cancer survival from population-based cancer registries in Europe in order to make reliable comparisons of survival in different European populations by performing standardized analyses (the EUROCARE studies). The first EUROCARE study, published in 1995, covered survival of cancer patients in 30 registries, and the second study, published in 1999, was extended to cover 44 cancer registries in 17 countries.[44,45] In the USA, population-based information on incidence of and survival from cancer is collected within the SEER program.[3]

Heading "Leukemias":

Figure 30.11 shows overall sex-specific, 1-year and 5-year survival rates for all leukemias combined in 17 European countries, 1985-89. The figure shows the relative survival (in %), as the mortality of the general population has been subtracted from the patients' mortality prior to the calculation of survival. This also implies that one minus the relative survival may be interpreted as the proportion of patients who die as a consequence of the cancer at the 1-year and 5-year points after diagnosis.

The survival analyses were based in some countries on few regions, in other countries on the entire population (Denmark, Estonia, Iceland, Scotland, Slovakia, and Slovenia). At the bottom of Figure 30.11, survival rates are shown for men and women in Europe, on the basis of all data available.[45]

Again, on the basis of all data available, Figure 30.12 gives the population-based relative survival rates for each of four major subtypes of leukemia in Europe. A marked variation in survival by subtype is evident in each sex.

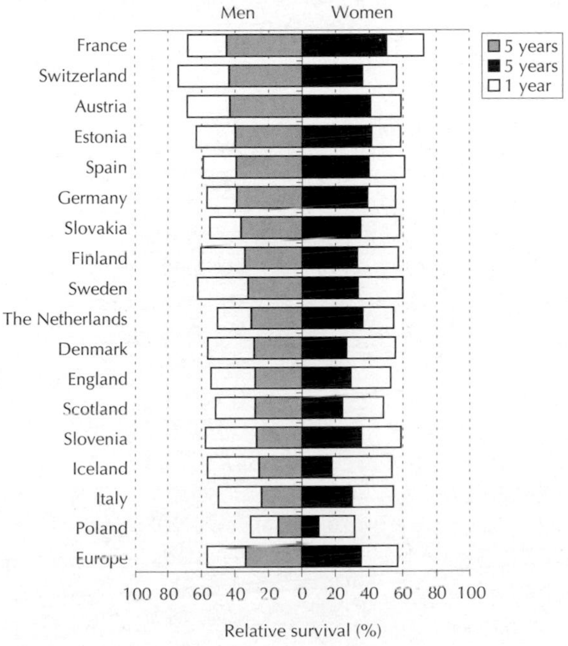

Figure 30.11 (a horizontal bar chart comparing Men and Women relative survival across European countries: France, Switzerland, Austria, Estonia, Spain, Germany, Slovakia, Finland, Sweden, The Netherlands, Denmark, England, Scotland, Slovenia, Iceland, Italy, Poland, Europe; x-axis "Relative survival (%)" from 100 to 100; legend shows 5 years, 5 years, 1 year).

Caption: "Figure 30.11 Relative 1-year and 5-year survival rates (age-standardized) from all types of leukemia combined among patients in the EUROCARE II study, 1985-89.[15]"

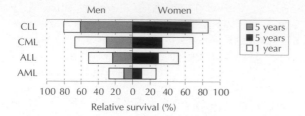

**Figure 30.12** Relative 1-year and 5-year survival rates (age-standardized) from chronic lymphocytic leukemia (CLL), chronic myeloid leukemia (CML), acute lymphoblastic leukemia (ALL), and acute myeloid leukemia (AML) among men and women in Europe.[15]

## Lymphomas

Figure 30.13 shows overall 1-year and 5-year survival rates for Hodgkin's disease and NHL, in European men and women diagnosed during 1985–89 (data on Hodgkin's disease were not available for Iceland and Spain). Considerable geographical variation in survival within Europe was reported, ranging from 41% (Estonia) to 85% (Austria) for 5-year survival after Hodgkin's disease, and from 21% (Estonia) to 61% (Austria) for 5-year survival after NHL.[45]

## Multiple myeloma

Finally, for the same areas of Europe and on the basis of the EUROCARE II study, Figure 30.14 shows the sex-specific relative survival rates for multiple myeloma (data on multiple myeloma were not available for France and Poland). Again, a marked variation is seen within Europe, some of which, however,

may be due to random variation due to small numbers of cases.

## Survival in European and US populations

A comparison was undertaken of population-based, age- and sex-adjusted cancer survival data from the adult population in the USA and Europe.[46] The study considered 12 types of cancers, Hodgkin's disease and NHL included, diagnosed during 1985–89 and reported to one of the 41 EUROCARE cancer registries of 17 European countries or to one of the nine SEER registries in the USA, covering the populations of the states of Connecticut, Iowa, Utah, New Mexico, and Hawaii, and the metropolitan areas of Atlanta, Detroit, Seattle, and San Francisco–Oakland, which add to approximately 10% of the US population.

Figure 30.15 shows the 5-year survival (in %) in Europe and the USA, respectively, in patients with one of 12 selected cancers. Cancer types are ordered according to decreasing survival probability. In general, European patients had significantly lower survival rates than American patients. The authors found that differences in the method of data collection, the quality of registration, and the type of analysis had only marginal effect on the difference in survival. They speculated that the observed differences in favor of patients in the USA could be due to three factors: earlier cancer detection, better response to treatment at an earlier disease stage, and more effective treatment protocols.[46] For Hodgkin's disease and NHL, in particular, the relative excess risks for dying before 5 years of follow-up were 1.15 and 1.11, respectively, to the disadvantage of Europe (Figure 30.15).

**(a)**

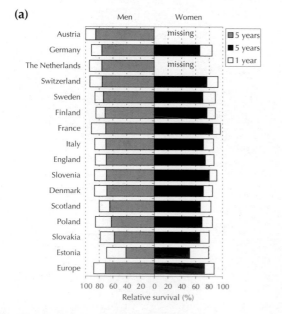

**(b)**

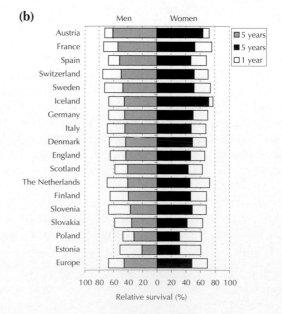

**Figure 30.13** Relative 1-year and 5-year survival rates (age-standardized) from (a) Hodgkin's disease and (b) non-Hodgkin lymphoma among patients in the EUROCARE II study 1985–89.[15]

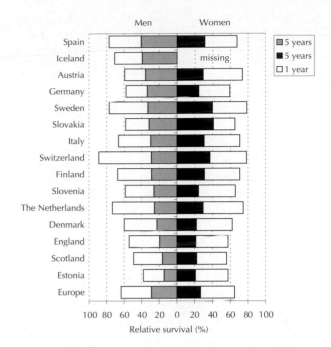

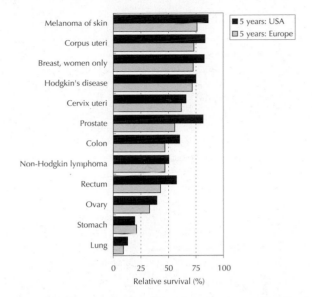

**Figure 30.14** Relative 1-year and 5-year survival rates (age-standardized) from multiple myeloma among patients in the EUROCARE II study 1985–89.[15]

**Figure 30.15** Standardized 5-year relative survival for 12 selected cancers in adult patients in Europe and the USA, 1985–89.[46]

## Conclusions

The hematological malignancies are a heterogeneous group of disorders, and their descriptive epidemiology as well as the identification of etiologies has been hampered by the many changes over time in diagnostic practice and disease classification. Some rather limited international variation is seen for each of the main diagnostic groups of leukemia, Hodgkin's disease, NHL, and multiple myeloma. Overall, the group of hematological malignancies represents approximately 8–9% of all cancers in men and 8% of all cancers in women in Australia, the USA, and Canada. The proportions appear to be slightly lower in the European Union. In these areas of the world, leukemias and NHL are the most prevalent hematological cancers, with markedly increasing time trends for the NHL. The group of NHL is relatively more frequent in Canada and among Whites in the USA than in other populations, while Black Americans clearly form a high-risk population with regard to multiple myeloma.

Little is known about the etiology of the hematological malignancies. Genetic factors as well as ionizing radiation (the leukemias), chemotherapeutic agents, viral and bacterial infections (the lymphomas), and a limited number of occupational exposures have been implicated. Population-based surveys of cancer patients in Europe, diagnosed in 1985–89, have shown 5-year survival rates from leukemia, Hodgkin's disease, NHL, and multiple myeloma of 34%, 71%, 45%, and 29%, respectively, among men, and 35%, 73%, 48%, and 27%, respectively, among women. Considerable geographical variation within Europe was reported for each of the main diagnostic groups. For a number of selected cancer types, Hodgkin's disease and NHL included, a comparison of the European rates with those of a similar population-based survey from the USA showed that American patients tended to have a markedly better survival than European patients, which is possibly due to a combination of earlier cancer detection, better response to treatment at an earlier disease stage, and more effective treatment protocols.

## REFERENCES

1. Parkin DM, Pisani P, Ferlay J. Estimates of the worldwide incidence of 25 major cancers in 1990. *Int J Cancer* 1999; **80**: 827–41.
2. Parkin DM, Whelan SL, Ferlay J et al (eds). *Cancer Incidence in Five Continents. IARC Scientific Publication 143*, Vol VII. Lyon: IARC, 1997.
3. *National Cancer Institute Surveillance and Epidemiology End Results Program. SEER Cancer Statistics Review, 1973–1999.* US Department of Health and Human Services: www. seer.cancer.gov, 20 August 2002.
4. Storm HH, Engholm G, Ferlay J (eds). *Cancer Incidence and Mortality in the Nordic Countries. NORDCAN,*

Version 1. Association of Nordic Cancer Registries (ANCR), 2002: dataset on CD ROM.

5. Ferlay J, Bray F, Pisani P et al. *Cancer Incidence, Mortality and Prevalence Worldwide. GLOBOCAN 2000.* Lyon: IARC, 2001: dataset on CD ROM.

6. Feraly J, Bray F, Sankila R et al. *Cancer Incidence, Mortality and Prevalence in the European Union. EUCAN 1997.* Lyon: IARC, 1999: dataset on CD ROM.

7. Devesa SS, Blot WJ, Stone BJ et al. Recent time trends in the United States. *J Natl Cancer Inst* 1995; **87**: 175–82.

8. Groves FD, Linet MS, Travis LB et al. Cancer Surveillance Series: non-Hodgkin's lymphoma incidence by histologic subtype in the United States from 1978 through 1995. *J Natl Cancer Inst* 2000; **92**: 1240–51.

9. Devesa SS, Fears T. Non-Hodgkin's lymphoma times trends: United States and international data. *Cancer Res* 1992; **52**(Suppl): 5432s–40s.

10. Holford TR, Zheng T, Mayne ST et al. Time trends of non-Hodgkin's lymphoma: Are they real? What do they mean? *Cancer Res* 1992; **52**(Suppl): 5443s–6s.

11. Brown P deN, Hertz H, Olsen JH et al. Incidence of childhood cancer in Denmark 1943–1984. *Int J Cancer* 1989; **18**: 546–55.

12. Parkin DM, Kramárová E, Draper GJ et al (eds). *International Incidence of Childhood Cancer. IARC Scientific Publication 144.* Lyon: IARC, 1998.

13. Rabkin CS, Ward MH, Manns A et al. Epidemiology of non-Hodgkin's lymphoma. In: Margarth IT (ed) *The Non-Hodgkin's Lymphomas.* New York: Oxford University Press, 1997: 171–88.

14. Thomatis L (ed). *Cancer: Causes, Occurrence and Control. IARC Scientific Publication 100.* Lyon: IARC, 1990: 81–2.

15. Holland WW, Doll R, Carter CO. The mortality from leukaemia and other cancers among patients with Down's syndrome and among their parents. *Br J Cancer* 1962; **16**: 177–84.

16. Hill DA, Gridley G, Cnattingius S. Mortality and cancer incidence among individuals with Down syndrome. *Arch Intern Med* 2003; **163**: 705–11.

17. Lindor NM, Green MH, The concise handbook of family cancer syndromes. *J Natl Cancer Inst* 1998; **90**: 1039–71.

18. Mettler FA, Upton AC. *Medical Effects of Ionizing Radiation,* 2nd edn. Philadelphia: WB Saunders, 1995.

19. Winther JF, Ulbak K, Dryer L et al. Radiation. *APMIS* 1997; **105**(Suppl 76): 83–99.

20. *Health Effects of Exposure to Low Levels of Ionizing Radiation (BEIR V).* Washington DC: National Academy Press, 1990.

21. *UNSCEAR. Sources, Effects and Risks of Ionizing Radiation.* New York: United Nations, Publ E.86.IX.9, 1988.

22. Gilbert ES, Omohundro E, Buchanon JA et al. Mortality of workers at the Hanford site: 1945–1986. *Health Phys* 1993; **64**: 577–90.

23. Carpenter L, Higgins C, Douglas A et al. Combined analysis of mortality in three United Kingdom nuclear industry workforces, 1946–1988. *Radiat Res* 1994; **138**: 224–38.

24. Schubrauer-Berigan MK, Wenzl TB. Leukaemia mortality among radiation-exposed workers. *Occup Med* 2001; **16**: 271–87.

25. Cardis E, Gilbert ES, Carpenter L et al. Effects of low doses and low dose rates of external ionizing radiation: cancer mortality among nuclear industry workers in three countries. *Radiat Res* 1995; **142**: 117–32.

26. Wertheimer N, Leeper E. Electrical wiring configurations and childhood cancer. *Am J Epidemiol* 1979; **109**: 273–84.

27. Milham S. Mortality from leukemia in workers exposed to electrical and magnetic fields. *N Engl J Med* 1982; **307**: 249.

28. Wright WE, Peters JM, Mack TM. Leukaemia in workers exposed to electrical and magnetic fields. *Lancet* 1982; **ii**: 1160–1.

29. *Non-Ionizing Radiation,* Part 1: *Static and Extremely Low-Frequency (ELF) Electric and Magnetic Fields. IARC Monographs on the Evaluation of Carcinogenic Risks to Humans,* Vol 80. Lyon: IARC, 2002.

30. *Overall Evaluations of Carcinogenicity: An Updating of IARC Monographs, Vols 1–42. IARC Monographs on the Evaluation of Carcinogenic Risks to Humans,* Suppl 7. Lyon: IARC, 1987.

31. Mueller N. Hodgkin's disease. In: Schottenfeld D, Fraumeni JF Jr (eds) *Cancer Epidemiology and Prevention,* 2nd edn. New York: Oxford University Press, 1996: 893–919.

32. *Wood Dust and Formaldehyde. IARC Monographs on the Evaluation of Carcinogenic Risks to Humans,* Vol 62. Lyon: IARC, 1995.

33. *Some Antiviral and Antineoplastic Drugs, and Other Pharmaceutical Agents. IARC Monographs on the Evaluation of Carcinogenic Risks to Humans,* Vol 76. Lyon: IARC, 2000.

34. *Schistosomes, Liver Flukes and* Helicobacter pylori. *IARC Monographs on the Evaluation of Carcinogenic Risks to Humans,* Vol 61. Lyon: IARC, 1994: 177–240.

35. Cerham JR, Walace RB, Folsom AR et al. Transfusion history and cancer risk in older women. *Ann Intern Med* 1993; **119**: 8–15.

36. Blomberg J, Möller T, Olsson H et al. Cancer morbidity in blood recipients – results of a cohort study. *Eur J Cancer* 1993; **29A**: 2101–5.

37. Memmon A, Doll R. A search for unknown bloodborn oncogenic viruses. *Int J Cancer* 1994; **58**: 366–8.

38. *Occupational Exposures in Insecticide Application, and Some Pesticides. IARC Monographs on the Evaluation of Carcinogenic Risks to Humans,* Vol 53. Lyon: IARC, 1991.

39. *Some Thyrotropic Agents. IARC Monographs on the Evaluation of Carcinogenic Risks to Humans,* Vol 79. Lyon: IARC, 2001: 379–604.

40. *Dry Cleaning, Some Chlorinated Solvents and Other Industrial Chemicals. IARC Monographs on the Evaluation of Carcinogenic Risks to Humans,* Vol 64. Lyon: IARC, 1995.

41. *Printing Processes and Printing Inks, Carbon Black and Some Nitro Compounds. IARC Monographs on the Evaluation of Carcinogenic Risks to Humans,* Vol 65. Lyon: IARC, 1996.

42. *Occupational Exposures of Hairdressers and Barbers and Personal Use of Hair Colourants; Some Hair Dyes, Cosmetic Colourants, Industrial Dyestuffs and Aromatic Amines. IARC Monographs on the Evaluation of Carcinogenic Risks to Humans,* Vol 58. Lyon: IARC, 1993.

43. Gregersen H, Mellemkjær L, Salling Ibsen J et al. Cancer risk in patients with monoclonal gammopathy of undetermined significance. *Am J Hematol* 2000; **63**: 1–6.

44. Sant M, Gatta G. The EUROCARE database. In: Berrino F, Sant M, Verdecchia A et al. (eds) *The Eurocare Study, IARC Scientific Publication 132.* Lyon: IARC, 1995: 15–31.

45.  Capocaccia R, Gatta G, Chessa E et al. Presentation of the EUROCARE-2 study. In: Berrino F, Capocaccia R, Estève J et al. (eds) *Survival of Cancer Patients in Europe: The EUROCARE-2 Study. IARC Scientific Publication 151.* Lyon: IARC, 1999: 1–26.

46.  Gatta G, Capocaccia R, Coleman MP et al. Toward a comparison of survival in American and European cancer patients. *Cancer* 2000; **89**: 893–900.

# 31 Lymphoid malignancies in children

Raul C Ribeiro and Ching-Hon Pui

## Introduction

Lymphoid malignancies are clonal disorders of the immune system that result from the transformation of immature lymphoid progenitor cells at a particular stage of differentiation. Because the lymphoid system is functionally diverse, has a wide anatomic distribution, interacts with other cellular systems, and, during childhood and adolescence, undergoes continuous remodeling, the clinical and biological characteristics of lymphoid malignancies in young patients vary substantially. Traditionally, pediatric lymphoid malignancies have been grouped in two broad categories: acute lymphoblastic leukemia (ALL) and non-Hodgkin lymphomas (NHL). These malignancies are further classified depending on the type of lymphoid lineage involved in the process. B-lineage malignancies account for more than 88% of cases of ALL and 50% of cases of NHL (Burkitt, lymphoblastic, and large B-cell lymphomas), whereas T-lineage malignancies account for about 12% of ALL cases and 50% of NHL cases (lymphoblastic and anaplastic large-cell lymphomas). Understanding the mechanisms by which the human lymphoid system develops and acquires functional diversity has led to an integrated view of the lymphoid malignancies that occur in childhood. From that perspective, childhood ALL and NHL represent a spectrum of the same disorder. Because a lymphoid malignancy is usually associated with a particular lymphoid compartment, each group of pediatric malignancies may be viewed in a functional context, as shown in Figure 31.1.

In this chapter we review the pathophysiology and clinical manifestations of ALL and NHL, re-examine the mechanisms of these disorders in the light of the new molecular genetic findings, and discuss the role of these findings in improving therapy for ALL and NHL.

## Epidemiology and risk factors

In the US, of the 12 400 new cases of cancer diagnosed per year in children, adolescents, and young adults

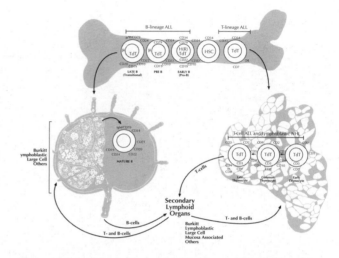

**Figure 31.1** Schematic representation of the origins of normal B and T cells and their routes of circulation in primary (bone marrow, lymph nodes, thymus) and secondary lymphoid organs (skin and lymphoid tissue associated with mucosa and the gastrointestinal tract; lymph nodes and thymus are both primary and secondary lymphoid organs). The CD antigens characteristic of each cell type are shown, and the types of leukemia and lymphoma that arise from each subset of cells are indicated. DR, leukocyte histocompatibility antigens; H(R), rearranged immunoglobulin heavy chain; HSC, hematopoietic stem cell; TdT, terminal deoxynucleotidyl transferase; μ, immunoglobulin heavy chain; ψ, pseudo-light chains.

less than 20 years old, 2400 (19.4%) are ALL and 800 (6.5%) NHL.[1,2] Together, ALL and NHL represent the most common types of pediatric malignancy and account for about one-third of all childhood cancers. Acute lymphoblastic leukemia represents 17% of all pediatric cancer affecting neonates and infants, 46% of cancer occurring in children between the ages of 2 and 3 years, and 9% of cancers occurring just before the age of 20 years. Non-Hodgkin lymphoma affects 3% of children less than 5 years old and 9% of those between the ages of 15 and 19 years (Figure 31.2). A

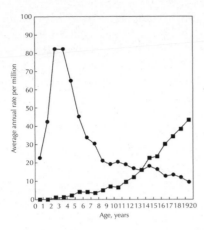

**Figure 31.2** Age-specific rates, for all races and both sexes, of acute lymphoblastic leukemia (ALL; circles) and non-Hogdkin lymphoma (NHL; squares). Data from the Surveillance Epidemiology End Results (SEER; with permission).[1,2]

prenatal origin of some cases of childhood ALL, first suggested by genetic studies of identical twins with concordant leukemia, was established by examining the neonatal blood (archived blood spots) of children who later developed leukemia. In this neonatal blood were cells that contained transcripts of leukemia-specific fusion genes or clonotypically rearranged genes at the loci encoding immunoglobulin or T-cell receptors. Because of the relatively low rate of concordance of some types of leukemia in identical twins, the sometimes long delay after birth before leukemia develops, the variety of presenting features and outcome, and the failure of fusion transcripts alone to induce leukemia in model systems, it is thought that additional postnatal events are required for full leukemic transformation.[3–7]

Over the past 20 years, there has been an apparent increase in the incidences of ALL and NHL in the US. It is estimated that between 1977 and 1995, the incidence of ALL increased by 0.9% per year. This increase in the rate of leukemia was not observed in black children. Similarly, the rates of other types of leukemia did not increase during this period. The incidence of NHL in children younger than 15 years remained stable from 1975 through 1995, but during this period the incidence of NHL in adolescents increased from 10.7 per million (1975–1979) to 16.3 per million (1990–1995).[1] The reasons for these increased incidences of ALL and NHL are not known. Some investigators have suggested that the apparent increase in incidence of ALL is a result of improvement in diagnostic specificity from the mid 1970s, which led to the recognition as ALL of forms of lymphoid leukemia that were previously not specified as ALL.[8]

The incidences of ALL and NHL are higher in boys than in girls, and the rates of ALL and NHL are markedly higher for white children than for black

children in all age groups. The incidence rate of ALL in white children younger than 5 years, which is a good measure of the incidence peak, is more than double that in black children (63.2 vs. 26.9 per million). Therefore, the difference in incidence reflects mainly the lower rates of ALL among black children younger than 5 years.

International variation in the incidences of ALL and NHL has been reported.[9,10] However, the lack of population registry makes comparison between countries difficult. The peak in ALL incidence noted in children in developed countries is absent or diminished for children in developing countries. This observation has been used to support the 'hygiene theory' in which the greater peak incidence in children aged between 2 and 5 years in industrialized countries compared with that in developing nations reflects the delayed exposure of children in developed countries to common childhood infectious diseases.[11] In NHL, there is a clear relation between Epstein–Barr virus (EBV) infection (with malaria as a cofactor) and the incidence of Burkitt lymphoma.[12] Moreover, acquired immunodeficiency syndrome (AIDS) resulting from human immunodeficiency virus (HIV) infection has been associated with an increased risk of NHL.[13] However, for the most part, the factors contributing to the increased incidence of NHL are unclear.

Causes of childhood lymphoid malignancies are largely unknown. Most children with ALL or NHL do not appear to have predisposing factors. Moreover, recent observations suggest that different subtypes of lymphoid malignancies may involve different etiologic factors. For example, ALL in infants, which is consistently associated with 11q23 chromosomal abnormalities, has epidemiological associations that are different from those of ALL in other age groups. Because this chromosomal region is also affected in cases of secondary acute myeloid leukemia AML due to the use of topoisomerase II inhibitors,[14] some investigators have proposed that nontherapeutic or naturally occurring topoisomerase II inhibitors may have a role in the etiology of infant ALL.[15–17]

Certain factors and specific constitutional syndromes have been associated with an increased predisposition to ALL or NHL.[18] Increased risk of ALL has been associated with Down syndrome,[19,20] neurofibromatosis,[21] Shwachman syndrome,[22] Bloom syndrome,[23] ataxia telangiectasia,[24,25] and Klinefelter syndrome.[26] Patients with congenital immunodeficiencies such as Wiskott–Aldrich syndrome,[27] X-linked lymphoproliferative syndrome, and severe combined immunodeficiency[28,29] have a significantly higher risk of developing NHL than do individuals in the general population. Exposure to ionizing radiation has been implicated in the development of childhood ALL.[30,31] Less clear is the association between electromagnetic fields (EMF) and the development of ALL; a recent analysis of pooled data from several studies found little or no association between the risk of ALL and EMF.[32]

Pharmacogenetics, a rapidly advancing biological field that investigates the genetic basis for inherited differences among individual responses to specific drugs or environmental xenobiotics,[33] has the potential to provide clues to the different incidences of ALL and NHL that occur across diverse ethnic groups and geographic regions. The implication is that individuals with altered drug-metabolizing enzyme activities resulting from genetic polymorphisms are more susceptible to carcinogens. Indeed, a higher prevalence of polymorphisms that result in inactive detoxifying enzymes has been associated with de novo ALL in infants and children, AML in adults, and therapy-related leukemia.[34,35] Other xenobiotic-metabolizing enzymes have also been implicated in the development of leukemia.[36] New methods, such as the use of microchip arrays and genome-wide DNA analysis, are now being applied to the interpretation of several of the genes encoding drug- and xenobiotic-metabolizing enzymes to elucidate the roles of these enzymes in drug response and disease production.

# Diagnosis and classification

The examination of bone marrow or tumor mass (nodal or extranodal) is mandatory for the definitive diagnosis of ALL or NHL, respectively. Occasionally, the bone marrow can be difficult to aspirate because of fibrosis, necrosis, or tightly packed marrow. Sampling of the most accessible, representative nodal or extranodal tumor is the best approach in patients suspected to have NHL. In patients with a large mediastinal mass, who are at very high risk of complications during anesthesia, pleural effusion can provide an adequate number of tumor cells for diagnosis. Alternatively, needle biopsy of regional lymph nodes, which can be performed without general anesthesia, may also yield adequate material for diagnosis of primary mediastinal NHL.

The diagnosis of acute leukemia is established by morphologic criteria, from Romanowsky-stained bone marrow films. The arbitrary proportion of 25% or more blast cells is required for the diagnosis of leukemia. Further characterization of the leukemic cells by a panel of cytochemical stains separates lymphoid and myeloid leukemias. Approximately 80% to 85% of cases of childhood ALL have the bone marrow totally replaced by lymphoblasts. Acute lymphoblastic leukemias have been classified according to the criteria of the French–American–British (FAB) Cooperative Group as L1 (80%), L2 (18%), or L3 (2%),[37] but this system has largely been abandoned due to the lack of correlation with immunophenotypic or genetic features. The ALL blasts are always negative for myeloperoxidase (MPO) activity and rarely positive for Sudan black B staining. The periodic acid-Schiff stain, which detects glycogen deposits, is positive in about 70% of cases of ALL. Flow cytometric analysis, using antibodies to lymphoid and myeloid antigens, is crucial for the precise classification of lymphoid leukemias and recognition of hybrid or mixed-lineage leukemia.[38]

About 88% of childhood ALL is of B-cell origin. Of these B-lineage cases, less than 2% are leukemias arising from the expansion of mature B cells and are classified as Burkitt leukemia; the remaining B-lineage cases comprise ALL derived from B-precursor cells. T-cell ALL accounts for about 12% of cases of ALL. There is a loose association between these main immunophenotypic groups and the clinical features present at the time of diagnosis. For example, patients with mature B-cell leukemia usually have an abdominal mass or other extranodal tumor deposits at the time of initial examination. Patients with T-cell ALL tend to be adolescent (median age, 10.5 years) males with a mediastinal mass, leukocytosis, an elevated serum lactate dehydrogenase (LDH) concentration, and central nervous system (CNS) leukemia.[39] Patients with precursor B-cell ALL tend to be younger (median age, 4.6 years) and to have a small tumor burden at the time of diagnosis.

Until recently, the main contribution of the immunophenotypic classification was to reveal that the standard treatment of ALL was not adequate for certain immunophenotypic subgroups.[40–42] Therefore, for treatment purposes, grouping cases into mature B-cell, T-cell, and precursor B-cell (pre- and pro-B) categories is necessary.[43] A caveat to this approach is that, in rare situations, there are morphologically typical lymphoblasts that express lineage-specific myeloid markers. These lymphoblasts can express a combination of MPO and either B-cell or T-cell markers. Recent experimental evidence suggests that there are separate myeloid and lymphoid progenitors for B and T cells.[44] The prognosis is usually poor in this type of leukemia, and treatment has not been standardized.[45] Another important contribution of the immunophenotype is to the parametric flow cytometric analysis that defines the unique combination of antigens expressed by the leukemic cells in each case.[46] This unique profile provides a very sensitive tool with which to follow the kinetics of blast cell clearance during treatment and enables the detection of minimal residual disease.[47]

Cytogenetic characterization of the leukemic cells is an integral part of the initial evaluation of childhood ALL.[42,47,48] In virtually all cases of ALL, a genetic abnormality can be detected.

Numerical chromosome abnormalities, which occur in about 50% of cases of ALL, can be determined directly, by conventional cytogenetic analysis, or indirectly, by quantifying the DNA content of the leukemic cells by using flow cytometric methods to obtain the DNA index.[49] By convention, normal diploid (46 chromosomes) cells have a DNA index of 1. Numerical chromosome abnormalities in ALL are classified into four subgroups. The frequency of each subgroup of ALL, classified on the basis of numeric chromosomal abnormalities, is listed in Table 31.1. Structural rearrangements or translocations that can be detected by using conventional cytogenetic or molecular methods are present in about 40% of cases. The most common structural abnormalities found in ALL are listed in Table 31.2. Lately, the combination of advanced computer and optical technology has added another dimension to conventional cytogenetic analysis and is providing important insights into the pathobiology of the disease. Routine methods now available for the genetic characterization of ALL, such as spectral karyotyping or chromosome painting, provide reliable and precise information on the chromosomal location of material involved in leukemia-associated gene rearrangements.[50]

Although the classification of NHL in general is very complex and still evolving,[51] the classification of pediatric NHL is relatively simple and straightforward. Virtually all childhood NHL can be classified into one of three groups, each of which exhibits dif-

fuse histologic characteristics: Burkitt, lymphoblastic, and large-cell lymphomas. In one series, histology revealed only 17 (1.3%) cases of follicular (nodular) NHL among 1336 children or adolescents.[52] Burkitt lymphoma is composed of sheets of monomorphic lymphoid cells. Commonly, macrophages dispersed throughout the tumor give it the classic 'starry sky' appearance. In the bone marrow or blood, the Burkitt cells (in FAB L3 subtype ALL) are relatively uniform

**Table 31.1 Frequency of abnormal numbers of chromosomes in lymphoblastic leukemia in children**

| Blast cell ploidy | Frequency (%) |
|---|---|
| 46, Diploid (normal) | 10–20 |
| 46, Pseudodiploid (structural abnormalities) | 30–40 |
| <45, Hypodiploid | 7–8 |
| 23–29, Near haploid | <1 |
| 30–44, Low hypodiploid | <1 |
| >46, Hyperdiploid | 40–50 |
| 47–50, Low hyperdiploid | 10–15 |
| 51–65, High hyperdiploid | 30–55 |
| 66–80, Near triploid | 1 |
| >80, Near tetraploid | 1 |

**Table 31.2 Frequency of the most common structural abnormalities of chromosomes in lymphoblastic leukemia in children**

| Cytogenetic abnormality | Immunophenotype | Fusion gene | Frequency (%) |
|---|---|---|---|
| t(12;21)(p13;q22) | B-lineage | TEL-AML1 | 20–25 |
| t(1;19)(q23;p13) | B-lineage | PBX1-E2A | 5 |
| t(9;22)(p34;q11) | B-lineage | BCR-ABL | 4 |
| t(4;11)(q21;q23) | B-lineage | MLL-AF4 | 3 |
| t(8;14)(q24;q32) | B-lineage (mature) | MYC-IgH | 2–3 |
| t(17;19)(q22;p13) | B-lineage | HLF-E2A | <1 |
| t(11;19)(q23;p13.3) | B-lineage | MLL-ENL | <1 |
| t(8;22)(q24;q11) | B-lineage (mature) | MYC-IgL | <1 |
| t(2;8)(p12;q24) | B-lineage (mature) | MYC-IgK | <1 |
| t(1;14)(p32;q11) | T-lineage | TAL1-TCRδ | <1 |
| t(1;7)(p32;q34) | T-lineage | TAL1-TCRβ | <1 |
| t(1;7)(p34;q34) | T-lineage | LCK-TCRβ | <1 |
| t(7;9)(q34;q32) | T-lineage | TAL2-TCRβ | <1 |
| t(7;9)(q34;q34) | T-lineage | TAN1-TCRβ | <1 |
| t(8;14)(q24;q11) | T-lineage | MYC-TCRα/δ | <1 |
| t(11;14)(p15;q11) | T-lineage | LMO1-TCRδ | <1 |
| t(11;14)(p13;q11) | T-lineage | LMO2-TCRδ | <1 |
| t(7;10)(q34;q24) | T-lineage | HOX11-TCRβ | <1 |
| t(7;11)(q34;p13) | T-lineage | RHOM2-TCRβ | <1 |
| t(7;9)(q34;p13) | T-lineage | LYL1-TCRβ | <1 |
| t(10;14)(q24;q11) | T-lineage | HOX11-TCRδ | <1 |

with a moderate amount of deeply basophilic cytoplasm containing sharply defined, clear vacuoles and with round nuclei containing coarsely reticular chromatin. The cells express monotypic surface IgM (either κ or λ, light chains) and harbor specific chromosomal translocations involving the C-*MYC* oncogene. The most common of these cytogenetic abnormalities, present in 80% of cases, is the t(8;14)(q24;q32) translocation. The t(2;8)(p12;q24) and t(8;22)(q24;q11) account for the remaining cases.[53]

Lymphoblastic NHL arises from transformed, immature T or B cells. The T-cell immunophenotype, which accounts for more than 80% of all lymphoblastic NHL, expresses an immunophenotypic profile similar to that of normal thymocytes at an intermediate or late stage of differentiation. As with Burkitt NHL, T-cell malignancies involve several cytogenetic abnormalities that lead to the activation of transcription factors, as a result of specific translocations in the T-cell receptor genes. Typically, these translocations are juxtaposed with a small number of developmentally important transcription factor genes, including *HOXll (TLX1), TAL1 (SCL), TAL2, LYL1, BHLHB1, LMO1,* and *LMO2*.[54]

Large-cell NHL is the most heterogeneous group of all subtypes of pediatric NHL. Immunophenotypic analysis of large-cell NHL reveals that the neoplastic cells can be of T-cell or B-cell lineage or have no lineage-specific markers (null cells). Regardless of the immunophenotype, about 40% of large-cell NHL cases express the CD30 (Ki-1) antigen.[55] In a classification system adopted by the World Health Organization, large-cell NHL is divided into diffuse B-cell and anaplastic large-cell lymphoma (ALCL). Classification as ALCL requires the coexpression of CD30 and the membrane epithelial antigen (MEA) in lymphoma cells expressing T-cell or null-cell markers.[51] About 80% of ALCL cases identified by this criterion harbor the t(2;5)(p23;q35) chromosomal rearrangement.[56] The result of this translocation is the fusion of the gene encoding anaplastic lymphoma kinase (ALK) with regulatory elements of the gene encoding nucleophosmin (NPM), a nonribosomal nucleolar phosphoprotein.[57] Fusion of the *ALK* gene can also result from other translocations, including t(1;2), t(2;3), inv(2), and t(2;22). Importantly, ALK protein can be detected by immunohistochemistry with polyclonal and monoclonal antibodies on paraffin sections, which aids diagnosis.

## Clinical manifestations

The initial clinical manifestations of ALL in children vary widely. The symptoms and signs are determined by the degree of bone marrow failure and the propensity of the leukemic cells to infiltrate extramedullary

sites. In addition, the leukemic cells are metabolically active and produce numerous pro-inflammatory mediators, which can make the presenting features even more varied. Fever resulting from infection or, more commonly, inflammatory mediators is one of the most common signs, occurring in about 60% of patients. Pallor, fatigue, lethargy, petechiae, ecchymosis, and bone pain are also common. Other frequent findings disclosed by physical examination include liver, spleen, and lymph node enlargement. Subclinical involvement of the testis is very common in ALL.[58] However, clinically detected testicular enlargement occurs in approximately 2% of male patients. Bone pain and arthralgia are very common presenting features of ALL.[59] Stretching of the periosteum as a result of expansion of the medullary cavity is thought to be the mechanism underlying bone pain. Central nervous system manifestations are very rarely present at the time of initial examination. The signs and symptoms of CNS involvement are related to increased intracranial pressure and include irritability, lethargy, headaches, nausea, and vomiting. Cranial nerve palsies, most commonly of the seventh cranial nerve, may be present. Examination of the optic fundus can reveal papilledema and, occasionally, leukemic infiltration of the optic nerve and retina. Patients with T-cell ALL can present with a large, anterior mediastinal mass, sometimes with large pleural effusions (Figure 31.3). These patients may have a brassy cough, dyspnea, stridor, cyanosis,

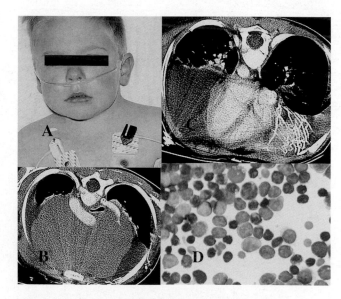

**Figure 31.3** (A) A 5-year-old boy with respiratory distress and clinical signs of superior vena cava syndrome (note the facial edema and plethora). A CT scan of the chest revealed (B) an anterior mediastinal mass (10 × 8 × 10 cm) that compressed the trachea and (C) bilateral pleural effusion and collateral venous flow to the intercostal vessels. Examination of the pleural effusion revealed a WBC count of 37 × 10⁹/L and 80% lymphoblasts (D). Immunophenotyping confirmed that the child had ALL of T-cell lineage.

facial and upper torso edema (Figure 31.3A), and venous engorgement resulting in collateral venous circulation over the chest and abdomen (Figure 31.3B). In addition, a mediastinal mass can compress the trachea and superior vena cava, to various degrees. Mediastinal involvement represents a medical emergency and an early management challenge (see below).

Similarly to ALL, the presenting features of childhood NHL are extremely diverse. The dominant clinical manifestations depend on the tumor's location and the extent of the disease. Virtually any lymphoid tissue can be involved, including peripheral lymph nodes, tonsils, thymus, spleen, and intestinal lymphoid aggregates (Peyer's patches). In addition, extralymphatic extension to include the bone marrow, CNS, bone, and skin is also common in childhood NHL.

Painless enlargement of the cervical lymph nodes is the most common clinical presentation. In a St Jude review,[60] one-third of children with NHL had palpable lymph nodes in the head and neck region. One-third of patients with NHL presents with primary mediastinum involvement, which is commonly associated with supraclavicular and axillary adenopathy. The clinical presentation of patients with a large mediastinal mass is described above. Abdominal presentation of childhood NHL is associated with a palpable mass. Tumors in the gastrointestinal tract usually affect the distal ileum, cecum, and mesenteric nodes. Retroperitoneal and renal extension is also common. Patients complain of intermittent pain in

the periumbilical region or right iliac fossa. Nausea, vomiting, and weight loss are also common features. Occasionally, signs of an acute abdomen due to intussusception are the dominant feature. Generally, the primary tumor site is associated with a particular histologic subtype. An abdominal mass is most common in Burkitt NHL; mediastinal and peripheral lymph node tumors are most common in lymphoblastic or diffuse, large B-cell NHL; and skin, bone, and soft tissue tumors are most common in ALCL. In disseminated cases it is often impossible to determine the tumor's primary site. Less common presentations of NHL include subcutaneous lesions, thyroid and parotid enlargement, proptosis, and spinal cord compression. Spinal cord compression, albeit rare, should be considered a medical emergency and be treated urgently to prevent permanent neurologic deficits. The histologic, immunophenotypic, and cytogenetic characteristics of childhood NHL are listed in Table 31.3.

## Laboratory findings

Almost all cases of childhood ALL have one or more abnormalities of the blood counts. Abnormalities of two or more hematologic lineages should raise high suspicion of leukemia in a child. Because anemia develops over a relatively long period, it usually does not compromise the cardiovascular system. Patients with T-cell ALL tend to have normal or minimally abnormal hemoglobin levels. The WBC count is elevated in more than 50% of cases, and is above 50 ×

**Table 31.3 Clinically relevant histologic types, immunophenotype, and cytogenetic features of non-Hodgkin lymphoma (NHL) in children**

| Histologic type* | Immunophenotype | Cytogenetic abnormality | Fusion gene |
|---|---|---|---|
| Burkitt | B-cell (mature) | t(8;14)(q24;q32) | MYC-IgH |
| | | t(8;22)(q24;q11) | MYC-IgL |
| | | t(2;8)(p12;q24) | MYC-IgK |
| Lymphoblastic | T-cell | Same as T-cell ALL† | |
| | Pre-B | Same as pre-B ALL† | |
| Large-cell | B-cell | | |
| Anaplastic large-cell | T-cell, null | t(2;5)(p23;q32) | NPM-ALK |
| | | t(1;2)(q21;p23) | TPM3-ALK |
| | | t(2;3)(p23;q21) | TFG-ALK |
| | | Inv(2)(p23;q35) | ATIC-ALK |
| | | t(2;22)(p23;q11) | CTCL-ALK |
| | | t(X;2)(q11;p23) | MOESIN-ALK |
| | | t(2;19)(p23;13) | TPM4-ALK |

* World Health Organization classification; † ALL, acute lymphoblastic lymphoma.

$10^9$/L in 20% of cases. About 45% of patients have a WBC count lower than $10 \times 10^9$/L. Lymphocytes and lymphoblasts account for most cells in the differential count. Neutropenia is a common finding. Thrombocytopenia is a very common finding in ALL. About 70% of patients have platelet counts below $100 \times 10^9$/L; some patients present with apparent isolated thrombocytopenia. Overt bleeding is rare, even in patients with platelet counts less than $20 \times 10^9$/L. Coagulation parameters are usually normal, and plasma fibrinogen concentrations tend to be elevated, reflecting a systemic inflammatory response. Mild coagulopathy with slightly increased prothrombin time and partial thromboplastic time and a low fibrinogen concentration is a relatively common finding in T-cell ALL and generally has no clinical consequences.[61] Disseminated intravascular coagulation (DIC) has been associated with pre-B ALL and the rare t(17;19)(q22;p13) chromosomal abnormality.[62]

Elevated serum urate concentrations and increased urinary excretion of uric acid, which are common presenting features, reflect an increased rate of purine metabolism. Serum LDH concentrations are increased, particularly in patients with a large leukemic cell burden. Hypercalcemia, which is present in less than 1% of patients with ALL, results from the release by the leukemic cells of parathyroid hormone-related peptide or other cytokines. These patients may have multiple osteolytic lesions. Hyperphosphatemia is a relatively common presenting feature of ALL and usually indicates renal impairment resulting from dehydration or tumor lysis. Chest radiography is required and easily identifies a mediastinal mass and pleural effusion. Skeletal involvement, which is very common in ALL, includes metaphysical bands, periosteal reactions, osteolytic lesions, osteosclerosis, and osteopenia. However, a routine skeletal survey or bone scintillography is not warranted in these patients because these abnormalities do not have clinical or prognostic implications and resolve with treatment. However, rarely, osteopenia can be severe and lead to vertebral collapse and severe back pain.[63] Lumbar puncture and examination of the cerebrospinal fluid (CSF) are integral components of the initial evaluation of a child with ALL. About 3% of these patients have overt CNS leukemia, which is defined as a WBC count of 5 or more per microliter of CSF, with leukemic cells confirmed by morphologic examination of a cytocentrifuge preparation; CNS leukemia may also be suspected from the presence of cranial nerve palsies. Even in the absence of pleocytosis, the presence of leukemic cells in cytocentrifuge preparations has clinical implications: these patients have an increased risk of CNS relapses[64] and require more intensive CNS-directed therapy. Recently, there has been a concern that the lumbar puncture itself can seed leukemic cells into an otherwise clean CNS (traumatic tap) and thus increase the risk of CNS relapse.[65]

In patients with NHL, the blood counts are usually normal. Anemia, thrombocytopenia, and circulating lymphomatous cells are present in patients with bone marrow involvement. As in patients with ALL, serum concentrations of uric acid and LDH can be elevated. Although CNS involvement is rare at presentation of NHL, particularly in those with large-cell lymphoma, lumbar puncture and CSF examination should be performed in all patients. An expeditious radiologic investigation is required to demonstrate areas of tumor involvement and is used in monitoring the tumor's response to therapy. Whole-body computerized tomography (CT) is the imaging modality of choice to determine the extent of the tumor, and radionuclide scanning with both technetium-99 and gallium-67 is generally performed in all patients. The roles of magnetic resonance imaging (MRI), photon emission CT, and thallium scanning in childhood NHL have not yet been defined. Bone marrow examination is mandatory in the initial evaluation of NHL. Bone marrow biopsy may disclose tumor involvement that is not clear from examination of the bone marrow aspirate and is, therefore, recommended by most investigators as part of the work-up to determine disease stage.

## Differential diagnosis

Because of their varied clinical and laboratory manifestations, childhood ALL and NHL can mimic several nonmalignant and malignant diseases. Rheumatoid arthritis is commonly misdiagnosed in patients with ALL who present with bone and joint pain. The inflammatory process in the joints of patients with ALL can be migratory, as in rheumatoid arthritis, and quiescent for days or weeks. Of interest, these patients usually have near-normal blood counts. In addition, they tend to have persistent fever, a prolonged erythrocyte sedimentation rate, and increased serum concentrations of C-reactive protein. If patients are given steroids or methotrexate, two drugs commonly used in the treatment of rheumatoid arthritis, the diagnosis of leukemia can be delayed for several months. Aplastic or hypoplastic anemia followed by spontaneous remission can precede ALL. Typically, at the time of initial examination, patients have pancytopenia and hypocellular bone marrow, to varied extents, and no leukemic cells; they improve within 1 to 4 weeks with supportive care only. Sometimes this process is referred to as preleukemia because overt ALL, usually of B-cell lineage, is frequently diagnosed within 3 to 9 months of the initial insult.[66] Hypereosinophilia, which is usually associated with several benign disorders, can also be the first sign of ALL. The leukemic cells sometimes harbor the t(5;14)(q31;q32).[67] Rarely, patients with solid tumors (including neuroblastoma and rhabdomyosarcoma) present with pancytopenia and circulating blasts.

Most often, however, other presenting features and the immunophenotype of the malignant cells indicate the correct diagnosis. Immune thrombocytopenic purpura (ITP) is also frequently the presumptive misdiagnosis of childhood ALL. However, a detailed analysis of blood counts reveals at least one or more abnormalities of the blood counts if the diagnosis is ALL,[68] whereas the blood counts are, except for the platelet count, completely normal in ITP. Infectious mononucleosis and other viruses produce severe hematologic responses that are occasionally confused with leukemia. Careful characterization of the circulating cells will establish the correct diagnosis.

Differentiating between a reactive lymphoproliferative process and NHL rarely presents a difficulty. Delay in diagnosis of NHL occasionally occurs in patients with localized, painless adenopathy because histologic studies of the lymph nodes were inconclusive for the presence of malignancy. Patients with persistent, painless enlargement of the lymph nodes after a trial of antibiotic therapy for 10 to 14 days should undergo a lymph node biopsy, preferably surgically, to provide adequate tissue for immunophenotyping, molecular, and conventional studies. Persistently enlarged lymph nodes in patients with acquired or congenital immunodeficiency represent a significant diagnostic dilemma. Collectively, these abnormalities have been classified as lymphoproliferative disorders (LPD) and range from reactive polyclonal hyperplasia to true monoclonal malignant lymphomas. Children presenting with an isolated mediastinal mass present a diagnostic challenge. Several malignant and nonmalignant conditions, including histoplasmosis, sarcoidosis, Hodgkin disease, germ cell tumor, thymic carcinoma, neuroblastoma, and myeloblastoma, may present with a mediastinal mass. Results of serologic studies may provide evidence for some of these diseases, but usually, CT-guided needle biopsy is necessary to provide tissue for diagnosis. Primary lymphoma of the bone is commonly misdiagnosed. Indeed, in a St Jude study, 10 of the 11 patients with primary lymphoma of the bone had received an alternative initial diagnosis.[69] To differentiate between primary lymphoma of the bone and other small blue cell tumors, immunohistochemical studies with an extensive panel of markers are required in addition to histologic studies.

## Prognostic factors

Despite effective treatment of childhood lymphoid malignancies, about 20 to 25% of children with lymphoid malignancies die from their diseases. In general, the presenting features of patients who have a poor outcome tend to differ from those whose disease is cured by current treatment modalities. Prognostic factor analysis is an attempt to disclose subgroups of patients who have dissimilar outcomes. Factors found to be associated with poor outcome in patients with ALL include age less than 1 year or more than 10 years, hyperleukocytosis or clinical evidence of massive leukemia burden, CNS involvement, T-cell immunophenotype, certain genetic abnormalities in the leukemic cells, and persistence of leukemia after induction therapy.[42] Treatment can modify the prognostic value of certain variables. For example, hyperleukocytosis, which is a common presenting feature of leukemia in infants, T-lineage leukemia, and subsets of B-lineage leukemia, is a strong predictor of poor outcome in many studies of childhood ALL. However, with new, effective strategies to treat T-cell leukemia, hyperleukocytosis is no longer an adverse prognostic indicator for this subset of leukemia, but continues to be a strong prognostic indicator in B-lineage leukemia. Prognostic factor analysis has also led to the identification of subtypes of leukemia that can be treated less intensively. For example, patients with subtypes of ALL in which the leukemic cells are hyperdiploid (>50 chromosomes) or have the TEL-AML1 fusion have a very good outcome with standard therapy. Recently, a highly favorable outcome was observed in T-cell ALL with HOX11 expression of MLL-ENL fusion.[54] Conversely, some subtypes of ALL, such as ALL with any 11q23 chromosomal abnormality in infants or ALL with the Philadelphia chromosome, have poor outcome regardless of treatment strategy.[70,71]

However, there is clinical heterogeneity even among specific genetic subtypes of ALL. For example, among patients with ALL and the Philadelphia chromosome, those 1 to 9 years old with a low leukocyte count at the time of the initial examination have a relatively favorable outcome.[71] Infants with 11q23 abnormalities fare worse than do children 1 or more years old with this type of abnormality.[70] The predictive value of presenting features can be improved by including information on the patient's response to initial therapy. For example, molecular and flow cytometric methods can be used to follow the kinetics of leukemic cell clearance and to check for the persistence of leukemia after induction or consolidation therapy. Approximately 20 to 25% of patients for whom induction therapy has achieved complete remission by morphologic criteria have evidence of leukemia, shown by flow cytometric and molecular methods, with the bone marrow containing between 0.001% and 4% mononuclear cells. The use of these methods has disclosed that rapid, early clearance of leukemic cells is associated with a good prognosis, whereas persistence of leukemia after remission induction therapy is associated with an increased risk of relapse.[72] Patients who have less than 0.01% leukemic cells after 2 weeks of remission induction treatment have a particularly favorable prognosis. An integrated model for using prognostic features is depicted in Figure 31.4. Prognostic factor analysis of

ALL may improve further with the use of gene expression profiling, a method used recently[73] to accurately identify patients at high risk of relapse (Figure 31.5).

In NHL, staging systems have been used to identify groups of patients with diverse prognoses. The most used of these systems, introduced by St Jude, is applicable to all subtypes of NHL (Table 31.4).[60] The

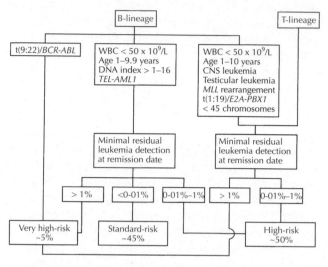

Figure 31.4 Risk classification in the current (Total Therapy Study XV) St Jude Children's Research Hospital ALL trial. Infants (12 months or younger) are treated on a separate treatment protocol. Estimated proportions of patients classified in each of the three risk groups are shown in the respective boxes. (Reproduced with permission, from *Lancet Oncology* 2002; **10**: 597.)

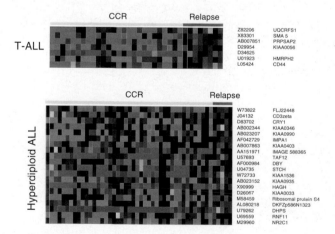

Figure 31.5 Expression pattern of genes (on an Affymetrix array) that were selected as discriminant of relapse in patients with T-cell ALL (*7* genes) and hyperdiploid (>*50* chromosomes) ALL (20 genes). The Gene-Bank accession number and the gene symbol or DNA sequence name are listed on the right side of each panel. (From Yeoh EJ, Ross ME, Shurtleff SA et al. Classification, subtype discovery, and prediction of outcome in pediatric acute lymphoblastic leukemia by gene expression profiling. *Cancer Cell* 2002; **2**: 133–143, with permission.)

## Table 31.4 The St Jude staging system for non-Hodgkin lymphoma (NHL) in children

| Stage | Description |
|---|---|
| I | A single tumor (extranodal) or single anatomic area (nodal), excluding mediastinum or abdomen |
| II | A single tumor (extranodal) with regional node involvement on same side of diaphragm:<br>(a) Two or more nodal areas<br>(b) Two single (extranodal) tumors with or without regional node involvement<br>A primary gastrointestinal tract tumor (usually ileocecal) with or without associated mesenteric node involvement, grossly completely resected |
| III | Two or more tumors on both sides of the diaphragm:<br>(a) Two single tumors (extranodal)<br>(b) Two or more nodal areas<br>All primary intrathoracic tumors (mediastinal, pleural thymic)<br>All extensive primary intraabdominal disease; unresectable<br>All primary paraspinal or epidural tumors regardless of other sites |
| IV | Any of the above with initial CNS or bone marrow involvement (<25%) |

main value of this classification scheme is in separating patients with localized disease from those with advanced disease. More recently, information on immunophenotype and molecular findings has been incorporated into classification schemes. This approach established the foundations on which investigators can develop treatment regimens specific to immunophenotype and disease stage. As in ALL, response to therapy has been used to make treatment decisions in NHL as well. French investigators proposed using imaging studies to estimate the reduction in tumor mass after one week of cyclophosphamide, vincristine, and prednisone (COP) treatment in patients with B-cell lymphoma. Patients whose primary tumor was reduced by less than 20% received a more intensive treatment strategy.[74] Recently, gene chip arrays have been developed to identify the molecular features associated with NHL.[75] Whether this method will add meaningful prognostic information remains to be determined.

## Treatment

### Acute lymphoblastic leukemia

#### Lessons from the past

The treatment of childhood ALL is one of the major successes of modern medicine. Current treatments are expected to cure about 80% of newly diagnosed ALL.[42] Over the years, several treatment principles have endured. First, a combination of several chemotherapeutic agents is superior to a single agent in inducing remission of ALL.[76] Second, certain classes of drugs are appropriate to induce remission, whereas others are appropriate to maintain it.[77] Third, after remission is achieved by induction therapy, combination chemotherapy is required for a prolonged period to eradicate leukemic cells.[78] Fourth, the complete elimination of leukemic cells requires that specific components of the therapy be targeted to subclinical leukemic involvement of the CNS.[79] Fifth, it must be recognized that ALL is a heterogeneous disorder with many subtypes that respond differently to specific treatment strategies.[80] Finally, properly conducted clinical trials on the efficacy of risk-directed therapy for ALL are important.[41,81] For example, contemporary clinical trials have similar overall outcome (Table 31.5), but different trials have disclosed diverse treatment facets. Some trials have proved particular treatment components to be more effective in certain subtypes of leukemia and others to be associated with unique complications. Careful analysis of these data has enabled investigators to combine components of these trials to increase efficacy and reduce morbidity.

## Induction of remission (early therapy)

The first objective in the treatment of childhood ALL is to induce complete remission. To achieve complete remission, the leukemic burden has to be reduced by 99%, or from $10^{12}$ to $10^{10}$ leukemic cells. Treatment with a combination of glucocorticoids (prednisone, prednisolone, dexamethasone) and vincristine can induce complete remission of ALL in about 85% of children. Prednisone and prednisolone have been the most used types of steroids. Dexamethasone appears to be more potent and penetrates the CNS better, but its use may be associated with higher mortality rates.[82] The addition of L-asparaginase to the treatment regimen, with or without an anthracycline, increases the rate of complete remission to above 95% within 4 to 6 weeks. The role of L-asparaginase in prolonging remission has been documented.[83] Delaying L-asparaginase administration to the postremission phase does not jeopardize the rate of complete remis-

### Table 31.5 Results of studies of lymphoblastic leukemia in children*

| Study† | Year | Number of patients | 5-year event-free survival rate % (SE) Overall | B-lineage‡ Standard risk | High risk | T-lineage |
|---|---|---|---|---|---|---|
| AIEOP-91 | 1991–95 | 1194 | 70.8 (1.3) | 79.9 (1.5) | 61.5 (2.9) | 40.4 (4.1) |
| BFM-90 | 1990–95 | 2178 | 78.0 (0.9) | 87.4 (1.0) | 66.3 (2.1) | 61.1 (2.9) |
| CCG-1800 | 1989–95 | 5121 | 75 (1) | 80 (1) | 67 (2) | 73 (2) |
| COALL-CLCG-92 | 1992–97 | 538 | 76.9 (1.9) | 82.1 (2.4) | 75.7 (3.9) | 71.2 (5.1) |
| DCLSG-7 | 1988–91 | 218 | 65.3 (3.2) | 69.3 (4.1) | 66.6 (7.6) | 57.7 (8.6) |
| DFCI-91-01 | 1991–95 | 377 | 83 (2) | 85 (2) | 82 (4) | 79 (8) |
| EORTC-58881 | 1989–98 | 2065 | 70.9 (1.1) | 78.4 (1.3) | 57.3 (2.4) | 64.4 (2.9) |
| NOPHO-III | 1992–98 | 1143 | 776. (1.4) | 85.2 (1.5) | 67.9 (3.3) | 61.3 (4.9) |
| POG | 1986–94 | 3828 | 70.9 (0.8) | 77.4 (0.9) | 55.3 (1.6) | 51.0 (2.4) |
| SJCRH-13A | 1991–94 | 165 | 76.9 (3.3) | 88.1 (3.6) | 70.4 (6.2) | 60.9 (10.2) |
| TCCSG-L92-13 | 1992–95 | 347 | 63.4 (2.7) | 67.8 (3.4) | 56.7 (5.4) | 59.3 (8.6) |
| UKALL-XI | 1990–97 | 2090 | 63 (1.1) | 74 (2.2) | 59 (4.1) | 51 (3.5) |

* Results were taken from a series of articles on long-term results of pediatric ALL clinical trials published by 12 major study groups or institutions (*Leukemia* 2000; **14**: 2196–2204).

† AIEOP, Associazione Italiana di Ematologia ed Oncologia Pediatrica; BFM. Berlin-Frankfurt-Münster Study Group; CCG, Children's Cancer Group; COALL, Cooperative All Study Group; DCLSG, Dutch Childhood Leukemia Study Group; DFCI, Dana-Farber Cancer Institute ALL consortium; EORTC-CLCG, European Organization for Research on the Treatment of Cancer, Children's Leukaemia Cooperative Group; NOPHO, Nordic Society of Pediatric Hematology and Oncology; POG, Pediatric Oncology Group; SJCRH, St Jude Children's Research Hospital; TCCSG, Tokyo Children's Cancer Study Group; UKALL, UK Medical Research Council Working Party on Childhood Leukaemia.

‡ The standard-risk group included children 1–9 years old with leukocyte count $<50 \times 10^9/L$; all others (except infants) were placed in the high-risk group. The differences in 'overall' results are partly related to the disproportion of high-risk cases referred to some institutions.

SE, standard error.

sion or event-free survival and is associated with fewer thrombotic complications.[84,85] CNS-directed therapy, which begins concomitantly with the administration of these systemic agents, is described later in this chapter. After the induction of remission is achieved, many treatment regimens prescribe additional chemotherapeutic components. These have been used early in the induction process[86] or after 4 weeks of standard chemotherapy.

### Consolidation and intensification therapy

The concept of consolidation and intensification of therapy is widely accepted as essential components of the overall treatment of ALL. This strategy was pioneered by investigators in the Berlin–Münster–Frankfurt (BFM) consortium.[87] Consolidation therapy is delivered immediately after induction therapy, when bone marrow function has been restored, and intensification (re-induction) therapy, between 2 and 4 months later, during maintenance therapy. There are many different ways to intensify postremission therapy. For example, investigators at the Dana-Farber Cancer Institute demonstrated that postremission therapy with L-asparaginase and doxorubicin was associated with an improved outcome in patients with T-cell leukemia.[88,89] Investigators of the Children's Cancer Group (CCG), like the BFM investigators, found that two phases of delayed intensification ('double delayed intensification') also improved the outcome of patients with high-risk leukemia.[90,91] The availability of these data has allowed St Jude investigators to develop an innovative approach to early therapy (about the first 4 months after remission). All patients receive high-dose methotrexate as consolidation therapy. Very high-dose (Sg/m$^2$) methotrexate has been shown to improve outcome in T-cell ALL.[92,93] Patients with T-cell leukemia also receive extended and intensive L-asparaginase and doxorubicin therapy following consolidation therapy, as in the Dana-Farber protocol. Re-induction phases (essentially a repetition of the induction therapy) occur on weeks 7 and 17 of postremission therapy, as proposed by BFM and CCG investigators. Patients with persistent disease after induction and consolidation therapy or ALL with the Philadelphia chromosome receive a block of intensive chemotherapy consisting of cytarabine, etoposide, dexamethasone, and L-asparaginase followed by hematopoietic stem cell transplantation (HSCT); patients with low-risk ALL receive postremission therapy that is of relatively low intensity and well tolerated.

### Maintenance therapy

Because the early postremission therapy – consolidation and intensification therapy and interim chemotherapy – extends through the first 2 to 6 months, maintenance therapy, which follows these phases of therapy, can be considered the final phase of treatment. The mechanism of the eradication of the leukemic clone after remission is poorly understood; the drugs and schedules prescribed in this phase have evolved over five decades and remain largely based on empiric evidence. In most protocols, this phase of therapy continues for 2 to 3 years from the time of remission. In the current St Jude study, girls receive chemotherapy for a total of 2.5 years and boys for 3 years. Attempts to reduce the duration of remission induction therapy have not been successful the few times they have been tried.[94,95] Similarly, there has been no evidence that prolonging the duration of maintenance therapy beyond 3 years has any added benefit. Daily oral doses of 6-mercaptopurine (6-MP), preferably taken at night on an empty stomach, and weekly doses of parenteral methotrexate constitute the framework of maintenance chemotherapy. Adjusting the dosage of these agents on the basis of the absolute neutrophil count is associated with a better prognosis.[96] However, the tolerance of 6-MP depends on the function of thiopurine S-methyltransferase, an enzyme produced by several autosomal codominant alleles. About 10% of patients with ALL have an inherited deficiency of this enzyme, which results in poor tolerance of 6-MP. To avoid prolonged myelosuppression, many patients with this enzyme deficiency need to be given lower 6-MP doses commensurate with their level of enzymatic activity.[97,98] Recently, it has become possible to determine, from the patient's genotype, which patients are at higher risk of toxicity from 6-MP, and thus require a lower dose. The addition of intermittent pulses of vincristine plus dexamethasone to the regimen has been shown to decrease the rate of relapse and is widely accepted.[99] Further intensification of therapy, usually for patients at high risk of relapse, can be attained by adding other drug pairs. Because of the need for prolonged maintenance therapy, the possible benefit of further intensification has to be weighed against the potential long-term side-effects of this strategy. These side-effects include secondary AML, infertility, and cardiac dysfunction.

### Central nervous system involvement

Overt CNS involvement at the time of diagnosis of ALL is relatively rare, affecting about 3 to 5% of newly diagnosed patients. Features that are associated with overt CNS leukemia at the time of diagnosis include age less than 1 year, the presence of T-cell markers, a hypodiploid karyotype, presence of the Philadelphia chromosome, and high WBC counts. These features and the presence of any amount of leukemic cells in the CSF (including those introduced iatrogenically into the spinal canal during a diagnostic spinal tap) increase the risk of CNS relapse.[65] Even patients who have no discernible adverse presenting features are at risk of CNS leukemia if they do not receive appropriate CNS-directed therapy. In the mid

1960s, St Jude investigators elegantly demonstrated that 2400 cGy delivered to the cranium and 1500 cGy to the spine reduced the rate of CNS relapse from 50% to 5%. Subsequently, they showed that intrathecal methotrexate could replace spinal radiotherapy. Because the toxicity associated with radiotherapy is substantial, several modifications aiming to reduce neurological toxicity have been tested during the past 30 years. First, it was found that the dose and fields of irradiation can be reduced when appropriate intrathecal and systemic therapies are provided.[87] Second, radiation therapy can be eliminated completely for patients with low-risk ALL.[100] Third, preventive CNS-directed therapy is not necessary beyond 1 year after complete remission. Fourth, intensive use of intrathecal therapy is effective in preventing CNS leukemia in more than 80% of children with ALL.[101,102] Finally, in high-risk cases, the radiation dose can be reduced to 1200 cGy without increasing the risk of CNS relapse, provided that effective systemic chemotherapy is used.[87] We and Dutch investigators are testing the hypothesis that in the context of intensive systemic and intrathecal therapy, cranial irradiation can be omitted, irrespective of the adverse prognostic features present at the time of the initial examination.

## Non-Hodgkin lymphoma

Progress in the treatment of children and adolescents with NHL parallels that of ALL. Results of most contemporary clinical trials are revealing survival rates approaching 90%.[74,103,104] Moreover, the use of risk-adapted strategies specific for disease stage and immunophenotype in conjunction with a wide range of effective agents, which are largely responsible for the improved survival rates, has practically eliminated the relevance of clinical and biologic prognostic factors. Treatment has emerged as the single most important determinant of successful outcome for patients with NHL. Clinical and biologic features that guide the therapeutic strategy include the extent of the disease at the time of diagnosis, sites of involvement, immunophenotype, morphology and immunohistochemistry of tumor cells, and early response to therapy.

### Lower-risk non-Hodgkin lymphoma (localized disease)

Patients with low-risk NHL, which accounts for about 10 to 20% of pediatric NHL, are those that after treatment with only two or three courses of chemotherapy have an excellent prognosis, with a probability of survival of more than 90%. Typically, these chemotherapy courses consist of a combination of corticosteroids, cyclophosphamide, vincristine, and doxorubicin (CHOP, COPAD) at standard dosages and given every 3 weeks. The Pediatric Oncology Group has conducted several studies[105] on patients with

stage I or II NHL, the results of which can be summarized as follows: (1) local radiotherapy can be safely omitted; (2) chemotherapy cycles of moderate intensity (4 agents) are sufficient for the eradication of NHL; (3) the duration of chemotherapy should be no longer than 6 months for these patients; (4) CNS-directed therapy is indicated only for patients with primary tumors in the head and neck region; (5) lymphoblastic lymphoma, which accounts for only 10 to 15% of disease of limited extent, requires maintenance chemotherapy with daily 6-MP and weekly methotrexate administration. Similar results have been achieved by other pediatric cooperative groups using modified versions of the St Jude staging system.

### Higher-risk non-Hodgkin lymphoma (advanced-stage disease)

Patients who are not classified as having limited or low-risk disease are collectively grouped as high-risk patients. Naturally, patients placed in this category have a wide range of tumor burdens and are likely to have diverse prognoses. Because of this diversity, there are large discrepancies between treatments given depending on the staging system used. For example, a patient with Burkitt lymphoma without CNS involvement and <25% blast cells in the bone marrow is considered to have disease stage IV according to the St Jude system, but is placed in group B in the SFOP staging system (the SFOP system stipulates 70% or more of bone marrow involvement for group C). Treatment of group C disease is much more intensive than that of group B.[106] Other investigators define risk categories among patients with advanced-stage disease on the basis of serum LDH concentrations.[107]

The highly successful protocol developed by French investigators, the LMB89,[74] for patients with B-cell NHL (Burkitt, Burkitt-like, and large B-cell lymphomas) has become the benchmark for other protocols. Intensive, high-dose treatment of short total duration (5 to 8 months) and a reduced interval between treatment cycles are the hallmark of all effective combinations for patients with B-cell (Burkitt, Burkitt-like, small noncleaved-cell, large B-cell) NHL. CNS-directed therapy is mandatory and is intensive in patients with evidence of CNS involvement or those in the high-risk category. In developing treatment for advanced-stage lymphoblastic NHL, it has been assumed that this form of the disease behaves the same as does T-cell ALL. This observation is derived from the seminal Children's Cancer Group study, reported about 20 years ago, showing that the $LSA_2L_2$ regimen, an ALL-type therapy, was significantly more effective than pulse chemotherapy (COMP) for patients with lymphoblastic NHL.[108] However, because most lymphoblastic NHL is of T-cell immunophenotype, ALL regimens that have not been particularly successful in treating T-cell ALL are expected to yield poor results in treating lymphoblastic NHL as well. The BFM-90 protocol for NHL represents one of those treatment strategies that incorporated treatment components found to be effective in T-cell ALL. This treatment was associated with a 5-year event-free survival (EFS) rate of 92% in more than 100 patients with lymphoblastic lymphoma – a truly remarkable achievement.

The third largest group of childhood NHL, comprising about 15% of all pediatric NHL, is ALCL. By definition, this includes tumors with T-cell markers or a null-cell immunophenotype.[109] Because the clinical and biologic characterization of this subtype of NHL is still evolving, the interpretation of treatment programs for this disease is difficult. B-cell and ALL-type treatment strategies for ALCL have been reported. Only a few pediatric cooperative treatment groups have reported their results in patients selected by the contemporary definition of ALCL-co-expression of CD30 and the epithelial membrane antigen in cells with T-cell or null immunophenotype. Remarkably, the results, albeit inferior to those noted in pediatric B-cell or lymphoblastic NHL, have shown that about 60 to 80% survival rates can be achieved with either treatment strategy. The SFOP used a protocol[110] based on the treatment of B-cell NHL that prescribes two cycles of COPAD plus high-dose methotrexate followed by 5 to 7 months of maintenance chemotherapy. Complete responses were achieved in 95% of the patients; 21 patients experienced an adverse event. BFM investigators using a strategy developed for B-cell NHL have reported improved results. The 5-year EFS rates for 55 patients with stage III and 6 patients with stage IV NHL were 76% and 50%, respectively. The duration of treatment was only 5 months in the BFM study, but 10 to 24 months in others.[103]

# Salvage therapy (partial responses or relapse)

The development of methods to detect the presence of minimal amounts of disease has revealed a new dimension to the concept of relapse in childhood lymphoid malignancies. Alternative therapeutic strategies or salvage therapy are now recommended for patients who have subclinical evidence of persistent disease. Because patients destined to experience a relapse of the disease are being identified early in the relapsing process, the actual number of patients in whom classic clinical and laboratory manifestations of relapse develop is becoming progressively small. Thus, patients who experience relapse after contemporary, effective, risk-adapted therapy present true medical challenges.

### Acute lymphoblastic leukemia

Traditionally, ALL relapse has been classified as hematologic, extramedullary, or combined.

Hematologic and bone marrow relapse are usually further defined as being early (during or <6 months after cessation of therapy) or late relapses. Poor prognostic factors at the time of relapse include a short first remission period, hematologic relapse rather than extramedullary relapse, high intensity primary therapy, T-cell immunophenotype, Philadelphia chromosome, and a high WBC count. A first remission lasting more than 30 months, an isolated extramedullary relapse, or presence of the *TEL-AML* gene fusion has been associated with a higher likelihood of achieving a second, durable remission.[111] Usually, the treatment used to obtain a second remission includes a combination of dexamethasone, vincristine, L-asparaginase, anthracycline, etoposide, high-dose cytarabine, and high-dose methotrexate. A second course of CNS-directed therapy is included during this phase. For many years, there was controversy over the best approach for second postremission therapy. Some investigators defended the use of intensive chemotherapy for patients who experienced late relapse, whereas others recommended HSCT.[112] At present, there is a consensus that patients with early hematologic relapse should proceed to HSCT after the achievement of a second remission.[113,114]

Isolated relapses in extramedullary sites usually involve the CNS or the testes. Although they are considered isolated, most of these cases are likely to have subclinical bone marrow involvement. The type and intensity of previous CNS therapy can influence the rate of CNS relapse. Investigators at the Dana-Farber Cancer Institute[86] showed that boys with standard-risk ALL who did not receive radiation therapy as part of their CNS-directed therapy had an unexpectedly high incidence of CNS relapse. The management of 'isolated' CNS relapse includes intensive intrathecal treatment along with systemic chemotherapy consisting of induction, consolidation, and maintenance therapies for at least 1 year from the event. Cranial radiotherapy is mandatory in these cases. There is controversy about the timing of delivery of cranial irradiation; it appears that systemic and intrathecal treatment for 4 to 6 months before definitive radiotherapy is associated with better long-term disease control. Intrathecal treatment should not be given after cranial radiotherapy because of an increased risk of neurotoxicity. Because of the high rate of success of salvage therapy for patients with isolated CNS relapse, HSCT is not recommended for these patients.

Isolated testicular relapse, a rarity with current treatment modalities, usually involves both testicles. Patients with clinical evidence of testicular involvement during therapy have a poor prognosis. Relapse occurring after completion of therapy is associated with a better prognosis. The principles of management are similar to those applied to CNS relapse: patients should receive intensive systemic therapy for at least 1 year and, after completion of induction therapy, irradiation of both testicles. Whether the use of testicular radiotherapy can be avoided by administering high-dose methotrexate remains to be determined. In patients with clinical evidence of unilateral testicular relapse, some investigations advocate orchiectomy of the testis involved and no irradiation of the 'uninvolved' testis, in an attempt to preserve testicular function.

## Non-Hodgkin lymphoma

Persistent or relapsed NHL presents serious management problems. Because contemporary, risk-directed therapies are usually very intensive, the overall prognosis for these patients is dismal. In patients with a residual mass after induction and consolidation therapy, persistent disease should be confirmed by biopsy, because imaging studies commonly detect nonviable tumor. When persistent disease during therapy or relapse is documented, the options for salvage therapy depend on the intensity and types of agents used in the primary therapy, histologic type of disease, and timing of the relapse. Because primary therapy for Burkitt lymphoma or large B-cell lymphoma includes most of the known effective agents, salvage therapy is usually based on regimens containing cisplatin or carboplatin. A widely used combination is ifosfamide, carboplatin, and etoposide (ICE). Monoclonal antibodies to B-cell antigens have been successfully used to treat B-cell lymphomas.[115–117] These antibodies have been used in combination with conventional chemotherapy or conjugated to radioisotopes.[118,119] The monoclonal anti-CD20 (rituximab), for example, has been widely used in combination with standard chemotherapy. Because a second complete response to non-cross-resistant chemotherapy regimens, if achieved, is usually short, HSCT is recommended. The principles of management of relapsed lymphoblastic NHL are similar to those of relapsed ALL. When a second remission is obtained, HSCT is also indicated. The outcome is very poor for patients who have residual disease after salvage therapy. Contrary to what is observed in Burkitt and lymphoblastic NHL, second remission is usually possible in ALCL. Salvage treatment has included intensive chemotherapy with or without HSCT. In a recent study by the SFOP, a second remission was achieved in 36 of 41 cases of relapsed ALCL.[120] It is noteworthy that 8 of 13 patients had prolonged remission with the use of a single agent, vinblastine (given weekly), which suggests that several relapses of ALCL do not preclude a long period of disease-free survival.

# Supportive care

Patients with lymphoid malignancies often present with respiratory, cardiovascular, neurologic, renal, hemorrhagic, infectious, and metabolic complications. Intense tissue remodeling – cell proliferation and cell death – results in a large tumor burden and rapid turnover of nucleoproteins, both of which are responsible for the dysfunction of these organ systems. Prompt recognition, careful clinical and laboratory evaluations to determine the presence of these complications, and early intervention have decreased the mortality rate resulting from these complications (i.e., deaths not due directly to the leukemia or lymphoma) to less than 1%.

White blood cell counts $>300 \times 10^9/L$ at the time of initial examination can be associated with leukostasis syndrome in ALL, although this complication is rare. Neurologic and pulmonary signs and symptoms sometimes observed include dizziness, visual blurring, tinnitus, ataxia, confusion, somnolence, stupor, coma, tachypnea, dyspnea, pulmonary infiltrates, and progression to frank respiratory failure. The management of leukostasis is controversial, but many investigators consider leukophoresis for patients with an initial leukocyte count approaching $300 \times 10^9/L$. It is also recommended that specific antileukemia chemotherapy should begin (with corticosteroid and vincristine) on the first day and the outcome closely monitored. As the patient improves clinically, other chemotherapeutic drugs are added. On the rare occasions in which coagulopathy is symptomatic at the time of diagnosis of ALL, platelet transfusions, plasma cryoprecipitate, and fresh frozen plasma should be given to keep platelet counts above $50.0 \times 10^9/L$ and fibrinogen concentration above 1.0 g/L. The use of heparin is not indicated in these instances because the coagulopathy usually resolves within 24 to 48 hours of starting antileukemic treatment.

Respiratory distress from compression of mediastinal structures is common in lymphoblastic NHL. Compression of the vessels of the mediastinum can lead to intraluminal thrombosis (Figure 31.6) and sudden death. In cases of severe compression, general anesthesia is not recommended, because of an increased risk of complete, irreversible airway block. In an emergency it is sometimes necessary, before diagnosis is made, to reduce the risk of airway compression by administration of corticosteroids or local radiotherapy (or both). Massive ascites and intra-abdominal involvement in Burkitt lymphoma can cause compression of the bowel and ureters. In addition, compression of abdominal blood and lymphatic vessels can occur, which results in reduced blood flow and lymphatic return and in edema of the lower extremities.

Patients with leukemia and NHL are at particularly high risk for biochemical complications because of the high rate of cell turnover and the high sensitivity of the malignant cells to chemotherapy. Often, biochemical abnormalities are present before the initiation of chemotherapy and are induced by fever,

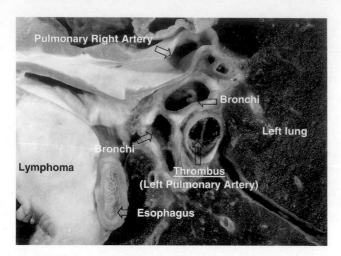

**Figure 31.6** Autopsy findings from a 12-year-old boy with non-Hodgkin lymphoma who died of cardiopulmonary arrest after sudden respiratory failure. A thrombus occluding the left pulmonary artery can be seen.

infection processes, dehydration, and even spontaneous cell lysis. These metabolic abnormalities, which include hyperuricemia, hyperphosphatemia, hypocalcemia, hyperkalemia, and azotemia, are characteristic of tumor lysis syndrome (TLS). The pathogenetic consequences of this syndrome result from the release of cellular breakdown products that exceed the hepatic and renal anabolic and catabolic capacities. The deposition of uric acid, its precursors (hypoxanthine and especially xanthine), or both, and phosphorus in the lumina of the renal tubules is believed to be central to the development of renal insufficiency. If these metabolic abnormalities become severe, renal failure, cardiac arrhythmia, respiratory distress, and death can follow.

Features associated with increased risk of TLS include hyperleukocytosis, massive organomegaly, renal enlargement, extrinsic compression of the genitourinary tract, and elevated serum LDH activity. Patients with established TLS or at high risk for TLS should be monitored carefully. Preferably, they should be admitted to an intensive care unit and cared for by a multidisciplinary team. Adequate urinary flow is the single most important measure to accomplish before chemotherapy is started. To determine the adequacy of renal function, a slightly hypotonic solution without potassium should be administered intravenously at a daily rate of 2 to 5 L/m² per day. Administration of fluids dilutes intravascular solutes such as urates and phosphates, increases renal blood flow and glomerular filtration, and flushes precipitated solutes from the renal tubules. The availability of recombinant urate oxidase (rasburicase) has dramatically facilitated the prevention and management of hyperuricemia.[121]

## REFERENCES

1. Smith MA, Ries LAG, Gurney JG et al. Leukemia. In: Ries LAG, Smith MA, Gurney JG et al., eds. *Cancer Incidence and Survival among Children and Adolescents: United States SEER Program 1975-1995*. Bethesda, MD: National Cancer Institute, 1999; 17–31.

2. Percy CL, Smith MA, Linet M et al. Lymphomas and reticuloendothelial Neoplasms. In: Ries LAG, Smith MA, Gurney JG et al., eds. *Cancer Incidence and Survival among Children and Adolescents: United States SEER Program 1975-1995*. Bethesda, MD: National Cancer Institute, SEER Program, 1999; 35–48.

3. Wheldon EG, Lindsay KA, Wheldon TE et al. A two-stage model for childhood acute lymphoblastic leukemia: application to hereditary and nonhereditary leukemogenesis. *Math Biosci* 1997; **139**: 1–24.

4. Smith MA, Chen T, Simon R. Age-specific incidence of acute lymphoblastic leukemia in U.S. children: in utero initiation model. *J Natl Cancer Inst* 1997; **89**: 1542–4.

5. Mori H, Colman SM, Xiao Z et al. Chromosome translocations and covert leukemic clones are generated during normal fetal development. *Proc Natl Acad Sci U S A* 2002; **99**: 8242–7.

6. Greaves M. Childhood leukaemia. *Br Med J* 2002; **324**: 283–7.

7. Taub JW, Konrad MA, Ge Y et al. High frequency of leukemic clones in newborn screening blood samples of children with B-precursor acute lymphoblastic leukemia. *Blood* 2002; **99**: 2992–6.

8. Miller RW, Young JL Jr, Novakovic B. Childhood cancer. *Cancer* 1995; **75**: 395–405.

9. Parkin DM, Stiller CA, Draper GJ et al. *International Incidence of Childhood Cancer* Lyon, France: IARC Scientific Publications No. 87, 1988.

10. McNally RJ, Cairns DP, Eden OB et al. Examination of temporal trends in the incidence of childhood leukaemias and lymphomas provides aetiological clues. *Leukemia* 2001; **15**: 1612–18.

11. Smith MA, Simon R, Strickler HD et al. Evidence that childhood acute lymphoblastic leukemia is associated with an infectious agent linked to hygiene conditions. *Cancer Causes Control* 1998; **9**: 285–98.

12. Magrath IT. Non-Hodgkin's lymphomas: epidemiology and treatment. *Ann N Y Acad Sci* 1997; **824**: 91–106.

13. Mueller BU. Cancers in children infected with the human immunodeficiency virus. *Oncologist* 1999; **4**: 309–17.

14. Pui CH, Relling MV. Topoisomerase II inhibitor-related acute myeloid leukaemia. *Br J Haematol* 2000; **109**: 13–23.

15. Ross JA. Maternal diet and infant leukemia: a role for DNA topoisomerase II inhibitors? *Int J Cancer Suppl* 1998; **11**: 26–8.

16. Ross JA, Potter JD, Robison LL. Infant leukemia, topoisomerase II inhibitors, and the MLL gene. *J Natl Cancer Inst* 1994; **86**: 1678–80.

17. Ross JA. Dietary flavonoids and the MLL gene: A pathway to infant leukemia? *Proc Natl Acad Sci USA* 2000; **97**: 4411–13.

18. Vessey CJ, Norbury CJ, Hickson ID. Genetic disorders associated with cancer predisposition and genomic instability. *Prog Nucleic Acid Res Mol Biol* 1999; **63**: 189–221.

19. Lange B. The management of neoplastic disorders of haematopoiesis in children with Down's syndrome. *Br J Haematol* 2000; **110**: 512–24.

20. Robison LL, Neglia JP. Epidemiology of Down syndrome and childhood acute leukemia. *Prog Clin Biol Res* 1987; **246**: 19–32.

21. Bader JL, Miller RW. Neurofibromatosis and childhood leukemia. *J Pediatr* 1978; 92: 925–9.

22. Woods WG, Roloff JS, Lukens JN et al. The occurrence of leukemia in patients with the Shwachman syndrome. *J Pediatr* 1981; 99: 425–8.

23. German J. Bloom's syndrome. XX. The first 100 cancers. *Cancer Genet Cytogenet* 1997; **93**: 100–6.

24. Swift M, Morrell D, Massey RB et al. Incidence of cancer in 161 families affected by ataxia-telangiectasia. *N Engl J Med* 1991; **325**: 1831–1836.

25. Taylor AM, Metcalfe JA, Thick J, Mak YF. Leukemia and lymphoma in ataxia telangiectasia. *Blood* 1996; **87**: 423–38.

26. Shaw MP, Eden OB, Grace E et al. Acute lymphoblastic leukemia and Klinefelter's syndrome. *Pediatr Hematol Oncol* 1992; **9**: 81–5.

27. Kersey JH, Shapiro RS, Filipovich AH. Relationship of immunodeficiency to lymphoid malignancy. *Pediatr Infect Dis J* 1988; **7**: S10–S12.

28. Filipovich AH, Mathur A, Kamat D et al. Primary immunodeficiencies: genetic risk factors for lymphoma. *Cancer Res* 1992; **52**: 5465s–5467s.

29. Knowles DM. Immunodeficiency-associated lymphoproliferative disorders. *Mod Pathol* 1999; **12**: 200–17.

30. Brill A, Tomonaga M, Hibi S. Leukemia in man following exposure to ionizing radiation. *Ann Intern Med* 1962; **56**: 590–609.

31. Evans JS, Wennberg JE, McNeil BJ. The influence of diagnostic radiography on the incidence of breast cancer and leukemia. *N Engl J Med* 1986; **315**: 810–15.

32. Ahlbom IC, Cardis E, Green A et al. Review of the epidemiologic literature on EMF and Health. *Environ Health Perspect* 2001; **109**: 911–33.

33. Pui CH, Relling, MV, Evans WE. Role of pharmacogenomics and pharmacodynamics in acute lymphoblastic leukemia. *Bailliere's Best Practice and Research in Clinical Haematology* (in press).

34. Relling MV, Dervieux T. Pharmacogenetics and cancer therapy. *Nat Rev Cancer* 2001; **1**: 99–108.

35. Krajinovic M, Labuda D, Richer C et al. Susceptibility to childhood acute lymphoblastic leukemia: influence of CYPIA1, CYP2D6, GSTMI, and GSTT1 genetic polymorphisms. *Blood* 1999; **93**: 1496–501.

36. Schwahn B, Rozen R. Polymorphisms in the methylenetetrahydrofolate reductase gene: clinical consequences. *Am J Pharmacogenomics* 2001; **1**: 189–201.

37. Bennett JM, Catovsky D, Daniel MT et al. Proposals for the classification of the acute leukaemias. French-American-British (FAB) co-operative group. *Br J Haematol* 1976; **33**: 451–8.

38. Pui CH, Behm FG, Crist WM. Clinical and biologic relevance of immunologic marker studies in childhood acute lymphoblastic leukemia. *Blood* 1993; **82**: 343–62.

39. Pui CH, Behm FG, Singh B et al. Heterogeneity of presenting features and their relation to treatment outcome in 120

40. children with T-cell acute lymphoblastic leukemia. *Blood* 1990; **75**: 174–9.

40. Pui CH, Raimondi SC, Hancock ML et al. Immunologic, cytogenetic, and clinical characterization of childhood acute lymphoblastic leukemia with the t(1;19) (q23; p13) or its derivative. *J Clin Oncol* 1994; **12**: 2601–6.

41. Pui CH, Campana D, Crist WM. Toward a clinically useful classification of the acute leukemias. *Leukemia* 1995; **9**: 2154–7.

42. Pui CH, Campana D, Evans WE. Childhood acute lymphoblastic leukaemia – current status and future perspectives. *Lancet Oncol* 2001; **2**: 597–607.

43. Pui CH, Evans WE. Acute lymphoblastic leukemia. *N Engl J Med* 1998; **339**: 605–15.

44. Katsura Y. Redefinition of lymphoid progenitors. *Nat Rev Immunol* 2002; **2**: 127–32.

45. Killick S, Matutes E, Powles RL et al. Outcome of biphenotypic acute leukemia. *Haematologica* 1999; **84**: 699–706.

46. Campana D, Coustan-Smith E. Detection of minimal residual disease in acute leukemia by flow cytometry. *Cytometry* 1999; **38**: 139–52.

47. Coustan-Smith E, Sancho J, Hancock ML et al. Clinical importance of minimal residual disease in childhood acute lymphoblastic leukemia. *Blood* 2000; **96**: 2691–6.

48. Raimondi SC. Current status of cytogenetic research in childhood acute lymphoblastic leukemia. *Blood* 1993; **81**: 2237–51.

49. Look AT, Roberson PK, Williams DL et al. Prognostic importance of blast cell DNA content in childhood acute lymphoblastic leukemia. *Blood* 1985; **65**: 1079–86.

50. Raimondi SC. Fluorescence in situ hybridization: molecular probes for diagnosis of pediatric neoplastic diseases. *Cancer Invest* 2000; **18**: 135–47.

51. Chan JK. The new World Health Organization classification of lymphomas: the past, the present and the future. *Hematol Oncol* 2001; **19**: 129–50.

52. Ribeiro RC, Pui CH, Murphy SB et al. Childhood malignant non-Hodgkin lymphomas of uncommon histology. *Leukemia* 1992; **6**: 761–5.

53. Reis A. Genetics and B-cell leukaemia. *Lancet* 1999; **353**: 3.

54. Ferrando AA, Neuberg DS, Staunton J et al. Gene expression signatures define novel oncogenic pathways in T cell acute lymphoblastic leukemia. *Cancer Cell* 2002; **1**: 75–87.

55. Sandlund JT, Pui CH, Santana VM et al. Clinical features and treatment outcome for children with CD30+ large-cell non-Hodgkin's lymphoma. *J Clin Oncol* 1994; **12**: 895–8.

56. Rimokh R, Magaud JP, Berger F et al. A translocation involving a specific breakpoint (q35) on chromosome 5 is characteristic of anaplastic large cell lymphoma ('Ki-1 lymphoma'). *Br J Haematol* 1989; **71**: 31–6.

57. Morris SW, Kirstein MN, Valentine MB et al. Fusion of a kinase gene, ALK, to a nucleolar protein gene, NPM, in non-Hodgkin's lymphoma. *Science* 1994; **263**: 1281–4.

58. Kim TH, Hargreaves HK, Chan WC et al. Sequential testicular biopsies in childhood acute lymphocytic leukemia. *Cancer* 1986; **57**: 1038–41.

59. Gallagher DJ, Phillips DJ, Heinrich SD. Orthopedic manifestations of acute pediatric leukemia. *Orthop Clin North Am* 1996; **27**: 635–44.

60. Murphy SB, Fairclough DL, Hutchison RE et al. Non-Hodgkin's lymphomas of childhood: an analysis of the

histology, staging, and response to treatment of 338 cases at a single institution. *J Clin Oncol* 1989; **7**: 186–93.

61. Ribeiro RC, Pui CH. The clinical and biological correlates of coagulopathy in children with acute leukemia. *J Clin Oncol* 1986; **4**: 1212–18.

62. Raimondi SC, Privitera E, Williams DL et al. New recurring chromosomal translocations in childhood acute lymphoblastic leukemia. *Blood* 1991; **77**: 2016–22.

63. Ribeiro RC, Pui CH, Schell MJ. Vertebral compression fracture as a presenting feature of acute lymphoblastic leukemia in children. *Cancer* 1988; **61**: 589–92.

64. Mahmoud HH, Rivera GK, Hancock ML et al. Low leukocyte counts with blast cells in cerebrospinal fluid of children with newly diagnosed acute lymphoblastic leukemia. *N Engl J Med* 1993; **329**: 314–19.

65. Gajjar A, Harrison PL, Sandlund JT et al. Traumatic lumbar puncture at diagnosis adversely affects outcome in childhood acute lymphoblastic leukemia. *Blood* 2000; **96**: 3381–4.

66. Breatnach F, Chessells JM, Greaves ME The aplastic presentation of childhood leukaemia: a feature of common-ALL. *Br J Haematol* 1981; **49**: 387–93.

67. Meeker TC, Hardy D, Willman C et al. Activation of the interleukin-3 gene by chromosome translocation in acute lymphocytic leukemia with eosinophilia. *Blood* 1990; **76**: 285–9.

68. Dubansky AS, Boyett JM, Falletta J et al. Isolated thrombocytopenia in children with acute lymphoblastic leukemia: a rare event in a Pediatric Oncology Group Study. *Pediatrics* 1989; **84**: 1068–71.

69. Furman WL, Fitch S, Hustu HO et al. Primary lymphoma of bone in children. *J Clin Oncol* 1989; **7**: 1275–80.

70. Pui CH, Gaynon PS, Boyett JM et al. Outcome of treatment in childhood acute lymphoblastic leukaemia with rearrangements of the l 1q23 chromosomal region. *Lancet* 2002; **359**: 1909–15.

71. Arico M, Valsecchi MG, Camitta B et al. Outcome of treatment in children with Philadelphia chromosome-positive acute lymphoblastic leukemia. *N Engl J Med* 2000; **342**: 998–1006.

72. Coustan-Smith E, Sancho J, Behm FG et al. Prognostic importance of measuring early clearance of leukemic cells by flow cytometry in childhood acute lymphoblastic leukemia. *Blood* 2002; **100**: 52–8.

73. Yeoh EJ, Ross ME, Shurtleff SA et al. Classification, subtype discovery, and prediction of outcome in pediatric acute lymphoblastic leukemia by gene expression profiling. *Cancer Cell* 2002; **1**: 133–43.

74. Patte C, Auperin A, Michon J et al. The Societe Francaise d'Oncologie Pediatrique LMB89 protocol: highly effective multiagent chemotherapy tailored to the tumor burden and initial response in 561 unselected children with B-cell lymphomas and L3 leukemia. *Blood* 2001; **97**: 3370–9.

75. Rosenwald A, Wright G, Chan WC et al. The use of molecular profiling to predict survival after chemotherapy for diffuse large-B-cell lymphoma. *N Engl J Med* 2002; **346**: 1937–47.

76. DeVita VT, Schein PS. The use of drugs in combination for the treatment of cancer: rationale and results. *N Engl J Med* 1973; **288**: 998–1006.

77. Pinkel D. Five-year follow-up of 'total therapy' of childhood lymphocytic leukemia. *JAMA* 1971; **216**: 648–52.

78. George SL, Aur RJ, Mauer AM et al. A reappraisal of the results of stopping therapy in childhood leukemia. *N Engl J Med* 1979; **300**: 269–73.

79. Aur RJ, Simone J, Hustu HO et al. Central nervous system therapy and combination chemotherapy of childhood lymphocytic leukemia. *Blood* 1971; **37**: 272–81.

80. Simone JV, Verzosa MS, Rudy JA. Initial features and prognosis in 363 children with acute lymphocytic leukemia. *Cancer* 1975; **36**: 2099–108.

81. Manera R, Ramirez I, Mullins J et al. Pilot studies of species-specific chemotherapy of childhood acute lymphoblastic leukemia using genotype and immunophenotype. *Leukemia* 2000; **14**: 1354–61.

82. Hurwitz CA, Silverman LB, Schorin MA et al. Substituting dexamethasone for prednisone complicates remission induction in children with acute lymphoblastic leukemia. *Cancer* 2000; **88**: 1964–69.

83. Mauer AM. Treatment of acute leukaemia in children. *Clin Haematol* 1978; **7**: 245–58.

84. Harms DO, Janka-Schaub GE. Co-operative study group for childhood acute lymphoblastic leukemia (COALL): long-term follow-up of trials 82, 85, 89 and 92. *Leukemia* 2000; **14**: 2234–9.

85. Silverman LB, Declerck L, Gelber RD et al. Results of Dana-Farber Cancer Institute Consortium protocols for children with newly diagnosed acute lymphoblastic leukemia (1981–1995). *Leukemia* 2000; **14**: 2247–56.

86. LeClerc JM, Billett AL, Gelber RD et al. Treatment of childhood acute lymphoblastic leukemia: results of Dana-Farber ALL Consortium Protocol 87-01. *J Clin Oncol* 2002; **20**: 237–46.

87. Schrappe M, Reiter A, Ludwig WD et al. Improved outcome in childhood acute lymphoblastic leukemia despite reduced use of anthracyclines and cranial radiotherapy: results of trial ALL-BFM 90. German-Austrian-Swiss ALL-BFM Study Group. *Blood* 2000; **95**: 3310–22.

88. Schorin MA, Blattner S, Gelber RD et al. Treatment of childhood acute lymphoblastic leukemia: results of Dana-Farber Cancer Institute/Children's Hospital Acute Lymphoblastic Leukemia Consortium Protocol 85-01. *J Clin Oncol* 1994; **12**: 740–7.

89. Silverman LB, Gelber RD, Dalton VK et al. Improved outcome for children with acute lymphoblastic leukemia: results of Dana-Farber Consortium Protocol 91-01. *Blood* 2001; **97**: 1211–18.

90. Lange BJ, Bostrom BC, Cherlow JM et al. Double-delayed intensification improves event-free survival for children with intermediate-risk acute lymphoblastic leukemia: a report from the Children's Cancer Group. *Blood* 2002; **99**: 825–33.

91. Nachman JB, Sather HN, Sensel MG et al. Augmented post-induction therapy for children with high-risk acute lymphoblastic leukemia and a slow response to initial therapy. *N Engl J Med* 1998; **338**: 1663–71.

92. Schrappe M, Reiter A, Zimmermann M et al. Long-term results of four consecutive trials in childhood ALL performed by the ALL-BFM study group from 1981 to 1995. Berlin-Frankfurt-Munster. *Leukemia* 2000; **14**: 2205–22.

93. Pin CH, Sallan S, Relling MV et al. International Childhood Acute Lymphoblastic Leukemia Workshop: Sausalito, CA, 30 November-1 December 2000. *Leukemia* 2001; **15**: 707–15.

94. Chessells JM, Harrison G, Lilleyman JS et al. Continuing (maintenance) therapy in lymphoblastic leukaemia: lessons from MRC UKALL X. Medical Research Council

Working Party in Childhood Leukaemia. *Br J Haematol* 1997; **98**: 945–51.

95. Tsuchida M, Ikuta K, Hanada R et al. Long-term follow-up of childhood acute lymphoblastic leukemia in Tokyo Children's Cancer Study Group 1981-1995. *Leukemia* 2000; **14**: 2295–306.

96. Relling MV, Hancock ML, Boyett JM et al. Prognostic importance of 6-mercaptopurine dose intensity in acute lymphoblastic leukemia. *Blood* 1999; **93**: 2817–23.

97. Dibenedetto SP, Guardabasso V, Ragusa R et al. 6-Mercaptopurine cumulative dose: a critical factor of maintenance therapy in average risk childhood acute lymphoblastic leukemia. *Pediatr Hematol Oncol* 1994; **11**: 251–8.

98. Relling MV, Hancock ML, Rivera GK et al. Mercaptopurine therapy intolerance and heterozygosity at the thiopurine S-methyltransferase gene locus. *J Natl Cancer Inst* 1999; **91**: 2001–8.

99. Lange BJ, Blatt J, Sather HN et al. Randomized comparison of moderate-dose methotrexate infusions to oral methotrexate in children with intermediate risk acute lymphoblastic leukemia: a Childrens Cancer Group study. *Med Pediatr Oncol* 1996; **27**: 15–20.

100. Kamps WA, Bokkerink JP, Hakvoort-Cammel FG et al. BFM-oriented treatment for children with acute lymphoblastic leukemia without cranial irradiation and treatment reduction for standard risk patients: results of DCLSG protocol ALL-8 (1991–1996). *Leukemia* 2002; **16**: 1099 111.

101. Pui CH, Mahmoud HH, Rivera GK et al. Early intensification of intrathecal chemotherapy virtually eliminates central nervous system relapse in children with acute lymphoblastic leukemia. *Blood* 1998, **92**: 411 15.

102. Pui CH, Boyett JM, Rivera GK et al. Long-term results of Total Therapy studies 11, 12 and 13A for childhood acute lymphoblastic leukemia at St Jude Children's Research Hospital. *Leukemia* 2000; **14**: 2286–94.

103. Seidemann K, Tiemann M, Schrappe M et al. Short-pulse B-non-Hodgkin lymphoma-type chemotherapy is efficacious treatment for pediatric anaplastic large cell lymphoma: a report of the Berlin-Frankfurt-Munster Group Trial NHL-BFM 90. *Blood* 2001; **97**: 3699–706.

104. Reiter A, Schrappe M, Ludwig WD et al. Intensive ALL-type therapy without local radiotherapy provides a 90% event-free survival for children with T-cell lymphoblastic lymphoma: a BFM group report. *Blood* 2000; **95**: 416–21.

105. Link MP, Shuster JJ, Donaldson SS et al. Treatment of children and young adults with early-stage non-Hodgkin's lymphoma. *N Engl J Med* 1997; **337**: 1259–66.

106. Patte C. Non-Hodgkin's lymphoma. *Eur J Cancer* 1998; **34**: 359–62.

107. Reiter A, Schrappe M, Tiemann M et al. Improved treatment results in childhood B-cell neoplasms with tailored intensification of therapy: A report of the Berlin-Frankfurt-Munster Group Trial NHL-BFM 90. *Blood* 1999; **94**: 3294–306.

108. Anderson JR, Wilson JF, Jenkin DT et al. Childhood non-Hodgkin's lymphoma. The results of a randomized therapeutic trial comparing a 4-drug regimen (COMP) with a 10-drug regimen (LSA2-L2). *N Engl J Med* 1983; **308**: 559–65.

109. Jaffe ES. Anaplastic large cell lymphoma: the shifting sands of diagnostic hematopathology. *Mod Pathol* 2001; **14**: 219–28.

110. Brugieres L, Deley MC, Pacquement H et al. CD30(+) anaplastic large-cell lymphoma in children: analysis of 82 patients enrolled in two consecutive studies of the French Society of Pediatric Oncology. *Blood* 1998; **92**: 3591–8.

111. Seeger K, Adams HP, Buchwald D et al. TEL-AML1 fusion transcript in relapsed childhood acute lymphoblastic leukemia. The Berlin-Frankfurt-Munster Study Group. *Blood* 1998; **91**: 1716–22.

112. Mielcarek M, Sandmaier BM, Maloney DG et al. Nonmyeloablative hematopoietic cell transplantation: status quo and future perspectives. *J Clin Immunol* 2002; **22**: 70–4.

113. Bunin N, Carston M, Wall D et al. Unrelated marrow transplantation for children with acute lymphoblastic leukemia in second remission. *Blood* 2002; **99**: 3151–7.

114. Woolfrey AE, Anasetti C, Storer B et al. Factors associated with outcome after unrelated marrow transplantation for treatment of acute lymphoblastic leukemia in children. *Blood* 2002; **99**: 2002–8.

115. Grillo-Lopez AJ, Hedrick E, Rashford M et al: Rituximab ongoing and future clinical development. *Semin Oncol* 2002; **29**: 105–12.

116. Leonard JP, Link BK. Immunotherapy of non-Hodgkin's lymphoma with hLL2 (epratuzumab, an anti-CD22 monoclonal antibody) and Hu1D10 (apolizumab). *Semin Oncol* 2002; **29**: 81 6.

117. Coiffier B, Haioun C, Ketterer N et al. Rituximab (anti-CD20 monoclonal antibody) for the treatment of patients with relapsing or refractory aggressive lymphoma: a multicenter phase II study. *Blood* 1998; **92**: 1927–32.

118. Gordon LI, Witzig TE, Wiseman GA et al. Yttrium 90 ibritumomab tiuxetan radioimmunotherapy for relapsed or refractory low-grade non-Hodgkin's lymphoma. *Semin Oncol* 2002; **29**: 87–92.

119. Behr TM, Griesinger F, Riggert J et al. High-dose myeloablative radioimmunotherapy of mantle cell non-Hodgkin lymphoma with the iodine-131-labeled chimeric anti-CD20 antibody C2B8 and autologous stem cell support. Results of a pilot study. *Cancer* 2002; **94**: 1363–72.

120. Brugieres L, Quartier P, Le Deley MC et al. Relapses of childhood anaplastic large-cell lymphoma: treatment results in a series of 41 children – a report from the French Society of Pediatric Oncology. *Ann Oncol* 2000; **11**: 53–8.

121. Pui CH, Mahmoud HH, Wiley JM et al. Recombinant urate oxidase for the prophylaxis or treatment of hyperuricemia in patients With leukemia or lymphoma. *J Clin Oncol* 2001; **19**: 697–704.

# 32 Acute lymphoblastic leukemia in adults

Dieter Hoelzer and Nicola Gökbuget

## Introduction

### Incidence

Acute lymphoblastic leukemia (ALL) is a malignant disease characterized by a clonal proliferation of malignant lymphoblasts. It is a rare disease in adults. According to the most recent report of the National Cancer Institute (NCI) the incidence per 100 000 is 1.5 in whites and 0.8 in blacks. The male to female ratio was 1.6:0.8. After a first peak in children younger than 5 years of age (6.7/100 000) the incidence decreases continuously. There is a slight increase after the age of 50 years and a second minor peak in the age group of 80–84 years (1.5/100 000). In the period from 1973 to 2000, a slight increase in age-adjusted incidence rates from 1.2 to 1.4/100 000 was observed.[1]

### Etiology

#### Genetics

Children with rare disorders such as Down syndrome, Klinefelter syndrome, Fanconi's anemia, Bloom syndrome, ataxia telangiectasia, and neurofibromatosis have an increased risk of developing acute leukemias, preferentially acute myeloid leukemias (AML), but also ALL. Genetic predisposition may also be inferred from simultaneous development of ALL in identical twins, but this is mainly indicative of an intrauterine event affecting both twins.

#### Irradiation

The incidence of acute leukemia was increased 20-fold in survivors of the atomic bomb explosions (>1 Gy exposure) in Japan. Emission from nuclear power stations has also been raised as a possible leukemogenic risk. Whether the Cherbonyl accident led to an increased incidence of leukemia is still controversial.

#### Chemicals

It has been known for a considerable time that chemical agents such as benzene, chloramphenicol and others causing bone marrow aplasia can eventually lead to the development of acute leukemias. More recently, secondary therapy-related leukemias have become an appreciable problem. Acute myeloid leukemias have occurred after exposure to alkylating agents such as cyclophosphamide, epipodophyllotoxins, topoisomerase II inhibitors and (rarely) anthracyclines that are used extensively in the treatment of ALL. Secondary ALL occurs rarely as a second neoplasm.

#### Viral

There is no direct evidence that a virus causes human ALL, but there are indirect suggestions for its involvement. In the endemic African type of Burkitt lymphoma, the Epstein–Barr virus (a DNA virus of the herpes family) has been implicated as a potential causative agent (see also Chapter 14). Endemic infection with human T-cell leukemia/lymphoma virus type I (HTLV-I) in Japan and in the Caribbean is an etiologic factor for adult T-cell leukemia/lymphoma (see also Chapter 13).

## Diagnosis

For classification of leukemic blast cells in ALL, morphological and cytochemical studies, immunophenotyping, and cytogenetic and molecular genetic analysis are required.

### Morphology

Morphology remains the means by which acute leukemia is initially detected, and, together with cytochemical reactions, it can distinguish between ALL and AML. The French–American–British (FAB) classification which classifies leukemic blast cells by their cytological features (L1, small monomorphic type; L2, large, heterogeneous type; L3, Burkitt cell type) is of no prognostic value except for the identification of the L3 subtype, which is indicative of B-lineage ALL (B-ALL).

## Immunophenotype

Immunophenotyping of ALL blast cells is the major classification of ALL subtypes (Table 32.1). ALL blast cells can be subdivided into B-lineage or T-lineage by detection of lineage-specific antigens. Within the B-lineage or T-lineage ALL, the subtypes are defined according to their stage of differentiation.

### B-lineage ALL

**Pro-B-ALL** (also termed early pre-B-ALL or pre-pre-B-ALL) expresses HLA-DR, TdT and CD19, but shows no expression of other differentiation B-cell antigens. It occurs in about 11% of adult and 5% of childhood ALL.

**Common ALL** is the major immunological subtype in childhood as well as in adult ALL. It comprises about 50% of cases of adult ALL. Common ALL is characterized by the presence of CD10 (formerly CALLA).

**Pre-B-ALL** is identical to common ALL, except for the expression of cytoplasmatic immunoglobulin. Only very rarely, CD10 may be absent in this subtype. Pre-B-ALL comprises nearly 10% of adult ALL.

**Mature B-ALL** is found in about 4% of adult ALL patients. The blast cells express surface antigens of mature B cells, including surface membrane immunoglobulin. CD10 may be present and occasionally also cytoplasmic immunoglobulin.

### T-lineage ALL

Approximately 25% of adult ALL cases have blast cells with a T-cell phenotype. All cases express the T-cell antigen gp40 (CD7), and in addition they may, according to their degree of T-cell differentiation, express other T-cell antigens, for example CD2 and/or the cortical thymocyte antigen CD1. A minority of T-ALL blast cells may also express CD10 together with T-cell antigens. In most cases of T-ALL, one or more of the T-cell receptor genes is rearranged. These properties make it possible to classify T-cell ALL according to their stage of differentiation.

**Early T-precursor ALL** accounts for 6% of adult ALL. It shows characteristic T-cell markers (cyCD3 and CD7) but no further differentiation markers.

**Thymic (cortical) T-ALL** is the most frequent subtype of T-ALL (10%). It is characterized particularly by the expression of CD1a. Surface CD3 may be present. Since this subtype is associated with a better prognosis, it's identification is of particular importance.

**Mature T-ALL** has a frequency of 6%. The blast cells do not express CD1a but they are positive for surface CD3.

### Cytogenetics

Cytogenetic abnormalities are independent prognostic variables for predicting the outcome of adult ALL.

---

**Table 32.1 Immunologic classification, corresponding cytogenetic and molecular aberrations and frequencies in adult acute lymphoblastic leukemia (ALL)**

| | EGIL | Adults (%)* | Surface marker | Cytogenetics** | Molecular genetics** |
|---|---|---|---|---|---|
| **B-lineage** | | | HLA-DR+, TdT+, CD19+ and/or CD79a+ and/or CD22+ | | |
| Pro B-ALL | B-I | 11 | No further differentiation markers | t(4;11) | ALL1(MLL)-AF4 |
| Common-ALL | B-II | 50 | CD10+ | t(9;22) | BCR-ABL |
| Pre B-ALL | B-III | 12 | CD10+/-, cytoplasmic immunoglobulin (cyIgM+) | t(9;22), t(1;19) | BCR-ABL; E2A-PBX1 |
| B-ALL | B-IV | 5 | CD10+/-, surface immunoglobulin (sIgM+) | t(8;14) | CMYC-IgH |
| **T-lineage*** | | | TdT+, cytoplasmic CD3 (cyCD3+) or surface CD3 (sCD3+) | | |
| Early T-ALL | T-I T-II | 6 | cyCD3+, CD7+, CD5+/-, CD2+/- | | |
| Cortical T-ALL (Thy ALL) | T-III | 10 | cyCD3+, CD7+, CD1a+, sCD3+/- | t(11;14) | LMO1/-TCRα/δ |
| Mature T-ALL | T-IV | 6 | sCD3+, CD1a- | t(10;14) | HOX-11-TCRα/δ |

* Frequencies according to central immunophenotyping of the GMALL Study group; personal communication of Prof. Dr. E. Thiel and Dr. S. Schwartz, Free University of Berlin, Germany and EGIL[2]; ** most frequent, typical aberrations; *** The EGIL classification subdivides T-ALL into four subgroups; however, only the differentiation between early, mature and thymic T-ALL is of clinical relevance.

In three recent studies, clonal chromosomal aberrations could be detected in about 62–85% of adult ALL patients.[3,4,5] Between 15% and 38% of the cases had normal metaphases.

The major cytogenetic abnormalities in ALL are clonal translocations such as t(9;22), t(4;11), t(8;14), t(1;19) or t(10;14) and other structural abnormalities such as 9p, 6q or 12p abnormalities. In addition, the abnormalities can be classified according to the modal chromosomal number (<46, 46 with other structural abnormalities, 47–50, >50).

The demonstration of chromosomal abnormalities in ALL is relevant for several reasons: the presence of such defects may confirm the diagnosis if a karyotype specific for ALL is found; chromosomal abnormalities are closely correlated with clinical features and immunological subtypes; and they are independent prognostic variables for predicting leukemia-free survival.

### Molecular genetics

Molecular analyses – detecting gene rearrangements in ALL by the polymerase chain reaction (PCR), Southern blot analysis, or fluorescent in-situ hybridization (FISH) with chromosome-specific DNA probes – are useful approaches to establish more precise diagnosis and to define the quality of remission, and may also give insights into the pathophysiology of the leukemic process (e.g. the mechanisms of leukemic cell stimulation by BCR–ABL fusion proteins).

The most frequent molecular markers in ALL are BCR–ABL and ALL1–AF4. The Philadelphia (Ph) chromosome t(9;22)(q34;q11) results from a translocation involving the breakpoint cluster region of the BCR gene on chromosome 22 and the ABL gene on chromosome 9. The BCR–ABL gene rearrangement can be demonstrated by molecular techniques. PCR analyses have revealed an incidence of 20–30% BCR–ABL[+] ALL in adults[6] compared with 3% in childhood ALL patients. One-third of adult ALL patients with a Ph chromosome show M-BCR rearrangements (resulting in a 210 kDa protein), similar to patients with chronic myeloid leukemia (CML), whereas two-thirds have M-BCR rearrangements (resulting in a 190 kDa protein). It is noteworthy that BCR–ABL is more frequently detected than the corresponding chromosome abnormality t(9; 22), owing to occasional difficulties in obtaining sufficient material for cytogenetic analysis.

t(4;11)(q21;q23) is the most frequent form of 11q23 abnormality in ALL. The involved gene on chromosome 11 is named MLL (for mixed-lineage leukemia). Synonyms are ALL-1, HRX and HTRX1. The MLL gene is fused to a gene located on chromosome 4 that is named AF-4 (also referred to as FEL). The fusion gene ALL1–AF4 is frequently detected in infant leukemia and in patients with pro B-ALL (CD10−). The overall incidence in adults is about 6%.

Other molecular aberrations occur more rarely and are alocated to specific subtypes as shown in Table 32.1.

# Clinical manifestations

Most adult patients initially present with clinical symptoms resulting from bone marrow failure. Pallor, tachycardia, weakness and fatigue are due to anemia; petechiae or other hemorrhagic manifestations are attributable to thrombocytopenia; infectious complications are due to neutropenia. Clinical signs of leukemia are related directly to infiltration of organs with leukemic blasts, such as lymphadenopathy, splenomegaly and hepatomegaly, are present in most patients, but are infrequently problems for which the patient first seeks medical advice.

### Patient characteristics and clinical symptoms

Characteristic symptoms and clinical manifestations are given in Table 32.2. There is a male preponderance in T-ALL and mature B-ALL. In T-ALL, there is a higher proportion of adolescent patients and a significantly lower frequency of patients above 50 years. One-third of ALL patients had infection or fever at presentation, and one-third presented with hemorrhagic episodes. Hepatomegaly and splenomegaly was observed in about half of the patients; lymphadenopathy was more often seen in T-ALL, as well as mediastinal tumor and central nervous system (CNS) involvement. Massive thymic enlargement can cause dyspnea, especially when associated with pleural effusions. CNS involvement at presentation was seen overall in 3% of adult ALL patients with higher incidences in T-ALL (8%) and in mature B-ALL (13%). Less than half of these patients initially had CNS symptoms such as headache, vomiting, lethargy, nuchal rigidity, and cranial nerve or peripheral nerve dysfunction. In the remaining patients, the diagnosis of CNS involvement was made by demonstration of leukemic blast cells in the cerebrospinal fluid. Very rarely there is leukemic CNS involvement without lymphoblasts in the CSF, but verified by computed tomography (CT scan) or related clinical symptoms only.

Virtually any organ can be infiltrated by ALL blast cells; 15% of T-ALL and one-third of mature B-ALL patients had such organ involvement (Table 32.2).

# Laboratory evaluation

The peripheral blood-cell values at diagnosis in a large cohort of patients are shown in Table 32.3. The

**Table 32.2  Patient characteristics and clinical parameters in subgroups of adult acute lymphoblastic leukemia (ALL)\***

|  |  | T-lineage ALL n = 158 | B-lineage ALL n = 423 | Mature B-ALL n = 59 |
|---|---|---|---|---|
| **Patient characteristics** |  |  |  |  |
| Sex | male | 73% | 54% | 78% |
|  | female | 27% | 46% | 22% |
| Age | 15–20 years | 22% | 19% | 8% |
|  | 20–50 years | 67% | 58% | 64% |
|  | >50 years | 11% | 24% | 27% |
| **Clinical symptoms and manifestations** |  |  |  |  |
| Bleeding |  | 28% | 28% | 30% |
| Infections |  | 22% | 29% | 37% |
| Hepatomegaly |  | 45% | 41% | 56% |
| Splenomegaly |  | 55% | 43% | 47% |
| Mediastinal tumor |  | 62% | 1% | 5% |
| CNS involvement |  | 8% | 3% | 13% |
| Other organ involvement |  | 15% | 4% | 32% |

\* Data from GMALL trials 03/87–04/89

**Table 32.3  Laboratory findings at time of diagnosis of ALL in 938 adult patients**

|  |  | Patients (%) |
|---|---|---|
| Bone marrow aspirable |  | 84 |
| Leukemic blast cells in bone marrow | <50% | 3 |
|  | 51–90% | 51 |
|  | >90% | 46 |
| Leukemic blast cells in peripheral blood | Present | 92 |
|  | Not present | 8 |
| White blood cell count (×10$^6$/L) | <5000 | 27 |
|  | 5000–10 000 | 14 |
|  | 10 000–50 000 | 31 |
|  | 50 000–100 000 | 12 |
|  | >100 000 | 16 |
| Neutrophils (×10$^6$/L) | <500 | 23 |
|  | 500–1000 | 14 |
|  | 1000–1500 | 9 |
|  | >1500 | 54 |
| Platelets (×10$^6$/L) | <25 000 | 30 |
|  | 25 000–50 000 | 22 |
|  | 50 000–150 000 | 33 |
|  | >150 000 | 15 |
| Hemoglobin (g/dL) | <6 | 8 |
|  | 6–8 | 20 |
|  | 8–10 | 27 |
|  | 10–12 | 24 |
|  | >12 | 21 |
| Fibrinogen (mg/dL) | <100 | 4 |
|  | >100 | 96 |
| LDH | <240 | 16 |
|  | >240 | 84 |

elevated leukocyte count in more than half of the patients should be noted; leukopenia can also be found, but most patients had leukemic blast cells in the peripheral blood, and 'aleukemic leukemias' are rare. In patients with normal or decreased leukocyte counts, the diagnosis may be missed by automated blood cell assay, and thus the importance of microscopic examination of blood smears is stressed. Neutropenia and thrombocytopenia in a third or less of the patients correspond roughly with symptoms of infection and bleeding.

An initial lumbar puncture should be done to determine whether the CNS is involved. It should, however, be postponed as long as there is a risk of bleeding due to a very low platelet count, or a risk of blast cell contamination due to leukemic blast cells in the peripheral blood. When the leukocyte count in the spinal fluid is low or the morphological detection of blasts is inconclusive, demonstration of an immunologically defined blast cell population can confirm a diagnosis of CNS involvement.

# Therapy

## Initial evaluation and supportive therapy

At diagnosis, the evaluation of an adult with ALL should include a history and a careful physical examination. Speed in clinical evaluation and diagnosis is important in order to initiate supportive measures and to decide on appropriate therapy. In only a few cases is the leukemic process so far advanced that immediate treatment of leukemia is necessary – for example, in patients with symptoms due to a large mediastinal mass and pleural effusions or to a rapidly progressing B-ALL.

A few general measures should be initiated at once. Sufficient fluid intake to guarantee urine production of 100 ml/h throughout induction therapy should be maintained to reduce the danger of uric acid formation. Parenteral fluid administration may be required when the patient's oral intake is inadequate owing to nausea or difficulty in swallowing. Placement of an implantable port system is advantageous when anticipating a long period of induction therapy or when part of the therapy will be carried out on an outpatient basis.

Patients should receive allopurinol to reduce the formation of uric acid and avoid the danger of urate nephropathy. Allopurinol should be given at a dose of 300 mg/day, which may be increased to 600 mg/day if high leukocyte counts or organomegaly persist. The dose of allopurinol has to be reduced when 6-mercaptopurine (6-MP) is given, since it potentiates the action of 6-MP. Rasburicase is a new recombinant urate oxidase enzyme which catalyzes the oxidation of uric acid to allantoin.[7] Recently it has been demon-

strated that rasburicase can reduce high uric acid faster and safer than allopurinol thereby preventing a tumor lysis syndrome in almost all cases.[8] It might, therefore, be an alternative in patients with high risk of tumor lysis syndrome.

During the induction period, patients are at high risk of infections and hemorrhagic complications, since thrombocytopenia and granulocytopenia are aggravated by chemotherapy.

### Bleeding prevention

In general, platelet transfusions should be given in response to bleeding episodes and to prevent bleeding when platelet counts fall below $20\,000 \times 10^6$/L, especially during febrile periods. Most often, daily platelets are given until bleeding ceases. HLA-matched platelets are given to patients who become refractory to random donor platelets. The incidence of fatal hemorrhage during induction therapy has been significantly lowered by these measures.

### Infection prophylaxis

The use of more intense cytostatic regimens has resulted not only in improved response rates of malignancies but also in higher infection-associated morbidity and mortality.[9] Long-term neutropenia is the most important risk factor, but CD4 lymphopenia, antibody deficiency, and multiple immunosuppression in allogeneic stem cell transplantation also lead to severe and lethal infections. Whereas formerly gram-negative microorganisms were the leading cause of febrile neutropenia, in the last decade gram-positive bacterial infections, mostly caused by staphylococci, have increased and are frequently correlated to indwelling central venous access. Invasive fungal infections are, however, the most dangerous development with an increasing frequency particularly of mold infections.[10] The successful management of febrile neutropenia is based on hygienic procedures including body hygiene, germ-reduced food, reverse isolation or high-efficiency particulate air filtration, antibiotic prophylaxis, sufficient diagnostics, and consequent empirical antimicrobial therapy.

For antibacterial prophylaxis, sulfamethoxazole–trimethoprim or fluoroquinolones, both mainly directed against gram-negative organisms, have mostly been used.[11] Co-trimoxazole also reduces the incidence of *Pneumocystis carinii* pneumonia, which occurs in approximately 20% of ALL patients without prophylaxis.[12] Although antifungal prophylaxis with oral amphotericin B solution or triazoles may successfully reduce candida colonization and prevent local candida infections, the prophylactic procedures for reducing systemic mycoses are disappointing. Fluconazole has been reported to reduce only systemic *Candida albicans* infections in stem cell transplantation (SCT) patients, but non-*albicans* infections, especially by fluconazole-resistant *Candida krusei*, are emerging. Because of its high lethality and difficult diagnostic approval, *Aspergillus* infection is a particular problem. Attempts to prevent aspergilloses have included prophylaxis with itraconazole, intravenous low-dose amphotericin B, liposomal amphotericin B, and inhalation of aerosolized amphotericin B, but in randomized studies no clear benefit could be shown.[13]

In febrile neutropenia consequent and early diagnostic procedures are necessary. They include physical examination, microbiological investigations, imaging procedures and biopsies. Cultures of blood, urine, sputum, and other infected areas are mandatory. Aspergillus galactomannan antigen test (Platelia) may be advantageous in supporting diagnostic efforts in suspected aspergillosis. Furthermore PCR methods are investigated for early detection of fungal infections.[14] Imaging procedures such as chest X-ray or abdominal ultrasound are routine diagnostic tools. High-resolution computed tomography of the lungs is one of the most important diagnostic steps for the early diagnosis of Aspergillus pneumonia. Fungal pneumonias also may be microbiologically proven with bronchoalveolar lavage or biopsy.

Successful treatment of febrile neutropenia is based on immediate empirical administration of broad-spectrum antibiotics. As initial therapy, combinations such as β-lactam antibiotics plus aminoglycosides or monotherapy (e.g. with carbapenems, piperacillin-tazobactam or cephalosporins of class 3 and 3a) are actual standard.[15] Considering the increasing problems of invasive fungal infections, empiric antimycotic treatment with amphotericin B or fluconazole for patients with refractory fever or pulmonary infiltration has been established.[15] So far, conventional amphotericin B, amphotericin lipid formulations, 5-flucytosine, fluconazole and itraconazole represented antimycotic standard treatment in proven or suspected invasive mycoses. This standard, however, is now changing by introduction of highly potent new antimycotics such as voriconazole (effective in the treatment particularly of aspergillosis, but also of fluconazole-resistant candidosis or fusariosis) and caspofungin (successful treatment for candidoses and aspergilloses).[16]

### Hematopoietic growth factors

The use of hematopoietic growth factors such as granulocyte colony-stimulating factor (G-CSF) and granulocyte–macrophage colony-stimulating factor (GM-CSF) is a valuable component of supportive therapy during the treatment of ALL. There is no indication that these CSFs stimulate leukemic cell growth in a clinically significant manner.

The majority of clinical trials have demonstrated that the prophylactic administration of G-CSF signifi-

cantly accelerates neutrophil recovery,[17–20] and several prospective randomized studies have also shown that this is associated with a substantially reduced incidence and duration of febrile neutropenia and of severe infections.[19,20] The enhanced marrow recovery allows closer adherence to the dose and schedule of chemotherapeutic regimens. However, it still remains an open question whether the increased dose intensity translates into an improved leukemia-free survival (LFS).

The advantage of G-CSF administration is particularly evident in selected high-risk patients receiving multiple treatment cycles, whereas clinical effects appear to be negligible in patients at low risk of infectious complications. The scheduling of G-CSF is of great importance. It is noteworthy that G-CSF can be given in parallel with chemotherapy without aggravating the myelotoxicity of these specific regimens.[20–22] Since patients with initial neutrophil count $<500/\mu l$ had an increased rate of severe infections in an ongoing German multicenter trial for adult ALL (GMALL), all patients with this feature receive G-CSF already on the first day of chemotherapy.

On the other hand, it was demonstrated that after short consolidation cycles G-CSF application may be postponed. Therefore, in the context of a regimen based on high-dose cytarabine/mitoxantrone, the G-CSF application could be postponed from day 12 to day 17 without negative effects on duration of neutropenia.[23] Similar results were reported for consolidation therapy with the hyper-CVAD (cyclophosphamide, vincristine, Adriamycin [doxorubicin], dexamethasone) regimen.[24]

See also Chapter 20 on the use of hematopoietic growth factors.

## Chemotherapy

The chemotherapy of ALL is generally divided into several phases, beginning with remission induction. The objective of induction chemotherapy is to achieve complete remission (CR), that is, eradication of leukemia as determined by morphological criteria and recently also by molecular markers. Whereas the induction phase of therapy is usually well defined, postremission therapy can be subdivided into intensification/consolidation and maintenance phases. Usually a prophylactic treatment of the CNS is added (Table 32.4).

### Remission induction therapy

Exact diagnosis and management of initial complications are the prerequisites for successful induction therapy. A cautious cell reduction phase is recommended for patients with a large leukemic tumor

**Table 32.4 Overall treatment results in adult acute lymphoblastic leukemia (ALL) in larger studies***

| Group | Year | Number | Age | Induction | Consolidation | Maintenance | CR (%) | LFS % at (years) |
|---|---|---|---|---|---|---|---|---|
| MDACC[34,35] | 1990,95 | 112 | 30 | V,AD,DX,C | M,A,AD,**HDAC**,V,P,D,MP,**HDM** | AD,V,AC,P/auto SCT, **HDM**,D,V,MP,P | 82 | 26 (3) |
| GATLA[36] | 1991 | 137 | 30 | V,P,D | – | MP,M,V,P | 80 | 20 (5) |
| GATLA[36] | 1991 | 145 | 29 | V,P,D,A,C,AC,MP | AD,V,DX,A,AC,C,MP | M,,MP,V,P | 78 | 34 (6) |
| CALGB 8011[37] | 1991 | 277 | 33 | V,P,A,D | MP,M,[AC,D] | MP,M,V,P | 64 | 29 (9) |
| CALGB 8513[38] | 1991 | 164 | 32 | V,P,Mi/D,**HDM** | V,P,Mi/D,**HDM**,AC,MP,A | – | 64 | 18 (3) |
| BALSG[39] | 1997 | 109 | 15–50 | V,P,D,A | V,P,A,D,**IDM**,VM,AC | M,MP | 88 | 42 (5) |
| EORTC[40] | 1992 | 106 | 27 | V,P,AD,[**HDAC**] | A,**HDC**,[M,TG,AC] | MP,M,P,V,AD,BCNU,C | 74 | 40 (8) |
| L+B+V[41] | 1992 | 212 | 27 | V,P,A,AD[C;**HDAC**] | | MP,M,C | 71 | 32 (10) |
| FGTALL[42] | 1993 | 581 | 33 | V,P,D/R,C,[amsa,AC] | D/R,AC,A | MP,M,V,C,P,D/R,DT,BCNU | 76 | 17 (5) |
| GMALL 01[43] | 1993 | 368 | 25 | V,P,A,D,C,AC,M,MP | V,DX,AD,AC,C,TG | MP,M | 74 | 35 (10) |
| GMALL 02[43] | 1993 | 562 | 28 | V,P,A,D,C,AC,M,MP | V,DX,AD,AC,C,TG,VM,AC | MP,M | 75 | 39 (7) |
| UKALL IX[44] | 1993 | 266 | | V,P,A,(MP,M)/D | | MP,M,V,P | 68 | 22 (8) |
| Lyon + other[45] | 1995 | 135 | 31 | V,P,A,D:C,AC,MP | **HDM**,ARC, allo/auto SCT | [Il-2] | 93 | 44 (3) |
| CALGB 8811[46] | 1995 | 197 | 32 | V,P,A,D,C | C,MP,AC,V,A,M,AD,DX,TG | MP,M,V,P | 85 | 30 (5) |
| GIMEMA 0183[47] | 1996 | 358 | 31 | V,P,A,D | V,IDM,IDAC,P,VM,AC | MP,M,V,P[A,AC,VM,IDAC] | 79 | 25 (10) |
| HOVON[48] | 1997 | 130 | 35 | V,P,A,D | **HDAC**,amsa,MP,VP | – | 73 | 28 (5) |
| SAKK[49,50] | 1994,97 | 140 | 31 | V,P,D,M,A,**HDAC**,VP | allo/auto SCT; >50y: **HDC** | – | 69 | 21 (5) |
| UKALL XA[51] | 1997 | 618 | >15 | V,P,D,A | [AC,VP,D,TG] | MP,MTX,V,P | 82 | 28 (5) |
| PETHEMA[52] | 1998 | 108 | 28 | V,P,D,A,C | **HDM**,V,D,P,A,C,VM,AC | MP,M[VD,P,Mi,A,C,VM,AC] | 86 | 41 (4) |
| CALGB[22] | 1998 | 198 | 35 | C, D,V,P,A | C,MP,AC,V,A,MP,M,AD,DX,TG,P | MP,M,V,P | 85 | 40 (3) |
| MDACC[32] | 2000 | 204 | 39 | V,AD,DX,C | **HDM**, **HDAC**,P | M,,MP,V,P | 91 | 38 (5) |
| SWEDEN[27] | 2002 | 120 | 44 | **HDAC**,C,D,V,BM | AM,**HDAC**,V,BM,C,D,VP +/– SCT | MP,M,D,V,P,AC,TG | 86 | 36 (3) |
| GIMEMA[31] | 2002 | 794 | 28 | V,P,A,D,C,[**HDAC**,Mi] | V,**HDM**,**HDAC**,DX,VM | MP,M,V,[AC,Mi,VM,**HDAC**,**HDM**,DX] | 82 | 29 (9) |

* since 1990, >100 patients, follow-up >3 years; Bold text = high dose cycles

Abbreviations: [N,M], with or without; N/M, either/or; A, L-asparaginase; amsa, Amascrine; ARC, AC, cytarabine; AD, doxorubicin; BCNU, carmustine; C, cyclophosphamide; CR, rate of complete remission; D, daunorubicin; DT, dactinomycin; DX, dexamethasone; HDC, high-dose cyclophosphamide; HDAC, high dose cytarabine; HDM, high dose methotrexate; IDAC, intermediate dose cytarabine; IDM, intermediate dose methotrexate; IL-2, Interleukin 2; LFS, leukemia-free survival; M, methotrexate; Mi, mitoxantrone; MP, 6-mercaptopurine; MRD, median remission duration; P, prednisone; R, rubidazone; TG, thioguanine; V, vincristine; VD, vindesine; VM, teniposide; VP, etoposide

BALSG, Bay Area Leukemia Study Group; CALGB, Cancer and Leukemia Group B; EORTC, European Organisation for Research and Treatment of Cancer; FGTALL, French Group for Treatment of Adult Acute Leukemia; GATLA, Argentine Group for Treatment of Acute Leukemia; GIMEMA, Gruppo Italiano Malattie Ematologiche Maligne Adupo; GMALL, German multicenter trials in Adult ALL; HOVON, Dutch Hemato-Oncology Group; L+B+V, London (St. Bartholomew's Hospital) + Bergamo (Ospedale Riuniti) + Vicenza (Ospedale San Bartolo); MDACC, M.D. Anderson Cancer Center; SAKK, Swiss Group for Epidemiologic and Clinical Cancer Research; UKALL, U. K. Medical Research Council ALL trials mass and/or a high leukocyte count (>30 000 × 10⁶/L). Patients with extreme leukocytosis (>100 000 × 10⁶/L) have been treated initially with leukapheresis. However, these patients can also be managed with vincristine and prednisone in nearly all cases without complications. For mature-B-ALL, initial treatment with cyclophosphamide and prednisone for one week usually results in safe reduction of large tumor masses.[25]

Standard induction therapy for ALL in most studies consists of vincristine, prednisone, asparaginase and an anthracycline. Prednisone and prednisolone have been most frequently administered, although dexamethasone shows a higher antileukemic activity in vitro and a better penetration to the cerebrospinal fluid.[26] The addition of the anthracyclines daunorubicin or doxorubicin (Adriamycin) results in a CR rate of 80–85%. Whereas formerly daunorubicin was mostly administered at a weekly schedule, recently many trials include dose intensification with doses of 30 to 60 mg/m² at a 2–3 day schedule.[22,27,28]

Asparaginase does not affect the CR rate, but probably improves LFS and if not used during induction therapy it is often included as part of the consolidation treatment. Evidence comes from pediatric studies where the addition of asparaginase to vincristine and prednisone has led to improved CR rates in relapsed ALL patients. Leukemia-free survival has also been improved by the administration of post-induction doses of asparaginase. The addition of asparaginase to conventional induction therapy did not improve the CR rate in one trial in adult ALL, but there was a trend towards a higher LFS.[29] Three different asparaginase preparations with significantly different half-lives are available: Native Escherichia coli (1.2 days), Erwinia (0.65 days) and PEG-E. coli (5.7 days).[30] The availability may vary between different countries. In order to reach equal efficacy the application schedule has to be adapted according to half-life.

The next step in improving induction therapy was the addition of cyclophosphamide and cytosine arabinoside (AC, cytarabine). This does not raise the overall CR rate, but possibly improves the remission quality. Cyclophosphamide and cytarabine therapy is particularly useful as initial treatment for special ALL subgroups such as T-ALL. A randomized study by the Italian GIMEMA group comparing a three drug induction with and without cyclophosphamide did not show a difference in terms of CR rate (81% vs. 82%).[31] However, in several non-randomized trials, high CR rates (85–91%) were achieved with regimens including cyclophosphamide pretreatment,[22,32] particularly in adult T-ALL.[33]

### High-dose treatment

Another strategy is to add high-dose cytarabine (HDAC; 1–3 g/m², usually for 12 doses) before or after the standard induction therapy. This approach has resulted in a median CR rate of 79%, which is not superior to that obtained with conventional treatment, and it remains uncertain whether and for which subgroups it may be beneficial for LFS.[53] Up-front application before conventional chemotherapy yielded higher CR rates[27,40,54–56] than application after induction therapy,[32,41,57] which was in part related to a higher induction mortality. Furthermore, any type of induction therapy with HDAC may lead to an increased incidence of severe neutropenia after subsequent chemotherapy cycles (Table 32.5). So far there are no data demonstrating that LFS can be improved by the use of HDAC during induction.

In conclusion, all approaches for induction therapy – including high dose treatment – result in a CR rate of approximately 80% in adult ALL. However the molecular CR rate is clearly lower (see chapter on MRD) and the addition of new therapeutic approaches – other than chemotherapy – such as molecular targeting or antibody treatment may be the future approach to increase the molecular CR rate.

### Failure during induction therapy or refractory ALL

Between 15% and 20% of adult ALL patients will not achieve CR after induction therapy, in contrast to fewer than 5% of children with ALL. Less than 10% of adult ALL patients die during the induction period. Mortality during induction is age-dependent, increasing with age from less than 3% in adolescents to 20% in patients over 60 years of age. The main cause of death is infection, particularly fungal infection. The remaining nonresponders may achieve a partial remission or may be refractory to standard treatment. The number of patients (approximately 10%) who are refractory to chemotherapy is steadily decreasing with the use of more intensive induction regimens, which do, however, lead more frequently to aplasia or toxic death. This stresses the need for optimal supportive treatment. All patients who are refractory to induction therapy are candidates for stem cell transplantation whenever possible.

### Intensification therapy

Consolidation therapy refers to high-dose chemotherapy, to the use of new agents or to readministration of the induction regimen. These measures are aimed at eliminating clinically undetectable residual leukemia after induction chemotherapy, and thereby preventing relapse as well as the emergence of drug-resistant cells.

Intensification schedules include teniposide, etoposide, m-amsacrine, mitoxantrone, idarubicin and HDAC, and intermediate- or high-dose methotrexate. There is evidence that intensification therapy can prolong LFS in adult ALL (Table 32.5).

**Table 32.5** High-dose cytarabine in induction of adult acute lymphoblastic leukemia (ALL)

| Author | Year | Age | Induction | N | CR (%) |
|---|---|---|---|---|---|
| **Before conventional induction** | | | | | |
| Stryckmans et al[40] | 1992 | 27 (16–65) | **R: HDAC** 1.4 g/m$^2$ × 1 V,P,AD | 106 | 74 both arms |
| Hallbook et al[58] | 1999 | 44 (16–82) | **HDAC** 3 g/m$^2$ × 3 (3d) C, D, V, BX | 120 | 85 |
| Ifrah et al[54] | 1999 | 31 (16–55) | **HDAC** 1 g/m$^2$ × 6 (3 d) I, P | 64 | 72 |
| Weiss et al [55] | 1996 | 39 (18–76) | **HDAC** 3 g/m$^2$ × 5 (5d) Mi | 37 | 84 |
| Willemze et al [56] | 1995 | 31 (17–61) | **HDAC** 1 g/m$^2$ × 12 (6d) VP, amsa, P | 26 HR | 72 |
| **After conventional induction 'Secondary'** | | | | | |
| Bassan et al[41] | 1992 | 32 (14–59) | V,P,AD,A **HDAC** 2 g/m$^2$ × 12 (6d)* | 57 | 67 |
| Cassileth et al[57] | 1992 | 31 (16–65) | V,P,D **HDAC** 3 g/m$^2$ × 12 (6d)* | 89 | 69 |
| Kantarjian et al[32] | 2000 | 39 (16–79) | C, V, AD, DX HDM, P **HDAC** 3 g/m$^2$ × 4 (2d) | 204 | 91 |

*for CR/PR

Abbreviations: ( ) estimate from published remission duration curve; AD, adriamycin; amsa, amsacrine; BX, betamethasone; C, cyclophosphamide; DX, dexamethasone; HDAC, high-dose cytarabine; HDM, high-dose methotrexate; HR, high risk; I, idarubicin; Mi, mitoxantrone; n.r., not reported; OS, overall survival; P, prednisone; V, vincristine; VP, VP16

Randomized trials have failed to demonstrate a clear advantage of any particular consolidation regimen. In two earlier studies by the Italian GIMEMA group, focusing on the impact of intensified versus conventional maintenance treatment, no advantage could be demonstrated for the intensified regimen.[31,47] In a Cancer and Leukemia Group B study using consolidation courses of AML-like therapy with daunorubicin and cytarabine in addition to 6-mercaptopurine and methotrexate, the outcome was not superior to conventional maintenance alone.[37] Also in a GIMEMA study an AML-like regimen yielded no benefit. In a randomized trial by the British Medical Research Council (MRC), however, there was a reduction in the risk of relapse in patients receiving early and/or late intensification.[51] Additional evidence for the value of intensification therapy comes from childhood ALL studies.

### High-dose chemotherapy

High-dose chemotherapy in consolidation has been used mainly to overcome drug resistance or to achieve therapeutic drug levels in the cerebrospinal fluid.

***High-dose cytarabine (HDAC):*** Although there is wide experience with HDAC for the treatment of ALL,[53,59,60] it still remains uncertain what dose is optimal and if there is actually a benefit. Usually doses ranging from 1 to 3 g/m$^2$ every 12 hours for 4–5 days are given within combinations. It has been included in several trials in adult de novo ALL as part of consolidation therapy[48,57,61,62] or during induction and consolidation treatment[32,56]. With a weighted mean for the LFS of 30% (26–50%), the results are not superior to trials without HDAC.

It is possible that specific subgroups of ALL may profit from HDAC treatment; thus excellent results are achieved for pediatric B-ALL with LFS of greater than 80%,[63] for adult mature B-ALL,[64] and apparently for adult pro-B-ALL with LFS of 50–60%.[65] For other adult poor-risk groups such as late responders, Ph+ ALL or pre-T-ALL, the value of HDAC was not demonstrated.

***High-dose methotrexate (HDM):*** The use of HDM has been extensively studied for the treatment of childhood ALL and, to a lesser extent, adult ALL.[66] A wide range of doses (0.5–8 g/m$^2$) has been used. HDM appears to be effective in preventing systemic and testicular relapses in childhood ALL.[67] The effect of HDM on CNS leukemia may contribute to the favorable results reported with its use. Overall the intensive use of HDM may have had a major role in improvement of outcome in pediatric B-ALL. Several studies have investigated the efficacy of HDM in adult ALL – as consolidation[68–70] or during consolidation and induction treatment.[38,71] The weighted mean for LFS of six studies, which also comprised a variety of other drugs, is 41%, with a wide range (31–56%). Most favorable results have been achieved in small trials with HDM as part of intensive multidrug consolidation regimens.

**HDAC together with HDM:** The combination of cycles having HDAC with cycles having HDM during consolidation was reported from six trials with a weighted mean for LFS of 32% (17–48%).[31,32,39,47,72] Therefore, there is some evidence that the inclusion of HDAC and HDM as part of multidrug consolidation treatment may improve overall results.

## Maintenance therapy

The optimal duration and form of maintenance therapy in adult ALL is unknown. Because the aim of maintenance or continuation therapy is to eliminate minimal residual disease (MRD), the optimal form of maintenance therapy may be identified with reliable methods for the detection of MRD (see Chapter 32). Standard maintenance is based on combination treatment with 6-mercaptopurine and methotrexate. The potential effects of further intensification cycles for specific subgroups of ALL remain open. In a large Italian multicenter study (GIMEMA 0183), the randomized comparison of intensive and conventional maintenance showed no difference.[47] However, attempts to omit maintenance altogether after induction and consolidation therapy have resulted in inferior results.[38,48,49,73] There is a need for prospective trials with maintenance schedules adapted to immunological subtypes of ALL (e.g. longer for common ALL, shorter for T-ALL, and none for B-ALL) and particularly adapted to MRD.

## Prophylaxis of central nervous system leukemia

Adult ALL patients without initial CNS involvement who do not receive specific prophylactic CNS treatment had a CNS relapse rate of 30% (29–32%) in early studies. Thus treatment and prophylaxis of CNS leukemia is an important part of ALL treatment. Several options are available: intrathecal methotrexate alone or in combination with cytarabine or prednisone/dexamethasone, cranial irradiation, or systemic treatment with HDAC or HDM (reviewed in [74]). Rarely, CNS directed therapy is administered as intraventricular therapy in adult ALL.

With intrathecal chemotherapy alone, the rate of isolated and combined CNS relapses could be reduced to 13% (8–19%). In many adult ALL trials, additional prophylactic CNS irradiation (24 Gy) has been included. This combined approach further reduces the CNS relapse rate to 9% (3–19%). It is questionable whether systemic high-dose treatment alone provides sufficient CNS prophylaxis, since the CNS relapse rate is about 14% (10–16%). For high-dose chemotherapy together with intrathecal therapy, the rate of CNS relapses was 7% (2–16%); with additional CNS irradiation, it was 6% (1–13%). Therefore, the combination of several CNS-active measures is preferable. This is also evident from a retrospective analysis from the MD Anderson Cancer Center, where the lowest CNS relapse rate (2%) was achieved in a recent trial with early high-dose chemotherapy and intrathecal therapy but without CNS irradiation for all patients.[35]

Prophylactic treatment of the CNS may result in acute or chronic neurotoxicity. Adverse effects include febrile reactions, arachnoiditis, leukoencephalopathy, and subclinical dysfunctions, including learning disabilities. In adult ALL patients chemical meningitis after intrathecal therapy (e.g. indicated by headache) occurs often and may even lead to reduction of the planned schedule.

## Therapy for relapsed and resistant leukemia

Patients who fail to achieve CR or those who relapse subsequently have been treated with a variety of protocols (summarized in [75] and [76]). The repetition of regimens including vincristine, anthracyclines and steroids similar to standard induction treatment in earlier studies led to CR rates of 61%. This is a reasonable approach particularly in patients with preceding remission duration of more than 18 months.[77]

In patients with a first remission duration below 18 months the CR rate is clearly below 50%, again with a wide variation that may be attributed to patient selection and non-uniform intensity of pretreatment. Therefore, new combinations with idarubicin (46–64% CR rate) or fludarabine (67–83% CR rate) have been evaluated. Other new approaches, such as antibody therapy, Imatinib in Ph/BCR–ABL positive ALL or new cytostatic drugs such as Nelarabine in T-ALL, are currently under investigation and may lead to better CR rates in relapsed ALL.

For all chemotherapy regimens, the duration of second remission is usually short (<6 months), and long-term survival with chemotherapy alone is less than 5%. Consequently, the only curative chance for adult patients with relapsed or resistant ALL is SCT. The major aim of relapse treatment is the induction of a second CR or good partial remission and to proceed immediately to a SCT.

# Stem cell transplantation

Stem cell transplantation (SCT) from peripheral blood and, to a lesser extent, from bone marrow is the major postremission strategy for eradication of residual disease in adult ALL and can replace consolidation/maintenance treatment (reviewed in references [78] and [79]). Prognostic factors for remission duration after chemotherapy (i.e. age, WBC count, immunophenotype, BCR–ABL status) are also predictive for the outcome after SCT.

## Allogeneic SCT from sibling donors

In a total of 1100 adult patients in first CR, LFS after allogeneic SCT was 50%, with an RI of 24% and a TRM of 27% (Table 32.6). In the International and European bone marrow transplant registries (IBMTR and EBMT), a substantial number of adult ALL patients has been collected. Among recipients of HLA-identical sibling transplants in first remission, reported to the IBMTR between 1994 and 1999, the survival after 3 years was 61% for 561 patients <20 years of age and 48% for 909 patients >20 years of age.[81] Age is a risk factor for TRM and RI, which were 28% and 29% respectively in patients below 40 years compared with 37% TRM and 38% RI in older ones.[82] Relapse incidence is reduced in patients with limited graft-versus-host disease (GvHD) compared with those without GvHD or with extensive GvHD, probably owing to a graft-versus-leukemia (GvL) effect resulting in a better LFS in the former patients.

After allogeneic SCT beyond first CR or relapsed/refractory ALL, LFS is 34% and 20% respectively (Table 32.6). The RI of 47% and 71% is still high.

## Matched unrelated SCT

Only one-third of potential SCT candidates with ALL will have an HLA-identical sibling donor. To extend the possibilities of allogeneic SCT by enlarging the number of potential donors, matched SCT from unrelated donors (MUD) and to a smaller extent mismatched SCT from related donors (MM) is increasingly being employed. The lower relapse rate with both approaches is probably due to the more pronounced GvL reaction, which is, however, outweighed by the high TRM of approximately 40%.[80,83] Matched SCT from unrelated donors can result in long-term survival of about 39% for patients transplanted in first CR and 27% for patients in CR2 (Table 32.6). Among 223 patients >20 years of age who received unrelated donor transplants for ALL in first remission reported to the IBMTR, the probability of survival after 3 years was 40%.[81]

This might be increased by improved donor selection, less toxic preparative regimens, better management of GvHD and improved supportive care. Overall the results of MUD SCT in ALL seem encouraging. MUD SCT is the treatment of choice for high-risk patients in CR1 if a sibling donor is not available. For patients with Ph/BCR–ABL positive ALL the results of MUD SCT are already approaching those of sibling SCT. Mismatched or haploidentical SCT in adult ALL is still experimental and an option only for rare cases; it is explored by few very experienced SCT centers.

**Table 32.6 Recent results of stem cell transplantation (SCT) in adult acute lymphoblastic leukemia (ALL)**

| SCT | Disease Stage | N | LFS/OS[a] (%) | Relapse Incidence[a] (%) | TRM[a] (%) |
|---|---|---|---|---|---|
| Allogeneic sibling | CR1 | 1100 | 50 | 24 | 27 |
| | CR2 | 1019 | 34 | 48 | 29 |
| | Rel./refr. | 216 | 18 | 75 | 47 |
| MUD | CR1 | 318 | 39 | 10 | 47 |
| | ≥CR2 | 231 | 27 | 8[b] | 75[b] |
| | Rel/refr | 47 | 5[b] | 31[b] | 64[b] |
| Autologous | CR1 | 1369 | 42 | 51 | 5 |
| | CR2 | 258 | 24 | 70 | 18[c] |
| NMSCT | All stages | 132 | 23 | 47 | 42 |

[a] weighted mean and range of published studies
[b] one study[80]
[c] one study
Abbreviations: LFS, leukemia-free survival; MUD, matched unrelated donor; NMSCT, nonmyeloablative SCT; OS, overall survival; Rel, relapsed; refr, refractory; TRM, transplant related mortality

## Autologous SCT

Autologous SCT is a readily available alternative, and can be performed in patients up to 65 years of age owing to its low TRM (2–8%) (Table 32.6). The major disadvantage is the high relapse rate (51%), probably caused to some extent by the reinfusion of leukemic blasts but more by the lack of GvL effects. Purging of the marrow graft with chemotherapeutic agents (e.g. mafosfamide) or monoclonal antibodies may reduce the leukemia cell burden. Thus purging with immunomagnetic beads can reduce tumor load by 2 log in Ph/BCR–ABL positive ALL.[84] Purging is however not routinely used.

The LFS of 42% for autologous SCT in first remission is inferior to that for allogeneic SCT, although it may be better than chemotherapy. In advanced stages, the results are again inferior (24% LFS) to those of allogeneic SCT, but still superior to chemotherapy (Table 32.6).

The administration of maintenance treatment (e.g. with 6-mercaptopurine/methotrexate) after autologous SCT may contribute to a reduction in RI.[85] Collection of peripheral blood stem cells is now the major stem cell source for autologous SCT and bone marrow is only used if mobilization fails.

## Nonmyeloablative SCT

Nonmyeloablative SCT (NMSCT) or reduced intensity conditioning regimens is a new approach, which deserves evaluation in ALL and may lead to an extension of indications for allogeneic SCT. In contrast to conventional SCT, which mainly relies on cell kill by high-dose chemotherapy and total body irradiation (TBI), NMSCT aims at the utilization of GvL effects. Immunosuppression (e.g., with purine analogs, other cytostatic drugs and/or low-dose TBI) is followed by the infusion of donor stem cells from siblings or MUD with adapted immunosuppression to establish host tolerance.[86]

So far, in more than 100 adult ALL patients with high median age and poor prognostic features the probabilities for survival after NMSCT was around 23% with relapse rate of 47% and TRM of 42%[87] (Table 32.6). Overall, it seemed to be of some benefit in patients in CR1.[88,89] In patients with advanced refractory or relapsed ALL due to a high TRM rate, this form of SCT is at present not successful.

## Indications for SCT in first complete remission

The overall LFS of 50% after allogeneic SCT is superior to that obtained with chemotherapy alone and also to that of autologous SCT.[45,90,91] Several study groups failed, however, to demonstrate a significant advantage in terms of overall survival for allogeneic or autologous SCT in first CR compared with chemotherapy.[42,92–95] As autologous SCT seems to produce similar results to chemotherapy, the argument that autologous SCT requires a shorter duration of treatment compared with chemotherapy may be made.

In high-risk patients, however, LFS and overall survival was superior after allogeneic SCT (39%) compared with the control group including autologous SCT and chemotherapy patients (14%).[96]

Therefore, at present it appears advisable that low-risk patients having an LFS of about 50% after chemotherapy should receive a SCT only after relapse. For high-risk adult ALL patients, allogeneic SCT in first CR is advisable. In very high-risk cases (such as Ph/BCR–ABL positive ALL) without a compatible family donor, MUD SCT is recommended in younger patients. Older patients should receive autologous SCT or NMSCT.

# Prognostic factors

The major risk factor for attaining a CR is advanced age and Ph+ ALL. Prognostic factors are of greater importance for duration of remission and survival (Tables 32.7 and 32.8).

### Table 32.7  Outcome of adult acute lymphoblastic leukemia (ALL) according to subgroups

| Subgroup | Patient number | CR rate[a] (%) | LFS[a] (%) |
|---|---|---|---|
| Overall | 5413 | 83 (75–91) | 34 (29–49) |
| **Age** | | | |
| 15–20 yrs | | 82–95 | 32–65[b] |
| 20–50 yrs | | 80 | 35–40 |
| 50–60 yrs | | 60–70 | 20–30 |
| >60 yrs | | 20–50 | 10–20 |
| **Immunologic subtype** | | | |
| T-ALL | 621 | 65–85 | 30–50 |
| Thymic | | 90 | 50–60 |
| Early/mature | | 65–80 | 30 |
| Pro-B-ALL | 57 | 75 | 40–50 |
| Common ALL | 881 | 80 | 30–50[c] |
| B-ALL | 89 | 77 | >50 |
| **Cytogenetics** | | | |
| Ph/BCR-ABL+ ALL | 352 | 66 | 15–20[d] |

[a] pooled data from published studies; [b] results from pediatric studies; [c] depending on risk factors; [d] without SCT
Abbreviations: CR, complete remission; LFS, leukemia free survival

**Table 32.8 Adverse prognostic factors for remission duration in adult acute lymphoblastic leukemia (ALL)***

- High WBC in B-lineage ALL; >30.000, >100.000/µl
- Advanced age; >35 - >50 - >60 years
- Immunologic subtypes; early T, mature T, pro B
- Chromosomal abnormalities and corresponding molecular markers
    Ph⁺ ALL [t(9;22) BCR–ABL]
    t(4;11), ALL1-AF4
- Treatment response
    Late achievement of complete remission; >3–4 wks
    MRD detection >10⁻⁴ after induction therapy, increase of MRD

* as they emerged from more than 3000 adult ALL patients treated in the GMALL (German Multicenter Studies for Adult ALL) trials[97,98]
MRD, minimal residual disease

## Age

There is a continuous decline in CR rate from 95% in children to 40–60% in patients over 50–60 years of age.[99] Most trials demonstrate that increasing age is also associated with shorter remission duration and survival and that LFS is inferior in patients over 50–60 years.

## Immunophenotype, cytogenetics, and molecular genetics

The immunophenotype is an independent prognostic variable in ALL, despite the fact that with modern treatment strategies the previously poor prognosis of phenotypes such as T-ALL and mature B-ALL has been changed. In ongoing recent trials, there is a tendency to use the immunophenotype to adjust treatment regimens accordingly (e.g. for mature B-ALL).

### T-lineage ALL

Results for T-ALL have recently improved, with CR rates of greater than 80% and LFS of 46% compared with earlier results with remission duration of less than 10 months and survival rates below 10%. The addition of cyclophosphamide and cytarabine to the usual cytostatic drugs for ALL is mainly responsible for this improvement.[33,100] There is, however, a substantial difference in outcome for the T-ALL subtypes. Thymic T-ALL, which accounts for half of the adult T-ALL patients, has a favorable outcome with CR rates of 85–90% and survival >50% at 5 years. Early T-ALL and mature T-ALL have a poorer outcome with CR rates of 70% and LFS rates of approximately 30%.[101]

High-dose methotrexate (HDM) contributed to the improvement of survival in children with T-ALL,[102,103] as did HDAC,[104] which improved the prognosis for adult ALL patients with high WBC counts and T-cell ALL.[104,105] For adults, the benefit of HDM in T-ALL has to be confirmed in larger trials. New treatment approaches in adult T-ALL include purine analogs such as cladribine and compound GW506U78 (Nelarabine)[106,107] or antibody therapy such as anti-CD52. Also SCT for early/mature T-ALL patients in CR 1 seems promising.[108]

### B-lineage ALL

In *common and pre-B-ALL*, CR rates in adult trials have improved to 80% or more, but patients still relapse in most studies over a period of up to 5–6 years, and only one-third survive. This may in part be explained by the fact that approximately 30% of adult patients with common/pre-B-ALL are Ph/BCR–ABL positive and their prognosis remains poor. But the results are also not encouraging for adult patients with Ph-negative common/pre-B-ALL. Higher doses of anthracyclines given in induction and reaching a certain cumulative amount may be beneficial.[109] The outcome for patients with *pre-B-ALL* seems to be similar to that for common ALL.

Within common/pre-B-ALL prognostic factors are decisive for outcome; high-risk patients with adverse prognostic features such as high WBC (>30 000/µl) and/or late achievement of CR (>3–4 weeks) (Table 32.8) have a survival of 25% or less whereas standard risk without any of those features have a 5-year survival of >50%.[110]

*Ph/BCR–ABL⁺ ALL* (Ph⁺ ALL) as a subtype of common/pre-B-ALL has the worst prognosis in children as well as in adults. In 13 studies with a total of 384 patients, the mean CR rate is 67% (44–76%). The median remission duration in all series is short (5–11 months), and the survival, from 0% to 20% at 3–5 years, is extremely poor in all reports. The only curative chance for adult Ph+ ALL patients is SCT – including allogeneic sibling and matched unrelated SCT. The introduction of the ABL-tyrosine kinase inhibitor Imanitib (formerly STI571) leads to a promising new treatment modality for Ph⁺ ALL.

Adults with the subtype *pro-B-ALL* or the t(4; 11) translocation, which nearly exclusively occurs in this subgroup, had a poor prognosis, as did infant ALL patients.[111] With intensive regimens including HDAC and mitoxantrone as consolidation therapy, the results for adults seem to improve.[65] Pro-B-ALL patients have also a benefit from allogeneic SCT in CR1 with survival rates of 60%,[112] as well as from autologous SCT.

A decade ago, CR rates for adults with *mature B-ALL* were low (<50%), and remission duration and survival were short (11 months). A change was brought about by innovative childhood B-ALL studies, which significantly improved outcome, with CR rates of 80–94% and LFS of 63% (weighted mean). The most important drugs for this improvement are apparently high doses of fractionated cyclophosphamide or ifosfamide, HDM (0.5–8 g/m²) and HDAC, in conjunction with the conventional drugs for remission induction in ALL, given in short cycles at frequent intervals over 6 months. The application of these childhood B-ALL protocols in original or modified form also brought about a substantial improvement for adult patients with B-ALL. Complete remission rate is now approximately 75% (62–83%) and the LFS 55% (20–71%).[25,64,113]

B-cell ALL has a higher incidence of CNS involvement at diagnosis and of CNS relapse. Therefore, effective measures against CNS disease, such as HDM and HDAC as well as intrathecal therapy, are important components of treatment regimens. On the other hand, maintenance treatment has been omitted. Because relapses occur almost exclusively within the first year in childhood as well as in adult B-cell ALL studies, patients thereafter can be considered as cured.

Recent treatment protocols include antibody therapy with anti-CD20 (rituximab), since more than 80% of the patients are CD20⁺, with quite promising preliminary results.[60,114,115]

In mature B-ALL, because of too small patient cohorts it is difficult to extract significant prognostic factors, but older age (>50 years), high WBC (>30 000/µl), bone lesions, and mediastinal involvement are associated with inferior outcome.

## Other prognostic factors

Chromosomal abnormalities correlate markedly with outcome in ALL, independently of other features. Hypodiploidy and translocations, particularly t(9;22) Ph⁺, are unfavorable findings in adults. The prognostic impact of cytogenetic aberrations may, however, differ between protocols since it depends on the applied treatment. This is evident for the t(4;11) translocation, a formerly extremely unfavorable group, which has now an improved outcome in some protocols. The translocations t(8;14), t(2;8) and t(8;22) are present in most cases of mature B-ALL and in Burkitt lymphoma and have lost their poor prognostic impact owing to the improved treatment for patients with B-ALL or Burkitt lymphoma.

Extensive organ involvement at presentation (e.g. hepatomegaly, splenomegaly, CNS leukemia and mediastinal involvement) has been found in some studies to have an adverse influence on remission duration. CNS leukemia is considered an adverse prognostic factor in some reports. However, in other studies, the LFS for patients with initial CNS involvement was not inferior. Mediastinal mass, although indicative of a large tumor burden, had no adverse influence on either CR rate or remission duration in several adult ALL series. Most ALL patients with mediastinal tumors have the T-ALL subtype, so that any adverse influence of mediastinal mass is probably outweighed by the recent improvement in treatment of T-ALL.

# Future directions

## Minimal residual disease

Recent advances in molecular and immunological techniques have allowed the detection of minimal residual disease (MRD), defined as leukemic cells undetectable by morphological examination (see Chapter 17). The most relevant methods for ALL are flow cytometry and PCR analysis, with sensitivities ranging between $10^{-4}$ and $10^{-6}$ (summarized in references[116–118]). Flow cytometry allows the detection of characteristic constellations of two or more cell-surface antigens. PCR methods – and nowadays real-time PCR – are directed towards the detection of fusion proteins resulting from specific translocations (e.g. BCR–ABL, E2A–PBX1, MLL–AF4 and TEL–AML1). These are present in 20–30% of adult ALL patients. In addition, PCR methods target clonal rearrangements of immunoglobulin chain genes (IgH, IgK) or T-cell receptor genes (TCR-β, -δ, -λ, -γ). IgH rearrangements can be detected in 96% and 20% of B- and T-lineage ALL patients respectively. The frequency of detectable TCR rearrangements is 36–57% and 25–93% respectively.[119] A prerequisite is the identification of individual rearrangements at the time of diagnosis in each patient, which is possible in more than 90% of ALL patients with combinations of two or three targets.

Clinical MRD studies in childhood ALL (reviewed in [116–118]), mostly evaluating MRD by PCR analysis, have shown a widespread pattern. A considerable proportion of patients have detectable MRD after induction treatment, despite morphological CR. This only partly limits the predictive value of MRD evaluation, since the quantitative amount of MRD is correlated with relapse risk. Patients with MRD above the threshold of $10^{-3}$–$10^{-4}$ have a significantly lower LFS compared with those below. Not all patients with positive MRD, however, eventually relapse, and so the kinetics of MRD are apparently another prognostic parameter. The continuous decrease of MRD or very low levels are associated with a low relapse risk. Thus, in patients remaining in continuous CR, the incidence of MRD positivity decreased from initially 36% to 10% after more than 24 months (Table 32.9). On the other hand, in patients with final relapse, the proportion of positive MRD results remained consistently high (78%) during month 1 to 24 of therapy.

Table 32.9  Kinetics of MRD detection and outcome in adult and childhood ALL

| Studies | Patient outcome after CR | Time after complete remission (months) | | | | | |
| --- | --- | --- | --- | --- | --- | --- | --- |
| | | 1–6 | | 7–24 | | >24 | |
| N | | N[1] | MRD[+2] | N[1] | MRD[+2] | N[1] | MRD[+2] |
| 20 | CCR | 343 | 36% | 260 | 18% | 257 | 10% |
| 10 | Relapse | 140 | 78% | 51 | 78% | 72 | 58% |

[1] Number of patients analyzed for MRD
[2] Percentage of patients with positive MRD status

In adult ALL, the results in childhood ALL were overall confirmed – but with some specific differences.[120] A very good response as indicated by an early and rapid decrease of MRD already during induction may be associated with a very low relapse risk.[121] However, in general the decrease of MRD occurs more slowly in adults and fewer patients reach a negative MRD status. This applies particularly for patients with low MRD immediately after induction, who still show a considerable relapse rate of approximately 50%.[122–124] Thus the longitudinal course of MRD may be more important in adults compared with children. High MRD at any time-point after induction is associated with a higher relapse risk,[125,126] and the predictive value increases at later time-points (months 6–9).[127]

The predictive value of MRD evaluation depends on the technical quality, such as sensitivity or number of target genes, and on the frequency of evaluations in individual patients. In a retrospective study of the GMALL a broad spectrum of target genes (IgH, IgK, and TCR rearrangements) was measured quantitatively with high sensitivity ($<10^{-4}$).[128] Based on these results MRD-based risk groups could be defined[129] for the ongoing GMALL study.

There is a need for larger prospective studies to evaluate the potential of MRD determination and to justify therapeutic decisions based on MRD detection. Such decisions could be various: the redefinition of CR in patients who are in morphological CR but with detectable MRD, or the evaluation of the effectiveness of specific treatment elements (e.g. MRD evaluation before and after high-dose cycles or bone marrow purging chemotherapy, antibody treatment, molecular therapy, SCT).[120,129] Furthermore, in patients with repeatedly negative MRD, treatment could be stopped earlier, whereas in those with high levels or continuously positive MRD, alternative treatment approaches such as SCT could be considered. Thus in the ongoing GMALL study in patients with low risk according to MRD treatment is stopped after 1 year, whereas in MRD high-risk patients intensification with SCT or experimental treatment is intended. It is unclear at present how to proceed with MRD intermediate-risk patients, who cannot be allocated to either group and form a rather large patient cohort.[130]

## Treatment with monoclonal antibodies

Targeted therapy with monoclonal antibodies (MoAbs) is a new treatment option in adult ALL. Acute lymphocytic leukemia blasts express a variety of specific antigens – such as CD19, CD20, and cyCD22 for B-lineage ALL; or CD25, CD7, CD3 for T-lineage ALL and CD52 or CD33 for both – which may serve as targets for treatment with monoclonal antibodies (MoAbs). The presence of the target antigen on at least 20–30% of the blast cells is generally considered as a prerequisite for MoAb therapy. First results with the combination of chemotherapy and rituximab are promising in mature B-ALL. Other MoAbs such as anti-CD52 (Campath-1H), B43(Anti-CD19)-Genistein, B43(Anti-CD19)-PAP; Anti-B4-bR (Anti-CD19) in B-Lineage ALL and Anti-CD7-Ricin in T-lineage ALL have been investigated in phase I-II pilot trials in ALL.[131]

### Anti-CD20

The inclusion of rituximab, which is a chimeric MoAb to CD20 lead to an improvement of results in B-cell non-Hodgkin lymphoma (NHL). CD20, defined as expression on more than 20% of the blast cells is, however, also present on one-third of B-precursor ALL blasts, particularly in elderly patients (40–50%), and the majority of mature B-ALL blast cells (80–90%). This provides a rationale to explore rituximab in B-precursor ALL, mature B-ALL and Burkitt lymphoma. Favorable results were observed in two trials where rituximab was used in combination with intensive chemotherapy. Nineteen patients with newly diagnosed Burkitt NHL or mature B-ALL received anti-CD20 together with the hyper-CVAD regimen for a total of 8 doses. Eighty-nine percent complete responses (CR) were observed.[132] In a GMALL study with 53 patients (mature B-ALL, Burkitt and other high-grade NHL) the remission rate was 91% in mature B-ALL and in Burkitt NHL a response rate of 96% (PR, CR) was achieved after 2 cycles.[115] The interim results indicate that there was apparently no additional toxicity compared with the previous protocol with chemotherapy only. The GMALL study group has recently started prospective trials with a combination of anti-CD20 and chemotherapy for patients with B-precursor ALL.

### Anti-CD52

The CD52 antigen is expressed in most lymphatic cells and to a higher degree in T-lymphoblasts compared with B-lymphoblasts. CD52 antibodies were first used for ex-vivo T-cell depletion of allogeneic bone marrow grafts in order to prevent GvHD. The humanized antibody Campath-1H showed antitumor activity in chronic lymphocytic leukemia, T-cell prolymphocytic leukemia and other T-NHL. In ALL only case reports are available. Nevertheless several studies with Campath-1H in ALL are ongoing, for those in relapse (also in combination with chemotherapy), in status of positive MRD, or even in de novo ALL as consolidation treatment.

### ABL tyrosine kinase inhibitors in Ph/BCR–ABL positive ALL

In Ph/BCR–ABL positive (Ph[1]) leukemia the BCR–ABL fusion gene is causally involved in leukemogenesis and is considered to be essential for leukemic transformation. With an inhibitor of the ABL tyrosine kinase (STI571, Imatinib) cellular proliferation of BCR–ABL+ CML and ALL cells can be inhibited selectively.[133]

### Clinical experience with Imatinib in advanced Ph+ ALL

First studies in relapsed or refractory Ph+ ALL patients yielded a hematologic response rate of 60% and a CR rate of 19% with an Imatinib monotherapy at a daily dose of 600 mg orally. Rapid blast cell clearance occurred within 1 week of treatment in the majority of patients, but this PB response did not necessarily correspond with a bone marrow response. The median time to progression was short for ALL patients (2 months).[134] Hematologic toxicity of grades III and IV was frequent, but was rarely associated with serious infectious or hemorrhagic complications. Non-hematologic toxicity attributed to Imatinib consisted primarily of mild-to-moderate gastrointestinal

discomfort, peripheral and facial edema, and muscle cramps, and was readily manageable. Thus Imatinib was well tolerated even in heavily pretreated patients. One important issue is probably that, owing to a low penetration to the CSF, prophylaxis of CNS relapse should be given in parallel to Imatinib therapy.[135]

### Imatinib and allogeneic stem cell transplantation in Ph+ ALL

The efficacy of Imatinib was also explored in patients with Ph+ ALL who relapsed after allogeneic SCT. The CR rate in 20 patients was 50%.[136] Donor cell chimerism increased to above 96% in both BM and PB within the first 4 weeks of Imatinib in responding patients, indicating a selective expansion of Ph- donor cells over the leukemic clone. Disease-free survival after 2 years is approximately 20% and overall survival 40%, due to subsequent salvage therapy.[137] Therefore, Imatinib as a single agent induces remissions in a substantial proportion of patients relapsing after allogeneic SCT and, in a few cases, even molecular remission can be achieved.

### Current concepts for Imatinib treatment in de novo Ph+ ALL

As a consequence of the results in relapsed/refractory ALL, Imatinib has now entered trials in de novo ALL. Imatinib was given for 4 weeks after induction therapy in de novo Ph+ ALL with CR. The BCR–ABL level after induction therapy decreased by more than 0.5 log in half of the cases, remained unchanged or increased in 40%, and approximately 10% of the patients achieved a molecular CR. In a subsequent study, Imatinib was given in parallel with the second phase of induction therapy.[138] Preliminary encouraging results of a combination regimen have also been shown by the group at MD Anderson. Patients with Ph+ ALL received Imatinib parallel to intensive chemotherapy (hyper-CVAD regimen) for several cycles without serious unexpected toxicity.[139] Imatinib as first line therapy in patients with newly diagnosed Ph+ ALL is also currently being tested by the GMALL Study Group in a randomized trial in elderly (≥55 years) patients with de novo Ph+ ALL. First results show that this combination is safe, that complete remissions can be achieved by a Imatinib monotherapy, and that the combination of Imatinib and chemotherapy is feasible.[140]

## REFERENCES

1. Seer*Stat Database: Incidence - SEER 9 Regs Public Use, Nov 2002 Sub (1973–2000). National Cancer Institute, DCCPS, Surveillance Research Program, Cancer Statistics Branch, released April 2003, based on the November 2002 submission. 2003.

2. Bene MC, Castoldi G, Knapp W et al. Proposal for the immunological classification of acute leukemias. Leukemia 1995; 9: 1783–6.

3. Secker-Walker LM, Prentice HG, Durrant J et al. Cytogenetics adds independent prognostic information in

adults with acute lymphoblastic leukaemia on MRC trial UKALLL XA. *Br J Haematol* 1997; **96:** 601–10.

4. Charrin C. Cytogenetic abnormalities in adult acute lymphoblastic leukemia: Correlations with hematologic findings and outcome. A collaborative study of the Groupe Francais de Cytogénétique Hématologique. *Blood* 1996; **87:** 3135–42.

5. Wetzler M, Dodge RK, Mrozek K et al. Prospective karyotype analysis in adult acute lymphoblastic leukemia: The Cancer and Leukemia Group B experience. *Blood* 1999; **93:** 3983–93.

6. Gleissner B, Gökbuget N, Bartram CR et al. Leading prognostic relevance of the BCR–ABL translocation in adult acute B-lineage lymphoblastic leukemia: a prospective study of the German Multicenter Trial Group and confirmed polymerase chain reaction analysis. *Blood* 2002; **99:** 1536–43.

7. Navolanic PM, Pui CH, Larson RA et al. Elitek(TM)-rasburicase: an effective means to prevent and treat hyperuricemia associated with tumor lysis syndrome, a Meeting Report, Dallas, Texas, January 2002. *Leukemia* 2003; **17:** 499–514.

8. Pui CH, Mahmoud HH, Wiley JM et al. Recombinant urate oxidase for the prophylaxis or treatment of hyperuricemia in patients with leukemia or lymphoma. *J Clin Oncol* 2001; **19:** 697–704.

9. Pizzo PA. Management of fever in patients with cancer and treatment- induced neutropenia. *N Engl J Med* 1993; **328:** 1323–52.

10. Meunier F. Targeting fungi: a challenge. *Am J Med* 1995; **99:** 60–7.

11. Rogers TR. Prevention of infection during neutropenia. *Br J Haematol* 1991; **79:** 544–9.

12. Hughes WT, Rivera GK, Schell MJ et al. Successful intermittent chemoprophylaxis for Pneumocystis carinii pneumonitis. *N Engl J Med* 1987; **316:** 1627–32.

13. Cornely OA, Ullmann AJ, Karthaus M. Evidence-based assessment of primary antifungal prophylaxis in patients with hematologic malignancies. *Blood* 2003; **101:** 3365–72.

14. Buchheidt D, Skladny H, Baust C, Hehlmann R. Systemic infections with Candida sp. and Aspergillus sp. in immunocompromised patients with hematological malignancies: current serological and molecular diagnostic methods. *Chemotherapy* 2000; **46:** 219–28.

15. Hughes WT, Armstrong D, Bodey GP et al. Guidelines for the use of antimicrobial agents in neutropenic patients with cancer. *Clin Infect Dis* 2002; **34:** 730.

16. Ruhnke M, Maschmeyer G. Management of mycoses in patients with hematologic disease and cancer – review of the literature. *Eur J Med Res* 2002; **7:** 227–35.

17. Kantarjian HM, Estey E, O'Brien S et al. Granulocyte-stimulating factor supportive treatment following intensive chemotherapy in acute lymphocytic leukemia first remission. *Cancer* 1993; **72:** 2950–5.

18. Scherrer R, Geissler K, Kyrle PA et al. Granulocyte colony-stimulating factor (G-CSF) as an adjunct to induction chemotherapy of adult acute lymphoblastic leukemia (ALL). *Ann Hematol* 1993; **66:** 283–9.

19. Ottmann OG, Hoelzer D, Gracien E et al. Concomitant granulocyte colony-stimulating factor and induction chemoradiotherapy in adult acute lymphoblastic leukemia: a randomized phase III trial. *Blood* 1995; **86:** 444–50.

20. Geissler K, Koller E, Hubmann E et al. Granulocyte colony-stimulating factor as an adjunct to induction chemotherapy for adult acute lymphoblastic leukemia – a randomized phase- III study. *Blood* 1997; **90:** 590–6.

21. Ottmann OG, Hoelzer D. Do G-CSF and GM-CSF contribute to the management of acute lymphoblastic leukemia? *Leukemia* 1996; **10:** S52–7.

22. Larson RA, Dodge RK, Linker CA et al. A randomized controlled trial of filgrastim during remission induction and consolidation chemotherapy for adults with acute lymphoblastic leukemia: CALGB study 9111. *Blood* 1998; **92:** 1556–64.

23. Hofmann WK, Seipelt G, Langenhan S et al. Prospective randomized trial to evaluate two delayed granulocyte colony stimulating factor administration schedules after high-dose cytarabine therapy in adult patients with acute lymphoblastic leukemia. *Ann Hematol* 2002; **81:** 570–4.

24. Weiser MA, O'Brien S, Thomas DA et al. Comparison of two different schedules of granulocyte-colony-stimulating factor during treatment for acute lymphocytic leukemia with a hyper- CVAD (cyclophosphamide, doxorubicin, vincristine, and dexamethasone) regimen. *Cancer* 2002; **94:** 285–91.

25. Hoelzer D, Ludwig W-D, Thiel E et al. Improved outcome in adult B-cell acute lymphoblastic leukemia. *Blood* 1996; **87:** 495–508.

26. Balis FM, Lester CM, Chrousos GP et al. Differences in cerebrospinal fluid penetration of corticosteroids: possible relationship to the prevention of meningeal leukemia. *J Clin Oncol* 1987; **5:** 202–7.

27. Hallbook H, Simonsson B, Ahlgren T et al. High-dose cytarabine in upfront therapy for adult patients with acute lymphoblastic leukaemia. *Br J Haematol* 2002; **118:** 748–54.

28. Todeschini G, Tecchio C, Meneghini V et al. Estimated 6-year event-free survival of 55% in 60 consecutive adult acute lymphoblastic leukemia patients treated with an intensive phase II protocol based on high induction dose of daunorubicin. *Leukemia* 1998; **12:** 144–9.

29. Nagura E. Nation-wide randomized comparative study of doxorubicin, vincristine and prednisolone combination therapy with and without L-asparaginase for adult acute lymphoblastic leukemia. *Cancer Chemother Pharmacol* 1994; **33:** 359–65.

30. Asselin BL. The three asparaginases. Comparative pharmacology and optimal use in childhood leukemia. *Adv Exp Med Biol* 1999; **457:** 621–9.

31. Annino L, Vegna ML, Camera A et al. Treatment of adult acute lymphoblastic leukemia (ALL): long-term follow-up of the GIMEMA ALL 0288 randomized study. *Blood* 2002; **99:** 863–71.

32. Kantarjian HM, O'Brien S, Smith TL et al. Results of treatment with hyper-CVAD, a dose-intensive regimen, in adult acute lymphocytic leukemia. *J Clin Oncol* 2000; **18:** 547–61.

33. Hoelzer D, Thiel E, Löffler H et al. Intensified Chemotherapy and Mediastinal Irradiation in Adult T-Cell Acute Lymphoblastic Leukemia. In: Gale RP, Hoelzer D, eds. *Acute Lymphoblastic Leukemia.* New York: Alan R.Liss; 1990, pp. 221–9.

34. Kantarjian HM, Walters RS, Keating MJ et al. Results of the Vincristine, Doxorubicin, and Dexamethasone Regimen in Adults With Standard- and High-Risk Acute Lymphocytic Leukemia. *J Clin Oncol* 1990; **8:** 994–1004.

35. Cortes J, O'Brien SM, Pierce S et al. The value of high-dose systemic chemotherapy and intrathecal therapy for central nervous system prophylaxis in different risk groups of adult acute lymphoblastic leukemia. *Blood* 1995; **86:** 2091–7.

36. Lluesma-Gonalons M, Pavlovsky S, Santarelli MT et al. Improved results of an intensified therapy in adult acute lymphocytic leukemia. *Ann Oncol* 1991; **2:** 33–9.

37. Ellison RR, Mick R, Cuttner J et al. The Effects of Postinduction Intensification Treatment With Cytarabine and Daunorubicin in Adult Acute Lymphocytic Leukemia: A Prospective Randomized Clinical Trial by Cancer and Leukemia Group B. *J Clin Oncol* 1991; **9:** 2002–15.

38. Cuttner J, Mick R, Budman DR et al. Phase III Trial of Brief Intensive Treatment of Adult Acute Lymphocytic Leukemia Comparing Daunorubicin and Mitoxantrone: A CALGB Study. *Leukemia* 1991; **5:** 425–31.

39. Linker CA. Risk-adapted treatment of adult acute lymphoblastic leukemia (ALL). *Leukemia* 1997; **11:** S24–7.

40. Stryckmans P, de Witte T, Marie JP et al Therapy of adult ALL: overview of 2 successive EORTC studies: (ALL-2 & ALL-3). *Leukemia* 1992; **6:** 199–203.

41. Bassan R, Battista R, Rohatiner AZS et al. Treatment of adult acute lymphoblastic leukaemia (ALL) over a 16 year period. *Leukemia.* 1992; **6:** 186–90.

42. Fiere D, Lepage E, Sebban C et al. Adult Acute Lymphoblastic Leukemia. A Multicentric Randomized Trial Testing Bone Marrow Transplantation as Postremission Therapy. *J Clin Oncol* 1993; **11:** 1990–2001.

43. Hoelzer D, Thiel E, Ludwig WD et al. Follow-up of the first two successive German multicentre trials for adult ALL (01/81 and 02/84). *Leukemia* 1993; **7:** Suppl 2: 130–4.

44. Durrant IJ. Results of Medical Research Council trial UKALL IX in acute lymphoblastic leukaemia in adults: report from the Medical Research Council Working Party on Adult Leukaemia. *Br J Haematol* 1993; **85:** 84–92.

45. Attal M, Blaise D, Marit G et al. Consolidation treatment of adult acute lymphoblastic leukemia: a prospective, randomized trial comparing allogeneic versus autologous bone marrow transplantation and testing the impact of recombinant interleukin-2 after autologous bone marrow transplantation. *Blood* 1995; **86:** 1619–28.

46. Larson RA, Dodge RK, Burns CP et al. A five-drug remission induction regimen with intensive consolidation for adults with acute lymphoblastic leukemia: Cancer and Leukemia Group B study 8811. *Blood* 1995; **85:** 2025–2037.

47. Mandelli F, Annino L, Rotoli B. The GIMEMA ALL 0183 trial: analysis of 10-year follow-up. *Br J Haematol* 1996; **92:** 665–72.

48. Dekker AW, van't Veer MB, Sizoo W et al. Intensive postremission chemotherapy without maintenance therapy in adults with acute lymphoblastic leukemia. *J Clin Oncol* 1997; **15:** 476–82.

49. Wernli M, Tichelli A, von Fliedner V et al. Intensive induction/consolidation therapy without maintenance in adult acute lymphoblastic leukaemia: a pilot assessment. *Br J Haematol* 1994; **87:** 39–43.

50. Wernli M, Abt A, Bargetzi M et al. A new therapeutic strategy in adult acute lymphoblastic leukemia: intensive induction/consolidation, early transplant, maintenance-type therapy in relapse only. *Proc Am Soc Clin Oncol* 1997; **16:** 6a.

51. Durrant IJ, Prentice HG, Richards SM. Intensification of treatment for adults with acute lymphoblastic leukaemia: results of U.K. Medical Research council randomized trial UKALL XA. *Br J Haematol* 1997; **99:** 84–92.

52. Ribera JM, Ortega J, Oriol A et al. Treatment of high-risk acute lymphoblastic leukemia. Preliminary results of the protocol PETHEMA ALL-93. In: Hiddemann et al, ed. *Acute leukemias VII. Experimental approaches and novel therapies.* Berlin: Springer-Verlag; 1998, pp. 755–65.

53. Gökbuget N, Hoelzer D. The role of high-dose cytarabine in induction therapy for adult ALL. *Leuk Res* 2002; **26:** 473–6.

54. Ifrah N, Witz F, Jouet JP et al. Intensive short term therapy with granulocyte-macrophage-colony stimulating factor support, similar to therapy for acute myeloblastic leukemia, does not improve overall results for adults with acute lymphoblastic leukemia. GOELAMS Group. *Cancer* 1999; **86:** 1496–1505.

55. Weiss M, Maslak P, Feldman E et al. Cytarabine with high-dose mitoxantrone induces rapid complete remission in adult acute lymphoblastic leukemia without the use of vincristine or prednisone. *J Clin Oncol* 1996; **14:** 2480–5.

56. Willemze R, Zijlmans JMJM, den Ottolander GJ et al. High-dose Ara-C for remission induction and consolidation of previously untreated adults with ALL or lymphoblastic lymphoma. *Ann Hematol* 1995; **70:** 71–4.

57. Cassileth PA, Andersen JW, Bennett JM et al. Adult acute Lymphocytic Leukemia: the Eastern Cooperative Oncology Group experience. *Leukemia* 1992; **6:** 178–81.

58. Hallbook H, Simonsson B, Bjorkholm M et al. High dose ara-c as upfront therapy for adult patients with acute lymphoblastic leukemia (ALL). *Blood* 1999; **94:** 1327a.

59. Hoelzer D. High-dose chemotherapy in adult acute lymphoblastic leukemia. *Semin Hematol* 1991; **28:** 84–9.

60. Hoelzer D, Gökbuget N. New approaches in acute lymphoblastic leukemia in adults: Where do we go? *Semin Oncol* 2000; **27:** 540–59.

61. Hoelzer D, Arnold R, Aydemir U et al. Results of intensified consolidation therapy in four consecutive German multicentre studies for adult ALL. *Blood* 1993; **82:** 193a.

62. Daenen S, van Imhoff GW, Haaxma-Reiche H et al. Acute lymphoblastic leukemia: single center experience with modified chemotherapy. *Blood* 1995; **86:** 754a.

63. Patte C, Auperin A, Michon J et al. The Societe Francaise d'Oncologie Pediatrique LMB89 protocol: highly effective multiagent chemotherapy tailored to the tumor burden and initial response in 561 unselected children with B-cell lymphomas and L3 leukemia. *Blood* 2001; **97:** 3370–9.

64. Thomas DA, Cortes J, O'Brien S et al. Hyper-CVAD program in Burkitt's-type adult acute lymphoblastic leukemia. *J Clin Oncol* 1999; **17:** 2461–70.

65. Ludwig W-D, Rieder H, Bartram CR et al. Immunophenotypic and genotypic features, clinical characteristics, and treatment outcome of adult pro-B acute lymphoblastic leukemia: results of the German multicenter trials GMALL 03/87 and 04/89. *Blood* 1998; **92:** 1898–1909.

66. Gökbuget N, Hoelzer D. High-dose methotrexate in the treatment of adult acute lymphoblastic leukemia. *Ann Hematol* 1996; **72:** 194–201.

67. Freeman AI, Weinberg V, Brecher ML et al. Comparison of intermediate methotrexate with cranial irradiation for the post-induction treatment of acute lymphocytic leukemia in children. *N Engl J Med* 1983; **308:** 477.

68. Wiernik PH, Dutcher JP, Paietta E et al. Long-term follow-up of treatment and potential cure of adult acute lymphocytic leukemia with MOAD: a non-anthracycline containing regimen. *Leukemia* 1993; **7:** 1236–41.

69. Evensen SA, Brinch L, Tjonnfjord G, Stavem P, Wisloff F. Estimated 8-year survival of more than 40% in a population-based study of 79 adult patients with acute lymphoblastic leukaemia. *Br J Haematol* 1994; **88**: 88–93.

70. Ribeira JM, Ortega JJ, Fontanillas M et al. Late reinduction chemotherapy has no value in adult acute lymphoblastic leukemia (ALL). Results of the Pethema ALL-89 protocol. *Blood* 1996; **10**: 213a.

71. Elonen E, Almqvist A, Hänninen A et al. Intensive treatment of acute lymphatic leukaemia in adults: ALL86 protocol. *Haematologica* 1991; **76**: 133.

72. Elonen E, for the Finnish Leukaemia Group. Long-term survival in acute lymphoblastic leukaemia in Adults. A prospective study of 51 patients. *Eur J Haematol* 1992; **48**: 75–82.

73. Cassileth PA, Andersen JW, Hoagland HC et al. High-dose cytarabine therapy in adult acute lymphocytic leukemia. In: Gale RP, Hoelzer D, eds. *Acute Lymphoblastic Leukemia.* New York: Alan R Liss; 1990, pp.197–203.

74. Blaney SM, Poplack DG. Neoplastic meningitis: diagnosis and treatment considerations. *Med Oncol* 2000; **17**: 151–62.

75. Welborn JL. Impact of reinduction regimens for relapsed and refractory acute lymphoblastic leukemia in adults. *Am J Hematol* 1994; **45**: 341–4.

76. Bassan R, Lerede T, Barbui T. Strategies for the treatment of recurrent acute lymphoblastic leukemia in adults. *Haematologica* 1996; **81**: 20–36.

77. Freund M, Diedrich H, Ganser A et al. Treatment of Relapsed or Refractory Adult Acute Lymphocytic Leukemia. *Cancer* 1992; **69**: 709–16.

78. Forman SJ. The role of allogeneic bone marrow transplantation in the treatment of high-risk acute lymphocytic leukemia in adults. *Leukemia* 1997; **11**: 18–19.

79. Rowe JM, Liesveld JL. Hematopoietic growth factors in acute leukemia. *Leukemia* 1997; **11**: 328–41.

80. Cornelissen JJ, Carston M, Kollman C et al. Unrelated marrow transplantation for adult patients with poor-risk acute lymphoblastic leukemia: strong graft-versus-leukemia effect and risk factors determining outcome. *Blood* 2001; **97**: 1572–7.

81. IMBTR. Summary slides 2002. *IMBTR/ABMTR Newsletter* 2002; **9**: 4.

82. Cahn J-Y, Labopin M, Schattenberg A et al. Allogeneic bone marrow transplantation for acute leukemia in patients over the age of 40 years. *Leukemia* 1997; **11**: 416–19.

83. Sierra J, Radich J, Hansen JA et al. Marrow transplants from unrelated donors for treatment of Philadelphia chromosome-positive acute lymphoblastic leukemia. *Blood* 1997; **90**: 1410–14.

84. Atta J, Martin H, Bruecher J et al. Residual disease and immunomagnetic bead purging in patients with BCR-ABL-positive acute lymphoblastic leukemia. *Bone Marrow Transplant* 1996; **18**: 541–8.

85. Powles R, Sirohi B, Treleaven J et al. The role of posttransplantation maintenance chemotherapy in improving the outcome of autotransplantation in adult acute lymphoblastic leukemia. *Blood* 2002; **100**: 1641–7.

86. Slavin S, Nagler A, Naparstek E et al. Nonmyeloablative stem cell transplantation and cell therapy as an alternative to conventional bone marrow transplantation with lethal cytoreduction for the treatment of malignant and nonmalignant hematologic disorders. *Blood* 1998; **91**: 756–63.

87. Gökbuget N, Hoelzer D. Non-myeloablative conditioning before allogeneic stem cell transplantation in adult acute lymphoblastic leukemia. *Haematologica* 2003; **88**: 484–6.

88. Arnold R, Massenkeil G, Bornhauser M et al. Nonmyeloablative stem cell transplantation in adults with high-risk ALL may be effective in early but not in advanced disease. *Leukemia* 2002; **16**: 2423–8.

89. Martino R, Giralt S, Caballero MD et al. Allogeneic hematopoietic stem cell transplantation with reduced-intensity conditioning in acute lymphoblastic leukemia: a feasibility study. *Haematologica* 2003; **88**: 555–60.

90. Vey N, Stoppa AM, Faucher C et al. Long-term results of bone marrow transplantation (BMT) as post- remission therapy in adult acute lymphoblastic leukemia: experience of a single institution in 88 patients. *Br J Haematol* 1996; **93**: 61.

91. Carey PJ, Proctor SJ, Taylor P, Hamilton PJN. Autologous bone marrow transplantation for high-grade lymphoid malignancy using melphalan/irradiation conditioning without purging or cryopreservation. *Blood* 1991; **77**: 1593–8.

92. Zhang MJ, Hoelzer D, Horowitz MM et al. Long-term follow-up of adults with acute lymphoblastic leukemia in first remission treated with chemotherapy or bone marrow transplantation. The Acute Lymphoblastic Leukemia Working Committee. *Ann Intern Med* 1995; **123**: 428–31.

93. Oh H, Ohno R, Tanimoto M et al. Is chemotherapy or HLA-identical sibling bone marrow transplantation better in adults with acute lymphoblastic leukemia (ALL) in first remission? *Blood* 1995; **86**: 617a.

94. Forman SJ, Chao N, Niland JC et al. Intensive chemotherapy or bone marrow transplantation for adult ALL in first complete remission. *Blood* 1995; **86**: 616a.

95. de Witte T, Awwad B, Boezeman J et al. Role of allogeneic bone marrow transplantation in adolescent or adult patients with acute lymphoblastic leukemia or lymphoblastic lymphoma in first remission. *Bone Marrow Transplant* 1994; **14**: 767–74.

96. Sebban C, Lepage E, Vernant J-P et al. Allogeneic bone marrow transplantation in adult acute lymphoblastic leukemia in first complete remission: a comparative study. *J Clin Oncol* 1994; **12**: 2580–7.

97. Gökbuget N, Hoelzer D, Arnold R et al. Treatment of Adult ALL According to the Protocols of the German Multicenter Study Group for Adult ALL (GMALL). *Hemat Oncol Clin North Am* 2000; **14**: 1307–25.

98. Ludwig WD, Raghavachar A, Thiel E. Immunophenotypic classification of acute lymphoblastic leukemia. *Bailliere's Clinical Haematology* 1994; **7**: 235.

99. Hoelzer D. Which factors influence the different outcome of therapy in adults and children with ALL ? *Bone Marrow Transplant* 1989; **4**: 98–100.

100. Clarkson B, Gaynor J, Little C et al. Importance of Long-Term Follow-up in Evaluating Treatment Regimens for Adults with Acute Lymphoblastic Leukaemia. *Haematol Blood Trans* 1990; **33**: 397.

101. Hoelzer D, Arnold R, Freund M et al. Characteristics, outcome and risk factors in adult T-lineage acute lymphoblastic leukemia (ALL). *Blood* 1999; **94**: 2926a.

102. Schorin MA, Blattner S, Gelber RD et al. Treatment of childhood acute lymphoblastic leukemia: results of Dana-Farber Cancer Institute/Children's Hospital acute lymphoblastic leukemia consortium protocol 85-01. *J Clin Oncol* 1994; **12**: 740–7.

103. Feickert HJ, Bettoni C, Schrappe M et al. Event-free survival of children with T-cell acute lymphoblastic leukemia after introduction of high dose methotrexate in multicenter trial ALL-BFM 86. *Proc ASCO* 1993; **12**: 317.

104. Arico M, Basso G, Mandelli F et al. Good steroid response in vivo predicts a favourable outcome in children with T-cell acute lymphoblastic leukemia. *Cancer* 1995; **75**: 1684–93.

105. Rohatiner AZS, Bassan R, Battista R et al. High- dose cytosine arabinoside in the initial treatment of adults with acute lymphoblastic leukemia. *Br J Cancer* 1992; **62**: 454–8.

106. Kurtzberg J, Keating M, Moore JO et al. 2-amino-9-B-D-arabinosyl-6-methoxy-9H-guanine (GW506U; Compound 506U) is highly active in patients with T-cell malignancies: Results of a phase I trial in pediatric and adult patients with refractory hematological malignancies. *Blood* 1996; **88**: 2666a.

107. Gökbuget N, Al-Ali H, Atta J et al. Improved outcome of poor prognostic relapsed/refractory T-ALL and T-lymphoblastic lymphoma (LBL) with compound GW506U78 followed by immediate stem cell transplantation (SCT). *Hematol J* 2003; **4**: 266 (abstract 891).

108. Arnold R, Beelen D, Bunjes D et al. Phenotype Predicts Outcome after Allogeneic Stem Cell Transplantation in Adult High Risk ALL Patients. *Blood* 2003; **102** (abstract 1719).

109. Todeschini G, Meneghini V, Pizzolo G et al. Relationship between daunorubicin dosage delivered during induction therapy and outcome in adult acute lymphoblastic leukemia. *Leukemia* 1994; **8**: 376–81.

110. Gökbuget N, Arnold R, Buechner TH et al. Intensification of induction and consolidation improves only subgroups of adult ALL: Analysis of 1200 patients in GMALL study 05/93 [abstract]. *Blood* 2001; **98**: 802a.

111. Pui C-H, Behm F, Downing JR et al. 11q23/MLL rearrangement confers a poor prognosis in infants with acute lymphoblastic leukemia. *J Clin Oncol* 1994; **12**: 909–15.

112. Arnold R, Bunjes D, Ehninger G et al. Allogeneic stem cell transplantation from HLA-identical sibling donor in high risk ALL patients is less effective than transplantation from unrelated donors. *Blood* 2002; **100**: 77a (abstract 279).

113. Lee EJ, Petroni GR, Schiffer CA et al. Brief-duration high-intensity chemotherapy for patients with small non-cleaved-cell lymphoma or FAB L3 acute lymphocytic leukemia: results of cancer and leukemia group B study 9251. *J Clin Oncol* 2001; **19**: 4014–22.

114. Thomas D, Cortes J, Giles F et al. Rituximab and Hyper-CVAD for adult Burkitt's (BL) or Burkitt's-Like (BLL) Leukemia or Lymphoma [abstract]. *Blood* 2001; **98**: 804a.

115. Hoelzer D, Baur K-H, Giagounidis A et al. Short Intensive Chemotherapy with Rituximab Seems Successful in Burkitt NHL, Mature B-ALL and Other High-Grade B-NHL. *Blood* 2003; **102**: abstract 236.

116. Foroni L, Harrison CJ, Hoffbrand AV, Potter MN. Investigation of minimal residual disease in childhood and adult acute lymphoblastic leukaemia by molecular analysis. *Br J Haematol* 1999; **105**: 7–24.

117. Campana D, Pui C-H. Detection of minimal residual disease in acute leukemia: methodological advances and clinical significance. *Blood* 1995; **85**: 1416–34.

118. Szczepanski T, Orfao A, van dV, V, San Miguel JF, van Dongen JJ. Minimal residual disease in leukaemia patients. *Lancet Oncol* 2001; **2**: 409–17.

119. Beishuizen A, van Wering E, Breit TM et al. Molecular biology of acute lymphoblastic leukemia: implications for detection of minimal residual disease. In: Hiddemann et al, eds. *Acute leukemias V. Experimental approaches and management of refractory disease.* Berlin: Springer-Verlag; 1996, p. 460.

120. Gökbuget N, Kneba M, Raff T et al. Risk-adapted treatment according to minimal residual disease in adult ALL. *Best Pract Res Clin Haematol* 2002; **15**: 639-52.

121. Brueggemann M, Raff T, Gökbuget N, Hoelzer D, Kneba M. Early Tumor Kinetics in Adult Acute Lymphoblastic Leukemia (ALL) Has High Prognostic Impact. *Blood* 2003; **102**: abstract 215.

122. Brisco MJ, Hughes E, Neoh SH et al. Relationship between minimal residual disease and outcome in adult acute lymphoblastic leukemia. *Blood* 1996; **87**: 5251–6.

123. Preudhomme C, Grardel N, Huyghe P et al. Evaluation of Minimal Residual Disease (MRD) by Competitive Quantitative PCR Using IgH/TCR Rearrangements Has Prognostic Value in Adult Acute Lymphoblastic-Leukemia (ALL): A Single Center Study. *Blood* 2001; **98**: 1331a.

124. Vidriales MB, Perez JJ, Lopez-Berges MC et al. Minimal residual disease (MRD) in adolescent (>14 years) and adult acute lymphoblastic leukaemias (ALL): Early immunophonotypical evaluation has high clinical value. *Blood* 2003; **101**: 4695–4700.

125. Ciudad J, San Miguel JF, López-Berges MC et al. Prognostic value of immunophenotypic detection of minimal residual disease in acute lymphoblastic leukemia. *J Clin Oncol* 1998; **16**: 3774–81.

126. Brueggemann M, Droese J, Scheuring U et al. Minimal residual disease in adult patients with acute lymphoblastic leukemia during the first year of therapy predicts clinical outcome. *Hematol J* 2001; **1**: 700a.

127. Mortuza FY, Papaioannou M, Moreira IM et al. Minimal residual disease tests provide an independent predictor of clinical outcome in adult acute lymphoblastic leukemia. *J Clin Oncol* 2002; **20**: 1094–104.

128. Brueggemann M, Droese J, Raff TH et al. The prognostic significance of minimal residual disease in adult standard risk patients with acute lymphoblastic leukemia [abstract]. *Blood* 2001; **98**: 314a.

129. Hoelzer D, Gökbuget N, Brüggemann M et al. Clinical impact of minimal residual disease (MRD) in trial design for adult ALL [abstract]. *Blood* 2001; **98**: 584a.

130. Gökbuget N, Raff T, Brueggemann M et al. Prospective Risk Stratification Based on Minimal Residual Disease (MRD) Is Feasible in Adult ALL but Limited by a High Proportion of MRD-Intermediate Risk. *Blood.* 2003; **102**: abstract 1373.

131. Gökbuget N, Hoelzer D. Treatment with monoclonal antibodies in acute lymphoblastic leukemia: current knowledge and future prospects. *Ann Hematol* 2003; **83**: 201–5.

132. Thomas DA, Cortes J, Giles FJ et al. Rituximab and Hyper-CVAD for Adult Burkitt's (BL) or Burkitt's-Like (BLL) Leukemia or Lymphoma. *Blood* 2002; **100**: 3022.

133. Druker BJ, Sawyers C, Kantarjian H et al. Activity of a specific inhibitor of the BCR-ABL tyrosine kinase in the blast crisis of chronic myeloid leukemia and acute lymphoblastic leukemia with the Philadelphia chromosome. *N Engl J Med.* 2001; **344**: 1038–42.

134. Ottmann OG, Druker BJ, Sawyers CL et al. A phase II study of Imatinib Mesylate (Glivec) in Patients with Relapsed or

Refractory Philadelphia Chromosome-Positive Acute Lymphoid Leukemias. *Blood* 2002; **100:** 1965–71.

135. Pfeifer H, Wassmann B, Hofmann WK et al. Risk and prognosis of central nervous system leukemia in patients with Philadelphia chromosome-positive acute leukemias treated with imatinib mesylate. *Clin Cancer Res* 2003; **9:** 4674–81.

136. Wassmann B, Pfeifer H, Scheuring U et al. In molecular relapse after stem cell transplantation (SCT) for Ph+ALL, Imantib can induce sustained molecular remissions. *Blood.* 2003; 1378a.

137. Wassmann B, Scheuring UJ, Pfeifer H et al. Imatinib mesylate induces sustained molecular remissions in Philadelphia-chromosome positive acute lymphoblastic leukemia (Ph ALL) following molecular relapse after stem cell transplantation (SCT). *Hematol J* 2003; **4:** 146 (abstract 474).

138. Pfeifer H, Wassmann B, Scheuring UJ et al. In De Novo Ph+ALL Imatinib, Given Intermittently or Simultaneously with Chemotherapy, Can Effectively Reduce the Leukemic Cell Burden but Induces Molecular Remissions in Only a Subset of Patients. *Blood* 2003; **102:** abstract 3273.

139. Thomas DA, Faderl S, Cortes J et al. Treatment of Philadelphia chromosome-positive acute lymphocytic leukemia with hyper-CVAD and imatinib mesylate. *Blood* 2003; **102:** 790a.

140. Ottmann OG, Wassmann B, Gökbuget N et al. A Randomized Trial of Imatinib Versus Chemotherapy Induction Followed by Concurrent Imatinib and Chemotherapy as First-Line Treatment in Elderly Patients with De Novo Philadelphia-Positive Acute Lymphoblastic Leukemia. *Blood* 2003; **102:** abstract 791

# 33 Chronic lymphoid leukemias

**Emili Montserrat**

## Introduction

Chronic lymphoid leukemias are lymphoproliferative disorders due to the proliferation of lymphoid cells arrested at a mature stage of their differentiation pathways. These diseases have in common the mature (peripheral) origin of the lymphoid cells from which they arise and that neoplastic cells, besides involving lymphoid tissues such as lymph nodes or spleen, are also present in bone marrow and peripheral blood.

## Classification and diagnosis

Chronic lymphoid leukemias are classified as shown in Table 33.1. Morphology, immunophenotype, cytogenetics and molecular characteristics contribute to the classification of these diseases (Tables 33.2 and 33.3). The diagnosis is based on a careful review of peripheral blood films and immunophenotyping. Nevertheless, the histopathological study of lymph nodes, spleen and bone marrow, as well as any other tissue involved by the disease, can be essential for the diagnosis. Moreover, in some cases, cytogenetics and molecular biological studies contribute important information.

## Chronic lymphocytic leukemia

Galton and Dameshek made, in 1966 and 1967 respectively, seminal descriptions of chronic lymphocytic leukemia (CLL), in which this disease was considered as being due to the progressive accumulation (rather than to an abnormal rapid proliferation) of immunoincompetent small lymphocytes.[1,2] Since then, important progress has been made in the understanding of CLL, and different entities have been sorted out from what was formerly known as CLL.[3–6] In the World Health Organization (WHO) classification, CLL is considered the leukemic counterpart of the small lymphocytic lymphoma.[7]

---

**Table 33.1  Chronic lymphoid leukemias. Classification.**

**B-cell origin**
Chronic lymphocytic leukemia
Prolymphocytic leukemia
Hairy-cell leukemia
- classical
- variant
Non-Hodgkin lymphoma with leukemic expression
- splenic lymphoma with villous lymphocytes
- follicular lymphomas
- lymphoplasmacytic/Waldenström's macroglobulinemia
- mantle-cell lymphoma
- others

**T/NK-cell origin**
Prolymphocytic leukemia
- classical
- small variant
Lymphoproliferative disease of granular lymphocytes
- T-cell type
- NK-cell type
Sézary syndrome
Adult T-cell leukemia–lymphoma
Peripheral T-cell lymphomas (others)

---

### Epidemiology

The median age of patients at diagnosis is about 70 years.[3,4] Chronic lymphocytic leukemia is rare in people under the age of 40. The overall incidence is about 5 cases per 100 000 people per year and increases with age,[3–6] and it is the most frequent form of leukemia in Western countries, where it accounts for 30% of all leukemias. In contrast, CLL constitutes only 10% of all leukemias in Asian populations; this variation reflects real differences in the incidence of the disease among different races.[8] In most series, CLL is more frequent in males than in females.[3–6]

## Table 33.2 Immunophenotype, cytogenetic and molecular features of B-cell chronic lymphoid leukemias

| Disease | SmIg | CD5 | CD43 | CD22 | CD23 | CD25 | FMC7 | CD103 | CD11c | CD10 | CD79b | Other features |
|---|---|---|---|---|---|---|---|---|---|---|---|---|
| CLL | -/+ | + | + | -/+ | + | +/- | -/+ | - | -/+ | - | - | +12, del13q14, 6q-, 11q+, 14q+ |
| Lymph | ++ | -/+ | +/- | + | - | -/+ | + | - | -/+ | - | +/- | (CIg+, 100%), +12, 13q-, 14q+, 11q+, t(9;14), PAX-5 |
| PL | ++ | -/+ | + | + | -/+ | - | + | - | - | -/+ | + | t(11;14)(q13;q32), cyclin D1, 14q+, +12 |
| HCL | ++ | - | + | + | - | + | + | + | + | - | -/+ | HC2+, +5, Annexin A1 |
| SLVL | ++ | -/+ | + | + | +/- | -/+ | + | -/+ | +/- | -/+ | + | +3, t(11;14)(q13;q32), del/t7q22-35, 2p11, |
| MCL | ++ | + | + | +/- | - | - | ÷ | - | - | -/+ | + | t(11;14)(q13;q32), cyclin D1 |
| FL | ++ | -/+ | - | +/- | -/+ | - | + | - | - | +/- | + | t(14;18)(q32;q21), bcl-2 |

All express pan-B cell markers (e.g. CD19, CD20) and HLA-DR class II antigens.
CLL = chronic lymphocytic leukemia; Lymph = lymphoplasmacytoid lymphoma/immunocytoma; PL = prolymphocytic leukemia; HCL = hairy-cell leukemia; SLVL = splenic lymphoma with villous lymphocytes; MCL = mantle-cell lymphoma; FL = follicular lymphoma; CIg = cytoplasmic immunoglobulin.

**Table 33.3  Immunophenotypic, cytogenetic and molecular characteristics of T-cell and NK-cell chronic lymphoid leukemias**

| Disease | CD2 CD3 CD5 | CD4 | CD8 | CD56 | Cytogenetic and molecular features |
|---------|-------------|-----|-----|------|-------------------------------------|
| T-PL | +++ | ++ | −/+ | − | inv(14), trisomy 8, t(14;14), TCL-1(+), del(11q)/ATM gene TCR genes rearranged |
| Sézary | +++ | ++ | − | − | TCR genes rearranged |
| CD3⁺ LDGL | CD3⁺ CD2⁺ | − | ++ | − | TCRβ gene rearranged |
| NK⁺ LDGL | CD3⁻ CD2⁻ | − | − | + | Germinal TCR genes |
| ATLL | +++ | ++ | −/+ | − | TCR genes rearranged, HTLV-I⁺ |

T-PL: T-cell prolymphocytic leukemia; LDGL: lymphoproliferative disease of granular lymphocytes; ATLL: adult T-cell leukemia-lymphoma.

## Etiology

The etiology of CLL is unknown. It is not associated with exposure to radiation or other cytotoxic agents.[9] Familial cases of CLL support the existence of a genetic basis for this disease.[10] An interesting observation is the so-called 'anticipation phenomenon' whereby, in younger members of the affected family, CLL presents, on average, 20 years earlier than in the older members.[11] In about 5% of first-degree relatives of patients with CLL, it is possible to demonstrate in peripheral blood a population immunophenotypically identical to that of CLL; the clinical significance of this observation is still unclear.[12]

### Biology

The CD5⁺ B cells from which CLL arises constitute a small subpopulation of B lymphocytes with a characteristic immunophenotype that resembles that of lymphocytes normally present in the mantle zone of lymphoid follicles; these cells may also be found in the peripheral blood of a small proportion (2–3%) of normal subjects, a finding of uncertain clinical significance.[13] Chronic lymphocytic leukemia results from the neoplastic transformation and accumulation of such B lymphocytes. The majority of these cells are arrested in the $G_0$ phase of the cell cycle. They also express large amounts of anti-apoptotic BCL2 proteins whereas the pro-apoptotic BCLX proteins are decreased. This, together with the interaction of neoplastic and stromal cells through a number of chemokines, leads to the accumulation of leukemic cells.[3–6]

Immunophenotypically, the neoplastic lymphocytes from CLL express surface membrane immunoglobulin (SmIg), usually of IgM or both IgM and IgD types, in small amounts ('weak' SmIg expression), and a single Ig light chain (κ or λ). They also express CD5, HLA-DR and B-cell antigens (e.g. CD19, CD20); in most cases they are CD23⁺ whereas CD22 and CD79b are infrequently or weakly expressed.

From the cytogenetic standpoint, in approximately 90% of the patients it is possible to demonstrate chromosomal abnormalities by fluorescent in-situ hybridization (FISH).[14–17] The most frequent abnormalities are del(13q), del(11q), trisomy 12 and del(6q). Karyotypic evolution is observed in around 20% of the patients, usually in relation to disease progression.[18,19]

No genes have been consistently associated with CLL. Putative oncogenes have been identified in the band 13q14.[20,21] In cases of disease progression, del(11q), overexpression of the c-*myc* oncogene, deletions of the *Rbl* gene, and mutations of the p53 tumor-suppressor gene have been reported.[18,19]

Chronic lymphocytic leukemia has long been considered a homogeneous disease of naïve CD5⁺ B cells, pre-germinal cells not exposed to antigenic stimulation. In 1999, two different groups made an important breakthrough in the understanding of CLL by showing that whereas in some cases IgV$_H$ genes are unmutated in others IgV$_H$ genes are mutated.[22,23] As discussed later, these two forms have different clinical behavior. Since somatic mutation takes place in the germinal centre of lymphoid follicles, CLL can be either a tumor of pre-germinal-center B cells or a tumor of post-germinal-center B cells. These two forms, however, share the same genetic signature as determined by microarrays and, because of this, CLL is considered to be a single disease with two variants (i.e. mutated, unmutated).[24]

## Clinical features

About 70% of CLL patients are diagnosed in an asymptomatic phase on the occasion of a routine medical examination. In symptomatic patients, the most frequent findings are generalized lymphadenopathy, fatigue, and weight loss. A history of repeated infections in the months preceding the diagnosis is not infrequent. Infections are primarily due to hypogammaglobulinemia. Most of the infections are caused by common bacteria such as *Streptococcus pneumoniae, Staphylococcus* and *Haemophilus influenzae.* Herpes zoster is also a common complication. The use of new treatment agents with a highly immunosuppressive effect has led to the observation of infections due to opportunistic organisms such as *Legionella pneumophila, Pneumocystis carinii, Listeria monocytogenes,* and cytomegalovirus (CMV). *Candida* and *Aspergillus* species are also of concern.[25,26]

The infiltration of extralymphatic tissues (e.g. pleura, lung, skin, and the CNS) is extremely rare.[27,28] In addition, vasculitis,[27] hypercalcemia,[29] and nephrotic syndrome[30] have occasionally been described. In rare cases (<1% of patients), spontaneous remissions may be observed at some time during the course of the disease.[31,32]

Some cytogenetics abnormalities correlate with particular clinical features. Thus, del(11q) is particularly frequent in young males with bulky disease; trisomy 12 is commonly associated with atypical morphology of the lymphocytes in peripheral blood; del(6q) may be more common in cases with lymphoplasmacytoid cells; finally, del(17p) with mutations of *p53* are observed in transforming disease conveying refractoriness to treatment.[14,18]

## Laboratory features

The hallmark of the disease is the presence of an increased white blood cell (WBC) count with more than 90% small, mature-appearing lymphocytes (Figure 33.1). Usually, the more advanced the disease is, the higher is the WBC count. About 20% of patients present with anemia or thrombocytopenia. Autoimmune phenomena are frequent. For example, a positive direct antiglobulin test may be found in less than 2% to up to 35% of patients, depending on the series analyzed.[33–36] The antibodies are typically warm antibodies of the IgG class. Autoimmune hemolytic anemia occurs in 10–25% of patients, and may be triggered by cytotoxic agents used to treat the

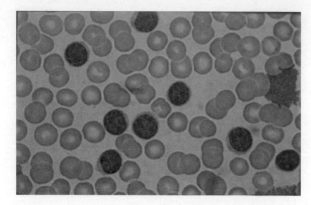

**Figure 33.1** Chronic lymphocytic leukemia (peripheral blood).

disease. Immune thrombocytopenia is observed in only 2% of cases. Pure red-cell aplasia and immune neutropenia are even less frequent, and, as it occurs with immune thrombocytopenia, can be difficult to document.

Hypogammaglobulinemia, which is rare at diagnosis, may eventually occur in about 60% of patients during the course of the disease.[37] On the other hand, a marked monoclonal (M) immunoglobulin component, usually of IgM type, can be found in about 5% of cases,[38] but a small M component can be detected in the serum or urine of 80% of patients using high-resolution techniques.[39]

## Disease transformation

In approximately 3–10% of patients the disease undergoes a transformation into a more aggressive type, most commonly large-cell lymphoma (Richter syndrome).[40] In such cases, fever, weight loss, night sweats, enlarged lymphadenopathy, increased lactate dehydrogenase (LDH) serum levels, anemia, hypercalcemia, thrombocytopenia, and monoclonal gammopathy are the most frequent features.[41] Diagnosis is not always easy, since the histological transformation may be a phenomenon localized in an isolated organ (e.g. spleen, lymph nodes of a given territory, extralymphatic tissue) rather than a generalized event. The immunological, cytogenetic and molecular characteristics of the lymphoma may be the same as or different from those of the original CLL.[42] In some cases disease transformation is associated with the presence of Epstein–Barr virus (EBV) in the tumor. The prognosis in cases of transformation into large-cell lymphoma is poor, with a median survival of less than 6 months.[40] Transformation into prolymphocytic leukemia can also be observed.[43] Chronic lymphocytic leukemia can also transform into Hodgkin lymphoma, which is considered as a variety of Richter syndrome.[40,44]

## Second malignancies

Patients with CLL have an increased risk of suffering other cancers.[45–47] However, risk assessment is not easy owing to the variability in the criteria used to evaluate it. In a study based on data from population-based cancer registries, the observed/expected ratio was 1.20, with an increased risk for Kaposi sarcoma, malignant melanoma, larynx cancers, lung cancer, and also bladder and gastric cancer in men. No relationship was found between the characteristics of the disease and its treatment and the incidence of secondary cancers.[47]

## Diagnostic criteria

The National Cancer Institute/Working Group[48] and the International Workshop on CLL[49] independently proposed criteria for the diagnosis of CLL. These criteria are summarized in Table 33.4. Nevertheless, CLL can be diagnosed whenever there is an absolute increase in the number of lymphocytes in the blood that are morphologically and immunophenotypically consistent with the diagnosis (i.e. SmIg$^{+/-}$ CD5$^+$, CD 19$^+$, CD20$^+$, CD23$^+$, FMC7$^-$). Bone marrow examination should no longer be considered a necessary diagnostic criterion, although it may provide important information regarding tumor burden and the origin of cytopenias (central vs. peripheral).

Chronic lymphocytic leukemia has been divided into different morphological variants on the basis of the proportion of atypical cells in peripheral blood. The FAB Group distinguished the following types (Table 33.4)[50]:

- *Typical,* in which most lymphocytes are small and mature in appearance, with less than 10% being atypical
- *CLL/prolymphocytoid (CLL/PL),* when the proportion of prolymphocytes (larger lymphocytes with prominent nucleolus) is between 11% and 54%
- *Mixed* form, which is a more vaguely defined variety in which there is a variable proportion of atypical lymphocytes but less than 10% prolymphocytes.

The most recent WHO classification only refers to *typical CLL,* with less than 10% prolymphocytes, and to *CLL with increased prolymphocytes* (CLL/PL), defined as those cases with more than 10% and less than 55% prolymphocytes.[7] In practice, the diagnosis of atypical CLL should not be accepted unless other diagnostic possibilities are carefully discarded.

## Prognosis

The median survival of patients with CLL is about 10 years. Besides patients who have a survival not different from that of the general population, there are others who have a rapidly fatal course. Clinical stages (early vs. advanced), degree of bone marrow infiltration (non-diffuse vs. diffuse histopathological pattern, or <80% vs. >80% lymphocytes in bone marrow aspirate), blood lymphocyte levels (low vs. high), lymphocyte doubling time (>12 months vs. ≤12 months), lymphocyte morphology (typical vs. atypical) and cytogenetic abnormalities [normal karyotype, de(13q) as single anomaly vs. complex abnormalities, del(11q), del(17p)] are good predictors of survival.[51–53] Thymidine kinase, LDH, B2-microglobulin, CD23, CD25, and CD20 serum levels have also been found to be of prognostic value in some studies.[54–58] Overexpression of *MDR-1* and *MDR-3* genes and P-glycoprotein detection on neoplastic cells, as well as mutations of the *p53* tumor suppressor gene, have been correlated with resistance to therapy and poor prognosis.[59] Finally, response to therapy is associated with a better outcome.[60]

Clinical stages have been the most useful prognostic parameters in CLL (Table 33.5; Figure 33.2). They do, however, have some limitations. For example, progressive and indolent forms of the disease are not identified. Moreover, the mechanisms accounting for cytopenias are not taken into consideration, yet there is some indication that patients with cytopenias of immune origin may have a better outcome than those in whom the cytopenia is caused by a massive infil-

---

### Table 33.4 Diagnostic criteria for chronic lymphocytic leukemia[81–85]

1. Absolute lymphocytosis in peripheral blood
   >5 × 10$^9$/L (NCI/Working Group)
   >10 × 10$^9$/L (IWCLL)
2. The majority of lymphocytes should be small and mature in appearance
   Morphological subtypes:
   2.1. *Typical or classic CLL:* <10% atypical lymphocytes
   2.2. *CLL/PL:* prolymphocytes in blood between 11% and 54%
   2.3. *Mixed:* variable proportion of atypical lymphocytes; <10% prolymphocytes
3. Characteristic immunophenotype
   SmIg$^{+/-}$, CD5$^+$, CD19$^+$, CD20$^+$, CD23$^+$, FMC7$^{-/+}$, CD22$^{+/-}$, CD79b$^-$
4. Bone marrow infiltration
   >30% lymphocytes in bone marrow aspirate
   or consistent pattern in bone marrow biopsy

CLL: chronic lymphocytic leukemia; IWCLL: International Workshop for Chronic Lymphocytic Leukemia; NCI: National Cancer Institute; PL: prolymphocytoid

### Table 33.5  Staging systems used for chronic lymphocytic leukemia

| Staging system | Stage | Clinical features | Median survival (years) |
|---|---|---|---|
| **Rai** | | | |
| Low-risk | 0 | Lymphocytosis alone | 14.5 |
| Intermediate-risk | I | Lymphocytosis Lymphadenopathy | |
| | II | Lymphocytosis Spleen or liver enlargement | 7.5 |
| High-risk | III | Lymphocytosis Hemoglobin <11 g/dL | |
| | IV | Lymphocytosis Platelet <100 000/microliter) | 2.5 |
| **Binet** | | | |
| Low-risk | A | No anemia, no thrombocytopenia <3 lymphoid areas* enlarged | 15.5 |
| Intermediate-risk | B | No anemia, no thrombocytopenia ≥3 lymphoid areas enlarged | 5.5 |
| High-risk | C | Hemoglobin <10 g/dL or Platelets <100 000 microliter | 3 |

* The Binet staging system[52] takes into consideration the following lymphoid areas: lymph nodes (whether unilateral or bilateral) in the head and neck, axillae, groin, spleen and liver.

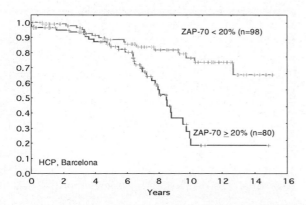

**Figure 33.2** Survival probability of 685 patients with chronic lymphocytic leukemia (CLL) followed up at the Department of Hematology/Postgraduate School of Hematology 'Farreras-Valenti' of Barcelona according to Binet's stages.

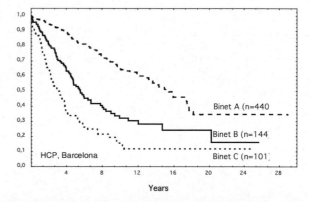

**Figure 33.3** Survival probability of 178 patients with chronic lymphocytic leukemia (CLL) followed up at the Department of Hematology/Postgraduate School of Hematology 'Farreras-Valenti' of Barcelona according to the expression of ZAP-70 on neoplastic lymphocytes as detected by cytofluorometry.

tration of the bone marrow by neoplastic cells.[61] Furthermore, clinical stages are a mere reflection of the biological diversity of the disease. In this regard, the correlation of certain cytogenetic abnormalities, as well as that of the mutational status of $IgV_H$ genes, with the clinical outcome has signified an important progress in the understanding of the natural history of CLL. The mutational status of $IgV_H$ genes separates CLL into two forms with distinct presenting features and outcome. Thus, compared with those who have $IgV_H$ mutations, patients who have unmutated $IgV_H$ genes have a more malignant disease, including evidence of advanced, progressive disease, atypical cell morphology, adverse cytogenetic features, and resistance to therapy.[22,23] Unfortunately, studying $IgV_H$ mutations is not possible on a routine basis. CD38 expression correlates, although not absolutely, with

$IgV_H$ mutations; moreover, CD38 expression may vary over time[62] Recently, it has been demonstrated that ZAP-70 expression, as evaluated by cytofluorometry or polymerase chain reaction (PCR), strongly correlates with $IgV_H$ mutations and has important prognostic significance by itself[63,64] (Figure 33.3).

## Treatment

There is not a curative therapy for CLL, and the impact of the disease on patients' survival is highly variable. Therefore, not all patients with CLL require treatment. Therapy is considered justified when any of the following features is present:

- General symptoms (i.e. weight loss, extreme fatigue, night sweats or fever without evidence of infection)
- Increasing anemia or thrombocytopenia due to bone marrow failure
- Bulky or progressive lymphadenopathy
- Massive or progressive splenomegaly
- Autoimmune cytopenias not responsive to corticosteroids
- Rapidly increasing lymphocyte counts in peripheral blood.

Marked hypogammaglobulinemia or increased WBC counts, in the absence of any of the above criteria, are not sufficient to initiate treatment.[49]

### Treatment approaches

Patients with low-risk disease

Treatment of patients in early stage (Binet A; Rai 0) has resulted in a delay in the rate of disease progression but no survival benefit.[65,66] It should be noted, however, that this notion derives from studies in which the treatment employed was chlorambucil or other alkylating agents. Whether patients with CLL in early stage might gain benefit from early intervention with the newer and more effective therapies is being addressed in clinical trials.

Patients with intermediate- and high-risk disease

A proportion of patients in intermediate stage (Binet B; Rai I and II) have indolent disease; these patients may be followed with no therapy, as for those with low-risk disease. However, the majority of patients with intermediate stage of the disease and virtually all patients with advanced stage (Binet C; Rai III and IV) due to bone marrow infiltration require therapy.

Over the last two decades, chlorambucil has been the treatment of choice. The number of complete responses obtained with chlorambucil is low (10%) and, besides symptoms palliation, it is doubtful that it has any impact on the natural history of the disease. Because of this, chlorambucil is usually given to patients not likely to tolerate more intensive therapies

due to associated comorbidity. Likewise, radiation therapy has a limited role in the treatment of CLL, although it may be useful to treat bulky lymphadenopathy or splenomegaly causing compressive problems in patients not suitable for chemotherapy.[3–6]

Purine analogs, particularly fludarabine, are the most effective agents to treat CLL. Treatment with fludarabine results in a much higher complete remission (CR) rate than chlorambucil or alkylating based chemotherapies (20–40% vs. 10%) and a longer disease-free interval, although survival is not prolonged.[66–69] Fludarabine (given intravenously or orally) is now considered the treatment of choice for most patients with CLL. The efficacy of fludarabine may be improved by combining it with other agents (e.g. cyclophosphamide, mitoxantrone, rituximab).[70–73] There are already data indicating that the combination of fludarabine plus cyclophosphamide not only results in a superior response rate than fludarabine alone but also a longer freedom from progression and, perhaps, a longer survival.[71,72]

The most important side-effects of purine analogs are myelosuppression and infections. Infections due to opportunistic organisms may be observed. This seems to be more frequent in patients receiving corticosteroids and, particularly, in those who have been heavily pretreated.[20,26,74] Although the cause is not clear, the risk of contracting opportunistic infections is attributed in part to the decrease in CD4 lymphocytes caused by purine analogs. Owing to the risk of infection, it is reasonable to employ antibiotic and antiviral prophylaxis (e.g. sulfamethoxazole–trimethoprim, acyclovir) in patients receiving purine analogs. Another side-effect of concern is the triggering of autoimmune hemolytic anemia (AIHA), which in some cases can be fatal.[75,76] Because of this, purine analogs should be avoided in patients with AIHA or a positive Coombs' test.

Anecdotal cases of pulmonary toxicity[77,78] and tumor lysis syndrome[79] have been reported. In addition, several cases of transfusional acute graft-versus-host disease have been described.[80,81] As far as long-term complications are concerned, several reports of myelodysplasia in heavily pretreated patients have been reported.[82,83]

Patients with cytopenias due to an immune mechanism (e.g. stage C (III, IV) immune)

These patients should initially be treated with corticosteroids, with cytotoxic agents added only when there is no response after 2–4 weeks of treatment. In patients with AIHA that is not responding to or is difficult to control with corticosteroids plus cytotoxic agents, high-dose immunoglobulin, cyclosporine, or rituximab may be tried. A proportion of these patients, however, will eventually require splenectomy.[84] Purine analogs should be avoided in patients with AIHA as well in those with a positive Coombs' test. Pure red-cell aplasia (PRCA) may occasionally be associated with CLL; the treatment of choice is cyclosporine; rituximab can also be effective.[3–6,85]

Patients with hypersplenism

In such cases, splenectomy or low-dose radiotherapy over the spleen may be of benefit.

Patients with systemic complications

Hypogammaglobulinemia is frequent in CLL and is the major cause of infections, which are the major cause of death and a significant cause of morbidity. In a number of studies, high and intermediate doses of immunoglobulin have been found to be of some value in preventing infections.[86,87] Cost/benefit considerations, however, make the routine use of immunoglobulin in all patients with hypogammaglobulinemia questionable.[88] Hematopoietic growth factors (i.e. GM-CSF, G-CSF) may overcome treatment-related neutropenia.[89] Finally, erythropoietin may be useful to treat anemia unresponsive to other measures.[90]

Disease transformation

Although the prognosis of such an event is usually poor (median survival <6 months), patients responding to aggressive lymphoma-type chemotherapy may have long survival.

### New treatment approaches

Monoclonal antibodies

Alemtuzumab (Campath-1H) is an anti-CD52 antibody of which antigen is present on most B and T cells. In a number of studies, response rates of about 50% have been reported, with these being higher in peripheral blood and bone marrow than in lymph nodes and spleen. In fact, alemtuzumab has been used in patients who have achieved a good partial response to improve the response and to clear peripheral blood from leukemic cells before autologous transplantation. Interestingly, alemtuzumab has proved to be effective in patients refractory to fludarabine. Toxicity includes rigors, chills, fever, immunosuppression, and lymphocytopenia. Opportunistic infections can be observed. Cytomegalovirus (CMV) reactivation is a problem that deserves monitoring and preemptive therapy.[90–94] Different trials are underway to evaluate the optimal dose, schedule, and route of administration (i.e. subcutaneous vs. intravenous), as well as the combination of alemtuzumab with other agents (e.g. fludarabine, rituximab).

Rituximab is an anti-CD20 antibody. In CLL the amount of CD20 on the surface of neoplastic cells is moderate, this being a possible reason for the low response rate to rituximab when given alone.[90,95] However, rituximab acts synergistically with fludarabine and cyclophosphamide, with impressive preliminary treatment results having been reported.[72,73,91] Patients with high WBC counts (i.e. higher than 50 000/μL) may develop the so-called cytokine-release syndrome characterized by fever, rigors, skin rash, nausea, vomiting, hypotension, and dyspnea, upon rituximab administration.

Stem cell transplants

An increasing number of subjects with CLL are being offered stem cell transplants.[96–100] Autologous transplants do not cure the disease but may prolong survival in selected patients (i.e. sensitive to chemotherapy, without unfavorable prognostic factors, and transplanted early in the course of the disease). In contrast, allogeneic transplants can cure about 40% of the patients, but at the cost of a high toxicity and mortality (25–50%). Because of this, and the advanced age of most patients with CLL, the role of allotransplants with reduced intensity conditioning regimens is being intensively investigated; preliminary results are encouraging, with TRM of 10–20% (at 1 year) and an overall survival of about 60% (at 1 year).[98]

Other treatments

Other more experimental treatments include the protein kinase C inhibitor UCN-O1, the protein kinase C activator bryostatin, the cyclin-dependent kinase inhibitor flavopiridol, the topoisomerase-I inhibitor 9-aminocamptothecin, depsipeptide and bcl-2 antisense oligonucleotides, as well as new monoclonal antibodies (e.g. anti-CD23, anti-HLA-DR).[3–6]

# B-cell prolymphocytic leukemia

Prolymphocytic leukemia (PL) was described by Galton et al in 1974 as an entity that should be separated from CLL and other forms of leukemia.[101] This is an extremely infrequent disease (less than 1% of all leukemias), characterized by a high WBC count and the presence in peripheral blood of a high number of large lymphocytes with prominent nucleolus (prolymphocytes). Clinically, the most frequent feature is a huge splenomegaly. The disease predominates in males, and its prognosis is poor. Although recognized in the WHO classification as an entity on its own, it is extremely likely that many cases of B-cell PL, as diagnosed in the past, actually corresponded to other diseases such as mantle-cell lymphoma with leukemic expression.

## Biology

The normal counterpart of prolymphocyte has not been fully identified. The presence of mutated $IgV_H$ genes in a proportion of cases suggests that, at least in some cases, prolymphocytes are post-germinal cells that have undergone antigen-driven selection.[102] The neoplastic cells of B-cell PL express strong SmIg (as opposed to CLL, in which SmIg is weak) and pan-B-cell markers (e.g. CD19, CD20); they are usually negative for CD11c and CD23, variably positive for CD5, and may show weak expression of CD10. In contrast to the small lymphocytes of CLL, prolymphocytes express FMC7 and CD22.

A marker chromosome 14q+, which has a breakpoint at 14q32, the locus for the IgV$_H$ gene, is found in two-thirds of patients. The translocations involving chromosome 14 are not always well defined, although the most frequent is t(11;14)(q13;q32). Most cases of B-cell PL with t(11;14), however, are likely to represent mantle-cell lymphoma with leukemic expression.[103] In half of the cases, *p53* mutations are observed.

### Clinical features

The median age of patients at diagnosis is about 70 years, and males predominate over females (4:1). The diagnosis is often made because of the discomfort caused by a massive splenomegaly. In all cases, the WBC is high and usually exceeds 100 000/µL. Anemia and thrombocytopenia may be observed in up to 30% of patients. The majority of them (90%) have splenomegaly that can be of huge size. Lymphadenopathy is rare or absent.

### Diagnosis

A marked increase in WBC count is a constant feature of the disease. The diagnosis is based on the finding of a large proportion of prolymphocytes in the peripheral blood. Morphologically, prolymphocytes are usually larger than the small lymphocytes of CLL, and also have a more abundant cytoplasm with moderate basophilia; the nucleus is round with a clumped chromatin pattern, and the presence of a prominent vesicular nucleolus is a prominent feature (Figure 33.4). Conventionally, more than 55% of prolymphocytes

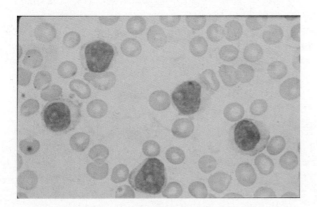

**Figure 33.4** B-cell prolymphocytic leukemia (peripheral blood).

are required to make the diagnosis, although in most instances the percentage is 70–80%. B-cell PL must be differentiated from CLL with 'prolymphocytoid' transformation, as well as the so-called CLL/PL, in which patients with CLL have a variable proportion (<55%) of prolymphocytes in the peripheral blood at diagnosis; CLL/PL is closer to CLL than to PL.[104] The disease should also be differentiated from marginal zone lymphoma with leukemic expression (splenic lymphoma with villous lymphocytes). Finally, cases of B-cell PL with t(11;14) constitute a confusing area since most of these cases actually correspond to mantle-cell lymphoma.[103] The immunophenotype of B-cell PL is shown in Table 33.2.

### Prognosis

The prognosis is poor, with a median survival of approximately two years. There are patients, however, in which the disease has a more benign, smoldering course.

### Treatment

Patients with B-cell PL are usually refractory to treatment. Splenectomy may be useful to control the disease for variable periods of time. Fludarabine alone or associated to other agents (e.g. cyclophosphamide) may produce a significant number of responses. Alemtuzumab has been shown to be highly effective in T-cell PL, the experience in B-cell PL being less. In younger patients with aggressive disease, stem cell transplantation should be considered.

## Hairy-cell leukemia

Hairy-cell leukemia (HCL) was first recognized by Bouroncle et al in 1958, and given the name 'leukemic reticuloendotheliosis'.[105] The disease was rediscovered in the 1970s, and was called hairy-cell leukemia because of the 'hairy' aspect of the cells that proliferate in this disease. It is an infrequent disease, accounting for only 2–4% of all leukemias, in which hairy-cells infiltrate the bone marrow and the spleen.

### Biology

In most cases, HCL has its origin in mature, memory B cells. However, on rare instances cases displaying T-cell markers have been reported. The cyclin D1 gene is overexpressed at mRNA and protein levels in a high proportion of patients. Nonetheless, the levels of expression are much lower than in mantle-cell lymphomas, and this overexpression is not associated with *BCL1* rearrangements or *CCND1* gene amplification.[106] The growth of malignant cells is regulated by cytokines (e.g. tumor necrosis factor (TNF)-α, interleukin (IL)-2, IL-4 and IL-6, and B-cell growth factor

(BCGF)), probably through both autocrine and paracrine pathways.[107] Cytogenetically, trisomy 5, structural abnormalities involving the pericentromeric regions of chromosomes 5 and 2, and 1q42 abnormalities have been reported.[108]

### Clinical features

The median age of patients at diagnosis is about 60 years. The disease clearly predominates in males (5:1). The majority of patients manifest symptoms secondary to severe pancytopenia (i.e. bacterial infections, bleeding) and weakness. Sometimes, HCL presents with opportunistic infections secondary to the severe cellular immunodeficiency and monocytopenia. It is not unusual, however, to diagnose HCL in asymptomatic patients undergoing routine laboratory examinations. Splenomegaly is found in 80% of cases. In rare instances, HCL may present with osseous involvement, vasculitis, nephrotic syndrome, and arthritis.[109,110] Although peripheral lymphadenopathy is not observed, a proportion of cases present with or develop abdominal lymph adenopathy, a feature that has been associated with a poor response to therapy.[111]

### Diagnosis

Laboratory features frequently seen in HCL include anemia, neutropenia, and thrombocytopenia. Monocytopenia is a constant feature. Other laboratory features include elevation of the leukocyte alkaline phosphatase (LAP) level and high mean corpuscular volume (MCV) (>100 fL) of erythrocytes. Hypergammaglobulinemia and moderate abnormalities of the liver enzymes may also be observed. In some cases, monoclonal M components can be found.[109,110]

In most cases (but not in all), a variable proportion of hairy cells are present in the peripheral blood (Figure 33.5). Almost always, hairy cells display tartrate-resistant alkaline phosphatase (TRAP) activity, but this finding is not specific for HCL. Immuno-

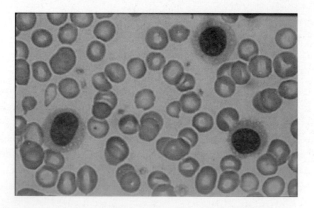

**Figure 33.5** Hairy-cell leukemia (peripheral blood).

phenotypically, hairy cells have SmIg and are positive for pan-B-cell markers (e.g. CD19, CD20 and CD22); the most characteristic markers of HCL are positivity for CD11c, CD103, CD25 and Annexin A1 (ANXA1), this latter being highly specific.[112] (See Table 33.2).

Frequently, the bone marrow cannot be aspirated ('dry tap'). Therefore, a bone marrow biopsy is important to establish the diagnosis. Usually, the bone marrow is hypercellular. A patchy infiltration by hairy cells and a significant increase in reticulin fibers (which explains the difficulties in performing bone marrow aspiration) are the most characteristic features. However, some cases with hypocellular bone marrow, posing the differential diagnosis with aplastic anemia, have been reported. In these cases, immunohistochemical studies can be of great help in making the diagnosis. The spleen is also infiltrated. The fact that the red pulp of the spleen is primarily involved may be of help in differentiating HCL from other lymphoproliferative disorders that basically involve the white pulp of the spleen (e.g. splenic lymphoma with villous lymphocytes).[109,110]

In the so-called HCL variant, there are a number of distinctive features separating it from classical HCL.[113] The morphology of the leukemic cells is intermediate between those of hairy cells and prolymphocytes, with abundant basophilic cytoplasm with villous projections, and a centrally located nucleus with a prominent nucleolus. The cells are acid-phosphatase positive, but, in contrast to classical HCL, they are tartrate-sensitive. The immunophenotype is intermediate between those of HCL, PL, and splenic lymphoma with villous lymphocytes. CD25 and HC2 are usually negative. Moreover, the WBC is high and neither monocytopenia nor neutropenia are present; LAP and MCV are normal. HCL variant is resistant to treatment.

### Prognosis

The prognosis of HCL has improved over the last decade as a result of its earlier diagnosis and better treatments. The 4-year survival from diagnosis is currently about 80%, as compared with 60% in patients diagnosed in the 1970s. In most studies, anemia, increased WBC counts, and degree of spleen enlargement predict survival.[109,110]

### Treatment

Not all patients with HCL need treatment. About 10% have an indolent or totally asymptomatic disease, and may be followed with no therapy until progression is observed. The criteria for giving treatment include[109]:

- Anemia (Hb <10 g/dL)
- Neutropenia (granulocyte count <1000/μL)
- Thrombocytopenia (platelets <100 000/μL)

- Symptomatic splenomegaly
- Recurrent infections
- Extralymphatic disease
- Autoimmune complications
- Presentation in the leukemic phase of the disease

Treatments for HCL have increased in the last few years.[114,115] Splenectomy and interferon alfa-2a (IFN-$\alpha_{2a}$), which have been standard treatments for HCL, are being replaced by cladribine (2-chlorodes-oxyadenosine) and pentostatin (2'-deoxycoformycin). Nevertheless there is still place for surgery in some patients with massive spleen enlargement. In patients requiring treatment, complete responses are obtained in 75–85% of cases treated with cladribine and in 33–89% of patients receiving pentostatin.[116,118]

In a randomized study in which pentostatin was compared with IFN-$\alpha_{2a}$, in untreated patients, response rates were significantly higher with pentostatin than IFN-$\alpha_{2a}$ (79% vs. 38%; $p$ <0.001); relapse-free survival was also longer in those patients treated with pentostatin ($p$ <0.001). Hemoglobin level, young age, and no or small splenomegaly were associated with response achievement.[118] Cladribine given in 2-hour infusion or subcutaneously seems to be as effective as when given by continuous infusion.[119] Nevertheless, even in cases in which CR is achieved according to conventional clinical and hematological criteria, residual disease may be often identified in bone marrow by means of immunohistochemical studies.[120]

# Non-Hodgkin lymphomas with leukemic expression

Non-Hodgkin lymphomas differ from chronic lymphoid leukemias in that the primary site of the disease is usually the lymph nodes and other lymphoid tissues rather than the bone marrow and peripheral blood. Although all the lymphomas have the potential for spreading to bone marrow and peripheral blood, there are a number of them in which this is a relatively frequent event[121–123] (see also Chapter 31 on non-Hodgkin lymphomas).

# Splenic lymphoma with villous lymphocytes/marginal zone lymphoma of the spleen

Splenic lymphoma with villous lymphocytes (SLVL) and marginal zone lymphoma of the spleen are considered equivalent terms. SLVL presents with a variable number of circulating 'villous' lymphocytes in the peripheral blood, which also infiltrate the bone marrow and the spleen, and usually has a benign clinical course.[124–126]

## Biology

Tumor cells have surface IgM and IgD and are CD20$^+$ and CD79b$^+$. CD5, CD10, CD23, CD43, Bcl-6 and Cyclin D1 are typically absent. Immunoglobulin heavy and light changes are rearranged and somatic mutations can be observed in about half of the cases. In addition, intraclonal variation has been observed, suggesting ongoing mutations. Allelic loss of chromosome 7q31-32 has been reported in up to 40% of the patients. Cases with 7q loss tend to show a more aggressive behavior, with more frequent tumoral progression.[127] Deletion of 17p has been observed in approximately 10% of the cases. Cases associated to hepatitis C virus have been described, particularly in Italy.[126]

## Clinical features

At diagnosis, the majority of patients are elderly (median 70 years), and usually present with massive splenic enlargement; lymphadenopathy is absent or limited to the splenic hilar lymph nodes. In many cases, the diagnosis is made on the occasion of a routine medical examination. The lymphocyte count is usually only moderately elevated (10 000–30 000/μL). Other features at diagnosis can be anemia and thrombocytopenia (in less than 20% of the patients), as well as monoclonal gammopathy (particularly of the IgM type), which can be found in up to 30% of cases. Autoimmune hemolytic anemia and immune thrombocytopenia may be also observed. Disease transformation into aggressive lymphoma occurs in 10% of cases.[124–126]

## Diagnosis

The diagnosis is usually made in the course of routine laboratory studies or when investigating a splenomegaly causing compressive problems. The WBC count rarely exceeds 30 000/μL. The proportion of villous lymphocytes (Figure 33.6) is variable.

In terms of differential diagnosis, the negativity of CD5 is useful in excluding chronic lymphocytic leukemia, absence of CD103 in ruling out hairy cell leukemia, and absence of CD10 in excluding follicular lymphoma. Sometimes, the diagnosis is eventually made after splenectomy. In contrast to HCL, in SLVL the white pulp rather than the red pulp is involved.[127]

## Prognosis

Median survival of patients with SLVL is around 10 years, and 5-year overall survival is about 80%. In many cases the disease runs an indolent clinical course. Increasing age, anemia, thrombocytopenia, high WBC count (i.e. >15 000/μL), autoimmune hemolytic anemia, serum M component, high beta-2

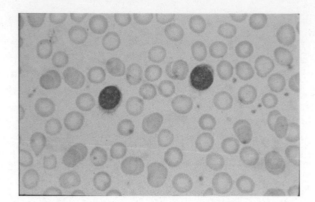

**Figure 33.6** Splenic lymphoma with villous lymphocytes (peripheral blood).

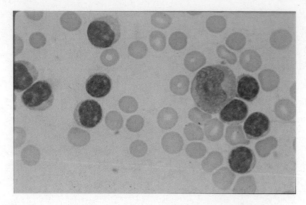

**Figure 33.7** Follicular lymphoma in leukemic phase (peripheral blood).

microglobulin serum levels and p53 overexpression by neoplastic cells have been associated with a poorer outcome.[128,129]

### Treatment

Asymptomatic patients do not require treatment. Splenectomy may be useful not only to confirm the diagnosis but also to correct the anemia or thrombocytopenia caused by hypersplenism. Fludarabine can be useful in patients requiring systemic chemotherapy. In cases of SLVL associated to hepatitis C virus, interferon alone or associated to ribavirin may induce the regression of the disease.[130]

## Follicular lymphomas

A significant proportion of patients with follicular (centroblastic/centrocytic) lymphomas present with circulating lymphoma cells in the peripheral blood at diagnosis, and others develop a leukemic phase during the course of the disease. Overall, 10–30% of patients, depending on the series analyzed, show circulating neoplastic cells either at diagnosis or during the disease evolution. The proportion is higher if peripheral blood involvement is assessed by cytofluorometry or PCR, but the clinical significance of this latter finding is unsettled.

Bone marrow infiltration is present in a large number of patients (40–60%), frequently in the form of aggregates or nodules in paratrabecular position.

The lymphocyte count varies from moderately increased to very high levels. The cytological features of the atypical cells may also vary. There are cases in which most cells are small and cleaved cells (centrocytes) (Figure 33.7), whereas in others a mixture of small and large cells (centroblasts) is observed. Immunophenotypically, these cells usually express CD10, pan-B-cell antigens (e.g. CD19, CD20, CD22),

and in most cases are CD5⁻ and CD43⁻ (see Table 33.2).[121–123] These cells can display the t(14;18) and express *BCL2*. Whereas the presence of atypical cells in peripheral blood has no prognostic significance by itself, the proportion of large circulating cells does correlate with poor prognosis; this is most likely due to the fact that large cells in blood indicate disease transformation.

## Lymphoplasmacytic lymphoma/Waldenström's macroglobulinemia

Lymphoplasmacytic lymphoma/Waldenström's macroglobulinemia (LPL/WM) is a rare disorder (1.5% of lymphomas) characterized by a monoclonal lymphoplasmacytic proliferation accompanied by a serum monoclonal IgM. It is a disease of the elderly, the median age of patients at diagnosis being 65.[131] In the WHO classification LPL and WM are considered equivalent diseases, although not all patients with LPL present with the classical syndrome described by Jan G Waldenström in 1944, consisting of anemia, lymphadenopathy, epistaxis, and hypergammaglobulinemia.

### Biology

The disease has its origin in post-germinal center B cells that have undergone somatic mutations. Immunophenotypically, besides markers present in other B-cell lymphomas, some antigens typical of plasma cells (e.g. CD38 and CD71) may be observed. Intracytoplasmic immunoglobulin (cIg) is also present. Other typical markers include IgM⁺, IgD⁻, CD19⁺, CD20⁺, CD5⁻, CD10⁻, and CD23⁻. No specific cytogenetic features or molecular abnormalities have been identified, although del(6q) can be detected in about 50% of the patients.[132] Expression of PAX50 due to t(9;14)(p13;q32) has been reported in about 50% of lymphoplasmacytic lymphomas, although it seems to be restricted to cases without a serum monoclonal protein.[133]

## Clinical features

Clinical features are variable. Some patients are asymptomatic, whereas others present with constitutional symptoms, lymphadenopathy, splenomegaly, and hematologic abnormalities. The IgM paraprotein may cause hyperviscosity syndrome (i.e. mucosal hemorrhage, visual disturbances, headache, vertigo, somnolence), although this is only observed in 15% of patients. The physical characteristics of the IgM paraprotein may result in cryoglobulinemia, although most cases of type II mixed cryoglobulinemia are associated with hepatitis C infection, even in patients with LPL/WM. The IgM paraprotein may also function as an autoantibody and may produce cold-agglutinin hemolysis, autoimmune thrombocytopenia, acquired von Willebrand's disease or polyneuropathy. The WBC count is usually only moderately increased, and the proportion of atypical cells is variable (30–50%). The most usual phenotype is CD5-, CD10-, CD43+/-, CD19+, CD20+, CD22+, CD79b+/- (see Table 33.2).[84] Progression into aggressive lymphoma (e.g. immunoblastic) may be observed. Light-chain associated amyloidosis may also occur.[131]

## Diagnosis

In patients with a classical presentation, evidence of mature lymphocytosis, or plasmacytoid cells in bone marrow, peripheral blood (Figure 33.8), and a serum monoclonal IgM protein, diagnosis is straightforward. There is no agreement on the minimum protein concentration needed for diagnosis, although it is usually >30 g/L. in cases of typical WM. The diagnosis can be complicated by the fact that a serum monoclonal IgM protein can be observed in diseases other than LPL/WM, such as monoclonal gammopathy of unknown significance, multiple myeloma, marginal zone lymphoma, and CLL.

## Prognosis

The median overall survival is around 6 years, although it may vary among series depending on the diagnostic criteria employed. The individual prognosis is highly variable. Unfavorable prognostic factors include advancing age, cytopenia, low albumin, and increased serum beta-2 microglobulin. Several prognostic systems have been proposed. Morel et al associated an increased risk with: patients who are 65 years or older, albumin <40 g/L, and cytopenia (hemoglobin <120 g/L, platelet count <150 000/μL, WBC count <4000/μL (with 1 cytopenia given 1 point and 2

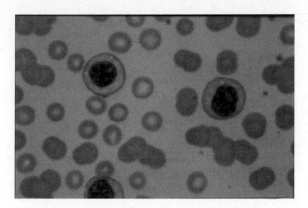

**Figure 33.8** Lymphoplasmacytic lymphoma with leukemic expression (peripheral blood).

or 3 cytopenias given 2 points). Patients were divided into low-risk (0 or 1 point and 87% 5-year survival), intermediate-risk (2 points and 62% 5-year survival), and high-risk (3 or 4 points and 25% 5-year survival).[134]

Dhodapkar et al proposed a prognostic model based on 3 factors: serum beta-2 microglobulin, hemoglobin, and serum IgM concentration. Patients with low beta-2 microglobulin had the best 5-year survival (87% if hemoglobin was 120 g/L and 64% if hemoglobin was <120 g/L). Patients with a high beta-2 microglobulin level had the worst 5-year survival; 53% if they had an IgM ≤40 000 mg/L and 22% if the IgM was >40 000 mg/L.[135]

## Treatment

Since LPL/WM is incurable, patients without symptoms should be only monitored, and treatment given only in case of disease progression. The basis for LPL/WM treatment consists of: plasmapheresis to treat the hyperviscosity syndrome, alkylating agents, purine analogs, and rituximab.

Alkylating agents convey the risk of myelodysplasia and because of this should be avoided, particularly in younger patients. Purine analogs (i.e. fludarabine, cladribine) are highly effective, although responses can be delayed. Rituximab is also useful. In patients receiving rituximab, however, IgM may increase during the first months of therapy to decrease thereafter, a fact of which treating physicians should be aware. The possibility of combining purine analogs with other agents (e.g. cyclophosphamide, rituximab) is appealing. Autologous stem-cell transplants may be considered in younger patients failing to respond to initial therapy; at present, allogeneic stem cell transplantation is considered an experimental procedure in LPL/WM.

# Mantle-cell lymphomas in leukemic phase

Mantle-cell lymphomas (MCL) are neoplasias that arise in the mantle zone of lymph nodes and that account for 5–10% of all lymphomas. In 40–80% of the cases, neoplastic cells from MCL involve the bone marrow and peripheral blood.[136]

## Biology

The t(11;14)(q13;q32), with overexpression of the *cyclin D1 gene*, is a highly characteristic feature of MCL.[137] Mutations of *p53* and deletions of the cyclin-dependent kinase inhibitors *p21^{Waf1}* and *p16^{INK4a}* have been associated with atypical morphology and poor outcome.[138,139] In about one-third of the patients $V_H$ genes are mutated. Immunophenotypically, MCL is CD5[+], a marker also found in CLL. In contrast to CLL, however, SmIg expression is strong and in most instances MCL lymphocytes do not express CD23 and can be FMC7[+] (see Table 33.2).

## Clinical features

Mantle-cell lymphomas usually affect older males. Although a prominent splenomegaly is the most relevant feature, extranodal involvement is also common. In 40–80% of the eases, MCL involves the bone marrow and the peripheral blood, with this leading to a leukemic picture (MCL 'leukemia'), which may be confounded with CLL and other lymphomas in leukemic phase.[140]

## Diagnosis

The neoplastic cells characteristic of MCL are small to medium-sized, have an irregular, slightly indented or cleaved nucleus (Figure 33.9). Three morphological varieties are recognized: typical, small-cell, and blastoid. In the blastoid variant, the lymphocytes are larger and highly atypical. Although MCL in leukemic phase may be suspected from the examination of peripheral blood films, immunophenotyping, as well as cytogenetic and molecular studies, are necessary to confirm the diagnosis (see Table 33.2).

## Prognosis

Mantle-cell lymphoma has a poor prognosis, with a median survival of 3–5 years. Blastic forms have a worse prognosis than the others. As mentioned above, mutations of p53 and deletions of *p21^{Waf1}* and *p16^{INK4a}* have been associated with atypical morphology and poor outcome.[138,139] Patients with mutated $V_H$ genes may have a relatively better prognosis than those with unmutated $V_H$ genes.[141] Leukemic expression has also been associated with a poor prognosis. Well-recognized prognostic factors for lymphoma patients (e.g.,

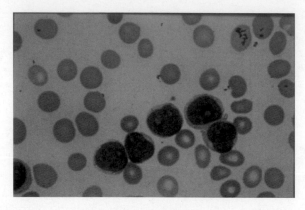

**Figure 33.9** Mantle-cell lymphoma (blastic variant) with leukemic expression (peripheral blood).

serum LDH and the International Prognostic Index) also apply to this disease.

## Treatment

Mantle-cell lymphoma is refractory to standard lymphoma regimens. Chemoimmunotherapy (e.g. rituximab + CHOP; rituximab + FCM [fludarabine, cyclophosphamide, mitoxantrone]) offers the highest possibility of achieving a response, although most patients eventually relapse.[142] Autologous transplantation may prolong survival but does not cure the disease. Allogeneic transplantation has been effective in some cases, and deserves further investigation.[143] Encouraging results have been reported with allotransplants with reduced intensity conditioning regimens.[144]

# T-cell prolymphocytic leukemia

T-cell prolymphocytic leukemia (T-cell PL) is one of the most frequent form of T-cell chronic lymphoproliferative disorder leukemic expression. This is a disease of adult people and predominates in males.

## Biology

The neoplastic cells are TdT(-) and express pan-T-cell antigens (e.g. CD2, CD3, and CD5). CD7 is expressed in over 90% of patients. In approximately 70% of cases, the prolymphocytes express a helper-cell phenotype (CD4[+], CD8[-]). The most consistent cytogenetic abnormality involves chromosome 14, usually inv(14) with breakpoints at q11 (the locus for T-cell a and b receptors) and q32, this leading to the overexpression of the *CTL-1* gene. Trisomy 8 is observed in half of the cases. Deletions of chromosome 11, namely del(11q), where the ataxia telangiectasia gene (*ATM*) is located, are found in a high proportion of patients. Finally, serology for HTLV-I is negative.[145–147]

## Clinical features

The majority of the patients have constitutional symptoms and abdominal discomfort caused by a large spleen. In contrast to B-cell PL, lymphadenopathy and hepatomegaly may be present. Skin involvement is not rare. In the advanced phases of the disease pleural effusion, ascites, and CNS involvement may be observed. The WBC is high, with counts above 100 000 not being infrequent. Anemia and thrombocytopenia may be found in 30% of the patients.

## Diagnosis

From the morphological point of view, a mixture of small and large atypical cells can be observed. The nuclei are regular or oval in half of the cases, and irregular with convolutions and folds in the other half. The cytoplasm shows protrusions or blebs. T prolymphocytes stain strongly with α-naphthyl acetate esterase. Under electron microscopy, the most important feature of the prolymphocyte is the presence of a large, centrally placed nucleolus, which is usually surrounded by a halo of heterochromatin. This can be useful to identify prolymphocytes of small size not easily identifiable by light microscopy. The immunophenotype of T-cell PL is shown in Table 33.3.

## Prognosis

The prognosis is poor, the median survival being around 6 months.

## Treatment

Alemtuzumab is the most effective single agent to treat T-cell PL.[148] Fludarabine-based therapies (e.g. fludarabine, cyclophosphamide, prednisone) followed by alemtuzumab have given promising results. Pentostatin can be also of benefit.[149] In younger patients, bone marrow transplantation should be considered.

# Lymphoproliferative diseases of granular lymphocytes

Lymphoproliferative diseases of granular lymphocytes (LDGL), also known as large granular lymphocyte leukemias (LGL), are a heterogeneous group of disorders that result from the chronic proliferation of large granular lymphocytes. Formerly, these diseases had been known by terms such as chronic T-cell lymphocytosis with neutropenia, T8 chronic lymphocytic leukemia, and T-suppressor cell CLL, among others. The term 'lymphoproliferative diseases of granular lymphocytes' is better, since in most cases these disorders are not malignant, truly leukemic conditions. These diseases account for less than 5% of all chronic lymphoproliferative disorders and predominate in the adulthood.[150–153]

## Biology

Lymphoproliferative diseases of granular lymphocytes may have either a CD3+ (T-cell) or a CD3− (NK-cell) phenotype. The etiology of LDGL is unknown, although in some cases the Epstein–Barr virus might be implicated.[154] Also, a higher frequency of the DR4 haplotype has been claimed in some studies, indicating some genetic predisposition.[153]

## Clinical features

The median age of patients at diagnosis is 60 years. The clinical presentation of T-cell LDGL is quite different from that of NK-cell LDGL.

T-cell LDGL, which accounts for up to 80% of cases of LDGL, has a chronic course with symptoms primarily resulting from the neutropenia, which can be severe. Recurrent bacterial infections (primarily involving skin, sinuses, and perirectal areas) are common. In addition, rheumatoid arthritis, as well as a number of serological abnormalities (e.g. hyper- or, more rarely, hypo-gammaglobulinemia, circulating immune complexes, positive tests for rheumatoid factor, antinuclear antibodies, antineutrophil antibodies, and antiplatelet antibodies), occur very frequently in T-cell LDGL. Pure red-cell aplasia and autoimmune (Coombs-positive) hemolytic anemia may be also encountered.[154] The course of the disease is stable or slowly progressive; few patients present with widespread disease and transformation into large cell lymphoma is exceedingly rare.

In about half of the patients, an enlarged spleen is found. Other less frequent features are hepatomegaly (about one-third of patients) and lymphadenopathy (less than 20% of cases); skin involvement is observed in less than 5% of patients.

In contrast, NK-cell LDGL usually presents as a disseminated disease, with fever without evidence of infection, night sweats, weight loss, and a rapid and aggressive clinical course.

## Diagnosis

Currently, two different forms of LDGL are recognized (see Table 33.3):

- *T-cell LDGL*, in which the most frequent phenotype is CD3+, CD8+' TIA-1+, CD4− with rearrangement of the T-cell receptor β (TCRβ) and, more rarely, T-cell receptor γ (TCRγ).
- *NK-cell LDGL* with the phenotype CD3−, CD4−, CD8−, CD16+, CD11b+ CD56+, CD57− (this entity is considered an aggressive leukemia).

Among the laboratory findings, the presence of granular lymphocytes in peripheral blood is the hallmark of the disease (Figure 33.10). In addition, severe neutropenia is frequent, and anemia and thrombocytopenia may also be observed. Bone marrow shows infiltration by atypical lymphocytes in about 80% of cases, although it is usually barely detectable or moderate. In some instances hypoplasia or the erythroid precursors, as well as 'maturation arrest' of myeloid precursors, may be found.

The existence of a granular lymphocytosis greater than 5000/μL lasting for more than 6 months in the peripheral blood has been considered as diagnostic criterion. However, there are cases in which the diagnosis can be established in patients presenting with a lower level of granular lymphocytes, provided that other important diagnostic criteria (i.e. cytogenetic and molecular analysis), as well as the clonality of the population, are demonstrated.[156] The latter is particularly difficult in CD3$^-$ cases (NK-cell LDGL) owing to the lack of clonal markers; these cells do not rearrange TCRα, -γ or -δ genes. Cytogenetic abnormalities, if present, can be useful to demonstrate clonality. Among the monoclonal antibodies used to make the diagnosis, positivity of CD16 plays a central role. Since the CD3$^+$/CD16$^+$ subset accounts for less than 5% of normal cells in healthy subjects, the increase in that population is highly suggestive of CD3$^+$ LDGL. Nevertheless, the differential diagnosis between LDGL (particularly those that are CD3$^-$) and lymphocytosis reactive to infections, autoimmune disorders, or other clinical situations may be extremely difficult.

### Treatment

Patients with T-cell LDGL may run a chronic course for years, not needing therapy or only requiring treatment because of recurrent infections or severe anemia. Treatment is indicated in patients with severe neutropenia leading to recurrent bacterial infections.

Corticosteroids, followed by oral cyclophosphamide in steroid-refractory or steroid-dependent cases,

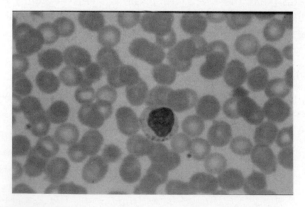

**Figure 33.10** Large granular lymphocyte in peripheral blood.

result in an overall response rate of approximately 70%. In patients not responding to these measures, cyclosporine A or G-CSF can be effective.[157,158]

In contrast to the good prognosis of patients with T-cell LDGL, those with NK-cell LDGL usually die of disseminated disease within a few months of presentation, and this must be treated as an aggressive leukemia, including stem-cell transplantation whenever possible.

# Sézary syndrome

Cutaneous T-cell lymphomas (CTCL) have a wide spectrum of presenting and evolving forms. Mycosis fungoides is an indolent lymphoma that primarily involves the skin in early stages of the disease. Nevertheless, after a variable period of time, it may progress and involve visceral sites and lymph nodes. Sézary syndrome, an entity described in 1938, is an erythrodermic variant of CTCL associated with the presence of circulating tumor cells in the peripheral blood.[159] Primary CTCL should be distinguished from other peripheral T-cell lymphomas that may involve the skin.[160–162]

### Biology

The similarities between the skin lesions of mycosis fungoides and Sézary syndrome and those of adult T-cell leukemia–lymphoma has led to the consideration of a possible etiological role for a retrovirus (e.g. HTLVI/II); human herpes viruses (e.g. herpes simplex virus) have also been implicated, although with inconclusive results.[160–162]

### Clinical features

Sézary syndrome is mainly seen in elderly patients, with a median age at diagnosis of 65 years, and is more common in males. The disease may present either de novo or as part of the evolution of mycosis fungoides. The major cutaneous manifestation of Sézary syndrome is a generalized pruritic erythrodermia. Other features include edema, lymphadenopathy, hepatomegaly, alopecia, ectropion, onychodystrophy and palmar–plantar keratoderma. Characteristically, circulating Sézary cells are found. Sézary cells may be infrequent or very numerous. The neoplastic cells may all be small or may be a mixture of small and large cells. Cells have a highly infolded, complex nuclear form that is usually described as cerebriform or convoluted (see Figure 33.10). Cytogenetic studies show multiple chromosome abnormalities.

### Diagnosis

The coexistence of cutaneous lesions, characterized histologically by the presence of atypical lymphocytes in the epidermis, either singly in lacune or more definitively in clusters (Darier–Pautrier microabscesses), and Sézary cells in the blood (Figure 33.11) are essential requirements to make the diagnosis of Sézary syndrome. Nevertheless, in the early phases of the disease, CTCL may be difficult to differentiate from chronic inflammatory dermatoses. In turn, Sézary cells may be difficult to identify and to differentiate from reactive lymphocytes. Cytogenetic analysis and demonstration of aneuploidy by flow-cytometric quantification of DNA are useful for detecting peripheral blood involvement in CTCL. Ultrastructural studies are useful to define precisely the morphology of neoplastic cells. Immunophenotypically, Sézary cells express several T markers, particularly CD2, CD3, CD5 and, less consistently, CD7. The most common phenotype is CD4+, CD8− (see Table 33.3).

## Prognosis

The prognosis of patients with Sézary syndrome is variable. Kim et al identified a number of prognostic factors in mycosis fungoides/Sézary syndrome[163]: age at presentation of 65 years or more, T classification, and presence of extracutaneous disease. Survival may range from less than 2 years (in patients with disseminated disease) to more than 10 years (in those with localized disease).

## Treatment

Treatment of CTCL depends on whether the disease is limited to the skin or whether there is systemic involvement.[161,164,165] Several types of therapy including radiotherapy and phototherapy (e.g. PUVA, psoralen followed by UVA irradiation), as well as extracorporeal photochemotherapy, may be effective to improve the skin lesions. However, patients with advanced disease such as those with Sézary syndrome require systemic chemotherapy such as that used in aggressive lymphomas. Interferon alfa-a2, pentostatin, cladribine, and alemtuzumab may be useful. Unfortunately, however, responses are usually partial and transient.

# Adult T-cell leukemia–lymphoma

Adult T-cell leukemia–lymphoma (ATLL) was recognized in 1977 as a new clinicopathological entity.[166,167] In 1980, the etiological relationship between the human T-cell leukemia virus I (HTLV-I) and ATLL was established.[168] Adult T-cell leukemia–lymphoma is endemic in Japan, the Caribbean basin, Africa, South America, and the South Eastern USA. It is increasingly seen in Europe among the population originating from Afro-Caribbean areas, and also, although sporadically, in Caucasians.[169,170] Besides rapidly evolving forms, there are others that run a more indolent, chronic course. Treatment has to be individualized based on the risk of each patient.[171] This disorder is discussed in detail in Chapter 13.

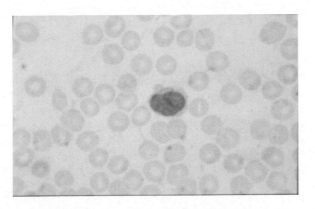

**Figure 33.11** Sézary cell in peripheral blood.

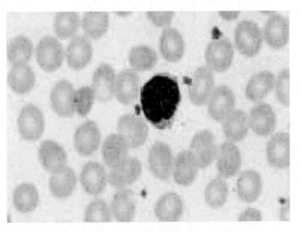

**Figure 33.12** Adult T-cell leukemia–lymphoma (peripheral blood).

## REFERENCES

1. Galton DAG. The pathogenesis of chronic lymphocytic leukemia. *Can Med Assoc J* 1966; **94**: 1005–10.
2. Dameshek W. Chronic lymphocytic leukemia: an accumulative disease of immunologically incompetent lymphocytes. *Blood* 1967; **29**: 566–84.
3. Rozman C, Montserrat E. Chronic lymphocytic leukemia. *N Engl J Med* 1995; **333**: 1052–57.
4. Montserrat E, Bosch F, Rozman C. Chronic lymphocytic leukemia: recent progress in biology, diagnosis, and therapy. *Ann Oncol* 1997; **8**: (Suppl 1): 93–101.

5. Kipps TJ. Chronic lymphocytic leukemia. *Curr Opin Hematol* 2000; **7**: 223–34.

6. Keating MJ, Chiorazzi N, Messmer B et al. Biology and treatment of chronic lymphocytic leukemia. *Hematology* 2003 (American Society of Hematology Education Program Book): 153–75.

7. Jaffe ES, Harris NL, Stein H et al. *Tumours of Haematopoietic and Lymphoid Tissues.* Lyon: IARC Press, 2001.

8. Nishiyarna H, Mokuno J, lnoue T. Relative frequency and mortality rate of various types of leukemia in Japan. *Jap J Cancer Res* 1969; **60**: 71–81.

9. Finch SC, Linet MS. Chronic leukaemias. *Bailliere's Clin Haematol* 1992; **5**: 27–56.

10. Cuttner J. Increased incidence of hematologic malignancies in first-degree relatives of patients with chronic lymphocytic leukemia. *Cancer Invest* 1992; **10**: 103–9.

11. Goldin LR, Sgambati M, Marti GE et al. Anticipation in familial chronic lymphocytic leukemia. *Am J Hum Genet.* 1999 **65**: 265–69.

12. Rawstron C, Yuille R, Fuller R et al. Inherited predisposition to CLL is detectable as sub-clinical monoclonal B-lymphocyte expansion. *Blood* 2002; **100**: 2289–90.

13. Rawstron AC, Green MJ, Kuzmicki A et al. Monoclonal B lymphocytes with the characteristics of 'indolent' chronic lymphocytic leukemia are present in 3.5% of adults with normal blood counts. *Blood* 2002; **100**: 635–39.

14. Dohner H, Stilgenbauer S, Benner A et al. Genomic aberrations and survival in chronic lymphocytic leukemia. *N Engl J Med* 2000; **343**: 1910–16.

15. Dohner H, Stilgenbauer S, Dohner K et al. Chromosome aberrations in B-cell chronic lymphocytic leukemia: reassessment based on molecular cytogenetic analysis. *J Mol Med* 1999; **77**: 266–81.

16. Dohner H, Stilgenbauer S, Fischer K et al. Cytogenetic and molecular cytogenetic analysis of B cell chronic lymphocytic leukemia: specific chromosome aberrations identify prognostic subgroups of patients and point to loci for candidate genes. *Leukemia* 1997; **11**: S19–24.

17. Stilgenbauer S, Bullinger L, Benner A et al. Incidence and clinical significance of 6q deletions in B cell chronic lymphocytic leukemia. *Leukemia* 1999; **13**: 1331–34.

18. Oscier O, Fitchett M, Herbert T et al. Karyotypic evolution in B-cell chronic lymphicytic leukemia. *Gene Chromosomes Cancer* 1991; **3**: 16–20.

19. Fegan C, Robinson H, Thompson P et al. Karyotypic evolution in CLL: identification of a new subgroup of patients with deletions of llq and advanced or progressive disease. *Leukemia* 1995; **9**: 2003–8.

20. Migliazza A, Bosch F, Komatsu H et al. Nucleotide sequence, transcription map, and mutation analysis of the 13q14 chromosomal region deleted in B-cell chronic lymphocytic leukemia. *Blood* 2001; **97**: 2098–104.

21. Bullrich F, Fujii H, Calin G et al. Characterization of the 13q14 tumor suppressor locus in CLL: identification of ALT1, an alternative splice variant of the LEU2 gene. *Cancer Res.* 2001; **61**: 6640–48.

22. Hamblin TJ, Davis Z, Gardiner A et al. Unmutated Ig V(H) genes are associated with a more aggressive form of chronic lymphocytic leukemia. *Blood* 1999; **94**: 1848–54.

23. Damle RN, Wasil T, Fais F et al. Ig V gene mutation status and CD38 expression as novel prognostic indicators in chronic lymphocytic leukemia. *Blood* 1999; **94**: 1840–47.

24. Rosenwald A, Alizadeh AA, Widhopf G et al. Relation of gene expression phenotype to immunoglobulin mutation genotype in B cell chronic lymphocytic leukaemia. *J Exp Med* 2001; **194**: 1639–47.

25. Molica S. Infections in chronic lymphocytic leukemia: risk factors and impact on survival, and treatment. *Leuk Lymphoma* 1994; **13**: 203–14.

26. Morrison VA. The infectious complications of chronic lymphocytic leukemia. *Semin Oncol* 1998; **25**: 98–106.

27. Bonvalet D, Foldes C, Civatte J. Cutaneous manifestations in chronic lymphocytic leukemia. *J Dermatol Surg Oncol* 1984; **10**: 278–82.

28. Lopez Guillermo A, Cervantes F, Blade J et al. Central nervous system involvement demonstrated by immunological study in prolymphocytic variant of chronic lymphocytic leukemia. *Acta Haematol* 1989; **81**: 109–11.

29. Van de Casteele M, Verhoef GEG, Demuynck H et al. Hypercalcemia, monoclonal protein, and osteolytic bone lesions in chronic lymphocytic leukemia. *Ann Hematol* 1994; **69**: 79–80.

30. Seney FD, Federgreen WR, Stein H et al. A review of nephrotic syndrome associated with chronic lymphocytic leukemia. *Arch Intern Med* 1986; **146**: 137–41.

31. Ribera JM, Vinolas N, Urbano Ispizua A et al. 'Spontaneous' complete remissions in chronic lymphocytic leukemia: report of three cases and review of the literature. *Blood Cells* 1987; **12**: 471–9.

32. Thomas R, Ribeiro I, Shepherd P et al. Spontaneous clinical regression in chronic lymphocytic leukaemia. *Br J Haematol* 2002; **116**: 34.

33. Duhrsen U, Augener W, Zwingers T et al. Spectrum and frequency of autoimmune derangements in lymphoproliferative disorders: analysis of 637 cases and comparison with myeloproliferative diseases. *Br J Haematol* 1987; **67**: 235–39.

34. Kipps TJ, Carson DA. Autoantibodies in chronic lymphocytic leukemia and related systemic autoimmune diseases. *Blood* 1993; **81**: 2475–87.

35. Hamblin TJ, Oscier DG, Young BJ. Autoimmunity in chronic lymphocytic leukemia. *J Clin Pathol* 1986; **39**: 713–16.

36. Ward JH. Autoimmunity in chronic lymphocytic leukemia. *Curr Treat Options Oncol* 2001; **2**: 253–257.

37. Rozman C, Montserrat E, Vinolas N. Serum immunoglobulins in B-chronic lymphocytic leukaemia. Natural history and prognostic significance. *Cancer* 1988; **61**: 279–83.

38. Pangalis GA, Moutsdopoulos HM, Papadopoulos NM et al. Monoclonal and oligoclonal immunoglobulins in the serum of patients with B-chronic lymphocytic leukemia. *Acta Haematol* 1988; **80**: 23–27.

39. Beaume A, Brizard A, Dreyfus B et al. High incidence of serum monoclonal IgS detected by a sensitive immunoblotting technique in B-cell chronic lymphocytic leukemia. *Blood* 1994; **84**: 1216–19.

40. Richter MN. Generalized reticular cell sarcoma of lymph nodes associated with lymphatic leukaemia. *Am J Pathol* 1928; **4**: 285–92.

41. Robertson LE, Pugh W, O'Brien S et al. Richter's syndrome: a report on 39 patients. *J Clin Oncol* 1993; **11**: 1985–9.

42. Cherepakhin V, Baird SM, Meisenholder GW et al. Common clonal origin of chronic lymphocytic leukemia and high-grade lymphoma of Richter's syndrome. *Blood* 1993; **82**: 3141–7.

43. Enno A, Catovsky D, O'Brien M et al. 'Prolymphocytoid' transformation of chronic lymphocytic leukemia. *Br J Haematol* 1979; **41**: 9–18.

44. Choi H, Keller RH. Coexistence of chronic lymphocytic leukemia and Hodgkin's disease. *Cancer* 1981; **48**: 48–57.

45. Greene MH, Hoover RN, Fraumeni JF. Subsequent cancer in patients with chronic lymphocytic leukemia. A possible immunologic mechanism. *J Natl Cancer Inst* 1978; **61**: 337–40.

46. Travis LB, Curtis RE, Hankey BF et al. Second cancers in patients with chronic lymphocytic leukemia. *J Natl Cancer Inst* 1992. **84**: 1422–7.

47. Hisada M, Biggar RJ, Greene MH et al. Solid tumors after chronic lymphocytic leukemia. *Blood* 2001; **98**: 1979–81.

48. International Workshop on Chronic Lymphocytic Leukemia. Chronic lymphocytic leukemia: recommendations for diagnosis, staging, and response criteria. *Ann Intern Med* 1989; **110**: 236–8.

49. Cheson BD, Bennett JM, Grever M et al. National Cancer Institute-sponsored working group guidelines for chronic lymphocytic leukemia: revised guidelines for diagnosis and treatment. *Blood* 1996; **87**: 4990–7.

50. Bennett JM, Catovsky D, Daniel MT et al. Proposals for the classification of chronic (mature) B and T lymphoid leukemias. *J Clin Pathol* 1989; **42**: 567–84.

51. Rai KR, Sawitsky A, Cronkite EP et al. Clinical staging of chronic lymphocytic leukemia. *Blood* 1975; **46**: 219–34.

52. Binet JL, Auquier A, Dighiero G et al. A new prognostic classification of chronic lymphocytic leukemia derived from a multivariate survival analysis. *Cancer* 1981; **48**: 198–206.

53. Montserrat E. Classical and new prognostic factors in chronic lymphocytic leukemia: where to now? *Hematol J* 2002; **3**: 7–9.

54. Montserrat E, Vinolas N, Reverter JC et al. Natural history of chronic lymphocytic leukemia: on the progression and prognosis of early clinical stages. *Nouv Rev Franc* 1988; **30**: 359–61.

55. Hallek M, Langenmayer I, Nerl C et al. Elevated serum thymidine kinase levels identify a subgroup at high risk of disease progression in early, nonsmoldering chronic lymphocytic leukemia. *Blood;* 1999; **93**: 1732–7.

56. Reinisch W, Wiliheim M, Hilgarth M et al. Soluble CD23 reliably reflects disease activity in B-cell chronic lymphocytic leukemia. *J Clin Oncol* 1994; **12**: 2146–52.

57. Lavabre-Bertrand T, Exbrayat C, Bourquard P et al. CD23 antigen density is related to gamma globulin level, bone marrow reticulin pattern, and treatment in B chronic lymphocytic leukemia. *Leuk Lymphoma* 1994; **13**: 89–94.

58. Manshouri T, Do KA, Wang X et al. Circulating CD20 is detectable in the plasma of patients with chronic lymphocytic leukaemia and is of prognostic significance. *Blood* 2003; **101**: 2507–13.

59. El Rouby S, Thomas A, Costin D et al. p53 gene mutation in B-cell chronic lymphocytic leukemia is associated with drug resistance and is independent of MDR1/MDR3 gene expression. *Blood* 1993; **82**: 3452–9.

60. Catovsky D, Fooks I, Richards S (a report from the MRC CLL 1 trial), Prognostic factors in chronic lymphocytic leukaemia: the importance of age, sex, and response to treatment in survival. *Br J Haematol* 1989; **72**: 141–9.

61. Mauro FR, Foa R, Cerretti R et al. Autoimmune hemolytic anemia in chronic lymphocytic leukemia: clincial, therapeutic, and prognostic features. *Blood* 2000; **95**: 2788–92.

62. Hamblin TJ, Orchad JA, Ibbotson RE et al. CD38 expression and immunoglobulin variable region mutations are independent prognostic variables in chronic lymphocytic leukemia, but CD38 expression may vary during the course of the disease. *Blood* 2002; **99**: 1023–9.

63. Crespo M, Bosch F, Villamor N et al. ZAP-70 expression as a surrogate for immunoglobulin-variable-region mutations in chronic lymphocytic leukemia. *N Engl J Med* 2003; **348**: 1764–75.

64. Wiestner A, Rosenwald A, Barry TS et al. ZAP-70 expression identifies a chronic lymphocytic leukemia subtype with unmutated immunoglobulin genes, inferior clinical outcome, and distinct gene expression profile. *Blood* 2003; **101**: 4944–51.

65. Dighiero G, Maloum K, Desablens B et al. Chlorambucil in indolent chronic lymphocytic leukemia. *N Engl J Med* 1998; **338**: 1506–11.

66. Chemotherapeutic options in chronic lymphocytic leukemia: a meta-analysis of the randomized trials. CLL Trialists' Collaborative Group. *J Natl Cancer Inst* 1999; **91**: 861–8.

67. Johnson S, Smith AG et al. The French Cooperative Group on CLL. Multicentre prospective randomized trial of fludarabine versus cyclophosphamide, doxorubicin, and prednisone (CAP) for treatment of advanced-stage chronic lymphocytic leukemia. *Lancet* 1996; **347**: 1432–8.

68. Rai KR, Peterson BL, Appelbaum FR et al. Fludarabine compared with chlorambucil as primary therapy for chronic lymphocytic leukemia. *N Engl J Med* 2000; **343**: 1750–7.

69. Leporrier M, Chevret S, Cazin B et al. Randomized comparison of fludarabine, CAP, and ChOP in 938 previously untreated stage B and C chronic lymphocytic leukemia patients. *Blood* 2001; **98**: 2319–25.

70. Bosch F, Ferrer A, Lopez-Guillermo A et al. Fludarabine, cyclophosphamide and mitoxantrone in the treatment of resistant or relapsed chronic lymphocytic leukaemia. *Br J Haematol* 2002; **119**: 976–84.

71. Eichorst BF, Busch R, Hopfinger G et al. Fludarabine plus cyclophosphamide (FC) induces higher remission rates and longer progression free survival than fludarabine (F) alone in first line therapy of advanced chronic lymphocytic leukemia (CLL): results of a phase III study (CLL4 protocol) of the German Study Group (GCLLSG). *Blood* 2003; **102**: abstract # 243.

72. Wierda W, O'Brien S, Faded S et al. Improved survival in patients with relapsed - refractory chronic lymphocytic leukemia (CLL) treated with fludarabine, cyclophosphamide, and rituximab (FCR) combination. *Blood* 2003; **102**: abstract # 373.

73. Byrd JC, Peterson BL, Morrison VA et al. Randomized phase 2 study of fludarabine with concurrent versus sequential treatment with rituximab in symptomatic, untreated patients with B-cell chronic lymphocytic leukemia: results from Cancer and Leukemia Group B 9712 (CALGB 9712). *Blood* 2003; **101**: 6–14.

74. Cheson BD. Infectious and immunosuppresive complications of purine analog therapy. *J Clin Oncol* 1995; **13**: 2431–48.

75. Bastion Y, Coiffier B, Dumontet C et al. Severe autoimmune hemolytic anemia in two patients treated with fludarabine for chronic lymphocytic leukemia. *Ann Oncol* 1992; **3**: 171–3.

76. Di Raimondo F, Giustolisi R, Cacciola E et al.

Autoimmune hemolytic anemia in chronic lymphocytic leukemia patients treated with fludarabine. *Leuk Lymphoma* 1993; **11**: 63–8.

77. Hurst PG. Habib MP, Garewall H et al. Pulmonary toxicity associated with fludarabine monophosphate. *Invest New Drugs* 1987; **5**: 207–210.

78. Cervantes F, Salgado C, Montserrat E et al. Fludarabine for prolymphocytic leukaemia and risk of interstitial pneumonitis. *Lancet* 1990; **2**: 1130.

79. Frame JN, Dahut WL, Crowley S. Fludarabine and acute tumor lysis in chronic lymphocytic leukemia. *N Engl J Med* 1992; **327**: 1396.

80. Maung ZT, Wood AC, Jackson GH et al. Transfusion-associated graft-versus-host disease in fludarabine-treated B-chronic lymphocytic leukaemia. *Br J Haematol* 1994; **88**: 649–52.

81. Briz M, Cabrera R, Sanjuan I et al. Diagnosis of transfusion-associated graft versus-host disease by polymerase chain reaction in fludarabine treated B-chronic lymphocytic leukaemia. *Br J Haematol* 1995; **91**: 409–11.

82. Morrison VA, Rai KR, Peterson BL et al. Therapy-related leukemias are observed in patients with chronic lymphocytic leukemia after treatment with fludarabine and chlorambucil: results of an intergroup study of the Cancer and Leukemia Group B 9011. *J Clin Oncol* 2002; **20**: 3878–84.

83. Orchad JA, Bolam S, Oscier DG. Association of myelodysplastic syndromes with purine analogues. *Br J Haematol* 1998; **100**: 677–9.

84. Majumdar C, Singh AK. Role of splenectomy in chronic lymphocytic leukaemia with massive splenomegaly and cytopenia. *Leuk Lymphoma* 1992; **7**: 131–4.

85. Chikkappa G, Pasquale D, Zarrabi MH et al. Cyclosporine and prednisone therapy for pure red cell aplasia in patients with chronic lymphocytic leukemia. *Am J Hematol* 1992; **41**: 5–12.

86. Cooperative Group for the Study of Immunoglobulin in Chronic Lymphocytic Leukemia, Intravenous immunoglobulin for the prevention of infection in chronic lymphocytic leukemia. A randomized, controlled clinical trial. *N Engl J Med* 1988; **319**: 902–7.

87. Chapel H, Dicato M, Gamin H et al. Immunoglobulin replacement in patients with chronic lymphocytic leukaemia: a comparison of two dose regimes. *Br J Haematol* 1994; **88**: 209–12.

88. Weeks JC, Tiemey MR, Weinstein MC. Cost effectiveness of prophylactic intravenous immune globulin in chronic lymphocytic leukemia. *N Engl J Med* 1991; **325**: 81–6.

89. Hollander AAMJ, Kluin-Nelemans HC, Haak HR et al. Correction of neutropenia associated with chronic lymphocytic leukemia following treatment with granulocyte-macrophage colony stimulating factor. *Ann Hematol* 1991; **62**: 32–4.

90. Pozlopoulos Ch, Panayiotidis P, Angelopoulos MK et al. Treatment of anaemia in B-chronic lymphocytic leukaemia (B-CLL) with recombinant human erythropoietin (r-HuEPO) (abst). *Br J Haematol* 1994; **87**: 232.

91. Tallman MS. Monoclonal antibody therapies in leukemias. *Semin Hematol* 2002; **39**: 12–19.

92. Osterborg A, Dyer MJ, Bunjes D et al. Phase II multicenter study of human CD52 antibody in previously treated chronic lymphocytic leukemia. European Study Group of CAMPATH-1H Treatment in Chronic Lymphocytic Leukemia. *J Clin Oncol.* 1997; **4**: 1567–74.

93. Osterborg A, Fassas AS, Anagnostopoulos A et al. Humanized CD52 monoclonal antibody Campath-1H as first line treatment in chronic lymphocytic leukemia. *Br J Haematol.* 1996; **93**: 151–3.

94. Dyer MJ, Kelsey SM, Mackay HJ et al. In vivo 'purging' of residual disease in CLL with Campath-1H. *Br J Haematol.* 1997; **97**: 669–72.

95. Huhn D, von Schilling C, Wilhelm M et al. Rituximab therapy of patients with B-cell chronic lymphocytic leukemia. *Blood* 2001; **98**: 1326–31.

96. Dreger P, Montserrat E. Autologous and allogeneic stem cell transplantation for chronic lymphocytic leukemia. *Leukemia* 2002; **16**: 985–92.

97. Esteve J, Villamor N, Colomer D et al. Stem cell transplantation for chronic lymphocytic leukemia: different outcome after autologous and allogeneic transplantation and correlation with minimal residual disease status. *Leukemia* 2001; **15**: 445–51.

98. Dreger P, Brand R, Hansz J et al. Treatment-related mortality and graft-versus-leukemia activity after allogeneic stem cell transplantation for chronic lymphocytic leukemia using intensity-reduced conditioning. *Leukemia* 2003; **17**: 841–8.

99. Ritgen M, Lange a, Stilgenbauer S et al. Unmutated immunoglobulin variable heavy-chain gene status remains an adverse prognostic factor after autologous stem cell transplantation for chronic lymphocytic leukemia. *Blood* 2003; **101**: 2049–53.

100. Dreger P, Stilgenbauer S, Benner A et al. The prognostic impact of autologous stem cell transplantation in patients with chronic lymphocytic leukemia: a risk-matched analysis based on the $V_H$ gene mutational status Blood 2004; **103**: 2850–58.

101. Galton DAG, Goldman JM, Wiltshaw E et al, Prolymphocytic leukaemia. *Br J Haematol* 1974; 27: 7–23.

102. Davi F, Maloum K, Michell A et al, High frequency of somatic mutations in the VH genes expressed in prolymphocytic leukaemia. *Blood* 1996; **88**: 3953–61.

103. Schlette F, Bueso-Ramos C, Giles F et al. Mature B-cell leukemias with more than 55% prolymphocytes. A heterogeneous group that includes an unusual variant of mantle cell lymphoma. *Am J Clin Pathol* 2001; **115**: 571–81.

104. Melo J, Robinson DSF, Catovsky D. The differential diagnosis between chronic lymphocytic leukemia and other B-cell lymphoproliferative disorders: morphological and immunological studies. In: Polliack A, Catovsky D, eds. *Chronic Lymphocytic Leukemia* Chur: Harwood Academic Publishers, 1988, pp. 85–103.

105. Bouroncle BA, Wiseman BK, Doak CA. Leukemic reticuloendotheliosis. *Blood* 1958; **13**: 609–29.

106. Bosch F, Campo E, Jares P et al. Increased expression of the *PRAD-1/CCNDl* gene in hairy cell leukaemia. *Br J Haematol* 1995; **91**: 1025–30.

107. Schmid M, Porzsolt F. Autocrine and paracrine regulation of neoplastic cell growth in hairy cell leukemia. *Leuk Lymphoma* 1995; **17**: 401–10.

108. Haglund U, Juliusson C, Stellan B et al. Hairy cell leukemia is characterized by clonal chromosome abnormalities clustered to specific regions. *Blood* 1994; **83**: 2637–45.

109. Platanias LC, Colomb HM. Hairy cell leukaemia. *Bailliere's Clin Haematol* 1993; **6**: 887–98.

110. Frassoldati A, Lamparelli T, Federico M et al. Hairy cell leukemia: a clinical review based on 725 cases of the

Italian Cooperative Group (ICGHCL). *Leuk Lymphoma* 1994; **13**: 307–16.

111. Mercieca J, Matutes E, Emmett E et al. 2-Chlorodeoxy-adenosine in the treatment of hairy cell leukaemia: differences in response in patients with and without abdominal lymphadenopathy. *Br J Haematol* 1996; **93**: 409–11.

112. Falini B, Tiacci E, Liso A et al. Simple diagnostic assay for hairy cell leukaemia by immunocytochemical detection of annexia A1 (ANXA1). *Lancet* 2004; **363**: 1869–70.

113. Cawley JC, Bums GF, Hayhoe FGJ. A chronic lymphoproliferative disorder with distinctive features: a distinct variant of hairy-cell leukaemia. *Leuk Res* 1980; **4**: 547–59.

114. Goodman GR, Bethel KJ, Saven A. Hairy cell leukemia: an update. *Curr Opin Hematol* 2003; **10**: 258–66.

115. May U, Strehl J, Gorschluter M et al. Advances in the treatment of hairy-cell leukemia. *Lancet Oncol* 2003; **4**: 86–94.

116. Saven A, Piro LD. Complete remissions in hairy cell leukemia with 2-chlorodeoxyadenosine after failure with 2'-deoxycoformycin. *Ann Intern Med* 1993; **119**: 278–83.

117. Seymour JF, Kurzrock R, Freireich E et al. 2-Chlorodeoxyadenosine induces durable remissions and prolonged suppression of CD4+ lymphocyte counts in patients with hairy-cell leukemia. *Blood* 1994; **83**: 2906–11.

118. Grever M, Kopecky K, Foucar MK et al. Randomized comparison of Pentostatin versus 'interferon alfa-2a in previously untreated patients with hairy cell leukemia: an intergroup study. *J Clin Oncol* 1995; **13**: 974–82.

119. Juliusson G, Heldal D, Hippe E et al. Subcutaneous injections of 2-chlorodeoxyadenosine for symptomatic hairy-cell leukemia. *J Clin Oncol* 1995; **13**: 989–95.

120. Wheaton S, Tailman MS, Hakimian D et al. Minimal residual disease may predict bone marrow relapse in patients with hairy cell leukemia treated with 2-chlorodeoxyadenosine. *Blood* 1996; **87**: 1556–60.

121. Bain BJ, Catovsky D. The leukaemic phase of non-Hodgkin's lymphoma. *J Clin Pathol* 1995; **48**: 189–93.

122. Kroft SH, Finn WG, Peterson LC. The pathology of the chronic lymphoid leukaemias. *Blood Rev* 1995; **9**: 234–50.

123. Pileri SA, Zinzani PL, Went P. Indolent lymphoma: the pathologist's viewpoint. *Ann Oncol* 2004; **15**: 12–18.

124. Mulligan SP, Catovsky D. Splenic lymphoma with villous lymphocytes. *Leuk Lymphoma* 1992; **6**: 97–105.

125. Dogan A, Isaacson PG. Splenic marginal zone lymphoma. *Semin Diagn Pathol* 2003; **20**: 121–27.

126. Thieblemont C, Felman P, Callet-Bauchu E et al. Splenic marginal-zone lymphoma: a distinct clinical and pathological entity. *Lancet Oncol* 2003; **4**: 95–103.

127. Boonstra R, Bosga-Bouwer A, Van Imhoff GW et al. Splenic marginal lymphomas presenting with splenomegaly and typical immunophenotype are characterized by allelic loss in 7q31-32. *Mod Pathol* 2003; **16**: 1210–17.

128. Troussard X, Valensi F, Duchayne E et al. Splenic lymphoma with villous lymphocytes: clinical presentation, biology and prognostic factors in a series of 100 patients. *Br J Haematol* 1996; **93**: 731–6.

129. Parry-Jones N, Matutes E, Gruzka-Westwood AM et al. Prognostic features of splenic lymphoma with villous lymphocytes. *Br J Haematol* 2003; **120**: 759–64.

130. Hermine O, Lefrere F, Bronowickj JP et al. Regression of splenic lymphoma with villous lymphocytes after treatment of hepatitis C infection. *N Engl J Med* 2002; **347**: 89–94.

131. Ghobrial IM, Gertz M, Fonseca R. Waldenstrom macroglobulinaemia. *Lancet Oncol* 2003; **4**: 679–85.

132. Offit K, Louie DC, Parsa NZ et al. del(7)(q32) is associated with a subset of small lymphocytic lymphoma with plasmacytoid features. *Blood* 1995; **86**: 2365–70.

133. Iida S, Rao P, Nallasivam P et al. The t(9;14)(q13;q32) chromosomal translocation associated with lymphoplasmacytoid lymphoma involves the PAX-S gene. *Blood* 1996; **88**: 4110–17.

134. Morel P, Moncoduit M, Jacomy D et al. Prognostic factors in Waldenstrom macroglobulinemia: a report of 232 patients with the description of a new scoring system and its validation on 253 other patients. *Blood* 2000; **96**: 852–8.

135. Dhodapkar MV, Jacobson JL, Gertz MA et al. Prognostic factors and response to fludarabine therapy in patients with Waldenstrom macroglobulinemia: results of United States intergroup trial (Southwest Oncology Group 59003). *Blood* 2001; **98**: 41–48.

136. Weisenburger D, Armitage JO. Mantle cell lymphoma: an entity comes of age. *Blood* 1996; **87**: 4483–94.

137. Bosch F, Jares P, Campo E et al. PRAD-1/CYCLIN Dl gene overexpression in chronic lymphoproliferative disorders: a highly specific marker of mantle cell lymphoma. *Blood* 1994; **84**: 2726–32.

138. Greiner TC, Moynihan MJ, Chan WC et al. p53 mutations in mantle cell lymphoma are associated with variant cytology and predict poor prognosis. *Blood* 1996; **87**: 4302–10.

139. Pinyol M, Hernandez L, Cazorla M et al. Deletions and loss of expression of p16INK4a and jwafl genes are associated with aggressive variants of mantle cell lymphomas *Blood* 1997. **89**: 272–80.

140. Velders GA, Kluin-Nelemans JC, De Boer CJ et al. Mantle-cell lymphoma: a population-based clinical study. *J Clin Oncol* 1996; **14**: 1269–74.

141. Orchad J, Garand R, Davis Z et al. A subset of t(11;14) lymphoma with mantle cell features displays mutated Ig VH genes and includes patients with good prognosis, nonnodal disease. *Blood* 2002: **101**: 4975–81.

142. Dreyling MH, Forstpointner R, Repp R et al. Combined immuno-chemotherapy (R-FCM) results in superior remission and survival rates in recurrent and follicular and mantle cell lymphoma. Final results of a prospective randomized trial of the German Low Grade Lymphoma Study Group (abstract # 351). *Blood* 2003; **102**: 103a.

143. Haas R, Brittinger G, Meusers P et al. Myeloablative therapy with blood stem cell transplantation is effective in mantle-cell lymphoma. *Leukemia* 1996; **10**: 1975–9.

144. Khouri IF, Lee M-S, Saliba RM et al. Nonablative allogeneic stem cell transplantation for advanced/recurrent mantle-cell lymphoma. *J Clin Oncol* 2003; **21**: 4407–4412.

145. Brunning RD, T-prolymphocytic leukemia. *Blood* 1991; **78**: 3111–13.

146. Matutes E, Brito-Babapulle V, Swansbury J et al. Clinical and laboratory features of 78 cases of T-prolymphocytic leukemia. *Blood* 1991; **78**: 3269–74.

147. Yullie MAR, Coignet LJA, Abraham SM et al. ATM is usually rearranged in T-cell prolymphocytic leukemia. *Oncogene* 1998; **16**: 789–96.

148. Deardren CE, Matutes E, Cazin B et al. High remission rate in T-cell prolymphocytic leukemia with CAMPATH-1H. *Blood* 2001; **98**: 1721–6.

149. Mercieca J, Matutes E, Dearden C et al. The role of

Pentostatin in the treatment of T-cell malignancies: analysis of response rate in 145 patients according to the disease subtype. *J Clin Oncol* 1994; **12**: 2588–93.

150. Sokol L, Loughran TP Jr. Large granular lymphocyte leukemia and natural killer cell leukemia/lymphomas. *Curr Treat Options Oncol* 2003; **4**: 289–96.

151. Jaffe ES. Classification of natural killer (NK) cell and NK-like T-cell malignancies. *Blood* 1996; **87**: 1207–10.

152. Semenzato G, Zambello R, Starkebaum C et al. The lymphoproliferative disease of granular lymphocytes: updated criteria for diagnosis. *Blood* 1997; **89**: 250–60.

153. Matutes E., Catovsky D. Mature T-cell leukemias and leukemia/lymphoma syndromes: review of our experience in 175 cases. *Leuk Lymphoma* 1991; **4**: 81–91.

154. Pellenz M, Zambello R, Semenzato G et al. Detection of Epstein-Barr virus by PCR in lymphoproliferative disease of granular lymphocytes. *Leuk Lymphoma* 1996; **23**: 371–4.

155. Gentile TC, Wener MH, Starkebaum G et al. Humoral immune abnormalities in T-cell large granular lymphocyte leukemia. *Leuk Lymphoma* 1996; **23**: 365–70.

156. Semenzato G, Zambello R, Starkebaum C et al. The lymphoproliferative disease of granular lymphocytes: updated criteria for diagnosis. *Blood* 1997; **89**: 250–60.

157. Jakubowski A, Winton EF, Gencarelli A et al. Treatment of chronic neutropenia associated with large granular lymphocytosis with cyclosporine A and filgrastim. *Am J Hematol* 1995; **50**: 288–91.

158. Bible KC, Tefferi A. Cyclosporine A alleviates severe anaemia associated with refractory large granular lymphocytic leukaemia and chronic natural killer cell lymphocytosis. *Br J Haematol* 1996; **93**: 406–8.

159. Sezary A, Bouvram Y. Erythrodermie avec presence de cellules monstreuses dans derme et sang circulant. *Bull Soc Fr Dermatol Syph* 1938; **45**: 254–60.

160. Woods GS, Greenberg HL. Diagnosis, staging, and monitoring of cutaneous T-cell lymphoma. *Dermatol Ther* 2003; **16**: 269–75.

161. Querfeld C, Rosen ST, Kuzel TM et al. Cutaneous T cell lymphomas: a review with emphasis on current treatment approaches. *Semin Cutan Med Surg* 2003; **22**: 150–61.

162. Kim YH, Liu HL, Mraz-Gernhard S et al. Long-term outcome of 525 patients with mycosis fungoides/Sezary syndrome: clinical prognostic factors and risk for disease progression. *Arch Dermatol* 2003; **139**: 857–66.

163. Rosen ST. Foss FM. Chemotherapy for mycosis fungoides and the Sezary syndrome. *Hematol Oncol Clin North Am* 1995; **9**: 1109–16.

164. Kuzel TM, Hurria A, Samuelson E et al. Phase II trial of 2-chlorodeoxyadenosine for the treatment of cutaneous T-cell lymphoma. *Blood* 1996; **87**: 906–11.

165. Takatsuki K, Uchiyama T, Sagawa K et al. Adult T cell leukemia in Japan. In: Seno S, Takaku F, Irino S, eds. *Topics in Hematology*. Amsterdam: Excerpta Medica, 1977, pp. 73–77.

166. Uchiyama T, Yodoi J, Sagawa K et al, Adult T cell leukemia: clinical and hematologic features in 16 cases. *Blood* 1977; **50**: 481–92.

167. Poiesz BJ, Ruscetti FW, Gazdar AF et al. Detection and isolation of type C retrovirus particles from fresh and cultured lymphocytes of patients with cutaneous T-cell lymphoma. *Proc Natl Acud Sci USA* 1980; **77**: 7415–19.

168. Catovsky D, Greaves MF, Rose M et al. Adult T-cell lymphoma in Blacks from the West Indies. *Lancet* 1982; **i**: 639–43.

169. Cunningham D, Gilchrist NG, Jack A et al. T-lymphoma associated with HTLV-I outside the Caribbean and Japan. *Lancet* 1985; **ii**: 337–38.

170. Ishikawa T. Current status of therapeutic approaches to adult T-cell leukemia. *Int J Hematol* 2003; **78**: 304–11.

# 34 Multiple myeloma

Nikhil C Munshi and Kenneth C Anderson

## Introduction

Multiple myeloma is a clonal B-cell malignancy characterized by the accumulation of bone marrow plasma cells. The critical step in malignant transformation occurs late in B-cell differentiation after antigen selection and somatic hypermutation. These transformed cells then migrate to the bone marrow, where critical interactions between the malignant cell, extracellular matrix proteins, and bone marrow stromal cells promotes tumor cell growth, survival, and drug resistance.[1]

The malignant plasma cells in myeloma generally produce one of the five major classes of immunoglobulins. IgG is the commonest variety, followed by IgA (Table 34.1). Other classes of immunoglobulins produced include IgM, IgD, and IgE. Except for IgM, produced in a variant of plasma cell disorder and in Waldenström's macroglobulinemia, the other types are only rarely observed. In a small number of patients, only the light chains of the immunoglobulin molecules are produced (i.e. Bence Jones proteinuria); rarely myeloma may be totally non-secretory by virtue of a lack of any immunoglobulin-related proteins.[2]

The majority of myeloma patients have disseminated disease at diagnosis; however, a small number may present with localized myelomatous involvement (plasmacytoma). The type and nature of the myelomatous involvement, as well as associated cytokines produced, determines its manifestations. Specifically, the presenting symptoms are related to the extent of bone marrow involvement, the amount and type of immunoglobulins produced (especially with regard to renal manifestations), the immune reactivity of the monoclonal antibodies, and tumor cell microenvironmental interactions, with production of critical cytokines driving bone resorption. Presenting features may include bone marrow-related symptoms such as anemia, osteolytic lesions with pain, pathological fractures or development of vertebral collapse, immune deficiency with susceptibility to infections, and renal dysfunction. Especially in an early-stage myeloma, the disease is diagnosed in an asymptomatic setting on routine laboratory examination.

Due to recent advances in our understanding of the disease biology, therapeutic options are not limited to cytotoxic agents; both interactions between the malignant cells and microenvironment and factors in the bone marrow milieu are potential targets for novel therapies.

## Epidemiology

Multiple myeloma is a relatively uncommon malignancy, accounting for only 1% of all cancers in the Caucasian population. However, it is the second most common hematological cancer, comprising 10% of malignancies. The median age at diagnosis is 71 years, with 14 600 new cases in the USA in 2003. The estimated annual US mortality was 10 900 in 2002. In the USA, the average annual age-adjusted incidence rates per 100 000 are 6.7 for men and 4.2 for women among Whites, and 12.9 for men and 10.4 for women among Blacks. There is a significant association with advancing age. As seen in Figure 34.1, there is a sharp

**Table 34.1 Frequency of different types of monoclonal proteins produced by plasma cell tumors**

| Type of monoclonal protein | % |
|---|---|
| IgG | 52 |
| IgA | 21 |
| IgD | 2 |
| IgE | <0.01 |
| IgM (Waldenström's) | 12 |
| Light chain only (κ or λ) | 11 |
| Heavy chain only (α, γ, μ) | <1 |
| Two or more | 0.5 |
| None detected | 1 |

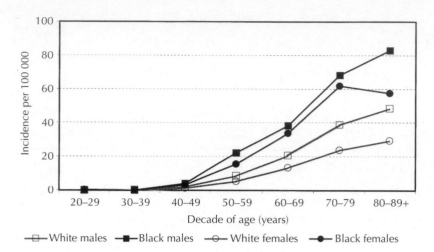

**Figure 34.1** Multiple myeloma: average annual age-, sex-, and race-specific incidence per 100 000 in the USA, 1997–2000. An increase in incidence is noted with advancing age, and a higher incidence is observed in males than females and in African-American than Caucasian populations.

increase in the incidence of myeloma beyond 50 years of age. The incidence is higher in men and twofold higher in Blacks in all age groups. A substantially lower incidence is observed in Chinese and Japanese populations, whereas the incidence in other ethnic groups, including Native Hawaiians, Americans, and Alaskans is higher than in US Caucasians in the same geographical area. The reason for the higher incidence of myeloma in African-Americans remains unclear, since social or economic conditions, household size, and family income cannot account for this.[3]

# Risk factors

The etiology of multiple myeloma and monoclonal gammopathy remains obscure. However, a number of environmental and familial risk factors have been described.

## Environmental exposures

The strongest single factor linked to an increased risk of myeloma is exposure to ionizing radiation.[4] Evidence from atomic bomb survivors and people exposed to low levels of radiation (including radiologists and those handling radioactive materials) suggests an increased incidence of myeloma after a latent period of up to 20 years.[5,6] There have been some reports of a potential risk of myeloma from exposure to metals (especially nickel), agricultural chemicals, benzene and petroleum products, other aromatic hydrocarbons, and silicones. However, the overall risk of developing myeloma following such exposure remains unclear.[4,7–12] Alcohol and tobacco consumption has not been clearly linked to myeloma. Among medications, only mineral oil used as a laxative has been reported to be associated with an increased risk of myeloma in some patients.[13,14]

## Familial and genetic factors

Direct genetic linkage has not been established in myeloma;[15] however, familial occurrence has been reported.[16,17] It remains unclear whether these occurrences are a result of genetic factors or due to shared environmental conditions. The risk of developing myeloma appears to be enhanced in the setting of HLA-B5 and HLA-Cw2 in both African-American and Caucasian populations.[18]

## Relationship with other medical conditions

A number of case–control studies have examined the relationship between myeloma and certain other medical conditions. Repeated infections or antigenic stimulation of the plasma cell compartment have been proposed as possible predisposing conditions for myeloma. A relationship between viral and bacterial infections, allergies, and autoimmune conditions has been studied; to date, conclusive evidence of an association is lacking.

## Premyeloma conditions

The presence of a monoclonal protein at low levels without any other manifestations of myeloma occurs in 3% of the population older than 50 years. Although such monoclonal gammopathy of undetermined significance (MGUS) has been considered to be a premalignant condition, the rate of conversion to myeloma associated with additional genetic changes remains extremely low.[19,20] MGUS in mice is dependent on the strain of mice, ageing, pre-existing immune status, and antigenic stimulation. In humans, MGUS is correlated with age and associated with immune disorders and infectious diseases. In one report, of 57 patients with MGUS who had undergone evaluation for *Helicobacter pylori* infection for various gastrointestinal symptoms, 39 (68%) had evidence of *H. pylori* infection and 11 of these 39 (28%) had normalization of the serum paraproteins following eradication of *H. pylori* infection.[21] Seroprevalence of *H. pylori*, however, has not been consistently associated with MGUS.[22] The development of MGUS has also been reported in the setting of T-cell deficiency, i.e. in AIDS.[23]

# Myeloma cells

## Phenotype

The identification of myeloma cells is based on morphological characteristics observed with Wright–Giemsa staining as shown in Figure 34.2. Morphologically, it is difficult to distinguish myeloma cells from normal plasma cells, except for dysmorphic characteristics, including multinucleate forms, cells in clusters and sheets, and plasmablastic characteristics in myeloma. Myeloma cells express monoclonal light and heavy chains, evidenced by staining for cytoplasmic κ and λ light chain. Additionally, myeloma cells are CD138+, CD38+, and CD45-. Details of other markers are shown in Table 34.2.

## Karyotypic abnormalities

Conventional chromosomal analysis is limited owing to the low mitotic activity of plasma cells, detecting abnormalities in only 20–30% of cases. This is a significant under-representation, as a majority of malignant cells are aneuploid on flow cytometry. However, newer techniques of multicolor fluorescence in situ hybridization (FISH) and spectral karyotyping (SKY), as well as refined G-banding techniques, have identified many non-random changes in a large fraction of patients.[24,25]

Karyotypic abnormalities identified by FISH can already be detected in individuals with MGUS. Chromosomal abnormalities in myeloma are typically complex, with an average of 11 numerical and structural abnormalities per cell, and increase with disease progression.[26–28] Structural abnormalities frequently include translocations involving 14q32 at the switch regions. Southern blot assay detects translocations that are not detectable by conventional karyotypic

| Table 34.2 Expression of cell surface molecules on normal plasma cells and myeloma cells | | |
|---|---|---|
| Cell surface molecule | Normal plasma cell | Myeloma cell |
| CD11a | + | − |
| CD11b | − | − |
| CD44 | + | + |
| CD54 | + | + |
| CD56 | − | + |
| CD58 | − | + |
| LFA-1 | − | −/+ |
| VLA-4 | + | + |
| VLA-5 | + | + |
| MPC-1 | + | + |
| RHAMM | − | + |
| CD138 | + | + |
| CD19 | + | − |
| CD28 | − | − |
| CD38 | + | + |
| CD40 | + | + |
| CD45 | + | −[a] |

[a] CD45 on immature myeloma cells.

analysis; these translocations induce dysregulation of several oncogenes and are hypothesized to be initiating events.[24] Spectral karyotyping affords additional help in defining these translocations.[25]

## Molecular abnormalities

Translocations involving the immunoglobulin heavy-chain gene at 14q32 are detected in 20–30% of myeloma cases by conventional cytogenetics and in a higher percentage of patients using molecular techniques.[26,27,29] These abnormalities are also present in MGUS, suggesting a role in the initial steps of the transformation.[30] The most frequent abnormality involving 14q32 is t(11;14), involving cyclin D1 on chromosome 11[29,31] (Table 34.3).

The 4p16 region contains the fibroblast growth factor receptor 3 (FGFR3) and MMSET genes. FGFR3 is an oncogenic receptor tyrosine kinase, which may be activated by the Ig switch region translocation t(4;14)(p16.3;q32) in myeloma patients.[32–35] Activating mutations of FGFR3 trigger mitogen-activated protein kinase (MAPk) cascade signaling, resulting in growth of myeloma cells.[36] Mutated FGFR3 has also been shown to confer resistance to caspase-3-mediated apoptosis.[32,37] Spectral karyotyping has identified another non-random translocation, t(14:16) (q32:q22−23), involving the Ig switch region and the c-MAF oncogene.[38] The additional translocations t(9;14) and t(6;14) involve the PAX5 and IRF4

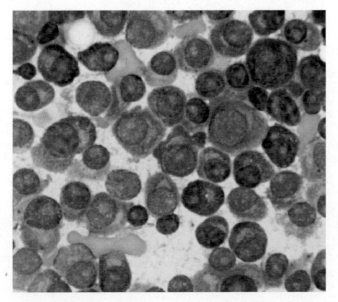

**Figure 34.2** Morphological characteristics of myeloma cells stained with Wright–Giemsa stain.

**Table 34.3 Non-Ig sites for illegitimate switch recombination**

| Chromosome | Frequency | Gene(s) | Function |
|---|---|---|---|
| 11q13 | 30 | *Cyclin D1* | Induces growth |
| 4p16 | 25 | *FGFR3, MMSET* | Growth factor |
| 8q24 | 5 | *c-MYC* | Growth/apoptosis |
| 16q23 | 1 | *c-MAF* | Transcription factor |
| 6p25 | <1 | *IRF4* | Transcription factor |

genes, respectively;[39,40] however, the translocating partner chromosome locus is not identified in the majority of cases. Furthermore, although 14q32 is commonly involved in translocations, its significance in myelomagenesis remains unclear owing to the variety of partner chromosomes involved and its lack of prognostic significance.

Cytogenetic abnormalities involving loss of either part or the whole of chromosome 13, or deletion of chromosome 11q, have been reported to predict poor outcome in a cohort of patients treated with high-dose melphalan and stem cell rescue.[41] Perez-Simon et al[25] have confirmed the association of chromosome 13 abnormalities as assessed by deletion of the retinoblastoma gene (*RB1*) with advanced disease and poor outcome in a cohort of patients treated with conventional therapy. Using the *RB1* gene as a probe, FISH analysis reveals *RB1* deletion in over 40% of these patients.[42] Additionally, constitutive phosphorylation of the retinoblastoma protein (pRB) in myeloma cells can be further enhanced by interleukin-6 (IL-6).[43] Abnormalities in *p16* and *p15* have been reported in 75% and 67% of myeloma patients, respectively, suggesting an important defect in the pRB regulatory pathway.[44–47]

## Microenvironment

Myeloma cells express adhesion molecules that mediate interaction with the microenvironment, including both bone marrow stromal cell elements and extracellular matrix proteins (Table 34.4). Adhesion plays a significant role in the migration and localization of myeloma cells in the bone marrow and also induces tumor cell growth and survival. For example syndecan-1, a myeloma cell surface transmembrane heparan sulfate proteoglycan regulates growth of myeloma cells via interaction with type-I collagen; and mediates increased osteoclast activity.[48–50] Elevated serum levels of syndecan-1 correlate with increased tumor mass, and poor prognosis.[48] Besides the adhesion-induced signaling mediating growth, survival, and anti-apoptosis, binding of myeloma

**Table 34.4 Expression of adhesion molecules on the surface of myeloma cells and their interacting counterparts on bone marrow stromal cells (BMSC) or extracellular matrix (ECM)**

| Myeloma cell | BMSC | ECM |
|---|---|---|
| NCAM (CD56) | HSP[a] | |
| LFA-1 (CD11a) | ICAM-1 (CD54) | |
| VLA-4 | VCAM-1 (CD106) | |
| VLA-5 | | Fibronectin |
| Syndecan-1 (CD138) | | Fibronectin Type I collagen |

[a] HSP, heparan sulfate proteoglycan.

cells to bone marrow stromal cells also induces transcription and secretion of cytokines. As seen in Figure 34.3, adhesion of myeloma cell to bone marrow stromal cells triggers production of IL-6, insulin-like growth factor I (IGF-I), vascular endothelial growth factor (VEGF), stromal cell-derived factor 1 (SDF-1), and tumor necrosis factor $\alpha$ (TNF-$\alpha$),[51–55] which mediate tumor cell growth, survival drug resistance, and migration.

The biological and clinical relevance of increased angiogenesis, have only recently been evaluated in multiple myeloma. Increased bone marrow microvessel density (MVD) has been reported in patients with multiple myeloma compared with individuals with MGUS.[56–58] Moreover, in patients with myeloma, the degree of MVD has been correlated with prognosis.[59,60] Immunohistochemical studies show that VEGF, an important angiogenic factor, is expressed by myeloma cells.[61] Hepatocyte growth factor, which also promotes angiogenesis, is increased in the serum of myeloma patients and predicts a negative outcome, especially in patients with increased $\beta_2$-microglobulin levels.[62] Finally, novel agents that can overcome drug resistance in myeloma, such as thalidomide, inhibit angiogenesis.

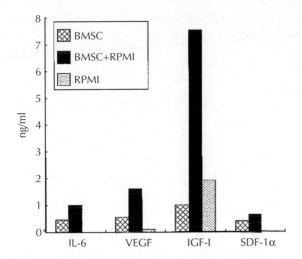

**Figure 34.3** Induction of cytokine secretion triggered by myeloma cell binding to bone marrow stromal cells (BMSC): IL-6, interleukin-6; VEGF, vascular endothelial growth factor; IGF-I, insulin-like growth factor I; SDF-1α, stromal cell-derived factor 1α.[51,53–55]

# Role of cytokines

Myeloma cells and bone marrow stromal cells through their interaction produces cytokines, including IL-6,[51] IGF-I,[55] VEGF,[53] SDF-1,[54] TNF-α,[52] transforming growth factor β (TGF-β),[63] IL-21,[64] and others that mediate tumor cell growth, survival, anti-apoptosis, migration, and development of drug resistance.

## Interleukin 6

IL-6 is an essential growth and survival factor for myeloma. The IL-6 receptor (IL-6R), composed of two polypeptide components: the α chain (gp80, IL-6Rα) and the signal transducing element, the β chain (gp130), is expressed by myeloma cells. The gp130 component is shared by a family of cytokines, including oncostatin M (OSM) and leukemia inhibitory factor (LIF). Interaction of IL-6 with its receptor activates the RAS/RAF/MEK/ERK pathway mediating proliferation, JAK/STAT pathway modulating anti-apoptosis, and PI3K/AKT signaling pathway mediating cell cycle in development of drug resistance (Figure 34.4). IL-6 is mainly produced by stromal cells following binding of myeloma cells and is also triggered by other cytokines including TNF-α,[52] IL-1β and VEGF in the bone marrow milieu.[53] IL-6 increases the proportion of myeloma cells in S phase, prevents apoptosis of malignant plasma cells, and confers resistance to antitumor agents such as dexamethasone. Dexamethasone induced apoptosis is mediated by caspase-9 and -3 activation; IL-6 blocks caspase-9 activation, thereby protecting cells. Soluble IL-6Rα, can amplify the responses of myeloma cells to IL-6; interestingly, both high serum IL-6Rα levels and high serum IL-6 levels are associated with poor prognosis. IL-6 and soluble IL-6Rα also mediate enhanced bone resorption by osteoclasts. IL-6 has been targeted therapeutically by antibodies specific for IL-6 or IL-6R, as well as by using an IL-6 superantagonist (SANT-7), which binds IL-6R but does not trigger downstream signaling. These treatment approaches have failed to show significant responses. Neutralizing anti-IL-6 murine monoclonal antibodies have been administered either locally (malignant pleural effusions) or intravenously in patients with advanced myeloma; although clinical responses were not seen, therapy reduced the survival and proliferation of malignant

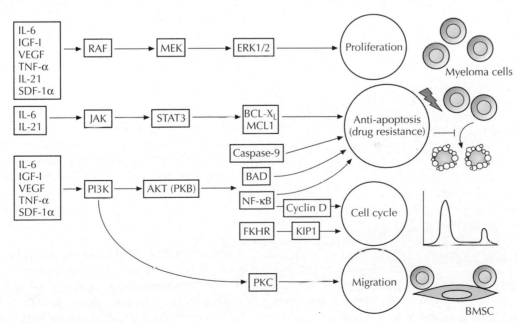

**Figure 34.4** Cytokine-mediated signaling cascades inducing growth, anti-apoptosis (drug resistance), and migration in myeloma.

plasma cells, confirming a role for IL-6 in mediating myeloma growth in vivo.

### Insulin-like growth factor I

IGF-I is also a growth and survival factor in myeloma. It activates the phosphoinositol 3′-kinase (PI3K) and MAPK signaling pathways mediating myeloma cell proliferation and anti-apoptosis.[65,66] It induces more potent anti-apoptotic activity against dexamethasone, than does IL-6. IGF-I enhances tumor cell growth and survival by upregulating FLIP, XIAP, and A1/Bfl1,[65] and by increasing telomerase activity.[67] We have recently shown that IGF-I mediates adhesion and migration of myeloma cells via $\beta_1$-integrin.[55,68] These studies have provided a rationale for the use of IGF-I as a therapeutic target, and both anti-IGF-I antibodies and small-molecule inhibitors of IGF-I show promise in preclinical studies.

### Vascular endothelial growth factor

VEGF has only modest direct effects on myeloma cells; however, it plays a significant role in triggering tumor cell migration and angiogenesis.[69,70] Its production is upregulated both by myeloma cell adhesion to stromal cells and by IL-6.[71] It is a specific endothelial cell mitogen, and elevated VEGF levels in myeloma may account, at least in part, for increased angiogenesis.[61] Myeloma cells express VEGF receptor FLT1, and VEGF triggers its phosphorylation and the consequent activation of downstream MEK (MAPK/ERK kinase) and PKCα (protein kinase Cα) signaling. These data have provided the preclinical rationale to evaluate VEGF as a therapeutic target. PTK787, a potent inhibitor of the VEGF receptor, has shown antimyeloma activity[72] and is being evaluated in early clinical trials.

### Other cytokines

A number of other cytokines play an important role in myeloma biology. TNF-α, secreted by myeloma cells, has little direct effect on myeloma cell growth and survival. However, it induces secretion of IL-6 by bone marrow stromal cells. It is also a strong inducer of NFκB activation, thereby upregulating adhesion molecules, binding to the bone marrow stroma, and cell adhesion-mediated drug resistance (CAMDR). Although thalidomide and its IMiD analogs, which have potent anti-TNF-α activity, are effective in novel treatments, specific antibody inhibitors of TNF-α have not shown a clinical response.

SDF-1α is expressed by bone marrow stromal cells, and its receptor CXCR4 is expressed by myeloma cells. It induces only a minimal proliferative effect; however, it mediates migration and adhesion, thereby inducing IL-6 secretion and drug resistance.

IL-21 directly induces proliferation and anti-apoptosis independent of IL-6 signaling. TNF-α upregulates expression of both IL-21 and IL-21R. IL-21 triggers phosphorylation of Jak1, STAT3, and ERK1/2 (p44/p42 mitogen-activated protein kinases).

TGF-β is produced by myeloma cells and induces secretion of IL-6 by bone marrow stromal cells. It also mediates the immunosuppression characteristic of myeloma.

# Signaling pathways

### Drug resistance

As a result of intrinsic and acquired resistance to conventional chemotherapy only 50% of patients with multiple myeloma achieve a partial response, with only few complete responses. There are several drug resistance mechanisms operative in myeloma.[73] First, altered intracellular drug concentration due to overexpression of the multidrug resistance (MDR1) gene, which functions as an ATP-dependent drug efflux pump. Cyclosporine (cyclosporin A) and verapamil inhibit this function and have been tested as chemosensitizers, with only modest short-term benefit.[74] PSC833, a non-immunosuppressive and non-nephrotoxic derivative of cyclosporine D, has also been evaluated in a phase II trial, with limited success.[75,76] Second, multidrug resistance-associated protein (MRP), a member of the ATP-binding cassette (ABC) transporter gene superfamily, may also be partially responsible for clinical drug resistance.[77] Third, expression of lung resistance related protein (LRP), a member of vault proteins (MVP), localized to the nuclear membrane and involved in the transport of substances such as alkylating agents to the nucleus is associated with poor response and shortened survival.[78] However, dose intensification of melphalan has been shown to overcome the resistance due to increased LRP expression.[79]

# Clinical features

The most frequent presenting symptom of multiple myeloma is bone pain, especially back pain, usually caused by lytic bone lesions or pathological compression fractures of one or more vertebrae. A radiographic survey of the entire skeleton, including both femora and humeri, identifies either osteopenia or lytic lesions in 80% of patients with myeloma. As the bone disease in myeloma is mainly lytic, due to increased osteoclastic activity and minimal osteoblastic activity, a bone scan is not useful in diagnosis or follow-up. More recently, magnetic resonance imaging (MRI) with inversion recovery imaging (STIR) has provided greater sensitivity to detect bone disease, as well as bone marrow infiltration that is not detected on plain radiographs. Interestingly, the incidence of back pain as a presenting feature decreased from 68% in the 1960s and 1970s to 37% in the 1980s, and about 20% of myeloma patients are asymptomatic and are diagnosed by chance during routine laboratory examinations.

Acute or chronic renal failure is detected in about 20% of myeloma patients at presentation, and it increases during the course of the disease. Bence Jones proteinuria, with light-chain deposition disease or cast nephropathy, and hypercalcemia are responsible for more than 95% of renal impairment. Other causes of renal compromise include hyperuricemia, amyloidosis, pyelonephritis, and the use of non-steroidal anti-inflammatory drugs (NSAIDs) for pain control.

A normochromic anemia is present in about 60% of cases at diagnosis; this is usually due to bone marrow infiltration with plasma cells, other contributing factors being renal failure with decreased erythropoietin production, and plasma volume expansion.

Myeloma patients are susceptible to bacterial infections due to both the profound reduction of normal immunoglobulin production and the inadequate response to antigenic stimuli. The mechanism of immunosuppression is multifactorial. Pneumonia is the most common infection, followed by urinary tract infection.

The deposition of immunoglobulin produced by the myeloma cells may lead to organ dysfunction. This deposition may be predominantly localized to the kidney or may be systemic in the form of amyloidosis. Amyloidosis is diagnosed based on the demonstration of AL amyloid deposit in abdominal fat (sensitivity 80%), rectum (sensitivity 75%), or other target organs including kidney, liver, and heart. Clinical presentation of AL amyloidosis may include proteinuria, nephritic syndrome, renal failure, congestive heart failure, and hepatomegaly.

## Diagnosis

The initial evaluation of myeloma includes a hemogram, serum and urine protein electrophoresis and immunofixation, quantitative serum immunoglobulin levels, urinary protein and Bence Jones protein excretion in 24 hours, complete skeletal radiographic survey, and bone marrow aspiration and biopsy. The diagnostic criteria for MGUS, smoldering and indolent myeloma, and multiple myeloma are based on the presence of monoclonal immunoglobulins in serum and/or urine, bone marrow plasmacytosis, and lytic bone lesions. The precise well-defined diagnostic criteria are shown in Table 34.5. Following establishment of diagnosis, more detailed cellular

and molecular studies (Table 34.6) are required to stage myeloma and evaluate prognostic variables that may help to both plan appropriate therapy and predict patient outcome.

---

**Table 34.5 Diagnostic criteria for multiple myeloma, myeloma variants, and monoclonal gmmopathy of unknown significance (MGUS)**

**Multiple myeloma**

*Major criteria*

I. Plasmacytoma on tissue biopsy

II. Bone marrow plasmacytosis with >30% plasma cells

III. Monoclonal globulin spike on serum electrophoresis exceeding 3.5 g/dl for IgG or 2 g/dl for IgA ≥1 g/24 h of $\kappa$ or $\lambda$ light-chain excretion on urine electrophoresis in the presence of amyloidosis

*Minor criteria*

a. Bone marrow plasmacytosis 10–30%

b. Monoclonal globulin spike present but less than the level defined above

c. Lytic bone lesions

d. Suppressed uninvolved immunoglobulins; IgM <50 mg/dl, IgA <100 mg/dl, or IgG <600 mg/dl

Diagnosis is confirmed when any of the following features are documented in symptomatic patients with clearly progressive disease:

- I + b, I + c, I + d (I + a not sufficient)
- II + b, II + c, II + d
- III + a, III + c, III + d
- a + b + c, a + b + d

(i.e. three minor criteria must include a + b)

**Indolent myeloma**

Same as myeloma, except:

- No bone lesions or only limited bone lesion (≤3 lytic lesions): no compression fractures
- M-component levels: (a) IgG <7 g/dl; (b) IgA <5 g/dl
- No symptoms or associated disease features, i.e.
- Performance status >70%
- Hemoglobin >10 g/dl
- Serum calcium normal
- Serum creatinine <2 mg/dl
- No infections

**Smoldering myeloma**

Same as indolent myeloma, except:

- No bone lesions
- Bone marrow plasma cells ≤30%

**Monoclonal gammopathy of unknown significance**

- Monoclonal gammopathy
- M-component level:
  IgG ≤3.5 g/dl
  IgA ≤2 g/dl
- Bence Jones protein ≤1 g/24 h
- Bone marrow plasma cells <10%
- No bone lesions
- No symptoms

### Table 34.6  Laboratory investigations of myeloma

**Identification and quantitation of monoclonal protein**
- Serum protein electrophoresis
- Quantitative immunoglobulin
- 24-hour urine: total protein and Bence Jones protein
- Immunofixation of urine and serum
- Serum-free light chain

**Radiological evaluation**
- Skeletal survey
- MRI with STIR images
- Bone densitometry

**Morphological evaluation**
- Bone marrow aspirate and biopsy
  - Cytogenetics
  - Flow cytometry (DNA-CIg)
  - Plasma cell Labeling index
- Solitary lytic lesion biopsy

**Prognostic factor evaluation**
- Chemistry panel (creatinine, calcium, albumin, lactate dehydrogenase)
- $\beta_2$-microglobulin
- C-reactive protein

**Specialized studies for selected patients**
- Serum viscosity if IgM component or high IgA levels or serum M-component >7 g/dl
- Abdominal fat pad or rectal biopsy for amyloid

## Therapy

Combination chemotherapy has been used for the treatment of multiple myeloma for over 30 years. The advent of high-dose chemotherapy and autologous stem cell transplantation, combined with the recent development of novel biologically based therapies, has changed the way in which myeloma is managed. An important question is when to start treatment in a patient with myeloma, since early diagnosis and treatment do not form the basis of successful therapy in myeloma. A patient with asymptomatic or smoldering myeloma is currently not treated, since a randomized study in early-stage myeloma showed no difference in remission duration or overall survival in groups of patients promptly treated with early induction therapy versus initiation of chemotherapy only at the time of progression of disease.[80] Therapy can be safely deferred in the absence of symptomatic disease or signs of progression, including a rise in M-component in serum and/or urine, increase in number or size of the lytic bone lesions, anemia, renal failure, and hypercalcemia.

### Response evaluation

Serum immunoglobulin levels, as well as monoclonal protein (M-protein) levels detected in serum or urine by protein electrophoresis, provide an easy and reliable method to evaluate response to therapy. In the past, various degrees of reduction in serum M-protein levels (>25% to >75%) were classified as partial responses (PR), while a complete response (CR) required the total disappearance of serum M-proteins. Due to higher renal catabolism, urine Bence Jones proteinuria is reduced more quickly, and response criteria have therefore required higher levels of reduction (>90%) to achieve partial response. At present, the European Group for Blood and Marrow Transplantation (EBMT) criteria are most commonly utilized.[81] A CR requires the disappearance of M-protein in serum and urine confirmed by negative immunofixation, with normalization of bone marrow on two determinations 6 weeks apart. A PR requires a 50% reduction in serum or a 90% reduction in urine paraproteins, again on two determinations 6 weeks apart.

It should be noted that molecular evaluation using sensitive allele-specific polymerase chain reaction (PCR) techniques can detect minimal residual disease in patients otherwise considered in complete remission by the conventional criteria described above. Moreover, an early reduction in M-component by more than 50% during the first or second course of combination chemotherapy may be reflective of myeloma cells with higher proliferative potential and paradoxically portend a poor prognosis.[82–85]

Although improvement in bone lesions is not traditionally considered a response criterion since bony defects rarely heal, the appearance of new bone lesions is indicative of progressive disease. Disappearance of lesions observed on MRI and positron emission tomography (PET) scans have been described; however, this criterion has not yet been incorporated into the definition of complete response.

Measurement of free light chains in serum is a new test that provides an accurate measurement of disease burden, especially in patients with light- chain-only disease, with non-secretory or oligosecretory myeloma, and in AL amyloid. Due to the shorter half-life of free light chains, the degree of change in serum levels of free light chains, as well as the change in the $\kappa:\lambda$ ratio of the free light chains, required for achieving PR or CR, have not yet been defined.

### Standard-dose chemotherapy

Melphalan in combination with prednisone (MP) has been a standard regimen with convenient oral dosing for over 30 years. Melphalan is administered orally at 0.25 mg/kg on days 1–4, and prednisone at 60–100 mg on days 1–4. Due to unpredictable absorption, the dosage of oral melphalan is modified if the patient does not develop cytopenia. A partial response, defined by a greater than 50% reduction in M-protein, has been observed in over 50% of patients, but CR is rare. Patients achieving stable disease with MP also have improved survival. Subsequently, combinations of vincristine and doxorubicin with oral dexamethasone (VAD) were demonstrated to achieve more rapid responses in a significant fraction of patients. This regimen achieves 40–60% responses, with a median remission duration of 18 months and have extended the overall survival beyond 3 years.

Intensification of these regimens by adding other agents may result in higher response rates, but does not increase survival. The common chemotherapeutic combinations used in myeloma are listed in Table 34.7. A meta-analysis of 18 published randomized trials comprising 3814 patients comparing MP with other combination regimens failed to show any survival advantage over MP. Selection of initial combination therapy has therefore been determined based on toxicity and plans for future high-dose therapy and stem cell transplantation regimens. Since melphalan and other alkylating agents cause stem cell damage, these agents are avoided in patients who are potential candidates for stem cell transplantation.

## High-dose therapy and stem cell transplantation

Conventional chemotherapy achieves a CR in no more than 5% of patients. Based on a log–linear dose–response effect in killing tumor cells in vitro by most alkylating agents, McElwain and Powles first reported on the ability of high doses of intravenous melphalan to overcome relative drug resistance and induce CR in previously treated myeloma patients.[86,87] The Intergroupe Français du Myelome was the first to conduct a randomized clinical trial (IFM-90) comparing 1 year of standard-dose chemotherapy consisting of VMCP (vincristine, melphalan, cyclophosphamide, and prednisone) alternating with BVAP (carmustine, vincristine, doxorubicin, and prednisone) with a short course of the same standard-dose induction chemotherapy followed by consolidation with high-dose therapy (HDT) consisting of melphalan with total body irradiation (TBI) followed by autologous bone marrow transplantation.[88] An updated analysis of this randomized trial presented by Attal et al[88] confirmed the benefits of HDT in terms of higher CR rate (22% versus 5%), event-free survival (EFS) time (median 28 months versus 18 months), and overall survival (OS) time (median 57 months versus 44 months) than observed in patients treated with standard-dose chemotherapy (Figure 34.5).

**Table 34.7 Commonly used standard-dose combination regimens for multiple myeloma**

| Chemotherapy | Drugs[a] | Days | | | | | | | Interval (days) |
| | | 1 | 2 | 3 | 4 | 5 | 6 | 7 | |
|---|---|---|---|---|---|---|---|---|---|
| VAD | DOX 9 mg/m²/24 h | X | X | X | X | | | | 28 |
| | VCR 0.4 mg/m²/24 h | X | X | X | X | | | | |
| | DEX 40 mg p.o. | X | X | X | X | | | | |
| VMCP/VBAP | VCR 0.03 mg/kg i.v. | X | | | | | | | 28 |
| | L-PAM 5 mg/m² p.o. | X | X | X | X | X | X | X | |
| | CTX 100 mg/m² p.o. | X | X | X | X | X | X | X | |
| | P 60 mg/m² p.o. | X | X | X | X | X | X | X | |
| | *alternated with* | | | | | | | | |
| | VCR 0.03 mg/kg i.v. | X | | | | | | | |
| | BCNU 30 mg/m² i.v. | X | | | | | | | |
| | DOX 30 mg/m² i.v. | X | | | | | | | |
| | P 60 mg/m² p.o. | X | X | X | X | X | X | X | |
| NOP | VCR 2 mg i.v. | X | | | | | | | 28 |
| | MITOX 16 mg/m² i.v. | X | | | | | | | |
| | PRED 250 mg/m² p.o. | X | X | X | X | | | | |
| MOD | VCR 2 mg i.v. | X | X | X | X | | | | 28 |
| | MITOX 16 mg/m² i.v. | X | X | X | X | | | | |
| | DEX 40 mg p.o. | X | X | X | X | | | | |

[a] DOX, doxorubicin; VCR, vincristine; DEX, dexamethasone; L-PAM, melphalan; CTX, cyclophosphamide; P, prednisone; BCNU, carmustine; MITOX, mitoxantrone; PRED, prednisolone.

A similar response and survival benefit has been reported more recently from the Medical Research Council (MRC)-VII trial, which randomized 407 patients to either standard-dose chemotherapy or HDT with stem cell transplantation.[89] A Spanish trial of 164 patients treated with HDT versus conventional therapy also showed a superior CR rate in the HDT arm, with a trend for prolonged EFS and OS in the HDT arm (Table 34.8).[90] In contrast, the MAG trial by Fermand et al[91] of 190 newly diagnosed myeloma patients failed to show superiority of HDT. More recently, the US Intergroup study randomizing patients between HDT versus conventional therapy followed by delayed HDT at relapse failed to show superiority of HDT for either achievement of CR or overall survival.[92] In this study, a significant fraction of patients received HDT as salvage therapy after relapsing in the conventional-therapy cohort. In this group, 52% of 161 patients failing conventional therapy received HDT as salvage; their response rate was 59% and their survival post relapse was 30 months versus 23 months for those not receiving salvage HDT (*p*=0.05). Although three out of five studies show a benefit of HDT (Table 34.8), the duration of benefit after HDT remains limited. The improvement in EFS and OS after HDT versus conventional-dose therapy has ranged from 4 to 12 months and from 1 to >23 months, respectively.

**Table 34.8 Results of large randomized studies comparing standard-dose therapy versus high-dose therapy (HDT)**

| Ref | | No. of patients | CR rate (%) | EFS (median, months) | OS (median, months) |
|---|---|---|---|---|---|
| 88 | Conventional | 100 | 5[a] | 18* | 37[a] |
| | HDT | 100 | 22 | 27 | 52% at 60 |
| 91 | Conventional | 96 | — | 18.7[a] | 50.4 |
| | HDT | 94 | — | 24.3 | 55.3 |
| 90 | Conventional | 83 | 11[a] | 34.3[a] | 66.9 |
| | HDT | 81 | 30 | 42.5 | 67.4 |
| 89 | Conventional | 200 | 8.5[a] | 19.6[a] | 42.3[a] |
| | HDT | 201 | 44 | 31.6 | 54.8 |
| 92 | Conventional | 252 | 15 | 21[a] | 53 |
| | HDT | 258 | 17 | 25 | 58 |

CR, complete response; EFS, event-free survival; OS, overall survival.
[a] Significant difference.

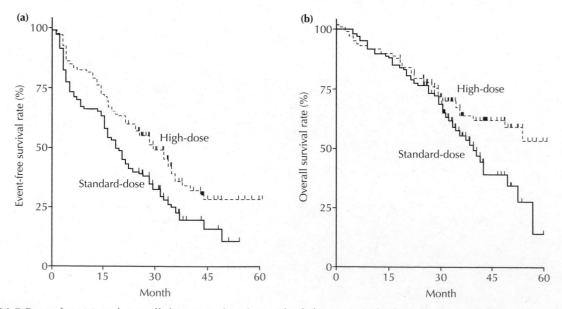

**Figure 34.5** Event-free (a) and overall (b) survival with standard-dose versus high-dose chemotherapy. IFM-90 randomized study.

## Conditioning regimen

Melphalan with or without TBI is the most commonly employed regimen. Regimens commonly used in leukemia or lymphoma (namely, busulfan–cyclophosphamide, cyclophosphamide–TBI; BEAM (carmustine, etoposide, cytarabine, and melphalan), or CBV (cyclophosphamide, carmustine, and etoposide)) have also been tested in myeloma.[93,94] None of these regimens has shown superiority over melphalan alone in the analysis of EBMT or American Bone Marrow Transplant Registry data.[95] Importantly, the addition of TBI adds significant morbidity without benefit. Data from retrospective studies – both single-center[96] and the EBMT Registry[97] – show that patients receiving a regimen containing TBI fared poorly compared with those receiving melphalan alone. In a randomized study in 282 newly diagnosed patients by the Intergroupe Francophone du Myelome, patients receiving melphalan (200 mg/m²) had statistically superior survival compared with those receiving melphalan (140 mg/m²) with TBI (8 Gy). Patients on the melphalan-only arm also had significantly less toxicity. The response rates and EFS rates were identical in the two arms of the study.[98]

## Tandem transplants

Attempts to further improve the results of autologous stem cell transplantation have included intensification with tandem transplants. Harousseau et al[99] were the first to report the feasibility of tandem autologous bone marrow transplantation, with a 69% CR in a small select group of patients. Barlogie et al[100] investigated a sequential non-cross-resistant remission induction regimen, followed by tandem autologous transplantations ('total therapy'), in 231 newly diagnosed patients; 41% patients achieved CR after two transplants, and the median EFS and OS times were 43 months and 68 months, respectively.

Attal et al[101] from the Intergroupe Français du Myelome have recently reported a randomized comparison (IFM-94) of single HDT (melphalan 140 mg/m² and TBI 8 Gy) versus double HDT (melphalan 200 mg/m², followed by melphalan 140 mg/m² and TBI 8 Gy) in 399 newly diagnosed patients. This study reports no significant improvement in CR or a very good PR rate between the two arms (42% versus 50%, respectively; $p=0.10$); however, there was a significant improvement in the probability of EFS at 7 years (10% versus 20%; $p=0.03$) and in the estimated OS rate at 7 years (21% versus 42%; $p=0.01$) in favor of the double-HDT arm (Figure 34.6). The Myeloma Autogreffe Group (MAG) ($n=193$), Dutch–Belgian Hematology–Oncology Cooperative Group (HOVON) ($n=255$), and Bologna ($n=178$) trials have a median follow-up of 27–30 months, and have not yet shown a significant benefit for tandem transplantation.

## Timing of high-dose therapy

Multi-institutional trials demonstrating that HDT as initial therapy prolongs remission duration and survival but is not curative have led to the exploration of the question whether HDT should be used early after diagnosis versus delayed as a treatment for relapsed myeloma. To evaluate this important question, Fermand et al[91] randomized 185 newly diagnosed patients to undergo three or four cycles of VAMP (vinblastine, doxorubicin, methotrexate, and prednisone)

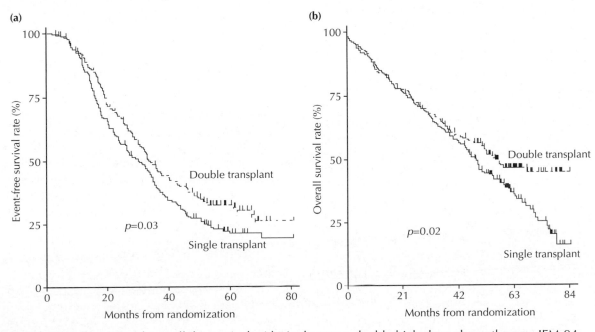

**Figure 34.6** Event-free (a) and overall (b) survival with single versus double high-dose chemotherapy. IFM-94 randomized study.

followed by early HDT and autotransplantation (n=91), or conventional chemotherapy with VMCP for 1 year. The latter group of patients were offered HDT if they had primary refractory disease or upon relapse (n=94). Although patients who underwent early transplantation had significantly longer EFS times (39 months versus 13 months), the overall survival was identical in both arms (median 64.6 months and 64 months). Importantly, the time without symptoms and treatment analysis reflecting quality of life (mean 27.8 months versus 22.3 months) showed superior results for the early-HDT arm. Vesole et al[102] have confirmed the effectiveness of high-dose chemotherapy as salvage therapy, achieving EFS and OS times of 21 months and >43 months, respectively, in 135 patients with advanced refractory myeloma. In this study, patients with primary unresponsive disease had superior outcomes to patients with resistant relapse (progression on last-salvage chemotherapy), with EFS times of 37 months versus 17 months, respectively (p=0.0004), and OS times of ≥43 months versus 21 months, respectively (p=0.0003). Gertz et al[103] from the Mayo Clinic have also reported a similar experience in 64 patients undergoing elective delayed transplant at the time of progression following standard therapy.

## Hematopoietic stem cell source and purging

Compared with bone marrow stem cells (BMSC), mobilized peripheral blood stem cells (PBSC) provide more rapid engraftment, and have therefore become the favored source of stem cells. For example, the IFM-94 study demonstrated more rapid hematopoietic recovery with PBSC support compared with BMSC support,[101] with similar EFS and OS durations. Successful mobilization of adequate numbers of stem cells depends on the duration and type of prior chemotherapy, especially stem cell-damaging agents, and radiation to bone marrow-containing areas. As the duration of prior standard-dose chemotherapy increases, the ability to collect adequate numbers of stem cells decreases. In one study, 86% of patients who received less than 12 months of prior therapy successfully mobilized $2 \times 10^6$ or more CD34+ cells/kg, compared with 48% of patients with more than 24 months of prior therapy.[104] Additionally, myeloma patients who had received less than 1 year of prior therapy had more rapid granulocyte and platelet recovery after PBSC.

Virtually all stem cell products have detectable myeloma cells as evaluated by immunofluorescence techniques or PCR assays.[105] Purging of tumor cells using a monoclonal antibody cocktail containing CD10 (the common acute lymphoblastic leukemia antigen, CALLA), CD20 (a pan-B-cell antigen), plasma cell-associated antigen 1 and complement lysing, or using peanut agglutinin and anti-CD19 antibodies,

has not improved outcomes. Positive selection of CD34+ cells to deplete myeloma cells results in 3–5 log reductions in contamination.[106,107] However, the success in obtaining a tumor-free graft has not translated into any significant advantage in response or survival time. A large, multicenter, randomized study comparing CD34-selected cells versus unselected PBSC in 131 patients failed to show any significant differences in EFS or OS times.[107] Finally, a pilot study selecting very early hematopoietic stem cells (CD34+ Thy1+ Lin−) devoid of any clonal B-cell contamination[108] resulted in delayed hematopoietic engraftment and prolonged immune suppression. Due to these results, emphasis is now on strategies to improve responses to HDT rather than purging autografts.

## Management of older patients

As the incidence of myeloma increases with age, the role of HDT has been evaluated in patients over 65 years old. Older age has not been reported to affect stem cell mobilization or engraftment.[109] The feasibility and efficacy of HDT with PBSC transplantation in patients aged 70 years or older has been evaluated in 70 patients (median age 72 years, range 70–83 years) treated with melphalan (200 or 140 mg/m²).[110] In this study, the treatment-related mortality rate was higher (16%) in the initial 25 patients receiving melphalan at 200 mg/m². Although CR was achieved in 27%, the median CR duration was only 1.5 years, with 3-year EFS and OS rates projected at 20% and 31%, respectively. Although this study confirms the feasibility of HDT in older patients with myeloma, it also indicates a higher risk in this patient population, and highlights the need for strict patient selection based on clinical status.

## Management of patients with renal dysfunction

Although one-third of patients with symptomatic myeloma present with renal insufficiency, hydration, control of hypercalcemia and effective therapy, can reverse it in 50% of cases. Renal dysfunction of less than 6 months' duration, with rapid initiation of therapy and a reduction in M-protein, is associated with a higher likelihood of improving renal function. Improvement in renal function is mainly observed in patients with light-chain cast nephropathy and light-chain deposition disease; therefore, renal biopsy is used to identify these reversible conditions, where there is a need for aggressive treatment. Based on the observation that the pharmacokinetics of melphalan are unaltered by renal failure,[111] high-dose melphalan and PBSC transplantation was used to treat 81 patients with myeloma and renal failure (creatinine >2 mg/dl).[112] In this setting, renal failure had no impact on the quality of stem cell collection and/or engraftment. However, treatment-related mortality rates were 6% and 13% after the first and second autologous stem cell transplants, respectively, and melphalan at 200 mg/m² caused excessive toxicity. A CR was achieved in 31 patients (38%) after tandem transplantation, and the probabilities of EFS and OS to 3 years were 48% and 55%, respectively. Dose reduction and close monitoring are needed to ensure the safety of the procedure, and the role of transplantation in the setting of renal failure remains investigational.

Recent developments in novel therapies have provided alternative strategies for the treatment of myeloma in the setting of renal failure. Thalidomide, bortezomib, and arsenic trioxide have all been evaluated in this setting. Ease of administration, limited toxicity, and effectiveness make these primary modes of therapy for myeloma patients with renal failure.

## Maintenance therapy

Despite improvements in remission rates, there is no clear plateau in the survival curves following conventional therapy or HDT. Although the proportion of patients achieving CR has increased, all patients eventually relapse. Various maintenance therapies have been evaluated in myeloma in an effort to sustain remission. Interferon-α (IFN-α), the most widely evaluated agent as maintenance therapy, have only demonstrated modest improvements in EFS and OS times (5–12 months) in randomized studies in patients achieving remission with standard-dose therapy. The role of IFN-α following HDT has not been confirmed.[113] Low-dose prednisone administered on alternate days has prolonged remission duration following standard-dose therapy in a single randomized study.[114] Thalidomide and its analog IMiD3 (with and without added dexamethasone), bisphosphonates, and immune manipulations such as idiotype vaccination and protein-pulsed dendritic cell-based vaccination strategies are under evaluation as maintenance strategies to prolong EFS and OS in myeloma.

## Allogeneic transplantation

### Syngeneic transplantation

Bensinger et al[115] have reported their experience with 11 patients receiving syngeneic transplants. Five patients achieved a CR and three achieved a PR. The most recent update shows one patient from either remission group alive 9 and 15 years after transplantation respectively. The EMBT Registry experience was reviewed by Gahrton et al.[116] Twenty-five patients undergoing syngeneic transplantation were compared with 125 case-matched patients undergoing autologous or allogeneic transplantation. Although the CR rate (syngeneic 68%, autologous 48%, and allogeneic 58%) was not significantly different between the three grafts, patients undergoing syngeneic transplantation had a significantly superior median survival time compared with autologous (72 months versus 25 months; $p=0.009$) or allogeneic (72 months versus 16 months; $p=0.008$) transplantation.

### Allogeneic transplantation

The older myeloma patient population with limited donor availability, coupled with frequent renal impairment, has restricted use of allogeneic transplantation in myeloma. Additionally, the almost 50% 1-year mortality rate has limited the use of this procedure to a high-risk patient population. Importantly, the allogeneic graft-versus-myeloma (GVM) effect may result in a favorable long-term outcome after allogeneic transplantation. A retrospective case-matched analysis of EBMT registry data compared 189 patients receiving allografts with an equal number of patients from the same time period receiving autografts. This study showed a superior median survival outcome for patients undergoing autologous compared with allogeneic transplantation (34 versus 18 months, respectively).[117] The 1-year treatment-related mortality rate was significantly higher following allogeneic transplantation (41% with allografts and 13% with autografts). However, interestingly, patients undergoing allogeneic transplantation and surviving the first year had a tendency towards better progression-free survival and OS.

In a single-center experience from the Dana-Farber Cancer Institute a low transplant-related mortality rate of 10% has been reported with selective depletion of CD6+ T cells as the sole form of graft-versus-host-disease (GVHD) prophylaxis.[118] However, the median progression-free survival time of 12 months, and the median OS time of 22 months was inferior to their previous experience with autologous transplantation. Another case-matched comparative single institution study has also failed to show a survival advantage for allogeneic transplants.[119]

### Donor lymphocyte infusions

A GVM effect has been demonstrated by the induction of CR with donor lymphocyte infusion (DLI) following relapse after allogeneic transplantation.[120] Lokhorst et al[121] have reported 6 CR and 8 PR following DLI in 27 patients after allogeneic transplantation. Five of these patients remained disease-free more than 30 months after DLI. However, DLI was associated with significant toxicity including acute GVHD in 55% and chronic GVHD in 26% of patients, five patients experiencing bone marrow aplasia, which was fatal in two cases. Strategies to reduce GVHD after DLI have included lowering the number of T cells infused, selective depletion of CD8+ T cells, and use of herpes simplex virus thymidine kinase gene (HSV-Tκ) transduction of DLI, which allows the use of ganciclovir to deplete T cells if significant GVHD develops.[123–124] Immunizing donors with idiotype vaccine may allow selective transfer of T cells specific for GVM without increasing the incidence of GVHD.

### Non-myeloablative transplants

Based on the canine model experience,[125] coupled with reduced day-100 transplant-related mortality in pilot studies in patients, allogeneic matched sibling transplantation in patients who were otherwise considered poor risk for the standard allogeneic preparative regimen has been performed. Badros et al first reported on 16 patients undergoing allogeneic transplantation following non-myeloablative conditioning with melphalan (100 mg/m²). The transplant-related mortality rate in the first 120 days was low (6%). Five CR were reported; however, acute GVHD developed in 10 patients (63%) and chronic GVHD was seen in 7 patients (44%) living beyond 4 months. Giralt et al[127] have used reduced-intensity conditioning with fludarabine and melphalan in 16 patients. Successful engraftment was observed in all patients; however, the 100-day mortality rate was 20% and the 1-year mortality rate was 40%, with only six patients alive after a median follow-up period of 15 months.

A combination of initial autologous transplantation for tumor cytoreduction followed by non-myeloablative matched sibling transplantation was evaluated by Maloney et al[128] in 54 patients. The treatment was performed in an outpatient setting, with a low 100-day mortality rate (2%). The overall response rate was 83%, with 53% CR. With a median post allograft follow-up of 552 days, the overall survival rate was 78%. However, GVHD remains a problem, with 38% of patients developing acute GVHD and 46% chronic GVHD requiring therapy.

While the early clinical results with non-myeloablative transplants are encouraging, this strategy is associated with significant morbidity due to acute and chronic GVHD and a mortality rate of up to 20% at 1 year. It should therefore only be utilized in the context of clinical trials.

### Idiotype vaccinations

Myeloma is a clonal proliferation of B cells producing a monoclonal immunoglobulin. The unique idiotypic structures are expressed on the surfaces of myeloma cells, making them an attractive target for eliciting a tumor-specific immune response. Osterborg et al[129] have elicited tumor-specific T- and B-cell responses after repeated administration of monoclonal immunoglobulin mixed with alum and granulocyte–macrophage colony-stimulating factor (GM-CSF). Similarly, specific T-cell responses has been reported by Kwak et al[130] in patients receiving post-transplant

immunization. Vaccination with idiotype pulsed dendritic cells have also been successful in eliciting T-cell immune responses.[131] It remains to be seen whether such immune responses translate into better survival.

### Novel biologically based therapies

In the past three years, we and others have used in vitro systems and in vivo animal models to characterize novel therapeutic agents directed at targets specific to both the myeloma cell and its microenvironment. Improved understanding of myeloma cell survival in its microenvironment has provided such new targets. Myeloma cells adhere to the extracellular matrix and to bone marrow stromal cells, allowing myeloma cells to grow, survive, and have anti-apoptotic effects against conventional chemotherapies. These effects are mediated partly through adhesion-mediated signaling and partly through various cytokines, including IL-6, VEGF, TNF-$\alpha$, and IGF-I. The molecular mechanisms mediating these effects include the RAS/RAF/MAPK, JAK–STAT, and PI3K/Akt pathways. The later pathway through NK$\kappa$B provides drug resistance signals. This understanding has translated from bench to bedside in related clinical trials. Thalidomide and its analog immunomodulatory agents (IMiDs), the proteasome inhibitor Bortezomib, and arsenic trioxide ($As_2O_3$) are three agents that have already demonstrated marked clinical anti-myeloma activity even in patients with refractory relapsed myeloma, thus confirming the utility of our preclinical models for identifying and validating novel therapies.

### Thalidomide

Although the first use of thalidomide in myeloma was based on its anti-angiogenic activity along with reports of increased angiogenesis in myeloma bone marrow, subsequent studies have demonstrated its effect both directly on myeloma cells as well as on their microenvironment.[132] Thalidomide and the more potent analog IMiDs abrogate the adhesion of myeloma cells to bone marrow stromal cells and block the secretion of myeloma growth and survival factors such as IL-6, TNF-$\alpha$, VEGF, and fibroblast growth factor (FGF), which are triggered by the binding of myeloma cells to bone marrow stromal cells (Figure 34.7). These agents also induce immune responses by improving antigen presentation by dendritic cells through inhibition of VEGF, expansion of the number and function of natural killer (NK) cells,[133] and providing T-cell costimulatory signals through the B7–CD28 pathway.[134,135]

The first phase II study in 169 patients with advanced post-transplant relapsed myeloma investigated thalidomide in incremental doses of 200–800 mg, demonstrating at least partial responses in 26% of

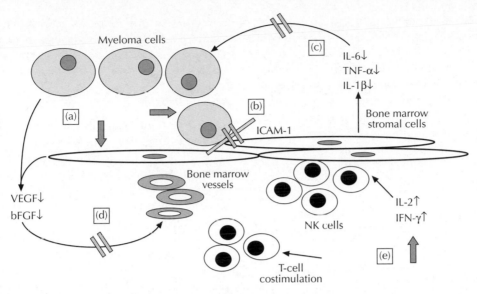

**Figure 34.7** Mechanism of action of thalidomide. (a) Direct effect on myeloma cells. (b) Effect on expression of adhesion molecules and adhesion of myeloma cells to bone marow stromal cells (ICAM-1, intercellular adhesion molecule 1). (c) Decrease in cytokines produced by stromal cells and myeloma cells in response to their interaction (IL, interleukin; TNF-α, tumor necrosis factor α); (d) Anti-angiogenic effect due to a decrease in angiogenesis-promoting cytokines produced by myeloma cell–stromal cell interaction (VEGF, vascular endothelial growth factor; bFGF, basic fibroblast growth factor). (e) Immunomodulatory effects on T cells and natural killer (NK) cells (IFN-γ, interferon-γ).[133]

patients, with an overall response rate of 34%.[136,137] The efficacy of thalidomide was subsequently confirmed in several phase II studies, showing responses in 25–40% patients with relapsed myeloma.[138–146] The major toxicities of thalidomide are somnolence, constipation, neurological symptoms, fatigue, and deep venous thrombosis.[136,147] Based on in vitro results showing synergism as well as reversal of resistance, thalidomide has been combined with dexamethasone. This combination has achieved a response rate of over 50% in relapsed patients and a rate of 70% in newly diagnosed patients (Table 34.9).[148,149] Excitingly, thalidomide is now being evaluated in combination with conventional therapies. Preliminary evidence suggests achievement of

high CR rates. The study by Weber et al[148] showed a 16% CR rate with a combination of thalidomide and dexamethasone; other combinations with high CR rates include melphalan, prednisone, plus thalidomide, giving a 22% CR,[150] and pegylated doxorubicin, vincristine, reduced-frequency dexamethasone, plus thalidomide, giving a 46% CR or near CR rate.[151]

Based on in vitro and in vivo animal data, the thalidomide analog CC-5013 (IMiD3) has been evaluated in a derived phase I clinical trial and has shown at least a 25% reduction in paraprotein levels (minimal response) in 15 of 24 (63%) patients, including 11 patients who had received prior thalidomide. Stable disease (<25% reduction in paraprotein) was

**Table 34.9 Results of combination of thalidomide (T) plus dexamethasone (D) in relapsed and newly diagnosed multiple myeloma**

| Ref | Patient population | No. of patients | Therapy/dosing | Response rate (%) |
|---|---|---|---|---|
| Palumbo[150] 2003 | Relapsed | 120 | 100 mg/d T + 40 mg D | 52 |
| Dimopoulos[150a] 2001 | Refractory | 44 | 200–400 mg/d T + 20 mg/m² D | 55 |
| 148 | Newly diagnosed | 40 | 200–800 mg/d T + 20 mg D | 72 |
| 149 | Newly diagnosed | 50 | 200–400 mg/d T + 40 mg D | 64 |

observed in an additional 2 (8%) patients.[152] Therefore, 17 (71%) of 24 patients demonstrated benefit from treatment. Although myelosuppression was the dose-limiting toxicity observed at the highest dose level, no significant somnolence, constipation, or neuropathy was seen in this study. These results therefore provide the basis for the evaluation of CC-5013, either alone or in combination, to treat patients with myeloma at earlier stages of the disease. A phase II trial of CC-5013 in patients with relapsed/refractory myeloma has achieved 10% CR, 25% PR and 40% stable disease rates. A formal evaluation of thalidomide or CC-5013, alone and/or with dexamethasone, is ongoing in newly diagnosed patients and as maintenance therapy.

## Bortezomib

Bortezomib (Velcade), a boronic acid dipeptide and a novel proteasome inhibitor, has demonstrated significant activity against myeloma. Bortezomib blocks NFκB activation and mediates anti-myeloma activity by inhibiting paracrine IL-6 production in bone marrow stromal cells. It also acts directly to induce apoptosis of myeloma cells resistant to conventional therapies, overcomes the protective effects of IL-6, and synergizes with dexamethasone for anti-myeloma effects. Importantly, it acts in the microenvironment to inhibit the binding of myeloma cells to bone marrow stromal cells, to inhibit the transcription and secretion of IL-6 triggered by adhesion of myeloma cells to stromal cells and to inhibit bone marrow angiogenesis.[153–158] Based on exciting animal model results and a confirmed safety profile in a phase I study that in fact showed responses in both of two myeloma patients, a multicenter phase II trial of bortezomib in myeloma was completed in 2002. In this trial, 202 patients with refractory relapsed myeloma were treated with 1.3 mg of bortezomib per square meter of body-surface area twice weekly for 2 weeks, followed by 1 week without treatment, for up to eight cycles (24 weeks). Dexamethasone (20 mg orally daily for 4 days) was added to the regimen in patients with a suboptimal response. Among 193 evaluable patients, a 35% response rate was observed, including 7 CR and 12 near-CR with only immunofixation positivity.[159] The median duration of response was 12 months, and the median overall survival was 16 months. Grade 3 adverse events included thrombocytopenia (28%), fatigue (12%), peripheral neuropathy (12%), and neutropenia (11%). The drug was approved by the US Food and Drug Administration (FDA) for clinical application in patients with relapsed and refractory myeloma based on this study. Addition of dexamethasone in this study improved responses in 19% patients, confirming synergism between these two agents. A randomized study comparing bortezomib versus dexamethasone in relapsed myeloma was recently closed prematurely due to superior results with bortezomib. Evaluation of this agent in newly diagnosed patients and in combination with other agents is underway.[160]

## Arsenic trioxide

Arsenic trioxide is another agent that targets myeloma cells as well as the bone marrow microenvironment, and is available commercially. It induces apoptosis of drug-resistant myeloma cell lines and patient cells via activation of caspase-9 and decreases binding of myeloma cells to bone marrow stromal cells, thereby inhibiting secretion of IL-6 and VEGF induced by adhesion of myeloma cells to stromal cells.[161,162] It also induces immune effects and inhibits telomerase. A phase I clinical study of arsenic trioxide showed at least a minimal response in 3 of 14 patients with refractory relapsed disease.[163] The most common toxicities include myelosuppression, neuropathy, and QT interval prolongation. An additive effect of arsenic trioxide with dexamethasone and ascorbic acid has been observed in vitro.[161] Based on these results, an ongoing phase I/II study is evaluating the safety and efficacy of arsenic trioxide in combination with dexamethasone and ascorbic acid in patients with relapsed myeloma.[164]

## Bisphosphonates

Bisphosphonates have been extremely useful in reducing skeletal complications and bone pain in myeloma.[165,166] Bisphosphonates, and specifically the aminobisphosphonates, have a direct effect on the bone marrow microenvironment, thereby decreasing IL-6 production and downregulating osteoclast activity. Furthermore, they activate $\gamma/\delta$ T cells with antimyeloma activity, and induce apoptosis of osteoclasts through inhibition of farnesyl and geranylgeranyl transferase activity.[167,168] In addition to a reduction in skeletal events ($p=0.016$), a significant survival advantage was observed (21 months versus 14 months; $p=0.041$) in patients receiving salvage chemotherapy and pamidronate versus chemotherapy alone.[165,169] In vitro cytotoxic effects of bisphosphonates have been observed in myeloma cell lines,[170,171] patient cells in vitro, and tumor specimens in the SCID–hu model.[172] In one report, pamidronate administered alone every 2 weeks showed a response or a delay in disease progression in occasional patients.[173] Zoledronic acid is one of the most potent bisphosphonates, and in animal studies it has been found to be superior to pamidronate in inducing osteoclast apoptosis.[172] Pamidronate 90 mg, and zoledronic acid 4 mg are equipotent in reducing bone-related problems in myeloma; however, zoledronic acid has a more convenient schedule of administration over 15 minutes (compared to 1–2 hours for pamidronate). Patients may occasionally develop mild hypocalcemia and need to be closely

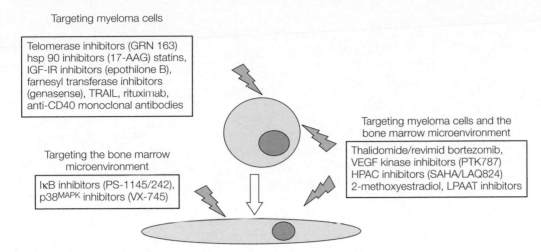

Targeting myeloma cells

Telomerase inhibitors (GRN 163)
hsp 90 inhibitors (17-AAG) statins,
IGF-IR inhibitors (epothilone B),
farnesyl transferase inhibitors
(genasense), TRAIL, rituximab,
anti-CD40 monoclonal antibodies

Targeting myeloma cells and the
bone marrow microenvironment

Thalidomide/revimid bortezomib,
VEGF kinase inhibitors (PTK787)
HPAC inhibitors (SAHA/LAQ824)
2-methoxyestradiol, LPAAT inhibitors

Targeting the bone marrow
microenvironment

IκB inhibitors (PS-1145/242),
p38$^{MAPK}$ inhibitors (VX-745)

**Figure 34.8** Novel therapies targeting myeloma cells in the bone marrow microenvironment.

observed for changes in renal function while on long-term bisphosphonate therapy.

## Other potential agents

With improvements in our understanding of myeloma cell–bone marrow stromal cell interactions and of adhesion-mediated and cytokine-mediated signaling, both in vitro systems and in vivo animal models have been developed to characterize mechanisms that promote myeloma cell growth, survival, drug resistance, and migration in the bone marrow milieu. These model systems have allowed the development of several promising biologically based therapies that can target both the myeloma cell and the bone marrow microenvironment. Drugs with potential efficacy in myeloma and undergoing clinical evaluation include those that predominantly target myeloma cells (such as the telomerase inhibitor GRN 163, the heat-shock protein 90 (hsp90) inhibitor 17-AAG, TRAIL, statins, IGF-I receptor (IGF-IR) inhibitors, and farnesyl transferase inhibitors), those that target both myeloma cells and the microenvironment (such as thalidomide/revimid, bortezomib, the VEGF kinase inhibitor PTK787, the HPAC inhibitors SAHA and LAQ824, 2-methoxyestradiol, arsenic trioxide, and LPAAT inhibitors), and those that target only the bone marrow microenvironment (such as IκB kinase inhibitors and p38$^{MAPK}$ inhibitors) (Figure 34.8).

Based on ongoing proteomic and genomic studies, these novel agents will be combined in a biologically rational approach in clinical trials to overcome drug resistance and improve patient outcome. For example, genomic studies have demonstrated the induction of hsp90, a molecular chaperone, in myeloma cells following exposure to a proteasome inhibitor. Preclinical results have shown synergistic effects with a combination of bortezomib and the hsp90 inhibitor 17-AAG, providing the rationale for molecularly based combination of these two agents. Similarly, these studies have defined the preclinical rationale for combining bortezomib with conventional DNA-damaging agents.[160] Ultimately, it may be possible to carry out gene profiling to define targets of sensitivity versus resistance in order to develop the next generation of more potent and less toxic therapeutics and to select combinations of targeted therapies.

## REFERENCES

1. Hallek M, Bergsagel PL, Anderson KC. Multiple myeloma: increasing evidence for a multistep transformation process. *Blood* 1998; **91**: 3–21.
2. Pruzanski W, Ogryzlo MA. Abnormal proteinuria in malignant diseases. *Adv Clin Chem* 1970; **13**: 335–82.
3. Cohen HJ, Crawford J, Rao MK et al. Racial differences in the prevalence of monoclonal gammopathy in a community-based sample of the elderly. *Am J Med* 1998; **104**: 439–44 [Erratum 1998; **105**: 362].
4. Riedel DA, Pottern LM. The epidemiology of multiple myeloma. *Hematol Oncol Clin North Am* 1992; **6**: 225–47.
5. Ichimaru M, Ishimaru T, Mikami M, Matsunaga M. Multiple myeloma among atomic bomb survivors in Hiroshima and Nagasaki, 1950–76: relationship to radiation dose absorbed by marrow. *J Natl Cancer Inst* 1982; **69**: 323–8.
6. Omar RZ, Barber JA, Smith PG. Cancer mortality and morbidity among plutonium workers at the Sellafield plant of British Nuclear Fuels. *Br J Cancer* 1999; **79**: 1288–301.
7. Bergsagel DE, Wong O, Bergsagel PL et al. Benzene and multiple myeloma: appraisal of the scientific evidence. *Blood* 1999; **94**: 1174–82.
8. Lundberg I, Milatou-Smith R. Mortality and cancer incidence among Swedish paint industry workers with

long-term exposure to organic solvents. *Scand J Work Environ Health* 1998; **24**: 270−5.

9.  Salmon SE, Kyle RA. Silicone gels, induction of plasma cell tumors, and genetic susceptibility in mice: a call for epidemiologic investigation of women with silicone breast implants. *J Natl Cancer Inst* 1994; **86**: 1040−1.

10. Tricot GJ, Naucke S, Vaught L et al. Is the risk of multiple myeloma increased in patients with silicone implants? *Curr Top Microbiol Immunol* 1996; **210**: 357−9.

11. Cuzick J, De Stavola B. Multiple myeloma − a case−control study. *Br J Cancer* 1988; **57**: 516−20.

12. Fritschi L, Siemiatycki J. Lymphoma, myeloma and occupation: results of a case−control study. *Int J Cancer* 1996; **67**: 498−503.

13. Doody MM, Linet MS, Glass AG et al. Risks of non-Hodgkin's lymphoma, multiple myeloma, and leukemia associated with common medications. *Epidemiology* 1996; **7**: 131−9.

14. Linet MS, Harlow SD, McLaughlin JK. A case−control study of multiple myeloma in whites: chronic antigenic stimulation, occupation, and drug use. *Cancer Res* 1987; **47**: 2978−81.

15. Watanabe T, Suzuki Y, Murakami S, Komatsu M. [Multiple myeloma in siblings]. *Rinsho Ketsueki [Jpn J Clin Hematol]* 1999; **40**: 135−9.

16. Brown LM, Linet MS, Greenberg RS et al. Multiple myeloma and family history of cancer among Blacks and Whites in the U.S. *Cancer* 1999; **85**: 2385−90.

17. Grosbois B, Jego P, Attal M et al. Familial multiple myeloma: report of fifteen families. *Br J Haematol* 1999; **105**: 768−70.

18. Ludwig H, Mayr W. Genetic aspects of susceptibility to multiple myeloma. *Blood* 1982;**59**:1286−91.

19. Kyle RA. Monoclonal gammopathy of undetermined significance. *Am J Med* 1978; **64**: 814−26.

20. Avet-Loiseau H, Facon T, Daviet A et al. 14q32 translocations and monosomy 13 observed in monoclonal gammopathy of undetermined significance delineate a multistep process for the oncogenesis of multiple myeloma. Intergroupe Francophone du Myelome. *Cancer Res* 1999; **59**: 4546−50.

21. Malik AA, Ganti AK, Potti A et al. Role of *Helicobacter pylori* infection in the incidence and clinical course of monoclonal gammopathy of undetermined significance. *Am J Gastroenterol* 2002; **97**: 1371−4.

22. Rajkumar SV, Kyle RA, Plevak MF et al. *Helicobacter pylori* infection and monoclonal gammopathy of undetermined significance. *Br J Haematol* 2002; **119**: 706−8.

23. Konrad RJ, Kricka LJ, Goodman DB et al. Myeloma-associated paraprotein directed against the HIV-1 p24 antigen in an HIV-1-seropositive patient. *N Engl J Med* 1993; **328**: 1817−19.

24. Sawyer JR, Lukacs JL, Munshi N et al. Identification of new nonrandom translocations in multiple myeloma with multicolor spectral karyotyping. *Blood* 1998; **92**: 4269−78.

25. Perez-Simon JA, Garcia-Sanz R, Tabernero MD et al. Prognostic value of numerical chromosome aberrations in multiple myeloma: a FISH analysis of 15 different chromosomes. *Blood* 1998; **91**: 3366−71.

26. Sawyer J, Waldron J, Jagannath S, Barlogie B. Cytogenetics findings in 200 patients with multiple myeloma. *Cancer Genet Cytogenet* 1995; **82**: 41−9.

27. Dewald GW, Kyle RA, Hicks GA, Greipp PR. The clinical significance of cytogenetic studies in 100 patients with multiple myeloma, plasma cell leukemia, or amyloidosis. *Blood* 1985; **66**: 380−90.

28. Gould J, Alexanian R, Goodacre A et al. Plasma cell karyotype in multiple myeloma. *Blood* 1988; **71**: 453−6.

29. Hallek M, Bergsagel LP, Anderson KD. Multiple myeloma: increasing evidence for a multistep transformation process. *Blood* 1998; **91**: 3−21.

30. Avet-Loiseau H, Li JY, Morineau N et al. Monosomy 13 is associated with the transition of monoclonal gammopathy of undetermined significance to multiple myeloma. Intergroupe Francophone du Myelome. *Blood* 1999; **94**: 2583−9.

31. Chesi M, Bergsagel PL, Brents LA et al. Dysregulation of cyclin D1 by translocation into an IgH γ switch region in two multiple myeloma cell lines. *Blood* 1996; **88**: 674−81.

32. Chesi M, Nardini E, Brents LA et al. Frequent translocation t(4;14)(p16.3;q32.3) in multiple myeloma is associated with increased expression and activating mutations of fibroblast growth factor receptor 3. *Nat Genet* 1997; **16**: 260−4.

33. Li Z, Zhu YX, Plowright EE et al. The myeloma-associated oncogene fibroblast growth factor receptor 3 is transforming in hematopoietic cells. *Blood* 2001; **97**: 2413−19.

34. Chesi M, Brents LA, Ely SA et al. Activated fibroblast growth factor receptor 3 is an oncogene that contributes to tumor progression in multiple myeloma. *Blood* 2001; **97**: 729−36.

35. Plowright EE, Li Z, Bergsagel PL et al. Ectopic expression of fibroblast growth factor receptor 3 promotes myeloma cell proliferation and prevents apoptosis. *Blood* 2000; **95**: 992−8.

36. Hart KC, Robertson SC, Kanemitsu MY et al. Transformation and Stat activation by derivatives of FGFR1, FGFR3, and FGFR4. *Oncogene* 2000; **19**: 3309−20.

37. Chesi M, Nardini E, Lim RS et al. The t(4;14) translocation in myeloma dysregulates both *FGFR3* and a novel gene, *MMSET*, resulting in *IgH/MMSET* hybrid transcripts. *Blood* 1998; **92**: 3025−34.

38. Chesi M, Bergsagel PL, Shonukan OO et al. Frequent dysregulation of the c-*maf* proto-oncogene at 16q23 by translocation to an Ig locus in multiple myeloma. *Blood* 1998; **91**: 4457−63.

39. Iida S, Rao PH, Butler M et al. Deregulation of *MUM1/IRF4* by chromosomal translocation in multiple myeloma. *Nat Genet* 1997; **17**: 226−30.

40. Mahmoud MS, Huang N, Nobuyoshi M et al. Altered expression of *Pax-5* gene in human myeloma cells. *Blood* 1996; **87**: 4311−15.

41. Tricot G, Sawyer JR, Jagannath S et al. The unique role of cytogenetics in the prognosis of patients with myeloma receiving high-dose therapy and autotransplants. *J Clin Oncol* 1997; **15**: 2659−66.

42. Dao DD, Sawyer JR, Epstein J et al. Deletion of the retinoblastoma gene in multiple myeloma. *Leukemia* 1994; **8**: 1280−4.

43. Urashima M, Ogata A, Chauhan D et al. Interleukin-6 promotes multiple myeloma cell growth via phosphorylation of retinoblastoma protein. *Blood* 1996; **88**: 2219−27.

44. Ng MH, Chung YF, Lo KW et al. Frequent hypermethylation of *p16* and *p15* genes in multiple myeloma. *Blood* 1997; **89**: 2500−6.

45. Tasaka T, Berenson J, Vescio R et al. Analysis of the *p16*$^{INK4A}$, *p15*$^{INK4B}$ and *p18*$^{INK4C}$ genes in multiple myeloma. *Br J Haematol* 1997; **96**: 98−102.

46. Urashima M, Teoh G, Ogata A et al. Characterization of p16$^{INK4A}$ expression in multiple myeloma and plasma cell leukemia. *Clin Cancer Res* 1997; **3**: 2173–9.

47. Kawano MM, Mahmoud MS, Ishikawa H. Cyclin D1 and p16$^{INK4A}$ are preferentially expressed in immature and mature myeloma cells, respectively. *Br J Haematol* 1997; **99**: 131–8.

48. Dhodapkar MV, Kelly T, Theus A et al. Elevated levels of shed syndecan-1 correlate with tumour mass and decreased matrix metalloproteinase-9 activity in the serum of patients with multiple myeloma [published erratum appears in Br J Haematol 1998 May;101(2):398]. *Br J Haematol* 1997; **99**: 368–71 [Erratum 1998; **101**: 398].

49. Dhodapkar MV, Weinstein R, Tricot G et al. Biologic and therapeutic determinants of bone mineral density in multiple myeloma. *Leuk Lymphoma* 1998; **32**: 121–7.

50. Yang Y, Yaccoby S, Liu W et al. Soluble syndecan-1 promotes growth of myeloma tumors in vivo. *Blood* 2002; **100**: 610–17.

51. Chauhan D, Uchiyama H, Urashima M et al. Regulation of interleukin-6 in multiple myeloma and bone marrow stromal cells. *Stem Cells* 1995; **15**: 35–9.

52. Hideshima T, Chauhan D, Schlossman R et al. The role of tumor necrosis factor α in the pathophysiology of human multiple myeloma: therapeutic applications. *Oncogene* 2001; **20**: 4519–27.

53. Dankar B, Padro T, Leo R et al. Vascular endothelial growth factor and interleukin-6 in paracrine tumor–stromal cell interactions in multiple myeloma. *Blood* 2000; **95**: 2630–6.

54. Hideshima T, Chauhan D, Hayashi T et al. The biological sequelae of stromal cell-derived factor-1α in multiple myeloma. *Mol Cancer Ther* 2002; **1**: 539–44.

55. Tai YT, Podar K, Catley L et al. Insulin-like growth factor-1 induces adhesion and migration in human multiple myeloma cells via activation of β$_1$-integrin and phosphatidylinositol 3′-kinase/AKT signaling. *Cancer Res* 2003; **63**: 5850–8.

56. Vacca A, Ribatti D, Roncali L et al. Bone marrow angiogenesis and progression in multiple myeloma. *Br J Haematol* 1994; **87**: 503–8.

57. Rajkumar SV, Fonseca R, Witzig TE. Bone marrow angiogenesis in patients achieving complete response after stem cell transplantation for multiple myeloma. *Leukemia* 1999; **13**: 469–72.

58. Rajkumar SV, Mesa RA, Fonseca R et al. Bone marrow angiogenesis in 400 patients with monoclonal gammopathy of undetermined significance, multiple myeloma, and primary amyloidosis. *Clin Cancer Res* 2002; **8**: 2210–16.

59. Munshi NC, Wilson C. Increased bone marrow microvessel density in newly diagnosed multiple myeloma carries a poor prognosis. *Semin Oncol* 2001; **28**: 565–9.

60. Kumar S, Fonseca R, Dispenzieri A et al. Bone marrow angiogenesis in multiple myeloma: effect of therapy. *Br J Haematol* 2002; **119**: 665–71.

61. Bellamy WT, Richter L, Frutiger Y, Grogan TM. Expression of vascular endothelial growth factor and its receptors in hematopoietic malignancies. *Cancer Res* 1999; **59**: 728–33.

62. Seidel C, Borset M, Turesson I et al. Elevated serum concentrations of hepatocyte growth factor in patients with multiple myeloma. The Nordic Myeloma Study Group. *Blood* 1998; **91**: 806–12.

63. Urashima M, Ogata A, Chauhan D et al. Transforming growth factor-β1: differential effects on multiple myeloma versus normal B cells. *Blood* 1996; **87**: 1928–38.

64. Brenne AT, Baade Ro T, Waage A et al. Interleukin-21 is a growth and survival factor for human myeloma cells. *Blood* 2002; **99**: 3756–62.

65. Mitsiades CS, Mitsiades N, Poulaki V et al. Activation of NF-κB and upregulation of intracellular anti-apoptotic proteins via the IGF-1/Akt signaling in human multiple myeloma cells: therapeutic implications. *Oncogene* 2002; **21**: 5673–83.

66. Qiang YW, Kopantzev E, Rudikoff S. Insulinlike growth factor-I signaling in multiple myeloma: downstream elements, functional correlates, and pathway crosstalk. *Blood* 2002; **99**: 4138–46.

67. Akiyama M, Hideshima T, Hayashi T et al. Cytokines modulate telomerase activity in a human multiple myeloma cell line. *Cancer Res* 2002; **62**: 3876–82.

68. Qiang YW, Yao L, Tosato G, Rudikoff S. Insulin-like growth factor I induces migration and invasion of human multiple myeloma cells. *Blood* 2004; **103**: 301–8.

69. Podar K, Tai YT, Davies FE et al. Vascular endothelial growth factor triggers signaling cascades mediating multiple myeloma cell growth and migration. *Blood* 2001; **98**: 428–35.

70. Podar K, Tai YT, Lin BK et al. Vascular endothelial growth factor-induced migration of multiple myeloma cells is associated with β$_1$ integrin- and phosphatidylinositol 3-kinase-dependent PKCα activation. *J Biol Chem* 2002; **277**: 7875–81.

71. Gupta D, Treon SP, Shima Y et al. Adherence of multiple myeloma cells to bone marrow stromal cells upregulates vascular endothelial growth factor secretion: therapeutic applications. *Leukemia* 2001; **15**: 1950–61.

72. Lin B, Podar K, Gupta D et al. The vascular endothelial growth factor receptor tyrosine kinase inhibitor PTK787/ZK222584 inhibits growth and migration of multiple myeloma cells in the bone marrow microenvironment. *Cancer Res* 2002; **62**: 5019–26.

73. Gieseler F, Nussler V. Cellular resistance mechanisms with impact on the therapy of multiple myeloma. *Leukemia* 1998; **12**: 1009–12.

74. Pilarski LM, Yatscoff RW, Murphy GF, Belch AR. Drug resistance in multiple myeloma: cyclosporin A analogues and their metabolites as potential chemosensitizers. *Leukemia* 1998; **12**: 505–9.

75. Sonneveld P, Marie JP, Huisman C et al. Reversal of multidrug resistance by SDZ PSC 833, combined with VAD (vincristine, doxorubicin, dexamethasone) in refractory multiple myeloma. A phase I study. *Leukemia* 1996; **10**: 1741–50.

76. Sikic BI. Pharmacologic approaches to reversing multidrug resistance. *Semin Hematol* 1997; **34**(4 Suppl 5): 40–7.

77. Abbaszadegan MR, Futscher BW, Klimecki WT et al. Analysis of multidrug resistance-associated protein (MRP) messenger RNA in normal and malignant hematopoietic cells. *Cancer Res* 1994; **54**: 4676–9.

78. Filipits M, Drach J, Pohl G et al. Expression of the lung resistance protein predicts poor outcome in patients with multiple myeloma. *Clin Cancer Res* 1999; **5**: 2426–30.

79. Raaijmakers HG, Izquierdo MA, Lokhorst HM et al. Lung-resistance-related protein expression is a negative predictive factor for response to conventional low but not to intensified dose alkylating chemotherapy in multiple myeloma. *Blood* 1998; **91**: 1029–36.

80. Hjorth M, Hellquist L, Holmberg E et al. Initial versus deferred melphalan–prednisone therapy for asymptomatic multiple myeloma stage I – a randomized study. Myeloma Group of Western Sweden. *Eur J Haematol* 1993; **50**: 95–102.

81. Blade J, Samson D, Reece D et al. Criteria for evaluating disease response and progression in patients with multiple myeloma treated by high-dose therapy and haemopoietic stem cell transplantation. Myeloma Subcommittee of the EBMT. European Group for Blood and Marrow Transplantation. *Br J Haematol* 1998; **102**: 1115–23.

82. Boccadoro M, Marmont F, Tribalto M et al. Early responder myeloma: kinetic studies identify a patient subgroup characterized by very poor prognosis. *J Clin Oncol* 1989; **7**: 119–25.

83. Latreille J, Barlogie B, Johnston D et al. Ploidy and proliferative characteristics in monoclonal gammopathies. *Blood* 1982; **59**: 43–51.

84. Boccadoro M, Marmont F, Tribalto M et al. Multiple myeloma: VMCP/VBAP alternating combination chemotherapy is not superior to melphalan and prednisone even in high-risk patients. *J Clin Oncol* 1991; **9**: 444–8.

85. Durie BG, Salmon SE, Moon TE. Pretreatment tumor mass, cell kinetics, and prognosis in multiple myeloma. *Blood* 1980; **55**: 364–72.

86. McElwain T, Powles R. High-dose intravenous melphalan for plasma-cell leukemia and myeloma. *Lancet* 1983; **i**: 822–4.

87. McElwain TJ, Gore ME, Meldrum M et al. VAMP followed by high dose melphalan and autologous bone marrow transplantation for multiple myeloma. *Bone Marrow Transplant* 1989; **4**(Suppl 4): 109–12.

88. Attal M, Harousseau JL, Stoppa AM et al. A prospective, randomized trial of autologous bone marrow transplantation and chemotherapy in multiple myeloma. Intergroupe Français du Myelome. *N Engl J Med* 1996; **335**: 91–7.

89. Child JA, Morgan GJ, Davies FE et al. High-dose chemotherapy with hematopoietic stem-cell rescue for multiple myeloma. *N Engl J Med* 2003; **348**: 1875–83.

90. Blade J, Surenda A, Diaz-Mediavilla J et al. High-dose therapy autotransplantation/intensification vs continued conventional chemotherapy in multiple myeloma patients responding to initial treatment chemotherapy. Results of a prospective randomized trial from the Spanish Cooperative group PETHEMA. *Blood* 2001; **98**: 815a.

91. Fermand JP, Ravaud P, Chevret S et al. High-dose therapy and autologous peripheral blood stem cell transplantation in multiple myeloma: up-front or rescue treatment? Results of a multicenter sequential randomized clinical trial. *Blood* 1998; **92**: 3131–6.

92. Barlogie B, Kyle RA, Anderson KC et al. Comparable survival in multiple myeloma (MM) with high dose therapy (HDT) employing mel 140 mg/m² + TBI 12 Gy autotransplants versus standard dose therapy VBMCP and no benefit from interferon (IFN) maintenance: results of Intergroup trial S9321. *Blood* 2003; **102**: 42a.

93. Ventura GJ, Barlogie B, Hester JP et al. High dose cyclophosphamide, BCNU and VP-16 with autologous blood stem cell support for refractory multiple myeloma. *Bone Marrow Transplant* 1990; **5**: 265–8.

94. Adkins DR, Salzman D, Boldt D et al. Phase I trial of dacarbazine with cyclophosphamide, carmustine, etoposide,

and autologous stem-cell transplantation in patients with lymphoma and multiple myeloma. *J Clin Oncol* 1994; **12**: 1890–901.

95. Bjorkstrand B. European Group for Blood and Marrow Transplantation Registry studies in multiple myeloma. *Semin Hematol* 2001; **38**: 219–25.

96. Desikan KR, Tricot G, Dhodapkar M et al. Melphalan plus total body irradiation (MEL-TBI) or cyclophosphamide (MEL-CY) as a conditioning regimen with second autotransplant in responding patients with myeloma is inferior compared to historical controls receiving tandem transplants with melphalan alone. *Bone Marrow Transplant* 2000; **25**: 483–7.

97. Bjorkstrand B, Ljungman P, Bird JM et al. Autologous stem cell transplantation in multiple myeloma: results of the European Group for Bone Marrow Transplantation. *Stem Cells* 1995; **13**(Suppl 2): 140–6.

98. Moreau P, Facon T, Attal M et al. Comparison of 200 mg/m² melphalan and 8 Gy total body irradiation plus 140 mg/m² melphalan as conditioning regimens for peripheral blood stem cell transplantation in patients with newly diagnosed multiple myeloma: final analysis of the Intergroupe Francophone du Myelome 9502 randomized trial. *Blood* 2002; **99**: 731–5.

99. Harousseau JL, Milpied N, Laporte JP et al. Double-intensive therapy in high-risk multiple myeloma. *Blood* 1992; **79**: 2827–33.

100. Barlogie B, Jagannath S, Desikan KR et al. Total therapy with tandem transplants for newly diagnosed multiple myeloma. *Blood* 1999; **93**: 55–65.

101. Attal M, Harousseau JL, Facon T et al. Single versus double autologous stem-cell transplantation for multiple myeloma. *N Engl J Med* 2003; **349**: 2495–502.

102. Vesole DH, Barlogie B, Jagannath S et al. High-dose therapy for refractory multiple myeloma: improved prognosis with better supportive care and double transplants. *Blood* 1994; **84**: 950–6.

103. Gertz MA, Lacy MQ, Inwards DJ et al. Early harvest and late transplantation as an effective therapeutic strategy in multiple myeloma. *Bone Marrow Transplant* 1999; **23**: 221–6.

104. Desikan KR, Barlogie B, Jagannath S et al. Comparable engraftment kinetics following peripheral blood stem cell infusion mobilized with G-CSF with or without cyclophosphamide in multiple myeloma. *J Clin Oncol* 1998; **14**: 1547–53.

105. Gazitt Y, Tian E, Barlogie B et al. Differential mobilization of myeloma cells and normal hematopoietic stem cells in multiple myeloma after treatment with cyclophosphamide and granulocyte–macrophage colony-stimulating factor. *Blood* 1996; **87**: 805–11.

106. Anderson KC, Andersen J, Soiffer R et al. Monoclonal antibody-purged bone marrow transplantation therapy for multiple myeloma. *Blood* 1993; **82**: 2568–76.

107. Stewart AK, Vescio R, Schiller G et al. Purging of autologous peripheral-blood stem cells using CD34 selection does not improve overall or progression-free survival after high-dose chemotherapy for multiple myeloma: results of a multicenter randomized controlled trial. *J Clin Oncol* 2001; **19**: 3771–9.

108. Tricot G, Gazitt Y, Leemhuis T et al. Collection, tumor contamination, and engraftment kinetics of highly purified hematopoietic progenitor cells to support high dose therapy in multiple myeloma. *Blood* 1998; **91**: 4489–95.

109. Siegel DS, Desikan KR, Mehta J et al. Age is not a prognostic variable with autotransplants for multiple myeloma. *Blood* 1999; **93**: 51–4.

110. Badros A, Barlogie B, Siegel E et al. Autologous stem cell transplantation in elderly multiple myeloma patients over the age of 70 years. *Br J Haematol* 2001; **114**: 600–7.

111. Tricot G, Alberts DS, Johnson C et al. Safety of autotransplants with high-dose melphalan in renal failure: a pharmacokinetic and toxicity study. *Clin Cancer Res* 1996; **2**: 947–52.

112. Badros A, Barlogie B, Siegel E et al. Results of autologous stem cell transplant in multiple myeloma patients with renal failure. *Br J Haematol* 2001; **114**: 822–9.

113. Browman G, Bergsagel D, Sicheri D et al. Randomized trial of interferon maintenance in multiple myeloma: a study of the National Cancer Institute of Canada Clinical Trials Group. *J Clin Oncol* 1995; **13**: 2354–60.

114. Berenson JR, Crowley JJ, Grogan TM et al. Maintenance therapy with alternate-day prednisone improves survival in multiple myeloma patients. *Blood* 2002; **99**: 3163–8.

115. Bensinger WI, Demirer T, Buckner CD et al. Syngeneic marrow transplantation in patients with multiple myeloma. *Bone Marrow Transplant* 1996; **18**: 527–31.

116. Gahrton G, Svensson H, Bjorkstrand B et al. Syngeneic transplantation in multiple myeloma – a case matched comparison with autologous and allogeneic transplantation. *Bone Marrow Transplant* 1999; **24**: 741–5.

117. Bjorkstrand B, Ljungman P, Svensson H et al. Allogenic bone marrow transplantation versus autologous stem cell transplantation in multiple myeloma: a retrospective case-matched study from the European Group for Blood and Marrow Transplantation. *Blood* 1996; **88**: 4711–18.

118. Alyea EP, Anderson KC. Allotransplantation for multiple myeloma. *Cancer J* 2001; **7**: 166–74.

119. Mehta J, Tricot G, Jagannath S et al. Salvage autologous or allogeneic transplantation for multiple myeloma refractory to or relapsing after a first-line autograft? *Bone Marrow Transplant* 1998; **21**: 887–92.

120. Tricot G, Vesole DH, Jagannath S et al. Graft-versus-myeloma effect: proof of principle. *Blood* 1996; **87**: 1196–8.

121. Lokhorst HM, Schattenberg A, Cornelissen JJ et al. Donor lymphocyte infusions for relapsed multiple myeloma after allogeneic stem-cell transplantation: predictive factors for response and long-term outcome. *Blood* 2000; **18**: 3031–7.

122. Salama M, Nevill T, Marcellus D et al. Donor leukocyte infusions for multiple myeloma. *Bone Marrow Transplant* 2000; **26**: 1179–84.

123. Munshi NC, Govindarajan R, Drake R et al. Thymidine kinase (TK) gene-transduced human lymphocytes can be highly purified, remain fully functional and are killed efficiently with ganciclovir. *Blood* 1997; **89**: 1334–40.

124. Soiffer RJ, Alyea EP, Hochberg E et al. Randomized trial of CD8+ T-cell depletion in the prevention of graft-versus-host disease associated with donor lymphocyte infusion. *Biol Blood Marrow Transplant* 2002; **8**: 625–32.

125. Storb R, Yu C, Zaucha JM et al. Stable mixed hematopoietic chimerism in dogs given donor antigen, CTLA4Ig, and 100 cGy total body irradiation before and pharmacologic immunosuppression after marrow transplant. *Blood* 1999; **94**: 2523–9.

126. Badros A, Barlogie B, Morris C et al. High response rate in refractory and poor-risk multiple myeloma after allotrans-

127. Giralt S, Aleman A, Anagnostopoulos A et al. Fludarabine/melphalan conditioning for allogeneic transplantation in patients with multiple myeloma. *Bone Marrow Transplant* 2002; **30**: 367–73.

128. Maloney DG, Molina AJ, Sahebi F et al. Allografting with nonmyeloablative conditioning following cytoreductive autografts for the treatment of patients with multiple myeloma. *Blood* 2003; **102**: 3447–54.

129. Osterborg A, Yi Q, Henriksson L et al. Idiotype immunization combined with granulocyte–macrophage colony-stimulating factor in myeloma patients induced type I, major histocompatibility complex-restricted, CD8- and CD4-specific T-cell responses. *Blood* 1998; **91**: 2459–66.

130. Kwak LW, Sternas L, Jagannath S et al. T-cell responses elicited by immunization of multiple myeloma patients with idiotypic M-protein plus GM-CSF in remission after autologous transplantation (PSCT). *Blood* 1997; **90**: 579a.

131. Yi Q, Desikan KR, Barlogie BB, Munshi NC. Optimizing dendritic cell-based immunotherapy in multiple myeloma. *Br J Hematol* 2002; in Press.

132. Hideshima T, Chauhan D, Shima Y et al. Thalidomide and its analogs overcome drug resistance of human multiple myeloma cells to conventional therapy. *Blood* 2000; **96**: 2943–50.

133. Raje N, Anderson K. Thalidomide – a revival story. *N Engl J Med* 1999; **341**: 1606–9.

134. LeBlanc R, Hideshima T, Catley LP et al. Immunomodulatory drug (Revamid) co-stimulates T cells via the B7–CD28 pathway. *Blood* 2003; in press.

135. Hayashi T, Hideshima T, Akiyama M et al. Ex vivo induction of multiple myeloma-specific cytotoxic T lymphocytes. *Blood* 2003; **102**: 1435–42.

136. Barlogie B, Desikan R, Eddlemon P et al. Extended survival in advanced and refractory multiple myeloma after single-agent thalidomide: identification of prognostic factors in a phase 2 study of 169 patients. *Blood* 2001; **98**: 492–4.

137. Singhal S, Mehta J, Desikan R et al. Antitumor activity of thalidomide in refractory multiple myeloma. *N Engl J Med* 1999; **341**: 1565–71.

138. Thomas DA, Estey E, Giles FJ et al. Single agent thalidomide in patients with relapsed or refractory acute myeloid leukaemia. *Br J Haematol* 2003; **123**: 436–41.

139. Schey SA, Cavenagh J, Johnson R et al. An UK Myeloma Forum phase II study of thalidomide; long term follow-up and recommendations for treatment. *Leuk Res* 2003; **27**: 909–14.

140. Abdalla SH, Mahmoud S. Thalidomide in relapsed or refractory multiple myeloma: How much and for how long? *Leuk Lymphoma* 2003; **44**: 989–91.

141. Buchler T, Hermosilla M, Ferra C et al. Outcome and toxicity of salvage treatment on patients relapsing after autologous hematopoietic stem cell transplantation – experience from a single center. *Hematology* 2003; **8**: 145–50.

142. Mileshkin L, Biagi JJ, Mitchell P et al. Multicenter phase 2 trial of thalidomide in relapsed/refractory multiple myeloma: adverse prognostic impact of advanced age. *Blood* 2003; **102**: 69–77.

143. Kumar S, Gertz MA, Dispenzieri A et al. Response rate, durability of response, and survival after thalidomide

therapy for relapsed multiple myeloma. *Mayo Clin Proc* 2003; **78**: 34–9.

144. Neben K, Moehler T, Benner A et al. Dose-dependent effect of thalidomide on overall survival in relapsed multiple myeloma. *Clin Cancer Res* 2002; **8**: 3377–82.

145. Johnston RE, Abdalla SH. Thalidomide in low doses is effective for the treatment of resistant or relapsed multiple myeloma and for plasma cell leukaemia. *Leuk Lymphoma* 2002; **43**: 351–4.

146. Ahmad I, Islam T, Chanan-Khan A et al. Thalidomide as salvage therapy for VAD-refractory multiple myeloma prior to autologous PBSCT. *Bone Marrow Transplant* 2002; **29**: 577–80.

147. Zangari M, Anaissie E, Barlogie B et al. Increased risk of deep-vein thrombosis in patients with multiple myeloma receiving thalidomide and chemotherapy. *Blood* 2001; **98**: 1614–15.

148. Weber D, Rankin K, Gavino M et al. Thalidomide alone or with dexamethasone for previously untreated multiple myeloma. *J Clin Oncol* 2003; **21**: 16–99.

149. Rajkumar SV, Hayman S, Gertz MA et al. Combination therapy with thalidomide plus dexamethasone for newly diagnosed myeloma. *J Clin Oncol* 2002; **20**: 4319–23.

150. Palumbo A, Bertola A, Musto P et al. Oral melphalan, prednisone and thalidomide for newly diagnosed myeloma. *Blood* 2003; **102**: 148a.

150a. Dinopoulos, MA, Zervas K, Kouvatseas G et al. Thalidomide and dexamethasone combination for refractory multiple myeloma. *Ann Oncol* 2001; **12**: 991–5.

151. Agrawal NR, Hussein MA, Elson P et al. Pegylated doxorubicin (D), vincristine (V), reduced frequency dexamethasone (D) and thalidomide (T) (DVd-T) in newly diagnosed (Nmm) and relapsed/refractory (Rmm) multiple myeloma patients. *Blood* 2003; **102**: 831a.

152. Richardson PG, Schlossman RL, Weller E et al. Immunomodulatory drug CC-5013 overcomes drug resistance and is well tolerated in patients with relapsed multiple myeloma. *Blood* 2002; **100**: 3063–7.

153. Hideshima T, Anderson KC. Molecular mechanisms of novel therapeutic approaches for multiple myeloma. *Nat Rev Cancer* 2002; **2**: 927–37.

154. Hideshima T, Chauhan D, Richardson P et al. NF-κB as a therapeutic target in multiple myeloma. *J Biol Chem* 2002; **277**: 16639–47.

155. Hideshima T, Richardson P, Chauhan D et al. The proteasome inhibitor PS-341 inhibits growth, induces apoptosis, and overcomes drug resistance in human multiple myeloma cells. *Cancer Res* 2001; **61**: 3071–6.

156. Hideshima T, Richardson P, Chauhan D et al. The proteosome inhibitor PS341 overcomes apoptotic resistance mechanisms in human multiple myeloma cells. Submitted.

157. Mitsiades N, Mitsiades CS, Poulaki V et al. Molecular sequelae of proteasome inhibition in human multiple myeloma cells. *Proc Natl Acad Sci USA* 2002; **99**: 14374–9.

158. Mitsiades N, Mitsiades CS, Poulaki V et al. Biologic seque-lae of nuclear factor-κB blockade in multiple myeloma: therapeutic applications. *Blood* 2002; **99**: 4079–86.

159. Richardson PG, Barlogie B, Berenson J et al. A phase 2 study of bortezomib in relapsed, refractory myeloma. *N Engl J Med* 2003; **348**: 2609–17.

160. Mitsiades N, Mitsiades CS, Richardson PG et al. The proteasome inhibitor PS-341 potentiates sensitivity of multiple myeloma cells to conventional chemotherapeutic agents: therapeutic applications. *Blood* 2003; **101**: 2377–80.

161. Hayashi T, Hideshima T, Akiyama M et al. Arsenic trioxide inhibits growth of human multiple myeloma cells in the bone marrow microenvironment. *Mol Cancer Ther* 2002; **1**: 851–60.

162. McCafferty-Grad J, Bahlis NJ, Krett N et al. Arsenic trioxide uses caspase-dependent and caspase-independent death pathways in myeloma cells. *Mol Cancer Ther* 2003; **2**: 1155–64.

163. Munshi NC, Tricot G, Desikan R et al. Clinical activity of arsenic trioxide for the treatment of multiple myeloma. *Leukemia* 2002; **16**: 1835–7.

164. Bahlis NJ, McCafferty-Grad J, Jordan-McMurry I et al. Feasibility and correlates of arsenic trioxide combined with ascorbic acid-mediated depletion of intracellular glutathione for the treatment of relapsed/refractory multiple myeloma. *Clin Cancer Res* 2002; **8**: 3658–68.

165. Berenson JR, Lichtenstein A, Porter L et al. Efficacy of pamidronate in reducing skeletal events in patients with advanced multiple myeloma. *N Engl J Med* 1996; **334**: 488–93.

166. Apperley JF, Croucher PI. Bisphosphonates in multiple myeloma. *Pathol Biol* 1999; **47**: 178–81.

167. Berenson JR, Lipton A. Bisphosphonates in the treatment of malignant bone disease. *Annu Rev Med* 1999; **50**: 237–48.

168. Shipman CM, Croucher PI, Russell RG et al. The bisphosphonate incadronate (YM175) causes apoptosis of human myeloma cells in vitro by inhibiting the mevalonate pathway. *Cancer Res* 1998; **58**: 5294–7.

169. Berenson JR, Lichtenstein A, Porter L et al. Long-term pamidronate treatment of advanced multiple myeloma patients reduces skeletal events. Myeloma Aredia Study Group. *J Clin Oncol* 1998; **16**: 593–602.

170. Aparicio A, Gardner A, Tu Y et al. In vitro cytoreductive effects on multiple myeloma cells induced by bisphosphonates. *Leukemia* 1998; **12**: 220–9.

171. Shipman CM, Rogers MJ, Apperley JF et al. Anti-tumour activity of bisphosphonates in human myeloma cells. *Leuk Lymphoma* 1998; **32**: 129–38.

172. Yaccoby S, Pearse RN, Johnson CL et al. Myeloma interacts with the bone marrow microenvironment to induce osteoclastogenesis and is dependent on osteoclast activity. *Br J Haematol* 2002; **116**: 278–90.

173. Dhodapkar MV, Singh J, Mehta J et al. Anti-myeloma activity of pamidronate in vivo. *Br J Haematol* 1998; **103**: 530–2.

# 35 Hodgkin lymphoma

**Karolin Behringer, Volker Diehl, and Andreas Engert**

## Introduction

Hodgkin lymphoma (HL, Hodgkin's disease) is a malignant hematopoietic disease with annual incidence of 2.2 per 100 000 for women and 3.3 per 100 000 for men.[1] Histomorphologically, HL is characterized by Hodgkin (H) and Reed–Sternberg (RS) cells surrounded by a variety of reactive bystander cells such as lymphocytes, macrophages, neutrophils, histiocytes, and plasma cells. For more than a century, HL was regarded as a chronic inflammatory disorder, which is reflected in the old term 'lymphogranulomatosis'. After the detection of aneuploidy and monoclonality and the successful transplantation of H-RS cells into immunocompromised animals, HL is now considered a truly malignant disease.

The origin of the characteristic H-RS cells has been the subject of debate for a long time. Immunophenotyping and genetic analyses have demonstrated that up to 90% of cases have lymphocytic markers.[2,3] H-RS cells consistently express activation antigens such as CD25, which forms the light chain of the interleukin (IL)-2 receptor, and CD30, originally detected by the monoclonal antibody Ki-1. Cloning of the CD30 molecule and its ligand CD30L demonstrated CD30/CD30L as new members of the tumor necrosis factor (TNF) receptor and ligand superfamily.[4] Taken together, these data point towards a lymphoid origin of H-RS cells. This was further underlined by single-cell DNA sequence analysis of immunoglobulin (Ig) gene rearrangements amplified from single, micromanipulated H-RS cells, which showed that these cells largely represent clonal populations. The Ig gene rearrangements in H-RS cells strongly suggest B cells as their precursors.[5]

A possible etiological role of the Epstein–Barr virus (EBV) in HL has been discussed for many years. Data indicate that EBV is present in approximately 40% of cases[6,7] (see Chapter 16). Thus, chronic viral infection, activation of cellular oncogenes, loss of tumor suppressor genes, and deregulation of cytokines may be factors involved in the pathogenesis of this disease.[8,9]

## Histopathology and correlation with age

The diagnosis of HL is based on morphological and immunohistochemical investigations. One of the most important criterion is the detection of H-RS cells in histological sections. In addition to the classical H-RS cells, another characteristic feature is the composition of the surrounding lymphoid and histiocytic cells. Usually, H-RS cells, which are considered the true tumor cells, represent less than 1% of the whole infiltrate. Lymphocytes, histiocytes, and other reactive cells constitute the overwhelming cell population.

According to histopathology, the bulk of classical HL can be subdivided into nodular sclerosis (NS) and mixed-cellularity (MC). NSHL shows sclerotic bands surrounding nodules in which lacunar cells are visible. These lacunar cells are variants of H-RS cells. NSHL occurs at a higher frequency among young adults and remains constant at a significantly lower level in the group over 30 years of age. According to the World Health Organization (WHO) classification, the new HL subtype lymphocyte-rich classical HL (LRCHL) and nodular lymphocyte-predominant HL (LPHL) are diagnosed at a frequency of 3–5%, and lymphocyte-depleted HL (LDHL) even less, at a frequency of less than 1%. Cases that do not fit into LP, NS, or LD subtypes or show partial infiltration are termed MCHL; their occurrence increases with age.[10,11]

LPHL is now generally recognized as a distinct clinicopathological entity. Histologically, LPHL is characterized by large nodules composed of small lymphoid cells, usually mixed with groups of epitheloid cells. Classical H-RS cells are rare, whereas a variety of similar cells referred to as L&H cells are scattered in the nodular infiltrations. In addition to L&H and a few H-RS cells, the cellular composition, including the nodular destruction of lymph node architecture, forms a characteristic tumor mass relatively sharply demarcated from the reactive tissue. Most LPHL cases are of the nodular form. The rare cases of completely or almost completely diffuse infiltration can cause difficulties in the differential diagnosis between LPHL, T-cell-rich large B-cell lymphoma, peripheral T-cell lymphoma, and classical HL. LPHL cells express the CD20 antigen in up to 98% of cases and the CD79a antigen in 80%. In contrast, classical HL cells stain positive for CD30 in nearly all cases and for CD15 in 74% of cases.

## Staging

A clinical-stage classification serves as a guide in determining the prognosis and treatment of the disease. The extent of HL is classified using the four-stage Ann Arbor classification. The absence (A) or presence (B) of systemic symptoms (fever, weight loss, and night sweats), introduced in 1965 by the Rye staging classification, is also used for staging HL.

At the Ann Arbor meeting, it was decided to classify limited direct extension from an adjacent nodal site as local extranodal extension (E).[12] The classification assumes that the local extension has a prognosis equivalent to that of nodal disease of the same anatomical extent.[13] Patients with several extranodal sites are classified in stage IV. At the time of the Ann Arbor meeting, staging laparotomy was used routinely. Since then, staging laparotomy has been omitted from most diagnostic procedures. Thus, clinical staging has become the mainstay for staging this disease. Clinical stages (CS) are based on the results of physical examination, chest X-ray, contrast-enhanced computed tomography (CT) scan (neck, chest, and abdomen), abdominal ultrasound, skeletal and/or bone marrow radionuclide imaging, and bone marrow biopsy. A few additional recommendations were made at the Cotswold meeting in 1989.[14] The classification included prognostic factors such as mediastinal mass, other bulky nodal disease, and the extent of subdiaphragmatic disease (Table 35.1).

Table 35.2 outlines the recommended staging procedures. Recommendations for staging should emphasize a careful history and physical examination to identify the presence of B symptoms and to determine whether palpable adenopathy is present. Diagnostic imaging methods must include chest X-ray, and CT scans of the neck, thorax, abdomen, and pelvis. Hematological studies require a complete blood count. All patients should have bone marrow aspiration and biopsy as well as bone marrow and/or skeletal radionuclide imaging performed. Biochemical tests should include liver function and renal function tests. Additional optional procedures, which may also be of value in selected cases, include positron-emission tomography (PET) and magnetic resonance imaging (MRI).

### Table 35.1 The 'Cotswold' staging classification

| Stage | Defining features |
|---|---|
| I | Involvement of a single lymph node region or lymphoid structure (e.g. spleen, thymus, Waldeyer's ring) |
| II | Involvement of two or more lymph node regions or lymphoid structures on the same side of the diaphragm |
| III | Involvement of lymph node regions or lymphoid structures on both sides of the diaphragm: |
| | III$_1$ with or without splenic hilar, celiac, or portal nodes |
| | III$_2$ with para-aortic, iliac, mesenteric nodes |
| IV | Involvement of extranodal site(s) beyond that designated 'E' |

**Modifying characteristics**

| | |
|---|---|
| A | No symptoms |
| B | Fever, drenching sweats, weight loss |
| X | Bulky disease: >one-third widening of mediastinum >10 cm maximum dimension of nodal mass |
| E | Involvement of single extranodal site, contiguous with or proximal to known nodal site |
| CS | Clinical stage |
| PS | Pathological stage |

### Table 35.2 Recommended procedures for staging of patients with Hodgkin lymphoma

**History and examination**

B symptoms: weight loss >10% during 6 months, documented fever, night sweats

**Hematology**
Complete blood count
Erythrocyte sedimentation rate (ESR)
Bone marrow biopsy

**Radiographic procedures**
Chest X-ray
CT of neck and chest
CT of abdomen and pelvis
Ultrasound scanning
Bone scans

**Under special circumstances**
Magnetic resonance imaging (MRI)
Gallium scan
Positron-emission tomography (PET)

# Staging laparotomy

In the past, staging laparotomy was routinely performed in supradiaphragmatic clinical stage I and II patients. It was restricted to those patients for whom management decisions depended on the identification of subdiaphragmatic disease. Many centers found that after laparotomy 20–30% of patients had to be upstaged.[15,16] For the majority of patients, it became apparent that laparotomy had disclosed occult disease in the spleen, which underlined the inaccuracy of the radiological methods at that time in assessing the spleen. Arguments against staging laparotomy included the severe side-effects of the procedure. The overall mortality rate ranged from 1.5% to 3.0% after splenectomy, including deaths from overwhelming sepsis (OPSI syndrome). The procedure became less frequently used with the introduction of effective chemotherapy programs for the majority of patients in early stages.

The routine use of laparotomy for staging has subsequently become obsolete.[17]

# Treatment groups and prognostic factors

Disease stage is the principal factor in selecting treatment strategies for patients with HL. Since the identification of generally applicable risk factors at diagnosis would allow a more individually tailored treatment strategy, several analyses assessing risk factors have been performed. Based on these data, the German Hodgkin Lymphoma Study Group (GHSG) defines three prognostic groups:

1.  *Early stages:* patients in stages I and II without risk factors such as large mediastinal mass, extranodal disease, ESR ≥50 in A stages or >30 in B stages, or three or more lymph node areas involved.
2.  *Intermediate stages:* patients in stages I and IIA with one or more of the following risk factors: large mediastinal mass, extranodal disease, ESR ≥50 in A stages or >30 in B stages, or three or more involved lymph node areas. Patients in stage IIB with ESR ≥30 and/or three or more involved lymph-node areas are also stratified into the intermediate-risk group.
3.  *Advanced stages:* all patients in stages III and IV, and selected IIB patients having large mediastinal mass and/or extranodal disease.

In an attempt to more precisely define the risk of patients with advanced disease treated with COPP/ABVD-based regimens, Hasenclever and Diehl[18] analyzed a variety of clinical and laboratory parameters to construct a prognostic index. The International Prognostic Score (IPS) consists of serum albumin <4 g/dl, hemoglobin < 10.5 g/dl, male sex, stage IV disease, age 45 years or older years or older, white blood cell count (WBC) 15 000/mm³ or higher, and lymphocyte count less than 600/mm³ or less than 8% of WBC.

# Treatment

## Early stages

Radiotherapy using the extended-field (EF) technique was until recently considered the treatment of choice for patients with early-stage HL. As long-term follow-up has increased, it has become clear that EF radiotherapy results in significant long-term toxicity. Those who receive mediastinal radiation have an increased risk of experiencing a fatal myocardial infarction.[19] Radiotherapy is also associated with an increased risk of second solid tumors in or adjacent to radiation fields. The cumulative risk varies between 7.8% and 23.3% at 15 to 25 years after first-line treatment; and shows no signs of leveling off even into the third decade after treatment.[20–23]

Thus, in order to avoid long-term toxicities of the EF irradiation and to reduce the rate of relapse after irradiation alone, it was the aim of randomized clinical studies to evaluate the addition of chemotherapy in order to reduce the extent of radiotherapy.[24]

Kaplan[25] demonstrated that the likelihood of disease recurrence at an irradiated site was inversely related to dose, with recurrence rates of less than 5% if 35 Gy was given and 2% at doses of 40 Gy. As a consequence of this analysis, a total dose of 40 Gy was regarded as standard in the radiotherapy of HL for many years. In the HD4 trial of the GHSG, a standard therapy consisting of 40 Gy radiotherapy delivered using the EF technique was then randomly compared with a radiotherapy of 30 Gy EF plus 10 Gy involved field (IF) in pathologically staged PS I/II patients. After a median follow-up of 86 months, there were no significant differences between the two groups in terms of relapse-free and overall survival rates.[26]

Radiotherapy using the EF technique can induce complete remission (CR) rates of 90–98% in patients with early-stage favorable disease.[27,28] but 30–40% will relapse and about 63–74% of these patients are alive after 10 years.[29,30] Due to the high relapse rate after radiotherapy alone and the increased risk of secondary cancers, EF radiotherapy has been abandoned by most study groups.

Combined-modality treatment has been compared with EF radiotherapy alone in another study conducted by the GHSG, randomizing 617 favorable clinically staged CS IA–IIB patients to subtotal nodal and splenic irradiation alone or to two courses of ABVD (Table 35.3) following radiotherapy (the HD7 trial).[31] The final analysis of this study revealed at a median follow-up of 7 years an advantage in terms of freedom

## Table 35.3  The ABVD chemotherapy regimen

| Drug | Dose | Route | Days |
|------|------|-------|------|
| Doxorubicin ('Adriamycin') | 25 mg/m² | i.v. | 1, 15 |
| Bleomycin | 10 U/m² | i.v. | 1, 15 |
| Vinblastine | 6 mg/m² | i.v. | 1, 15 |
| Dacarbazine | 375 mg/m² | i.v. | 1, 15 |
| Recycle from day 29 | | | |

from treatment failure (FFTF) in patients receiving ABVD (96%) compared with those treated with irradiation alone (87%).

Other studies compared combined-modality treatment followed by IF radiotherapy with EF radiation alone. In the EORTC H7F trial, six cycles of EBVP (epirubicin, bleomycin, vinblastine, and prednisone) and IF irradiation was tested against mantle and paraaortic–splenic irradiation (subtotal nodal irradiation, STNI) for favorable-prognosis CS IA–IIA patients. The relapse-free survival rate after 5 years was significantly higher for patients receiving combined-modality treatment (90% versus 81%), whereas survival rates did not differ.[32] Another study by the EORTC (H8F) randomized patients with early-stage favorable disease to two arms: three cycles of MOPP/ABV (mechlorethamine, vincristine, procarbazine, and prednisone/doxorubicin, bleomycin, and vinblastine; see below) with IF irradiation were compared with mantle and paraaortic-splenic irradiation. The relapse-free survival of the two groups differed significantly (99% versus 80%, respectively).[33] Hence, these observations underline the role of the combined-modality treatment as the new standard.

Today, most groups in the USA and Europe prefer combined treatment such as two cycles of ABVD followed by IF radiotherapy using 20–30 Gy. An exclusion is the LPHL subtype in favorable stage IA without risk factors, which can be treated by excision followed by a 'wait and see' strategy or IF radiotherapy with 20–30 Gy.

The main aim of currently ongoing studies is to reduce the long-term complications while retaining the good response. One example is the recently closed HD10 trial of the GHSG evaluating the optimal intensity of therapy for both chemotherapy and IF radiotherapy. Patients were randomized to either two or four cycles of ABVD followed by either 20 or 30 Gy IF radiotherapy.

### Intermediate (early unfavorable) stages

It has become common practice to treat patients in early unfavorable stages with risk factors with a combined-modality approach using both chemotherapy and radiation. Radiotherapy alone cannot sufficiently control disease activity in this group. A combined-modality treatment consisting of four to six cycles of MOPP or ABVD (Table 35.3) plus EF radiation was for a long time regarded as standard treatment. Many European countries preferred COPP over MOPP (with the former containing cyclophosphamide instead of mechlorethamine).

A French group has compared IF versus EF irradiation with 40 Gy in a sandwich regimen using three to six cycles of MOPP in CS I, II, and IIIA patients. This study could not detect a significant difference in either disease-free on overall survival between the two treatment groups.[34]

In the HD1 study of the GHSG, patients in CS/PS I, II, and IIIA with risk factors were treated with two cycles of COPP/ABVD followed by radiation (40 Gy EF versus 20 Gy EF plus 20 Gy bulk). The CR rate was 87%, showing no differences between the three risk groups having large mediastinal mass, extranodal involvement, or massive spleen involvement.[35]

## Table 35.4  The BEACOPP-baseline and escalated BEACOPP chemotherapy regimens

| Drug | Dose[a] | Route | Days |
|------|---------|-------|------|
| Bleomycin | 10 U/m² | i.v. | 8 |
| Etoposide | 100 (200) mg/m² | i.v. | 1–3 |
| Doxorubicin ('Adriamycin') | 25 (35) mg/m² | i.v. | 1 |
| Cyclophosphamide | 650 (1250) mg/m² | i.v. | 1 |
| Vincristine ('Oncovin') | 1.4 mg/m²[b] | i.v. | 8 |
| Procarbazine | 100 mg/m² | p.o. | 1–7 |
| Prednisone | 40 mg/m² | p.o. | 1–14 |
| Recycle from day 22 | | | |

[a] Doses for escalated BEACOPP in parentheses.
[b] The vincristine dose may be capped at 2 mg.

Survival and FFTF of the 148 patients randomized were identical after a median follow-up of 48 months.

A reduction in the intensity of therapy might be possible for both chemotherapy and radiotherapy within the combined modality in order to minimize treatment-related side-effects. A possible reduction of toxicity might be achieved by a reduced radiation volume. In a large trial by the GHSG (HD8), patients with intermediate-stage disease were randomly assigned to four cycles of COPP alternating with ABVD plus 30 Gy EF or IF radiotherapy.[36] There were no significant differences between the two groups in terms of FFTF, overall survival (OS) at 5 years, or CR. Based on these results and the better tolerability, a combined-modality approach of four cycles of ABVD followed by IF radiotherapy is the current standard for most trials.

Since the results in intermediate stages are not yet satisfying, most current clinical trials explore more effective chemotherapy. BEACOPP-baseline (Table 35.4) as a novel chemotherapy regimen for patients with intermediate stages was introduced in the recently closed HD11 trial of the GHSG. Patients were randomized between four cycles of ABVD or four cycles of BEACOPP-baseline followed by an IF radiation with 20 or 30 Gy.

## Advanced stages

Advanced-stage HL was fatal until the development of effective polychemotherapy regimens. The first four-drug combination chemotherapy for HL, using vincristine, methotrexate, cyclophosphamide, and prednisone (MOMP), produced remission rates of 80%.[37] In 1964, this regimen was modified, with the substitution of procarbazine for methotrexate and mechlorethamine (nitrogen mustard) for cyclophosphamide, and the duration was lengthened to 6 months.[38] The resulting MOPP regimen became the gold standard at that time for the treatment of advanced disease.[39] In Europe, some groups used COPP instead of MOPP (replacing mechlorethamine by cyclophosphamide) or ChlVPP (chlorambucil, vinblastine, procarbazine, and prednisone), with very similar results to those achieved with MOPP. In 1979, the Milan group[40] reported a combination that was effective in MOPP-resistant cases, namely ABVD (Table 35.3). ABVD was subsequently used together with MOPP in alternating monthly cycles (MOPP/ABVD). This combination, as well as ABVD alone, has demonstrated superior effects as compared with MOPP alone.[41,42]

A possible strategy to improve treatment results is to develop time- or dose-intensified regimens of effective cytostatic drugs. This notion is based on retrospective data showing that the treatment outcome in HL is correlated with the dose intensity of cytostatic drugs.[43]

There are two principal ways in which to enhance dose intensity:

- dose escalation of drugs on a constant time schedule;
- application of the same dose over a shorter period of time.

One example of a time-intensified protocol was reported by Klimo and Connors.[44] In their study, impressive results were obtained using a MOPP/ABV hybrid aimed at rapid alternation of cytostatic drugs. These data from a non-randomized pilot study were, however, not reproduced in a randomized multicenter trial comparing MOPP/ABVD with the MOPP/ABV hybrid.[40] Promising treatment results have been achieved with the brief Stanford V chemotherapy regimen in advanced HL.[45]

In the three-armed HD9 trial of the GHSG, the new BEACOPP regimen,[46] given in standard and escalated doses (Table 35.4), was compared with the alternating COPP/ABVD regimen in a multicenter setting.[47] Radiotherapy was applied after eight cycles of chemotherapy to sites of initial bulky disease or residual disease after chemotherapy. The second interim analysis of this study identified superior outcome in both BEACOPP arms compared with COPP/ABVD. Thus, the COPP/ABVD arm was closed prematurely.[48] The final analysis of this study showed significant improvement at 5 years' median observation in terms of FFTF rate (69% for COPP/ABVD, 76% for BEACOPP-baseline, and 87% for escalated BEACOPP) (Figure 35.1) and OS rate (83% for COPP/ABVD, 88% for BEACOPP-baseline, and 91% for escalated BEACOPP).

As an example of a time-intensified chemotherapy, the GHSG evaluated the BEACOPP-14 schedule which is BEACOPP-baseline, but given in 14-day instead of 21-day intervals. The aim is to achieve effective tumor control with reduced toxicity. The regimen was tested in a multicenter pilotstudy, with the final analysis showing an estimated FFTF rate of 90% and an OS rate of 97% at 34 months median observation time. The acute hematotoxicity ranged between that of escalated and baseline BEACOPP-21. Consequently, eight cycles of BEACOPP-14 are included in the current HD15 trial of the GHSG.[49]

With the advent of more effective treatment for patients in advanced stages, the role of additional radiation has become more questionable. The duration of chemotherapy is also still controversial. In a study by the Southwestern Oncology Group (SWOG), patients were randomized after three cycles of MOPP/ABVD between radiotherapy or no further treatment. The results were superior for irradiated patients.[50] In the HD3 study by the GHSG, patients who were in CR after three cycles of COPP/ABVD were randomized between additional radiotherapy or a fourth COPP/ABVD course. There was no significant

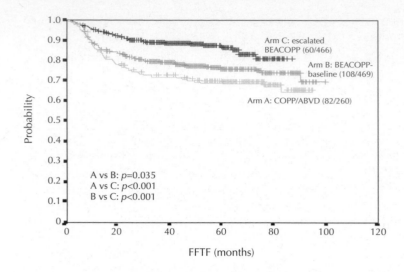

**Figure 35.1** Freedom from treatment failure (FFTF) by treatment arm. Results of the HD9 trial of the German Hodgkin Lymphoma Study Group (GHSG).

difference between the two arms.[51] Other studies addressing this question include the HD12 and HD15 trials of the GHSG, in which patients received either radiation to sites of initial bulky disease and residual disease after eight cycles of chemotherapy or no further treatment (HD12). Radiation in the HD15 trial is only given on PET-positive residual tumors. In the H34 (20884) trial of the EORTC, patients in CR after MOPP/ABV received further two cycles of chemotherapy followed by either radiotherapy with the IF technique or observation. The results showed that the additional radiotherapy did not improve relapse-free survival or OS in patients who had already achieved a CR with MOPP/ABV. In contrast, those patients who had a partial remission and additional IF irradiation had a similar overall outcome compared with those who had reached a CR after chemotherapy.[52,53,54]

## Salvage treatment

### Treatment of relapses after radiotherapy

Patients who relapse after radiotherapy can be treated with standard chemotherapy such as six or eight cycles of ABVD or eight cycles of escalated BEACOPP, depending on stage. Radiation is additionally applied to outfield relapses.

### Treatment of relapses after chemotherapy

Relapses after chemotherapy occur in about one-third of patients in CR. The optimal salvage therapy for these patients depends on the initial treatment and the duration of the response. Three risk groups can be identified (Figure 35.2):

- patients with no initial CR;
- patients with a short initial CR (<12 months);
- patients with a long initial CR (>12 months).

Due to the disappointing results of conventional chemotherapy, high-dose chemotherapy (HDCT) followed by autologous stem cell transplantation (ASCT) is the treatment of choice for most patients with progressive, early, and late relapsed disease. Patients with primary progressive HL have a particularly poor prognosis. Treatment consists of salvage chemotherapy, radiotherapy, and HDCT followed by ASCT.

Conventional chemotherapy in patients with late relapse can induce remission in up to 55% of cases.

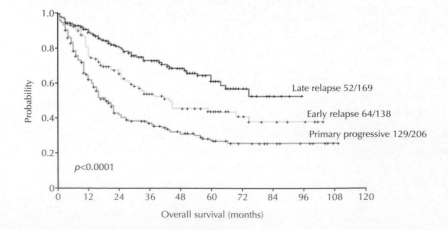

**Figure 35.2** Overall survival in patients with primary progressive, early, and late relapsed Hodgkin lymphoma after first-line polychemotherapy. GHSG 1988–99.

However, several studies, including the randomized HDR1 trial of the GHSG, demonstrated an improved FFTF after HDCT compared with conventional chemotherapy, even for late relapses. Another option is salvage radiotherapy for strictly localized relapses without B symptoms in previously non-irradiated areas.

More than 50% of highly selected patients who undergo HDCT achieve a CR.[55] The OS rate reported at 8 years is 25%. The data indicate that patients who responded to a previous salvage chemotherapy ('sensitive relapse') have a better prognosis with HDCT than patients who did not respond ('resistant relapse'). Thus, HDCT with ASCT has become the standard treatment for patients with chemotherapy-sensitive relapses. Since peripheral blood SCT (PBSCT) is more convenient than autologous bone marrow transplantation (ABMT),[56] this approach has become the standard procedure. A significantly improved outcome in patients treated with HDCT at relapse has been shown in two randomized studies, performed by the British National Lymphoma Investigation (BNLI) and the GHSG/EBMT (HDR-1).[55,58]

In a large multicenter phase II trial, patients with either relapsed or refractory HL were enrolled, receiving initially two cycles of DHAP (dexamethasone, cytarabine, and cisplatin) followed by sequential high-dose chemotherapy (BEAM: carmustine, etoposide, cytarabine, and melphalan), and PBSCT. In the last interim analysis of this study, the response rate was 77% (68% complete and 9% partial), and freedom from second failure (FF2F) and overall survival (OS) were 59% and 79%, respectively, for all patients. Toxicity was tolerable.[59]

These data demonstrate the feasability and high effectivity of this protocol in a large multicenter setting, and led to the GHSG randomized follow-up study (HDR2). Patients with early and late relapsed HL are randomized after two cycles of DHAP between BEAM or additional sequential high-dose chemotherapy followed by BEAM.

In several studies on patients with relapsed disease, prognostic factors were evaluated. In a retrospective analysis performed by the GHSG, early relapse, stage III or IV at relapse and hemoglobin (<10.5 g/dl female or <12 g/dl male) were associated with a particularly poor prognosis in multivariate analysis.[60]

### Rituximab for relapsed CD20+ Hodgkin lymphoma

Fourteen patients with relapsed LPHL or other CD20+ subtypes were enrolled in a phase II trial of the GHSG. Treatment consisted of the chimeric monoclonal anti-CD20 antibody rituximab given as a 4-weekly intravenous infusion. The results show an overall response rate of 86%, eight patients with CR, four with partial response, and two with progressive disease. Thus, rituximab is a safe and effective treatment with mild to moderate adverse events in the subgroub of CD20+ HL.[61] Similar results in small cohorts of patients have been reported from other groups.

## Treatment-related complications

The most serious long-term side-effect in patients successfully treated for HL is the development of second malignancies. Investigations of an international database covering 12 411 patients calculated a cumulative incidence rate for second tumors of 11.2% after 15 years,[25] including 2.2% acute leukemias, 1.8% non-Hodgkin lymphomas, and 7.5% solid tumors. In another study including 1253 HL patients, the 25-year cumulative risk of solid tumors was 23.3%, of leukemia and MDS 3.3%, and NHL 3.5%.[62] Secondary lung cancer, breast cancer, and gastrointestinal cancer are most commonly observed.[63] Acute myeloid leukemias usually developed within 5 years after treatment.[64] The prognosis is generally poor, with remission rates of 30–40% and survival rates of less than 5%. Non-malignant sequelae include gonadal dysfunction. Male patients treated with COPP/ABVD show azoospermia rates of up to 86%.[65,66] However, the majority of patients suffer from disease-related gonadal dysfunction, such as oligo-, astheno- or teratospermia prior to the initiation of treatment.[67,68] The azoospermia in ABVD-treated patients appears to be less pronounced and reversible, developing in about 50% of cases. A more recent analysis including a total of 84 female patients with HD and Non-Hodgkin lymphoma treated with at least three cycles of chemotherapy with an alkylating agent or six cycles with procarbazine reported 34(40.5%) women with premature ovarian failure.[69] Furthermore the likelihood of amenorrhoea after treatment for HL is age-related. Other sequelae are thyroidal dysfunction, interstitial fibrosis, radiation-induced pneumonitis, cardiomyopathy, and ischemic coronary heart disease.[70]

The risk of developing pneumonitis is two- to three-fold greater for patients with large mediastinal masses who receive combined-modality treatment including mantle field radiotherapy.[71] In addition, radiotherapy can cause radiation pneumonitis and chronic fibrosis of the lung. Bleomycin may further increase this toxicity.

## Future developments

Approaches with biological agents aiming at the selective destruction of residual tumor cells are being investigated. HL is a very good candidate for antibody-based immunotherapy because H-RS cells express in high copy numbers on their cell surfaces lymphoid activation markers (CD25 and CD30) that are sparse on normal tissue.[72] These are potential targets for antibody-based immunotherapy. A combined-modality treatment might be feasible using standard chemotherapy or radiotherapy regimens to reduce bulky disease and then using immunotherapy to destroy possible residual tumor cells.

Current monoclonal antibody-based experimental strategies involve immunotoxins, bispecific monoclonal antibodies,[73] radioimmunoconjugates, and completely human antibodies directed at CD30.[74] Ongoing clinical trials in patients with resistant HL indicate therapeutic effects of radioimmunoconjugates and human monoclonal antibodies.

## REFERENCES

1. Correa P, O'Connor GT. Epidemiologic patterns of Hodgkin's disease. *Int J Cancer* 1971; **8**: 192.

2. Kadin M. The Reed–Sternberg cell, an activated T-cell? The evidence has come full circle. *Leuk Lymphoma* 1992; **1**: 281.

3. Stein H, Schwarting R, Dallenbach F, Dienemann D. Immunology of Hodgkin and Reed–Sternberg cells. *Rec Res Cancer Res* 1989; **117**: 14.

4. Smith CA, Gruss HJ, Davis T et al. CD30 antigen, a marker for Hodgkin's lymphoma, is a receptor whose ligand defines an emerging superfamily of cytokines with homology to TNF. *Cell* 1993; **73**: 1349.

5. Kuppers R, Rajewsky K. The origin of Hodgkin and Reed/Sternberg cells in Hodgkin's disease. *Annu Rev Immunol* 1998; **16**: 471–93.

6. Stein H, Mason DY, Gerdes J et al. The expression of the Hodgkin's disease associated antigen Ki-1 in reactive and neoplastic lymphoid tissue: evidence that Reed–Sternberg cells and histiocytic malignancies are derived from activated lymphoid cells. *Blood* 1985; **4**: 848.

7. Jarrett RF, MacKenzie J. Epstein–Barr virus and other candidate viruses in the pathogenesis of Hodgkin's disease. *Semin Hematol* 1999; **36**: 260–9.

8. Dürkop H, Latza U, Hummel M et al. Molecular cloning and expression of a new member of the nerve growth factor receptor family that is characteristic for Hodgkin's disease. *Cell* 1992; **68**: 421.

9. Skinnider BF, Kapp U, Mak TW. The role of interleukin 13 in classical Hodgkin lymphoma. *Leuk Lymphoma* 2002; **43**: 1203–10.

10. Stein H, Delsol G, Pileri S et al. Hodgkin lymphoma. In: Jaffe ES, Harris NL, Stein H (eds) *World Health Organization Classification of Tumours. Pathology and Genetics of Tumours of Haematopoietic and Lymphoid Tissues.* Lyon: IARC Press, 2001: 237–53.

11. Crowther DSS, Bonadonna G. Hodgkin's disease in adults. In: Peckham MPH, Veronesi U (eds) *Oxford Textbook of Oncology.* Oxford: Oxford University Press, 1995: 1720–5.

12. Carbone PP, Kaplan HS, Musshoff K et al. Report of the Committee on Hodgkin's Disease Staging Classification. *Cancer Res* 1971; **3**: 1860.

13. Musshoff K. Prognostic and therapeutic implications of staging extranodal Hodgkin's disease. *Cancer Res* 1971; **31**: 1814.

14. Lister TA, Crowther D. Staging for Hodgkin's disease. *Semin Oncol* 1990; **17**: 696.

15. Leibenhaut MH, Hoppe RT, Efrom B et al. Prognostic indicators of laparatomy findings in clinical stage I–II supradiaphragmatic Hodgkin's disease. *J Clin Oncol* 1989; **7**: 81.

16. Mauch P, Larson D, Osteen R et al. Prognostic factors for positive surgical staging in patients with Hodgkin's disease. *J Clin Oncol* 1990; **2**: 257–65.

17. Carde P, Hagenbeek A, Hayat M et al. Clinical staging versus laparotomy and combined modality with MOPP versus ABVD in early stage Hodgkin's disease. The H6 randomised trials from the European Organisation for Research and Treatment of Cancer Lymphoma Cooperative Group. *J Clin Oncol* 1993; **11**: 2258.

18. Hasenclever D, Diehl V. A prognostic score for advanced Hodgkin's disease. International Prognostic Factors Project on Advanced Hodgkin's Disease. *N Engl J Med* 1998, **339**: 1506–14.

19. Hancock SL, Tucker MA, Hoppe RT. Factors affecting late mortality from heart disease after treatment of Hodgkin's disease. *JAMA* 1993; **270**: 1949.

20. Tucker MA, Coleman CN, Cox RS et al. Risk of second cancers after treatment for Hodgkin's disease. *N Engl J Med* 1988; **318**: 76.

21. Henry-Amar M. Second cancer after the treatment for Hodgkin's disease: a report from the International Database on Hodgkin's Disease. *Ann Oncol* 1992; **3**(Suppl 4): 117.

22. van Leeuwen FE, Klokman WJ, Veer MB, et al. Long-term risk of second malignancy in survivors of Hodgkin's disease treated during adolescence or young adulthood. *J Clin Oncol* 2000; **18**: 487–97.

23. Swerdlow AJ, Barber JA, Hudson GV, et al. Risk of second malignancy after Hodgkin's disease in a collaborative British cohort: the relation to age at treatment. *J Clin Oncol* 2000; 18: 498–509.

24. Mauch PM. Management of early stage Hodgkin's disease: the role of radiation therapy and/or chemotherapy. *Ann Oncol* 1996; **7**(Suppl 4): 79.

25. Kaplan HD. *Hodgkin's Disease.* Cambridge, MA: Harvard University Press, 1980.

26. Duhmke E, Franklin J, Pfreundschuh M et al. Low-dose radiation is sufficient for the noninvolved extended-field treatment in favorable early-stage Hodgkin's disease: long-term results of a randomized trial of radiotherapy alone. *J Clin Oncol* 2001; **19**: 2905–14.

27. Jones E, Mauch P. Limited radiation therapy for selected patients with stages IA and IIA Hodgkin's disease. *Semin Radiat Oncol* 1996; **6**: 162–71.

28. Biti G, Cimino G, Cartoni C et al. Extended-field radiotherapy is superior to MOPP chemotherapy for the treatment of pathologic stage I–IIA Hogkin's disease: eight-year update of an Italian prospective randomized study. *J Clin Oncol* 1992; **10**: 378–82.

29. Specht L, Horwich A, Ashley S. Salvage of relapse of

patients with Hodgkin's disease in clinical stages I or II who were staged with laparotomy and initially treated with radiotherapy alone. A report from the International Database on Hodgkin's Disease. *Int J Radiat Oncol Biol Phys* 1994; **30**: 805–11.

30. Horwich A, Specht L, Ashley S. Survival analysis of patients with clinical stages I or II Hodgkin's disease who have relapsed after initial treatment with radiotherapy alone. *Eur J Cancer* 1997; **33**: 848–53.

31. Sieber M, Franklin J, Tesch H et al. Two cycles ABVD plus extended field radiotherapy is superior to radiotherapy alone in early stage Hodgkin's disease: results of the German Hodgkin's Lymphoma Study Group (GHSG) trial HD7. *Blood* 2002; **100**: A341.

32. Carde P, Noordijk E, Hagenbeek A. Superiority of EBVP chemotherapy in combination with involved field irradiation over subtotal nodal irradiation in favorable clinical stage I–II Hodgkin's disease: the EORTC–GPMC H7F randomized trial. *Proc Am Soc Clin Oncol* 1997; **16**: 13.

33. Hagenbeek A, Eghbali H, Fermé C et al. Three cycles of MOPP/ABV hybrid and involved-field irradiation is more effective than subtotal nodal irradiation in favorable supradiaphragmatic clinical stages I–II Hodgkin's disease: preliminary results of the EORTC–GELA H8-F randomized trial in 543 patients. *Blood* 2000; **96**: A575.

34. Zittoun R, Audobort A, Hoerni B et al. Extended versus involved fields irradiation combined with MOPP chemotherapy in early clinical stages of Hodgkin's disease. *J Clin Oncol* 1985; **3**: 207.

35. Löffler M, Rühl U, Rüffer U et al. Irradiation with 20, 30 or 40 Gy is equally effective in non-bulky areas after two double cycles of COPP–ABVD polychemotherapy in intermediate-stage Hodgkin's disease. *Blood* 1994; **84**(Suppl 1): 921.

36. Engert A, Schiller P, Josting A, Herrmann R, Koch P, Sieber M, Boissevain F, de Wit M, Mezger J, Dühmke E, Willich N, Müller RP, Schmidt BF, Renner H, Müller-Hermelink HK, Pfistner B, Wolf J, Hasenclever D, Löffler M, Diehl V. Involved-field radiotherapy is equally effective and less toxic compared with extended-field radiotherapy after four cycles of chemotherapy in patients with early-stage unfavorable Hodgkin's Lymphoma: Results of the HD8 trial of the German Hodgkin's Lymphoma Study Group. *J Clin Oncol*, 2003; **21**: 3601–3608.

37. DeVita VT, Serpick A. Combination chemotherapy in the treatment of advanced Hodgkin's disease. *Proc Am Assoc Cancer Res* 1967; **8**: 13.

38. De Vita VT, Serpick A, Carbone PP. Combination chemotherapy in the treatment of advanced Hodgkin's disease. *Ann Intern Med* 1970; **73**: 891.

39. Longo DL, Young RRC, Wesley M et al. Twenty years of MOPP therapy for Hodgkin's disease. *J Clin Oncol* 1986; **4**: 1295.

40. Santoro A, Bonadonna G. Prolonged disease-free survival in MOPP-resistant Hodgkin's disease after treatment with Adriamycin, bleomycin, vinblastine and dacarbazine (ABVD). *Cancer Chemother Pharmacol* 1979; **2**: 101.

41. Santoro J, Bonadonna G, Valagussa P et al. Long-term results of combined chemotherapy–radiotherapy approach in Hodgkin's disease: superiority of ABVD plus radiotherapy versus MOPP plus radiotherapy. *J Clin Oncol* 1987; **5**: 27.

42. Canellos GP, Anderson JR, Propert KJ et al. Chemotherapy of advanced Hodgkin's disease with MOPP, ABVD, or MOPP alternating with ABVD. *N Engl J Med* 1992; **327**: 1478.

43. Gribben JG, Vaughan-Hudgson B, Linch DC. The potential value of very intensive therapy with autologous bone marrow rescue in the treatment of malignant lymphomas. *Hematol Oncol* 1987; **5**: 281.

44. Klimo P, Connors JM. An update on the Vancouver experience in the management of advanced Hodgkin's disease treated with the MOPP/ABV hybrid program. *Semin Hematol* 1988; **25**: 34.

45. Connors JM. MOPP/ABV hybrid versus alternating MOPP/ABVD for advanced Hodgkin's disease. *Proc Am Soc Clin Oncol* 1992; **11**: 1073a.

46. Barlett NL, Rosenberg SA, Hoppe RT et al. Brief chemotherapy, Stanford V, and adjuvant radiotherapy for bulk or advanced-stage Hodgkin's disease: a preliminary report. *J Clin Oncol* 1995; **13**: 1080.

47. Diehl V, Sieber M, Rüffer U et al. BEACOPP: an intensified chemotherapy regimen in advanced Hodgkin's disease. *Ann Oncol* 1997; **8**: 1.

48. Diehl V, Franklin J, Hasenclever C et al. BEACOPP, a new dose-escalated and accelerated regimen, is at least as effective as COPP/ABVD in patients with advanced-stage Hodgkin's lymphoma: interim report from a trial of the German Hodgkin's Lymphoma Study Group. *J Clin Oncol* 1998; **16**: 3810–21.

48. Diehl V, Franklin J, Pfreundschuh M, Lathan B, Paulus U, Hasenclever D, et al. Standard and increased-dose BEACOPP chemotherapy compared with COPP-ABVD for advanced Hodgkin's disease. *N Engl J Med*, 2003; **348**: 2386–95.

49. Sieber M, Bredenfeld H, Josting A, et al. 14-day variant of the bleomycin, etoposide, doxorubicin, cyclophosphamide, vincristine, procarbazine, and prednisone regimen in advanced-stage Hodgkin's lymphoma: results of a pilot study of the German Hodgkin's Lymphoma Study Group. *J Clin Oncol* 2003; **21**: 1734–9.

50. Fabian CJ, Mansfield CM, Dahlberg S et al. Low-dose involved field radiation after chemotherapy in advanced Hodgkin's disease. A Southwest Oncology Group randomized study. *Ann Intern Med* 1994; **120**: 903.

51. Diehl V, Löffler M, Pfreundschuh M et al. Further chemotherapy versus low-dose involved-field radiotherapy as consolidation of complete remission after six cycles of alternating chemotherapy in patients with advanced Hodgkin's disease. *Ann Oncol* 1995; **6**: 901.

52. Raemaekers J, Burgers M, Henry-Amar M et al. Patients with stage III/IV Hodgkin's disease in partial remission after MOPP/ABV chemotherapy have excellent prognosis after additional involved-field radiotherapy: interim results from the ongoing EORTC-LCG and GPMC phase III trial. The EORTC Lymphoma Cooperative Group and Groupe Pierre-et-Marie-Curie. *Ann Oncol* 1997; **8**(Suppl 1): 111–14.

53. Raemaekers J, Kluin-Nelemans H, Teodorovic I et al. The achievements of the EORTC Lymphoma Group. European Organisation for Research and Treatment of Cancer. *Eur J Cancer* 2002; **38**(Suppl 4): 107–13.

54. Aleman BM, Raemaekers JM, Tirelli U, et al. Involved-field radiotherapy for advanced Hodgkin's lymphoma. *N Engl J Med* 2003; 348:2396-406.

55. Kessinger A, Biermann PJ, Vose JM et al. High dose cyclophosphamide, carmustine and etoposide followed

by autologous peripheral stem cell transplantation for patients with relapsed Hodgkin's disease. *Blood* 1991; **77**: 2322.

56. Bierman P, Vose J, Anderson J et al. Comparison of autologous bone marrow transplantation (ASCT) with peripheral stem cell transplantation for patients with Hodgkin's disease. *Blood* 1993; **82**(Suppl 1): 445a.

57. Linch D, Winfield D, Goldstone A et al. Dose intensification with autologous bone-marrow transplantation in relapsed and resistant Hodgkin's disease: results of a BNLI randomised trial. *Lancet* 1993; **341**: 1051–4.

58. Schmitz N, Sextro M, Pfistner B. HDR-1: high-dose therapy (HDT) followed by hematopoietic stem cell transplantation (HSCT) for relapsed chemosensitive Hodgkin's disease (HD): final results of randomized GHSG and EBMT trial (HD-R1). *Proc Am Soc Clin Oncol* 1999; **18**: 18.

59. Josting A, Rudolph C, Mapara M et al. Cologne high-dose sequential chemotherapy in relapsed and refractory Hodgkin lymphoma – results of a large multicenter study for the prospective randomized HDR-2 trial of the German Hodgkin Lymphoma Study Group (GHSG). *Blood* 2002; **100**: A812.

60. Josting A, Franklin J, May M et al. New prognostic score based on treatment outcome of patients with relapsed Hodgkin's lymphoma registered in the database of the German Hodgkin's Lymphoma Study Group. *J Clin Oncol* 2002; **20**: 221–30.

61. Rehwald U, Schulz H, Reiser M et al. Treatment of relapsed CD20+ Hodgkin lymphoma with the monoclonal antibody rituximab is effective and well tolerated: results of a phase 2 trial of the German Hodgkin Lymphoma Study Group. *Blood* 2003; **101**.

62. van Leeuwen FE, Klokman WJ, Veer MB, et al. Long-term risk of second malignancy in survivors of Hodgkin's disease treated during adolescence or young adulthood. *J Clin Oncol* 2000; **18**: 487–97.

63. Behringer K, Josting A, Schiller P, et al. Solid Tumors in Patients Treated for Hodgkin's Disease: A Report from the German Hodgkin Lymphoma Study Group. *Ann Oncol* 2004; **15**: 1079–85.

64. Josting A, Wiedenmann S, Franklin J et al. Secondary myeloid leukemia and myelodysplastic syndromes in patients treated for Hodgkin's disease: A report from the German Hodgkin's Lymphoma Study Group. *J Clin Oncol* 2003; **21**.

65. Kreuser ED, Felsenberg D, Behles C et al. Long-term gonadal dysfunction and its impact on bone mineralization in patients following COPP/ABVD chemotherapy for Hodgkin's disease. *Ann Oncol* 1992; **3**(Suppl 4): 111.

66. Kreuser E, Felsenberg D, Behles C, et al. Long-term gonadal dysfunction and its impact on bone mineralization in patients following COPP/ABVD chemotherapy for Hodgkin's disease. *Ann Oncol* 1992; **3**(Suppl 4): 105–10.

67. Rueffer U, Breuer K, Josting A et al. Male gonadal dysfunction in patients with Hodgkin's disease prior to treatment. *Ann Oncol* 2001; **12**: 1307–11.

68. Fitoussi, Eghbali H, Tchen N et al. Semen analysis and cryoconservation before treatment in Hodgkin's disease. *Ann Oncol* 2000; **11**: 679–84.

69. Franchi-Rezgui P, Rousselot P, Espie M et al. Fertility in young women after chemotherapy with alkylating agents for Hodgkin and non-Hodgkin lymphomas. *Hematol J* 2003; **4**: 116–20.

70. Valagussa P, Santoro A, Bonadonna G. Thyroid, pulmonary, and cardiac sequelae after treatment for Hodgkin's disease. *Ann Oncol* 1992; **3**(Suppl 4): 111.

71. Tarbell N, Thompson L, Mauch P. Thoracic irradiation in Hodgkin's disease: disease control and long-term complications. *Int J Radiat Oncol Biol Phys* 1990; **18**: 275–81.

72. Engert A, Burrows F, Jung W et al. Evaluation of ricin A-chain containing immunotoxins directed against CD30 as potential reagents for the treatment of Hodgkin's disease. *Cancer Res* 1990; **50**: 6944.

73. Engert A, Pohl C, Diehl V. Experimental therapy in Hodgkin's disease. *Ann Oncol* 1992; **3**(Suppl 4): 97.

74. Borchmann P, Schnell R, Fuss I et al. *Wickenhauser C, Schiller P, Diehl V, Engert A* Phase 1 trial of the novel bispecific molecule H22×Ki-4 in patients with refractory Hodgkin lymphoma. *Blood* 2002; **100**: 3101–7.

# 36 Non-Hodgkin lymphomas

**Anton Hagenbeek and Philip M Kluin**

## Introduction

Non-Hodgkin lymphomas (NHLs) form a heterogeneous group of approximately 50 different clinicopathologic entities (Tables 36.1–3). In western countries, the incidence of NHL is approximately 10/100 000 females per year and 14/100 000 males per year. In some countries, it has shown a steady trend to increase in recent decades. However, this increase may be partially artificial in view of the changes in diagnostic tools and criteria, and the change in the age distribution of the general population. The latter has a major impact, since NHL generally represents a disease of the elderly. Since most NHLs show hematogenic spread, and conversely some leukemia patients present with or develop lymphadenopathy during the

---

### Table 36.1  B-cell lymphomas and leukemias (WHO Classification)

|  | Site of presentation |
|---|---|
| **Primary leukemic disorders** | |
| Precursor B-cell lymphoblastic leukemia/lymphoma | Bm, bl, ln, spl |
| BCLL/small lymphocytic lymphoma | Bm, bl, ln, spl |
| B-cell prolymphocytic leukemia (PLL) | Spl, bl, bm |
| Mantle-cell lymphoma | Ln, bm, bl, spl, extranodal |
| Splenic marginal zone B cell lymphoma | Spl, bl, bm |
| Plasma cell leukemia | Bm, bl |
| **Primary nonleukemic disorders** | |
| Burkitt lymphoma/leukemia | extranodal/ln, bm, bl |
| Follicular lymphoma | Ln, bm, bl |
| Nodal marginal zone lymphoma | Ln, bm |
| *Diffuse large B-cell lymphoma* | Ln/extranodal |
| Mediastinal large B-cell lymphoma | Mediastinum/thymus |
| Extranodal marginal zone (MALT) lymphoma | Stomach, lung, salivary glands, etc. |
| Lymphoplasmacytic lymphoma | Bm, spl, ln |
| **Plasma cell disorders** | |
| Plasma cell myeloma | Bm |
| Plasmacytoma | (Para)nasal |
| Monoclonal immunoglobulin deposition diseases (amyloidosis) | Bm, kidney, other organs |
| **Very uncommon disorders** | |
| Lymphomatoid granulomatosis | Lung |
| Primary effusion lymphoma | Pleura, ascites |
| Intravascular large B-cell lymphoma | Skin, CNS |
| Monoclonal light and/or heavy chain diseases | Bm, kidney |

BM, bone marrow; bl: blood; ln: lymph node; spl: spleen; CNS: central nervous system.

## Table 36.2 T/NK cell lymphomas and leukemias (WHO classification)

| | Site of presentation |
|---|---|
| **Primary leukemic disorders** | |
| Precursor T lymphoblastic leukemia/lymphoma | Bm, bl, mediastinum |
| T-cell prolymphocytic leukemia | Bm, bl, spl, liver, skin |
| T-cell large granular lymphocytic leukemia | Bm, bl, spl |
| **Primary nonleukemic disorders** | |
| Angioimmunoblastic T-cell lymphoma | Ln, bm, spl, liver, bl |
| Anaplastic large cell lymphoma | Ln/extranodal |
| Peripheral T-cell lymphoma unspecified | Ln/extranodal |
| Extranodal NK/T-cell lymphoma, nasal type | Nose, palate, testis, intestine |
| Enteropathy type T-cell lymphoma | Small intestine |
| Hepatosplenic T-cell lymphoma | Liver, spl, bm |
| **Primary cutaneous disorders** | |
| Blastic NK cell lymphoma | Skin, bm |
| Mycosis fungoides | Skin |
| Sézary syndrome | Skin, bl, ln |
| Primary cutaneous CD30+ T-cell lymphoproliferative disorders | Skin |
| Anaplastic large cell lymphoma | Skin |
| Lymphomatoid papulosis | Skin |
| Subcutaneous panniculitis type T-cell lymphoma | Subcutis |
| **Very uncommon disorders** | |
| Adult T-cell leukemia/lymphoma | Dependent on subtype: skin, ln, bl, bone, bm, liver, spl |
| Aggressive NK-cell leukemia | Bm, bl |

Bm: bone marrow; bl: blood; ln: lymph node; spl: spleen.

course of the disease, the boundaries between certain NHLs and leukemias are not very distinct. Examples are lymphocytic lymphoma and chronic lymphocytic leukemia, and Burkitt lymphoma and its leukemia variant, previously called acute lymphoblastic leukemia type L3.

In western countries, B-cell lymphomas make up approximately 85–90% of all NHLs. Approximately 65% of NHLs are primary nodal, and present at pre-existent lymphoid sites such as lymph nodes and tonsils. Lymphomas that arise in the mucosa-associated lymphoid tissues and in sites without pre-existing lymphoid tissue such as the stomach, soft tissues, testis and brain are mostly called primary extranodal. The clinical presentation of NHL largely depends on the primary localization and spread of tumor cells. The significance of the site of presentation is particularly salient in primary extranodal lymphomas. Apart from mechanical discomfort, other features such as bone marrow failure caused by lymphomatous infiltration may contribute to the clinical presentation. Furthermore, B-cell lymphomas with a high content of plasma cells or plasmacytoid cells such as lymphoplasmacytic lymphoma may produce large quantities of paraprotein, leading to clinical symptoms. Tumor-derived immunoglobulins (Igs) may show reactivity to auto-antigens, resulting in hemolytic anemia, thrombocytopenia, cryoglobinemia, peripheral neuropathy, etc. Other symptoms such as fever and the occurrence of eosinophilia may be related to the production of cytokines by tumor cells or reactive bystander cells. These latter phenomena are particularly prominent in peripheral T-cell lymphomas and Hodgkin lymphoma.

## Etiology and pathogenesis

The following etiological factors play a major role in the genesis of NHL:

1. Infection by oncogenic viruses
2. Inflammation and persistent proliferation
3. Illegitimate gene recombination
4. Impaired immunity of the host.

As in other malignancies, the etiology of malignant lymphoma is multifactorial. The best-documented example is African Burkitt lymphoma (see later). In approximately 50% of B-cell lymphomas, recurrent chromosomal translocations such as a t(14;18) can

**Table 36.3  Immunodeficiency-associated lymphoproliferative disorders (WHO classification)**

| | Remarks |
| --- | --- |
| Lymphoproliferative diseases in primary immune disorders | |
| Fatal infectious mononucleosis | Mainly in XLP and SCID |
| DLBCL | EBV+, in all types |
| Lymphomatoid granulomatosis | EBV+, mainly in Wiskott–Aldrich syndrome |
| T-cell lymphomas/leukemias | Mainly in ataxia telangiectasia |
| Various | Ln ALPS |
| | |
| HIV-related lymphomas | |
| Burkitt lymphoma | 30% EBV+ +/– plasmacytoid |
| Diffuse large B-cell lymphoma | EBV+ |
| Plasmablastic lymphoma | EBV+ oral & other mucosa |
| Primary effusion lymphoma | Pleura, ascites; EBV+, HHV8+ |
| PTLD-like lymphoproliferations (polymorphic) | |
| Extranodal marginal zone B-cell lymphoma | Extremely rare |
| Peripheral T-cell lymphoma NOS | |
| Hodgkin lymphoma | Rare |
| | |
| Post-transplant lymphoproliferative disorders | |
| Infectious mononucleosis-like | Ln, Waldeyer, primary infect; young children; polyclonal |
| Early plasmacytic hyperplasia | Ln, Waldeyer, children, EBV+; polyclonal |
| Polymorphic PTLD | Extranodal, graft, Waldeyer, Ln; poly-/oligo/monoclonal |
| DLBCL | Extranodal, graft, Waldeyer, Ln; monoclonal |
| Plasmacytoma-like PTLD/plasma cell myeloma | Intestine, other extranodal sites; bm, may be EBV negative; late lesions |
| T-PTLD | EBV+/– monoclonal |
| Hodgkin (like) PTLD | EBV+, CD30+, 15+ |

Ln: lymph node; bm: bone marrow; XLPL: X-linked lymphoproliferative disease; SCID: severe combined immuno-deficiency; ALPS: auto-immune lymphoproliferative syndrome.

be identified. In at least three entities (Burkitt lymphoma, follicular lymphoma and mantle-cell lymphoma), specific translocations affect the majority of cases and hence are critical events. In most translocations, juxtapositions of Ig genes or T-cell receptor (TCR) genes (in B- and T-cell lymphomas, respectively) lead to deregulation of the involved (onco)genes and (over)production of otherwise-normal oncoproteins. In contrast to myeloid leukemias, the generation of fusion genes and abnormal protein products is relatively exceptional, and so far only documented in T-cell anaplastic large cell lymphoma and extranodal marginal-zone lymphoma of mucosa-associated lymphoid tissue (MALT) type (see later). In general, translocations involving Ig genes are more frequent in mature B-cell lymphomas than in precursor B-cell leukemias, whereas translocations involving TCR genes are more frequent in precursor T-cell leukemias than in mature T-cell lymphomas. This difference has not been fully explained, but may be related to the fact that T-cells undergo only one wave of T-cell receptor gene rearrangements,

while B cells undergo three major waves: after the initial *V(D)J* recombinations of the immunoglobulin genes in precursor B cells, the mature germinal center B cells also undergo hypermutations and immunoglobulin class switch recombinations (Figure 36.1). Mechanistically, all recombinations in early B and T cells including the hypermutations and class

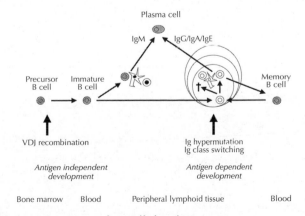

**Figure 36.1** Normal B-cell development.

switch represent events that include the generation of double-strand DNA breaks, and in consequence they are potentially at risk to undergo erroneous recombinations, including chromosomal translocations. Many additional aspects have to be understood to fully appreciate the role of oncogenes and translocations in lymphomas:

- *The nature of the gene involved.* Genes involved in translocations are nuclear transcription factors (often affected in precursor B- and T-cell malignancies like acute lymphoblastic leukemia, ALL), cell cycle regulators (such as cyclin DI), anti-apoptotic genes (such as *BCL2*), and genes coding for cytokines.

- *Their role in normal B- and T-cell development.* For instance, the effect of deregulation of the *BCL2* gene by t(14;18) can only be understood knowing the expression pattern and function of the BCL2 protein during normal B-cell ontogeny (the effect of the deregulation is restricted to germinal center B cells; see Figures 36.2 and 36.3).

- *Interaction with other genes or gene products.* For instance in the E2A/Rb pathway, cyclin D1 interacts with numerous other proteins, including many activators and repressors. This cascade ultimately leads to the release of E2A involved in $G_1$/S-phase transition. The balance between type D cyclins, CDK4 and inhibitors and activators is crucial in normal cell cycle control, while disbalances may lead to both early $G_1$ transition and/or apoptosis.

- *The moment at which a translocation takes place during B- or T-cell ontogeny.* For instance, the translocation t(11;14)(q13;q32) is characteristic of mantle-cell lymphoma. In this lymphoma, it occurs during the first Ig gene rearrangements in early precursor B cells of the bone marrow. A t(11;14) with involvement of *cyclin D1* is occasionally found in multiple myeloma. However,

the latter breakpoints at 14q32 localize at Ig switch sites, suggesting a later origin during Ig class switching in germinal center B cells.

The current knowledge of oncogenes, viruses, cell adhesion molecules and cytokines is of tremendous help in understanding many aspects of lymphomagenesis. However, the mechanisms by which the tumor cells are blocked at a certain level of maturation is still incompletely understood. This block in maturation in particular forms the basis of all current classification systems, the so-called 'frozen stage model' of neoplasia describing the more or less strict maturation block of tumor cells. It may be almost absolute, such as in mantle-cell lymphoma, or less strict, such as in follicular lymphoma and marginal-zone B-cell lymphoma (see later).

Initial tumorigenesis must be discerned from tumor progression. There is increasing evidence that progression in NHL is caused by gene alterations that differ from the original events. These 'secondary' events include inactivation of tumor-suppressor genes such as *p53* and *p16*, amplification of genes such as *REL*, genomic instabilities leading to trisomy and disturbances in gene dosage, and less frequently translocations such as t(8;14) involving the MYC oncogene.

Many lymphomas present at sites that are normally devoid of lymphoid tissue. One explanation is that these lymphomas develop from chronic inflammation and subsequent induction of lymphoid tissue. Examples are the development of gastric extranodal marginal-zone type (MALT) B-cell lymphomas against a background of *Helicobacter pylori*-induced chronic gastritis with induction of MALT, and the development of B-cell lymphomas against a background of autoimmune-mediated inflammation in Sjögren disease.

Depending on the stage of differentiation, normal B and T cells circulate in the peripheral blood, and home to distinct peripheral lymphoid sites such as the peripheral lymph nodes, the spleen or the MALT. Circulation and homing are guided by the presence of many molecules, such as CD44, selectins and integrins on lymphocytes, and their specific ligands on (high) endothelial cells, stroma, etc. Lymphocytes are directed into specific lymphoid tissues by the presence of homing receptors and addressins on high endothelial cells. Spread after invasion in the lymphoid compartments is directed by chemokine receptors on lymphocytes and their ligands. Expression of these receptors is often inducible and dependent on (local) maturation of lymphocytes, and thus on the local microenvironment, including the presence of T cells, cytokines, etc. Many of these properties, which are retained in NHL, may explain not only the presence of different homing properties in NHL but also the presence of intratumor heterogeneity and the sometimes dramatic morphological and phenotypic alterations during the course of the disease.

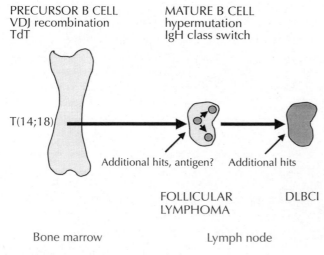

**Figure 36.2** Molecular origin of follicular lymphoma and t(14;18).

# A biological basis of classification

Previous classifications were mainly based on morphology (the Rappaport classification[1] and the International Working Formulation, WF[2] or on morphology and normal lymphoid development (the Kiel and Lukes–Collins classification[3–5]). Most importantly, none of these classifications received worldwide support. Ideally, classifications should be based on the distinction of clinicopathologic entities defined by morphology, immunophenotype, genetic abnormalities, clinical presentation including pattern of dissemination and prognosis. Furthermore, they should be based on consensus amongst expert pathologists, immunologists, molecular biologists and hemato-oncologists. From this point of view, the REAL and more recently introduced World Health Organization (WHO) classifications[6–8] are major achievements. It should be underlined that the WHO classification represents an update of the REAL classification, and that such a process of updating will remain necessary in the future as well.

# Grading of malignant lymphoma

NHL represent a large number of distinct clinicopathological entities, each with a distinct presentation, behavior and prognosis. In the Kiel classification, grading was a histologic feature and exclusively based on the presence of blasts. In contrast, grading according to the WF was based on morphology and clinical outcome according to the therapeutic options in 1970–80. According to the current WHO and REAL classifications, grading is again an exclusively histologic feature, and only used for those entities in which the (variable) percentage of blasts might have clinical (prognostic) significance. So far, official proposals for grading have only been made for follicular lymphoma.[8–10]

# B-cell lymphomas

In western countries, the great majority of NHLs are B-cell lymphomas (Table 36.1). For most of these lymphomas, normal counterparts can be identified, and hence a 'frozen stage model' can be applied. In some subtypes, leukemic spread may occur at the onset of disease or may develop during its course, making distinction between leukemic NHL and primary leukemia rather arbitrary.

## Lymphocytic lymphoma/B-CLL

Lymphocytic lymphoma/B-CLL (chronic lymphocytic leukemia) is defined as a lymphoma or leukemia that consists of small B lymphocytes with or without plasmacytoid cells. Lymphocytic lymphoma and CLL are lumped, since the borderline is equivocal. For instance, different numerical criteria ($>4$ to $>15 \times 10^9$ lymphocytes/L) are used in different classification systems.[11,12] In western countries, lymphocytic lymphoma/CLL has an incidence of approximately 3.2 cases/100 000 inhabitants/year, but it shows a continuous increase in incidence with age, up to an incidence of approximately 75/100 000 inhabitants/year for people over 80 years old. Autoimmune phenomena, including autoimmune hemolytic anemia, occur in 10–20% of CLLs.

### Genetics, etiology and pathogenesis

Using refined analysis with fluorescent in situ hybridization (FISH) and comparative genomic hybridization, the most common genetic abnormalities in lymphocytic lymphoma/CLL are del 13q14 in approximately 50% (so far no tumor-suppressor gene has been identified),[13,14] deletions involving the ATM gene at 11q23 in 20–30% and trisomy 12 in 10–15% of cases. While initial studies on CLL showed that as many as 35% of all CLLs may have trisomy 12,[15–20] later studies showed that this percentage is much too high, and more essentially, that this abnormality is associated with an atypical morphology and phenotype, as well a relatively poor prognosis. Other genetic abnormalities like t(11;14)(q13;q32), t(14;18)(q32;q21) and rearrangements centromeric of the BCL2 gene at 18q21 occur in less than 5% of cases.[21–24] Rearrangements of the Ig heavy- and light-chain genes and mutational patterns have been extensively studied. Most studies suggest a preferential use of certain $V_H$ gene segments, especially 51p1, $V_H 4.21$ $V_H 4.18$ and VH251.[25–33]

In normal mature B cells, particularly follicle-center B cells, hypermutations affect the recombined $V_H$, $D_H$ and $J_H$ gene segments, especially at the CDR2 and CDR3 regions. Hypermutations are implicated in the process of affinity maturation of B cells, necessary for the generation of monospecific, high-affinity antibodies. Originally it was thought that, like their putative normal counterparts (immature CD5 positive B cells), most CLLs lack hypermutations[26,34–36] and produce low-affinity multireactive antibodies like rheumatoid factor.[37] However, more recent investigations show that approximately half of all CLLs contain hypermutations, albeit at a lower level than in follicular lymphoma.[38,39] This suggests two entities: one CLL that is pregerminal center B-cell derived and one CLL that is postgerminal center cell derived. The occurrence of hypermutations is strongly associated with the absence of ZAP-70, a protein with an unknown function in B cells, but in analogy to its function in normal T cells, it is likely involved in B-cell receptor (BCR)-mediated signaling. Most importantly, CLL with hypermutations or with low ZAP-70 expression have a relatively favorable prognosis, which is independent from other prognostic parameters.[30,40–42] The presence of these unmutated and mutated forms of CLL supports the idea of two entities. However, hypermutations are not correlated with expression of activation-induced cytidine deaminase (AID – essential in the genesis of these mutations) neither with the occurrence of immunoglobulin class switching or class switch attempts. Furthermore, gene expression profiles as assessed by gene array analysis show only limited differences between unmutated and hypermutated CLL.[43,44]

### Morphology and immunophenotype

At the cytologic level, circulating cells show a typical nuclear morphology with round or indented nuclei and coarse chromatin. The cytoplasm may show some plasmacytoid differentiation. Smudge cells ('Gumprechtse Schollen') may be numerous. Less than 10% prolymphocytes are present in blood smears. The presence of nuclear clefts in some CLLs hinders distinction from leukemic NHL, particularly mantle-cell and follicular lymphoma. Lymph node histology often reveals the presence of so-called pseudo-follicles with accumulation of prolymphocytes. These structures can be mistaken for follicle centers, especially in the case of poor fixation, leading to a wrong diagnosis of follicular lymphoma. Their presence also excludes a diagnosis of immunocytoma and mantle-cell lymphoma, both potential differential diagnoses of CLL. Bone marrow aspirates and biopsies are positive in almost all cases. In bone marrow biopsies, the pattern is interstitial, nodular, nodular and interstitial, or diffuse. The presence of a diffuse pattern is independently associated with a poor prognosis.[45] Immunophenotypically, lymphocytic lymphoma/CLL can be confidently diagnosed on the basis of expression of faint Ig (mostly IgM), CD5, CD23 and BCL2 with lack of CD10, BCL6 and cyclin D1 (Table 36.4).[45]

### Progression

Approximately one-third of patients show morphological tumor progression during the course of the disease. Other patients will suffer from progressive disease due to resistance to chemotherapy, whereas approximately 50% of patients succumb to intercurrent infections, cancer or unrelated disorders. The most common type of morphological progression is prolymphocytoid transformation, defined by the presence of between 10% and 55% circulating prolymphocytes, progressive lymphadenopathy, splenomegaly and refractoriness to chemotherapy. Rare forms of progression are Richter syndrome showing progression to immunoblastic lymphoma or a Hodgkin-like lymphoma,[46–49] so-called 'para-immunoblastic' lymphoma,[50] and the very rare occurrence of a TdT+ lymphoblastic leukemia.[51–52] CLL patients are at risk in developing secondary malignancies that might include secondary, clonally unrelated malignant lymphomas. Indeed in a significant part of the cases with Richter transformation, no clonal relationship could be demonstrated by any molecular means.

## Mantle-cell lymphoma

The clinicopathological entity mantle-cell lymphoma (MCL) was first described in 1992.[53–56] In western countries, it makes up approximately 5% of all NHLs. In the Kiel classification, MCL was called centrocytic lymphoma because it was originally thought to be a follicle-center- rather than a mantle-zone-related lymphoma. American authors previously called it intermediately differentiated lymphocytic lymphoma (ILL), lymphocytic lymphoma of intermediate differentiation, and mantle-zone lymphoma (MZL).[57–59] MCL has not been recognized as a distinct entity in the WF.

MCL is a disorder of elderly patients, with a median age of at least 65 years. Most patients present with generalized disease and involvement of lymph nodes, spleen, liver and bone marrow. Approximately one-third of these patients present with extranodal disease, especially of the gastrointestinal tract. In 'lymphomatous polyposis', numerous intestinal (especially ileocecal) polyps with extensive nodular infiltrates are formed. These tumor cells express lymphocyte Peyer patch adhesion molecule (LPAM), i.e. $\alpha_4\beta_7$ integrins, also expressed by normal intraepithelial T cells of the gut.[60] Some patients present with pronounced splenomegaly and a leukemic picture without lymphadenopathy.[61–63] The leukemic cells may have a blastic appearance with prominent nucleoli. This variant may therefore be easily mixed up with either splenic marginal-zone lymphoma or prolymphocytic leukemia. In contrast to lymphomas and leukemias that may form a differential diagnosis, almost all MCL patients have a very poor prognosis, with a median survival of 2–3 years, unless they are treated with aggressive chemotherapy in combination with anti-CD20 monoclonal antibody therapy and autologous stem cell rescue, or allogeneic stem cell transplantation.[56,64–67] This necessitates the use of firm criteria to distinguish these lymphoproliferative disorders.

### Genetics, etiology and pathogenesis

In general, IgH genes are unmutated and have not undergone any attempts to class switching, however, approximately 15–20% of all cases show a low level of hypermutation, and this hypermutation seems to be associated with a preferential usage of certain VH gene segments. So far, and opposite to the situation in CLL, there is no obvious clinical difference between

**Table 36.4  Immunophenotype of chronic B-cell leukemias, lymphomas and myeloma**

| | Mantle-cell lymphoma | Chronic lymphocytic leukemia | Follicular lymphoma | Nodal marginal zone lymphoma | Lymphoplasmacytic lymphoma | Splenic marginal zone lymphoma | Extranodal marginal zone lymphoma | Hairy-cell leukemia | Myeloma |
|---|---|---|---|---|---|---|---|---|---|
| SmIg | + | ± | + | + | + | + | + | + | − |
| CyIg | − | minority | − | ± | + | ± | −/+ | − | + |
| IgH-isotype | μδ | μ,μδ,γ | μ,μδ,γ,neg | μ,μδ | μ,γ,α | μ,μδ,γ | μ,μδ,γ,α | μ,μδ,γ,α | γ,α(δ,μ,ε) |
| CD20 | + | ± | + | + | + | + | + | + | −/+ (20%) |
| CD79 | + | + | + | + | + | + | + | + | variable |
| CD5 | + | +/± | − | − | − | − | − | − | − |
| CD10 | − | − | + (gr 3 variable) | − | − | − | − | minority | − |
| CD11c | − | − | − | ? | ? | + | variable | ++ | − |
| CD21 | minority | variable | minority | − | − | minority | variable | − | − |
| CD23 | − | variable | minority | − | − | minority | − | − | − |
| CD25 | − | + | − | ? | ? | minority | ? | + | − |
| CD35 | − | minority | − | − | − | − | variable | − | − |
| CD43 | − | + | − | − | ? | − | − | + | − |
| CD103 | − | − | − | − | − | minority | − | + | − |
| CD138 | − | − | − | − | +/− (heterogeneous) | − | variable | − | + |
| BCL2 | + | + | + (gr 3 variable) | + | + | + | + | + | variable |
| BCL6 | − | − | + | − | − | − | − | − | − |
| CyclinD1 | + | − | − | − | − | − | − | ± | variable |

+: strong; ±/': weak; −: negative; variable: >25% of cases positive; minority: <25% of cases positive; heterogeneous: heterogeneity in tumor.

unmutated and hypermutated cases.[68–71] At the cytogenetic level, t(11;14)(q13;q32) can be detected in two-thirds of MCLs.[72] Since the BCL-1 breakpoint on chromosome 11q13 involves an area of at least 220 kb, FISH analysis is the best method to detect all t(11;14) breakpoints.[73–79] Using FISH, a BCL-1 breakpoint can be detected in at least 95% of the cases and due to the translocation, the *cyclin D1 (CCND1)* gene is overexpressed in all these cases. This can be demonstrated by immunohistochemistry or quantitative RT-PCR,[78,80–82] especially since *cyclin D1* is not expressed in normal B cells and most other B-cell neoplasias (Hairy-cell leukemia is a regular exception with a weak expression but no translocation.[83,84]) Of note, PCR is not appropriate for 11q13/BCL1 breakpoint detection, since only 30–40% of all 11q13/BCL1 breakpoints can be detected. In very few, MCL not cyclin D1 but cyclin D2 or D3 proteins may be overexpressed, leading to a similar deregulation of the cell cycle.[85] It should be noted that the t(11;14) is rarely, if not at all, found in other B-cell lymphomas and leukemias, except for 15–20% of multiple myelomas (MMs), in which the molecular make up of the breakpoints differs, however.[86–90] Possibly, the rare cases of CLL[21,22,57–59] and splenic lymphoma with villous lymphocytes (SLVL)[60] with a t(11;14), in fact represent variant MCL.[91–94]

Similar to CLL, other (secondary?) genetic events include loss of 13q14.3 (up to 40%) and deletion of *ATM* at 11q23. In many CLLs and MCLs with these deletions, *ATM* has undergone truncating or missense mutations, small deletions or insertions.[95–98] In MCL but not in CLL, ATM mutations are associated with an increased number of chromosomal imbalances and tumor progression. Other abnormalities in MCL are associated with tumor progression as well: approximately 25% of the so-called blastic and pleomorphic variants carry p53 mutations.[99,100] Bi-allelic deletions of p16 have also been identified.[101,102] Very recent cDNA microarray-based gene expression studies in MCL have shown that especially the proliferation status of the tumor as assessed by (over) expression of genes involved in proliferation is a very important denominator of prognosis.[85]

### Morphology and immunophenotype

Histologically, three growth patterns of MCL can be seen: mantle-zone, nodular and diffuse. All patterns are associated with the same poor prognosis. At the cytomorphologic level, three variants have been described:

1. *Classical type*, with small to intermediately sized cleaved cells
2. *Blastoid variant,* mimicking lymphoblastic lymphoma with a relatively dispersed chromatin
3. *Pleomorphic variant* with large cleaved or ovoid nuclei and often prominent nucleoli.

The immunophenotype of MCL is remarkably homogeneous: all MCLs represent B-cell lymphomas with strong expression of surface IgM and Ig light chains, CD5 and lack of CD10, CD23 and BCL6.[103,104] Approximately 5% of the cases may lack CDS expression and extremely rare cases have both CD5 and CD10 expression. Virtually all MCLs express nuclear cyclin D1, however the intensity may vary considerably as detected by sensitive immunohistochemistry or RT-PCR.[78,105,106] Another adjunct in its diagnosis is the demonstration of numerous dendritic reticulum cells (DRCs) with antibodies against CD21 or CD35. Ki-67/Mib-1 as a marker of proliferation fraction may be used as a prognostic marker.[56,107–109]

### Lymphoplasmacytic lymphoma

Lymphoplasmacytic lymphoma is a relatively rare B-cell disorder, with an estimated incidence of 0.5/100 000 cases/inhabitants/year in western countries. It comprises less than 5% of all NHLs. In the REAL classification, the disorder has erroneously been designated as 'immunocytoma lymphoplasmacytoid', giving rise to much confusion, since this term was previously used for a subset of CLL with some plasmacytoid differentiation. Most patients with immunocytoma present with stage IV disease and localization in the bone marrow, lymph nodes and spleen. Although not synonymous, many cases of immunocytoma have a clinical picture of Waldenström disease with IgM paraproteinemia and symptoms of hyperviscosity. Furthermore, chronic, cold agglutinin-mediated, immune hemolytic anemia is a common feature.[110,111] This is almost invariably associated with anti-i/I antibodies and Ig gene rearrangement to the $V_H4.24$ gene segment.[112] Clinically related disorders are the Ig heavy-chain disorders, µHCD and γHCD. These disorders may be associated with specific morphological aspects of tumor cells, such as highly vacuolated plasma cells in µHCD.[113]

### *Genetics, etiology and pathogenesis*

Although previous genetic studies suggested a t(9;14)(p13;q32) or breakpoints at 9p13 with juxtaposition to other loci, involving the PAX-5 gene in approximately half of the cases, this could not be confirmed in a large series of cases.[114–117] PAX-5 or BSAP is a nuclear transcription factor involved in proliferation and especially plasma-cell differentiation of B cells and myeloma cells.[118–121] All reported four cases with the translocation presented as a lymphocytic lymphoma with plasmacytoid differentiation but without any paraprotein. Therefore, the translocation is most likely absent in bona fide lymphoplasmacytic lymphoma as defined by the World Health Organization (WHO) classification.

## Morphology and immunophenotype

In almost all patients, the diagnosis is made by means of a bone marrow biopsy. The infiltrate may be patchy or diffuse, but not typically nodular-like in lymphocytic lymphoma/CLL. The tumor consists of a mixture of small lymphocytes, plasmacytoid cells and mature plasma cells. In some cases small, cleaved cells are also present. In a few cases there is a prominent plasmacytic differentiation imitating myeloma. Abnormally processed immunoglobulins may be visible as so-called Russell or Dutcher bodies. Immuno-histochemistry for B-cell and plasma-cell markers, especially intracytoplasmic immunoglobulins, is indispensable to establish the diagnosis – also because the aggregates may be very small. In the spleen, tumor cells typically tend to cluster in the red pulp. Immunohistochemistry shows the presence of CD20, CD45, CD79a and cytoplasmic immunoglobulins, mostly IgM, with absence of CD5, CD10 and BCL6; CD138 is present on the mature plasma cells only.[122]

## Follicular lymphoma

This lymphoma was called follicle-center lymphoma in the REAL classification. In western countries, follicular lymphomas represent approximately 20–30% of all NHLs. It usually presents in multiple lymph nodes, but extranodal sites may also be involved. The bone marrow is involved in approximately 55% of cases. Approximately 10% of patients present with stage I disease. Particular clinical subtypes are primary cutaneous follicular lymphomas and primary mesenteric and/or retroperitoneal follicular lymphomas with sclerosis.

## Genetics, etiology and pathogenesis

Almost all follicular lymphomas carry the t(14;18)(q32:q21) involving the BCL2 gene at 18q21 and the Ig gene complex at 14q32.[123] All translocations leave the coding domain of the BCL2 gene intact. Three breakpoint clusters can be identified: approximately 60–70% of breakpoints occur downstream of the gene in the major breakpoint region (MBR), 10–15% in the minor breakpoint cluster (mcr) approximately 20 kb further downstream, and 5–15% in between the MBR and mcr. Few cases have a breakpoint at the other 5′ side of the gene. Approximately two-thirds of all breakpoints within the MBR and mcr can be detected by standard PCR. No data are available for the occurrence of this translocation in the so called 'diffuse follicle-center lymphomas'.

As shown in Figure 36.3, the t(14;18) translocation results in deregulation of one of the antagonists of apoptosis, the BCL2 gene. This effect is most apparent during the follicle-center cell reaction: in normal follicle-center B cells, BCL2 protein is downregulated and most B cells will not survive this 'killing field'

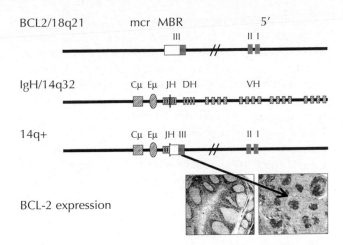

**Figure 36.3** Deregulation of BCL-2 by chromosomal translocation t(14;18) in follicular lymphoma.

associated with proliferation and apoptosis necessary for affinity maturation of the BCR. However, t(14;18)-carrying B cells have a strong survival advantage. Most likely, deregulation of BCL2 is essential but not sufficient for tumorigenesis, and deregulation of other genes as well as BCR-mediated stimulation of proliferation and survival may play an important additional role. The latter possibility is supported by the molecular analysis of the Ig genes in follicular lymphoma (evidence for ongoing hypermutations, over-representation of replacement mutations in the antigen recognition sites, and especially the presence of dominant subclones).[124,125] As expected, some follicular lymphomas have already undergone complete or abortive Ig class switching.[126]

Follicular lymphoma was the first malignancy to demonstrate that cells with a tumor-specific translocation are circulating in normal individuals. Using sensitive PCR experiments and appropriate control experiments, t(14;18) translocations were demonstrated in one of $10^4$–$10^5$ B cells of approximately 50% of all individuals with an increased incidence in elderly people as well as smokers.[127–131] Single individuals may carry more than one independent clone. This suggests that the t(14;18) is generated in a more or less random way and that additional events ultimately lead to expansion of a single clone. Alternatively, these sporadic translocation-carrying cells do not overexpress the BCL2 protein, and therefore, do not have any advance over normal cells.

## Morphology and immunophenotype

By definition, follicular lymphomas show a block in maturation at the level of normal follicle-center B cells, i.e. centroblasts and centrocytes. The neoplastic follicles closely mimic normal follicle centers in architecture and cellular composition. In most cases, a diagnosis can easily be made, whereas in other cases, it may be very difficult to diagnose this tumor without the help of immunohistochemistry or molecular analysis. In some cases, follicular lymphoma seems to start against a background of follicular hyperplasia, making the diagnosis extremely difficult. In rare lymphomas, unusual growth patterns or extensive plasma-cell differentiation occurs.[132,133] In the Kiel classification, follicular lymphomas were called follicular centroblastic-centrocytic or follicular centroblastic lymphoma, depending on the fraction of centroblasts in the tissue section.

Very few follicular lymphomas have a completely diffuse growth pattern ('diffuse follicle center cell lymphoma'). This variant has been overestimated in the past and many cases would currently have been classified as mantle-cell or marginal-zone lymphoma. Most likely the remaining cases represent follicular lymphomas with a big diffuse component or diagnoses obtained in relatively small biopsies such as needle biopsies with a high chance of sampling error.

For bone marrow staging of follicular lymphoma, a bone marrow biopsy is obligatory, since aspirates frequently give false-negative results. This is explained by the localization of tumor cells in especially seams along the trabecular surface in combination with deposition of reticulin fibers. In the few patients who have a leukemic type of follicular lymphoma (occurring in 10% of patients), the marrow may also contain many small lymphocytes with 'notched' nuclei.

Although it seems to be one disease, follicular lymphoma may be heterogeneous as well. The great majority of follicular lymphomas have a relatively monomorphic appearance with domination of centrocytes over centroblasts (grades 1, 2 and 3A lymphomas, see later). A small minority of the cases (probably 5% or less), however, mainly consist of centroblasts (grade 3B). The immunophenotype of the grade 1, 2 and 3A lymphomas is relatively consistent: approximately 90% of the cases express CD10, BCL6 and BCL2. Therefore, immunohistochemistry for the BCL2 protein is a very useful adjunct but not an absolute tool to distinguish follicular lymphoma from follicular hyperplasia.[134–136] Note that BCL2 staining should *not* be used to discriminate follicular lymphoma from other B-cell neoplasias, which are often BCL2 positive as well. Most cases express IgM, sometimes with coexpression of IgD, whereas other cases have undergone class switching to IgG or IgA. The lack of Ig expression in approximately 10% of the cases must not be interpreted as lack of evidence of malignancy. This lack of expression is apparently caused by either double translocations affecting both IgH alleles at 14q32 or the occurrence of secondary mutations introducing stop codons in the Ig genes.[137] Since the tumor cells are often fragile and may form a minority, data obtained by cell suspension analysis should also be interpreted cautiously. In all lym-

phomas, aggregates of dendritic cells stained by antibodies against CD21 or CD35 are present; in many, there are residual follicle mantle-zone B cells and numerous T cells. In contrast to the lower grades, grade 3B follicular lymphoma often does not express CD10 and BCL2, and often does not contain a translocation t(14;18), supporting the idea that it represents a different disease.

### Grading and tumor progression in follicular lymphoma

Follicular lymphomas are graded histologically according to the number of blasts or 'large transformed' cells. Different systems and cut-off levels have been used in the various classification systems. In the REAL classification, no definite system was proposed, however the WHO proposed to use the Berard grading system, as this is the single system that has been clinically validated.[9,10,138] In brief, counting in 10 unselected high-power fields of 0.159 mm$^2$ each, grade 1 contains 0–5, grade 2 contains 6–15 and grade 3 contains more than 15 (centro- or immuno-) blasts per high-power field. Using this system, grade 1 and 2 lymphomas can be lumped, whereas grade 3 lymphomas should be considered as more aggressive ones. In spite of the strict rules of the grading system, it remains difficult to use, even in hands of highly experienced hematopathologists. This is caused by the difficulties in classifying large, small blasts and large centrocytes, the bias to select areas with an increase in blasts, and the current tendency to take small (needle) biopsies that do not allow to count in a sufficiently large tissue area. Moreover, as shown earlier, several studies suggest that the current distinction is artificial and that a distinction should be made between grade 1, 2 and 3A versus grade 3B. The reported difference in clinical outcome between grades 2 and 3 might be mainly dependent on other parameters such as the presence of diffuse areas in the lymphoma. In summary, grading of follicular lymphomas remains highly controversial, and probably it is most appropriate to wait for better, biologically supported and reproducible criteria. As an alternative for grading, assessment of the proliferation index as measured with the Ki-67/MIB 1 antibody has been proposed, however, although this seems to have some prognostic significance, it does not necessarily match with the histological grading.[10,139]

Tumor progression occurs in at least 25% of patients and probably in more than 50%.[140] It is often characterized by histological transformation to large-cell lymphoma. A histological spectrum of centroblastic, immunoblastic or small noncleaved (non)Burkitt morphology has been described,[141] whereas a few patients develop overt acute leukemia with or without expression of terminal transferase (TdT).[142,143] Some cases contain many small blasts that mimic lymphoblasts, which express immunoglobulin and lack TdT. These cells are called 'blastoid'.[144] Tumor progression may occur at the start of or during the course of the disease, and is independent of treatment.

## Extranodal marginal-zone lymphomas of MALT

Primary extranodal marginal-zone B-cell lymphomas make up approximately 2–3% of all NHLs. The big majority of these lymphomas represent primary gastric lymphoma. Only this subtype will be described here. In contrast to the intestine, however, the normal stomach does not contain MALT, but MALT is induced by *Helicobacter pylori* (HP)-associated chronic inflammation. The normal intestinal MALT consists of several compartments:

1.  The lamina propria contains a mixture of T cells and (IgA-expressing) plasma cells. T cells are found as mainly CD4+ lamina propria lymphocytes and CD8+ or CD4−CD8− intraepithelial lymphocytes (IELs). A proportion of exclusively the IELs expresses the TCRγδ receptor. Both the intraepithelial and stromal T cells are expanded in celiac disease.
2.  Peyer patches consist of follicles with prominent follicle centers surrounded by a distinct mantle zone and marginal zone. In contrast to the other zones, marginal-zone cells express IgM, CD21 and CD35, but no CD5 or CD10 and no or weak IgD. The surface epithelium above the follicle may be populated with specialized intraepithelial B lymphocytes giving rise to the so-called lymphoepithelial lesions. Intra-epithelial B cells exclusively express a recently identified FcR-related molecule, IRTA1.[145]

The first MALT lymphomas were described for the stomach. Subsequently, similar lymphomas were recognized at other mucosal and even nonmucosal sites such as the salivary glands,[141,146] thyroid,[148,149] orbit,[150–152] breast,[153–155] skin,[156–160] thymus,[161] bladder,[162] and dura.[163] Later on, the analogy with the normal marginal zone of the spleen and lymph nodes and with the rare lymphomas primarily presenting in these organs (monocytoid B-cell lymphoma and splenic lymphoma with villous lymphocytes) led to the concept that there is one type of marginal-zone lymphoma that can present in the spleen, lymph node or at extranodal sites. However, there are many strong arguments against this concept, and most likely these three entities have nothing to do with each other. For instance, there is no clinical overlap or transition between the three disorders, and genetic abnormalities of the three types of marginal-zone lymphomas are entirely different. For that reason, they have been again separated in the WHO classification.

### Genetics, etiology and pathogenesis

The current genetic data for gastric marginal-zone lymphomas are fascinating but still incomplete.

Gastric MALT lymphomas are monoclonal neoplastic disorders with a very indolent behavior. Most likely they start as an oligoclonal and subsequently monoclonal expansion of marginal-zone B cells that are growth and cell survival dependent on inflammatory Th$_2$-type T cells. This process is triggered and maintained by HP-induced gastritis and induction of local MALT tissue. Early MALT lymphoma cells remain dependent on this HP-specific T-cell help, and eradication of HP leads to regression of these early lymphomas.[164–168] At this early stage of the disease, no specific genetic alterations are known. However, because of the genetic instability in the proliferating cells, many tumors will acquire genetic abnormalities. The most common and specific translocation is the t(11;18)(q21;q21) involving the *MALT1/MLT* and *AP12* gene leading to a chimeric transcript of both genes[169–177] *MALT1* is a paracaspase and binds to BCL10, which itself is also involved in the t(1;14)(p22;q32) translocation rarely observed in gastric MALT lymphomas as well. Both *MALT1* and *BCL10* are involved in a specific signaling pathway, where *MALT1* is downstream of *BCL10*. *MALT1* is essential to induce NFkappaB upon B-cell activation by T cells. Constitutive activation of *MALT1* by chromosomal translocation t(11;18) will, therefore, lead to constitutive NFkappaB activation and result in enhanced proliferation and resistance to apoptosis.[178] Indeed MALT lymphomas with this translocation have a more aggressive behavior with transmural growth, and most essentially, they are often resistant to antibiotic treatment aiming at HP eradication.[172,179,180] Therefore, patients with a t(11;18)-positive gastric MALT lymphoma probably should be treated with HP eradication supplemented with conventional (chemo)therapy. Interestingly, MALT lymphomas without these translocations seem to be more prone to acquire other genetic alterations such as trisomy 3. Progression to large cell lymphoma may be associated with p53 mutation or t(8;14) involving MYC.[181–183]

Concomitant with their continuous T-cell mediated stimulation, re-entry in and recruitment from MALT-associated germinal centers, gastric MALT lymphoma tumor cells contain (ongoing) hypermutations associated with a (post-)follicle-center cell genotype.[184–187]

Normal mature B cells, and especially memory B cells, show extensive circulation and re-circulation in the peripheral blood. B cells of the MALT show a limited pattern of circulation and specific homing to other MALT sites, including the draining (mesenteric) lymph nodes. This specific homing seems to be determined by specific homing receptors on lymphocytes and addressins on the high endothelial venules in lymphoid tissues, and may partly explain the limited dissemination of the lymphomas.[188] For instance, alpha4beta7 integrin may play a role in this process.[189,190]

## Morphology and immunophenotype

Macroscopically, MALT lymphomas of the stomach mostly present in the antrum with one or more small ulcerations or flat infiltrative lesions. In cases with large tumor masses, the appearance may be similar to carcinoma. In some cases, the lymphoma presents at multiple sites in the stomach, or even simultaneously or metachronously in the stomach, intestine, lungs or tonsils. Histologically, MALT lymphomas may be highly heterogeneous. Some lymphomas show a typical monomorphous appearance caused by expansion of 'centrocyte-like' B cells. In other cases, the cells are mixed with small lymphocytes, mature plasma cells and blasts. Cases with prominent plasma cell differentiation were previously interpreted as solitary plasmacytoma. In many cases, tumor cells tend to invade the epithelial lining and crypts, giving rise to 'lymphoepithelial lesions'. However, it should be noted that the presence of these lesions is not sufficient to call it malignant. Some MALT lymphomas additionally show 'follicular colonization', i.e. invasion of reactive follicles by tumor cells; in the past, this phenomenon was interpreted either as follicular lymphoma or as a sign of benignity.

## Grading and tumor progression

Based on the percentage of blast cells, a clinically relevant grading system has been proposed.[191,192] This system was originally based on a retrospective analysis in patients treated with radiotherapy alone and not with antibiotic treatment as presently used. The system also bears prognostic significance for the clinical response to HP eradication. However, it should be noted that grading of these lymphomas is severely impeded by the fact that almost all patients with gastrointestinal MALT lymphoma currently undergo endoscopic examination with biopsy and not a (partial) gastrectomy. Sampling error may occur, especially if few biopsies are taken.

Approximately half of all primary B-cell lymphomas of the stomach are dominated by blasts and lack features of MALT lymphomas such as lymphoepithelial lesions. Although many authors believe that these tumors represent progressed indolent MALT lymphomas, this has only been proved in a limited number of patients.[193] Of note, these tumors lack the chromosomal translocations t(11;18) or t(1;14) (Figure 36.4). In consequence, these large-cell tumors can only be lumped in the 'wastebasket' category of diffuse large B-cell lymphomas (DLBCLs).

## Diffuse large B-cell lymphoma

In western countries, DLBCLs comprise approximately 30–40% of all NHLs. Clinically, morphologically and genetically, DLBCL is a heterogeneous disorder, comprising multiple separate entities that share a large-cell morphology. Approximately half of the lymphomas arise within lymph nodes, and the other half at extranodal sites such as the thymic region, stomach, small and large bowel, skin, thyroid, testis, bone, soft tissues, and brain. According to the WHO classification, primary mediastinal and primary intravascular DLBCLs have already been designated as distinct clinicopathological entities. According to the EORTC classification for primary cutaneous lymphomas, primary cutaneous large B-cell lymphomas should be separated as well, and even further distinguished according to the localization in the

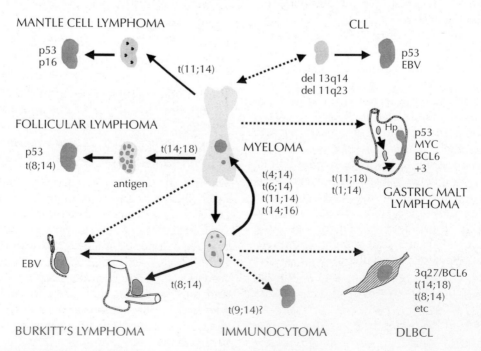

**Figure 36.4** Chromosomal translocations and their origin in B-cell neoplasia.

skin.[159,194,195] Primary mediastinal DLBCL mainly affects young adults, and often presents with a very bulky mediastinal mass and a superior vena cava syndrome. It tends to remain localized, without dissemination to lymph nodes or bone marrow. Intravascular lymphoma is mostly encountered in the skin or brain. Tumor cells are localized within the lumina of blood vessels, but do not overtly circulate in the peripheral blood. Intracerebral intravascular DLBCL results in severe brain dysfunction.

Just as at primary presentation, DLBCL may also be very heterogeneous in dissemination upon relapse. For instance, nodal lymphomas tend to spread to other lymph nodes and the tonsils, DLBCL of the stomach to regional lymph nodes or other MALT sites, testicular lymphoma to the contralateral testis and cerebrum, and bone lymphoma to other skeletal sites. Primary cutaneous lymphomas of the head and trunk often lack any propensity to disseminate, and hence may be cured by local radiotherapy. Most likely, these patterns reflect the presence or absence of specific adhesion molecules involved in invasion, circulation, adherence to endothelial cells, etc.[190,196,197] Thus, as in T-cell lymphomas, there is a strong tendency to distinguish DLBCL according to tumor site.

### Genetics, etiology and pathogenesis

So far, DLBCL seems to be a genetic wastebasket. Genetic alterations often comprise complex abnormalities, including translocations, deletions, trisomies, amplifications and the presence of many marker chromosomes. The most frequent chromosomal breakpoint is at the BCL6 gene at 3q27.[198–210] These breakpoints are found in at least one-third of the cases, including acquired immunodeficiency syndrome (AIDS)-related lymphomas,[211,212] but also occur in 5–10% of follicular lymphomas.[213–215] Most BCL6 breakpoints cluster in a small (regulatory) region of 10kb just upstream of the gene, however, an additional breakpoint cluster far upstream of the gene has recently been identified.[216] By translocation, BCL6 is juxtaposed to a large number of different translocation partners (a 'promiscuous gene'). Most translocations will lead to promoter-substitution of BCL6. Notably, mutations in the same regulatory region of BCL6 occur at high frequency in all lymphomas of (post)follicular origin and even in myelomas, but most frequently in DLBCL.[147,148] Exclusively in DLBCL, a part of these mutations affects regulatory elements and in consequence leads to activation of the gene.[217–219] The BCL6 gene codes for a zinc-finger protein with homology to Drosophila transcription factors, whereas it functions as a repressor of many other genes. BCL6 plays an essential role in the formation and maintenance of normal germinal centers. Possibly, it controls the ability of B cells to interact with T cells by preventing CD40-induced expression of CD80, an essential costimulatory molecule in T–B-cell interaction.[210] Indeed, the bcl6 protein

is present in all normal follicle center cells, all follicular lymphomas and in 75–80% of all DLBCLs, but not or only weakly in mantle-cell lymphomas, lymphocytic lymphomas/CLLs and postgerminal center B-cell lymphomas. In contrast to the original report,[204] BCL6 rearrangement is not associated with a favorable prognosis.[208,220]

The second most frequent (15%) translocation in DLBCL is the t(14;18), with a breakpoint in BCL2. Interestingly, this translocation is mainly present in primary nodal DLBCL.[221,222] Most likely, t(14;18)-positive DLBCL represents progressed subclinical follicular lymphoma. Unlike the situation in follicular lymphoma, there is a poor correlation between the presence of t(14;18) and expression of BCL2 protein in DLBCL. In fact many cases without any detectable translocation show expression of the protein and this expression is associated with a relatively poor survival, especially a poor disease-free survival.[223–226] Recent gene expression studies suggest that this overexpression (that is not caused by a t(14;18)) is specifically found in the subset of DLBCL with an activated B-cell profile (see later).

The third most common (5–10%) translocation in DLBCL is the t(8;14), with involvement of MYC at 8q24.[221,227] Most breakpoints are 5' or in the first intron of MYC, and at IgH switch sites of 14q32. In a very few DLBCLs, a combination of t(14;18) and t(8;14) has been identified, and molecular analysis of these cases suggests that the t(8;14) is secondary to the t(14;18).[228] Most DLBCLs with t(8;14) present at extranodal sites, especially the gastrointestinal tract. In primary extranodal DLBCL and especially primary mediastinal large B-cell lymphoma, a high frequency of amplification of the REL gene at chromosome 2p is found.[229–231] This abnormality has gained much recent interest, especially since it leads to activation of NFkappaB and since a similar amplification is present in classical Hodgkin lymphomas.[232–235] Discussion of the rapidly increasing number of chromosomal and specific gene alterations in DLBCL is beyond the scope of this chapter. They include a very frequent but thus far nonspecific deletion at 6q.[236–238]

Since the first publication in 2000,[239] much attention has been paid to gene expression analysis using cDNA or oligonucleotide array analysis. Several hundreds of DLBCLs, mainly of nodal origin, have been studied so far, whereas studies on specific categories of extranodal lymphomas have been done or are underway.[240,241] Most essentially, these studies show that nodal DLBCL can at least be distinguished in two types of lymphomas: one type has a gene expression profile of germinal center B cells (GCs); in the other type gene expression resembles that of activated B-cells (ABCs). These patterns corroborate expression of several markers of germinal center and post-germinal center B cells such as CD10 and MUM-1/IRF-4, respectively. Furthermore, as expected, t(14;18) is almost exclusively found in DLBCL with a GC profile.[242] NFkappaB activation was especially observed in the DLBCL with an ABC profile.[243] Clinically most relevant, DLBCLs with this ABC profile have a far worse prognosis than DLBCLs with a GC expression profile. In multivariate analysis, this prognostic factor is independent of the International Prognostic Index (IPI) prognostic index. Gene expression studies have also been used in reverse, i.e. to investigate whether DLBCL with a favorable vs. a poor response to standard chemotherapy has differences in gene expression.[244]

### Morphology and immunophenotype

Large B-cell lymphomas are highly heterogeneous in morphology. Several attempts have been made to describe the various cells and subtypes, such as *monomorphic, polymorphic* or *multilobated centroblastic* and *immunoblastic*. Additionally, an *anaplastic* variant of DLBCL mimicking T-cell anaplastic large cell lymphoma and sometimes also expressing CD30 (see later) has been described. Finally, comparable with Hodgkin lymphoma, some DLBCLs contain a very dominant population of reactive cells, and dependent on the predominant component, these DLBCLs are called T-cell-rich B-cell lymphoma, histiocyte-rich B-cell lymphoma or epithelioid-cell-rich B-cell lymphoma. At first glance, this extensive subtyping of DLBCL looks absurd, but the significance becomes apparent if one considers that, from a pathologist's point of view, each subtype may have a completely different and often difficult differential diagnosis. For instance, even with additional immunophenotyping, the monomorphic centroblastic subtype may be very difficult to distinguish from Burkitt lymphoma; immunoblastic lymphoma may be impossible to distinguish from plasmacytoma, whereas T-cell-rich and histiocyte-rich B-cell lymphomas may be very difficult to differentiate from the diffuse variant of lymphocyte-predominant Hodgkin lymphoma.

### Other aspects of DLBCL

Approximately 10–30% of all DLBCLs have bone marrow localization, and a so-called 'discordant morphology' is observed in approximately half of these patients. Discordant lymphomas are lymphomas with different appearances at different sites – for instance DLBCL in a lymph node and predominantly centrocytes with a few centroblasts in the bone marrow biopsy. Most likely (but formally not proven), these lymphomas represent progressed low-grade (follicular) lymphomas. The clinical implications of this finding are obvious. Some studies have shown that after complete remission, patients with discordant disease follow the course of indolent follicle-center lymphomas, i.e. they have a short disease-free survival but a favorable overall survival.[245–247] This may parallel the described effect of t(14;18) on disease-free survival. Therefore, bone marrow biopsies should always be analyzed carefully for the presence of tiny paratrabecular aggregates of abnormal lymphoid cells.

## Burkitt lymphoma

Burkitt lymphoma was originally described as a clinical entity in equatorial Africa, with endemic malaria and other infections. The Epstein–Barr virus (EBV) was identified in 1964 and the characteristic t(8;14)(q24;q32) translocation in 1972[248] (see Chapter 16). A specific localization of the breakpoints at 8q24 at the *MYC* locus (see later) further substantiated that these lymphomas are an entity. These lymphomas are called 'African type' or 'endemic' Burkitt lymphoma. Later on, lymphomas with a similar morphology and translocations (but different at the molecular level – see later) but with a different clinical context, and mostly without EBV infection, were identified elsewhere, including the USA and Europe. These lymphomas are called 'Burkitt lymphoma, non-African type' or 'sporadic Burkitt lymphoma', and represent approximately 2–5% of all NHL in western countries. Burkitt Lymphomas are extremely fast growing tumors with in some cases a doubling time of less than 24 h.

There is a very strong, so far unexplained male predominance, and especially male patients show a bimodal age distribution with a peak between 5 and 15 years of age. Pediatric Burkitt lymphomas mainly present at extranodal sites, whereas adult lymphomas tend to present more in the lymph nodes. The best-known example is mesenteric/ileocecal Burkitt lymphoma in children. More recently, an increase in incidence has been observed due to the emergence of human immunodeficiency virus (HIV) infection and AIDS. Also, these lymphomas are mostly EBV negative, and of the 'non-African' type. Confusingly, some (non-African) Burkitt lymphomas, especially in adult patients, cannot be easily discerned from lymphomas with a variant morphology or DLBCL with a very high proliferation rate. A part of these lymphomas have been called 'Burkitt-like lymphoma' in the REAL classification, and are called 'atypical Burkitt lymphoma' in the WHO classification. Even very experienced hematopathologists have classification problems in this grey zone between DLBC and Burkitt lymphomas,[249] and it certainly will be necessary to redefine Burkitt lymphoma on the basis of biologically relevant parameters such as specific gene alterations or gene expression patterns.

### Genetics, etiology and pathogenesis

Using conventional banding analysis, almost all Burkitt lymphomas contain a t(8;14)(q24;q32), a t(2;8)(p12;q24) or a t(8;22)(q24;q11). The latter variant translocations involve the Ig light-chain loci. In

African Burkitt lymphoma, the frequency is up to 100%. In African Burkitt lymphomas, breakpoints mainly involve the $J_H$ or $D_H$ genes at 14q32 of the IgL genes at 2p12 and 22q11, and may have an origin from IgH hypermutations. In non-African Burkitt lymphoma, the breakpoints are more common at $S_\mu$ and $S_\alpha$, indicating an origin from class-switching follicle-center B-cells. Within the 8q24 region, breakpoints are found within or immediately 5′ of *MYC* (mostly in sporadic types), or far 5′ and far (several hundreds of kb) 3′ of *MYC* (mostly African types).[250–255] Most likely, breakpoints can be best detected using FISH analysis.[77,256] Studies on hypermutations in Ig genes in African Burkitt Lymphoma cell lines showed extensive hypermutations, indicating that the cells do represent mature B cells.[257,258]

### Morphology and immunophenotype

Most Burkitt lymphomas present with large and extremely rapidly growing tumor masses. The prototype of the non-African-type Burkitt lymphoma is a large mass in the ileocecal mesenteric region, with extension in the intestinal wall and generation of ascites. Polypoid masses in the submucosa may give rise to invagination. Tumor cells may be found in the peripheral blood and bone marrow, giving the appearance of an acute leukemia previously called ALL L3. Most characteristically, the tumor cells show a diffuse, cohesive growth pattern with interspersed tingible body macrophages stuffed with apoptotic tumor cells. This combination creates the typical 'starry sky' pattern under low-level microscopy. Cytologically and immunophenotypically, Burkitt lymphoma cells resemble early blasts (small centroblasts) in normal follicle centers. This explains why a distinction between Burkitt lymphoma and the monomorphic centroblastic variant of DLBCL may be difficult (see earlier). To prevent autolysis and poor morphology, it is extremely important to speed up transfer of surgical material to the pathology laboratory. Cytological preparations (imprints or smears of ascites) are extremely helpful, since they may show diagnostic details such as lipid-containing vacuoles. Immunophenotypically, Burkitt lymphoma cells show strong expression of surface IgM. Like normal follicle-center cells and follicular lymphomas, almost all Burkitt lymphomas express CD 10 and BCL6, whereas TdT is consistently absent. BCL2 expression should be absent as well. The variant-type Burkitt lymphoma in elderly patients discussed earlier exhibits more pleomorphism, anisonucleosis, bigger nucleoli, and often plasmacytic differentiation with cytoplasmic staining in immunofluorescence for immunoglobulins.[176]

### Other B-cell lymphomas

As shown in Table 36.1, there are many other lymphomas that may be conceived as a clinicopathological entity. Splenic marginal-zone lymphoma either with or without villous lymphocytes (SLVLs) is a rare clinicopathological entity that, like other indolent B-cell lymphomas, has been associated with hepatitis C virus infection.[259–261] In one study antiviral therapy appeared to be effective in only those lymphomas that were associated with the virus. In contrast to earlier reports that suggested a heterogeneous phenotype, this lymphoma should be characterized by the consistent absence of CD5, CD10 and cyclinD1 expression. Splenectomy preparations show a distinct infiltration of the white pulp with aggregates of tumor cells in the red pulp, which is different from the pattern in HCL, variant HCL and prolymphocytic leukemia (PLL).

## Immune-deficiency-associated EBV-positive lymphomas

In the WHO classification, three main subgroups have been proposed (Table 31.3):

1. Immunoproliferative diseases associated with primary immune disorders (PIDs)
2. Lymphomas associated with infection by HIV
3. Post-transplant lymphoproliferative disorders (PTLDs)

There is a large number of primary immune disorders with an increased incidence of lymphoproliferative disorders, including diseases that present early during life such as severe combined immune deficiency (SCID) and disorders that present later on such as the autoimmune lymphoproliferative syndrome (ALPS). The incidence differs depending on the underlying disorder and the genetic background.[262–264] Many disorders are X-linked and, therefore, preferentially present in males (SCID, X-linked lymphoproliferative syndrome, hyper IgM syndrome). With the exception of the lymphomas in ALPS, many of these lymphoproliferative disorders present at extranodal sites and almost all cases are EBV driven. In ALPS, that is caused by mutations in FAS/CD95, CD95 ligand/FADD, caspase 8 or caspase 10, a wide variety of lymphoproliferative disorders including Hodgkin lymphoma have been described.[265–269] In common variable immunodeficiency, chronic antigenic stimulation rather than EBV may lead to the development of lymphomas. Large B-cell lymphoma is the most common type in PID, with the exception of T-cell lymphomas in ataxia teleangiectasia, as well as a very heterogeneous range of lymphomas in ALPS.

Lymphomas associated with infection by HIV comprise a wide range of disorders. Most cases are diffuse large B-cell lymphomas, but they also include Burkitt lymphoma, plasmablastic tumors, primary effusion lymphoma, peripheral T-cell lymphomas and Hodgkin lymphoma. Again many lymphomas involve extranodal sites, especially the mucosal sites, lungs, pleural cavities, brain, and bone marrow.[270-274] Most lymphomas are EBV driven and such lymphomas frequently lack expression of several lymphoid markers such as CD45 and CD20.[275] This implies that the lymphoid nature may be missed if other markers (CD30, CD79a, CD138, Ig) are omitted. One example is the primary effusion lymphoma; these EBV-positive and human herpes virus type 8 (HHV-8)- or Kaposi sarcoma virus (KSV)-positive tumor cells lack almost all lymphoid markers, but contain monoclonal rearrangements of the Ig genes.[276-278] Interestingly, the incidence of these lymphomas has dramatically decreased, which is caused by the currently very effective antiviral therapy in western countries, whereas some of the current patients present with disorders that have more analogy to PTLD, especially the polymorphic lymphoproliferative disorder.

PTLDs also have a highly varying clinical and pathologic picture, which is very much dependent on the clinical context, age, and level of immune suppression. In some transplant patients and especially children, generalized disease with circulating tumor cells may be present. In some patients, the tumor preferentially involves the transplanted organ itself.[279-284] Histologically, these lymphomas have a variable morphology, leading to a number of different classifications. Again, most disorders are EBV positive, but especially lymphomas that occur relatively late after transplant, including the so-called plasmacytomas, can be EBV negative. Immunophenotypically, the tumors often show cytoplasmic Ig, which is detectable in formalin-fixed and paraffin-embedded tissue. Depending on mainly host factors, especially the level of immune deficiency and time after transplant, immunoglobulin expression can be polyclonal, oligoclonal or monoclonal. This may reflect the evolution of these tumors from polyclonal B-cell infection by EBV, clonal evolution, and overgrowth by a single clone. The variable clonality status of the tumor cells is also observed using molecular analysis (Southern blot analysis or PCR) of Ig gene rearrangements. Depending especially on host factors, different types of EBV infection may be seen: latency type 1, but especially types 2 or 3, and even lytic infection may occur. Of note, many patients will respond to a combination therapy aiming at (temporarily) alleviating the immune suppression, to allow the patient to restore the immune status, in combination with monoclonal antibodies against the infected B cells (e.g. anti CD20). Furthermore, the current strategies to continuously monitor the EBV load in the peripheral blood and to start therapy as soon as possible will probably lead to the decrease and altered pathology of these disorders.

# T-cell lymphomas

T-cell lymphomas comprise approximately 9–15% of all NHLs in western countries, but are far more frequent in Asian countries. This is probably not due to the presence of HTLV-I-related T-cell lymphomas in parts of Japan, but rather to the relatively low incidence of some B-cell lymphomas in combination with a relatively high frequency of EBV-positive nasal-type T/NK-cell lymphomas. Perhaps even more than B-cell lymphomas, T-cell lymphomas show a restricted presentation at specific sites of the body. Grossly, they can be categorized as primary nodal T-cell lymphomas such as angio-immunoblastic T-cell lymphoma, and other mainly extranodal lymphomas. Distinct examples of lymphomas with a restricted extranodal presentation and dissemination are mycosis fungoides (MF), Sézary syndrome, cutaneous anaplastic large-cell lymphoma/lymphomatoid papulosis, panniculitic-like T-cell lymphoma, nasal (type) T/NK-cell lymphomas, intestinal T-cell lymphoma associated with enteropathy, and hepatosplenic $\gamma\delta$T-cell lymphoma. Phenotypically, most T-cell lymphomas represent malignancies of mature TCR$\alpha\beta^+$ T-cells, and in some cases NK cells.[285] Tumor cells in angio-immunoblastic T-cell lymphoma and MF/ Sézary syndrome are mainly CD4$^+$ and lack cytotoxic molecules, however, many other lymphomas, especially the primary extranodal tumors have properties of cytotoxic T cells with expression of TIA-1 and granzyme B, either or not in combination with CD8 or CD4. These include the majority of anaplastic large-cell lymphomas (ALCLs).[286,287] Only a few lymphomas, in particular the EBV-positive nasal lymphomas, are derived from true CD56$^+$ NK cells.[288] In consequence, these tumors do not harbor clonal TCR gene rearrangements.

## T-lymphoblastic lymphoma/T-ALL

T-lymphoblastic lymphoma is part of a spectrum of neoplasms derived from precursor T cells. In many patients, the tumor extends from the thymic region into the mediastinum, pleural cavities, cervical lymph nodes, blood and bone marrow. Therefore, differentiation between primary lymphoma and leukemia is arbitrary. There is a preference to affect young boys and adolescents. Because of the localization and extremely rapid growth, stenosis of the trachea may become life threatening within a few days or even hours, necessitating an extremely rapid diagnosis. In some patients, it is only possible to get a cytological aspirate and to perform limited immunocytochemistry before the start of therapy. Like their normal counterparts, the tumor cells are extremely sensitive to irradiation and corticosteroids.

### Genetics, etiology and pathogenesis

T-ALL and lymphoblastic lymphoma are very interesting with respect to possible genetic alterations. This is discussed extensively in Chapter 18. In brief, a large number of different nuclear transcription factors can be activated by juxtaposition with TCR genes, but, surprisingly, these translocations result in a similar phenotype.[289,290]

## Morphology and immunophenotype

In most patients, the tumor cells look like lymphoblasts as seen in ALL. The tumor cells show a high mitotic activity and sometimes a high degree of apoptosis. They may extensively infiltrate soft tissues. All lymphomas and acute leukemias should be immunophenotyped appropriately to determine the cell lineage and immaturity of tumor cells, the latter always by TdT. By further typing, the exact stage of maturation can be determined. For instance, the presence of CD1 with coexpression of CD4 and CD8 indicates a phenotype of cortical thymocytes.

## Angio-immunoblastic lymphoma

Angio-immunoblastic lymphoma (AIL) is a clinico-pathological entity mostly affecting elderly patients.[291,292] Patients present with a syndrome that is characterized by generalized lymphadenopathy and many of the following features: initial skin rash, fever, hepatosplenomegaly, Coombs-positive hemolytic anemia, eosinophilia and polyclonal hypergammaglobulinemia. Almost all patients succumb to the disease, either due to progression to overt immunoblastic lymphoma or to secondary infections. Secondary infections seem to be caused by a severe cellular immune deficiency in combination with treatment. On the basis of strict histological and sometimes also molecular criteria (see later), especially early forms of AIL have to be differentiated from abnormal immune reactions. Originally, the disorder was thought to be a reactive process and was named immunoblastic lymphadenopathy (IBL) or angio-immunoblastic lymphadenopathy with dysproteinemia (AILD). After the introduction of strict histological criteria and the finding that at least 60% of these lesions harbor clonal TCR rearrangements, the name AILD-like T-cell lymphoma or its contraction AIL should be used.

### Genetics, etiology and pathogenesis

Infection and hypersensitivity have been proposed but never proven to be etiological agents in AILD and AIL. Cytogenetic abnormalities, including trisomy 3 and oligoclonal abnormalities, have been reported.[293] Studies of Ig and TCR gene rearrangements show that at least 60% have clonal TCR rearrangements. Approximately 20% have clonal Ig rearrangements without TCR rearrangement, and in fact some AILD lymphomas develop into immunoblastic B-cell lymphomas instead of a T-cell lymphoma. This is explained by secondary EBV infection of B cells due to depressed immune surveillance in these severely immune-deficient patients.[294,295] This can be detected using RNA in situ hybridization for EBER and immunohistochemistry for LMP-1.

## Morphology and immunophenotype

Lymph nodes involved by AIL show atrophy of follicles ('burned-out' follicles) and expansion of T-cell areas with extension in perinodal fatty tissues and obliteration of sinuses. Clusters of 'clear' blast cells should be identified. Tumor cells are present against an impressive background of numerous arborizing high endothelial venules, plasma cells, eosinophils, neutrophils and clusters of epithelioid histiocytes. The presence of large and very irregular aggregates of follicular (CD21+ and CD35+) dendritic reticulum cells is almost diagnostic for the disease. Recent studies have shown an aberrant expression of CD10 on many tumor cells.[296] Possibly, the pleomorphic background in almost all cases is evoked by a cascade of cytokines. There may be an additional infiltrate of EBV-positive atypical immunoblasts (and plasma cells), which can be poly-, oligo- or monoclonal upon immunohistochemistry and molecular analysis. AIL often presents in the bone marrow as small, loosely arranged aggregates. A reticulin stain and immunohistochemistry are extremely helpful in unmasking these aggregates. Additionally, the skin is often involved by AIL.

## Anaplastic large cell lymphoma

Anaplastic large cell lymphoma (ALCL) or large-cell anaplastic lymphoma (LCAL), previously also called Ki-1-positive lymphoma, may present in two different forms: primary cutaneous (see later) and primary systemic. The latter will be described here. Most ALCLs occur in children or young adults. Together with Burkitt lymphoma and T-lymphoblastic lymphoma, ALCL forms the great majority of NHLs of childhood. ALCLs can be misdiagnosed as Hodgkin lymphoma, metastatic carcinoma or melanoma because of incomplete phenotyping or an aberrant phenotype (see later). Some cases may mimic a reactive lymphadenopathy. B-cell lymphomas with anaplastic morphology should be excluded and classified as DLBCL. Finally, there is a distinct trend to restrict the term ALCL to those lymphomas that express the ALK protein (see later). This is supported by the observation that especially the patients with ALK-positive ALCL have a relatively very good outcome.[297–301] Primary nodal ALCL may disseminate to the skin and bones, and in approximately 10–20% of cases to the bone marrow. Note that secondary skin involvement must be differentiated from primary cutaneous ALCL, since exclusively cutaneous ALCL has an excellent prognosis (see later).

### Genetics, etiology and pathogenesis

Approximately 60% or more of all nodal ALCLs contain a translocation with production of a fusion gene between anaplastic large cell lymphoma kinase (*ALK*) and other genes.[302-305] This frequency is even higher in ALCL of childhood. The translocation is absent in primary cutaneous ALCL as well as enteropathy-associated T-cell lymphomas with anaplastic morphology and CD30 expression (see later). The fusion protein can be visualized by RT-PCR or FISH, but also with an antibody against the ALK protein. After the first description of the classical t(2;5) involving *ALK* and nucleophosmin (*NPM*), many other fusion partners have been identified. In general approximately 70% of all breakpoints involve *NPM*, whereas in the remaining 30%, other translocations are identified. One peculiar type of B-cell lymphoma, *ALK*-positive diffuse large B-cell lymphoma is, however, also associated with chromosomal translocations involving the *ALK* gene, especially the t(2;7)(p23;q23) involving *CLATHRIN*.[306-308] Analysis of Ig and TCR gene rearrangements are of little help in ALCL. Results are highly variable, and in many cases too few tumor cells are present to be detected by PCR and Southern blot analysis. In cases with clonal rearrangements, mostly monoclonal TCR but also Ig gene rearrangements have been reported.

## Morphology and immunophenotype

Lymph nodes with the classical form of ALCL show a typical morphology: large, polymorphic so-called 'hallmark cells' with round, kidney-shaped or doughnut-like nuclei and often prominent nucleoli, are tightly clustered within afferent lymph vessels and sinuses, giving the appearance of metastic carcinoma, melanoma or malignant histiocytosis. Other forms form tumor nodules or accumulations along high endothelial venules. Small-cell, giant-cell and Hodgkin-like variants of ALCL, as well as lymphohistiocytic and granulocyte-rich subtypes have been described.[304] However, Hodgkin-like ALCL has been overemphasized in the literature, and most cases can now be assigned to the syncytial variant of the nodular sclerosing subtype of Hodgkin lymphoma. Many ALCLs evoke a pleomorphic background of reactive lymphocytes, plasma cells, eosinophils, neutrophils and especially histiocytes similar to Hodgkin lymphoma. Immunohistochemistry of these systemic ALCLs shows that approximately half of all ALCLs lack CD45, whereas epithelial membrane antigen (EMA) is present in approximately half of the cases, allowing the possibility of a misdiagnosis of metastatic carcinoma. Other positive markers are CD30 and CD25. Incomplete T-cell markers are present in more than 50% of the cases, as are cytotoxic molecules such as TIA-1 and granzyme B. In approximately 60% of the cases, ALK protein is easily found. Interestingly, highly dependent on the underlying chromosomal translocation, ALK may be present in the cytoplasm and nucleus (in case of the classical t(2;5) involving nucleophosmin, translocating the ALK protein to the nucleus) or in distinct cytoplasmic compartments. In contrast to Hodgkin lymphoma, CD15 is commonly negative.

## Nasal-type T/NK-cell lymphoma

Nasal-type T/NK-cell lymphoma[288,309-313] has previously been described as 'lethal midline granuloma', 'polymorphic reticulosis' or 'lymphomatoid granulomatosis'. It is especially common in some Asian regions. Almost all tumors present in the nasal cavity with ulcerative lesions or polypoid masses. This may lead to a suspicion of Wegener granulomatosis. The tumors show a locally destructive growth, sometimes with erosion of bone and even permeation into the base of the skull. Other unusual sites of primary presentation are the testis and intestine. Lymph node metastasis is uncommon, but metastasis may occur at extranodal sites. Histology often reveals extensive necrosis, and sometimes invasion of the walls of blood vessels – therefore termed 'angiocentric lymphoma'. Since this feature is not present in all nasal-type lymphomas, and can also be seen in some B-cell lymphomas, this latter name has been omitted. Almost all lymphomas are CD2$^+$, cytoplasmic CD3$\zeta^+$, CD56$^+$, TIA-1$^+$ and granzyme-B$^+$, and are often also CD8$^+$. No clonal T-cell receptor gene rearrangement is found. This corroborates a phenotype of NK or cytotoxic T-cells. Thus the presence of cytoplasmic CD3$\zeta$ should not be interpreted as proof of T-cell origin. As demonstrated by immunohistochemistry, in situ hybridization, and other molecular studies, almost all (>90%) lymphomas are EBV positive.

## Intestinal T-cell lymphoma

Intestinal T-cell lymphoma is a disease of the elderly, and is closely associated with enteropathy or overt celiac disease.[314-320] Clinically, it may present with a period of increased abdominal discomfort and malresorption. Other patients present with perforation of the jejunum or ileum with peritonitis. Surgical intervention shows one or more perforations and often multiple foci of tumor or ulcers. Histological examination may show large tumor masses, usually with a high degree of pleomorphism, but sometimes also very extensive multifocal ulceration without easily recognizable tumor cells. Extensive sampling may reveal only small tumor foci, often with an aberrant phenotype. In some cases there is an extensive eosinophilia that masks the tumor cells. At the cytological level, the tumor cells may vary from small to large, the large cell type often exhibiting anaplastic and pleomorphic nuclei. They have a phenotype of activated cytotoxic T cells (granzyme-B$^+$). Approximately half of the cases show strong expression of CD30 mimicking ALCL, and in some cases the tumor cells have an anaplastic morphology including the presence of so-called 'hallmark cells', as well.

However, these tumors should not be considered as ALCL, which is supported by a consistent absence of the ALK protein. Small-celled types may show expression of CD56.[321] In view of the relationship with enteropathy, especially celiac disease, the adjacent mucosa of all specimens should be thoroughly examined for any increase in intraepithelial lymphocytes (IELs) or overt villous atrophy.

## Peripheral T-cell lymphomas not otherwise specified

This group of lymphomas is more or less a wastebasket of lymphomas, including the so-called 'Lennert lymphoma'. The latter often presents with generalized lymphadenopathy and splenomegaly. Histologically, it is dominated by clusters of epithelioid histiocytes, interspersed small- and medium-sized T-cells, and few blasts. Most importantly, using additional stainings, pathologists should exclude a reactive process (Whipple disease and mycobacterial infection), angioimmunoblastic T-cell lymphoma, mixed-type Hodgkin lymphoma, immunocytoma and epithelioid/T-cell-rich B-cell lymphoma.

## Cutaneous T-cell lymphomas: MF and Sézary syndrome

Mycosis fungoides and Sézary syndrome are the most common cutaneous T-cell lymphomas (CTCLs). However, other primary CTCLs should be recognized: pleomorphic and immunoblastic lymphomas, as well as CD30[+] anaplastic large cell lymphoma and the 'borderline' condition lymphomatoid papulosis. Clinically, MF often presents on the trunk ('swimming-suit localization'). Dermatological presentations may be in the form of patches, plaques and tumors. Especially in the tumor-forming stage, tumor cells may disseminate to local lymph nodes, followed by internal localizations. Based on lymph-node histology, a specific staging may be used.[322,323] Variant forms of MF comprise (large) parapsoriasis en plaque, MF with mucinosis follicularis, follicular MF, Pagetoid reticulosis/Woringer-Kolopp disease and the extremely rare granulomatous slack skin disease.[324–326]

No consistent cytogenetic data are available for MF. Monoclonal TCR gene rearrangements are easily identified during the placque- and tumor-forming stages, however, clonality is difficult to demonstrate in the early patch stage, especially because of the presence of very few tumor cells that are admixed with reactive T-cells.[327]

In its classical form, the patch stage of MF is difficult to diagnose. Skin biopsies show a band-like infiltrate of T-cells with a few atypical large, so-called cerebriform nuclei in the dermal papillae, and especially in the lower part of the epidermis, where they may form Pautrier abcesses.

Immunophenotypically, the cells are CD2[+], CD3[+], CD4[+], CD5[+] and CD8[-]. In approximately 10–20% of cases, loss of both CD4 and CD8, and/or loss of CDS, may be of help in differentiating MF from reactive dermatitis. Occasional cases with CD8 expression have been described, and these neoplasias seem to have a more aggressive course.[328–330] These CD8[+] malignancies must be differentiated from actinic reticuloid. In the plaques, the lesions are more extensive and far easier to recognize. In the tumor lesions, extensive infiltration of the dermis is present. These deeper infiltrates often show extensive atypia, with presence of blast cells that show loss of T-cell markers. In some patients, the blasts may be very anaplastic and CD30[+].

Epidermotropism may be lost in these lesions, and hence a diagnosis of MF can only be made in combination with previous or simultaneous biopsies of other, less advanced lesions. Involvement of lymph nodes develops along a certain sequence, and starts with dermatopathic lymphadenopathy, slight infiltration of tumor cells and partial infiltration, and ends with complete destruction of structures.

Sézary syndrome is an extremely rare disorder.[331] It is often lumped with MF; however, its clinical presentation is different, as well as its relatively poor prognosis. Clinically, patients present with red skin, palmar and plantar scaling, and extreme itching. Draining lymph nodes and blood are often involved from the start of the disease. Cerebriform tumor cells should be identified in blood smears or sections made from buffy coats. According to most criteria used, the blood should contain more than $1 \times 10^9$ abnormal (cerebriform) cells per liter and an abnormally high CD4/CD8 ratio. Sézary syndrome must be differentiated from reactive conditions, especially extreme forms of eczema and hypersensitivity to light.

Skin biopsies may show a picture similar to the patch or plaque of MF, but in many cases the infiltrate is more restricted to the dermis. Phenotypically, the tumor cells are CD4[+]. Lymph-node biopsies should always be taken, since the histology may differentiate between reactive processes and Sézary syndrome. In contrast to MF, sinuses and T-cell areas are infiltrated by abnormal cerebriform cells.

## CD30[+] cutaneous ALCL and lymphomatoid papulosis

Apart from the classical cutaneous T-cell lymphomas MF and Sézary syndrome, other T-cell lymphomas can be recognized. Most frequently, they present as a solitary or multiple nodules or tumors. Some tumors, especially those containing CD30[+] tumor cells, cutaneous ALCL, show signs of (spontaneous) regression. Since these ALCL have an excellent prognosis as compared with the CD30[-] lymphomas, and show overlap with lymphomatoid papulosis (LP), they should be separately diagnosed and treated.[332–338]

Cutaneous ALCL and LP have an unidentified etiology and pathogenesis. In contrast to the nodal counterpart, the t(2;5) translocation or any variant translocation involving the ALK gene is consistently absent. Clonal TCR gene rearrangements have been identified in both ALCL and LP. Metachronous ALCL and LP may develop in single patients. Histologically, these tumors show infiltrates of large pleomorphic cells (see earlier). Especially during regression, edema, fibrosis and infiltration by eosinophils and neutrophils may be prominent. LP is defined by the presence of (multiple) small papules that show a spontaneous tendency to 'come and go' in an asynchronous pattern. Histologically, LP can show a similar picture to ALCL or a picture more reminiscent of MF, or a mixture of both. In both ALCL and LP, immunohistochemistry invariably shows a strong staining for CD30 and variable staining for T-cell markers including CD4, but absence of CD15, ALK and EMA as well as all B-cell markers. Cytotoxic molecules such as TIA-1 and granzyme-B are present in 50% (ALCL) to 100% (LP). Since all lymphomas with CD30 expression on more than 75% of the tumor cells have a similar behavior, and the presence of CD30 seems to overrule morphology. It is strongly advised to stain for CD30 antigen in all primary cutaneous T-cell lymphomas.

### Other primary extranodal T-cell lymphomas

Other distinct but uncommon T-cell lymphomas – surprisingly all associated with an (activated) cytotoxic phenotype – are the T-cell large granular lymphocytic leukemia, sometimes associated with rheumatoid arthritis, splenomegaly, granulocytopenia and (pseudo) Felty syndrome, subcutaneous panniculitis-like T-cell lymphoma, associated with hemophagocytosis, and hepatosplenic γδT-cell lymphoma. The latter mainly affects young, male patients, and is associated with cytopenias, especially thrombocytopenia.

## Treatment

### Staging and treatment evaluation

After the histological diagnosis has been made on a lymph-node biopsy, including appropriate immunophenotyping and (if indicated) cytogenetic and/or molecular biological investigations, the staging procedure is initiated, including:

- Patient's history
- A thorough physical examination
- Measurement of the sizes of enlarged lymph nodes, liver and/or spleen, and extranodal localizations, if present

- Inspection of Waldeyer ring by an ear, nose and throat specialist, with biopsies if doubtful lesions are observed
- CT scans of the neck, thorax and abdomen
- A bone marrow biopsy, including immunopathology
- Routine blood hematology and chemistry investigations, including the $\beta_2$-microglobulin and the serum lactate dehydrogenase serum levels and serum immunoelectrophoresis to detect paraproteins.

In recent years [67]Ga scintigraphy and [18]FDG photon emission tomography (PET) have been increasingly introduced as methods of nuclear diagnostics in NHL. It has become clear that [67]Ga scintigraphy does not offer additional value as compared to conventional staging by CT scans.[339–341] However, [18]FDG appears to be at least complementary to conventional staging, but may in 10–15% of patients detect additional localizations of NHL, thereby changing the stage and treatment strategy.[342–344] Obviously, site-specific investigations should be performed based on specific symptomatology, e.g. a work-up of the gastrointestinal tract, lumbar puncture, nuclear magnetic resonance imaging (MRI) of the central nervous system and/or spinal cord, and other extranodal sites, and X-rays of bones. While performing the staging procedure, one should be aware that NHL can manifest itself at various exotic locations such as the orbits, conjunctivae, thyroid gland, mammae, skin, kidney, urinary bladder, testicles, cervix uteri and bone. In cases where anemia, granulocytopenia and/or thrombocytopenia are present, it should be remembered that, apart from bone marrow infiltration with NHL or hypersplenism in the case of splenomegaly, autoimmune phenomena might be the underlying cause as a consequence of a disordered immune system.

In general, for NHL, the Ann Arbor staging system that was developed for Hodgkin lymphoma is still in use (Table 36.5). The absence or presence of fever, night sweats and/or unexplained loss of 10% or more of body weight in the 6 months preceding admission are to be denoted in all cases by the suffix letters A or B, respectively. Only 20% of all patients with NHL present in stage I. In most patients, disseminated disease is present at diagnosis. In this respect, the Ann Arbor staging seems to be less relevant for NHL as compared with Hodgkin lymphoma, which shows a more contiguous spread. Certain subtypes of NHL have their own staging nomenclature (MALT lymphoma and NHL of the skin; see later).

To assess the response to treatment, complete restaging after the completion of treatment is of utmost importance, employing the relevant methods mentioned earlier. The following response criteria were assessed by an International Working Group as summarized in Table 36.6.[345]

**Table 36.5  Ann Arbor staging***

| Stage | Definition |
|---|---|
| I | Involvement of a single lymph node region (I) or of a single extralymphatic organ or site (I$_E$) |
| II | Involvement of two or more lymph node regions on the same side of the diaphragm (II), or localized involvement of an extralymphatic organ or site and of one or more lymph node regions on the same side of the diaphragm (II$_E$) |
| III | Involvement of lymph node regions on both sides of the diaphragm (III), which may also be accompanied by involvement of the spleen (III$_S$) or by localized involvement of an extralymphatic organ or site (III$_E$) or both (III$_{SE}$) |
| IV | Diffuse or disseminated involvement of one or more extralymphatic organs or tissues, with or without associated lymph node involvement |

* Adopted at the Workshop on the Staging of Hodgkin Disease held at Ann Arbor, MI, USA in April 1971.

In particular, problems may arise in judging whether a patient is in complete or partial remission when small residual masses are left after therapy. In general, one should try to obtain material for cytology/immunophenotyping or histopathology to determine if lymphoma is still there. Residual masses, which occur in 40–60% of treated patients, quite often do not contain vital lymphoma tissue.[346] Again here, there is a role for nuclear diagnostics to determine whether vital lymphoma is still present in these residual lesions. In particular [18]FDG PET scanning has demonstrated a low percentage of false positivity and a high specificity (>90%). In 83 patients with aggressive NHL the 2-years disease-free survival rate was 85% in patients with a negative PET scan after chemotherapy was completed vs. 4% in those with persistent [18]FDG uptake.[347] Due to the high physiological uptake below the diaphragm in liver, spleen and colon [67]GA scintigraphy is particular valuable to investigate residual masses in the mediastinum. Currently, prospective clinical studies are being performed to define the impact of these new tools in restaging the patient.

In summary, after the histopathological diagnosis of NHL has been made, it has now become feasible without invasive procedures to accurately stage the disease at the time of presentation, with methods ranging from physical examination to molecular diagnostics. In performing prospective (randomized) clinical trials, it should be emphasized that all participants must use the same staging procedures and employ similar response criteria to guarantee the interpretation of the results.

An extensive review of advanced methods to detect minimal residual disease in lymphoid malignancies is presented in Chapter 21. In general, it is obvious that establishing the immunological/molecular biological phenotype at diagnosis allows the specific detection of small numbers of NHL cells that might have survived treatment.

**Prognostic factors**

A first impression on the prognosis of a patient with NHL is provided at the time of histological diagnosis. Although the WHO classification of B- and T-cell lymphomas does not include malignancy grades, based on the knowledge of biological behavior, a global estimate can be given of the course of the disease if current appropriate treatment can be given according to the NHL subtype, i.e. of indolent, aggressive or very aggressive nature (Tables 36.1–36.3). However, based on results from staging procedures in large cohorts of patients and final treatment outcome, a more refined predictive model was developed in 1993 – in the first place applicable to aggressive NHL subtypes. The major prognostic factors include age, stage, serum lactate dehydrogenase level, performance status and number of extranodal disease sites. In this way, four risk groups could be predicted with different survival rates (Table 36.7).[348] Later, this IPI also proved to be valid for patients with low-grade, malignant, indolent NHLs.[349,350] Recently a prognostic model for follicular, low-grade malignant NHL has been developed. This Follicular Lymphoma International Prognostic Index (FLIPI) is based on slightly different parameters at diagnosis as compared with the IPI for the aggressive lymphomas, i.e. age, stage, serum lactate dehydrogenase level, hemoglobin level and number of nodal disease sites involved.[351] By employing these prognostic indices, a new era of NHL treatment is entered, with the initiation of prognostic factor-tailored treatment strategies, just as has been introduced earlier in the treatment of Hodgkin lymphoma, and are now being evaluated in other hematological malignancies such as the acute leukemias. This new development should prevent under- and overtreatment, limiting at the same time unnecessary (late) side effects.

Apparently, a new set of prognostic factors appears during the course of therapy, such as the dose intensity of the cytostatic drugs administered, the response to initial treatment, the time to relapse, and the sensitivity to second-line chemotherapy.

To date, several International Working Groups are evaluating the prognostic significance of cytogenetic abnormalities, aberrant expression of oncogenes and a number of other biological markers both in patients with indolent NHL and aggressive NHL (see also Chapter 18). This should obviously lead to a further refinement of the currently employed IPI for aggressive NHL as well as the FLIPI for follicular NHL.[352] In

**Table 36.6 Response criteria based on criteria assessed by an International Working Group**[345]

**Complete response (CR) requires:**
1. Complete disappearance of all detectable clinical and radiographic evidence of disease and disappearance of all disease-related symptoms if present before therapy.
2. Normal LDH (i.e. upper level of normal-ULN). An elevated LDH detracts from a CR unless it is attributable to causes not related to NHL, e.g. hemolysis.
3. • All nodes and nodal masses must have reduced in size to 1.0 cm in greatest transverse diameter, or
   • If some nodes have regressed to a size between 1.0 and 1.5 cm in greatest transverse diameter from a size over 1.5 cm, while none have a size over 1.5 cm, the SPD (sum of the product of the largest perpendicular diameters) of the indicator lesions must have regressed by more than 75%.
4. The spleen, if considered to be enlarged before therapy on the basis of a CT scan, must have regressed in size and must not be palpable and/or no longer considered enlarged on physical examination. however, no normal size can be specified, because of the difficulties in accurately evaluating splenic size. Similarly, other organs considered to be enlarged before therapy due to involvement by lymphoma, such as liver and kidneys, must have decreased in size.
5. Any nodules in liver or spleen must have disappeared.
6. If the bone marrow was involved by lymphoma before treatment, the infiltrate must be cleared on repeat bone marrow aspirate and biopsy of the same site.

**CR/unconfirmed (CRu)** includes those patients who fulfill criteria 1, 2, 4 and 5 above, but with one or more of the following features/exceptions:
1. A residual lymph node mass 1.5 cm in greatest transverse diameter that has regressed by more than 75% as regards the product of the largest perpendicular diameters. Individual nodes that were previously confluent must have regressed by more than 75% in their size compared with the size of the original mass. The SPD size of the indicator lesions must have regressed by more than 75%.
2. Indeterminate bone marrow (increased number or size of aggregates without cytologic or architectural atypia).

In case of apparent CRu it is recommended to perform, if possible, a cytological aspiration or biopsy of a residual lymph node mass to determine the cytopathological status. It is also recommended in case of CRu to repeat CT or ultrasound of the residual lesions after 2–4 months.

**Partial response (PR) requires:**
1. ≥50% decrease in SPD of the indicator lesions.
2. ≥50% decrease in SPD of splenic and hepatic nodules if present and bi-dimensionally measurable at the start of treatment.
3. No increase in the size of any single node, nodule, liver, or spleen by more than 25%.
4. No new sites of disease.
5. All patients who meet criteria for CR of CRu except for:
   • an LDH>ULN that is not attributable to other causes than NHL, or
   • with remaining but decreased number of nodules in liver or spleen, or
   • with remaining assessable disease
   are classified as PR.

**Stable disease (SD)**
1. Is defined as less than PR (see above) but is not progressive disease (see below).

**Progressive disease (PD) requires:**
1. ≥50% increase in the product of the largest perpendicular diameters of any at baseline identified abnormal node, nodal mass or nodule.
2. Appearance of any new lesion during or at the end of therapy.

particular RNA expression patterns in NHL as assessed by microarray technology (see also Chapter 20) have yielded within a distinct histological entity of NHL subgroups with significantly different prognoses. For example, in diffuse large B-cell NHL, as described before, two subtypes were recognized: germinal center B-like lymphoma and activated B-like lymphoma. Independent of the IPI, there was a remarkable differ-ence in overall survival rate at 5 years: 76% vs. 16%, respectively.[353] Subsequently, immunostains based on the specific gene expression profile predicted similar overall survival as compared to the DNA microarray-based prognostic factors.[354] Similar data are currently becoming available for a variety of other subtypes of NHL. The prognostic roles of these new factors under-line the biological heterogeneity of patients with NHL.

**Table 36.7  International Prognostic Index predicting the outcome of treatment in patients with aggressive NHL***

| Index (n = 2031) | No. of risk factors | % of patients | CR† rate (%) | RFS‡ at 5 years (%) | OS§ at 5 years (%) |
|---|---|---|---|---|---|
| Low | 0 or 1 | 35 | 87 | 70 | 73 |
| Low intermediate | 2 | 27 | 67 | 50 | 51 |
| High intermediate | 3 | 22 | 55 | 49 | 43 |
| High | 4 or 5 | 16 | 44 | 40 | 26 |

* According to Shipp et al[348]; † CR = complete remission; ‡ RFS = relapse-free survival; § OS = overall survival.

# Treatment of indolent NHL

## Stages I and II

Follicular NHL, the most frequent type of indolent NHL, representing 20–30% of all patients with NHL, presents at diagnosis with stage I or II localized disease in only 10–20% of patients. Local treatment, e.g. involved-field radiotherapy, is generally accepted as the treatment of choice. Usually radiation doses of 30–36 Gy are employed. Results from four retrospective studies in large cohorts of patients with significant follow up are presented in Table 36.8.[355–358] From these, it appears that relapse-free survival at 10–12 years after radiotherapy ranges from 44–56%. If patients have remained free of disease for a least 10 years, their chance of relapse is very low. It may be concluded that about half of the patients were understaged at the time of diagnosis, since they relapsed later on, usually in nonirradiated areas. In this respect, it is noteworthy that in up to 75% of patients, with a t(14;18)-positive follicular NHL, who are clinically staged stage I or II, t(14;18)-positive cells are detected the peripheral blood and bone marrow, which may indicate that the disease is indeed already disseminated.[359]

Circulating lymphocytes with the t(14;18) translocation have been observed in patients for many years after treatment without signs of a clinical relapse.[360] It has been hypothesized that these cells represent a premalignant clone that does not lead to clinical overt disease.

Finally, more extensive radiotherapy (e.g. total lymphoid irradiation) or adjuvant chemotherapy in addition to local radiotherapy showed an improved relapse-free survival in some studies, although no effect on overall survival was noted.[361–363]

In conclusion, there is certainly a need to add new treatment modalities (e.g. monoclonal antibodies) to radiotherapy alone to decrease the significant relapse rate in these early stage patients.

## Stages III and IV

The treatment of patients with disseminated indolent NHL (stages III and IV) is a major challenge in hematooncology today. Currently available treatment modalities in follicular NHL are summarized in Table 36.9.

## Wait and see approach vs. chemotherapy

Despite numerous treatment efforts ranging from single-agent chlorambucil therapy to low-dose total-body irradiation or (aggressive) combination chemotherapy, the median survival time of 7–9 years, reflecting the biological behavior of the disease, has not really changed over the past 30 years.[364,365]

**Table 36.8  Results of radiotherapy for stages I and II indolent NHL**

| No. of patients | Median follow up (years) | Years of observation | RFS* (%) | OS† (%) | Ref No. |
|---|---|---|---|---|---|
| 124 | 5.5 | 10 | 54 | 68 | 355 |
| 190 | 9.1 | 12 | 53 | 58 | 356 |
| 144 | 8.7 | 10 | 56 | 69 | 357 |
| 177 | 7.7 | 10 | 44 | 64 | 358 |

* RFS = relapse-free survival; † OS = overall survival.

## Table 36.9  Treatment modalities in follicular NHL

Wait and see policy
Mono- or combination chemotherapy
Radiotherapy
Marrow ablative chemo-radiotherapy followed by autologous peripheral blood stem-cell transplantation
Immunotherapy
- Interferons
- Allogeneic stem-cell transplantation
- Monoclonal antibodies
- Radio-immunotherapy
- Vaccination strategies

Although aggressive upfront chemotherapy has shown a significant increase in disease-free survival, the overall survival was not different from that obtained in patients in which the 'wait and see' approach was followed.[366] In a recent follow-up study in 151 patients, in the 'wait-and-see' arm of a randomized trial by the British National Lymphoma Investigation (BNLI) Group, it was observed that 72% of patients subsequently received systemic chemotherapy at a median time of 2.7 years after diagnosis, 16% died without receiving systemic chemotherapy from other causes than NHL at a median time of 3.8 years after diagnosis, and 12% of the patients had still not received any systemic treatment and were still alive at a medium observation time of more than 15 years (D Linch, personal communication). It is now generally recommended to treat patients who do not participate in prospective clinical trials with mild chemotherapy (chlorambucil), courses of CVP (i.e. cyclophosphamide, vincristine, prednisone) or fludarabine (see later) if clinically indicated. Criteria to start treatment after a period of watchful waiting are the occurrence of 'B' symptoms (including pyrexia, nightsweats and weight loss), pruritus and general malaise for which there is no other cause, progressive disease over a 3-month period, or critical organ involvement such as ureteric, esophageal or bronchial obstruction or evidence of bone marrow failure.

### Interferons

In the late 1970s and 1980s, results from phase II clinical studies on the efficacy of natural and, later, recombinant interferons (IFNs) in low-grade malignant NHL were published.[367–369] Response rates ranging from 30–55% were reported in patients who had previously been treated with chemotherapy, with responses lasting from 3–12 months. In addition, it appeared from preclinical and clinical studies that biological response modifiers are most efficacious if applied when the tumor load is small, i.e. during the phase of minimal residual disease. Several large,

prospective randomized studies have been published since then. Two studies addressing the role of IFN – α maintenance treatment – after first-line remission induction chemotherapy, yielded quite similar results in terms of a prolongation of the median failure-free survival to about 2 years in the IFN-α arm vs. 1–1.5 years in the 'no further treatment' arm.[370,371] However, so far, there are no indications that overall survival is significantly influenced. In two other trials, IFN-α treatment was combined with combination chemotherapy, and, apart from (again) an increase in failure-free survival, in one study a significant prolongation of overall survival was reported, namely 61.1 months for the chemotherapy group and 83.1 months for the chemotherapy/IFN-α group.[372,373] In their new studies, only a few collaborative groups have now adopted IFN-α treatment as one of the standard components of the conventional treatment arm. In a recent meta-analysis performed on the results from 10 phase III prospective randomized clinical trials in 1939, newly diagnosed patients with follicular NHL with a median follow up of 7 years the following conclusions were drawn. When IFN is given in the context of relatively intensive initial chemotherapy including anthracyclines and at a dose $36 \times 10^6$ units per month with at least 5 million units per dose, IFN prolongs remission duration and overall survival.[374] However, in conclusion IFN has not been included as a component of first-line treatment in follicular NHL, mainly because of its significant side effects, leading to both patients' and doctors' reluctance.

### Fludarabine

Recently, purine analogues such as fludarabine and 2-chlorodeoxyadenosine (2-CdA) have been introduced in the treatment of indolent NHL. In phase II studies in previously untreated patients, response rates varying from 30% to 70% have been reported.[375,376] From a recently analyzed prospective randomized EORTC (European Organisation for Research and Treatment of Cancer) study comparing fludarabine monotherapy with CVP chemotherapy as first-line treatment in stages III/IV patients with follicular NHL, it appeared that fludarabine induces more than twice as many complete remissions: 38% vs. 15%. However, there were no differences between both arms as regards progression-free survival and overall survival.[377] Despite significant T-cell depletion by fludarabine, no increase in (opportunistic) infections was noted. However, in heavily pretreated patients, prolonged administration of purine analogues might increase the risk of opportunistic infections. Prophylactic administration of antibiotics might then be indicated. In recent years different combinations of fludarabine with other cytostatic drugs such as mitoxantrone and/or cyclophosphamide have been explored with response rates of up to 80–95%, including up to 80% complete remissions.[378] In up to 80% of patients, a molecular remission was achieved as defined as PCR negativity for bcl-2 in the peripheral blood and this corresponded to an enhanced failure-free survival and overall survival.[379]

## Autologous stem cell transplantation

Encouraging data have recently been reported from a number of phase II clinical studies employing marrow-ablative treatment followed by autologous stem cell transplantation in patients with (relapsed) low-grade malignant NHL. Disease-free survival rates have been reported to range from 60% to 85% at a median follow-up of 3–7 years.[380–382] Several centers have introduced methods to purge autologous stem cell grafts employing monoclonal antibodies, and have reported an improved disease-free survival.[383] Obviously, the potential beneficial effect of purging should be proven in randomized trials. From a recently published study in a small series of relapsed patients, purging of the autologous marrow graft with a cocktail of monoclonal antibodies did not yield an improvement in failure-free survival and overall survival as compared to unpurged marrow grafts.[384] In summary, the positive results reported for stem cell transplantation so far should be looked at with some caution, because of possible selection biases that might have occurred in these phase II studies. Obviously, given the biology of growth of low-grade malignant NHL, it is too early to judge the influence on the median survival time in this patient category. Treatment-related mortality in these studies was below 5%. However, in addition, secondary myelodysplastic syndromes/acute myeloid leukemia have been reported after autologous stem-cell transplantation in patients with NHL.[385] The exact role of marrow ablative treatment in patients with disseminated indolent NHL is currently being explored in ongoing prospective randomized clinical trials. At the most, a prolongation of progression-free survival is achieved; however, in a recently reported study from the French–Belgian Lymphoma Collaborative Group (GELA) a significant increase in overall survival was noted after autologous stem-cell transplantation applied in first remission as compared with prolonged chemotherapy in combination with IFN, i.e. 81% vs. 74% overall survival at 5 years.[386] Obviously, these data need to be confirmed.

## Allogeneic stem cell transplantation

So far, allogeneic stem cell transplantation seems to be the only curative treatment modality in patients with follicular NHL. About 50% of patients enjoy a prolonged disease-free survival with evidence for a plateau of the survival curve.[387] Until recently, this approach has only been available for younger patients with an HLA-identical sibling donor. Obviously, given the relatively high median age of follicular NHL

patients, most patients were not eligible to undergo marrow-ablative chemo-radiotherapy and allogeneic stem-cell transplantation. Besides, the rate of treatment-related mortality has been substantial (20–40%), mainly due to acute graft-versus-host disease, infections and organ toxicity. Recently, reduced intensity conditioning was introduced, employing low doses of cytostatic drugs and low-dose total-body irradiation. In combination with immunosuppressive agents, an allogeneic graft can be established and the observed anti-lymphoma effect is therefore mainly due to graft-versus-lymphoma activity exerted by the allogeneic donor lymphocytes. The first preliminary data show that there may be less treatment-related mortality and 50% survival with the first signs of a plateau in the survival curve.[388] Most centers, so far, do not perform allogeneic stem-cell transplantation in first remission, but rather in a later phase of the disease. Relapse after allogeneic SCT is usually treated by a donor lymphocyte infusion to profit again from the graft-versus-lymphoma effect. Finally, if no HLA-identical sibling is available, a matched unrelated donor transplant may be an option. Additional information is given in Chapter 29.

Of particular importance in the group of patients who present with a follicular NHL is the increasing chance of progressing to an NHL of higher malignancy grade. As described earlier, incidence rates between 25% and 50% have been reported.[389] As soon as this de-differentiation occurs, the outlook is poor. In this subgroup of patients, marrow-ablative treatment followed by autologous or allogeneic stem-cell transplantation may be envisaged to be of benefit. Aggressive chemotherapy alone is not effective in the long run.

## Monoclonal antibodies, radio-immunotherapy

Immunotherapy with anti-CD20 antibodies has been one of the most promising treatment modalities that has entered the treatment arena in NHL during the past years. In particular, the human–mouse chimeric monoclonal antibody MabThera (Rituximab) appears to be most efficacious. In previously treated patients MabThera monotherapy induces a response in 40–50% of the patients, with a median time to progression of slightly more than 1 year.[390–394] A somewhat lower response rate is achieved upon retreatment with the antibody.[392] Currently, the role of MabThera maintenance treatment as part of the first- or second-line treatment is explored as well as its efficacy in combination with a variety of chemotherapy regimens. Currently available data point at a significant increase in progression-free survival with negligible additional toxicity from the monoclonal antibody treatment. In the years to come, it is expected that monoclonal antibodies will become an integral part of first-line and subsequent treatment regimens in follicular NHL.

In addition, radio-immunotherapy has been introduced, conjugating anti-CD20 antibodies to radioisotopes such as $^{131}$I and $^{90}$Y. Significant response rates have been achieved.[393,394] However, this type of intravenous targeted radiotherapy leads to significant hematological toxicity as compared to the virtually nontoxic treatment with cold antibodies. The exact role of radio-immunotherapy in bulky vs. minimal residual disease is currently being investigated in prospective randomized studies. Chapter 25 provides a more detailed description of the currently available data on (radio-)immunotherapy in NHL.

### Treatment of relapse in patients with indolent NHL

No standard treatment strategies are defined for patients with relapsed indolent NHL. Second-line chemotherapy regimens, monoclonal antibodies alone or in combination with chemotherapy, radio-immunotherapy, autologous or allogeneic stem cell transplantation, preferably in the setting of a clinical trial, local radiotherapy in particular for palliative purposes, or new treatment modalities (see later) are options in that situation, which is met in virtually all patients, given the rather long overall survival time.

### Vaccination treatment

As regards new treatment modalities, it is of particular importance to mention the development of vaccination strategies employing NHL-specific idiotype vaccines in the treatment of patients with B-cell NHL. Preliminary data show that if a specific immune response occurs in vivo against the immunoglobulin expressed by the lymphoma cells, this is clearly related to a more favorable outcome in terms of an increase in progression-free survival and possibly even overall survival.[395–397] Several prospective randomized clinical trials are ongoing to test the efficacy of vaccination strategies in the phase of minimal residual disease. Conclusive data are not yet available. Chapter 26 summarizes in more detail current achievements as well as perspectives on T-cell-mediated immunotherapy of cancer.

### MALT lymphoma

In the group of indolent NHLs, lymphomas of the MALT require separate consideration. As stated before, these primary extranodal marginal-zone B-cell lymphomas make up approximately 2–3% of all NHLs. A special staging system for the most frequent localization of this type of NHL in the stomach has been introduced.[398] The role of *H. pylori* (HP) has been discussed before. By eradicating this micro-organism, biopsy-proven remissions can be achieved in up to 70% of these patients.[399] However, it may take 1 year or more before a complete regression of the lymphoma has taken place. Therefore endoscopic follow-up at regular times is of the utmost importance. MALT lymphomas characterized by a t(11;18) are usually resistant to HP eradication treatment and show a more aggressive growth.[400] If no response is observed, involved-field radiotherapy may be given with curative intent to lesions limited to the stomach or its direct environment. Currently, there is no role for surgical intervention in this specific type of NHL. Disseminated MALT lymphoma is treated with chemotherapy with similar regimens as employed in follicular NHL.

### Mycosis fungoides

Mycosis fungoides is one of the more frequent indolent lymphomas of the T-cell type. As mentioned before, a special staging system has been developed for this particular manifestation of NHL, based on the extent of cutaneous disease, type of cutaneous lesion, presence of nodal disease and involvement of other extranodal sites.[401] Depending on the stage at presentation, a variety of treatment modalities are recognized, including topical therapy (steroids, nitrogen mustard, ultraviolet light), local radiotherapy, systemic chemotherapy and total skin electron-beam irradiation. In general, high response rates are achieved, but, particularly in disseminated disease, the duration of complete remission is relatively short.[402]

### CD30⁺ anaplastic large cell lymphoma of the skin

Finally, as a representative of the group of indolent NHLs, CD30⁺ anaplastic large cell lymphoma limited to the skin should be mentioned. Primary cutaneous localizations lack the translocation in which the ALK gene is involved, as mentioned before. When this lymphoma is present as a primary cutaneous lesion, the prognosis is excellent. Management should be conservative, and a 'wait and see' policy after surgical excision is justified.[403]

## Treatment of aggressive NHL

### Diffuse large B-cell lymphoma

#### Localized disease

Approximately 10% of this most frequent representative of the group of aggressive lymphomas present in stage I. From the extensive literature that is available on treatment outcome, it emerges that a limited number of chemotherapy courses followed by involved-field radiotherapy is the treatment of choice, yielding a complete remission rate of more than 90% and a cure rate of 80–90%.[404] With radiotherapy alone, there appears to be a higher relapse rate. As regards chemotherapy, an anthracycline-containing regimen appears to be most appropriate. Three courses of the CHOP chemotherapy regimen (cyclophosphamide,

Adriamycin, vincristine and prednisone) remain the gold standard. This is followed by involved-field radiotherapy, e.g. 30 Gy if complete remission is achieved with chemotherapy and 40 Gy if three courses of CHOP lead to a partial remission.

## Disseminated disease

Before the IPI was developed, patients presenting with stages II, III or IV of diffuse large B-cell lymphoma were all treated according to the same guidelines. The CHOP regimen was one of the first effective regimens to treat aggressive lymphomas, resulting in 50% complete remissions, 60% of whom remained disease-free, so that overall about 30% of the patients could be cured. In the 1980s, various single-center studies were published on the results of second- and third-generation chemotherapy regimens, which are characterized by adding more active drugs to the original CHOP regimen and reducing the total duration of treatment.[403,406] This would lead to an increase in the relative dose intensity, which was thought to be important to improve the results. Complete remission rates of up to 85% were achieved, followed by a significant increase in disease-free survival. However, when collaborative groups took these regimens into multicenter studies, the results were less good and approached those obtained with CHOP. Apparently, a selection bias in the phase II single-center studies must have played a role. Finally, a prospective randomized study comparing conventional CHOP chemotherapy with the new-generation regimens MBACOD, MACOP-B and ProMACE-CytaBOM revealed no differences as regards complete remission rate, disease-free and overall survival (Table 36.10).[407] In addition, the more aggressive regimens were more toxic. These results clearly illustrate the importance of performing randomized studies. Only with this methodological approach can a new more effective treatment strategy be reliably developed. This requires many patients to be enrolled in studies in a short time, and this can only be done if collaborative groups embark on intergroup studies. Fortunately,

this is occurring with increasing frequency throughout the world.

Since the introduction of a predictive model for aggressive NHL, modern therapeutic approaches incorporate prognostic-factor tailored treatment strategies. The International Prognostic Index appears to be a better tool to predict treatment outcome as compared with the classical Ann Arbor staging (Table 36.5). As stated before, the introduction of new biological prognostic markers and gene expression profiling of NHL is expected to further refine the prognostic index, thereby leading to a combination of the highest possible treatment efficacy and the lowest degree of toxicity. The ultimate goal of prognostic indices beyond the IPI should be tailor-made treatment for each individual patient. If this is achieved, prospective, randomized phase III clinical trials will no longer be necessary. Under- and overtreatment will thus be prevented.

Given CHOP as standard baseline chemotherapy, several studies have been published in which either dose escalation of cyclophosphamide and Adriamycin, or shortening of the usual 3-week interval between CHOP courses were explored. As regards dose escalation, prospective randomized studies employing hematopoietic growth factors are currently ongoing. So far, no definite data can be reported. Dose escalation without growth factors has not shown any significant benefit. Reducing the interval between CHOP courses to 2 weeks did not show an advantage in studies in younger patients with a favorable IPI score (Pfreundschuh, personal communication).

## High-dose chemotherapy followed by autologous peripheral blood stem-cell transplantation in first remission

In a number of phase III randomized clinical trials the efficacy of high-dose chemotherapy followed by autologous peripheral blood stem-cell transplantation in first partial or complete remission was investigated.[408–411]

---

**Table 36.10 The SWOG/ECOG randomized trial comparing CHOP with second- and third-generation chemotherapy regimens in aggressive NHL***

| Regimen | No. of patients | CR† rate (1) | DFS‡ at 3 years | OS§ at 3 years |
|---|---|---|---|---|
| CHOP | 225 | 44 | 41 | 54 |
| mBACOD | 223 | 48 | 46 | 52 |
| MACOP-B | 218 | 51 | 41 | 50 |
| ProMACE–CytaBOM | 233 | 56 | 46 | 50 |

* According to Fisher et al[407]; † CR = complete remission; ‡ DFS = disease-free survival; § OS = overall survival.

In general, these studies have not yielded an advantage in favor of high-dose, marrow-ablative treatment in first remission. From subgroup analyses it seems that IPI high-risk patients might possibly benefit from autologous stem-cell transplantation early in the phase of the disease.[412] However, prospective randomized studies need to confirm this statistically non-valid analysis. In summary, introducing this treatment modality as a standard treatment in first remission outside clinical trials is not recommended. The role of allogeneic stem-cell transplantation is less clear. Although some patients show a graft-versus-aggressive NHL effect, allogeneic transplantation is at the moment performed in only relatively few patients. For further reading, see Chapter 29.

### Treatment of relapse in patients with aggressive NHL

Approximately 50% of patients relapsing from an aggressive NHL will respond to second-line chemotherapy. However, the majority of these patients will subsequently relapse and ultimately die from their disease. Many regimens, employing drugs that are non-cross-resistant with the CHOP regimen, have been tested in the past years. All appear to have similar efficacy.[413–415] A pivotal study at this stage of the disease appears to be the PARMA study, which addressed the question of the value of high-dose chemotherapy followed by autologous bone marrow transplantation in patients at relapse but still responding to second-line chemotherapy (responsive relapse). Patients responding to two courses of DHAP chemotherapy (dexamethasone, cytosine arabinoside and cisplatin) were prospectively randomized to receive either bone marrow transplantation or further DHAP courses. The outcome was significantly better for those patients receiving a marrow graft: the event-free survival at 5 years was 46% in the transplant arm and 12% in the conventional chemotherapy arm, with percentages of actuarial overall survival of 53% and 32%, respectively.[416] Thus, in patients younger than 65 years with a chemosensitive relapse, high-dose therapy with autologous stem-cell transplantation should be the standard approach. A possible role of involved-field radiotherapy in addition to chemotherapy or stem-cell transplantation is unclear as this has not been investigated in a prospective phase III clinical study.

### Elderly patients with aggressive NHL

As more than 50% of patients with aggressive NHL are above the age of 60, this group poses a special challenge to the hemato-oncologist. As discussed before, in the IPI, age is an unfavorable prognostic factor. This is particularly due to the greater vulnerability of elderly patients when treated with aggressive chemotherapy. Impaired function of vital organs, altered metabolism of cytostatic drugs and severe myelosuppression preclude optimal dose intensity.

However, if adequate treatment can be administered, complete remission rates as well as disease-free survival are quite similar to those achieved in younger patients.[417] In this patient category, CHOP is regarded as standard treatment. Recently, several collaborative groups have focused on the combination of chemotherapy with a hematopoietic growth factor (G-CSF) in an attempt to lower the incidence of granulocytopenia, with a subsequent reduction in the number of infections. In a recently published, prospective randomized trial, this was proven to be the case.[418] In a randomized Dutch HOVON study, adding G-CSF led to a significant increase in relative dose intensity, but no improvements were noted in the complete remission rate or in overall survival.[419]

Shortening of the interval between CHOP courses was recently investigated in elderly patients. Results suggest that CHOP every 2 weeks is superior to CHOP every 3 weeks (Pfreundschuh, personal communication).

A major breakthrough in current NHL treatment occurred following the publication of Coiffier et al in January 2002 on the efficacy of CHOP chemotherapy in combination with MabThera in elderly patients with diffuse large B-cell NHL. In patients above 60 years of age, CHOP + MabThera induced a higher complete remission rate as compared to CHOP alone (76% vs. 63%) and with a median follow-up of 2 years, survival was significantly better for patients treated with CHOP + MabThera vs. patients treated with CHOP alone (70% vs. 57%).[420] These differences are well maintained after 4 years of follow-up, as appeared from subsequently reported analyses (Coiffier, personal communication). Based on these results addition of MabThera to first-line CHOP chemotherapy has now become standard treatment in elderly patients with aggressive NHL in most treatment centers worldwide. Whether this will also hold for younger patients remains to be established.

### Primary NHL of the brain

Primary NHL of the brain is a rare tumor, representing 1–2% of all NHLs. Most of these lymphomas are of the aggressive B-cell type. In general, the survival is poor, with a 5-year survival rate below 10%. In recent years, several phase II studies have been published, reporting an improved overall survival rate (median survival: 3 years) when either high-dose methotrexate or high-dose cytosine arabinoside, passing the blood–brain barrier, were introduced in the chemotherapy regimens and combined with whole-brain irradiation.[421–423] However, these improved results go hand in hand with an increase in neurotoxicity.

### Mantle-cell lymphoma

As stated before, this particular subtype of NHL, has a poor prognosis. From a retrospective clinicopathological comparison with other NHL subtypes, it appears that patients with mantle-cell lymphoma have a similar overall survival and response rate as patients with aggressive NHL, but a shorter duration of response and progression-free survival. Compared with patients with indolent NHL, their response rate, duration of response and progression-free survival showed no difference, while their overall survival was nearly half as long.[424]

In other words, in terms of survival, mantle-cell lymphoma behaves like aggressive NHL, while progression-free survival is quite similar to that observed in indolent NHL. At present, there is still no clue as to which combination of cytostatic drugs would be the treatment of choice. From retrospective analyses it appears that there is no major difference between treatment with alkylating agents or anthracycline-containing combinations. Both types of treatment induce complete remissions in 30–50% of the patients. However, most patients relapse within 12 months, with a median survival of 30 months.[425–427] Phase II studies with Fludarabine, MabThera, high-dose methotrexate and cytosine arabinoside as well as marrow ablative chemotherapy followed by autologous peripheral blood stem-cell transplantation lead to complete remission rates of 60% in previously untreated patients with mantle-cell lymphoma.[428–430] However, the real value of these regimens has to be established through properly designed randomized studies.

### Peripheral T-cell lymphoma

As compared to diffuse large B-cell NHL, the prognosis of patients with a peripheral T-cell lymphoma (all types as indicated in the WHO classification) is less favorable.[431] Effective chemotherapy is lacking and most of the cases are treated with CHOP chemotherapy. The efficacy of anti-T-cell monoclonal antibodies is currently being investigated.

# Treatment of very aggressive NHL

## Lymphoblastic lymphoma/Burkitt lymphoma

Several entities are recognized in this group: lymphoblastic lymphoma of precursor B or T origin, Burkitt lymphoma, the acute form of adult T-cell lymphoma leukemia and most of the immunodeficiency-associated EBV-positive lymphomas (see later). Their highly aggressive nature, including a strong tendency to localize in the central nervous system (CNS), calls for very aggressive chemotherapy, including prophylactic treatment of the CNS. As regards the lymphoblastic/Burkitt lymphomas, usually similar treatment regimens are applied as in acute lymphoblastic leukemia. These are discussed in Chapter 32 and will not be repeated here.

### Immunodeficiency-associated lymphomas

Post-transplantation lymphoproliferative disease (PTLD) usually is of B-cell origin and positive for EBV. Treatment consists of reduction or withdrawal of immunosuppressive agents and anti-CD20 monoclonal antibodies (MabThera). Up to 80% remissions can be achieved with a 1-year survival rate of 50–60%. Frequent monitoring of the serum EBV DNA load after allogeneic stem-cell transplantation and subsequent pre-emptive treatment with MabThera as soon as the EBV load increases appears to be very effective in preventing PTLD.[432] Finally, infusions of donor buffy coat cells directed against EBV antigens, have yielded remarkable remissions.[433] Chemotherapy does not seem to play a major role, resulting only in short-lasting responses. Thus, humoral and/or cellular immunotherapy of these types of NHL appears to be promising.

AIDS-related NHL shows in 60–70% the histology of diffuse large B-cell NHL. The remainder is for the greater part of the Burkitt type. Standard CHOP in combination with highly active antiretroviral therapy (HAART) is the treatment of choice. In 50% of patients a complete remission is obtained, which may last longer than 1 year.[434,435] In addition to progressive NHL, opportunistic infections are the major causes of death.

In conclusion, in general, the tools to accurately diagnose, stage and treat NHL have step-by-step become more refined during recent years. This has resulted in improved perspectives for many patients. Only by continuing carefully planned clinical studies can further improvements in today's lymphoma treatment be anticipated.

## REFERENCES

1. Rappaport H. *Tumors of the Hematopoietic System.* Washington: Armed Forces Institute of Pathology; 1966.
2. The Non-Hodgkin's lymphoma pathologic classification project. National Cancer Institute sponsored study of classifications of non-Hodgkin's lymphomas. Summary and description of a working formulation for clinical use. *Cancer* 1982; 49: 2112.
3. Lennert K, Mohri N, Stein H, Kaiserling E et al. In: Lennert K, ed. *Malignant Lymphoma Other than Hodgkin's Disease.* Berlin: Springer-Verlag, 1978.
4. Lennert K, Feller AC. *Histopathologie der Non-Hodgkin-Lymphoma.* 2nd edn. Berlin: Springer-Verlag, 1990.
5. Lukes RJ, Collins RD. Immunologic characterization of

human malignant lymphomas. *Cancer* 1974; **34**: 1488–1503.

6. Harris NL, Jaffe ES, Stein H et al. A revised European-American classification of lymphoid neoplasms: A proposal from the International Lymphoma Study Group. *Blood* 1994; **84**: 1361–92.

7. Harris NL, Jaffe ES, Diebold J et al. World Health Organization Classification of Neoplastic Disease of the Hematopoietic and Lymphoid Tissues: Report of the Clinical Advisory Committee Meeting – Arlie House, Virginia, November 1997. *J Clin Oncol* 1999; **17**: 3835–49.

8. Jaffe ES, Harris NL, Stein H et al. *Tumours of Hematopoietic and Lymphoid Tissues. Pathology and Genetics.* Lyon: IARC Press, 2001.

9. Hans CP, Weisenburger DD, Vose JM et al. A significant diffuse component predicts for inferior survival in grade 3 follicular lymphoma, but cytologic subtypes do not predict survival. *Blood* 2003; **101**: 2363–7.

10. Martin AR, Weisenburger DD, Chan WC et al. Prognostic value of cellular proliferation and histologic grade in follicular lymphoma. *Blood* 1995; **85**: 3671–8.

11. Bennett JM, Catovsky D, Daniel M-T et al. Proposals for the classification of chronic mature) B and T lymphoid leukaemias. *J Clin Pathol* 1989; **42**: 567–84.

12. Bain BJ. *Leukemia diagnosis. A guide to the FAB classification.* London: Lippincott Company; 1990.

13. Stilgenbauer S, Lichter P, Dohner H. Genetic features of B-cell chronic lymphocytic leukemia. *Rev Clin Exp Hematol* 2000; **4**: 8–72.

14. Hawthorn LA, Chapman R, Oscier D et al. The consistent 13q14 translocation breakpoint seen in chronic B-cell leukaemia (BCLL) involves deletion of the D13S25 locus which lies distal to the retinoblastoma predisposition gene. *Oncogene* 1993; **8**: 1415–9.

15. Juliusson G, Oscier DG, Fitchett M. Prognostic subgroups in B-cell chronic lymphocytic leukemia defined by specific chromosomal abnormalities. *N Engl J Med* 1990; **323**: 720–4.

16. Anastasi J, Le Beau MM, Vardiman JW et al. Detection of trisomy 12 in chronic lymphocytic leukemia by fluorescence in situ hybridization to interphase cells: A simple and sensitive method. *Blood* 1992; **79**: 1796–1801.

17. Perez Losada A, Wessman M, Tiainen M et al. Trisomy 12 in chronic lymphocytic leukemia: An interphase cytogenetic study. *Blood* 1991; **78**: 775–9.

18. Raghoebier S, Kibbelaar RE, Kleiverda JK et al. Mosaicism of trisomy 12 in chronic lymphocytic leukemia detected by non-radioactive in situ hybridization. *Leukemia* 1992; **6**: 1220–6.

19. Criel A, Wlodarska I, Meeus P et al. Trisomy 12 is uncommon in typical chronic lymphocytic leukaemias. *Br J Haematol* 1994; **87**: 523–8.

20. Que TH, Marco JG, Ellis J et al. Trisomy 12 in chronic lymphocytic leukemia detected by fluorescence in situ hybridization: Analysis by stage, immunophenotype, and morphology. *Blood* 1993; **82**: 571–5.

21. Adachi M, Tefferi A, Greipp PR et al. Preferential linkage of BCL-2 to immunoglobulin light chain gene in chronic lymphocytic leukemia. *J Exp Med* 1990; **171**: 559–64.

22. Rechavi G, Katzir N, Brok-Simoni F et al. A search for bcll, bcl2 and c-myc oncogene rearrangements in chronic lymphocytic leukemia. *Leukemia* 1989; **3**: 57–60.

23. Raghoebier S, Van Krieken JHJM, Kluin-Nelemans JC et al. Oncogene rearrangements in chronic B-cell leukemia. *Blood* 1991; **77**: 1560–4.

24. Gaidano G, Newcomb EW, Gong JZ et al. Analysis of alterations of oncogenes and tumor suppressor genes in chronic lymphocytic leukemia. *Am J Pathol* 1994; **144**: 1312–9.

25. Kipps TJ, Tomhave E, Pratt LF et al. Developmentally restricted immunoglobulin heavy chain variable region gene expressed at high frequency in chronic lymphocytic leukemia. *Proc Natl Acad Sci USA* 1989; **86**: 5913–7.

26. Pratt LF, Rassenti L, Larrick J et al. Ig V region gene expression in small lymphocytic lymphoma with little or no somatic hypermutation. *J Immunol* 1989; **143**: 699–705.

27. Tobin G, Thunberg U, Johnson A et al. Chronic lymphocytic leukemias utilizing the VH3-21 gene display highly restricted Vlambda2-14 gene use and homologous CDR3s: implicating recognition of a common antigen epitope. *Blood* 2003; **101**: 4952–7.

28. Garand R, Sahota SS, Avet-Loiseau H et al. IgG-secreting lymphoplasmacytoid leukaemia: a B-cell disorder with extensively mutated VH genes undergoing Ig isotype-switching frequently associated with trisomy 12. *Br J Haematol* 2000; **109**: 71–80.

29. Johnson TA, Rassenti LZ, Kipps TJ. Ig VH1 genes expressed in B cell chronic lymphocytic leukemia exhibit distinctive molecular features. *J Immunol* 1997; **158**: 235–46.

30. Efremov DG, Ivanovski M, Siljanovski N et al. Restricted immunoglobulin VH region repertoire in chronic lymphocytic leukemia patients with autoimmune hemolytic anemia. *Blood* 1996; **87**: 3869–76.

31. Efremov DG, Ivanovski M, Siljanovski N et al. Restricted immunoglobulin VH region repertoire in chronic XX lymphocytic leukemia patients with autoimmune hemolytic anemia. *Blood* 1996; **87**: 3869–76.

32. Johnson TA, Rassenti LZ, Kipps TJ. Ig VH1 genes expressed in B cell chronic lymphocytic leukemia exhibit distinctive molecular features. *J Immunol* 1997; **158**: 235–46.

33. Tobin G, Thunberg U, Johnson A et al. Chronic lymphocytic leukemias utilizing the VH3-21 gene display highly restricted Vlambda2-14 gene use and homologous CDR3s: implicating recognition of a common antigen epitope. *Blood* 2003; **101**: 4952–7.

34. Kipps TJ, Tomhave E, Chen PP et al. Autoantibody-associated kappa light chain variable region gene expressed in chronic lymphocytic leukemia with little or no somatic mutation. *J Exp Med* 1988; **167**: 840–52.

35. Meeker T, Grimaldi JC, O'Rourke R et al. Lack of detectable somatic hypermutation in the V region of the IgH chain gene of a human chronic B lymphocytic leukemia. *J Immunol* 1988; **141**: 3994–8.

36. Rassenti LZ, Kipps TJ. Lack of extensive mutations in the $V_H S$ genes used in common B cell chronic lymphocytic leukemia. *J Exp Med* 1993; **177**: 1039–46.

37. Jahn S, Schwab J, Hansen A et al. Human hybridomas derived from CDS+ B lymphocytes of patients with chronic lymphocytic leukemia B-CLL) produce multi-specific natural IgM (kappa) antibodies. *Clin Exp Immunol* 1991; **83**: 413–7.

38. Oscier DG, Thompsett A, Zhu D et al. Differential rates of somatic hypermutation in V(H) genes among subsets of chronic lymphocytic leukemia defined by chromosomal abnormalities. *Blood* 1997; **89**: 4153–60.

39. Sakai A, Marti GE, Caporaso N et al. Analysis of expressed immunoglobulin heavy chain genes in familial B-CLL. *Blood* 2000; **95**: 1413–19.

40. Chen L, Widhopf G, Huynh L et al. Expression of ZAP-70 is associated with increased B-cell receptor signaling in chronic lymphocytic leukaemia. *Blood* 2002; **100**: 4609–14.

41. Wiestner A, Rosenwald A, Barry TS et al. ZAP-70 expression identifies a chronic lymphocytic leukemia subtype with unmutated immunoglobulin genes, inferior clinical outcome, and distinct gene expression profile. *Blood* 2003; **101**: 4944–51.

42. Crespo M, Bosch F, Villamor N et al. ZAP-70 expression as a surrogate for immunoglobulin-variable-region mutations in chronic lymphocytic leukemia. *N Engl J Med* 2003; **348**: 1764–75.

43. Rosenwald A, Alizadeh AA, Widhopf G et al. Relation of gene expression phenotype to immunoglobulin mutation genotype in B cell chronic lymphocytic leukemia. *J Exp Med* 2001; **194**: 1639–47.

44. Klein U, Tu Y, Stolovitzky GA et al. Gene expression profiling of B cell chronic lymphocytic leukemia reveals a homogeneous phenotype related to memory B cells. *J Exp Med* 2001; **194**: 1625–38.

45. Rozman C, Montserrat E, Rodriguez Fernandez JM et al. Bone marrow histologic pattern – the best single prognostic parameter in chronic lymphocytic leukemia: a multivariate survival analysis of 329 cases. *Blood* 1984; **64**: 642–8.

46. Armitage JO, Dick FR, Corder MP. Diffuse histiocytic lymphoma complicating chronic lymphocytic leukemia. *Cancer* 1978; **41**: 422–7.

47. Foucar K, Rydell RE. Richter's syndrome in chronic lymphocytic leukemia. *Cancer* 1980; **46**: 118–34.

48. Delsol G, Laurent G, Kuhlein E et al. Richter's syndrome. Evidence for the clonal origin of the two proliferations. *Am J Clin Pathol* 1981; **76**: 308–15.

49. Brecher M, Banks PM. Hodgkin's disease variant of Richter's syndrome: Report of eight cases. *Am J Clin Pathol* 1990; **93**: 333–9.

50. Pugh WC, Manning JT, Butler JJ. Paraimmunoblastic variant of small lymphocytic lymphoma/leukemia. *Am J Surg Pathol* 1988; **12**: 907–17.

51. Archimbaud E, Charrin C, Gentilhomme O et al. Initial clonal acute lymphoblastic transformation of chronic lymphocytic leukemia with t(11; 14) and t(8; 12) chromosome translocations and acquired homozygosity. *Acta Haematol (Basel).* 1988; **79**: 168–73.

52. Pistoia V, Roncella S, Di Celle PF et al. Emergence of a B-cell lymphoblastic lymphoma in a patient with B-cell chronic lymphocytic leukemia: Evidence for the single-cell origin of the two tumors. *Blood* 1991; **78**: 797–804.

53. Banks PM, Chan J, Cleary ML et al. Mantle cell lymphoma: A proposal for unification of morphologic, immunologic, and molecular data. *Am J Surg Pathol* 1992; **16**: 637–40.

54. Shivdasani RA, Hess JL, Skarin AT et al. Intermediate lymphocytic lymphoma: Clinical and pathologic features of a recently characterized subtype of non-Hodgkin's lymphoma. *J Clin Oncol* 1993; **11**: 802–11.

55. Zucca E, Stein H, Coiffier B. European lymphoma task force (ELTF): report of the workshop on mantle cell lymphoma (MCL). *Ann Oncol* 1994; **5**: 507–11.

56. Velders GA, Kluin-Nelemans JC, De Boer CJ et al. Mantle cell lymphoma: a population based clinical study. *J Clin Oncol* 1996; **14**: 1269–74.

57. Duggan MJ, Weisenburger DD, Ye YL et al. Mantle zone lymphoma: A clinicopathologic study of 22 cases. *Cancer* 1990; **66**: 522–9.

58. Weisenburger DD, Sanger WG, Armitage JO et al. Intermediate lymphocytic lymphoma: immunophenotypic and cytogenetic findings. *Blood* 1987; **69**: 1617–21.

59. Palutke M, Eisenberg L, Mirchandani I, Tabaczka P et al. Malignant lymphoma of small cleaved lymphocytes of the follicular mantle zone. *Blood* 1982; **59**: 317–22.

60. Pals ST, Drillenburg P, Dragosics B et al. Expression of the mucosal homing receptor alpha 4 beta 7 in malignant lymphomatous polyposis of the intestine. *Gastroenterology* 1994; **107**: 1519–23.

61. Pittaluga S, Verhoef G, Criel A et al. 'Small' B-cell non-Hodgkin's lymphomas with splenomegaly at presentation are either mantle cell lymphoma or marginal zone cell lymphoma. A study based on histology, cytology, immunohistochemistry, and cytogenetic analysis. *Am J Surg Pathol* 1996; **20**: 211–23.

62. Molina TJ, Delmer A, Cymbalista F et al. Mantle cell lymphoma, in leukaemic phase with prominent splenomegaly. A report of eight cases with similar clinical presentation and aggressive outcome. *Virchows Arch* 2000; **437**: 591–8.

63. Angelopoulou MK, Siakantariz MP, Vassilakopoulos TP et al. The splenic form of mantle cell lymphoma. *Eur J Haematol* 2002; **68**: 12–21.

64. Pittaluga S, Bijnens L, Teodorovic I et al. Clinical analysis of 670 cases in two trials of the European Organization for the Research and Treatment of Cancer Lymphoma Cooperative Group subtyped according to the Revised European–American Classification of Lymphoid Neoplasms: a comparison with the Working Formulation. *Blood* 1996; **87**: 4358–67.

65. Argatoff LH, Connors JM, Klasa RJ et al. Mantle cell lymphoma: a clinicopathologic study of 80 cases. *Blood* 1997; **89**: 2067–78.

66. Hiddemann W, Dreyling M. Mantle cell lymphoma: therapeutic strategies are different from CLL. *Curr Treat Options Oncol* 2003; **4**: 219–26.

67. Berinstein NL, Mangel J. Integrating monoclonal antibodies into the management of mantle cell lymphoma. *Semin Oncol* 2004; **31** (Suppl 2): 2–6.

68. Nodit L, Bahler DW, Jacobs SA et al. Indolent mantle cell lymphoma with nodal involvement and mutated immunoglobulin heavy chain genes. *Hum Pathol* 2003; **34**: 1030–4.

69. Babbage G, Garand R, Robillard N et al. Mantle cell lymphoma with t(11; 14) and unmutated or mutated VH genes expresses AID and undergoes isotype switch events. *Blood* 2003 **103**: 2795–8.

70. Walsh SH, Thorselius M, Johnson A et al. Mutated VH genes and preferential VH3-21 use define new subsets of mantle cell lymphoma. *Blood* 2003; **101**: 4047–54.

71. Orchard J, Garand R, Davis Z et al. A subset of t(11; 14) lymphoma with mantle cell features displays mutated IgVH genes and includes patients with good prognosis, nonnodal disease. *Blood* 2003; **101**: 4975–81.

72. De Boer CJ, Van Krieken JHJM, Schuuring E et al. BCL1/cyclin Dl in malignant lymphoma. *Ann Oncol* 1997; **8**(Suppl 2): 109–17.

73. Vaandrager JW, Schuuring E, Zwikstra E et al. Direct visualization of dispersed 11q13 chromosomal translocations

in mantle cell lymphoma by multi-color DNA fiber FISH. *Blood* 1996; **88**: 1177–82.

74. Monteil M, Callanan M, Dascalescu C et al. Molecular diagnosis of t(11; 14) in mantle cell lymphoma using two-colour interphase fluorescence in situ hybridization. *Br J Haematol* 1996; **93**: 656–60.

75. Avet-Loiseau H, Garand R, Gaillard F et al. Detection of t(11; 14) using interphase molecular cytogenetics in mantle cell lymphoma and atypical chronic lymphocytic leukemia. *Genes Chromosomes Cancer* 1998; **23**: 175–82.

76. Siebert R, Matthiesen P, Harder S et al. Application of interphase cytogenetics for the detection of t(11; 14)(q13; q32) in mantle cell lymphomas. *Ann Oncol* 1998; **9**: 519–26.

77. Haralambieva E, Kleiverda K, Mason DY et al. Detection of three common translocation breakpoints in non-Hodgkin's lymphomas by fluorescence in situ hybridization on routine paraffin-embedded tissue sections. *J Pathol* 2002; **198**: 163–70.

78. Belaud-Rotureau MA, Parrens M, Dubus P et al. A comparative analysis of FISH, RT-PCR, PCR, and immunohistochemistry for the diagnosis of mantle cell lymphomas. *Mod Pathol* 2002; **15**: 517–25.

79. Coignet LJ, Schuuring E, Kibbelaar RE et al. Detection of 11q13 rearrangements in hematologic neoplasias by double-color fluorescence in situ hybridization. *Blood* 1996; **87**: 1512–19.

80. De Boer CJ, Schuuring E, Dreef EJ et al. Cyclin D1 protein analysis in the diagnosis of mantle cell lymphoma. *Blood* 1995; **86**: 2715–23.

81. Swerdlow SH, Yang WI, Zukerberg LIZ et al. Expression of cyclin D1 protein in centrocytic/mantle cell lymphomas with and without rearrangement of the BCL1/cyclin D1 gene. *Hum Pathol* 1995; **26**: 999–1004.

82. Yang WI, Zukerberg LR, Motokura T et al. Cyclin Dl (Bcl-1, Pradl) protein expression in low grade B-cell lymphomas and reactive hyperplasia. *Am J Pathol* 1994; **145**: 86–96.

83. de Boer CJ, Kluin-Nelemans JC, Dreef E et al. Involvement of the CCND1 gene in hairy cell leukemia. *Ann Oncol* 1996; **7**: 251–6.

84. Bosch F, Campo E, Jares P et al. Increased expression of the Prad-1/Ccndl gene in hairy-cell leukemia. *Br J Haematol* 1995; **91**: 1025–30.

85. Rosenwald A, Wright G, Wiestner A et al. The proliferation gene expression signature is a quantitative integrator of oncogenic events that predicts survival in mantle cell lymphoma. *Cancer Cell* 2003; **3**: 185–97.

86. VandenBerghe H, Vermaelen K, Louwagie A et al. High incidence of chromosome abnormalities in IgG3 myeloma. *Cancer Genet Cytogenet* 1984; **11**: 381–7.

87. Weh HJ, Gutensohn K, Selbach J et al. Karyotype in multiple myeloma and plasma cell leukaemia. *Eur J Cancer* [A] 1993; **29A**: 1269–73.

88. Fiedler W, Weh HJ, Hossfeld DK. Comparison of chromosome analysis and BCL-1 rearrangement in a series of patients with multiple myeloma. *Br J Haematol* 1992; **81**: 58–61.

89. Vaandrager JW, Kluin PM, Schuuring E. The t(11; 14)(q13; q32) in multiple myeloma cell line KMS12 has its 11q13 breakpoint 330 kb centromeric from the cyclin D1 gene. *Blood* 1997; **89**: 349–50.

90. Janssen JWG, Vaandrager JW, Heuser T. Concurrent activation of a novel putative transforming gene, MYEOV, and

91. cyclin D1 in a subset of multiple myeloma cell lines with t(11; 14)(q13; q32). *Blood* 2000; **95**: 2691–8.

91. Cuneo A, Balboni M, Piva N et al. Atypical chronic lymphocytic leukaemia with t(11; 14)(q13; q32): karyotype evolution and prolymphocytic transformation. *Br J Haematol* 1995; **90**: 409–16.

92. Bird ML, Ueshima Y, Rowley JD et al. Chromosome abnormalities in B cell chronic lymphocytic leukemia and their clinical correlations. *Leukemia* 1989; **3**: 182–91.

93. Juliusson G, Oscier DG, Fitchett M et al. Prognostic subgroups in B-cell chronic lymphocytic leukemia defined by specific chromosomal abnormalities. *N Engl J Med* 1990; **323**: 720–4.

94. Jadayel D, Matutes E, Dyer MJS et al. Splenic lymphoma with villous lymphocytes: analysis of BCL-1 rearrangements and expression of the cyclin D1 gene. *Blood* 1994; **83**: 3664–71.

95. Stilgenbauer S, Schaffner C, Winkler D et al. The ATM gene in the pathogenesis of mantle-cell lymphoma. *Ann Oncol* 2000; **11**: 127–30.

96. Schaffner C, Idler I, Stilgenbauer S et al. Mantle cell lymphoma is characterized by inactivation of the ATM gene. *Proc Natl Acad Sci USA* 2000; **97**: 2773–8.

97. Camacho E, Hernandez L, Hernandez S et al. ATM gene inactivation in mantle cell lymphoma mainly occurs by truncating mutations and missense mutations involving the phosphatidylinositol-3 kinase domain and is associated with increasing numbers of chromosomal imbalances. *Blood* 2002; **99**: 238–44.

98. Fang NY, Greiner TC, Weisenburger DD et al. Oligonucleotide microarrays demonstrate the highest frequency of ATM mutations in the mantle cell subtype of lymphoma. *Proc Nat Acad Sci U S A* 2003; **100**: 5372–7.

99. Hernandez L, Fest T, Cazorla M et al. p53 gene mutations and protein overexpression are associated with aggressive variants of mantle cell lymphoma. *Blood* 1996; **87**: 3351–9.

100. Greiner TC, Moynihan MJ, Chan WC et al. p53 mutations in mantle cell lymphoma are associated with variant cytology and predict a poor prognosis. *Blood* 1996; **87**: 4302–10.

101. Dreyling MH, Bullinger L, Ott G et al. Alterations of the cyclin Dl/p16-pRB pathway in mantle cell lymphoma. *Cancer Res* 1997; **57**: 4608–14.

102. Pinyol M, Hernandez L, Cazorla M et al. Deletions and loss of expression of p16(INK4a) and p21(Wafl) genes are associated with aggressive variants of mantle cell lymphomas. *Blood* 1997; **89**: 272–80.

103. Segal GH, Masih AS, Fox AC et al. CDS-expressing B-cell non-Hodgkin's lymphomas with bcl-1 gene rearrangement have a relatively homogeneous immunophenotype and are associated with an overall poor prognosis. *Blood* 1995; **85**: 1570–9.

104. Segal GH, Fishleder AJ, Stoler MH et al. Frozen sections of cellular lymphoid proliferations provide adequate DNA for routine gene rearrangement analysis. *Am J Clin Pathol* 1991; **96**: 360–3.

105. Specht K, Kremer M, Muller U et al. Identification of cyclin D1 mRNA overexpression in B-cell neoplasias by real-time reverse transcription-PCR of microdissected paraffin sections. *Clin Cancer Res* 2002; **8**: 2902–11.

106. Hui P, Howe JG, Crouch J et al. Real-time quantitative RT-PCR of cyclin D1 mRNA in mantle cell lymphoma: com-

parison with FISH and immunohistochemistry. *Leuk Lymphoma* 2003; **44**: 1385–94.

107. Raty R, Franssila K, Joensuu H et al. Ki-67 expression level, histological subtype, and the International Prognostic Index as outcome predictors in mantle cell lymphoma. *Eur J Haematol* 2002; **69**: 11–20.

108. Hashimoto Y, Nakamura N, Kuze T et al. The evaluation of the biological behavior and grade among cases with mantle cell lymphoma. *Leuk Lymphoma* 2002; **43**: 523–30.

109. Raty R, Franssila K, Jansson SE et al. Predictive factors for blastoid transformation in the common variant of mantle cell lymphoma. *Eur J Cancer* 2003; **39**: 321–9.

110. Heinz R, Stacher A, Pralle H et al. Lymphoplasmacytic/ lymphoplasmacytoid lymphoma: a clinical entity distinct from chronic lymphocytic leukaemia? *Blood* 1981; **43**: 183–92.

111. Crisp D, Pruzanski W. B-cell neoplasms with homogeneous cold-reacting antibodies (cold agglutinins). *Am J Med* 1982; **72**: 915–22.

112. Kraj P, Friedman DF, Stevenson F et al. Evidence for the overexpression of the VH4-34 (VH4.21) Ig gene segment in the normal adult human peripheral blood B cell repertoire. *J Immunol* 1995; **154**: 6406–20.

113. Franklin EC. Mu-chain disease. *Arch Intern Med* 1975; **135**: 71–2.

114. Offit K, Parsa NZ, Filippa D et al. t(9; 14)(p13; q32) denotes a subset of low-grade non-Hodgkin's lymphoma with plasmacytoid differentiation. *Blood* 1992; **80**: 2594–9.

115. Iida S, Rao PH, Nallasivam P et al. The t(9; 14)(p13; q32) chromosomal translocation associated with lymphoplasmacytoid lymphoma involves the PAX-5 gene. *Blood* 1996; **88**: 4110–7.

116. Schop RF, Kuehl WM, Van Wier SA et al. Waldenstrom macroglobulinemia neoplastic cells lack immunoglobulin heavy chain locus translocations but have frequent 6q deletions. *Blood* 2002; **100**: 2996–3001.

117. Schop RF, Fonseca R. Genetics and cytogenetics of Waldenstrom's macroglobulinemia. *Semin Oncol* 2003; **30**: 142–5.

118. Mahmoud MS, Huang N, Nobuyoshi M et al. Altered expression of Pax-5 gene in human myeloma cells. *Blood* 1996; **87**: 4311–5.

119. Kudo A. Pax-5, a transcription factor controlling B cell differentiation. *Tanpakushitsu Kakusan Koso* 1996; **41**: 1058–66.

120. Nutt SL, Thevenin C, Busslinger M. Essential functions of Pax-5 (BSAP) in pro-B cell development. *Immunobiology* 1997; **198**: 227–35.

121. Hagman J, Wheat W, Fitzsimmons D et al. Pax-5/BSAP: regulator of specific gene expression and differentiation in B lymphocytes. *Curr Top Microbiol Immunol* 2000; **245**: 169–94.

122. Chilosi M, Adami F, Lestani M et al. CD138/syndecan-1: a useful immunohistochemical marker of normal and neoplastic plasma cells on routine trephine bone marrow biopsies. *Mod Pathol* 1999; **12**: 1101–6.

123. Horsman DE, Gascoyne RD, Coupland RW et al. Comparison of cytogenetic analysis, southern analysis, and polymerase chain reaction for the detection of t(14; 18) in follicular lymphoma. *Am J Clin Pathol* 1995; **103**: 472–8.

124. Bahler DW, Levy R. Clonal evolution of a follicular lymphoma: Evidence for antigen selection. *Proc Natl Acad Sci USA* 1992; **89**: 6770–4.

125. Zelenetz AD, Chen TT, Levy R. Clonal expansion in follicular lymphoma occurs subsequent to antigenic selection. *J Exp Med* 1992; **176**: 1137–48.

126. Vaandrager JW, Schuuring E, Kluin Nelemans JC et al. DNA fiber FISH analysis of immunoglobulin class switching in B cell neoplasia: aberrant CH gene rearrangements in follicle center cell lymphoma. *Blood* 1998; **92**: 2871–8.

127. Ji W, Qu G-Z, Ye P et al. Frequent detection of BCL2/JH translocations in human blood and organ samples by a quantitative polymerase chain reaction assay. *Cancer Res* 1995; **55**: 2876–82.

128. Limpens J, De Jong D, Van Krieken JHJM et al. Bcl-2/JH Rearrangements in benign lymphoid tissues with follicular hyperplasia. *Oncogene* 1991; **6**: 2271–6.

129. Limpens J, Stad R, Vos C et al. Lymphoma associated translocation t(14; 18) in blood B cells of normal individuals. *Blood* 1995; **85**: 2528–36.

130. Liu Y, Hernandez AM, Shibata D, Cortopassi GA. BCL2 translocation frequency rises with age in humans. *Proc Natl Acad Sci USA* 1994; **91**: 8910–4.

131. Bell DA, Liu Y, Cortopassi GA. Occurrence of bcl-2 oncogene translocation with increased frequency in the peripheral blood of heavy smokers. *J Natl Cancer Trust* 1995; **87**: 223–4.

132. Cong P, Raffeld M, Teruya-Feldstein J. In situ localization of follicular lymphoma: description and analysis by laser capture microdissection. *Blood* 2002; **99**: 3376–82.

133. Keith TA, Cousar JB, Glick AD et al. Plasmacytic differentiation in follicular center cell (FCC) lymphomas. *Am J Clin Pathol* 1985; **84**: 283–90.

134. Gaulard P, D'Agay M-F, Peuchmaur M et al. Expression of the bcl-2 gene product in follicular lymphoma. *Am J Pathol* 1992; **140**: 1089–95.

135. Ben-Ezra JM, King BE, Harris AC et al. Staining for Bcl-2 protein helps to distinguish benign from malignant lymphoid aggregates in bone marrow biopsies. *Mod Pathol* 1994; **7**: 560–4.

136. Krajewski S, Bodrug S, Gascoyne R et al. Immunohistochemical analysis of Mcl-1 and Bcl-2 proteins in normal and neoplastic lymph nodes. *Am J Pathol* 1994; **145**: 515–25.

137. De Jong D, Voetdijk BMH, Ommen van GJB et al. Translocation t(14; 18) in B cell lymphomas as a cause for defective immunoglobulin production. *J Exp Med* 1989; **169**: 613–24.

138. Anderson JR, Vose JM, Bierman PJ et al. Clinical features and prognosis of follicular large-cell lymphoma: A report from the Nebraska Lymphoma Study Group. *J Clin Oncol* 1993; **11**: 218–24.

139. Cibull ML, Heryet A, Gatter KC et al. The utility of Ki67 immunostaining, nuclear organizer region counting, and morphology in the assessment of follicular lymphomas. *J Pathol* 1989; **158**: 189–93.

140. Garvin AJ, Simon RM, Osborne CK et al. An autopsy study of histologic progression in non-Hodgkin's lymphomas. 192 cases from the National Cancer Institute. *Cancer* 1983; **52**: 393–8.

141. Sham RL, Pradyamna P, Carignan J et al. Progression of follicular large cell lymphoma to Burkitt's lymphoma. *Cancer* 1989; **63**: 700–2.

142. Gauwerky CE, Hoxie J, Nowell PC et al. Pre-B-cell leukemia with a t(8; 14) and a t(14; 18) translocation is preceded by follicular lymphoma. *Oncogene* 1988; **2**: 431–5.

143. De Jong D, Voetdijk BMH, Beverstock GC et al. Activation of the c-*myc* oncogene in a precursor-B-cell blast crisis of follicular lymphoma, presenting as composite lymphoma. *N Engl J Med* 1988; **318**: 1373–8.

144. Natkunam Y, Warnke RA, Zehnder JL et al. Blastic/blastoid transformation of follicular lymphoma: immunohistologic and molecular analyses of five cases. *Am J Surg Pathol* 2000; **24**: 525–34.

145. Falini B, Tiacci E, Pucciarini A et al. Expression of the IRTA1 receptor identifies intraepithelial and subepithelial marginal zone B cells of the mucosa-associated lymphoid tissue (MALT). Blood 2003; **102**: 3684–92.

146. Wolvius EB, Van der Valk P, van der Wal JE et al. Primary non-Hodgkin's lymphoma of the salivary glands. An analysis of 22 cases. *J Oral Pathol Med* 1996; **25**: 177–81.

147. Takahashi H, Cheng J, Fujita S et al. Primary malignant lymphoma of the salivary gland: a tumor of mucosa-associated lymphoid tissue. *J Oral Pathol Med* 1992; **21**: 318–325.

148. Anscombe AM, Wright DH. Primary malignant lymphoma of the thyroid – a tumour of XX mucosa-associated lymphoid tissue: review of seventy-six cases. *Histopathol* 1985; **9**: 81–97.

149. Isaacson PG, Androulakis-Papachristou A, Diss TC et al. Follicular colonization in thyroid lymphoma. *Am J Pathol* 1992; **141**: 43–52.

150. Ohshima K, Kikuchi M, Sumiyoshi Y et al. Clonality of benign lymphoid hyperplasia in orbit and conjunctiva. *Pathol Res Pract* 1994; **190**: 436–43.

151. Jakobiec FA, Iwamoto T, Patell M et al. Ocular adnexal monoclonal lymphoid tumors with a favorable prognosis. *Ophthalmology* 1986; **93**: 1547–57.

152. Knowles DM, Jakobiec FA, McNally L et al. Lymphoid hyperplasia and malignant lymphoma occurring in the ocular adnexa (orbit, conjunctiva, and eyelids): A prospective multiparametric analysis of 108 cases during 1977 to 1987. *Hum Pathol* 1990; **21**: 959–73.

153. Mattia AR, Ferry JA, Harris NL. Breast lymphoma: A B-cell spectrum including the low grade B-cell lymphoma of mucosa associated lymphoid tissue. *Am J Surg Pathol* 1993; **17**: 574–87.

154. Bobrow LG, Richards MA, Happerfield LC et al. Breast lymphomas: A clinicopathologic review. *Hum Pathol* 1993; **24**: 274–8.

155. Kuper-Hommel MJ, Snijder S, Janssen-Heijnen ML et al. Treatment and survival of 38 female breast lymphomas: a population-based study with clinical and pathological reviews. *Ann Hematol* 2003; **82**: 397–404.

156. Willemze R, Rijlaarsdam JU, Meijer CJ. Are most primary cutaneous B-cell lymphomas 'marginal cell lymphomas'? [comment]. *Br J Dermatol* 1995; **133**: 950–2.

157. Bailey EM, Ferry JA, Harris NL et al. Marginal zone lymphoma (low-grade B-cell lymphoma of mucosa-associated lymphoid tissue type) of skin and subcutaneous tissue: a study of 15 patients. *Am J Surg Pathol* 1996; **20**: 1011–23.

158. Cerroni L, Signoretti S, Hofler G et al. Primary cutaneous marginal zone B-cell lymphoma: a recently described entity of low-grade malignant cutaneous B-cell lymphoma [see comments]. *Am J Surg Pathol* 1997; **21**: 1307–15.

159. Willemze R, Kerl H, Sterry W et al. EORTC classification for primary cutaneous lymphomas: a proposal from the cutaneous lymphoma study group of the European Organization for Research and Treament of Cancer. *Blood* 1997; **90**: 354–71.

160. Storz MN, Van de Rijn M, Kim YH et al. Gene expression profiles of cutaneous B cell lymphoma. *J Invest Dermatol* 2003; **120**: 865–70.

161. Isaacson PG, Chan JKC, Tang C et al. Low-grade B-cell lymphoma of mucosa-associated lymphoid tissue arising in the thymus: A thymic lymphoma mimicking myoepithelial sialadenitis. *Am J Surg Pathol* 1990; **14**: 342–51.

162. Pawade J, Banerjee SS, Harris M et al. Lymphomas of mucosa-associated lymphoid tissue arising in the urinary bladder. *Histopathol* 1993; **23**: 147–51.

163. Kumar S, Kumar D, Kaldjian EP et al. Primary low-grade B-cell lymphoma of the dura: a mucosa associated lymphoid tissue-type lymphoma. *Am J Surg Pathol* 1997; **21**: 81–7.

164. Hussell T, Isaacson PG, Crabtree JE et al. The response of cells from low-grade B-cell gastric lymphomas of mucosa-associated lymphoid tissue to *Helicobacter pylori*. *Lancet* 1993; **342**: 571–4.

165. Wotherspoon AC, Doglioni C, Diss TC et al. Regression of primary low-grade B-cell gastric lymphoma of mucosa-associated lymphoid tissue type after eradication of *Helicobacter pylori*. *Lancet* 1993; **342**: 575–7.

166. Parsonnet J, Hansen S, Rodriguez L. *Helicobacter pylori* infection and gastric lymphoma. *N Engl J Med* 1994; **330**: 1267–71.

167. Roggero E, Zucca E, Pinotti G et al. Eradication of *Helicobacter pylori* infection in primary low-grade gastric lymphoma of mucosa-associated lymphoid tissue (see comments). *Ann Intern Med* 1995; **122**: 767–9.

168. Bayerdorffer E, Neubauer A, Rudolph B et al. Regression of primary gastric lymphoma of mucosa-associated lymphoid tissue type after cure of *Helicobacter pylori* infection. MALT Lymphoma Study Group (see comments). *Lancet* 1995; **345**: 1591–4.

169. Horsman D, Gascoyne R, Klasa R et al. t(11; 18)(q21; q21.1): A recurring translocation in lymphomas of mucosa-associated lymphoid tissue (MALT)? *Gen Chrom Cane* 1992; **4**: 183–7.

170. Kalla J, Schaffner C, Ott G et al. The API2-MALT 1 fusion gene characteristic for MALT-type lymphoma: Tumor specific gene rearrangement detected in *Helicobacter pylori* associated gastritis. *Blood* 2000; **96**: 88A.

171. Kalla J, Stilgenbauer S, Schaffner C et al. Heterogeneity of the AP12-MALT1 gene rearrangement in MALT-type lymphoma. *Leukemia* 2000; **14**: 1967–74.

172. Liu H, Ye H, Dogan A et al. T(11; 18)(q21; q21) is associated with advanced mucosa-associated lymphoid tissue lymphoma that expresses nuclear BCL10. *Blood* 2001; **98**: 1182–7.

173. Ott G, Katzenberger T, Greiner A et al. The t(11; 18)(q21; q21) chromosome translocation is a frequent and specific aberration in low-grade but not high-grade malignant non-Hodgkin's lymphomas of the mucosa-associated lymphoid tissue (MALT) type. *Cancer Res* 1997; **57**: 3944–8.

174. Stilgenbauer S, Kalla J, Wildenberger K et al. Characterization of the l 1q21 breakpoint of the t(11; 18)(q21; q2i) associated with MALT-type lymphoma. *Blood* 1998; **92**: 70A.

175. Rosenwald A, Ott G, Stilgenbauer S et al. Exclusive detection of the t(11; 18)(q21; q21) in extranodal marginal zone B cell lymphomas (MZBL) of MALT type in contrast to other MZBL and extranodal large B cell lymphomas. *Am J Pathol* 1999; **155**: 1817–21.

176. Dierlamm J, Baens M, Wlodarska I et al. The apoptosis

inhibitor gene API2 and a novel 18q gene, MLT, are recurrently rearranged in the t(11; 18)(q21; q21) associated with mucosa-associated lymphoid tissue lymphomas. *Blood* 1999; **93**: 3601–9.

177. Dierlamm J, Baens M, Stefanova-Ouzounova M et al. Detection of t(11; 18)(q21; q21) by interphase fluorescence in situ hybridization using API2 and MLT specific probes. *Blood* 2000; **96**: 2215–8.

178. Ruefli-Brasse AA, French DM, Dixit VM. Regulation of NF-(kappa) B-dependent lymphocyte activation and development by paracaspase. *Science* 2003 **302**: 1581–4.

179. Liu H, Ruskon-Fourmestraux A, Lavergne-Slove A et al. Resistance of t(11; 18) positive gastric mucosa-associated lymphoid tissue lymphoma to *Helicobacter pylori* eradication therapy. *Lancet* 2001; **357**: 39–40.

180. Liu H, Ye H, Ruskone-Fourmestraux A et al. T(11; 18) is a marker for all stage gastric MALT lymphomas that will not respond to *H. pylori* eradication. *Gastroenterology* 2002; **122**: 1286–94.

181. Van Krieken JHJM, Raffeld M, Raghoebier S et al. Molecular genetics of gastrointestinal non-Hodgkin's lymphomas: Unusual prevalence and pattern of c-myc rearrangements in aggressive lymphomas. *Blood* 1990; **76**: 797–800.

182. Ott G, Katzenberger T, Kalla J et al. A chromosomal profile of large cell B-cell lymphomas: data from 83 nodal and primary extranodal cases studied at a single institution. (Abstract). *Path Res Pract* 1997; **193**: 109.

183. Du M, Peng H, Singh N, Isaacson PG, Pan L. The accumulation of p53 abnormalities is associated with progression of mucosa-associated lymphoid tissue lymphoma. *Blood* 1995; **86**: 4587–93.

184. Du M, Diss TC, Xu C et al. Ongoing mutation in MALT lymphoma immunoglobulin gene suggests that antigen stimulation plays a role in the clonal expansion. *Leukemia* 1996; **10**: 1190–7.

185. Qin Y, Greiner A, Trunk MJ et al. Somatic hypermutation in low-grade mucosa-associated lymphoid tissue-type B-cell lymphoma. *Blood* 1995; **86**: 3528–34.

186. Thiede C, Alpen B, Morgner A et al. Ongoing somatic mutations and clonal expansions after cure of *Helicobacter pylori* infection in gastric mucosa-associated lymphoid tissue B-cell lymphoma. *J Clin Oncol* 1998; **16**: 3822–31.

187. Nardini E, Rizzi S, Menard S et al. Molecular phenotype distinguishes two subsets of gastric low-grade mucosa-associated lymphoid tissue lymphomas. *Lab Invest* 2002; **82**: 535–41.

188. Moller P, Eichelmann A, Mechtersheimer G et al. Expression of bl-integrins, H-CAM (CD44) and LECAM-1 in primary gastro-intestinal B-cell lymphomas as compared to the adhesion receptor profile of the gut-associated lymphoid system, tonsil and peripheral lymph node. *Int J Cancer* 1991; **49**: 846–55.

189. Drillenburg P, vanderVoort R, Koopman G et al. Preferential expression of the mucosal homing receptor integrin alpha(4)beta(7) in gastrointestinal non-Hodgkin's lymphomas. *Am J Pathol* 1997; **150**: 919–27.

190. Drillenburg P, Pals ST. Cell adhesion receptors in lymphoma dissemination. *Blood* 2000; **95**: 1900–10.

191. De Jong D, Boot H, Van Heerde P et al. Histological grading in gastric lymphoma: pretreatment criteria and clinical relevance. *Gastroenterology* 1997; **112**: 1466–74.

192. De Jong D, Vyth-Dreese F, Dellemijn T et al. Histological and immunological parameters to predict treatment outcome of *Helicobacter pylori* eradication in low-grade gastric MALT lymphoma. *J Pathol* 2001; **193**: 318–24.

193. Chan JKC, Ng CS, Isaacson PG. Relationship between high-grade lymphoma and low-grade B-cell mucosa-associated lymphoid tissue lymphoma (MALToma) of the stomach. *Am J Pathol* 1990; **136**: 1153–64.

194. Grange F, Bekkenk MW, Wechsler J et al. Prognostic factors in primary cutaneous large B-cell lymphomas: a European multicenter study. *J Clin Oncol* 2001; **19**: 3602–10.

195. Vermeer MH, Geelen FA, van Haselen CW et al. Primary cutaneous large B-cell lymphomas of the legs. A distinct type of cutaneous B-cell lymphoma with an intermediate prognosis. Dutch Cutaneous Lymphoma Working Group. *Arch Dermatol* 1996; **132**: 1304–8.

196. Horst E, Meijer CJLM, Radaszkiewicz T et al. Adhesion molecules in the prognosis of diffuse large-cell lymphoma: Expression of a lymphocyte homing receptor (CD44), LFA-1 (CD lla/18), and ICAM-1 (CD54). *Leukemia* 1990; **4**: 595–9.

197. Joensuu H, Ristamaki R, Klemi PJ et al. Lymphocyte homing receptor (CD44) expression is associated with poor prognosis in gastrointestinal lymphoma. *Br J Cancer* 1993; **68**: 428–32.

198. Deweindt C, Kerckaert JP, Tilly H et al. Cloning of a breakpoint cluster region at band 3q27 involved in human non-Hodgkin's lymphoma. (See comments). *Genes Chromosomes Cancer* 1993; **8**: 149–54.

199. Kerckaert J-P, Deweindt C, Tilly H et al. GAZ3, a novel zinc-finger encoding gene, is disrupted by recurring chromosome 3q27 translocations in human lymphomas. *Nature Genet* 1993; **5**: 66–70.

200. Ye BH, Rao PH, Chaganti RSK et al. Cloning of bcl-6, the locus involved in chromosome translocations affecting band 3q27 in B-cell lymphoma. *Cancer Res* 1993; **53**: 2732–5.

201. Dal la-Favera R, Ye BH, Lo Coco F et al. Identification of genetic lesions associated with diffuse large-cell lymphoma. (Review). *Ann Oncol* 1994; **5**(Suppl 1): 55–60.

202. Kawamata N, Miki T, Fukuda T et al. The organization of the BCL6 gene. *Leukemia* 1994; **8**: 1327–30.

203. Miki T, Kawamata N, Arai A et al. Molecular cloning of the breakpoint for 3q27 translocation in B-cell lymphomas and leukemias. *Blood* 1994; **83**: 217–22.

204. Offit K, Lo Coco F, Douie DC. Rearrangement of the BCL-6 gene as a prognostic marker in diffuse large-cell lymphoma. *N Engl J Med* 1994; **331**: 74–80.

205. Onizuka T, Moriyama M, Yamochi T et al. BCL-6 gene product, a 92- to 98-kD nuclear phosphoprotein, is highly expressed in germinal center B cells and their neoplastic counterparts. *Blood* 1995; **86**: 28–37.

206. I'e BH, Lo Coco F, Chang CC et al. Alterations of the BCL-6 gene in diffuse large-cell lymphoma. *Curr Top Microbiol Immunol* 1995; **194**: 101–8.

207. Ye BH, Cattoretti G, Shen Q et al. The BCL-6 proto-oncogene controls germinal-centre formation and Th2-type inflammation. *Nat Genet* 1997; **16**: 161–70.

208. Kramer MHH, Hermans J, Wijburg E et al. Clinical relevance of BCL2, BCL6, MYC rearrangements in diffuse large B-cell lymphoma. *Blood* 1998; **92**: 3152–62.

209. Dalla-Favera R, Migliazza A, Chang CC et al. Molecular pathogenesis of B cell malignancy: the role of BCL-6. *Curr Top Microbiol Immunol* 1999; **246**: 257–63.

210. Niu H, Cattoretti G, Dalla-Favera R. BCL6 controls the expression of the B7-1/CD80 costimulatory receptor in germinal center B cells. *J Exp Med* 2003; **198**: 211–21.

211. Gaidano G, Lo Coco F, Ye BH et al. Rearrangements of the BCL-6 gene in acquired immunodeficiency syndrome-associated non-Hodgkin's lymphoma: association with diffuse large-cell subtype. *Blood* 1994; **84**: 397–402.

212. Gaidano G, Carbone A, Pastore C et al. Frequent mutation of the 5′ noncoding region of the BCL-6 gene in acquired immunodeficiency syndrome-related non-Hodgkin's lymphomas. *Blood* 1997; **89**: 3755–62.

213. Akasaka T, Lossos IS, Levy R. BCL6 gene translocation in follicular lymphoma: a harbinger of eventual transformation to diffuse aggressive lymphoma. *Blood* 2003; **102**: 1443–8.

214. Daudignon A, Bisiau H, Le Baron F et al. Four cases of follicular lymphoma with t(14; 18)(q32; q21) and t(3; 4)(q27; p13) with LAZ3 (BCL6) rearrangement. *Cancer Genet Cytogenet* 1999; **111**: 157–60.

215. Capello D, Vitolo U, Pasqualucci L et al. Distribution and pattern of BCL-6 mutations throughout the spectrum of B-cell neoplasia. *Blood* 2000; **95**: 651–9.

216. Butler MP, Iida S, Capello D et al. Alternative translocation breakpoint cluster region 5′ to BCL-6 in B-cell non-Hodgkin's lymphoma. *Cancer Res* 2002; **62**: 4089–94.

217. Wang X, Li Z, Naganuma A, Ye BH. Negative autoregulation of BCL-6 is bypassed by genetic alterations in diffuse large B cell lymphomas. *Proc Natl Acad Sci USA* 2002; **99**: 15018–23.

218. Artiga MJ, Saez AI, Romero C et al. A short mutational hot spot in the first intron of BCL-6 is associated with increased BCL-6 expression and with longer overall survival in large B-cell lymphomas. *Am J Pathol* 2002; **160**: 1371–80.

219. Jardin F, Bastard C, Contentin N et al. Intronic BCL-6 mutations are preferentially targeted to the translocated allele in t(3; 14)(q27; q32) non-Hodgkin B-cell lymphoma. *Blood* 2003; **102**: 1872–6.

220. Muramatsu M, Akasaka T, Kadowaki N et al. Rearrangement of the BCL6 gene in B-cell lymphoid neoplasms: comparison with lymphomas associated with BCL2 rearrangement. *Br J Haematol* 1996; **93**: 911–20.

221. Raghoebier S, Kramer MHH, Van Krieken JHJM et al. Essential differences in oncogene involvement between primary nodal and extranodal large cell lymphoma. *Blood* 1991; **78**: 2680–5.

222. Jacobson JO, Wilkes BM, Kwiatkowski DJ et al. bcl-2 rearrangements in de novo diffuse large cell lymphoma: Association with distinctive clinical features. *Cancer* 1993; **72**: 231–6.

223. Offit K, Koduru PRK, Hollis R et al. 18q21 Rearrangement in diffuse large cell lymphoma: Incidence and clinical significance. *Br J Haematol* 1989; **72**: 178–83.

224. Kramer MH, Hermans J, Parker J et al. Clinical significance of bc12 and p53 protein expression in diffuse large B-cell lymphoma: a population-based study. *J Clin Oncol* 1996; **14**: 2131–8.

225. Hermine O, Haioun C, Lepage E et al. Prognostic significance of bcl-2 protein expression in aggressive non-Hodgkin's lymphoma. *Blood* 1996; **87**: 265–72.

226. Hill ME, MacLennan KA, Cunningham DC et al. Prognostic significance of BCL-2 expression and BCL-2 major breakpoint region rearrangement in diffuse large cell non-Hodgkin's lymphoma: A British National Lymphoma Investigation study. *Blood* 1996; **88**: 1046–51.

227. Ladanyi M, Offit K, Jhanwar SC et al. *MYC* rearrangement and translocations involving band 8q24 in diffuse large cell lymphomas. *Blood* 1991; **77**: 1057–63.

228. Yano T, Jaffe ES, Longo DL et al. *MYC* rearrangements in histologically progressed follicular lymphomas. *Blood* 1992; **80**: 758–67.

229. Houldsworth J, Mathew S, Rao PH et al. REL proto-oncogene is frequently amplified in extranodal diffuse large cell lymphoma. *Blood* 1996; **87**: 25–9.

230. Joos S, Otano-Joos MI, Ziegler S et al. Primary mediastinal (thymic) B-cell lymphoma is characterized by gains of chromosomal material including 9p and amplification of the REL gene. *Blood* 1996; **87**: 1571–8.

231. Lu D, Thompson JD, Gorski GK et al. Alterations at the rel locus in human lymphoma. *Oncogene* 1991; **6**: 1235–41.

232. Joos S, Menz CK, Wrobel G et al. Classical Hodgkin lymphoma is characterized by recurrent copy number gains of the short arm of chromosome 2. *Blood* 2002; **99**: 1381–7.

233. Wessendorf S, Schwaenen C, Kohlhammer H et al. Hidden gene amplifications in aggressive B-cell non-Hodgkin lymphomas detected by microarray-based comparative genomic hybridization. Oncogene 2003; **22**: 1425–9.

234. Barth TF, Martin-Subero JI, Joos S et al. Gains of 2p involving the REL locus correlate with nuclear c-Rel protein accumulation in neoplastic cells of classical Hodgkin lymphoma. *Blood* 2003; **101**: 3681–6.

235. Joos S, Granzow M, Holtgreve-Grez H et al. Hodgkin's lymphoma cell lines are characterized by frequent aberrations on chromosomes 2p and 9p including REL and JAK2. *Int J Cancer* 2003; **103**: 489–95.

236. Offit K, Parsa NZ, Gaidano G et al. 6q deletions define distinct clinico-pathologic subsets of non-Hodgkin's lymphoma. *Blood* 1993; **82**: 2157–62.

237. Scaravaglio P, Saglio G, Geuna M et al. Isochromosome 6p and deletion of 6q characterize two related cytogenetic clones in a patient with immunoblastic lymphoma *Cancer Genet Cytogenet* 1995; **81**: 179–81.

238. Zhang YM, Matthiesen P, Harder S et al. A 3-cM commonly deleted region in 6q21 in leukemias and lymphomas delineated by fluorescence in situ hybridization. *Genes Chromosomes Cancer* 2000; **27**: 52–8.

239. Alizadeh AA, Eisen MB, Davis RE et al. Distinct types of diffuse large B-cell lymphoma identified by gene expression profiling. *Nature* 2000; **403**: 503–11.

240. Rosenwald A, Wright G, Chan WC et al. The use of molecular profiling to predict survival after chemotherapy for diffuse large-B-cell lymphoma. *N Engl J Med* 2002; **346**: 1937–47.

241. Rosenwald A, Wright G, Leroy K et al. Molecular diagnosis of primary mediastinal B cell lymphoma identifies a clinically favorable subgroup of diffuse large B cell lymphoma related to Hodgkin lymphoma. *J Exp Med* 2003; **198**: 851–62.

242. Huang JZ, Sanger WG, Greiner TC et al. The t(14; 18) defines a unique subset of diffuse large B-cell lymphoma with a germinal center B-cell gene expression profile. *Blood* 2002; **99**: 2285–90.

243. Davis RE, Brown KD, Siebenlist U et al. Constitutive nuclear factor kappaB activity is required for survival of activated B cell-like diffuse large B cell lymphoma cells. *J Exp Med* 2001; **194**: 1861–74.

244. Shipp MA, Ross KN, Tamayo P et al. Diffuse large B-cell lymphoma outcome prediction by gene-expression profil-

ing and supervised machine learning. *Nat Med* 2002; **8**: 68–74.

245. Fisher DE, Jacobson JO, Ault KA et al. Diffuse large cell lymphoma with discordant bone marrow histology: Clinical features and biological implications. *Cancer* 1989; **64**: 1879–87.

246. Robertson LE, Redman JR, Butler JJ et al. Discordant bone marrow involvement in diffuse large-cell lymphoma: A distinct clinical-pathologic entity associated with a continuous risk of relapse. *J Clin Oncol* 1991; **9**: 236–42.

247. Yan Y, Chan WC, Weisenburger DD et al. Clinical and prognostic significance of bone marrow involvement in patients with diffuse aggressive B-cell lymphoma. *J Clin Oncol* 1995; **13**: 1336–42.

248. Manolov G, Manolova Y. Marker band in one chromosome 14 from Burkitt lymphoma. *Nature* 1972; **237**: 33–4.

249. A clinical evaluation of the International Lymphoma Study Group classification of non-Hodgkin's lymphoma. The Non-Hodgkin's Lymphoma Classification Project. *Blood* 1997; **89**: 3909–18.

250. Neri A, Barriga F, Knowles DM et al. Different regions of the immunoglobulin heavy-chain locus are involved in chromosomal translocations in distinct pathogenetic forms of Burkitt lymphomas. *Proc Natl Acad Sci USA* 1988; **85**: 2748–52.

251. Joos S, Haluska FG, Falk MH et al. Mapping chromosomal breakpoints of Burkitt's t(8;14) translocations far upstream of c-myc. *Cancer Res* 1992; **52**: 6547–52.

252. Joos S, Falk MH, Lichter P et al. Variable breakpoints in Burkitt lymphoma cells with chromosomal t(8;14) translocation separate c-myc and the IgH locus up to several hundred kb. *Hum Mol Genet* 1992; **1**: 625–32.

253. Gutierrez MI, Bhatia K, Barriga F et al. Molecular epidemiology of Burkitt's lymphoma from South America: differences in breakpoint location and Epstein–Barr virus association from tumors in other world regions. *Blood* 1992; **79**: 3261–66.

254. Zeidler R, Joos S, Delecluse H-J et al. Breakpoints of Burkitt's lymphoma t(8; 22) translocations map within a distance of 300 kb downstream of MYC. *Gen Chromosome Cancer* 1994; **9**: 282–7.

255. Basso K, Frascella E, Zanesco L et al. Improved long-distance polymerase chain reaction for the detection of t(8; 14)(q24; q32) in Burkitt's lymphomas. *Am J Pathol* 1999; **155**: 1479–85.

256. Haralambieva E, Banham AH, Bastard C et al. Detection by the fluorescence in situ hybridization technique of MYC translocations in paraffin-embedded lymphoma biopsy samples. *Br J Haematol* 2003; **121**: 49–56.

257. Chapman CJ, Mockridge CI, Rowe M et al. Analysis of VH genes used by neoplastic B cells in endemic Burkitt's lymphoma shows somatic hypermutation and intraclonal heterogeneity. *Blood* 1995; **85**: 2176–81.

258. Tamaru J, Hummel M, Marafioti T et al. Burkitt's lymphomas express VH genes with a moderate number of antigen-selected somatic mutations. *Am J Pathol* 1995; **147**: 1398–1407.

259. Luppi M, Longo G, Ferrari MG et al. Additional neoplasms and HCV infection in low-grade lymphoma of MALT type. *Br J Haematol* 1996; **94**: 373–5.

260. Hermine O, Lefrere F, Bronowicki JP et al. Regression of splenic lymphoma with villous lymphocytes after treatment of hepatitis C virus infection. *N Engl J Med* 2002; **347**: 89–94.

261. Rabkin CS, Tess BH, Christianson RE et al. Prospective study of hepatitis C viral infection as a risk factor for subsequent B-cell neoplasia. *Blood* 2002; **99**: 4240–2.

262. Sander CA, Medeiros LJ, Weiss LM et al. Lymphoproliferative lesions in patients with common variable immunodeficiency syndrome. *Am J Surg Pathol* 1992; **16**: 1170–82.

263. Filipovich AH, Mathur A, Kamat D et al. Primary immunodeficiencies: Genetic risk factors for lymphoma. *Cancer Res* 1992; **52**(Suppl 1): 5465s–7s.

264. Levine AM. Lymphoma complicating immunodeficiency disorders. *Ann Oncol* 1994; **5**(Suppl 2): 29–35.

265. Sneller MC, Wang J, Dale JK et al. Clinical, immunologic, and genetic features of an autoimmune lymphoproliferative syndrome associated with abnormal lymphocyte apoptosis. *Blood* 1997; **89**: 1341–8.

266. Lim MS, Straus SE, Dale JK et al. Pathological findings in human autoimmune lymphoproliferative syndrome. *Am J Pathol* 1998; **153**: 1541–50.

267. Chun HJ, Zheng L, Ahmad M et al. Pleiotropic defects in lymphocyte activation caused by caspase-8 mutations lead to human immunodeficiency. *Nature* 2002; **419**: 395–9.

268. van den Berg A, Maggio E, Diepstra A et al. Germline FAS gene mutation in a case of ALPS and NLP Hodgkin lymphoma. *Blood* 2002; **99**: 1492–4.

269. Rieux-Laucat F, Le Deist F, Fischer A. Autoimmune lymphoproliferative syndromes: genetic defects of apoptosis pathways. *Cell Death Differ* 2003; **10**: 124–33.

270. Raphael BG, Knowles DM. Acquired immunodeficiency syndrome-associated non-Hodgkin's lymphoma. *Semin Oncol* 1990; **17**: 361–6.

271. Ioachim HL, Dorsett B, Cronin W et al. Acquired immunodeficiency syndrome-associated lymphomas: Clinical, pathologic, immunologic, and viral characteristics of 111 cases. *Hum Pathol* 1991; **22**: 659–73.

272. Levine AM. Acquired immunodeficiency syndrome-related lymphoma. *Blood* 1992; **80**: 8–20.

273. Hamilton-Dutoit SJ, Delecluse HJ, Raphael M et al. Detection of Epstein–Barr virus genomes in AIDS related lymphomas: Sensitivity and specificity of in situ hybridisation compared with Southern blotting. *J Clin Pathol* 1991; **44**: 676–80.

274. Hamilton-Dutoit SJ, Rea D, Raphael M et al. Epstein–Barr virus-latent gene expression and tumor cell phenotype in acquired immunodeficiency syndrome-related non-Hodgkin's lymphoma. Correlation of lymphoma phenotype with three distinct patterns of viral latency. *Am J Pathol* 1993; **143**: 1072–85.

275. Delecluse HJ, Anagnostopoulos I, Dallenbach F et al. Plasmablastic lymphomas of the oral cavity: a new entity associated with the human immunodeficiency virus infection. *Blood* 1997; **89**: 1413–20.

276. Cesarman E, Nador RG, Aozasa K et al. Kaposi's sarcoma-associated herpesvirus in non-AIDS related lymphomas occurring in body cavities. *Am J Pathol* 1996; **149**: 53–7.

277. Nador RG, Cesarman E, Chadburn A et al. Primary effusion lymphoma: a distinct clinicopathologic entity associated with the Kaposi's sarcoma-associated herpes virus. *Blood* 1996; **88**: 645–56.

278. Schulz TF. KSHV/HHV8-associated lymphoproliferations in the AIDS setting. *Eur J Cancer* 2001; **37**: 1217–26.

279. Nalesnik MA, Jaffe R, Starzi TE et al. The pathology of posttransplant lymphoproliferative disorders occurring in

the setting of cyclosporine A–prednisone immunosuppression. *Am J Pathol* 1988; **133**: 173–92.

280. Yousem SA, Randhawa P, Locker J et al. Posttransplant lymphoproliferative disorders in heart–lung transplant recipients: Primary presentation in the allograft. *Hum Pathol* 1989; **20**: 361–9.

281. Swerdlow SH. Post-transplant lymphoproliferative disorders: a morphologic, phenotypic and genotypic spectrum of disease. *Histopathol* 1992; **20**: 373–85.

282. Knowles DM, Cesarman E, Chadburn A et al. Correlative morphologic and molecular genetic analysis demonstrates three distinct categories of posttransplantation lymphoproliferative disorders. *Blood* 1995; **85**: 552–65.

283. Capello D, Cerri M, Muti G et al. Molecular histogenesis of posttransplantation lymphoproliferative disorders. *Blood* 2003; **102**: 3775–85.

284. Loren AW, Porter DL, Stadtmauer EA et al. Post-transplant lymphoproliferative disorder: a review. *Bone Marrow Transplant* 2003; **31**: 145–55.

285. Mum PM, Feller A, Gaulard P et al. Peripheral T/NK-cell lymphoma: a report of the IXth Workshop of the European Association for Haematopathology. *Histopathol* 2001; **38**: 250–70.

286. De Bruin PC, Kummer JA, Van der Valk P et al. Granzyme B-expressing peripheral T-cell lymphomas: neoplastic equivalents of activated cytotoxic T cells with preference for mucosa-associated lymphoid tissue localization. *Blood* 1994; **84**: 3785–91.

287. Foss HD, Anagnostopoulos I, Araujo I et al. Anaplastic large-cell lymphomas of T-cell and null-cell phenotype express cytotoxic molecules. *Blood* 1996; **88**: 4005–11.

288. Kanavaros P, Lescs MC, Briere J et al. Nasal T-cell lymphoma: a clinicopathologic entity associated with peculiar phenotype and with Epstein–Barr virus. *Blood* 1993; **81**: 2688–95.

289. Rabbitts TH. Chromosomal translocations in human cancer. *Nature* 1994; **372**: 143–9.

290. Heerema NA, Sather HN, Sense MG et al. Frequency and clinical significance of cytogenetic abnormalities in pediatric T-lineage acute lymphoblastic leukemia: a report from the Children's Cancer Group. *J Clin Oncol* 1998; **16**: 1270–8.

291. Ferry JA. Angioimmunoblastic T-cell lymphoma. *Adv Anat Pathol* 2002; **9**: 273–9.

292. Dogan A, Attygalle AD, Kyriakou C. Angioimmunoblastic T-cell lymphoma. *Br J Haematol* 2003; **121**: 681–91.

293. Schlegelberger B, Zhang Y, Weber-Matthiesen K et al. Detection of aberrant clones in nearly all cases of angioimmunoblastic lymphadenopathy with dysproteinemia-type T- cell lymphoma by combined interphase and metaphase cytogenetics. *Blood* 1994; **84**: 2640–8.

294. Anagnostopoulos I, Hummel M, Finn T et al. Heterogeneous Epstein–Barr virus infection patterns in peripheral T-cell lymphoma of angioimmunoblastic lymphadenopathy type. *Blood* 1992; **80**: 1804–12.

295. Weiss LM, Jaffe ES, Liu X-F et al. Detection and localization of Epstein–Barr viral genomes in angioimmunoblastic lymphadenopathy and angioimmunoblastic lymphadenopathy-like lymphoma. *Blood* 1992; **79**: 1789–95.

296. Attygalle A, Al Jehani R, Diss TC et al. Neoplastic T cells in angioimmunoblastic T-cell lymphoma express CD10. *Blood* 2002; **99**: 627–33.

297. Falini B, Pileri S, Zinzani PL et al. ALK+ lymphoma: clinico-pathological findings and outcome. *Blood* 1999; **93**: 2697–706.

298. Stein H, Foss HD, Durkop H et al. CD30(+) anaplastic large cell lymphoma: a review of its histopathologic, genetic, and clinical features. *Blood* 2000; **96**: 3681–95.

299. Jaffe ES. Anaplastic large cell lymphoma: The shifting sands of diagnostic hematopathology. *Mod Pathol* 2001; **14**: 219–28.

300. Weisenburger DD, Anderson JR, Diebold J et al. Systemic anaplastic large-cell lymphoma: results from the non-Hodgkin's lymphoma classification project. *Am J Hematol* 2001; **67**: 172–8.

301. ten Berge RL, Oudejans JJ, Ossenkoppele GJ et al. ALK-negative systemic anaplastic large cell lymphoma: differential diagnostic and prognostic aspects – a review. *J Pathol* 2003; **200**: 4–15.

302. Morris SW, Kirstein MN, Valentine MB et al. Fusion of a kinase gene, ALK, to a nucleolar protein gene, NPM, in non-Hodgkin's lymphoma. *Science* 1994; **263**: 1281–4.

303. Wellmann A, Otsuki T, Vogelbruch M et al. Analysis of the t(2; 5)(p23; q35) translocation by reverse transcription polymerase chain reaction in CD30+ anaplastic large cell lymphomas, in other non-Hodgkin's lymphomas of T-cell type, and in Hodgkin's disease. *Blood* 1995; **86**: 2321–8.

304. Benharroch D, Meguerian Bedoyan Z, Lamant L et al. ALK-positive lymphoma: a single disease with a broad spectrum of morphology. *Blood* 1998; **91**: 2076–84.

305. Falini B, Bigerna B, Fizzotti M et al. ALK expression defines a distinct group of T/null lymphomas ('ALK lymphomas') with a wide morphological spectrum. *Am J Pathol* 1998; **153**: 875–86.

306. Delsol G, Lamant L, Mariame B et al. A new subtype of large B-cell lymphoma expressing the ALK kinase and lacking the t(2; 5) translocation. *Blood* 1997; **89**: 1483–90.

307. Gascoyne RD, Lamant L, Martin-Subero JI et al. ALK-positive diffuse large B-cell lymphoma is associated with Clathrin-ALK rearrangements: report of 6 cases. *Blood* 2003; **102**: 2568–73.

308. De Paepe P, Baens M, van Krieken H et al. ALK activation by the CLTC-ALK fusion is a recurrent event in large B-cell lymphoma. *Blood* 2003; **102**: 2638–41.

309. Tsang WY, Chan JK, Yip TT et al. In situ localization of Epstein–Barr virus encoded RNA in non-nasal/nasopharyngeal CD56-positive and CD56-negative T-cell lymphomas. *Hum Pathol* 1994; **25**: 758–65.

310. Weiss LM, Arber DA, Strickler JG. Nasal T-cell lymphoma. *Ann Oncol* 1994; **5**(Suppl 1): 39–42.

311. Mori N, Yatabe Y, Oka K et al. Expression of perforin in nasal lymphoma. Additional evidence of its natural killer cell derivation. *Am J Pathol* 1996; **149**: 699–705.

312. Chan JK, Sin VC, Wong KF et al. Nonnasal lymphoma expressing the natural killer cell marker CD56: a clinicopathologic study of 49 cases of an uncommon aggressive neoplasm. *Blood* 1997; **89**: 4501–13.

313. Ohshima K, Suzumiya J, Shimazaki K et al. Nasal T/NK cell lymphomas commonly express perform and Fas ligand: important mediators of tissue damage. *Histopathol* 1997; **31**: 444–50.

314. Spencer J, Cerf Bensussan N, Jarry A et al. Enteropathy-associated T cell lymphoma (malignant histiocytosis of the intestine) is recognized by a monoclonal antibody (HML-1) that defines a membrane molecule on human mucosal lymphocytes. *Am J Pathol* 1988; **132**: 1–5.

315. Isaacson PG. Histopathology of the complications of celiac disease: Enteropathy-associated T cell lymphoma and ulcerative jejunitis. *Front Gastrointest Res* 1992; **19**: 194–212.

316. De Bruin PC, Jiwa NM, Oudejans JJ et al. Epstein–Barr virus in primary gastrointestinal T cell lymphomas. Association with gluten-sensitive enteropathy, pathological features, and immunophenotype. *Am J Pathol* 1995; **146**: 861–7.

317. Ashton Key M, Diss TC, Pan L et al. Molecular analysis of T-cell clonality in ulcerative jejunitis and enteropathy-associated T-cell lymphoma. *Am J Pathol* 1997; **151**: 493–8.

318. Wright DH. Enteropathy associated T cell lymphoma. *Cancer Surv* 1997; **30**: 249–61.

319. Bagdi E, Diss TC, Munson P et al. Mucosal intra-epithelial lymphocytes in enteropathy-associated T-cell lymphoma, ulcerative jejunitis, and refractory celiac disease constitute a neoplastic population. *Blood* 1999; **94**: 260–4.

320. Baumgartner AK, Zettl A, Chott A et al. High frequency of genetic aberrations in enteropathy-type T-cell lymphoma. *Laboratory Investigation* 2003; **83**: 1509–16.

321. Chott A, Haedicke W, Mosberger I et al. Most CD56+ intestinal lymphomas are CD8+CD5-T-cell lymphomas of monomorphic small to medium size histology. *Am J Pathol* 1998; **153**: 1483–90.

322. Scheffer E, Meijer CJLM, Vloten van WA. Dermatopathic lymphadenopathy and lymph node involvement in mycosis fungoides. *Cancer* 1980; **45**: 137–48.

323. Scheffer E, Meijer CJ, Willemze R et al. Lymph node histopathology in mycosis fungoides and Sézary's syndrome. *Curr Probl Dermatol* 1990; **19**: 105–13.

324. Wood GS, Bahler DW, Hoppe RT et al. Transformation of mycosis fungoides: T-cell receptor b gene analysis demonstrates a common clonal origin for plaque-type mycosis fungoides and CD30+ large-cell lymphoma. *J Invest Dermatol* 1993; **101**: 296–300.

325. Shapiro PE, Pinto FJ. The histologic spectrum of mycosis fungoides/Sézary syndrome (cutaneous T-cell lymphoma). A review of 222 biopsies, including newly described patterns and the earliest pathologic changes. *Am J Surg Pathol* 1994; **18**: 645–67.

326. van Doorn R, van Haselen CW, Voorst Vader PC et al. Mycosis fungoides: disease evolution and prognosis of 309 Dutch patients. *Arch Dermatol* 2000; **136**: 504–10.

327. Bakels V, Van Oostveen JW, Geerts M-L et al. Diagnostic and prognostic significance of clonal T-cell receptor beta gene rearrangements in lymph nodes of patients with mycosis fungoides. *J Pathol* 1993; **170**: 249–55.

328. Santucci M, Pimpinelli N, Massi D et al. Cytotoxic/natural killer cell cutaneous lymphomas. Report of EORTC Cutaneous Lymphoma Task Force Workshop. *Cancer* 2003; **97**: 610–27.

329. Vermeer MH, van Doorn R, Dukers D et al. CD8+ T cells in cutaneous T-cell lymphoma: expression of cytotoxic proteins, Fas ligand, and killing inhibitory receptors and their relationship with clinical behavior. *J Clin Oncol* 2001; **19**: 4322–9.

330. Bekkenk MW, Vermeer MH, Jansen PM et al. Peripheral T-cell lymphomas unspecified presenting in the skin: analysis of prognostic factors in a group of 82 patients. *Blood* 2003; **102**: 2213–9.

331. Vonderheid EC, Bernengo MG, Burg G et al. Update on erythrodermic cutaneous T-cell lymphoma: report of the International Society for Cutaneous Lymphomas. *J Am Acad Dermatol* 2002; **46**: 95–106.

332. Beljaards RC, Meijer CJLM, Scheffer E et al. Prognostic significance of CD30 (Ki-1/Ber-H2) expression in primary cutaneous large-cell lymphomas of T-cell origin: A clinico- opathologic and immunohistochemical study in 20 patients. *Am J Pathol* 1989; **135**: 1169–78.

333. Kaudewitz P, Stein H, Dallenbach F et al. Primary and secondary cutaneous K1-I' (CD30+) anaplastic large cell lymphomas: Morphologic, immunohistologic, and clinical characteristics. *Am J Pathol* 1989; **135**: 359–67.

334. Beljaards RC, Kaudewitz P, Berti E et al. Primary cutaneous CD30-positive large cell lymphoma: Definition of a new type of cutaneous lymphoma with a favorable prognosis: A European multicenter study of 47 patients. *Cancer* 1993; **71**: 2097–104.

335. De Bruin PC, Beljaards RC, Van Heerde P et al. Differences in clinical behaviour and immunophenotype between primary cutaneous and primary nodal anaplastic large cell lymphoma of T-cell or null cell phenotype. *Histopathol* 1993; **23**: 127–135.

336. DeCoteau JF, Butmarc JR, Kinney MC et al. The t(2; 5) chromosomal translocation is not a common feature of primary cutaneous CD30+ lymphoproliferative disorders: comparison with anaplastic large-cell lymphoma of nodal origin. *Blood* 1996; **87**: 3437–41.

337. Kummer JA, Vermeer MH, Dukers D et al. Most primary cutaneous CD30-positive lymphoproliferative disorders have a CD4-positive cytotoxic T-cell phenotype. *J Invest Dermatol* 1997; **109**: 636–40.

338. Kadin ME, Carpenter C. Systemic and primary cutaneous anaplastic large cell lymphomas. *Seminars in Hematology* 2003; **40**: 244–56.

339. Delcambre C, Reman O, Henry-Amar M et al. Clinical relevance of gallium-67 scintigraphy in lymphoma before and after therapy. *Eur J Nucl Med* 2000; **27**: 176–84.

340. Ha CS, Choe JG, Kong JS et al. Agreement rates among single photon emission computed tomography using gallium-67, computed axial tomography and lymphangiography for Hodgkin's disease and correction of image findings with clinical outcome. *Cancer* 2000; **89**: 1371–9.

341. Wirth A, Seymour JF, Hicks RJ et al. Fluorine-18 fluorodeoxyglucose positron emission tomography, gallium-67 scintigraphy, and conventional staging for Hodgkin's disease and non-Hodgkin's lymphoma. *Am J Med* 2002; **112**: 262–8.

342. Sasaki M, Kuwabara Y, Koga H et al. Clinical impact of whole body FDG-PET on the staging and therapeutic decision making for malignant lymphoma. *Ann Nucl Med* 2002; **16**: 337–45.

343. Moog F, Bangerter M, Kotzerke J et al. 18-F-fluorodeoxyglucose-positron emission tomography as a new approach to detect lymphomatous bone marrow. *J Clin Oncol* 1998; **16**: 603–9.

344. Buchmann I, Moog F, Schirrmeister H et al. Positron emission tomography for detection and staging of malignant lymphoma. *Recent Results Cancer Res* 2000; **156**: 78–89.

345. Cheson BD, Horning SJ, Coiffier B et al. Report of an international workshop to standardize response criteria for non-Hodgkin's lymphomas. NCI Sponsored International Working Group. *J Clin Oncol* 1999; **17**: 1244–53.

346. Surbone A, Longo DL, DeVita VT Jr et al. Residual abdominal masses in aggressive non-Hodgkin's lymphoma after combination chemotherapy: Significance and management. *J Clin Oncol* 1988; **6**: 1832–7.

347. Spaepen K, Stroobants S, Dupont P et al. Prognostic value of positron emission tomography (PET) with fluorine-18 fluorodeoxyglucose (18FDG) after first-line chemotherapy

in non-Hodgkin's lymphoma: Is [18]FDG-PET a valid alternative to conventional diagnostic methods? *J Clin Oncol* 2001; **19**: 414–19.

348. Shipp MA, Harrington DP, Anderson JR et al. A predictive model for aggressive non-Hodgkin's lymphoma. *N Engl J Med* 1993; **329**: 987–94.

349. López-Guillermo A, Montserrat E, Bosch F et al. Applicability of the International Index for aggressive lymphomas to patients with low-grade lymphoma. *J Clin Oncol* 1994; **12**: 1343–8.

350. Hermans J, Krol ADG, van Groningen K et al. International Prognostic Index for aggressive non-Hodgkin's lymphoma is valid for all malignancy grades. *Blood* 1995; **86**: 1460–3.

351. Solal-Celigny P. Follicular Lymphoma International Prognostic Project. *Ann Oncol* 2002; **13**: 18 (abstract).

352. Kersten MJ, De Jong D, Raemaekers JJM et al. Beyond the International Prognostic Index: New prognostic factors in follicular lymphoma and diffuse large cell lymphoma. A meeting report of the Second International Lunenburg Lymphoma Workshop. *The Hematology Journal* 2004; in press.

353. Alizadeh AA, Eisen MB, Davis RE et al. Distinct types of diffuse large B-cell lymphoma identified by gene expression profiling. *Nature* 2000; **403**: 503–11.

354. Hans CP, Weisenburger DD, Greiner TC et al. Confirmation of the molecular classification of diffuse large B-cell lymphoma by immunohistochemistry using a tissue microarray. *Blood* 2004; **103**: 275–82.

355. Paryani SB, Hoppe RT, Cox RS et al. Analysis of non-Hodgkin's lymphomas with nodular and favorable histologies, stages I and II. *Cancer* 1983; **52**: 2300–7.

356. Gospodarowicz MK, Bush RS, Brown TC et al. Prognostic factors in nodular lymphomas: A multivariate analysis based on the Princess Margaret Hospital experience. *Int J Rad Oncol Biol Phys* 1984; **10**: 489–97.

357. Besa PC, McLaughlin PW, Cox JD et al. Long term assessment of patterns of treatment failure and survival in patients with stage I or II follicular lymphoma. *Cancer* 1995; **75**: 2361–7.

358. MacManus MP, Hoppe RT. Is radiotherapy curative for stage I and II low-grade follicular lymphoma? Results of a long-term follow-up study of patients treated at Stanford University. *J Clin Oncol* 1996; **14**: 1282–90.

359. Lambrechts AC, Hupkes PE, Dorssers LCJ et al. Translocation (14;18)-positive cells are present in the circulation of the majority of patients with localized (stage I and II) follicular non-Hodgkin's lymphoma. *Blood* 1993; **82**: 2510–16.

360. Price CGA, Meerabaux J, Murtagh S et al. The significance of circulating cells carrying t(14;18) in long remission from follicular lymphoma. *J Clin Oncol* 1991; **9**: 1527–32.

361. Monfardini S, Banfi A, Bonadonna C et al. Improved five-years survival after combined radiotherapy-chemotherapy for stage I and II non-Hodgkin's lymphoma. *Int J Rad Oncol Biol Phys* 1980; **6**: 125–34.

362. Carde P, Burgers JMV, Van Glabbeke M et al. Combined radiotherapy-chemotherapy for early stage non-Hodgkin's lymphoma: The 1975–1980 EORTC Controlled Lymphoma Trial. *Radiation Oncol* 1984; **2**: 301–12.

363. Kelsey SM, Newland AC, Hudson GV et al. A British National Lymphoma Investigation randomized trial of single-agent chlorambucil plus radiotherapy versus radiotherapy alone in low-grade localized non-Hodgkin's lymphoma. *Radiation Oncol* 1994; **11**: 19–25.

364. Portlock CS. Management of the low-grade non-Hodgkin's lymphomas. *Seminars Oncol* 1990; **17**: 51–9.

365. Lister TA. The management of follicular lymphoma. *Ann Oncol* 1991; **2**: 131–5.

366. Young RC, Longo DL, Gladstein E et al. The treatment of indolent lymphomas: watchful waiting versus aggressive combined modality treatment. *Seminars Hematol* 1988; **25**: 11–16.

367. Merigan TC, Sikora, K, Breeden JH et al. Preliminary observations of the effect of human leucocyte interferon in non-Hodgkin's lymphoma. *N Engl J Med* 1978; **299**: 1449–53.

368. Foon KA, Sherwin SA, Abrams PG et al. Treatment of advanced non-Hodgkin's lymphoma with recombinant leucocyte A interferon. *N Engl J Med* 1984; **311**: 1148–52.

369. O'Connell MJ, Colgan JP, Oken MM et al. Clinical trial of recombinant leucocyte A inferferon as initial therapy for favourable histology non-Hodgkin's lymphomas and chronic lymphocytic leukaemia. An Eastern Cooperative Oncology Group pilot study. *J Clin Oncol* 1986; **4**: 128–36.

370. Hagenbeek A, Carde P, Meerwaldt JH et al. Maintenance of remission with human recombinant interferon alfa-2a in patients with stages III and IV low-grade malignant non-Hodgkin's lymphoma. *J Clin Oncol* 1998; **16**: 41–7.

371. Unterhalt M, Herrmann R, Nahler M et al. Significant prolongation of disease free survival in advanced low grade non-Hodgkin lymphomas (NHL) by interferon alpha maintenance. *Blood* 1995; **86**: 439A (abstract).

372. Smalley RV, Andersen JW, Hawkins MJ et al. Interferon-α combined with cytotoxic chemotherapy for patients with non-Hodgkin's lymphoma. *N Engl J Med* 1992; **327**: 1336–41.

373. Solal-Celigny P, Lepage E, Brousse N et al. Recombinant interferon alfa-2b combined with a regimen containing doxorubicin in patients with advanced follicular lymphoma. *N Engl J Med* 1993; **329**: 1608–14.

374. Rohatiner A, Gregory W, Peterson B et al. A meta-analysis of randomized studies evaluating the role of interferon α as treatment for follicular lymphoma. *Proc Am Soc Clin Oncol* 2002; **18**: 264A (abstract).

375. Saven A, Emanuele S, Kosty M et al. 2-Chlorodeoxyadenosine activity in patients with untreated, indolent non-Hodgkin's lymphoma. *Blood* 1995; **86**: 1710–16.

376. Solal-Celigny P, Brice P, Brousse N et al. Phase II trial of fludarabine monophosphate as firstline treatment in patients with advanced follicular lymphoma: A multicenter study by the Groupe d'Etude des Lymphomes de l'Adulte. *J Clin Oncol* 1996; **14**: 514–19.

377. Hagenbeek A, Eghbali H, Monfardini S et al. Fludarabine versus conventional CVP chemotherapy in newly diagnosed patients with stages III and IV low grade follicular malignant non-Hodgkin's lymphoma. Preliminary resulsts from a prospective, randomized phase III clinical trial in 381 patients. *Blood* 1998; **92**: 1294A (abstract).

378. McLaughlin P, Hagemeister FB, Romaguera JE et al. Fludarabine, mitoxantrone, and dexamethasone: An effective new regimen for indolent lymphoma. *J Clin Oncol* 1996; **14**: 1262–8.

379. Tsimberidou AM, McLaughlin P, Younes A et al. Fludarabine, mitoxantrone, dexamethasone (FND) compared with an alternating triple (ATT) regimen in patients with stage IV indolent lymphoma. *Blood* 2002; **100**: 4351–7.

380. Rohatiner AZS, Johnson PWM, Price CGA et al.

Myeloablative therapy with autologous bone marrow transplantation as consolidation therapy for recurrent follicular lymphoma. *J Clin Oncol* 1994; **12**: 1177–84.

381. Bastion Y, Brice P, Haioun A et al. Intensive therapy with peripheral blood progenitor cell transplantation in 60 patients with poorprognosis follicular lymphoma. *Blood* 1995; **86**: 3257–62.

382. Haas R, Moos M, Mbhle R et al. High-dose therapy with peripheral blood progenitor cell transplantation in low-grade non-Hodgkin's lymphoma. *Bone Marrow Transplant* 1996; **37**: 149–55.

383. Freedman AS, Ritz J, Neuberg D et al. Autologous bone marrow transplantation in 69 patients with a history of low-grade B-cell non-Hodgkin's lymphoma. *Blood* 1991; **77**: 2524–9.

384. Schouten HC, Qian W, Kvalay S et al. High-dose therapy improves progression-free survival and survival in relapsed follicular non-Hodgkin's lymphoma: Results from the randomized European CUP trial. *J Clin Oncol* **21**: 2003: 3918–27.

385. Darrington DL, Vose JM, Anderson JR et al. Incidence and characterization of secondary myelodysplastic syndrome and acute myelogenous leukemia following high-dose chemoradiotherapy and autologous stem cell transplantation for lymphoid malignancies. *J Clin Oncol* 1994; **12**: 2527–34.

386. Sebban C, Coiffier B, Belanger C et al. A randomized trial in follicular lymphoma comparing a standard chemotherapy regimen with 4 courses of CHOP followed by autologous stem cell transplant with TBI: The GELF94 tiral from GELA. *The Hematology Journal* 2003; **4**: 486 (abstract).

387. Hunault-Berger M, Ifrah N, Solal-Celigny P, Intensive therapies in follicular non-Hodgkin's lymphomas. *Blood* 2002; **100**: 1141–52.

388. Robinson SP, Goldstone AH, Mackinnon S et al. Chemoresistant or aggressive lymphoma predicts for a poor outcome following reduced-intensity allogeneic progenitor cell transplantation: An analysis from the Lymphoma Working Party of the European Group for Blood and Bone Marrow Transplantation. *Blood* 2002; **100**: 4310–16.

389. Aisenberg AS. Coherent view of non-Hodgkin's lymphoma. *J Clin Oncol* 1995; **13**: 2656–75.

390. Maloney DG, Grillo-Lopez AJ, White CA et al. IDEC-C2B8 (Rituximab)anti-CD20 monoclonal antibody therapy in patients with relapsed low-grade non-Hodgkin's lymphoma. *Blood* 1997; **90**: 2188–95.

391. McLaughlin P, Grillo-Lopez AJ, Link BK et al. Rituximab chimeric anti-CD20 monoclonal antibody therapy for relapsed indolent lymphoma: Half of patients respond to a four-dose treatment program. *J Clin Oncol* 1998; **16**: 2825–33.

392. Davis TA, Grillo-Lopez AJ, White CA et al. Rituximab anti-CD20 monoclonal antibody therapy in non-Hodgkin's lymphoma: Safety and efficacy of re-treatment. *J Clin Oncol* 2000; **18**: 3135–43.

393. Kaminski MS, Zelenetz AD, Press OW et al. Pivotal study of Iodine I[131] Tositumomab for chemotherapy-refractory low-grade or transformed low-grade B-cell non-Hodgkin's lymphoma. *J Clin Oncol* 2001; **19**: 3918–28.

394. Witzig TE, White CA, Gordon LI et al. Safety of Yttrium[90] Ibritumomab Tiuxetan radioimmunotherapy for relapsed low-grade, follicular, or transformed non-Hodgkin's lymphoma. *J Clin Oncol* 2003; **21**: 1263–70.

395. Barrios Y, Cabrera R, Yanez R et al. Anti-idiotypic vaccination in the treatment of low-grade B-cell lymphoma. *Haematologica* 2002; **87**: 400–7.

396. Timmerman JM, Czerwinski DK, Davis TA et al. Idiotype-pulsed dendritic cell vaccination for B-cell lymphoma: Clinical and immune responses in 35 patients. *Blood* 2002; **99**: 1517–26.

397. Bendandi M, Gocke CD, Kobrin CD et al. Complete molecular remissions induced by patient-specific vaccination plus granulocyte-monocyte colony-stimulating factor against lymphoma. *Nat Med* 1999; **5**: 1171–77.

398. Rohatiner A, d'Amore F, Coiffier B et al. Report on a workshop convened to discuss the pathological and staging classifications of gastrointestinal tract lymphoma. *Ann Oncol* 1994; **5**: 397–400.

399. Zucca El, Roggero E. Biology and treatment of MALT lymphoma: The state of the art in 1996. *Ann Oncol* 1996; **7**: 787–92.

400. Liu H, Ruskon-Fourmestraux, Lavergne-Slove A et al. Resistance of t(11;18) positive gastric mucosa-associated lymphoid tissue lymphoma to Heliobacter pylori eradication therapy. *Lancet* 2001; **357**: 39–40.

401. Foss FM, Sausville EA. Prognosis and staging of cutaneous T-cell lymphoma. *Hematol Oncol Clin North Am* 1995; **9**: 1011–19.

402. Koh H, Foss F. Cutaneous T-cell lymphoma. *Hematol Oncol Clin North Am* 1995; **9**: 5–14.

403. Beljaards RC, Kaudewitz P, Berti E et al. Primary cutaneous CD30-positive large cell lymphoma: Definition of a new type of cutaneous lymphoma with a favorable prognosis: A European multicenter study of 47 patients. *Cancer* 1993; **71**: 2097–104.

404. Miller T, Dahlberg S, Cassady J et al. Chemotherapy alone compared with chemotherapy plus radiotherapy for localized intermediate- and high-grade non-Hodgkin's lymphoma. *N Engl J Med* 1998; **339**: 21–6.

405. Coleman M, Gerstein G, Topilow A et al. Advances in chemotherapy for large cell lymphoma. *Seminars Hematol* 1987; **24**: 8–20.

406. DeVita VR jr, Hubbard SM, Young RC et al. The role of chemotherapy in diffuse aggressive lymphomas. *Seminars Hematol* 1988; **25**: 2–10.

407. Fisher RI, Gaynor ER, Dahlberg S et al. Comparison of a standard regimen (CHOP) with three intensive chemotherapy regimens for advanced non-Hodgkin's lymphoma. *N Engl J Med* 1993; **32**: 1002–6.

408. Kluin-Nelemans HC, Zagonel V, Anastasopoulou A et al. Standard chemotherapy for aggressive non-Hodgkin's lymphoma: Randomized phase III EORTC study. *J Natl Cancer Inst* 2001; **93**: 22–30.

409. Verdonck LF, Van Putten WL, Hagenbeek A et al. Comparison of CHOP chemotherapy with autologous bone marrow transplantation for slowly responding patients with aggressive non-Hodgkin's lymphoma. *N Engl J Med* 1995; **332**: 1045–51.

410. Haioun C, Lepage E, Gisselbrecht C et al. Comparison of autologous bone marrow transplantation with sequential chemotherapy for intermediate-grade and high-grade non-Hodgkin's lymphoma in first complete remission: A study of 484 patients. Group d'Etude des Lymphomes de l'Adulte. *J Clin Oncol* 1994; **12**: 2543–51.

411. Santini G, Salvagno L, Leoni P et al. VACOP-B versus VACOP-B plus autologous bone marrow transplantation for advanced diffuse non-Hodgkin's lymphoma: Results of

a prospective randomized trial by the non-Hodgkin's Lymphoma Cooperative Study Group. *J Clin Oncol* 1998; **16**: 2796–802.

412. Haioun C, Lepage E, Gisselbrecht C et al. Benefit of autologous bone marrow transplantation over sequential chemotherapy in poor-risk aggressive non-Hodgkin's lymphoma: Updated results of the prospective study LNH87-2. Groupe d'Etude des Lymphomes de l'Adulte. *J Clin Oncol* 1997; **15**: 1131–7.

413. Cabanillas F, Hagemeister FB, Bodey GP et al. IMVP-16: an effective regimen for patients with lymphoma who have relapsed after initial combination chemotherapy. *Blood* 1982; **60**: 693–7.

414. Velasquez WS, McLaughlin P, Tucker S et al. ESHAP – an effective chemotherapy regimen in refractory and relapsing lymphoma: a 4-year follow-up study. *J Clin Oncol* 1994; **12**: 1169–76.

415. Chopra R, Linch DC, McMillan AK et al. Mini-BEAM followed by BEAM and ABMT for very poor risk Hodgkin's disease. *Br J Haematol* 1992; **81**: 197–202.

416. Philip T, Guglielmi C, Hagenbeek A et al. Autologous bone marrow transplantation as compared with salvage chemotherapy in relapses of chemotherapy-sensitive non-Hodgkin's lymphoma. *N Engl J Med* 1995; **333**: 1540–5.

417. O'Reilly SE, Connors JM, Howdle S et al. In search of an optimal regimen for elderly patients with advanced stage diffuse large-cell lymphoma: Results of a phase II study of P/DOCE chemotherapy. *J Clin Oncol* 1993; **11**: 2250–7.

418. Zinzani PLI, Pavone E, Storti S et al. Randomized trial with or without granulocyte colony-stimulating factor as adjunct to induction VNCOP-B treatment of elderly high-grade non-Hodgkin's lymphoma. *Blood* 1997; **89**: 3974–9.

419. Doorduijn JK, Van der Holt B, Van Imhoff GW et al. CHOP compared with CHOP plus granulocyte colony-stimulating factor in elderly patients with aggressive non-Hodgkin's lymphoma. *J Clin Oncol* 2003; **21**: 3041–50.

420. Coiffier B, Lepage E, Brière J et al. CHOP chemotherapy plus Rituximab compared with CHOP alone in elderly patients with diffuse large B-cell lymphoma. *N Engl J Med* 2002; **346**: 235–42.

421. Abrey LE, Yahalom J, DeAngelis LM. Treatment for primary CNS lymphoma: The next step. *J Clin Oncol* 2000; **18**: 3144–50.

422. Brada M, Hjiyiannakis D, Hines F et al. Short intensive primary chemotherapy and radiotherapy in sporadic primary CNS lymphoma (PCL). *Int J Radiat Oncol Biol Phys* 1998; **40**: 1157–62.

423. O'Brien P, Roos D, Pratt G et al. Phase II multicenter study of brief single-agent methotrexate followed by irradiation in primary CNS lymphoma. *J Clin Oncol* 2000; **18**: 519–26.

424. Teodorovic I, Pittaluga S, Kluin-Nelemans JC et al. Efficacy of four different regimens in 64 mantle-cell lymphoma cases: Clinicopathologic comparison with 498 other non-Hodgkin's lymphoma subtypes. *J Clin Oncol* 1995; **13**: 2819–26.

425. Meusers P, Engelhard M, Bartels H et al. Multicenter randomized therapeutic trial for advanced centrocytic lymphoma: Anthracycline does not improve the prognosis. *Hematol Oncol* 1989; **7**: 365–80.

426. Andersen NS, Jensen MK, De Nully Brown P et al. A Danish population-based analysis of 105 mantle cell lymphoma patients: Incidences, clinical features, response, survival and prognostic factors. *Eur J Cancer* 2002; **38**: 401–8.

427. Hiddemann W, Unterhalt M, Hermann R et al. Mantle-cell lymphomas have more widespread disease and a slower response to chemotherapy compared with follicle-center lymphomas: Results of a prospective comparative analysis of the German Low-Grade Lymphoma Study Group. *J Clin Oncol* 1998; **16**: 1922–30.

428. Foran JM, Rohatiner AZ, Cunningham D et al. European phase II study of Rituximab (chimeric anti-CD20 monoclonal antibody) for patients with newly diagnosed mantle-cell lymphoma and previously treated mantle-cell lymphoma, immunocytoma, and small B-cell lymphocytic lymphoma. *J Clin Oncol* 2000; **18**: 317–24.

429. Howard OM, Gribben HG, Neuberg DS et al. Rituximab and CHOP induction therapy for newly diagnosed mantle-cell lymphoma: Molecular complete responses are not predictive of progression-free survival. *J Clin Oncol* 2000; **20**: 1288–94.

430. Khouri IF, Romaguera J, Kantarjian H et al. Hyper-CVAD and high-dose methotrexate/cytarabine followed by stem cell transplantation: An active regimen for aggressive mantle-cell lymphoma. *J Clin Oncol* 1998; **16**: 3803–9.

431. Gisselbrecht C, Gaulard P, Lepage E et al. Prognostic significance of T-cell phenotype in aggressive non-Hodgkin's lymphomas. *Blood* 1998; **92**: 76–82.

432. Van Esser JWJ, Neisters HGM, Van der Holt B et al. Prevention of Epstein-Barr virus-lymphoproliferative disease by molecular monitoring and preemptive Rituximab in high-risk patients after allogeneic stem cell transplantation. *Blood* 2002; **99**: 4364–9.

433. Papadopoulos EB, Ladanyi M, Emanuel D et al. Infusions of donor leukocytes to treat Epstein–Barr virus-associated lymphoproliferative disorders after allogeneic bone marrow transplantation. *N Engl Med* 1994; **330**: 1185–91.

434. Ratner L, Lee J, Tang S et al. Chemotherapy for human immunodeficiency virus-associated non-Hodgkin's lymphoma in combination with highly active antitretroviral therapy. *J Clin Oncol* 2001; **19**: 2171–8.

435. Vaccher E, Spina M, Di Gennaro G et al. Concomitant Cyclophosphamide, Doxorubicin, Vincristine, and Prednisone chemotherapy plus highly active antiretroviral therapy in patients with human immunodeficiency virus-related, non-Hodgkin's lymphoma. *Cancer* 2001; **91**: 155–63.

# 37 Acute myeloid leukemia in children and adolescents

## GJL Kaspers and Y Ravindranath

## Introduction

Today the cure rate in childhood acute lymphoblastic leukemia (ALL) has approached nearly 80% while that for acute myeloid leukemia (AML) continues to be between 35% and 50%, which is one of the lowest in all childhood cancers.[1] More recent studies suggest that survival rates above 50% are possible.[2–5] Factors contributing to the low results are the heterogeneous features of AML, with multiple morphologic subtypes and distinct cytogenetic associations and a high frequency of extramedullary involvement at diagnosis compared with ALL. This heterogeneity precluded, until recently, identification of clearly definable subgroups of patients with defined outcome. An additional contributing factor was the prior strategy of using a uniform therapy regardless of the morphologic/cytogenetic variant. However within the last 15 years, the inclusion of high-dose cytarabine (cytosine arabinoside, Ara-C) has permitted the identification of distinct subgroups of AML patients with superior outcome: children with Down syndrome[6] and AML with molecular lesions of the core binding factor complex (CBF) – i.e. AML with inv(16) and t(8;21).[7–9] An additional major advance in treatment has been the demonstration of the unique sensitivity of acute promyelocytic leukemia (APL) with the t(15;17) to retinoid-based therapy.[10–13] These discoveries clearly raise the hope that with proper risk group-based definitions and risk-based therapeutic strategies, further improvements can be achieved in the treatment of all subgroups of patients with AML. In this chapter, we will explore the unique features of AML in children compared with adults, and review the treatment results of large pediatric studies within the last two decades and the lessons derived from these regarding future strategies.

## Biology and classification

Unlike ALL, the incidence of AML is relatively uniform throughout the pediatric age group (Figure 37.1).[14] Moreover, in contrast to ALL, the morphologic and cytogenetic variants in AML appear to be the same in both adults and children, except for the frequency of certain subgroups. For example, Down syndrome and AML is unique to children and there is a higher frequency of t(8;21) and 11q 23 abnormalities compared with adults.[15,16] In contrast, the incidence of *FLT3* gene internal tandem duplications and mutations are lower.[17–22] Furthermore, within the last

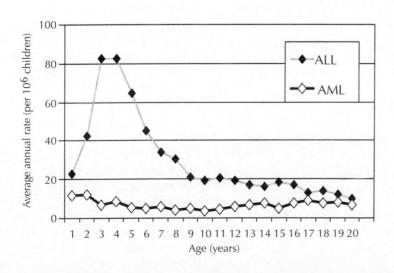

**Figure 37.1** Age-specific incidence rates for acute lymphoblastic and acute myeloid leukemias (ALL and AML) in childhood. From reference 14, with permission.

several years, it has been recognized that the previous FAB (French–American–British) classification excludes certain groups of de novo AML patients who might benefit from intensive chemotherapy because of the requirement of the presence of 30% blast cells for a diagnosis of AML.[23,24] The recent modification to the FAB system suggested by the WHO clearly addresses these issues.[25,26] These changes in classification are reviewed in Chapter 38. Other presentations needing special attention are cases of so-called isolated granulocytic sarcoma, as some of these cases may in fact represent FAB type M2 AML with t(8;21) with a low blast percentage or acute megakaryocytic leukemia (AMKL), which in infants can present with chloromatous lesions and may even mimic neuroblastoma.[27] In each case, cytogenetic evaluation of the biopsy of the chloroma and bone marrow with appropriate histochemical stains and the use of platelet-specific markers should help resolve the diagnostic dilemma. Urinary catecholamine metabolites and abdominal ultrasound may be necessary in doubtful cases to exclude neuroblastoma.

A unique subgroup in childhood AML are those with Down syndrome. In Down syndrome, AML can present as transient myeloproliferative disorder (TMD) in the neonatal period or as AMKL or acute erythroleukemia (AEL) in later infancy.[6,28–30] Interestingly, the AMKL in Down syndrome is not associated with the t(1;22) cytogenetic marker found in AMKL in non-Down children.[31,32] Regardless, the outcome is excellent – spontaneous recovery is the rule in TMD,[33,34] and in later infancy AML in Down syndrome children is highly responsive to therapy, as initially reported by the Pediatric Oncology Group (POG).[6,29,30,32,35–40]

Additional unique subgroups in children are cases of AML developing in children with constitutional aplastic anemias (notably Fanconi anemia and those with paroxysmal nocturnal hemoglobinuria, which is often associated with monosomy 7), children receiving granulocyte colony-stimulating factor (G-CSF)[41–43] and AML with 11q23 abnormalities following epipodophyllotoxin therapy.[44–46] Further, de novo 11q23 AML in neonates has been linked to maternal exposure to flavinoids.[47] We will explore further some of these unique features of childhood AML in relation to prognostic features, drug resistance, and treatment results.

## Risk group definitions and prognostic features

As noted earlier, distinctive subgroups with differing outcome began to emerge with the introduction of high-dose cytarabine in the treatment of AML. It had been recognized for a long time, however, that patients with monocytic features have a poor outcome, while the M4Eo subgroup with abnormal eosinophils and inv(16) have a better outcome.[48] Subsequent large adult studies in the mid to late 1980s showed the importance of cytogenetics in the prognosis of AML and led to the identification of three cytogenetically based risk groups: good risk or favorable cytogenetics with inv(16), t(8;21), and t(15;17); an intermediate-risk group with normal cytogenetics; and those with all other genetic abnormalities, comprising a poor-risk (unfavorable cytogenetics) group.[7,8,16] On the other hand, the Berlin–Frankfurt–Münster (BFM) group used different strategies for risk group definition in pediatric patients. The BFM group did not include cytogenetics, but did include a centrally reviewed FAB morphology and centrally reviewed assessment of response to induction therapy.[49,50] In a multivariate analysis, bone marrow blasts present on day 15, morphologically defined risk groups, and hyperleukocytosis proved to be of prognostic value. Since the specific karyotypes t(8;21), t(15;17), and inv(16) were closely associated with the favorable morphologic types M2, M3, and M4, respectively, the outcome was in the same range for these cytogenetic and FAB subgroups. The BFM group suggested that the standard-risk group should be defined by favorable morphology (M2 with Auer rods, M3, and M4Eo) and a significant blast reduction on day 15 (not required for the FAB type M3), comprising 31% of all patients. This risk group had an estimated 5-year survival rate of 73%, and an event-free survival (EFS) rate of 68% for patients treated on the BFM87 regimen.[50] The remainder of the AML patients would comprise the poor-prognosis group. Investigators from the UK Medical Research Council (MRC) combined cytogenetics and response to the first course of chemotherapy and identified three groups: good, comprising those with t(8;21), inv(16), or M3 AML, irrespective of response status or presence of additional abnormalities; standard (neither good or poor); and poor, comprising those with cytogenetic abnormalities other than t(8;21), inv(16), and t(15;17) or normal cytogenetics or resistant disease.[51] The survival rates for these three groups were 70%, 48%, and 15%, respectively, and the relapse rates were 33%, 50%, and 78% (both with $p < 0.0001$). In newer treatment strategies, most adult and pediatric patients with APL are being treated on protocols that use all-*trans*-retinoic acid (ATRA, which is not used in other AML cases), and there is an attempt at reducing therapy for Down syndrome children with AML. The POG conducted a recursive partitioning analysis of prognostic factors in a large cohort with complete cytogenetics and excluding patients with Down syndrome or APL.[15,52] In this comprehensive study of 478 childhood AML cases, once again cytogenetics emerged as the most reliable predictor of outcome. In a multivariate analysis, patients with FAB type M5 had a poorer outcome, while those with inv(16) had the best outcome, followed by t(8;21) and those with normal cytogenetics; the difference between t(8;21) and normal cytogenetic subgroups was not statistically significant. In the partitioning analysis, three groups emerged: female patients with t(8;21), inv(16), or a normal karyotype had the best prognosis (the 4-year EFS rate was 55.1±5.7%); male patients with t(8;21), inv(16), or normal chromosomes had an intermediate prognosis (4-year EFS rate 38.1% ± 5.3%); the third group comprised the remainder (4-year EFS rate 27% ± 3.2%). Only one other pediatric study suggested a better outcome in female patients.[40] Non-Down syndrome FAB type M7 AML patients, relatively rare, seem to have a poor prognosis.[53]

Another cytogenetic feature with prognostic significance is the t(9;11), occurring more frequently in children aged less than 1–2 years.[54] Investigators at St Jude Children's Research Hospital reported that children with AML and a t(9;11), most often associated with FAB type M5 and younger age, had significantly better outcome than other cases with an *MLL* gene rearrangement and than other FAB type M5 cases. In fact, this subgroup had the best overall prognosis compared with all other subgroups of AML.[55] Other groups have also reported that infants with AML have a relatively favorable prognosis.[35,40,56]

In the past few years, another marker, the *FLT3* internal tandem duplication (ITD) has emerged as another important independent prognostic variable.[17–22,57] In a select group of children with AML treated on the Children's Cancer Group (CCG) 2891 study in whom *FLT3* ITD determinations could be done, the results for *FLT3* ITD emerged as the single most important prognostic variable.[21] It should be recognized that not all of the patients included in this evaluation had complete cytogenetic information. On the other hand, the MRC group evaluated the role of *FLT3* ITD patients treated on the MRC AML10 and 12 trials, with a higher proportion with cytogenetic information.[17,20] Both the CCG study and the MRC studies

suggest that *FLT3* ITD may be present in about 20–27% of patients, and are associated with hyperleukocytosis and a high percentage of bone marrow blast cells. Complete remission was lower in patients with *FLT3* ITD, and there was a higher induction death rate in both studies, resulting in adverse EFS and overall survival. The MRC studies also confirmed the findings of the CCG 2891 study and showed that *FLT3* ITD was the most important significant prognostic factor. The MRC studies found no evidence that the relative effect of *FLT3* ITD differed between the cytogenetic risk groups. The conclusion was that the presence of *FLT3* ITD is an additive risk factor.

It is clear from the above that prognosis in AML is determined by biologic markers of blast cells – be they cytogenetics and thereby specific alterations of genes involved in leukemogenesis such as the *CBF* complex, constitutional events such as Down syndrome, or expression of certain myeloid proliferation signaling genes (*FLT3*) (Table 37.1). These observations raise the hope that more rationally designed therapeutic strategies will be developed for each of the AML variants, with their own set of cytogenetic and molecular aberrations. Recent technical advances, such as gene expression profiling and proteomic studies, will be helpful in identifying novel subgroup-specific treatment targets. Such targeted strategies, as opposed to the current practice of a single treatment protocol for the average patient, should pave the way for improved results of all cases of AML.

## Treatment of AML

The modern treatment of AML started with the development of the now classic '3+7' combination of daunorubicin and cytarabine by Yates et al[58,59] and subsequently the concept of intensification of treatment by Weinstein et al.[60] Thereafter, treatment concepts focused on further intensification of either the induc-

### Table 37.1  Prognostic factors in pediatric AML at initial diagnosis

| Factor | Good | Poor |
| --- | --- | --- |
| Age | < 1–2 years | > 10 years |
| Sex | Female | Male |
| White blood cell count | < 100 | > 100 |
| Extramedullary disease | Absent | Present (skin, chloroma) |
| Initial treatment response | CR after first course | No complete response after first course |
| FAB type | M1/2 with Auer rods, M3, M4Eo | M0, M1, M5, M7 (non-Down) |
| Cytogenetics | t(15;17), inv(16), t(8;21), t(9;11), constitutional trisomy 21 | *FLT3* internal tandem duplication, chromosome 5/7 abnormalities, 3q abnormalities, complex karyotype without good-risk cytogenetics |

tion regimen or postremission therapy using high-dose cytarabine, allogeneic bone marrow transplantation (BMT), and autologous BMT in first remission. These strategies have resulted in improved control of AML both in adults and in children, but with the results in pediatric age groups being significantly better than in adults. The major reasons for the better results in children are: (i) general better tolerance of therapy in this age group compared with adults and (ii) a somewhat higher frequency of true de novo AML in children, particularly those with core binding factor leukemias, namely t(8;21) and inv(16).[15,16] It is now possible to achieve remission in 80–90% of children with AML, and the long-term EFS (with remission failures, relapses, and deaths in remissions included) rate varies between 38% and 50%, or even higher.[4,5,35,40,49,50,61–66] Within the last decade, the treatment of children with APL has been virtually identical to that in adults with APL (see Chapter 39). Further, as noted above, Down syndrome children with AML represent a unique subgroup, and the treatment strategies in these children will be described separately below. Regardless, it should be noted that, in general, the treatment of AML is very intensive compared with the therapy used in ALL. The period of myelosuppression is longer and therefore a higher risk for fatal complications from bleeding or infections. The risk for sepsis for α-hemolytic streptococcal infections is high, particularly after the use of high-dose cytarabine,[67] and there is a higher incidence of fungal infection. Thus, referral of these children to specialized treatment centers should be considered if such special support services are not available.

## Remission induction therapy

Daunorubicin for 3 days and cytarabine for 7–10 days is the backbone of therapy in most protocols. In several treatment regimens, a third or fourth drug has been added – thioguanine in POG studies,[62,68] thioguanine, etoposide, and dexamethasone in the DCTER regimen used by the CCG,[64] and etoposide instead of thioguanine in the MRC[5] and BFM[69] trials. Other strategies that have been used to improve outcome are the use of high-dose cytarabine in the POG 9421 protocol,[70] the concept of intensified-timing DCTER by the CCG,[64] the use of mitoxantrone instead of daunorubicin by the French Society of Pediatric Hematology and Immunology (SHIP),[2,66] and idarubicin in place of daunorubicin.[4,71] What are the lessons from these strategies? How can these be applied for development of new therapies? In Table 37.2, we have summarized the results from these various studies in relation to drug dosage for daunorubicin and cytarabine with the first induction course and the duration of exposure to cytarabine. Caution needs to be exercised in the interpretation of the results as summarized in Table 37.2 because of the significant differences among the studies with relation to the eligibility criteria, such as the upper limit of age (e.g. up to age 21 years in the US studies versus up to 15 years in the MRC studies, and 17 years in the BFM group), inclusion or exclusion of secondary AML cases, the ethnicity/race-based heterogeneity of the population served, and the treatment center size. Another variable is the definition of complete remission; for example, the POG 8821 study[35] included patients with so-called M2A marrow (<15% blasts) as well as those with classic M1 marrow (<5% blasts), while the CCG, MRC and BFM studies required M1 marrow and 'normalization' of peripheral blood counts. Despite these limitations, some general conclusions can be drawn from these studies: (1) a total daunorubicin dosage of less than 100 mg/m² as in CCG 2891 standard timing is associated with lower remission rates as well as lower EFS and overall survival; (2) a total dose of cytarabine in excess of

---

**Table 37.2 Dose intensity of daunorubicin/cytarabine induction therapy in pediatric AML and outcome**

| Study | DNR (mg/m²) | Ara-C (mg/m²) | Days of Ara-C | ED (%) | RD (%) | CR (%) | EFS3 (%) | EFS5 (%) | OS3 (%) | OS5 (%) | Ref |
|---|---|---|---|---|---|---|---|---|---|---|---|
| POG 8821 | 135 | 700 | 7 | 4 | 10.9 | 85 | 34±2.5 | | 42±2.6 | | 35 |
| CCG 2891-S | 80 | 800 | 4 | 4 | 26 | 70 | 27±7 | | 39±7 | | 64,65 |
| CCG 2891-I | 160 | 1600 | 8 | 11 | 14 | 75 | 42±7 | | 51±7 | | 64,65 |
| BFM87 | 180 | 1200 | 7 | 9 | 16 | 75 | | 41±3 | | 49±3 | 71 |
| BFM87 | 180 | 1200 | 7 | 7 | | 82 | | 51±2 | | 60±3 | 71 |
| AML10 | 150 | 2000 | 10 | 5 | 5 | 91 | | 49 | | 59 | 5 |
| NOPHO88 | 75 | 1000 | 5 | 11.8 | 3.5 | 84 | | 42 | | | 40 |
| LAME | Mitox 60 mg | 1400 | 7 | 5 | 5 | 90 | | 48 | | 53 | 2 |

DNR, daunorubicin; Ara-C, cytarabine; Mitox, mitoxantrone; ED, early deaths; RD, resistant disease; CR, complete response rate; EFS, event-free survival rates at 3 years (EFS3) and at 5 years (EFS5); OS, overall survival rates at 3 years (OS3) and at 5 years (OS5).

1 g/m$^2$ or a total exposure of 10 days is superior to the standard dose of 100 mg/m$^2$ for 7 days. In fact, with regard to the cytarabine, there appears to be a dose/duration of exposure-dependent effect on EFS. For example, CCG 2891 standard-timing DCTER had only 4 days of exposure to cytarabine with the initial induction course and a 27% EFS rate at 3 years,[64] compared with the 42% 3-year EFS rate in POG 8821, and the 49% EFS rate at 5 years in the MRC AML10 trial,[5] which used 2 g/m$^2$ of cytarabine over 10 days. Daunorubicin administration schedules also differ among the protocols. In the POG 8821 DAT induction regimens, daunorubicin was given on days 1, 2, and 3 as a bolus, while it was given as a continuous infusion in the CCG 2891 regimen, as a 90-minute infusion in two split doses in the BFM regimen,[4,49] and as a 6-hour infusion on days 3, 5, and 7 in the MRC protocols. The known pharmacokinetic properties of daunorubicin and time to intercalation of daunorubicin with DNA suggest that a minimal infusion time of 90 minutes is required for the optimal binding of daunorubicin to DNA.[72] Consistent with this, the results in the BFM87/93 and MRC AML10 studies are superior to those obtained in the POG 8821 study, which used a bolus schedule. The intensive-timing DCTER regimen in part compensated for this by administering two courses of DCTER on days 1 and 10, with a total of 160 mg of daunorubicin and 8 days of cytarabine in the first 2 weeks of therapy.[64,65] Not unexpectedly, as the intensity of the treatment increased, the percentage of children with treatment-related complications increased from a low of 4% in the POG 8821 study to a high of 11% in the intensified-timing DCTER.

Another feature of interest in the induction therapy is the role of a third drug besides the anthracycline and cytarabine. Both the POG and CCG studies included thioguanine, while the CCG, BFM, and MRC groups included etoposide during induction. The exact contribution from the third drug is not clear, although the rationale for the addition of etoposide is its effect on monocytic leukemia.[73,74] In a direct comparison within the MRC AML10 trial, the difference in remission induction rates between the etoposide regimen and the thioguanine regimen was not statistically significant, nor was there any difference in event-free or overall survival, but subgroup analyses (e.g. within monocytic leukemia) were not shown.[5]

The POG 9421 studies tested standard-dose cytarabine 100 mg/m$^2$ × 7 versus 1 g/m$^2$ twice daily for 14 doses for intensification of treatment. In this study, which excluded Down syndrome and APL cases, preliminary results show no appreciable improvement in results based on this induction intensity.[70] This contrasts with the results obtained by increasing the intensity of cytarabine for induction in the adult studies of the Southwest Oncology Group (SWOG) and the Australian investigators.[75,76] One reason for an apparent lack of effect of high-dose cytarabine for induction

in children versus adults is the relatively high remission induction rate with standard-dose cytarabine in children.

Two current trials are exploring the role of idarubicin versus daunorubicin during induction in pediatric AML. Of these, the results of the BFM93 study have been published,[4,71] while those from CCG 2961, in which idarubicin was substituted for daunorubicin in the DCTER regimen, are yet to be published. Idarubicin has the theoretical advantage over daunorubicin of a longer intracellular half-life and greater in vitro cytotoxicity. Further, the metabolite of idarubicin appears to be somewhat less susceptible to multidrug resistance-mediated efflux. In adult trials, there appears to be a slight advantage with idarubicin or daunorubicin.[77,78]

The BFM93 results showed that idarubicin induction led to a significantly better blast cell reduction in the marrow on day 15.[71] Event-free and overall survival in BFM93 were superior to those in BFM87, but the benefit from idarubicin appeared to be restricted to high-risk patients only. The toxicity of the BFM93 regimen, which included idarubicin for induction and high-dose cytarabine and mitoxantrone (IIAM) in consolidation therapy, was somewhat higher compared with the previous BFM87 study. Thus, the results of the CCG 2961 trial are of interest in determining whether any significant improvement can be demonstrated with idarubicin. The SHIP used mitoxantrone in place of daunorubicin in the LAME 89–91 trial, with an 87% remission induction rate and a 48% disease-free survival rate for the chemotherapy group.[2]

# Postremission therapy

The POG, CCG and MRC AML10 trials compared autologous BMT in first remission with intensive chemotherapy. In the POG[35] and CCG trials,[65] no advantage could be shown for autologous BMT, while in the MRC AML10 trial,[5] there was a reduced relapse rate with autologous BMT, but this did not translate into a significant overall benefit. An earlier pediatric Italian study from the pre-high-dose cytarabine era also failed to show any survival benefit with autologous BMT in first remission.[79] These results contrast with those for adults in the European (EORTC) and MRC AML10 trials.[80,81] Both the EORTC and MRC trials showed an advantage for adult AML patients with autologous BMT versus no further therapy. On the other hand, an intergroup adult trial in the USA[82] showed no significant difference in 4-year survival rates among patients randomly assigned to high-dose cytarabine or autologous BMT. The exact reasons for the differences observed in these results are not clear. It is worth comparing the two pediatric US trials and the EORTC and MRC trial. For example, in both of the US pediatric AML studies, randomization occurred immediately after achieving remission and patients assigned to chemotherapy received several additional courses of therapy. In the EORTC and MRC trials, all patients received equal numbers of courses prior to randomization and the comparison was between high-dose chemotherapy plus autologous BMT rescue versus no further therapy in the control group. It can be argued that the advantage seen for autologous BMT in the MRC AML10 and EORTC trials was simply due to an extra course of chemotherapy (preparative regimen), i.e. more therapy is better than less therapy, since a graft-versus-leukemia effect is not expected from autologous marrow infusion. In fact, in gene marking studies, relapse post autologous infusion of marrow in AML has been shown to be due to residual leukemic cells contaminating the harvested marrow.[83]

Thus, what are the important components of the postremission chemotherapy strategy? In brief, most studies have included several courses of high-dose cytarabine, for example a six-dose schedule in the POG 8821 study and an eight-dose timed split-dose schedule in the CCG and Nordic trials.[40,64,84,85] The MRC group included the combination of amsacrine, cytarabine, and etoposide (MACE), mitoxantrone/cytarabine, and cytarabine/L-asparaginase (CLASP). Of these drug combinations, amsacrine is not available in the USA either commercially or as an investigational agent. Mitoxantrone is widely available, and appears to be an effective agent when used in combination with cytarabine or other agents in relapsed pediatric patients.[86,87] The results from the LAME 89/91 studies[2,66] and as well the recent BFM93 trial[4] with the HAM (high-dose cytarabine and mitoxantrone) combination suggest that there may be some benefit from including this combination in the postremission phase of AML.

## Maintenance therapy

The role of maintenance therapy remains controversial. Two studies suggest that maintenance does not result in added benefit after intensive consolidation.[2,88] BFM AML studies continue therapy up to 1 year total.

## CNS-directed therapy

It is of interest that despite a higher incidence of blasts in the cerebrospinal fluid (CSF) at diagnosis in AML than in ALL cases, central nervous system (CNS) relapse as a primary site is less common in AML. Perhaps this is due to the somewhat lower EFS and the early bone marrow relapse in AML compared with ALL. From 5% to 20% of children with AML have been reported to have blasts in the CSF at diagnosis.[5,62,89] The CNS-directed therapy in AML has included four to six intrathecal doses of methotrexate or cytarabine (not concurrent or within 72 hours of systemic high-dose cytarabine) or cranial irradiation.

The US studies used chemotherapeutic agents, whereas the BFM and MRC groups have given cranial irradiation for patients with CNS disease at diagnosis.[5,89] Whether these particular features account for the differences between the BFM and MRC trials versus the US trials is uncertain.

## Treatment for hyperleukocytosis

Abnormal clinical findings related to hyperviscosity from high leukocyte counts are uncommon.[90–2] However, a portion of patients might demonstrate leukostasis in the CNS (Figure 37.2). Radiation has been used on occasion, as well as exchange transfusion or leukopheresis. In general, early institution of induction therapy appears to be the most efficient method of controlling hyperleukocytosis. However, it may be decided to give short-term single-agent low-dose cytarabine in these situations.

## Treatment of CNS extramedullary disease (EMD)

Isolated granulocytic chloromatous presentation is most commonly seen with monocytic leukemia, patients with t(8;21), and those with megakaryocytic leukemia. In general, most chloromatous lesions respond to chemotherapy, and if imaging studies show complete remission of the lesion then there appears to be no benefit from local irradiation. For lesions that cause organ dysfunction, such as compression of the spinal cord or the optic nerve, radiotherapy should be considered. Whether EMD contributes to an adverse prognosis remains controversial. It is of interest that patients with t(8;21) may

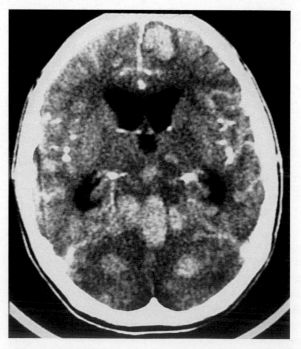

**Figure 37.2** Computed tomography (CT) image of brain in a child with monocytic leukemia, showing infiltrates.

present with chloromatous lesions, a group of patients whose prognosis appears to be the same as those patients with t(8;21) without EMD. A high frequency of chloromatous lesions in t(8;21) has been linked to coexpression of CD56 (neural cell adhesion molecule, NCAM) in this AML variant with good prognosis.[93,94] In the previously cited report from POG,[52] EMD did not add to a risk in either the favorable or the adverse cytogenetics group. A similar conclusion was reached by the Dutch investigators.[95]

## Down syndrome and AML

One of the more remarkable developments in childhood AML in the last decade and a half is the recognition that AML in Down syndrome (DS) is highly curable.[6] In the original publication from the POG investigators, all 12 children with AML and DS survived, compared with an overall survival rate of 33% in non-DS children treated on the same protocol – a striking difference from earlier publications, in which DS children had similar or poorer outcome compared with non-DS children.[96] Since then, the POG, as well as other groups, have shown that over 75% of DS children with AML achieve long-term remission with current therapy.[29,30,32,36–38,40,97,98] This improved outcome in DS children coincided with the inclusion of high-dose cytarabine in the treatment protocols, as children with DS treated on less intensive regimens or given no treatment fared poorly.[32,40] On the other hand, there is some concern that treating DS AML cases on the present AML protocols with further intensification of induction and consolidation may expose these children to excessive toxicity and a high risk of treatment-related death. Hence, sufficient time must be allowed for full recovery of blood counts prior to the initiation of the next course of chemotherapy.[30,97]

AML with DS and core binding factor (CBF) AML cases (inv(16) and t(8;21)) constitute a unique group highly sensitive to high-dose cytarabine-containing regimens. There are several genes on chromosome 21 that alter the sensitivity not only to cytarabine but also to anthracyclines in both a specific and a non-specific manner.[98–100] Increased activity of cystathionine β-synthase (CBS: 21q22.1) has been linked to the low levels of homocysteine, methionine and S-adenosylmethionine and the relative folate deficiency in DS. Further, it has long been proposed that the dysmorphology in DS is primarily from increased activity of CBS. Carbonyl reductase (CBR) is involved in the metabolism of anthracyclines, converting the parent drugs to less potent but longer-lasting alcohol derivatives (e.g. daunorubicinol). The neuronal damage in DS has been linked to increased oxygen radical generation,[101] which may be altered by the chromosome 21-localized gene SOD1 (superoxide dismutase 1).

The relative folate deficiency on account of CBS potentially primes the cells for cytarabine cytotoxicity. The net effect of increased CBS activity is decreased generation of deoxythymidine (dTTP): low dTTP results in feedback inhibition of deoxycytidine deaminase; therefore the levels of dCMP and dCTP will decrease, while deoxycytidine kinase (dCK) activity is upregulated because of low dCMP. In this setting, administration of cytarabine would result in a net increase in the generation of cytarabine triphosphate (Ara-CTP) and there is less competition from dCTP for binding to DNA and RNA polymerase.[98] In studies by the Wayne State group, DS AML cells have low endogenous dCTP and are significantly more sensitive to Ara-C in in vitro MTT assays;[99] there was a positive correlation of Ara-CTP values with CBS transcript levels (which were increased up to tenfold), and the $IC_{50}$ values, as expected, had an inverse relationship with the CBS expression level.[102]

In addition to this unique endogenous modulation of cytarabine metabolism, DS AML cells are also unusually sensitive to daunorubicin and other drugs.[100,103–105] These observations suggest that while there is a specific endogenous modulation of cytarabine metabolism in DS, the DS cells may be primed to undergo drug-induced apoptosis, presumably due to the well-known increased generation of oxygen radicals in DS cells.[97,101,106]

## Treatment of relapsed AML

The incidence of relapsed AML has significantly decreased recently, with more effective upfront therapy. However, relapses still occur in at least 30–40% of patients. This implies a rough incidence of 2–3 cases of relapsed AML in 1 million children annually.

The literature on systematic studies of the treatment of relatively unselected groups of children with relapsed AML is limited. There is general agreement, however, that without high-dose chemotherapy and allogeneic BMT few relapsed children will be cured. Table 37.3 summarizes the results of several larger studies on pediatric relapsed AML. An older paper reported a probability of 6 years' survival after a bone marrow relapse of only 4%, and a median survival of less than 6 months.[107] The results of some recent studies are summarized below. Wells et al[86] reported preliminary data of a group of 37 evaluable patients with relapsed or refractory AML. CR was achieved in 73% of patients, with a 2-year DFS of 41%. Leahey et al[108] reported a CR rate of 66% in 15 children with refractory or recurrent AML, using idarubicin with continuous-infusion fludarabine and cytarabine. Dahl et al[87] reported a 35% CR rate in 66 children with refractory or recurrent AML using mitoxantrone, etoposide, and cyclosporine for reversal of increased drug efflux via MDR1 (see below). Stahnke et al[109] report the most

**Table 37.3  Clinical studies including longer follow-up in pediatric relapsed AML**

| Ref | No. of Patients | CR (%) | Long-term outcome |
| --- | --- | --- | --- |
| 86 | 37 | 73 | pDFS (2-yr) 0.41 |
| 110 | 125 | 69 | pDFS (3-yr) 0.44 |
| | | | pOS (3-yr) 0.24 |
| 111 | 23 | 74 | 9 out of 17 DFS |
| | | | 9 out of 23 OS |
| 112 | 48 | – | pDFS (7-yr) 0.42 from autologous SCT |
| 109 | 102 | 51 | pOS (5-yr) 0.21 |

CR, complete response rate; pDFS, probability of disease-free survival; pOS, probability of overall survival; SCT, stem cell transplantation.

recent experiences of the BFM AML group. In about two-thirds of children with first-relapsed AML, intensive reinduction was applied, consisting of mitoxantrone, etoposide, and high-dose cytarabine in most patients. The overall CR rate was 51%. The 5-year probability of survival from relapse was 21%±5%. Children with an early relapse, defined as occurring within 1.5 years from diagnosis, did significantly worse than children with a late relapse, with probabilities of 5-year survival from relapse of 10% and 40%, respectively. In fact, time until relapse was the only significant prognostic factor. None of the patients who did not achieve second CR after reinduction chemotherapy survived, irrespective of further treatment. Post-reinduction therapy consisted of allogeneic and autologous stem cell transplantation, but 12 patients received chemotherapy only, and 5 of these were reported to be alive. The MRC group reported their experiences recently in patients who relapsed after initial treatment on the AML10 trial.[110] Results in relapsed patients were not the result of a formal treatment protocol, and in about one-third of cases further treatment was withheld. With different types of reinduction chemotherapy, the overall complete remission rate was 69%. The majority of patients (about two-thirds) achieving a second CR later received a stem cell transplant, including autografts and matched unrelated and matched family donor allografts. Overall (including patients not further treated), the probability of survival at 3 years was 24%, and the probability of disease-free survival at 3 years from second CR was 44%. As in ALL, the length of first CR was the most significant predictor of outcome. If it was less than 1 year then the CR rate was 36% and the probability of 3-year survival 11%, compared with 75% and 49%, respectively, for patients who relapsed at least 1 year after achieving a first CR. Ida-FLAG (idarubicin with fludarabine, cytosine, and G-CSF) is another regimen that has been tried. In one study, Ida-FLAG was given to 23 patients, with a CR rate of 74%. A total of 9 patients were in continuous CR for 10–39 months (median 18 months), i.e. 40% of the total group.[111] Although not the subject of the study, Ida-FLAG was more myelotoxic than FLAG. Vignetti et al[112] reported that autologous BMT in 48 children in second CR resulted in an EFS rate of 42% at 7 years from diagnosis, with equal results in case of conditioning regimens with and without total body irradiation. Although this obviously concerns a selected group of patients who remained long enough in continuous CR, this series again illustrates that long-term survival in relapsed AML can be achieved in some patients without allogeneic stem cell transplantation. However, it should be recognized that most relapsed patients are already heavily pretreated, the options for reinduction therapy are limited by the degree of prior exposure to anthracylines, and organ function may be significantly compromised. Thus, the question should be raised as to whether a child with relapsed AML should be offered intensive treatment with curative intent. For children with a late-relapsed AML, occurring at least 1 year from diagnosis, the answer will normally be yes in view of the a priori chance of 50% for long-term survival. However, for children with early-relapsed AML, this chance is about 10%, and for these patients the individual situation will have a greater impact. The wish of the child and parents, the previously experienced side-effects, and perhaps remaining late effects, and other information unique to that patient should be taking into account. One may argue that if the condition of the patient allows it, an attempt at reinduction chemotherapy should be made in all patients. If the first course of intensive chemotherapy does not give a major response, arbitrarily defined as less than 20% leukemic cells in the bone marrow 4–6 weeks after the start of chemotherapy, it can always be decided at that time that further treatment is not indicated because of the very low chance of cure in this subset is patients.

# Clinical relevance of cellular drug resistance testing

Cellular drug resistance is one of the main determinants of the success of chemotherapy, together with pharmacokinetics and the kinetics of minimal residual disease and its potential to relapse. Drug resistance itself is determined by a number of factors, including pharmacodynamics and pharmacogenomics, and the intrinsic properties of leukemic cells. Cellular drug resistance can be measured by several techniques. In the past, clonogenic assays were mostly used, with the assumption that measuring effects of anticancer agents on the clonogenic cells was of utmost importance. Total cell kill and apoptosis assays are now being used more frequently. Here, the results of both types of assays will be summarized, without any explicit statement regarding the value of one or the other. In general, cellular drug resistance testing does seem to provide clinically relevant information, and should ideally be included as add-on study in clinical trials.

## Relation to cell biological features: FAB type, Down syndrome, and cytogenetics

In two publications, the group from Amsterdam reported on a comparison between pediatric ALL and AML samples obtained at initial diagnosis.[103,113] In the largest series, it appeared that AML samples were significantly more resistant in vitro to several drugs, including glucocorticoids, vincristine, L-asparaginase, anthracyclines, etoposide, and other drugs. For some drugs, especially cytarabine and thiopurines, AML and ALL samples were similarly sensitive. The only drug that was more cytotoxic towards AML cells was 2-chlorodeoxyadenosine (cladribine), and this was largely due to its increased activity towards FAB type M5 samples.[103] For methotrexate, AML cells were significantly more resistant upon short-term exposure, but this difference disappeared upon long-term (21 hours) exposure to methotrexate.[114] FAB type M5 samples displayed a remarkably sensitive profile, with increased sensitivity to most drugs as compared with non-M5 samples.[103] These drugs included cytarabine, etoposide, and anthracyclines. However, FAB type M5 samples were also more sensitive to the more typical ALL drugs vincristine, L-asparaginase, and methotrexate, and this sensitivity was in the same range as that of ALL samples.[103,114] The favorable prognosis of AML in children with Down syndrome could be explained by a remarkably increased sensitivity of the AML cells to several drugs, including cytarabine and daunorubicin, as first reported by the Detroit group.[100] However, also for other drugs, AML cells of these patients appeared to be more sensitive, at least in vitro.[115] These drugs included vincristine, etoposide, and thiopurines, which confirmed the data of a

small pilot study by a Scandinavian group.[105] More recently, it was reported that leukemia-specific cytogenetic abnormalities also correlated with cellular drug resistance.[104] Especially, samples with abnormalities (monosomy or deletions) of chromosome 5 or 7 demonstrate a significantly increased resistance to cytarabine (borderline to daunorubicin), while samples with the t(9;11) showed a remarkable sensitive profile, with significantly increased sensitivity to most drugs tested, including etoposide, daunorubicin, and amsacrine.

## Resistance mechanisms for anthracyclines

Active outward transport of anthracyclines as a mechanism of resistance was recognized in the early 1970s.[116] Subsequent work[117] linked this anthracycline efflux with the expression of a 170 kDa glycoprotein (P-gp), the product of the *MDR1* gene, now localized to chromosome 7q21.1. Since then other members of the same ABC (ATP-binding cassette) transporter family have been discovered, including the multidrug resistance-related protein (MRP1)[118] and the breast cancer resistance protein (BCRP, chromosome 4q22).[119] In addition, a non-ABC family protein has been found to be associated with multidrug resistance: the lung resistance-related protein (LRP), also known as the major vault protein (MVP).[120] P-gp, MRP1, and BCRP are expressed at the cell surface, while LRP/MVP is predominantly cytosolic.

With regard to childhood AML, few studies have prospectively compared the relevance of expression of these drug-resistance proteins to outcome. Preliminary results of the studies that have been completed to date show that P-gp expression in the pediatric age group is lower than what has been encountered in adult studies. It appears that P-gp expression in diagnostic blast cell samples increases with age. Thus, in pediatric patients, P-gp expression is detectable in about 15–17% of cases of de novo AML,[121–123] consistent with values in adults aged 20–35 years, compared with 27% for those between the ages of 35 and 49, 39% for those 50–65, and up to 70% in those aged over 65 years.[124,125] Since P-gp expression can be induced by exposure to xenobiotics, including anthracyclines, as well as certain natural products such as grapefruit juice,[126,127] it is conceivable that with age, there is a non-specific induction of P-gp in certain individuals. These data suggest that the level of P-gp expression may not be intrinsic to the leukemic cells (i.e. it might reflect the P-gp status in the somatic environment as a whole) and may not always be linked to a specific leukemic cytogenetic event. This is further illustrated by observations in AML with monosomy 7/7q–, which is associated with poor prognosis, and the contrasting superior outcome in AML with inv(16). Van den Heuvel-Eberink et al[128] found no evidence for decreased expression or activity of *MDR1* in monosomy 7/7q– cases, contrary to what one may have expected from the localization of *MDR1* on 7q. A similar lack of loss of function of MRP in *MRP1*-deleted inv(16) cases (*MRP* and *LRP/MVP* are localized to 16p31–32) has also been demonstrated,[129] suggesting that the good prognosis of inv(16) may not be linked to decreased anthracycline efflux as originally proposed.[130] Van den Heuvel-Eberink et al[131] also looked critically at P-gp expression in paired samples in the same patients from diagnosis and relapse, and found no evidence of increased expression/efflux or evidence for *MDR1* gene-related clonal selection at relapse.

Of considerable importance is the concept that *MDR1* expression in AML may not necessarily have a negative implication. For example, *MDR1*-overexpressing cells exhibit increased collateral sensitivity to nucleoside analogs.[132,133] Supporting this finding are the clinical observations that *MDR1* is overexpressed in AML1 with t(8;21)[134] and in AML blasts from Down syndrome patients.[97] Both AML with t(8;21)[93] and AML in Down syndrome[6,93] are highly sensitive to high-dose cytarabine containing regimens and are associated with a superior outcome.

It is not surprising from the foregoing discussion that studies with the drug-reversal agents cyclosporine and PSC833 for improving treatment response and long-term outcome have produced mixed results.[87,135,136] In the SWOG 9126 trial, higher doses of cyclosporine (16 mg/kg/day), yielding a mean blood concentration exceeding 1600 ng/ml (a dose sufficient for modulation of P-gp-mediated efflux) produced a decrease in induction resistance and possibly increased relapse-free and overall survival.[135] Cyclosporine-treated patients had higher mean values for daunorubicin concentration, but response rates were different in patients with comparable daunorubicin concentrations whether or not they had received cyclosporine. These data would suggest that the cyclosporine may have a non-Pgp-linked beneficial effect on the response rate by increasing the cytotoxicity of daunorubicin.

A preliminary review of the large prospective randomized trial of cyclosporine during consolidation by the POG (9421) also demonstrated a probable nonspecific benefit from this agent.[70] In the POG 9421 study, the patients were randomized to receive standard-dose cytarabine during induction versus high-dose cytarabine during induction and post remission; both groups were randomized to receive drug combinations with or without cyclosporine. The control arm with standard '3+7' daunorubicin and cytarabine and no cyclosporine had an inexplicably low remission induction rate. Nonetheless, a positive effect was noted when the two cyclosporine arms were compared with those not receiving this agent. Correlations

with P-gp expression are not yet available from this study, but the low expression of P-gp in pediatric patients suggests that any benefit may not all be P-gp-linked. Cyclosporine can also block MRP- and BCRP-related drug efflux in a dose-dependent fashion. As suggested by List et al,[135] it is possible that some of the benefit is through the total blockade of efflux rather than the one mediated by P-gp alone. Alternatively, through its interaction with cyclophilin, cyclosporine may suppress angiogenic responses to vascular endothelial growth factor (VEGF), a cytokine that is implicated in myeloblast cell renewal and that confers an adverse prognosis in AML. Another possibility is that cyclosporine may potentiate the cytotoxicity of several drugs through augmentation of ceramide-mediated apoptosis, by inhibiting glycosylation of ceramide via the glucoceramide synthase pathway.[137] Several MDR-reversal agents appear to inhibit glucoceramide synthase, suggesting that their clinical effect may be partly related to this mechanism.

## Drug resistance as a prognostic factor

There is relatively little data on the prognostic significance of in vitro cellular drug resistance in childhood AML. However, the studies that have been reported all strongly suggest a correlation between increased resistance of AML cells and a worse initial treatment response, as reviewed by Kaspers et al.[138] Data on the prediction of long-term clinical outcome, which was reported to be feasible in childhood ALL,[138a,139] are less convincing in AML.[104,140] Apparently, the AML cells responsible for a relapse are not always being tested appropriately by the current cellular drug resistance assays. Several studies have addressed the issue of differences in drug resistance profiles between untreated and relapsed AML samples of children. Hongo et al[141] reported that within the FAB type M4 and M5 groups, relapsed samples were more resistant to cytarabine and also to etoposide. Similarly, Klumper et al[142] reported a threefold increased resistance to cytarabine, but not to etoposide, in relapsed AML samples. Of potential interest, the group in Amsterdam have reported that although relapsed AML samples were more resistant to cytarabine, this was not seen for cladribine.[143] This was mainly explained by an increased antileukemic activity of cladribine in FAB type M5 samples, which is in agreement with data from clinical studies performed at St Jude's Children Research Hospital.[144]

In conclusion, cellular drug resistance may be helpful in identifying novel agents as good AML agents, and may especially identify subgroups of AML patients that are more or less sensitive to certain drugs. Using these data enables a more rational design of subgroup-directed tailored treatment. This does, however, require a major change in the design of future treatment protocols. Instead of distinguishing two or three subgroups, treatment will become much more individualized, based on information from pharmacogenomic, oncogenomic, and cellular drug resistance studies, and on the measurement of minimal residual disease as the ultimate test of response. To move from giving the average treatment to the average patient towards individualized treatment will be one of the biggest challenges in the coming few years.

## Future directions

Numerous developments suggest that the study and treatment of pediatric AML will change in the future. Some interesting areas are briefly discussed below.

### Genomics

In order to unravel the etiology of leukemia, and to identify novel drug targets, further studies on the molecular characterization of leukemic (and normal) cells are of the utmost importance.[145] Recent developments such as high-throughput gene expression profiling and proteomic studies will be helpful in this respect – but not sufficient. Functional studies will remain necessary. In the same area of oncogenomics, pharmacogenomic studies will be helpful in individualizing drug treatment, taking more account of the unique characteristics of the host.

### New drugs

New drugs may be old drugs in a new coat, or real novel agents. An example of an old drug in a relatively new formula is liposomal daunorubicin (DaunoXome). This agent has mainly been used to treat Kaposi sarcoma. Out of 979 Kaposi sarcoma patients treated with DaunoXome, 1 patient developed cardiotoxicity with clinical symptoms (Summary of Product Characteristics, Gilead Sciences, 5 June 2001). In general, liposomal anthracyclines cause less cardiotoxicity at higher cumulative doses than conventional anthracyclines.[146] Animal solid tumor studies showed that at equivalent daunorubicin dosages, DaunoXome had significantly increased antitumor activity and less toxicity compared with free daunorubicin.[147] Another drug that is clinically available but is not being used often is cladribine. Both preclinical and clinical studies suggest that this agent has marked antileukemic activity in acute monoblastic leukemia.[103,143,144] A study performed in 17 relapsed AML patients demonstrated that single agent cladribine induced complete hematologic remissions in 47% of them.[148]

Perhaps even more exciting are the vast number of truly novel drugs that are emerging.[149] Targeted agents mediated by or consisting of monoclonal antibodies (e.g. anti-CD33 linked to calicheamicin (gemtuzumab ozogamicin, Mylotarg®) and anti-CD20 (rituximab®)) or drugs directly targeted at leukemia-specific targets such as gene fusion proteins (e.g. imatinib (STI571, Gleevec/Glivec®)) or mutated tyrosine kinases (e.g. drugs targeted at FLT3, c-KIT, or VEGF) are promising agents with at least theoretically major selectivity towards the leukemic cells. The latter aspect is important in order to minimize side-effects in the short and long term. Other new types of drugs include farnesyl transferase inhibitors, histone deacetylase inhibitors, and proteasome inhibitors. Future clinical studies will have to teach us how to use these agents, on their own and, more importantly, in combination chemotherapy. The pressure on pharmaceutical companies to study their novel agents in the pediatric population will be helpful in this respect. All these developments will have the consequence, however, that our approach will have to change from giving the average treatment to the average patient towards a much more individualized approach taking into account the uniqueness of each leukemia and each patient. We will have to adjust the design of our randomized clinical studies in order to accomplish this, which will be a major but necessary challenge.

### Minimal residual disease (MRD)

Data from measurements of minimal residual disease in ALL and in subgroups of AML have clearly demonstrated the prognostic significance of this information.[150–152] For the majority of patients with AML, however, molecular biological studies are not applicable to measure minimal residual disease. Flow-cytometric identification of so-called leukemia-aberrant phenotypes is a good, perhaps cheaper, and certainly less labor-intensive alternative, and will be applicable in more than 90% of patients with AML to monitor minimal residual disease. The main question that should be addressed, however, is whether the sensitivity of this method will be high enough to detect low numbers of minimal residual disease. At least in ALL, most studies suggest that it is important to detect low levels of minimal residual disease (e.g. less than 1 in 10 000 cells) to identify good-risk patients.[152] It seems likely that monitoring minimal residual disease in AML will become routine at some point, which will allow us to identify patients at low or high risk for a subsequent relapse and to adjust treatment. Another theoretical application is to quantify minimal residual disease for comparing the antileukemic effect of two or more different treatment regimens in patients in 'complete remission'.

## Conclusions

In conclusion, with the use of intensive chemotherapy regimens that combine currently available drugs, and with improved supportive care, the prognosis for

AML in children and adolescents has improved considerably. Survival rates above 50% have been reported recently by several groups. The awareness of the uniqueness of each individual and his or her AML, together with significant technical improvements in genomic studies and drug development, raise justified hope that this prognosis can improve further. Other innovative research, such as studies on cellular drug resistance, apoptosis and cell death regulators, and minimal residual disease monitoring, will stimulate and support this expected rise in the number of children and adolescents who will be cured of their AML in the near future.

## REFERENCES

1. Greenlee RT, Hill-Harmon MB, Murray T. Cancer statistics, 2001. *CA CancerJ Clin* 2001; **51**: 15–36.
2. Perel Y, Auvrignon A, Leblanc T. Impact of addition of maintenance therapy to intensive induction and consolidation chemotherapy for childhood acute myeloblastic leukemia: results of a prospective randomized trial, LAME 89/91. *J Clin Oncol* 2002; **20**: 2774–82.
3. Behar C, Suciu S, Benoit Y. Mitoxantrone-containing regimen for treatment of childhood acute leukemia (AML) and analysis of prognostic factors: results of the EORTC Children Leukemia Cooperative Study 58872. *Med Pediatr Oncol* 1996; **26**: 173–9.
4. Creutzig U, Berthold F, Boos J. Improved treatment results in high-risk pediatric acute myeloid leukemia patients after intensification with high-dose cytarabine and mitoxantrone: results of study Acute Myeloid Leukemia–Berlin–Frankfurt–Munster 93. *J Clin Oncol* 2001; **19**: 2705–13.
5. Stevens RF, Hann IM, Wheatley K. Marked improvements in outcome with chemotherapy alone in paediatric acute myeloid leukemia: results of the United Kingdom Medical Research Council's 10th AML trial. MRC Childhood Leukaemia Working Party. *Br J Haematol* 1998; **101**: 130–40.
6. Ravindranath Y, Abella E, Krischer JP. Acute myeloid leukemia (AML) in Down's syndrome is highly responsive to chemotherapy: experience on Pediatric Oncology Group AML Study 8498. *Blood*, 1992; **80**: 2210–14.
7. Bloomfield CD. Prognostic factors for selecting curative therapy for adult acute myeloid leukemia. *Leukemia* 1992; **6**(Suppl 4): 65–7.
8. Bloomfield CD, Lawrence D, Byrd JC. Frequency of prolonged remission duration after high-dose cytarabine intensification in acute myeloid leukemia varies by cytogenetic subtype. *Cancer Res* 1998; **58**: 4173–9.
9. Löwenberg B, Downing JR, Burnett A. Acute myeloid leukemia. *N Engl J Med* 1999; **341**: 1051–62.
10. Degos L. Differentiating agents in the treatment of leukemia. *Leuk Res* 1990; **14**: 717–19.
11. Degos L, Wang ZY. All *trans* retinoic acid in acute promyelocytic leukemia. *Oncogene* 2001; **20**: 7140–5.
12. Tallman MS, Nabhan C, Feusner JH. Acute promyelocytic leukemia: evolving therapeutic strategies. *Blood* 2002; **99**: 759–67.
13. Warrell RP Jr, de The H, Wang ZY. Acute promyelocytic leukemia. *N Engl J Med* 1993; **329**: 177–89.
14. Smith MG, Gurney JG, Ross JA. *Cancer Incidence and Survival among Children and Adolescents: United States SEER Program 1975–1995*. Bethesda, MD: Cancer Statistics Branch, NCI.
15. Raimondi SC, Chang MN, Ravindranath Y. Chromosomal abnormalities in 478 children with acute myeloid leukemia: clinical characteristics and treatment outcome in a cooperative Pediatric Oncology Group study – POG 8821. *Blood* 1999; **94**: 3707–16.
16. Grimwade D, Walker H, Oliver F. The importance of diagnostic cytogenetics on outcome in AML: analysis of 1,612 patients entered into the MRC AML 10 trial. The Medical Research Council Adult and Children's Leukaemia Working Parties. *Blood* 1998; **92**: 2322–33.
17. Abu-Duhier FM, Goodeve AC, Wilson GA. FLT3 internal tandem duplication mutations in adult acute myeloid leukaemia define a high-risk group. *Br J Haematol* 2000; **111**: 190–5.
18. Iwai T, Yokota S, Nakao M. Internal tandem duplication of the *FLT3* gene and clinical evaluation in childhood acute myeloid leukemia. The Children's Cancer and Leukemia Study Group, Japan. *Leukemia* 1999; **13**: 38–43.
19. Kondo M, Horibe K, Takahashi Y. Prognostic value of internal tandem duplication of the *FLT3* gene in childhood acute myelogenous leukemia. *Med Pediatr Oncol* 1999; **33**: 525–9.
20. Kottaridis PD, Gale RE, Frew ME. The presence of a FLT3 internal tandem duplication in patients with acute myeloid leukemia (AML) adds important prognostic information to cytogenetic risk group and response to the first cycle of chemotherapy: analysis of 854 patients from the United Kingdom Medical Research Council AML 10 and 12 trials. *Blood* 2001; **98**: 1752–9.
21. Meshinchi S, Woods WG, Stirewalt DL. Prevalence and prognostic significance of *Flt3* internal tandem duplication in pediatric acute myeloid leukemia. *Blood* 2001; **97**: 89–94.
22. Xu F, Taki T, Yang HW. Tandem duplication of the *FLT3* gene is found in acute lymphoblastic leukaemia as well as acute myeloid leukaemia but not in myelodysplastic syndrome or juvenile chronic myelogenous leukaemia in children. *Br J Haematol* 1999; **105**: 155–62.
23. Head DR. Revised classification of acute myeloid leukemia. *Leukemia* 1996; **10**: 1826–31.
24. Head DR. Proposed changes in the definitions of acute myeloid leukemia and myelodysplastic syndrome: Are they helpful? *Curr Opin Oncol* 2002; **14**: 19–23.
25. Bennett JM. World Health Organization classification of the acute leukemias and myelodysplastic syndrome. *Int J Hematol* 2000; **72**: 131–3.
26. Jaffe ES, Harris NL, Stein H et al (eds). *World Health Organization Classification of Tumours. Pathology and Genetics of Tumours of Haematopoietic and Lymphoid Tissues.* Lyon: IARC Press, 2001: Chap 4.
27. Pui CH, Rivera G, Mirro J. Acute megakaryoblastic leukemia. Blast cell aggregates simulating metastatic tumor. *Arch Pathol Lab Med* 1985; **109**: 1033–5.

28. Zipursky A, Poon A, Doyle J. Leukemia in Down syndrome: a review. *Pediatr Hematol Oncol* 1992; **9**: 139–49.

29. Lange BJ, Kobrinsky N, Barnard DR. Distinctive demography, biology, and outcome of acute myeloid leukemia and myelodysplastic syndrome in children with Down syndrome: Children's Cancer Group Studies 2861 and 2891. *Blood* 1998; **91**: 608–15.

30. Lange B. The management of neoplastic disorders of haematopoiesis in children with Down's syndrome. *Br J Haematol* 2000; **110**: 512–24.

31. Lion T, Haas OA, Harbott J. The translocation t(1;22)(p13;q13) is a nonrandom marker specifically associated with acute megakaryocytic leukemia in young children. *Blood* 1992; **79**: 3325–30.

32. Creutzig U, Ritter J, Vormoor J. Myelodysplasia and acute myelogenous leukemia in Down's syndrome. A report of 40 children of the AML-BFM Study Group. *Leukemia* 1996; **10**: 1677–86.

33. Zipursky A, Thorner P, De Harven E. Myelodysplasia and acute megakaryoblastic leukemia in Down's syndrome. *Leuk Res* 1994; **18**: 163–71.

34. Zipursky A, Brown E, Christensen H. Leukemia and/or myeloproliferative syndrome in neonates with Down syndrome. *Semin Perinatol* 1997; **21**: 97–101.

35. Ravindranath Y, Yeager AM, Chang MN. Autologous bone marrow transplantation versus intensive consolidation chemotherapy for acute myeloid leukemia in childhood. Pediatric Oncology Group. *N Engl J Med* 1996; **334**: 1428–34.

36. Slordahl SH, Smeland EB, Holte H et al. Leukemic blasts with markers of four cell lineages in Down's syndrome ('megakaryoblastic leukemia'). *Med Pediatr Oncol* 1993; **21**: 254–8.

37. Craze JL, Harrison G, Wheatley K et al. Improved outcome of acute myeloid leukaemia in Down's syndrome. *Arch Dis Child* 1999; **81**: 32–7.

38. Kojima S, Kato K, Matsuyama T et al. Favorable treatment outcome in children with acute myeloid leukemia and Down syndrome. *Blood* 1993; **81**: 3164.

39. Lie SO. Acute myelogenous leukaemia in children. *Eur J Pediatr* 1989; **148**: 382–8.

40. Lie SO, Jonmundsson G, Mellander L et al. A population-based study of 272 children with acute myeloid leukaemia treated on two consecutive protocols with different intensity: best outcome in girls, infants, and children with Down's syndrome. Nordic Society of Paediatric Haematology and Oncology (NOPHO). *Br J Haematol* 1996; **94**: 82–8.

41. Freedman MH, Alter BP. Risk of myelodysplastic syndrome and acute myeloid leukemia in congenital neutropenias. *Semin Hematol* 2002; **39**: 128–33.

42. Freedman MH, Bonilla MA, Fier C et al. Myelodysplasia syndrome and acute myeloid leukemia in patients with congenital neutropenia receiving G-CSF therapy. *Blood* 2000; **96**: 429–36.

43. Alter BP, Caruso JP, Drachtman RA et al. Fanconi anemia: myelodysplasia as a predictor of outcome. *Cancer Genet Cytogenet* 2000; **117**: 125–31.

44. Felix CA. Secondary leukemias induced by topoisomerase-targeted drugs. *Biochim Biophys Acta* 1998; **1400**: 233–55.

45. Pui CH, Relling MV, Rivera GK et al. Epipodophyllotoxin-related acute myeloid leukemia: a study of 35 cases. *Leukemia* 1995; **9**: 1990–6.

46. Winick NJ, McKenna RW, Shuster JJ et al. Secondary acute myeloid leukemia in children with acute lymphoblastic leukemia treated with etoposide. *J Clin Oncol* 1993; **11**: 209–17.

47. Ross JA, Potter JD, Reaman GH et al. Maternal exposure to potential inhibitors of DNA topoisomerase II and infant leukemia (United States): a report from the Children's Cancer Group. *Cancer Causes Control* 1996; **7**: 581–90.

48. Kalwinsky DK, Mirro J Jr, Dahl GV. Biology and therapy of childhood acute nonlymphocytic leukemia. *Pediatr Ann* 1988; **17**: 172–6, 179–90.

49. Creutzig U, Ritter J, Schellong G. Identification of two risk groups in childhood acute myelogenous leukemia after therapy intensification in study AML-BFM-83 as compared with study AML-BFM-78. AML-BFM Study Group. *Blood* 1990; **75**: 1932–40.

50. Creutzig U, Zimmermann M, Ritter J et al. Definition of a standard-risk group in children with AML. *Br J Haematol* 1999; **104**: 630–9.

51. Wheatley K, Burnett AK, Goldstone AH et al. A simple, robust, validated and highly predictive index for the determination of risk-directed therapy in acute myeloid leukaemia derived from the MRC AML10 trial. United Kingdom Medical Research Council's Adult and Childhood Leukaemia Working Parties. *Br J Haematol* 1999; **107**: 69–79.

52. Chang M, Raimondi SC, Ravindranath Y et al. Prognostic factors in children and adolescents with acute myeloid leukemia (excluding children with Down syndrome and acute promyelocytic leukemia): univariate and recursive partitioning analysis of patients treated on Pediatric Oncology Group (POG) Study 8821. *Leukemia* 2000; **14**: 1201–7.

53. Athale UH, Razzouk BI, Raimondi SC et al. Biology and outcome of childhood acute megakaryoblastic leukemia: a single institution's experience. *Blood* 2001; **97**: 3727–32.

54. Pui CH, Raimondi SC, Srivastava DK et al. Prognostic factors in infants with acute myeloid leukemia. *Leukemia* 2000; **14**: 684–7.

55. Rubnitz JE, Raimondi SC, Tong X et al. Favorable impact of the t(9;11) in childhood acute myeloid leukemia. *J Clin Oncol* 2002; **20**: 2302–9.

56. Kawasaki H, Isoyama K, Eguchi M et al. Superior outcome of infant acute myeloid leukemia with intensive chemotherapy: results of the Japan Infant Leukemia Study Group. *Blood* 2001; **98**: 3589–94.

57. Kiyoi H, Naoe T, Nakano Y et al. Prognostic implication of *FLT3* and N-*RAS* gene mutations in acute myeloid leukemia. *Blood* 1999; **93**: 3074–80.

58. Yates JW, Wallace HJ, Ellison RR et al. Cytosine arabinoside (NSC-63878) and daunorubicin (NSC-83142) therapy in acute nonlymphocytic leukemia. *Cancer Chemother Rep* 1973; **57**: 485–8.

59. Yates J, Glidewell O, Wiernik P et al. Cytosine arabinoside with daunorubicin or Adriamycin for therapy of acute myelocytic leukemia: a CALGB study. *Blood* 1982; **60**: 454–62.

60. Weinstein HJ, Mayer RJ, Rosenthal DS et al. Treatment of acute myelogenous leukemia in children and adults. *N Engl J Med* 1980; **303**: 473–8.

61. Ritter J, Creutzig U, Schellong G. Treatment results of three consecutive German childhood AML trials: BFM-78, -83, and -87. AML-BFM-Group. *Leukemia* 1992; **6**(Suppl 2): 59–62.

62. Ravindranath Y, Steuber CP, Krischer J et al. High-dose cytarabine for intensification of early therapy of childhood acute myeloid leukemia: a Pediatric Oncology Group study. *J Clin Oncol* 1991; **9**: 572–80.

63. Hann IM, Stevens RF, Goldstone AH et al. Randomized comparison of DAT versus ADE as induction chemotherapy in children and younger adults with acute myeloid leukemia. Results of the Medical Research Council's 10th AML trial (MRC AML10). Adult and Childhood Leukaemia Working Parties of the Medical Research Council. *Blood* 1997; **89**: 2311–18.

64. Woods WG, Kobrinsky N, Buckley JD et al. Timed-sequential induction therapy improves postremission outcome in acute myeloid leukemia: a report from the Children's Cancer Group. *Blood* 1996; **87**: 4979–89.

65. Woods WG, Neudorf S, Gold S et al. A comparison of allogeneic bone marrow transplantation, autologous bone marrow transplantation, and aggressive chemotherapy in children with acute myeloid leukemia in remission. *Blood* 2001; **97**: 56–62.

66. Michel G, Baruchel A, Tabone MD et al. Induction chemotherapy followed by allogeneic bone marrow transplantation or aggressive consolidation chemotherapy in childhood acute myeloblastic leukemia. A prospective study from the French Society of Pediatric Hematology and Immunology (SHIP). *Hematol Cell Ther* 1996; **38**: 169–76.

67. Gamis AS, Howells WB, DeSwarte-Wallace J et al. Alpha hemolytic streptococcal infection during intensive treatment for acute myeloid leukemia: a report from the Children's Cancer Group study CCG-2891. *J Clin Oncol* 2000; **18**: 1845–55.

68. Steuber CP, Culbert SJ, Ravindranath Y et al. Therapy of childhood acute nonlymphocytic leukemia: the Pediatric Oncology Group experience (1977–1988). *Hamatol Bluttransfus* 1990; **33**: 198–209.

69. Creutzig U, Ritter J, Riehm H et al. The childhood AML studies BFM-78 and -83: treatment results and risk factor analysis. *Hamatol Bluttransfus* 1987; **30**: 71–5.

70. Becton D, Dahl GV, Berkow RL et al. A phase III study of intensive cytarabine (Ara-C) induction followed by cyclosporine (CSA) modulation of drug resistance in de novo pediatric AML: POG 9421. *Blood* 2001; 311a.

71. Creutzig U, Ritter J, Zimmermann M et al. Idarubicin improves blast cell clearance during induction therapy in children with AML: results of study AML-BFM 93. AML-BFM Study Group. *Leukemia* 2001; **15**: 348–54.

72. Gieseler F, Nussler V, Brieden T et al. Intracellular pharmacokinetics of anthracyclines in human leukemia cells: correlation of DNA-binding with apoptotic cell death. *Int J Clin Pharmacol Ther* 1998; **36**: 25–8.

73. Odom LF, Gordon EM. Acute monoblastic leukemia in infancy and early childhood: successful treatment with an epipodophyllotoxin. *Blood* 1984; **64**: 875–82.

74. Odom LF, Lampkin BC, Tannous R et al. Acute monoblastic leukemia: a unique subtype – a review from the Childrens Cancer Study Group. *Leuk Res* 1990; **14**: 1–10.

75. Weick JK, Kopecky KJ, Appelbaum FR et al. A randomized investigation of high-dose versus standard-dose cytosine arabinoside with daunorubicin in patients with previously untreated acute myeloid leukemia: a Southwest Oncology Group study. *Blood* 1996; **88**: 2841–51.

76. Bishop JF, Matthews JP, Young GA et al. Intensified induction chemotherapy with high dose cytarabine and etoposide for acute myeloid leukemia: a review and updated results of the Australian Leukemia Study Group. *Leuk Lymphoma* 1998; **28**: 315–27.

77. AML Collaborative Group. A systematic collaborative overview of randomized trials comparing idarubicin with daunorubicin (or other anthracyclines) as induction therapy for acute myeloid leukaemia. *Br J Haematol* 1998; **103**: 100–9.

78. Wiernik PH, Banks PL, Case DC et al. Cytarabine plus idarubicin or daunorubicin as induction and consolidation therapy for previously untreated adult patients with acute myeloid leukemia. *Blood* 1992; **79**: 313–19.

79. Amadori S, Ceci A, Comelli A et al. Treatment of acute myelogenous leukemia in children: results of the Italian Cooperative Study AIEOP/LAM 8204. *J Clin Oncol* 1987; **5**: 1356–63.

80. Burnett AK, Goldstone AH, Stevens RM et al. Randomised comparison of addition of autologous bone-marrow transplantation to intensive chemotherapy for acute myeloid leukaemia in first remission: results of MRC AML10 trial. UK Medical Research Council Adult and Children's Leukaemia Working Parties. *Lancet* 1998; **351**: 700–8.

81. Zittoun RA, Mandelli F, Willemze R et al. Autologous or allogeneic bone marrow transplantation compared with intensive chemotherapy in acute myelogenous leukemia. European Organization for Research and Treatment of Cancer (EORTC) and the Gruppo Italiano Malattie Ematologiche Maligne dell'Adulto (GIMEMA) Leukemia Cooperative Groups. *N Engl J Med* 1995; **332**: 217–23.

82. Cassileth PA, Harrington DP, Appelbaum FR et al. Chemotherapy compared with autologous or allogeneic bone marrow transplantation in the management of acute myeloid leukemia in first remission. *N Engl J Med* 1998; **339**: 1649–56.

83. Brenner MK, Rill DR, Moen RC et al. Gene-marking to trace origin of relapse after autologous bone-marrow transplantation. *Lancet* 1993; **341**: 85–6.

84. Capizzi RL, Powell BL. Sequential high-dose ara-C and asparaginase versus high-dose ara-C alone in the treatment of patients with relapsed and refractory acute leukemias. *Semin Oncol* 1987; **14**(2 Suppl 1): 40–50.

85. Capizzi RL, Davis R, Powell B et al. Synergy between high-dose cytarabine and asparaginase in the treatment of adults with refractory and relapsed acute myelogenous leukemia – a Cancer and Leukemia Group B study. *J Clin Oncol* 1988; **6**: 499–508.

86. Wells RJ, Odom LF, Gold SH et al. Cytosine arabinoside and mitoxantrone treatment of relapsed or refractory childhood leukemia: initial response and relationship to multidrug resistance gene 1. *Med Pediatr Oncol* 1994; **22**: 244–9.

87. Dahl GV, Lacayo NJ, Brophy N et al. Mitoxantrone, etoposide, and cyclosporine therapy in pediatric patients with recurrent or refractory acute myeloid leukemia. *J Clin Oncol* 2000; **18**: 1867–75.

88. Wells RJ, Woods WG, Buckley JD et al. Treatment of newly diagnosed children and adolescents with acute myeloid leukemia: a Childrens Cancer Group study. *J Clin Oncol* 1994; **12**: 2367–77.

89. Creutzig U, Ritter J, Zimmermann M et al. Does cranial irradiation reduce the risk for bone marrow relapse in acute myelogenous leukemia? Unexpected results of the Childhood Acute Myelogenous Leukemia Study BFM-87. *J Clin Oncol* 1993; **11**: 279–86.

90. Bunin NJ, Kunkel K, Callihan TR. Cytoreductive procedures in the early management in cases of leukemia and hyperleukocytosis in children. *Med Pediatr Oncol* 1987; **15**: 232–5.

91. Bunin NJ, Pui CH. Differing complications of hyperleukocytosis in children with acute lymphoblastic or acute non-lymphoblastic leukemia. *J Clin Oncol* 1985; **3**: 1590–5.

92. Creutzig U, Ritter J, Budde M et al. Early deaths due to hemorrhage and leukostasis in childhood acute myelogenous leukemia. Associations with hyperleukocytosis and acute monocytic leukemia. *Cancer* 1987; **60**: 3071–9.

93. Byrd JC, Dodge RK, Carroll A et al. Patients with t(8;21)(q22;q22) and acute myeloid leukemia have superior failure-free and overall survival when repetitive cycles of high-dose cytarabine are administered. *J Clin Oncol* 1999; **17**: 3767–75.

94. Tallman MS, Hakimian D, Shaw JM et al. Granulocytic sarcoma is associated with the 8;21 translocation in acute myeloid leukemia. *J Clin Oncol* 1993; **11**: 690–7.

95. Bisschop MM, Revesz T, Bierings M et al. Extramedullary infiltrates at diagnosis have no prognostic significance in children with acute myeloid leukaemia. *Leukemia* 2001; **15**: 46–9.

96. Levitt GA, Stiller CA, Chessells JM. Prognosis of Down's syndrome with acute leukaemia. *Arch Dis Child* 1990; **65**: 212–16.

97. Ravindranath Y, Taub JW. Down syndrome and acute myeloid leukemia. Lessons learned from experience with high-dose Ara-C containing regimens. *Adv Exp Med Biol* 1999; **457**: 409–14.

98. Taub JW, Ravindranath Y. Treatment of childhood acute myeloid leukaemia. *Baillières' Clin Haematol* 1996; **9**: 129–46.

99. Taub JW, Matherly LH, Stout ML et al. Enhanced metabolism of 1-β-D-arabinofuranosylcytosine in Down syndrome cells: a contributing factor to the superior event free survival of Down syndrome children with acute myeloid leukemia. *Blood* 1996; **87**: 3395–403.

100. Taub JW, Stout ML, Buck SA et al. Myeloblasts from Down syndrome children with acute myeloid leukemia have increased in vitro sensitivity to cytosine arabinoside and daunorubicin. *Leukemia* 1997; **11**: 1594–5.

101. Busciglio J, Yankner BA. Apoptosis and increased generation of reactive oxygen species in Down's syndrome neurons in vitro. *Nature* 1995; **378**: 776–9.

102. Taub JW, Huang X, Matherly LH et al. Expression of chromosome 21-localized genes in acute myeloid leukemia: differences between Down syndrome and non-Down syndrome blast cells and relationship to in vitro sensitivity to cytosine arabinoside and daunorubicin. *Blood* 1999; **94**: 1393–400.

103. Zwaan CM, Kaspers GJL, Pieters R et al. Cellular drug resistance profiles in childhood acute myeloid leukemia: differences between FAB types and comparison with acute lymphoblastic leukemia. *Blood* 2000; **96**: 2879–86.

104. Zwaan ChM, Kaspers GJL, Pieters R et al. Cellular drug resistance in childhood acute myeloid leukemia is related to chromosomal abnormalities. *Blood* 2002; **100**: 3352–60.

105. Frost BM, Gustafsson G, Larsson R et al. Cellular cytotoxic drug sensitivity in children with acute leukemia and Down's syndrome: an explanation to differences in clinical outcome? *Leukemia* 2000; **14**: 943–4.

106. Bar-Peled O, Korkotian E, Segal M et al. Constitutive overexpression of Cu/Zn superoxide dismutase exacerbates kainic acid-induced apoptosis of transgenic-Cu/Zn superoxide dismutase neurons. *Proc Natl Acad Sci USA* 1996; **93**: 8530–5.

107. Buckley JD, Chard DL, Baehner RL et al. Improvement in outcome for children with acute nonlymphocytic leukemia. A report from the Children's Cancer Study Group. *Cancer* 1989; **63**: 1457–65.

108. Leahey A, Kelly K, Rorke LB et al. A phase I/II study of idarubicin (Ida) with continuous infusion fludarabine (F-ara-A) and cytarabine (ara-C) for refractory or recurrent pediatric acute myeloid leukemia (AML). *J Pediatr Hematol Oncol* 1997; **19**: 304–8.

109. Stahnke K, Boos J, Bender-Gotze C, Ritter J et al. Duration of first remission predicts remission rates and long-term survival in children with relapsed acute myelogenous leukemia. *Leukemia* 1998; **12**: 1534–8.

110. Webb DK, Wheatley K, Harrison G et al. Outcome for children with relapsed acute myeloid leukaemia following initial therapy in the Medical Research Council (MRC) AML 10 trial. MRC Childhood Leukaemia Working Party. *Leukemia* 1999; **13**: 25–31.

111. Fleischhack G, Hasan C, Graf N et al. IDA-FLAG (idarubicin, fludarabine, cytarabine, G-CSF), an effective remission-induction therapy for poor-prognosis AML of childhood prior to allogeneic or autologous bone marrow transplantation: experiences of a phase II trial. *Br J Haematol* 1998; **102**: 647–55.

112. Vignetti M, Rondelli R, Locatelli F et al. Autologous bone marrow transplantation in children with acute myeloblastic leukemia: report from the Italian National Pediatric Registry (AIEOP-BMT). *Bone Marrow Transplant* 1996; **18**(Suppl 2): 59–62.

113. Kaspers GJ, Kardos G, Pieters R et al. Different cellular drug resistance profiles in childhood lymphoblastic and non-lymphoblastic leukemia: a preliminary report. *Leukemia* 1994; **8**: 1224–9.

114. Rots MG, Pieters R, Jansen G et al. A possible role for methotrexate in the treatment of childhood acute myeloid leukaemia, in particular for acute monocytic leukaemia. *Eur J Cancer* 2001; **37**: 492–8.

115. Zwaan CM, Kaspers GJ, Pieters R et al. Different drug sensitivity profiles of acute myeloid and lymphoblastic leukemia and normal peripheral blood mononuclear cells in children with and without Down syndrome. *Blood* 2002, **99**: 245–51.

116. Dano K. Active outward transport of daunomycin in resistant Ehrlich ascites tumor cells. *Biochim Biophys Acta* 1973; **323**: 466–83.

117. Kartner N, Riordan JR, Ling V. Cell surface P-glycoprotein associated with multidrug resistance in mammalian cell lines. *Science* 1983; **221**: 1285–8.

118. Cole SP, Bhardwaj G, Gerlach JH et al. Overexpression of a transporter gene in a multidrug-resistant human lung cancer cell line. *Science* 1992; **258**: 1650–4.

119. Doyle LA, Yang W, Abruzzo LV et al. A multidrug resistance transporter from human MCF-7 breast cancer cells. *Proc Natl Acad Sci USA* 1998; **95**: 15665–70.

120. Scheper RJ, Broxterman HJ, Scheffer GL et al. Overexpression of a *M*(r) 110 000 vesicular protein in non-P-glycoprotein-mediated multidrug resistance. *Cancer Res* 1993; **53**: 1475–9.

121. Sievers EL, Smith FO, Woods WG et al. Cell surface expression of the multidrug resistance P-glycoprotein (P-170) as detected by monoclonal antibody MRK-16 in

pediatric acute myeloid leukemia fails to define a poor prognostic group: a report from the Childrens Cancer Group. *Leukemia* 1995; **9**: 2042–8.

122. den Boer ML, Pieters R, Kazemier KM et al. Relationship between major vault protein/lung resistance protein, multidrug resistance-associated protein, P-glycoprotein expression, and drug resistance in childhood leukemia. *Blood* 1998; **91**: 2092–8.

123. Ravindranath Y, Becton D, Buck S et al. Multidrug resistance gene (MDR1) expression and cytotoxicity to daunorubicin and cytarabine in childhood acute myeloid leukemia (AML). *Med Ped Oncol* 1999; 148a.

124. Leith CP, Kopecky KJ, Godwin J et al. Acute myeloid leukemia in the elderly: assessment of multidrug resistance (MDR1) and cytogenetics distinguishes biologic subgroups with remarkably distinct responses to standard chemotherapy. A Southwest Oncology Group study. *Blood* 1997; **89**: 3323–9.

125. Leith CP, Kopecky KJ, Chen IM et al. Frequency and clinical significance of the expression of the multidrug resistance proteins MDR1/P-glycoprotein, MRP1, and LRP in acute myeloid leukemia: a Southwest Oncology Group Study. *Blood* 1999; **94**: 1086–99.

126. Soldner A, Christians U, Susanto M et al. Grapefruit juice activates P-glycoprotein-mediated drug transport. *Pharm Res* 1999; **16**: 478–85.

127. Broxterman HJ, Giaccone G, Lankelma J. Multidrug resistance proteins and other drug transport-related resistance to natural product agents. *Curr Opin Oncol* 1995; **7**: 532–40.

128. van den Heuvel-Eibrink MM, Wiemer EA, de Boevere MJ et al. *MDR1* expression in poor-risk acute myeloid leukemia with partial or complete monosomy 7. *Leukemia* 2001; **15**: 398–405.

129. van Der Kolk DM, Vellenga E, van Der Veen AY et al. Deletion of the multidrug resistance protein *MRP1* gene in acute myeloid leukemia: the impact on MRP activity. *Blood* 2000; **95**: 3514–19.

130. Kuss BJ, Deeley RG, Cole SP et al. Deletion of gene for multidrug resistance in acute myeloid leukaemia with inversion in chromosome 16: prognostic implications. *Lancet* 1994; **343**: 1531–4.

131. van den Heuvel-Eibrink MM, Wiemer EA, de Boevere MJ et al. *MDR1* gene-related clonal selection and P-glycoprotein function and expression in relapsed or refractory acute myeloid leukemia. *Blood* 2001; **97**: 3605–11.

132. Bergman AM, Munch-Petersen B, Jensen PB et al. Collateral sensitivity to gemcitabine (2′,2′-difluorodeoxycytidine) and cytosine arabinoside of daunorubicin- and VM-26-resistant variants of human small cell lung cancer cell lines. *Biochem Pharmacol* 2001; **61**: 1401–8.

133. Martin-Aragon S, Mukherjee SK, Taylor BJ et al. Cytosine arabinoside (ara-C) resistance confers cross-resistance or collateral sensitivity to other classes of anti-leukemic drugs. *Anticancer Res* 2000; **20**(1A): 139–50.

134. Pearson L, Leith CP, Duncan MH et al. Multidrug resistance-1 (*MDR1*) expression and functional dye/drug efflux is highly correlated with the t(8;21) chromosomal translocation in pediatric acute myeloid leukemia. *Leukemia* 1996; **10**: 1274–82.

135. List AF, Kopecky KJ, Willman CL et al. Benefit of cyclosporine modulation of drug resistance in patients with poor-risk acute myeloid leukemia: a Southwest Oncology Group study. *Blood* 2001; **98**: 3212–20.

136. Sonneveld P, Burnett A, Vossebeld P et al. Dose-finding study of valspodar (PSC 833) with daunorubicin and cytarabine to reverse multidrug resistance in elderly patients with previously untreated acute myeloid leukemia. *Hematol J* 2000; **1**: 411–21.

137. Senchenkov A, Litvak DA, Cabot MC. Targeting ceramide metabolism – a strategy for overcoming drug resistance. *J Natl Cancer Inst* 2001; **93**: 347–57.

138. Kaspers GJ, Zwaan CM, Veerman AJ et al. Cellular drug resistance in acute myeloid leukemia: literature review and preliminary analysis of an ongoing collaborative study. *Klin Padiatr* 1999; **211**: 239–44.

138a. Kaspers GJ et al. In vitro cellular drug resistance and prognosis in childhood acute lymphoblastic leukemia. *Blood*; **90**: 2723–9.

139. Hongo T, Yajima S, Sakurai M et al. In vitro drug sensitivity testing can predict induction failure and early relapse of childhood acute lymphoblastic leukemia. *Blood* 1997; **89**: 2959–65.

140. Yamada S, Hongo T, Okada S et al. Clinical relevance of in vitro chemoresistance in childhood acute myeloid leukemia. *Leukemia* 2001; **15**: 1892–7.

141. Hongo T, Fujii Y, Yajima S. In vitro chemosensitivity of childhood leukemic cells and the clinical value of assay directed chemotherapy. In: Kaspers GJ (ed) *Drug Resistance in Childhood Leukemia and Lymphoma I.* Chur: Harwood Academic Publishers, 1993: 313–19.

142. Klumper E, Pieters R, Kaspers GJ et al. In vitro chemosensitivity assessed with the MTT assay in childhood acute non-lymphoblastic leukemia. *Leukemia* 1995; **9**: 1864–9.

143. Zwaan ChM, Pieters R, Huismans DR et al. Circumvention of cytarabine resistance by 2-chlorodeoxyadenosine in pediatric acute myeloid and acute lymphoblastic leukemia: an in vitro study. *Blood* 2000; gb(Suppl I): 307a.

144. Krance RA, Hurwitz CA, Head DR et al. Experience with 2-chlorodeoxyadenosine in previously untreated children with newly diagnosed acute myeloid leukemia and myelodysplastic diseases. *J Clin Oncol* 2001; **19**: 2804–11.

145. Ramaswamy S, Tamayo P, Rifkin R et al. Multiclass cancer diagnosis using tumor gene expression signatures. *Proc Natl Acad Sci USA* 2001; **98**: 15149–54.

146. Levitt G. Cardioprotection. *Br J Haematol* 1999; **106**: 860–9.

147. Corbett TH, Griswold DP, Roberts BJ et al. Biology and therapeutic response of a mouse mammary adenocarcinoma (16/C) and its potential as a model for surgical adjuvant chemotherapy. *Cancer Treat Rep* 1978; **62**: 1471–88.

148. Santana VM, Mirro J, Kearns C et al. 2-Chlorodeoxyadenosine produces a high rate of complete hematologic remission in relapsed acute myeloid leukemia. *J Clin Oncol* 1992; **10**: 364–70.

149. Zwiebel JA. New agents for acute myelogenous leukemia. *Leukemia* 2000; **14**: 488–90.

150. Sievers EL, Lange BJ, Buckley JD et al. Prediction of relapse of pediatric acute myeloid leukemia by use of multidimensional flow cytometry. *J Natl Cancer Inst* 1996; **88**: 1483–8.

151. Sievers EL, Radich JP. Detection of minimal residual disease in acute leukemia. *Curr Opin Hematol* 2000; **7**: 212–16.

152. Szczepanski T, Orfao A, van der Velden VH et al. Minimal residual disease in leukaemia patients. *Lancet Oncol* 2001; **2**: 409–17.

# 38 Acute myeloid leukemia in adults

Bob Löwenberg and Alan K Burnett

## Cell of origin

Acute myeloid leukemia (AML) is a malignant clonal disorder of immature hematopoietic cells and is characterized by aberrant hematopoietic cellular proliferation and maturation. Leukemic blasts may express abilities for maturation to a variable degree, which leads to morphologic heterogenoity. Generally, the transformed leukemic stem cell is committed to the granulocytic lineage, but sometimes a predominance of blast cells from the erythroid or megakaryocytic lineage may be observed. The leukemic transformation may occur at the level of a pluripotent or a less primitive hematopoietic cell.[1,2]

In certain patients, peripheral blood polymorphonuclear cells, erythroid cells, and platelets exhibit the clonal features characteristic of the leukemic cells, indicating that the leukemia originates from early precursor cells with pluripotential differentiation abilities.[1,3,4] This is apparent from the presence of genetic markers in several blood cell lineages, for example unique cytogenetic abnormalities.[4] Multilineage involvement is frequently seen in elderly patients with AML. In others, particularly children and younger adults, the erythroid cells and platelets often originate from normal stem cells.[1,3] A possible explanation for this observation is that in such patients, leukemic transformation has occurred at the level of a more mature primitive progenitor cell that is monopotent and committed to myeloid differentiation only. Even when overt leukemia has been eradicated with chemotherapy and apparently normal hematopoiesis has been reinstituted (complete hematologic remission), clonal marrow or blood hematopoiesis may persist in a subset of patients. The fact that clonal hematopoiesis may be found during clinical remission suggests that, following therapy, the disease has reverted to an earlier evolutionary phase of its development. Most likely, preleukemic hematopoietic cells dominate the marrow and blood during those clonal remissions. These data are entirely consistent with the multistep pathogenesis of AML.

## Cellular heterogeneity

Human AML is characterized by a heterogeneous cellular composition. This heterogeneity is an expression of hierarchical subpopulations of cells of different maturational stages within the neoplasm. The cellular hierarchy is apparent from morphologic examination, immunologic phenotyping, cytogenetics, and cell culture analysis.[2] The successive stages of maturation of AML cells can be ranked according to phenotype as well as proliferative potential. For instance, cells with high proliferative abilities (forming large colonies) may be distinguished from cells with low proliferative abilities (forming small colonies or clusters), or 'end' cells (non-proliferative in vitro). The colony-forming cells (AML-CFU) act as progenitors giving rise to in vitro colonies of daughter cells that are phenotypically more mature. However, in general, AML cells are unable to develop towards terminally differentiated cells[5] – they only generate partially and abnormally maturing progeny.[6] Thus, the maturation block is not always absolute. Both the variable cellular stages at which cell transformation has taken place and the variable residual maturational abilities retained by these transformed cells probably determine the phenotypic diversity of clinical AML.

## Concept of AML stem cells

The concept of tumor stem cells postulates that some cells in a tumor have the capacity to maintain long-term growth of the tumor. The progeny derived from these malignant stem cells lack these abilities for self-renewal. The in vivo significance of in vitro AML colony-forming cells is difficult to define, but in vitro observations indicate that in vitro colony-formers are relatively mature progenitors and do not function to maintain and expand the malignancy.[6,7] Human AML cells may engraft in severe combined immunodeficient (SCID) mice or the variant non-obese diabetic SCID/NOD mice following intravenous injection.[8–11]

The finding that human leukemia can be sustained in these immunodeficient mice for several months suggests that primitive AML progenitor cells are responsible for AML growth in these animals. The cell type that initiates outgrowth of human leukemia in vivo in these murine recipients has been characterized as a cell that may be discriminated from the AML in vitro colony-forming cell. It expresses a phenotype strikingly similar to that of primitive normal hematopoietic stem cells.[11–14] For instance, the cell initiating AML in SCID animals appears to be CD34+, CD38-, HLA-DR- and 5-flurouracil (5-FU)-resistant. The repopulating AML cell in SCID mice is quiescent. It currently represents one of the best available approximations of the AML stem cell. Stroma-dependent cultures that permit the establishment of human hematopoiesis in vitro for a few months have recently also been applied to human leukemia. These long-term cultures of AML have been extrapolated from initial studies in the mouse. One of these methods, the cobblestone area-forming cell (CAFC) assay has proved convenient for both quantitative and qualitative studies of primitive AML progenitors (cobblestone area formation late in culture, i.e. beyond 6 weeks). These late-appearing CAFC mimic cells with repopulating abilities and express primitive progenitor phenotypes. Thus, for example, stroma-supported late-CAFC represent a subset of AML cells that are CD38- CD34+ and 5-Fu-resistant.[13,14]

## Leukemogenesis

It is generally accepted that leukemia is the result of a multistep process.[15,16] According to this idea, the transformed hematopoietic progenitor cells initially acquire a single genetic lesion resulting in only slight variations in cell survival, proliferation, or maturational abilities as compared with their normal counterparts. Additional genetic lesions may result in full leukemic transformation. The search for the targets of the oncogenic events has indicated various mechanisms that may lead to leukemia. Genetic lesions may result in the activation of genes that contribute to leukemogenesis (oncogenes) or loss of activity of genes that prevent tumor growth (tumor suppressor genes).[17] The genes involved in leukemia development affect specific cellular regulatory mechanisms: growth factor receptor function (e.g. the granulocyte colony-stimulating factor receptor (G-CSFR[18,19] and FLT3[20,21]; see below), signal transduction (e.g. the RAS family[22]), and transcription (e.g. c-MYC[23]). As a consequence, these processes may dysregulate critical biologic functions, in particular the abilities of proliferation (e.g. tyrosine kinase mutations) and differentiation (e.g. PML–RAR α[24]), and programmed cell death (e.g. TP53).[25] Proliferation of AML cells is controlled by hematopoietic growth factors. In vitro, leukemic cells in some cases exhibit spontaneous

proliferative activity. This may be caused by the autocrine production of hematopoietic growth factors or by the constitutional activation of metabolic pathways that are otherwise activated only when a growth factor activates its receptor.[26,27] It has been shown that autonomous proliferation of AML cells in short-term culture predicts a comparatively high probability of relapse and poor survival.[28]

### Abnormal receptor complex formation and function in hematopoietic disorders

Mutations in hematopoietic growth factors receptor genes that interfere with normal receptor complex formation and function may play a role in the pathophysiology of hematopoiesis.[26] In murine models, it has been demonstrated that mutations in the extracellular domain of the macrophage colony-stimulating factor receptor (M-CSFR, CSF1R)[29] or in the erythropoietin receptor (EPOR)[27,30] result in ligand-independent activation of these receptors and induce leukemia. On the other hand, structural abnormalities might also impair receptor function, and as a consequence hematocytopenia of one or more cell lineages may evolve. In particular, mutations have been found in the hematopoietic growth factor receptors FLT3[20,21,31–39] and c-KIT.[40–42]

### FLT3 mutations

Internal tandem duplications (ITDs) and activating point mutations have been reported in the part of the FLT3 gene coding for the juxtamembrane (JM) segment of the receptor. Elongation of the JM domain causes ligand-independent dimerization resulting in constitutive activation of STAT5 and MAPK in cell lines.[35] Primary AML blasts show a reduced responsiveness to stromal support in long-term culture.[33] FLT3 ITDs have been reported to occur in approximately 13−20% of cases of AML[20,34,36–39,43–47] and D835 point mutations in 5−7% of cases.[21]

The 5-year event-free survival (EFS) rate for patients with an FLT3 ITD was 14%, which compared with a rate of 69% for patients without mutations.[38] In another study, the low response probability of childhood AML with FLT3 ITD (40%, versus 74% in wild-type FLT3 cases) and an EFS rate of only 7% were confirmed.[36] In several adult series of patients with AML, FLT3 mutations conferred a poor prognosis.[31,34,39,43,45,46] FLT3 mutations express adverse prognostic significance independent of other prognostic variables. Of particular note is that among cytogenetically defined good-risk and intermediate-risk patients, a notably poor-risk subset can be distinguished according to the presence of FLT3 mutations.[34,36,43,46] FLT3 mutations have also been associated with leukocytosis (an established unfavorable prognostic indication) in acute promyelocytic leukemia (APL) and with leukemic transformation of myelodysplasia (MDS). In a study in 201 newly diagnosed patients, 46 had *FLT3* mutations of both (*n*=3) or one (*n*=43) allele and in addition independent N-*RAS* mutations in 25 cases. *FLT3* mutation correlated with reduced survival independently of other prognostic parameters and was the most significant negative predictor of outcome.

### c-KIT mutations

The receptor tyrosine kinase c-KIT (which is the receptor for stem cell factor/Steel factor (SCF)) is expressed in the majority of cases of AML and also in patients with chronic myeloid leukemia (CML), but is uncommon in acute lymphoblastic leukemia (ALL). Levels of expression are of the same order as on normal hematopoietic precursors. These receptors have the ability to bind ligand, and are functional, as exposure to ligand will raise a proliferative or survival response. Mutations of c-KIT were initially identified in human mast cell lines. These mutations are usually located in the JM intracytoplasmic region of the receptor and involve point mutations leading to constitutive phosphorylation (in the absence of ligand). Mutant c-KIT receptors, upon transduction to cell lines, confer factor independence as well as tumorigenicity. A variable number of mutations have been reported, among which the D816V (aspartate to valine) and D816Y (aspartate to tyrosine) substitutions are comparatively common. These mutations may result in altered growth abilities not only as the result of receptor activation but also due to altered intracellular substrate specificity. It is currently assumed that c-*KIT* mutations might contribute to leukemogenesis, particularly in cooperation with other coexistent oncogenic events, as has been shown in a c-*MYB* transformation model.[48] In a minority of cases of human AML, c-*KIT* mutations have been identified.[40,41,49] These and other mutations, including point mutations of the extracellular domain, have also been reported in patients with myeloproliferative syndromes as well as patients with AML.[40,49,50] AML with c-*KIT* mutations may show increased levels of mast cell infiltration.[50] c-*KIT* mutations are commonly seen in AML with t(8;21) and inv(16) cytogenetics, the so-called core binding factor leukemias,[40] and recent evidence suggests that in the case of c-*KIT* mutations these leukemias show a greater tendency of relapse.[42]

### G-CSF, G-CSFR mutations

Patients with severe congenital neutropenia (SCN) or Kostmann's disease typically present in infancy with a quantitative lack of circulating granulocytes and an arrest of granulocytic maturation at the promyelocytic stage in the marrow, and suffer from recurrent and severe bacterial infections. They are predisposed to the development of AML. SCN was the first clinical condition in which structural hematopoietic receptor mutations in relation to leukaemia were revealed.[18,19] These mutations generally represent nonsense mutations of the *G-CSFR* gene that encode for a receptor from which the cytoplasmic C-terminal part has been deleted. Approximately 10% of cases of SCN carry *G-CSFR* mutations, usually localized within a narrow stretch and resulting in a receptor lacking approximately 82–98 amino acids at its intracytoplasmic end. Patients with SCN and mutated *G-CSFR* have an approximately 30-fold increased risk to transform to AML.[51] Thus SCN with mutated *G-CSFR* apparently represent preleukemic conditions. Cells transduced with the truncated G-CSFR show numerous molecular and biochemical abnormalities in signaling following activation by the ligand, resulting in abnormal biological responses as well. These abnormalities relate to altered cell survival and apoptosis, granulocytic cellular maturation, as well as cell cycling and proliferation rate.

*G-CSFR* variant mutations have also been reported – some in the extracellular domain resulting in normal binding affinity of the receptor for ligand but loss of responsiveness to ligand stimulation.[52] *G-CSFR* mutations have been described in sporadic cases of de novo AML.[18] These point mutations in the *G-CSFR* gene may cause overexpression of non-functional G-CSFR splice variants that could interfere with normal G-CSFR function in a dominant negative fashion. The fact that mutations in the C-terminal region of G-CSFR, specifically disrupting the maturation signaling function of the receptor, may be involved in the pathogenesis of AML might suggest that signaling molecules that are specifically activated through the C-terminal domain of G-CSFR could be additional potential targets for transforming mutations leading to AML. The true frequency of *G-CSFR* mutations in primary AML or MDS remains to be settled, as current analysis has been based upon relatively small series.

## Diagnosis and classification of AML

The diagnosis of AML is primarily based on morphological and cytochemical criteria. These criteria constitute the basis of the French–American–British (FAB) classification that is commonly used to distinguish subtypes of AML.[53–56] These subtypes (see Table 38.1) include the categories M0 through M7. Immunophenotyping, cytogenetic analysis and molecular examination are employed to add specific information for a more precise diagnosis. Immunophenotyping using a panel of monoclonal antibodies adds further precision and objectivity to the diagnosis.

In recent years, it has become essential to add genetic and molecular information to the diagnostic process.

**Table 38.1 Cytological criteria for the diagnosis of acute myeloid leukemia: French–American–British (FAB) classification**

| FAB subtype | Microscopy | Cytochemistry/immunology |
|---|---|---|
| M0 | • Blasts ≥30% of bone marrow nucleated cells<br>• <3% of blasts positive for Sudan black B or peroxidase<br>• Myeloperoxidase positivity by ultrastructural cytochemistry | Myeloid immunological markers (e.g. CD13, CD33, myeloperoxidase) |
| M1 | • Blasts ≥90% of bone marrow non-erythroid cells (i.e. excluding also lymphocytes, plasma cells, macrophages, and mast cells from the count)<br>• ≥3% of blasts positive for Sudan black B or peroxidase<br>• Maturing granulocytic cells (i.e. promyelocytes towards polymorphonuclear cells) ≤10% of non-erythroid cells<br>• (Pro)monocytes ≤10% of non-erythroid marrow cells | |
| M2<br>with maturation | • Blasts 30–89% of bone marrow non-erythroid cells<br>• Maturing granulocytic cells (i.e. promyelocytes to polymorphonuclear cells) >10% of non-erythroid cells<br>• Monocytic cells (i.e., monoblasts to monocytes) <20% of non-erythroid cells and not meeting other criteria for M4 | |
| M3<br>(acute hypergranular promyelocytic leukemia) | • Promyelocytes (most hypergranular) >30% of bone marrow nucleated cells | |
| M3 variant | • Promyelocytes (hypogranular or microgranular) >30% of bone marrow nucleated cells | |
| M4<br>(acute myelomonocytic leukemia) | • Blasts ≥30% of bone marrow nucleated cells<br>• Granulocytic cells (myeloblasts to polymorphonuclear cells) ≥20% of non-erythroid cells<br>• Monocytic cells (monoblasts to monocytes) ≥20% of non-erythroid cells and peripheral blood monocytes ≥5 × $10^9$/l<br>(or)<br>• Monocytic cells ≥20% of non-erythroid cells and confirmed by cytochemistry or urinary lysozymes elevated<br>(or)<br>• Marrow resembling M2, but blood monocytes ≥5 × $10^9$/l and confirmed by cytochemistry or elevated urine lysozymes | Positive for Sudan black B, peroxidase chloroesterase (granulocyte linage) plus α-naphthyl esterase (monocyte lineage) |
| M5A<br>(acute monoblastic leukemia) | • Blasts ≥30% of bone marrow non-erythroid cells<br>• Bone marrow monocytic component ≥80% of non-erythroid cells<br>• Monoblasts <80% of bone marrow monocytic component | |
| M5B<br>(acute monoblastic monocytic leukemia) | • Blasts ≥30% of bone marrow non-erythroid cells<br>• Bone marrow monocytic component ≥80% of non-erythroid cells<br>• Monoblasts <80% of bone marrow monocytic component | |
| M6<br>(acute erythroleukemia) | • Erythroblasts ≥50% of bone marrow nucleated cells<br>• Blasts ≥30% of bone marrow non-erythroid cells | |
| M7<br>(acute megakaryoblastic leukemia) | • Blasts ≥30% of bone marrow nucleated cells | Blasts demonstrated to be megakaryoblasts by immunological markers, ultrastructural morphology or cytochemistry |

This provides information that may have crucial implications for choice of treatment and prognosis. For example, the FAB M3 subtype is strongly associated with the t(15;17) reciprocal translocation resulting in the PML/RARα fusion protein. This signifies a unique sensitivity to retinoic acid.

The AML M0 subtype is characterized by small to medium-sized blasts with a high nuclear–cytoplasmic ratio, open chromatin, multiple nucleoli, and moderately basophilic cytoplasm. Myeloperoxidase (MPO)-positive cells constitute less than 3% of the blast population. The blasts may be positive for anti-MPO, anti-CD33, anti-CD13, anti-CD7, and anti-TdT (terminal deoxynucleotidyl transferase) antibody staining. The cells may also be MPO-positive at the ultrastructural level. FAB M0 leukemia is considered

to represent a poor-risk subtype of AML. Other special morphological variants of AML include AML with basophilia, especially associated with the translocation t(6;9)(p23;q34), AML with natural killer (NK)-cell phenotype, AML with erythrophagocytosis (especially those associated with the translocation t(8;16)(p11;p13)). Not infrequently AML at initial presentation may show trilineage myelodysplasia. These myelodysplastic abnormalities include nuclear abnormalities of the erythroblasts, hypogranulated neutrophils, and mononuclear megakaryocytes, which might indicate the development of AML from an antecedent myelodysplasia. AML with trilineage morphological abnormalities generally indicate a poor prognosis. Immunophenotyping of the leukemia may contribute to establishing the diagnosis of AML and distinguish the disease from ALL or other undifferentiated malignancies.

The impact of cytogenetics on prognosis will be discussed below, but the inclusion of this information has highlighted the heterogeneity of AML and has enabled distinct molecular entities to be identified. This has contributed to the newer WHO classification of AML[57,58] (Table 38.2) whereby distinct molecular genetic entities, i.e. t(15;17), t(8;21), inv(16), and abnormalities of 11q23 (MLL gene) are grouped together as AML with recurrent abnormalities. In this category, there is uniquely no threshold for the marrow blast count. The second category is defined by the addition of multilineage dysplasia. The third category is defined by whether the disease is secondary to alkylating agents or to MDS. The fourth category, which is designated as AML not otherwise categorized, contains the remaining FAB categories, i.e. M0, M1, M2, M4, M5a, M5b, M6a, M6b, and M7. The point of this classification is to give greater recognition to the etiological, molecular genetic, and prognostic information that is now available. As more such information emerges, so the definitions will need to be altered.

## Table 38.2 WHO classification of acute myeloid leukemia[57,58]

**Acute myeloid leukemia with recurrent genetic abnormalities**
Acute myeloid leukemia with t(8;21)(q22;q22) (AML1–ETO)
Acute myeloid leukemia with abnormal bone marrow eosinophils and inv(16)(p13q22) or t(16;16)(p13;q22) (CBFβ–MYH11)
Acute promyelocytic leukemia with t(15;17)(q22;q22) (PML RARα) and variants
Acute myeloid leukemia with 11q23 (MLL) abnormalities

**Acute myeloid leukemia with multilineage dysplasia**
Following myeloid dysplastic syndrome (MDS) or MDS/myeloproliferative disorder (MPD)
Without antecedent MDS or MDS/MPD, but with dysplasia in at least 50% of cells in two or more myeloid lineages

**Acute myeloid leukemia and myelodysplastic syndromes, therapy-related**
Alkylating agent/radiation-related type
Topoisomerase II inhibitor-related type (some may be lymphoid)
Others

**Acute myeloid leukemia, not otherwise categorized**
Acute myeloid leukemia, minimally differentiated
Acute myeloid leukemia without maturation
Acute myeloid leukemia with maturation
Acute myelomonocytic leukemia (AMML)
Acute monoblastic/acute monocytic leukemia
Acute erythroid leukemia (erythroid/myeloid and pure erythroleukemia)
Acute megakaryoblastic leukemia
Acute basophilic leukemia
Acute panmyelosis with myelofibrosis
Myeloid sarcoma

# Immunocytology and cytogenetics

The immunophenotypes are exponents of the heterogeneous cellular composition of the neoplasm.[59] The following markers are commonly applied for classifying AML: the progenitor cell markers CD34, CD117 (c-KIT), TdT, and HLA-DR, the myeloid markers anti-MPO, CD13, CD33, and CD14, the monocytic markers CD15, CD11b, CD11c, and CD68, the megakaryocytic markers CD61 and CD14, and the erythroid marker glycophorin A. Acquired cytogenetic abnormalities are frequently apparent in patients with AML. These abnormalities may include balanced translocations, inversions, or insertions without gain or loss of chromosome, or unbalanced aberrations (see also Chapter 17). In children and young adults, a predominance of balanced translocations is seen. At an older age and in secondary leukemias, it is mainly numerical and unbalanced abnormalities (e.g. deletions of chromosomes 5 or 7) that are seen. Patients with secondary leukemia may present with complex abnormalities, which are generally defined as the presence of more than three distinct chromosome abnormalities. The chromosome abnormalities occur non-randomly and are therefore useful to distinguish specific subtypes of AML. They are also of value as indicators of AML with favorable, intermediate, or poor-risk prognosis. Molecular techniques to demonstrate molecular abnormalities by fluorescence in situ hybridization (FISH) and to detect hidden mutations or fusion genes by polymerase chain reaction (PCR) are rapidly gaining applicability in the clinical diagnosis of patients with AML, and can provide genetic information when cytogenetics has failed.

## Remission induction treatment

It is well established that achieving a complete remission is a prerequisite for improved survival. Modern schedules will achieve remissions in about 75–80% of patients younger than 60 years[60] and around 50–55% in older patients (see below). There is a continuous decline in remission rate from childhood (90%) to old age (30%), with a reciprocal increase in resistant disease as a cause of induction failure. Some of the reasons for this age-related response will be discussed later. The mainstay drugs have been daunorubicin and cytosine arabinoside (cytarabine, Ara-C) given as a 7- or 10-day schedule. There appears to be little extra benefit in increasing the daunorubicin dose beyond around 50 mg/m$^2$, although higher doses are currently in clinical trial.[61] Comparative studies of daunorubicin dose have been rare. In a comparison between 30 and 45 mg/m$^2$, there was a higher complete response (CR) rate (72% versus 59%) in the 45 mg/m$^2$ patients, but there was no survival advantage.[62]

A third drug, such as thioguanine, has often been added. The addition of etoposide to a standard 7-day cytarabine with 3-day anthracycline has shown benefit in one study.[63] Although etoposide did not improve the CR rate, it did prolong remission. A very large (1600 patients) prospective comparison of thioguanine versus etoposide as the third drug showed no difference.[64] Combinations of cytarabine and daunorubicin with etoposide or thioguanine or a combination of mitoxantrone plus cytarabine did not result in relapse or survival advantages in older patients.[65]

There have been a number of attempts to intensify induction by increasing the dose of cytarabine, which appear to be beneficial.[66–68] This has been confirmed in randomized studies.[69,70]

A number or trials have prospectively compared daunorubicin with an alternative anthracycline: idarubicin[71–76] or mitoxantrone.[65,77–79] In the six randomized comparisons of idarubicin, there was fairly consistent evidence to suggest that idarubicin could achieve a higher CR rate, but some of these studies had a control arm that was inferior to what could reasonably be expected. The overall advantage for idarubicin may be less clear in older patients. Four randomized comparisons of mitoxantrone also suggested that it could improve the CR rate, but not survival. Both of these newer drugs tend to produce more prolonged cytopenia, and if used in consecutive courses will require some dose reduction – which has raised questions about how superior they are on a dose-equivalent basis.

The possibility to apply growth factors in conjunction with chemotherapy as an approach to prime the leukemia for the cytotoxic action of the chemotherapeutic agents and thereby enhance the efficacy of remission induction therapy will be discussed below[212] (see below modulation of resistance to chemotherapy with hematopoietic growth factors).

The message appears to be that more intensive treatment of younger patients will increase the remission rate. There is fairly convincing evidence that with a more intensive approach to induction, even though a higher remission rate may not be achieved, remissions will be achieved more promptly and there is a beneficial effect on long-term outcome.[69,76,80] The MRC AML12 trial has recently been completed comparing a standard daily dose of cytarabine (200 mg/m$^2$) with an intermediate dose (400 mg/m$^2$), both over 10 days, or high-dose cytarabine in induction and consolidation. Neither has shown an improved outcome.[81]

## Response evaluation after induction therapy

Attaining a CR is a prerequisite for long-term disease-free and overall survival. Therefore the assessment of CR is an important step in the management of patients with AML. CR has traditionally been defined as a cellular marrow with less than 5% blasts, no circulating blasts, no evidence of extramedullary leukemia, and recovery of granulocyte (PMN 1.5 x 10$^9$/L) and platelet (100 x 10$^9$/L) counts. Since the NCI criteria for CR were published in 1990, treatment, however, has changed quite considerably, and this has challenged the current validity of the definition of CR. Chemotherapy has become more dose intensive. This directly impacts on the cellularity of the marrow following chemotherapy and the ability for prompt hematological recovery. Furthermore, the next cycle of treatment often follows before full hematological recovery. In a recent analysis (still unpublished) in 1200 patients treated with contemporary strategies in 3 successive AML study protocols from HOVON (Dutch-Belgian Cooperative Hemato-Oncology) and SAKK (Swiss Cancer) Cooperative Groups, the prognostic impact of each of the definition elements of CR following cycle I was assessed. The analysis shows that % marrow blasts and extramedullary leukemia after induction therapy are powerful predictive hematological determinants of outcome (relapse, disease-free survival). It also reveals that the cutoff value of 5% is still valid. Thus, of the traditional CR parameters, % marrow blasts, absence of extramedullary leukemia and haematological recovery continue to stand out as predictors of outcome. In clinical management it has become quite common to conduct an "early" bone marrow assessment (at approximately days 7-10 after the first cycle) to identify those with refractory disease at an early point post-therapy. Recently, a group of experts have revisited the definition of CR and updated the scoring methodology for CR.[214] For reasons of international intercomparability between studies and standardization, they recommend to define CR in operational terms and distinguish morphological CR, CR with incomplete blood count recovery (CRi), cytogenetic CR (CRc), and molecular CR (CRm). Immunological approaches based on multiple parameter flow cytometry and quantitative (real-time) reverse transcriptase polymerase chain reactions for fusion genes in t(8;21) and inv(16) show promise as regards further refinement of the assessment of CR.

## Postremission chemotherapy

As previously mentioned, remission induction treatment independently influences long-term outcome and it is therefore difficult to separate the impact of these two phases of treatment. While it is clear that further treatment is necessary after remission has been achieved, exactly what and how much is less clear. While there is at least one modern study that shows the benefit of maintenance,[82,83] the fashion for younger patients has been to limit the duration of treatment, but to make it more intensive. For younger patients, the traditional concept of consolidation as a phase of treatment, perhaps with the same drugs but at lower dosage, should probably be consigned to history. It is now appropriate to administer treatment courses at an induction level of intensity. The question then is how many courses, and is there a best-choice schedule?

There has been much interest in recent years in dose escalation of cytarabine. It certainly appears that a single course is superior to a maintenance approach.[84,85] One of the most influential studies was carried out by the Cancer and Leukemia Group B (CALGB), who compared three dose levels of cytarabine given for four courses.[86] They reported a dose–response effect for patients under 60 years, with a 3 $g/m^2$ schedule being superior to a 100 or 400 mg group. Such a high dose was not found to be tolerable for older patients, and compliance was poor. Within the limits of analysis imposed by the small numbers involved, it was not possible to show a dose effect in older patients. The overall benefit of high-dose cytarabine has been confirmed by another major trial group.[70] The MRC AML10 protocol was primarily designed to assess the value of adding a stem cell transplant (i.e. a fifth course) to four courses of intensive treatment, which in themselves were able to deliver a 40% 7-year survival rate. While the interpretation of the outcome is a little complicated, it was clear that adding the extra course achieved a very substantial further reduction in relapse risk.[87] This provided the rationale for the MRC AML12 trial, which compared a total of four versus five courses. An initial analysis shows no benefit for the extra course of treatment. No high-dose cytarabine was included in this trial, which produced similar results to high-dose cytarabine schedules.[88,203] Several older studies attempted to address the question of how many consolidation courses should be given, but it is probable that such studies are no longer relevant in the context of the more intensive approach given nowadays. There is some evidence to suggest that patients with favorable cytogenetics derive most benefit from high-dose cytarabine,[89] but in general evidence to match a particular schedule to a risk group is sparse.

## Stem cell transplantation

In younger patients, it has become accepted practice to offer allogeneic bone marrow transplantation (BMT) to patients who have an HLA-matched donor (see also Chapter 29). This is based on consistent data from several centers that projected a long-term survival rate of around 55%,[90,91] which was a lot more hopeful than contemporary chemotherapy schedules offering about 25% survival. Some early prospective comparative studies confirmed the superiority of this approach in spite of the increased procedural mortality and morbidity.[91,92] No truly randomized trials were attempted. A number of concerns have been expressed about whether patients who received a transplant (allograft or autograft) have been selected as already being at a reduced risk of relapse. This is clearly the case, because they have spent a period of time either receiving consolidation treatment or awaiting transplant arrangements to be made. They are therefore patients who have avoided relapse or other treatment-related toxicities during this time period. In similarly 'time-censored' cohorts of patients treated with chemotherapy alone, the outcome is better than the 25% referred to above, and more similar to the transplant results.[93]

Since the general adoption of BMT as a standard treatment, chemotherapy results have improved as well, particularly in children. This has happened generally by deploying the skills developed from managing the transplant cases, thereby enabling much more intensive schedules to be given. It is clear that some of the prognostic factors referred to below also affect the outcome of transplantation. In particular, patients with an adverse karyotype have a poorer survival after allograft than other cases, mostly due to an increased risk of relapse.[94] In one prospective analysis taking into account risk factors, and evaluating allografts on the basis of donor availability versus inavailability, there was no advantage in good- or poor-risk patients, but there was an advantage for patients of standard risk.[87]

Good-risk patients who relapse can fairly reliably be returned to a second remission, so it is probably appropriate to reserve transplant for second remission, particularly if other factors such as cost and patient morbidity and quality of life are taken into account. This has been supported by further analysis of the MRC AML10 trial, where the significant reduction in relapse risk in the favorable karyotype group was entirely due to the t(15;17) subset, who are now treated with retinoic acid, but not in the t(8;21) or inv(16) patients.[87] In two other donor/no donor comparisons, no significant advantages were noted with regard to disease-free survival or overall survival in any of the risk groups.[95,96] The MRC AML12 trial did not prescribe transplant in good-risk cytogenetic groups. This did not result in a change in survival.[88]

Autologous BMT has been widely used as a means of consolidation therapy for first remission.[97-101] The advantages of this approach are that it is an option for patients who do not have a sibling donor and it will avoid some of the morbidity associated with allograft and therefore has the potential to be safely given to patients aged up to 60 years. Numerous single-center studies and registry data all confirm an expected outcome of 45–55%,[102] i.e. not that different from what can be achieved with an allograft.

However, the same points about patient selection as mentioned above apply, and therefore it was realized that prospective trials were required to establish what role autografting may have. A substantial proportion of entrants to these trials are children, who by virtue of age and favorable karyotype preponderance already have a more favorable outlook. In this context, autografting has been shown to have limited if any benefit, particularly[103,104] when the morbidity of the procedure is taken into account (e.g. growth retardation) and the fact that this subgroup of patients can be salvaged if they relapse is recognized. A large adoles-

cent and pediatric trial reported by the Children's Cancer Study Group[105] did provide evidence that allogeneic transplantation improved results in children, but some concerns have been raised about the analysis of that trial.[106,107] In any event, there is also evidence that the results of chemotherapy in children have improved greatly – probably again as a result of more successful supportive care.

Of the major trials reported in adults, in those conducted by the EORTC–GIMEMA, UK MRC, the GOELAM group in France, and the US Intergroup, around 1000 patients were randomized to compare autografting with further chemotherapy, or in the case of the MRC AML10 study to compare the addition of transplantation with intensive treatment.[87,108–110] The EORTC and MRC trials showed a substantial reduction in relapse risk and a significant advantage in disease-free survival. An overall survival advantage was less convincing, because a proportion of the patients (particularly in the EORTC trial) who relapsed could be salvaged. The GOELAM group observed no survival advantage, while the MRC study showed a survival advantage that emerged late. The US Intergroup study did not show any advantage for either transplant approach when compared with high-dose cytarabine. In all of these studies – but most particularly the MRC and US Intergroup studies – there was a problem of substantial non-compliance with randomization and of delivering the autograft even when randomization was achieved.

The procedure has a higher mortality rate (up to 15%) than anticipated from the previous single-center studies (around 6–8%). This is often due to the consequences of poor engraftment. Were this to be rectified then autologous BMT would be much more clearly advantageous. This raises the issue of whether peripheral blood stem cells (PBSC) could be a better source for transplants. Collected data within the European Group for Blood and Marrow Transplantation suggest that hematopoietic recovery may be better for neutrophil recovery but less clear for platelets. There is no evidence to support the use of PBSC to reduce the risk of relapse. Augmentation of autologous marrow with PBSC seems to be capable of enhancing engraftment of neutrophils and platelets,[111] but it remains to be seen whether this modification of the technique has an impact on survival.[204]

It is emerging that transplantation for good-risk disease and children could reasonably be applied as a second-line option. There are no prospective studies comparing transplantation with chemotherapy in second remission, but a retrospective database analysis has indicated that allografting is better than chemotherapy for younger patients (below 30 years) and for patients with longer first remission (over 1 year) and, paradoxically, older patients with shorter first remissions (less than 1 year). Although there are data to support the use of transplantation as first treatment of relapse,[112] on the basis that patients are not lost during reinduction therapy, this has not been widely adopted.

Allogeneic transplantation from unrelated donors is being more widely used, but it is largely untested in AML in prospective studies. Until the technique improves substantially, its role in AML is likely to be limited to areas where current treatment is inadequate, such as for the first-line treatment of young patients who are identified as being at high risk or as an option in second remission. Non-intensive transplantation protocols are now being explored. While they are feasible, the antileukemic effect is not yet clear.

## Overall results of treatment

In an historical review of patients treated on MRC protocols for more than 25 years, there has been a steady improvement in outcome with time. While there may be a number of explanations, and there may be differences between the patients treated, it is likely that this reflects the more intensive approach that has been taken, which has been permitted by improved supportive care. For older patients, there is little sign of any improvement in outcome (Figure 38.2).

## Factors determining treatment outcome

From what has already been said, several factors have been identified in recent years as reliable predictors of whether patients will respond to treatment and whether they are likely to relapse (Table 38.3).

## Age

Age is a major determinant of what therapeutic options can be offered to patients, and will also have a major influence on how they respond to the treatment and whether or not they will subsequently relapse. There is a steady decline in success from remission induction treatment and an increase in the risk of relapse with age. Both effects are only partially explained by the uneven distribution of favorable or unfavorable karyotype or poorer performance score at diagnosis. In contemporary studies, remission rates of 90% for children under 15 years, 80% for patients aged 16–60 years, and around 50% for older patients are now the norm. The true position in older patients is not absolutely clear, since the figures are derived from patients who enter clinical trials. It is well known that this is the minority of older patients. Poorer outcome with age can be explained in part by the tendency for favorable karyotypes to occur in younger patients while the opposite is true for older patients, but the general medical health of older patients tends to be less robust and therefore they can withstand intensive chemotherapy less well (see below).

### Cytogenetics and molecular genetics

Cytogenetic abnormalities are seen in approximately 60% of cases of AML and are highly predictive of response to therapy as well as probability of relapse.[113–116] The translocations t(8;21), inv16 or t(16;16), and t(15;17) generally carry a relatively favorable prognosis and are more commonly seen among younger patients with AML. The fusion genes of each of these translocations have been identified and can be detected with molecular probes in reverse transcriptase (RT)–PCR. Among patients with these chromosomal abnormalities or the corresponding

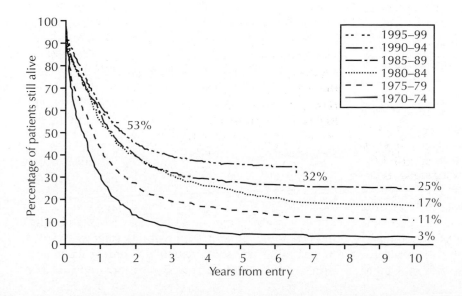

**Figure 38.1** Survival in MRC AML trials: age 15–59 years.

**Table 38.3 Unfavorable prognostic factors for outcome of chemotherapy in adult patients with AML**

| | Predictive for complete response | Predictive for relapse following response or for overall survival |
|---|:---:|:---:|
| **Young and middle-aged adults (15–60 years)** | | |
| Greater age | + | + |
| Cytogenetics (chromosomes 5 or 7 or complex abnormalities | + | + |
| Immunophenotype (CD34+) | + | + |
| Multidrug-resistance phenotype | + | + |
| High white blood cell count | + | + |
| Autonomous cell growth in culture | + | + |
| **Elderly (>60 years)** | | |
| Greater age | + | – |
| Abnormal cytogenetics | + | + |
| Poor performance | + | + |
| High white blood cell count | + | + |
| Secondary AML or prior MDS | + | – |

The above listed factors have been identified to express negative prognostic value in two or more prospective studies. The following specific favorable cytogenetic abnormalities have been distinguished: t(8;21), inv(16), and t(15;17).

molecular genetic abnormalities (*AML1–ETO*, *CBFβ–MYH11*, and *PML–RARα*), the response to induction therapy is 80% or greater and for those entering remission the probability of relapse is approximately 30%, resulting in 5-year survival rates of 60–70%. The latter molecular or cytogenetic subsets of AML correlate with cytomorphological categories. For instance, t(8;21) correlates mainly with FAB subtype M2, while inv(16) correlates with FAB M4 with eosinophils. However, the cytogenetics and molecular genetics of a particular case, rather than the FAB subtype, possess the overriding prognostic significance.

In contrast, patients with monosomies of chromosomes 7 (−7) or 5 (−5), 11q23 (*MLL* gene) abnormalities,[117] abnormalities of the long arm of chromosome 3 (abn3q), t(6;9), t(9;22), or Philadelphia chromosome and complex cytogenetic abnormalities (four or more different cytogenetic aberrations) generally have a distinctively poor prognosis. Among these individuals (when aged 60 years or younger), the average complete response to induction treatment is 60% with a majority of patients (approximately 80%) relapsing within 2 years, so that the survival rate at 5 years is approximately 15%.[118] These cytogenetic and molecular indicators have led to the definition of prognostic groups: favorable risk (favorable molecular

genetics or cytogenetics), unfavorable risk (poor-risk cytogenetics), and intermediate risk (all others). Usually, these risk classifications are refined by considering selected additional prognostic determinants that enhance the value of the cytogenetic or molecular distinctions. Risk-scoring systems based upon multiple prognostic factors may permit more precise approximations of prognosis in individual cases. For the sake of practicality, most collaborative groups have restricted the use of these additional risk factors, and only take into account a limited number of covariables with considerable prognostic impact. As an example, the MRC group has considered rapid versus late attainment of complete response (i.e. after cycle 1 versus cycle 2) in their risk score in order to enhance the separation between intermediate-risk and poor-risk patients.[119] The Dutch–Belgian HOVON and Swiss SAKK groups have required a white blood cell count of less than $20 \times 10^9/l$ in addition to favorable cytogenetics for the good-risk category (risk of relapse 24% at 5 years).[120] Another recent study has confirmed the white blood cell index as a prognostic factor in t(8;21) AML.[121]

Various studies have suggested that AML with *FLT3* internal tandem duplications (ITD), seen in 15–30% of pediatric and adult patients, predicts for significantly greater risk of relapse and for reduced survival.[31,34,36,39,43] Other studies with large numbers of patients have not yet unquestionably reproduced the prognostic value of *FLT3* ITD for survival.[122–124] More recently, it has been suggested that a high mutant/wild-type *FLT3* ratio enhances the predictive power of *FLT3* for survival as well.[122,125] Interestingly, *FLT3* mutations are mainly seen in the largest category of intermediate-cytogenetic-risk AML. Hence, *FLT3* ITD offer important additional molecular markers to distinguish a new subset of poor-risk AML. Another recurrent D835 point mutation of the *FLT3* receptor, seen in approximately 5–10% of de novo AML, has not yet been convincingly correlated with prognosis.

Mutations of the tumor suppressor gene *TP53* predict negative outcome.[126] In addition, high levels of *BCL2* and *WT1* expression have also been suggested to define AML with poor risk.[127] Tandem repeats of the *MLL* gene also appear to confer inferior outcome.[128] *EVI1* is an oncogene overexpressed in AML with translocations of 3q26. *EVI1* mRNA overexpression also characterizes AML with poor-risk outcome when associated with 3q26 abnormalities. Recently, it was shown that *EVI1* expression in AML in the absence of 3q26 cytogenetic abnormality also predicts notably bad prognosis.[129] In contrast, *CEBPα* mutations define AML with relatively good risk.[130,131]

These cases, hidden among the intermediate-cytogenetic-risk subset of AML patients, can now be separated. Each of these molecular defined groups is of relatively small size, confirming the genetic heterogeneity of AML. With the introduction of high-throughput analysis for molecular abnormalities and gene expression profiling, it will probably in the near future be possible to define new classes of AML (Table 38.4). The introduction of expression array chips (Chapter 20) may yield composite mRNA signatures of AML cells with prognostic value.[205,206] These distinctions, when properly validated, are likely to provide powerful tools for guiding treatment strategies in AML in the future.

## Immunophenotyping

There is at present no clear picture as to what contribution immunophenotyping at diagnosis makes to prognosis. Some of the inconsistency of the evidence can be attributed to technical differences, for example methods, antibodies, and thresholds of positivity, as well as the inherent heterogeneity of the disease. There seems to be general agreement that immunological definition is helpful in endorsing the FAB subgroups known to have an impact on prognosis, for example M6, M7 biphenotypic (adverse), M3 (favorable). In general, lack of DR or CD34 expression will be favorable.[132,133] MDR1/P-glycoprotein (P-gp) positivity (multidrug-resistance phenotype) will be unfavorable.[133–137]

## Initial morphological response to treatment

The appearance of the bone marrow in response to initial treatment is increasingly being recognized in both ALL and AML as predictive of outcome. Failure to substantially clear blasts within a few days of treatment has been taken in some chemotherapy protocols as an indication to give more treatment at that time. When the blast count has not been reduced below 15% after hematopoietic recovery from the first course, the prospect of achieving CR with the next course diminishes, but even for those who do achieve CR, the relapse risk is high compared with those with less than 20% blasts at that point. The conventional definition of CR depends on observing less than 5% blasts in the bone marrow, but in the MRC AML10 trial there was little difference between patients at less than 5% or between 5% and 15% who subsequently entered CR on long-term survival.[119] The morphological response to treatment can identify a subgroup of patients who are failed by present approaches to treatment and need novel approaches. Such patients who receive a transplant also do less well. Dysplasia of all lineages in remission may indicate a pre-existing myelodysplasia, and is thought to have a less good outcome.

## Table 38.4 Molecular markers additional to cytogenetics with prognostic significance for remission duration or survival in adult AML

| Marker | Frequency | Predictive for relapse | Survival | Ref |
|---|---|---|---|---|
| *TP53* mutation | 9/200 (4.5%) | — | Unfavorable | 126 |
| High *BCL2* and *WT1* mRNA expression | 35/98 (36%) | Unfavorable | Unfavorable | 127 |
| *MLL* partial tandem duplication | 18/221[a] (8%) | Unfavorable | NS | 128 |
| High *EVI1* mRNA expression | 32/319 (10%) | Unfavorable | Unfavorable | 129 |
| *CEBPα* mutation | 15/135 (11%) | Favorable | Favorable | 130 |

[a] Normal cytogenetics only. NS, not significant.

### Other factors

Poor performance score, male sex, high leukemic cell burden (i.e. high white blood cell count or organomegaly) and raised lactate dehydrogenase (LDH) have all been recognized for a long time as being associated with poor treatment outcome (Table 38.3). Markers of chemoresistance, such as PgP expression[133–137] and function, as discussed above, are now being more consistently shown to be individual predictors of response. Clearly there is a tendency for functional resistance (which has been associated with PgP expression), adverse karyotype, and age to be associated in the same patient. However, each has been identified as an individually powerful predictor of outcome. The cells in some cases of AML can be demonstrated to proliferate in a cytokine-free culture system. In a study where patients were stratified into three categories (low, intermediate, and high) based on in vitro proliferative response, differences in outcome were noted.[207] The respective CR rates were 68%, 62%, and 39%, while the relapse rates were 51%, 71%, and 89%. This translated into a major difference in survival difference (high 4% verses low 44%). The biological explanation for the heterogeneity of in vitro responses may relate to autonomous generation of growth factors and prevention of apoptotic death.

In summary, there are a number of powerful prognostic factors in AML that have potential as guides towards appropriate treatment, and away from ineffective or inappropriate lines of management. The most important in these respects are patient age (where a division around 60 years can be made), karyotype (which has both a favorable and an unfavorable subgroup), and initial response to treatment (where persisting with similar therapy to what has already been tried is unproductive). Prognostic values used to direct treatment are at present most relevant in younger patients, in whom more treatment options, particularly stem cell transplantation, can be considered.

## Minimal residual disease

The genetic abnormalities seen in a significant proportion of cases of AML provide unique markers of minimal residual disease, which in some instances can be detected with molecular methods. Such markers have been used to monitor the disappearance of leukemic cells during treatment and during remission (see also Chapter 22), or to asses their re-emergence following remission. Conventional cytogenetic analysis, FISH, and Southern blot analysis provide relatively insensitive measurements (1 leukemic cell per $10^2$ cells). RT–PCR measures transcripts of fusion genes at much greater sensitivity ($10^{-3}$ to $10^{-6}$), and more recently real-time PCR has been introduced for quantitative measurements of fusion gene transcripts. As yet, these techniques have been applied mainly to the most common fusion genes: *AML1–ETO* (t(8;21)), *CBFβ–MYH11* (inv(16) and t(16;16)), *BCR–ABL* (t(9;22)), and a few others.

In AML with t(8;21), *AML1–ETO* fusion transcripts have been detected in patients in long-term remission, indicating that their persistence does not necessarily predict relapse.[138–141] A proportion of the long-term survivors did become negative for such transcripts.[142] More recently, quantitative PCR techniques have permitted individuals at high risk of relapse to be distinguished from those in stable remission.[143,144] These studies are based upon small series of cases, emphasizing the need for more information regarding the predictive value of quantitative PCR measurements. Studies of real-time PCR are in progress. In AML with inv(16) or t(16:16), *CBFβ–MYH11* transcripts have been followed. There are at least eight variant transcripts. Most studies conducted so far have only assessed the common type A transcript (present in more than 80% of patients with this abnormality) in limited numbers of patients, and therefore cannot provide definite conclusions regarding the clinical value of this marker.[144–146] Both PCR-positive and PCR-negative cases have been reported among long-term survivors. Studies with quantitative PCR have as yet provided only preliminary (but promising) data.[147–151] Especially when PCR negativity appears after completion of therapy, it may predict continuous remission.[147–151] Another significant proportion of patients with AML present with *MLL* gene rearrangements (abn (11q23)).[152] One of many *MLL* abnormalities is the *MLL–AF9* fusion gene in patients with the t(9;11) translocation, but the value of molecular methods for the detection of this genetic abnormality remains uncertain.[153,154]

## Targeted leukemic cell killing

An appealing concept in AML treatment is to direct therapeutic agents specifically to the leukemic cell population while sparing normal hematopoietic progenitors and normal tissue. Antibodies and growth factors conjugated to a cytotoxic agent can be used to deliver drugs to the site of the malignant cell (see also Chapter 25). For instance, the granulocyte–macrophage colony-stimulating factor (GM-CSF)–cholera toxin and the GM-CSF–*Pseudomonas* toxin have shown significant activity against leukemic progenitor cells in colony assays as well as in vivo repopulation assays.[155,156] The CD33 antigen is a 67 kDa glycoprotein that functions as a sialic acid-dependent adhesion protein. It is expressed on most AML cells, including leukemic clonogenic precursors, but is not expressed on normal pluripotent hematopoietic stem cells. The CD33 antigen is absent from non-hematopoietic tissue. Because of these properties of selective binding and the fact that upon binding of specific antibody the CD33 antigen is internalized, anti-CD33 antibodies are suitable for delivering cytotoxic agents to leukemic cells.[157,158,201] Several other interesting immunoconjugates (e.g. anti-CD45 antibodies and G-CSF–toxin conjugates) are under development. Clinical studies with a humanized anti-CD33 antibody conjugated with the chemotherapeutic antitumor antibiotic calicheamicin (gemtuzumab ozogamicin, Mylotarg) show that approximately 30% of cases with AML in relapse may enter complete remission after one or two injections of this agent.[157,201] Currently, the use of this drug as a single agent is being evaluated in patients of younger age and with newly diagnosed disease. See also Chapter 25.

The targeting of disease alleles (e.g. mutated signaling molecules and transcription factors) remains a promising challenge. The paradigms of retinoic acid therapy in PML–RARα+ leukemia and of imatinib in BCR–ABL+ leukemia have demonstrated the applicability of this concept. There are many potential targets in AML, and it will be important to target those involved in the multistep leukemogenic cascade on which AML growth continues to depend, and preferably those with a broad range of activity affecting common pathways of development of multiple AML types. Current research is concentrating on a variety of principles. Examples of these include the development of kinase inhibitors (e.g. FLT3 inhibitors),[159,208] inhibitors of activated RAS processing,[160] and inhibitors of transcription repressors (histone deacetylase inhibitors[161]) (see also Chapter 27).

# Treatment of the patient of older age with AML

AML is seen at all ages, but more than half of patients are aged 60 years or older.[162,163] Because of demographic changes and the projected increase in the number of elderly people among the total population in the next decade, a significant increase in the incidence of cases of AML is foreseen.[164] Intensified cytotoxic therapy and stem cell transplantation have improved the prognosis of AML in recent years in young and middle-aged adults. However, these modern approaches to therapy have as yet provided little benefit to individuals with AML older than 60 years. Elderly people suffer from AML that in general is resistant to chemotherapy. Furthermore, aged individuals have greater difficulties in tolerating the toxicity and morbidity that accompany intensive chemotherapy.

Should older patients with AML actually be submitted to remission induction chemotherapy, or is it better to refrain from this and offer palliative support to these individuals? A purely supportive approach results in short survival and is associated with frequent hospitalization and a poor quality of life.[165]The prevailing opinion today is that intensive chemotherapy is the treatment of choice for elderly patients suffering from AML – provided they are fit. Remission induction chemotherapy usually involves a combination of the chemotherapeutic agents cytarabine and an anthracycline (daunorubicin or idarubicin) or an anthracenedione (mitoxantrone). Following one or two cycles of chemotherapy, approximately 50% of patients aged 60 years or more enter complete remission. Thus, the elderly population of patients respond significantly less favorably to induction treatment. The inverse relationship between age and CR rate is also apparent from a number of studies that enrolled patients covering a broad range of ages. These results are indicative of a progressive decline in the response to chemotherapy with increasing age. Patients aged 0–39, 40–59, 60–84, and 70–84 years show average response rates of about 78%, 66%, 45%, and 35%, respectively.[166] Independent prognostic factors that express an additional negative impact on the probability of attaining CR are poor performance status of older patients at diagnosis, high blast or white blood cell counts, and abnormal cytogenetics (Table 38.3).[79,167,168]

## Complications and mortality during remission induction therapy in the elderly

Approximately 30% of patients do not enter remission, owing to early death or death during the hypoplastic phase post chemotherapy. Death occurs during hospitalization in spite of supportive care, including antibiotics as well as red blood cell and platelet transfusions. A majority of the deaths among these individuals are due to infections. The greater death rate indicates that elderly individuals are less able to tolerate the consequences of severe infections, including hemodynamic dysfunction and the associated negative effects on cardiac, pulmonary, and renal function.[166] There are also age-related changes that might affect the pharmacokinetics and pharmacodynamics of antineoplastic agents, resulting in more intense or prolonged exposure. Reduced marrow regenerative abilities, the reduced tolerance of other organs to handle the toxic effects of drugs, as well as the reduced elimination and metabolism of drugs might all explain why elderly patients are at increased risk of hematopoietic and other complications from intensive chemotherapy. The incidence of severe infections in elderly patients with AML on induction therapy is approximately 20%.[169] Approximately 10% of patients die during or within the week following completion of chemotherapy.[170] Those who have experienced significant toxicity following the first cycle of chemotherapy are generally prematurely withdrawn from additional efforts of treatment. Thus, the obstacles to offering adequate therapy to older patients with AML are still quite formidable.

## Outcome of treatment and prognosis in elderly AML

Patients aged over 60 years, once induced into remission, are usually consolidated with additional cycles of chemotherapy, but rarely with stem cell transplantation or high-dose chemotherapy. Stem cell transplants are currently applied to patients aged 60 years and above only infrequently. Allogeneic transplants employing reduced-intensity conditioning regimens and associated with less organ toxicity are currently in clinical trial[209–211]. As discussed earlier, it will not be possible to give substantial amounts of intensive treatment anyway. Among patients aged 60 years and older treated with chemotherapy, survival at 2 years has been estimated as approximately 20%[79,168,169,171] and at 4–5 years as 10% or less.[79,168,170,171] The median disease-free survival is approximately 9 months[79,167,168,170] and approximately 30% of patients survive free of leukemia at 2 years. The disease-free survival rate at 4–5 years is about 5–15%.[79,86,168,170,171] Apparently, only a minor fraction of elderly patients submitted to intensive chemotherapy at the end become long-term survivors (Figure 38.2). These results probably represent an overestimate of the true outcome of elderly individuals with AML. Many patients are not referred to hospital for chemotherapy, or are ineligible for chemotherapy for medical reasons. Taking account of these patients, the overall prognosis of elderly patients with AML is even more dismal than indicated by the results of prospective studies.

One report estimated that only about one-third of elderly patients were selected to enter treatment protocols, and this is confirmed from the UK MRC databases.[171] In fact, the variability of patient selection leading to the inclusion of patients with variable risks in individual studies might also explain the differing outcomes of treatment in study reports. In one study of more than 400 cases, an additional 196 patients were identified as not having entered the trial. The most important reasons for exclusion of patients from trial therapy were their old age and poor clinical condition. The median age of non-trial patients (67 years) was significantly greater than that (53 years) of the trial group.

Based on these considerations, it can be estimated that the real 4-year survival rate of elderly patients is 5% or less. Therefore, the choice to treat or not to treat is critical in these individuals. A poor performance status and high white blood cell count and unfavorable cytogenetics at diagnosis have been identified as powerful prognostic factors for survival.[79,167–169] It makes sense to select patients for induction treatment only if they are in reasonable good clinical condition. Further, it makes sense to continue treatment only if they respond to and tolerate the first cycle of treatment with no major complications. The aim of this prognostic approach is to attempt to avoid treatment that has no benefit.

# Randomized studies in AML to enhance hematopoietic recovery after chemotherapy

The rationale for applying hematopoietic growth factors to the treatment of adult patients with AML is mainly twofold.[172] First, the introduction of these factors may hasten hematopoietic regeneration following chemotherapy and thus reduce morbidity and mortality. Second, in vitro studies have shown that hematopoietic growth factors might sensitize AML

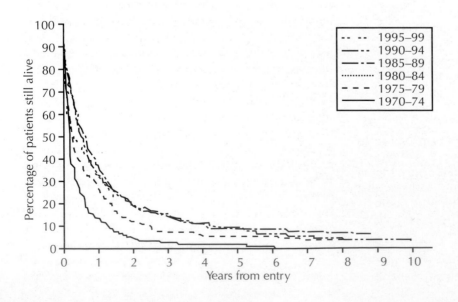

**Figure 38.2** Survival in MRC AML trials: age over 60 years.

cells to chemotherapy, and their coadministration with chemotherapy might enhance the antileukemic efficacy of treatment. The results of a limited number of randomized studies that were concerned with evaluating the role of G-CSF or GM-CSF after completion of chemotherapy have been reported. Several studies have been conducted in previously untreated patients. Some studies were done in patients with relapsed or refractory AML, and included some patients with CML in blast crisis.[172–174] These studies were all done in a relatively aged population, as the median ages of the patient groups in each of the trials varied between 43 and 71 years. In all studies, the application of G-CSF or GM-CSF after chemotherapy resulted in a reduction of the duration of severe neutropenia, although it varied from 2 to 12 days.

Beneficial effects of G-CSF or GM-CSF treatment on the number of severe infections and the need for antibiotic treatment have been reported. In one of the randomized G-CSF studies,[175] fewer documented infections were observed and patients in the G-CSF arm had fewer days with fever – and fewer days of antibiotic treatment in another study.[176] Application of GM-CSF reduced WHO grade 4–5 infections significantly in one of the three GM-CSF studies.[177] However, a consistent reduction of infection-related morbidity and mortality that would justify the general application of G-CSF or GM-CSF to patients with AML undergoing intensive chemotherapy has not been noted. Thus, the results of currently available studies do not establish a role for G-CSF or GM-CSF in modifying the response to induction chemotherapy or survival. An explanation for the lack of clinical utility could relate to the fact that the enhanced hematopoietic recovery results in a reduction of neutropenia of only a few days following a prolonged period of neutropenia.

# Refractory disease

Resistance of AML to chemotherapy is still the major cause of treatment failure in patients of all ages with AML (see also Chapter 23). The proportion of patients showing primary resistance to chemotherapy as the cause of remission induction failure may be estimated as 15% or more. Others may first achieve a CR, but after variable periods of time encounter recurrence of the leukemia. Why should AML in a fraction of individuals be relatively unresponsive to chemotherapy? The answers to this question are still open. M0 cytological FAB subtype, unfavorable cytogenetic abnormalities (e.g. chromosome 5 and 7 abnormalities), MDR1 surface marker expression, BCL2 positivity, CD34 immunophenotype, and high levels of autonomous proliferation in culture have all been shown to be adverse cellular predictors of treatment outcome. Overexpression of the membrane P-glyco-

protein (P-gp) is a typical phenotypic marker of drug resistance. P-gp belongs to a group of phosphorylated glycoproteins first described in hamster ovary cells. The classical form of multidrug resistance (MDR) was established when similar increased P-gp expression was found in a large range of cell lines.[178] Primary or acquired resistance to chemotherapy in patients is also associated with P-gp expression. In addition, there are several other proteins that are responsible for a form of pleiotropic resistance shown in multidrug-resistant cell lines that do not express P-gp, but do express the multidrug resistance-related protein (MRP) or lung resistance related protein/major vault protein (LRP/MVP). Intracellular concentrations at adequate levels of the antileukemic chemotherapeutic agents daunomycin, mitoxantrone, and etoposide are critical for achieving cell kill of leukemia cells. Several cellular escape mechanisms have been defined that counteract chemotherapy cytotoxicity and confer drug resistance. High P-gp expression results in enhanced P-gp pumping activity and reduced intracellular drug concentrations in MDR-positive cells. Since the recognition of MDR as an independent mechanism of drug resistance, attempts have been made to downregulate P-gp or inhibit its function, using oligonucleotides and protein kinase C (PKC) inhibitors such as staurosporine. Another approach to modulating P-gp is to inhibit its interaction with cytostatic drugs by the use of competitor agents. It is currently accepted that various reversal agents can restore drug accumulation by competing with cytostatic drugs for P-gp-binding sites. These agents include calcium channel blockers, calmodulin inhibitors, immunosuppressive agents, quinolines, indole alkaloids, detergents, steroids, and antiestrogens.[179,180]

There is only limited experience with reversing MDR in AML in vivo[181,182] with mitoxantrone/etoposide, to which cyclosporine was added. Although several responses were noted, the toxicity of this regimen was considerable. In another small study, quinine was used as a reversing agent in refractory AML, and was well tolerated.[183] Two studies evaluated the cyclosporine analog PSC833 as a modulator of drug resistance and showed more induction deaths but reduced late relapse and mortality.[184,213] One of the largest studies to date[185] included 226 patients with refractory and/or relapsed AML. They were treated with daunorubicin plus high-dose cytarabine, to which cyclosporine was added in a dose-escalation design. The toxicity of cyclosporine was dose-dependent and included prolongation of myelosuppression, nausea, and hyperbilirubinemia. The plasma levels of daunorubicin were elevated in patients who received a high dose of cyclosporine. The rate of complete remission was not significantly improved in this group, but both overall and relapse-free survival were significantly increased with the cyclosporine. The results of this study indicate that it is possible to combine a drug-reversal agent such as cyclosporine with combination chemotherapy in AML patients without unacceptable toxicity and with clinical benefit, but additional confirmatory studies are clearly needed.

## Modulation of resistance to chemotherapy with hematopoietic growth factors

Cytarabine is one of the most effective cytotoxic agents included in the induction therapy of AML. It is an analog of 2′-deoxycytidine. It is metabolized to Ara-CTP, the active form. Ara-CTP is incorporated into DNA. This results in slowing of elongation of the nucleotide chain and a defect in the ligation of newly synthesized fragments of DNA. Ara-CTP also acts as an inhibitor of DNA polymerase in competition with deoxycytidine triphosphate (dCTP).

Cytarabine cytotoxicity is S-phase-dependent and related to the rate of DNA synthesis. Reasons for treatment failure of AML patients in response to cytarabine may relate to pharmacological resistance of the leukemia (due, for example, to a deletion of deoxycytidine kinase) or kinetic resistance (cells not in S phase may escape cell killing). Enhanced cytotoxicity of cytarabine against AML colony-forming cells (AML-CFU) following incubation of the cells with G-CSF, interleukin-3 (IL-3), or GM-CSF has been demonstrated by various investigators.[186–188] There is an average threefold increase in the cytotoxicity of cytarabine to AML clonogenic cells in the context of stimulation with GM-CSF (range 2.2- to 229-fold) and IL-3 (range 1.5- to 63.2-fold), corresponding to an additional cell kill at a magnitude of 1–1.5 log on the cytarabine dose–response curve.[189] Costimulation of AML cells with a variety of hematopoietic growth factors in culture enhances the incorporation of Ara-CTP into cellular DNA.[189] GM-CSF may enhance DNA polymerase activity in leukemic cells, and this increased activity is related to augmented cytarabine incorporation and AML cell cytotoxicity[190] G-CSF or GM-CSF has been applied simultaneously with chemotherapy in order to sensitize leukemic cells to the cytotoxic effects of chemotherapy. At present, results from uncontrolled prospective studies[191–193] and several randomized studies of relatively small size (and therefore limited statistical power) are available.[194–197] In two larger studies, GM-CSF was applied both during and after chemotherapy.[168,198] Although these studies were conducted in patients of older age, thus representing poor-prognosis AML, in one of them G-CSF sensitization improved disease-free survival.[198] In one large phase III study, specially and selectively designed to assess the value of growth factor priming, G-CSF was given concomitantly with chemotherapy only and not continued until neutrophil recovery.[212] This study was conducted in adults aged 15–60 years with newly diagnosed AML, and showed a reduced relapse rate and better disease-free survival for those treated with G-CSF. The advantage was apparent mainly in patients with AML of intermediate prognosis (according to cytogenetics).[212] Clearly, the therapeutic concept of growth factor priming in AML deserves further clinical trial.

## Novel treatment approaches

The limitations of conventional approaches to treatment using various chemotherapy schedules have been described in this chapter. Intensification of treatment has brought better results in younger patients. This in turn has exposed more clearly the risk factors that are valuable in predicting the risk of relapse and has enabled a degree of targeting of treatment (e.g. transplantation). There still remains the major problem of preventing relapse. Allogeneic stem cell transplantation has consistently been shown to be the best modality to prevent relapse, but it continues to be limited by procedural morbidity and mortality and the need for a matched donor. The time-censoring benefit also applies to the transplanted cohorts, while it does not to chemotherapy schedules. The Holy Grail of capturing the graft-versus-host leukemia effect of allografting will continue to be pursued.

It may be, however, that the limits of conventional intensive chemotherapy have been reached, and there is no doubt that, for many patients, (particularly those with high-risk disease or older patients), novel approaches are needed. Over the next few years, targeted treatment will become available aimed at the molecular lesions and/or their consequences that are thought to play key roles in disease causation (see also Chapter 27). Preliminary studies have been initiated of, for example, farnesyl transferase inhibitors aimed at counteracting the effect of *RAS* mutations and kinase inhibitors abrogating the FLT3 receptor mutations.[199,208] Several agents are under development, each of which has provided enticing preclinical data. It will, however, take a significant time before such agents are fully assessed. As the molecular mechanisms unfold, so new targeted drugs will become available. These will be aimed at small groups of patients, and this brings the additional challenge of developing clinical trials that are of sufficient size for the usual statistical rigor. It seems likely that novel approaches to trial statistics are also needed. Another potential way to improve the therapeutic ratio of treatment is by immune targeting. The concept of the 'magic bullet' is not new, but clinical opportunities have only arisen relatively recently. In the context of AML, the CD33 antigen has become the focus of attention. It is expressed in 90% of cases of AML, and, as far as is known, is not expressed on normal tissues. It is expressed on normal hematopoietic precursors, but not stem cells. This is a favorable profile, but might also be a limitation if leukemic stem cells also do not express CD33.

Naked antibodies, whether or not humanized to enable repeated use, have met with little success as single agents.[200] However, the coupling of a toxic agent to the antibody is an attractive concept, particularly as the CD33 antigen–antibody complex is rapidly internalized to the cell, thus providing an ideal drug delivery system. Gemtuzumab ozogamicin has been developed as such an agent. This is a humanized anti-CD33 monoclonal antibody that is coupled to the powerful antitumor antibiotic calicheamicin (see the section on targeted leukemic cell killing earlier in this chapter). Early clinical trials demonstrated a favorable side-effect profile and efficacy in that 30% of relapsed patients achieved second remission.[157,201]

On this basis, the drug received regulatory approval in the USA for the treatment of relapse in patients over 60 years. There are a number of situations in which this agent could find a role. Several studies are using it as a component of an overall treatment plan, either in sequence with courses of chemotherapy or giving it coincidentally with chemotherapy. This latter approach must be introduced with care and with a reduced dose of the immunoconjugate, since preliminary studies suggest that coincidental use will result in important hepatotoxicity.[202] Careful clinical trials of these new approaches will require patience, but may well open the way to many more directed treatment approaches.

Modern laboratory techniques (see also Chapter 20) such as expression profiling and proteomics promise much in relation to diagnostics, prognostication, treatment choices, and the development of molecularly targeted treatments.[205,206]

## REFERENCES

1. Fialkow PJ, Singer JW, Adamson JW et al. Acute non-lymphatic leukemia: heterogenity of stem cell origin. *Blood* 1981; **57**: 1068–73.
2. Griffin JD, Löwenberg B. Clonogenic cells in acute myeloblastic leukemia. *Blood* 1986; **68**: 1185–95.
3. Fialkow PJ, Singer JW, Raskind WH et al. Clonal development, stem cell differentiation, and clinical remission in acute nonlymphocytic leukemia. *N Engl J Med* 1987; **317**: 468–73.
4. Keinänen M, Griffin JD, Bloomfield CD et al. Clonal chromosomal abnormalities showing multiple-cell-lineage involvement in acute myeloid leukemia. *N Engl J Med* 1988; **318**: 1153–8.
5. Salem M, Delwel R, Mahmoud LA et al. Maturation of human acute myeloid leukemia in vitro: the response to five recombinant haematopoietic factors in a serum free system. *Br J Haematol* 1989; **71**: 363–70.
6. Touw I, Löwenberg B. Variable differentiation of human acute myeloid leukemia during colony formation in vitro: a membrane marker analysis with monoclonal antibodies. *Br J Haematol* 1985; **59**: 37–44.
7. Chang LJA, Till JE, McCulloch EA. The cellular basis of self-renewal in culture by human acute myeloblastic leukemia blast cell progenitors. *J Cell Physiol* 1980; **102**: 217–22.
8. De Lord C, Clutterbuck R, Titley J et al. Growth of primary human acute leukemia in severe combined immunodeficient mice. *Exp Hematol* 1991; **19**: 991–3.
9. Sawyers CL, Gishizky ML, Quan S et al. Propagation of human blastic myeloid leukemias in the SCID mouse. *Blood* 1992; **79**: 2089–98.
10. Namikawa R, Ueda R, Kyoizumi S. Growth of human myeloid leukemias in the human marrow environment of the SCID-hu mice. *Blood* 1993; **82**: 2526–36.
11. Lapidot T, Sirard C, Vormoor J et al. A cell initiating human acute myeloid leukemia after transplantation into SCID mice. *Nature* 1994; **367**: 645–8.
12. Bonnet D, Dick JE. Human acute myeloid leukemia is organised as a hierarchy that originates from a primitive hematopoietic cell. *Nat Med* 1997; **3**: 730–7.
13. Terpstra W, Prins A, Ploemacher RE et al. Long-term leukemia-initiating capacity of a CD34 subpopulation of acute myeloid leukemia. *Blood* 1996; **87**: 2187–94.
14. Terpstra W, Ploemacher RE, Prins A et al. Fluorouracil selectively spares acute myeloid leukemia cells with long-term growth abilities in immunodeficient mice and in culture. *Blood* 1996; **88**: 1944–50.
15. Sawyers C, Denny CT, Witte ON. Leukemia and the disruption of normal hematopoieis. *Cell* 1991; **64**: 337–50.
16. Hunter T. Cooperation between oncogenes. *Cell* 1991; **64**: 249–70.
17. Cline MJ. The molecular basis of leukemia. *N Engl J Med* 1994; **330**: 328–36.
18. Dong F, Hoefsloot LH, Schelen AM et al. Identification of a nonsense mutation in the G-CSF receptor in severe congenital neutropenia. *Proc Natl Acad Sci USA* 1994; **91**: 4480–4.
19. Dong F, Brynes RK, Tidow N, Welte K et al. Mutations in the gene for the G-CSF receptor in patients with AML preceded by congenital neutropenia. *N Engl J Med* 1995; **333**: 487–93.
20. Nakao M, Yokota S, Iwai T et al. Internal tandem duplication of the *Flt-3* gene found in acute myeloid leukemia. *Leukemia* 1996; **10**: 1911–18.
21. Yamamoto Y, Kiyoi H, Nakano Y et al. Activating mutation of D835 within the activation loop of *FLT3* in human hematologic malignancies. *Blood* 2001; **97**: 2434–9.
22. Bos JL, Toksoz D, Marshall CJ et al. Amino acid substitution at codon 13 of the N-*ras* oncogene in human myeloid leukemia. *Nature* 1985; **315**: 726–30.
23. Croce CM, Nowell PC. Molecular basis of human B-cell neoplasia. *Blood* 1985; **65**: 1–7.
24. Kakizuka A, Miller WH Jr, Umesono K et al. Chromosomal translocation t(15;17) in human acute promyelocytic leukemia fuses *RARα* with a novel putative transcription factor *PML*. *Cell* 1991; **66**: 663–74.

25. Fenaux P, Preudhomme C, Quiquandon I et al. Mutations of the *p53* gene in acute myeloid leukemia. *Br J Haematol* 1992; **80**: 178–83.

26. Löwenberg B, Touw IP. Hematopoietic growth factors and their receptors in acute leukemia. *Blood* 1993; **81**: 281–92.

27. Longmore GD, Lodish HF. An activating mutation in the murine erythropoietin receptor induces erythroleukemia in mice: a cytokine receptor superfamily oncogene. *Cell* 1991; **67**: 1089–102.

28. Löwenberg B, Van Putten WLJ, Touw IP et al. Autonomous proliferation of leukemic cells in vitro as a determinant of prognosis in adult acute myeloid leukemia. *N Engl J Med* 1993; **328**: 614–19.

29. Roussel MF, Downing JR, Sherr CJ. Transforming activities of human CSF-1 receptors at codon 301 in their extracellular domaine. *Oncogene* 1990; **5**: 25–30.

30. Yoshimura A, Longmore G, Lodish HF. Point mutation in the exoplasmic domain of the erythropoietin receptor resulting in hormone-independent activation and tumorgenicity. *Nature* 1990; **348**: 647–9.

31. Kiyoi H, Naoe T, Nakano Y et al. Prognostic implication of *Flt3* and N-*ras* gene mutations in acute myeloid leukemia. *Blood* 1999; **93**: 3074–80.

32. Yokota S, Kiyoi H, Nakao M et al. Internal tandem duplication of the *Flt-3* gene is preferentially seen in acute myeloid leukemia and myelodysplastic syndrome among various hematological malignancies: a study on a large series of patients and cell lines. *Leukemia* 1997; **11**: 1605–9.

33. Rombouts WC, Broyl A, Martens ACM et al. Human acute myeloid leukemia cells with internal tandem duplications in the *Flt-3* gene show reduced proliferative ability in stroma supported long-term cultures. *Leukemia* 1999; **13**: 1071–8.

34. Rombouts WJC, Blokland I, Löwenberg B, Ploemacher R. Biological characteristics and prognosis of adult acute myeloid leukemia with internal tandem duplications in the *Flt3* gene. *Leukemia* 2000; **14**: 675–83.

35. Hayakawa F, Towatari M, Kiyoi H et al. Tandem duplicated *Flt3* constitutively activates STAT5 and MAP kinase and introduces autonomous cell growth in IL3 dependent cell lines. *Oncogene* 2000; **19**: 624–31.

36. Meshinchi S, Woods WG, Stirewalt DL et al. Prevalence and prognostic significance of *FLT3* internal tandem duplication in pediatric acute myeloid leukemia. *Blood* 2001; **97**: 89–94.

37. Xu F, Yang HW, Hanada R et al. Tandem duplication of the *FLT3* gene is found in acute lymphoblastic leukaemia as well as acute myeloid leukaemia but not in myelodysplastic syndrome or juvenile chronic myelogenous leukaemia in children. *Br J Haematol* 1999; **105**: 155–62.

38. Kondo M, Horibe K, Takahashi Y et al. Prognostic value of internal tandem duplications of the *FLT3* gene in childhood acute myelogenous leukemia. *Med Pediatr Oncol* 1999; **33**: 525–9.

39. Abu-Duhier FM, Goodeve AC, Wilson GA et al. *FLT3* internal tandem duplications mutations in adult acute myeloid leukaemia define a high-risk group. *Br J Haematol* 2000; **111**: 190–5.

40. Berghini A, Larizza I, Cairoli R, Morra E. c-*kit* activating mutations and mast cell proliferation in human leukemia. *Blood* 1998; **92**: 701–2.

41. Berghini A, Peterlongo P, Ripamonti CB et al. c-*kit* mutations in core binding leukemias. *Blood* 2000; **95**: 726–7.

42. Care RS, Valk PJM, Goodeve AC et al. Incidence and prognosis of c-*kit* and *flt3* mutations in core binding factor (CBF) acute myeloid leukaemias. *Br J Haematol* 2003; **121**: 775–7.

43. Kottaridis PD, Gale RE, Frew ME et al. The presence of a *FLT3* internal tandem duplication in patients with acute myeloid leukemia (AML) adds important prognostic information to cytogenetic risk group and response to the first cycle of chemotherapy: analysis of 854 patients from the United Kingdom Medical Research Council AML10 and 12 trials. *Blood* 2001; **98**: 1752–9.

44. Thiede C, Steudel C, Mohr B et al. Analysis of *FLT3*-activating mutations in 979 patients with acute myelogenous leukemia: association with FAB subtypes and identification of subgroups with poor prognosis. *Blood* 2002; **99**: 4326–36.

45. Liang DC, Shih LY, Hung IJ et al. Clinical relevance of internal tandem duplication of the *FLT3* gene in childhood acute myeloid leukemia. *Cancer* 2002; **94**: 3292–8.

46. Fröhling S, Schlenk RF, Breitruck J et al. Prognostic significance of activating *FLT3* mutations in younger adults (16–60 yrs) with acute myeloid leukemia and normal cytogenetics: a study of the Acute Myeloid Leukemia Study Group Ulm. *Blood* 2002; **100**: 4372–80.

47. Schnittger S, Schoch C, Dugas M et al. Analysis of *FLT3* length mutations in 1003 patients with acute myeloid leukemia: correlation to cytogenetics, FAB subtype, and prognosis in the AMLCG study and usefulness as a marker for the detection of minimal residual disease. *Blood* 2002; **100**: 59–66.

48. Ferrao P, Macmillan EM, Ashman LK, Gonda TJ. Enforced expression of full length c-Myb leads to density-dependent transformation of murine haemapoietic cells. *Oncogene* 1995; **11**: 1631–8.

49. Gari M, Goodeye A, Wilson G et al. c-*kit* proto-oncogene exon 8 in-frame deletion plus insertion mutations in acute myeloid leukaemia. *Br J Haematol* 1999; **105**: 894–900.

50. Smith FO, Broudy VC, Zsebo KM et al. Cell surface expression of c-kit receptors by childhood acute myeloid leukemia blasts is not of prognostic value: a report from the Childrens Cancer Group. *Blood* 1994; **84**: 847–52.

51. Dong F, Dale DC, Bonilla MA et al. Mutations in the granulocyte colony-stimulating factor receptor gene in patients with severe congenital neutropenia. *Leukemia* 1997; **11**: 120–5.

52. Ward AC, Van Aesch YM, Gits J et al. A point mutation in the extracellular domain of the granulocyte colony-stimulating factor (G-CSF) receptor in a case of severe congenital neutropenia hyporesponsive to G-CSF treatment. *J Exp Med* 1999; **190**: 497–507.

53. Bennett JM, Catovsky D, Daniel MT et al. Proposals for the classification of the acute leukaemias (FAB cooperative group). *Br J Haematol* 1976; **33**: 451–8.

54. Bennett JM, Catovsky D, Daniel MT et al. A variant form of acute hypergranular promyelocytic leukaemia (M3). *Br J Haematol* 1980; **44**: 169–70.

55. Bennett JM, Catovsky D, Daniel MT et al. Criteria for the diagnosis of acute leukemia of megakaryocytic lineage (M7): a report of the French–American–British cooperative group. *Ann Intern Med* 1985; **103**: 460–2.

56. Bennett JM, Catovsky D, Daniel MT et al. Proposed revised criteria for the classification of acute myeloid leukemia. *Ann Intern Med* 1985; **103**: 620–9.

57. Vardiman JW, Harris NL, Brunning RD. World Health

Organization (WHO) classification of the myeloid neoplasms. *Blood* 2002; **100**: 2292–302.

58. Jaffe ES, Harris NL, Stein N, Vardiman (eds). *World Health Organization Classification of Tumours. Pathology and Genetics of Tumours of Haematopoietic and Lymphoid Tissues.* Lyon: IARC Press, 2001: Chap 4.

59. Sanz MA, Sempere A. Immunophenotyping of AML and MDS and detection of residual disease. *Clin Haematol* 1996; **9**: 35–55.

60. Löwenberg B, Downing JR, Burnett AK. Acute myeloid leukemia. *N Engl J Med* 1999; **341**: 1051–62.

61. Berman E. Chemotherapy in acute myelogenous leukemia: higher dose, higher expectations? *J Clin Oncol* 1995; **13**: 1–4.

62. Yates J, Glidewell O, Wiernik P et al. Cytosine arabinoside with daunomycin or Adriamycin for therapy of acute myelocytic leukemia: a CALGB study. *Blood* 1982; **60**: 454–63.

63. Bishop JF, Lowenthal PM, Joshua D et al. Etoposide in acute non-lymphoblastic leukemia. *Blood* 1990; **75**: 27–32.

64. Hann IM, Stevens RF, Goldstone AH et al. Randomized comparison of DAT versus ADE as induction chemotherapy in children and younger adults with acute myeloid leukaemia. Results of the Medical Research Council's 10th AML trial (MRC AML 10). *Blood* 1997; **89**: 2311–18.

65. Goldstone AH, Burnett AK, Wheatley K et al. Attempts to improve treatment outcomes in acute myeloid leukemia (AML) in older patients: the results of the United Kingdom Medical Research Council AML11 trial. *Blood* 2001; **98**: 1302–11.

66. Mitus AJ, Miller KB, Schenkein DP et al. Improved survival for patients with acute myelogenous leukemia. *J Clin Oncol* 1995; **13**: 560–9.

67. Philips GL, Reece DE, Shepherd JD et al. High-dose cytarabine and daunorubicin induction and postremission chemotherapy for the treatment of acute myelogenous leukemia in adults. *Blood* 1991; **77**: 1429–35.

68. Forman SJ, Nademanee AP, O'Donnell MR et al. High dose cytosine arabinoside and daunorubicin as primary therapy for adults with acute non-lymphoblastic leukemia: a pilot study. *Semin Oncol* 1985; **12**: 114–16.

69. Bishop JF, Matthews JP, Young GA et al. A randomised study of high-dose cytarabine in induction in acute myeloid leukemia. *Blood* 1996; **87**: 1710–17.

70. Weick JK, Kopecky KJ, Appelbaum FR et al. A randomized investigation of high-dose versus standard dose cytosine arabinoside with daunorubicin in patients with previously untreated acute myeloid leukemia: a Southwest Oncology Group study. *Blood* 1996; **88**: 2841–51.

71. Gonzalez-Llaven J, Rubio-Borja KE, Martinez O. Efficacy of idarubicin plus Ara-C in induction remission of de novo adult acute non-lymphoblastic leukemia. *Haematologica* 1991; **76**: 128.

72. Reiffers J, Hurteloup P, Stoppa AM et al. A prospective controlled study comparing idarubicin and daunorubicin as induction treatment for acute non-lymphoblastic leukemia in the elderly. *Haematologica* 1988; **73**(Suppl 1): 126.

73. Vogler WR, Velez-Garcia E, Weiner RS et al. A phase III trial comparing idarubicin and daunorubicin in combination with cytarabine in acute myelogenous leukemia: a Southeastern Cancer Study Group study. *J Clin Oncol* 1992; **10**: 1103–11.

74. Wiernik PH, Banks PLC, Case DC Jr et al. Cytarabine plus idarubicin or daunorubicin as induction and consolidation therapy for previously untreated adult patients with acute myeloid leukemia. *Blood* 1992; **79**: 313–19.

75. Mandelli F, Petti MC, Ardia A et al. A multicentric study from the Italian Cooperative Group GIMEMA. *Eur J Cancer* 1991; **27**: 750–5.

76. Berman E, Heller G, Santorsa J et al. Results of a randomized trial comparing idarubicin and cytosine arabinoside in adult patients with newly diagnosed acute myelogenous leukemia. *Blood* 1991; **77**: 1666–74.

77. Arlin Z, Case DC, Moore J et al. Randomized multicenter trial of cytosine arabinoside with mitoxantrone or daunorubicin in previously untreated adult patients with acute non-lymphoblastic leukemia (ANLL). *Leukemia* 1990; **4**: 177–83.

78. Wahlin A, Hornstein P, Hedenus M, Malm C. Mitoxantrone and cytarabine versus daunorubicin and cytarabine in previously treated patients with acute myeloid leukemia. *Cancer Chemother Pharmacol* 1991; **28**: 480–3.

79. Löwenberg B, Suciu S, Archimbaud E et al. Mitoxantrone versus daunorubicin in induction-consolidation chemotherapy, the value of low-dose cytarabine for maintenance of remission and an assessment of prognostic factors in acute myeloid leukemia in the elderly: final report of the Leukemia Cooperative Group of the European Organization for the Research and Treatment of Cancer and the Dutch–Belgian Hemato-Oncology Cooperative HOVON Group. Randomized phase III study AML-9. *J Clin Oncol* 1998; **16**: 872–81.

80. Roos JKH, Gray RG, Wheatley K. Dose intensification in acute myeloid leukaemia: greater effectiveness at lower cost. Principal report of the Medical Research Council's AML9 study. MRC Leukaemia in Adults Working Party. *Br J Haematol* 1996; **94**: 89–98.

81. Burnett AK, Wheatley K, Goldstone AH et al. MRC AML12: a comparison of ADE vs MAE and S-DAT vs H-DAT + retinoic acid for induction and four vs five total courses using chemotherapy or stem cell transplant in consolidation in 3459 patients under 60 years with AML. *Blood* 2002; **100**: 155a.

82. Kobayashi T, Miyawaki S, Tanimoto M et al. Randomized trials between behenoyl cytarabine and cytarabine in combination induction and consolidation therapy, and with or without ubenimex after maintenance/intensification therapy in adult acute myeloid leukemia. *J Clin Oncol* 1996; **14**: 204–13.

83. Büchner TH, Urnbanitz D, Hiddemann W et al. Intensified induction and consolidation with or without maintenance chemotherapy for acute myeloid leukemia (AML): two multicenter studies of the German AML Cooperative Group. *J Clin Oncol* 1985; **3**: 1583–9.

84. Cassileth PA, Lynch E, Hines JD et al. Varying intensity of postremission therapy in acute myeloid leukemia. *Blood* 1992; **79**: 1924–30.

85. Wolff SN, Herzig RH, Fay JW et al. High-dose cytarabine and daunorubicin as consolidation therapy for acute myeloid leukemia in first remission: long-term follow up and results. *J Clin Oncol* 1989; **7**: 1260–7.

86. Mayer RJ, Davis RB, Schiffer CA et al. Intensive postremission chemotherapy in adults with acute myeloid leukemia. *N Engl J Med* 1994; **331**: 896–903.

87. Burnett AK, Wheatley AH, Goldstone RF et al. The value

of allogeneic bone marrow transplant in patients with acute myeloid leukaemia at differing risk of relapse: results of the UK MRC AML10 trial. *Br J Haematol* 2002; **118**: 385–400.

88. Wheatley K, Burnett AK, Gibson B et al. Optimising consolidation therapy: four versus five courses SCT versus chemotherapy – preliminary results of MRC AML12. *Hematol J* 2002; **3**: 159–60.

89. Bloomfield CD, Lawrence D, Byrd JC et al. Frequency of prolonged remission duration after high-dose cytarabine intensification in acute myeloid leukemia varies by cytogenetic subtype. *Cancer Res* 1998; **58**: 4173–9.

90. Appelbaum FR, Fisher LD, Thomas D et al. Chemotherapy versus marrow transplantation for adults with acute non-lymphoblastic leukemia: a five-year follow up. *Blood* 1988; **72**: 179–84.

91. McGlave PB, Haake RJ, Bodstrom BC et al. Allogeneic bone marrow transplantation for acute non-lymphocytic leukemia in first remission. *Blood* 1988; **72**: 1512–17.

92. Reiffers J, Gaspard MH, Maraninchi D et al. Comparison of allogeneic or autologous bone marrow transplantation and chemotherapy in patients with acute myeloid leukemia in first remission: a prospective controlled trial. *Br J Haematol* 1989; **72**: 57–63.

93. Gray R, Wheatley K. How to avoid bias when comparing bone marrow transplantation with chemotherapy. *Bone Marrow Transplant* 1991; **7**: 9–12.

94. Gale RP, Horowitz MM, Weiner RS et al. Impact of cytogenetic abnormalities on outcome of bone marrow transplants in acute myelogenous leukemia in first remission. *Bone Marrow Transplant* 1995; **16**: 203–8.

95. Keating S, de Witte T, Suciu S et al. The influence of HLA-matched sibling donor availability on treatment outcome for patients with AML: an analysis of the AML 8A study of the EORTC Leukaemia Cooperative Group and GIMEMA. *Br J Haematol* 1998; **102**: 1344–53.

96. Slovak ML, Kopecky J, Cassileth PA et al. Karyotypic analysis predicts outcome of preremission and postremission therapy in adult acute myeloid leukemia: a Southwest Oncology Group/Eastern Cooperative Group study. *Blood* 2000; **96**: 4075–83.

97. Burnett AK, Tansey P, Watkins R et al. Transplantation of unpurged autologous bone marrow in acute myeloid leukemia in first remission. *Lancet* 1984; **ii**: 1068–70.

98. Löwenberg B, Abels J, Van Bekkum DW et al. Transplantation of non-purified autologous bone marrow in patients with AML in first remission. *Cancer* 1984; **54**: 2840–3.

99. Stewart R, Buckner C, Bensinger W et al. Autologous marrow transplantation in patients with acute non-lymphocytic leukemia in first remission. *Exp Hematol* 1985; **13**: 267–72.

100. Goldstone AH, Anderson CC, Linch DC et al. Autologous bone marrow transplantation following high dose therapy for the treatment of adult patients with acute myeloid leukaemia. *Br J Haematol* 1986; **64**: 529–37.

101. Löwenberg B, Verdonck LJ, Dekker AW et al. Autologous bone marrow transplantation in acute myeloid leukemia in first remission: results of Dutch prospective study. *J Clin Oncol* 1990; **8**: 287–94.

102. Gorin NC, Labopin M, Meloni G et al. Autologous bone marrow transplantation for acute myeloid leukemia in Europe: further evidence of the role of marrow purging by mafosfamide. *Leukemia* 1997; **5**: 896–904.

103. Amadori S, Testi AM, Arico M et al. Prospective comparative study on bone marrow transplantation and post-remission chemotherapy for childhood acute myelogenous leukemia. *J Clin Oncol* 1993; **11**: 1046–54.

104. Ravindranath Y, Yeager AM, Chang MN et al. Autologous bone marrow transplantation versus intensive consolidation chemotherapy for acute myeloid leukemia in childhood. *N Engl J Med* 1996; **334**: 1428–34.

105. Woods WG, Neudorf S, Gold S et al. A comparison of allogeneic bone marrow transplantation, autologous bone marrow transplantation, and aggressive chemotherapy in children with acute myeloid leukemia in remission: a report from the Children's Cancer Group. *Blood* 2000; **97**: 56–62.

106. Burnett AK. Transplantation in first remission of acute myeloid leukemia. *N Engl J Med* 1998; **339**: 1698–1700.

107. Woods et al. Intensive Chemotherapy vs BMT in pediatric AML – a matter of controversies. *Blood* 2001–2002 Letter.

108. Zittoun RA, Mandelli F, Willemze R et al. Autologous or allogeneic bone marrow transplantation compared with intensive chemotherapy in acute myelogenous leukemia. *N Engl J Med* 1995; **332**: 217–23.

109. Harousseau JL, Pignon B, Dufour P et al. Autologous bone marrow transplantation vs intensive chemotherapy in first complete remission: interim results of GOELAM study in AML. *Leukemia* 1992; **6**: 120–3.

110. Cassileth PA, Harrington DP, Appelbaum F et al. Chemotherapy compared with autologous or allogeneic bone marrow transplantation in the management of acute myeloid leukemia in first remission. *N Engl J Med* 1998; **339**: 1649–56.

111. Demirer T, Buckner CD, Appelbaum FR et al. Rapid engraftment after autologous transplantation utilizing marrow and recombinant granulocyte colony-stimulating factor-mobilized peripheral blood stem cells in patients with acute myelogenous leukemia. *Bone Marrow Transplant* 1995; **15**: 915–22.

112. Gale RP, Horowitz MM, Rees JKH et al. Chemotherapy versus transplants for acute myelogenous leukemia in second remission. *Leukemia* 1996; **10**: 13–19.

113. Yunis JJ, Brunning RD, Howe RB, Lobell M. High-resolution chromosomes as an independent prognostic indicator in adult acute nonlymphocytic leukemia. *N Engl J Med* 1984; **311**: 812–18.

114. Keating MJ, Smith TL, Kantarjian H et al. Cytogenetic pattern in acute myelogenous leukemia: a major reproducible determinant of outcome. *Leukemia* 1988; **2**: 403–12.

115. Mrozek K, Heinonen K, de la Chapelle A, Bloomfield CD. Clinical significance of cytogenetics in acute myeloid leukemia. *Semin Oncol* 1997; **24**: 17–31.

116. Grimwade D, Walker H, Oliver F et al. The importance of diagnostic cytogenetics on outcome in AML: analysis of 1,612 patients entered into the MRC AML 10 trial. *Blood* 1998; **92**: 2322–33.

117. DiMartino JF, Cleary ML. *MLL* rearrangements in haematological malignancies: lessons from clinical and biological studies. *Br J Haematol* 1999; **106**: 614–26.

118. Stevens RF, Hann IM, Wheatley K, Gray RG. Marked improvements in outcome with chemotherapy alone in paediatric acute myeloid leukaemia: results of the United Kingdom Medical Research Council's 10th AML trial. *Br J Haematol* 1998; **101**: 130–40.

119. Wheatley K, Burnett AK, Goldstone AH et al. A simple,

robust, validated and highly predictive index for the determination of risk-directed therapy in acute myeloid leukemia derived from the MRC AML 10 trial. *Br J Haematol* 1999; **107**: 69–79.

120. Löwenberg B. Prognostic factors in acute myeloid leukemia. *Baillière's Clin Haematol* 2001; **14**: 65–706.

121. Nguyen S, Leblanc T, Fenaux P et al. A white blood cell index as the main prognostic factor in t(8;21) acute myeloid leukemia (AML): a survey of 161 cases from the French AML Intergroup. *Blood* 2002; **99**: 3517–23.

122. Thiede C, Steudel C, Mohr B et al. Analysis of *FLT3*-activating mutations in 979 patients with acute myelogenous leukemia: association with FAB subtypes and identification of subgroups with poor prognosis. *Blood* 2002; **99**: 4326–36.

123. Schnittger S, Schoch C, Dugas M et al. Analysis of *FLT3* length mutations in 1003 patients with acute myeloid leukemia: correlation to cytogenetics, FAB subtype, and prognosis in the AMLCG study and usefulness as a marker for the detection of minimal residual disease. *Blood* 2002; **100**: 59–66.

124. Liang DC, Shih LY, Hung IJ et al. Clinical relevance of internal tandem duplication of the *FLT3* gene in childhood acute myeloid leukemia. *Cancer* 2002; **94**: 3292–8.

125. Whitman SP, Archer KJ, Feng L et al. Absence of the wild type allele predicts poor prognosis in adult de novo acute myeloid leukemia: a Southwest Oncology Group/Eastern Cooperative Oncology Group study. *Blood* 2000; **96**: 4075–83.

126. Nakano Y, Naoe T, Kiyoi H et al. Prognostic value of *p53* gene mutations and the product expression in de novo acute myeloid leukemia. *Eur J Haematol* 2000; **65**: 23–31.

127. Karakas T, Miething CC, Maurer U et al. The coexpression of the apoptosis-related genes *bcl-2* and *wt1* in predicting survival in adult acute myeloid leukemia. *Leukemia* 2002; **16**: 846–54.

128. Döhner K, Tobis K, Ulrich R et al. Prognostic significance of partial tandem duplications of the *MLL* gene in adult patients 16 to 60 years old with acute myeloid leukemia and normal cytogenetics: a study of the Acute Myeloid Leukemia Study Group Ulm. *J Clin Oncol* 2002; **20**: 3254–61.

129. Van Waalwijk van Doorn-Khosrovani SB, Erpelinck C, Van Putten WLJ et al. High *EVI1* expression predicts poor survival in acute myeloid leukemia: a study of 319 de novo AML patients. *Blood* 2003; **101**: 837–45.

130. Preudhomme C, Sagot Ch, Boissel N et al. Favorable prognostic significance of *CEPPA* mutations in patients with de novo acute myeloid leukemia: a study from the Acute Leukemia French Association (ALFA). *Blood* 2002; **100**: 2717–23.

131. Van Waalwijk van Doorn-Khosrovani SB, Erpelinck C, Meijer J et al. Biallelic mutations in the *CEBPA* gene and low *CEBPA* expression levels as prognostic markers in intermediate-risk AML. *Hematol J* 2002; **3**: 324.

132. Geller RB, Zuhurak M, Hurwitz CA et al. Prognostic importance of immunophenotyping in adults in acute myelocytic leukaemia: The significance of the stem cell glycoprotein CD-34 (MY10). *Br J Haematol* 1990; **76**: 340–7.

133. Priker R, Wallner J, Geissler K et al. *MDR1* gene expression and treatment outcome in acute myeloid leukemia. *J Natl Cancer Inst* 1991; **83**: 708–12.

134. Marie JP, Zittoun R, Sikic BI. Multidrug resistance *(MDR1)* gene expression in adult acute leukemias: correlations with treatment outcome and in vitro drug sensitivity. *Blood* 1991; **78**: 586–92.

135. Campos L, Guyotat D, Archimbaud F, et al. Clinical significance of multidrug resistance P-glycoprotein expression on acute nonlymphoblastic leukemia cells at diagnosis. *Blood* 1992; **79**: 473–6.

136. Te Boekhorst PAW, De Leeuw K, Schoester et al. Predominance of functional multidrug resistance (MDR-1) phenotype in CD34+ leukemia cells. *Blood* 1993; **82**: 3157–62.

137. Ino T, Miyazaki H, Tsogai M et al. Expression of P-glycoprotein in de novo acute myelogenous leukemia at initial diagnosis: results of molecular and functional assays, and correlation with treatment outcome. *Leukemia* 1994; **8**: 1492–7.

138. Nucifora G, Larson RA, Rowley JD. Persistence of the 8;21 translocation in patients with acute myeloid leukemia type M2 in long-term remission. *Blood* 1993; **82**: 712.

139. Kusec R, Laczika K, Knobl P et al. *AML1/ETO* fusion mRNA can be detected in remission blood samples of all patients with t(8;12) acute myeloid leukemia after chemotherapy or autologous bone marrow transplantation. *Leukemia* 1994; **8**: 735–9.

140. Saunders MJ, Tobal K, Liu Yin JA. Detection of t(8;12) by reverse transcriptase polymerase chain reaction in patients in remission of acute myeloid leukaemia type M2 after chemotherapy or bone marrow transplantation. *Leuk Res* 1994; **18**: 891.

141. Jurlander J, Caliguri MA, Ruutu T et al. Persistence of the *AML1/ETO* fusion transcript in patients treated with allogeneic bone marrow transplantation for t(8;21) leukemia. *Blood* 1996; **88**: 2183–91.

142. Morschhauser F, Cayenla JM, Martinieta S. Evaluation of minimal residual disease using reverse-transcription polymerase chain reaction in t(8;21) acute myeloid leukemia: a multicenter study of 51 patients. *J Clin Oncol* 2000; **18**: 788–95.

143. Muto A, Mori S, Matsushita H et al. Serial quantiation of minimal residual disease of t(8;21) acute myelogenous leukemia with RT-competitive PCR assay. *Br J Haematol* 1996; **95**: 85–94.

144. Claxton DF, Liu P, Hsu HB et al. Detection of fusion transcripts generated by the inversion 16 chromosome in acute myelogenous leukemia. *Blood* 1994; **83**: 1750–6.

145. Hebert J, Cayuela J, Daniel MT et al. Detection of minimal residual disease in acute myelomonocytic leukemia with abnormal marrow eosinophils by nested polymerase chain reaction with allele specific amplification. *Blood* 1994; **84**: 2291–6.

146. Tobal K, Johnson PR, Saunders MJ et al. Detection of *CBFβ/MYH11* transcripts in patients with inversion and other abnormalities of chromosome 16 at presentation and remission. *Br J Haematol* 1995; **91**: 104–8.

147. Guerrasio A, Pilatrino C, De Micheli D et al. Assessment of minimal residual disease (MRD) in *CBFβ/MYH11*-positive acute myeloid leukemias by qualitative and quantitative RT–PCR amplification of fusion transcripts. *Leukemia* 2002; **16**: 1176–81.

148. Van der Reijden BA, Simons A, Luiten E et al. Minimal residual disease quantification in patients with acute myeloid leukaemia and inv(16)/*CBFβ–MYH11* gene fusion. *Br J Haematol* 2002; **118**: 411–18.

149. Marcucci G, Caligiuri MA, Dohner H et al. Quantification of *CBFβ/MYH11* fusion transcript by real time RT–PCR in patients with inv(16) acute myeloid leukemia. *Leukemia* 2001; **15**: 1072–80.

150. Evans PA, Short MA, Jack AS et al. Detection and quantitation of the *CBFβ/MYH11* transcripts associated with the inv(16) in presentation and follow-up samples from patients with AML. *Leukemia* 1997; **11**: 364–9.

151. Buonamici S, Ottaviani E, Testoni N et al. Real-time quantitation of minimal residual disease in inv(16)-positive acute myeloid leukemia may indicate risk for clinical relapse and may identify patients in a curable state. *Blood* 2002; **99**: 443–9.

152. Matino JF, Cleary ML. *MLL* rearrangements in haematological malignancies: lessons from clinical and biological studies. *Br J Haematol* 1999; **106**: 614–26.

153. Mitterbauer G, Zimmer C, Fonatch C et al. Monitoring of minimal residual leukemia in patients with *MLL–AF9* positive acute myeloid leukemia by RT–PCR. *Leukemia* 1999; **13**: 1519–26.

154. Lin Yin LA, Tobal K. Detection of minimal residual disease in acute myeloid leukaemia: methodologies, clinical and biological significance. *Br J Haematol* 1999; **106**: 578–90.

155. Rozemuller H, Terpstra W, Rombouts EJC et al. GM-CSF receptor targeted treatment of primary AML in SCID mice using *Diphtheria* toxin fused to huGM-CSF. *Leukemia* 1998; **12**: 1962–70.

156. Terpstra W, Rozemuller H, Breems DA et al. *Diphtheria* toxin fused to GM-CSF eliminates AML cells with the potential to initiate leukemia in immunodeficient mice, but spares normal hemopoietic stem cells. *Blood* 1997; **90**: 3735–42.

157. Sievers EL, Appelbaum FR, Spielberger RT et al. Selective ablation of acute myeloid leukemia using antibody-targeted chemotherapy: a phase I study of an anti-CD33 calicheamicin immunoconjugate. *Blood* 1999; **93**: 3678–84.

158. Scheinberg DA, Lovett D, Diugi CR et al. A phase I trial of monoclonal antibody M195 in acute myelogenous leukemia: specific bone marrow targeting and internalization of radionuclide. *J Clin Oncol* 1991; **9**: 478.

159. Levis M, Allebach J, Tse KF, et al. A FLT3-targeted tyrosine kinase inhibitor is cytotoxic to leukemia cells in vitro and in vivo. *Blood* 2002; **99**: 3885–92.

160. Thuy Le D, Shannon KM. Ras processing as a therapeutic target in hematologic malignancies. *Curr Opin Hematol* 2002; **9**: 308–16.

161. Melnick A, Licht JD. Histone deacetylases as therapeutic targets in hematologic malignancies. *Curr Opin Hematol* 2002; **9**: 322–33.

162. Brinker H. Population-based age and sex specific incidence rates in the 4 main types of leukemia. *Scand J Haematol* 1982; **29**: 241–9.

163. Brinker H. Estimate of overall treatment results in acute non-lymphocytic leukemia based on age specific rates of incidence and complete remission. *Cancer Treat Rep* 1985; **65**: 5–11.

164. Liu Yin JA. Acute myeloid leukaemia in the elderly: biology and treatment. *Br J Haematol* 1993; **83**: 1–6.

165. Löwenberg B, Zittoun R, Kerkhofs H et al. On the value of intensive remission-induction chemotherapy in elderly patients of 65+ years with acute myeloid leukemia: a randomised phase III study of the EORTC Leukemia Group. *J Clin Oncol* 1989; **7**: 1268–74.

166. Löwenberg B. Treatment of the elderly patient with acute leukaemia. *Baillière's Clin Haematol* 1996; **9**: 147–60.

167. Bow EJ, Sutherland JA, Kilpatrick MG et al. Therapy of untreated acute myeloid leukemia in the elderly: remission-induction using a non-cytarabine-containing regimen of mitoxantrone plus etoposide. *J Clin Oncol* 1996; **14**: 1345–52.

168. Löwenberg B, Suciu S, Archimbaud E et al. Use of recombinant granulocyte–macrophage colony-stimulating factor during and after remission induction chemotherapy in patients aged 61 years and older with acute myeloid leukemia (AML): final report of AML-11, a phase III randomized study of the Leukemia Cooperative Group of European Organisation for the Research and Treatment of Cancer (EORTC-LCG) and the Dutch Belgian Hemato-Oncology Cooperative Group (HOVON). *Blood* 1997; **20**: 2952–61.

169. Stone RM, Berg DT, George SL et al. Granulocyte–macrophage colony-stimulating factor after initial chemotherapy for elderly patients with primary acute myelogenous leukemia. *N Engl J Med* 1995; **332**: 1671–7.

170. Liu Yin JA, Johnson PRE, Davies JM et al. Mitozantrone and cytosine arabinoside as first-line therapy in elderly patients with acute myeloid leukemia. *Br J Haematol* 1991; **79**: 415–20.

171. Rees JKH, Gray RG, Swirsky D, Hayhoe FGF. Principal results of the Medical Research Council's 8th Acute Myeloid Leukemia trial. *Lancet* 1986; **ii**: 1236–41.

172. Terpstra WE, Löwenberg B. Application of myeloid growth factors in the treatment of acute myeloid leukemia. *Leukemia* 1997; **11**: 315–27.

173. Schiffer CA. Hematopoietic growth factors as adjuncts to the treatment of acute myeloid leukemia. *Blood* 1996; **88**: 3675–85.

174. Rowe JM, Liesveld JL. Hematopoietic growth factors in acute leukemia. *Leukemia* 1997; **11**: 328–41.

175. Ohno R, Tomonaga M, Kobayashi T et al. Effect of granulocyte colony-stimulating factor after intensive induction therapy in relapsed or refractory acute leukemia. *N Engl J Med* 1990; **323**: 871–7.

176. Godwin JR, Kopecky KJ, Head DR et al. A double blind placebo controlled trial of G-CSF in elderly patients with previously untreated acute myeloid leukemia. *Blood* 1995; **86**(Suppl 1): 434a.

177. Rowe JM, Andersen J, Mazza JJ et al. A randomized placebo-controlled study of granulocyte–macrophage colony-stimulating factor in adult patients (>55–70 years of age) with acute myelogenous leukemia (AML): a study of the Eastern Cooperative Oncology Group (E1490). *Blood* 1995; **86**: 457–62.

178. Kartner N, Riordan JR, Ling V. Cell surface P-glycoprotein associated with multidrug resistance in mammalian cell lines. *Science* 1983; **221**: 1285–8.

179. Beck WT. Multidrug resistance and its circumvention. *Eur J Cancer* 1990; **26**: 513–15.

180. Sonneveld P. Mulidrug resistance in acute leukemia. *Baillière's Clin Haematol* 1996; **9**: 185–205.

181. Sonneveld P, Nooter K. Reversal of drug-resistance by cyclosporin-A in a patient with acute myelocytic leukemia. *Br J Haematol* 1990; **75**: 208–11.

182. Marie JP, Bastie JN, Colana F et al. Cyclosporin A as a modifier agent in the salvage treatment of acute leukemia (AL). *Leukemia* 1993; **7**: 821–4.

183. Solary E, Caillot D, Chauffert B et al. Feasibility of using quinine, a potential multidrug resistance-reversing agent, in combination with mitoxantrone and cytarabine for the treatment of acute leukemia. *J Clin Oncol* 1992; **10**: 1730–6.

184. Baer MR, George SL, Dodge RK, et al. Phase 3 study of the multidrug resistance modulator PSC833 in previously untreated patients of 60 years of age and older with acute myeloid leukemia: Cancer and Leukemia Group B study 9720. *Blood* 2002; **100**: 1224–32.

185. List A, Kopecky K, Willman C et al. Benefit of cyclosporine modulation of drug resistance in patients with poor-risk acute myeloid leukemia: a Southwest Oncology Group study. *Blood* 2001; **98**: 3212–20.

186. Te Boekhorst PAW, Löwenberg B, Vlastuin M, Sonneveld P. Enhanced chemosensitivity of clonogenic blasts from patients with acute myeloid leukemia by G-CSF, IL-3 or GM-CSF stimulation. *Leukemia* 1993; **7**: 1191–8.

187. Lista P, Porcu P, Avanzi GC, Pegoraro L. Interleukin-3 enhances the cytotoxic ability of 1-β-arabino-furanosyl-cytosine (ara-C) on acute myeloblastic leukemia (AML) cell. *Br J Haematol* 1988; **69**: 121–3.

188. Lista P, Brizzi MF, Rossi M et al. Different sensitivity of normal and leukaemic progenitor cells to Ara-C and IL-3 combined treatment. *Br J Haematol* 1990; **76**: 21–6.

189. Hiddemann W, Kiehl M, Zühlsdorf M et al. Granulocyte–macrophage colony-stimulating factor and interleukin-3 enhance the incorporation of cytosine arabinoside into the DNA of leukemic blasts and the cytotoxic effects on clonogenic cells from patients with acute myeloid leukemia. *Semin Oncol* 1992; **19**(Suppl 1): 31–7.

190. Reuter C, Auf der Landwehr U, Schleyer E et al. Modulation of intracellular metabolism of cytosine arabinoside in acute myeloid leukemia by granulocyte–macrophage colony-stimulating factor. *Leukemia* 1994; **8**: 217–25.

191. Rossi HA, O'Donnell J, Sarcinelli F et al. Granulocyte–macrophage colony-stimulating factor (GM-CSF) priming with successive concomitant low-dose Ara-C for elderly patients with secondary/refractory acute myeloid leukaemia or advanced myelodysplastic syndrome. *Leukemia* 2002; **16**: 310–15.

192. Frenette PS, Desforges JF, Schenkein DP et al. Granulocyte–macrophage colony stimulating factor (GM-CSF) priming in the treatment of elderly patients with acute myelogenous leukaemia. *Am J Hematol* 1995; **49**: 48–55.

193. Estey E, Thall P, Kantarjian H et al. Treatment of newly diagnosed acute myelogenous leukemia with granulocyte–macrophage colony-stimulating factor (GM-CSF) before and during continuous infusion high-dose ara-C + daunorubicin: comparison to patients treated without GM-CSF. *Blood* 1992; **79**: 2246–55.

194. Ohno R, Naoe T, Kanamaru A et al. A double-blind controlled study of granulocyte colony-stimulating factor started two days before induction chemotherapy in refractory acute myeloid leukemia. *Blood* 1994; **83**: 2086–92.

195. Zittoun R, Suciu S, Mandelli F et al. Granulocyte–macrophage colony-stimulating factor associated with induction treatment of acute myelogenous leukemia: a randomized trial by the European Organization for Research and Treatment of Cancer and Leukemia Cooperative Group. *J Clin Oncol* 1996; **14**: 2150–9.

196. Löwenberg B, Boogaerts MA, Daenen SMGJ et al. Value of different modalities of granulocyte macrophage colony-stimulating factor applied during or after induction therapy of acute myeloid leukemia. *J Clin Oncol* 1997; **15**: 3496–506.

197. Estey EH, Thall PF, Pierce S et al. Randomized phase II study of fludarabine + cytosine arabinoside + idarubicin ± all-*trans* retinoic acid ± granulocyte colony-stimulating factor in poor prognosis newly diagnosed acute myeloid leukemia and myelodysplastic syndrome. *Blood* 1999; **93**: 2478–84.

198. Witz F, Sadoun A, Perrin MC et al. A placebo-controlled study of recombinant human granulocyte–macrophage colony-stimulating factor administered during and after induction treatment for de novo acute myelogenous leukemia in elderly patients. *Blood* 1998; **91**: 2722–30.

199. Gilliland DG, Griffin JD. The roles of FLT3 in hematopoiesis and leukemia. *Blood* 2002; **100**: 1532–42.

200. Caron PC, Scheinberg DA. Anti-CD33 monoclonal antibody M195 for the therapy of myeloid leukemia. *Leuke Lymphoma* 1993; **11**: 1–6.

201. Sievers EL, Larson RA, Stadtmauer EA et al. Efficacy and safety of gemtuzumab ozogamicin in patients with CD33-positive acute myeloid leukemia in first relapse. *J Clin Oncol* 2001; **19**: 3244–54.

202. Giles FJ, Kantarjian HM, Kornblau SM et al. Mylotarg (gemtuzumab ozogamicin) therapy is associated with hepatic venoocclusive disease in patients who have not received stem cell transplantation. *Cancer* 2001; **92**: 406–13.

203. Burnett AK, Wheatley K, Stevens R et al. Further data to question the use of alloBMT in AML CR1 in addition to intensive chemotherapy: the MRC experience in 715 patients under 44 years with donors available. *Blood* 2002; **10**(11): 269a.

204. Suciu S, Mandelli F, De Witte T et al. Allogeneic compared to autologous stem cell transplantation in the treatment of patients <46 years old with acute myeloid leukemia (AML) in first complete remission (CR1): an intention to treat analysis of the EORTC/GIMEMA AML-10 trial. *Blood* 2003; **102**: 1232–40.

205. Valk PJM, Verhaak RGW, Beijnen MA et al. Prognostically useful gene-expression profiles in acute myeloid leukemia. *N Engl J Med* 2004; **350**: 1617–28.

206. Bullinger L, Döhner K, Bair E et al. Use of gene-expression profiling to identify prognostic subclasses in adult acute myeloid leukemia. *N Engl J Med* 2004; **350**: 1605–16.

207. Löwenberg B, Putten WLJ van, Touw IP et al. Autonomous proliferation of leukemic cells in vitro as a determinant of prognosis in adult acute myeloid leukemia. *N Engl J Med* 1993; **328**: 614–9.

208. Douglas Smith B, Levis M, Beran M et al. Single-agent CEP-701, a novel FLT3 inhibitor, shows biologic and clinical activity in patients with relapsed or refractory acute myeloid leukemia. *Blood* 2004; **103**: 3669–76.

209. Feinstein LC, Sandmaier BM, Hegenbart U et al. Non-myeloablative allografting from human leucocyte antigen-identical sibling donors for treatment of acute myeloid leukemia in first remission. *Br J Haematol* 2003; **120**: 281–8.

210. Martino R, Dolores Caballero M, Pereze Simon JA et al. Evidence for a graft-vesus-leukemia effect after allogeneic peripheral blood stem cell transplantation with reduced-intensity conditioning in acute myelogenous leukemia

and myelodysplastic syndromes. *Blood* 2002; **100**: 2243–5.

211. Bertz H, Potthoff K and Finke J. Allogeneic stem-cell transplantation from related and unrelated donors in older patients with myeloid leukemia. *J Clin Oncol* 2003; **21**: 1480-4.

212. Löwenberg B, Putten W van, Theobald M et al. Effect of priming with granulocyte colony-stimulating factor on the outcome of chemotherapy for acute myeloid leukemia. *N Engl J Med* 2003; **349**: 743–52.

213. Greenberg PL, Lee SJ, Advani R et al. Mitoxantrone, Etoposide, and Cytarabine with or without Valspodar in patients with relapsed or refractory acute myeloid leukemia and high-risk myelodysplastic syndrome: a phase III trial (E2995). *J Clin Oncol* 2004; **22**: 1078–86.

214. Cheson BD, Bennett JM , Kopecky KJ et al. Revised recommendations of the International Working Group for diagnosis, standardization of response criteria, treatment outcomes, and reporting standards for therapeutic trials in acute myeloid leukemia. *J Clin Oncol* 2003; **21**: 4642–9.

# 39 Acute promyelocytic leukemia

**Laurent Degos**

## Introduction

Acute promyelocytic leukemia (APL) was recognized as a distinct subset of acute myeloid leukemia (AML) in the 1950s,[1] distinguished by morphological features categorized as M3 in the French-American-British (FAB) nomenclature,[2,3] and by an associated coagulopathy with a bleeding diathesis,[4] often exacerbated by cytotoxic chemotherapy,[5] leading to a relatively high rate of early mortality, mainly due to intracranial hemorrhage.

APL is relatively uncommon, the frequency being estimated as 10% of acute leukemias. The mean incidence in Europe is about 2–3 cases per million inhabitants per year. In the USA there are up to 800 new cases every year. The frequency seems to be higher in southern Europe (Italy and Spain: 15% of AML) than in central Europe (Germany: 7% of AML). A particularly high incidence of APL is found in Latin America (Mexico), accounting for one-third of AML.[6] Both sexes are equally vulnerable to APL, and there is a wide range in age at first presentation. However, APL is a rare disease in children.

## Definition

APL was initially defined morphologically. In 1977, it was found to be consistently associated with a balanced and reciprocal translocation between the long arms of chromosomes 15 and 17: t(15;17).[7–9] Ten years later, a collaborative study by Chinese and French groups demonstrated the in vivo and in vitro effects of all-trans retinoic acid (ATRA; tretinoin) in the differentiation of malignant cells from APL patients. At the same time, the gene encoding the retinoic acid receptor alpha (RARα) was mapped to chromosome 17q21.[10] Because ATRA was found to be clinically effective in this disease, rearrangements of the RARα gene in the translocation were assumed.[11] The breakpoint of the translocation disrupted the RARα gene on chromosome 17 and a previously unknown gene, initially called myl[12] and renamed PML (for ProMyelocytic Leukemia),[13,14] on chromosome 15. The two genes PLM and RARα are fused, leading to the transcription of a fusion product PML–RARα that has been found in all patients studied, and is considered as the signature of the disease.[15–17]

Thus APL is defined not only by morphological and clinical features but also by the specific translocation t(15;17) resulting in the fusion of two genes PML and RARα, generating a disease-specific fusion protein that is potentially involved in the carcinogenesis.

## Clinical features and laboratory findings

Usually, the first symptoms of APL are consequences of bleeding diathesis. Hemorrhages of the skin and mucosae prompt physicians to perform a hemogram. Sometimes severe hemorrhage (intracranial) leads to early death. Usually, no tumor, bone pain, adenopathy, or spleno- or hepatomegaly are recorded. Patients with APL share many of the symptoms of acute non-lymphocytic leukemia, such as pallor, fatigue, weakness, palpitations, dyspnea on exertion, and fever.

In contrast to other subtypes of leukemia, in the hemogram, the majority of patients (approximately 95%) have a total white blood cell (WBC) count of less than $5 \times 10^9$/L. Marked thrombocytopenia ($<50 \times 10^9$/L) is usually found. The anemia is variable, often related to hemorrhage. However, about 5% of patients, usually those having a variant form called the microgranular form, present with an elevated WBC count of up to $100 \times 10^9$/L)

In the common form, with a low WBC count, few malignant cells are found in the blood, most of them being the bone marrow.

The diagnosis of APL is made morphologically on bone marrow smears. In the bone marrow, the majority of cells are abnormal, having some similarities with promyelocytes (size of cell, nucleus/cytoplasm ratio, and nuclear aspect). The malignant cells bear numerous large granules and several Auer rods. Bone marrow aspirates are also taken at presentation for cytogenetic evaluation and for reverse transcriptase polymerase chain reaction (RT–PCR) assays in order to detect the t(15;17) translocation and the PML–RARα mRNA respectively.

A microgranular variant (M3v) of the disease is characterized by a bilobed nucleus and very small granules that are not visible with light microscopy. Patients with M3v have a high WBC count and a poor prognosis (early death and risk of relapse).

Immunophenotyping confirms the myeloid lineage (CD13-CD33) with association in some cases with CD19 and/or CD2 antigens usually found in lymphoid lineages.

## Coagulation disorders

The coagulopathy in APL can provoke a life-threatening hemorrhage, which rapidly induces a course in untreated patients. The risk of early mortality necessitates treatment of the patient immediately after diagnosis. The coagulopathy is characterized by severe fibrinopenia and thrombocytopenia. The mechanisms of fibrinopenia result from at least three distinct syndromes due to the release of procoagulant activators, plasminogen activators, and lysozymal neutrophil enzymes from leukemic cells.[18,19] The procoagulant effect activates thrombin, leading to diffuse intravascular coagulation (DIC). The plasminogen activation induces a primary fibrinogenolysis, whereas the lysozymal neutrophil enzymes (human leukocyte elastase, cathepsin G, and proteinase 3, also called myeloblastin) provoke a leukocyte-mediated proteolysis that cleaves various substrates, including fibrinogen itself and von Willebrand factor. On one hand, the primary fibrinolysis theory is supported by the high level of annexin II detected on APL leukemic cells (and not on other types of leukemic cells); annexin II is a cell surface receptor for plasminogen, as well as for one of its activators, the tissue plasminogen activator, tPA.[20] On the other hand, the DIC theory is supported by the presence of tissue factor release by APL cells.[21] Tissue factor serves to initiate coagulation by an interaction with Factor VII. The relative extent of these mechanisms in APL patients is still debated, and recommendations for the management of hemostatic disorders (heparin, antifibrinolytic drugs, plasma, or nothing) in APL patients treated with chemotherapy, therefore, vary from one group to another.[22–27] Two parameters are usually evaluated during the treatment: the plasma level of fibrinogen and the number of platelets. In order to follow the DIC, factor V, fibrinogen degradation products, and soluble complexes are serially tested.

The rule for treating patients with APL is to transfuse platelets in order to have more than $50 \times 10^9$/L permanently during the treatment until complete remission.

A rapid normalization of fibrinogen level is observed in APL patients treated with ATRA; this normalization is related to the disappearance of plasmin-dependent primary fibrinogenolysis (see below) more than to the control of the DIC. Patients treated by ATRA are still susceptible to thrombosis, which is prevented by low molecular weight heparin. Conversely, chemotherapy exacerbates the fibrinopenia and the DIC.

## Molecular genetics of APL

As mentioned above, Rowley and colleagues[7,8] discovered in the mid-1970s that APL was always[9] associated with a balanced and reciprocal translocation between the long arms of chromosomes 15 and 17: t(15;17)(q23;q21). Two reciprocal fusion transcripts result from this translocation: PML–RARα which is found in all patients with APL and contains the functional parts of the RARα and PML genes, and a small RARα–PML transcript that is detected in only about two-third patients.

RARα belongs to the retinoid receptors – members of a superfamily of nuclear receptors that act as ligand-dependent transcription factors. Retinoid receptors bind to specific sites in DNA (called RA responsive elements) on the promoter region of some genes and act as transcription factors controlling the expression of target genes. Two families of nuclear retinoid receptors RAR (α, β, and γ) and RXR (α, β, and γ) have been identified.[28–33] These receptors contain two binding sites: one domain that binds to DNA on the promoting region of a target gene, and another domain that binds to the retinoids that switch on the transcription activity. These receptors have the capacity to dimerize, which markedly increases the DNA-binding affinity and the activation of a target gene. Almost all the domains are present in the PML–RARα fusion protein: only the first domain of RARα is missing – this is a domain involved in the activation of the target gene. The natural ligand of RAR is ATRA, while the ligand of RXR is 9-cis retinoic acid,[34,35] a metabolite and isomer of ATRA. The 9-cis isomer is also able to bind to RAR. Usually heterodimers, made of one RAR and one RXR, bind to DNA on two adjacent responsive elements. The expression of the genes targeted by RAR subtypes α, β, and γ differs in the tissue distribution – for example, RARγ in the skin. Other types of receptors bind to similar responsive elements on DNA, and also dimerize with RXR, such as vitamin D3 receptors (VD3R), the thyroid hormone receptor (TR) and RXR itself. However, the heterodimers RXR–RXR, VD3R–RXR, TR–RXR and RAR–RXR bind to different target gene promoters according to the number (1 to 5 respectively) of nucleotides inserted between the two DNA-responsive elements.

PML was discovered with the cloning of the translocation t(15;17) and belongs to a family of nine proteins that share a ring finger (an atypical zinc finger domain) and another large domain implicated in dimmer formation.[36] All these domains are present in the PML–RARα fusion product; only a small portion of the molecule is missing.

In fact, the breakpoint on *RARα* gene is always in the same region (second intron, leaving the A domain outside of the fusion *PLM–RARα*) while the breakpoint on *PML* could localized on three different regions leading to three isoforms of PML–RARα fusion protein: bcr1 the longest, bcr3 the shortest, and less frequently a bcr2 isoform similar to bcr3.

The fusion gene *PML–RARα* is under the control of the promoter of the *PML* gene.

Immunostaining with anti-PML antibodies has demonstrated that PML is normally localized on discrete subnuclear structure[37] previously identified by electron microscopy and called PML nuclear bodies. However, prior to the cloning of *PML*, these structures were identified using a subset of auto-antibodies from patients with primary biliary cirrhosis (PBC).[38] Most of these auto-antibodies recognized a molecule called SP100.[39] Other proteins (NDP55, SUMO, DaXX, BLM) are also present together with SP100 and PML on these nuclear bodies.[40] PML nuclear bodies are parts of the nuclear matrix, a biochemically defined scaffold that has been proposed to play an important role in intranuclear biology. PML localization is regulated in the cell cycle (diffuse nuclear fluorescence during S phase and a subsequent reformation of bodies).[41]

In APL patients, the nuclear body is disrupted, and the PML molecules as well as PML–RARα molecules, are spread out in the nucleus and in the cytoplasm[37] taking with them normal PML/PML and RXR/RAR molecules through PML and RXR dimerization respectively.

The transforming potential of the fusion-gene products has been tested by cotransfection assays in cell lines. These experiments demonstrated an alteration (repression or overactivation) of transactivation of target genes of retinoic acid receptors.[13,14] Retinoic acid-mediated differentiation of the HL60 cell line is also blocked by the presence of the PML–RARα fusion product.[42] The fusion protein seems to block the activity of retinoic acid receptors, mainly in the differentiation of the granulocytic lineage.

In the presence of high concentrations of ATRA, all these abnormalities are reversed. Retinoic acid-induced reporter genes blocked by PML–RARα are activated, and HL60 transfected with *PML–RARα* can be differentiated in the presence of retinoic acid. The normal allele of *RARα* (on the non-translocated chromosome 17) is transiently upregulated while *RXR*

gene expression is downregulated under ATRA treatment. In a second step, RARα molecules are cleared. On the other hand, after ATRA treatment, the nuclear body is rebuilt, PML relocalized in 24 hours in vitro and in five days in vivo and PML–RAR degraded.

At the molecular level, it was reported that the fusion protein PML–RARα inhibits the exchanges of corepressor with coactivators of transcription of *RARα* target gene. In fact, RAR–RXR dimers are attached to corepressors which are linked to histone deacetylase (HDAC).

Histone deacetylases compact DNA on histone, blocking the transcription process. In presence of retinoic acid, RXR–RAR dimers exchange corepressors to coactivators, which are linked to histone acetylase, decompacting the DNA from histones, allowing by this fact the transcription. High doses of retinoic acid are capable to reverse the inhibition of PML–RARα in this exchange of corepressor–coactivators.

In conclusion, the fusion protein PML–RARα on the one hand induces an arrest of differentiation of the granulocytic lineage through an abnormal RARα, and on the other hand alters the nuclear biology and probably the natural apoptosis through an abnormal PML. ATRA restores these two abnormalities.

Another agent, arsenic (as the trioxide $As_2O_3$) is also able to induce complete remission by way of differentiation effect (promyelocyte to abnormal myelocyte) and apoptosis. Arsenic targets its effects on the PML moiety of the fusion protein PML–RARα. Arsenic induces first a relocalization of PML in the nucleus, and on the nuclear bodies, and second, a degradation of PML as well as PML–RARα inside the nuclear bodies through a sumoylation (due to a link with the SUMO molecule) by the proteasome. Thus, under treatment by arsenic, the PML–RARα fusion proteins as well as PML molecules are relocalized in the nucleus and rapidly degraded.

## Treatment

### Results of intensive chemotherapy

Several studies demonstrates the sensitivity of APL to anthracycline treatment.[5] The complete remission (CR) rate was improved progressively (reaching 80% of patients), due to better management of the coagulopathy and thus to a reduction of the fatal bleeding, using intensive platelet support during the induction phase associated with a potential beneficial role of heparin and/or antifibrinolytic agents.[23–25] With consolidation chemotherapy, the median disease-free survival ranges from 11 to 25 months, and approximately 35% of the patients who achieved a CR (25% of patients at diagnosis) could probably be cured of the disease. In contrast to the situation in other acute non-lymphocytic leukemia, cytarabine (cytosine arabinoside; Ara-C) at standard doses does not appear to be beneficial in combination with anthracyclines.[43] High dose of Ara-C could reduce the number of relapses.

Adverse prognostic factors for CR with chemotherapy are greater age, microgranular APL variant, high leukocyte count, and severe coagulopathy at diagnosis; a shorter disease-free survival (relapse rate) was observed in patients with a high leukocyte count at diagnosis.[22,43–46]

### Results obtained with ATRA

Retinoids are able to induce a terminal differentiation of leukemic cell lines, such as HL60 and U937, and of short-term culture APL cells from humans.[47,48] In 1985, a first informal meeting in Paris, Wang and Degos pointed out the differentiation activity of retinoids on APL cells. In fact, at that time the only available retinoid in Europe, the ethyl ester retinoid (etretinate) was not effective on APL cells.[47] The differentiation effect on fresh cells is restricted to patients with the APL subtype of non-lymphoblastic leukemia and the sensitivity of the malignant cells depend on the specific derivative, with ATRA being the most efficient drug.[49]

All trans retinoic acid was produced in Shanghai and first used to treat patients there.[50] Following a second collaborative meeting (French and Chinese) in Shanghai in 1987, the Chinese drug was kindly provided to subsequently treat French patients.[51]

### Differentiative effect obtained with ATRA alone

Treatment with ATRA (daily dose 45 mg/m$^2$) was proposed for newly diagnosed patients in Shanghai[50] and for patients in first or subsequent relapse in Paris,[51] with the CR rate reaching 90% in both studies. The clinical features were unusual for a chemotherapy inducing a CR of leukemia. Instead of the initial worsening observed with conventional chemotherapy, coagulopathy (fibrinogenopenia) rapidly improved. No primary resistance, no aplastic phase, no hairless, and few infectious episodes were observed. The most remarkable features was the progressive change of malignant cells in bone marrow, with signs of their terminal differentiation and with Auer rods being sometimes observed in mature cells.[51] The differentiation process was confirmed by serial fluorescence in situ hybridization (FISH) and clonality was demonstrated using X chromosome-linked polymorphism.[52] Clonal malignant cells carrying the t(15;17) translocation are replaced by polyclonal hematopoiesis. Correction of neutrophils and platelets occurred first, after 1 month of treatment, while low hemoglobin levels and monocytopenia persisted for a few days after treatment, most likely in relation to the inhibitory effect of retinoic acid on BFU-E burst-forming units, erythroid) and CFU-M (colony-forming units, monocyte-macrophage).[53]

### Two major adverse effects: retinoic acid syndrome and secondary resistance

Treatment with ATRA alone showed two adverse effects: one during treatment (retinoic acid syndrome) and one following it (secondary resistance to ATRA). An activation of leukocytes inducing an increase in WBC count is observed during treatment with ATRA alone,[51] and one-third of patients develop fever, dyspnea and even renal failure corresponding to the well described and so-called ATRA syndrome.[54]

The 'ATRA syndrome' corresponding to a leukocyte activation syndrome, combines fever, respiratory distress, weight gain, pleural or pericardial effusions, and, sometimes, renal failure. The incidence of this syndrome is lower in China compared with Europe or America,[55] and the syndrome is frequently preceded by an increase in WBC counts in peripheral blood. The pathophysiology is not clearly understood and appears to be related to cytokine release by differentiating cells.[56] Two approaches have been attempted to counteract this syndrome: the *European attitude* is to prevent the syndrome using chemotherapy when WBC counts increase; the *American attitude* is to treat the syndrome with high-dose intravenous corticosteroids. The current consensus is to use chemotherapy in combination with ATRA and to add corticosteroids either from the onset of treatment, if patients have a high WBC count, or when patients show symptoms of ATRA syndrome during treatment.

Following treatment with ATRA alone, patients experience an induction of a secondary resistance to ATRA.

Secondary resistance occurs in all patients treated with ATRA.[57] Thus, patients receiving ATRA alone achieved CR for only a short time, usually relapsing within 6 months. Patients treated with ATRA become refractory to this treatment for a period of 6–12 months and the acquired resistance is usually reversible after this period. Since all patients acquire a resistance and because that resistance is usually reversible, it appears that a secondary genetic charge is not involved in this process, in contrast to the phenomenon occurring in artificial ATRA-resistant cell lines.

The observed resistance is likely to be related to feedback mechanisms aimed at reducing ATRA concentrations in the organism. A significant decrease of ATRA levels in plasma is observed after only a few days of treatment and ATRA remains at lower, sometimes undetectable, levels even if the dose is doubled.[58] On one hand, ATRA treatment increases the activity of cytochrome P450 implicated in the catabolism of ATRA itself, which reduces the plasma level of the drug,[58] and on the other, ATRA increases the transcription of the cytoplasmic retinoic acid binding protein II (CRABP II), trapping the ATRA and thereby inducing a reduction of nucleic concentration of the drug.[59]

## Other side-effects

Dryness of lips and mucosae are usual, but these can be alleviated by symptomatic treatment. Increase in transaminases and triglycerides and bone pain are common, but they have never required discontinuation of treatment in our experience. Headache, due to intracranial hypertension, is generally moderate in adults but may be severe in children, and associated with signs of pseudotumor cerebri.[60] Lower ATRA doses (25 mg/m²/day) in children reduce this side-effect, and this dose seems to be as effective as conventional doses of 45 mg/m²/day.[60] Monitoring of hemostatic parameters in APL patients treated with ATRA alone shows that primary fibrinogenolysis disappears during the first days of treatment, while DIC and leukocyte-mediated proteolysis seem to persist for the first 2 or 3 weeks of ATRA therapy.[19,61,62] This could lead to a transient period of hypercoagulability not compensated by fibrinolytic activity, and a few well-documented cases of thromboembolic events in APL patients treated with ATRA have been reported.[63,64]

## ATRA in combination with chemotherapy: a step towards the cure of APL

The occurrence of secondary resistance to ATRA in APL patients led us (French trials) to administer a treatment combining ATRA with intensive chemotherapy.

*Non-randomized studies.* In the first studies,[65] 26 newly diagnosed cases of APL, treated with ATRA (45 mg/m²/day) until CR, followed by three courses of chemotherapy (daunorubicin and cytarabine), were compared with an historical control group treated with chemotherapy alone (Figure 39.1). Initial results showed that ATRA followed by chemotherapy dramatically reduces the number of relapses (occurring within 24 months after the onset of the disease). These results have now been largely confirmed.[66,67]

*Randomized trials: ATRA followed by chemotherapy.* A European trial (APL 91) comparing three courses of chemotherapy (daunorubicin and cytarabine) to initial ATRA treatment followed by the same chemotherapy in newly diagnosed APL patients was prematurely stopped after 18 months because the event-free survival (EFS) was significantly better in the ATRA group. The analysis at 4 years confirmed the higher actuarial EFS (63% vs. 17%; $p<0.0004$), mainly due to a reduction in relapse rate (13% vs. 78%; $p <0.03$).[68,69] In a 3-year American inter-group study, started in 1992 and closed in 1995, three courses of chemotherapy were compared with ATRA treatment followed by two courses of chemotherapy.[70] The incidence of relapse was significantly reduced in patients who received ATRA (33% vs. 68% at 3 years; $p <0.01$).

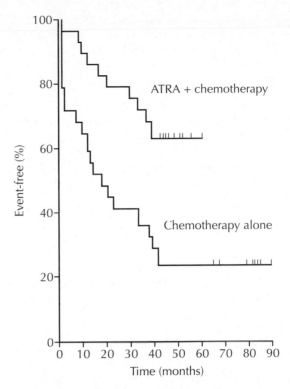

**Figure 39.1** Event-free survival: pilot study (ATRA + conventional chemotherapy) compared with historical series.

*Randomized trials: ATRA given simultaneously with chemotherapy.* Initially ATRA was used alone until CR followed by chemotherapy. The European group (APL 93 trial) compared two combination regimens including ATRA and chemotherapy, ATRA being given either prior to chemotherapy or simultaneously with chemotherapy. In the latter combination, ATRA was started 3 days before chemotherapy in order to maintain the beneficial effect on coagulation disorders. Relapses at 2 years are significantly less frequent (6% vs. 16%) when ATRA is given simultaneously to chemotherapy.[71]

### Treatment after remission

A retrospective Chinese study conducted by the Chinese Cooperative Study Group summarizing 5-year survival probability in 423 APL patients treated with ATRA as induction of remission, followed by ATRA alone or ATRA plus chemotherapy as maintenance therapy, has shown that the alternating use of chemotherapy and ATRA could yield a longer survival time.[55]

Two randomized studies[70,71] strongly suggest that maintenance treatment with ATRA has a beneficial effect in newly diagnosed APL. The American inter-group trial[70] compared continuous ATRA treatment as maintenance (45 mg/m²/day) for 1 year with no maintenance. The frequency of relapse was reduced in patients who received ATRA (10 of 46 vs. 24 of 54 patients). However, liver toxicity limits the use of continuous maintenance with ATRA. Patients who received no ATRA during induction therapy also benefited from ATRA maintenance.

The European APL group (APL 93 trial)[71] randomized patients who achieved CR into groups with no maintenance and maintenance with ATRA 15 days every 3 months, continuous low-dose chemotherapy with 6-mercaptopurine and methotrexate (MTX), or both (ATRA and low-dose chemotherapy) for 2 years using a 2 × 2 factorial design. The frequency of relapse at 2 years was reduced in patients who received ATRA compared with those who did not (13% vs. 25%; $p$ <0.002) and was also reduced in patients who received low-dose chemotherapy compared with those who did not (11% vs. 27%; $p$ <0.03). An additive effect of low-dose chemotherapy and ATRA maintenance therapies was also observed (7% of relapse at 2 years). Furthermore, patients with higher rise of relapse because of high blood cell counts at diagnosis seemed to benefit particularly from both low-dose chemotherapy and ATRA maintenance (10% vs. 30% of relapse rate at 2 years).

*Standard treatment.* The conclusion of these randomized trials suggests that APL patients should be treated with ATRA and chemotherapy including anthracyclines simultaneously, as induction treatment; two courses of chemotherapy (including anthracyclines or similar drugs), for consolidation; and ATRA in combination with low-dose chemotherapy for 2 years, as maintenance therapy. Under these conditions we can achieve a CR rate over 90% and a relapse rate lower than 10% at 2 years. If few delayed relapses occur, we hope that more than 75% of APL patients will actually be cured.

### Prognostic factors

White blood cell count

High WBC counts at diagnosis (more than 5000–10 000 mm³, according to the various group protocols) increase the risk of early mortality and relapses. The M3v hypogranular form is often associated with a high WBC count which increases the risks of leukocyte activation syndrome and relapse. Simultaneous administration of ATRA, chemotherapy with dexamethasone reduces the risk of leukocyte activation syndrome and mortality. In addition maintenance therapy (ATRA plus chemotherapy) reduces the risk of relapse.[71]

Age

Patients older than 65 years have a higher risk of early death (17% vs. 6% in younger patients).[71] New treatment combinations, such as the association of ATRA and arsenic trioxide ($As_2O_3$), which exclude or reduce anthracyclines, have yet to be tested.

Other types of APL

Therapy-related APL (t-APL) has a similar outcome as non t-APL.[72] Several other translocations including RARα as a partner are actually registered. Some are sensitive to ATRA, others are not (see Table 39.1). In case of the t(11;17) translocation involving the PLZF–RARα fusion protein, G-CSF appears to be beneficial when associated with ATRA.[73]

*Immunophenotype.* APL blasts have a different immunophenotype from those of other forms of AML. Although, like other AML, APL blasts are positive for CD13 and CD33, they lack HLA-DR antigens and are usually negative for CD34 and CD7, indicating that they derive from a more mature progenitor cell than other AML cells. Sometimes they also carry lymphocyte markers such as the B-cell marker CD19, or the T-cell marker CD2. This latter marker is mainly found in cases of M3v and in patients with PML–RARα/bcr3 breakpoint. CD19 seems to be associated with high WBC counts.[74] The presence or not of CD56 is suspected to affect survival.[75,76]

*Karyotype and molecular biology.* Additional karyotype abnormalities do not appear to influence prognosis in APL.[77,78] The type of PML–RARα isoform has

---

**Table 39.1 Acute promyelocytic leukemia (APL) and APL-like acute leukemia with a translocation involving *RARα* (17q21)**

| Gene | Location | Name | Function | Sensitive to ATRA (tretinoin) | Reference |
|------|----------|------|----------|-------------------------------|-----------|
| *PML* | 15q22 | Promyelocytic leukemia | Apoptosis | Yes | |
| *PZLF* | 11q23 | Promyelocytic leukemia zinc finger | Morphogenesis (limbs, skeleton) | No | Chen et al, 1993[91] |
| *NPM* | 5q35 | Nucleophosmin | Ribosome biogenesis | Yes | Redner et al, 1996[92] |
| *NuMA* | 11q13 | Nuclear mitotic apparatus | Chromatic compaction | Yes | Wells et al, 1997[93] |
| *STAT 5b* | 17q11 | Signal transducer Activ. Transcript. | Transcription factor for EPO, G-CSF, IL2, IL3, IL7 | No | Arnould et al, 1999[94] |

been suggested as a prognostic factor, with bcr1, the longest isoform, giving a better prognostic index.[79] In a recent clinical trial using ATRA plus chemotherapy as maintenance therapy, the bcr type is no longer considered to be a prognostic factor.[71]

Molecular remission is an endpoint for a better survival. However, the definition of molecular remission depends upon the sensitivity of the RT–PCR technique. Quantitative RT–PCR provides threshold value for prognostic estimates after combination chemotherapy/ATRA treatment. Some patients have shown a delayed molecular CR without early relapse (personal observations). A conversion from negative to positive PCR result is consistently associated with subsequent hematological relapse.[80–83]

*Cellular (in vitro) assay. Sensitivity to ATRA using short-term culture.* The sensitivity of the leukemic clone from fresh bone marrow cells to ATRA at diagnosis is an independent criterion of long-term patient outcome, in terms of better EFS, few relapses and better overall survival.[84] It has been demonstrated previously that primary cultures of blast cells are correlated with CR.[49] Thus, the efficacy of differentiation therapy in vivo would appear to be correlated with the in vitro sensitivity, in contrast to classical chemotherapy where in vitro experiments cannot predict in vivo results.

### Unresolved issues

Management of patients with high WBC at diagnosis

Patients with high WBC at diagnosis are still at high risk of early mortality and of relapse once they have achieved CR. These patients usually have severe coagulopathy at diagnosis and bleeding symptoms, and have an increased incidence of early death with chemotherapy alone. Our results suggest that the

addition of ATRA to chemotherapy, by providing more rapid reversal of coagulopathy, has further improved prognosis.[85,86] Furthermore, the addition of intravenous steroids is recommended in these patients as well as low molecular weight heparin. A maintenance therapy (ATRA and low-dose chemotherapy) reduces the incidence of relapses.

The role of bone marrow transplantation

Because more than 75% of patients treated with ATRA, intensive chemotherapy and maintenance therapy have prolonged remissions of their disease, the roles of allogeneic bone marrow transplantation (BMT) in first CR in these patients is not recommended, even if the results of allogeneic BMT seem to be better in APL than in other AML.[87] Our more recent results, however, suggest that patients presenting with high WBC counts treated by ATRA plus chemotherapy (without maintenance therapy) are still at risk of relapse, and could be candidates for allogeneic BMT. Patients with positive RT–PCR findings for *PML–RARα* rearrangements during follow-up in first CR could also be candidates, when we will have more data on the exact threshold of positivity by quantitative RT–PCR.

Because only limited experience of autologous BMT in APL is available, its place in this disease after ATRA plus chemotherapy is unknown. The fact that, in some cases, APL blasts are negative for CD34 antigen[88] suggests a possible role for autologous BMT using marrow or circulating progenitors collected after CD34+ selection.

Usually, allogeneic and autologous BMT are proposed after relapse in APL patients.

### Arsenic treatment

Two teams from Harbin (Manchuria, China) reported at the Chinese Society of Hematology (Da Lian,

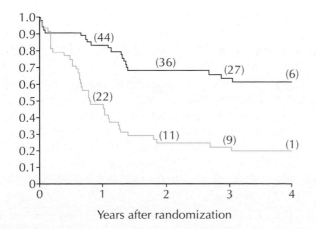

**Figure 39.2** Event-free survival according to randomized treatment (APL91 study). Thick line: ATRA plus chemotherapy, 54 patients, 20 events. Thin line: chemotherapy alone, 47 patients, 38 events. $p = 0.0001$, log-rank test.

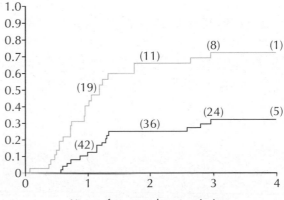

**Figure 39.3** Relapse according to randomized treatment (APL91 study). Thick line: ATRA plus chemotherapy, 49 patients, 15 relapses. Thin line: chemotherapy alone, 38 patients, 24 relapses. $p = 0.0001$, log-rank test.

September 1995) the beneficial effect of arsenic (as $As_2O_3$) given daily at a dose of 10 mg intravenously until complete remission (30–60 days). The first trials started in 1971 and included 60 patients: 30 de novo patients and 30 relapse patients, with 75% and 53% CR respectively. The second team included 72 patients: 30 de novo patients, with 73% achieving CR, 17% partial remission, and 10% resistance; and 42 refractory and relapse patients, with 52% achieving CR, 12% partial remission, and 36% non-response.

Arsenic trioxide has been confirmed to be effective in the treatment of APL mainly by groups of Shanghai (China)[89] but also in Europe (Paris, France), in USA (New York), and in Japan. In vitro, $As_2O_3$ exerts a dose-dependent dual effect: it triggers apoptosis at relatively high concentrations (0.5–2.0 μmol/L) and induces partial and mild differentiation at low concentrations (0.1–0.5 μmol/L). $As_2O_3$ induces a degradation of the PML–RARα molecule as well as the wild-type PML. In vivo, $As_2O_3$ (10 mg intravenous infusion daily) induces a high complete remission rate in patients with both primary and relapsed APL (around 90%), Side-effects, such as skin reaction, gastrointestinal symptoms, electrocardiographic changes (QT elongation), peripheral neuropathy, and liver dysfunction, are mild-to-moderate in relapsed patients. However, severe hepatic adverse effects have been found in de novo patients (one death and one severe liver failure among 10 de novo patients in the Shanghai Chinese series). Therefore, arsenic is not actually included in front line treatment in de novo APL and is preferentially proposed in consolidation causes. In relapsed patients, after CR obtained using arsenic, the combination of $As_2O_3$ with chemotherapy as postremission therapy has yielded better survival than treatment with $As_2O_3$ alone, and subsequently a bone marrow transplantation (allogeneic or autologous) is proposed as an intensification treatment. The in vivo effect of $As_2O_3$ seems to be related to the

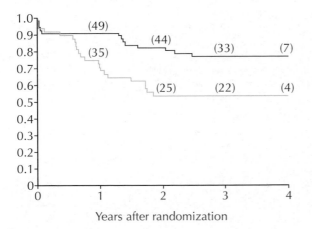

**Figure 39.4** Survival according to randomized treatment (APL91 study). Thick line: ATRA plus chemotherapy, 54 patients, 13 deaths. Thin line: chemotherapy alone, 47 patients, 22 deaths. $p = 0.013$, log-rank test.

expression of APL specific PML–RARα oncoprotein. A synergistic effect between $As_2O_3$ and ATRA has been shown in the APL mouse model.[90] Besides $As_2O_3$, other arsenic compounds such as $As_4S_4$ also show a therapeutic effect in APL. The toxic effects of arsenic treatment in de novo APL patients restrict its use to multidrug postremission therapy consolidation or as a rescue for relapsed APL patients.

## Conclusion

### Acute promyelocytic leukemia as a model for malignancies

Acute promyelocytic leukemia[95] is the first model of a malignant disease treated by differentiation agents. ATRA, in vitro and in vivo, induces a terminal differentiation (followed by natural apoptosis) of malignant cells. Therefore, ATRA is the principal model of a cell modifier in the treatment of malignancies. Other cell modifiers are actually proposed in leukemia, for instance, arsenic for the treatment of APL, and antikinase, which has shown promising results in chronic myeloid leukemia.

Acute promyelocytic leukemia is also the first model of an acquired genetic disease specifically treated by a drug (ATRA). In fact, ATRA is active in APL and not in other leukemias. APL is characterized by the translocation t(15;17) with a fusion of a large part of the *RARα* gene on chromosome 17 to a part of the promyelocytic leukemia (*PML*) gene on chromosome 15. A pharmacologic dose of ATRA overcomes the blockage of exchange between corepressors and coactivators of *RARα* caused by the fusion with the partner *PML*.

In addition, because ATRA is effective in the leukemia-bearing specific chromosome aberration t(15;17) with *PML–RARα* fusion gene, the treatment of APL with ATRA constitutes the first successful model for gene-targeting therapy.

Acute promyelocytic leukemia gives the opportunity to better understand leukemogenesis. The *PML–RARα* fusion gene is sufficient to induce leukemia in mice. In fact, RARα is a nuclear receptor acting as a ligand-dependent transcription factor.[96] RARα binds to DNA on specific responsive elements located in the promoter region of a set of genes. These genes are transcribed when ATRA is present. Several of these genes are involved in the myeloid differentiation. A defect of RARα induces an arrest of myeloid differentiation at the promyelocytic stage. The partner of fusion protein PML is not a DNA-binding protein. PML proteins located on nuclear bodies seem to be involved in apoptotic events of the cell. Thus, a defect of PML proteins could induce long survival and accumulation of the malignant cells. In conclusion, the leukemic process is caused by an arrest of differentiation (RARα defect) and a long survival (PML defect).

A new–old drug, arsenic (As$_2$O$_3$ and arsenic sulfide) also has a specific activity in APL. In fact, arsenic clears the PML molecule and thus also clears the oncogenic molecule PML–RAR. In vitro, arsenic mainly activates the apoptotic events of APL cells; in vivo, both differentiation and apoptosis are observed.

Two drugs, ATRA and As$_2$O$_3$ are now available for the treatment of APL. These drugs have different mecha-

nisms of action – one acts on RARα the other on PML – that cleans the oncogene molecule and cures the two abnormalities, differentiation arrest and defect of apoptosis. In mice transplanted with cells bearing the *PML–RARα* transgene, the induced leukemia is cured by the association of ATRA with As$_2$O$_3$, whereas the use of one of these drugs on its own prolongs survival but does not produce complete cure. The cure of one of the most dramatic leukemias, APL, is now reachable.

## REFERENCES

1. Hillestad LK. Acute promyelocytic leukemia. *Acta Med Scand* 1957; **159**: 189–94.

2. Bennett JM, Catowsky D, Daniel MT et al. Proposals for the classification of the acute leukemias. *Br J Haematol* 1976; **33**: 451–8.

3. Bennett JM, Catowsky D, Daniel MT et al. A variant form of hypergranular promyelocytic leukemia (M3). *Ann Intern Med* 1980; **92**: 261–262.

4. Gralnick HR, Sultan C. Acute promyelocytic leukemia: haemorrhagic manifestation and morphologic criteria. *Br J Haematol* 1975; **29**: 373–376.

5. Marty M, Ganem G, Fisher J et al. Leucémie aiguë promyelocytaira: etude retrospective de 119 malades traits par Daunorubicine. *Nouv Rev Fr Hematol* 1984; **26**: 371–378.

6. Chang E, Levine AM, Douer D. Distribution of PML breakpoint cluster region in the PML-RARα fusion transcripts in acute promyelocytic leukemia of Latino patients. *Blood* 1995, ASH abstract 673.

7. Golomb HM, Rowley J, Vardiman J et al. Partial deletion of long arm chromosome 17: a specific abnormality in acute promyelocytic leukemia? *Arch Intern Med* 1976; **136**: 825–8.

8. Rowley JD, Golomb HM, Dougherty C. 15/17 translocation: a consistent chromosomal change in acute promyelocytic leukaemia. *Lancet* 1977; **1**: 549–550.

9. Larson RA, Kondon K, Vardiman JW et al. Evidence for a 15;17 translocation in every patient with acute promyelocytic leukemia. *Am J Med* 1984; **76**: 827–841.

10. Mattei MG, Petkovich M, Mattei JF et al. Mapping of the human retinoic acid receptor to the q21 band of chromosome 17. *Hum Genet* 1988; **80**: 186–188.

11. Chomienne C, Ballerini P, Balitrand N et al. The retinoic acid receptor alpha gene is rearranged in retinoic acid sensitive promyelocytic leukemias. *Leukemia* 1990; **45**: 802–807.

12. De Thé H, Chomienne C, Lanotte M et al. The t(15;17) translocation of acute promyelocytic leukaemia fuses the retinoic acid receptor alpha gene to a novel transcribed locus. *Nature* 1990; **347**: 558–561.

13. De Thé H, Lavau C, Marchio A et al. The PML RAR alpha fusion mRNA generated by the t(15;17) translocation in acute promyelocytic leukemia encodes a functionally altered RAR. *Cell* 1991; **66**: 675–184.

14. Kakizuka A, Miller WH Jr, Umesono K et al. Chromosomal translocation t(15;17) in human acute promyelocytic leukemia fuses RAR alpha with a novel putative transcription factor, PML. *Cell* 1991; **66**: 663–674.

15. Borrow J, Goddard AD, Sheer D, Solomon E. Molecular analysis of acute promyelocytic leukemia breakpoint clus-

ter region on chromosome 17. *Science* 1990; **249**: 1577–1580.

16. Alcalay M, Angrilli D, Pandolfi PP et al. Translocation breakpoint of acute promyelocytic leukemia likes within the retinoic acid receptor alpha locus. *Proc Natl Acad Sci USA* 1991; **88**: 1977–1981.

17. Chen SJ, Zhu YJ, Tong JH et al. Rearrangements in the second intron of the RAR alpha gene are present in a large majority of patients with acute promylocytic leukemia and are used as molecular marker for retinoic acid induced leukemia cell differentiation. *Blood* 1991; **78**: 2696–2701.

18. Speiser W, Pabinger-Fasching I, Kyrle PA et al. Hemostatic and fibrinolytic parameters in patients with acute myeloid leukemia: Activation of blood coagulation, fibrinolysis and unspecific proteolysis. *Blut* 1990; **61**: 298–302.

19. Dombret H, Scrobohaci ML, Daniel M et al. In vivo thrombin and plasmin activities in patients with acute promyelocytic leukemia (APL): effect of all-trans retinoic acid (ATRA) therapy. *Leukemia* 1995; **9**: 19–24.

20. Menell JS, Cesarman GM, Jocovina A et al. Annexin II and bleeding in acute promyelocytic leukemia. *N Engl J Med* 1999; **340**: 994–1004.

21. Zhu J, Guo WM, Yao YY et al. Tissue factors on acute promyelocytic leukemia and endothelial cells are differently regulated by retinoic acid, arsenic trioxide and chemotherapeutic agents. *Leukemia* 1999; **13**: 1062–1070.

22. Kantarjian H, Keating M, Walters R. Acute promyelocytic leukemia. MD Anderson Hospital Experience. *Am J Med* 1986; **80**: 789–797.

23. Rodighiero F, Avvisati G, Castaman G et al. Early deaths and anti-hemorrhagic treatments in acute promyelocytic leukemia. A GIMEMA retrospective study in 268 consecutive patients. *Blood* 1990; **11**: 2112–2117.

24. Hoyle C, Swirsky D, Freedman L, Hayhoe F. Beneficial effect of heparin in the management of patients with APL. *Br J Haematol* 1988; **68**: 283–289.

25. Goldberg MA, Ginsburg D, Mayer RJ et al. Is heparin administration necessary during induction chemotherapy for patients with acute promyelocytic leukemia? *Blood* 1987; **69**: 187–191.

26. Schartz BS, Williams EC, Conlan MG, Mosher DF. Epsilon-aminocaproic acid in the treatment of patients with acute promyelocytic leukemia and acquired alpha-2-plasmin inhibitor deficiency. *Ann Intern Med* 1986; **105**: 873–877.

27. Avvisati G, Ten Cate JW, Buller HR, Mandelli F. Tranexamic acid for control of haemorrhage in acute promyelocytic leukaemia. *Lancet* 1989; **2**: 121–124.

28. Evan RM. The steroid and thyroid hormone receptor superfamily. *Science* 1988; **240**: 889–895.

29. Petkovich M, Brand NJ, Krust A, Chambon P. A human retinoic acid receptor which belongs to the family of nuclear receptors. *Nature* 1987; **330**: 444–450.

30. Giguere V, Ong ES, Segui P, Evants RM. Identification of a receptor for the morphogen retinoic acid. *Nature* 1987; **330**: 624–629.

31. De Thé H, Marchio A, Tiollais P, Dejean A. A novel steroid thyroid hormone receptor-related gene inappropriately expressed in human hepato-cellular carcinoma. *Nature* 1987; **330**: 667–670.

32. Mangelsdorf DJ, Ong ES, Dyck A, Evans RM. Nuclear receptor that identifies a novel retinoic acid response pathway. *Nature* 1990; **345**: 224–229.

33. Leid M, Kastner P, Lyons R et al. Purification, cloning and RXR identity of the HeLa cell factor with which RAR or TR heterodimerizes to bind target sequences efficiently. *Cell* 1992; **68**: 377–395.

34. Levin AA, Sturzenbecker LJ, Kazmer S et al. 9-cis retinoic acid stereo-isomer binds and activates the nuclear receptor RXR alpha. *Nature* 1992; **355**: 359–361.

35. Heyman TRA, Mangelsdorf DJ, Dyck JA et al. 9-cis retinoic acid in a high affinity ligand for the retinoid X receptor. *Cell* 1992; **68**: 397–406.

36. Goddard AD, Borrow J, Freemont P, Solomon E. Characterization of a zinc finger gene disrupted by the t(15;17) in acute promyelocytic leukemia. *Science* 1991; **254**: 1371–1374.

37. Daniel MT, Koken M, Romangne O et al. PML protein expression in haematopoietic and APL cells. *Blood* 1993; **82**: 1858–1867.

38. Szostecki C, Guldner H, Netter H, Will H. Isolation and characterization of cDNA encoding a human nuclear antigen predominantly recognized by autoantibodies of patients with primary biliary cirrhosis. *J Immunol* 1990; **145**: 4338–47.

39. Sternsdorf T, Guldner HH, Szostecki C et al. Two nuclear dot-associated proteins, PML and Sp100, are often co-autoimmunogenic in patients with primary biliary cirrhosis. *Scand J Immunol* 1995; **42**: 257–268.

40. Korioth F, Gieffers C, Maul GG, Frey J. Molecular characterization of NDP52, a novel protein of the nuclear domain 10, which is redistributed upon virus infection and interferon treatment. *J Cell Biol* 1995; **130**: 1–13.

41. Koken M, Linares-Cruz G, Quignon F et al. The PML growth-suppressor has an altered expression in human oncogenesis. *Oncogene* 1995; **10**: 1315–1324.

42. Rousselot P, Hardas B, Castaigne S et al. The PML-RAR alpha gene product of the t(15;17)translocation inhibits retinoic acid induced granulocytic differentiation. *Oncogene* 1994; **9**: 545–551.

43. Cunningham I, Gee T, Reich L. Acute promyelocytic leukemia: treatment results during a decade at Memorial Hospital. *Blood* 1989; **73**: 1116–22.

44. Cordonnier C, Vernant JP, Brun B. acute promyelocytic leukemia in 57 previously untreated patients. *Cancer* 1988; **61**: 7–13.

45. Fenaux P, Pollet JP, Vandenbossche L et al. Treatment of acute promyelocytic leukemia: a report on 70 cases. *Leuk Lymphoma* 1991; **4**: 249–256.

46. Thomas W, Archimbaud E, Treille-Ritouet D, Fiere D. Prognostic factors in acute promyelocytic leukemia: a retrospective study of 67 cases. *Leuk Lymphoma* 1991; **4**: 249–256.

47. Breitman TR, Collings SJ, Keene BR. Terminal differentiation of human promyelocytic leukemia cells in primary culture in response to retinoic acid. *Blood* 1981; **57**: 1000–1008.

48. Chomienne C, Balitrand N, Cost H, Degos L et al. Structure-activity relationships of the aromatic retinoids on the differentiation of the human histiocytic lymphoma cell line U-937. *Leuk Res* 1986; **1**: 1301–1305.

49. Chomienne C, Ballerini P, Balitrand N et al. All-trans retinoic acid in promyelocytic leukemias. II. In vitro studies structure function relationship. *Blood* 1990; **76**: 1710–1717.

50. Huang M, Yu-Chen Y, Shu-Rong C et al. Use of all trans retinoic acid in the treatment of acute promyelocytic leukemia. *Blood* 1988; **72**: 567–572.

51. Castaigne S, Chomienne C, Daniel MT et al. All-trans retinoic acid as a differentiating therapy for acute promyelocytic leukemias. I. Clinical results. *Blood* 1990; **76**: 1704–1709.

52. Warrell RP, Frankel SR, Miller WH et al. Differentiation therapy of acute promyelocytic leukemia with tretinoin (all trans retinoic acid). *N Engl J Med* 1991; **324**: 1385–1393.

53. Miclea JM, Chomienne C. Effect of all-trans retinoic acid on CD34+ human myeloid cells. *Leukemia* 1994; **8**: 214–215.

54. Frankel SR, Eardley A, Lauwers G et al. The 'retinoic acid syndrome' in acute promyelocytic leukemia. *Ann Intern Med* 1992; **117**: 292–296.

55. Wang ZY, Sun GL, Shen ZX. *Chin Med J* 1999; **112**: 963–967 (quoted by L Degos, Z Y Wang. *Oncogene* 2001; **20**: 7140–5.

56. Dubois C, Schlageter MH, de Gentile A et al. Modulation of IL-6 and IL-1β and G-CSF secretion by all trans retinoic acid in acute promyelocytic leukemia. *Leukemia* 194; **8**: 1750–1757.

57. Warrell RP, Maslak P, Eardley A et al. Treatment of acute promyelocytic leukemia with all-trans retinoic acid: an update of the New York experience. *Leukemia* 1994; **8**: 926–933.

58. Muindi J, Frankel SR, Miller WH et al. Continuous treatment with all-trans retinoic acid causes a progressive reduction in plasma drug concentrations: implications for relapse and retinoid 'resistance' in patients with acute promyelocytic leukemia. *Blood* 1992; **79**: 299–303.

59. Cornic M, Delva L, Guidez F et al. Induction of retinoic acid binding protein in normal and malignant human myeloid cells by retinoic acid in AML3 patients. *Cancer Res* 1992; **52**: 3329–3334.

60. Mahmoud HH, Hurwitz CA, Roberts WM et al. Tretinoin toxicity in children with acute promyelocytic leukaemia. *Lancet* 1993; **342**: 1394–1395.

61. Stadler M, Ganser A, Hoelzer D. Acute promyelocytic leukemia. *N Engl J Med* 1994; **330**: 140–141.

62. Dombret H, Scrobohaci ML, Ghorra P et al. Coagulation disorders associated with acute promyelocytic leukemia: corrective effect of all-trans retinoic acid treatment. *Leukemia* 1993; **7**: 2–9.

63. Runde V, Aul C, Sudhoff T et al. Retinoic acid in the treatment of acute promyelocytic leukemia: Inefficacy of the 13cis isomer and induction of complete remission by the all-trans isomer complicated by thromboembolic events. *Ann Hematol* 1992; **64**: 270–272.

64. Hashimoto S, Koike T, Tatewaki W et al. Fatal thromboembolism in acute promyelocytic leukemia during all-trans retinoic acid therapy combined with antifibrinolytic therapy for prophylaxis of hemorrhage. *Leukemia* 1994; **8**: 1394–1395.

65. Fenaux P, Castaigne S, Dombret H et al. All-trans retinoic acid followed by intensive chemotherapy gives a high complete remission rate and may prolong remissions in newly diagnosed acute promyelocytic leukemia: A pilot study on 26 cases. *Blood* 1992; **80**: 2176–2181.

66. Warrell RP, Maslak P, Eardley A et al. Treatment of acute promyelocytic leukemia with all-trans retinoic acid: an update of the New York experience. *Leukemia* 1994; **8**: 926–933.

67. Kanamaru A, Takemoto Y, Tanimot M et al. All-trans retinoic acid for the treatment of newly diagnosed acute promyelocytic leukemia. *Blood* 1995; **85**: 1202–1206.

68. Fenaux P, Le Deley MC, Castaigne S et al, and the European APL91 group. Effect of all trans retinoic acid in newly diagnosed acute promyelocytic leukemia. Results of a multicenter randomized trial. *Blood* 1993; **82**: 3241–3249.

69. Fenaux P, Chevret S, Guerci A et al. Long term follow-up confirms the benefit of all trans retinoic acid in acute promyelocytic leukemia. *Leukemia* 2000; **14**: 1371–1377.

70. Tallman MS, Andersenn JW, Schiffer CA et al. All trans retinoic acid in acute promyelocytic leukemia. *N Engl J Med* 1997; **337**: 1021–1028.

71. Fenaux P, Chastang C, Chevret S et al. A randomised comparison of all trans retinoic acid (ATRA) followed by chemotherapy and ATRA plus chemotherapy and the role of maintenance therapy in newly diagnosed acute promyelocytic leukemia. *Blood* 1999; **94**: 1191–1200.

72. Beaumont M, Laï JL, Simonnet Z et al. Therapy related acute promyelocytic leukemia (APL) increasing incidence, especially after non Hodgkin's lymphoma (NHL) treated intensively. *Blood* 2000; **96**: 321a (abstract 1385).

73. Jansen JH, de Ridder MC, Geertsma WM et al. Complete remission of t(11;17) positive acute promyelocytic leukemia induced by all trans retinoic acid and granulocyte colony-stimulating factor. *Blood* 1999; **94**: 39–45.

74. Guglielmi C, Martelli MP, Diverio D et al. Immunophenotype of adult and childhood acute promyelocytic leukemia: correlation with morphology, type of PML gene breakpoint and clinical outcome. A cooperative Italian study on 196 cases. *Br J Haematol* 1998; **102**: 1035–1041.

75. Murray CK, Estey E, Paietta E et al. CD56 expression in acute promyelocytic leukemia: a possible indicator of poor treatment outcome. *J Clin Oncol* 1999; **17**: 293–297.

76. Ferrera F, Morabito F, Martino B et al. CD56 expression is an indicator of poor clinical outcome in patients with acute promyelocytic leukemia treated with simultaneous all trans retinoic acid and chemotherapy. *J Clin Oncol* 2000; **18**: 1295–1300.

77. Schoch C, Haase D, Haferlach T et al. Incidence and implication of additional chromosome aberrations in acute promyelocytic leukemia with translocation t(15;17) (q22;q21): a report on 50 patients. *Br J Haematol* 1996; **94**: 493–500.

78. Slack JL, Arthur DC, Lawrence D et al. Secondary cytogenetic changes in APL – prognostic importance in patients treated with chemotherapy alone and association with the

79. Vahdat L, Maslak P, Miller WH et al. Early mortality and the retinoic acid syndrome in acute promyelocytic leukemia: Impact of leukocytosis, low-dose chemotherapy, PML-RAR alpha isoform, and CD13 expression in patients treated with all trans retinoic acid. *Blood* 1994; **84**: 3843–3849.

80. Biondi A, Rambaldi A, Pandolfi PP et al. Molecular monitoring of the myl/retinoic acid receptor alpha fusion gene in APL by polymerase chain reaction. *Blood* 1992; **80**: 492–497.

81. Castaigne S, Balitrand N, de Thé H et al. A PML/RAR alpha fusion transcript is constantly detected by RNA based polymerase chain reaction in acute promyelocytic leukemia. *Blood* 1992; **79**: 3110–3118.

82. Huang W, Sun GL, Li XS et al. Acute promyelocytic leukemia: relevance of two major PML-RARα isoforms and detection of minimal residual disease by retrotransferase-polymerase chain reaction. *Blood* 1993; **82**: 1264–1269.

83. Lo Coco F, Diverio D, Avvisati G et al. Therapy of molecular relapse in acute promyelocytic leukemia. *Blood* 1999; **94**: 2225–2229.

84. Cassinat B, Chomienne C. Future perspectives for acute promyelocytic leukemia therapy. *Semin Haematol* 2001; **38**: 86–91.

85. Degos L, Dombret H, Chomienne C et al All trans retinoic acid as a differentiating agent in the treatment of acute promyelocytic leukemia. *Blood* 1995; **85**: 2643–2653.

86. Dombret H, Sutton L, Duarte M et al. Combined therapy with all trans retinoic acid and high-dose chemotherapy in patients with hyperleukocytic acute promyelocytic leukemia and severe visceral hemorrhage. *Leukemia* 1992; **6**: 1237–1242.

87. Mandelli F, Labopin M, Granean A et al, and EBMT. European survey of bone marrow transplantation in acute promyelocytic leukemia (M3). *Bone Marrow Transplantation* 1994; **14**: 293–298.

88. Paietta E, Andersen J, Gallagher R et al. The immunophenotype of acute promyelocytic leukemia (APL): an ECOG study. *Leukemia* 1992; **8**: 1108–1112.

89. Chen Z, Chen GQ, Shen ZX, Wang ZY. Treatment of acute promyelocytic leukemia with arsenic compounds: in vitro and in vivo studies. *Semin Hematol* 2001; **38**: 26–36.

90. Llallemand-Breitenbach V, Guillemin MC, Janin A et al. Retinoic acid and arsenic synergize to eradicate leukemic cells in a mouse model of acute promyelocytic leukemia. *J Exp Med* 1999; **7**: 1043–1052.

91. Chen ZC, Brand NJ, Chen A et al. Fusion between a novel Krüppel-like zinc finger gene and the retinoic acid receptor-alpha locus due to a variant t(11;17) translocation associated with acute promyelocytic leukaemia. *EMBO J* 1993; **12**: 1161–1167.

92. Redner RL, Rush EA, Faas S et al. The t(15;17) variant of acute promyelocytic leukemia expresses a nucleophosmin-retinoic acid receptor fusion. *Blood* 1996; **87**: 882–886.

93. Wells RA, Catzavelos C, Kamel-Reid S. Fusion of retinoic acid alpha to NuMA, the nuclear mitotic apparatus protein, by a variant translocation in acute promyelocytic leukaemia. *Nat Genet* 1997; **17**: 109–113.

94. Arnould C, Philippe C, Bourdon V et al. The signal transducer and activator of transcription STAT5b gene is a new partner of retinoic acid receptor alpha in acute promyelocytic-like leukaemia. *Hum Mol Genet* 1999; **8**: 1741–1749.

95. Special issued on APL: Acute Promyelocytic Leukemia. Guest editor L. Degos. *Semin Hematol* 2001; **28**(1).

96. Ten years of Molecular APL: from RARalpha to PML nuclear bodies. Guest editors M. Chelbi-Alix and H. de Thé. *Oncogene* 2001; **20**(49).

# 40 Myelodysplastic syndromes

**Pierre Fenaux and Claude Gardin**

## Introduction

Myelodysplastic syndromes (MDSs) are clonal disorders of pluripotent hematopoietic stem cells, of generally unknown etiology, occurring predominantly in the elderly. They are characterized by ineffective hematopoiesis leading to blood cytopenias, a high incidence of progression to acute myeloid leukemia (AML) and overall by a limited response to most available treatments.

## Epidemiology

### Incidence, age and sex[1–5]

MDS is a disorder of elderly people, occurring at a median age of about 70 years.[1–3] Childhood MDS is rare,[4] relatively often familial and often associated with monosomy 7[5] in those in that age range. Among adults, only 8–10% of the patients are younger than 50 years at diagnosis.[2] The incidence of MDS is about 3–5/100 000 per year, reaching 30/100 000 per year in patients aged over 70. The incidence does not seem to have increased over the last 20 years. A male predominance is seen in all series (with a M:F ratio of 1.5:2).

### Etiology

The etiology of MDS is generally unknown ('de novo' MDS). However about 20% of MDSs are 'secondary' to exogenous factors – mostly to antineoplastic chemo- or radiotherapy, less often to occupational or environmental exposure to various chemicals. Finally genetic predisposition to MDS includes constitutional disorders of childhood[3] and possibly genetic polymorphisms for enzymes involved in the detoxification of potential carcinogenic substances.[6]

#### *Exogenous factors*

Antineoplastic drugs (therapy-related MDS)[7,8]

A majority of cases of AML occurring after exposure to antineoplastic drugs are preceded by a phase of MDS. The most frequently incriminated drugs are alkylating agents, especially when used for prolonged periods. Some alkylating agents, such as cyclophosphamide, could induce fewer cases of MDS than others, especially when used in pulsed injections such as in CHOP cycles. Mechlorethamine (used in MOPP protocol) or prolonged use of melphalan, on the contrary, induces more cases of MDS. The nature of the primary tumor seems to have an impact on the incidence of therapy-related MDS, which is for example with chlorambucil less than 1% after CLL, but reaches 10% after polycythemia vera. Likewise, therapy-related MDS after hydroxyurea and pipobroman has only been reported in myeloproliferative disorders.

The epipodophyllotoxin agents etoposide (VP16) and teniposide (VM26) and, to a lesser extent, anthracyclines, have also been incriminated in the development of secondary AML, but these AMLs are generally not preceded by a preleukemic phase of MDS, and carry other genetic abnormalities, mainly balanced translocations involving 11q23, t(8;21), t(15;17), inv 16).[7,8]

After autologous marrow or stem cell transplantation, especially in lymphoma, an incidence of MDS of 3–5% has been reported.[9] Some studies have shown that the MDS clone was generally present prior to the conditioning regimen, and was rather due to prior treatment, especially prolonged alkylating agents, than to the conditioning regimen itself. On the other hand, total-body irradiation in the conditioning regimen is also associated with a higher risk of MDS.

Therapy-related MDS usually develops 3–7 years after exposure to chemotherapy and is associated to complete or partial loss of chromosome 7 in more than half of the cases, often with complex cytogenetic abnormalities.

Occupational and environmental exposure to chemicals[10–14]

Exposure to benzene and its derivatives has clearly been associated with the development of MDS, or AML generally preceded by MDS.[10,11]

For other compounds, data are less clear. The few case–control studies performed in MDS suggest a higher incidence of MDS not only in persons exposed to petroleum derivatives and exhausts from diesel engines (which contain benzene derivatives among others) but also in persons using insecticides, pesticides and weedkillers.[14] Those findings might possibly explain the higher incidence of MDS observed in agricultural workers and factory workers in some studies. A higher incidence of MDS was also present in smokers or ex-smokers in several experiences.[13,14] This could be due to the polycyclic aromatic hydrocarbons that are present in tobacco smoke.[14] Evidence for an association between MDS (or AML) and other exposures, including professional exposure to radiation, work in nuclear plants and high magnetic fields, has not been demonstrated.

### Immunological disorders in MDS

The increased incidence of immunological abnormalities in MDS, the favorable response to immunosuppressive drugs in some cases of MDS (see later) and the fact that 10–15% of cases of aplastic anemia (a disorder generally of autoimmune origin) evolve to MDS suggest a pathogenic role of immune effectors in some subsets of MDS.[15,16] Evolution to MDS, in aplastic anemia, is strongly associated to immunosuppressive treatment (as compared to allogeneic BMT), and possibly to high-dose or prolonged uses of G-CSF.

In addition, a significant association has been observed between MDS and some immunological disorders, including relapsing polychondritis, seronegative arthritis, vasculitis and possibly Crohn's disease.[17–19]

### Genetic predisposition in MDS

A high incidence of antecedent constitutional disorders (about 35%) is seen in childhood MDS.[20–22] These include Fanconi anemia, Noonan syndrome, Schwachman-Diamond syndrome, Down syndrome, mitochondrial cytopathies and neurofibromatosis. A large proportion of MDS occurring in these situations have monosomy 7.[3,4,23] In addition, families with several cases of MDS have been reported, both in children and adults.[24,25] In more than one family, a linkage to the 16q22 region has been suggested, by lodscore analysis.[24]

# Biology of MDS

## Cytogenetic abnormalities[26–36]

Clonal cytogenetic abnormalities in marrow cells are seen in about 50–60% of cases of MDS (Table 40.1).[26,27] In contrast to some other hematological malignancies, MDSs are not associated with any specific chromosomal abnormality. However, the rare

occurrence of translocations and the high incidence of complete or partial chromosomal loss or (less often) chromosomal gain is typical of MDS and distinguishes MDS from AML. The most frequent abnormalities are, in decreasing order, del 5q monosomy 7, trisomy 8, del 20q and loss of the Y chromosome, the latter being clearly a clonal anomaly. Among translocations, unbalanced translocations, leading to loss of chromosomal material are relatively frequent. For example, unbalanced t(5;17)(p11;p11) and t(7;17)(p11;p11) translocations lead to 17p deletion. These translocations are more frequent in therapy-related MDS than in de novo MDS.[7,8,29] Complex cytogenetic findings (i.e. with at least three chromosome abnormalities) are seen in 15–20% of MDS and 50% of therapy-related MDS (Table 40.1).

The fluorescence in situ hybridization (FISH) technique, performed on cytogenetic preparations (metaphase or interphase nuclei) or on bone marrow

### Table 40.1 Main cytogenetic abnormalities encountered in MDS

| | Approximate incidence (%) | |
| --- | --- | --- |
| | De novo MDS | Secondary MDS |
| **Partial chromosomal deletion** | | |
| del 5q | 20 | 20 |
| del 20q | 3–4 | <1 |
| del 7q | 1–2 | 10 |
| del or del 11q | 2–3 | <1 |
| del or del 12p | 1–2 | 3–4 |
| del 13q | 1 | <1 |
| **Chromosome loss** | | |
| Monosomy 7 | 10–15 | 50 |
| Loss of Y chromosome | 3–4 | 10 |
| Monosomy 17 | 3 | 5–7 |
| **Chromosome gain** | | |
| Trisomy 8 | 10–15 | 10 |
| Trisomy 11 | 3 | 1 |
| Trisomy 21 | 2 | 1 |
| **Translocations** | | |
| t(3;3)(q21;q26) | 1-2 | 3 |
| t(1;7)(p11;p11) | <1 | 4–5 |
| t(5;17)(q11;p11) | 1-2 | 4–5 |
| t(5;7)(q11;p11) | <1 | 2 |
| t(5;12) | <1 | <1 |
| **Other findings** | | |
| iso(17q) | <1 | 3–4 |
| inv(3)(q12;q26) | <1 | 3 |
| **Complex finding** | | |
| (≥ 3 chromosome abnormalities) | 15–20 | 50 |

slides, appears to be more sensitive than conventional cytogenetic analysis in some situations, especially for the detection of monosomy 7 and trisomy 8.[30–34] It is useful when low numbers of mitoses are obtained or when only one or two abnormal mitoses are found, questioning the clonality of the anomaly. Multiplex FISH or spectral karyotype (SKY) techniques,[34] whereby each chromosome pair is stained by a different color, can be useful in complex karyotypes, where they generally show the involvement of a larger number of chromosomes than expected from conventional studies, and often reveal unsuspected translocations.

The role of cytogenetic findings in the diagnosis of MDS – but more importantly for prognosis – will be stressed later.[27,35,36]

## Molecular abnormalities

Few genes involved in the pathogenesis of MDS have been identified (Table 40.2). This is certainly due in part to the fact that recurring chromosomal translocations are rarely seen in MDS – as translocation breakpoints indicate precisely the chromosomal regions of interest for the discovery of involved genes.

### RAS, NF1, PTPN11 mutations in MDS

Point mutations involving codons 12 or 13 or 61 of members of the RAS gene family (mainly N-RAS, less

often K-RAS and rarely H-RAS), leading to an activated RAS protein, constitute the most frequent known molecular anomaly identified in MDS.[37–40] Incidence of RAS mutations of about 30% in MDS were reported in early series, but that often included patients with advanced MDS. The incidence of RAS mutations at diagnosis in MDS is more likely to be in the range of 10–15%, with a higher incidence in chronic myelomonocytic leukemia (CMML) by comparison with other MDS subgroups. RAS mutations often appear during the course of the disease, as shown by longitudinal studies. Cases of MDS occurring in children with neurofibromatosis are associated with NF1 gene deletions and with a decrease in neurofibromin, the product of NF1 gene.[41] Neurofibromin is active in the RAS pathway, and inactivation of neurofibromin, like RAS gene mutations, leads to RAS activation.[42] This suggests the importance of a deregulated RAS pathway in the pathogenesis of MDS. This is further substantiated by the fact that RAS mutations often occur in the absence of chromosomal abnormalities, suggesting the involvement of a limited number of genetic defects in pathogenesis. On the other hand, no abnormalities of the NF1 gene have been found in adult MDS.[43]

Recently, point mutations of the PTPN11 gene, another gene involved in the RAS pathway and encoding for the SHP-2 phosphatase have been described in childhood MDS or AML.[44] These muta-

### Table 40.2  Known molecular abnormalities in MDS

| Gene | Type of anomaly | Incidence (%) |
|---|---|---|
| p15 | Hypermethylation | 0–60 |
| RAS (N or K) | Point mutation (codon 12,13 or 61) | 10–30 |
| p53 | Point mutation + deletion of other allele | 5 |
| FMS | Point mutation (codon 969 or rarely 301) | 5–10 |
| Flt3 | Deletion (ITD) point mutation D835 | 5–20 |
| AML1 | Point mutations Point mutations (tMDS) | 2.7 >15 |
| PTPN11 | Point mutations | 10 (children) |
| NF1 | Deletions | 5 (children only) |
| TEL | Fusion to PGDF-R gene (t(5;12) translocation) | <1 |
| MDS1– EVI1 EVI1 | Fusion to AML1 gene (t(3;21) translocation) | <1 |

tions differ from the germline mutations present in patients with Noonan syndrome, and are associated with a gain of function of SHP-2. These mutations are frequent (35%) in sporadic juvenile CMML, not associated with Noonan syndrome.

### FMS, p53, and AML1 mutations in MDS

The FMS gene encodes for the macrophage colony-stimulating factor (M-CSF) receptor. It has been reported to be mutated in about 10% of MDS cases, with a predominance in CMML, as for RAS mutations.[38,45] However, most mutations involve codon 969, a mutation that does not lead to activation of the M-CSF receptor. Some mutations involve codon 301, leading to activation of the receptor, but they only account for 10–15% of FMS gene mutations. The role of FMS mutations in MDS therefore still has to be more precisely established.

P53 gene mutations occur in about 5% of MDS cases.[46–48] As in other malignancies they predominate in exons 5–8 of the gene, and are generally missense mutations inactivating p53. They can be detected by single-stranded conformation polymorphism (SSCP) analysis of exons 5–8 of the gene, or immunocytochemistry on bone marrow slides (which detects p53 overexpression, almost synonymous with p53 missense mutation). p53 mutations are almost exclusively seen in refractory anemia with excess blasts (RAEB), refractory anemia with excess blasts in transformation (RAEB-T) and CMML, and are generally associated with deletion of the nonmutated allele, through deletion of chromosome 17p (resulting from t(5;17) or other unbalanced translocations involving 17p, monosomy 17 or, less often, iso 17q).[47,48] Most MDS cases with p53 mutations have complex cytogenetic abnormalities. It is unknown whether this is secondary to the p53 mutation, since p53 inactivation can lead to chromosomal instability. In the current authors' experience, p53 mutations in MDS (and AML) have always been found at diagnosis and are not acquired during the course of the disease. However, this does imply that they constitute an 'early' event in pathogenesis.

Missense mutations of the AML1 gene, have been identified at low frequency in de novo MDS,[49] but found in five of 13 patients with therapy-related MDS and six of 13 atomic bomb survivors in Hiroshima, diagnosed with MDS. All mutations but one were dominant-negative AML1 mutations,[50] as the germline mutations, described in the familial platelet disorder predisposing to AML (FDP/AML).[51]

Mutations of flt3, either D835 mutations or internal tandem duplications (ITDs) of the juxtamembrane region, have been described in MDS but their frequency is lower than in AML[52,54] and they seem restricted to advanced-stage MDS or MDS having progressed to AML.[54]

Finally, it should be noted that deletion and/or decreased expression of the retinoblastoma gene is very rare in MDS.[55]

### p15 hypermethylation[56–61]

Abnormal hypermethylation of gene promoter regions is a ubiquitous mechanism of reduced gene expression in tumor cells, as are irreversible missense mutations or gene deletions. In MDS, hypermethylation of the p15 gene, a cell cycle inhibitor, has been well studied.[56,57] Hypermethylation of p15 may be an early event in MDS,[60] but is also more frequently found (60%) in advanced-stage MDS.[56] Sequential studies have confirmed the association of abnormal methylation of p15 with clinical progression.[59]

The use of demethylating agents, such as 5azacytidine or its analog decitabine, have yielded major responses in MDS patients (see later). Reactivation of hypermethylated gene expression, such as p15,[61] is the rationale of the clinical use of demethylating agents, at low dose, although several mechanisms of action of these drugs in the clinical setting (cytotoxicity and differentiation through demethylation) have been demonstrated.

### Other well-characterized molecular anomalies in MDS

A few other gene abnormalities have been well characterized in MDS, but they occur in very small subgroups of MDS. They have generally been found in the rare cases of MDS with balanced translocations, molecular analysis of which has led to the discovery of fusion genes between a known gene and a new gene of interest, which could be subsequently cloned.

### MDS with t(5;12)(q31;p13)[62–64]

A few cases of MDS generally having features of atypical CMML with, in particular, eosinophilia have been reported. Cloning of the translocation breakpoint allowed the identification in 12p13 of TEL gene, a member of the ETS gene family.[62] In this translocation, the TEL gene was fused to the PDGF receptor gene (PDGF-R) at 5q31, the fusion product having constitutive tyrosine kinase activity. Importantly, the tyrosine kinase inhibitor, imatinib, has in vitro inhibitory activity on the fusion product, and is associated in vivo with a favorable clinical response.[63] Other translocations in rare CMML patients involve the fusion of the PDGF-R to other genes than TEL. Some new partners of PDGF-R have been even identified.[63,64]

### MDS with t(3;21)(q26;q22) or t(1;3)(p36;q21)[65]

A small number of MDS with t(3;21), generally occurring after antineoplastic drugs, has been reported. In these cases, the AML1 gene situated in 21q22 is fused to one of the following genes identified at 3q26: EVI1, MDS1, EAP or both (AML MDS1 – EVI1 complex fusion). In patients with high-risk MDS, a t(1;3) (p36;q21) translocation has also been described. The fusion involves an EVI 1-like gene, named MEL1, and RPN1, a housekeeping gene.

## MDS with t(3;5)(q25;q34)[66]

Patients with MDS and t(3;5)(q25;q34) have been described. The chimeric fusion gene involves the NPM gene, a regulator of p53, also frequently involved in anaplastic lymphoma subtypes, and a new gene: MLF1. In vitro expression of the fusion gene in cell lines is associated with increased apoptosis.[67,68]

## Unidentified genes: from cytogenetics to molecular biology of specific 'entities' in MDS

In AML, specific morphological-cytogenetic entities such as M2 AML with t(8;21), M4 eosino AML with inv(16), M3 AML with t(15;17) have been described. As in AML, specific entities with morphological–cytogenetic characteristics have been identified in MDS, including the '5q syndrome' and 17p deletions with dysgranulopoiesis (see later). In AML, specific gene abnormalities are being found in a growing number of these 'entities'. This search has been more difficult in MDS – to a large extent because translocations, which offer a good opportunity to identify new genes, are so rare in MDS. Because chromosomal deletions are frequent in MDS, the role of inactivation of tumor-suppressor gene(s) situated on deleted chromosomal fragments is strongly suspected in the pathogenesis of MDS. However, discovering new genes whose abnormalities could specifically be involved in MDS in these large chromosomal segments has so far proved difficult, in spite of cytogenetic, FISH and molecular techniques.

In the case of del 5q, the deletion is always interstitial, but of variable extent.[69–72] Analysis of large numbers of del 5q cases, however, showed two main commonly deleted segments in 5q31 and 5q32, respectively. The next step was to analyze known genes located in this region. However, none of the genes coding for growth factors or growth factor receptors situated in this region were found to be part of the common deleted segment. A third step was to identify new genes in those segments, one allele of which was deleted through del 5q and the other allele inactivated on the remaining chromosome 5 (by deletion or mutation). By positional FISH and molecular biology techniques, several genes, candidate genes, were shown to play a possible role, but no consensus has been reached. In fact, several genes could be involved in the pathogenesis of MDS with del 5q. Another possibility is that loss of one allele of one or several genes could lead to impaired hematopoiesis (haplo-insufficiency).

For other chromosome deletions, including del 20q, monosomy 7 and del 7q, common deleted segments have been identified in 20q11 and 7q31.[72–76] Several groups are also looking for tumor-suppressor genes; some candidate genes have been identified.

## Gene-expression profiles using microassay technique in MDS

Preliminary results of gene-expression profiles using the microarray technique in MDS have been published. Studies were complicated by the heterogeneity of the clonal cells in MDS, and the difficulty in comparing them to normal counterparts. Most groups have studied purified CD34+ populations. Among the genes overexpressed in MDS, the DLK1 gene, involved in stem cell and adipocyte differentiation, has been identified by at least two different groups.[77,78]

## Clonality in MDS

The first demonstration that MDSs were clonal disorders came from studies of $G_6PD$ isoenzymes in hematopoietic cells, although clonality was already strongly suspected when an abnormal clone was seen by chromosome findings. More recently, X-linked gene polymorphisms have been used to study clonality in female patients.[79,80] The main genes studied were the PGK, M27β and HUMARA genes. Their polymorphisms allow these genes to be informative in 50% (PGK gene) or almost all females (M27β and HUMARA genes).[80] Although there is still some controversy, it appears that in the majority of MDS cases, only myeloid but not lymphoid cells are part of the neoplastic clone; in some cases, however, B and/or T cells may also be clonal.[70,81]

Studies combining chromosome analysis (e.g. by FISH) and cell-lineage determination (e.g. by immunophenotype) have been performed both on marrow progenitors and circulating cells. In the former, the Scandinavian group found in MDS with del 5q, the chromosomal abnormality in early CD34+, CD38- progenitors.[82] By contrast, in MDS with +8, this cytogenetic abnormality was not found in CD34+, CD38- marrow progenitors.[83] Blood studies also showed that, in many cases of MDS, chromosome abnormalities such as monosomy 7 or trisomy 8 were present in only part of the circulating granulocytes.[84] In a study of MDS with del 20q, circulating granulocytes were shown not to carry the deletion.[85] All these findings could reflect the persistence of some non-clonal granulopoiesis in MDS in some patients with monosomy 7 or trisomy 8. However, in some well-studied examples, it was demonstrated by X-linked polymorphisms that granulocytes that did not carry the mutation were clonal. Likewise, in one study CD34+ and CD38- marrow cells that did not carry +8 behaved as MDS cells.[83] This suggests that chromosome abnormalities may be late genetic events, in many cases of MDS. In the case of childhood MDS, several findings show that monosomy 7 is a secondary event, and could constitute a 'common final pathway' to different conditions predisposing to MDS.[5]

## Immunological abnormalities in MDS

Associations between autoimmune disorders (including Crohn disease, ulcerative colitis, rheumatic disease, glomerulopathy, systemic lupus erythematosus, vasculitis, and seronegative arthritis) and MDS have been reported, especially in CMML.[17,18] The association may be stronger for relapsing polychrondritis (RP).[18,19] Indeed, in a series of 18 RP cases, five had clinical MDS. In a systematic study of bone marrow samples in seven cases of RP, three had morphological signs of MDS. This suggests a pathophysiological link beetween the two disorders. MDS could be a consequence of the immune disorder. Alternatively, granulocyte and/or monocyte dysfunction in MDS could lead to impaired disposal of immune complexes and subsequent deposition in small blood vessels, allowing the local activation of inflammatory mediators. Abnormalities of B cells including hypergammaglobulinemia, a higher incidence of monoclonal immunoglobulins and a higher incidence of autoantibodies than in a control age-matched population, are seen in CMML but not in other MDSs.[18] Irrespective of the type of MDS, the number of circulating T cells is generally diminished, and their function is reduced. Recently, several works have shown in MDS a skewed oligoclonal pattern in the T-cell repertoire, with preferential use of some V$\beta$ chain rearrangements, as seen in immunological disorders.[86–88] In some MDS patients, circulating clonal large granular T cells are also present.[89] An inhibition of CFU-GM growth by T cells has also been demonstrated in MDS.[87] Importantly, response to antithymocyte globulin (ATG) was associated to normalization of the T-cell repertoire and of CFU-GM growth in the presence of T cells. Impaired NK activity and dramatic reduction in the generation of NK cells from CD34+ cells in the presence of IL15 are also found.[90,91] Monocytes in MDS are derived from the abnormal clone, but only subtle functional impairment is generally seen.

Finally, a higher than expected incidence of lymphoid neoplasms, especially of immunoglobulin-secreting tumors, is seen in MDS.[18]

A particular situation where autoimmunity could be implicated is MDS with thrombocytopenia. Indeed, specific auto-antibodies directed against platelets are seen in 20% of MDSs,[92] and some responses are observed in this situation with therapeutic agents that are active in idiopathic thrombocytopenic purpura (ITP) (danazol steroids, high-dose immunoglobulins). In some of those patients, platelet lifespan was reduced and splenectomy improved platelet counts.[93,94,95]

The relationship between impaired immunity and clonal proliferation in MDS is therefore still uncertain. In some cases, abnormal lymphoid function could be explained in cases where lymphocytes are part of the abnormal clone. In other more frequent MDS cases, an immune attack on bone marrow progenitors could lead to destruction of most of them and genetic instability of the remaining progenitors.[96] This could lead to aplastic anemia evolving, after subsequent genetic events, in MDS.[16] Another model gives a major role to monocytes, which in MDS are part of the abnormal clone. Disordered monocyte/macrophage function could lead to persistent immune stimulation, by poor clearance of bacterial antigens, overactive antigen presentation, upregulated cytokine expression or a mixture of all three. This in turn would lead to B-cell hyperplasia, hypergammaglobulinemia, production of auto-antibodies and a greater risk of genetic errors in proliferating B cells, leading to neoplastic changes in some cases. This model could explain why CMML is the MDS subtype with the greatest immune disturbances.

## Cellular proliferation, differentiation and death in MDS

### Erythropoiesis in MDS

Ferrokinetic study of erythropoiesis with $^{59}$Fe demonstrates in MDS high marrow iron turnover (MIT) but low iron incorporation in erythrocytes, which is a characteristic feature of ineffective erythropoiesis.[97] A high proliferation of early erythroblasts, about 30% of erythroblasts being in S phase, has also been demonstrated. However, moderately shortened red cell lifespan is also often present in MDS. Finally, with evolution to RAEB and RAEB-T, MIT and percentage of ineffective erythropoiesis fall and a component of quantitative failure of erythropoiesis emerges.[97]

Growth of mature erythroid progenitors (burst-forming units erythroid [BFU-E] and colony-forming units erythroid [CFU-E]) from bone marrow and peripheral blood is suboptimal in most cases of MDS and absent in 30–75% of cases.[98] Long-term bone marrow cultures show reduced progenitor recovery in MDS patients. Overall, MDS erythroid progenitors appear to have reduced self-renewal capability, reduced capacity to generate BFU-E from blast colonies, and a deficiency of BFU-E relative to CFU-E in most patients.

### Growth factors and growth factor receptors in MDS

Because cytopenias in MDS could have been due in part to a lack of growth factors (GFs) or of response to GFs, serum levels of GF were measured and an analysis of GF receptors was performed.[99] Overall, very few abnormalities were found. In a recent report, expression of G-CSF receptors at the cell's surface was found to be variable in MDS.[100] Erythropoietin (EPO) concentration is usually appropriate for the degree of anemia, but sometimes low or high. In patients with low levels for the degree of anemia, response to treatment with EPO is often observed.[101] No rearrangements or abnormal expression of FMS, IL3 and GM-CSF genes (all situated in 5q) were seen, and no mutation of the c-KIT gene (which encodes for the SCF receptor) was observed.[102]

### Apoptosis in MDS

Increased apoptosis (programmed cell death) of myeloid cells would provide an explanation of the ineffective hematopoiesis leading to blood cytopenias observed in MDS, despite normal or increased numbers of bone marrow precursor cells. Quantitative studies in thin-section bone marrow biopsies support this assumption in most cases of MDS, although apoptosis of MDS cells is generally less important in bone marrow aspirates.[103,104] The importance of apoptosis measured in these studies is variable, from modestly increased to massive.[105] In some studies apoptosis predominates in immature cells, in others in more mature cells (high- vs. light-density cells). The increased tendency of MDS cells to undergo apoptosis can be demonstrated by morphological analysis, showing typical apoptotic features, by ISEL or similar techniques, DNA fragmentation (DNA laddering), or Annexin V labeling.[106,107]

Increased apoptosis is more important in less advanced stages of MDS, when compared to MDS with higher blast counts,[106,108,109] the escape of clonal cells from apoptosis could therefore be associated with progression of MDS and transformation.

Mechanisms of increased apoptosis in MDS remain uncertain.[108,110–112] Activation of cell death receptor signaling, including elevated TNF-α levels, TNF-related apopotosis inducing ligand (TRAIL), Fas and Fas ligand overexpression, are found in MDS bone marrows and/or plasma, especially in low risk patients (RA or RARS).[113–117] Direct activation of the mitochondrial apoptotic pathway has also been found. Increased ratios between proapoptotic (bad, bax) and antiapoptotic (bcl2, bclXL) molecules of the bcl2 family have been observed in early MDS, whereas this ratio tended to diminish with disease evolution.[113] Some MDS cells appear to be more sensitive to Fas-mediated cytotoxicity, such as MDS cells with trisomy 8 when compared to MDS cells with monosomy 7.[118]

What triggers the increased apoptosis in MDS is unknown: intrinsic defects of the clonal cells, including mitochodrial dysfunction,[119] may predominate in some MDS subtypes such as RARS or alternatively extrinsic apoptotic inducing signals from stromal cells, monocytes or T cells may play a major role in other patients, more likely to respond to anti TNF-α therapeutics or immune suppression.

# Diagnosis of MDS[120]

The diagnosis of MDS is, in the majority of cases, relatively easily made by the combined examination of blood and bone marrow aspirate – at least if the latter is examined by an experienced morphologist. Aplastic anemia and some diseases accompanied by marrow dysplasia, including vitamin $B_{12}$ and/or folate deficiency, exposure to heavy metals, recent cytotoxic therapy, ongoing inflammation (including HIV, and chronic liver disease/alcohol use), should, however be ruled out before concluding that MDS is present. Bone marrow trephine biopsy and karyotype, and less often, other tests may be useful to ascertain diagnosis in difficult cases.

Recently, flow cytometry studies in MDS have been reported, using various myeloid antigens on blast cells and/or more mature myeloid cells. Although these immunophenotypic studies are not yet standardized, they could improve the diagnosis and quantification of dysplasia, and could be of independent prognostic value.[121–124]

### Clinical findings

They are nonspecific and are usually the consequences of cytopenias, including:

- Symptoms of anemia
- Infections due to neutropenia but also to the frequently associated defect in neutrophil function. As in other types of neutropenia, infections are mainly due to Gram-negative bacilli or Gram-positive cocci, and less often to deep fungal infections
- Bleeding due to thrombocytopenia; this is usually seen in patients with very low platelet counts (however, bleeding may also occur in moderately thrompocytopenic patients or even in patients with normal platelets counts, because of thrombocytopathy, with abnormal platelet function).

No organomegaly is generally found in MDS, except in CMML, where splenomegaly is found in one-third of cases, sometimes associated to hepatomegaly. Specific infiltration of other organs is also observed in some cases of CMML – particularly infiltration of serous cavities (leading to pleural, pericardial or less often peritoneal effusions) or infiltration of the skin.

### Peripheral blood findings

MDSs are characterized by cytopenias of variable importance, involving one or several myeloid lineages.

### Red cells

Anemia is present in about 85% of the cases and is usually macrocytic. The mean corpuscular volume (MCV) rarely exceeds 120 μm³, however, contrary to what is frequently observed in megaloblastic anemias. Red cell shape abnormalities are frequent, including elliptocytosis and sometimes schizocytosis, and nucleated red cells can be found in about 10% of cases. Qualitative defects of erythrocytes, reflecting abnormal erythropoiesis, can be observed, including increased Hb F (or less often Hb H), decreased red cell enzyme activities (especially of pyruvate kinase), a paroxysmal nocturnal hemoglobinurea (PNH)-like disorder, and modification of red cell group antigens.

### Granulocytes and monocytes

Neutropenia is present in about 50% of the cases at diagnosis, and is often associated to morphological anomalies of neutrophils, including hypogranulation and less often hypolobulation with, in its extreme form pseudo-Pelger-Hüet anomaly. Qualitative neutrophil defects include decreased myeloperoxidase, and impaired chemotactic and bactericidal capability, which can potentiate, as described earlier, the risk of infections associated with neutropenia. The proportion of monocytes may be increased, and absolute circulating monocytosis (>1000/mm³) defines the CMML subtype of MDS.

### Platelets

Thrombocytopenia is present at diagnosis in about 30% of cases. Thrombocytosis can be observed, although rarely. Platelets may be abnormally large, and may have poor granulation or large, fused central granulation. Platelet dysfunction, reflected by prolonged bleeding time and decreased aggregation to collagen or adrenaline, and secondary to dysthrombopoiesis, can be observed. It may clinically increase the bleeding tendency.

Lymphocytes

As described earlier, T-cell lymphopenia and abnormal T-cell function can be observed.

### Bone marrow aspirate

The bone marrow aspirate is usually normo- or hypercellular, but is sometimes hypocellular, due to marrow fibrosis, poor aspiration, or true hypocellularity.

Myelodysplastic features are a characteristic finding of MDS. The different types of morphological abnormalities of myeloid precursors that can be observed are listed in Table 40.3. Among the most typical changes are megaloblastoid changes in erythroblasts, the presence of ringed sideroblasts (after Prussian blue staining), hypogranulation and hypolobulation of granulocytes, micromegakaryocytes, and large mononuclear megakaryocytes. It is notable that myelodysplastic features do not always involve all three myeloid lineages, and that the megaloblastoid changes observed in erythroblasts in MDS are generally less pronounced than in vitamin $B_{12}$ or folate deficiency. This characteristic and the hyperlobulation of granulocytes seen in vitamin deficiencies allow strong diagnostic orientation by morphology alone. On the other hand, none of the dysplastic features observed in MDS is specific.

| Table 40.3 Myelodysplastic features in MDS | |
|---|---|
| **MDS** | **Bone marrow and/or peripheral blood findings** |
| Dyserythropoiesis | Bone marrow: |
| |     Multinuclearity |
| |     Nuclear fragments |
| |     Megaloblastoid changes |
| |     Cytoplasmic abnormalities |
| |     Ringed sideroblasts |
| | Peripheral blood: |
| |     Poikilocytosis |
| |     Anisocytosis |
| |     Nucleated red blood cells |
| Dysgranulopoiesis | Nuclear abnormalities, including: |
| |     Hypolobulation |
| |     Ring-shaped nuclei |
| |     Hypogranulation |
| Dysmegakaryopoiesis | Micromegakaryocytes |
| |     Large mononuclear forms |
| |     Multiple small nuclei |

Prussian blue staining for iron should be systematically performed to reveal ringed sideroblasts where iron is stored in (abnormal) mitochondria, giving ring-shaped staining around the nucleus.

An increased percentage of marrow blasts (defined by marrow blasts >5%) is seen in about 50% of MDS, and is very specific of MDS, in the context of myelodysplastic features of the myeloid precursors. Because the percentage of marrow blasts forms the basis of the FAB classification of MDS, it is important to clearly identify marrow blasts and to distinguish them from more mature myeloid cells, especially promyelocytes. For this purpose, the FAB group distinguishes type I blasts, which have no cytoplasmic granules, from type II blasts, which have a few primary azurophilic granules, and are termed 'myeloblasts' by others. The blast percentage used for FAB and by the recent WHO classification should include type I and type II blasts. Marrow blasts of MDS usually have morphological and immunological features of myeloid blasts (CD13$^+$, CD14$^+$, CD33$^+$, peroxidase$^+$) but pure lymphoid (TdT$^+$, CD19$^+$, CD10$^+$) and biphenotypic patterns have been noted. They express CD34, a marker of stem cells, more often than blasts of AML. Expression of P-glycoprotein, the product of the multidrug resistance (MDR) gene is found in blast cells of MDS at diagnosis in 50% of the cases of MDS with an excess of marrow blasts (RAEB and RAEB-T), as compared to 20–30% in de novo AML. This higher incidence of P-glycoprotein expression in MDS could explain in part the lower response rate to chemotherapy seen in MDS, in comparison with de novo AML (see later).

## Bone marrow biopsy[125–127]

Because, in many cases, blood examination and bone marrow aspirate are sufficient for a diagnosis of MDS, the current authors feel bone marrow biopsy should not be systematically performed in elderly MDS patients, especially if it does not lead to any treatment modification. However it is obviously important in cases of difficult diagnosis, and it could bring additional prognostic information in some cases.

Bone marrow biopsy obviously assesses bone marrow cellularity better than bone marrow aspirate in MDS. Normal or increased cellularity is seen in 85–90% of cases, but authentic hypocellularity can be observed in 10–15% of cases (hypocellular MDS). Provided that care is taken to fix and process the specimen properly, myelodysplastic features can be analyzed very well in marrow biopsies, and for many authors this method is superior to marrow aspirate for the analysis of dysmegakaryopoiesis.

Marrow biopsy can also allow the detection of clusters of immature granulocytes in the intertrabecular region, away from their normal sites along the osseous surface, termed abnormal localization of immature precursors (ALIP).[125–127] ALIP has been linked to an increase of intracellular vascular endothelial growth factor (VEGF) with coexpression of one of its receptors, flt1, suggesting autocrine cytokine interaction, in patients with CMML, but also in other types of advanced MDS.[126] The presence of ALIP, even when it coexists with a normal percentage of blasts on bone marrow aspirates, might predict a poor outcome.[125,127] However, it may be difficult to distinguish true ALIP from clusters of early erythroblasts or megakaryocytes.[127]

Finally, biopsy is needed to assess fibrosis in MDS. A mild degree of reticulin fibrosis has been reported in up to 50% of patients with MDS, but only 15–20% show a significant increase in reticulin fibers, and collagen formation is rarely seen.

## Other tests for diagnosis

Apart from tests aimed at ruling out differential diagnoses, other tests are rarely indicated.

### Bone marrow karyotype

This allows the diagnosis of MDS in difficult cases, with moderate cytopenias and/or myelodysplastic features, by showing a clonal abnormality typical of MDS, especially monosomy 7, trisomy 8, del 5q or del 20q. When the number of mitoses obtained is low, FISH analysis of those chromosomes may also be useful to demonstrate the anomaly.

### Bone marrow progenitor cultures[99,128]

Colony-forming unit granulocyte-macrophage (CFU-GM) growth is characteristic of MDS when the number of colonies is diminished and small aggregates (clusters) predominate. A marked decrease of BFU-E and CFU-E is almost always observed in MDS.

### Magnetic resonance imaging[129]

A few studies have shown that magnetic resonance imaging (MRI) of the spine or femur gave atypical marrow patterns in MDS that could be differentiated from those observed in aplasia. MRI could therefore be useful in some cases of difficult diagnosis.

### Isotopic studies

Normal platelet lifespan study using $^{111}$In-labeled platelets may be useful to demonstrate MDS and rule out autoimmune destruction in cases with isolated thrombocytopenia.

Isotopic study of erythropoiesis can sometimes be useful, by demonstrating ineffective erythropoiesis, which is typical of MDS.[98]

## Differential diagnosis[130]

Megaloblastic anemias, due to vitamin $B_{12}$ and/or folate deficiency should always be ruled out, by measuring serum and erythrocyte levels of those compounds.

When an excess of marrow blasts is present, diagnosis of MDS is generally easy, the only question being the border with AML, which is defined by a percentage of marrow blasts greater than 30% in the French–American–British (FAB) classification and 20% in the World Health Organization (WHO) classification.

In cases with numerous ringed sideroblasts, other sideroblastic anemias (due to alcohol abuse, lead poisoning, copper deficiency or, very rarely, congenital sideroblastic anemias) can be ruled out relatively easily.

Chronic blood monocytosis is almost diagnostic of CMML, but causes of transient monocytosis should be eliminated.

In cytopenias without excess of marrow blasts, ringed sideroblasts and blood monocytosis, MDS is a diagnosis of exclusion. In particular, one should exclude several causes of myelodysplastic features of marrow precursors:

- Vitamin $B_{12}$ and folate deficiency
- Recent cytotoxic therapy
- Inflammation, including viral infections and particularly human immunodeficiency virus (HIV) infection, which can lead to myelodysplastic features in the bone marrow, probably resulting from infection of myeloid cells, nutritional factors, autoimmunity and drug effects
- Chronic liver disease and alcohol use.

Aplastic anemia should be ruled out in hypocellular MDS.

In MDS with isolated neutropenia or thrombocytopenia, other causes of neutropenia and peripheral thrombocytopenia should be excluded.

# Classification of MDS

## FAB Classification[131]

The FAB classification of MDS, proposed in 1982, has been widely adapted by hematologists for almost 20 years (Table 40.4). It is based on a small number of variables (blood and marrow blasts, ringed sideroblasts and blood monocytes) and is easy to apply, although discordances between groups have arisen, due to a large extent to the interpretation of the blast category on marrow smears. Some authors, for example, until recently did not categorize type II blasts among the blasts' cell population, but counted them as promyelocytes.

### RAEB and RAEB-T

RAEB and RAEB-T account for about 30% and 10% of MDSs, respectively. Pancytopenia is usually present. Cytogenetic abnormalities, present in 60% of cases, are often of the unfavorable type (monosomy 7, trisomy 8, complex findings). About one-half of the patients progress to AML, and survival is short, with a median survival of about 9 months for RAEB-T and 15 months for RAEB.

### Refractory anemia with ringed sideroblasts

Refractory anemia with RARS constitutes about 10% of MDS. The median age is older than in other MDSs

## Table 40.4  FAB classification of MDS[65]

| FAB type[*] | Frequency[†] Circulating blasts (%) | Marrow blasts (%) | Ringed sideroblasts (%) | Blood monocytes (× $10^9$/l) |
|---|---|---|---|---|
| RA | <1 | <5 | >15 | <1 |
| RARS | <1 | <5 | ≥15 | <1 |
| RAEB | <5 | 5–20 | Variable | <1 |
| RAEB-T | >5 | 21–30 or Auer rods | Variable | <1 |
| CMML | <5 | >30[‡] | Variable | ≥1 |

[*]RA: refractory anemia; RARS: refractory anemia with ringed sideroblasts; RAEB: refractory anemia with excess blasts; RAEB-T: refractory anemia with excess blasts in transformation; CMML: chronic myelomonocytic leukemia.
[†]Underlining indicates the important feature of some subtypes; [‡]Some authors classify patients with features of CMML but 21–30% blasts or >5% circulating blasts among RAEB-T.

(with the exception of CMML). Anemia is usually not associated with neutropenia or thrombocytopenia, and, in contrast, thrombocytosis is seen in 25–30% of cases. Cytogenetic abnormalities are less frequent than in RAEB and RAEB-T and, when present, are generally not unfavorable. Progression to AML occurs in only 10% of cases, and survival ranges between 5 and 10 years. The main complication of RARS is repetitive anemia, requiring frequent RBC transfusions, which expose the patient to the long-term risk of iron overload.

### Chronic myelomonocytic leukemia

Chronic myelomonocytic leukemia (CMML), like RARS, occurs at an older age than most MDSs, and has a more significant male predominance than other MDSs. It has characteristics of both MDS and myeloproliferative disorders (MPDs). Characteristics of MPD result from the granulocytic and monocytic proliferation, which tends to increase during the disease evolution, leading to high leukocyte counts and immature circulating granulocytes, in addition to monocytosis, splenomegaly and sometimes visceral involvement (particularly of the skin and serous cavities). Some authors have attempted to make a distinction between 'myelodysplastic' CMML, with no hyperleukocytosis and no organomegaly from 'myeloproliferative' CMML, with hyperleukocytosis and frequent splenomegaly. However, the former often evolves to the latter and the disorder should be seen as a continuum rather than as composed of clear-cut entities. About 25% of CMMLs progress to AML, and median survival is about 2.5 years.

### Refractory anemia or refractory cytopenias

This group is a diagnosic of exclusion among MDS, characterized by negative findings (no excess of marrow blasts, no blood monocytosis, no significant numbers of ringed sideroblasts). Although it is termed 'refractory anemia' (RA), this group is relatively heterogeneous: it also includes patients with pancytopenia, and patients without anemia but with neutropenia and/or thrombocytopenia. Therefore the term 'refractory cytopenia(s)' would appear preferable to "refractory anemia". About 20% of patients included in this group progress to AML, and median survival ranges from 4–6 years.

### WHO classification of MDS[132]

Published in 1999, the WHO classification is largely inspired from the FAB classification, but with several important modifications (Table 40.5):

- RAEB-T no longer exists, and MDS with marrow blasts from 20–30% are classified in AML.
- RA and RARS are divided each into two groups, based on the absence or presence of myelodysplastic features in the granulocytic and

---

**Table 40.5  WHO classification of myeloid neoplasms relevant to MDS according to the WHO classification, 1999**

**Myelodysplastic/myeloproliferative diseases**
  Chronic myelomonocytic leukemia
  Atypical chronic myelogenous leukemia
  Juvenile myelomonocytic leukemia
**Myelodysplastic syndromes**
  Refractory anemia
  With ringed sideroblasts
  Without ringed sideroblasts
  Refractory cytopenia (myelodysplastic syndrome) with multilineage dysplasia
  Refractory anemia (myelodysplastic syndrome) with excess blasts
  5q-syndrome
  Myelodysplastic syndrome, unclassifiable
**Acute myeloid leukemias***
  AML with multilineage dysplasia
  With prior myelodysplastic syndrome
**AML and myelodysplastic syndromes, therapy related**
  Alkylating agent related
  (Epipodophyllotoxin related (some may be lymphoid))**

*de novo AMLs are not included in this table.
**are generally not preceded by MDS

---

megakaryocytic lineage. When they are absent and MDS features are confined to the erythrocytic lineage, they are classified as having 'pure refractory anemia' (PRA) and 'pure refractory sideroblastic anemia' (PSA); when they are present, patients are classified as having 'refractory cytopenias with multilineage dysplasia' (RCMD) and 'refractory sideroblastic cytopenias with multilineage dysplasia' (RSMD).
- CMMLs are reclassified into a group of 'myeloproliferative/myelodysplastic disorders' or MPSs.
- The '5q- syndrome' (i.e. MDS with isolated del 5q) is classified separately.
- RAEBs are divided in RAEB 1 (with fewer than 10% marrow blasts) and RAEB 2 (with 10% blasts or greater).

Discussion has arisen after publication of those WHO proposals. In particular, there can be some interobserver variability in differentiating PRA from RCMD, and PSA from RSMD, as this differentiation is only based on morphological criteria. Furthermore, many patients with marrow blasts between 20–30% blasts can remain stable for months, and it is difficult to classify them among AMLs. Also, many CMMLs, at least at diagnosis, have limited features of MPD (high WBC counts, splenomegaly etc.) and never acquire them or acquire them after prolonged evolution. On the other hand, the prognostic value of multilineage dysplasia, in RA and RAS (according to FAB classification) has been shown.[133,134] Likewise, for RAEB, the cut-off point of 10% for marrow blasts appears to have important prognostic value. It has also been shown that RAEB-T had almost similar response to chemotherapy as AML, at least after adjustment on other features (especially cytogenetics).

## Atypical forms of MDS[131]

Most MDS cases can be classified according to FAB or WHO criteria. However, several types of MDS, with relatively specific features, were recognized after the FAB classification was proposed.

### MDS with myelofibrosis[135]

These probably include about 5% of MDSs, and are more frequently seen in therapy-related MDS. They can only be recognized well by marrow biopsy, which generally shows prominent dysmegakaryopoiesis. They can be distinguished from agnogenic myeloid metaplasia by the absence of splenomegaly, the absence of teardrop-shaped RBCs and the absence of leukoerythroblastosis, and from acute megakaryoblastic leukemia by the absence or small percentages of blasts of megakaryocytic origin.

### Hypocellular MDS[131]

These include cases with bone marrow cellularity below 30% (or below 20% in patients older than 60 years) and represent about 10% of de novo MDS, but are more frequent in therapy-related MDS. They are often associated to chromosome abnormalities, especially to monosomy 7, which helps distinguish them from aplastic anemia (AA). However, the borderline between hypoplastic MDS and AA may not always be clear-cut, as suggested for example by the therapeutic response to antilymphocyte globulin in well-documented cases of hypoplastic MDS.

### MDS with erythroblastopenia[131]

In some cases of MDS, anemia may be associated with erythroblastopenia on marrow samples, confirmed by ferrokinetic studies of erythropoiesis. When other lineages are not involved, these cases should be distinguished from erythroblastopenia of autoimmune origin, particularly associated to thymoma. del 5q is often observed in MDS with erythroblastopenia.

### MDS with features of MPD

As seen earlier, CMMLs often have features of MPD. Another disorder at the MDS/MPD interface is 'atypical CMML', characterized in the blood by moderate hyperleukocytosis, granulocytic dysplasia with a moderate number of immature granulocytes, usually between 3% and 10% of monocytes, no basophilia, no Philadelphia (Ph1) chromosome and no BCR rearrangement.

Finally, thrombocytosis is observed in some MDS, especially in RARS, and in MDS with 3q21, 3q26 abnormalities, del 5q or less often del 20q. Some cases of RARS or RA with del 20q can evolve to a typical MPD with myelofibrosis.[136]

## Specific morphological-cytogenetic 'entities' in MDS

As mentioned earlier, the identification of morphological–cytogenetic subgroups in AML such as M2 with t(8;21), M3 with t(15;17) and M4 eosino with inv(16) has allowed the discovery of specific cancer genes, which in at least one case (M3 with t(15;17)) is indicative of a response to a specific form of treatment. A few similar entities have also been identified in MDS, although no specific gene abnormality has as yet been identified in most of them, as seen earlier.

### 5q- (del 5q) syndrome[69]

del 5q may be associated with other chromosomal abnormalities or with an important excess of marrow blasts, and in those cases no typical features are generally seen. However, isolated del 5q in patients with RA (or RAEB) generally has very typical features, and can be recognized before cytogenetic results: most cases occur in elderly females, who have severe anemia, prominent macrocytosis, erythroblastopenia, normal leukocyte counts, thrombocytosis, and typical hypolobulated megakaryocytes in the bone marrow. The 5q deletion generally involves bands 5q13 to 5q33, progression to AML is rare, and survival is prolonged.

### MDS with 17p deletion[137]

MDS with 17p deletion have characteristics of RAEB or RAEB-T, and are often therapy related. They generally have a specific type of dysgranulopoiesis, with small granulocytes having prominent pseudo-Pelger-Hüet anomaly and cytoplasmic vacuoles, an association almost never seen in the current authors' experience in MDS or AML without 17p deletion. In three-quarters of cases, those patients have mutation of the nondeleted p53 allele (since the p53 gene is situated in 17p13 and one p53 allele is deleted in patients with 17p deletion). Although p53 inactivation may play an important role, it is suspected that other genes are involved in the pathogenesis of this syndrome.

### MDS with t(3;3)(q21;q26) or inv(3)(q21;q26)[138]

These are typically RAEB or RAEB-T, often therapy related, with thrombocytosis and micromegakaryocytes in the bone marrow. The gene(s) involved in these MDS variants are not yet identified, but the EVI1 and/or MDS1/EVI genes, located in 3q26, are inappropriately expressed after these rearrangements.

## Other entities

Two of these, namely MDS with t(5;12) and MDS with t(3;21) are very rare, but their analysis has led to the discovery of new genes whose disruption seems to play a role in pathogenesis, as seen earlier.

No other chromosomal abnormality is associated with specific hematological features in MDS.

# Childhood MDS[4,5,20–22]

Childhood MDSs are rare, accounting for about 2–3% of all MDSs. In about 35% of the cases, they occur in a background of constitutional abnormalities, including Down syndrome, Fanconi anemia, Noonan syndrome, mitochondrial cytopathies, neurofibromatosis and Schwachman-Diamond syndrome. They occur mainly in young children and are often not classifiable in the FAB or adult WHO classifications.

Recently, a modified WHO classification of childhood MDS has been proposed (Table 40.6).[4] Besides juvenile chronic myeloid leukemia (JMML) and transient myeloproliferations or AML associated with Down syndrome, de novo MDSs are split into refractory cytopenias (RCs), RAEB and RAEB-T. Therapy-related or secondary JMMLs are separately recognized (see Table 40.6).

The most frequent entity in childhood MDS is JMML, which has many features in common with adult CMML, including hepatosplenomegaly, high leukocyte counts and monocytosis. It is also characterized

by frequent elevation of Hb F. In mitochondrial cytopathies, the FAB type of MDS is usually RARS. The most frequent chromosomal abnormality in childhood MDS, including JCML, is monosomy 7, present in about 40% of cases. Point mutations of ras, PTPN11 or mutations of NF1 are present in the majority of these patients, and appear to be mutually exclusive. Interestingly, these gene mutations all lead to activation of the RAS pathway in leukemic cells.

In JMML, spontaneous colony-forming unit granulocyte-macrophage (CFU-GM) growth, which appears to be due to hypersensivity of CFU-GM to GM-CSF, has been observed.[5] Because GM-CSF is particularly produced by monocytes, this phenomenon could be involved in the myeloid proliferation, through an autocrine mechanism.

On the whole, childhood MDSs have a poor prognosis. Chemotherapy, in particular gives limited results and allogeneic bone marrow transplantation (BMT) should be proposed whenever possible. Its results, as for other hematological malignancies, are somewhat better in childhood than in adult MDS.

# Prognostic factors in MDS[36,138–142]

Although a large number of prognostic factors have been reported in MDS, a small number of them are generally sufficient in clinical practice. The most important factors are the percentage of marrow blasts, the number and extent of blood cytopenias and cytogenetic data; these factors can be grouped together in prognostic 'scores', mainly the International Prognostic scoring" (see Table 40.7).

### Prognostic factors

These include prognostic factors for survival, but also for progression to AML.

### Survival

Female sex and lower age are associated to more prolonged survival. However when the death rate in MDS is adjusted to that of a sex- and age-matched population (standard mortality ratio), it appears that MDS per se is not less aggressive in females and younger patients, and that their better survival rate is related to a lower incidence of death from other causes.[142]

Bone marrow blast percentage is certainly the most important prognostic factor, and is inversely proportional to survival. The number and extent of cytopenias also has major prognostic value, independent of that of marrow blasts. The FAB classification, largely based on marrow and circulating blasts, therefore has strong prognostic value, with RAEB and RAEB-T having short survival, RA and RARS relatively prolonged survival, and CMML an intermediate outcome. The

---

**Table 40.6 Diagnostic categories of myelodysplastic and myeloproliferative diseases in children (Hasle et al, 2003)**

I Myelodysplastic/myeloproliferative diseases
Juvenile myelomonocytic leukemia (JMML)
Chronic myelomonocytic leukemia (CMML) (secondary only)
BCR-ABL negative chronic myelogenous leukemia (Ph-CML)

II Down syndrome (DS) disease
Transient abnormal myelopoiesis (TAM)
Myeloid leukemia of DS

III Myelodysplastic syndromes
Refractory cytopenia (RC)
  PB blasts <2% and BM blasts <5%
Refractory anemia with excess blasts (RAEB)
  PB blasts 2–19% and BM blasts 5–19%
Refractory anemia with excess blasts in transformation (RAEB-T)
  BM blasts 20–29%

WHO classification further refines prognosis, with RCMD and RSMD having significantly poorer prognosis than PRA and PSA, RAEB 2 than RAEB 1 and the 5q- syndrome having a more favorable outcome.

Apart from bone marrow blasts and cytopenias, the only factor having clearly shown independent prognostic value is cytogenetic analysis. Three main prognostic groups can be identified by cytogenetics.[26,27,35] Complex cytogenetic abnormalities have a very poor prognosis, with survival rarely exceeding a few months; monosomy 7 also has a poor prognosis, although usually yields a longer survival when isolated. Isolated del 5q and probably isolated del 20q and loss of Y chromosome (although this is more disputed[76]) are a favorable subgroup with prolonged survival; patients with normal karyotype or with other single abnormalities have an intermediate prognosis.

Other parameters have been associated with a short survival, including ALIP,[125–127,143] importance of myelodysplastic features on marrow analysis (included in the WHO classification), CD34 expression by marrow blasts,[122,123] serum lactate dehydrogenase (LDH) levels,[144] results of marrow progenitor cultures,[128] presence of RAS[37,38] and p53 mutations,[38,145] and P-glycoprotein expression by marrow blasts.[146] Hyperexpression of WT1 has also been shown to be of prognostic value in some studies, although not shown to be independent of other widely known prognostic variables such as blast counts or IPSS score.[147]

## Progression to AML

Prognostic factors for progression to AML are generally similar to those associated with survival, in particular increased bone marrow blast percentage and the presence of complex cytogenetic rearrangements, which are associated with very high rates of progression to AML.

## Prognostic factors in treated patients

Most prognostic factors have been established in cohorts of MDS that received supportive care only. Other prognostic factors could appear with the application of specific treatments. For example, P-glycoprotein expression, which was an unfavorable factor in cases with MDS who received intensive chemotherapy, had no prognostic value on results of treatment with low-dose cytosine arabinoside (Ara C) in the current authors' experience.[146] Likewise, RAEB-T, according to the FAB classification, was the best prognostic subgroup in patients who received intensive chemotherapy, in contrast to patients treated by supportive care only.[148] Prognostic factors associated with response to ATG or G-CSF-Epo will be discussed later.

On the other hand, 'unfavorable' karyotypes are associated with a poor response to all available treatments, including intensive or low-dose chemotherapy, growth factors and immunosuppressive drugs, although it has been suggested that response to decitabine, a hypomethylating agent, could be independent of cytogenetic features.

## Prognostic scores in MDS[36,37,139–142]

These are based on parameters that have demonstrated prognostic value by multivariate analysis, and their purpose is to provide useful guidelines to the clinician for the choice of a therapeutic approach. Several prognostic scores for survival and progression to AML mainly based on bone marrow blasts, number

### Table 40.7 International Prognostic Scoring System (IPSS) for myelodysplastic syndrome (MDS)

| Prognostic variable | Survival and AML Evolution Score Value | | | | |
| --- | --- | --- | --- | --- | --- |
| | 0 | 0.5 | 1 | 1.5 | 2 |
| Marrow blasts (%) | <5 | 10 | | 11–20 | 20–30 |
| Karyotype * | Good | Intermediate | Poor | | |
| Cytopenias † | 0–1 | 2–3 | | | |

| Risk category | Combined score |
| --- | --- |
| Low | 0 |
| Int-1 | 0.5–1 |
| Int-2 | 1.5–2 |
| High | >2.5 |

AML: acute myeloid leukemia. *Good: normal, Y, del(5q), del(20q); Poor: complex (three abnormalities) or chromosome seven abnormalities; Intermediate: other abnormalities. †Neutrophils <1800/μL, hemoglobin <10 g/dL, platelets <100 000/μL.

of cytopenias and cytogenetic features have been designed, mainly the International Prognostic Scoring System (IPSS), adapted after meetings of major groups involved in MDS (summarized in Table 40.7). It has been suggested that a few other factors could be of value and yield additional prognostic value independent of the IPSS. They include in particular the presence of RAS or p53 mutations,[145] and immune phenotypes of blast and myeloid cells,[124] shown to be a predictor independent of the IPSS score in one recent study. Ongoing studies using microarrays will most likely be powerful tools to uncover new biologically relevant predictors of survival or response to various therapies.

## Treatment of MDS

Overall, it remains disappointing. The only really potentially curative treatment available so far is allogeneic stem cell transplantation, which can, however, only be performed in a small proportion of patients, given the usual age of MDS cases, although the advent of nonmyeloablative regimens may increase this proportion. Other treatments include chemotherapy, demethylating agents, growth factors, other agents aimed at reducing apoptosis, immunosuppressive drugs and new targeted treatment such as farnesyl transferase inhibitors. Supportive care remains an important component of the treatment.

### Response criteria in MDS

Because, in MDS, treatment generally cannot eradicate the disease but can at best improve cytopenias, response criteria used in clinical trials in MDS have been recently adapted to take into account all types of responses. Response criteria proposed by an International Working Group (IWG)[149] are summarized in Table 40.8. They include, as for AML, CR and PR, but also take into account 'hematological improvement' (HI) of one or several lineages. They also encourage the use of quality-of-life parameters in evaluating results of therapies.

### Allogeneic stem cell transplantation (SCT)[150-156]

Most reported series concern allogeneic SCT with standard conditioning regimens, bone marrow stem cells and from familial donors. Combination of published literature showed that about 40% of the patients were alive in first long-term remission, 30% relapsed and 30% died from the procedure. The high incidence of transplant-related mortality, by comparison to allogeneic SCT in other blood malignancies, is probably due to the age of the transplanted patients, a high proportion of cases being older than 40 and to the fact that those retrospective series often included a large proportion of patients allografted some 10–15

years ago. Relapses occured mainly in patients with an excess of marrow blasts and in patients with cytogenetic abnormalities. In order to prevent them, some authors advocated the use of intensive anthracycline – Ara C chemotherapy before allogeneic BMT in RAEB and RAEB-T. This hypothesis is being investigated in randomized trials. Another approach has been to reinforce the conditioning regimen. This does indeed lead to lower relapse rates – but also to higher transplant-related mortality. A last approach to reduce the relapse rate is the use of peripheral stem cells, which in a recent experience was shown to reduce the relapse rate post-transplant, with only moderate increase in chronic GVHd incidence, and survival improvement, by comparison to historical controls using bone marrow stem cells.

Several experiences of allogeneic SCT using a non-myeloablative regimen, aimed at reducing toxicity, have been reported, although with limited follow-up.[156] The mortality rate during the first years of follow-up is about 25%, but it is too early to evaluate the incidence of relapse after the procedure. As the GVL effect induced by nonmyeloablative allo SCT can probably be effective on a small tumor burden, it is suggested that, in patients with increased marrow blast percentage, nonmyeloablative allo SCT should be preceded by chemotherapy in order to reduce the leukemic burden. Nonmyeloablative allo SCT appears especially suitable for patients older than 50, i.e. the great majority of MDS patients.

Large reports of unrelated-donor marrow transplantation in patients with MDS have also been published. The 2-year disease-free survival, relapse and transplant-related mortality were of about 25%, 25% and 45%.[88] As for other hematological malignancies, results have however improved over the last years due to better donor-recipient HLA matching with molecular biology techniques.

### Intensive chemotherapy with or without autologous stem cell transplantation

Large series of MDS treated with intensive chemotherapy, in MDS phase or after progression to AML, have been published in the last few years.[157-164] They clearly show that the complete remission (CR) rates obtained are lower than in de novo AML, and range between 40% and 60%. Furthermore, median CR duration is only about 1 year and fewer than 10–15% of patients have prolonged remission.

On the other hand, several of those studies have shown that some subgroups of patients, including patients younger that 60, patients with RAEB-T at diagnosis and patients with normal karyotype had better results with intensive chemotherapy and that their survival rates could be prolonged with this approach, although probably only a small proportion

## Table 40.8 Measurement of response/treatment effect in MDS (International Working Group)

Altering disease natural history
1. Complete remission (CR)
   - *Bone marrow evaluation*:
     Repeat bone marrow showing less than 5% myeloblasts with normal maturation of all cell lines, with no evidence for dysplasia*. When erythroid precursors constitute less than 50% of bone marrow nucleated cells, the percentage of blasts is based on all nucleated cells; when there are 50% or more erythroid cells, the percentage blasts should be based on the nonerythroid cells.

   - *Peripheral blood evaluation* (absolute values must last at least 2 months):
     Hemoglobin greater than 11 g/dL (untransfused, patient not on erythropoietin)
     Neutrophils 1500/mm 3 or more (not on a myeloid growth factor)
     Platelets 100 000/mm 3 or more (not on a thrombopoetic agent)
     Blasts, 0%
     No dysplasia*

2. Partial remission (PR) (absolute values must last at least 2 months)†:
   All the CR criteria (if abnormal before treatment), except:
   - *Bone marrow evaluation*:
     Blasts decreased by 50% or more over pretreatment, or a less advanced MDS FAB classification than pretreatment. Cellularity and morphology are not relevant.

3. Stable disease
   Failure to achieve at least a PR, but with no evidence of progression for at least 2 months.

4. Failure
   Death during treatment or disease progression characterized by worsening of cytopenias, increase in the percentage bone marrow blasts, or progression to an MDS FAB subtype more advanced than pretreatment.

5. Relapse after CR or PR one or more of the following:
   Return to pretreatment bone marrow blast percentage.
   Decrement of 50% or greater from maximum remission/response levels in granulocytes or platelets.
   Reduction in hemoglobin concentration by at least 2 g/dL or transfusion dependence.

6. Disease progression
   For patients with less than 5% blasts: a 50% or more increase in blasts to more than 5% blasts.
   For patients with 5% to 10% blasts: a 50% or more increase to more than 10% blasts.
   For patients with 10% to 20% blasts: a 50% or more increase to more than 20% blasts.
   For patients with 20% to 30% blasts: a 50% or more increase to more than 30% blasts.
   One or more of the following: 50% or greater decrement from maximum remission/response levels in granulocytes or platelets, reduction in hemoglobin concentration by at least 2 g/dL, or transfusion dependence.

7. Disease transformation
   Transformation to AML (30% or more blasts).

8. Survival and progression-free survival.

Cytogenic response
(Requires 20 analyzable metaphases using conventional cytogenetic techniques)

*Major*: No detectable cytogenetic abnormality, if preexisting abnormality was present.
*Minor*: 50% or more reduction in abnormal metaphases.

Fluorescent in situ hybridization may be used as a supplement to follow a specifically defined cytogenetic abnormality.

Quality of life
Measured by an instrument such as the FACT questionnaire.
Clinically useful improvement in specific domains:
   Physical
   Functional
   Emotional
   Social
   Spiritual

Hematological improvement (HI)

(Improvements must last at least 2 months in the absence of ongoing cytotoxic therapy.)

Hematologic improvement should be described by the number of individual, positively affected cell lines
(e.g. HI-E; HI-E + HI-N; HI-E + HI-P + HI-N):

1. Erythroid response (HI-E)

*Major response*: For patients with pretreatment hemoglobin less than 11 g/dL, greater than 2 g/dL increase in hemoglobin; for RBC transfusion-dependent patients, transfusion independence.

*Minor response*: For patients with pretreatment hemoglobin less than 11 g/dL, 1–2 g/dL increase in hemoglobin; for RBC transfusion-dependent patients, 50% decrease in transfusion requirements.

2. Platelet response (HI-P)

*Major response*: For patients with a pretreatment platelet count less than 100 000/mm³, an absolute increase of 30 000/mm³ or more; for platelet transfusion-dependent patients, stabilization of platelet counts and platelet transfusion independence.

*Minor response*: For patients with a pretreatment platelet count less than 100 000/mm³, a 50% or more increase in platelet count with a net increase greater than 10 000/mm³ but less than 30 000/mm³.

3. Neutrophil response (HI-N)

*Major response*: For absolute neutrophil count (ANC) less than 1500/mm³ before therapy, at least a 100% increase, or an absolute increase of more than 500/mm³, whichever is greater.

*Minor response*: For ANC less than 1500/mm³ before therapy, ANC increase of at least 100%, but absolute increase less than 500/mm³.

4. Progression/relapse after HI: One or more of the following‡:
   a 50% or greater decrement from maximum response levels in granulocytes or platelets, a reduction in hemoglobin concentration by at least 2 g/dL, or transfusion dependence.

For a designated response (CR, PR, HI), all relevant response criteria must be noted on at least 2 successive determinations at least 1 week apart after an appropriate period following therapy (e.g. 1 month or longer).

*The presence of mild megaloblastoid changes may be permitted if they are thought to be consistent with treatment effect. However, persistence of pretreatment abnormalities (e.g. pseudo-Pelger-Hüet cells, ringed sideroblasts, dysplastic megakaryocytes) are not consistent with CR. †In some circumstances, protocol therapy may require the initiation of further treatment (e.g. consolidation, maintenance) before the 2-month period. Such patients can be included in the response category into which they fit at the time the therapy is started. ‡ In the absence of another explanation such as acute infection, gastrointestinal bleeding, hemolysis, and so on.

could be cured.[148, 160] By contrast, the presence of an abnormal, or worse a complex karyotype, p53 mutation and of P-glycoprotein expression predicts poor response to chemotherapy and long-term outcomes.[146,165,166]

Although several drugs (including fludarabine and topotecan) have been tested for induction treatment in combination to Ara C, generally at high dose, it appears that anthracyclin high-dose Ara C combinations (especially with idarubicin) remain the most effective induction regimens.[159,164] G-CSF and GM-CSF can significantly reduce the duration of aplasia after intensive chemotherapy. This effect is important to consider because the duration of aplasia after chemotherapy is longer in MDS than in de novo AML, and addition of G or GM-CSF could also reduce the incidence of deaths due to myelosuppression. However, their overall impact on CR rate and survival is unproven.[161,163] The current authors results suggest that agents reverting MDR gene expression, such as quinine, can increase the CR rate in P-glycoprotein-positive cases but they will have to be confirmed.[162]

In order to prevent relapse, several groups performed autologous bone marrow transplantation (ABMT) or peripheral stem cell transplantation (APSCT) after achievement of CR. The fact that, in a majority of MDS patients, lymphocytes do not appear to be part of the clone suggests the persistence of normal non-clonal hematopoietic cells that could reconstitute hematopoiesis after myeloablative treatment. Furthermore, it has been shown that circulating progenitors obtained after mobilization with chemotherapy and growth factors MDSs in hematological remission after chemotherapy were polyclonal,[167] although those findings rest on limited numbers of cases. More than 400 autografted MDS cases have been reported so far.[168-170] Hematological reconstitution does not seem to differ from that observed in AML, and is shorter after APSCT than ABMT.[169,170] However, the incidence of post-transplant relapse is high, and it is uncertain whether this approach will cure a significantly greater fraction of MDS patients, than intensive chemotherapy alone.[170] An ongoing trial compares intensive post-remission chemotherapy and autologous transplantation in CR.

## Low-dose chemotherapy and demethylating agents

Low-dose chemotherapy has been initially advocated in MDS on the basis of potentially 'differentiating' effects. The most frequently used drug has been low-dose Ara C (3–10 mg/m$^2$/12 h during 2–3 weeks),[171,172] while a few studies have used other drugs including hexamethylene bisacetamide (HMBA).[173] It is in fact unclear whether these drugs have a differentiating effect; in the case of Ara C (at least at 10 mg/m$^2$/12 h), a cytotoxic effect is obvious and pancytopenia is generally observed.

Response rates are usually in the range of 30–40%, about one-half being CR and one-half partial responses (PRs). Myelotoxicity is important, however, at Ara C 10 mg/m$^2$/12 h,[171] and regimens combining low-dose Ara C and G or GM-CSF do not seem superior to low-dose Ara C alone in terms of response and survival.[172] Most responses to low-dose Ara C do not exceed 12–18 months. A higher response rate to low-dose Ara C has been reported in patients with normal karyotype. Although, in a randomized trial, treatment with low-dose Ara C showed no superiority over supportive care only;[171] this treatment is probably beneficial to some MDS patients.

Two pyrimidine analogs other than cytarabine have also been used at low dose in MDS, i.e. 5 azacytidine and 3'5' deoxyazacytidine (decitabine). In vitro and in vivo data strongly suggest that, at least in part they may be active through gene demethylation. As seen earlier, hypermethylation of genes such as p15, leading to its inactivation, appear to be a major pathogenetic mechanism of progression of MDS and demethylation could restore their tumor-suppressive effect. Response rates of 50–60% have been reported with both 5 azacytidine and decitabine, with approximately 20% showing a complete response.[174-176] Furthermore, in a randomized study, treatment with 5 azacytidine was associated with significantly longer time to evolution to AML and improved quality of life and, a trend for improved survival[174,175] as compared to supportive care alone, despite the crossover of most patients allocated to supportive care. Following these studies, the use of 5azacytidine in the treatment of MDS has been approved by the American FDA.[177]

## Growth factors

### Erythropoietin

Erythropoietin (Epo), even at a very high dose (150 U/kg three times a week subcutaneously) can improve transfusion requirements in only about 25% of cases. However, in patients whose transfusion requirements are less than two red blood cell (RBC) units per month, and who have a serum Epo level of less than 200–500 U/ml, however, the response rate reaches 40–45%.[101] For responders, drug doses and/or frequency may be reduced, according to tolerance. For nonresponders to Epo alone after 4–6 weeks, the addition of G-CSF or GM-CSF to EPO increases the overall response rate to 40% and to at least 70% in patients with low serum Epo levels, limited transfusion requirement, or RARS.[178-183]

Trials are ongoing with darbepoetin, a modified form of Epo, with a 3-fold longer half-life.

### Granulocyte colony-stimulating factor and granulocyte-macrophage colony-stimulating factor

G-CSF and GM-CSF can correct neutropenia in about 75% of cases of MDS, using conventional doses of

5 μg/kg/d, and there is no evidence that they increase the incidence of progression to AML.[184] However no study has shown that growth factors, by potentially reducing the risk of infection, could improve survival.

Furthermore, G-CSF and GM-CSF are expensive treatments, especially if they have to be applied for prolonged periods in patients where, as in MDS, neutropenia is chronic. It has been shown that low-dose G-CSF or GM-CSF (i.e. 0.25–0.5 μg/kg/d) are almost as efficient as conventional doses in correcting neutropenia.[185]

In addition to improving neutropenia, granulocytic growth factors improve granulocytic function. Their stimulating effect on granulopoiesis seems to exert itself on both clonal and nonclonal hematopoiesis in MDS.

### Growth factors for megakaryocytic lineage

No trials of thrombopoietin, the specific platelet growth factor, or of its truncated form M-GDF, have been reported in MDS. Other growth factors with thrombopoietic (although nonspecific) activity have been used in MDS. Some platelet responses have been reported with IL3 and IL6, but with relatively important toxicity. More recently, platelet responses have been observed with IL11, but also with important toxicity.[186] The latter could be reduced with lower doses of IL11, which can still increase platelet counts.

Finally, no experience of treatment of MDS with growth factors active at the multipotent stem cell level, including stem cell factor or FLT3 ligand has been reported.

### Immunosuppressive drugs

Initial case reports of responses to ATG and/or cyclosporine A (CsA) in hypoplastic forms of MDS, have led to phase II trials of ATG or CsA in MDS patients, all RBC transfusion dependent. CsA alone, despite an early encouraging report, seems to have limited efficacy. ATG, with or without CsA, can yield major erythroid responses, or ever trilineage responses in about 35% of the patients, in several ATG trials.[187–189] Responses are more frequent in patients with RA. Of interest, patients with RA and normal or increased cellularity can obtain a meaningful response to ATG. Responses are durable, estimated to be 75% at 2 years in the largest cohort reported to date.[187]

Prognostic factors of response, initially identified by the NIH investigators were: younger age, low blast count, normal cytogenetics, presence of other cytopenias, presence of a PNH clone or DR2/15 subtype, and duration of previous RBC transfusion dependence. In a multivariate analysis of an expanded cohort of MDS patients treated with ATG and/or CsA at the NIH, DR2/15, age and shorter duration of previous RBC dependence, were the only significant prognostic factors of response to immunosuppressive therapy.[187,190]

The combined use of ATG and CsA in MDS was not associated with a higher response rate when compared to ATG alone, in the NIH studies.[190]

### Other drugs in MDS

Many drugs have been proposed in MDS over the last 20 years, based on their potential mechanism of action, or sometimes empirically.

Interferon-α, IL-2 and vitamin D derivatives have shown very limited efficacy, if any, in MDS.[191] Retinoids alone appear to improve cytopenias in limited numbers of patients,[192] but a preliminary report suggests they could have synergistic activity with EPO.[193]

Danazol and other androgens also appear to significantly improve thrombocytopenia in about one-third of MDS patients with no major excess of blasts. Their mechanism of action is uncertain but probably includes stimulation of megakaryopoiesis.[194,195] Low-dose melphalan can also yield responses, including CRs, in one-third of 'high-risk' patients.[196]

More recently, drugs supposedly active through their antiapoptotic or antiangiogenic activity have been used in MDS. Thalidomide has both antiangiogenic and antiapoptotic activity, the latter through its anti-TNF properties. Cytopenias are improved in about one-third of MDS patients, mainly those without excess of marrow blasts, but many patients stop treatment due to side-effects (constipation, fatigue, sleepiness), which are often prominent in this elderly population.[197,198] Therefore trials using lower thalidomide daily doses (200–300 mg) have been started. Thalidomide derivatives with fewer side-effects are in development. Promising early results, using the thalidomide analog CC 5013 have been reported with higher response rates, including a high incidence of complete responses in RA or 5q- patients.[199] An anti-VEGF antibody, bevacizumab is currently under study in phase II trials.[200] Other treatments aimed at reducing TNF-α levels in MDS, using soluble TNF-α, anti TNF-α have been tested in a few patients, some of whom improved their cytopenias.[201–203]

Amifostine is capable of reducing increased apoptosis of MDS precursors but, after a first favorable experience where it was shown to improve cytopenias in about two-thirds of the patients,[204] subsequent results have generally been more disappointing.[205] Other drugs being currently investigated included arsenic trioxide, which gives significant responses in 25–30% of the patients,[206,207] and farnesyl transferase inhibitors (FTIs). The latter have been designed to inhibit proteins such as activated ras, but probably also inhibit other proteins involved in the pathogenesis of MDS, such as the MAP kinase pathway.[208] They are active in about one-third of the patients, and CR has been reported, including in RAEB and RAEB-T. CMML may be particularly sensitive to FTIs.[209] Furthermore, presence of ras mutations does not appear to be a prognostic factor of response to FTIs. Arsenic trioxyde can also improve cytopenias in 20 to 25% of both low risk and high risk MDS. Its mechanisms of action includes triggering of apoptosis (in high risk MDS), differentiation induction and angiogenesis inhibition (in low risk MDS).

In 'proliferative' CMML with hyperleukocytosis, and sometimes splenomegaly or visceral involvement, the most frequently used cytotoxic drugs used are hydroxyurea and 6-mercaptopurine. Although preliminary reports suggested that (VP16) gave better response rates than those two drugs, especially in cases of visceral involvement, this was not confirmed in a randomized study in advanced CMML, where hydroxyurea gave both higher response rates and more prolonged survival than VP16.[210]

Finally, and importantly, reports show favorable response to imatinib in the rare cases of CMML with t(5;12) translocation[63] with TEL-PDGF-R rearrangement further stressing the importance of cytogenetic analysis in MDS. On the other hand, imatinib appears to be ineffective in CMML without t(5;12), including with those with other 12p abnormalities.

## Supportive care in MDS

Supportive care remains a major component in the management of MDS.

Repeated RBC cell transfusions expose patients to the risk of iron overload, which, as in thalassaemias, can be efficiently prevented in patients who require frequent transfusions by prolonged subcutaneous infusions of desferroxamine during several nights every week. Two reports strongly suggest that slow direct subcutaneous injections of desferroxamine (0.5–1 g) once or twice daily are as effective in MDS as prolonged subcutaneous infusion with similar daily dosage.[211] The oral chelator L1 appears somewhat less effective than desferroxamine. Other oral iron chelators are currently tested in MDS, including the ICL 670 agent.

Platelet transfusions can be useful in the case of severe bleeding episodes. Broad-spectrum antibiotics should be administered for all infectious episodes in neutropenic cases.

## Therapeutic strategy in MDS

There is no clear consensus over the therapeutic strategy in MDS in many situations, given the limited number of efficient available treatments in these disorders. The therapeutic strategy is generally based on age, IPSS (and/or bone marrow blasts infiltration) and donor availability for an allograft. The current authors have summarized in Figure 40.1 the approach currently used by the French MDS group. In patients aged less than 50–55 years with an HLA-identical family donor, who constitute fewer than 5% of MDS cases, allogeneic BMT is certainly the best treatment. However, it should probably not be performed in MDS with low or int1 IPSS until progression occurs.[212] When decided, the current authors suggest that it should not be preceded by intensive chemotherapy except in patients who present with a high marrow blast percentage (especially RAEB2 and RAEB-T) and do not have an unfavorable karyotype (i.e. patients who have a good chance to achieve CR with chemotherapy). The source of stem cells (marrow or peripheral stem cells) is also a matter of debate but currently available data favors the use of peripheral blood stem cells in patients with an excess of marrow blasts, who remain at high risk of relapse. In patients aged between 55 and 65, allogeneic BMT using nonmyeloablative regimens is currently under study. This approach has not yet demonstrated to be curative in MDS but, as seen earlier, preliminary results are encouraging.

In other patients, the current authors suggest the following attitude, also based on age, FAB or WHO classification, and/or IPSS.

### In patients with low or int1 IPSS (or if kanyotype is not available, marrow blasts <10%)

No treatment is useful in the absence of symptoms. Supportive care (transfusions, antibiotics) should be administered whenever required. In case of anemia, requiring transfusions, a trial of EPO ± G-CSF is warranted, if baseline serum EPO level is low (<500 U/l). Treating with epo ± G-CSF may also be discussed in patients with anemia not requiring transfusions as it may, by correcting anemia, improve the quality of life. In case of failure of epo + G-CSF, subcutaneous desferroxamine should be proposed, as soon as ferritinemia rises above 1500–2000 ng/ml and/or important hepatic or cardiac iron infiltration occurs. Investigational drugs (ATG, thalidomide, and other drugs) can then be proposed. ATG may be especially indicated early in the disease, when several cytopenias or a small PNH clone are present, or if the patient is HLA DR2/15. CC5013 may be particularly indicated in patients with 5q⁻ syndrome.

In the case of repeated infections in severely neutropenic cases, low-dose G-CSF or GM-CSF can be envisaged, at least during infectious episodes and if a neutrophil response is observed, in combination with antibiotics. In patients with platelets below 50–60 × 10⁹/l or in the presence of bleeding symptoms, the

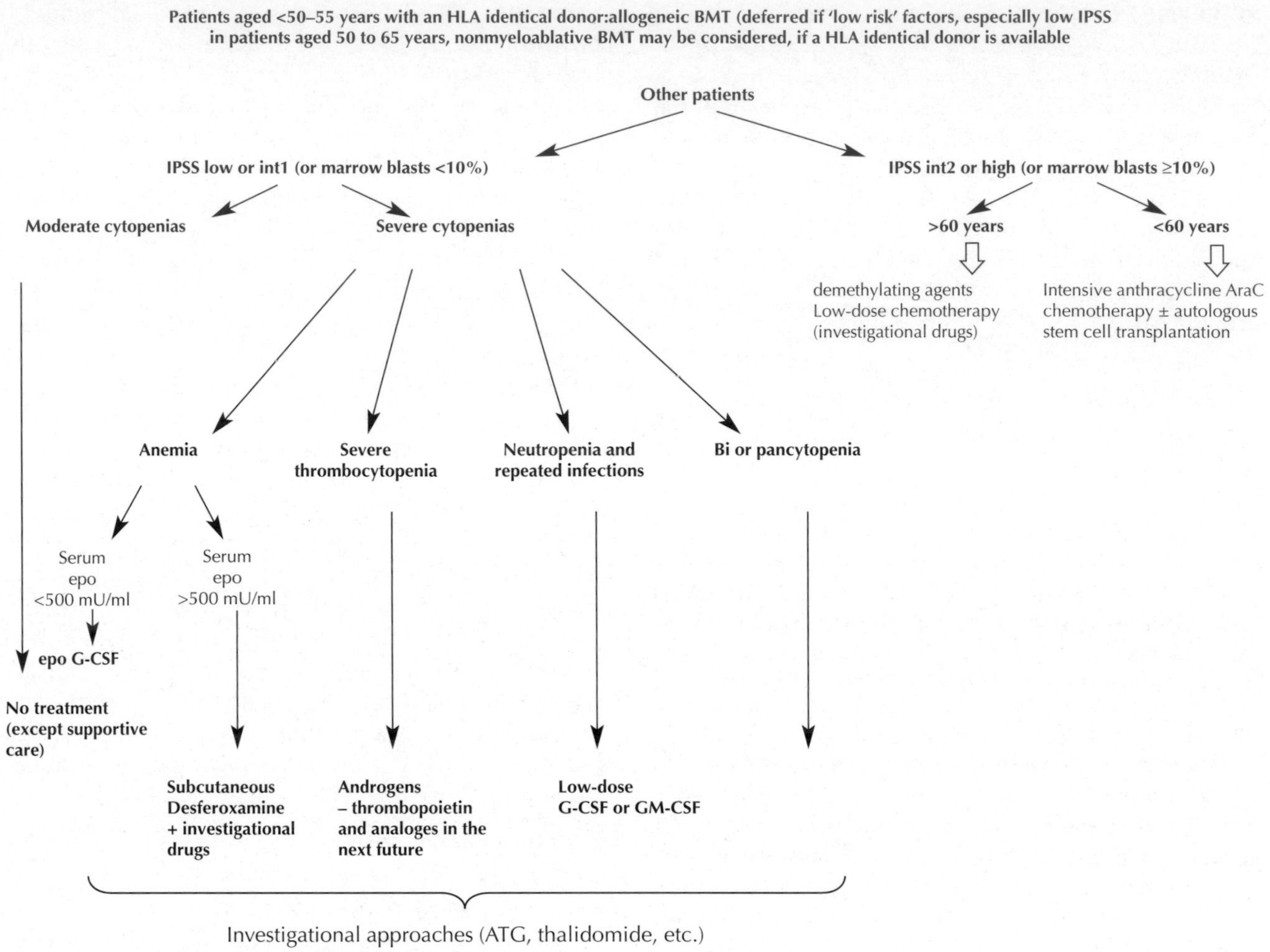

Patients aged <50–55 years with an HLA identical donor:allogeneic BMT (deferred if 'low risk' factors, especially low IPSS in patients aged 50 to 65 years, nonmyeloablative BMT may be considered, if a HLA identical donor is available

Other patients

IPSS low or int1 (or marrow blasts <10%)

IPSS int2 or high (or marrow blasts ≥10%)

Moderate cytopenias

Severe cytopenias

>60 years

demethylating agents
Low-dose chemotherapy
(investigational drugs)

<60 years

Intensive anthracycline AraC
chemotherapy ± autologous
stem cell transplantation

Anemia

Severe
thrombocytopenia

Neutropenia and
repeated infections

Bi or pancytopenia

Serum
epo
<500 mU/ml

Serum
epo
>500 mU/ml

epo G-CSF

No treatment
(except supportive
care)

Subcutaneous
Desferoxamine
+ investigational
drugs

Androgens
– thrombopoietin
and analoges in the
next future

Low-dose
G-CSF or GM-CSF

Investigational approaches (ATG, thalidomide, etc.)

**Figure 40.1** Proposed therapeutic strategy in MDS.

current authors suggest a trial of danazol at a daily dose of 600–800 mg for at least 3 months. Trials with thrombopoietin or IL11 should be starting. In case of severe neutropenia, anemia or thrombocytopenia not responding to those approaches, or in case of bi- or tri-cytopenia, investigational approaches should be tried.

### In patients with int2 or high IPSS (or if kanyotype is not available marrow blasts >10%)

Some kind of treatment aimed at reducing the blastic proliferation is required. In patients aged less than 60 years, capable of receiving intensive chemotherapy, the current authors suggest an anthracycline–Ara C course, followed, in the case of CR achievement, by consolidation chemotherapy and possibly autologous peripheral blood SCT. In older patients, several multi-center trials with demethylating agents are starting; low-dose Ara C, with or without growth factors can be efficient in some patients, especially with normal karyotype. Preliminary results with FTIs are also encouraging.

## Conclusion

MDS are frequent disorders of the elderly whose pathophysiology remains poorly known. However, knowledge of the role of alkylating agents in the etiology of MDS has already led to a reduction in their prolonged use, and this should translate into fewer cases of therapy-related MDS. Better knowledge of other occupational and environmental factors could also lead to preventive measures.

Further improvement in understanding the mechanisms of ineffective hematopoiesis should lead to the design of new therapeutic approaches that, for instance, could reduce apoptosis.

In cases with a major excess of blasts, the major goal, as in AML, remains the eradication of blast cells.

As in AML, progress will probably be also achieved by overcoming drug resistance, the possibility of separating nonclonal from clonal cells for autologous stem cell transplantation and improvements in allogeneic stem cell transplantation procedures.

# REFERENCES

1. Aul C, Gattermann N, Schneider W. Epidemiological and etiological aspects of myelodysplastic syndromes. *Leuk Lymphoma* 1995; **16**: 247–62.

2. Aul C, Giagounidis A, Germing U. Epidemiological features of myelodysplastic syndromes: Results from regional cancer surveys and hospital-based statistics. *Int J Hematol* 2001; **4**: 405–10. (Review)

3. Williamson PJ, Kruger AR, Reynolds PJ et al. Establishing the incidence of myelodysplastic syndrome. *Br J Haematol* 1994; **87**: 743–5.

4. Hasle H, Niemeyer CM, Chessells JM et al. A pediatric approach to the WHO classification of myelodysplastic and myeloproliferative diseases. *Leukemia* 2003; **2**: 277–82. (Review)

5. Luna-Fineman S, Shannon KM, Lange BJ. Childhood monosomy 7: Epidemiology, biology, and mechanistic implications. *Blood* 1995; **85**: 1985–9.

6. Morgan GJ, Smith MT. Metabolic enzyme polymorphisms and susceptibility to acute leukemia in adults. *Am J Pharmacogenomics* 2002; **2**: 79–92. (Review)

7. Levine EG, Bloomfield CD. Leukemias and myelodysplastic syndromes secondary to drug, radiation and environmental exposure. *Semin Oncol* 1992; **19**: 47–84.

8. Smith SM, Le Beau MM, Huo D et al. Clinical-cytogenetic associations in 306 patients with therapy-related myelodysplasia and myeloid leukemia: The University Of Chicago Series. *Blood* 2003; Mar 6 (Epub Ahead Of Print)

9. Armitage JO, Carbone PP, Connors JM et al. Treatment-related myelodysplasia and acute leukemia in non-Hodgkin's lymphoma patients. *J Clin Oncol* 2003; **5**: 897–906. (Review)

10. Aksoy M. Malignancies due to occupational exposure to benzene. *Am J Med* 1985; **2**: 217–45.

11. Stillman WS, Varella-Garcia M, Irons RD. The benzene metabolite, hydroquinone, selectively induces 5q31– and –7 in human CD34+CD19– bone marrow cells. *Exp Hematol* 2000; **2**: 169–76.

12. Farrow A, Jacobs A, West RR. Myelodysplasia, chemical exposure, and other environmental factors. *Leukemia* 1989; **3**: 33–5.

13. West RR, Stafford DA, White AD et al. Cytogenetic abnormalities in the myelodysplastic syndromes and occupational or environmental exposure. *Blood* 2000; **6**: 2093–7.

14. Nisse C, Haguenoer JM, Grandbastien B et al. Occupational and environmental risk factors of the myelodysplastic syndromes in the north of France. *Br J Haematol* 2001; **4**: 927–35.

15. Socie G, Henry-Amar M, Bacigalupo A et al. The European Bone Marrow Transplant Registry – Severe Aplastic Anemia Working Party malignant tumors occurring after treatment of aplastic anemia. *N Engl J Med* 1993; **329**: 1152–60.

16. Maciejewski JP, Risitano A, Sloand EM et al. Distinct clinical outcomes for cytogenetic abnormalities evolving from aplastic anemia. *Blood* 2002; **9**: 3129–313.

17. Hamblin TJ. Immunological abnormalities in myelodysplastic syndromes. *Sem Hematol* 1996; **33**: 150–62.

18. Mufti GJ, Figes A, Hamblin TJ et al. Immunological abnormalities in myelodysplastic syndromes. I. Serum immunoglobulins and autoantibodies. *Br J Hematol* 1986; **63**: 143–7.

19. Hebbar M, Brouillard M, Wattel E et al. Association of myelodysplastic syndrome and relapsing polychondritis: Further evidence. *Leukemia* 1995; **9**: 731–3.

20. Passmore SJ, Hann IM, Stiller CA et al. Pediatric syelodysplasia: A study of 68 children and a new prognostic scoring system. *Blood* 1995; **85**: 1742–50.

21. Bader-Meunier B, Mielot F, Tchernia G et al. Myelodysplastic syndromes in childhood: Report of 49 patients from a French multicenter study. *Br J Haematol* 1996; **92**: 344–50.

22. Sasaki H, Manabe A, Kojima S et al. Myelodysplastic syndrome in childhood: A retrospective study of 189 patients in Japan. *Leukemia* 2001; **11**: 1713–20.

23. Minelli A, Maserati E, Giudici G. Familial partial monosomy 7 and myelodysplasia: different parental origin of the monosomy 7 suggests action of a mutator gene. *Cancer Genet Cytogenet* 2001; **2**: 147–51.

24. Gao O, Horwitz M, Roulston D et al. Susceptibility gene for familial acute myeloid leukemia associated with loss of 5q and/or 7q is not localized on the commonly deleted portion of 5q. *Genes Chromosomes Cancer* 2000; **2**: 164–72.

25. Mandla SG, Goobie S, Kumar RT et al. Genetic analysis of familial myelodysplastic syndrome: Absence of linkage to chromosomes 5q31 and 7q22. *Cancer Genet Cytogenet* 1998; **2**: 113–18.

26. Fenaux P. Chromosome and molecular abnormalities in myelodysplastic syndromes. *Int J Hematol* 2001; **4**: 429–37. (Review)

27. Sole F, Espinet B, Sanz GF et al. Incidence, characterization and prognostic significance of chromosomal abnormalities in 640 patients with primary myelodysplastic syndromes. Grupo Cooperativo Espanol De Citogenetica Hematologica. *Br J Haematol* 2000; **2**: 346–56.

28. Christiansen DH, Andersen MK, Pedersen-Bjergaard J. Mutations with loss of heterozygosity of p53 are common in therapy-related myelodysplasia and acute myeloid leukemia after exposure to alkylating agents and significantly associated with deletion or loss of 5q, a complex karyotype, and a poor prognosis. *J Clin Oncol* 2001; **5**: 1405–13.

29. Takeyama K, Seto M, Uike N et al. Therapy-related leukemia and myelodysplastic syndrome: A large-scale Japanese study of clinical and cytogenetic features as well as prognostic factors. *Int J Hematol* 2000; **2**: 144–52.

30. Flactif M, Lai JL, Preudhomme C et al. Fluorescence in situ hybridization improves the detection of monosomy 7 in myelodysplastic syndromes. *Leukemia* 1994; **8**: 1012–18.

31. Wyandt HE, Chinnappan D, Loannidou S et al. Fluorescence in situ hybridization to assess aneuploidy for chromosomes 7 and 8 in hematologic disorders. *Cancer Genet Cytogenet* 1998; **2**: 114–24.

32. Rigolin GM, Bigoni R, Milani R et al. Clinical importance of interphase cytogenetics detecting occult chromosome lesions in myelodysplastic syndromes with normal karyotype. *Leukemia* 2001; **12**: 1841–7.

33. Ketterling RP, Wyatt WA, Vanwier SA et al. Primary myelodysplastic syndrome with normal cytogenetics: Utility of 'FISH panel testing' and M-FISH. *Leuk Res* 2002; **3**: 235–40.

34. Mohr B, Bornhauser M, Thiede C et al. Comparison of spectral karyotyping and conventional cytogenetics in 39

patients with acute myeloid leukemia and myelodysplastic syndrome. *Leukemia* 2000; **6**: 1031–8.

35. Morel P, Hebbar M, Lai JL et al. Cytogenetic analysis has strong independent prognostic value in de novo myelodysplastic syndromes and can be incorporated in a new scoring system: A report on 408 cases. *Leukemia* 1993; **7**: 1315–23.

36. Greenberg P, Cox C, Lebeau MM et al. International Scoring System for evaluating prognosis in myelodysplastic syndromes. *Blood* 1997; **6**: 2079–88.

37. Paquette RL, Landaw EM, Pierre RV. Et ALN-Ras mutations are associated with poor prognosis and increased risk of leukemia in myelodysplastic syndrome. *Blood* 1993; **82**: 590–9.

38. Padua RA, Guinn BA, AI-Sabah AI et al. RAS, FMS and p53 mutations and poor clinical outcome in myelodysplasias: A 10-year follow-up. *Leukemia* 1998; **6**: 887–92.

39. Mitani K, Hangaishi A, Imamura N et al. No concomitant occurrence of the N-Ras and p53 gene mutations in myelodysplastic syndromes. *Leukemia* 1997; **6**: 863–5.

40. Horiike S, Misawa S, Nakai H et al. N-Ras mutation and karyotypic evolution are closely associated with leukemic transformation in myelodysplastic syndrome. *Leukemia* 1994; **8**: 1331–6.

41. Shannon KM, O'connell P, Martin GA et al. Loss of the normal NF1 allele from the bone marrow in children with type 1 neurofibromatoses and malignant myeloid disorders. *N Engl J Med* 1994; **330**: 587–601.

42. Largaespada DA, Brannan CI, Jenkins NA et al. NF1 deficiency causes Ras-mediated granulocyte/macrophage colony stimulating factor hypersensitivity and chronic myeloid leukaemia. *Nature Genet* 1996; **12**: 137–46.

43. Preudhomme C, Vachee A, Quesnel B et al. Rare occurrence of mutations of the FLR exon of the neurofibromatosis 1 (NF1) gene in myelodysplastic syndromes (MDS) and acute myeloid leukemia (AML). *Leukemia* 1993; **7**: 1071.

44. Tartaglia M, Niemeyer CM, Fragale A et al. Somatic mutations in PTPN11 in juvenile myelomonocytic leukemia, myelodysplastic syndromes and acute myeloid leukemia. *Nat Genet* 2003 Apr 28. (Epub ahead of print)

45. Ridge SA, Worwood M, Oscier D et al. FMS mutations in myelodysplastic, leukemic and normal subjects. *Proc Natl Acad Sci USA* 1990; **87**: 1377–80.

46. Jonveaux P, Fenaux P, Pignon JM et al. Mutation in the p53 gene in myelodysplastic syndromes oncogene. *Oncogene* 1991; **6**: 2243–7.

47. Lai JL, Preudhomme C, Zandecki M et al. Myelodysplastic syndromes and acute myeloid leukemia with 17p deletion. An entity characterized by specific dysgranulopoiesis and a high incidence of p53 mutations. *Leukemia* 1995; **9**: 370–81.

48. Christiansen DH, Andersen MK, Pedersen-Bjergaard J. Mutations with loss of heterozygosity of p53 are common in therapy-related myelodysplasia and acute myeloid leukemia after exposure to alkylating agents and significantly associated with deletion or loss of 5q, a complex karyotype, and a poor prognosis. *J Clin Oncol* 2001; **5**: 1405–13.

49. Imai Y, Kurokawa M, Izutsu K et al. Mutations of the AML1 gene in myelodysplastic syndrome and their functional implications in leukemogenesis. *Blood* 2000; **9**: 3154–60.

50. Harada H, Harada Y, Tanaka H et al. Implications of somatic mutations in the AML1 gene in radiation-associated and therapy-related myelodysplastic syndrome/acute myeloid leukemia. *Blood* 2003; **2**: 673–80.

51. Song WJ, Sullivan MG, Legare RD et al. Haploinsufficiency of CBFA2 causes familial thrombocytopenia with propensity to develop acute myelogenous leukaemia. *Nat Genet* 1999; **2**: 166–75.

52. Yokota S, Kiyoi H, Nakao M et al. Internal tandem duplication of the FLT3 gene is preferentially seen in acute myeloid leukemia and myelodysplastic syndrome among various hematological malignancies. A study on a large series of patients and cell lines. *Leukemia* 1997; **10**: 1605–9.

53. Yamamoto Y, Kiyoi H, Nakano Y et al. Activating mutation of D835 within the activation loop of FLT3 in human hematologic malignancies. *Blood* 2001; **8**: 2434–9.

54. Horiike S, Yokota S, Nakao M et al. Tandem duplications of the FLT3 receptor gene are associated with leukemic transformation of myelodysplasia. *Leukemia* 1997; **9**: 1442–6.

55. Preudhomme C, Vachee A, Lepelley P et al. Inactivation of the retinoblastoma gene appears to be very uncommon in myelodysplastic syndromes. *Br J Haematol* 1994; **87**: 61–7.

56. Quesnel B, Guillerm G, Vereecque R et al. Methylation of the P15(INK4b) gene in myelodysplastic syndromes is frequent and acquired during disease progression. *Blood* 1998; **8**: 2985–90.

57. Preisler HD, Li B, Chen H et al. P151NK4B gene methylation and expression in normal, myelodysplastic, and acute myelogenous leukemia cells and in the marrow cells of cured lymphoma patients. *Leukemia* 2001; **10**: 1589–95.

58. Au WY, Fung A, Man C et al. Aberrant P15 gene promoter methylation in therapy-related myelodysplastic syndrome and acute myeloid leukaemia: Clinicopathological and karyotypic associations. *Br J Haematol* 2003; **6**: 1062–5.

59. Tien HF, Tang JH, Tsay W et al. Methylation of the P15(INK4B) gene in myelodysplastic syndrome: It can be detected early at diagnosis or during disease progression and is highly associated with leukaemic transformation. *Br J Haematol* 2001; **1**: 148–54.

60. Teofili L, Martini M, Di Mario A et al. Expression of P15(Ink4b) gene during megakaryocytic differentiation of normal and myelodysplastic hematopoietic progenitors. *Blood* 2001; **2**: 495–7.

61. Daskalakis M, Nguyen TT, Nguyen C et al. Demethylation of a hypermethylated P15/INK4B gene in patients with myelodysplastic syndrome by 5-Aza-2'-deoxycytidine (decitabine) treatment. *Blood* 2002; **8**: 2957–64.

62. Golub TR, Barker GF, Lovett M, Gilliland DG. Fusion of PDGF receptor beta to a novel Ets-like gene, Tel, in chronic myelomonocytic leukemia with T(5;12) chromosomal translocation. *Cell* 1994; **2**: 307–16.

63. Apperley JF, Gardembas M, Melo JV et al. Response to imatinib mesylate in patients with chronic myeloproliferative diseases with rearrangements of the platelet-derived growth factor receptor beta. *N Engl J Med* 2002; **7**: 481–7.

64. Baxter EJ, Kulkarni S, Vizmanos JL et al. Novel translocations that disrupt the platelet-derived growth factor receptor beta (PDGFRB) gene in BCR-ABL-negative chronic myeloproliferative disorders. *Br J Haematol* 2003; **2**: 251–6.

65. Nucifora G, Rowley JD. AML1 and the 8;21 and 3;21 translocations in acute and chronic myeloid leukemia. *Blood* 1995; **86**: 1–14.

66. Mochizuki N, Shimizu S, Nagasawa T et al. A novel gene,

MEL1, mapped to 1 p36.3 is highly homologous to the MDS1/EVI1 gene and is transcriptionally activated in T(1; 3)(P36;021)-positive leukemia cells. *Blood* 2000; **9**: 3209–14.

67. Matsumoto N, Yoneda-Kato N, Iguchi T et al. Elevated MLF1 expression correlates with malignant progression from myelodysplastic syndrome. *Leukemia* 2000; **10**: 1757–65.

68. Yoneda-Kato N, Fukuhara S, Kato J. Apoptosis induced by the myelodysplastic syndrome – associated NPM-MLF1 chimeric protein. Oncogene 1999; **25**: 3716–24.

69. Van Den Berghe H, Vermaelen K, Mecucci C et al. The 5q-anomaly. *Cancer Genet Cytogenet* 1985; **17**: 189–255.

70. Boultwood J, Fidler C, Strickson AJ et al. Narrowing and genomic annotation of the commonly deleted region of the 5q-syndrome. *Blood* 2002; **12**: 4638–41.

71. Horrigan SK, Arbieva ZH, Xie HY et al. Delineation of a minimal interval and identification of 9 candidates for a tumor suppressor gene in malignant myeloid disorders on 5q31. *Blood* 2000; **7**: 2372–7.

72. Castro PD, Liang JC, Nagarajan L. Deletions of chromosome 5q13.3 and 17p loci cooperate in myeloid neoplasms. *Blood* 2000; **6**: 2138–43.

73. Dohner K, Brown J, Hehmann U et al. Molecular cytogenetic characterization of a critical region in bands 7q35-Q36 commonly deleted in malignant myeloid disorders. *Blood* 1998; **11**: 4031–5.

74. Liang H, Fairman J, Claxton DF et al. Molecular anatomy of chromosome 7q deletions in myeloid neoplasms: Evidence for multiple critical loci. *Proc Natl Acad Sci U S A* 1998; **7**: 3781–5.

75. Velloso ER, Michaux L, Ferrant A et al. Deletions of the long arm of chromosome 7 in myeloid disorders: loss of band 7q32 implies worst prognosis. *Br J Haematol* 1996; **3**: 574–81.

76. Bench AJ, Nacheva EP, Hood TL et al. Chromosome 20 deletions in myeloid malignancies: Reduction of the common deleted region, generation of a PAC/BAC contig and identification of candidate genes. UK Cancer Cytogenetics Group (UKCCG).*Oncogene* 2000; **34**: 3902–13.

77. Miyazato A, Ueno S, Ohmine K et al. Identification of myelodysplastic syndrome-specific genes by DNA microarray analysis with purified hematopoietic stem cell fraction. *Blood* 2001; **2**: 422–7.

78. Hofmann WK, De Vos S, Komor M et al. Characterization of gene expression of CD34+ cells grom normal and myelodysplastic bone marrow. *Blood* 2002; **10**: 3553–60.

79. Van Kamp H, Fibbe WE, Jansen RPM et al. Clonal involvement of granulocytes and monocytes, but not of T and B lymphocytes and natural killer cells in patients with myelodysplasia: Analysis by X-linked restriction fragment polymorphisms and polymerase chain reaction of the phosphoglycerate kinase gene. *Blood* 1992; **80**: 1774–80.

80. Anan K, Ito M, Misawa M et al. Clonal analysis of peripheral blood and haemopoietic colonies in patients with aplastic anaemia and refractory anaemia using the polymorphic short tandem repeat on the human androgen-receptor (HUMARA) gene. *Br J Haematol* 1995; **89**: 838–44.

81. Preudhomme C, Vachee A, Morschauser F et al. Immunoglobulin and T cell receptor delta gene rearrangements are rarely found in myelodysplastic syndromes in chronic phase. *Leukemia* 1994; **18**: 365–71.

82. Kroef MJ, Fibbe WE, Mout R et al. Myeloid but not lymphoid cells carry the 5q deletion: polymerase chain reaction analysis of loss of heterozygosity using mini-repeat sequences on highly purified cell fractions. *Blood* 1993; **7**: 1849–54.

83. Nilsson L, Astrand-Grundstrom I, Anderson K et al. Involvement and functional impairment of the CD34(+)CD38(–)Thy-1(+) hematopoietic stem cell pool in myelodysplastic syndromes with trisomy 8. *Blood* 2002; **1**: 259–67.

84. Soenen V, Fenaux P, Flactif M et al. Combined immunophenotyping and in situ hybridization (FICTION): A rapid method to study cell lineage involvement in myelodysplastic syndromes. *Br J Haematol* 1995; **90**: 701–6.

85. Wattel E, Lai JL, Hebbar M et al. Deletion 20q in MDS is associated with distinct hematological and prognostic features. *Leuk Res* 1993; **17**: 921–6.

86. Kook H, Zeng W, Guibin C et al. Increased cytotoxic T cells with effector phenotype in aplastic anemia and myelodysplasia. *Exp Hematol* 2001; **11**: 1270–7.

87. Molldrem JJ, Jiang YZ, Stetler-Stevenson M et al. Haematological response of patients with myelodysplastic syndrome to antithymocyte globulin is associated with a loss of lymphocyte-mediated inhibition of CFU-GM and alterations in T-cell receptor Vbeta profiles. *Br J Haematol* 1998; **5**: 1314–22.

88. Kochenderfer JN, Kobayashi S, Wieder ED et al. Loss of T-lymphocyte clonal dominance in patients with myelodysplastic syndrome responsive to immunosuppression. *Blood* 2002; **10**: 3639–45.

89. Saunthararajah Y, Molldrem JL, Rivera M et al. Coincident myelodysplastic syndrome and T-cell large granular lymphocytic disease: Clinical and pathophysiological features. *Br J Haematol* 2001; **1**: 195–200.

90. Zeng W, Maciejewski JP, Chen G et al. Selective reduction of natural killer T cells in the bone marrow of aplastic anaemia. *Br J Haematol* 2002; **3**: 803–9.

91. Bourgeois E, Fenaux P, Bourhis JH et al. Altered NK cell function and differentiation in myelodysplastic syndromes (MDS). *Blood* 2002; **11**: 360A.

92. Hebbar M, Kaplan C, Caulier MT et al. Low incidence of specific anti-platelet antibodies detected by the MAIPA assay in the serum of thrombocytopenic MDS patients and lack of correlation between platelet autoantibodies, platelet lifespan and response to danazol therapy. *Br J Haematol* 1996; **94**: 112–15.

93. Wattel E, Cambier N, Caulier MT et al. Androgen therapy in myelodysplastic syndromes with thrombocytopenia: A report on 20 cases. *Br J Haematol* 1994; **87**: 205–8.

94. Bourgeois E, Caulier MT, Rose C et al. Role of splenectomy in the treatment of myelodysplastic syndromes with peripheral thrombocytopenia: A report on six cases. *Leukemia* 2001; **6**: 950–3.

95. Peddie CM, Wolf CR, Mclellan LI et al. Oxidative DNA damage in CD34+ myelodysplastic cells is associated with intracellular redox changes and elevated plasma tumour necrosis factor – alpha concentration. *Br J Haematol* 1997; **3**: 625–31.

96. Rosenfeld C, List A. A hypothesis for the pathogenesis of myelodysplastic syndromes: implications for new therapies. *Leukemia* 2000; **1**: 2–8. (Review)

97. Cazzola M, Barosi G, Berzuini C et al. Quantitative evaluation of erythropoietic activity in dysmyelopoietic syndromes. *Br J Haematol* 1982; **50**: 55–62.

98. Coutinho LH, Geary CG, Chang J et al. Functional studies of bone marrow haematopoietic and stromal cells in the myelodysplastic syndromes (MDS). *Br J Haematol* 1990; **75**: 16–25.

99. Zwierzina H, Schollenberger S, Herold M et al. Endogenous serum levels and surface receptor expression of Gm-Csf and Il-3 in patients with myelodysplastic syndromes. *Leuk Res* 1992; **16**: 1181–6.

100. Sultana TA, Harada H, Ito K et al. Expression and functional analysis of granulocyte colony-stimulating factor receptors on CD34++ cells in patients with myelodysplastic syndrome (MDS) and MDS-acute myeloid leukaemia. *Br J Haematol* 2003; **1**: 63–75.

101. Hellstrom-Lindberg E. Efficacy of erythropoietin in the myelodysplastic syndromes: A meta-analysis of 205 patients from 17 studies. *Br J Haematol* 1995; **89**: 67–71.

102. Mareni C, Sessarego M, Montera M et al. Expression and genomic configuration of GM-CSF, IL-3, M-CSF receptor (C-FMS), early growth response gene-1 (EGR-1) and M-CSF genes in primary myelodysplastic syndromes. *Leuk Lymphoma* 1994; **15**: 135–41.

103. Raza A, Gezer S, Mundle S et al. Apoptosis in bone marrow biopsy samples involving stromal and hematopoietic cells in 50 patients with myelodysplastic syndromes. *Blood* 1995; **1**: 268–76.

104. Mundle SD, Venugopal P, Cartlidge JD et al. Indication of an involvement of interleukin-1 beta converting enzyme-like protease in intramedullary apoptotic cell death in the bone marrow of patients with myelodysplastic syndromes. *Blood* 1996; **7**: 2640–7.

105. Shetty V, Hussaini S, Broady-Robinson L et al. Intramedullary apoptosis of hematopoietic cells in myelodysplastic syndrome patients can be massive: Apoptotic cells recovered from high-density fraction of bone marrow aspirates. *Blood* 2000; **4**: 1388–92.

106. Parker JE, Fishlock KL, Mijovic A et al. 'Low-risk' myelodysplastic syndrome is associated with excessive apoptosis and an increased ratio of pro- versus anti-apoptotic Bcl-2-related proteins. *Br J Haematol* 1998; **4**: 1075–82.

107. Bouscary D, Chen YL, Guesnu M et al. Activity of the caspase-3/CPP32 enzyme is increased in "early stage" myelodysplastic syndromes with excessive apoptosis, but caspase inhibition does not enhance colony formation in vitro. *Exp Hematol* 2000; **7**: 784–91.

108. Mundle S, Venugopal P, Shetty V et al. The relative extent and propensity of CD34+ vs. CD34- cells to undergo apoptosis in myelodysplastic marrows. *Int J Hematol* 1999; **3**: 152–9.

109. Gupta P, Niehans GA, Leroy SC et al. Fas ligand expression in the bone marrow in myelodysplastic syndromes correlates with FAB subtype and anemia, and predicts survival. *Leukemia* 1999; **1**: 44–53.

110. Claessens YE, Bouscary D, Dupont JM et al. In vitro proliferation and differentiation of erythroid progenitors from patients with myelodysplastic syndromes: Evidence for Fas-dependent apoptosis. *Blood* 2002; **5**: 1594–601.

111. Tehranchi R, Fadeel B, Forsblom AM et al. Granulocyte colony-stimulating factor inhibits spontaneous cytochrome C release and mitochondria-dependent apoptosis of myelodysplastic syndrome hematopoietic progenitors. *Blood* 2003; **3**: 1080–6.

112. Parker JE, Mufti GJ, Rasool F et al. The role of apoptosis, proliferation, and the Bcl-2-related proteins in the myelodysplastic syndromes and acute myeloid leukemia secondary to MDS. *Blood* 2000; **12**: 3932–8.

113. Allampallam K, Shetty V, Mundle S et al. Biological significance of proliferation, apoptosis, cytokines, and monocyte/macrophage cells in bone marrow biopsies of 145 patients with myelodysplastic syndrome. *Int J Hematol* 2002; **3**: 289–97.

114. Fontenay-Roupie M, Bouscary D, Guesnu M et al. Ineffective erythropoiesis in myelodysplastic syndromes: Correlation with Fas expression but not with lack of erythropoietin receptor signal transduction. *Br J Haematol* 1999; **2**: 464–73.

115. Mundle SD, Ali A, Cartlidge JD et al. Evidence for involvement of tumor necrosis factor-alpha in apoptotic death of bone marrow cells in myelodysplastic syndromes. *Am J Hematol* 1999; **1**: 36–47.

116. Gersuk GM, Beckham C, Loken MR et al. A role for tumour necrosis factor-alpha, Fas and Fas-ligand in marrow failure associated with myelodysplastic syndrome. *Br J Haematol* 1998; **1**: 176–88.

117. Zang DY, Goodwin RG, Loken MR et al. Expression of tumor necrosis factor-related apoptosis-inducing ligand, Apo2L, and its receptors in myelodysplastic syndrome: effects on in vitro hemopoiesis. *Blood* 2001; **10**: 3058–65.

118. SIoand EM, Kim S, Fuhrer M et al. Fas-mediated apoptosis is important in regulating cell replication and death in trisomy 8 hematopoietic cells but not in cells with other cytogenetic abnormalities. *Blood* 2002; **13**: 4427–32.

119. Gattermann N. From sideroblastic anemia to the role of mitochondrial DNA mutations in myelodysplastic syndromes. *Leuk Res* 2000; **2**: 141–51. (Review)

120. Kouides PA, Bennett JM. Morphology and classification of the myelodysplastic syndromes and their pathologic variants. *Semin Hematol* 1996; **33**: 95–110.

121. Stetler-Stevenson M, Arthur DC, Jabbour N et al. Diagnostic utility of flow cytometric immunophenotyping in myelodysplastic syndrome. *Blood* 2001; **4**: 979–87.

122. Ogata K, Nakamura K, Yokose N et al. Clinical significance of phenotypic features of blasts in patients with myelodysplastic syndrome. *Blood* 2002; **12**: 3887–96.

123. Maynadie M, Picard F, Husson B et al. Immunophenotypic clustering of myelodysplastic syndromes. *Blood* 2002; **7**: 2349–56.

124. Wells DA, Benesch M, Loken MR et al. Myeloid and monocytic dyspoiesis as determined by flow cytometric scoring in myelodysplastic syndromes correlates with the IPSS and with outcome after hemopoietic stem cell transplantation. *Blood* 2003; Mar 20 (Epub ahead of print])

125. Bellamy WT, Richter L, Sirjani D et al. Vascular endothelial cell growth factor is an autocrine promoter of abnormal localized immature myeloid precursors and leukemia progenitor formation in myelodysplastic syndromes. *Blood* 2001; **5**: 1427–34.

126. Mangi MH, Mufti GJ. Primary myelodysplastic syndromes: Diagnostic and prognostic significance of immuno-histochemical assessment of bone marrow biopsies. *Blood* 1992; **79**: 198–205.

127. Tricot G, De Wolf-Peeters C, Vlietinck R et al. Bone marrow histology in myelodysplasic syndromes. II. Prognostic value of abnormal localization of immature precursors in MDS. *Br J Haematol* 1984; **58**: 217–25.

128. Greenberg PL. Biological and clinical implications of marrow culture studies in the myelodysplastic syndromes. *Semin Hematol* 1996; **33**: 163–75.

129. Takagi S, Tanaka O, Miura Y. Magnetic resonance imaging of femoral marrow in patients with myelodysplastic syndromes or leukemia. *Blood* 1995; **86**: 316–22.

130. Rosati S, Anastasi J, Vardiman J. Recurring diagnostic problems in the pathology of the myelodysplastic syndromes. *Semin Hematol* 1996; **33**: 111–126.

131. Bennett JM, Catovsky D, Daniel MT et al. Proposals for the classification of the myelodysplastic syndromes. *Br J Haematol* 1982; **51**: 189–99.

132. Vardiman JW, Harris NL, Brunning RD. The World Health Organization (WHO) classification of the myeloid neoplasms. *Blood* 2002; **7**: 2292–302. (Review)

133. Nosslinger T, Reisner R, Koller E et al. Myelodysplastic syndromes, from French–American–British to World Health Organization: Comparison of classifications on 431 unselected patients from a single institution. *Blood* 2001; **10**: 2935–41.

134. Germing U, Gattermann N, Strupp C, Aivado M, Aul C. Validation of the WHO proposals for a new classification of primary myelodysplastic syndromes: A retrospective analysis of 1600 patients. *Leuk Res* 2000; **12**: 983–92; 1993; **17**: 921–6.

135. Lambertenghi-Deliliers G, Annaloro C, Oriani A et al. Myelodysplastic syndrome associated with bone marrow fibrosis. *Leuk Lymphoma* 1992; **8**: 51–5.

136. Wattel E, Lai JL, Hebbar M et al. Deletion of the long arm of chromosome 20 in de novo myelodysplastic syndromes is associated with distinct hematological and prognostic features. *Leuk Res* 1993; **17**: 921–6.

137. Lai JL, Preudhomme C, Zandecki M et al. Myelodysplastic syndromes and acute myeloid leukemia with 17p deletion. An entity characterized by specific dysgranulopoiesis and a high incidence of p53 mutations. *Leukemia* 1995; **9**: 370–8.

138. Nucifora G. The EVI1 gene in myeloid leukemia. *Leukemia* 1997; **11**: 2022–31.

139. Mufti GJ, Stevens JR, Oscier DG et al. Myelodysplastic syndromes: A scoring system with prognostic significance. *Br J Haematol* 1985; **59**: 425–33.

140. Sanz GF, Sanz MA, Vallespi T et al. Two regression models and a scoring system for predicting survival and planning treatment in myelodysplastic syndromes: A multivariate analysis of prognostic factors in 370 patients. *Blood* 1989; **74**: 395–408.

141. Aul C, Gattermann N, Heylla et al. Primary myelodysplastic syndromes: Analysis of prognostic factors in 235 patients and proposals for an improved scoring system. *Leukemia* 1992; **6**: 52–9.

142. Morel P, Declercq C, Hebbar M et al. Prognostic factors in myelodysplastic syndromes: Critical analysis of the impact of age and gender and failure to identify a very-low risk group using standard mortality ratio techniques. *Br J Haematol* 1996; **94**: 116–19.

143. Verburgh E, Achten R, Maes B et al. Additional prognostic value of bone marrow histology in patients subclassified according to the international prognostic scoring system for myelodysplastic syndromes. *J Clin Oncol* 2003; **2**: 273–82.

144. Aul C, Gattermann N, Germing U et al. Risk assessment in primary myelodysplastic syndromes: validation of the Dusseldorf score. *Leukemia* 1994; **11**: 1906–13.

145. Kita-Sasai Y, Horiike S, Misawa S et al. International Prognostic Scoring System and TP53 mutations are independent prognostic indicators for patients with myelodysplastic syndrome. *Br J Haematol* 2001; **2**: 309–12.

146. Lepelley P, Soenen V, Preudhomme C et al. Expression of the multidrug resistance P glycoprotein and its relationship to hematological characteristics and response to treatment in myelodysplastic syndromes. *Leukemia* 1994; **8**: 998–1005.

147. Cilloni D, Gottardi E, Messa F et al. Significant correlation between the degree of WTi expression and the International Prognostic Scoring System score in patients with myelodysplastic syndromes. *J Clin Oncol* 2003; **10**: 1988–95.

148. Fenaux P, Morel P, Rose C et al. Prognostic factors in adult de novo myelodysplastic syndromes treated by intensive chemotherapy. *Br J Haematol* 1991; **77**: 497–501.

149. Cheson BD, Bennett JM, Kantarjian H et al. Report of an international working group to standardize response criteria for myelodysplastic syndromes. *Blood* 2000; **12**: 3671–4.

150. Guardiola P, Runde V, Bacigalupo A et al. Retrospective comparison of bone marrow and granulocyte colony-stimulating factor-mobilized peripheral blood progenitor cells for allogeneic stem cell transplantation using HLA identical sibling donors in myelodysplastic syndromes. *Blood* 2002; **12**: 4370–8.

151. Sierra J, Perez WS, Rozman C et al. Bone marrow transplantation from HLA-identical siblings as treatment for myelodysplasia. *Blood* 2002; **6**: 1997–2004.

152. Deog HJ, Storer B, Slattery JT et al. Conditioning with targeted busulfan and cyclophosphamide for hemopoietic stem cell transplantation from related and unrelated donors in patients with myelodysplastic syndrome. *Blood* 2002; **4**: 1201–7.

153. Anderson JE, Anasetti C, Appelbaum FR et al. Unrelated donor marrow transplantation for myelodysplasia (MDS) and MDS-related acute myeloid leukaemia. *Br J Haematol* 1996; 93: 59–67.

154. Castro-Malaspina H, Harris RE, Gajewski J et al. Unrelated donor marrow transplantation for myelodysplastic syndromes: outcome analysis in 510 transplants facilitated by the national marrow donor program. *Blood* 2002; **6**: 1943–51.

155. De Witte T, Pikkemaat F, Hermans J et al. Genotypically nonidentical related donors for transplantation of patients with myelodysplastic syndromes: Comparison with unrelated donor transplantation and autologous stem cell transplantation. *Leukemia* 2001; **12**: 1878–84.

156. Parker JE, Shafi T, Pagliuca A et al. Allogeneic stem cell transplantation in the myelodysplastic syndromes: Interim results of outcome following reduced-intensity conditioning compared with standard preparative regimens. *Br J Haematol* 2002; **1**: 144–54.

157. Hoyle C, De Bastos C, Wheatley K et al. AML associated with previous chemotherapy MDS or myeloproliferative disorders: Results from the MRC's 9th AML Trial. *Br J Haematol* 1989; **72**: 45–53.

158. Gajewski J, Ho W, Nimer S et al. Efficacy of intensive chemotherapy for acute myelogenous leukemia associated with a preleukemic syndrome. *J Clin Oncol* 1989; **7**: 1637–45.

159. Estey EH, Kantarjian HM, O'Brien S et al. Comparison of idarubicin + Ara-C-, fludarabine + Ara-C-, and topotecan + Ara-C-based regimens in treatment of newly diagnosed acute myeloid leukemia, refractory anemia with excess blasts in transformation, or refractory anemia with excess blasts. *Blood* 2001; **13**: 3575–83.

160. Estey EH, Kantarjian HM, O'Brien S et al. High remission rate, short remission duration in patients with refractory anemia with excess blasts (RAEB) in transformation (RAEB-T) given acute myelogenous leukemia (AML)-type chemotherapy in combination with granulocyte-CSF (G-CSF). *Cytokines Mol Ther* 1995; **1**: 21–8.

161. Estey EH, Thall PF, Pierce S et al. Randomized phase II study of fludarabine + cytosine arabinoside + idarubicin +/− all-trans retinoic acid +/− granulocyte colony-stimulating factor in poor prognosis newly diagnosed acute myeloid leukemia and myelodysplastic syndrome. *Blood* 1999; **8**: 2478–84.

162. Wattel E, Solary E, Hecquet B et al. Quinine improves the results of intensive chemotherapy in myelodysplastic syndromes expressing P glycoprotein: Results of a randomized study. *Br J Haematol* 1998; **4**: 1015–24.

163. Ossenkoppele GJ, Van Der Holt B, Verhoef GE et al. A randomized study of granulocyte colony-stimulating factor applied during and after chemotherapy in patients with poor risk myelodysplastic syndromes: A report from the HOVON Cooperative Group. Dutch–Belgian Hemato-Oncology Cooperative Group. *Leukemia* 1999; **8**: 1207–13.

164. Beran M, Shen Y, Kantarjian H et al. High-dose chemotherapy in high-risk myelodysplastic syndrome: Covariate-adjusted comparison of five regimens. *Cancer* 2001; **8**: 1999–2015.

165. Estey EH, Pierce S, Keating MJ. Identification of a group of AMUMDS patients with a relatively favorable prognosis who have chromosome 5 and/or 7 abnormalities. *Haematologica* 2000; **3**: 246–9.

166. Wattel E, Preudhomme C, Hecquet B et al. P53 mutations are associated to resistance to chemotherapy and short survival in hematologic malignancies. *Blood* 1994; **84**: 3148–58.

167. Delforge M, Demuynck H, Vandenberghe P et al. Polyclonal primitive hematopoietic progenitors can be detected in mobilized peripheral blood from patients with high-risk myelodysplastic syndromes. *Blood* 1995; **86**: 3660–7.

168. De Witte T, Hermans J, Vossen J et al. Haematopoietic stem cell transplantation for patients with myelo-dysplastic syndromes and secondary acute myeloid leukaemias: A report on behalf of the chronic leukaemia working party of the European Group For Blood And Marrow Transplantation (EBMT). *Br J Haematol* 2000; **3**: 620–30.

169. De Witte T, Suciu S, Verhoef G et al. Intensive chemotherapy followed by allogeneic or autologous stem cell transplantation for patients with myelodysplastic syndromes (Mdss) and acute myeloid leukemia following MDS. *Blood* 2001; **8**: 2326–31.

170. Oosterveld M, Muus P, Suciu S et al. Chemotherapy only compared to chemotherapy followed by transplantation in high risk myelodysplastic syndrome and secondary acute myeloid leukemia; Two parallel studies adjusted for various prognostic factors. *Leukemia* 2002; **9**: 1615–21.

171. Cheson BD, Jasperse DM, Simon R et al. A critical appraisal of low-dose Ara C in patients with acute non lymphocytic leukemia and myelodysplastic syndromes. *J Clin Oncol* 1986; **4**: 1857–64.

172. Miller KB, Kyungmann K, Morrison FS et al. The evaluation of low-dose cytarabine in the treatment of myelodysplastic syndromes: A phase III intergroup study. *Ann Hematol* 1992; **65**: 162–8.

173. Stone R, Michaeli J et al. Hexamethylene bisacetamide in myelodysplastic syndrome and acute myelogenous leukemia: A phase II clinical trial with a differentiation-inducing agent. *Blood* 1992; **80**: 2604–9.

174. Silverman LR, Demakos EP, Peterson BL et al. Randomized controlled trial of azacitidine in patients with the myelodysplastic syndrome: A study of the cancer and leukemia group B. *J Clin Oncol* 2002; **10**: 2429–40.

175. Kornblith AB, Herndon JE 2nd, Silverman LR et al. Impact of azacytidine on the quality of life of patients with myelodysplastic syndrome treated in a randomized phase III trial: A cancer and leukemia group B study. *J Clin Oncol* 2002; **10**: 2441–52.

176. Wijermans P, Lubbert M, Verhoef G et al. Low-dose 5-Aza-2′-deoxycytidine, A DNA hypomethylating agent, for the treatment of high-risk myelodysplastic syndrome: A multicenter phase II study in elderly patients. *J Clin Oncol* 2000; **18**: 956–62.

177. Lubbert M, Wijermans P, Kunzmann R et al. Cytogenetic responses in high-risk myelodysplastic syndrome following low-dose treatment with the DNA methylation inhibitor 5-Aza-2′-deoxycytidine. *Br J Haematol* 2001; **2**: 349–57; **5**: 956–62.

178. Hellstrom-Lindberg E for The Scandinavian MDS Group. A combination of granulocyte-colony-stimulating factor and erythropoietin may synergistically improve the anemia in patients with myelodysplastic syndromes. *Leuk Lymphoma* 1993; **11**: 221–4.

179. Hellstrom-Lindberg E, Ahlgren T, Beguin Y et al. Maintenance treatment of the anemia of myelodysplastic syndromes with recombinant human granulocyte colony-stimulating factor and erythropoietin: Evidence for in vivo synergy. *Blood* 1996; **10**: 4076–81.

180. Kanter G, Lewensohn L, Linder O et al. Treatment of anemia in myelodysplastic syndromes with granulocyte colony-stimulating factor plus erythropoietin: Results from a randomized phase II study and long-term follow-up of 71 patients. *Blood* 1998; **1**: 68–75.

181. Mantovani L, Lentini G, Hentschel B et al. Treatment of anaemia in myelodysplastic syndromes with prolonged administration of recombinant human granulocyte colony-stimulating factor and erythropoietin. *Br J Haematol* 2000; **2**: 367–75.

182. Terpos E, Mougiou A, Kouraklis A et al. Prolonged administration of erythropoietin increases erythroid response rate in myelodysplastic syndromes: A phase II trial in 281 patients. *Br J Haematol* 2002; **1**: 174–80.

183. Hellstrom-Lindberg E, Gulbrandsen N, Lindberg G et al. A validated decision model for treating the anaemia of myelodysplastic syndromes with erythropoietin + granulocyte colony-stimulating factor: Significant effects on quality of life. *Br J Haematol* 2003; **6**: 1037–46.

184. Ganser A, Hoelzer D. Clinical use of hematopoietic growth factors in the myelodysplastic syndromes. *Semin Hematol* 1996; **3**: 186–95. (Review)

185. Rose C, Wattel E, Bastion Y et al. Treatment with very low-dose GM-CSF in myelodysplastic syndromes with neutropenia. A report on 29 cases. *Leukemia* 1994; **8**: 1458–62.

186. Kurzrock R, Cortes J, Thomas DA et al. Pilot study of low-dose interleukin-11 in patients with bone marrow failure. *J Clin Oncol* 2001; **21**: 4165–72.

187. Molldrem JJ, Leifer E, Bahceci E et al. Antithymocyte globulin for treatment of the bone marrow failure associated

with myelodysplastic syndromes. *Ann Intern Med* 2002; **3**: 156–63.

188. Aivado M, Rong A, Stadler M et al. Favourable response to antithymocyte or antilymphocyte globulin in low-risk myelodysplastic syndrome patients with a 'non-clonal' pattern of X-chromosome inactivation in bone marrow cells. *Eur J Haematol* 2002; **4**: 210–16.

189. Killick SB, Mufti G, Cavenagh JD et al. A pilot study of antithymocyte globulin (ATG) in the treatment of patients with 'low-risk' myelodysplasia. *Br J Haematol* 2003; **4**: 679–84.

190. Saunthararajah Y, Nakamura R, Nam JM et al. HLA-DR15 (DR2) is overrepresented in myelodysplastic syndrome and aplastic anemia and predicts a response to immunosuppression in myelodysplastic syndrome. *Blood* 2002; **5**: 1570–4.

191. Hofmann WK, Ganser A, Seipelt G et al. Treatment of patients with low-risk myelodysplastic syndromes using a combination of all-trans retinoic acid, interferon alpha, and granulocyte colony-stimulating factor. *Ann Hematol* 1999; **3**: 125–30.

192. Hofmann WK, Kell WJ, Fenaux P et al. Oral 9-Cis retinoic acid (alitretinoin) in the treatment of myelodysplastic syndromes: Results from a pilot study. *Leukemia* 2000; **9**: 1583–8.

193. Stasi R, Brunetti M, Terzoli E et al. Sustained response to recombinant human erythropoietin and intermittent all-trans retinoic acid in patients with myelodysplastic syndromes. *Blood* 2002; **5**: 1578–84.

194. Wattel E, Cambier N, Caulier MT et al. Androgen therapy in myelodysplastic syndromes with thrombocytopenia: A report on 20 cases. *Br J Haematol* 1994; **1**: 205–8.

195. Chan G, Divenuti G, Miller K, Danazol for the treatment of thrombocytopenia in patients with myelodysplastic syndrome. *Am J Hematol* 2002; **3**: 166–71.

196. Omoto E, Deguchi S, Takaba S et al. Low-dose melphalan for treatment of high-risk myelodysplastic syndromes. *Leukemia* 1996; **4**: 609–14.

197. Raza A, Meyer P, Dutt D et al. Thalidomide produces transfusion independence in long-standing refractory anemias of patients with myelodysplastic syndromes. *Blood* 2001; **4**: 958–65.

198. Strupp C, Germing U, Aivado M et al. Thalidomide for the treatment of patients with myelodysplastic syndromes. *Leukemia* 2002; **1**: 1–6.

199. List AF, Kurtin SE, Glinsmann-Gibson BJ et al. Erythropoietic remitting activity of the immunomodulatory thalidomide analog, CC5013, in patients with myelodysplastic syndrome (MDS). *Blood* 2002; **11**: 96A.

200. Gotlib J, Jamieszon CHM, List A et al. Phase II study of bevacizumzb (Anti-VEGF humanized monoclonal antibody) in patients with myelodysplastic syndromes (MDS):

Early results. 7th International Symposium on Myelodysplastic Syndromes. *Leuk Res* 2003; **S1**: 115.

201. Deeg HJ, Gotlib J, Beckham C et al. Soluble TNF receptor fusion protein (Etanercept) for the treatment of myelodysplastic syndrome: A pilot study. *Leukemia* 2002; **2**: 162–4.

202. Maciejewski JP, Risitano AM, Sloand EM et al. A pilot study of the recombinant soluble human tumour necrosis factor receptor (P75)-Fc fusion protein in patients with myelodysplastic syndrome. *Br J Haematol* 2002; **1**: 119–26.

203. Stasi R, Amadori S. Infliximab chimaeric anti-tumour necrosis factor alpha monoclonal antibody treatment for patients with myelodysplastic syndromes. *Br J Haematol* 2002; **116**(2): 334–7.

204. List AF, Brasfield F, Heaton R et al. Stimulation of hematopoiesis by amifostine in patients with myelodysplastic syndrome. *Blood* 1997; **9**: 3364–9.

205. Bowen DT, Denzlinger C, Brugger W et al. Poor response rate to a continuous schedule of amifostine therapy for 'low/intermediate risk' myelodysplastic patients. *Br J Haematol* 1998; **3**: 785–7.

206. AF List, Schiller GJ, Mason J et al. (Arsenic trioxyde) in patients with myelodysplastic syndromes (MDS): Prelimininary findings in a phase 2 clinical study. 7th International Symposium On Myelodysplastic Syndromes. *Leuk Res* 2003; **S1**: 110.

207. Vey N, Dreyfus F, Guerci A et al. (Arsenic trioxyde) in patients with myelodysplastic syndromes (MDS): Prelimininary findings in a phase 1/2 study. 7th International Symposium On Myelodysplastic Syndromes. *Leuk Res* 2003; **S1**.

208. Cortes JE, Kurzrock R, Kantarjian HM. Farnesyltransferase inhibitors: Novel compounds in development for the treatment of myeloid malignancies. *Semin Hematol* 2002; **3** (Suppl 2): 26–30.

209. R Kurzrock, Kantarjian HM, Cortes JE et al. Farnesyl protein transferase inhibitor (FTI) Zarnestra TM (R1157777) in patients with myelodsyplastic syndromes (MDS): Clinical and biological aspects. 7th International Symposium on Myelodysplastic. Syndromes. *Leuk Res* 2003; **S1**: 105.

210. Wattel E, Guerci A, Hecuet B et al. A randomized trial of hydroxyurea versus VP 16 in adult chronic myelomonocytic leukemia. *Blood* 1996; **88**: 2480–7.

211. Di Gregorio F, Romeo MA, Pizzarelli G et al. An alternative to continuous subcutaneous infusion of desferrioxamine in thalassaemic patients. *Br J Haematol.* 1997; 601–2.

212. Cutler CS, Lee SJ, Greenberg P et al. A decision analysis of allogeneic bone marrow transplantation for the myelodysplastic syndromes: delayed transplantation for low-risk myelodysplasia is associated with improved outcome. *Blood* 2004; **104**: 579–85.

# 41 Chronic myeloid leukemia

François Guilhot and Lydia Roy

## Introduction

Chronic myeloid leukemia (CML) is a hematopoietic stem cell disease characterized by neoplastic proliferation of hematopoietic stem cells and their progeny within the bone marrow and in extramedullary hematopoietic sites. This leukemic disease was classified in the group of myeloproliferative disorders, which also include polycythemia vera, agnogenic myeloid metaplasia, and essential thrombocythemia.[1] CML was then distinguished from other myeloproliferative diseases by the presence in the hematopoietic stem cells of a reciprocal translocation between chromosomes 9 and 22 in over 90% of patients. The first description of the marker was given by Nowell and Hungerford,[2] who reported in 1960 two cases with an apparent loss of the long arm of chromosome 21 or 22. This abnormality was confirmed and designated the Philadelphia (Ph) chromosome.[3–5] Later, with the availability of more sensitive banding techniques, the Ph chromosome was identified as a modified chromosome 22 and part of a reciprocal translocation.[6,7] As the result of this translocation, a new chimeric tyrosine-specific protein kinase gene is generated. This new gene is a fusion of the cellular oncogene, ABL, located on chromosome 9, with a segment of chromosome 22, designated the breakpoint cluster region BCR.[8–11]

The Philadelphia chromosome was the first example of a specific cytogenetic abnormality consistently associated with a human cancer. Although approximately 10% of patients are Ph-, it is generally accepted that, at a molecular level, the fusion gene is invariably found in CML. The expansion of the myeloid compartment explains the main clinical and biological features of the disease. In the early stage of the disease, this expansion can easily be controlled by standard chemotherapy. However, the disease will inexorably progress from this early indolent chronic stage to a more aggressive accelerated stage and will finally terminate in blast crisis. The modern approach to the treatment of patients with CML in chronic phase includes the use of imatinib and interferon-α (alone or in combination), allogeneic bone marrow transplantation or autografting, each option being undertaken with the aim of re-establishing normal hematopoiesis.

## Etiology and epidemiology

The reason why the Philadelphia translocation occurs is still unknown. The most frequent environmental agent associated with CML is exposure to ionizing radiation. Since 1950, a cohort of 120 000 atomic bomb survivors from Japan and their controls have represented an important source of information regarding radiation leukemogenesis. Most of the radiation to which these people were exposed was relatively low-energy γ radiation. The earliest cases of radiation-induced leukemia occurred 3−4 years following exposure, with the peak incidence 4 years later. People who were less than 15 years old at the time of exposure had the highest risk of radiation-induced leukemia. The radiation effect disappeared 15 years following exposure for all age groups.[12–14] An increased risk of 4.61 for CML has been recorded in patients with ankylosing spondylitis treated with spinal irradiation.[15] The relative risk for CML was also increased in women treated with X-rays for cervical carcinoma.[16] Diagnostic X-ray exposure has been associated with an increased occurrence of CML.[17] A similar observation was reported for patients receiving intravenous thorium dioxide for diagnostic X-ray contrast studies.[18] In contrast to the high incidence of therapy-related myelodysplastic syndrome and acute myeloid leukemia, therapy-related CML is less frequent. CML has been described after treatment for Hodgkin disease[19,20] or after high-dose chemotherapy with subsequent autologous stem cell transplantation.[21,22]

In vitro, high-dose ionizing irradiation of hematopoietic cell lines can induce the formation of the BCR–ABL fusion gene with corresponding mRNA transcripts.[23,24] Although ionizing radiation is a physical mutagen known to induce DNA double-strand breaks, little is known of the molecular mechanisms by which it generates leukemia-specific fusion genes.

In several large studies, no relationship was found between benzene exposure and CML.[25,26] In general, no chemical or petrochemical products have been recognized as factors that could increase the occurrence of CML.

There is no evidence of a genetic predisposition although multiple occurrence of CML in a family has been reported.[27]

Chromosomal polymorphism studies in Ph+ leukemic patients and their parents have suggested that the chromosome 22 involved in the t(9;22) translocation is of maternal origin, whereas the chromosome 9 is preferentially of paternal origin. This indicated that parental imprinting could be involved in the formation of the fusion gene.[28] However, additional studies demonstrated that in leukocytes from normal individuals, both the paternal and maternal copies of the *ABL* gene are expressed at similar levels, and that there is no random allelic exclusion of *ABL* at the level of single hematopoietic progenitor cells.[29,30] Other reports showed that the *BCR* gene is not imprinted either.[31,32] Moreover, using Southern blot analysis and two intragenic polymorphisms located in the major breakpoint cluster region (M-*bcr*), the *BCR* gene was shown to be of paternal origin in three CML patients.[33]

It has been claimed that the *BCR–ABL* products are the prime cause of Ph+ leukemia. However, epidemiological data suggest that at least two stem cell mutations are necessary for the generation of CML chronic phase.[34]

There is no strong evidence for a significant association between HLA antigens and CML, although an increased frequency of HLA-CW3 and -CW4 has been found in CML patients.[35]

CML accounts for 7–20% of all leukemias, with an incidence estimated at between 1 and 2 per 100 000 persons.[36,37] Although the incidence increases with age, CML occurs in all age groups, with presentation being most common among those aged 40–60 years.[38] However, less than 10% of cases occur in patients under 20 years of age. The median age at diagnosis is 55–60 years. There is a small predisposition to CML in men, with a male-to-female ratio of 1.4–2.2 : 1. The clinical course is similar in males and females,[39] and CML is slightly more common in Whites and Blacks than in other races.

## Pathogenesis

### The *BCR–ABL* gene and its variants

The *BCR–ABL* gene is a consequence of the Ph translocation and occurs in a primitive hematopoietic stem cell. The breaks in chromosomes 9 and 22 transpose the proto-oncogene *ABL* (c-*ABL*) from its normal location on chromosome 9 to a new position on chromosome 22 (Figure 41.1). The *ABL* gene is the cellular homolog of a transforming element (v-*abl*) of the Abelson murine leukemia virus, and its 5′ end is oriented towards the centromere at band q34.[9] *ABL* has two alternative first exons, 1b and 1a, separated by 175 kb, and 10 other exons, which are more closely spaced.[40] The *ABL* locus thus spans 230 kb. The *ABL* gene is transcribed into two mRNA of either 6 or 7 kb. This gene encodes a 145 kDa tyrosine kinase.[40] Exon 11 encodes the nuclear localization signals and the actin-binding and DNA-binding domains of the ABL protein[41–43] (Figure 41.2. See color plate).

The *BCR* gene is located on chromosome 22, band q11; the locus spans 134 kb and encompasses 23 exons. The first intron, between exons 1 and 2, is described as the minor breakpoint cluster region (m-*bcr*), which contains chromosomal breakpoints found in acute lymphoblastic leukemia (ALL). The other breakpoints have been shown to occur in introns 13 and 14 in a region referred to as the major breakpoint cluster region (M-*bcr*).[44,45] The *BCR* gene is transcribed into two mRNA of either 4.5 or 6.7 kb. The gene encodes a 160 kDa serine/threonine kinase that phosphorylates several protein substrates[46] (Figure 41.3. See color plate).

Both *BCR* and *ABL* are expressed ubiquitously,[47,48] and their normal cellular functions have been investigated using null mutant mice. *ABL*-null mice have thymic and splenic atrophy with a reduction in developing B- and T-cell progenitor compartments,[49,50] which may indicate a role for the ABL protein in progression in pre-B cells. *BCR*-null mice develop septic

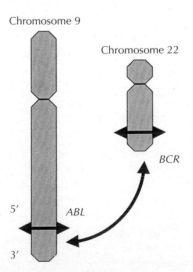

**Figure 41.1** Schematic diagram of chromosomes 9 and 22. The *ABL* from chromosome 9 is transposed to chromosome 22, and the terminal portion of chromosome 22 is transposed to the long arm of chromosome 9.

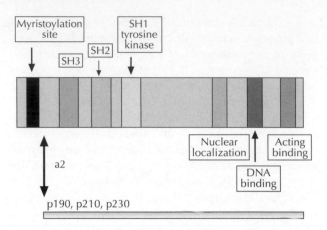

**Figure 41.2** Structure of *ABL*, with its domains. (See Plate 8)

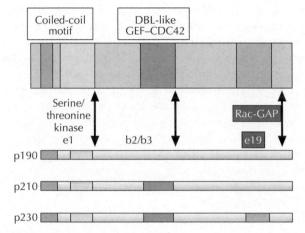

**Figure 41.3** Structure of *BCR*, with its domains. (See Plate 8)

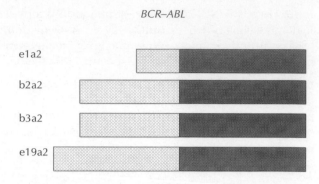

**Figure 41.4** Structure of the four *BCR–ABL* mRNA transcripts.

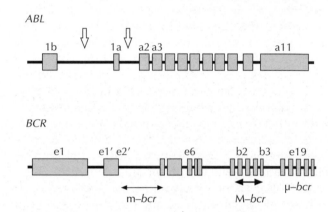

**Figure 41.5** Structure of the *ABL* and *BCR* genes, with their exons and introns. (See Plate 8)

shock, with a defect in neutrophil function that suggests a role for the BCR protein in the normal myeloid lineage.[51]

In the *ABL* gene, breakpoints can occur anywhere at the 5′ end of the gene upstream of the first exon 1b, between exons 1b and 1a, between 1a and a2, and in intron 2. In the *BCR* gene, breakpoints are found in three areas (Table 41.1; Figures 41.4 and 41.5, see Plate 8). In the vast majority of patients, the breakpoints are clustered in the M-*bcr* region, which spans 5.8 kb with the five exons, 12, . . ., 16, previously termed b1, . . ., b5. In this region, the position of the breakpoints vary

and may generate fusion transcripts with a b2a2 or a b3a2 junction. Such transcripts encode a p210 fusion protein.

m-*bcr* is located upstream of M-*bcr*, between the two alternative exons e2′ and e2. The *BCR–ABL* mRNA molecule resulting from a breakpoint within this region contains the e1a2 junction and is translated into a smaller 190 kDa BCR–ABL fusion protein.[40]

The third region is the most 3′ cluster region, and is termed the micro breakpoint cluster region (μ-*bcr*). Breakpoints in this region result in *BCR–ABL* tran-

| Table 41.1 The three regions of the *BCR* gene | | | |
|---|---|---|---|
| | m-*bcr* (minor *bcr*) | M-*bcr* (major *bcr*) | μ-*bcr* (micro *bcr*) |
| Site and location of the breaks within *BCR* | 5′, between exons e1′ and e2′ | A 5.8 kb region between e13 and e15 | 3′ |
| Size of transcript(s) | 7 kb | 8.5 kb | |
| Type of junction(s) | e1a2 | e13a2 (b2a2) e14a2 (b3a2) | e19a2 (c3a2) |
| Protein | p190[BCR–ABL] | p210[BCR–ABL] | p230[BCR–ABL] |

scripts with an e19a2 junction (previously termed c3a2). This *BCR–ABL* hybrid gene is the largest and is responsible for the production of a p230 protein with tyrosine kinase activity.[52]

The vast majority of the Ph+ CML patients have a p210-encoding *BCR–ABL* gene exhibiting mRNA transcripts with a b3a2 or b2a2 junction and sometimes both b3a2 and b2a2 (5–10% of cases). Several studies have attempted to correlate the position of the breakpoint within the M-*bcr* region and the duration of survival or the frequency of lymphoid blast crisis.[53,54] However, no such correlation was found when large series of patients were considered.[55] It has been claimed that a possible link may exist between the type of *BCR–ABL* fusion transcript and platelet count. Some groups reported that patients with 3'M-*bcr* breakpoints had significantly higher numbers of platelets,[56] although this was not confirmed by two other studies.[57] However, it is possible to select a subgroup of patients in whom the b3a2 transcript is associated with a higher platelet count.[58] Hematologic disorders associated with the production of the p190[BCR–ABL] protein are usually of ALL type, but very rare cases of CML and AML may have a similar molecular rearrangement. The various cases of CML with the production of the p230[BCR–ABL] protein are considered as less aggressive myeloproliferative disorders and are now described as chronic neutrophilic leukemia.

### The role of *BCR–ABL* in leukemic stem cell dysfunction

CML is characterized by genetic mutation that deregulates cell growth and its distribution. There are several mechanisms that may explain the myeloid expansion in CML: more rapid proliferation of leukemic cells, increased self-renewal of the progenitor, prolonged lifespan of leukemic leukocytes, and reduction of the cell death by apoptosis.

Various in vitro studies have been used to demonstrate the mitogenetic effect of *BCR–ABL*. When the *BCR–ABL* gene is transfected into hematopoietic cell lines, they become grow factor-independent with an increased proliferative capacity. The mitogenetic ability of *BCR–ABL* is mediated through activation of Ras, Raf, and MAPK leading to increased levels of c-Myc and c-Fos and subsequent increased gene transcription. When these *BCR–ABL*-containing cells are treated with antisense oligonucleotides against the *ras* or *raf* genes, the *BCR–ABL*-induced growth factor independence is abrogated. Most of these in vitro studies suggest that *BCR–ABL* acts as a mitogene by activating Ras and Myc.[59–61]

The myeloid expansion of leukemic cells is not explained by more rapid proliferation of these cells. Several kinetic studies performed during chronic phase have suggested that the leukemic precursors have lower mitotic indices, a smaller fraction of cells in DNA synthesis, longer generation times, and longer transit times in the maturation compartment compared with normal precursors.[62,63] When the leukocyte count is decreased by chemotherapy, these proliferative parameters return to normal. There is no evidence that cytokines that regulate cell growth either positively or negatively are overproduced in the microenvironment.[64] Thus, the proliferation of CML progenitors could be related to defects in the adhesive interaction that regulates the growth of normal hematopoietic progenitors. Several studies have suggested that adhesive interactions between CML cells and the marrow microenvironment are defective. This defect may, in part, explain the proliferation of hematopoietic progenitors.[65]

*BCR–ABL* mutants have been used to identify the *BCR–ABL* domains required for the transforming activity. In order to determine the possible role of the BCR–ABL oncoprotein SH3 domain, the properties of a BCR–ABL SH3 deletion mutant (ΔSH3 BCR–ABL) constitutively expressed in murine hematopoietic cells have been studied. ΔSH3 BCR–ABL can activate BCR–ABL-dependent downstream effector molecules (Ras, PI3K, MAPK, JNK, Myc, Jun, STATs, and Bcl-2). Leukemic growth from cells expressing ΔSH3 BCR–ABL was significantly delayed in SCID (severe combined immunodeficient) mice compared with that of cells expressing the wild-type protein. In vitro as well in vivo, ΔSH3 BCR–ABL-expressing cells showed a decreased interaction with collagen IV- and laminin-coated plates and a reduced capacity to invade the stroma. Such results suggest that the SH3 domain of BCR–ABL is important for in vitro transformation of hematopoietic cells and essential for full leukemogenic potential in vivo.[66]

Another mechanism by which myeloid expansion can be explained is a decreased cell death rate. Apoptotic cell death is dysregulated by *BCR–ABL*. This has been demonstrated in vitro using cell lines transfected with *BCR–ABL*: such cells are protected from apoptosis. An interaction between p210[BCR–ABL] and Bcl-2 has also been suggested: in cells transfected with *BCR–ABL* the removal of Bcl-2 with antisense oligonucleotides to the *bcl-2* gene abrogates the transforming ability of *BCR–ABL*.[67]

The CML blast crisis K562 cell line, which expresses p210[BCR–ABL], is resistant to antileukemic drug-induced apoptosis and overexpresses the antiapoptotic Bcl-$x_L$ but not Bcl-2.[68] Studies have indicated that a variety of apoptotic stimuli cause the pre-apoptotic mitochondrial release of cytochrome *c* into the cytosol. This release mediates the cleavage and activity of caspase-3, which is involved in the execution of apoptosis. BCR–ABL exerts its antiapoptotic affect upstream to the cleavage and activation of caspase-3. More precisely, BCR–ABL blocks apoptosis by preventing the cytosolic accumulation of cytochrome *c* and by inhibiting the activation of caspase-3.[69] Thus, altered adhesion to stroma cells and the extracellular matrix constitutively active mitogenetic signaling, reduced apoptosis, and proteasome-mediated degradation of ABL-inhibitory proteins are the four major mechanisms implicated in malignant transformation by *BCR–ABL*.

It is accepted that CML involves a pluripotent stem cell, which explains the presence of the Ph chromosome in the precursors of the myeloid, monocytic, lymphoid, and megakaryocytic lineages.[70] The clonal origin of the disease has also been suggested in the past by the demonstration of a presence of a single glucose-6-phosphate dehydrogenase isoenzyme in the erythroid, myeloid, and megakaryocytic compartments but not in fibroblasts in women with CML who are heterozygotes for isoenzymes A and B.[71] The same conclusion came from studies using DNA hybridation–methylation analysis of heterozygotic women with restriction fragment length polymorphisms (RFLP) at the X-linked locus for hypoxanthine phosphoribosyltransferase.[72]

The role of the *BCR–ABL* oncogene has been examined using transformed cells in murine models. The introduction into the germline of $p189^{BCR–ABL}$ cDNA is responsible for B-cell ALL. The same experiment using $p210^{BCR–ABL}$ cDNA transcriptionally regulated by a metallothionein promoter led to the development of late-onset AML, T-cell ALL, or T-lymphoblastic lymphoma.[73]

The transplantation of mouse marrow cells transduced with *BCR–ABL* cDNA into syngeneic animals induces a CML-like disease within a few months after transplant. When secondary transplants are reformed with marrow obtained from animals that developed a CML-like disorder more than 6 months after transplant, a fraction of secondary recipients develop a form of AML or ALL.[74–76] More recently, reproducible and sustained engraftment of SCID mice with intravenously transplanted chronic phase cells has been obtained using large numbers of cells from patients with high white blood cell count and high-dose irradiation for the conditioning regimen.[77] Using this model, it has been demonstrated that Ph⁻ and Ph⁺ cells coexist and that Ph⁻ progenitors engraft preferentially. By comparison with the SCID model, engraftment of NOD (non-obese diabetic) SCID mice with multiple types of normal and leukemic human cells is higher and can be achieved with lower numbers of CD34⁺ cell-enriched populations.[78]

# Clinical and biological features of the disease

## Symptoms and physical examination of the chronic phase

At the beginning, CML is asymptomatic, although patients are now being diagnosed earlier in the course of the disease. In several countries, general practitioners routinely perform leukocyte and platelet measurements, which may explain a higher frequency of incidental diagnosis (20–40% of cases). Patients with symptoms have a gradual onset of fatigue, anorexia, weight loss, and sweats.[79] Left upper quadrant discomfort and early satiety attributable to splenomegaly are less frequent. In a series of 430 patients,[80] fatigue was the most frequent symptom (33%), followed by bleeding (21%), weight loss (21%), and splenic discomfort (18%). Less than 10% of the patients had bone pain, infection, or headache. The frequency of signs or symptoms of increased tumor burden has decreased. Rare patients may have manifestations of leukostasis or symptoms related to hyperuricemia: stupor, priapism, tinnitus, cerebrovascular accidents, or acute gouty arthritis. Other infrequent symptoms include splenic infarction and perisplenitis, or acute febrile neutrophilic dermatosis (Sweet syndrome).

Physical examination is frequently normal because of earlier diagnosis. Splenomegaly is the predominant sign, present in 50–70% of cases. The size of the spleen may be an indication of chronic phase duration and is also greater in patients with history of fatigue and sweats.[80] Because spleen size is an important prognostic factor, the length of the spleen below the costal margin should be determined precisely. Hepatomegaly and lymphadenopathy are less common in chronic phase CML. Sternal tenderness is sometimes noted in the lower portion.

## Laboratory findings

Elevated leukocytosis, anemia, and thrombocytosis are common features. The hematocrit is decreased in most patients, with a normal reticulocyte count. Some cases of erythrocytosis or erythroid aplasia have been reported. The white blood cell count (WBC) is usually above $25 \times 10^9$/l and half of the patients have total WBC over $100 \times 10^9$/l. The WBC differential shows granulocytes at all stages of development from blasts to mature granulocytes, which are normal in appearance. The blast prevalence is about 5%, with a range from 0% to 14%; promyelocytes, myelocytes, and metamyelocytes account for about 45%, and segmented neutrophils about 35% of total leukocytes. Basophils are usually elevated between 5% and 15%. This elevation in basophil count, which is always present when the total leukocyte count is over $10 \times 10^9$/l, is an important sign in the preliminary differential diagnosis. Eosinophils are also elevated, but to a lesser degree. The total lymphocyte count is increased as the result of an expansion of T lymphocytes, whereas natural killer (NK)-cell activity is defective in CML.[81,82] An absolute monocytosis is usual. The platelet count is elevated in about 50% of patients, and some may have a count above $1000 \times 10^9$/l. A low platelet count is occasionally seen in CML at diagnosis, and may be a sign of accelerated or blastic phase. It is generally considered a sign of poor prognosis. Platelet function is frequently abnormal, but is not associated with exaggerated bleeding. A decrease in the second wave of epinephrin (adrenaline)-induced platelet aggregation is the most common abnormality, and is associated with a deficiency of adenine nucleotides in the storage pool.[83] Some patients have wide cyclic variations of all cells derived from myeloid stem cells, including reticulocytes and platelets, with a periodicity of 50–70 days.[84]

The bone marrow is markedly hypercellular, with a cellularity of 75–90%, fat being reduced. Granulopoiesis is dominant, with a myeloid-to-erythroid ratio of between 10 : 1 and 30 : 1, rather than the normal 2:1–5:1. Basophils and eosinophils are increased in proportion to their increase in the blood. Megakaryocytic hyperplasia is usual, with dysplastic changes in all cell lines. Some rare patients will have lipid-laden macrophages resembling Gaucher cells or sea-blue histiocytes. There is no deficiency of glucocerebrosidase in CML, but the normal cellular glucocerebrosidase activity is not high enough to degrade the increased glucocerebroside load associated with markedly increased cell turnover. Melofibrosis is not usually present in early chronic phase. However, fibrosis may occur during the course of the disease; the rapid development of myelofibrosis is generally considered a poor prognostic feature.[85]

The Ph chromosome is present in the marrow and nucleated blood cells of 90–95% of patients with typical features of CML. In the remaining patients, molecular studies have revealed the presence of the translocation. This chromosomal abnormality can be found in all blood cell lineages (erythroblasts, granulocytes, monocytes, megakaryocytes, B cells, and macrophage precursors). Stimulated T cells may display the Ph translocation, but skin and marrow fibroblasts do not. The Ph chromosome is a shorter chromosome 22 (22q–) resulting from the reciprocal translocation t(9;22) in which the distal end of chromosome 22 is exchanged for a small portion of the long arm of chromosome 9 (9q+). The breakpoints in chromosomes 9 and 22 are at bands q34 and q11, respectively. Using high-resolution cytogenetic analysis, the translocation has been precisely defined as t(9;22)(q34.1;q11.2).

Variant Ph chromosome translocations occur in 5–12% of patients. These translocations are 'simple variant' when they involve chromosomes 22 and a chromosome other than 9 and 'complex variant' when they involve chromosomes 9 and 22 and one or more other chromosomes.[86] In rare cases, the 22q– is not detected by microscopic examination. This situation has been described as a 'masked Ph chromosome'.[87] In a large review of 327 variant Ph translocations reported in the literature, no significant difference was found in survival between patients with standard, simple, or complex Ph translocations.[88]

Cytogenetic analysis usually displays the t(9;22) in 100% of mitoses. However, about 5–10% of patients have evidence of normal diploid cells at diagnosis. This finding is associated with a better prognosis.[89] Also, these patients may have favorable prognostic features, with a lower WBC, no spleen enlargement, and no symptoms at presentation. They may also have better cytogenetic responses with interferon-α and a longer survival.[90] Additional cytogenetic abnormalities at the time of diagnosis have been associated with a poor outcome.[91,92] In one large series of patients, the median survival of patients with additional cytogenetic abnormalities was 28 months versus 41 months for those without abnormalities.[91] However, such additional abnormalities are uncommon in chronic phase, whereas they are more frequent during accelerated and blastic phases. In Ph– patients, using restriction enzymes and molecular probes for the breakpoint cluster region, a Southern blot analysis will detect rearrangement of fragments, leading to the conclusion that all cases of CML have an abnormal long arm of chromosome 22. Such Ph–, BCR+ CML patients can express the p210[BCR–ABL] tyrosine kinase and have a clinical course identical to that of Ph+ CML patients.[93]

Leukocyte alkaline phosphatase (LAP) activity is usually reduced in all patients at diagnosis.[94] The activity increases towards or to normal in cases of infection or inflammation, and also when the leukocyte count is normal after chemotherapy. LAP activity is restored after infusion of leukocytes into leukopenic patients, suggesting an effect of regulators or factors extrinsic to the neutrophils.[95] Although low LAP activity is a classical feature of CML at diagnosis, it is not specific. It may be seen in idiopathic myelofibrosis, congenital hypophosphatasia, and paroxysmal nocturnal hemoglobinuria.

Increased production of uric acid with hyperuricemia and hyperuricosuria is usual in untreated patients. Because initial therapy leads to rapid cell destruction, excretion of the additional purine load may produce urinary tract blockage or urate nephropathy. Formation of urate stones is common in CML, and patients with latent gout may develop uric acid nephropathy or acute gouty arthritis. Patients with CML have an increased serum level of vitamin $B_{12}$ up to 10 times normal levels, whereas transcobalamin II, the physiological $B_{12}$ carrier, is not increased. This biological feature is not specific, since a high vitamin $B_{12}$ level may occur in the case of any increase in the number of neutrophilic granulocytes. The serum lactic dehydrogenase level (LDH) is elevated. It is possible to observe pseudohyperkalemia due to the release of potassium from white cells during clotting, and false hypoxemia or pseudohypoglycemia from in vitro utilization of oxygen or glucose by leukocytes.

## Clinical and biologic characteristics of advanced phases

After an indolent phase lasting 2–6 years when patients are treated with conventional chemotherapy, the disease changes to a more aggressive phase. This accelerated phase or metamorphosis is characterized by an increase in tumor burden and a poor response to therapy. After 1–1.5 years, this accelerated phase is followed by the blastic phase, which results in the patient's death within 3–6 months. Different definitions of the accelerated and blastic phases have been established based on the occurrence of several different clinical and biological features (Table 41.2).[96,97]

### Accelerated phase

Several features may suggest progression from chronic to accelerated phase, including fever without infection, bone pain, weight loss, night sweats, and splenic enlargement unresponsive to previously successful chemotherapy. Anemia may worsen, with an uncontrolled increase in WBC. The proportion of blasts and/or basophils may increase in the blood and marrow. A decrease in the platelet count to below $100 \times 10^9$/l is usual. Some marked dysplastic changes may occur in the major cell lineages, with reticulin and collagen fibrosis. The presence of additional cytogenetic abnormalities is common. Three additional abnormalities are frequently observed: trisomy 8, duplication of the Ph chromosome, and iso(17q). A higher incidence of these changes has been reported after treatment with busulfan compared with hydroxyurea.[98] The death rate during this phase is between 20% and 25%. Accelerated phase is, however, a loosely defined condition. Clinically, it may be suspected in the presence of progressive splenomegaly,

splenic pain, fever, or night sweats. However, approximately 20% of patients are asymptomatic when the diagnosis of accelerated phase is made on the basis of peripheral blood counts or bone marrow findings.[97]

The clinical significance of cytogenetic clonal evolution (i.e. the appearance of new cytogenetic abnormalities in addition to the Ph chromosome) as a manifestation of accelerated phase is more controversial and probably not uniform. In a study of 264 patients with clonal evolution, the median survival from the onset of clonal evolution was 19 months.[99] However, multivariate analysis identified four groups of patients with clearly differing outcomes. The 'good' group included 37 patients with no chromosome 17 abnormality, a percentage of metaphases with clonal evolution below 16% and a time to clonal evolution of less than 25 months, with a median survival of 54 months. In contrast, the median survivals of the two 'worst' groups were 6 months (27 patients with chromosome 17 abnormality and 34% or more abnormal metaphases) and 7 months (22 patients with other features of accelerated phase and 16% or more abnormal metaphases). The median survival of the 'intermediate' group ranged from 13 to 24 months.

There is no consensus definition of the accelerated phase, and the existing definitions are not always precise. Several authors have proposed various classifications,[80,100–103] which have been developed empirically (Table 41.3).

However, the Houston criteria have been defined using multivariate prognostic factor analysis. Kantarjian et al.[97] followed up 357 patients with newly diagnosed CML treated between 1965 and 1984 with hydroxyurea or busulfan ($n$=206), intensive chemotherapy ($n$=97), or more recently with interferon-$\alpha$ ($n$=54). The prognostic value of features of accelerated phase (as reported in the prior literature) was assessed for survival and time to blast crisis.

In a multivariate analysis, five factors were found to be independtly associated with poor survival: cytogenetic evolution, peripheral blasts 15% or more, peripheral basophils 20% or more, peripheral blasts and promyelocytes 30% or more, and thromocytopenia (platelets $<100 \times 10^9$/l).[105] Each of these factors was associated with a median survival below 18 months (7, 9, 17, 5, and 16 months, respectively). The corresponding median time to blast crisis ranged from 2 to 15 months (Table 41.4).

Altogether, it appears from an examination of these diagnostic criteria that patients classified as in accelerated phase in the Sokal or IBMTR systems[92,104] may still be classified as being in chronic phase in the Houston system. Furthermore, whereas the occurrence of chloromas qualifies for an accelerated phase in the IBMTR system, it is more commonly considered as evidence of progression to blast crisis.

---

### Table 41.2  Signs of accelerated and blastic phases of CML

**Accelerated phase**
Persisting progressive splenomegaly
Increasing WBC resistant to treatment
Increasing marrow fibrosis
Additional cytogenetic abnormalities
Anemia or thrombocytopenia (platelets $< 100 \times 10^9$/l) unrelated to therapy
Marked thrombocytosis
Fever not otherwise explained
Peripheral basophils $\geq$20%
Peripheral blasts plus promyelocytes $\geq$30%
Peripheral blasts $\geq$15%

**Blastic phase**
Peripheral blasts $\geq$20%
Bone marrow blasts $\geq$30%
Extramedullary blastic infiltrates

## Table 41.3 Definitions of accelerated phase CML

| MD Anderson Cancer Center[97] | Sokal[92] | IBMTR[106] |
|---|---|---|
| PB blasts ≥15% | PB or BM blasts ≥5% | PB or BM blasts ≥10% |
| PB blasts+promyelocytes ≥30% | — | PB or BM blasts+promyelocytes ≥20% |
| PB basophils ≥20% | PB basophils ≥20% | PB basophils+eosinophils ≥20% |
| Platelets ≤100 ×10⁹/l unrelated to therapy | Thrombopenia unrelated to therapy | Thrombocytopenia unresponsive to BU or HU therapy |
| Cytogenetic karyotypic evolution | Cytogenetic karyotypic evolution | Cytogenetic karyotypic evolution |
| | Platelets ≥1000 ×10⁹/l despite adequate therapy | Persistent thrombocytosis |
| | Marrow collagen fibrosis | Myelofibrosis |
| | Anemia unrelated to therapy | Anemia unresponsive to BU or HU therapy |
| | Progressive splenomegaly | Progressive splenomegaly |
| | Leukocyte doubling time <5 days | Rapid doubling time of leukocytes <5 days |
| | Frequent Pelger–Hüet-like neutrophils; nucleated erythrocytes; megakaryocyte nuclear fragments | Leukocyte count difficult to control with BU or HU therapy |
| | Fever not otherwise explained | Development of chloromas |

IBMTR, International Bone Marrow Transplant Registry; PB, peripheral blood; BM, bone marrow; BU, busulfan; HU, hydroxyurea.

## Table 41.4 Houston staging system for CML[105]

| Phase | Clinical characteristics | Stage | Definition |
|---|---|---|---|
| Chronic | Age ≥60 years<br>Spleen ≥ 10 cm | 1 | 0 or 1 characteristic |
| | Blasts ≥3% in blood or ≥5% in marrow<br>Basophils ≥7% in blood or ≥3% in marrow | 2 | 2 characteristics |
| | Platelets ≥700 × 10⁹/l | 3 | ≥3 characteristics |
| Accelerated | Cytogenetic clonal evolution<br>Blasts ≥15% in blood<br>Blasts + promyelocytes ≥30% in blood<br>Basophils ≥20% in blood<br>Platelets <100 × 10⁹/l | 4 | >1 characteristic defines accelerated phase |

However, it is also noteworthy that all patients who qualify for accelerated phase in the Houston system will also qualify in the other systems. Taking the example of the threshold used for peripheral blood blasts (≥15%), the Houston system probably define a group of patients with a more advanced stage of the disease, as compared with the Sokal (≥5%) and IBMTR (≥10%) systems.

In conclusion, whereas the Houston criteria are likely to identify a population of patients with a more advanced disease (i.e. closer to progression to blast crisis), the other systems may be used for an earlier identification of signs of progression. However, it must be emphasized that both the Sokal and IBMTR systems lack precision in the definition of some criteria such as 'progressive splenomegaly', 'anemia or thrombocytopenia', or 'persistent thrombosis'. All of these differences must be carefully taken into account when comparing reports from different studies.

### Blastic phase

Blast crisis is usually defined by the appearance of 30% or more blasts in the peripheral blood or the bone marrow.[102,106] However, alternative definitions have been proposed, such as the presence of more than 15% or 20% blasts, or more than 30% or 50% of blasts plus promyelocytes in the peripheral blood or the bone marrow, respectively.[107,108] In particular, a clinical advisory committee of international hematologists and oncologists has reached a consensus to define AML as a disease presenting at least 20% of blast cells in the bone marrow. The specific impact of this new threshold on the interpretation of the results of previously published studies using the usual threshold of 30% bone marrow blasts remains to be determined. Nevertheless, this new cut-off should be considered for the definition of acute phase of CML in future trials.[108]

The blastic phase usually results in the patient's death within 3–6 months. It may occur after a period of accelerated phase or arise directly from the chronic phase, the latter in 20–25% of patients. In some cases, extramedullary blastic tumors may precede marrow involvement. Thus, these tumors are sometimes considered to be the first manifestation of metamorphosis. These leukemic infiltrates appear in the lymph nodes, breast, or gastrointestinal or genitourinary tracts. Most of the patients with extramedullary manifestations will develop acute leukemia with marrow and blood involvement within a few months. A combination of morphology, histochemistry, monoclonal antibodies specific for lymphoid or myeloid cells, and cytogenetic and molecular analysis must be used in order to classify the blast cells. Lymphoblasts, like myeloid blasts, are Ph+.[107,109]

The blastic phase is myeloid in about 50% of cases – usually myeloblastic or myelomonocytic. Promyelocytic, eosinophilic, or basophilic blast crises have also been described. Some cases are undifferentiated (15–25%), classified as erythroblastic, or occasionally as megakaryoblastic.[107,109] In these latter cases, myelofibrosis is not unusual and monoclonal antiplatelet antibodies (e.g. antiplatelet glycoprotein antibodies) are useful to identify the proliferation. The blastic phase is lymphoid in 25% of case, the B phenotype being predominant, although rare patients have blasts with a T-lymphocyte phenotype. In vitro studies may occasionally show a biphenotypic blast crisis with cells having myeloid and lymphoid markers. The presence of additional chromosome abnormalities is frequent at this stage of the disease. The principal additional abnormalities are duplication of the Ph chromosome and iso(17q) or trisomy 8. These changes occur frequently, being noted in 62–86% of patients. Other chromosome abnormalities have also been noted.

## Forms of the disease and atypical presentation

In some patients (10–15%), symptoms and signs of leukostasis are present at diagnosis, with extreme leukocytosis exceeding $500 \times 10^9/l$. Hyperviscosity of the blood and infiltration of tissues may explain priapism, visual difficulty with retinal bleeding, and mental confusion due to cerebral hypoxia.[110] Hyperleukocytosis is more prevalent in children with Ph+ CML. Other cases may mimic polycythemia vera, idiopathic myelofibrosis, or primary thrombocythemia.[111] Skeletal lesions are uncommon (between 3% and 10%) and may represent ectopic areas of myeloid metaplasia or the first sign of blastic phase.[112]

Coexistence or sequential development of CML with other proliferative disorders has been described. CML has been diagnosed after treatment including radiotherapy and/or chemotherapy for Hodgkin's disease or non-Hodgkin lymphoma.[113] Patients may have concurrent lymphoproliferative malignancies (chronic lymphocytic leukemia, CLL) or myeloma or Waldenström's macroglobulinemia. In some cases, it has been clearly established that two independent clonal disorders are present.[114–116]

Ph+ adult-type CML may occur in children, but is rare under the age of 5 years. CML in children has the typical manifestation and course of the adult disorder. However they may present with higher total leukocyte counts with leukostatic symptoms.

Chronic neutrophilic leukemia is a rare form of proliferative disorder, which can now be classified as a molecular variant of CML. A few well documented cases with Ph+ leukemia have been reported in association with a $p230^{BCR-ABL}$ gene. The course of the disease seems to be much more benign than that of typical CML. Patients may complain of anorexia and weakness; otherwise, the disease is discovered after a routine blood test. The spleen is frequently less prominent and lymphadenopathy is infrequent. The patients have lower WBC and a low proportion of circulating immature granulocytes, anemia is less severe, and blastic transformation occurs much later, if at all. Some of these cases have shown a marked thrombocytosis, with platelet counts between $762 \times 10^9/l$ and $1442 \times 10^9/l$.[117–119]

Ph– CML is a heterogenous group of disorders. Patients who are Ph– but BCR+ have a clinical course similar to those with Ph+ CML: these patients should receive the same therapeutic options.[120] A subgroup of patients are Ph– and BCR–. They present with higher WBC, neutrophilia, and basophilia, and occasionally with splenic enlargement and bone marrow hypercellularity. The natural history of these patients is characterized by increasing leukemia burden, with leukocytosis, organomegaly, extramedullary infiltrates, and bone marrow failure without excess of blasts.[121] However, some of these patients may have similar clinical and biological features of chronic myelomonocytic leukemia (CMML).[122] A few cases of AML (2–3%) have the Ph translocation. These may represent an early blast crisis of CML. These patients have marked spleen and liver enlargement, normal platelet counts, basophilia, and a breakpoint within the M-bcr region, with production of the usual 210 tyrosine kinase.[123] Their prognosis is very poor. However, some patients enter remission by converting to chronic phase CML. About 5% of children with ALL and 20% of adults with ALL have the Ph chromosome in their blast cells.[124] In children, the prognosis is worse than that of those without the translocation, although the clinical and biological features are similar to those of classic ALL. However, these patients may have higher WBC, a more frequent L2 blast cell morphology, and a high incidence of pre-B CALLA+ disease.[125] Remission rates and median survivals are lower in adults with Ph+ ALL.

# Prognosis

Since the 1970s, several studies have been conducted in order to set up prognostic models. Such models have been used to categorize patients into risk groups.[91,126–130] At the time of diagnosis, most of these models (Table 41.5) have selected several variables associated with the duration of chronic phase, such as age, spleen size, race, hemoglobin level, WBC, and platelet count.

Using these variables, patients usually segregate into three risk groups with significantly different survival times. Good-risk patients have a median survival of 50–60 months, intermediate-risk a survival of 39 months, and high-risk a survival of 25–32 months. A subsequent model has been proposed including five prognostic variables (Table 41.6), patients being distributed into four categories (the fourth category corresponding to patients with accelerated phase). The median survivals of patients were 56, 45, 30 and 30 months, respectively.[105] For a long time, these prognostic models were used for the evaluation of therapeutic trials, and they also played an important role in deciding the timing of bone marrow transplantation.

One of the most popular prognostic systems is that proposed by Sokal et al[130] in 1984 and subsequently called the 'Sokal model'. This widely used model was derived on a cohort of 813 patients treated with chemotherapy. It is based on the calculation of a score, taking into account simple clinical parameters such as age, spleen size, platelet counts, and the percentage of blasts in the peripheral blood (Table 41.7). Patients are then distributed into three risk groups: low-risk (score <0.8), high-risk (score >1.2), and intermediate-risk. This model, developed in a large cohort of patients treated essentially with chemotherapy, was highly efficient in predicting long-term survival. However, these staging systems were based on series of patients treated with chemotherapy (mainly hydroxyurea or busulfan), and there have been concerns that they may not be fully applicable with interferon-based therapies.

Until recently, the modern approach to the treatment of patients with CML included the use of interferon-α (IFN-α) alone or in combination with cytarabine (cytosine arabinoside, Ara-C), allogeneic bone marrow transplantation from related as well as unrelated donors, and autologous stem cell transplantation. Most of the prognostic models are not applicable to these new therapeutic strategies. For example, several trials comparing IFN-α versus busulfan or IFN-α versus hydroxyurea.[100,131,132] and a single-arm trial with IFN-α[173] did not found any association of the Sokal index with survival. Most of the patients treated with IFN-α achieved a complete hematological remission (60–80%). In addition, treatment with IFN-α induces cytogenetic responses that are complete in some patients. Several trials have demonstrated that achieving major (i.e. < 35% Ph+ residual cells) or complete cytogenetic responses significantly improved survival.[134,135] Some studies have not found an association between achievement of major or complete responses and survival – probably because the number of responders was too small.[132,133] However, using a multivariate analysis including major cytogenetic response as a time-dependent variable, the achievement of such a response was independently associated with prolonged survival. Therefore, the achievement of a cytogenetic response might be the most important prognostic feature for patients with CML treated with IFN-α alone or in combination with cytarabine.[136]

A survival improvement has also been demonstrated in patients who achieved sustained cytogenetic responses compared with those with transient responses.[137] Also, the patients who achieved rapid hematologic responses had a higher probability of cytogenetic responses. Patients with a complete hematologic response within 3 months had a major cytogenetic response rate of 82%, compared with 29% in those who were resistant at that time.[138] Other predictive factors of the cytogenetic response could be lymphokine-activated killer (LAK) cytotoxicity level and the occurrence of autoimmune complications.[139,140]

More recently, a new prognostic scoring system adapted to IFN-α-treated patients has been

## Table 41.5  Prognostic variables in CML

- Age
- Race
- Spleen size
- Liver size
- Hemoglobin level
- WBC
- Platelet count
- Nucleated red blood cells in peripheral blood
- Percentage of blasts in peripheral blood or bone marrow
- Percentage of basophils in peripheral blood or bone marrow
- Percentage of promyelocytes plus myelocytes in peripheral blood
- Percentage of eosinophils in peripheral blood

## Table 41.6 Prognostic models for patients with CML

| Ref | Prognostic features | Staging | Survival according to stage at 4 years |
|---|---|---|---|
| 128 | Spleen >0 cm BCM<br>Liver >0 cm BCM<br>PB normoblasts ≥1%<br>BM blasts >5% | Stage 1: 0–1 factor<br>Stage 2: 2 factors<br>Stage 3: >2 factors | Stage 1: 51%<br>Stage 2: 39%<br>Stage 3: 45% |
| 129 | Spleen ≥15 cm BCM<br>Liver ≥15 cm BCM<br>Platelets > 500 × 10⁹ or <150 × 10⁹/l<br>WBC ≥100 × 10⁹/l<br>PB blasts ≥1%<br>PB granulated precursors ≥20% | Stage 1: 0–1 factor<br>Stage 2: 2–3 factors<br>Stage 3: >3 factors | Stage 1: 65%<br>Stage 2: 40%<br>Stage 3: 38% |
| 126 | Leukocyte-count<br>Platelet count<br>Age<br>Sex<br>Hemoglobin | Low risk: <0.8<br>Middle risk: 0.8–1.4<br>High risk: <1.4 | Low risk: 72%<br>Middle risk: 36%<br>High risk: 28% |
| 125 | Age<br>PB blasts<br>Spleen size<br>Platelet count | Low risk: <0.8<br>Intermediate risk: 0.8–1.2<br>High risk: >1.2 | Low risk: 62%<br>Intermediate risk: 43%<br>High risk: 33% |
| 91 | Age ≥ 60<br>Race<br>Spleen 0, 1–4, 5–9, ≥10 cm<br>Platelets < 150 × 10⁹/l or >700 × 10⁹/l<br>PB basophils ≥7% | Stage 1: <0.8<br>Stage 2: 0.8–1.39<br>Stage 3: ≥1.4 | Stage 1: 62%<br>Stage 2: 45%<br>Stage 3: 13% |

BCM, below costal margin; PB, peripheral blood; BM, bone marrow; WBC, white blood cells.

developed.[141] This model utilizes age, spleen size, blast count, platelet count, eosinophil count, and basophil count (Table 41.7). Among 908 patients included in 14 studies involving 12 institutions, three distinct risk groups were identified, with median survival times of 98 months, 65 months, and 42 months. This meta-analysis has been updated, with 1400 patients being followed for up to 12.5 years, and showing median survival times of 100, 69 months and 45 months for low-, intermediate-, and high-risk groups.[142] The distribution of patients was 42%, 45%, and 13% in the low-, intermediate-, and high-risk categories. This score, usually referred to as either the 'Hasford score' or the 'Euro score', has been used in clinical trials only recently. The merits of one prognostic model over the other remain unclear, and both the Sokal and the Euro systems are now widely used.

The decision whether to offer an individual patient the option of treatment by allogeneic stem cell transplantation (allo-SCT) must be based in part on an assessment of the probability of success using the best available stem cell donor. Gratwohl et al[143] have defined five principal prognostic factors for survival after allo-SCT on the basis of data submitted to the European Group for Blood and Marrow

## Table 41.7 Sokal and Hasford prognostic scoring systems for CML

| Hasford[a] | Sokal[b] | |
|---|---|---|
| *Parameters considered* | | |
| Age (<50 vs ≥50 years) | Age (years) | |
| Spleen size[c] | Spleen size[c] | |
| Peripheral blood: | Peripheral blood: | |
| • Blasts (%) | • Blasts (%) | |
| • Eosinophils (%) | • Platelet count (10⁹/l) | |
| • Basophils (%) | | |
| • Platelet count (10⁹/l) | | |
| *Risk categories* | | |
| ≤780 | Low | <0.8 |
| >780–≤1480 | Intermediate | 0.8–1.2 |
| >1480 | High | >1.2 |

[a] Hasford score = (0.6666 Age + 0.042 Spleen + 0.0584 Blasts + 0.0413 Eosinophils + 0.2039 Basophils + 1.0956 Platelets) × 1000, with Age = 0 if <50 years, = 1 otherwise; Basophils = 0 if <3%, = 1 otherwise; Platelets = 0 if <1500 × 10⁹/l, = 1 otherwise.
[b] Sokal score = exp {0.011 (Age − 43.4) + 0.0345 (Spleen − 7.51) + 0.188 [(Platelet/700)² − 0.563] + 0.0887 (Blasts − 2.1)}.
[c] In cm below the costal margin.

Transplantation (Table 41.8). They allocated a score of 0, 1, or 2 to each of the five factors in accordance with the degree to which the influence of that factor was favorable or unfavorable for a particular patient. Thus, for each factor in a given transplant procedure, a patient's total score could be 0 (most favorable) or 2 (least favorable). The aggregate prognostic score calculated in this way correlated well with actual survival (Table 41.9). This approach is extremely useful for helping a clinician to make recommendations and the patient to decide whether or not to undergo allo-SCT. It must be conceded, however, that many of the factors to be considered in such decision-making are 'empirical'. There is a complete absence of prospective studies addressing the results of allo-SCT in CML – a point stressed in the report from the American Society of Hematology Committee on Practice Guidelines.[144]

The presence of deletions adjacent to the translocation breakpoints on the derivative chromosome 9 has been described in 10–15% of patients with CML. These deletions span the translocation breakpoint, often involve both chromosome 9 and 22 sequences, are large (sometimes measuring many megabases), and occur at the same time as the formation of the Ph translocation. They are associated with an extremely poor prognosis, with those patients who carry them having shorter length of chronic phase, earlier disease transformation, and shorter survival. Also, in a direct comparison, deletion status was a far more powerful prognostic indicator than either the commonly used Sokal or Hasford scores.[145]

The recent approval in the USA and Europe of imatinib represents the latest improvement of the treatment of patients with CML. It will likely change the current clinical treatment pathway, as clinical trial results have been positive.[140] Advances in the treatment of CML, as well as progress in supportive care, have significantly impacted the natural history of the disease and its prognosis. Historically, the median survival for patients with CML was 3 years, with a 5-year survival rate of less than 20%. Today, patients with chronic phase disease have a median survival of 5–7 years and 50–60% of patients are alive at 5 years, with more than 30% being alive at 10 years. Because

## Table 41.8 Risk score for individual transplant procedures in CML as established by the European Group for Blood and Marrow Transplantation

| Feature | Score |
|---|---|
| *Donor type* | |
| HLA-identical sibling | 0 |
| Unrelated/non identical | 1 |
| | |
| *Stage of disease* | |
| Chronic phase | 0 |
| Accelerated phase | 1 |
| Blast crisis | 2 |
| | |
| *Age* | |
| <20 years | 0 |
| 20–40 years | 1 |
| >40 years | 2 |
| | |
| *Donor/recipient sex combination* | |
| Other | |
| Female donor or male recipient | 1 |
| | |
| *Interval from diagnosis to transplant* | |
| <12 months | 0 |
| >12 months | 1 |

## Table 41.9 The 5-year probability of leukemia-free survival (LFS), survival, transplant-related mortality (TRM), and relapse incidence (RI) in CML

| Risk score | % of patients with score | Probability of outcome at 5 years (%)[a] | | | |
|---|---|---|---|---|---|
| | | LFS | Survival | TRM | RI |
| 0 | 2 | 60 (62) | 72 (76) | 20 (21) | 26 |
| 1 | 18 | 60 (61) | 70 (73) | 23 (21) | 23 |
| 2 | 28 | 47 (44) | 62 (59) | 31 (35) | 32 |
| 3 | 28 | 37 (34) | 48 (49) | 46 (47) | 31 |
| 4 | 15 | 35 (28) | 40 (38) | 51 (53) | 28 |
| 5 | 7 | 19 (37) | 18 (39) | 71 (45) | 41 |
| 6 | 2 | 16 (15) | 22 (19) | 73 (81) | 32 |
| 7 | 0.1 | — | — | — | — |

[a] The numbers in parentheses are the results of weighted Cox risk scores developed on the reference group and applied to the test group (*n*=1222).

various and highly divergent treatment options are available for patients with CML, it is becoming ever more important to determine the effect of baseline characteristics on the efficacy of a given therapy. Imatinib has only recently been introduced for the treatment of CML patients. Thus it seems too early to use a define prognostic model for imatinib-treated patients.

## Treatment

### Treatment of the chronic phase of the disease

Some two decades ago, the treatment of a patient with chronic phase CML was virtually restricted to the use of standard chemotherapy such as busulfan or hydroxyurea. These drugs have the ability to control the signs and symptoms of the disease. However, progression to blastic phase was constant. At that time, a combination of antileukemic drugs was used, unfortunately without success, and finally the patient died within a few months after a median survival of the disease of 3–6 years. For many years, the prognosis of patients with CML was poor. The expected median survival was 3 years, and less than 20% of patients were alive at 5 years. However, prognosis has improved because of earlier diagnosis, improved antileukemic therapy, and better supportive care. Currently, many therapeutic options are offered for the treatment of chronic phase, such as IFN-α-based regimens, homoharringtonine, stem cell transplantation, and, recently, imatinib, a very promising tyrosine kinase inhibitor.

### *Chemotherapy*

Busulfan, introduced in 1953, became in 1968 the treatment of choice when the results of the UK Medical Research Council (MRC) randomized trial comparing radiotherapy with busulfan demonstrated the superiority of the drug.[147] Although busulfan produces good control of blood cells for a long period, it does not alter the course of the disease. Also, it has potential side-effects, which may be serious. The prolonged use of busulfan has been associated with adrenal insufficiency, pulmonary fibrosis, skin pigmentation, and marrow fibrosis. Prolonged aplasia can occur, which may be a major cause of death. However, survival has sometimes been prolonged in such cases. Other drugs, including thioguanine, melphalan, dibromomannitol, chlorambucil, 6-mercaptopurine, and cyclophosphamide, were not considered to be more active compared with busulfan. Hydroxyurea was introduced later (in 1972), and has been extensively used.[148] Hematologic relapse is usual if hydroxyurea is stopped. Thus, the drug must be administered continuously. Although hydroxyurea and busulfan can both control the hematological manifestations of CML, hydroxyurea proved to be

superior. In a prospective trial, patients who received hydroxyurea had a significantly longer median survival (56 months versus 44 months) compared with those who were treated with busulfan.[149] These findings have been confirmed in a meta-analysis of 812 patients enrolled in three randomized trials.[150]

Because of its in vitro activity, cytarabine was tested in vivo as a single agent for the treatment of patients with CML in chronic phase. Treatment of two patients in chronic phase with low-dose cytarabine resulted in a significant reduction of Ph+ metaphases.[151] The cytarabine was administered by subcutaneous infusion at a dose rate of 20 mg/m²/day, with the aim of inducing and maintaining a granulocyte count of less than 2000/μl for at least 10 days. It was administered for 17–31 days, either continuously or with interruptions of 2–7 days because of hematological toxicity or side-effects. Cytogenetic analyses were performed 4–9 days after the end of the cytarabine infusion. After two or three successive cycles, Ph+ metaphases decreased from 100% to 2 of 27 and 3 of 26 metaphases in patients 1 and 2, respectively. In contrast, subsequent intensive chemotherapy with high-dose hydroxyurea in a dosage sufficient to maintain granulocytopenia and normal serum vitamin $B_{12}$ levels reduced the Ph positivity to only 46% and 72%, respectively. Thus, it was concluded that a selective antileukemic effect has been seen with cytarabine but not with hydroxyurea. Also, it was assumed that cytarabine exhibits significant antileukemic selectivity, while hydroxyurea is a non-specific inhibitor of granulopoiesis. Similar antileukemic activity of cytarabine was observed in five patients in chronic phase.[152]

Homoharringtonine (HHT), a plant alkaloid, is one of a group of cephalotoxin esters isolated in 1969. It has long been recognized as an antitumor agent in Chinese folk medecine. Preclinical studies indicated good antitumor activity in murine P388 lymphocytic leukemia and L-615 leukemia. Several phase I–II studies documented some degree of antileukemia activity in refractory AML. The use of HHT in CML was first reported by Chinese teams. Of 15 patients in chronic phase, 9 achieved a hematological remission with a dose of HHT of 5–7 mg/day for 7–10 days.[153] However, no cytogenetic evaluation was reported. The most important antileukemia activity of HHT is inhibition of protein synthesis. However, induction of apoptosis has also been demonstrated. In vitro, HHT is able to induce a dose-dependent cell growth inhibition. It exerts a synergistic effect with IFN-α, cytarabine, and IFN-α+ cytarabine in inhibiting CML hematopoietic progenitors. Such in vitro synergism is the rational for clinical trials using the three agents.[154]

HHT has been used as a low-dose continuous infusion of 2.5 mg/m² daily for 14 days for induction, then for 7 days every month, in patients with late chronic phase CML. It induced a complete hematologic remission in two-thirds of patients (more than 50% of whom had shown resistance to IFN-α) and a cytogenetic response in one-third (half of which were major responses).[155] HHT was then given for 6 cycles as remission induction, followed by IFN-α maintenance to patients with early chronic phase CML. The complete hematologic response rate was 92% and the cytogenetic response rate was 68%.[156]

### Interferons

Interferons are cellular glycoproteins with antiproliferative, antiviral, and immunoregulatory properties. They are produced by various cell types in response to viral infection. Both IFN-α and IFN-β are acid-stable, bind to the same receptors, and are produced primarily by leukocytes and fibroblasts, respectively. In contrast, IFN-γ is an acid-labile, structurally distinct molecule that binds to a different receptor, and is produced mainly by T lymphocytes. IFN-α, the molecule used in CML, initially prepared from human leukocytes, is now essentially produced by recombinant techniques.

IFN-α has the potential to control progression in the chronic phase and was the first non-myelotoxic drug to be shown to cause a marked reduction in Ph positivity in some patients. The use of IFN-α in CML was first evaluated by the Houston group some 15 years ago. They first used human IFN α in 51 patients in chronic phase treated with doses of 3–9 MIU daily. IFN-α resulted in satisfactory control of the disease in 36 patients (71%), with normalization of peripheral blood counts and a gradual decrease in bone marrow cellularity. Of greatest interest was the finding that serial cytogenetic studies showed a reduction in the percentage of Ph+ cells in 20 of the 36 patients in whom satisfactory control was established. The Ph suppression lasted in 7 patients for more than 39–62 months.[157]

The responses to IFN-α among these patients required the development of standardized criteria for complete hematologic response (CHR) and cytogenetic responses (Table 41.10).

Following the first reports from the Houston group, several small phase II studies were published (Table 41.11). Using recombinant IFN-α2a, 2b, 2c, several studies from single-institution or cooperative groups have subsequently confirmed the efficacy of IFN-α in CML.[133,158–163] The dose of 5 MIU/m² daily has been used at the MD Anderson Cancer Center, Houston for the treatment of 274 patients with early chronic phase CML.[158] Of these 80% achieved CHR and 58% had a cytogenetic response (26% complete and 38% major). The median survival was 89 months. Achieving a cytogenetic response after 12 months of therapy was associated with a statistically longer survival. At 5 years, the survival rates were 90% for complete, 88%

### Table 41.10  Hematologic and cytogenetic Houston response criteria for CML

**Complete hematologic response**

- No signs and symptoms
- No palpable splenomegaly
- WBC <10 × 10⁹/l
- No immature peripheral cells
- Platelets <350 × 10⁹/l

**Cytogenetic responses**

| Type | % Ph⁺ cells in bone marrow |
|---|---|
| Complete | 0 |
| Partial | <35 |
| Minor | 35–95 |
| None | 100 |

for partial response, and 76% for minor cytogenetic responses.

The relationship of the response to the dose and schedule of the treatment with IFN-α, as well as the duration of chronic phase and survival, were then the subjects of several randomized studies (Table 41.12).[100,131,132,135,164]

In the German CML study, IFN-α was superior to busulfan therapy, but it did not demonstrate a survival advantage after hydroxyurea.[132] In the UK trial, major responses have been associated with IFN-α doses between 2 and 6 MIU daily, and responsiveness did not appear to be associated with higher doses.[131] In the Japanese trial, the predicted 5-year survival rates were 54% and 32% for the IFN-α and busulfan arms, respectively.[100]

A survival advantage was also demonstrated in the Italian study, with a 6-year survival rate of 50% with IFN-α compared with 29% with chemotherapy.[135] However, in the Benelux study, the benefits of a better hematologic and cytogenetic response after IFN-α did not translate in a longer survival for the IFN-α-treated patients.[164]

Studies of combinations of IFN-α and chemotherapy were conducted in order to attempt to achieve CHR or cytogenetic responses in IFN-α-resistant patients. It was also assumed that a higher cytogenetic response rate might be achieved by increasing myelosuppression with a combination of myelotoxic drugs. In a pilot study, 24 patients received hydroxyurea 50 mg/kg/day and IFN-α2a at a starting dose of 5 MIU/m²/day. Courses of low-dose cytarabine were given to 11 patients at a dose of 10–20 mg/m²/day for 10–15 days per month.[165] A CHR was obtained in 18 patients, 8 achieving a major cytogenetic response. A rapid cytogenetic improvement was recorded in 6 out of 11 patients receiving low-dose cytarabine, with a complete Ph chromosome suppression in 4.

### Table 41.11  Phase II studies with IFN-α in CML

| Ref | No. of patients | IFN-α dose | CHR (%) | Cytogenetic responses | | |
|---|---|---|---|---|---|---|
| | | | | Any | Major | Complete |
| 134 | 274 | 5 MIU/m²/d | 80 | 58 | 38 | 26 |
| 138 | 52 | 5 MIU/m²/d | 81 | — | 49 | — |
| 133 | 107 | 5 MIU/m²/d | 59 | 21 | 18 | — |
| 159 | 40 | — | 56 | 40 | — | — |
| 160 | 63 | 5 and 2 MIU/m²hwk[a] | 46 | 70 | 2 | — |
| 161 | 10 | 5 MIU/m²/wk | 33 | 0 | 0 | 0 |
| 163 | 27 | 2 MIU/m²/d, then weekly | 70 | 33 | 22 | 7 |

CHR, complete hematologic response rate.
[a] In a randomized study of 5 versus 2 MIU/m²/wk.

### Table 41.12  Interferon-α versus chemotherapy for CML in randomized studies

| Ref | No. of patients | Survival (months) | | p |
|---|---|---|---|---|
| | | INF-α | Chemotherapy | |
| 135 | 322 | 72 | 52 | 0.002 |
| 132 | 513 | 66 | 45 (busulfan) | 0.008 |
| | | | 56 (hydroxurea) | 0.44 |
| 131 | 587 | 61 | 41 | <0.001 |
| 100 | 159 | 54% at 5 years | 32% at 5 years for busulfan | 0.029 |
| 164 | 195 | 64 | 68 (hydroxyurea) | |

Subsequently, two French multicenter trials were conducted in order to study the potential benefit of a combination of IFN-α with low-dose cytarabine as front-line treatment.[136,166] In the second of these, the CML91 study, the dose of cytarabine was increased to 20 mg/m²/day, the monthly courses being started within 2 weeks after randomization.[136] The trial enrolled 810 patients, and 721 were studied: 360 randomly assigned to the IFN-α/cytarabine group and 361 to the IFN-α group. An update of this trial shows that the probability of having a major cytogenetic response at 24 months was significantly higher in the IFN-α/cytarabine group (p = 0.006). Also, the patients in the IFN-α/cytarabine group survived significantly longer than those in the IFN-α group (p = 0.02). At 3 years, the estimated survival rates were 85.7% and 79.1% for the IFN-α/cytarabine and IFN-α groups, respectively (Figure 41.6). In this trial, a relationship was also noted between cytogenetic response and survival.

The Italian Cooperative Study Group on CML conducted a similar randomized trial. In this, 540 evaluable patients were randomized, 275 being assigned to IFN-α plus cytarabine and 265 to IFN-α alone. At 12 months, the combination resulted in a higher cytogenetic response rate (41% versus 34%) and a higher major cytogenetic response rate (17% versus 9%; p=0.01). Survival was also improved with the combination, the difference being significant only for patients with low-risk disease (p=0.01).[167] Other groups have reported similar observation of a potential benefit of IFN-α therapy combined with low-dose cytarabine.[168–171]

Cytarabine ocfosfate (YNK01), an oral formulation of cytarabine, has been tested in combination with IFN-α by several groups.[172–174] In the Italian and French trials, the study design was the same: IFN-α 5 MIU/m² daily and YNK01 600 mg daily, 14 days per month. The response rate was higher in the Italian study, with a major cytogenetic response rate at 12 months of 28%, whereas it was 16% in the French study. Doses of YNK01 were too high, and lower doses such as 200 mg daily should be tested in the future.

Patients' compliance with prolonged treatment with IFN-α in CML is an important factor for achieving

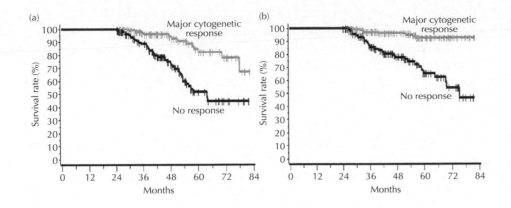

**Figure 41.6** Survival by cytogenetic response at 24 months in the CML91 study: (a) IFN-α; (b) IFN-α/cytarabine. Landmark analysis ($p < 10^{-4}$).

clinical benefit. In some studies, the antitumor efficacy appears to be related to higher-dose schedules of daily IFN-α therapy. Similarly, trials in CML suggest that an increased area under the curve (AUC), and associated prolonged tumor exposure to IFN-α, may be important in mediating the antileukemic effects. Therapy with IFN-α is cumbersome, and is associated with significant side-effects requiring dose reductions and temporary or permanent treatment interruptions in 10–50% of patients.

Polyethylene glycol (PEG) is a linear, hydrophobic, uncharged, flexible polymer available in a variety of molecular weights. A semisynthetic formulation (protein–polymer conjugate of IFN-α2b) was developed by attaching a single PEG 12 kDa molecule to the amino groups of selected lysine residues in the IFN-α2b molecule or the N-terminal amino acid. Twenty-seven adults with Ph+ CML in chronic or accelerated phases, in whom IFN-α treatment has failed, were included in a phase I study.[175] PEG IFN-α2b was given as a weekly subcutaneous injection starting at 0.75 μg/kg weekly and escalating to 1.5, 3, 4.5, 6, 7.5, and 9.0 μg/kg. The maximum tolerated dose was defined at 7.5–9 μg/kg; dose-limiting toxicities included severe fatigue, neurotoxicity, liver function abnormalities, and myelosuppression. The proposed phase II dose of PEG IFN-α2b was 6 μg/kg weekly. Among 19 patients with active disease, 7 (37%) achieved CHR; 2 (11%) had a cytogenetic response (complete).

A randomized study of PEG IFN-α2a versus IFN-α2a suggested a superiority of the pegylated form, with a higher response rate.[176] However, these results were not confirmed with PEG-IFN-α2b.[177]

There is accumulated evidence from randomized controlled trials that, compared with busulfan or hydroxyurea, IFN-α improves survival in chronic phase patients with favorable features: no or minimal prior treatment, relatively normal hemoglobin levels and platelet counts, less than 10% blasts in the blood, and especially beginning treatment within 6 months of diagnosis when IFN-α is coupled with other agents such as hydroxyurea or cytarabine.

## Results of clinical trials with imatinib

Through our understanding of signaling pathways regulating cellular growth, the cell cycle, and programmed cell death (apoptosis), numerous targets for anticancer agents have emerged. In this setting, the BCR–ABL rearrangement possesses many characteristics of an ideal therapeutic target. BCR–ABL functions as a constitutively activated tyrosine kinase, and mutagenic analysis has shown that this activity is essential for the transforming function of the protein. Consequently, an inhibitor of the BCR–ABL kinase would be predicted to be an effective and selective therapeutic agent for CML. Tyrosine kinases catalyze the transfer of phosphate from adenosine triphosphate (ATP) to tyrosine residues on substrate proteins. Because all protein kinases use ATP as a phosphate donor, it was thought that inhibitors of ATP binding would lack sufficient target specificity to be clinically useful. However, this turned out not to be the case, and a lead compound of the 2-phenylaminopyrimidine class rapidly emerged. One series of compounds, optimized against the platelet-derived growth factor receptor (PDGFR), showed equipotent activity against the ABL tyrosine kinase, of these, imatinib (imatinib mesylate, STI571, Gleevec/Glivec) emerged as a major compound for the treatment of CML. In vitro preclinical studies of imatinib showed specific inhibition of the proliferation of myeloid cell lines containing BCR–ABL. Colony-forming assays from CML patients showed a marked decrease (92–98%) in the number of BCR–ABL colonies, with little toxicity to normal stem cells. Further experiments showed that both p185[BCR/ABL]- and p210[BCR/ABL]-expressing cells were sensitive to imatinib and that dose-dependent inhibition of tumor growth was seen in animals inoculated with BCR–ABL-expressing cells.[178,179] Based on the efficacy of imatinib in these preclinical models and an acceptable animal toxicology profile, phase I and II trials were initiated, followed by a large phase III trial.

The first phase I/II trial included 83 patients in whom treatment with IFN-α had failed or who could not tolerate the drug.[180] Of these, 37 had hematologic resistance or relapse, 33 had cytogenetic resistance or relapse, and 13 could not tolerate IFN-α. The median duration of the therapy with IFN-α was 8.5 months (range 1 week – 8.5 years). Nineteen patients had had findings suggestive of accelerated disease. The median duration of treatment with imatinib was 310 days (range 17–607 days). Half of the patients assigned to receive daily doses of 25, 50, or 85 mg of imatinib were subsequently removed from the study within 2 months because of elevated white cell or platelet counts requiring therapy, which was not permitted by the protocol.

A subsequent phase II study enrolled 532 patients from December 1999 to May 2000.[181] After a central review of the data, the diagnosis of chronic phase CML was confirmed in 454 patients (85%). This diagnosis could not be confirmed for 78 (15%) patients, either because they had characteristics of accelerated (17 patients) or blastic (12 patients) phase or because of missing data (49 patients). Patients were eligible for this study if they were 18 years or older and had Ph+ CML in chronic phase that had failed prior IFN-α therapy according to one of the following criteria: hematologic failures were defined either as hematologic resistance (failure to achieve a CHR following at least 6 months of IFN-α treatment) or as relapse after achieving CHR, with WBC increased to $20 \times 10^9$/or more, while receiving IFN-α. In both cases, hydroxyurea was allowed for up to 50% of the IFN-α treatment duration. Cytogenetic failures were defined either as cytogenetic resistance (≥65% Ph positivity after at least 1 year of interferon) or as relapse from a major cytogenetic response (an increase in the percentage of Ph+ metaphases by at least 30%, or an increase to ≥65%). Intolerance of IFN-α was defined as any non-hematologic toxicity of grade 3 or more (as defined by NCI Common Toxicity Criteria) persisting for more than 1 month with IFN-α given at 25 MIU/week or higher.

In this single-arm multicenter phase II trial, patients received imatinib 400 mg orally daily. Dose escalation to 400 mg twice daily was permitted in patients who did not achieve a CHR after 3 months of treatment, whose disease relapsed within 3 months of a CHR, or who did not achieve a major cytogenetic response after 12 months of therapy. Imatinib induced major cytogenetic responses in 60% of the 454 patients with confirmed chronic phase CML and CHR in 95%. After a median follow-up of 18 months, CML had not progressed to the accelerated or blastic phases in an estimated 89% of patients, and 95% of the patients were alive. Grade 3 or 4 non-hematologic toxic effects were infrequent, and hematologic toxic effects were manageable. Only 2% of patients discontinued treatment because of drug-related adverse events, and no treatment-related deaths occurred (Table 41.13).

In order to demonstrate the benefit of imatinib compared with other IFN-α-based regimens, it was decided to set up a large international study. This study (IRIS: International Randomized Study of IFN + Ara-C vs STI571) was carried out in newly diagnosed patients with CML in chronic phase to compare the efficacy, safety, and tolerability of imatinib administered as monotherapy with that of standard treatment with IFN-α + cytarabine as the first-line treatment of the disease. The objective of the trial was to determine the progression-free survival in adult patients with newly diagnosed previously untreated Ph+ CML in chronic phase randomized to receive either imatinib as a single agent or a combination of IFN-α and cytarabine. The aim of the trial was also to assess the rates and durations of CHR and major cytogenetic responses as well as the quality of life and overall survival.[182]

In the imatinib arm, patients were treated with 400 mg/day. This dose was recommended for chronic phase patients following the results of the phase I and II studies. In the IFN-α arm, patients were treated with a target dose of IFN-α of 5 MIU/m²/day subcutaneously in combination with subcutaneous cytarabine 20 mg/m²/day for 10 days a month. Because of the high level of efficacy seen with imatinib given as second-line therapy in patients with chronic phase CML failing prior IFN-α therapy in the preceding phase II study 0110, patients showing lack of response (lack of CHR at 6 months, increasing WBC, no major cytogenetic response at 24 months), loss of response (loss of CHR or major cytogenetic response), or severe intolerance to treatment were allowed to cross over to the alternative treatment arm (Figure 41.7).

This multicenter phase III study included 1106 adult patients, 553 in each arm. The baseline characteristics of these patients were well balanced between the two arms and there were no differences between the two arms with regard to the distribution into the three subcategories of risk using a scoring system such as the Sokal score or the Euro score.

The median time from randomization to start of treatment was 3 days in both groups, ranging from 0 to 41 days in the imatinib arm and from 0 to 79 days in the IFN-α/cytarabine arm. After a median follow-up of 19 months, the estimated rate of a major cytogenetic response (0–35% of cells in metaphase positive for the Ph chromosome) at 18 months was 87.1% (95% confidence interval (CI) 84.1–90.0%) in the imatinib group and 34.7% (95% CI, 29.3–40.0%) in the group given IFN-α plus cytarabine ($p<0.001$). The estimated complete cytogenetic response rates were 76.2% (95% CI 72.5–79.9%) and 14.5% (95% CI 10.5–18.5%), respectively ($p<0.001$). At 18 months, the estimated rate of freedom from progression to accelerated phase or blast crisis CML was 96.7% in the imatinib group and 91.5% in the combination-therapy group ($p<0.001$) (Table 41.14).

**Table 41.13  Efficacy of imatinib in CML: summary of phase I and phase II trial results (numbers of patients, with percentages in parentheses)**

| | Phase I trials | | Phase II trials | | | | | | |
| --- | --- | --- | --- | --- | --- | --- | --- | --- | --- |
| | Chronic phase[a] 300–1000 mg/d (*n* = 54) | Blast crisis[b] 300–1000 mg/d (*n* = 58) | Chronic phase[a] 400 mg/d (*n* = 454) | Accelerated phase | | | Blast crisis[c] | | |
| | | | | Total (*n* = 181) | 400 mg/d (*n* = 62) | 600 mg/d (*n* = 119) | Total (*n* = 229) | 400 mg/d (*n* = 32) | 600 mg/d (*n* = 197) |
| HR | 54 (100) | 35 (60) | NR | 125 (69)[d] | 40 (65)[d] | 85 (71)[d] | 70 (31)[d] | 3 (9)[d] | 67 (34)[d] |
| CHR | 53 (98) | 8 (14) | 430 (95)[d] | 61 (34)[d] | 17 (27)[d] | 44 (37)[d] | 18 (8)[d] | 0 | 18 (9)[d] |
| Marrow response | NR | 27 (46) | NR | 22 (12)[d] | 6 (10)[d] | 16 (13)[d] | 10 (4)[d] | 1 (3)[d] | 9 (5)[d] |
| RCP | — | NR | — | 42 (23)[d] | 17 (27)[d] | 25 (21) | 42 (18)[d] | 2 (6)[d] | 40 (20)[d] |
| MCR | 17 (31) | 7 (12) | 272 (60) | 43 (24) | 10 (16) | 33 (28) | 37 (16) | 2 (6) | 35 (18) |
| CCR | 7 (13) | 5 (9) | 188 (41) | 30 (17) | 7 (11) | 23 (19) | 17 (7) | 1 (3) | 16 (8) |
| PCR | 10 (18) | 2 (3) | 84 (19) | 13 (7) | 3 (5) | 10 (8) | 20 (9) | 1 (3) | 19 (10) |
| mCR | 12 (22) | NR | 21 (5) | 12 (7) | 5 (8) | 7 (6) | 4 (2) | 1 (3) | 3 (2) |

HR, hematologic response; CHR, complete hematologic response; RCP, return to chronic phase; MCR, major cytogenetic response; CCR, complete cytogenetic response; PCR, partial cytogenetic response; mCR, minor cytogenetic response; NR, data not reported.

[a] Failing IFN-α therapy.

[b] Myeloid (*n* = 38) or lymphoid (*n* = 10) blast crisis or Ph+ acute lymphoblastic leukemia (*n* = 10).

[c] Myeloid blast crisis.

[d] Sustained response (≥4 weeks).

Discontinuation of first-line therapy was more frequent in the group of patients randomized to IFN-α, the most frequent reason for discontinuation being withdrawal of consent (13%). Importantly, in the USA, the rates of discontinuation of IFN-α due to withdrawal of consent, protocol violation, administrative problems, or loss of follow-up increased sharply around the time imatinib was introduced into the US market for the treatment of chronic phase patients failing prior IFN-therapy (May 2001). A similar pattern could not be observed outside the USA.

Further analysis using the Kaplan–Meier method has been performed, in which patients who crossed over or discontinued for reasons other than progression were censored. Using this approach, the estimated rate of CHR at 12 months in the imatinib arm was minimally affected (95.9%), whereas it increased to 66.5% in the IFN-α arm (*p*<0.001). Of interest, the rate of CHR to second-line imatinib for the 218 patients who crossed over was 83.5%, i.e. very similar to the reported rate of 88% in the phase II study 0110. Even when CHR was analyzed under the intention-to-treat

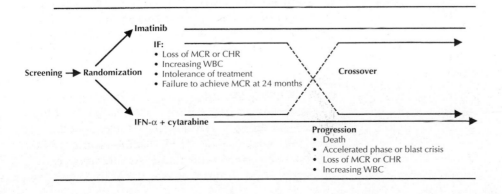

**Figure 41.7** IRIS trial design. MCR, major cytogenetic response; CHR, complete hematologic response; WBC, white blood cell.

**Table 41.14 Efficacy of imatinib as initial therapy for patients with newly diagnosed CML in chronic phase: best observed responses in the IRIS trial (percentages of patients)**

| Response | Imatinib (n = 553) | IFN-α + cytarabine (n = 553) | p |
|---|---|---|---|
| CHR | 95.3 | 55.5 | <0.001 |
| MCR | 85.2 | 22.1 | <0.001 |
| CCR | 73.8 | 8.5 | <0.001 |

CHR, complete hematologic response; MCR, major cytogenetic response; CCR, complete cytogenetic response.

(ITT) principle, the rate of CHR in the imatinib arm (94.6%) remained significantly higher than in the IFN-α arm (76.5%; $p<0.001$).

In patients who had a complete cytogenetic response, levels of BCR–ABL transcripts after 12 months of treatment had fallen by at least 3 log in 57% of those in the imatinib group and 24% of those in the group given IFN-α plus cytarabine ($p=0.003$).[183] On the basis of the complete cytogenetic response rates of 68% in the imatinib group and 7% in the group given IFN-α plus cytarabine at 12 months, an estimated 39% of all patients treated with imatinib but only 2% of all those given IFN-α plus cytarabine had a reduction in BCR–ABL transcripts levels of at least 3 log ($p<0.001$). For patients who had a complete cytogenetic response and a reduction in transcript levels of at least 3 log at 12 months, the probability of remaining progression-free was 100% at 24 months, as compared with 95% for such patients with a reduction of less than 3 log and 85% for patients who were not in complete cytogenetic remission at 12 months ($p<0.001$) (Figure 41.8).

Patients completed cancer-specific quality-of-life (QoL) (FACT-BRM) and utility (EQ-5D) questionnaires at baseline and during treatment ($n=1049$). The primary QoL endpoint was the Trial Outcome Index (TOI, a measure of physical function and well-being). Secondary endpoints included Social/Family Well-Being (SFWB), Emotional Well-Being (EWB), and the utility score. Primary analyses were ITT, with secondary analyses accounting for crossover. Multivariate mixed effects growth curve models and logistic and linear regression models were used. Patients on IFN-α plus cytarabine experienced a large decline in the TOI, while those on imatinib maintained their baseline level. Mean treatment arm differences at each visit were significant ($p<0.001$) and clinically relevant in favor of imatinib. Mean SFWB, EWB, and utility scores were also significantly better on imatinib. Patients who crossed over to imatinib experienced a large increase in TOI, and there were significant ($p<0.001$) differences between patients who did and did not cross over in favor of imatinib.[184] Tolerability of imatinib was good, serious adverse experiences being more frequent with IFN-α plus cytarabine (Tables 41.15 and 41.16).

### Stem cell transplantation

Allogeneic bone marrow transplantation (BMT) was first proposed for refractory leukemia and then for CML. The first results were published by the Seattle group, who demonstrated that, using an effective conditioning regimen, BMT could cure patients. The best BMT results are obtained using human leukocyte antigen (HLA)-matched sibling donors. However, unrelated BMT has improved recently.[185] Most patients are now transplanted in chronic phase (71%). Also, the proportion of patients who are offered BMT is higher. A study of 10 countries in Europe, North America, Australia, and New Zealand suggests that about 35% of persons with CML under the age of 55 years receive BMT.[186]

The best results are obtained when the transplant is performed during chronic phase and within the first year after diagnosis. Among 3409 recipients of HLA-identical transplants performed between 1989 and 1995 and reported to the International Bone Marrow Transplant Registry (IBMTR), the 3-year actuarial probabilities of relapse were 16% for 2753 patients transplanted in first chronic phase, 36% for 490 in accelerated phase, and 61% for 166 in blast phase. The 3-year probabilities of leukemia-free survival (LFS) were 59%, 37%, and 17%, respectively. Patients relapsing after an HLA-identical sibling transplant for CML often survive for long periods with conventional treatment. Many achieve durable remissions with donor lymphocyte infusions and some have succesful second BMTs. Consequently, 3-year survival rates after transplants are higher than LFS rates: 66% in chronic phase, 44% in accelerated

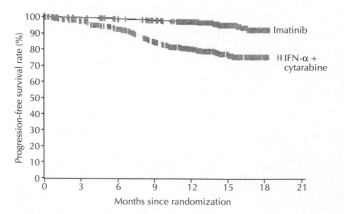

**Figure 41.8** Progression-free survival in the IRIS trial (vertical bars indicate censored observations).

**Table 41.15 Adverse experiences occurring in more than 10% of patients in the IRIS trial (percentages of patients)[a]**

| Event | All grades Imatinib (n = 551) | IFN-α + cytarabine (n = 533) | Grade 3 or 4 Imatinib (n = 551) | IFN-α + cytarabine (n = 533) |
|---|---|---|---|---|
| Superficial edema | 55.5 | 9.2 | 0.9 | 0.6 |
| Nausea | 43.7 | 61.4 | 0.7 | 5.1 |
| Muscle cramps | 38.3 | 11.1 | 1.3 | 0.2 |
| Musculoskeletal pain | 36.5 | 42.0 | 2.7 | 8.3 |
| Rash | 33.9 | 25.0 | 2.0 | 2.3 |
| Fatigue | 34.5 | 65.5 | 1.1 | 24.4 |
| Diarrhea | 32.8 | 41.7 | 1.8 | 3.2 |
| Headache | 31.2 | 42.6 | 0.4 | 3.2 |
| Joint pain | 28.3 | 39.6 | 2.4 | 7.3 |
| Abdominal pain | 27.0 | 24.6 | 2.4 | 3.9 |
| Nasopharyngitis | 22.0 | 8.3 | 0 | 0.2 |
| Myalgia | 21.4 | 38.8 | 1.5 | 8.1 |
| Hemorrhage | 20.9 | 20.6 | 0.7 | 1.5 |
| Vomiting | 16.9 | 27.4 | 1.5 | 3.4 |
| Dyspepsia | 16.2 | 9.2 | 0 | 0.8 |
| Pharyngolaryngeal pain | 16.0 | 13.3 | 0.2 | 0.2 |
| Cough | 14.5 | 22.3 | 0.2 | 0.6 |
| Dizziness | 14.5 | 23.8 | 0.9 | 3.4 |
| Upper respiratory tract infection | 14.5 | 8.3 | 0.2 | 0.4 |
| Weight gain | 13.4 | 1.7 | 0.9 | 0.2 |
| Pyrexia | 13.1 | 39.2 | 0.7 | 2.8 |
| Insomnia | 12.2 | 18.8 | 0 | 2.3 |
| Depression | 10.2 | 35.5 | 0.4 | 12.8 |
| Constipation | 8.5 | 14.3 | 0.7 | 0.2 |
| Anxiety | 7.3 | 11.4 | 0.2 | 2.6 |
| Dyspnea | 7.3 | 14.3 | 1.5 | 1.5 |
| Pruritus | 7.3 | 11.6 | 0.2 | 0.2 |
| Rigors | 7.3 | 33.8 | 0 | 0.8 |
| Influenza-like illness | 7.1 | 18.6 | 0 | 1.1 |
| Night sweats | 7.1 | 15.6 | 0.2 | 0.4 |
| Asthenia | 5.6 | 18.6 | 0.2 | 3.9 |
| Anorexia | 5.3 | 31.7 | 0 | 2.4 |
| Alopecia | 4.4 | 22.3 | 0 | 0.6 |
| Increased sweating | 3.6 | 14.8 | 0 | 0.4 |
| Weight loss | 3.1 | 17.1 | 0.2 | 1.3 |
| Stomatitis | 2.9 | 12.0 | 0 | 0.2 |
| Dry mouth | 2.2 | 10.3 | 0 | 0.2 |
| Mucosal inflammation | 0.7 | 10.3 | 0 | 3.2 |

[a] Adverse events regardless of relationship to therapy. The median follow-up period is 19 months. Adapted from Table 3 of reference 182.

phase, and 19% in blastic phase. In general, relatively few deaths after HLA-identical sibling transplants for chronic phase CML result from leukemia, particularly if the transplants are not T-cell-depleted. Most deaths are from transplant-related complications such as regimen-related toxicity, graft-versus-host disease (GVHD), and infection. An IBMTR study of HLA-identical sibling transplants for CML in first chronic phase performed between 1985 and 1990 identified prior treatment with hydroxyurea rather than busulfan and a short interval between diagnosis and transplant (less than 1 versus at least 1 year) as favorable prognostic factors. The 3-year probabilities of survival were 67% for patients treated with hydroxyurea and receiving transplant within 1 year of diagnosis, 59% for those treated with hydroxyurea and receiving transplant later, 54% for patients treated with busulfan and receiving transplant after 1 year after

**Table 41.16 Incidence of grade 3 or 4 hematologic and biochemical abnormalities in the IRIS trial (percentages of patients)**

| Event | Imatinib (*n* = 551) | IFN-α + cytarabine (*n* = 533) |
|---|---|---|
| Anemia | 3.1 | 4.3 |
| Neutropenia | 14.3 | 25.0 |
| Thrombocytopenia | 7.8 | 16.5 |
| Elevated serum ALT or AST levels | 5.1 | 6.8 |

ALT, alanine aminotransferase; AST, aspartate aminotransferase.

diagnosis, and 45% for those treated with busulfan and receiving transplant later.[187–189] A comparison was performed between a cohort of 548 patients of HLA-identical sibling transplants reported to the IMBTR and 196 patients receiving hydroxyurea (*n*= 121) or IFN-α (*n*= 75) in the German trial.[190] For the first 18 months after diagnosis, mortality was higher in the transplant than in the non-transplant cohort. From 18 to 56 months, mortality was similar, and after 56 months, mortality was lower in the transplant cohort.

Only 35% of patients with CML under the age of 55 years actually undergo an allogeneic transplant, primarily due to the lack of an appropriate tissue-compatible related donor. Alternative progenitor cell sources such as cord blood, mismatched related transplants, and matched unrelated donor transplants have been extensively explored as treatment options for patients with CML. CML is the most common indication for unerelated donor transplants, representing 35% of all unrelated donor transplants performed in the USA. With the increasing number and size of volunteer donor registries, the median time for identification of a suitable donor has decreased from 6.9 months to 5.5 months; however, only one of four searches actually culminates in transplantation. The

results of the largest series of unrelated donor transplantation for CML are summarized in Table 41.17.[185,191–193]

Acute GVHD and infectious complications remain the most important causes of morbidity and mortality of unrelated donor transplantation. The single most important prognostic factor for the development of acute GVHD is the degree of histocompatibility. Serologic typing underestimates the degree of mismatching in a large proportion of donor–recipient pairs. Modern molecular techniques have demonstrated that molecular mismatches in serologically matched donor–recipient pairs are common and correlate with transplant outcomes. In the Seattle study, young patients with CML (age <50 years) who receive a fully molecular matched unrelated donor and are transplanted within 1 year of diagnosis have an estimated 5-year survival rate of 74%, indistinguishable from recipients of fully matched sibling donor transplants.

The approach to patients with CML who lack an HLA-identical sibling donor has become increasingly complex. On the one hand, the availability of non-transplant strategies that can effectively achieve cytogenetic remission, such as imatinib, offers the possibility of long-term disease control for some patients without allogeneic transplantation. On the other hand, the increasing size and number of volunteer donor registries as well as improvements in tissue typing and supportive care have improved the outcomes of unrelated donor transplantation. The current challenge for physicians and patients is how to incorporate these strategies into the approach to each individual case and how to decide who should undergo unrelated donor transplantation as primary therapy or as salvage therapy for their disease. Transplant and non-transplant options should be viewed as complementary strategies in the treatment of CML, the goal being to obtain complete cytogenetic remissions in as many patients as possible with the minimum toxicity necessary for each patient.

One of the major causes of treatment failure is relapse, which occurs in 10–30% of patients who received unmanipulated donor marrow cells, but is considerably

**Table 41.17 Results of representative studies of unrelated donor transplantation for CML**

| Ref | *n* | Median age (years) | % survival | % GVHD II–IV | % GVHD III–IV | % relapse |
|---|---|---|---|---|---|---|
| 191 | 1423 | 35 | 37 (3 yr) | 43 | 33 | 8 |
| 192 | 115 | 33 | 46 (3 yr) | – | 24 | 23 |
| 185 | 196 | 35 | 57 (5 yr) | 77 | 35 | 10 |
| 193 | 27 | 32 | 52 (3 yr) | 39 | 8 | 9 |

more frequent in those who received marrow stem cells that have been depleted of T cells in an effort to minimize or eliminate GVHD. Patients who relapse may be treated with IFN-α[194] or by infusion of lymphocytes harvested from the original stem cell donor. The use of such donor lymphocyte infusions (DLI) was first reported in 1990, and many subsequent studies have confirmed their efficacy.[195,196] The benefit of the salvage treatment of post-transplant relapse with DLI can be estimated using a new definition of leukemia-free survival called 'current leukemia-free survival (CLFS)', which is defined as survival without evidence of leukemia at the time of the most recent assessment. Using this new statistical methodology, the 5-year estimate of conventional LFS was 36% in a cohort of 189 patients, but was 49% using the CLFS approach.[197] However, DLI are still associated with a high rate of acute and chronic GVHD. Current research is exploring the value of DLI, IFN-α, or imatinib in patients relapsing after BMT. Other approaches include new pretransplantation conditioning using non-myeloablative regimen.

High-dose chemotherapy followed by autologous stem cell infusion has also been considered as a therapeutic option that could improve survival.

Large prospective trials have recruited patients in order to address the question of whether autografting prolongs survival (Table 41.18). The observation that a substantial number of benign progenitors coexist with their malignant counterparts during early chronic phase provides the theoretical basis for the design of autologous transplantation trials. It is known that CML patients receiving high-dose chemotherapy or busulfan recover after a period of aplasia with predominantly Ph- hematopoiesis that is transient or occasionally long-lasting.[198] In several prospective trials, a significant proportion of patients treated with IFN-α achieved complete cytogenetic responses with restoration of Ph- hematopoiesis and prolongation of survival. In addition, it has been shown that Ph- progenitor cells can be successfully mobilized after high-dose chemotherapy with or without growth factor support.[198-205] In vitro data support the notion that Ph- cells are present in the bone marrow. It has been demonstrated that granulocyte–macrophage colony forming unit (CFU-GM) colonies from CML patients could be partially Ph-negative.[206]

Ex vivo culture of CML marrow in Dexter-type long-term bone marrow culture produces increasing numbers of Ph- hematopoietic cells.[207,208] Benign progenitors have also been selected on the basis of cell surface phenotype and have been shown to be polyclonal on the basis of the methylation pattern of the human androgen receptor gene located on the X chromosomes.[209] These observations support the hypothesis that Ph- hematopoietic cells are present in a significant proportion of patients with CML and that they are probably not part of the leukemic population.[210] These benign progenitors are suitable for reconstitution of hematopoiesis after high-dose chemotherapy and can be recovered from the marrow or peripheral blood in selected CML patients.

New approaches to select out benign progenitors from blood and marrow have been developed. However, the number of benign progenitors available for separation is often limited. There is also evidence that reduction of both normal and leukemic cells to low levels favors regeneration of normal stem cells, at

## Table 41.18 Results of autografting for CML

| Ref | Patients | Mobilization | Results Apheresis | Autografts |
|---|---|---|---|---|
| 203 | 23 CP1 (recently diagnosed) | CY: 5 g/m² G-CSF: 150 μg/m²/d | 21 patients collected (91%); 30% MCR | 0 patients |
| 202 | 40 CP1 (late chronic phase) | IDA+ HDAC G-CSF 263–300 μg/d | 59% MCR | 20 patients (high mortality) |
| 201 | 30 CP1 (recently diagnosed or late chronic phase) | IFN-α G-CSF 5 μg/kg/d | Collection on 29/30 patients; 5 MCR | 14 patients; 9 MCR |
| 199 | 22 recently diagnosed CP1 | mini-ICE + G-CSF | Collection on 22 patients; 63% CCR | 12 patients; 6 CCR, 7–15 months after graft |
| 260 | 8 CP1 | ICE G-CSF: 5–10 μg/kg IL-3: 5 μg/kg | Collection on 8 patients; 8 MCR | 8 patients; 8 MCR (FISH on blood) |

CP1, first chronic phase; CY, cyclophosphamide; G-CSF, granulocyte colony-stimulating factor; IDA, idarubicin; HDAC, high-dose cytarabine; IFN-α, interferon-α; (mini-)ICE, idarabicin, cytarabine, and etoposide; IL-3, interleukin-3; MCR, major cytogenetic response; CCR, complete cytogenetic response.

least in the short term. Thus, the sources of cells that have been used for autologous transplantation are unmanipulated peripheral blood stem cells (PBSC), or bone marrow cells, or in vitro manipulated cells, or mobilized PBSC following various regimens of chemotherapy, cytokines, and growth factors.

Autologous stem cell transplantations were performed first on CML patients with blastic transformation.[211,212] Subsequently, autografting has been used in chronic phase patients.[213,214] A retrospective analysis of the European Blood and Marrow Transplantation Registry (EBMTR) was performed on 174 patients who had undergone stem cell transplantation during their chronic phase[215] (and J Reiffers, personal communication, 2000). Patients received different conditioning regimens and most of them were treated with IFN-α after transplantation. The actuarial percentage of patients surviving at 5 years was 68.4% ± 11%, and was significantly higher for those who achieved a cytogenetic response.

McGlave et al[216] conducted an overview analysis of 200 patients autografted for CML with purged or unpurged marrow or PBSC at eight different transplant centers. At the time of publication, the survival time of 142 patients with chronic phase CML was not reached. However, as the data have matured, the outcome does not appear to be so good.

The crucial point is that these transplants are performed with leukemic stem cells included because the cryopreserved product is not manipulated. It has been demonstrated that progenitors released from the marrow into the circulation during the earliest stages of hematopoietic reconstitution following high-dose chemotherapy appear to be in part Ph−. Because these progenitors seem to have the capacity to reconstitute hematopoiesis, some groups have attempted to select these cells for the purpose of autografting.[217]

## Treatment of accelerated phase

In patients with accelerated phase CML, good hematologic control can be generally obtained by increasing the dose of IFN-α or hydroxyurea. However, the overall survival usually remains short, ranging from 8 to 18 months.[102]

In a cohort of 357 patients treated at the MD Anderson Cancer Center, Houston between 1965 and 1984, in which the majority of patients were managed with hydroxyurea, busulfan, or single-agent INF-α, the median survival after the onset of accelerated phase features was less than 18 months.[97] In a study of 20 patients treated with a combination of IFN-α and low-dose cytarabine (16 of whom had clonal evolution as the only evidence of accelerated phase), the CHR rate was 50%, and four patients (20%) achieved a partial or minor cytogenetic response. However, these responses were generally transient. The 3-year

survival rate for the 16 patients with clonal evolution was 74%. In contrast, it was only 22% for patients with accelerated phase features other than clonal evolution (4 from the present study and 9 from historical control series).[168]

Only two studies have evaluated the outcome of cohorts of more than 15 patients with accelerated phase CML treated with chemotherapy. In a study of 17 patients treated with decitabine, 9 (53%) achieved a response, with a median duration of 9 months. Six patients returned to chronic phase, two achieved a partial response, and one had a 'hematologic improvement' only, but no patients achieved a CHR. The median survival was 14 months, with a 2-year survival rate of 28%.[218] In another study of 24 patients treated with a combination of daunorubicin and high-dose cytarabine, 6 (25%) achieved a CHR and 4 (17%) returned to chronic phase. Five patients achieved a transient cytogenetic response. The median survival was 8 months, and the probability of survival at 18 months was 30%.[219]

Altogether, it appears that with chemotherapy and/or IFN-α, up to 50% of patients may achieve a response. However, these responses are usually short-lived, CHR are uncommon, and cytogenetic responses anecdotal. As consistently reported in these studies, the overall survival of patients with accelerated phase remains below 18 months.

The results of allogeneic BMT in patients with accelerated phase are intermediate between the results reported in patients with chronic phase or blast crisis. As with chemotherapy, the results may be significantly influenced by the criteria used to define accelerated phase CML. For example, in a study of 251 BMT patients from the Hammersmith Hospital in London, the proportion of patients transplanted in accelerated phase was 11% using the institution's criteria and 79% using the IBMTR criteria.[80] In a study by Clift et al,[101] 58 patients with accelerated phase (using criteria similar to the Sokal and IBMTR criteria) were transplanted at a single institution with HLA-matched sibling bone marrow donors. At 4-years, the overall and relapse-free survival rates were 49% and 43%, respectively. However, the rate of death not related to relapse was high, with 29 (50%) patients who died because of various complications of BMT (acute respiratory distress syndrome or other respiratory failures, cytomegelovirus infection, veno-occlusive disease, bacterial or fungal infection, or GVHD). Interestingly, the 4-year relapse rate was low, at 12%. In a multivariate analysis, factors associated with an improved survival were a young age (<38 years) and cytogenetic clonal evolution as the only manifestation of accelerated phase. The 4-year probability of survival for the 16 patients transplanted within 1 year of the diagnosis of CML and with cytogenetic clonal evolution as the only manifestation of accelerated phase was 74%. In contrast, the 4-year probability of survival for the 31 patients who were categorized as accelerated phase for reasons other than cytogenetic abnormalities was only 34%.

Data are also available from BMT registries. In one report of 1480 transplants from the EBMTR, 206 patients were grafted while in accelerated phase.[220] The 5-year LFS rate was only 22%. This low rate can be explained by a high relapse rate (42% at 2 years) and a high death rate. As in the study mentioned above, the transplant-related mortality rate was high: 47% at 2 years and 51% at 5 years. Similarly, in a report from the IBMTR, the 4-year LFS rate for the 408 patients transplanted in accelerated phase was 25%[221] (Figure 41.9). Among 3409 recipients of HLA-identical sibling transplants performed between 1989 and 1995, the 3-year actuarial relapse rate was 36% (30–42%) for 490 patients in accelerated phase. The 3-year LPS probability was 37% (35–39%). Patients relapsing after HLA-identical sibling transplant for CML often survive for long periods with conventional treatment. Many achieve durable remissions with DLI, and some have successful second BMT. Consequently, 3-year survival rates after transplants are somewhat higher than LFS rates: 44% (39–49%).[222]

## Imatinib

Imatinib has been tested on patients in accelerated phase in several phase I and II trials. In the first phase I study, imatinib showed relevant activity in a subset of patients with accelerated phase.[180] Of the 83 patients enrolled in this study, 19 had had findings suggestive of accelerated phase, and they responded favorably to the drug at a daily dose of 300 mg or higher. Therefore, a large phase II trial was conducted in order to confirm its observed activity and favorable safety profile.[223] The study was an open-label, non-randomized, multicenter, phase II trial designed to evaluate the clinical efficacy of imatinib as determined by the rate of sustained hematologic response.

Initially, enrolled patients received a daily dose of 400 mg. Following the availability of phase I dose-escalation data demonstrating the safety of prolonged treatment with higher doses, this initial daily dose was increased to 600 mg. For patients who had a relapse, dose escalation to a maximum of 400 mg twice daily was permitted. A total of 235 patients were enrolled in the study, of whom 181 had a confirmed diagnosis of accelerated phase.

Imatinib induced a hematologic response in 82% of the patients and sustained hematologic responses lasting at least 4 weeks in 69% (complete in 34%). The rate of major cytogenetic response was 24% (complete in 17%). Estimated 12-month progression-free and overall survival rates were 59% and 74%, respectively (see Table 41.13). In comparison, doses of 600 mg/day led to more cytogenetic responses (28% compared with 16%) and to longer duration of response (79% compared with 57% at 12 months) and time to disease progression (67% compared with 44% at 12 months), with no clinically relevant toxicity. A clear relationship between survival and cytogenetic response was observed using a landmark analysis at 3 months. Of 83 patients with an evaluation of cytogenetic response at 3 months after start of therapy, 20 (24%) had a major cytogenetic response at that time, and none of these 20 patients had died at the time of analysis. Of the 63 evaluated patients without major cytogenetic response after 3 months, 14 (22%) had died.

In multivariate analysis, the factors most strongly predictive of longer time to disease progression were hemoglobin levels of 100 g/l or higher and a starting dose of 600 mg. Female sex was marginally predictive in this analysis. In subgroup logistic regression analyses excluding patients without data for blasts in bone marrow or additional chromosomal abnormalities, neither variable added further to the prediction of hematologic response in multivariate analyses ($p > 0.10$). Further analyses indicated that varying the cutoff values used to define patient subgroups had little effect on most prognostic factors. Platelet counts below $40 \times 10^9/l$ were independently predictive of a shorter time to disease progression in exploratory analyses, but the reliability of this result was limited by the small number of patients in this subgroup. The use of different cutoff values for hemoglobin (<110 g/l) and blasts in peripheral blood (<5%) led to the elimination of male/female sex as a marginal prognostic factor in the final multivariate model, and to the inclusion of high platelet counts and low blast counts in peripheral blood as predictive of longer time to disease progression. In further exploratory multivariate analyses, a hemoglobin level of 100 g/l or higher was the sole factor significantly predictive for higher rates of sustained hematologic response. Exploratory multivariate analyses of prognostic factors for overall survival were limited by the small

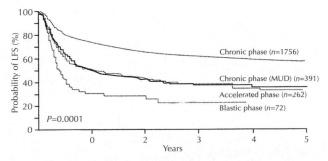

**Figure 41.9** Leukemia-free survival (LFS) after allogeneic bone marrow transplantation for CML: dotted lines, HLA-identical siblings; full line, matched unrelated donors. (Taken from International Bone Marrow Transplant Registry: 1990–1995)

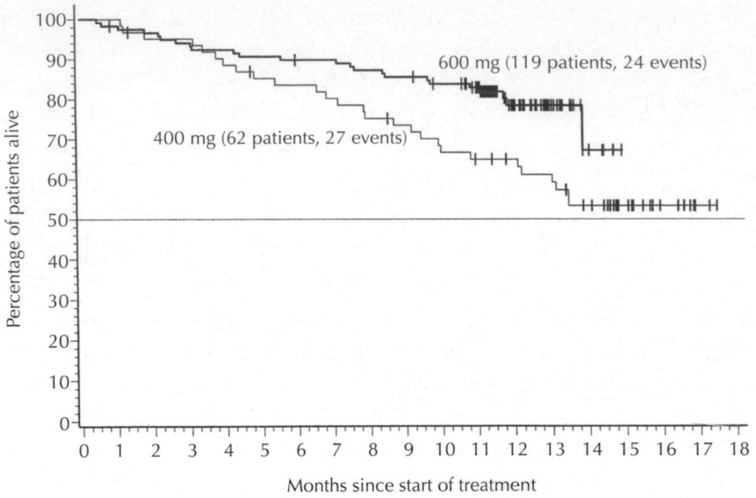


**Figure 41.10** Overall survival of CML patients in accelerated phase and treated with imatinib (vertical bars indicate censored observations).

number of patients who had died, but results identified three factors as predictive of longer survival: a starting dose of 600 mg, WBC $<30 \times 10^9/l$, and absence of splenomegaly (Figure 41.10).

The toxicity of imatinib in this trial was generally similar to that observed in a previous phase I study at comparable doses. The most frequently reported events were nausea, edema, vomiting, diarrhea, and muscle cramps. Grade 1 or 2 edema, dermatitis, vomiting, muscle cramps, myalgia, arthralgia, and weight increase/fluid retention were generally more frequent in the 600 mg dose group than for patients treated with imatinib at 400 mg per day, but the incidences of other grade 1 or 2 reactions, and of all grade 3 and 4 reactions, were similar in both dose groups. Routine laboratory tests revealed infrequent development of grade 3 abnormalities in aspartate aminotransferase (AST) (2% of patients), alanine aminotransferase (ALT) (3%), and bilirubin (2%) during treatment.

A comparison of the results of this study with historical reports suggests that imatinib may bring substantially increased efficacy to the treatment of patients in accelerated phase CML, compared with current alternative chemotherapy and biologic therapy. Among patients in the 600 mg dose group, the overall and complete hematologic response rates of 71% and 37%, respectively, compare favorably with the range of approximately 20–60% overall response rates in similar patients treated with single-agent therapies, IFN-α and low-dose cytarabine, or hydroxyurea and 6-mercaptopurine. The induction of major cytogenetic responses in 28% of patients treated with imatinib is encouraging, since fewer than 5% of patients with CML in accelerated phase achieve cytogenetic response with alternative therapies.The 12-month progression-free and overall survival rates of 67% and 78%, respectively, also compare favorably with the more transient responses observed with other therapies (Figure 41.11).

## Treatment of acute phase

### *High dose chemotherapy*

Patients with blast crisis are usually treated with combination chemotherapy regimens commonly

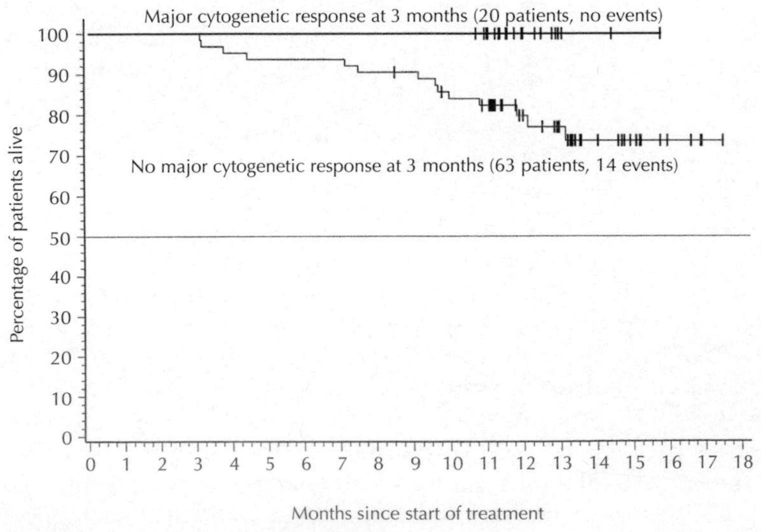


**Figure 41.11** Overall survival of patients in accelerated phase treated with imatinib by cytogenetic response at 3 months: landmark analysis (vertical bars indicate censored observations).

used in the treatment of acute myeloid or lymphoid leukemias, as appropriate. The drugs most often used are anthracyclins and cytarabine. However, only a limited number of studies have reported on the results of treatment of patients with blast crisis only. The information provided by these studies is limited as these reports are all small-scale phase I or II studies or single-institution series. Nevertheless, the response to chemotherapy is in the range of 22–65%.[109,224–231]

Responses are usually reported as complete response, partial response, return to chronic phase, or 'hematologic improvement'. Whereas the criteria for complete response are usually consistent, requiring the disappearance of blasts from the peripheral blood and the bone marrow and a complete recovery of peripheral blood counts, the criteria for partial response, return to chronic phase, or hematologic improvement vary greatly from study to study. Response criteria for blastic CML based on morphology and on cytogenetic or molecular markers have been proposed.[106] Improvement of marrow morphology defines either a complete (<5% blasts plus promyelocytes) or partial (5–15% blasts plus promyelocytes) response, but cytogenetic abnormalities are still present. Complete remission requires a loss of clonal progression. Disappearance of the $Ph^+$ cell population defines cytogenetic remission and polymerase chain reaction (PCR) negativity for Bcr–Abl rearrangement refers to biologic remission of CML. Less than 10% of patients are reported to achieve CHR.[232] In the largest series published to date, with 296 patients, lymphoid blast crisis appears to be more responsive to chemotherapy (with a 49% rate of complete response when treatment is given as first 'salvage', as compared with 19% and 12% for patients with myeloid and undifferentiated phenotypes).[109] Transient reductions in the proportion of $Ph^+$ cells are rarely reported.[225,230,232]

These responses are, however, invariably short-lived, with a median duration ranging from 1 to 8 months.[107,224,228–230,232,233] Overall, the survival of these patients is poor, averaging 3–6 months. Consistent with the suggestion that patients with a lymphoid phenotype may be more responsive to chemotherapy, in a large study of 296 patients from the Houston group, the median survivals were 3 and 9 months in patients with myeloid and lymphoid blast crisis, respectively.[109] Although the survival of responding patients remains short, responders had a significant prolongation of survival. For example, in one study,[231] patients who responded had a median survival of 231 days, whereas it was 73 days for the non-responders ($p = 0.008$). A retrospective analysis of prognostic factors was conducted in 90 patients in blast crisis.[234] The response to therapy was significantly better in lymphoid blast crisis and in patients without clonal evolution. In a multivariate analysis containing all significant variables of the univariate analysis, two parameters retained their prognostic significance: response to therapy and trisomy 8.

The toxicity of these combination chemotherapy regimens is typical of those used in the treatment of acute leukemias, and requires inpatient hospitalization. Common non-hematologic adverse events include nausea, vomiting, mucositis, and diarrhea. Myelosuppression is usual, and febrile neutropenias were reported in 80–94% of patients in one study with 162 patients.[232] In a series of 48 patients treated with a combination of daunorubicin and cytarabine, the median number of days with an absolute neutrophil count (ANC) below $0.5 \times 10^9/l$ was 28 (range 10–48), and the number of days with a profound thrombocytopenia below $30 \times 10^9/l$ was 19 (range 2–55).[219] In the study by Sacchi et al,[272] 5 out of the 90 patients who were treated with multiagent combination chemotherapy had early deaths that may be attributable to toxicity.

### Stem cell transplantation

BMT is usually performed only in patients with a good performance status, below 50 years of age, and with a suitable bone marrow donor. The outcome of patients receiving an allogeneic BMT while in overt blast crisis is very poor.[191] This poor outcome is usually related to a very high rate of transplant-related mortality and to a high rate of relapse. In a report of 1480 patients transplanted for CML from the EBMTR, 59 transplants were performed during blast crisis.[220] The transplant-related mortality rate was 62%, and the LFS rate at 2 years was only 17%. No patients were alive at 5 years of follow-up. These results are consistent with another report from the IBMTR of 1685 patients transplanted for CMC.[221] In this report, 113 patients were transplanted in blast crisis, and their LFS rate was approximately 15% at 2 years. Among 3049 patients who received an HLA-identical stem cell transplant between 1989 and 1995 and were reported to the IBMTR, 166 were in blastic phase. The 3-year LFS probability was 17% (10–24%), the 3-year actuarial probability of relapse was 61% (50–72%), and the 3-year survival rate was 19% (12–26%).[222] In a single-center study of 115 patients evaluating a preparative regimen with busulfan and cyclophosphamide but without total body irradiation, 27 patients were transplanted in blast crisis, and these patients had a relapse rate of 27% at 2 years. Furthermore, the presence of blast crisis at the time of transplant was identified as an independent negative prognostic factor for relapse and death in a multivariate analysis.[335]

The outcome of BMT performed with matched unrelated donors appears to be equally poor. In a report from the National Marrow Donor Program, the 2-year disease-free survival rate of 101 patients (out of 1423 with CML) transplanted while in blast crisis was approximately 10%.[236] In this report, in multivariate analyses, transplantation in advanced stage CML was significantly associated with a higher risk of graft failure, acute grade III/IV and chronic GVHD, leukemia relapse, and death.

High-dose chemotherapy followed by autologous stem cell transplantation has been used in order to restore a second chronic phase. Bone marrow or PBSC from these patients were cryopreserved during their chronic phase. Once the blast crisis was evident, the cells were infused following high-dose chemotherapy with or without total body irradiation. Although chronic phase CML could be re-established in most patients, it was usually short-lived, with recurrence of advanced disease and death occurring within 6 months to 1 year. In a few patients, cytogenetic responses were observed following transplantation, with a prolongation of survival.[237–239] McGlave et al[216] compiled the results of 200 consecutive autologous transplants performed with purged or unpurged bone marrow or PBSC grafts at eight different transplant centers in Europe and North America between 1984 and 1992. For patients transplanted in blastic phase, the median survival time was 4.1 months.

## Imatinib

A first phase I study included 58 patients with blastic phase CML and relapsed or refractory Ph+ ALL treated with a daily dose of 300–1000 mg imatinib.[240,241] The overall rates of response among patients with myeloblastic crisis and lymphoblastic crisis were 55% and 77%, respectively. Almost 80% of patients had a reduction of at least 50% in peripheral blasts, usually within the first week after the initiation of treatment. Of the subgroup of 38 patients who were receiving imatinib for myeloblastic crisis, 17 (45%) had a partial hematologic response (defined by a reduction in the marrow blast count to 15% or less) and 4 (11%) a complete response (<5% marrow blasts, neutrophils $>1 \times 10^9$/l, and platelets $>100 \times 10^9$/l). Three patients had a major cytogenetic response. Most responses were transient, but 7 patients (18%) remained in complete or partial remission for 3–12 months during treatment. The results for 10 patients with CML in lymphoblastic transformation and 10 with Ph+ ALL were similar. Of these 20 patients, 10 had a partial hematologic response and 4 a complete response. Two patients had a major cytogenetic response. Nevertheless, all patients who had a response relapsed within 4 months. Side-effects in patients who received imatinib for advanced leukemia were similar to those in patients with chronic-phase CML. Serious adverse events possibly due to imatinib occurred in 13 patients, usually at doses of 800–1000 mg/day. Only 3 patients had a febrile neutropenia, and no deaths were related to the use of the drug. Following these encouraging results, a large phase II trial was initiated in order to confirm the initial promising results of the phase I study.[242]

Male or female patients were eligible for inclusion in this study if they were at least 18 years of age and had Ph+ CML in myeloid blast crisis. The study was mainly designed to evaluate treatment in patients with newly diagnosed blast crisis, defined as patients who had not received specific therapy for advanced CML (either in blast crisis or in accelerated phase), with the exception of IFN-α and palliative therapy with hydroxyurea, or low-dose cytosine arabinoside (<30 mg/m² every 12–24 hours administered daily). However, enrollment was also open to patients who had received prior therapy for advanced CML, in order to allow a preliminary investigation of imatinib in a heavily pretreated population. Initially, the enrolled patients received treatment with orally administered imatinib at daily doses of 400 mg. Following the availability of phase I dose-escalation data demonstrating the safety of prolonged treatment with higher doses, this initial daily dose was increased by protocol amendment to 600 mg. For patients who relapsed, dose escalation (initially to 600 mg daily, and increased by protocol amendment to 400 mg twice daily) was permitted at the discretion of the investigator. Dose escalation was also permitted for patients who did not achieve hematologic response after at least 1 month of therapy. A total of 260 CML patients were enrolled in this phase II trial, of whom 229 had a confirmed diagnosis of CML in blast crisis. Of the 260 patients enrolled, 37 (14%) started therapy with imatinib at daily doses of 400 mg, which was the highest dose adequately tested for safety at the time of their enrollment. The remaining 223 (86%) patients started treatment at a daily dose of 600 mg, based on phase I data available after the start of this study, demonstrating that treatment with this higher dose was feasible and possibly associated with greater activity. At the time of data analysis, the median duration of treatment for all enrolled patients in the 400 and 600 mg dose groups was 3.7 months (25–75% quartiles: 1.5–7.6 months) and 4.0 months (25–75% quartiles: 1.9–9.3 months), respectively; 21% of the patients were treated for more than 1 year. The median actual dose intensities were 400 and 600 mg/day, as planned. About 50% of the patients in both dose groups reduced or interrupted treatment at least once, but 58% in the 400 mg dose group and 40% of the patients started with 600 mg had their dose escalated to 600 and 800 mg, respectively, at least once during the study. Of the 260 patients enrolled, 220 (85%) patients withdrew from treatment. The primary reasons for withdrawal were disease progression or unsatisfactory therapeutic effect for 151 (58%) patients, adverse events or laboratory test results for 23 (9%) patients, death during therapy for 24 (9%) patients, initiation of BMT for

14 (5%) patients, protocol violations for 3 (1%) patients, and withdrawal of consent for 5 (2%) patients.

After 1 month, more than 80% of the patients with available values had a blast count less than 15% in peripheral blood. Of the 229 patients, 119 (52%) had reductions in blast counts in peripheral blood and bone marrow features corresponding to hematologic response on at least one occasion; 35 (15%) patients had a CHR, 55 (24%) had a CHR or marrow response, and 64 (28%) met the criteria for return to chronic phase (RTC). Sustained hematologic responses, lasting at least 4 weeks, were reported for 31% of patients, including 8% of patients with CHR or 12% with either a CHR or a marrow response, and 18% with RTC. Responses usually occurred soon after the start of treatment: of the 70 patients with a sustained hematologic response, 45 (64%) achieved their first response within 1 month after starting imatinib therapy, corresponding to the first scheduled evaluation of response, and a further 15 (21%) responded within 2 months. In three patients, hematologic response was achieved only after their dose was escalated (one from 400 to 600 mg, and two from 600 to 800 mg). In a multivariate analysis, four factors were independently predictive of a higher likelihood of sustained hematologic response: initial dose of imatinib (34% with a dose of 600 mg and 9% with 400 mg), hemoglobin level of 100 g/l, or more, a patelet count of $100 \times 10^9$/l or more, and blood blasts less than 50%.

Major cytogenetic responses were reported for 37 (16%) patients, of which 7% were complete. Major, minor, or minimal cytogenetic response was reported in 71 (31%) patients. The median time to major cytogenetic response was approximately 3 months, corresponding to the first assessment of response in most patients. The initial dose of imatinib had a strong effect on response: major cytogenetic responses were reported for 18% of patients treated with 600 mg/day, and for 6% with 400 mg/day. The Kaplan–Meier esti-

mated median survival was 6.9 months (95% CI 5.7–8.7 months), and the estimated survival rate was 43% (9.5% CI 36–49%) at 9 months, 32% (25–38%) at 12 months, and 20% (15–27%) at 18 months. These estimates remained the same when survival data were included for the 10 patients who discontinued therapy to undergo BMT (4 of these 10 patients were still alive at the time of analysis). The estimated median survival was 7.5 months for previously untreated patients, and 5.6 months for patients who had received treatment for advanced CML (Figure 41.12).

## Ongoing and planned trials

### Imatinib in combination with other antileukemic agents

The rationale for the combination of imatinib with cytarabine is based on several observations. Cytarabine has well-described modest activity as a single agent in CML. In combination with IFN-α, it has been shown to significantly improve the rate of cytogenetic responses and survival in CML patients. Imatinib has shown significant activity in CML in all studies to date. In vitro studies examining the effects of imatinib plus cytarabine using CML cell lines and colony-forming assays of CML patient samples have shown synergistic antiproliferative effects of this combination.[243–246]

However, a concern with any single agent administered chronically is that resistant clones may emerge. Recent in vitro data suggest that cytarabine shows particular enhanced cytotoxic efficacy against potential imatinib-resistant CML cell lines. More recently, resistance has been associated, in some patients, with a single amino acid substitution in a threonine residue of the ABL kinase domain.[247] The majority of CML patients respond to imatinib. Relapse, however, is known to occur in a subset of patients, particularly those with advanced phase. While, to date, the relapse rate in the chronic phase is approximately

(a)

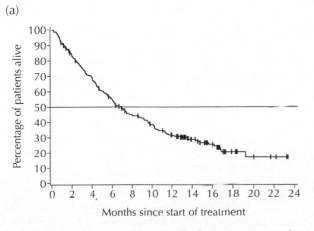

(b)

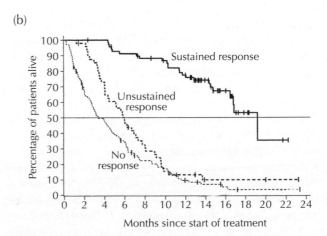

**Figure 41.12** (a) Overall survival of CML patients. (b) Overall survival of imatinib-treated by hematologic response. (Vertical bars indicate censored observations.)

15%, nearly 100% of advanced phase cases relapse despite continuation of imatinib at higher doses. When sensitive methods are used, BCR–ABL kinase domain mutations appear to be detectable in the majority of CML patients with acquired resistance to imatinib. A minority of patients exhibit genomic amplification of apparently non-mutated BCR–ABL. While it is possible that other mechanisms of resistance are contributing, future efforts to address imatinib resistance effectively must overcome the activity of BCR–ABL kinase domain mutants. The rapid rate of acquired resistance in the majority of advanced phase patients, coupled with the ability to occasionally detect kinase domain mutations prior to therapy, is supportive of a model in which mutant BCR–ABL isoforms exist at a variable rate prior to therapy.[248–251] Thus, new strategies using combination therapies are currently being explored.

A phase I study of the combination of imatinib plus low-dose cytarabine was initiated in CML chronic phase patients who failed IFN-α.[252] In this study, 22 patients were enrolled into four cohorts. Imatinib was given daily and cytarabine was administered on days 14–28, with cycles being repeated every 28 days.

In this study, the maximally tolerated dose was 400 mg of imatinib daily with 20 mg/m$^2$ of cytarabine given for 2 out of every 4 weeks. Myelosuppression at the highest dose level necessitated dose reductions in all patients such that no patient remained on treatment with 600 mg plus 20 mg/m$^2$ of cytarabine. Other toxicities that were more common with the combination as compared with imatinib alone included nausea (77% grade 1/2 and 14% Grade 3/4), diarrhea (36% grade 1/2), fluid retention (73% grade 1/2), and skin rashes (45% grade 1/2 and 9% grade 3/4). Grade 3/4 fatigue and elevations in aminotransferases were seen in 2 of 22 (9%) patients. With a median duration of follow-up of 300 days, the CHR rate was 86% and the major cytogenetic response rate was 32%. This compares favorably with the results reported in phase I and II studies of imatinib alone.

The CML French Group has recently conducted a phase II study to determine the safety and tolerability of a combination of imatinib and cytarabine. Other endpoints were rates and duration of major and complete cytogenetic responses at 6 and 12 months, 6-months CHR rate, level of molecular residual disease in patients in complete cytologic remission, and overall survival.[253, 254] Treatment was administered on 28-day cycles for 12 months. Patients received a continuous administration of imatinib orally at a dose of 400 mg daily. Cytarabine was given on days 14–28 of each cycle at an initial dose of 20 mg/m$^2$/day via subcutaneous injection, hydroxyurea being stopped at least 7 days before Imatinib. Thirty newly diagnosed CML patients in chronic phase (20 males and 10 females, median age 48 years, range 22–81 years) were recruited by 14 French centers. Adverse events were frequently observed, with grade 3 or 4 hematologic toxicities and non-hematologic toxicities in 53% (n=16) and 33% (n= 10) of patients, respectively. However, the CHR and complete cytologic response rates compared favorably with those previously obtained with imatinib alone. The cumulative incidence of complete cytologic response at 12 months was 83%, and at 6 months 100% of the patients achieved CHR. It was concluded that the combination was safe and promising, given the high response rate.

As imatinib and IFN-α are the two most active non-transplant therapies available for CML patients, this combination is an obvious choice for testing. In vitro data demonstrate additive or synergistic antiproliferative effects of the combination of imatinib with IFN-α using BCR–ABL$^+$ cell lines and in colony-forming assays using CML patient samples.[243,244] Based on these data, two phase I/II pilot studies with this combination are in progress – one using regular IFN-α and the other pegylated (PEG) IFN-α. By December 2001, 49 patients with chronic phase CML had been entered into PISCES (PEGIntron and Imatinib Combination Evaluation Study), with a median age 52.5 years, and of whom 32 were newly diagnosed (<6 months since diagnosis). After 6 months of treatment, the major cytogenetic response rate was 73.3% (n=22) overall and 82.4% (n=14) in the newly diagnosed patients (with complete responses is 36.7% and 41.2%, respectively). Of the 22 patients achieving a major cytogenetic response, 59% were taking 200 mg imatinib plus 0.25 µg/kg/wk PEG IFN-α (n=8), 200 mg imatinib plus 0.5 µg/kg/wk PEG IFN-α (n=4), or 400 mg imatinib plus 0.5 µg/kg/wk PEG IFN-α (n=1). All patients (n=35) achieved a CHR. Of 49 patients, 30 patients suffered grade 3/4 neutropenia within the first month on study while taking 400 mg imatinib plus 0.5 µg/kg/wk PEG IFN-α. Grade 1/2 adverse events were common; flu-like symptoms/fatigue (40.8%), increased liver aminotransferases (transient) (36.7%), edema (34.7%), on headache (28.6%). Grade 3/4 adverse events were rare, with febrile neutropenia and joint/muscle pain being experienced by 6.1%.[255] Additional studies are also evaluating the feasibility of administrating imatinib before or after BMT.

### SPIRIT study

The only known curative therapy for CML is allogeneic BMT, but the risks of this procedure are considerable and it is only available to a minority of patients with CML. Imatinib has produced remarkable results in the treatment of CML, although comparative data on long-term survival are not yet available.

In the light of recent evidence, patients and doctors increasingly consider imatinib to be the standard of care for newly diagnosed patients with CML. The

SPIRIT study is setting out to establish whether combining imatinib with other drugs or increasing the dose to 600 mg daily can improve survival when compared with imatinib 400 mg daily. It is a crucial long-term study attempting to improve the prognosis for patients with CML. SPIRIT is a phase III, multicenter, open-label, prospective randomized trial comparing imatinib alone versus imatinib plus cytarabine versus imatinib plus IFN-α in patients with chronic phase CML. Patients must be newly diagnosed (<6 months) and have been treated with only hydroxyurea and/or anagrelide.

It is expected that 3000 patients will be entered into the study, initially from the UK (MRC), USA (SWOG, ECOG, and CALGB), and France (FIφLMC). Additional countries may join later.

## Practical aspects of treatment

For young patients, the best treatment is still a matter of uncertainty – essentially because a stem cell transplant can be offered as first-line treatment. However, the transplant-related mortality should be considered and balanced with other treatments, such as imatinib.

The first step after a diagnosis of CML is to calculate risk factors. The two prognostic scoring systems – the Sokal and Euro scores – were validated for patients treated with standard chemotherapy or IFN-α-based regimens. Because a recent update of the IRIS study has suggested that patients treated with imatinib may respond differently according to the Sokal risk scoring system, this score could be used in the context of imatinib therapy. However, for young patients who are suitable for stem cell transplantation, the Gratwohl score is the appropriate scoring system.

Tolerance appears to be poor in the elderly, especially in terms of possible neurologic and psychiatric side-effects, such as depression. Although there is no firm evidence supporting this conclusion, caution is recommended. While no drugs have been identified to limit the side-effects of IFN-α, an effort has been made to modify IFN-α itself to make its administration easier and to minimize side-effects. The pegylation of IFN-α provides a pharmacokinetic profile that allows for weekly injections and is expected to limit toxicity, efficacy being equal.

Although therapy with imatinib is generally well tolerated, it is not devoid of side-effects. Particularly common side-effects include myelosuppresion, nausea, vomiting, edema, muscle cramps, arthralgias, diarrhea, and skin rashes. Elevated aminotransferases are observed less frequently, but occasionally necessitate discontinuance of therapy.

Myelosuppression is particularly common in CML patients treated with imatinib. In a phase II trial in chronic phase patients who had failed IFN-α, the protocol mandated interruption of therapy with imatinib for grade 3 myelosuppression. Using these guidelines, 25% of patients experienced grade 3 neutropenia (ANC $<1 \times 10^9$/l) and 16% developed grade 3 thrombocytopenia (platelets $< 50 \times 10^9$/l). In addition, 8% of patients developed grade 4 neutropenia (ANC $< 0.5 \times 10^9$/l). In advanced phase patients (accelerated and blastic phases), owing to the more life-threatening nature of the disease, treatment was not interrupted except for prolonged myelosuppression, and accordingly a higher percentage of patients developed grade 3 and 4 neutropenia and thrombocytopenia. In CML patients in blast crisis, almost 50% of patients developed grade 4 neutropenia. A number of deaths have been attributed to imatinib-induced myelosuppression, almost all of which were seen in advanced phase disease.[256]

Although myelosuppression can occur at any time during imatinib therapy, it generally occurs within the first 2–4 weeks in blastic phase patients, although slightly later in chronic and accelerated phase patients. Factors associated with myelosuppression besides advanced disease may include prior myelosuppression from IFN-α therapy or prior therapy with busulfan. The risk of developing myelosuppression may depend on the amount of residual normal hematopoiesis, and this may be negatively correlated with the above factors.

In CML patients in chronic phase, the recommended starting dose of imatinib is 400 mg. The complete blood count should be monitored weekly for the first month. Thereafter, the frequency of blood count monitoring depends on the stability and level of the blood count. Thus, if a patient's ANC falls to less than $1.5 \times 10^9$/l and/or the platelet count to less than $100 \times 10^9$/l, the CBC should be monitored weekly. If blood counts are higher than these levels, monitoring can be reduced to every 2 weeks until 12 weeks of treatment is reached, and, depending on the stability of the counts, the frequency of monitoring can be lengthened to monthly. For patients with advanced phase CML, a starting dose of 600 mg of imatinib is recommended. The CBC should be monitored at least weekly, or more often, depending on the clinical situation. Higher doses of imatinib are currently being explored with the aim that higher doses may reinduce hematologic response or improve the cytogenetic resistance to standard-dose imatinib.[257–259]

Imatinib is generally well tolerated, and the most common side-effects are mild and can be managed easily. However, therapy requires frequent and careful monitoring, particularly for myelosuppression, fluid retention, and hepatotoxicity, which are occasionally severe.

It has been estimated that in patients with overt clinical leukemia (at diagnosis or relapse), the total tumor burden represents approximately $10^{12}$ malignant cells or more. When clinical remission is achieved ('hematologic response'), the number of remaining leukemic cells may be as high as $10^{10}$–$10^{11}$. Therefore, the achievement of a hematologic response represents only one step in a continuum in the actual response to therapy. For this reason, the potential value of estimating the level of minimal residual disease (MRD), or the amount of persisting leukemic cells was recognized as early as the start of the 1980s.

Up to now, for patients achieving a CHR, the only tool that was routinely available was monitoring the cytogenetic response using standard karyotyping methods. The clinical value of achieving a cytogenetic response with IFN-α therapy has been strongly established, as discussed above. However, cytogenetic analysis is limited by the low number of cells analyzed (usually 20–30) and its consequent low sensitivity of about 5%, the need for dividing cells (excluding potential Ph+ 'quiescent' cells or cells with a low proliferative potential), and the need for invasive bone marrow aspirates. On the other hand, cytogenetic analysis is the only method that allows the detection of additional chromosomal abnormalities

('clonal evolution'), which is considered by some investigators to be suggestive of disease acceleration.

For these reasons, a number of techniques have been developed over the last 15 years to better monitor MRD, particularly in patients after BMT. Fluorescence in situ hybridization (FISH) reverse transcriptase PCR (RT-PCR), and quantitative PCR are the usual techniques for monitoring MDR.

Chromosome banding analysis is still the gold standard for the diagnosis and monitoring of CML. This technique is able to detect chromosomal abnormalities in addition to the Ph chromosome that may impact the outcome of the patients. However, the sensitivity of chromosome analysis is too low in good responders to detect residual disease. Hypermetaphase FISH (HM-FISH) is a new method that combines a modified preparation of metaphases with FISH. Recent data have confirmed the high sensitivity of this test compared with chromosome banding. Nested RT-PCR is more sensitive than HM-FISH, and is the method of choice for the detection of MRD after allogeneic BMT.

## REFERENCES

1. Dameshek W. Some speculations on the myeloproliferative syndromes. *Blood* 1951; **6**: 372–5.
2. Nowell PC, Hungerford DA. Chromosome studies on normal and leukemic human leukocytes. *J Natl Cancer Inst* 1960; **25**: 85–109.
3. Baikie AG, Court Brown WN, Bockton KE. A possible specific chromosome abnormality in human myeloid leukemia. *Nature* 1960; **188**: 1165–6.
4. Nowell PC, Hungerford DA, Chromosomes studies in human leukemia II chronic granulocytic leukemia. *J Natl Cancer Inst* 1961; **27**: 1013–35.
5. Tough IM, Court Brown WM, Buckton KE. Cytogenetic studies in chronic leukemia and acute leukemia associated with mongolism. *Lancet* 1961; **i**: 411–417.
6. Caspersson T, Gahrton G, Lindsten J, Zelh L. Identification of the Philadelphia chromosome on a number 22 by quinacrine mustard fluorescence analysis. *Exp Cell Res* 1970; **63**: 238–40.
7. Rowley JD. A new consistent chromosomal abnormality in chronic myelogenous leukemia identified by quinacrine, fluorescence and Giemsa staining. *Nature* 1973; **243**: 290–3.
8. Deklein A, Vankessel AG, Grosveld G. A cellular oncogene is translocated to the Philadelphia chromosome in chronic myelocytic leukemia. *Nature* 1982; **300**: 765–7.
9. Heisterkamp N, Groffen J, Stephenson J. Chromosomal localization of human cellular homologues of two viral oncogenes. *Nature* 1982; **299**: 747–9.
10. Bartram CR, Deklein A, Hagemeijer A et al. Translocation of c-*abl* oncogene correlates with the presence of a Philadelphia chromosome in chronic myelocytic leukaemia. *Nature* 1983; **306**: 277–80.
11. Groffen J, Stephenson JR, Heisterkamp N et al. Philadelphia chromosomal breakpoints are clustered within a limited region, *bcr*, on chromosome 22. *Cell* 1984; **36**: 93–9.
12. Ichimaru M, Ohkita T, Ishimaru T. Leukemia, multiple myeloma and malignant lymphoma. In: Shigimatsu I and Kagan A (eds) *Cancer in Atomic Bomb Survivors*. GANN Monograph on Cancer Research, No. 32, Tokyo:Japan Scientific Societies Press, 1986: 113–27.
13. Finch SC, Finch CA. *Summary of the Studies at ABCC–RERF Concerning the Late Hematologic Effects of Atomic Bomb Exposure in Hiroshima and Nagasaki*. RERF Technical Report 23–88. Hiroshima: Radiation Effects Research Foundation, 1988: 5–7.
14. Shimizv Y, Kato H, Schull W. Studies of the mortality of A-bomb survivors. Mortality 1950–85. Part 2. Cancer mortality based on the recently revised doses (D 586). *Radiat Res* 1990; **121**: 120–41.
15. Smith PG, Soll R. Mortality among patients with ankylosing spondylitis after a single treatment course with X-ray. *BMJ* 1982; **284**: 449–60.
16. Boice JDJR, Blettner M, Kleinerman RA et al. Radiation dose and leukemia risk in patients treated for cancer of the cervix. *J Natl Cancer Inst* 1987; **79**: 1295–311.
17. Preston-Martin S, Thomas DC, Yu MC et al. Diagnostic radiography as a risk factor for chronic myeloid and monocytic leukaemia. *Br J Cancer* 1989; **59**: 639–44.
18. National Research Council (Committee of the Biologic Effects of Ionizing Radiation). *The Effects on Populations of Exposure to Low Levels of Ionizing Radiation (BEIR V)*. Washington, DC: National Academy Press, 1990: 242–351.
19. Jackson GH, Latham JA, Lennard AL et al. Rapid onset of chronic granulocytic leukaemia after treatment for Hodgkin's disease. *Br J Haematol* 1994; **37**: 193–5.
20. Varady E, Deak B, Molnar ZS et al. Second malignancies

after treatment for Hodgkin's disease. *Leuk Lymphoma* 2001; **42**: 1275–81.

21. Numata A, Shimoda K, Gondo H et al. Therapy-related chronic myelogenous leukaemia following autologous stem cell transplantation for Ewing's sarcoma. *Br J Haematol* 2002; **117**: 613–16.

22. Aguiar RCT. Therapy related chronic myeloid leukemia: an epidemiological, clinical and pathogenetic appraisal. *Leuk Lymphoma* 1998; **29**: 17–26.

23. Ito T, Seyama T, Mizuno T et al, Induction of *BCR–ABL* fusion genes by in vitro X-irradiation. *Jpr J Cancer Res* 1993; **84**: 105–9.

24. Deininger MWN, Bose S, Gora-Tybor J et al. Selective induction of leukemia-associated fusion genes by high-dose ionizing radiation. *Cancer Res* 1998; **58**: 421–5.

25. Raabe GK, Wong O. Leukemia mortality by cell type in petroleum workers with potential exposure to benzene. *Environ Health Perspect* 1996; **104**(Suppl 6): 1381–92.

26. Dean MR. Chronic myeloid leukaemia and occupational exposure to benzene in a Royal Navy Submariner. *JR Nav Med Serv* 1996; **82**: 28–33.

27. Tokuhuta GK, Neely CL, Williams SC. Chronic myelocytic leukemia in identical twins and a sibling. *Blood* 1968; **31**: 216.

28. Haas OA, Argyriou-Tirita A, Lion T. Parental origin of chromosomes involved in the translocation t(q;22). *Nature* 1992; **359**: 414–16.

29. Melo JV, Yan X-H, Diamond J, Goldman JM. Lack of imprinting of the *ABL* gene. *Nat Genet* 1994; **8**: 318–19.

30. Melo JV, Yan X-H, Diamond J, Goldman JM. Balanced parental contribution to the *ABL* component of the *BCR–ABL* gene in chronic myeloid leukemia. *Leukemia* 1995; **9**: 734–45.

31. Riggings GJ, Zhang F, Warren ST. Lack of imprinting of *BCR*. *Nat Genet* 1994; **6**: 226.

32. Fioretos T, Heisterkamp N, Groffen J. No evidence for genomic imprinting of the human *BCR* gene. *Blood* 1994; **83**: 3441–4.

33. Litz CE, Copenhaver CM. Paternel origin of the rearranged major breakpoint cluster region in chronic myeloid leukemia. *Blood* 1994; **83**: 3445–8.

34. Vickers M. Estimation of the number of mutations necessary to cause chronic myeloid leukemia from epidemiological data. *Br J Haematol* 1996; **94**: 1–4.

35. Bortin MM, D'Amaro J, Bach FH et al. HLA association with leukemia. *Blood* 1987; **70**: 227–32.

36. Morrison VA. Chronic leukemias. *CA Cancer J Clin* 1994; **44**: 353–77.

37. German Federal Office of Statistics. *Sterbefalle, nach Todesursachen in Deutschland*, Wiesbaden: Statistischen Bundesamt, 1995.

38. Lee SJ. Chronic myelogenous leukemia. *Br J Haematol* 2000; **111**: 993–1009.

39. Cortes J, Talpaz M, Kantarjian H. Chronic myelogenous leukemia: a review. *Am J Med* 1996; **100**: 555–70.

40. Chissoe SL, Botenteich A, Wang Y-F et al. Sequence and analysis of the human *ABL* gene, the *BCR* gene and region involved in the Philadelphia chromosomal translocations. *Genomics* 1995; **27**: 67–82.

41. Kiprcds ET, Wang JY. Cell cycle-regulated binding of c-Abl tyrosine-kinase to DNA. *Science* 1992; **256**: 382–5.

42. McWhirter JR, Wang JY. An action binding functions contributes to transformation by the BCR–ABL oncoprotein of Philadelphia chromosome-positive human leukemias. *EMBO J* 1993; **12**: 1533–46.

43. Wen ST, Jackson PK, Vanetten RA. The cytostatic function of c-Abl is controlled by multiple nuclear localization signals, and requires the *p53* and *Rb* tumor suppressor gene products. *EMBO J* 1996; **15**: 1583–95.

44. Heisterkamp N, Stam K, Groffen J et al. Structural organization of the *bcr* gene and its role in the Ph translocation. *Nature* 1985; **315**: 758–61.

45. Gao LM, Goldman J. Long range mapping of the normal *BCR* gene. *Leukemia* 1991; **5**: 555–60.

46. Maru Y, Witte ON. The *BCR* gene encodes a novel serine/threonine kinase activity within a single exon. *Cell* 1991; **67**: 459–68.

47. Collins S, Coleman H, Grovedine M. Expression of *bcr* and *bcr–abl* transcripts in normal and leukemic cells. *Mol Cell Biol* 1987; **7**: 2870–6.

48. Renshaw MW, Capozza MA, Wang JY. Differential expression of type-specific c-abl mRNA in mouse tissues and cells. *Mol Cell Biol* 1988; **8**: 4547–51.

49. Schwartzberg PL, Stall AM, Hardin JD et al. Mice homozygous for the *abl* m1 mutation show poor viability and depletion of selected B and T cell population. *Cell* 1991; **65**: 1165–75.

50. Tybulewicz VLJ, Crawford CE, Jackson PK et al. Neonatal lethality and lymphopenia in mice with a homozygous disruption of the c-abl proto-oncogene. *Cell* 1991; **65**: 1153–63.

51. Voncken JW, Van Schaik H, Kaartinen V et al. Increased neutrophil respiratory burst in bcr-null mutants. *Cell* 1995; **80**: 719–28.

52. Wada H, Mizutani S, Nishimura J et al. Establishment and molecular characterization of a novel leukemic cell line with Philadelphia chromosome expressing p230^BCR/ABL fusion protein. *Cancer Res* 1995; **55**: 3192–6.

53. Mills KI, MacKenzie ED, Birnie GD. The site of the breakpoint within the *bcr* is a pronostic factor in Philadelphia-positive CML patients. *Blood* 1998; **72**: 1237–41.

54. Shtalrid M, Talpaz M, Kuzrock R et al. Analysis of breakpoints within the *bcr* gene and their correlation with the clinical course of Philadelphia positive chronic myelogenous leukemia. *Blood* 1998; **72**: 485–90.

55. Martinelli G, Chiamenti A, Gasparini P et al. *BCR* breakpoint subregions and blast crisis lineage in CML patients *Blood* 1992; **79**: 838–9.

56. Inokuchi K, Inoue T, Tojo A et al. A possible correlation between the type of *bcr–abl* hybrid messenger RNA and platelet count in Philadelphia positive chronic myelogenous leukemia. *Blood* 1991; **78**: 3125–27.

57. Opalka B, Wandl VB, Stuten Kemper R et al. No correlation between the type of *bcr-abl* hybrid messenger RNA and platelet counts in chronic myelogenous leukemia. *Blood* 1992; **80**: 1854–5.

58. Shepherd P, Suffolk R, Halsey J, Allan N. Analysis of molecular breakpoints and m-RNA transcripts in a prospective randomized trial of interferon in chronic myeloid leukemia: no correlation with clinical features, cytogenetic response, duration of chronic phase, or survival. *Br J Haematol* 1995; **89**: 546–54.

59. Sawyers CI. Molecular consequences of the *BCR-ABL* translocation in chronic myelogenous leukemia. *Leuk Lymphoma* 1993; **11**(Suppl 2): 101–3.

60. Sakai N, Ogiso Y, Fujita H et al. Induction of apoptosis by a dominant negative H-*Ras* mutant (116Y) in k562 cells. *Exp Cell Res* 1994; **215**: 131–6.

61. Sawyers CI, Callahan W, Witte ON. Dominant negative *MYC* blocks transformation by *ABL* oncogenes. *Cell* 1992; **70**: 901–10.

62. Clarkson B, Strife A. Linkage of proliferative and maturational abnormalities in chronic myelogenous leukemia and relevance to treatment. *Leukemia* 1993; **7**: 1638–721.

63. Stryckman P, Debussher L, Soquet M. Regulation of bone marrow myeloblast proliferation in chronic myeloid leukemia. *Cancer Res* 1976; **36**: 3034–8.

64. Wetzler M, Talpaz M, Lowe DG et al. Constitutive expression of leukemia inhibitory factor RNA by human bone marrow stromal cells and modulation by IL-1, TNF-α, and TGF-β. *Exp Hematol* 1991; **19**: 347–51.

65. Lundell BI, McCarthy JB, Kovach NL et al. Adhesion to fibronectin (FN) induced by the activating anti-integrin-β1 antibody, 8a2, restores adhesion mediated inhibition of CML progenitor proliferation. *Blood* 1996; **87**: 2450–2458.

66. Skorski T, Nieborowska-Skorska M, Wlodarski P et al. The SH3 domain contributes to BCR/ABL dependent leukemogenesis in vivo: role in adhesion, invasion and homing. *Blood* 1998; **91**: 406–18.

67. Medi A, Barder JP, Bedi GG et al. BCR–ABL mediated inhibition of apoptosis with delay of $G_2$/M transition after DNA damage: a mechanism of resistance to multiple anti cancer agents. *Blood* 1995; **86**: 1148–58.

68. Sanchez-Garcia I, Grutz G. Tumorigenic activity of the *BCR–ABL* oncogenes is mediated by BCL2. *Proc Natl Acad Sci USA* 1995; **92**: 5287.

69. Amarante-Mendes GP, Kim CN, Liu L et al. Bcr–Abl exerts its antiapoptotic effect against diverse apoptotic stimuli through blockage of mitochondrial release of cytochrome *c* and activation of caspase-3. *Blood* 1998; **91**: 1700–5.

70. Sandberg AA. The leukemias: chronic myelocytic leukemia: clonal origin in a stem cell common to granulocyte, erythrocyte, platelet and monocyte/macrophage. *Am J Med* 1997; **63**: 125–37.

71. Fialkow PJ, Garther SM, Yoshida A. Clonal origin of chronic myelocytic leukemia in men. *Proc Natl Acad Sci USA* 1967; **58**: 1468–71.

72. Yoffe G, Chinault AG, Talpaz M et al. Clonal nature of Philadelphia chromosome positive and negative chronic myelogenous leukemia by DNA hybridization analysis. *Exp Hematol* 1987; **15**: 725–8.

73. Voncken JW, Kaartinen V, Pattengale PK et al. BCR/ABL p210 and p190 cause distinct leukemia in transgenic mice. *Blood* 1995; **86**: 4603–11.

74. Daley CG, Van Etten RA, Baltimore D. Induction of chronic myelogenous leukemia in mice by the *p210$^{BCR–ABL}$* gene of the Philadelphia chromosome. *Science* 1990; **247**: 824–30.

75. Daley CG, Van Etten RA, Baltimore D. Blast crisis in a murine model of chronic myelogenous leukemia. *Proc Natl Acad Sci USA* 1991; **88**: 11335–8.

76. Gishizky ML, Johnson-White J, Witte ON. Efficient transplantation of *BCR-ABL*-induced chronic myelogenous leukemia-like syndrome in mice. *Proc Natl Acad Sci USA* 1993; **90**: 3755–59.

77. Sicard C, Lapidot T, Vormoor J et al. Normal and leukemic SCID-repopulating cells (SRC) coexist in the bone marrow and peripheral blood from CML patients in chronic phase, whereas leukemic SRC are detected in blast crisis. *Blood* 1996; **87**: 1539–48.

78. Wang JCY, Lapidot T, Cashman JD et al. High level engraftment of NOD/SCID mice by primitive normal and leukemic hematopoietic cells from patients with chronic myeloid leukemia in chronic phase. *Blood* 1998; **91**: 2406–14.

79. Spiers ASD. Clinical manifestations of chronic granulocytic leukemia. *Semin Oncol* 1995; **22**: 380–95.

80. Savage DG, Szjdlo RM, Goldman JM. Clinical features at diagnosis in 430 patients with chronic myeloid leukemia seen at a referral centre over a 16 year period. *Br J Haematol* 1997; **96**: 111–16.

81. Dowding C, Thing KH, Goldman JM, Galton DAG. Increased T-lymphocyte numbers in chronic granulocytic leukemia before treatment. *Exp Hematol* 1984; **12**: 811–15.

82. Fujimiya Y, Chang WC, Akke A et al. Natural killer cell immunodeficiency in patients with chronic myelogenous leukemia. *Cancer Immunol Immunother* 1987; **24**: 213–20.

83. Gerrard JM, Stoddard SF, Shapiro RS et al. Platelet storage pool deficiency and prostaglandin synthesis in chronic granulocytic leukemia. *Br J Haematol* 1978; **40**: 597–607.

84. Spiers ASD, Bain BJ, Turner J. The peripheral blood in chronic granulocytic leukemia. Study of 50 untreated Philadelphia-positive cases. *Scand J Haematol* 1977; **18**: 25–38.

85. Winfield D, Polacarz S. Bone marrow histology 3: value of bone marrow core biopsy in acute leukemia, myelodysplastic syndromes, and chronic myeloid leukemia. *J Clin Pathol* 1992; **45**: 855–859.

86. Mitelman F. The cytogenetic scenario of chronic myeloid leukemia. *Leuk lymphoma* 1993; **11**: 11–15.

87. Hagemeijer A, de Klein A, Godde-Saltz E et al. Translocation of c-*abl* to 'masked' Ph on chronic myeloid leukemia. *Cancer Genet Cytogenet* 1985; **18**: 95–104.

88. De Braekeleer M. Variant Philadelphia translocations, in chronic myeloid leukemia. *Cytogenet Cell Genet* 1987; **44**: 215–22.

89. Sakurai M, Hayata I, Sandberg A. Prognostic value of chromosomal finding in Ph-positive chronic myelocytic leukemia. *Cancer Res* 1976; **36**: 313–18.

90. O'Brien S, Thall PF, Siciliano MJ. Cytogenetics of chronic myelogenous leukemia. *Baillière's Clin Hematol* 1997; **10**: 259–76.

91. Kantarjian HM, Smith TL, McCredie KB et al. Chronic myelogenous leukemia: a multivariate analysis of the associations of patients characteristics and therapy with survival. *Blood* 1985; **66**: 1326–1335.

92. Sokal JE, Gomez GA, Baccarani M et al. Prognostic significance of additional cytogenetic abnormalities at diagnosis of Philadelphia chromosome-positive chronic granulocytic leukemia. *Blood* 1988; **72**: 294–8.

93. Kurzrock R, Blick MB, Talpaz M et al. Rearrangement in the breakpoint cluster region and the clinical course in Philadelphia-negative chronic myelogenous leukemia. *Ann Intern Med* 1986; **105**: 673–9.

94. Rosner F, Schreiber Z, Parise F. Leukocyte alkaline phosphatase. Fluctuations with disease status in chronic granulocytic leukemia. *Arch Intern Med* 1972; **130**: 892–4.

95. Rustin G, Goldman J, McCarthy D et al. An extrinsic factor controls neutrophil alkaline phosphatase synthesis in chronic granulocytic leukemia. *Br J Haematol* 1980; **45**: 381–387.

96. Kantarjian H, Keating M, Talpaz M et al. Chronic myelogenous leukemia in blast crisis. Analysis of 242 patients. *Am J Med* 1987; **83**: 445–454.

97. Kantarjian H, Dixon D, Keating M et al. Characteristics of accelerated disease in chronic myelogenous leukemia. *Cancer* 1988; **61**: 1441–6.

98. Alimena G, de Cuia MR, Diverio D et al. The Karyotype of blastic crisis. *Cancer Genet Cytogenet* 1987; **26**: 39–50.

99. Majlis A, Kantarjian H, SMITH T et al. What is the significance of cytogenetic clonal evolution (CE) in patients with philadephia chromosome positive chronic myelogenous leukemia? *Blood* 1994; **84**(Suppl 1): 150a.

100. Ohnishi K, Ohno R, Tomonaga M et al. A randomized trial comparing interferon-α with busulfan for newly diagnosed chronic myelogenous leukemia in chronic phase. *Blood* 1995; **86**: 906–16.

101. Clift RA, Buckner CD, Thomas ED et al. Marrow transplantation for patients in accelerated phase of chronic myeloid leukemia. *Blood* 1994; **84**: 4368–73.

102. Enright H, McGlave P. Chronic myelogenous leukemia. In: Hoffman R, Benz EJ, Shattil SJ et al (eds) *Hematology: Basic Principles and Practice*, 3rd edn. New York: Churchill Livingstone, 2000: 1155–71.

103. Larson RS, Wolff SN. Chronic myeloid leukemia. In: *Wintrobe's Clinical Hematology*, 10th edn, Vol 2, 2342–72. Philadelphia: Lea and Febiger, 1999: 2342–72.

104. Speck B, Bortin MM, Champlin R et al. Allogeneic bone marrow transplantation for chronic myelogenous leukemia. *Lancet* 1984; **i**: 665–8.

105. Kantarjian HM, Keating MJ, Smith TL et al. Proposal for a simple synthesis prognostic staging system in chronic myelogonous leukemia. *Am J Med* 1990; **88**: 1–8.

106. Arlin ZA, Silver RT, Bennett JM. Blastic phase of chronic myeloid leukemia: a proposal for standardization of diagnostic and response criteria. *Leukemia* 1990; **4**: 755–7.

107. Alimena C, Lazzarino M, Morra E et al. Clinical and cytologic characteristics of blastic phase in Ph-positive chronic myeloid leukemia treated with α-interferon. *Leukemia* 1996; **10**: 615–18.

108. Harris NL, Jaffe ES, Diebold J et al. World Health Organization classification of neoplastic diseases of the hematopoietic and lymphoid tissues: report of the Clinical Advisory Committee Meeting – Airlie House, Virginia, November 1997. *J Clin Oncol* 1999; **17**: 3835–49.

109. Derderian PM, Kantarjian H, Talpaz M et al. Chronic myelogenous leukemia in the lymphoid blastic phase: characteristics, treatment response and prognosis. *Am J Med* 1993; **94**: 69–74.

110. Hild OH, Myers TJ. Hyperviscosity in chronic granulocytic leukemia. *Cancer* 1980; **46**: 1418–21.

111. Stoll DB, Peterson P, Exten R et al. Clinical presentation and natural history of patients with essential thrombocythemia and the Philadelphia chromosome. *Am J Hematol* 1998; **27**: 77–83.

112. Martell RW, Myers HS, Jacobs P. Bone lesions in chronic granulocytic leukemia. *Br J Haematol* 1986; **62**: 31–5.

113. Berman E, Strife A, Wisniewski D et al. Duration of the preclinical phase of chronic myelogenous leukemia: a case report. *Blood* 1991; **78**: 2969–72.

114. Nanjangud GJ, Saikia TK, Chopra H et al. Development of Ph positive chronic myeloid leukemia treated with total body irradiation: a rare association. *Leuk Lymphoma* 1996; **22**: 355–9.

115. Djulbegovic B, Hadley T, Yen F. Occurrence of high grade T-cell lymphoma in a patient with Philadelphia chromosome-negative chronic myelogenous leukemia with break-

116. Martiat P, Mecucci C, Nizet Y et al. p190$^{BCR/ABL}$ transcript in a case of philadelphia-positive multiple myeloma. *Leukemia* 1990; **4**: 751–4.

117. Pane F, Frigeri F, Sindona M et al. Neutrophilic-chronic myeloid leukemia: a distinct disease with a specific molecular marker (BCR/ABL with C3/A2 junction). *Blood* 1996; **88**: 2410–14.

118. Melo JV. The diversity of BCR–ABL fusion protein and their relationship to leukemia phenotype. *Blood* 1996; **88**: 2375–84.

119. Yamagata T, Mitani K, Kanda Y et al. Elevated platelet count features the variant type of BCR/ABL junction in chronic myelogenous leukemia. *Br J Haematol* 1996; **94**: 370–372.

120. Cortes JE, Talpaz M, Beran M et al. Philadelphia chromosome-negative chronic myelogenous leukemia with rearrangement of the breakpoint cluster region. *Cancer* 1995; **75**: 464–470.

121. Kurzrock R, Kantarjian H, Shtalrid M et al. Philadelphia chromosome-negative chronic myelogenous leukemia without breakpoint cluster region rearrangement: a chronic myeloid leukemia with a distinct clinical course. *Blood* 1990; **75**: 445–452.

122. Martiat P, Michaux JL, Rodhain J, for the Groupe Français de Cytogénétique Hématologique. Philadelphia-negative (Ph-) chronic myeloid leukemia (CML): comparison with Ph+ CML and chronic myelomonocytic leukemia. *Blood* 1991; **78**: 205–11.

123. Kantarjian HM, Talpaz M, Chingra K et al. Significance of the p210 versus p190 molecular abnormalities in adults with Philadelphia chromosome positive acute leukemia. *Blood* 1991; **78**: 2411–18.

124. Anastasi J, Feng J, Dickstein JL et al. Lineage involvement by BCR/ABL in Ph+ lymphoblastic leukemias: chronic myelogenous leukemia presenting in lymphoid blast phase vs Ph+ acute lymphoblastic leukemia. *Leukemia* 1996; **10**: 795–802.

125. Schlieben S, Borkhardt A, Reinisch I et al. Incidence and clinical outcome of children with BCR/ABL-positive acute lymphoblastic leukemia (ALL). A prospective RT–PCR study based in 673 patients enrolled in the German Pediatric Multicenter Therapy Trials ALL-BFM-90 and CoALL-05-92. *Leukemia* 1996; **10**: 957–63.

126. Oguma S, Takatsuki K, Uchino H et al. Factors influencing survival in Philadelphia chromosome positive chronic myelocytic leukemia. *Cancer* 1982; **50**: 2928–34.

127. Cervantes F, Rozman C. A multivariate analysis of prognostic factors in chronic myeloid leukemia. *Blood* 1982; **60**: 1298–304.

128. Cervantes F, Robertson JE, Rozman C et al. Long-term survivors in chronic granulocytic leukemia: a study by the International CGL Prognosis Study Group. *Br J Haematol* 1994; **87**: 293–300.

129. Tura S, Baccarani M, Corbelli G et al. Staging of chronic myeloid leukemia. *Br J Haematol* 1981; **47**: 105–19.

130. Sokal JE, Cox EB, Baccarani M et al. Prognostic discrimination in 'good risk' chronic granulocytic leukemia. *Blood* 1984; **63**: 789–99.

131. Allan N, Richards S, Shepherd P et al. UK Medical Research Council randomized, multicentre trial of interferon-α n1 for chronic myeloid leukemia: improved survival irrespective of cytogenetic response. *Lancet* 1995; **345**: 1392–7.

132. Hehlmann R, Heimpel H, Hasford J et al. Randomized comparison of interferon-α with busulfan and hydroxyurea in chronic myelogenous leukemia (CML). *Blood* 1994; **84**: 4064–77.

133. Ozer H, George S, Schiffer C et al. Prolonged subcutaneous administration of recombinant α-2b interferon in patients with previously untreated Philadelphia chromosome-positive chronic-phase chronic myelogenous leukemia: effect on remission duration and survival: Cancer and Leukemia Group B study 8583. *Blood* 1993; **82**: 2975–84.

134. Kantarjian HM, Smith TL, O'Brien S et al. Prolonged survival in chronic myelogenous leukemia following cytogenetic response to α interferon therapy. *Ann Intern Med* 1995; **122**: 254–61.

135. Italian Cooperative Group on Chronic Myeloid Leukemia. Interferon-α-2b compared with conventional chemotherapy for the treatment of chronic myeloid leukemia. *N Engl J Med* 1994; **330**: 820–5.

136. Guilhot F, Chastang C, Michallet M et al. Interferon alfa-2b combined with cytarabine versus interferon alone in chronic myelogenous leukemia. *N Engl J Med* 1997; **337**: 223–9.

137. Talpaz M, Kantarjian H, Kurzrock R et al. Interferon α produces sustained cytogenetic responses in chronic myelogenous leukemia. *Ann Intern Med* 1991; **114**: 532–8.

138. Mahon F, Montastruc M, Faberes C, Reiffers J. Predicting complete cytogenetic response in chronic myelogenous leukemia patients treated with recombinant interferon-α. *Blood* 1996; **84**: 3592–4.

139. Meseri A, Delwail V, Brizard A et al. Endogenous lymphokine activated killer cell activity and cytogenetic response in chronic myelogenous leukemia treated with α-interferon. *Br J Haematol* 1993; **83**: 218–22.

140. Sacchi S, Kantajian H, O'Brien S et al. Immune-mediated and unusual complications during interferon α therapy in chronic myelogenous leukemia. *J Clin Oncol* 1995; **13**: 2401–7.

141. Hasford J, Pfirmann M, Hehlmann R et al. A new prognostic score for survival of patients with chronic myeloid leukemia treated with interferon alfa. *J Natl Cancer Inst* 1998; **90**: 850–8.

142. Hasford J, on behalf of the CML Collaborative Prognostic Factors Project Group. Prognosis of patients with CML: updated results of the collaborative CML prognostic factors project. *Blood* 2000; **96**(Suppl 1): 546a (Abst 2344).

143. Gratwohl A, Hermans J, Goldman JM et al. Risk assessment for patients with chronic myeloid leukaemia before allogeneic blood or marrow transplantation. *Lancet* 1998; **352**: 1087–92.

144. Silver RT, Woolf SH, Hehlmann R et al. An evidence-based analysis of the effect of busulfan, hydroxyurea, interferon and allogeneic bone marrow transplantation in treating the chronic phase of chronic myeloid leukemia: developed for the American Society of Hematology. *Blood* 1999; **94**: 1517–36.

145. Huntly BJ, Bench AJ, Delabesse E et al. Derivative chromosome 9 deletions in chronic myeloid leukemia: poor prognosis is not associated with loss of *ABL–BCR* expression, elevated BCR–ABL levels, or karyotypic instability. *Blood* 2002; **99**: 4547–53.

146. Huntly BJ, Guilhot F, Reid AG et al. Imatinib improves but may not fully reverse the poor prognosis of CML patients with derivative chromosome 9 deletions. *Blood* 2003; **102**: 2205–12.

147. Medical Research Council Working Party: Chronic granulocytic leukemia: comparison of radiotherapy and busulfan therapy. *BMJ* 1958; **i**: 201–8.

148. Kennedy BJ. Hydroxyurea therapy in chronic myelogenous leukemia. *Cancer* 1972; **29**: 1052–6.

149. Helmann R, Heimpel J, Hasford J et al. Randomized comparison of busulfan and hydroxyurea in chronic myelogenous leukemia: prolongation of survival by hydroxyurea. *Blood* 1993; **82**: 398–407.

150. Chronic Myeloid Leukemia Trialists' Collaborative Group. Interferon α versus chemotherapy for chronic myeloid leukemia: a meta analysis of seven randomized trials. *J Natl Cancer Inst* 1997; **89**: 1616–20.

151. Sokal JE, Gockerman JP, Bigner SH. Evidence for a selective antileukemic effect of cytosine arabinoside in chronic granulocytic leukemia. *Leukemia Res* 1988; **12**: 453–458.

152. Robertson MJ, Tantravahi R, Griffin JD et al. Hematologic remission and cytogenetic improvement after treatment of stable-phase chronic myelogenous leukemia with continuous infusion of low cytarabine. *Am J Hematol* 1993; **43**: 95–102.

153. Institute of Materia Medica, Chinese Academy of Medical Services and Chinese People's Liberation Army 187th Hospital. Studies on the antitumor constituents of *Cephalotaxus hainanesis* Li. *Acta Chim Sin* 1976; **34**: 283–287. [Chinese People's Liberation Army 187th Hospital. Homoharringtonine in the treatment of leukemias: clinical analysis of 72 cases. *Chin Med J* 1978; **3**: 163–6.]

154. Visani G, Russo D, Ottaviani E et al. Effects of homoharringtonine alone and in combination with interferon and cytosine arabinoside on in vitro growth and induction of apoptosis in chronic myeloid leukemia and normal hematopoietic progenitors. *Leukemia* 1997; **11**: 624–8.

155. O'Brien SM, Kantarjian H, Keating M et al. Homoharringtonine therapy induces responses in patients with chronic myelogenous leukemia in late chronic phase. *Blood* 1995; **86**: 3322–6.

156. O'Brien SM, Kantarjian H, Koller C et al. Sequential homoharringtonine and interferon α in the treatment of early chronic phase chronic myelogenous leukemia. *Blood* 1999; **93**: 4149–53.

157. Talpaz M, Kantarjian H, McCredie KB et al. Clinical investigation of human alpha interferon in chronic myelogenous leukemia. *Blood* 1987; **69**: 1280–8.

158. Kantarjian M, O'Brien S, Anderlini P et al. Treatment of chronic myelogenous leukemia: current status and investigational options. *Blood* 1996; **87**: 3069–81.

159. Niederle N, Kloke O, Wandl UB et al. Long-term treatment of chronic myelogenous leukemia with different interferons: results from three studies. *Leuk Lymphoma* 1993; **9**: 111–19.

160. Alimena G, Morra E, Lazzarino M et al. Interferon α-2b as therapy for Ph-positive chronic myelogenous leukemia: a study of 82 patients treated with intermittent or daily administration. *Blood* 1989; **72**: 642–7.

161. Freund M, Von Wussow P, Diedrich H et al. Recombinant human interferon (IFN) α2b in chronic myelogenous leukemia. Dose dependency of response and frequency of neutralizing anti-interferon antibodies. *Br J Haematol* 1989; **72**: 350–6.

162. Mahon FX, Montastruc M, Faberes C, Reiffers J. Predicting complete cytogenetic response in chronic myelogenous leukemia patients treated with recombinant interferon α. *Blood* 1994; **84**: 3592–4a.

163. Schofield JR, Robinson WA, Murphy JR, Rovira DK. Low doses of Interferon-α are as effective as higher doses in inducing remissions and prolonging survival in chronic myeloid leukemia. *Ann Intern Med* 1994; **121**: 736–44.

164. The Benelux CML Study Group. Randomized study on hydroxyurea alone versus hydroxyurea combined with low dose interferon-α2b for chronic myeloid leukemia. *Blood* 1998; **91**: 2713–21.

165. Guilhot F, Dreyfus B, Brizard A et al. Cytogenetic remissions in chronic myelogenous leukemia using interferon α2a and hydroxyurea with or without low dose cytosine-arabinoside. *Leuk Lymphoma* 1991; **4**: 49–55.

166. Guilhot F, Guerci A, Maloisel F et al. Follow-up of 1047 patients with chronic myelogenous leukemia treated with interferon or interferon with cytarabine. *Blood* 1997; **90**:(Suppl 1): Abst 2299.

167. Baccarani M, Rosti G, DE Vivo A et al. A randomized study of interferon-α and low-dose arabinosyl cytosine in chronic myeloid leukemia. *Blood* 2002; **99**: 1527–35.

168. Kantarjian HM, Keating MJ, Estey EH et al. Treatment of advanced stages of Philadelphia chrosomome-positive chronic myelogenous leukemia with interferon-α and low-dose cytarabine. *J Clin Oncol* 1992; **10**: 772–8.

169. Kantarjian H, O'Brien S, Beran M et al. Interferon α (IFN-A) and low-dose cytosine arabinoside (Ara-C) therapy in Philadelphia chromosome (Ph)-positive chronic myelogenous leukemia (CML). *Blood* 1995; **86**(Suppl 1): Abst 2105.

170. Arthur CK, Ma DDF. Combined interferon alfa-2a and cytosine arabinoside as first-line treatment for chronic myeloid leukemia. *Acta Haematol* 1993; **89**(Suppl 1): 15–21.

171. Thaler J, Hilbe W, Apfelbeck U et al. Interferon α2c and LD Ara-C for the treatment of patients with CML: results of the Austrian multicenter phase II study. *Leuk Res* 1997; **21**: 75–80.

172. Cervantes F, Sureda A, Hernandez-Boluda JC et al. Interferon plus intermittent oral Ara-C ocfosfate (YNK–01) in chronic myeloid leukemia primarily resistant or with minimal cytogenetic response to interferon. *Haematologica* 2001; **86**: 1281–6.

173. Maloisel F, Guerci A, Guyotat D et al. Results of a phase II trial of a combination or oral cytarabine ocfosfate (YNK01) and interferon-2b for treatment of chronic myelogenous leukemia patients in chronic phase. *Leukemia* 2002; **16**: 573–80.

174. Rosti G, Bonifazi F, Trabacchi E et al. A phase II study of α-interferon and oral arabinosyl cytosine (YNK01) in chronic myeloid leukemia. *Leukemia* 2003; **17**: 554–9.

175. Talpaz M, O'Brien S, Rose E et al. Phase I study of polyethylene glycol formulation of interferon α-2b (Schering 54031) in Philadelphia chromosome-positive chronic myelogenous leukemia. *Blood* 2001; **98**: 1708–13.

176. Lipton JH, Khoroshko ND, Golenkov AK et al. 2-year survival data from a randomized study of peginterferon alfa-2a (40KD) vs interferon alfa-2a in patients with chronic-phase chronic myelogenous leukemia. *Blood* 2003; **102**(Suppl 1): 904a.

177. Michallet M, Maloisel F, Delain M et al. Pegylated recombinant interferon α-2b vs recombinant interferon α-2b for the initial treatment of chronic-phase chronic myelogenous leukemia: a phase III study. *Leukemia* 2004; **18**: 309–15.

178. Buchdunger E, Zimmermann J, Mett H et al. Inhibition of the Abl protein-tyrosine kinase in vitro and in vivo by a 2-phenylaminopyrimidine derivative. *Cancer Res* 1996; **56**: 100–4.

179. Savage DG, Antman KH. Imatinib mesylate – a new oral targeted therapy. *N Engl J Med* 2002; **346**: 683–93.

180. Druker BJ, Talpaz M, Resta DJ et al. Efficacy and safety of a specific inhibitor of the BCR–ABL tyrosine kinase in chronic myeloid leukemia. *N Engl J Med* 2001; **344**: 1031–7.

181. Kantarjian H, Sawyers C, Hochhaus A et al. Hematologic and cytogenetic responses to imatinib mesylate in chronic myelogenous leukemia. *N Engl J Med* 2002; **346**: 645–52.

182. O'Brien SG, Guilhot F, Larson RA et al. Imatinib compared with interferon and low-dose cytarabine for newly diagnosed chronic-phase chronic myeloid leukemia. *N Engl J Med* 2003; **348**: 994–1004.

183. Hughes T, Kaeda J, Branford S et al. Frequency of major molecular responses to imatinib or interferon alfa plus cytarabine in newly diagnosed chronic myeloid leukemia. *N Engl J Med* 2003; **349**: 1423–32.

184. Hahn EA, Glendenning A, Sorensen MV et al. Quality of life in patients with newly diagnosed chronic phase chronic myeloid leukemia on imabinib versus interferon alfa plus low-dose cytarabine: results from the IRIS study. *J Clin Oncol* 2003; **21**: 2138–46.

185. Hansen JA, Gooleyta, Martin PJ et al. Bone marrow transplants from unrelated donors for patients with chronic myeloid leukemia. *N Eng J Med* 1998; **338**: 962–8.

186. Silberman G, Crosse MG, Peterson EA et al. Availability and appropriateness of allogenic bone marrow transplantation for chronic myeloid leukemia in 10 countries, *N Engl J Med* 1994; **331**: 1063–7.

187. Rowling PA. Current use and outcome of blood and marrow transplantation. *ABMTR Newsletter* 1996; **3**: 6–8.

188. Van Rhee F, Szydlo RM, Hermans J et al. Long term results after allogenic bone marrow transplantation for chronic myelogenous leukemia in chronic phase: a report from the Chronic Leukemia Working Party of the European Group for Blood and Marrow Transplantation. *Bone Marrow Transplant* 1997; **20**: 553–60.

189. Goldman JM, Szydlo RM, Horowitz MM et al. Choice of pretransplant treatment and timing of transplants for chronic myelogenous leukemia in chronic phase. *Blood* 1993; **82**: 2235–8.

190. Gale RP, Hehlmann R, Zhang MJ et al. Survival with bone marrow transplantation versus hydroxyurea or interferon for chronic myelogenous leukemia. *Blood* 1998; **91**: 1810–19.

191. McGlave, P, Verfaille CM (eds). *Biology and Therapy of Chronic Myelogenous Leukemia. Hematol Oncol Clin North Am* 1998; **12**: No. 1.

192. Spencer A, O'Brien S, Goldman J. Options for therapy in chronic myeloid leukaemia. *Br J Haematol* 1995; **91**: 2–7.

193. Drobyski WR, Ash RC, Casper JT et al. Effect of T-cell depletion as graft-versus-host disease prophylaxis on engraftment, relapse, and disease-free survival in unrelated marrow transplantation for chronic myelogenous leukemia. *Blood* 1994; **83**: 1980–87.

194. Higano CS, Chielens D, Raskind W et al. Use of α-2a-interferon to treat cytogentic relapse of chronic myeloid leukemia after marrow transplantation. *Blood* 1997; **90**: 2549–54.

195. Kolb HJ, Schattenberg A, Goldman JM et al. Graft-versus-leukemia effect of donor lymphocyte transfusions in marrow grafted patients. *Blood* 1995; **86**: 2041–50.

196. Dazzi F, Szydlo RM, Cross NCP et al. Durability of responses following donor lymphocyte infusions for patients who relapse after allogeneic stem cell transplantation for chronic myeloid leukemia. *Blood* 2000; **96**: 2712–16.

197. Craddock C, Szydlo RM, Klein JP et al. Estimating leukemia-free survival after allografting for chronic myeloid leukemia: a new method that takes into account patients who relapse and are restored to complete remission. *Blood* 2000; **96**: 86–90.

198. Cunningham I, Gee T, Dowling M et al. Results of treatment of Ph-negative chronic myelogenous leukemia with an intensive treatment regimen (L-5 protocol). *Blood* 1979; **53**: 375–95.

199. Carella AM, Cunningham I, Lerma E et al. Mobilization and transplantation of Philadelphia-negative peripheral-blood progenitor cells early in chronic myleogenous leukemia. *J Clin Oncol* 1997; **15**: 1575–82.

200. Carreras E, Sierra J, Rovira M et al. Successful autografting in chronic myeloid leukemia using Philadelphia-negative blood progenitor cells mobilized with rHug-CSF alone in patient responding to α-interferon. *Br J Haematol* 1997; **96**: 421–3.

201. Archimbaud E, Michallet M, Philip I et al. Granulocyte colony-stimulating factor given in addition to interferon-α to mobilize peripheral blood stem cells for autologous transplantation in chronic myeloid leukaemia. *Br J Haematol* 1997; **99**: 678–84.

202. Chalmers EA, Franklin IM, Kelsey S et al. Treatment of chronic myeloid leukemia in chronic phase with idarubicin and cytarabine: mobilisation of Ph-negative peripheral blood stem cells. *Br J Haematol* 1997; **96**: 617–34.

203. Hughes TP, Grigg A, Szer J et al. Mobilization of predominantly Philadelphia chromosome-negative blood progenitors using cyclophosphamide and rHUG-CSF in early chronic phase chronic myeloid leukemia: correlation with Sokal prognostic index and haematological control. *Br J Haematol* 1997; **96**: 635–40.

204. Johnson RJ, Owen RG, Child JA et al. Mobilization of Philadelphia-negative peripheral blood mononuclear cells in chronic myeloid leukemia using hydroxyurea and G-CSF (filgrastim). *Br J Haematol* 1996; **93**: 863–8.

205. Kantarjian HM, Talpaz M, Hester J et al. Collection of peripheral blood diploid cells from chronic myelogenous leukemia patients early in the recovery phase from myelosuppression induced by intensive chemotherapy. *J Clin Oncol* 1995; **13**: 553–9.

206. Carlo Stella C, Mangoni L, Piovani et al. Identification of Philadelphia-negative granulocyte–macrophage colony-forming units generated by stroma-adherent cells from chronic myelogenous leukemia patients. *Blood* 1994; **83**: 1373–80.

207. Coulombel L, Kalousek DK, Eaves CJ et al. Long-term marrow culture reveals chromosomally normal hematopoietic progenitor cells in patients with Philadelphia chromosome-positive chronic myelogenous leukemia. *N Engl J Med* 1983; **306**: 1493–8.

208. Dube ID, Kalousek DK, Coulombel L et al. Cytogenetic studies of early myeloid progenitor compartments on Ph¹-positive chronic myeloid leukemia. II. Long-term culture reveals the persistence of Ph¹-negative progenitors in treated as well as newly diagnosed patients. *Blood* 1984; **63**: 1172–7.

209. Verfaillie CM, Miller WJ, Boylan K, McGlave PB. Selection of benign primitive hematopoietic progenitors in chronic myelogenous leukemia on the basis of HLA-DR antigen expression. *Blood* 1992; **79**: 1003–10.

210. Dunbar CE, Stewart FM. Separating the wheat from the chaff: selection of benign hematopoietic cells in chronic myeloid leukemia. *Blood* 1992; **79**: 1107–10.

211. Buckner CD, Stewart P, Clift RA et al. Treatment of blastic transformation of chronic granulocytic leukemia by chemotherapy, total body irradiation and infusion of cryopreserved autologous marrow. *Exp Hematol* 1978; **6**: 96–109.

212. Korbling M, Burke P, Braine H et al. Successful engraftment of blood derived normal hemopoietic stem cells in chronic myelogenous leukemia. *Exp Hematol* 1981; **9**: 684–90.

213. Brito-Babapulle F, Bowcock SJ, Marcus RE et al. Autografting for patients with chronic myeloid leukaemia in chronic phase: peripheral blood stem cells may have a finite capacity for maintaining haemopoiesis. *Br J Haematol* 1989; **73**: 76–81.

214. Hoyle CF, Gray R, Goldman JM. Autografting for patients with CML in chronic phase: an update. *Br J Haematol* 1994; **86**: 76–81.

215. Reiffers J, Goldman JM, Meloni JM et al. Autologous stem cell transplantation on chronic myelogenous leukemia: a retrospective analysis of the European Group for Bone Marrow Transplantation. *Bone Marrow Transplant* 1994; **14**: 407–10.

216. McGlave PB, de Fabritiis P, Deisseroth A et al. Autologous transplants for chronic myelogenous leukemia: results from eight transplant groups. *Lancet* 1994; **343**: 1486–8.

217. Simonsson B, Oberg G, Killander A et al. Intensive treatment in order to minimize the Ph-positive clone in chronic myelogenic leukemia (CML). *Bone Marrow Transplant* 1994; **14**(Suppl 3): S55–6.

218. Kantarjian HM, O'Brien SM, Keating M et al. Results of decitabine therapy in the accelerated and blastic phases of chronic myelogenous leukemia. *Leukemia* 1997; **11**: 1617–20.

219. Kantarjian H, Talpaz M, Kontayiannis D et al. Treatment of chronic myelogenous leukemia in accelerated and blastic phase with daunorubicin, high-dose cytarabine and granulocyte macrophage colony stimulating factor. *J Clin Oncol* 1992; **10**: 398–405.

220. Gratwohl A, Hermans J, Niederwieser D et al. for the Chronic Myeloid Leukemia Working Party of the European Group for Bone Marrow Transplantation. Bone marrow transplantation for chronic myeloid leukemia: long term results. *Bone Marrow Transplant* 1993; **12**: 509–16.

221. McGlave P. Therapy of chronic myelogenous leukemia with related or unrelated donor bone marrow transplantation. *Leukemia* 1992; **6**(Suppl): 115–17.

222. Passweg JR, Rowling PA, Horowitz MM. Related donor bone marrow transplantation for chronic myelogenous leukemia. *Hematol Oncol Clin North Am* 1998; **12**: 81–92.

223. Talpaz M, Silver RT, Druker BJ et al. Imatinib induces durable hematologic and cytogenetic responses in patients with accelerated phase chronic myeloid leukemia: results of a phase 2 study. *Blood* 2002; **99**: 1928–37.

224. Dann EJ, Anastasi J, Larson RA. High dose Cladribine (2CDA) therapy for chronic myelogenous leukemia in blast phase (CML-BP). *Blood* 1996; **88**(suppl): 928.

225. Feldman E, Zorsky P, Armentrout S et al. Phase 1 trial of

short course, high-dose Mitoxantrone (M) in combination with high-dose Cytarabine (HIDAC) in patients (pts) with acute leukemia and blastic chronic myelogenous leukemia (BLCML). *Blood* 1990; **76**(Suppl): 1066.

226. Dutcher JP, Eudey L, Wiernik PH et al. Phase II study of mitoxantrone and 5-azacitidine for accelerated and blast crisis of chronic myelogenous leukemia: a study of the Eastern Cooperative Oncology Group. *Leukemia* 1992; **6**: 770–5.

227. Dutcher JP, Coletti D, Paietta E, Wiernik PH. A pilot study of α-interferon and plicamycin for accelerated phase of chronic myeloid leukemia. *Leuk Res* 1997; **21**: 375–80.

228. Dutcher JP, Lee S, Paietta E et al. Phase II study of carboplatin in blast crisis of chronic myeloid leukemia: Eastern Cooperative Oncology Group study E1992. *Leukemia* 1998; **12**: 1037–40.

229. Dann EJ, Anastasi J, Larson RA. High-dose cladribine therapy for chronic myelogenous leukemia in the accelerated or blast phase. *J Clin Oncol* 1998; **16**: 1498–504.

230. Montefusco E, Petti MC, Alimena G et al. Etoposide, intermediate-dose cytarabine and carboplatin (VAC): a combination therapy for the blastic phase of chronic myelogenous leukemia. *Ann Oncol* 1997; **8**: 175–9.

231. Schiffer CA, Debellis R, Kasdorf H, Wiernik PH. Treatment of the blast crisis of chronic myelogenous leukemia with 5-azaticidine and VP-16-213. *Cancer Treat Rep* 1982; **66**: 267–71.

232. Sacchi S, Katarjian HM, O'Brien S et al. Chronic myelogenous leukemia in nonlymphoid blastic phase. Analysis of the results of first salvage therapy with three different treatment approaches for 162 patients. *Cancer* 1999; **86**: 2632–41.

233. Walters RS, Kantarjian HM, Keating MJ et al. Therapy of lymphoid and undifferentiated chronic myelogenous leukemia in blast crisis with continuous vincristine and Adriamycin infusions plus high-dose decadron. *Cancer* 1987; **60**: 1708–12.

234. Griesshammer M, Heinze B, Hellmann R et al. Chronic myelogenous leukemia in blast crisis: retrospective analysis of prognostic factors in 90 patients. *Ann Hematol* 1996; **73**: 225–30.

235. Brodsky I, Biggs JC, Szer J et al. Treatment of chronic myelogenous leukemia with allogeneic bone marrow transplantation after preparation with busulfan and cyclophosphamide (BuCy2): an update. *Semin Oncol* 1993; **20**(Suppl 4): 27–31.

236. McGlave P, Ou Shu X, Wen W et al. Unrelated donor marrow transplantation for chronic myelogenous leukemia: 9 years' experience of the National Marrow Donor Program. *Blood* 2000; **95**: 2219–25.

237. Haines ME, Goldman JM, Worsley AM et al. Chemotherapy and autografting for chronic granulocytic leukemia in transformation: probable prolongation of survival in some patients. *Br J Haematol* 1984; **58**: 711–21.

238. Reiffers J, Trouette R, Marit G et al. Autologous stem cell transplantation for chronic granulocytic leukemia in transformation: a report of 47 cases. *Br J Haematol* 1991; **77**: 339–45.

239. Reiffers J, Mahon FX, Boiron JM et al. Autografting in chronic myeloid leukemia: an overview. *Leukemia* 1996; **10**: 385–8.

240. Druker BJ, Tamura S, Buchdunger E et al. Effects of a selective inhibitor of the Abl tyrosine kinase on the growth of Bcr–Abl positive cells. *Nat Med* 1996; **2**: 561–6.

241. Druker BJ, Sawyers CL, Kantarjian H et al. Activity of a specific inhibitor of the BCR–ABL tyrosine kinase in the blast crisis of chronic myeloid leukemia and acute lymphoblastic leukemia with the Philadelphia chromosome. *N Engl J Med* 2001; **344**: 1038–42.

242. Sawyers CL, Hochhaus A, Feldman E et al. Imatinib induces hematologic and cytogenetic responses in patients with chronic myelogenous leukemia in myeloid blast crisis: results of a phase II study. *Blood* 2002; **99**: 3530–9.

243. Kano Y, Akutsu M, Tsunoda S et al. In vitro cytotoxic effects of a tyrosine kinase inhibitor STI571 in combination with commonly used antileukemic agents. *Blood* 2001; **97**: 1999–2007.

244. Thiesing J, Ohno-Jones S, Kolibaba KS et al. Efficacy of imatinib mesylate, an Abl tyrosine kinase inhibitor, in conjunction with other antileukemic agents against Bcr–Abl-positive cells. *Blood* 2000; **96**: 3195–9.

245. Tipping AJ, Mahon FX, Zafirides G et al. Drug responses of STI571-resistant cells: synergism of STI571 with other chemotherapeutic drugs. *Leukemia* 2002; **16**: 2349–57.

246. Topaly J, Zeller WJ, Fruehauf S et al. Synergistic activity of the new ABL-specific tyrosine kinase inhibitor STI571 and chemotherapeutic drugs on BCR–ABL-positive chronic myelogenous leukemia. *Leukemia* 2001; **15**: 342–7.

247. Gorre ME, Mohammed M, Ellwood K et al. Clinical resistance to STI571 cancer therapy caused by BCR–ABL gene mutation or amplification. *Science* 2001; **293**: 876–80.

248. Branford S, Rudzki Z, Walsh S et al. High frequency of point mutations clustered within the adenosine triphosphate-binding region of BCR/ABL in patients with chronic myeloid leukemia or Ph-positive acute lymphoblastic leukemia who develop imatinib mesylate (STI571) resistance. *Blood* 2002; **99**: 3472–5.

249. Shah NP, Nicoll JM, Nagar B et al. Multiple BCR–ABL kinase domain mutations confer polyclonal resistance to the tyrosine kinase inhibitor imatinib mesylate (STI571) in chronic phase and blast crisis chronic myeloid leukemia. *Cancer Cell* 2002; **2**: 117–25.

250. Shah NP, Sawyers CL. Mechanisms of resistance to STI571 in Philadelphia chromosome-associated leukemias. *Oncogene* 2003; **22**: 7389–95.

251. Roche-Lestienne C, Soenen-Cornu V, Grardel-Duflos N et al. Several types of mutation of the *Abl* gene can be found in chronic myeloid leukemia patients resistant to STI571, and they can pre-exist to the onset of treatment. *Blood* 2002; **100**: 1014–18.

252. Druker BJ, Kantarjian HM, Talpaz M et al. A phase I study of Gleevec (imatinib mesylate) administered concomitantly with cytosine arabinoside (Ara-C) in patients with Philadelphia positive chronic myeloid leukemia (CML). *Blood* 2001; **98**: 3511a.

253. Guilhot F, Gardembas M, Rousselot Ph et al. Imatinib in combination with cytarabine for the treatment of Philadelphia-positive chronic myelogenous leukaemia chronic phase patients: rational and design of phase I/II trials. *Semin Hematol* 2003; **40**: 92–7.

254. Gardembas M, Rousselot Ph, Tulliez M et al. Results of a phase II study combining imatinib mesylate and cytarabine for the treatment of Philadelphia-positive chronic myelogenous leukaemia patients in chronic phase. *Blood* 2003; **102**: 4298–305.

255. O'Brien S, Vallance SE, Craddock C et al. PEGIntron and

STI571 combination evaluation study (PISCES) in chronic phase chronic myeloïd leukemia. *Blood* 2001; **98**: 3512.

256. Deininger M, O'Brien SG, Ford JM et al. Practical management of patients with chronic myeloid leukemia receiving imatinib. *J Clin Oncol* 2003; **21**: 1637–47.

257. Cortes J, Giles F, O'Brien S. Result of high-dose imatinib mesylate in patients with Philadelphia chromosome-positive chronic myeloid leukemia after failure of interferon-α. *Blood* 2003; **102**: 83–6.

258. Kantarjian HM, Talpaz M, O'Brien S et al. Dose escalation of imatinib mesylate can overcome resistance to standard-dose therapy in patients with chronic myelogenous leukemia. *Blood* 2003; **101**: 473–5.

259. Sneed TB, Kantarjian HM, Talpaz M. The significance of myelosuppression during therapy with imatinib mesylate in patients with chronic myelogenous leukemia in chronic phase. *Cancer* 2004; **100**: 116–21.

260. Heinzinger M, Waller CF, Rosenstiel A et al. Quality of IL-3 and G-CSF-mobilized peripheral blood stem cells in patients with early chronic phase CML. *Leukemia* 1998; **12**: 333–9.

# 42 Chronic myeloid disorders excluding CML

**Tiziano Barbui, Guido Finazzi, and Giovanni Barosi**

## Introduction

Chronic myeloproliferative disorders (MPD) are clonal diseases originating in a pluripotential hematopoietic stem cell. The clonal expansion results in increased and abnormal hematopoiesis and produces a group of interrelated syndromes, classified according to the predominant phenotypic expression of the myeloproliferative clone. Excluding chronic myeloid leukemia (CML), which is characterized by peculiar biological and clinical features and is described in Chapter 41, MPD include polycythemia vera (PV), essential thrombocythemia (ET), and myelofibrosis with myeloid metaplasia (MMM). Due to the underlying defect, which involves a common hematopoietic precursor cell, 'hybrid' phenotypes may be discovered at diagnosis and transitions among the syndromes may occur during the course of the disease. Nevertheless, the clinical course and management of the various syndromes is different, and this makes it essential to adopt clearly defined diagnostic criteria. In this chapter, we will briefly review the pathophysiological background, diagnostic approach, and natural history of MPD other than CML with the aim of offering the necessary background for up-to-date treatment.

## Polycythemia vera

### Pathophysiology

PV is an MPD characterized by generalized marrow hyperplasia with prevalent overproduction of the erythroid cell line that is independent of the physiological growth factor erythropoietin (EPO). This is manifested in vitro by 'spontaneous' colony formation in the absence of exogenous EPO. The molecular bases for these alterations are being actively studied, but still remain poorly understood.[1,2] An interesting finding from the molecular cloning of the EPO receptor (EPOR) made it possible to formulate the hypothesis that PV is caused by a mutation of the *EPOR* gene.

Actually, at least two different mutations of *EPOR* have been found in cases of congenital polycythemia,[3,4] but the search for these mutations has failed to reveal any abnormality in the majority of patients with familial erythrocytosis[2] or with PV.[5]

There are data showing that erythroid progenitors are hypersensitive to other growth factors, such as granulocyte–macrophage colony-stimulating factor (GM-CSF), interleukin-3 (IL-3),[6] insulin-like growth factor I (IGF-I),[7] and thrombopoietin (TPO).[8] This observation would seem to fit better with a more generalized intracellular defect (e.g. a shared signaling pathway) than with a selective receptorial defect. Moliterno et al reported that platelets from patients with PV displayed impaired tyrosine phosphorylation in response to TPO stimulation, whereas the response to thrombin remained intact.[9] The inability to transduce the TPO signal was due to a dramatic reduction or a complete absence of the TPO receptor, c-Mpl, in 34 of 34 PV patients. However, it is at present not clear how a loss of c-Mpl expression could contribute to the growth factor hypersensitivity of PV cells.

Interestingly, PV erythroid precursor cells express the anti-apoptotic protein Bcl-$x_L$ to a much higher proportion than normal precursor cells.[10] In addition, in PV, more mature cells, which normally show no Bcl-$x_L$ expression, still express high levels of the protein. Hematopoietic growth factors, such as IGF-I, act in part by suppressing apoptosis.[11] Thus, the observed growth factor hypersensitivity of PV cells could result from an intrinsic protection from apoptosis, thereby requiring less protection through growth factor stimulation.

Of particular interest is the cloning of PRV-1, a novel member of the uPAR receptor superfamily, which is overexpressed in granulocytes from patients with PV, but is not detectable in normal control granulocytes.[12] Moreover, PRV-1 is not expressed in granulocytes from patients with secondary erythrocytosis, whereas a more heterogeneous pattern was observed in patients with ET. Although PRV-1 is not expressed in resting granulocytes from normal controls, stimulation of these cells with granulocyte colony-stimulating factor (G-CSF) induces PRV-1 expression. Further studies are ongoing to establish whether this novel hematopoietic receptor may be useful in the differential diagnosis of PV and whether it may play a role in the pathophysiology of this MPD.

Even though pathognomonic chromosomal abnormalities have not been described so far, a deletion of the long arm of chromosome 20 can be found in 10–15% of patients with PV at diagnosis.[13] This abnormality does not seem to be restricted to this MPD phenotype, but is also present in patients with myelofibrosis or myelodisplastic syndromes. The fact that the 20q deletion is encountered in a spectrum of MPD suggests that this cytogenetic abnormality may mark the site of a tumor suppressor gene, or genes, possibly involved in the regulation of normal multipotent hematopoietic progenitors.[14]

## Diagnostic criteria

Several criteria have been used to establish a diagnosis of PV, with an elevated red blood cell mass (RCM) being the most important conventional parameter for distinguishing between true and apparent polycythemias. Secondary causes have to be ruled out by using previously formulated guidelines and algorithms. The Polycythemia Vera Study Group (PVSG) criteria[15] (Table 42.1) were initially formulated to enrol a uniform patient population with overt PV for studies on therapeutic intervention. Consequently, if these stringent criteria are adopted, patients in the initial stages of the disease may be excluded from this diagnosis. For such individuals, the new and more specific techniques include cytogenetic studies, endogenous colony formation and serum EPO assay.[16]

A revision of the PVSG criteria that takes into account these latter findings has been recently proposed by Pearson et al[17] (Table 42.2) and is based on the following considerations:

- The PVSG criteria included documenting a raised RCM based on normal ranges expressed in terms of milliliters per kilogram total body weight. This method is considered inappropriate for obese individuals, since adipose tissue is relatively avascular and does not contribute proportionally to the blood volume. In these cases, the presence of an absolute polycythemia in the initial phases can go undetected using the PVSG criteria. A more precise method of RCM measurement might be the use of formulae based on height and weight.[18] The proposed normal range for each prediction is +25% of the mean value, which includes 98% and 99% of normal males and females, respectively. Therefore, patients with a RCM more than 25% above their mean normal predicted value should be regarded as fulfilling the criterion of increased RCM.

- Cytogenetic abnormalities were not part of the list of PVSG criteria, but can now be identified in up to 20% of PV patients at diagnosis.[13] The most common changes are trisomies 1, 8, and 9, and deletions of 13q and 20q. The presence of karyotypic defects does not appear to affect prognosis,[19] but could be regarded as a major diagnostic criterion of PV; however, it should be borne in mind that an abnormal karyotype (e.g. a balanced translocation) can be found in less than 1% of phenotypically normal individuals.

- Patients with PV, but not those with secondary erythrocytosis, are able to generate spontaneous erythroid colonies without the addition of EPO to the culture medium. The EPO endogenous

---

**Table 42.1  Polycythemia Vera Study Group diagnostic criteria for polycythemia vera[15]**

| | |
|---|---|
| A1. Raised red cell mass:<br>Male > 36 ml/kg<br>Female > 32 ml/kg | B1. Thrombocytosis:<br>platelet count > 400 × 10⁹/l |
| A2. Normal arterial oxygen saturation > 92% | B2. Leukocytosis > 12 × 10⁹/l (no fever or infection) |
| A3. Splenomegaly | B3. Raised neutrophil alkaline phosphatase (score > 100) or raised vitamin $B_{12}$ (> 900 ng/l) or raised unsaturated vitamin $B_{12}$-binding capacity (>2200 ng/l) |

Diagnosis of polycythemia vera is acceptable if the following combinations are present:

   A1 + A2 + A3

or

   A1 + A2 + any two from category B

## Table 42.2 Proposed modified criteria for the diagnosis of polycythemia vera[17]

A1. Raised red cell mass
(> 25% above mean
normal predicted value)

A2. Absence of causes of
secondary polycythemia

A3. Palpable splenomegaly

A4. Clonality marker
(e.g. abnormal marrow karyotype)

B1. Thrombocytosis:
platelet count > $400 \times 10^9/l$

B2. Neutrophil leukocytosis
(neutrophil count > $10 \times 10^9/l$)

B3. Splenomegaly on isotope or
ultrasound scanning

B4. Characteristic BFU-E growth
or reduced serum erythropoietin

Diagnosis of polycythemia vera is acceptable if the following combinations are present:

A1 + A2 + A3 or A4

or

A1 + A2 + any two from category B

colonies (EEC) assay can now be considered reliable and reproducible,[20] but it still remains a complex and time-consuming test that is not readily available in most laboratories. Besides PV, EEC can also be observed in patients with apparently idiopathic thrombocythemia[21] and in some cases of CML or erythroleukemia.[22] The current role of the EEC assay in the diagnostic strategy of PV is to recognize incomplete or unusual presentations of the disease, for example in patients with rare sites of thrombosis who do not fulfill conventionally established criteria for a PV diagnosis.

- In vivo and in vitro bioassays, radio immunoassays (RIA), enzyme-linked immunoassays (ELISA), and immunoradiometric assays (IRMA) have been applied to measure serum EPO levels. These immunological techniques are specific, sensitive, reproducible, and easy to perform, and published studies show that normal individuals have values ranging from 6 to 32 IU/l. At diagnosis of PV, serum EPO levels are reduced or in the lower normal range, whereas normal or raised amounts are found in secondary polycythemia.[23,24] For this reason, EPO determination has been used in the differential diagnosis of PV, but the wide overlapping of results between PV and normal or secondary polycythemia patients limits the diagnostic value of this test, which at best should be considered among the minor criteria for PV diagnosis.

The modified criteria for diagnosis of PV represent a proposal that has the merit of summarizing the current state of knowledge in this field, and should also allow recognition of patients with an early disease presentation. Nevertheless, unusual cases with difficult-to-interpret clinical and laboratory characteristics still represent a diagnostic problem. If asymptomatic, these patients should be followed carefully and unnecessary therapeutic interventions avoided; if they present with serious symptoms, decisions about treatment should be made on the risk/benefit principle.

## Epidemiology and natural history

PV is a rare disease, the yearly incidence in Western Europe and the USA being approximately 5–16 cases per 1 million population.[25] The incidence was found to be higher in Jews and lower among Blacks and in Japan. However, these figures are probably underestimates in view of the difficulty in recognizing patients in the early stage of disease when only conventional criteria for diagnosis are applied.

PV usually appears during middle age and is slightly more prevalent in males. In a study carried out by the Gruppo Italiano Studio Policitemia (GISP),[26] the median age at diagnosis was 60 years in men and 62 years in women and the ratio of men to women was 1.2 : 1. Only a small number of PV patients have been reported in childhood, and these cases deserve careful investigation for the possible diagnosis of familial polycythemia, a rare but distinct nosological entity.[27]

PV has a natural history of slow progression into subsequent clinical and hematological phases. Its onset may be insidious, and symptoms may precede an overt diagnosis by years. During this 'developmental phase', patients may be asymptomatic or may present thrombotic complications, which are observed in up to 14% of cases before diagnosis of PV. In up to 20% of patients, thrombosis is the presenting symptom of disease; cerebral ischemia accounted for 70% of arterial thromboses at diagnosis in our study, and was as prevalent as myocardial infarction (30%) before diagnosis of PV.[23] These findings emphasize the importance of early diagnosis, and call for the implementation and validation of the new techniques discussed above. The 'polycythemic phase', clearly defined by conventional diagnostic criteria, may be either asymptomatic or characterized by thrombotic events of variable severity that also depend on the concomitant presence of other risk factors for vascular disease. Bleeding complications are less frequent than thrombosis, and are thought to account for 15–30% of cases. The 'spent phase' is the final stage, characterized by anemia, leukopenia, thrombocytopenia, and a leuko-erythroblastic peripheral blood picture. This transformation can be observed in up to 20% of PV patients after an average interval of 10 years from diagnosis, and its outcome is very poor, since no effective treatment is available. An attempt to improve prognosis was carried out in a small series of patients with transformed PV who underwent allogeneic bone marrow transplantation. Even though the results seem promising, this procedure should be considered only in selected young patients.[28]

Current treatments for PV have dramatically improved the natural history of patients in the pretransformed stages. Thus, the median life-expectancy has increased from 6–18 months in untreated patients to over 10 years in those receiving cytoreduction and antithrombotic drugs. Unfortunately, we now have to deal with complications chiefly related to the cytotoxic therapy, which are among the leading causes of death in these patients. The impact of the therapeutic guidelines provided by the PVSG on the natural history of PV has been investigated by the GISP in a retrospective cohort study of 1213 patients in Italy through an analysis of overall survival and incidence of thrombotic and neoplastic complications.[26] The cumulative median duration of survival exceeded 15 years, with an overall mortality rate of 2.94 deaths/100 patients per year. The age- and sex-standardized mortality rate was 1.7 times greater than that of the general Italian population. This finding contrasts with a previous study suggesting that expected survival in PV patients did not differ from the survival

of a control sample.[29] The most frequent causes of death were thrombosis (30% of cases) and cancer (15% of patients with acute leukemia and 15% with other cancers). These complications were analyzed in detail (Tables 42.3 and 42.4). The overall rate of fatal and non-fatal thrombotic events was 3.4 per 100 patients per year. The incidence of thrombosis increased significantly with age (<40 years, 1.8%; 40–57 years, 2.8%; 60–69 years, 4.0%; >70 years, 5.1% per year; $p<0.001$) and with a history of thrombosis (24.6% versus 17.3%; $p=0.001$), confirming previous data from the PVSG.[15] The risk of death for patients who had previously received radiophosphorus or alkylating or non-alkylating myelosuppressive agents was four times greater than that of those who had received phlebotomy or other pharmacological treatments (6.7% versus 1.6%; $p=0.06$). Thus, cytoreduction favorably affects the incidence of thrombotic events, but this treatment may be associated with an increased risk of secondary neoplasm. A reevaluation of the best approach with available drugs is therefore needed to improve the therapeutic profile.

## Therapy

At present, there is no known treatment that eradicates the abnormal clone. Consequently, therapy is aimed at reducing the incidence of vascular complications and limiting the progress of the myeloproliferative process. Available information for therapeutic recommendations in PV derives from a very limited number of randomized clinical trials and from a series of prospective and retrospective studies that have described the natural history of PV patients and indirectly evaluated the effect of different strategies on the main outcomes of the disease.[30] For practical purposes, we will discuss the results of strategies intended to reduce RCM and myeloid hyperplasia

**Table 42.3 Fatal and non-fatal thrombotic events (n=254) during follow-up in 1213 patients with polycythemia vera**

| Type of complication | No. of non-fatal events[a] | No. of fatal events[a] |
|---|---|---|
| Arterial thrombosis | 101 (50.5) | 44 (81.5) |
| Myocardial infarction | 28 (14.0) | 27 (50.0) |
| Ischemic stroke | 19 (9.5) | 17 (31.5) |
| Transient ischemic attack | 39 (19.5) | — |
| Peripheral arterial thrombosis | 15 (7.5) | — |
| Venous thromboembolism | 77 (38.5) | 10 (18.5) |
| Deep venous thrombosis | 35 (17.5) | — |
| Superficial thrombophlebitis | 37 (18.5) | — |
| Unknown | 5 (2.5) | — |
| Unknown | 22 (11.0) | — |
| Total | 200 (100) | 54 (100) |

[a] Percentages in parentheses.

## Table 42.4 Causes of death in 192 patients with polycythemia vera

| Cause of death | No. of patients[a] |
|---|---|
| Cardiovascular | 70 (36.4) |
| Arterial thrombosis | 46 (24.0) |
| Myocardial infarction | 14 (7.3) |
| Sudden death | 15 (7.8) |
| Ischemic stroke | 17 (8.8) |
| Venous thromboembolism | 10 (5.2) |
| Cerebral sinus thrombosis | 2 (1.0) |
| Pulmonary embolism | 6 (3.1) |
| Splanchnic thrombosis | 2 (1.0) |
| Other cardiovascular | 14 (7.3) |
| Hemorrhagic | 6 (3.1) |
| Gastrointestinal bleeding | 5 (2.6) |
| Cerebral hemorrhage | 1 (0.5) |
| Cancer | 57 (30.0) |
| Acute myeloid leukemia | 28 (14.6) |
| Breast cancer | 5 (2.6) |
| Colorectal cancer | 6 (3.1) |
| Lung cancer | 4 (2.1) |
| Other cancers | 14 (7.3) |
| Complications of polycythemia | 5 (2.6) |
| Myelodysplasia | 1 (0.5) |
| Spent phase | 4 (2.1) |
| Other causes | 54 (28.1) |
| Respiratory failure | 14 (7.3) |
| Hepatic failure | 4 (2.1) |
| Other | 36 (18.9) |
| Total | 192 (100) |

[a] Percentages in parentheses.

('cytoreductive' therapy) separately from those aimed at reducing the risk of thrombosis through the use of antithrombotic drugs.

## Cytoreduction

In the first study by the PVSG (the 01 trial),[15] 431 patients were randomized to one of the following treatments: (a) phlebotomy alone; (b) phosphorus-32 [32]P plus phlebotomy, and (c) chlorambucil plus phlebotomy. Patients treated with phlebotomy alone had an excess mortality within the first 2–4 years, principally due to thrombotic complications. In contrast, those randomized in the two myelosuppression arms of the study suffered from an increased rate of acute leukemia and other malignancies (non-Hodgkin lymphomas (NHL) and neoplasms of the gastrointestinal tract and skin), while the spent phase, with myelofibrosis and myeloid metaplasia, had virtually identical incidence in the three arms. Overall, the median survival was 8.9 years for patients receiving chlorambucil, 11.8 years for those receiving [32]P, and 13.9 years

for those undergoing phlebotomy only. The conclusion of this study was that myelosuppression could reduce the incidence of thrombosis and that chlorambucil had to be replaced by a new agent.

The search for a non-mutagenic myelosuppressive agent led the PVSG to investigate hydroxyurea (HU). This antimetabolite prevents DNA synthesis by inhibiting the enzyme ribonucleoside reductase. Because of its non-alkylating mechanism of action, it has been assumed that it would not be leukemogenic or carcinogenic in patients with PV. The PVSG experience with HU in PV was subsequently updated.[31] Fifty-one patients were followed for a median and a maximum of 8.6 and 15.3 years, respectively. The incidence of acute leukemia, myelofibrosis, and death were compared with the incidence in 134 patients treated with phlebotomy only in the PVSG-01 protocol. There were no statistically significant differences in any of the three parameters, although the HU group showed a tendency to more acute leukemias (9.8% versus 3.7%), less myelofibrosis (7.8% versus 12.7%), and fewer total deaths (39.2% versus 55.2%).

In a randomized clinical trial carried out in France, 292 PV patients aged below 65 years were given HU or pipobroman and were followed from 1980 until 1997.[32] Pipobroman is a bromide derivative of piperazine with a chemical structure related to that of the alkylating agents but whose mechanism of action also involves metabolic competition with pyrimidine bases. No significant differences between the two groups were observed in overall survival, rate of thrombotic complications, and incidence of secondary leukemia (about 5% at the 10th year and 10% at the 13th year). A significant increase in risk of progression to myelofibrosis was seen in the patients treated with HU (26 cases) compared with those treated with pipobroman (3 cases).

Another important issue regards patients who become resistant or develop significant side-effects while taking HU. Various studies, mainly in ET, showed that substituting either alkylating agents or [32]P for HU greatly increases the incidence of leukemic transformation.[33–35] Thus, some anxiety remains about the leukemogenic potential of HU, and this has prompted trials with other agents thought to be less toxic, such as interferon-α or anagrelide (described later in this chapter under ET).

Recombinant interferon-α (IFN-α) is an active agent in PV with antiproliferative activity that is virtually devoid of mutagenic risk.[36] The rationale for the use of this drug includes its myelosuppressive activity and its ability to antagonize the action of platelet-derived growth factor (PDGF), a product of megakaryopoiesis that initiates fibroblast proliferation. This observation would suggest that IFN-α could, theoretically, modify the natural history of PV and reduce or delay the development of myelofibrosis. IFN-α has been evaluated in some phase II studies.[37] The overall results indicate that RCM can be controlled within 6–12 months in up to 70% of cases, as seen by a reduction in the need for phlebotomy. In addition, IFN-α can reverse the associated splenomegaly, leukocytosis, and thrombocytosis in the majority of patients, and is particularly effective for the treatment of generalized pruritus. Side-effects are often a major problem with this drug, causing therapy withdrawal in approximately one-third of patients. Signs of chronic IFN-α toxicity include weakness, myalgia, weight and hair loss, severe depression, and gastrointestinal and cardiovascular toxicity.

These new drugs are of particular interest for the treatment of younger patients with PV, since their prolonged use could theoretically be devoid of leukemogenic risk. However, it should be emphasized that to date the demonstration of their efficacy is based only on secondary endpoints, such as reduction of RCM and platelet count. Their capacity to prevent vascular complications and secondary malignancies and, in turn, to improve the survival of PV patients remains to be established in appropriate clinical trials.

### Antithrombotic therapy

The use of aspirin or other antiplatelet agents in patients with PV and other MPD remains controversial, and the decision rests primarily on the clinical picture.[30] In fact, laboratory tests of platelet function (e.g. bleeding time and platelet aggregation studies), which have been generally unreliable in predicting the risk of bleeding and thrombosis,[38] are of little help.

Aspirin is generally recommended in PV patients who have had recurrent thrombotic complications, particularly those with digital or cerebrovascular occlusive syndromes. On the other hand, the risk of serious bleeding with aspirin use may be elevated in patients with prior histories of bleeding problems, especially of the gastrointestinal tract. Uncertainty reigns for those patients without a clear-cut prior history of bleeding or thrombosis, for whom the benefits and risks of aspirin or related drugs have not yet been evaluated.

The first trial in this field was carried out by the PVSG.[39] They randomized 163 PV subjects to be treated with [32]P or phlebotomy associated with aspirin 900 mg/day plus dipyridamole. After a median follow-up of 1.6 years, six bleeding episodes (mostly gastrointestinal) and seven thrombotic events were observed in the group assigned to antiplatelet therapy, while two thromboses and no bleeding episodes were observed in the other group. For this reason, the study was discontinued and the authors concluded that antiplatelet agents were both ineffective and potentially dangerous in PV patients. However, neither the excess of thrombosis nor that of bleeding was statistically significant, due to the low number of subjects recruited in the trial, and either mere chance or even a moderate imbalance between groups could have been responsible for the results. In addition, the excess of gastrointestinal bleeding was most likely related to the high dose of aspirin used in that study.

A new avenue for exploring the role of aspirin in preventing thrombosis in PV patients would be to decrease the dosage, since lower aspirin doses (30–250 mg/day) are thought to be at least as effective as higher ones and to be better tolerated.[40] With this in mind, the GISP completed a pilot study aimed at assessing the safety of low-dose aspirin (40 mg/day) in PV patients; 326 patients were considered and criteria for exclusion were clear indications (e.g. previous arterial thrombosis) for or against (e.g. gastrointestinal bleeding) aspirin. Thus, 112 (34%) patients were included and randomized to low-dose aspirin or placebo and were followed for more than 12 months. In this pilot study, no differences in side-effects or adverse events were apparent, showing the feasibility of a large-scale evaluation of low-dose aspirin in PV patients.[41]

### Current therapeutic recommendations and future directions

As a general rule, recommendations about the care of an individual patient outside the rigid criteria of clinical trials should derive from the best available evidence combined with clinical experience and practice. As briefly reviewed above, a sound scientific basis for making therapeutic decisions in PV patients is very limited due to the paucity of randomized clinical trials, and this causes uncertainty for the clinician when he or she must select the best available treatment for an individual patient.[42]

The possible leukemogenicity associated with the prolonged use of cytotoxic therapy suggests differentiating treatment primarily according to age.[15] In patients aged under 50 years, phlebotomy alone should be the choice, with the goal of maintaining the hematocrit below 46%. In patients over 70 years old, myelosuppressive therapy is indicated, and [32]P is probably the best therapeutic option. In patients between the ages of 50 and 70 years, there is room for individualization. The administration of HU seems to be justified in the case of frequent phlebotomies or when a previous history of thrombotic events confers a high probability of recurrence. The addition of low-dose aspirin or related drugs should always be considered in the case of cerebrovascular, coronary, or peripheral arterial ischemia.[30] Warfarin should be preferred in patients with recurrent venous thrombosis, even though a protective role for antiplatelet drugs cannot be excluded even in vascular occlusions of the venous tree.[43,44] These guidelines are shared by the majority of experts in this field,[25,45,46] but should be followed with caution in the light of a series of relevant considerations.

First, there are methodological limits to the PVSG-01 trial[15] that represents the cornerstone of the above recommendations. For instance, it was reported that 69 out of 156 patients died in the $^{32}$P group (44%) and 43 out of 132 (32%) died in the group allocated to phlebotomy. Since this difference was not statistically significant, the PVSG conclusion was that survival was the same in the two groups. However, the 28% relative reduction in mortality is not trivial, and one might wonder whether phlebotomy prolongs survival with respect to myelosuppression and whether the trial had the statistical power necessary to detect this potential advantage.[47]

Second, since the major problem with phlebotomy is patient acceptance of this procedure, one could argue about the actual feasibility of this treatment. This was assessed in a cohort of 75 patients randomized to receive only phlebotomy in the context of the PVSG-01 protocol by Najean et al,[48] who reported that phlebotomy had to be stopped after 9 years in almost all patients. The main reasons for this poor compliance were patient refusal, an increase in platelet count, or the development of cardiovascular problems. It is obvious that this observation weakens the conclusions reached in the phlebotomy arm of the PVSG-01 study.

Third, despite concerns about potential leukemogenicity, HU remains the myelosuppressive drug of choice. Unfortunately, at present, no other drugs have shown convincing evidence of efficacy on hard clinical endpoints, such as major thrombosis or survival. We advocate the organization of clinical trials aimed at assessing the role of the new drugs IFN-α or anagrelide in those patients most likely to be exposed to cytoreductive drugs for a long period, such as younger individuals, or in those who become resistant to HU.

Finally, a scientific answer about the efficacy and safety of low-dose aspirin in PV is expected from a large-scale, placebo-controlled clinical trial that is currently ongoing (European Collaboration on Low-Dose Aspirin – the ECLAP study). Until this trial has been completed, we recommend using aspirin in microvascular disturbances of PV, such as erythromelalgia, and in patients with a clear history of arterial thrombosis. This drug might be the cause of severe gastrointestinal bleeding in those individuals with previous episodes of bleeding, and should be considered with great caution in such cases.

# Essential thrombocythemia

## Pathophysiology

ET is a chronic myeloproliferative disorder characterized by sustained elevation of the platelet count, bone marrow hyperplasia, excessive proliferation of megakaryocytes, and a high incidence of thromboembolic complications. It has generally been assumed that ET is a clonal disease state. This was first demonstrated by Fialkow et al,[49] using the X-linked glucose-6-phosphate dehydrogenase (G6PD) locus as a cell marker for clonality. However, more recent studies using X-linked gene techniques such as the HUMARA polymorphism assay[50] showed a much more heterogeneous picture. In an elegant study of 46 patients classified as having ET on the basis of the PVSG diagnostic criteria,[51] HUMARA analysis and other X-chromosomal inactivation assays revealed polyclonal hematopoiesis in 13 patients (28%), clonal hematopoesis in 10 (22%), and an uninterpretable pattern in 23 patients (50%).[52] Patients with a polyclonal pattern had fewer thrombotic complications in comparison with those with monoclonal hematopoiesis. Others have confirmed this clinical correlation,[53] although the retrospective analysis and the small number of patients hitherto evaluated preclude any definite conclusions. These studies have raised serious doubts on the previous understanding of ET as a universally clonal disorder, and emphasize the considerable heterogeneity of this disease.[54]

The concept of 'polyclonal' ET suggests that persistent thrombocytosis may be due to elevation of thrombopoietin (TPO) or other thrombopoietic cytokines. However, serum TPO levels in ET are usually normal or only slightly elevated.[55] Furthermore, circulating TPO levels in ET are not significantly different from those in reactive thrombocytosis.[56] Similarly, mutations in either the TPO gene[57] or its receptor (c-mpl)[58] have not been identified in patients with sporadic ET. In contrast, some familial forms of thrombocytosis are associated with dominant mutations of the TPO gene (5′-untranslated regions of the TPO mRNA involving a donor splice site) that result in enhanced TPO production.[59-61] Several possibilities have been put forward to explain the 'inappropriately' normal or elevated TPO levels in ET. These include ineffective TPO clearance because of markedly reduced c-Mpl expression in platelets and megakaryocytes,[62] increased bone marrow stromal production of TPO,[63] and increased rate of TPO catabolism.[64] The clinical relevance of increased circulating TPO concentration and/or reduced c-Mpl expression is uncertain.[65] In a recent study in patients with ET, a weak heterogeneous expression pattern of c-Mpl in megakaryocytes correlated with thrombotic risk,[66] but this finding remains to be confirmed.

## Diagnostic criteria

The criteria generally accepted for the diagnosis of ET are those suggested by the PVSG[51] and subsequently updated.[33] They are mainly 'exclusion' criteria, developed to rule out other MPD with variable degrees of thrombocytosis, as well as reactive thrombocytosis secondary to chronic inflammatory diseases, malignancy, splenectomy, and iron deficiency. Several investigators have tried to improve the diagnostic criteria for ET by identifying positive markers of the disease. These include spontaneous megakaryocyte or erythroid colony formation, abnormal cytogenetics, and bone marrow histology.

### Spontaneous colony formation

The presence of spontaneous erythroid colony growth and/or colony formation of megakaryocyte progenitors is a strong indicator of ET. The diagnostic value of this test seems to be better when cultures containing plasma or serum are used. Spontaneous colony formation from bone marrow megakaryocyte progenitors was investigated in 24 patients with ET and 20 with reactive thrombocytosis using an in vitro assay containing 30% plasma.[67] Virtually all ET patients, but none of those with reactive thrombocytosis showed spontaneous bone marrow megakaryocyte colony-forming units (CFU-Meg). However, another study[68] demonstrated that a serum-free culture technique, combined with sensitive positive identification of CFU-Meg-derived cells, failed to discriminate between ET and reactive thrombocytosis.

### Cytogenetics

Non-stimulated metaphases obtained from marrow aspirates should be examined for cytogenetic abnormalities. Karyotypic analysis is primarily important in order to exclude the presence of the Philadelphia (Ph) chromosome, the genotypic hallmark of chronic myeloid leukemia (CML). There is some controversy over the proper classification of thrombocytosis associated with the Ph chromosome or its molecular equivalent, the BCR–ABL fusion gene.[69] However, most authors agree that such cases are not clearly distinguishable from CML and should be provisionally classified as CML.[65] Definite cytogenetic abnormalities are rare in Ph- ET, being observed in only 5% of patients at diagnosis. Karyotypic abnormalities generally arise upon transformation of ET to acute leukemia.[13] Deletions or elongations of the short arms of chromosomes 1, 2, 5, 17, 20, and 21 are the most frequent defects.[13] For the majority of these karyotypic abnormalities, the gene or genes responsible for the clinical phenotype in ET are not yet known.

### Bone marrow histology

It has been suggested that ET can be positively diagnosed by careful, quantitative examination of the bone marrow biopsy.[70,71] Typical clustering of enlarged megakaryocytes with multilobulated nuclei has been advocated to represent the hallmark feature of the disease. The histological background of hematopoiesis in ET features a discrete pattern of minimal or no prominence of erythropoiesis, no change in granulopoiesis, almost no fibrosis, and a reduction of stainable iron. A detailed evaluation of bone marrow features may also help to distinguish 'true' ET from the initial stages of idiopathic myelofibrosis[71] or myelodysplasia.[70] 'Early' myelofibrosis is characterized by increasing cellularity with prominent neutrophil granulopoiesis, borderline to slight reticulin fibrosis, and pronounced abnormalities of megakaryocyte differentiation, including hyperchromasia and marked nuclear–cytoplasmatic deviation. Notably, patients with these morphological features frequently develop an overt myelofibrosis and have a significantly worse life-expectancy. However, an experienced observer and a well-standardized procedure are required to diagnose ET by examination of the bone marrow biopsy. This is one of the major limits of the diagnostic classifications of ET based on bone marrow histology.

In summary, positive assays for establishing the presence of ET are promising but still insufficiently standardized to be recommended for diagnostic use in all patients. Despite current limitations, this is an expanding field and it is likely that in due course these tests will complement or substitute the time-honoured PVSG criteria.

### Prognostic factors for bleeding and thrombosis

The search for factors possibly associated with an increased risk of hemostatic complications in ET patients has formed the object of several studies (reviewed in reference 72). However, one limitation on the available information is that these studies are almost always retrospective and the data are generated by evaluation of a relatively small number of patients. This may explain the wide range in hemorrhage (13–63%) and thrombosis (8–84%) observed in cases reported in the literature.

### Bleeding

Risk factors predicting major bleeding and thrombosis were specifically looked for in a cohort study of 100 consecutive patients with ET diagnosed between 1978 and 1988 in our department at the Ospedali Riuniti, Bergamo, Italy and subsequently checked at least every 2 months.[73] The patients received busulfan when platelets exceeded $1000 \times 10^9/l$ and/or when a major thrombotic or hemorrhagic event occurred. Only four major bleeding episodes requiring hospital admission or blood transfusion (gastrointestinal tract and knee hemarthrosis) were registered (0.33%/patient-year (pt-yr)) in that study. Due to the low incidence of major hemorrhagic complications, any prognostic evaluation would be uncertain. In addition, there was no correlation between the broad array of specific structural, biochemical, and metabolic platelet defects and bleeding.[38] Thus, platelet functional tests are not considered good indicators for predicting the hemostatic disturbances in ET. In some particular cases, such as those with platelet counts above $1500 \times 10^9/l$, a decrease in high-molecular-weight multimers of von Willebrand factor may be detected and this might be associated with bleeding symptoms.[74]

## Thrombosis

At variance with a low incidence of major bleeding, 20 thrombotic episodes (17 arterial and 3 venous) were observed (6.6%/pt-yr) in our study.[73] When the incidence of thrombosis was analyzed in individuals at different ages, a rate of 1.7%/pt-yr was found in patients younger than 40 years, versus 6.3%/pt-yr in those aged between 40 and 60 and 15.1%/pt-yr in subjects aged over 60 ($p<0.001$ versus patients older than 40). The rate of thrombosis also increased progressively in relation to previous history of vascular occlusive episodes (from 3.4–31.4%/pt-yr), despite the fact that all these patients were treated with cytoreductive drugs (Table 42.5). Thus, a category of ET patients at increased risk for thrombosis was identified, namely those over 60 years old or with a history of thrombotic events.

## Clinical course of untreated, lower-risk ET patients

Withholding chemotherapy could be justifiable in asymptomatic ET patients under 60 years of age with a platelet count below $1500 \times 10^9/l$, due to their lower risk of developing major bleeding or thrombotic events.

The natural history of untreated, 'lower-risk' ET patients was evaluated in a prospective, controlled study.[75] In this study, 65 ET patients aged below 60 years, with no history of thrombosis or major bleeding and a platelet count below $1500 \times 10^9/l$ were compared with 65 age- and sex-matched normal controls. Patients were not treated with cytoreductive therapy

### Table 42.5 Risk factors for thrombosis in 100 patients with essential thrombocythemia

| Risk factor | Relative risk[a] | p |
|---|---|---|
| Age (years)[b] | | |
| 40–60 | 3.9 (0.7–21.5) | NS |
| >60 | 10.3 (2.1–51.5) | <0.001 |
| Previous thrombosis | 13.0 (4.1–41.5) | <0.0005 |
| Smoking | 0.9 | NS |
| Hyperlipidemia | 0.5 | NS |
| Hypertension | 0.95 | NS |

[a] 95% confidence intervals in parentheses.
[b] Reference category: age <40 years.

until the occurrence of major clinical events. After a median follow-up of 4.1 years, the incidence of thrombosis in patients and controls was 1.91 and 1.5%/pt-year, respectively. The age- and sex-adjusted risk rate ratio was 1.43 (95% confidence interval 0.37–5.4). No major bleeding was observed. This study indicates that the thrombotic risk of young, asymptomatic ET patients is not significantly increased compared with the normal population. These findings have been confirmed in another Italian cohort of 28 patients under 40 years of age followed for a median of 4 years.[76] However, it should be recognized that the number of patients included in these studies is relatively small and further data from large, currently ongoing clinical trials are warranted.

Thrombotic deaths have been reported occasionally in young ET patients,[77] but in general they seem very rare in 'lower-risk' subjects and there are no data showing that fatalities can be prevented by starting cytoreductive drugs early. This point should be considered in the risk/benefit evaluation of cytotoxic, potentially leukemogenic, drugs.

## Management of high-risk ET patients: benefits and risks

### Hydroxyurea

HU has emerged as the treatment of choice in patients with ET because of its convenience in use, its efficacy, and its low acute toxicity.[78] The drug is given at an initial dose of 15–20 mg/kg/day, with adjustments to maintain maximal reduction of platelet values without excessive lowering of white blood cell (WBC) counts. Continuous treatment with HU has been shown to reduce the platelet count to below $500 \times 10^9/l$ within 8 weeks in 80% of patients. Hematopoietic damage leading to leukopenia and megaloblastic anemia is the major short-term toxic effect of HU. Leukopenia is dose-related and quickly reversible if the drug is discontinued. Withdrawal is followed by a rebound of platelet counts, so that continuous treatment is necessary.

Lowering the platelet count by HU is associated with significant improvements in acute ischemic or hemorrhagic symptoms. In a randomized clinical trial, we demonstrated the efficacy of HU in preventing thrombosis in ET patients aged over 60 and/or with a history of previous thrombosis.[78] This trial randomized 114 (35 males and 79 females, median age 68, range 40–85; median platelet count $788 \times 10^9/l$, range $533–1240 \times 10^9/l$) to long-term treatment with HU ($n=56$) or no cytoreductive treatment ($n=58$). During a median follow-up of 27 months, two thromboses (one stroke and one myocardial infarction) were recorded in the HU-treated group (1.6%/pt-yr) versus 14 (one stroke, five transient ischemic attacks, five peripheral arterial occlusions, one deep vein thrombosis, and two superficial thrombophlebites) in the controls (10.7%/pt-yr; *p*=0.003).

It is not known whether ET patients have an inherent tendency to develop acute leukemia. A review of the literature from 1981 to 1994[79] identified a total of 40 Ph- ET cases transformed into acute leukemia after a mean time from presentation of 6.5 years. Two major factors appeared to facilitate blastic transformation: cytogenetic abnormalities[80] and cytotoxic treatments.[33–35] The role of cytotoxic drugs in enhancing the risk of developing hematological complications is one of the major issues currently under discussion in the question of using chemotherapy for ET. HU, as a non-alkylating agent, was initially thought to be non-mutagenic; however, long-term follow-up studies of HU-treated patients with PV and ET revealed that some cases did develope acute leukemia.[34] These reports cast doubts on the innocence of HU in the process of leukemogenicity. Even when used as a single agent in the treatment of PV and ET, the expected rate of acute leukemia is 5–10% and this fatal complication is encountered 4–8 years after the start of treatment. The rate of malignant events might be enhanced in patients given multiple cytotoxic drugs with different mechanisms of action (antimetabolites and alkylating agents).[33,35]

When balancing benefits and risks, one can conclude that there is convincing evidence for giving HU to ET patients at high risk for major thrombotic complications. In contrast, the risk of acute leukemia associated with the use of HU is more difficult to accept in young low-risk individuals. In these cases, thrombosis is expected to occur in 4–5% patients yearly, with only occasional fatal events, and there are no available data on the effectiveness of HU in reducing this rate. The place of new drugs in the management of ET will essentially depend on whether they can be proven to be equally effective and less leukemogenic than HU.

### Anagrelide

The efficacy of anagrelide in ET has been assessed in non-comparative clinical studies.[81] Response was defined as a platelet count under 500 or $600 \times 10^9/l$ or a 50% drop in platelet count. A response rate of 60–93% was reported, irrespectively of age, sex, spleen size, bleeding time, clinical symptoms, or prior treatment. The average dose required to control the platelet count was 2–2.5 mg/day and in most cases the median time for response was 3–4 weeks, although delayed responses up to 24 months were described. Patients refractory to HU responded to anagrelide in 68% of cases. Continuous therapy is required because the platelet count rebounds in a few days after withdrawal of the drug. The most common adverse side-effects of anagrelide are palpitations and tachycardia related to a vasodilative and positive

ionotropic effect. Transient neurological (headache and dizziness) or gastrointestinal (nausea and diarrhea) complications have also been reported. Sudden death was observed in two patients given anagrelide: one death was related to a pulmonary infiltrate and the other to congestive heart failure. Therefore, anagrelide should be used with caution in patients with a history of heart disease.

The long-term efficacy and safety of anagrelide have been analyzed in 37 consecutive young patients with ET (median age 40 years, range 18–49 years) followed in a single institution for a median follow-up period of 10.7 years (range 5.2–13.7 years).[82] The overall response rate was approximately 90% and the reduction of platelet count was sustained in more than 80% of patients. Four patients (11%) discontinued treatment because of toxicity. Most importantly, thrombotic complications while on therapy occurred in seven patients (19%) and major bleeding complications in six (16%). None of the patients developed acute leukemia. Thus, long-term therapy with anagrelide appears to be relatively well-tolerated, but thrombohemorrhagic complications continue to occur despite the control of thrombocytosis.

### Interferon-α

IFN-α is able to reduce the platelet count in patients with ET. With an average dose of about 3 M IU daily, the response rate was about 90%. During maintenance, the IFN-α dose could be tapered, but if IFN-α is suspended, the platelet count rebounds in the majority of patients. Long-term IFN-α treatment is limited by side-effects (see the discussion of therapy of PV above) and the mode of administration. A revision of 273 patients published in the literature[83] showed that IFN-α therapy had to be interrupted in 206 cases (75%). The most common reasons for withdrawal were IFN-α-related side-effects in 55% of cases and patient refusal or loss to follow-up in the other 20%. Thus far, no leukemogenic effects have been observed. As already mentioned for PV, these new drugs are promising cytoreductive agents, but further studies are required to identify their place in the therapy of MPD.

### Anti-aggregation therapy

The use of aspirin is widely accepted in ET patients with microvascular disturbances such as erythromelalgia or transient neurological and ocular ischemias.[84] For these patients, in the absence of contraindications and/or side-effects, the administration of aspirin at a dose of 100–300 mg/day is generally continued indefinitely, since its withdrawal is often associated with relapses of the clinical manifestations. The use of aspirin in ET patients with a history of arterial thrombosis is also becoming a widely accepted practice.[85] In the absence of clinical trials, this recommendation is largely based on the assumption that secondary prevention with aspirin is associated with a risk reduction comparable to that achievable in other clinical settings.[40] However, the enhanced risk of bleeding in ET patients should be appreciated and in each case the risk must be weighed against possible benefits. There is no evidence that other anti-aggregation agents are equally effective or that their addition to aspirin provides further benefit.

## Current therapeutic recommendations and future directions

Convincing evidence is emerging in the literature that the treatment of ET patients should be based primarily on the expected risk of major thrombotic complications. Young asymptomatic subjects with platelet counts in the range of $600-1500 \times 10^9/l$ are at lower risk and can be followed untreated. Nevertheless, it should be emphasized that major thrombotic events can also occur in a small percentage of these 'lower-risk' cases. Future studies should be directed toward identifying other parameters useful for predicting the vascular risk in this particular subset of patients. Furthermore, the risk/benefit ratio of low-dose aspirin in the primary prevention of thrombosis should be tested in appropriate clinical trials.

As far as 'higher-risk' patients are concerned, HU (plus aspirin in the case of ischemia and/or thrombosis) is the treatment of choice because its efficacy in preventing thrombotic complications has been clearly proven. However, the long-term leukemogenicity of this drug, as well as that of other effective cytoreductive agents such as busulfan and pipobroman, remains a major concern. Anagrelide and IFN-α could overcome this worry, but their efficacy has been hitherto demonstrated only in lowering the platelet count, and clinical studies aimed at documenting a clinical benefit as well in ET are urgently needed.

# Myelofibrosis with myeloid metaplasia

MMM is characterized by bone marrow fibrosis and neo-angiogenesis, immature myeloid and erythroid cells in the peripheral blood, anisopoikilocytosis with teardrop erythrocytes, and progressive splenomegaly due to myeloid metaplasia.

## Cellular and molecular pathogenesis

The clonal nature of MMM could be inferred from variable but not random patterns of chromosomal abnormalities and by isoenzyme expression for G6PD, mutations of the *ras* gene family, and restriction fragment X-chromosome DNA polymorphisms.[86] Clonality invariably involves erythroblasts, megakaryocytes, granulocytes, monocytes, and B lymphocytes, indicating that the disorder stems from a pluripotent progenitor.

Bone marrow fibrosis derives from fibroblastic proliferation and increased deposition of connective tissue proteins (collagens, non-collagenous glycoproteins, and basement membrane components). Proliferation of fibroblasts is a secondary event, because fibroblasts do not derive from a totipotent hematopoietic stem cell and because they display no intrinsic alteration.

Humoral factors released from the proliferating myeloid cells and responsible for increased collagen synthesis by bone marrow fibroblasts include platelet-derived growth factor (PDGF), fibroblast growth factors (FGF), platelet factor 4 (PF4), transforming growth factor β (TGF-β), and β-thromboglobulin. TGF-β release is thought to be pivotal, in that it induces the transcription of most of the observed connective tissue proteins.

Abnormalities of packaging and secretion of PDGF, PF4, and TGF-β in megakaryocytes and platelets[87] link megakaryocytes to the pathogenesis of myelofibrosis. The proliferating bone marrow population of monocytes–macrophages has been implicated by the observation that it is responsible for adhesion-mediated overproduction of two fibrogenic cytokines, IL-1 and TGF-β.[88]

Neo-angiogenesis is an integral component of the bone marrow stromal reaction in MMM. The hypothesis is that the bone marrow microenvironment in MMM hosts excess angiogenic cytokines.[89] In fact, increased serum levels of vascular endothelial growth factor (VEGF) in most patients with MMM were demonstrated,[90] and morphometric studies documented increased bone marrow vascularity. According to studies of microvessel density in bone marrow sections, MMM exhibits the most pronounced angiogenesis among MPD.[91] Since the extent of marrow angiogenesis correlates with hematopoietic cellularity and megakaryocyte clumping, neo-angiogenesis could be an integral part of the myeloproliferation in MMM.

The biological and molecular mechanisms responsible for the clonal proliferation in MMM are presently unknown. The characteristic exuberant in vitro 'spontaneous' growth of progenitor cells in the absence of exogenous growth factors classifies MMM as an autocrine-driven disease. A number of growth factor pathways have been investigated and a variety of anomalies detected; however, most of them are common to other MPD and affect a limited number of the cases investigated, suggesting that they are acquired abnormalities in the evolution of the neoplastic clone.

Elevated expression of the stem cell factor (SCF) receptor (c-Kit) and deregulation of the basic FGF (bFGF) pathway in circulating stem cells could provide the reason of the proliferative advantage to the affected clone in the disease. When compared with normal CD34+ progenitors, the expression of bFGF is significantly increased in MMM patients' CD34+ cells, and the density of bFGF type I and type II receptors is significantly augmented.[92] This increased bFGF expression is contrasted by a decreased expression of the receptor for TGF-β, a negative regulator of hematopoiesis.[92]

A truly autonomous megakaryocyte development occurs in MMM, which results neither from mutations or deletions in the coding region of the TPO receptor (c-*mpl*) nor from autocrine stimulation by TPO.[93] Reduced surface expression of the c-Mpl in MMM platelets has been reported, being due to a specific, incompletely processed form of platelet c-Mpl. The defect is associated with a failure to activate the kinase signaling system, with subsequent loss of phosphorylation of the proteins involved in signal transduction, JAK2 and STAT5.[9]

Among recurrent chromosomal abnormalities, deletion of 13q is one of the most frequent, suggesting deletion in a tumor suppressor locus.[94]

Myeloid metaplasia results from extramedullary diffusion of the neoplastic myeloid clone. The evidence that high numbers of CD34+ hematopoietic stem cells circulate in the bloodstream in patients with MMM has favored a model according which hemopoietic stem cells relocalize from bone marrow to extramedullary hematopoietic macroenvironment.[95]

## Clinical features and diagnosis

MMM is a rare disease, with an annual incidence of about 0.5 per 100 000. A slight male preponderance is usually reported and the median age at diagnosis ranges from 54 to 62 years. It has been described in children, and rarely may be familial.

Considerable variability is detected in the hematological features of the disease.[96–99] More than 50% of patients are anemic at diagnosis, and 25% have severe anemia (hemoglobin (Hb) < 8 g/dl). Normocytic anemia is the rule. Mechanisms of anemia include aregenerative, hemodilutional, hemolytic, folate deficiency and iron deficiency. The reticulocyte count is increased in 50% of patients, but ineffective reticulocytosis is present in many cases. In 15% of cases, a polycythemia is manifest, and if the RCM is measured, the percentage of patients with erythrocytosis is still higher.

Circulating erythroblasts range from 0% to 20% at diagnosis and they may constitute more than half of the nucleated cells in peripheral blood after splenectomy. WBC are increased in approximately half of the cases, and in more than 30% circulating blast cells are observed from the diagnosis. Elevated levels of plasma lactate dehydrogenase (LDH) correlate significantly with WBC counts. Thirthy-seven percent of cases present thrombocytopenia at diagnosis, while thrombocytosis is present in 13%. Thrombocytopenia is usually multifactorial in cause, due to both marrow failure and hypersplenism. Serious bleeding complicates MMM in approximately 16% of patients. This may be due to qualitative platelet dysfunctions, inapparent or manifest disseminated intravascular coagulation, or thrombocytopenia.

Fever, weight loss, nocturnal sweating, pruritus, and bone pain are the constitutional symptoms that accompany 40% of patients at diagnosis or during the course of the disease. Immune disorders with the presence of autoimmune phenomenona have been reported. Cutaneous vasculitis, dermatitis resembling Sweet syndrome, and pyoderma gangrenosum have been described. Plasma soluble IL-2 receptor levels were signficantly elevated, suggesting T-cell activation.[100]

Splenomegaly is the cardinal symptom of myeloid metaplasia. It occurs in 97–100% of patients at diagnosis, and is massive in about 10% of them. The liver enlargement is due to extramedullary hematopoiesis, which is associated with increased values of plasma alkaline phosphatase. A variety of symptoms may be due to myeloid metaplasia: intestinal hemorrhage, focal seizures, pulmonary failure, ascites, hematuria, spinal cord compression, testicular enlargement, and papular nodules of the skin.

Bone marrow histological pictures range from highly cellular with fewer fat cells and focal increase of reticulin stroma to absence of normal hematopoiesis with a dense or loose network of reticulin and collagenous fibers. Documentation of histological progression during the course of the disease is scanty, and on sequential studies a relatively constant pattern has been seen throughout the disease.[101] Bony changes that appear radiologically as sclerosis are characteristically seen in half of the patients. The axial skeleton is most frequently involved and osteolytic lesions occur rarely. Increased levels of circulating procollagen III peptide correlate with the extent of fibrosis and the degree of disease activity.

If analyzed singly, there is no one diagnostic finding that can be considered absolutely specific for MMM. Moreover, in MMM, the characteristic lineage proliferation that allows other MPD to be categorized with simple diagnostic criteria is lacking. Thus the PVSG originally identified diagnostic criteria of MMM in: myelofibrosis involving more than one-third of the sectional area of bone marrow biopsy, a leukoerythroblastic blood picture, splenomegaly and absence of the well established diagnostic criteria for the other CMPD (i.e. absence of increased red cell mass or Philadelphia chromosome), with systemic disorders excluded.[102]

More recently, Thiele et al[103] established a set of relevant criteria for the diagnosis of MMM with special regard to its early stages. The authors combined accepted clinical characteristics at diagnosis with corresponding histomorphological findings (the Cologne criteria), in the belief that bone marrow histology is an invaluable aid when attempting to define the different subtypes of MPDs. Megakaryocytes mark MMM by their characteristic bizarre shape with plump lobulation of nuclei and disturbances of nuclear cytoplasmic maturation that create a dysplastic appearance (Table 42.6). These criteria have been accepted in the WHO classification of MMM.[104]

The Italian Cooperative Group on Myeloproliferative Disorders[105] developed a definition of MMM using the evidence and a consensus methodology. This definition of the disease is shown in Table 42.7.

## Prognosis

The course of the disease is highly variable. One-quarter of patients are asymptomatic at diagnosis. Forty percent have progressive splenomegaly with worsening of anemia. A wide variety of complications and associated medical problems emerge during follow-up, including infections, heart failure, and cerebrovascular accidents.

The Median survival time from diagnosis ranges from 3.5 to 5.5 years, and most patients die from infections, hemorrhages, or evolution to acute leukemia. Between 5% and 30% of deaths are due to blastic transformation of the disease, with granulocytic, granulomonocytic, or megakaryocytic type blasts. Predictors of bad prognosis are severe anemia, a large number of immature myeloid cells in peripheral blood, and a clinical picture of erythroid failure. Increased angiogenesis correlates significantly with increased spleen size and has been found to be a significant and independent risk factor for overall survival.[91]

Dupriez et al[106] proposed a score (the LILLE scoring system) that was able to identify three distinct prognostic groups (Table 42.8). In the low-risk group (Hb

---

**Table 42.6  The Cologne criteria for the diagnosis and staging of myelofibrosis with myeloid metaplasia (idiopathic myelofibrosis, IMF)**

A. No preceding or allied other subtype of myeloproliferative disorder or myelodysplastic Syndrome

B. Splenomegaly (on palpation or >11 cm on ultrasound)

C. Thrombocythemia (platelet count $\geq 500 \times 10^9/l$)

D. Anemia (Hb < 12 g/dl)

E. Definite leuko-erythroblastic blood picture

F. Histopathology:
Granulocytic plus megakaryocytic myeloproliferation with large, multilobulated nuclei containing megakaryocytes that show abnormal clustering and definitive maturation defects and:
1. No reticulin fibrosis
2. Slight reticulin fibrosis
3. Marked increase (density) in reticulin fibers or collagen fibrosis (and)
4. Osteosclerosis (endophytic bone formation)

Diagnosis and classification of IMF is acceptable if the following combinations are present:
Stage 1. A+B+C+F$_1$ is consistent with a hypercellular (prefibrotic) stage clinically simulating essential thrombocythemia
Stage 2. A+B+C+D+F$_2$ is consistent with early IMF
Stage 3. A+B+D+F$_3$ is consistent with manifest IMF
Stage 4. A+B+D+E+F$_{3+4}$ is consistent with advanced IMF complicated by osteosclerosis (osteomyelosclerosis)

---

**Table 42.7  The Italian criteria for the diagnosis of myelofibrosis with myeloid metaplasia**

**Necessary criteria**
A. Diffuse bone marrow fibrosis

B. Absence of Philadelphia chromosome or BCR–ABL rearrangement in peripheral blood cells

**Optional criteria**
1. Splenomegaly of any grade
2. Anisopoikilocytosis with teardrop erythrocytes
3. Presence of circulating immature myeloid cells

4. Presence of circulating erythroblasts
5. Presence of clusters of megakaryoblasts and anomalous megakaryocytes in bone marrow sections
6. Myeloid metaplasia

Diagnosis of MMM is acceptable if the following combinations are present:
• The two necessary criteria plus any two optional criteria when splenomegaly is present
• The two necessary criteria plus any four optional criteria when splenomegaly is absent

**Table 42.8  The LILLE scoring system for predicting survival in myelofibrosis with myeloid metaplasia**

**Adverse prognostic factors**
Hb<10 g/dl
WBC <4 or >30 × 10⁹/L

**Scoring system** (number of adverse prognostic factors).

| No. of factors | Risk group | Median survival (months) |
|---|---|---|
| 0 | Low | 93 |
| 1 | Intermediate | 26 |
| 2 | High | 13 |

>10 g/dl and WBC between 4×10⁹/l and 30×10⁹/l), patients had a median survival of 93 months, whereas those in the intermediate-risk (Hb <10 g/dl or WBC < 4×10⁹/l or >30×10⁹/l) and high-risk (Hb <10 g/dl and WBC <4×10⁹/l or >30×10⁹/l) groups had median survivals of 26 and 13 months, respectively. A previously reported subgroup analysis of patients allowed Morel et al[107] to document that the disease was less frequently aggressive based on the LILLE score in patients younger than 55 years.

More recently, in a European collaboration study on 121 patients aged 55 years or less,[108] the median survival was 128 months, i.e. more than twice that reported in recent comprehensive series of MMM patients. Anemia, the presence of constitutional symptoms, and circulating blasts were the three presenting features associated with survival. These prognostic factors allowed separation of low-risk and high-risk groups among young patients. The former, with none or only one poor prognostic factor, included three-quarters of patients and had a median survival of more than 14 years, whereas the latter, with two or three poor prognostic factors, contained one-quarter of the patients, with a median survival of less than 3 years.

**Therapy**

At present, ablation of the abnormal hematopoietic clone with high-dose chemotherapy and allogeneic stem cell transplantation (SCT) is the only chance to achieve a cure in MMM. A report of a collaborative study including 55 patients (39 males and 16 females) evaluated the results of allogeneic SCT in patients with MMM on a larger scale.[109] An HLA-matched related donor was used in most cases, whereas in 6 cases the graft was harvested from HLA-mismatched related or three-loci-matched unrelated donors. Hematopoietic recovery was reached in 50 out of the

55 patients. Factors associated with a shorter time to reach the neutrophil engraftment endpoint (an absolute neutrophil count (ANC) of at least 0.5 × 10⁹/l) were splenectomy, absence of grade III myelofibrosis, and a high number of nucleated cells infused. Splenectomy and the absence of grade III myelofibrosis were also factors associated with a shorter time to achieve the platelet recovery endpoint (a platelet count of 50×10⁹/l). Out of 55 patients, 5 (9.1%) died early after SCT of primary graft failure, secondary graft failure, or transplantation-related complications. Among the 50 evaluable patients, 22 had grade 0–I, 15 grade II, and 13 grade III–IV acute graft-versus-heart disease (GVHD). Among 44 evaluable patients, 27 experienced chronic GVHD. Nineteen patients achieved complete histo-hematological remission. Resolution of myelofibrosis occurred between 21 days and 23 months after transplant. Seven patients showed evidence of relapse, which occurred at a median time of 12 months.

Overall, 43.6% of patients died, the causes of death being infections, chronic GVHD, acute GVHD, disease progression, solid organ failure, lymphoproliferative disorders, and graft failure. The Kaplan–Meier estimate of survival at 5 years was 49%, with a 57% survival rate for patients receiving an unmanipulated HLA-matched related graft (n=44). Hemoglobin greater than 10 g/dl at the time of transplant and the absence of grade III myelofibrosis were significantly associated with a better outcome.

No medical therapy has proven to have an effect on overall patient survival, and the therapeutic strategies are mainly aimed at maintaining quality of life. Patients with an intact quality of life and with no threatening erythrocytosis or thrombocytosis do not need any treatment.

Anemia deserves therapeutical consideration when it is symptomatic or progressively worsening. Aregenerative anemia responds to androgens (oxymetholone, fluoxymesterolone, methandrostenolone, testosterone enanthate, and danazol) in approximately 30–40% of cases.[110] Studies on the use of recombinant human erythropoietin (rHuEPO) in MMM have been reviewed in a total of 32 patients.[111] Overall, 53% of them responded to rHuEPO treatment, but the vast majority of responders were not transfusion-dependent and the doses required to achieve response varied from 300 to 1500 U/kg per week. Factors predicting response include serum erythropoietin level below 123 mU/ml, female gender, and none or mild transfusion requirement. In some patients, aggravation of splenomegaly due to stimulation of extramedullary erythropoiesis led to withdrawal of the drug.

An elevated platelet count (>600×10⁹/l), as after splenectomy, represents a major risk factor for thrombosis and hemorrhage. Therefore, patients with a number of platelets greater than $600 \times 10^9/l$ have to be treated. HU is the drug of first choice. The recommended starting dose is 1500 mg/day, and 500 mg/day as maintenance. The possible carcinogenic potential of HU becomes important in young people (<45 years old), who have the longest life-expectancy. In these cases (INF-$\alpha$) is a valuable alternative to cytostatic therapy.[112] Hematological responses have been seen in 50% of patients – usually those with a hyperproliferative type of disease. A reasonable starting dose is 5 MIU subcutaneously three to five times per week. Long-term control can be obtained with a well-tolerated lower dose.

With the aim of taking advantage mainly of its antiangiogenetic effect, and thus improving the microenvironment and hematopoietic cell maturation in the bone marrow and extramedullary sites, trials have determined the effect of thalidomide in patients with MMM. In a pooled analysis, updated data on 62 individual patients from five phase II trials were reported.[113] Overall, using a standard dose of thalidomide (i.e. starting with no less than 100 mg/day), 29% of patients with moderate to severe anemia showed an increase in hemoglobin or a reduction/abolition of blood transfusion requirements, 38% with moderate to severe thrombocytopenia had an increase in platelet count, and 41% with high-grade splenomegaly demonstrated a measurable reduction in spleen size. Major disease severity and high degrees of splenomegaly before therapy predicted response with a probability of 61.9%. However, 18% of the patients had a 'myeloproliferative reaction' with leukocytosis and/or thrombocytosis. Sixty-six percent of patients discontinued the drug before 6 months of treatment due to intolerance.

A progressively enlarging painful spleen with severe anemia and/or thrombocytopenia requires a choice between splenectomy and medical treatment. The decision depends on the trade-off between the risk of and the benefits from the operation, and at present no clear guidelines can be provided to help resolve this dilemma. Single-institution experiences in Italy[114] and the USA[115] (71 patients and 223 patients, respectively) showed 8.4–9% mortality and 31–39.3% morbidity rates. New hemorrhagic or thrombotic complications occurred in 16.9% of surviving patients, and were predicted by an age less than 50 years, a normal to high platelet count ($>200\times10^9/l$), and huge splenomegaly (>16 cm from the costal margin). There was a substantial improvement in anemia in 45% and 52% of patients at 3 months and 1 year, respectively, which was predicted by severe anemia, low platelet count ($<100\times10^9/l$), or normal to high WBC count ($>4\times10^9/l$). Postsurgical thrombocytosis of over $600 \times10^9/l$ or over $1000 \times 10^9/l$ was observed in 20.2% and 5.8% of patients, respectively, and was predicted by a platelet count greater than $50\times10^9/l$. Massive liver enlargement occurred in 24% of patients. An increased frequency of symptomatic or asymptomatic portal or splenic venous thrombosis warrants routine surveillance imaging with ultrasonography.

In a paper on 549 patients with primary MMM collected in a collaborative study group comprising 13 large hospitals in Italy,[116] splenectomy was reported to be an independent risk factor for blast transformation. The cumulative incidence of blast transformation was 27% in non-splenectomized patients and 55% in splenectomized patients 12 years after diagnosis. The overall median survival was 2.0 years (range 0–12.9) from the time of splenectomy.

## REFERENCES

1. Bench AJ, Green AR, Huntly BJP, Natcheva EP. The cellular and genetic pathology of polycythemia vera. In: *Hematology 2000, ASH Education Program Book*: 56–61.

2. Prchal JT. Pathogenetic mechanisms of polycythemia vera and congenital polycythemic disorders. *Semin Hematol* 2001; **38**(Suppl 2): 10–20.

3. De La Chapelle A, Traskelin AL, Juvonen E. Truncated erythropoietin receptor causes dominantly inherited benign human erythrocytosis. *Proc Natl Acad Sci USA* 1993; **90**: 4495–9.

4. Sokol L, Luhovi M, Yongli G et al. Primary familial polycythemia: a frameshift mutation in the erythropoietin receptor gene and increased sensitivity of erythroid progenitors to erythropoietin. *Blood* 1995; **86**: 15–22.

5. Hess G, Rose P, Gamm H et al. Molecular analysis of erythropoietin receptor system in polycythemia vera. *Br J Haematol* 1994; **88**: 794–802.

6. Dai CH, Krantz SB, Dessypris EN et al. Polychemia vera, II: hypersensitivity of bone-marrow erythroid, granulocyte–macrophage and megakaryocyte progenitor cells to interleukin-3 and granulocyte–macrophage colony-stimulating factor. *Blood* 1992; **80**: 891–9.

7. Correa PN, Eskinazi D, Axelrad AA. Circulating erythroid progenitors in polycythemia vera are hypersensitive to insulin-like growth factor-1 in vitro: studies in an improved serum-free medium. *Blood* 1994; **83**: 99–112.

8. Martin JM, Gandhi K, Jackson WR, Dessypris EN. Hypersensitivity of polycythemia vera megakaryocytes progenitors to thrombopoietin. *Blood* 1996; **88**: 94a.

9. Moliterno AR, Hankins WD, Spivak JL. Impaired expression of the thrombopoietin receptor by platelets from patients with polycythemia vera. *N Engl J Med* 1998; **338**: 572–80.

10. Silva M, Richard C, Benito A et al. Expression of Bcl-x in erythroid precursors from patients with polycythemia vera. *N Engl J Med* 1998; **338**: 564.

11. Lui Q, Schacher D, Hurth C et al. Activation of phosphatidylinositol 3'-kinase by insulin-like growth factor 1 rescues promyeloid cells from apoptosis and permits their differentiation into granulocytes. *J Immunol* 1997; **159**: 829.

12. Temerinac S, Klippel S, Strunck E et al. Cloning of PRV-1, a novel member of the uPAR receptor superfamily, which is overexpressed in polycythemia rubra vera. *Blood* 2000; **95**: 2569–76.

13. Bench AJ, Nacheva EP, Champion KM, Green AR. Molecular genetics and cytogenetics of myeloproliferative disorders. *Baillière's Clin Hematol* 1998; **11**: 819–48.

14. Asimakopoulos FA, White NJ, Nacheva E, Green AR. Molecular analysis of chromosome 20q deletions associated with myeloproliferative disorders or myelodysplastic syndromes. *Blood* 1994; **84**: 3086–94.

15. Berk PD, Goldberg JD, Donovan PB et al. Therapeutic recommendations in polycythemia vera based on Polycythemia Vera Study Group protocols. *Semin Hematol* 1986; **23**: 132–43.

16. Blacklock HA, Royle GA. Idiopathic erythrocytosis – a declining entity. *Br J Haematol* 2001; **115**: 774–81.

17. Pearson TC, Messinezy M, Westwood N. Evaluation of current diagnostic pathways in the erythrocytosis. In: *Hematology 2000, ASH Education Program Book*: 51–6.

18. Pearson TC, Guthrie DL, Simpson J et al. Interpretation of measured red cell mass and plasma volumes in adults. *Br J Haematol* 1995; **89**: 748–56.

19. Swolin B, Weinfeld A, Westin J. A prospective long-term cytogenetic study in polycythemia vera in relation to treatment and clinical course. *Blood* 1988; **72**: 386–95.

20. Lemoine F, Najman A, Baillou C et al. A prospective study of the value of bone marrow erythroid progenitor cultures in polycythemia. *Blood* 1986; **68**: 996–1002.

21. Shih LY, Lee CT. Identification of masked polycythemia vera from patients with idiopathic marked thrombocytosis by endogenous erythroid colony assay. *Blood* 1994; **83**: 744–8.

22. Najman A. The diagnostic value of erythoid progenitors culture in polycythemia vera. *Nouv Rev Fr Hematol* 1994; **36**: 177–8.

23. Cotes PM, Doré CJ, Liu Yin JA et al. Determination of serum immunoreactive erythropoietin in the investigation of erythrocytosis. *N Engl J Med* 1986; **315**: 283–7.

24. Najean Y, Schlageter MH, Toubert ME, Podgorniak MP. Radioimmunoassay of immunoreactive erythropoietin as a clinical tool for the classification of polycythemias. *Nouv Rev Fr Hematol* 1990; **32**: 237–40.

25. Bilgrami S, Greenberg BR. Polycythemia rubra vera. *Semin Oncol* 1995; **22**: 307–26.

26. Gruppo Italiano Studio Policitemia (GISP). Polycythemia vera: the natural history of 1213 patients followed over 20 years. *Ann Int Med* 1995; **123**: 656–64.

27. Gilbert HS. Familial myeloproliferative disease. *Baillière's Clin Hematol* 1998; **11**: 849–58.

28. Anderson JE, Sale G, Appelbaum FR et al. Allogenic bone marrow transplantation for primary myelofibrosis and myelofibrosis secondary to polycythemia vera or essential thrombocytosis. *Br J Haematol* 1997; **98**: 1010–16.

29. Rozman C, Giralt M, Feliu E et al. Life expectancy of patients with chronic nonleukemic myeloproliferative disorders. *Cancer* 1991; **67**: 2658–63.

30. Barbui T, Finazzi G. The basis of current management strategies and future perspectives in polycythemia vera. In: *Hematology 2000, ASH Education Program Book*: 61–8.

31. Fruchtman SM, Mack K, Kaplan ME et al. From efficacy to safety: a Polycythemia Vera Study Group report on hydroxyurea in patients with polycythemia vera. *Semin Hematol* 1997; **34**: 17.

32. Najean Y, Rain JD, for the French Polycythemia Study Group. Treatment of polycythemia vera: use of $^{32}$P alone or in combination with maintenance therapy using hydroxyurea in 461 patients greater than 65 years of age. *Blood* 1997; **89**: 2319–27.

33. Murphy S, Peterson P, Iland H et al. Experience of the Polycythemia Vera Study Group with essential thrombocythemia: a final report on diagnostic criteria, survival and leukemic transition by treatment. *Semin Hematol* 1997; **34**: 29–39.

34. Sterkers Y, Preudhomme C, Lai J-L et al. Acute myeloid leukemia and myelodysplastic syndromes following essential thrombocythemia treated with hydroxyurea: high proportion of cases with 17p deletion. *Blood* 1998; **91**: 616–22.

35. Finazzi G, Ruggeri M, Rodeghiero F, Barbui T. Second malignancies in patients with essential thrombocythemia treated with busulphan and hydroxyurea: long-term follow-up of a randomized clinical trial. *Br J Haematol* 2000; **110**: 577–83.

36. Silver RT. Interferon α2b: a new treatment for polycythemia vera. *Ann Intern Med* 1993; **119**: 1091–2.

37. Lengfelder E, Berger U, Hehlmann R. Interferon α in the treatment of polycythemia vera. *Ann Hematol* 2000; **79**: 103–9.

38. Finazzi G, Budde U, Michiels JJ. Bleeding time and platelet function in myeloproliferative disorders. *Leuk Lymphoma* 1996; **22**(Suppl 1): 87–94.

39. Tartaglia AP, Goldberg JD, Berk PD, Wasserman LR. Adverse effects of antiaggregating platelet therapy in the treatment of polycythemia vera. *Semin Hematol* 1986; **23**: 172–6.

40. Patrono C, Coller B, Dalen JE et al. Platelet-active drugs: the relationships among dose, effectiveness and side effects. *Chest* 2001; **119**(Suppl): 39S–63S.

41. Gruppo Italiano Studio Policitemia (GISP). Low-dose aspirin in polycythemia vera: a pilot study. *Br J Haematol* 1997; **97**: 453–6.

42. Streiff MB, Smith B, Spivak JL. The diagnosis and management of polycythemia vera in the era since the Polycythemia Vera Study Group: a survey of American Society of Hematology members' practice patterns. *Blood* 2002; **99**: 1144–9.

43. Pulmonary Embolism Prevention (PEP) Trial Collaborative Group. Prevention of pulmonary embolism and deep vein thrombosis with low-dose aspirin: Pulmonary Embolism Prevention (PEP) trial. *Lancet* 2000; **355**: 1295–302.

44. Antiplatelet Trialists' Collaboration. Collaborative overview of randomised trials of antiplatelet therapy – III: Reduction in venous thrombosis and pulmonary embolism by antiplatelet prophylaxys among surgical and medical patients. *BMJ* 1994; **308**: 235–46.

45. Tefferi A, Silverstein MN. Treatment of polycythemia vera and essential thrombocythemia. *Baillière's Clin Hematol* 1998; **11**: 769–86.

46. Spivak JL. The optimal management of polycythemia vera. *Br J Haematol* 2002; **116**: 243–54.

47. Marchioli R, Landolfi R, Barbui T, Tognoni G. Feasibility of randomized trials in rare diseases: the case of polycythemia vera. *Leuk Lymphoma* 1996; **22**(Suppl 1): 87–94.

48. Najean Y, Dresch C, Rain JD. The very long course of polycythemia: a complement to the previously published data of the Polycythemia Vera Study Group. *Br J Haematol* 1994; **86**: 233–5.

49. Fialkow PJ, Faguet GB, Jacobson RJ et al. Evidence that essential thrombocythemia is a clonal disorder with origin in a multipotent cell. *Blood* 1981; **58**: 916–19.

50. Gale RE, Mein CA, Linch DC. Quantification of X-chromosome inactivation patterns in haematological samples using the DNA-based HUMARA assay. *Leukemia* 1996; **10**: 362.

51. Murphy S, Iland H, Rosenthal D, Laszlo J. Essential thrombocythemia: an interim report from the Polycythemia Vera Study Group. *Semin Hematol* 1986; **23**: 177–82.

52. Harrison CN, Gale RE, Machin SJ, Linch DC. A large proportion of patients with a diagnosis of essential thrombocythemia do not have a clonal disorder and may be at lower risk of thrombotic complications. *Blood* 1999; **93**: 417–24.

53. Chiusolo P, La Barbera EO, Laurenti L et al. Clonal hemopoiesis and risk of thrombosis in young female patients with essential thrombocythemia. *Exp Hematol* 2001; **29**: 670–6.

54. Nimer SD. Essential thrombocythemia: another 'heterogeneous disease' better understood? *Blood* 1999; **93**: 417.

55. Wang JC, Chen C, Novetsky AD et al. Blood thrombopoietin levels in clonal thrombocytosis and reactive thrombocytosis. *Am J Med* 1998; **104**: 451–5.

56. Espanol I, Hernadez A, Cortes M et al. Patients with thrombocytosis have normal or slightly elevated thrombopoietin levels. *Haematologica* 1999; **84**: 312–16.

57. Harrison CN, Gale RE, Wiestner AC et al. The activation splice mutation in intron 3 of the thrombopoietin gene is not found in patients with non-familial essential thrombocythemia. *Br J Haematol* 1998; **102**: 1341–3.

58. Kiladijan JJ, El Kassar N, Hetet G et al. Study of the thrombopoietin receptor in essential thrombocythemia. *Leukemia* 1997; **11**: 1821–6.

59. Kondo T, Okabe M, Sanada M et al. Familial essential thrombocythemia associated with one-base deletion in the 5′-untranslated region of the thrombopoietin gene. *Blood* 1998; **92**: 1091–6.

60. Wiestner A, Schlemper RJ, van der Maas et al. An activating splice donor mutation in the thrombopoietin gene causes hereditary thrombocythemia. *Nat Genet* 1998; **18**: 49–52.

61. Ghilardi N, Wiestner A, Kikuchi M et al. Hereditary thrombocythemia in a Japanese family is caused by a point mutation in the thrombopoietin gene. *Br J Haematol* 1999; **107**: 310–16.

62. Horikawa Y, Matsamura I, Hashimoto K et al. Markedly reduced expression of platelet c-mpl receptor in essential thrombocythemia. *Blood* 1997; **90**: 4031–8.

63. Sakamaki S, Hirayama Y, Matsunaga T et al. Transforming growth factor-$\beta_1$ (TGF-$\beta_1$) induces thrombopoietin from bone marrow stromal cells, which stimulates the expression of TGF-$\beta$ receptor on megakaryocytes and, in turn, renders them susceptible to suppression by TGF-$\beta$ itself with high specificity. *Blood* 1999; **94**: 1961–70.

64. Axelrad AA, Eskinazi D, Correa PN et al. Hypersensitivity of circulating progenitor cells to megakaryocyte growth and development factor (PEG-rHuMGDF) in essential thrombocythemia. *Blood* 2000; **96**: 3310–21.

65. Steensma DP, Tefferi A. Cytogenetics and molecular genetic aspects of essential thrombocythemia. *Acta Haematol* 2002; **108**: 55–65.

66. Teofili L, Pierconti F, Di Febo A et al. The expression pattern of c-mpl in megakaryocytes correlates with thrombotic risk in essential thrombocythemia. *Blood* 2002; **100**: 714–17.

67. Rolovic Z, Basara N, Gotic M et al. The determination of spontaneous colony formation is an unequivocal test for discriminating between essential thrombocythemia and reactive thrombocytosis. *Br J Haematol* 1995; **90**: 326–31.

68. Sawyer BM, Westwood NB, Pearson TC. Circulating megakaryocyte progenitor cells in patients with primary thrombocythemia and reactive thrombocytosis: results using a serum-deprived culture assay and positive detection technique. *Eur J Hematol* 1994; **53**: 108–13.

69. Blickstein D, Aviram A, Luboshitz M et al. BCR–ABL transcripts in bone marrow aspirates of Philadelphia-negative essential thrombocythemia patients: clinical presentation. *Blood* 1997; **190**: 2768–71.

70. Annaloro C, Lambertenghi-Deliliers G, Oriani A et al. Prognostic significance of bone marrow biopsy in essential thrombocythemia. *Haematologica* 1999; **84**: 17–21.

71. Thiele J, Kvaniscka HM, Zankovich R et al. Relevance of bone marrow features in the differential diagnosis between essential thrombocythemia and early stage idiopathic myelofibrosis. *Haematologica* 2000; **85**: 1126–34.

72. Barbui T, Finazzi G. The management of essential thrombocythemia. *Crit Rev Oncol Hematol* 1999; **29**: 257–66.

73. Cortelazzo S, Viero P, Finazzi G et al. Incidence and risk factors for thrombotic complications in a historical cohort of 100 patients with essential thrombocythemia. *J Clin Oncol* 1990; **8**: 556–62.

74. van Genderen PJJ, Michiels JJ, van der Poel-van de Luytgaarde SCPAM, van Vliet HHDM. Acquired von Willebrand disease as a cause of recurrent mucocutaneous bleeding in primary thrombocythemia: relationship with platelet count. *Ann Hematol* 1994; **69**: 81–4.

75. Ruggeri M, Finazzi G, Tosetto A et al. No treatment for low risk thrombocythemia: results from a prospective study. *Br J Haematol* 1998; **103**: 772–7.

76. Randi ML, Luzzatto G, Fabris F. Low-risk thrombocythemia in patients younger than 40. *Br J Haematol* 1999; **104**: 928–36.

77. Mitus AJ, Barbui T, Shulman LN. Hemostatic complications in young patients with essential thrombocythemia. *Am J Med* 1990; **88**: 371–5.

78. Cortelazzo S, Finazzi G, Ruggeri M et al. Hydroxyurea in the treatment of patients with essential thrombocythemia at high risk of thrombosis: a prospective randomized trial. *N Engl J Med* 1995; **332**: 1132–6.

79. Shibata K, Shimamoto Y, Suga K et al. Essential thrombocythemia terminating in acute leukemia with minimal myeloid differentiation. A brief review of recent literature. *Acta Haematol* 1994; **91**: 84–8.

80. Lofvenberg E, Nordenson I, Walhlin A. Cytogenetic abnormalities and leukemic transformation in hydroxyurea-treated patients with Philadelphia chromosome negative chronic myeloproliferative disease. *Cancer Genet Cytogenet* 1990; **49**: 57–67.

81. Anagrelide Study Group. Anagrelide, a therapy for thrombocythemic states: experience in 577 patients. *Am J Med* 1992; **92**: 69–76.

82. Storen EC, Tefferi A. Long-term use of anagrelide in young patients with essential thrombocythemia. *Blood* 2001; **97**: 863–6.

83. Lengfelder E, Griesshammer M, Hehlmann R. Interferon-$\alpha$ in the treatment of essential thrombocythemia. *Leuk Lymphoma* 1996; **22**(Suppl 1): 135–42.

84. Michiels JJ, Koudstaal PJ, Mulder AH, van Vliet HHDM. Transient neurologic and ocular manifestations in primary thrombocythemia. *Neurology* 1993; **43**: 1107–10.

85. Landolfi R, Patrono C. Aspirin in polycythemia vera and essential thrombocythemia: current facts and perspectives. *Leuk Lymphoma* 1996; **22**(Suppl 1): 83–6.

86. Kreipe H, Jaquet K, Felgner J et al. Clonal granulocytes and bone marrow cells in the cellular phase of agnogenic myeloid metaplasia. *Blood* 1991; **78**: 1814–17.

87. Martyré MC, Magdelenat H, Bryckaert MC et al. Increased intrapletelet levels of platelet-derived growth factor and transforming growth factor-β in patients with myelofibrosis and myeloid metaplasia. *Br J Haematol* 1991; **77**: 80–6.

88. Rameshwar P, Denny TN, Stein D, Gascon P. Monocyte adhesion in patients with bone marrow fibrosis is required for the production of fibrogenic cytokines. Potential role for interleukin-1 and TGF-β. *J Immunol* 1994; **153**: 2819–30.

89. Pruneri G, Bertolini F, Soligo D et al. Angiogenesis in myelodysplastic syndromes. *Br J Cancer* 1999; **81**: 1398–401.

90. Di Raimondo F, Azzaro MP, Palumbo GA et al. Elevated vascular andothelial growth factor (VEGF) serum levels in idiopathic myelofibrosis. *Leukemia* 2001; **15**: 976–80.

91. Mesa RA, Hanson CA, Rajkumar SV et al. Evaluation and clinical correlations of bone marrow angiogenesis in myelofibrosis with myeloid metaplasia. *Blood* 2000; **96**: 3374–80.

92. Le Bousse-Kerdilès M-C, Chevillard S, Charpentier A et al. Differential expression of transforming growth factor-b, basic fibroblast growth factor, and their receptors in CD34+ hematopoietic progenitor cells from patients with myelofibrosis with myeloid metaplasia. *Blood* 1996; **88**: 4534–46.

93. Taksin AL, Le Couedic J-P, Dusanter-Fourt I et al. Autonomous megakaryocyte growth in essential thrombocythemia and idiopathic myelofibrosis is not related to a c-mpl mutation or to an autocrine stimulation by Mpl-L. *Blood* 1999; **93**: 125–39.

94. Pastore C, Nomdedeu J, Volpe G et al. Genetic analysis of chromosome 13 deletions in *BCR/ABL* negative chronic myeloproliferative disorders. *Genes Chromosomes Cancer* 1995; **14**: 106–11.

95. Barosi G, Viarengo G, Pecci A et al. Diagnostic and clinical relevance of the number of circulating CD34+ cells in myelofibrosis with myeloid metaplasia. *Blood* 2001; **98**: 3249–55.

96. Barosi G, Berzuini C, Liberato LN et al. A prognostic classification of myelofibrosis with myeloid metaplasia. *Br J Haematol* 1988; **70**: 397–401.

97. Visani G, Finelli C, Castelli U et al. Myelofibrosis with myeloid metaplasia: clinical and haematological parameters predicting survival in a series of 133 patients. *Br J Haematol* 1990; **75**: 4–9.

98. Hasselbalch H. Idiopathic myelofibrosis: a clinical study of 80 patients. *Am J Hematol* 1990; **34**: 291–300.

99. Rupoli S, Da Lio L, Sisti S et al. Primary myelofibrosis: a detailed statistical analysis of the clinicopathological variables influencing survival. *Ann Hematol* 1994; **68**: 205–12.

100. Wang JC, Wang A. Plasma soluble interleukin-2 receptor in patients with primary myelofibrosis. *Br J Haematol* 1994; **86**: 380–2.

101. Thiele J, Chen YS, Kvasnicka HM et al. Evolution of fibro-osteosclerotic bone marrow lesions in primary (idio-

pathic) osteomyelofibrosis. A histomorphometric study on sequential trephine biopsies. *Leuk Lymphoma* 1994; **14**: 163–9.

102. Laszlo J. Myeloproliferative disorders (MPD): myelofibrosis, myelosclerosis, extramedullary hematopoiesis, undifferentiated MPD, and hemorrhagic thrombocythemia. *Semin Hematol* 1975; **2**: 409–32.

103. Thiele J, Kvasnicka HM, Diehl V et al. Clinicopathological diagnosis and differential criteria of thrombocythemias in various myeloproliferative disorders by histopathology, histochemistry and immunostaining from the bone marrow. *Leuk Lymphoma* 1999; **33**: 207–18.

104. Thiele J, Pierre R, Imbert M et al. Chronic idiopathic myelofibrosis. In: Jaffe ES, Harris NL, Stein H, Vardiman JW (eds) *World Health Organization Classification of Tumours. Puthology and Genetics of Tumours of Haematopoietic and Lymphoid Tissues.* Lyon: IARC Press, 2001: 35–8.

105. Barosi G, Liberato LN, Grossi A et al. The Italian Consensus Conference on diagnostic criteria for myelofibrosis with myeloid metaplasia. *Br J Haematol* 1999; **104**: 730–7.

106. Dupriez B, Morel P, Demory JL et al. Prognostic factors in agnogenic myeloid metaplasia: a report on 195 cases with a new scoring system. *Blood* 1996; **88**: 1013–18.

107. Morel P, Demory JL, Dupriez B. Relevance of prognostic features in myeloid metaplasia to selection of patients for bone marrow transplantation. *Blood* 1997; **89**: 2219–28.

108. Cervantes F, Barosi G, Demory J-L et al. Myelofibrosis with myeloid metaplasia in young individuals: disease characteristics, prognostic factors and identification of risk groups. *Br J Haematol* 1998; **102**: 684–90.

109. Guardiola P, Anderson JE, Bandini G et al. Allogeneic stem cell transplantation for agnogenic myeloid metaplasia: a European Group for Blood and Marrow Transplantation, Societé Française de Greffe de Moelle, Gruppo Italiano per il Trapianto del Midollo Osseo, and Fred Hutchinson Cancer Research Center Collaborative Study. *Blood* 1999; **93**: 2831.

110. Cervantes F, Hernandez-Boluda JC, Alvarez A et al. Danazol treatment of idiopathic myelofibrosis with severe anemia. *Haematologica* 2000; **85**: 595–9.

111. Rodriguez JN, Martino ML, Dieguez JC et al. rHuEpo for the treatment of anemia in myelofibrosis with myeloid metaplasia. Experience in 6 patients and meta-analytical approach. *Haematologica* 1998; **83**: 616–21.

112. Gilbert HS. Long term treatment of myeloproliferative disease with interferon-α2b: feasibility and efficacy. *Cancer* 1998; **15**: 1205–13.

113. Barosi G, Elliott M, Canepa L et al. Thalidomide in myelofibrosis with myeloid metaplasia: a pooled-analysis of individual patient data from 5 studies. *Leuk Lymphoma* (in press).

114. Barosi G, Ambrosetti A Buratti A et al. Splenectomy for patients with myelofibrosis with myeloid metaplasia. Pretreatment variables and outcome prediction. *Leukemia* 1993; **7**: 200–6.

115. Tefferi A, Mesa RA, Nagorney DM et al. Splenectomy in myelofibrosis with myeloid metaplasia: a single-institution experience with 223 patients. *Blood* 2000; **95**: 2226–33.

116. Barosi G, Ambrosetti A, Centra A et al. Splenectomy and risk of blast transformation in myelofibrosis with myeloid metaplasia. *Blood* 1998; **91**: 3630–6.

# 43 Late effects after treatment for Hodgkin lymphoma

## Anthony J Swerdlow and Flora E van Leeuwen

## Introduction

As described elsewhere in this book (Chapter 35), the treatment of Hodgkin lymphoma (HL) has become extraordinarily successful over the last 40 years. One of the penalties of this success, however, has been the growing importance of late effects of treatment. The balance of early and late effects is especially critical in early-stage patients and after long follow-up. For instance, in stage I and II patients treated at Stanford during 1962–95, the cumulative probability of death from causes other than HL exceeded that due to the disease itself beyond about 12 years.[1] Beyond 20 years, indeed, mortality is virtually entirely due to causes other than HL.[2]

Some of the deaths occurring in long-term follow-up, of course, represent the mortality to be expected in any group of people as they grow older. Many, however, do not. In particular, patients with HL suffer large excesses of morbidity and mortality from second cancers and from cardiovascular disease (Table 43.1); this chapter concentrates on these major endpoints. In addition, treatment can have long-term effects on the lung, thyroid, bone and soft tissue, gastrointestinal system, urinary tract, immune system and infection, and on fertility. These have lesser effects on mortality, however, and are not reviewed here.

## Second malignancies

### Overall risk of second malignancy

Since the first reports of increased risk of second cancer in HL patients in the early 1970s,[5,6] nearly all major treatment centers have evaluated this risk in their patients. An excess of acute myeloid leukemia (AML) in chemotherapy-treated patients and an increased risk of solid tumors in radiotherapy-treated patients have been reported consistently in the literature.[7,8] The overall risk of selected second malignancies compared with the general population is given in Table 43.2, on the basis of results from two recent large studies, one from the UK[9] and one from a joint study in the USA, Canada, Scandinavia, and the Netherlands.[10]

The largest relative risk (10- to 15-fold) is observed for leukemia (with an even greater risk for AML: 22-fold),

## Table 43.1 Major causes of excess mortality in Hodgkin lymphoma (HL): selected large cohort studies

| Ref | No. in cohort | Age of cohort at treatment | Median follow-up (years) | Total no. of deaths | No. of deaths due to HL | No. of deaths due to 2nd cancer | No. of deaths due to cardiovascular disease | AER 2nd cancer | AER cardiovascular disease |
|---|---|---|---|---|---|---|---|---|---|
| 3 | 2498 | No age limits specified | –[a] | 754 | 333 | 160 | 117 (88 cardiac) | 43.5 | 28.0 (cardiac) |
| 4 | 1080 | ≤50 | 12 | 161 | 60 | 59 | 17 (cardiac) | 41.2 | 9.0 (cardiac) |
| 2 | 1261 | ≤40 | 18 | 534 | 291 | 116 | 50 | 41.3 | 17.8 |

AER, absolute excess risk = excess number of cases per 10 000 patients per year.
[a] Not specified, but maximum follow-up was approximately 35 years.

followed by a 6- to 14-fold increased risk for non-Hodgkin lymphoma (NHL), and 4- to 10-fold excesses for connective tissue, bone, and thyroid cancers. Moderately increased risks (2- to 4-fold) are observed for a number of solid tumors, such as cancers of the lung, stomach, esophagus, colon, breast, mouth and pharynx, and cervix, and melanoma. Because leukemia and NHL are diseases with a low incidence in the general population, even a high relative risk compared with the population may translate into a low cumulative (actuarial) risk. As shown in Figure 43.1, for the entire follow-up period the cumulative risk of solid tumors far exceeds that of leukemia or NHL. The absolute excess risk is the best measure to judge which subsequent tumors contribute most to the second cancer burden. Table 43.2 shows that, compared with the general population, HL patients in general experience an excess of about 45 malignancies per 10 000 person-years of observation, although, as discussed later, this varies with age at treatment and other factors. Solid tumors account for the majority of excess cancers (approximately 30 per 10 000 patients per year), with lung cancer contributing 10–12 excess cases per 10 000 person-years. Leukemia and NHL each account for about 8–9 cases per 10 000 person-years.

Temporal patterns of risk of second malignancy vary by tumor site, as illustrated in Table 43.3. In most studies, an increased risk of leukemia is observed as early as 2–4 years following initiation of chemotherapy, with peak occurrence between 5 and 9 years, and decreasing risks thereafter.[9–15] In studies with large numbers of long-term survivors, significantly increased relative risks are still observed for 15 years after first treatment.[9,10,13,15] The relative risk of NHL is already greatly increased in the first 5 years after treatment. In some studies, the risk remains rather constant over time,[10,12,16] whereas others report that risk increases with time since treatment.[13,17] The relative risk of solid tumors is minimally elevated in the 1- to 4-year follow-up period, and increases steadily with increasing follow-up time from 5 years since first treatment.[9,10,12,13,15–18] For some tumor sites (breast and thyroid), the excess risk does not become apparent until after 10 or even 15 years of observation. In studies that include data on 20-year survivors, the relative risk of solid tumors continued to increase through the 15- to 20-year follow-up period.[9,10,13–16,18–20] Only two recent studies have reported on the time course of risk 20 or more years after treatment.[10,15] In the international population-based study by Dores et al,[10] a downturn in the relative risk for all solid tumors com-

---

**Table 43.2  Relative risk of second cancers after Hodgkin lymphoma: results from two large studies[9,10]**

| Site or type | Swerdlow et al[9] (UK, 2000) (n=5519) | | | | Dores et al[10] (international, 2002) (n=32 591) | | | |
|---|---|---|---|---|---|---|---|---|
| | Obs | O/E | 95% CI | AER | Obs | O/E | 95% CI | AER |
| All cancers | 322 | 2.9 | 2.6–3.2 | 44.5 | 2153 | 2.3 | 2.2–2.4 | 47.2 |
| Leukemia | 45 | 14.6 | 10.7–19.2 | 8.9 | 249 | 9.9 | 8.7–11.2 | 8.8 |
| Non-Hodgkin lymphoma | 50 | 14.0 | 10.5–18.3 | 9.9 | 162 | 5.5 | 4.7–6.4 | 5.2 |
| Solid tumors | 227 | 2.2 | 1.9–2.5 | 25.7 | 1726 | 2.0 | 1.9–2.0 | 33.1 |
| Tongue, Mouth, Pharynx | 6 | 2.8 | 1.1–5.8 | 0.8 | 75 | 3.3 | 2.6–4.1 | 2.1 |
| Esophagus | 5 | 2.0 | 0.7–4.3 | 0.5 | 29 | 2.8 | 1.8–4.0 | 0.7 |
| Stomach | 13 | 2.2 | 1.2–3.6 | 1.5 | 80 | 1.9 | 1.5–2.4 | 1.5 |
| Colon | 18 | 2.3 | 1.4–3.6 | 2.2 | 129 | 1.6 | 1.4–1.9 | 2.0 |
| Rectum | 7 | 1.3 | 0.5–2.5 | 0.3 | 52 | 1.2 | 0.9–1.6 | 0.4 |
| Pancreas | 3 | 1.0 | 0.2–2.6 | 0 | 40 | 1.5 | 1.1–2.0 | 0.5 |
| Lung | 78 | 3.4 | 2.7–4.2 | 11.7 | 377 | 2.9 | 2.6–3.2 | 9.7 |
| Female breast | 19 | 1.4 | 0.9–2.1 | 3.1 | 234 | 2.0 | 1.8–2.3 | 10.5 |
| Uterine cervix | 7 | 2.1 | 0.9–4.1 | 0.8 | 37 | 2.0 | 1.4–2.7 | 1.6 |
| Prostate | 4 | 0.8 | 0.2–1.7 | −0.3 | 98 | 1.0 | 0.8–1.2 | −0.1 |
| Bladder | 5 | 0.8 | 0.3–1.8 | −0.2 | 66 | 1.4 | 1.1–1.8 | 0.8 |
| Central nervous system | 7 | 2.5 | 1.1–4.8 | 0.9 | 36 | 1.5 | 1.1–2.1 | 0.5 |
| Thyroid | 5 | 7.6 | 2.7–16.4 | 0.9 | 47 | 4.1 | 3.0–5.5 | 1.4 |
| Bone | 4 | 10.7 | 3.3–24.8 | 0.8 | 9 | 3.8 | 1.7–7.2 | 0.3 |
| Connective tissue | 3 | 3.9 | 1.0–10.1 | 0.5 | 32 | 5.1 | 3.5–7.2 | 1.0 |
| Melanoma | 6 | 2.3 | 0.9–4.6 | 0.7 | 52 | 1.7 | 1.3–2.3 | 0.9 |

Obs, observed number of cases; O/E, observed/expected; 95% CI, 95% confidence interval; AER, absolute excess risk = excess number of cases per 10 000 patients per year.

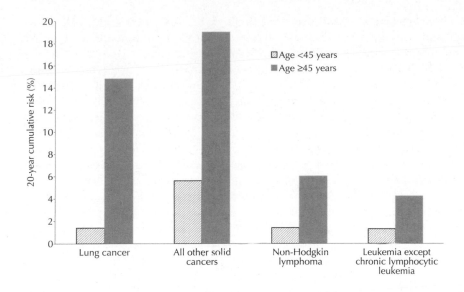

**Figure 43.1** BNLI cohort: 20-year cumulative risks of second primary cancer, by age at first treatment.[9]

bined was observed after 25 years of follow-up, with relative risks of 3.0 and 1.8 among patients in the 20- to 24-year interval and 25-year survivors, respectively (Table 43.3). A Dutch study in patients diagnosed with HL before the age of 40 years reported a relative risk for solid tumors of 5.3 among 25-year survivors, compared with a relative risk of 8.8 in the 20- to 24-year interval.[15] This suggests that the relative risk may decrease in very long-term survivors.

In accordance with the patterns of relative risks of leukemia, NHL, and solid tumors with time since first treatment, the absolute excess risks in long-term survivors differ greatly from those observed in the entire patient population. Table 43.3 clearly shows that the *absolute excess risks* of solid malignancies increase at a much steeper rate than the *relative risks*, due to the fact that, with longer follow-up, patients grow older and their background rate of cancer rises strongly.

**Table 43.3 Relative risks and absolute excess risks of second cancers after Hodgkin lymphoma, according to time since diagnosis[10]**

| Malignancy | Time since diagnosis (years) | | | | |
| --- | --- | --- | --- | --- | --- |
| | 1–9 (n=32 591) | 10–14 (n=11 326) | 15–19 (n=6195) | 20–24 (n=2861) | ≥25 (n=1111) |
| **All solid tumors** | | | | | |
| O/E (95% CI) | 1.6 (1.5–1.7) | 2.4 (2.2–2.7) | 2.5 (2.2–2.8) | 3.0 (2.5–3.5) | 1.8 (1.4–2.3) |
| AER | 19.2 | 50.2 | 63.5 | 109.6 | 62.4 |
| **Lung cancer** | | | | | |
| O/E (95% CI) | 2.7 (2.4–3.1) | 3.4 (2.7–4.3) | 2.9 (2.1–4.0) | 4.6 (3.2–6.5) | 0.8 (0.3–1.9) |
| AER | 8.1 | 12.2 | 11.6 | 27.7 | –2.4 |
| **Female breast cancer** | | | | | |
| O/E (95% CI) | 1.2 (1.0–1.5) | 2.7 (2.1–3.5) | 3.8 (2.9–4.9) | 3.0 (1.9–4.5) | 3.3 (2.0–5.2) |
| AER | 1.7 | 19.4 | 40.1 | 36.0 | 52.6 |
| **Stomach cancer** | | | | | |
| O/E (95% CI) | 1.3 (0.9–1.8) | 3.7 (2.4–5.5) | 2.6 (1.2–4.8) | 3.2 (1.3–6.6) | 2.1 (0.6–5.4) |
| AER | 0.5 | 4.1 | 2.8 | 5.2 | 4.0 |
| **Non-Hodgkin lymphoma** | | | | | |
| O/E (95% CI) | 4.9 (3.9–6.0) | 8.2 (6.0–11.0) | 4.7 (2.6–7.8) | 5.7 (2.6–10.8) | 4.4 (1.4–10.3) |
| AER | 4.1 | 9.0 | 5.3 | 8.0 | 7.4 |
| **Acute myeloid leukemia** | | | | | |
| O/E (95% CI) | 27.7 (23.3–32.7) | 17.2 (10.9–25.8) | 2.6 (0.3–9.4) | 10.1 (2.7–25.9) | 0 (0.0–11.5) |
| AER | 7.7 | 5.1 | 0.6 | 3.9 | –0.6 |

n, number of patients entering interval; O/E, observed/expected; 95% CI, 95% confidence interval; AER, absolute excess risk = excess number of cases per 10 000 patients per year.

Related to this phenomenon, the absolute excess risk amounts to about 100 excess cancer cases per 10 000 20-year survivors per year, as compared with 45/10 000/year in all patients (Table 43.2). Based on estimates from the study by Dores et al,[10] solid cancers contribute by far the most to the absolute excess risk in 20-year survivors, with 92 excess cases per 10 000 patients per year, followed by NHL (8/10 000/year), and AML (2/10 000/year). In females, breast cancer accounts for most of the absolute excess risk of solid tumors in 20-year survivors (42/10 000/year) (Table 43.3).[10] Lung cancer accounts for 17 excess cases per 10 000 patients per year in 20-year survivors of both sexes combined.

## Leukemia

For a number of second malignancies, the association with treatment factors has been investigated in detail. Leukemia following HL is certainly the most studied malignancy induced by treatment, and extensive knowledge of its risk factors has emerged.[8] Radiotherapy alone is associated with very little or no increased risk of leukemia,[9,12,17,18,21] while alkylating agent chemotherapy is linked with a greatly elevated risk. Several studies have compared the leuke-mogenicity of different chemotherapy regimens. The risk of AML rises sharply with an increasing number of MOPP (mechlorethamine, vincristine, procar-bazine, and prednisone) or MOPP-like cycles.[11,21] The risk associated with 10–12 MOPP cycles appears to be approximately three to five times higher than that following 6 MOPP cycles.[11,21] Since the 1980s, MOPP-only chemotherapy has been gradually replaced by ABV(D) (doxorubicin, bleomycin, vinblastine, and dacarbazine)-containing regimens in many centers. There are only a few reports on the occurrence of AML following ABV(D) alone. Patients treated with ABVD in the Milan Cancer Institute, where this regi-men was designed, were shown to have a significantly lower risk of AML than MOPP-treated patients (15-year cumulative risks of 0.7% and 9.5%, respec-tively).[22] Another study showed that HL patients treated with MOPP/ABV(D)-containing regimens in the 1980s had substantially lower risk of AML/ myelodysplastic syndrome (MDS) than patients treated in the 1970s with MOPP alone (10-year cumu-lative risks of 2.1% and 6.4%, respectively; $p$=0.07).[13] The German–Austrian Pediatric Hodgkin's Disease Group observed a low risk of AML (1.1% at 15 years) following regimens that contained relatively low doses of procarbazine, doxorubicin, and cyclophos-phamide, without mechlorethamine.[23]

An important question is whether radiotherapy adds to the risk of leukemia associated with chemotherapy. Evidence that combined-modality treatment results in greater risk than chemotherapy alone is provided by several reports,[18,22,24] whereas other large series indicate that the risk of AML after combined treat-ment is comparable to that after chemotherapy alone.[9,11–14,17,21,25] These inconsistent results may be due partly to differences in treatment regimens between studies, but also to lack of adjustment for type and amount of chemotherapy in some reports. The interaction between radiotherapy and chemotherapy was evaluated most rigorously in the large case–control study by Kaldor et al,[11] which included 163 cases of leukemia following HL. When examining the combined effects of radiation dose to the active bone marrow and the number of mechlorethamine–procarbazine-containing cycles, it was found that for each category of radiation dose (<10, 10–20, >20 Gy to the marrow), the risk of leukemia clearly increased with the number of chemotherapy cycles. In contrast, among patients with a given number of chemotherapy cycles, risk of leukemia did not consistently increase with higher radiation dose. Taken together, the preponderance of available data does not support the hypothesis that the combination of chemotherapy and radiotherapy confers a higher risk of leukemia than chemotherapy alone.

Intensification of therapy with autologous stem cell transplantation (ASCT) support is increasingly being used for relapsing lymphoma patients. Relatively high actuarial risks (4–15% at 5 years) of AML and MDS have been observed after ASCT for HL. Evidence suggests that much of the risk is related to intensive pretransplant chemotherapy.[26–29]

The influence of host-related factors such as age on the risk of leukemia in HL survivors has been exam-ined in a number of studies and has been reviewed elsewhere.[8] The reported higher *cumulative* risk of AML in older HL patients compared with younger ones mainly reflects the higher baseline incidence of the disease in older persons. In the few studies that have analyzed the *relative* risk of leukemia by age, based on comparisons with general population expectations, either no differences between age groups were observed[15–17] or the relative risk of AML was significantly greater at younger ages than at older.[9–11] The risk of AML in relation to treatment-associated acute and chronic bone marrow toxicity has been examined in only one study to date.[21] Significantly increased risks of leukemia were found among patients who developed thrombocytopenia, either in response to initial therapy or during fol-low-up. After adjustment for the type and amount of chemotherapy, patients who showed a decrease in platelet counts of 70% or more after initial treatment had an approximately fivefold higher risk of devel-oping leukemia than patients who showed a decrease of 50% or less. Severe acute thrombocy-topenia may indicate greater bioavailability of cyto-toxic drugs, which would be likely to contribute to the development of leukemia.

## Non-Hodgkin lymphoma

The literature consistently reports an increased risk of NHL following HL, but the causes of the excess risk are not well understood.[8] As increased risks of NHL occur in immunosuppressed patients, such as transplant recipients,[30] and as HL may be accompanied by immunosuppression,[31] several investigators have argued that the elevated risk of NHL may be attributed to HL itself rather than to its treatment. This view is supported by several studies in which risk did not vary appreciably between treatments.[9,12,16,17] However, in other studies, the risk of NHL was found to be lowest among patients treated with radiotherapy alone, and highest among patients who received intensive combined-modality treatment, both initially and for relapse.[13,18,32-34] The inconsistent results regarding the relation with treatment may be partly attributed to diagnostic misclassification, ie misdiagnosis of the primary tumor as HL while it represented NHL according to modern lymphoma classification schemes.[8,34] In only very few studies were diagnostic pathology slides of the second NHL and original HL reviewed in order to avoid such misclassification, however, and these did not give consistent results.[12,13,34] Although transformation to NHL may be part of the natural history of some types of HL, the role of intensive combined-modality treatment and its associated immunosuppression, and of the inherent immune deficiency associated with HL, should be explored further.

## Solid malignancies

### Role of radiation

Elevated risks of solid cancers following HL have generally been attributed to radiotherapy.[8,10,12-20,35] Excesses of melanoma, however, are more likely to be related to immunosuppression accompanying HL or its treatment, because elevated risks appear as early as in the 1- to 4-year follow-up interval.[9,36] Emergence of an increased risk of cervical cancer 10 years after the diagnosis of HL may also be related to defects in cellular immunity that may facilitate the progression of human papillomavirus-related neoplasia.[37] The other sites for which excess solid cancers have been reported (lung, breast, gastrointestinal tract, thyroid, bone, and connective tissue) are those for which elevated risks have also been described in other radiation-exposed cohorts.[38-40] Two case–control studies have examined lung cancer risk in relation to the radiation dose to the affected lung area, as well as the modifying effect of the patient's smoking habits.[41,42] In both studies, it was observed that the risk of lung cancer rose significantly with increasing radiation dose. In the largest study, which included 222 lung cancer patients and 444 matched controls, the relative risk (RR) was 7.2 (95% confidence interval (CI) 2.2–28) for patients who received 40 Gy or more (to the relevant

lung area) compared with those who received no radiation.[42] In the Dutch study, the increase in risk of lung cancer with increasing radiation dose was significantly greater among patients who smoked after diagnosis of HL than among those who refrained from smoking.[41] Travis and collaborators[42] observed that the increased relative risks from smoking appeared to multiply the elevated risks from radiation. Both studies imply that there are large absolute excess risks for lung cancer among irradiated patients who smoke.

The strongly elevated risk of breast cancer following radiotherapy for HL has become a major concern for female survivors.[10,15,43-47] A case–control study of breast cancer after HL in the Netherlands investigated the effects of radiation dose, chemotherapy, and reproductive factors.[48] The study included 48 patients who developed breast cancer 5 or more years after treatment for HL and 175 matched controls. The radiation dose to the area of the breast where the case's tumor had developed was estimated for each case–control set. The risk of breast cancer increased significantly with increasing radiation dose ($p_{trend}$=0.01), with an RR of 4.5 (95% CI 1.3–16.0) for patients who received 38.5 Gy or more, as compared with those who received less than 4 Gy. Patients who received chemotherapy and radiotherapy had significantly decreased risk compared with those treated with radiation alone (RR 0.45; $p$=0.009). For patients who never received chemotherapy, the risk of breast cancer increased more strongly with increasing radiation dose (RR 12.7 for patients receiving 38.5 Gy or more) than among patients also treated with chemotherapy. The substantial risk reduction associated with chemotherapy was attributable to its effect on menopausal age. Reaching menopause before age 36 (25% of the controls) was associated with a strongly reduced risk of breast cancer (RR 0.06; 95% CI 0.01–0.45). These results suggest that ovarian hormones are a crucial factor in promoting tumorgenesis once radiation has produced an initiating event.

### Role of chemotherapy

A very important question is whether chemotherapy for HL can also induce solid cancers, and, if so, at which sites. Several studies have indeed observed that chemotherapy significantly increased the risk of solid malignancy, in particular lung cancer.[9,12,49] The British National Lymphoma Investigation cohort study of 5519 patients[9] showed a significantly elevated risk of lung cancer following chemotherapy alone, with the RR (3.3; 95% CI 2.2–4.7) compared with the general population being of similar magnitude to that observed in patients treated with either radiotherapy (RR 2.9; 95% CI 1.9–4.1) or mixed-modality treatment (RR 4.3; 95% CI 2.9–6.2). Two large case–control studies have investigated the separate and joint roles of chemotherapy, radiation, and smoking in detail.[42,50] In both reports, there was a clear trend of increasing lung cancer risk with greater number of cycles of alkylating agent chemotherapy ($p_{trend}$<0.001)[42] or MOPP chemotherapy ($p_{trend}$ = 0.07[50] and $p_{trend}$ = 0.001[42]). In the largest study, in which individual radiation dosimetry was performed, the risk of lung cancer after treatment with alkylating agents and radiation together was as expected if individual excess relative risks were summed, with RRs of 4.2 (95% CI 2.1–8.8) for patients with alkylating agents alone, 5.9 (95% CI 2.7–13.5) for patients with radiotherapy alone (>5 Gy), and 8.0 (95% CI 3.6–18.5) for those with combined-modality treatment, compared with patients who received no alkylating agents and had a radiation dose of 5 Gy or less.[42] Among patients treated with MOPP chemotherapy, the risk of lung cancer rose with increasing cumulative dose of either mechlorethamine or procarbazine.[42] Both agents are carcinogenic to rodent lungs,[51] and mustard gas, from which mechlorethamine was originally derived, is also known to cause lung cancer in humans[52] – although of course after presumed inhalation in that circumstance. As was observed for the joint effects of smoking and radiotherapy, the risks from smoking appeared at least to multiply the risks from alkylating agent chemotherapy.[42,50] Smoking remains the major cause of lung cancer in patients treated for HL, as is evident from the observation that only 7 out of 222 cases included in the study by Travis and colleagues[42] occurred in patients who had never smoked.

In several series,[14,15,17,18,21] no increased risk of solid malignancy overall was observed following chemotherapy alone. However, the expected number of solid tumors 10 or more years after chemotherapy alone was less than two in nearly all negative studies, so a moderate increase in risk could not be excluded. If chemotherapy affects the risk of solid tumors, one might expect that patients receiving combined-modality treatment would have a greater relative risk than patients treated solely with radiotherapy, although this would depend on whether doses were comparable. Only one study to date has reported a significantly greater risk for solid cancers overall following chemo- and radiotherapy compared with irradiation alone,[16] whereas no such difference has been found in the majority of investigations.[1,12,14,17,18,21] For gastrointestinal tract cancers, however, larger risks were observed after combined-modality treatment than after irradiation alone.[9,15,20]

The inconsistent results reported with regard to the influence of chemotherapy on the risk of solid tumors may be partly related to the fact that most studies considered all solid tumors combined, whereas chemotherapy may differentially affect the risk of tumors at disparate sites. A recent study from the Netherlands Cancer Institute demonstrated that the addition of salvage chemotherapy to initial radiotherapy, as compared with initial irradiation alone, did not influence the risk of solid cancers overall, but significantly increased the risk of solid tumors other than breast cancer (RR 9.4, versus 4.7 for initial irradiation alone).[15] Conversely, patients who received salvage chemotherapy were found to experience significantly lower risks of breast cancer than patients treated with radiotherapy alone (RRs 2.8 and 7.6, respectively), probably related to premature ovarian failure due to intensive chemotherapy[15] (see also above).

## Effect of age at treatment

Several studies have shown that the relative risk of solid cancers increases strongly with decreasing age at first treatment.[9,10,15,20] The effect of age is most notable for breast cancer, with the risk increasing dramatically with younger age at first irradiation down to 10–14 years, but not younger. In a Dutch study, 15-year survivors who had radiation treatment before 20 years of age had an 18-fold increased risk of breast cancer; women irradiated at ages 20–29 had a 6-fold increased risk; and a small, non-significant increase was observed for women irradiated at age 30 or older (RR 1.7).[15] A similar trend, with even larger relative risks, was reported from Stanford University.[19] An approximately 100-fold increased risk of breast cancer has been observed after treatment at ages less than 16, with relative risks ranging from 17 to 458.[14,16,19,53] This huge variation in estimated risk is not surprising in view of the large differences between series in important variables such as the proportion of patients irradiated and the duration and completeness of follow-up. Generally, surveys with more complete follow-up have found lower relative risks of breast cancer[9,10,15,53,54] than those in which completeness of follow-up was less satisfactory or was not addressed.[14,16,55] Incomplete follow-up may lead to overestimation of the risk of second malignancy if patients who remain well lose contact with clinical follow-up, while those with second cancers come to attention because of this. The very high *actuarial* risks reported in two US studies (34% at 25 years after first treatment for women treated at ages under 20[55] and 35% at 40 years of age for those treated at ages under 16[14]) may well be exaggerated estimates, not only because of losses to follow-up but also because the actuarial method is less appropriate when including events that occur at follow-up intervals later than those at which data for most of the patients were censored.[43] In the Dutch study with (nearly) complete follow-up, the 25-year actuarial risk of breast cancer amounted to 16%, both for women first treated before age 20 and at ages 20–30.[15]

Several studies have demonstrated that age at treatment for HL is also a crucial determinant of increased relative risks for solid malignancies other than breast cancer.[9,10,15,20] Dores and colleagues[10] reported that the relative risk of lung cancer decreased from a 5.5-fold

**Table 43.4  Relative risks of various second malignancies, according to age at diagnosis of Hodgkin lymphoma (HL)[9,10]**

**Dores et al[10] (International, 2002)**

| Age at HL diagnosis | All 2nd cancers | All solid cancers | Female breast | Lung | GI tract | NHL | AML |
|---|---|---|---|---|---|---|---|
| <21 | 7.7[a] | 7.0[a] | 14.2[a] | 5.5[a] | 10.0[a] | 6.9[a] | 39.2[a] |
| 21–30 | 4.3[a] | 3.6[a] | 3.7[a] | 5.4[a] | 3.9[a] | 7.5[a] | 31.7[a] |
| 31–40 | 2.7[a] | 2.1[a] | 1.2 | 4.0[a] | 2.1[a] | 8.7[a] | 35.7[a] |
| 41–50 | 2.5[a] | 2.1[a] | 1.7[a] | 3.5[a] | 2.3[a] | 5.3[a] | 28.6[a] |
| 51–60 | 2.0[a] | 1.8[a] | 1.0 | 3.4[a] | 1.6[a] | 4.3[a] | 21.2[a] |
| ≥61 | 1.3[a] | 1.2[a] | 1.1 | 1.5[a] | 1.0 | 3.8[a] | 5.9[a] |

**Swerdlow et al[9] (UK, 2000)**

| Age at HL diagnosis | All 2nd cancers | All solid cancers | Female breast | Lung | GI tract | NHL | AML |
|---|---|---|---|---|---|---|---|
| <15 | 26.1[a] | – | 7.7[a,b] | 24.1[a] | 9.1[a,b] | 33.3[a] | 0 |
| 15–24 | 7.0[a] | – | – | 15.3[a] | – | 8.0[a] | 53.6[a] |
| 25–34 | 4.1[a] | – | 0.8[a,c] | 6.4[a] | 2.8[a,c] | 9.4[a] | 26.3[a] |
| 35–44 | 3.0[a] | – | – | 5.3[a] | – | 15.7[a] | 22.4[a] |
| 45–54 | 2.6[a] | – | 0.8 | 4.1[a] | 1.8 | 11.9[a] | 17.2[a] |
| ≥55 | 1.9[a] | – | 1.1 | 2.2[a] | 1.6[a] | 18.7[a] | 10.5[a] |

GI, gastrointestinal; NHL, non-Hodgkin lymphoma; AML, acute myeloid leukemia.
[a] $p < 0.05$.
[b] Joint category age at HL diagnosis <25 years.
[c] Joint category age at HL diagnosis 25–44 years.

increase (compared with the general population) for patients diagnosed before age 21 to a 1.5-fold increase for patients diagnosed at age 61 or above. In the UK study, the relative risks for lung cancer decreased from 20-fold among those diagnosed before age 25 to 2.2-fold for patients diagnosed at age 55 or above (Table 43.4). Table 43.4 demonstrates that a significantly greater relative risk with younger age at diagnosis of HL is also observed for digestive tract cancers[9,10,15,20] and for cancers of the thyroid, bone and soft tissue.[9,10] Despite the very high *relative risks at* younger ages, the *absolute excess* risks for all solid cancers except breast cancer are greater for those diagnosed at older ages, related to the much higher background rate of cancer among elderly patients.[9,10]

The strongly increased relative risks of solid tumors in patients treated for HL at a young age only become manifest after an extended follow-up period. This might point to a prolonged induction period, but it might also in principle relate to the attained age of the patients. Only three recent studies have distinguished the separate contributions of age at first treatment and attained age.[10,15,37] The relative risk of solid tumors was greatest among patients treated at a young age (≤20 years), but the largest relative risk emerged *before* the patients attained the age range at which solid tumors normally occur. Among patients first treated at age 20 or younger, in the largest study to date, the relative risk of developing a solid tumor at ages 40–59 was significantly lower than the relative

risk of solid tumor development before age 40 (RR 2.3 versus RR 10.5).[10,37] Table 43.5 shows that for breast cancer, the diminution in relative risk with increasing age is even more dramatic. Metayer et al[37] found that among female patients first treated at ages 17–20, the relative risk of developing breast cancer before age 30 was 84-fold increased, while the risk of breast cancer development after age 40 was only 4-fold elevated. It is notable that a similar finding has been reported with regard to the risk of breast cancer among atomic bomb survivors in Japan.[56]

**Table 43.5  Risk of breast cancer by age at diagnosis of Hodgkin lymphoma (HL) and attained age, in patients diagnosed before age 21 years[37]**

| | Age at HL diagnosis (years) | | | |
| | ≤16 (n=2674) | | 17–20 (n=3251) | |
| Attained age (years) | Obs | RR | Obs | RR |
|---|---|---|---|---|
| <30 | 6 | 125[a] | 8 | 84[a] |
| 30–34 | 7 | 47[a] | 8 | 30[a] |
| 35–39 | 6 | 28[a] | 9 | 16[a] |
| ≥40 | 1 | 2.0 | 7 | 4.0[a] |

Obs, observed number of cases; RR, relative risk.
[a] $p < 0.05$.

## Conclusions

In conclusion, the occurrence of treatment-related second cancers is a major problem in survivors of HL. The substantial increase in risk of solid tumors with time since diagnosis of HL necessitates careful, long-term medical surveillance of all patients. The greatly increased risk of NHL throughout follow-up demonstrates the importance of performing biopsies in recurrent HL. As the absolute excess risk of lung cancer is much greater among smokers than non-smokers, physicians should make a special effort to dissuade HL patients from smoking even before treatment starts. Women treated with mantle field irradiation before the age of 30 are at greatly increased risk of breast cancer. In many centers, from 8 years after irradiation, the follow-up program of these women now includes yearly breast palpation and mammography. Also, the importance of regular breast examinations is explained to survivors, and they are taught (monthly) breast self-examination. It should be emphasized, however, that the efficacy of these measures in this specific population has not been demonstrated. There is a strong need for research to evaluate the efficacy of programs aimed at reduction of breast cancer mortality in these high-risk women. Physicians should also be alert to the raised risk of gastrointestinal cancers in patients who have received para-aortic and pelvic radiation fields. Thorough examination of gastrointestinal complaints is indicated. Chemotherapy also appears to increase the risk of solid malignancies, in particular lung cancer. An important question to be answered in future research is whether modern chemotherapy regimens (ABV) also contribute to the risk of solid tumors, and if so, which cytotoxic drugs are responsible for the excess risk. One of the most devastating second malignancies to occur among patients cured of HL remains chemotherapy-related leukemia. As the poor prognosis of this complication cannot be changed by early diagnosis, it is promising that the risk of leukemia decreased dramatically with the introduction of ABV-based regimens in the 1980s. Hopefully, current treatment protocols that limit the dose and fields of radiotherapy will similarly reduce the late risk of solid cancers.

# Cardiovascular disease

Aside from second malignancies, cardiovascular disease is the most common cause of excess morbidity and mortality among long-term survivors of HL. The information available on the relation of cardiovascular disease to HL treatment is less extensive and detailed, however, than that for second malignancies. In general, also, the quality of epidemiological data available is poorer, and as a consequence the results are more difficult to interpret.

Two methodological points need especially to be borne in mind when considering the literature. First, because cardiovascular disease is such a common cause of morbidity and mortality in adults in Western countries, findings that substantial numbers of cardiovascular events, abnormalities, or deaths occur after treatment for HL does not in itself implicate the HL treatment as the cause; one needs to compare the numbers of events/deaths occurring with those to be expected in the general population of the same age and sex as the patients at the same calendar period, to conclude whether treatment has led to an increased risk. Unfortunately, much of the literature has not provided such 'expected' data, so that it is difficult to know to what extent the observed morbidity or mortality is in excess. This is particularly the case for incidence, because data on incidence of cardiovascular diseases such as pericarditis are scarce. Unlike the discussion of second malignancy, however, we have included such results in this chapter, faute de mieux.

A second methodological point, again unlike for second cancers, is that ascertainment of many cardiovascular endpoints, in particular subclinical disease, requires procedures that are beyond those needed for clinical care or treatment and are often invasive. As a consequence, usually only a modest proportion of eligible subjects undergo these procedures. There is therefore scope for selection bias in the subjects included, especially for long-term follow-up studies.

There have been three major potential cardiovascular late effects of HL treatment that have been of concern: the cardiac effects of radiation exposure to the heart, the cardiac effects of treatment with anthracyclines, and the potential ill-effects of carotid exposure to radiation.

## Cardiac effects of radiotherapy

Cardiac damage from chest radiotherapy is the most thoroughly investigated late cardiovascular effect of HL treatment. Electrocardiographic abnormalities are frequent (25% of patients or more) in many studies, but not all,[57,58] especially where radiation fields have been anterior or anteriorly weighted. In addition, however, mediastinal radiotherapy has been associated with a range of heart diseases, including acute and chronic constrictive pericarditis, valvular heart disease, ischemic heart disease, and myocardial infarction.

### Pericarditis

Pericarditis may be acute, occurring months or years after treatment, or chronic constrictive. The risk of pericarditis has been shown to increase with radiation dose[59–61] and with dose per fraction.[61] Subcarinal blocking can greatly decrease the incidence of pericarditis.[60] The risks of pericarditis have been greater when anterior field weighting was greatest, and radiation techniques were then modified to reduce the dose of radiation to the heart. In a French series of 499 patients treated during 1971–84 with mediastinal radiotherapy, mainly about 40 Gy, with anterior and posterior beams equally weighted, the 10-year cumulative incidence of pericarditis was 9.5%, whereas no cases of pericarditis occurred among 138 patients who did not receive mediastinal radiotherapy (p<0.005).[61] In a US series, carditis occurred within a year in 6.6% of 318 patients treated before 1970 with mediastinal radiotherapy, mainly 44 Gy.[59] In 590 patients treated during 1969–84 at Harvard with at least full mantle radiotherapy around 40 Gy, equally from anterior and posterior fields, however, and who were followed for at least 2 years (unless dying), pericarditis occurred in only 2.2%.[62] No comparison was made with expected numbers in the general population (see the introduction to this section).

### Heart valve injury

It is clear that radiation can cause heart valve injury in a substantial proportion of patients. In a study of 116 patients in Norway given mediastinal irradiation at ages under 50 years and examined by echocardiography 5–13 years later, aortic and/or mitral valvular regurgitation was found in 24% of patients. The prevalence was significantly greater in females (46%) than in males (16%),[63] and the lesions were more frequent and severe than expected from normal reference groups.[64] Age, period of follow-up, radiation dose, and chemotherapy were not found to be significant risk factors, however. In Zurich, echocardiography on 144 patients who had been treated with mediastinal irradiation for HL during 1964–92 showed that 29% had valvular thickening, although there was functional disturbance in only 3%.[65] The cumulative incidence of valvular thickening increased from 8% at 10 years after irradiation to 45% at 20 years. Furthermore, in patients who had echocardiography repeated 1–6 years after an initial such examination, 8% who were initially normal had developed valvular thickening at the second investigation and 37% of those whose valves were initially abnormal had deteriorated.

Valvular injury can lead to death, but is not a major cause – in a large HL cohort at Stanford, 7 out of 617 deaths were due to valvular heart disease or complications of valve replacement (expected number not stated).[66]

### Myocardial infarction and cardiac death

Myocardial infarction is an important late effect of mediastinal radiotherapy. The cumulative incidence of myocardial infarction in a French cohort receiving mediastinal irradiation, generally mantle, was 3.9% at 10 years,[61] while in a European Organization for Research and Treatment of Cancer (EORTC) cohort

who had received mantle radiotherapy, it was 2.4% at 10 years and 4.6% at 15 years.[67] In Swiss patients who had received mediastinal radiotherapy, the cumulative risk of ischemic events, sudden death, and congestive heart failure was 14% at 20 years.[65] In 145 patients treated with mantle irradiation at the MD Anderson Cancer Center, cumulative rates of cardiac complications (coronary artery disease, valvular stenosis, arrhythmia, and pericarditis) were 13% at 10 years and 35% at 20 years.[68]

In patients treated at ages under 21 years, mainly with mantle radiotherapy, the cumulative risk of myocardial infarction was 8.1% at 22 years.[58] The expected figures for the general population were not given in the above studies, however (see the introduction to this section).

Table 43.6 shows the relative risks of mortality from myocardial infarction and from cardiac death more broadly, in cohorts of patients most or all of whom were treated with mediastinal radiotherapy. The studies are highly heterogeneous with regard to age and sex distribution, dose distribution, duration of follow-up, calendar periods, and outcome, so it is unsurprising that the risks found vary, but in general relative risks for adults are around 3–10, and are far greater for child/adolescent-treated cohorts (≥20) than for all-age or adult cohorts. Absolute excess risks appear more similar between these groups, however, suggesting that the effect of radiation on risk may be closer to additive than multiplicative. This is also suggested by the one apparent outlier in the adult results: the relative risk from Mexico (where one would expect background rates to be low) is much greater than elsewhere, but the absolute excess risk is similar.

*Sex.* The relative risk of myocardial infarction or cardiac death has usually been found to be somewhat greater in men than in women,[65,66,71,75] although not always,[2,70] whereas absolute excess risks have been several times greater in men.[2,66,75] The more marked sex difference for absolute excess risks than for relative risks reflects higher background rates in men. For other cardiac disease mortality, relative risks have been similar between the sexes, but absolute excess risks have been greater in men.[66]

*Age at treatment.* As noted earlier, studies of patients treated as children and adolescents compared with those of patients treated as adults suggest much larger relative risks (but more similar absolute excess risks) for the former than the latter (Table 43.6). This is also true for comparisons within cohorts.[66,71,76]

Within adult ages, in a large cohort from Stanford,[66] relative risks of death due to myocardial infarction, and due to other cardiac diseases, decreased sharply with increasing age at irradiation, while absolute excess risks increased with age. A large Dutch cohort

**Table 43.6  Risks of mortality from cardiovascular disease after mediastinal irradiation in large cohorts of Hodgkin lymphoma patients**

| Ref | Country | No. in cohort | Years of treatment | Age range at treatment (years) | Type of treatment | Mortality endpoint | RR | AER |
|---|---|---|---|---|---|---|---|---|
| **All age or adult** | | | | | | | | |
| 69 | Europe | ~826[a] | 1963–86 | 'Adult' males[a] | Mantle RT or TNI or STNI ± CT | Myocardial infarction | 8.8 (5.1–14.1) | _[b] |
| 62 | USA | 590 | 1969–84 | 5–69 | Mantle or more extensive RT ± CT | Myocardial infarction | 6.7 (2.9–13.3) | 13.5 |
| 67[c] | Europe | 1660 | 1964–88 | Not stated | Mediastinal or more extensive RT ± CT | Cardiac failure | 10.2[d] | _[b] |
| 70 | N America | ~3368[e] | 1940–85 | All ages | Mediastinal RT | Coronary artery disease | 3.3 (1.4–8.0) | _[b] |
|  |  |  |  |  |  | Myocardial infarction | 4.1 (1.5–10.9) | _[b] |
| 66 | USA | 2232 | 1960–90 | 1–82 | 89% with mediastinal RT | Heart disease | 3.1 (2.4–3.7) | _[b] |
|  |  |  |  |  |  | Myocardial infarction | 3.2 (2.3–4.0) | 17.8 |
| 71 | USA | 326 | 1954–89 | 5–72 | Mantle RT ± CT | Myocardial infarction | 2.8 (0.7–4.9) | 10.4[f] |
| 65 | Switzerland | 352 | 1964–92 | Not stated | Mediastinal RT ± CT | Myocardial infarction | 4.2 (1.8–8.3) | _[b] |
| 72 | Canada | 611 | 1973–84 | 17–90 | 97% RT ± CT | Myocardial infarction | 1.5 (0.7–3.0) | 5.4 |
| 73 | Mexico | 2980 | 1970–95 | >18 | 63% RT ± CT | Cardiac | 29.8 (15.6–46.8) | 16.8 |
| 4[g] | USA | 1080 | 1969–97 | 3–50 | 97% RT ± CT; mainly extended-field | Cardiac | 3.2 (1.9–5.2) | _[b] |
| 2 | Netherlands | 1261 | 1965–87 | ≤40 | RT in 94% or more | Myocardial infarction | 4.0 (2.3–6.5) | 5.6 |
|  |  |  |  |  |  | Other cardiac disease | 9.1 (6.1–13.1) | 12.1 |
| **Young ages** | | | | | | | | |
| 58 | USA | 635 | 1961–91 | <21 | 89% with mediastinal RT, mainly ≥40 Gy | Myocardial infarction | 41.5 (18.1–82.1) | 10.4 |
|  |  |  |  |  |  | Other cardiac disease | 21.2 (7.8–47.2) | 7.3 |
| 74 | USA | 387 | 1968–90 | 3–25 | RT (mainly extended-field) ± CT | Cardiac disease | 22 (8–48) | _[b] |

RR, relative risk compared with general population rates (95% confidence limits in parentheses); AER, absolute excess risk = excess number of cases per 10 000 patients per year; TNI, total nodal irradiation; STNI, subtotal nodal irradiation; CT, chemotherapy; RT, radiotherapy.

[a] 1449 in cohort, but results not reported for females.
[b] Not stated in paper.
[c] Large overlap with subjects in reference 69.
[d] Elsewhere in the same paper stated as 8.6 (5.5–12.8).
[e] Cohort of 4665, of whom, based on a 10% sample, one can estimate that 3368 were given mediastinal irradiation.
[f] Estimated from data in the paper.
[g] Overlap with subjects in reference 62.

of patients aged 40 or younger at treatment showed similar effects for non-cerebrovascular cardiovascular disease.[2] EORTC data also indicate decreasing cardiac mortality with increasing age, dichotomizing the analysis at age 40.[61,69] In a large North American cohort, however, Boivin and colleagues[70] found greatest relative risks of death due to myocardial infarction after mediastinal irradiation at ages 60 and above, and in patients treated under age 40 and at ages 40–59 fairly similar to each other.

Relative risks of both myocardial infarction and other cardiac disease have been found to decrease with increasing attained adult age.[2,62,66,75]

*Calendar period.* The introduction of blocking should have diminished the rate of cardiac mortality in patients treated in subsequent years, but the evidence on this is not entirely consistent. At Stanford, in a large all-age cohort, the relative risk of death from cardiac diseases other than myocardial infarction decreased from 5.3 to 1.4 when left ventricular and subcarinal blocking were introduced (subsequently, there was also a reduction in fraction size and other modifications), but the relative risk of death from myocardial infarction barely changed (3.7 for patients treated before 1972 and 3.4 for those treated subsequently).[66] The authors suggested that this may have been because the blocking may not have shielded critical proximal coronary arteries. In patients treated under age 21 at Stanford, the risks of cardiac disease mortality overall, and of myocardial infarction specifically, were also similar for those treated before and after blocking was introduced,[58] and in the Netherlands, for patients treated under age 40, treatment-specific relative risks did not diminish with the introduction of shielding.[2] Boivin and colleagues,[70] however, found a relative risk of 6.3 (1.7–23.2) for myocardial infarction mortality in patients treated during 1940–66, when radiotherapy tended to be orthovoltage with anterior or predominantly anterior techniques, compared with 2.0 (0.7–5.2) for those treated in 1967–85, when megavoltage machines and improved techniques were used.

*Dose of radiation.* Investigation of the risk of cardiac death in relation to the dose of radiation has been limited by a lack of variation in dosage, because most patients treated with mantle radiotherapy have received around 40 Gy. In 2232 patients treated at Stanford, there was a relative risk of 2.6 (0.4–8.7) for those receiving 30 Gy or less to the mediastinum, and 3.5 (2.7–4.3) for those receiving more than this[58] – however, relatively few patients received the lower doses, with a correspondingly wide confidence interval. Cosset and colleagues,[61] in a follow-up of 637 French patients, stated that no 'dose–effect' could be detected for the incidence of myocardial infarction in relation to radiotherapy, but did not present risk data. In Sweden, the risk of mortality due to ischaemic heart disease was found to rise with an increasing dose to a larger volume fraction, but the statistical significance was not tested.[77]

*Duration since treatment.* Risks of cardiac mortality rise in the early years after mediastinal radiotherapy, and remain elevated for 20 years or more, although the literature is not consistent on when the peak relative risk is reached. At Stanford, for patients treated in 1960–90,[66] the relative risk of death due to myocardial infarction was significantly raised even 0–4 years after initial treatment (RR 2.0 (1.1–3.3)), and increased significantly and approximately progressively through 20 or more years after treatment. The absolute excess risks rose even more steeply. A similar pattern was present for other cardiac disease deaths. It should be noted, however, that the patients with longer follow-up were those treated during earlier calendar periods, when the radiation techniques gave less protection against myocardial damage. At Harvard, for patients treated in 1969–97, the relative risk of cardiac mortality was again raised in the first 5 years of follow-up and did not diminish even 20 and more years after first treatment.[4] Absolute excess risks of cardiac mortality rose steeply in long follow-up periods. In patients treated under age 21, risks of both myocardial infarction and other cardiac diseases have remained greatly elevated beyond 20 years of follow-up.[58] In a study in the Netherlands with exceptionally long follow-up, the peak of both relative and absolute excess risk of non-cerebrovascular cardiovascular disease mortality occurred at 20–24 years after treatment, and, based on modest numbers, there was a decrease thereafter.

Cosset and colleagues,[67] however, stated that in EORTC data, standardised mortality ratios for cardiac failure reached a peak 3–11 years after treatment, although data were not presented. North American data[70] also gave some suggestion of a similar pattern for myocardial infarction deaths.

*Interaction with other risk factors.* An important question is whether the effect of radiotherapy interacts with that of other risk factors for myocardial infarction. Data are limited and inconclusive. Glanzmann and colleagues[65] found that the risk of ischemic heart disease after mediastinal radiotherapy was greater in patients with cardiovascular risk factors in addition to radiotherapy than in those without, but this conclusion was based on small numbers and the difference between the groups was not significant. At Rochester, NY, the cardiovascular risk factor prevalence was greater in patients with cardiac events after radiotherapy than in the general population, but it was not stated how this compared with other radiotherapy-treated HL patients.[71] Boivin and colleagues[70] found inconsistent results on whether the risk of death due to myocardial infarction after mediastinal radiotherapy was greater in patients with certain other cardiovascular risk factors, and Hancock and colleagues[66] noted that 53% of 49 patients in their cohort who died of myocardial infarction after mediastinal irradiation and for whom smoking data were held were ever-smokers, compared with 47% of the cohort overall. It remains unclear, and needs investigation, how the increased risks from radiation interact with those from other cardiovascular risk factors – for instance, if they are additive or multiplicative.

## Chemotherapy with anthracyclines

### Cardiac effects of anthracyclines in cancer patients generally

A second potential source of long-term cardiac damage from treatment for HL is treatment with anthracyclines, notably doxorubicin. Doxorubicin can lead to an acute toxic cardiomyopathy, which has a peak onset at 1–3 months after cessation of treatment. Longer-term follow-up of such patients, however, has shown that there are also chronic cardiac complications.

Much of the evidence for this comes from studies following up children who were treated with anthracyclines for a range of childhood malignancies, mainly or entirely not HL. Abnormalities have been found in a high proportion of children, with the prevalence and/or severity greater in those with higher dose rates and higher cumulative doses and increasing with longer follow-up; and there is conflicting evidence on whether the prevalence and/or severity is greater with younger age of childhood treatment. Thus, Lipshultz and colleagues[78] performed echocardiograms on 120 patients (50% of those eligible) who had been treated at a median age of about 7 years with 244–550 mg/m$^2$ of doxorubicin, and found that all had echocardiographic abnormalities at follow-up 2 or more years after the end of treatment and 12 (10%) had congestive heart failure a year or more after treatment. Similarly, Steinherz and colleagues[79] evaluated by electrocardiograph 4–20 years after anthracycline treatment 201 patients treated at ages 2–23 years with 200–1275 mg/m$^2$ anthracycline (51 also with mediastinal radiotherapy), and found that 23% had abnormal cardiac function and 9 developed cardiac failure and dysrhythmia, of whom 3 died suddenly. Among 607 Dutch children treated with anthracyclines, clinical heart failure not attributable to other known causes was found in 2% after 2 years and 5% after 15 years, with a cumulative dose–response effect and 4 deaths from this complication.[80] Another large cohort study noted 6 deaths from doxorubicin-induced cardiomyopathy 5 or more years after childhood treatment.[81]

Few studies have furnished comparisons with expectations. Pihkala and colleagues[82] compared left ventricular contractility on echocardiogram at a median of 4 years after the end of treatment in children treated with anthracyclines and those not so treated. The prevalence of abnormality was greater in those receiving both anthracyclines and chest radiation (50% of 26 patients) or doxorubicin alone (32% of 53 patients) than in those treated with chest radiotherapy alone (8% of 12 patients) or in healthy children plus newly diagnosed untreated cancer patients (3% of 38 subjects). A greater cumulative dose of anthracycline was associated with decreased contractility ($p<0.05$). Green and colleagues,[83] in follow-up beyond 15 years of 474 patients treated for cancer at ages under 20, found that the relative risk of cardiac death in males was significantly associated with doxorubicin treatment in a univariate ($p=0.0015$, $n=5$) but not a multivariate analysis, while no cardiac deaths occurred in females.

In adults, anthracyclines can lead to late cardiac deaths, but the risk remains unquantified. Moreb and Oblon[84] noted that among a series of 19 adult cancer patients (none with HL) with anthracycline-induced heart failure, 7 died within weeks, but 4 more who had made a clinical recovery from their heart failure had a fatal relapse of it later during an intercurrent illness.

### Effect in patients with HL

Doxorubicin is commonly used in HL treatment – notably since the introduction of the ABVD regimen in 1973. Information on the effects of anthracyclines on cardiac disease in HL patients has been very limited, however. Large cohort studies have found no significant raised risk of mortality due to myocardial infarction or to coronary artery disease in relation to chemotherapy overall,[58,66,70] but they have not analyzed risks specifically in relation to anthracycline treatment.

In 39 children and adolescents treated with six cycles of A-COPP (doxorubicin, cyclophosphamide, vincristine, procarbazine, and prednisone) plus involved-field radiotherapy (IFR), probably followed for 6–14 years, Sullivan and colleagues[85] noted 1 death from cardiopathy, 1 case of late cardiac toxicity, plus 1 cardiac abnormality under treatment, whereas among 45 similar patients treated with MOPP and bleomycin plus IFR, no such episodes of toxicity occurred.

In patients treated as adults, several studies have assessed cardiac function in groups of about 20–40 patients treated with ABVD plus radiotherapy (± MOPP) 6 months to several years earlier, and have not found frequent serious abnormalities.[86–89] Because the assessments were for the subset of subjects who had survived and were willing to be tested, however, these represent a potentially biased evaluation of cardiac effects. Lund and colleagues[64] analyzed indices of myocardial function in relation to cumulative dose of doxorubicin in about 40 mainly adult patients and stated that there was 'no significant dose–response', but presented no data. Avilés and colleagues[90] investigated cardiac function at rest in adults 5–8 years after treatment with at least six cycles of chemotherapy but no mediastinal radiotherapy, and found an abnormal left ventricular ejection fraction (LVEF) in 40% of 45 patients treated with doxorubicin (ABVD), 31% of 51 treated with epirubicin (EVBD), and 42% of 40 treated with mitoxantrone (MVBD). It is unclear what proportion of the general population, or of other HL patients, would have been deemed abnormal on the basis of the same criteria. In Berlin pericardial thickening was found 2–10 years after treatment in 27% of 18 adult HL patients treated with COPP/ABVD without mediastinal irradiation and 45% of 31 treated with this chemotherapy plus mediastinal irradiation.[91] There was valvular thickening in 43% of the overall group of patients, but no significant difference in cardiac flow velocity between treated patients and controls.

With regard to major morbidity in adults, Avilés and colleagues,[73] in follow-up of 2980 patients with HL, stated that anthracycline treatment was 'associated' with cardiac events (occurrence of myocardial infarction, congestive heart failure, or LVEF abnormalities – mainly the first two categories, and including 27 deaths), but no denominator-based analyses of risk were presented.

## Cerebrovascular disease

Case reports have suggested that carotid artery disease and stroke might be late consequences of neck irradiation, and a cohort study of cancer (but not HL) patients treated with radiotherapy to the neck found a significantly raised incidence of stroke.[92] Evidence on cerebrovascular disease incidence or mortality in HL patients in relation to radiation treatment is scant, however. Elerding and colleagues,[93] in a cohort study of 910 patients who had survived at least 5 years after cervical irradiation for HL, NHL, or head and neck neoplasms (mainly the latter), found an incidence of stroke 66% (but not significantly) greater than expected for age, sex, and race, but the comparability of the expected data source is unclear. In 77 of the HL patients who underwent oculoplethysmography (but these were probably well under 50% of those approached to participate), 16% had significant

stenosis of the carotid/ophthalmic artery system (and 10% had carotid symptoms) – twice the frequency in a group of 25 age- and sex-similar patients referred to the authors' laboratory for evaluation of cardiovascular symptoms.[93] In a cohort of HL patients in the Netherlands almost all treated with radiotherapy – although this may not have been to the neck, a significantly raised relative risk of cerebrovascular accident mortality was found (3.3 (1.1–7.8)).[2]

## Conclusions

Mediastinal radiotherapy can cause a range of cardiac ill-effects, including pericarditis, valvular damage, ischemic heart disease, and myocardial infarction. Treatment strategies have been altered over time in order to try to reduce the risks of these ill effects, but the extent to which this has been achieved has not been well documented. There is extensive evidence that doxorubicin in high cumulative doses can cause cardiac damage in children, and data showing long-term cardiac mortality – although the risks of the latter have not been well quantified and the evidence is largely not from HL patients per se. There is a need for large cohort studies focused on the question of whether doxorubicin treatment for HL affects the risk of late mortality from cardiac disease, and whether the effects of mediastinal radiotherapy interact with any effects of doxorubicin. The possible effect of cervical irradiation on risks of stroke incidence and mortality also needs clarification.

While it would seem reasonable to reduce radiation doses to the heart within constraints of therapeutic needs, and to monitor and minimize cardiovascular risk factors in patients who have been treated with mediastinal radiotherapy, the evidence to show to what extent this will actually reduce cardiovascular disease and mortality risks is partial and inconclusive. There is a need for large-scale studies of long-term cardiovascular mortality and major morbidity in relation to the therapeutic modalities discussed above.

# Acknowledgments

We thank Mrs Margaret Snigorska for secretarial help.

## REFERENCES

1. Hancock SL, Hoppe RT. Long-term complications of treatment and causes of mortality after Hodgkin's disease. *Semin Radiat Oncol* 1996; **6**: 225–42.
2. Aleman BMP, van den Belt-Dusebout AW, Klokman WJ et al. Long-term cause-specific mortality of patients treated for Hodgkin's disease. *J. Clin Oncol* 2003; **21**: 3431–9.
3. Hoppe RT. Hodgkin's disease: complications of therapy and excess mortality. *Ann Oncol* 1997; **8** (Suppl 1): 115–18.
4. Ng AK, Bernardo MP, Weller E et al. Long-term survival and competing causes of death in patients with early-stage Hodgkin's disease treated at age 50 or younger. *J Clin Oncol* 2002; **20**: 2101–8.
5. Arseneau JC, Sponzo RW, Levin DL et al.

Nonlymphomatous malignant tumors complicating Hodgkin's disease. Possible association with intensive therapy. *N Engl J Med* 1972; **287**: 1119–22.

6.  Bonadonna G, De Lena M, Banfi A, Lattuada A. Secondary neoplasms in malignant lymphomas after intensive therapy. *N Engl J Med* 1973; **288**: 1242–3.

7.  van Leeuwen FE, Travis LB. Second cancers. In: DeVita VT Jr, Hellman S, Rosenberg SA (eds) *Cancer: Principles and Practice of Oncology*, 6th edn. Philadelphia: Lippincott Williams & Wilkins, 2001: 2939–60.

8.  van Leeuwen FE, Swerdlow AJ, Valagussa P, Tucker MA. Second cancers after treatment of Hodgkin's disease. In: Mauch PM, Armitage JO, Diehl V et al (eds) *Hodgkin's disease*. Philadelphia: Lippincott, Williams & Wilkins, 1999: 607–32.

9.  Swerdlow AJ, Barber JA, Vaughan Hudson G et al. Risk of second malignancy after Hodgkin's disease in a collaborative British cohort: the relation to age at treatment. *J Clin Oncol* 2000; **18**: 498–509.

10. Dores GM, Metayer C, Curtis RE et al. Second malignant neoplasms among long-term survivors of Hodgkin's disease: a population-based evaluation over 25 years. *J Clin Oncol* 2002; **20**: 3484–94.

11. Kaldor JM, Day NE, Clarke EA et al. Leukemia following Hodgkin's disease. *N Engl J Med* 1990; **322**: 7–13.

12. Swerdlow AJ, Douglas AJ, Vaughan Hudson G et al. Risk of second primary cancers after Hodgkin's disease by type of treatment: analysis of 2846 patients in the British National Lymphoma Investigation. *BMJ* 1992; **304**: 1137–43.

13. van Leeuwen FE, Klokman WJ, Hagenbeek A et al. Second cancer risk following Hodgkin's disease: a 20-year follow-up study. *J Clin Oncol* 1994; **12**: 312–25.

14. Bhatia S, Robison LL, Oberlin O et al. Breast cancer and other second neoplasms after childhood Hodgkin's disease. *N Engl J Med* 1996; **334**: 745–51.

15. van Leeuwen FE, Klokman WJ, Veer MB et al. Long-term risk of second malignancy in survivors of Hodgkin's disease treated during adolescence or young adulthood. *J Clin Oncol* 2000; **18**: 487–97.

16. Mauch PM, Kalish LA, Marcus KC et al. Second malignancies after treatment for laparotomy staged IA–IIIB Hodgkin's disease: long-term analysis of risk factors and outcome. *Blood* 1996; **87**: 3625–32.

17. Tucker MA, Coleman CN, Cox RS et al. Risk of second cancers after treatment for Hodgkin's disease. *N Engl J Med* 1988; **318**: 76–81.

18. Henry-Amar M. Second cancer after the treatment for Hodgkin's disease: a report from the International Database on Hodgkin's Disease. *Ann Oncol* 1992; **3** (Suppl 4): 117–28.

19. Hancock SL, Tucker MA, Hoppe RT. Breast cancer after treatment of Hodgkin's disease. *J Natl Cancer Inst* 1993; **85**: 25–31.

20. Birdwell SH, Hancock SL, Varghese A et al. Gastrointestinal cancer after treatment of Hodgkin's disease. *Int J Radiat Oncol Biol Phys* 1997; **37**: 67–73.

21. van Leeuwen FE, Chorus AM, Belt-Dusebout AW et al. Leukemia risk following Hodgkin's disease: relation to cumulative dose of alkylating agents, treatment with teniposide combinations, number of episodes of chemotherapy, and bone marrow damage. *J Clin Oncol* 1994; **12**: 1063–73.

22. Valagussa PA, Bonadonna G. Carcinogenic effects of cancer treatment. In: Peckham M, Pinedo H, Veronesi U (eds) *Oxford Textbook of Oncology*. Oxford: Oxford University Press, 1995; 2348–58.

23. Schellong G, Riepenhausen M, Creutzig U et al. Low risk of secondary leukemias after chemotherapy without mechlorethamine in childhood Hodgkin's disease. German–Austrian Pediatric Hodgkin's Disease Group. *J Clin Oncol* 1997; **15**: 2247–53.

24. Andrieu JM, Ifrah N, Payen C et al. Increased risk of secondary acute nonlymphocytic leukemia after extended-field radiation therapy combined with MOPP chemotherapy for Hodgkin's disease. *J Clin Oncol* 1990; **8**: 1148–54.

25. Boivin J-F, Hutchison GB, Zauber AG et al. Incidence of second cancers in patients treated for Hodgkin's disease. *J Natl Cancer Inst* 1995; **87**: 732–41.

26. Abruzzese E, Radford JE, Miller JS et al. Detection of abnormal pretransplant clones in progenitor cells of patients who developed myelodysplasia after autologous transplantation. *Blood* 1999; **94**: 1814–19.

27. Andre M, Henry-Amar M, Blaise D et al. Treatment-related deaths and second cancer risk after autologous stem-cell transplantation for Hodgkin's disease. *Blood* 1998; **92**: 1933–40.

28. Park S, Brice P, Noguerra ME et al. Myelodysplasias and leukemias after autologous stem cell transplantation for lymphoid malignancies. *Bone Marrow Transplant* 2000; **26**: 321–6.

29. Traweek ST, Slovak ML, Nademanee AP et al. Myelodysplasia and acute myeloid leukemia occurring after autologous bone marrow transplantation for lymphoma. *Leuk Lymphoma* 1996; **20**: 365–72.

30. Penn I. Cancers complicating organ transplantation. *N Engl J Med* 1990; **323**: 1767–9.

31. van Rijswijk RE, Sybesma JP, Kater L. A prospective study of the changes in immune status following radiotherapy for Hodgkin's disease. *Cancer* 1984; **53**: 62–9.

32. Krikorian JG, Burke JS, Rosenberg SA, Kaplan HS. Occurrence of non-Hodgkin's lymphoma after therapy for Hodgkin's disease. *N Engl J Med* 1979; **300**: 452–8.

33. Prosper F, Robledo C, Cuesta B et al. Incidence of non-Hodgkin's lymphoma in patients treated for Hodgkin's disease. *Leuk Lymphoma* 1994; **12**: 457–62.

34. Rueffer U, Josting A, Franklin J et al. Non-Hodgkin's lymphoma after primary Hodgkin's disease in the German Hodgkin's Lymphoma Study Group: incidence, treatment, and prognosis. *J Clin Oncol* 2001; **19**: 2026–32.

35. Hancock SL, Cox RS, McDougall IR. Thyroid diseases after treatment of Hodgkin's disease. *N Engl J Med* 1991; **325**: 599–605.

36. Tucker MA, Misfeldt D, Coleman CN, Clark WH Jr. Cutaneous malignant melanoma after Hodgkin's disease. *Ann Intern Med* 1985; **102**: 37–41.

37. Metayer C, Lynch CF, Clarke EA et al. Second cancers among long-term survivors of Hodgkin's disease diagnosed in childhood and adolescence. *J Clin Oncol* 2000; **18**: 2435–43.

38. Miller AB, Howe GR, Sherman GJ et al. Mortality from breast cancer after irradiation during fluoroscopic examinations in patients being treated for tuberculosis. *New Engl J Med* 1989; **321**: 1285–9.

39. United Nations Scientific Committee on the Effects of Atomic Radiation. *Sources and Effects of Ionizing Radiation: UNSCEAR 1994 Report to the General*

*Assembly with Scientific Annexes.* New York: United Nations 1994.

40. Boice JD Jr, Land CE, Preston DL. Ionizing radiation. In: Schottenfeld D, Fraumeni JF Jr (eds) *Cancer Epidemiology and Prevention.* Oxford: Oxford University Press, 1996: 319–54.

41. van Leeuwen FE, Klokman WJ, Stovall M et al. Roles of radiotherapy and smoking in lung cancer following Hodgkin's disease. *J Natl Cancer Inst* 1995; **87**: 1530–7.

42. Travis LB, Gospodarowicz M, Curtis RE et al. Lung cancer following chemotherapy and radiotherapy for Hodgkin's disease. *J Natl Cancer Inst* 2002; **94**: 182–92.

43. Donaldson SS, Hancock SL. Second cancers after Hodgkin's disease in childhood. *N Engl J Med* 1996; **334**: 792–4.

44. Wolf J, Schellong G, Diehl V. Breast cancer following treatment of Hodgkin's disease – more reasons for less radiotherapy? *Eur J Cancer* 1997; **33**: 2293–4.

45. Goss PE, Sierra S. Current perspectives on radiation-induced breast cancer. *J Clin Oncol* 1998; **16**: 338–47.

46. Neglia JP, Friedman DL, Yasui Y et al. Second malignant neoplasms in five-year survivors of childhood cancer: childhood cancer survivor study. *J Natl Cancer Inst* 2001; **93**: 618–29.

47. Wolden SL, Hancock SL, Carlson RW et al. Management of breast cancer after Hodgkin's disease. *J Clin Oncol* 2000; **18**: 765–72.

48. van Leeuwen FE, Klokman WJ, Storall M et al. Roles of radiation dose, chemotherapy and hormonal factors in breast cancer following Hodgkin's disease. *J Natl Cancer Inst* 2003; **95**: 971–80.

49. Kaldor JM, Day NE, Bell J et al. Lung cancer following Hodgkin's disease: a case-control study. *Int J Cancer* 1992; **52**: 677–81.

50. Swerdlow AJ, Schoemaker MJ, Allerton R et al. Lung cancer after Hodgkin's disease: a nested case-control study of the relation to treatment. *J Clin Oncol* 2001; **19**: 1610–18.

51. International Agency for Research on Cancer. Overall evaluations of carcinogenicity: an updating of IARC Monographs Volumes 1 to 42. *IARC Monogr Eval Carcinog Risks Hum Suppl* 1987; **7**: 1–440.

52. Easton DF, Peto J, Doll R. Cancers of the respiratory tract in mustard gas workers. *Br J Ind Med* 1988; **45**: 652–9.

53. Sankila R, Garwicz S, Olsen JH et al, for the Assocation of the Nordic Cancer Registries and the Society of Pediatric Hematology and Oncology. Risk of subsequent malignant neoplasms among 1,641 Hodgkin's disease patients diagnosed in childhood and adolescence: a population-based cohort study in the five Nordic countries. *J Clin Oncol* 1996; **14**: 1442–6.

54. Wolden SL, Lamborn KR, Cleary SF et al. Second cancers following pediatric Hodgkin's disease. *J Clin Oncol* 1998; **16**: 536–44.

55. Aisenberg AC, Finkelstein DM, Doppke KP et al. High risk of breast carcinoma after irradiation of young women with Hodgkin's disease. *Cancer* 1997; **79**: 1203–10.

56. Land CE. Studies of cancer and radiation dose among atomic bomb survivors. The example of breast cancer. *JAMA* 1995; **274**: 402–7.

57. Allavena C, Conroy T, Aletti P et al. Late cardiopulmonary toxicity after treatment for Hodgkin's disease. *Br J Cancer* 1992; **65**: 908–12.

58. Hancock SL, Donaldson SS, Hoppe RT. Cardiac disease following treatment of Hodgkin's disease in children and adolescents. *J Clin Oncol* 1993; **11**: 1208–15.

59. Stewart JR, Fajardo LF. Dose response in human and experimental radiation-induced heart disease. Application of the nominal standard dose (NSD) concept. *Radiology* 1971; **99**: 403–8.

60. Carmel RJ, Kaplan HS. Mantle irradiation in Hodgkin's disease: an analysis of technique, tumor eradication, and complications. *Cancer* 1976; **37**: 2813–25.

61. Cosset JM, Henry-Amar M, Pellae-Cosset B et al. Pericarditis and myocardial infarctions after Hodgkin's disease therapy. *Int J Radiat Oncol Biol Phys* 1991; **21**: 447–9.

62. Tarbell NJ, Thompson L, Mauch P. Thoracic irradiation in Hodgkin's disease: disease control and long-term complications. *Int J Radiat Oncol Biol Phys* 1990; **18**: 275–81.

63. Lund MB, Ihlen H, Voss BMR et al. Increased risk of heart valve regurgitation after mediastinal radiation for Hodgkin's disease: an echocardiographic study. *Heart* 1996; **75**: 591–5.

64. Lund MB, Kongerud J, Boe J et al. Cardiopulmonary sequelae after treatment for Hodgkin's disease: increased risk in females? *Ann Oncol* 1996; **7**: 257–64.

65. Glanzmann C, Kaufmann P, Jenni R et al. Cardiac risk after mediastinal irradiation for Hodgkin's disease. *Radiother Oncol* 1998; **46**: 51–62.

66. Hancock SL, Tucker MA, Hoppe RT. Factors affecting late mortality from heart disease after treatment of Hodgkin's disease. *JAMA* 1993; **270**: 1949–55.

67. Cosset JM, Henry-Amar M, Meerwaldt JH, for the EORTC Lymphoma Cooperative Group. Long-term toxicity of early stages of Hodgkin's disease therapy: the EORTC experience. *Ann Oncol* 1991; **2**(Suppl 2): 77–82.

68. Liao Z, Ha CS, Vlachaki MT et al. Mantle irradiation alone for pathologic stage I and II Hodgkin's disease: long-term follow-up and patterns of failure. *Int J Radiat Oncol Biol Phys* 2001; **50**: 971–7.

69. Henry-Amar M, Hayat M, Meerwaldt JH et al, for the EORTC Lymphoma Cooperative Group. Causes of death after therapy for early stage Hodgkin's disease entered on EORTC protocols. *Int J Radiat Oncol Biol Phys* 1990; **19**: 1155–7.

70. Boivin J-F, Hutchison GB, Lubin JH, Mauch P. Coronary artery disease mortality in patients treated for Hodgkin's disease. *Cancer* 1992; **69**: 1241–7.

71. King V, Constine LS, Clark D et al. Symptomatic coronary artery disease after mantle irradiation for Hodgkin's disease. *Int J Radiat Oncol Biol Phys* 1996; **36**: 881–9.

72. Brierley JD, Rathmell AJ, Gospodarowicz MK et al. Late effects of treatment for early-stage Hodgkin's disease. *Br J Cancer* 1998; **77**: 1300–7.

73. Avilés A, Neri N, Uadra I et al. Second lethal events associated with treatment for Hodgkin's disease: a review of 2980 patients treated in a single Mexican institute. *Leuk Lymphoma* 2000; **39**: 311–19.

74. Hudson MM, Poquette CA, Lee J et al. Increased mortality after successful treatment for Hodgkin's disease. *J Clin Oncol* 1998; **16**: 3592–600.

75. Mauch PM, Kalish LA, Marcus KC et al. Long-term survival in Hodgkin's disease. Relative impact of mortality, second tumors, infection, and cardiovascular disease. *Cancer J Sci Am* 1995; **1**: 33–42.

76. Lee CKK, Aeppli D, Nierengarten ME. The need for long-term surveillance for patients treated with curative radiotherapy for Hodgkin's disease: University of Minnesota experience. *Int J Radiat Oncol Biol Phys* 2000; **48**: 169–79.

77. Eriksson F, Gagliardi G, Liedberg A et al. Long-term cardiac mortality following radiation therapy for Hodgkin's disease: analysis with the relative seriality model. *Radiother Oncol* 2000; **55**: 153–62.

78. Lipshultz SE, Lipsitz SR, Mone SM et al. Female sex and higher drug dose as risk factors for late cardiotoxic effects of doxorubicin therapy for childhood cancer. *N Engl J Med* 1995; **332**: 1738–43.

79. Steinherz LJ, Steinherz PG, Tan CTC et al. Cardiac toxicity 4 to 20 years after completing anthracycline therapy. *JAMA* 1991; **266**: 1672–7.

80. Kremer LCM, van Dalen EC, Offringa M et al. Anthracycline-induced clinical heart failure in a cohort of 607 children: long-term follow-up study. *J Clin Oncol* 2001; **19**: 191–6.

81. Robertson CM, Hawkins MM, Kingston JE. Late deaths and survival after childhood cancer: implications for cure. *BMJ* 1994; **309**: 162–6.

82. Pihkala J, Saarinen UM, Lundström U et al. Myocardial function in children and adolescents after therapy with anthracyclines and chest irradiation. *Eur J Cancer* 1996; **32A**: 97–103.

83. Green DM, Hyland A, Chung CS et al. Cancer and cardiac mortality among 15-year survivors of cancer diagnosed during childhood or adolescence. *J Clin Oncol* 1999; **17**: 3207–15.

84. Moreb JS, Oblon DJ. Outcome of clinical congestive heart failure induced by anthracycline chemotherapy. *Cancer* 1992; **70**: 2637–41.

85. Sullivan MP, Fuller LM, Berard C et al. Comparative effectiveness of two combined modality regimens in the treatment of surgical stage III Hodgkin's disease in children. *Am J Pediatr Hematol Oncol* 1991; **13**: 450–8.

86. LaMonte CS, Yeh SDJ, Straus DJ. Long-term follow-up of cardiac function in patients with Hodgkin's disease treated with mediastinal irradiation and combination chemotherapy including doxorubicin. *Cancer Treat Rep* 1986; **70**: 439–44.

87. Santoro A, Bonadonna G, Valagussa P et al. Long-term results of combined chemotherapy-radiotherapy approach in Hodgkin's disease: superiority of ABVD plus radiotherapy versus MOPP plus radiotherapy. *J Clin Oncol* 1987; **5**: 27–37.

88. Brice P, Tredaniel J, Monsuez JJ et al. Cardiopulmonary toxicity after three courses of ABVD and mediastinal irradiation in favorable Hodgkin's disease. *Ann Oncol* 1991; **2** (Suppl): 73–6.

89. Salloum E, Tanoue LT, Wackers FJ et al. Assessment of cardiac and pulmonary function in adult patients with Hodgkin's disease treated with ABVD or MOPP/ABVD plus adjuvant low-dose mediastinal irradiation. *Cancer Invest* 1999; **17**: 171–80.

90. Avilés A, Arévila N, Maques JCD et al. Late cardiac toxicity of doxorubicin, epirubicin, and mitoxantrone therapy for Hodgkin's disease in adults. *Leuk Lymphoma* 1993; **11**: 275–9.

91. Kreuser E-D, Völler H, Behles C et al. Evaluation of late cardiotoxicity with pulsed Doppler echocardiography in patients treated for Hodgkin's disease. *Br J Haematol* 1993; **84**: 615–22.

92. Dorresteijn LDA, Kappelle AC, Boogerd W et al. Increased risk of ischemic stroke after radiotherapy on the neck in patients younger than 60 years. *J Clin Oncol* 2001; **20**: 282–8.

93. Elerding SC, Fernandez RN, Grotta JC et al. Carotid artery disease following external cervical irradiation. *Ann Surg* 1981; **194**: 609–15.

# 44 Late effects in children treated for acute leukemia

## Stuart Mucklow and Gill Levitt

## Introduction

A majority of pediatric patients who present with acute leukemia in a developed country will achieve long-term disease-free survival following intensive chemotherapy. Major developments of treatment regimens for pediatric leukemias have taken place over the last 30 years, validated through data obtained from large multicenter randomized clinical trials. Significant gains in rates of disease-free survival for successive cohorts of children with acute lymphoblastic leukemia (ALL) and acute myeloid leukemia (AML) have been achieved over this period (Figure 44.1). Advances in diagnostic techniques and disease classification, application of risk-stratified approaches to treatment, developments in combination chemotherapy therapies, and improvements in supportive care have all contributed to this survival benefit. Although further chemotherapy or allogeneic stem cell transplantation (alloSCT) can be successful in relapsed disease, most of the long-term survivors of pediatric leukemia are individuals who remain in first complete remission.[1]

However, the modalities used in the treatment of leukemia are associated with significant acute and long-term toxicities at therapeutic doses.[2,3] In children, dysfunction may arise either due to direct organ damage or through an impairment of the growth or maturation of an organ system. Toxicities are cumulative, so exposures to therapeutic agents that are accrued through retreatment of relapsed patients tend to be associated with greater organ damage.

An important aim of clinical trials of pediatric leukemia treatment is to seek to establish an optimal balance between the likelihood of achieving long-term disease remission through effective treatment, and minimizing treatment-associated morbidity in the disease-free survivors. Long-term follow-up is important to identify treatment-related morbidity, which may not appear until many years after the completion of therapy, and to assess its adverse impact on survivors' quality of life. This should be an important consideration in the process of reviewing and further developing treatment regimens for pediatric leukemia.

We believe that the correct setting for follow-up of child survivors of leukemia is in a dedicated age-specific 'long-term follow-up clinic'.[4,5] Here, surveillance for treatment-related morbidity can be part of a global assessment of the health and development of these individuals, in a supportive multidisciplinary environment that also addresses health promotion issues.

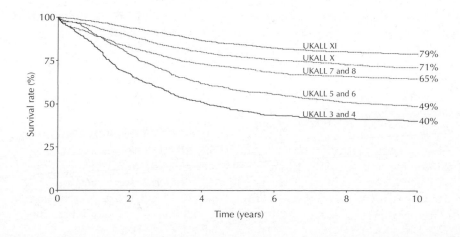

**Figure 44.1** Overall survival rates of children treated for acute lymphoblastic leukemia in successive UK MRC trials. Courtesy of S Richards and G Buck, MRC Clinical Trials Service Unit, University of Oxford, UK.

An essential basis for appropriate follow-up is an accurate end-of-treatment summary that clearly itemizes the relevant therapeutic exposures with potential toxicity. In this context, the original histological diagnosis is of less direct relevance. However, it can provide a useful means of categorization when a cohort of children who are being followed up in a long-term follow-up clinic have been treated according to a particular regimen and have accrued similar exposures. Debate continues over whether regular follow-up in a hospital-based clinic is necessary for all individuals who have been treated for leukemia in childhood, and the duration for which such follow-up remains appropriate.

The discussion of late effects of treatment for childhood leukemia in this chapter concentrates on four areas: cardiotoxicity, effects on growth and other endocrine dysfunction, cognitive and neuropsychological sequelae, and the increased risk of second primary neoplasms. This chapter is intended to complement the other chapters in this book on late effects associated with the treatment of Hodgkin lymphoma (HL) and alloSCT (Chapters 43 and 45). Our choice of areas that we consider to be clinically important is based on the selection of predominantly retrospective clinical studies of cohorts of survivors of childhood leukemia that have provided valuable data relating treatment modalities and long-term outcome. However, they are by no means the only ones that should be considered in the long-term follow-up of such individuals.[6–9] Systems that may be affected by therapeutic exposures to radiotherapy, chemotherapeutic or antimicrobial agents, or opportunistic infections are listed in detail in recent follow-up guidelines developed by the Children's Oncology Group.[10]

# Cardiotoxicity

Anthracycline drugs constitute an effective component of contemporary combination chemotherapy protocols for the treatment of AML and ALL in children. However, their use is limited by dose-related cardiotoxicity due to focal myocyte death and replacement fibrosis, which can result in acute or late cardiac dysfunction. Growth hormone insufficiency and obesity, which may also be consequences of childhood leukemia treatment, are additional independent risk factors for cardiac dysfunction in survivors. Two recent systematic reviews[11,12] have provided overviews of the risk factors for and incidence of heart failure and subclinical cardiotoxicity in survivors of childhood cancer who received anthracycline treatment.

An increased risk of cardiac dysfunction and ischemic heart disease following mantle irradiation that includes the heart, particularly with doses above 30 Gy, has been found following treatment for HL,[13,14] but no increased incidence of cardiac dysfunction has been demonstrated in ALL survivors who received craniospinal irradiation in addition to chemotherapy.

The cumulative total dose of anthracycline is the most important parameter associated with early cardiomyopathy and symptomatic heart failure.[15] An increased incidence of heart failure in children has been demonstrated with a cumulative exposure of more than 300 mg/m² of doxorubicin, while the rate increases rapidly above 450 mg/m².[16] Cumulative anthracycline exposure was also the most important factor identified in the retrospective analysis of children who had received chemotherapy on Pediatric Oncology Group protocols: a dose of more than 550 mg/m² increased the relative risk of congestive heart failure in this series reported by Krischer et al.[17] Other treatment factors included a maximum single anthracycline dose of over 50 mg/m², treatment with amsacrine, trisomy 21, female sex, and the ethnic origin of the child. Delivery of low or moderate anthracycline doses through continuous infusion rather than as a bolus does not appear to be cardioprotective in children.[18,19]

Cumulative anthracycline dose is also the strongest independent risk factor for developing late-stage cardiac dysfunction.[20–22] These late cardiotoxic effects of anthracycline exposure were identified initially through long-term surveillance of pediatric cancer survivors who had been treated in the late 1970s and received relatively high cumulative anthracycline doses. For example, the children described by Goorin et al[23] had been treated with between 390 and 450 mg/m² of doxorubicin.

Evidence of early cardiac dysfunction related to anthracycline treatment is also an important indicator of increased risk for developing late cardiac failure or asymptomatic dysfunction on echocardiography. A cross-sectional study of relapse-free ALL survivors,[20] who had been treated with cumulative doses of between 230 and 550 mg/m² of doxorubicin, found echocardiographic abnormalities of cardiac function in almost two-thirds of the patients at a median follow-up time of 6 years from remission. Of the children in this cohort, 11 (10%) had required treatment for acute congestive heart failure, and 5 of these suffered a recurrence, with 2 proceeding to cardiac transplant. Lipshulz et al[21] presented data that suggested an increasing prevalence of cardiac abnormalities with length of follow-up in ALL survivors, and more severe abnormalities were found in this study in female subjects.

The UK Medical Research Council (MRC) UKALL X Pilot and UKALL X clinical trials[24,25] were conducted in the 1980s to assess the value of intensification treatment in pediatric ALL. Patients were treated on a common treatment protocol with a cumulative total dose of 90, 180, or 270 mg/m² of daunorubicin, delivered through bolus infusions. Three samples, based on these doses, of 40 relapse-free patients from the combined trial cohorts, who were treated at a single institution, have been studied prospectively for more than a decade, and provided valuable data on long-term cardiotoxicity from exposure to lower cumulative anthracycline doses.[26,27]

Although all of the ALL survivors in the study were asymptomatic at the time of assessment, 23% were found to have echocardiographic abnormalities of cardiac function at a mean of 6 years post treatment, while 15% had abnormalities at 10 years.[26,27] In most individuals, the abnormality was increased left ventricular end-systolic wall stress, while a minority of the subjects also had a significant reduction in cardiac contractility. No association was found between cumulative dose, female sex, or age at presentation and the likelihood of an echocardiographic abnormality within this range of cumulative doses (90–270 mg/m² daunorubicin). Where deterioration was demonstrated in cardiac performance between the first and second assessments, this was more likely to be found in children who had received a cumulative dose of more than 240 mg/m². Significant improvements in functional echocardiographic parameters tended to be restricted to subjects who had received lower exposures. There was one sudden death – in a 16-year-old boy who had previously been shown to have mild echocardiographic abnormalities. Extensive myocardial fibrosis was found at autopsy. All other members of these sample cohorts remained asymptomatic.

Regular cardiac monitoring during and after anthracycline treatment is recommended practice.[5,8,10,28] However, Lipschultz et al[29] reviewed the evidence base for the Children's Cancer Study Group (CCSG) practice guidelines[28] and have disputed the value of echocardiographic screening, using chamber dimensions and fractional shortening as measures of left ventricular function, in reliably detecting early signs of anthracycline-related cardiotoxicity, or in providing prognostically relevant data with respect to long-term cardiac performance. More invasive tests, such as dobutamine stress testing, can increase the sensitivity of echocardiography, and may be appropriate for assessment in situations such as pregnancy or competitive sports.[5,30]

Angiotensin-converting enzyme (ACE) inhibitors have been used to treat anthracycline-related cardiac dysfunction in survivors of childhood leukemia with short-term improvement in echocardiographic cardiac function,[31] although the clinical benefit has been questioned.[32] The long-term benefit of ACE inhibitor treatment for such individuals is under investigation in a prospective clinical trial.[33]

A liposomal formulation of daunorubicin, Dauno-Xome, may offer equivalent efficacy with lower rates of acute or long-term cardiotoxicity and is under evaluation. Co-administration of dexrazoxane (ICRF-187) with an anthracycline has been shown to reduce the risk of acute cardiotoxicity,[34] but its effectiveness in avoiding late cardiac dysfunction has not been established.

# Endocrine dysfunction

Endocrine disturbances are present in up to 40% of childhood cancer survivors.[35] For survivors of childhood acute leukemia, the areas where late effects of treatment are particularly important are growth, obesity, skeletal changes, progression through puberty, and fertility. The deficits and adverse long-term outcomes that may be present depend on the nature and cumulative dose of the cytotoxic agents that were administered, and the dose and fields used for radiotherapy. They also relate to the age and developmental stage that the individual had reached at the time of treatment. A higher incidence of endocrine deficit is detected in studies where provocative testing is used as the investigational tool, rather than measurement of physiological parameters.

## Growth

Modern protocols for the treatment of childhood ALL do not use routine cranial or craniospinal irradiation to provide central nervous system (CNS)-directed therapy. Impaired growth is seen in some survivors after treatment with chemotherapy alone,[36–39] but the final height achieved is generally within the normal adult range. Growth hormone (GH) deficiency on laboratory testing is not found as frequently in these individuals as in survivors from earlier cohorts who received treatment for ALL that included low-dose cranial or craniospinal irradiation (18–24 Gy), where GH deficiency can be demonstrated in up to 50%.[40–45]

Some studies report a dose dependence of the deficit in GH production after 18 or 24 Gy cranial irradiation shown by GH stimulation testing,[40,44,46] but this relationship has not been observed by others.[47,48] In some individuals, the GH deficit was shown to evolve during the follow-up period,[42,45,49] and it may not become manifest until puberty, when the peak amplitude and periodicity of GH secretion may be adversely affected.[50]

Studies of long-term ALL survivors have also shown that spontaneous GH secretion over 24 hours is reduced both before and during puberty,[41,46,48,50] but a direct relationship between the mean 24-hour GH level and height or growth velocity has not been demonstrated.[41,51,52] Low-dose cranial irradiation may result in precocious puberty in girls,[53–56] but no effect on puberty has been demonstrated in boys. Precocious puberty may compound the effect of GH deficiency by reducing the time taken to reach final height.

Decreased final height relative to centile height at diagnosis has been demonstrated in several longitudinal and cross-sectional cohort studies of ALL survivors who received prophylactic low-dose cranial irradiation.[37,38,52,55,57–61] Davies et al[60] demonstrated that the short stature was disproportionate in their cohort of child survivors of ALL, who had relatively shorter backs than legs. Nevertheless, a majority still achieve an acceptable final height that lies within the normal adult range, and GH therapy[54,62] is not often required. However, survivors who require further cranial irradiation after a course of irradiation as primary CNS-directed therapy are often more severely affected.[40,63]

Secretion of GH is the most sensitive to disruption following low-dose cranial irradiation, and this does not commonly lead to a deficit in the production of other anterior pituitary hormones.[45] For example, a long-term follow-up study assessing thyroid hormone secretion found that prophylactic cranial irradiation for childhood ALL did not affect subsequent thyroid-stimulating hormone (TSH) secretion from the anterior pituitary in response to stimulation with exogenous thyroid-releasing hormone (TRH).[64] Low-dose craniospinal irradiation may lead to some direct thyroid damage, but the long-term risk of hypothyroidism after such treatment appears to be relatively low.

## Obesity

Survivors of childhood ALL show increased rates of obesity at all ages following treatment.[59,61,65–71] Effects on the timing of normal changes in body mass parameters, which influence adult obesity risk, are observed in young children following treatment for ALL.[73] Obesity may be a consequence of corticosteroid therapy or low-dose cranial irradiation, and may develop through treatment-related disturbances of the GH and leptin systems. Chronic changes in metabolic status could be exacerbated by the physical inactivity and reduced energy expenditure that have been documented in long-term survivors.[74,75]

The majority of long-term follow-up studies that have assessed obesity in survivors of childhood ALL have shown females to be at increased risk relative to male survivors.[67,70,71] However, some studies have not reproduced this observation.[66,69] Cranial irradiation has also been identified as a risk factor for weight gain or adiposity in most,[67,69,71] but not all,[66,73] reports. For example, Sklar et al[69] undertook a retrospective analysis of the body mass index (BMI) standard deviation (z) score, corrected for sex and height, from measurements recorded at diagnosis, at the end of treatment, and at the attainment of final adult height in 126 survivors treated for childhood ALL. They found that a significant increase in the mean BMI of the group treated with cranial radiotherapy could be observed at the completion of ALL treatment, and persisted to the completion of growth. Of the patients in this group, 40% were overweight when they attained their final height. No increase in BMI was seen for the group who had not been treated with cranial irradiation, and no association with cumulative corticosteroid dose, age at diagnosis, or sex was demonstrated in this study.

The largest retrospective cross-sectional study in this area to date, comprising almost 300 individuals, was based on cohorts drawn from the UK ALL X/XI clinical trials,[67] and compared survivors who had and had not received cranial irradiation. Both males and females treated with chemotherapy alone showed increased BMI z scores at more than 4 years from diagnosis. In individuals who had been treated with cranial irradiation, an increased BMI z score at final height was associated with female sex but not with age at diagnosis. Severe obesity (BMI z score >3) was only seen in females, with a prevalence of 8%.

## Skeletal changes

Osteopenia and osteoporosis are increased in incidence in survivors of childhood ALL.[76–82] The critical period for bone mineralization extends from childhood into early adulthood, with peak bone mineral density (BMD) reached by about age 25 years, and this process can be severely affected by treatment for acute leukemia in childhood.[83] Peak bone mass is the strongest predictor for risk of osteoporotic fracture in later life.

Changes in bone mineralization may be multifactorial:[83,84] causes may include craniospinal or cranial irradiation,[76,77,81,86] treatment with methotrexate[80,81,86] and corticosteroids,[87] deficiencies of hormones, including sex hormones and GH, nutritional deficiency during treatment, and reduced physical activity and biomechanical loading of the skeleton during and after treatment.[80] Most studies use dual-energy X-ray absorptiometry (DEXA) to assess BMD.[84]

Among ALL survivors, male sex and prophylactic cranial irradiation are risk factors for a reduced BMD, while age and pubertal status at treatment were not found to be associated with osteoporotic change.[81,82] However, a smaller study of a cohort of older children (mean age 16 years) treated for ALL with high-dose dexamethasone and methotrexate, but not cranial irradiation, found no long-term effect on BMD in either sex.[88] Children proceeding to bone marrow transplantation (BMT) may be more severely affected.[89,90]

## Gonadal function and fertility

In survivors of childhood acute leukemia, irradiation of the gonads and the cumulative dose of alkylating agents are the treatment modalities that have the greatest impacts on subsequent gonadal function and fertility in both sexes.[91,92]

Gonadal function in males is affected by relatively low doses of direct testicular irradiation.[92–96] The germinal epithelium appears to be exquisitely sensitive. Radiation doses less than 0.1 Gy can produce temporary oligospermia or azoospermia, while permanent azoospermia occurs with a dose above 2 Gy. Leydig cell damage following external radiation doses above 2 Gy can be detected biochemically through elevated luteinizing hormone (LH) levels, although testosterone levels are still maintained in many cases at this dose. With doses above 20 Gy, irreversible Leydig cell failure occurs in prepubertal boys, while older boys and adults can in some cases tolerate doses up to 30 Gy without loss of testosterone secretion.[92] Direct irradiation of the testes with a dose of 12 Gy to treat testicular involvement with leukemia has been shown to result in reduced testicular volume (<10 ml), permanent azoospermia, and elevated follicle-stimulating hormone (FSH) and reduced serum inhibin B levels, but testosterone replacement therapy is often not required.[91,97]

The effects are most marked in boys treated for ALL with testicular involvement or relapse who receive direct testicular irradiation,[94,97] and in those who proceed to high-dose therapy and BMT with total body irradiation (TBI) conditioning. There is also a risk of gonadal damage in males treated with craniospinal irradiation, due to scatter. In the cohort of ALL survivors investigated by Sklar et al[98] with FSH and testicular volume measurements, 55% of those who had been treated with craniospinal irradiation and 12 Gy direct testicular irradiation showed testicular failure; 13% who had received craniospinal irradiation alone were also affected, while none of the individuals treated with identical chemotherapy plus prophylactic cranial irradiation had signs of testicular failure.[98]

Cyclophosphamide and other alkylating agents damage the germinal epithelium of the testes, resulting in oligospermia or azoospermia and elevated FSH levels. At higher doses, Leydig cells may also be affected, leading to elevated LH levels, but testosterone levels often remain normal following primary chemotherapy for acute leukemia and most boys undergo normal progression through puberty.[91,92,99,100] However, spontaneous progression through puberty does not guarantee future fertility.

The degree of permanent damage to gonadal function is related to the cumulative dose of alkylating agents received: testicular failure and infertility is almost universal after exposure to more than 25 g/m$^2$ of cyclophosphamide, while normal function and fertility have been reported to be preserved in most males when the cumulative cyclophosphamide dose remains below 3.5 g/m$^2$.[101,102] It has been suggested

that prepubertal boys have a lower rate of testicular failure than adults at equivalent doses of cyclophosphamide. This may be based upon the finding of normal gonadotropin levels in prepubertal males despite gonadal damage, which is revealed in an elevation of LH and FSH levels as the child enters puberty. Kenney et al[102] found no effect of pubertal status in their cohort treated with high-dose cyclophosphamide.

Radiation damage to the ovaries due to scatter from low-dose craniospinal irradiation has been demonstrated in a significant proportion of female survivors of childhood ALL who received a dose of 10–15 Gy.[103] Direct abdominal irradiation is associated with a high rate of primary gonadal failure in survivors.[104] In a study of female ALL survivors in which ovarian function was assessed through measurement of FSH and LH levels, Hamre et al[105] found elevated levels indicating ovarian failure in 93% of individuals who had been treated with abdominal irradiation. Elevated levels were measured in 49% and 9% after identical chemotherapy and craniospinal or cranial irradiation, respectively. TBI with a single dose of 10 Gy causes ovarian failure in prepubertal girls,[63,106] but ovarian function can be preserved or can recover in many females with fractionated TBI to a cumulative dose of 12 Gy.[107,108]

With alkylating agent exposure in females, the cumulative dose again determines the risk of subsequent primary gonadal dysfunction. The combination chemotherapy treatments used for primary treatment of childhood leukemia do not often affect ovarian function or fertility.[103] The age at which the exposure occurs is important, and the ovaries of prepubertal girls appear to be relatively resistant to cytotoxic chemotherapy, probably due to the higher number of follicles that are present. Accelerated loss of follicles and cortical fibrosis have been observed directly in the ovaries of 10 girls following treatment for ALL.[109]

## Fertility

The majority of ALL survivors are fertile, and female survivors can have successful pregnancies.[110–113] Cryopreservation of semen from young postpubertal males is effective from the age of 14 years,[114,115] but gonadal tissue is not preserved from prepubertal males according to current recommended practice.

Although chemotherapy and irradiation could potentially damage DNA in germ cells, no excess risk for congenital malformations in the children of cancer survivors has been found.[110,116–120] To date, there has been no evidence of an excess risk of cancer being transmitted to the children of survivors of childhood leukemia, after exclusion of individuals suffering from familial cancer syndromes.[110,121]

# Cognitive and neuropsychological sequelae

There is considerable (although at times conflicting), evidence of impairment in cognitive or psychosocial functioning of survivors of childhood leukemia, although the methodology and evidence are of variable quality. Cognitive and psychosocial parameters are methodologically complex to assess, and changes may be multifactorial in etiology: the underlying disease itself, a direct effect of the modalities of treatment that were received, and the adverse impact of the experience of treatment for childhood leukemia on the individual and the family may all contribute to cognitive and psychosocial morbidity.

Cranial irradiation has been associated with long-term impairments in cognitive functioning and educational achievement in a number of studies of long-term survivors of childhood ALL. Cognitive deficits and neuropsychological morbidity are particularly severe in patients who received CNS irradiation with their primary course of treatment and subsequently require retreatment for CNS relapse or as part of TBI conditioning for alloSCT.[122] In contrast, intrathecal methotrexate does not appear to lead to a subsequent decrement in intelligence quotient (IQ) score in survivors[123] or in other areas of cognitive functioning.[124]

A meta-analysis of 30 earlier studies of cognitive function in long-term ALL survivors[125] concluded that individuals who had been treated with low-dose cranial or craniospinal irradiation showed a significant reduction in IQ relative to various control groups. This effect of CNS irradiation appeared to be inversely related to the individual's age at the time of exposure, and was more marked in females. Subsequent studies have generally supported these conclusions,[126–132] although it has not been established whether the IQ decrement remains stable with time.

The range of cognitive and educational deficits that have been described for survivors of childhood ALL who received CNS irradiation is wide. They include difficulties with attention or concentration, processing speed and abstract reasoning, short-term memory-dependent functions, and acquisition of language and numerical skills.[128,130,132–145]

For example, in a cohort of ALL survivors who were assessed in comparison with both sibling controls and survivors of childhood solid tumors,[135,140] persistent significant cognitive deficits were identified in the ALL survivors, who had received cranial irradiation with 18 or 24 Gy. No dose dependence was established. In a follow-up study, a memory deficit in tasks requiring strategic planning behavior was shown for the ALL group.[142] In another ALL cohort,[132] a significant reduction in cognitive and educational ability was found relative to solid tumor survivors and normal control subjects, with more severe deficits in tasks requiring language function, such as verbal IQ, reading, and spelling. Here, there was a trend towards a worse outcome following irradiation with a dose of 24 Gy compared to 18 Gy, with treatment given at a younger age. No sex differences in outcome were observed here, in contrast to other studies, where females have been found to be more severely affected than males.[131,146]

However, many of the relevant studies that consider these effects retrospectively assess relatively few subjects derived from cohorts of ALL survivors under long-term follow-up at single institutions, and compare them variously with siblings, parallel groups of relapse-free survivors of other childhood cancers, or controls drawn from the normal population. There are further methodological differences in ascertainment and analysis that make comparison of individual studies problematical. There is also considerable variation in the duration of relapse-free survival at follow-up. Prospective analyses of the long-term intellectual, cognitive, and educational achievements of survivors of childhood acute leukemia are rare. Such data would prove invaluable in determining the relative contributions of the leukemia and the adverse experience of being treated for a pediatric malignancy from the direct morbidity attributable to the various CNS-directed therapies used in contemporary treatment protocols for childhood ALL.

Valuable studies have also been undertaken on the psychosocial functioning of long-term survivors of childhood leukemia and other pediatric malignancies, with outcomes assessed against parameters such as social, educational, or occupational status, although the methodological considerations detailed above also apply to most of these studies. These may contribute to the inconsistent portrait of long-term psychosocial impairment reported by different groups for survivors of childhood leukemia.

Some studies report few psychological problems in relapse-free survivors of childhood leukemia and other malignancies,[147–151] and document normal social, academic, and vocational functioning relative to control groups.[152–155] In contrast, others report a higher prevalence of psychological distress, negative mood, poor coping skills, and poor body self-image,[156–161] and find greater deficits in social competence, increased behavioral problems, and poorer educational achievement in survivors of childhood cancer.[162–165] Cancer survivors are less likely to be married than individuals in the general population.[166]

Studies of the prevalence of psychiatric morbidity in survivors of childhood leukemia, including a recent population-based survey from Denmark, have not found an excess in this group.[159,167,168]

## Neurological changes

Structural changes in the brains of survivors of childhood leukemia may be seen in individuals treated with methotrexate or cranial irradiation.[169] Some subtle changes can be detected with sensitive imaging techniques, but may not be associated with any demonstrable functional impairment.

Several relatively small magnetic resonance (MR) studies have imaged the brains of survivors of childhood ALL treated with prophylactic cranial irradiation,[170–175] in which individuals were assessed up to 12 years from diagnosis. Various structural abnormalities were reported in some of the survivors, including periventricular white matter changes, cerebral atrophy, and calcification, but these findings were not accompanied by cognitive or neuropsychiatric assessments, and their significance is unclear. Cerebral atrophy may be a consequence of diffuse white matter injury resulting from cerebral irradiation.[169,175] In the MR angiography component of the study by Laitt et al,[173] changes in two subjects suggested the possibility of a radiation-induced large-vessel vasculopathy, although this is believed to be very rare with low-dose irradiation for CNS-directed therapy in ALL treatment.

Intrathecal methotrexate, which shows equivalent efficacy in preventing CNS relapse and has consequently replaced irradiation for CNS-directed therapy in contemporary treatment regimens for low-risk ALL patients, has also been found to produce cerebral white matter abnormalities on MR imaging.[176] Again, the clinical significance of these data has not been established. The neurotoxic effects of chemotherapeutic agents have been reviewed by Anderson et al,[143] Demopoulos and DeAngelis,[177] and Reddy and Witek.[178]

# Second malignancy

Survivors of childhood acute leukemia grow up with a lifelong increased risk of developing a second malignant neoplasm, but long-term follow-up of relapse-free survivors of ALL suggests that the cumulative incidence in this group is less than 4% at 20 years from diagnosis.[179–183] Histologically and clinically aggressive second neoplasms may present within the first few years of remission from ALL. Not all series include low-grade neoplasms such as basal cell carcinomas, which show a marked increase in incidence over longer follow-up periods.[183] Population-based studies may be more powerful than surveys based on a cohort from a single center.

There is a strong association between exposure to cranial or craniospinal irradiation in treatment for childhood ALL and an excess of second malignant neoplasms.[181,183–189] Many of the neoplasms reported in these series were solid tumors, frequently meningiomas, arising in or adjacent to radiotherapy fields. Asymptomatic meningiomas and other cerebral neoplasms have also been found in small MR imaging studies,[172,173] where the subjects were assessed at a median interval of more than 15 years from diagnosis. The thyroid gland is particularly radiosensitive, and may be at risk due to scatter in individuals who were treated with craniospinal irradiation, or who received TBI.[190]

Data have recently been presented by Pui et al[183] for the large cohort of patients treated in clinical trials at St Jude Children's Research Hospital between 1962 and 1992, who had achieved at least 10 years of event-free survival following remission induction and had been followed up for a median of over 18 years. These data demonstrate a significantly increased cumulative incidence of second neoplasms among individuals who had received low-dose cranial or craniospinal irradiation, of 4%, 7%, and 20% after 20, 25, or 30 years of event-free survival, respectively. Fellow survivors who were not treated with radiation had an incidence of less than 1% after 30 years from remission. Pui et al[183] reported that a majority of the second neoplasms diagnosed in irradiated individuals in this cohort were relatively benign or low-grade neoplasms, such as meningiomas and basal cell carcinomas, and this group had a non-significant small excess in mortality relative to the general population.

Registry-based case–control studies have provided an opportunity to investigate associations between exposures during childhood treatment for acute leukemia and the incidence of second malignant neoplasms in areas where registry data approach comprehensiveness. Klein et al[191] included survivors of AML and ALL in their case–control analysis of data from the German Childhood Cancer Registry. They were able to show a trend towards an increased incidence of second malignant neoplasms with radiotherapy, and established a dose-related excess risk for treatment with cyclophosphamide or other alkylating agents and mercaptopurine. No clear dose–response relationships were found in this study for methotrexate, cytarabine, or the topoisomerase II inhibitor etoposide. The association between secondary leukemia, often with a chromosomal translocation involving the *MLL* gene, and previous exposure to a topoisomerase II inhibitor has been established and risk estimates have been obtained in other studies.[192–194]

# Conclusions

In this chapter, we have provided an overview of four clinically important areas where there has been valuable research into subsequent adverse 'late effects' resulting from primary treatment of childhood leukemia. The selection of studies discussed above are necessarily of survivors who received historical rather than contemporary treatment for leukemia. Almost all are retrospective. One of the considerable strengths in this field has been the willingness of patients and clinicians to participate in meaningful large-scale clinical trials of childhood leukemia treatment, and some of the current clinical trial protocols now include long-term prospective studies of various late effects. Such data should prove valuable in confirming the results of previous investigators in this field, and will contribute to the further development of validated primary treatment regimens and the design of appropriate long-term follow-up systems for survivors.

Various models for long-term follow-up of childhood cancer survivors have been proposed,[4,8–10] and it is unlikely that any one can satisfy the needs of every individual in the context of disparate healthcare systems.

Nevertheless, we feel that a tiered model has considerable merit, and support the proposal for long-term follow-up of survivors of childhood cancer from the Late Effects Group of the UK CCSG[4] and developed by the Scottish Intercollegiate Guidelines Network (SIGN) authors as part of their practice guidelines.[5] In this model, most individuals who receive contemporary primary leukemia treatment could receive lifelong follow-up through annual or biennial assessments in an appropriately skilled primary care or specialist nurse-led setting, and be referred to a hospital-based multidisciplinary unit for specific treatment-related problems. However, the SIGN authors concede that the evidence base for this model has not yet been established. Other authors challenge whether lifelong follow-up is appropriate.[195]

Since childhood leukemia is relatively 'curable', and survivors can potentially enjoy a full lifespan, it is for this group, perhaps more than for any other group treated for hematological malignancy, that the 'weighting' that should be given to adverse late effects in selecting appropriate primary treatment is most important. We await with eager anticipation further high-quality data on late effects of childhood leukemia treatment upon which to consider modifications to current clinical practice.

## REFERENCES

1. Chessells JM, Veys P, Kempski H et al. Long-term follow-up of relapsed childhood acute lymphoblastic leukaemia. *Br J Haematol* 2003; **123**: 396–405.
2. Mardlin P, Chessells JM. Childhood leukaemia: the medical cost of cure. *Hosp Med* 2001; **62**: 200–4.
3. Jenney ME, Levitt GA. The quality of survival after childhood cancer. *Eur J Cancer* 2002; **38**: 1241–50.
4. Wallace WH, Blacklay A, Eiser C et al. Developing strategies for long term follow up of survivors of childhood cancer. *BMJ* 2001; **323**: 271–4.
5. Scottish Intercollegiate Guidelines Network. Long term follow up of survivors of childhood cancer. *SIGN Guideline 76.* Edinburgh: SIGN, 2004 (www.sign.ac.uk).
6. Liesner RJ, Leiper AD, Hann IM, Chessells JM. Late effects of intensive treatment for acute myeloid leukemia and myelodysplasia in childhood. *J Clin Oncol* 1994; **12**: 916–24.
7. Jenney ME, Faragher EB, Jones PH, Woodcock A. Lung function and exercise capacity in survivors of childhood leukaemia. *Med Pediatr Oncol* 1995; **24**: 222–30.
8. Langer T, Henze G, Beck JD. Basic methods and the developing structure of a late effects surveillance system (LESS) in the long term follow-up of pediatric cancer patients in Germany. For the German Late Effects Study Group in the German Society Pediatric Oncology and Hematology (GPOH). *Med Pediatr Oncol* 2000; **34**: 348–51.
9. Oeffinger KC, Eshelman DA, Tomlinson GE et al. Providing primary care for long-term survivors of childhood acute lymphoblastic leukemia. *J Fam Pract* 2000; **49**: 1133–46.
10. Children's Oncology Group. Childhood Cancer Survivor Long-Term Follow-Up Guidelines. Bethesda, MD, 2003 (www.childrensoncologygroup.org).
11. Kremer LC, van Dalen EC, Offringa M, Voute PA. Frequency and risk factors for anthracycline-induced clinical heart failure in children: a systematic review. *Ann Oncol* 2002; **13**: 503–12.
12. Kremer LC, van der Pal HJ, Offringa M et al. Frequency and risk factors of subclinical cardiotoxicity after anthracycline therapy in children: a systematic review. *Ann Oncol* 2002; **13**: 819–29.
13. Green DM, Gingell RL, Pearce J et al. The effect of mediastinal irradiation on cardiac function of patients treated during childhood and adolescence for Hodgkin's disease. *J Clin Oncol* 1987; **5**: 239–45.
14. Reinders JG, Heijmen BJ, Olofsen-van Acht MJ et al. Ischaemic heart disease after mantle field irradiation for Hodgkin's disease in long-term follow-up. *Radiother Oncol* 1999; **51**: 35–42.
15. Von Hoff DD, Rozencweig M, Layard M et al. Daunomycin-induced cardiotoxicity in children and adults. A review of 110 cases. *Am J Med* 1977; **62**: 200–8.
16. Kremer LC, van Dalen EC, Offringa M et al. Anthracycline-induced clinical heart failure in a cohort of 607 children: long-term follow-up study. *J Clin Oncol* 2001; **19**: 191–6.
17. Krischer JP, Epstein S, Cuthbertson DD et al. Clinical cardiotoxicity following anthracycline treatment for childhood cancer: the Pediatric Oncology Group experience. *J Clin Oncol* 1997; **15**: 1544–52.
18. Lipshultz SE, Giantris AL, Lipsitz SR et al. Doxorubicin administration by continuous infusion is not cardioprotective: the Dana Farber 91-01 Acute Lymphoblastic Leukemia protocol. *J Clin Oncol* 2002; **20**: 1677–82.
19. Levitt GA, Dorup I, Sorensen K, Sullivan I. Does anthracycline administration by infusion in children affect late cardiotoxicity? *Br J Haematol* 2004; **124**: 463–8.
20. Lipshultz SE, Colan SD, Gelber ED et al. Late cardiac

effects of doxorubicin therapy for acute lymphoblastic leukemia in children. *N Engl J Med* 1991; **324**: 808–15.

21. Lipshultz SE, Lipsitz SR, Mone SM et al. Female sex and higher drug doses as risk factors for late cardiotoxic effects of doxorubicin therapy for childhood cancer. *N Engl J Med* 1995; **332**: 1738–43.

22. Nysom K, Holm K, Lipsitz SR et al. Relationship between cumulative anthracycline dose and late cardiotoxicity in childhood acute lymphoblastic leukemia. *J Clin Oncol* 1998; **16**: 545–50.

23. Goorin AM, Chauvenet AR, Perez-Atayde AR et al. Initial congestive heart failure, six to ten years after doxorubicin chemotherapy for childhood cancer. *J Pediatr* 1990; **116**: 144–7.

24. Pinkerton CR, Bowman A, Holtzel H, Chessells JM. Intensive consolidation chemotherapy for acute lymphoblastic leukaemia (UKALL X pilot study). *Arch Dis Child* 1987; **62**: 12–18.

25. Chessells JM, Bailey C, Richards SM. Intensification of treatment and survival in all children with lymphoblastic leukaemia: results of UK Medical Research Council trial UKALL X. Medical Research Council Working Party on Childhood Leukaemia. *Lancet* 1995; **345**: 143–8.

26. Sorensen K, Levitt G, Bull C et al. Anthracycline dose in childhood acute lymphoblastic leukemia: issues of early survival versus late cardiotoxicity. *J Clin Oncol* 1997; **15**:61–8.

27. Sorensen K, Levitt G, Bull C et al. Late anthracycline cardiotoxicity after childhood cancer: a prospective longitudinal study. *Cancer* 2003; **97**: 1991–8.

28. Steinherz LJ, Graham T, Hurwitz R et al. Guidelines for cardiac monitoring of children during and after anthracycline therapy: report of the Cardiology Committee of the Children's Cancer Study Group. *Pediatrics* 1992; **89**: 942–9.

29. Lipshultz SE, Sanders SP, Goorin AN et al. Monitoring for anthracycline cardiotoxicity. *Pediatrics* 1994; **93**: 433–7.

30. Klewer SE, Goldberg SJ, Donnerstein RL et al. Dobutamine stress echocardiography: a sensitive indicator of diminished myocardial function in asymptomatic doxorubicin-treated long-term survivors of cancer. *J Am Coll Cardiol* 1992; **19**: 394–401.

31. Lipshultz SE, Lipsitz SR, Sallan SE et al. Long-term enalapril therapy for left ventricular dysfunction in doxorubicin-treated survivors of childhood cancer. *J Clin Oncol* 2002; **20**: 4517–22.

32. van Dalen ED, van der Pal HJ, van den Bos C et al. Treatment for asymptomatic anthracycline–induced cardiac dysfunction in childhood cancer survivors: the need for evidence. *J Clin Oncol* 2003; **21**: 3777.

33. Silber JH, Cnaan A, Clark BJ et al. Design and baseline characteristics for the ACE Inhibitor After Anthracycline (AAA) study of cardiac dysfunction in long-term pediatric cancer survivors. *Am Heart J* 2001; **142**: 577–85.

34. Wexler LH, Andrich MP, Venzon D et al. Randomized trial of the cardioprotective agent ICRF-187 in pediatric sarcoma patients treated with doxorubicin. *J Clin Oncol* 1996; **14**: 362–72.

35. Oberfield SE, Sklar CA. Endocrine sequelae in survivors of childhood cancer. *Adolesc Med* 2002; **13**: 161–9.

36. Katz JA, Chambers B, Everhart C et al. Linear growth in children with acute lymphoblastic leukemia treated without cranial irradiation. *J Pediatr* 1991; **118**: 575–8.

37. Katz JA, Pollock BH, Jacaruso D, Morad A. Final attained height in patients successfully treated for childhood acute lymphoblastic leukemia. *J Pediatr* 1993; **123**: 546–52.

38. Moell C, Marky I, Hovi L et al. Cerebral irradiation causes blunted pubertal growth in girls treated for acute leukemia. *Med Pediatr Oncol* 1994; **22**: 375–9.

39. Birkebaek NH, Fisker S, Clausen N et al. Growth and endocrinological disorders up to 21 years after treatment for acute lymphoblastic leukemia in childhood. *Med Pediatr Oncol* 1998; **30**: 351–6.

40. Shalet SM, Beardwell CG, Pearson D, Jones PH. The effect of varying doses of cerebral irradiation on growth hormone production in childhood. *Clin Endocrinol (Oxf)* 1976; **5**: 287–90.

41. Costin G. Effects of low-dose cranial radiation on growth hormone secretory dynamics and hypothalamic-pituitary function. *Am J Dis Child* 1988; **142**: 847–52.

42. Brennan BM, Rahim A, Mackie EM et al. Growth hormone status in adults treated for acute lymphoblastic leukaemia in childhood. *Clin Endocrinol (Oxf)* 1998; **48**: 777–83.

43. Melin AE, Adan L, Leverger G et al. Growth hormone secretion, puberty and adult height after cranial irradiation with 18 Gy for leukaemia. *Eur J Pediatr* 1998; **157**: 703–7.

44. Adan L, Trivin C, Sainte-Rose C et al. GH deficiency caused during cranial irradiation during childhood: factors and markers in young adults. *J Clin Endocrinol Metab* 2001; **86**: 5245–51.

45. Darzy KH, Shalet SM. Radiation-induced growth hormone deficiency. *Horm Res* 2003; **59**(Suppl 1): 1–11.

46. Stubberfield TG, Byrne GC, Jones TW. Growth and growth hormone secretion after treatment for acute lymphoblastic leukemia in childhood. 18-Gy versus 24-Gy cranial irradiation. *J Pediatr Hematol Oncol* 1995; **17**: 167–71.

47. Clayton PE, Shalet SM, Morris-Jones PH, Price DA. Growth in children treated for acute lymphoblastic leukaemia. *Lancet* 1988; **i**: 460–2.

48. Lannering B, Rosberg S, Marky I et al. Reduced growth hormone secretion with maintained periodicity following cranial irradiation in children with acute lymphoblastic leukaemia. *Clin Endocrinol (Oxf)* 1995; **42**: 153–9.

49. Clayton PE, Shalet SM. Dose-dependency of time of onset of radiation-induced growth hormone deficiency. *J Pediatr* 1991; **118**: 226–8.

50. Crowne EC, Moore C, Wallace WH et al. A novel variant of growth hormone (GH) insufficiency following low dose cranial irradiation. *Clin Endocrinol (Oxf)* 1992; **36**: 59–68.

51. Shalet SM, Price DA, Beardwell CG et al. Normal growth despite abnormalities of growth hormone secretion in children treated for acute leukemia. *J Pediatr* 1979; **94**: 719–22.

52. Hata M, Ogino I, Aida N et al. Prophylactic cranial irradiation of acute lymphoblastic leukemia in childhood: outcomes of late effects on pituitary function and growth in long-term survivors. *Int J Cancer* 2001; **96**(Suppl): 117–24.

53. Leiper AD, Stanhope R, Kiching P, Chessells JM. Precocious and premature puberty associated with treatment for acute lymphoblastic leukaemia. *Arch Dis Child* 1987; **62**: 1107–12.

54. Leiper AD, Stanhope R, Preece MA et al. Precocious or early puberty and growth failure in girls treated for acute lymphoblastic leukaemia. *Horm Res* 1988; **30**: 72–6.

55. Uruena M, Stanhope R, Chessells JM, Leiper AD. Impaired

pubertal growth in acute lymphoblastic leukaemia. *Arch Dis Child* 1991; **66**: 1403–7.

56. Ogilvy-Stuart AL, Clayton PE, Shalet SM. Cranial irradiation and early puberty. *J Clin Endocrinol Metab* 1994; **78**: 1282–6.

57. Berglund G, Karlberg J, Marky I, Mellander L. A longitudinal study of growth in children with acute lymphoblastic leukemia. *Acta Paediatr Scand* 1985; **74**: 530–3.

58. Robison LL, Nesbit ME, Sather HN et al. Height of children successfully treated for acute lymphoblastic leukemia: a report from the Late Effects Study Committee of Children's Cancer Study Group. *Med Pediatr Oncol* 1985; **13**: 14–21.

59. Dacou-Voutetakis C, Kitra V, Grafakos S et al. Auxologic data and hormonal profile in long-term survivors of childhood acute lymphoid leukemia. *Am J Pediatr Hematol Oncol* 1993; **15**: 277–83.

60. Davies HA, Didcock E, Didi M et al. Disproportionate short stature after cranial irradiation and combination chemotherapy for leukaemia. *Arch Dis Child* 1994; **70**: 472–5.

61. Davies HA, Didcock E, Didi M et al. Growth, puberty and obesity after treatment for leukaemia. *Acta Paediatr Suppl* 1995; **411**: 45–51.

62. Leung W, Rose SR, Zhou Y et al. Outcomes of growth hormone replacement therapy in survivors of childhood acute lymphoblastic leukemia. *J Clin Oncol* 2002; **20**: 2959–64.

63. Leiper AD, Stanhope R, Lau T et al. The effect of total body irradiation and bone marrow transplantation during childhood and adolescence on growth and endocrine function. *Br J Haematol* 1987; **67**: 419–26.

64. Lando A, Holm K, Nysom K et al. Thyroid function in survivors of childhood acute lymphoblastic leukaemia: the significance of prophylactic cranial irradiation. *Clin Endocrinol (Oxf)* 2001; **55**: 21–5.

65. Odame I, Reilly JJ, Gibson BE, Donaldson MD. Patterns of obesity in boys and girls after treatment for acute lymphoblastic leukaemia. *Arch Dis Child* 1994; **71**: 147–9.

66. van Dongen-Melman JE, Hokken-Koelega AC, Hahlen K et al. Obesity after successful treatment of acute lymphoblastic leukemia in childhood. *Pediatr Res* 1995; **38**: 86–90.

67. Craig F, Leiper AD, Stanhope R et al. Sexually dimorphic and radiation dose dependent effect of cranial irradiation on body mass index. *Arch Dis Child* 1999; **81**: 500–4.

68. Nysom K, Holm K, Michaelsen KF et al. Degree of fatness after treatment for acute lymphoblastic leukaemia in childhood. *J Clin Endocrinol Metab* 1999; **84**: 4591–6.

69. Sklar CA, Mertens AC, Walter A et al. Changes in body mass index and prevalence of overweight in survivors of childhood acute lymphoblastic leukaemia: role of cranial irradiation. *Med Pediatr Oncol* 2000; **35**: 91–5.

70. Warner JT, Evans WD, Webb DK, Gregory JW. Body composition of long-term survivors of acute lymphoblastic leukaemia. *Med Pediatr Oncol* 2002; **38**: 165–72.

71. Oeffinger KC, Mertens AC, Sklar CA et al. Obesity in adult survivors of childhood acute lymphoblastic leukemia: a report from the Childhood Cancer Survivor Study. *J Clin Oncol* 2003; **21**: 1359–65.

72. Reilly JJ, Kelly A, Ness P et al. Premature adiposity rebound in children treated for acute lymphoblastic leukemia. *J Clin Endocrinol Metab* 2001; **86**: 2775–8.

73. Birkebaek NH, Clausen N. Height and weight pattern up to 20 years after treatment for acute lymphoblastic leukaemia. *Arch Dis Child* 1998; **79**: 161–4.

74. Reilly JJ, Blacklock CJ, Dale E et al. Resting metabolic rate and obesity in childhood acute lymphoblastic leukaemia. *Int J Obes Relat Metab Disord* 1996; **20**: 1130–2.

75. Warner JT, Bell W, Webb DK, Gregory JW. Daily energy expenditure and physical activity in survivors of childhood malignancy. *Pediatr Res* 1998; **43**: 607–13.

76. Gilsanz V, Carlson ME, Roe TF, Ortega JA. Osteoporosis after cranial radiation for acute lymphoblastic leukemia. *J Pediatr* 1990; **117**: 238–44.

77. Arikoski P, Komulainen J, Voutilainen R et al. Reduced bone mineral density in long-term survivors of childhood acute lymphoblastic leukemia. *J Pediatr Hematol Oncol* 1998; **20**: 234–40.

78. Nysom K, Holm K, Michaelsen KF et al. Bone mass after treatment for acute lymphoblastic leukaemia in childhood. *J Clin Oncol* 1998; **16**: 3752–60.

79. Brennan BM, Rahim A, Adams JA et al. Reduced bone mineral density in young adults following cure of acute lymphoblastic leukaemia in childhood. *Br J Cancer* 1999; **79**: 1859–63.

80. Warner JT, Evans WD, Webb DK et al. Relative osteopenia after treatment for acute lymphoblastic leukaemia. *Pediatr Res* 1999; **45**: 544–51.

81. Kaste SC, Jones-Wallace D, Rose SR et al. Bone mineral decrements in survivors of childhood acute lymphoblastic leukemia: frequency of occurrence and risk factors for their development. *Leukemia* 2001; **15**: 728–34.

82. Tillmann V, Darlington AS, Eiser C et al. Male sex and low physical activity are associated with reduced spine bone mineral density in survivors of childhood lymphoblastic leukemia. *J Bone Miner Res* 2002; **17**: 1073–80.

83. Leiper AD. Osteoporosis in survivors of childhood malignancy. *Eur J Cancer* 1998; **34**: 770–772.

84. Leonard MB. Assessment of bone health in children and adolescents with cancer: promises and pitfalls of current techniques. *Med Pediatr Oncol* 2003; **41**: 198–207.

85. van der Sluis IM, van den Heuvel-Eibrink MM, Hahlen K et al. Bone mineral density, body composition, and height in long-term survivors of acute lymphoblastic leukemia in childhood. *Med Pediatr Oncol* 2000; **35**: 415–20.

86. Schwartz AM, Leonidas JC. Methotrexate osteopathy. *Skeletal Radiol* 1984; **11**: 13–16.

87. Strauss AJ, Su JT, Dalton VM et al. Bony morbidity in children treated for acute lymphoblastic leukaemia. *J Clin Oncol* 2001; **19**: 3066–72.

88. Lequin MH, van der Shuis IM, van Rijn RR et al. Bone mineral assessment with tibial ultrasonometry and dual-energy X-ray absorptiometry in long-term survivors of acute lymphoblastic leukemia in childhood. *J Clin Densitom* 2002; **5**: 167–73.

89. Bhatia S, Ramsay NK, Weisdorf D et al. Bone mineral density in patients undergoing bone marrow transplantation for myeloid malignancies. *Bone Marrow Transplant* 1998; **22**: 87–90.

90. Nysom K, Holm K, Michaelsen KF et al. Bone mass after allogeneic BMT for childhood leukaemia or lymphoma. *Bone Marrow Transplant* 2000; **25**: 191–6.

91. Muller HL, Klinkhammer-Schalke M, Seelbach-Gobel B et al. Gonadal function of young adults after therapy of malignancies during childhood or adolescence. *Eur J Pediatr* 1996; **155**: 763–9.

92. Sklar C. Reproductive physiology and treatment-related loss of sex hormone production. *Med Pediatr Oncol* 1999; **33**: 2–8.

93. Shalet SM, Horner A, Ahmed SR, Morris-Jones PH. Leydig cell damage after testicular irradiation for lymphoblastic leukaemia. *Med Pediatr Oncol* 1985; **13**: 65–8.

94. Leiper AD, Grant DB, Chessells JM. Gonadal function after testicular radiation for acute lymphoblastic leukaemia. *Arch Dis Child* 1986; **61**: 53–6.

95. Siimes MA, Rautonen J, Makipernaa A, Sipila I. Testicular function in adult males surviving childhood malignancy. *Pediatr Hematol Oncol* 1995; **12**: 231–41.

96. Grundy RG, Leiper AD, Stanhope R, Chessells JM. Survival and endocrine outcome after testicular relapse in acute lymphoblastic leukaemia. *Arch Dis Child* 1997; **76**: 190–6.

97. Castillo LA, Craft AW, Kernahan J et al. Gonadal function after 12-Gy testicular irradiation in childhood acute lymphoblastic leukaemia. *Med Pediatr Oncol* 1990; **18**: 185–9.

98. Sklar CA, Robison LL, Nesbit ME et al. Effects of radiation on testicular function in long-term survivors of childhood acute lymphoblastic leukemia: a report from the Children Cancer Study Group. *J Clin Oncol* 1990; **8**: 1981–7.

99. Shalet SM, Hann IM, Lendon M et al. Testicular function after combination chemotherapy in childhood for acute lymphoblastic leukaemia. *Arch Dis Child* 1981; **56**: 275–8.

100. Mustieles C, Munoz A, Alonso M et al. Male gonadal function after chemotherapy in survivors of childhood malignancy. *Med Pediatr Oncol* 1995; **24**: 347–51.

101. Nicholson HS, Byrne J. Fertility and pregnancy after treatment for cancer during childhood or adolescence. *Cancer* 1993; **71**: 3392–9.

102. Kenney LB, Laufer MR, Grant FD et al. High risk of infertility and long term gonadal damage in males treated with high dose cyclophosphamide for sarcoma during childhood. *Cancer* 2001; **91**: 613–21.

103. Wallace WH, Shalet SM, Tetlow LJ, Morris-Jones PH. Ovarian function following the treatment of childhood acute lymphoblastic leukaemia. *Med Pediatr Oncol* 1993; **21**: 333–9.

104. Wallace WH, Shalet SM, Crowne EC et al. Ovarian failure following abdominal irradiation in childhood: natural history and prognosis. *Clin Oncol (R Coll Radiol)* 1989; **1**: 75–9.

105. Hamre MR, Robison LL, Nesbit ME et al. Effects of radiation on ovarian function in long-term survivors of childhood acute lymphoblastic leukemia: a report from the Children's Cancer Study Group. *J Clin Oncol* 1987; **5**: 1759–65.

106. Byrne J, Fears TR, Gail MH et al. Early menopause in long-term survivors of cancer during adolescence. *Am J Obstet Gynecol* 1992; **166**: 788–93.

107. Spinelli S, Chiodi S, Bacigalupo A et al. Ovarian recovery after total body irradiation and allogeneic bone marrow transplantation: long term follow up of 79 females. *Bone Marrow Transplant* 1994; **14**: 373–80.

108. Sarafoglou K, Boulad F, Gillio A, Sklar C. Gonadal function after bone marrow transplantation for acute leukemia during childhood. *J Pediatr* 1997; **130**: 210–16.

109. Marcello MF, Nuciforo G, Romeo R et al. Structural and ultrastructural study of the ovary in childhood leukemia after successful treatment. *Cancer* 1990; **66**: 2099–104.

110. Green DM, Hall B, Zevon MA. Pregnancy outcome after treatment for acute lymphoblastic leukemia during childhood or adolescence. *Cancer* 1989; **64**: 2335–9.

111. Wallace WH, Shalet SM, Lendon M, Morris-Jones PH. Male fertility in long-term survivors of childhood acute lymphoblastic leukaemia. *Int J Androl* 1991; **14**: 312–19.

112. Wallace WH, Shalet SM, Tetlow LJ, Morris-Jones PH. Ovarian function following the treatment of childhood acute lymphoblastic leukaemia. *Med Pediatr Oncol* 1993; **21**: 333–9.

113. Bath LE, Wallace WH, Critchley HO. Late effects of the treatment of childhood cancer on the female reproductive system and the potential for fertility preservation. *Br J Obstet Gynaecol* 2002; **109**: 107–14.

114. Kliesch S, Behre HM, Jurgens H, Nieschlag E. Cryopreservation of semen from adolescent patients with malignancies. *Med Pediatr Oncol* 1996; **26**: 20–7.

115. Muller J, Sonksen J, Sommer P et al. Cryopreservation of semen from pubertal boys with cancer. *Med Pediatr Oncol* 2000; **34**: 191–4.

116. Li FP, Fine W, Jaffe N et al. Offspring of patients treated for cancer in childhood. *J Natl Cancer Inst* 1979; **62**: 1193–7.

117. Hawkins MM. Is there evidence of a therapy-related increase in germ cell mutation among childhood cancer survivors? *J Natl Cancer Inst* 1991; **83**: 1643–50.

118. Kenney LB, Nicholson HS, Brasseux C et al. Birth defects in offspring of adult survivors of childhood acute lymphoblastic leukemia. A Children's Cancer Group/National Institutes of Health Report. *Cancer* 1996; **78**: 169–76.

119. Green DM, Fiorello A, Zevon MA et al. Birth defects and childhood cancer in offspring of survivors of childhood cancer. *Arch Pediatr Adolesc Med* 1997; **151**: 379–83.

120. Byrne J, Rasmussen S, Steinhorn SC et al. Genetic diseases in offspring of long-term survivors of childhood and adolescent cancer. *Am J Hum Genet* 1998; **62**: 45–52.

121. Hawkins MM, Draper GJ, Winter DL. Cancer in the offspring of survivors of childhood leukaemia and non-Hodgkin lymphomas. *Br J Cancer* 1995; **71**: 1335–9.

122. Christie D, Battin M, Leiper AD et al. Neuropsychological and neurological outcome after relapse of lymphoblastic leukaemia. *Arch Dis Child* 1994; **70**: 275–80.

123. Kingma A, van Dommelen RI, Mooyaart EL et al. No major cognitive impairment in young children with acute lymphoblastic leukemia using chemotherapy only: a prospective longitudinal study. *J Pediatr Hematol Oncol* 2002; **24**: 106–14.

124. Rodgers J, Marckus R, Kearns P, Windebank K. Attentional ability among survivors of leukaemia treated without cranial irradiation. *Arch Dis Child* 2003; **88**: 147–50.

125. Cousens P, Waters B, Said J, Stevens M. Cognitive effects of cranial irradiation in leukaemia: a survey and meta-analysis. *J Child Psychol Psychiatry* 1988; **29**: 839–52.

126. Said JA, Waters BG, Cousens P, Stevens MM. Neuropsychological sequelae of central nervous system prophylaxis in survivors of childhood acute lymphoblastic leukemia. *J Consult Clin Psychol* 1989; **57**: 251–6.

127. Bleyer WA, Fallavollita J, Robison L et al. Influence of age, sex, and concurrent intrathecal methotrexate therapy on intellectual function after cranial irradiation during childhood: a report from the Children's Cancer Study Group. *Pediatr Hematol Oncol* 1990; **7**: 329–38.

128. Halberg FE, Kramer JH, Moore IM et al. Prophylactic cranial irradiation dose effects on late cognitive function in children treated for acute lymphoblastic leukemia. *Int J Radiat Oncol Biol Phys* 1992; **22**: 13–16.

129. Mulhern RK, Ochs J, Fairclough D. Deterioration of

intellect among children surviving leukemia: IQ test changes modify estimates of treatment toxicity. *J Consult Clin Psychol* 1992; **60**: 477–80.

130. Jankovic M, Brouwers P, Valsecchi MG et al. Association of 1800 cGy cranial irradiation with intellectual function in children with acute lymphoblastic leukaemia. ISPACC. International Study Group on Psychosocial Aspects of Childhood Cancer. *Lancet* 1994; **344**: 224–7.

131. Christie D, Leiper AD, Chessells JM, Vargha-Khadem F. Intellectual performance after presymptomatic cranial radiotherapy for leukaemia: effects of age and sex. *Arch Dis Child* 1995; **73**: 136–40.

132. Smibert E, Anderson V, Godber T, Ekert H. Risk factors for intellectual and educational sequelae of cranial irradiation in childhood acute lymphoblastic leukaemia. *Br J Cancer* 1996; **73**: 825–30.

133. Eiser C, Lansdown R. Retrospective study of intellectual development in children treated for acute lymphoblastic leukaemia. *Arch Dis Child* 1977; **52**: 525–9.

134. Meadows AT, Gordon J, Massari DJ et al. Declines in IQ scores and cognitive dysfunctions in children with acute lymphocytic leukaemia treated with cranial irradiation. *Lancet* 1981; **ii**: 1015–18.

135. Twaddle V, Britton PG, Craft AW et al. Intellectual function after treatment for leukaemia or solid tumours. *Arch Dis Child* 1983; **58**: 949–952.

136. Brouwers P, Riccarde R, Poplack D, Fedio P. Attentional deficits in long term survivors of acute lymphoblastic leukemia (ALL). *J Clin Neurol* 1984; **6**: 325–34.

137. Schlieper AE, Esseltine DW, Tarshis MA. Cognitive function in long-term survivors of childhood acute lymphoblastic leukemia. *J Pediatr Hematol Oncol* 1989; **6**: 1–9.

138. Eiser C. Cognitive deficits in children treated for leukaemia. *Arch Dis Child* 1991; **66**: 164–8.

139. Mulhern RK, Fairclough D, Ochs J. A prospective comparison of neuropsychologic performance of children surviving leukemia who received 18-Gy, or 24-Gy, or no cranial irradiation. *J Clin Oncol* 1991; **9**: 1348–56.

140. Rodgers J, Britton PG, Kernahan J, Craft AW. Cognitive function after two doses of cranial irradiation for acute lymphoblastic leukaemia. *Arch Dis Child* 1991; **66**: 1245–6.

141. Brown TR, Madan-Swain A, Pais R et al. Cognitive status of children treated with central nervous system prophylactic chemotherapy for acute lymphocytic leukemia. *Arch Clin Neuropsychol* 1992; **7**: 481–97.

142. Rodgers J, Britton PG, Morris RG et al. Memory after treatment for acute lymphoblastic leukaemia. *Arch Dis Child* 1992; **67**: 266–8.

143. Anderson V, Smibert E, Ekert H, Godber T. Intellectual, educational and behavioural sequelae after cranial irradiation and chemotherapy. *Arch Dis Child* 1994; **70**: 476–83.

144. Davidson A, Childs J, Hopewell JW, Tait D. Functional neurological outcome in leukaemic children receiving repeated cranial irradiation. *Radiother Oncol* 1994; **31**: 101–9.

145. Waber DP, Tarbell NJ, Fairclough D et al. Cognitive sequelae of treatment in childhood acute lymphoblastic leukemia: cranial radiation requires an accomplice. *J Clin Oncol* 1995; **13**: 2490–6.

146. Waber DP, Gioia G, Paccia J et al. Sex differences in cognitive processing in children treated with CNS prophylaxis for acute lymphoblastic leukemia. *J Pediatr Psychol* 1990; **15**: 105–22.

147. Greenberg HS, Kazak AE, Meadows AT. Psychologic functioning in 8- to 16-year old cancer survivors and their parents. *J Pediatr* 1989; **114**: 488–93.

148. Gray RE, Doan BD, Shermer P et al. Psychologic adaptation of survivors of childhood cancer. *Cancer* 1992; **70**: 2713–21.

149. Apajasalo M, Sintonen H, Siimes MA et al. Health-related quality of life of adults surviving malignancies in childhood. *Eur J Cancer* 1996; **32A**: 1354–8.

150. Elkin TD, Phipps S, Mulhern RK, Fairclough D. Psychological functioning of adolescent and young adult survivors of pediatric malignancy. *Med Pediatr Oncol* 1997; **29**: 582–8.

151. Maggiolini A, Grassi R, Adamoli L et al. Self-image of adolescent survivors of long-term childhood leukemia. *J Pediatr Hematol Oncol* 2000; **22**: 417–21.

152. Kelaghan J, Myers MH, Mulvihill JJ et al. Educational achievement of long-term survivors of childhood and adolescent cancer. *Med Pediatr Oncol* 1988; **16**: 320–6.

153. Spirito A, Stark LJ, Cobiella C et al. Social adjustment of children successfully treated for cancer. *J Pediatr Psychol* 1990; **15**: 359–71.

154. Green DM, Zevon MA, Hall B. Achievement of life goals by adult survivors of modern treatment for childhood cancer. *Cancer* 1991; **67**: 206–13.

155. Hays DM, Landsverk J, Sallan SE et al. Educational, occupational, and insurance status of childhood cancer survivors in their fourth and fifth decades of life. *J Clin Oncol* 1992; **10**: 1397–406.

156. Lesko LM. Surviving hematological malignancies: stress responses and predicting psychological adjustment. *Prog Clin Biol Res* 1990; **352**: 423–37.

157. Zeltzer LK, Chen E, Weiss R et al. Comparison of psychologic outcome in adult survivors of childhood acute lymphoblastic leukemia versus sibling controls: a Cooperative Children's Cancer Group and National Institutes of Health Study. *J Clin Oncol* 1997; **15**: 547–56.

158. Hobbie WL, Stuber M, Meeske K et al. Symptoms of posttraumatic stress in young adult survivors of childhood cancer. *J Clin Oncol* 2000; **18**: 4060–6.

159. Mackie E, Hill J, Kondryn H, McNally R. Adult psychosocial outcomes in long-term survivors of acute lymphoblastic leukaemia and Wilms' tumour: a controlled study. *Lancet* 2000; **355**: 1310–14.

160. Hudson MM, Mertens AC, Yasui Y et al. Health status of adult long-term survivors of childhood cancer: a report from the Childhood Cancer Survivor Study. *JAMA* 2003; **290**: 1583–92.

161. Waters EB, Wake MA, Hesketh KD et al. Health-related quality of life of children with acute lymphoblastic leukaemia: comparisons and correlations between parent and clinician reports. *Int J Cancer* 2003; **103**: 514–18.

162. Mulhern RK, Wasserman AL, Friedman AG et al. Social competence and behavioural adjustment of children who are long-term survivors of cancer. *Pediatrics* 1989; **83**: 18–25.

163. Haupt R, Fears TR, Robison LL et al. Educational attainment in long-term survivors of childhood acute lymphoblastic leukemia. *JAMA* 1994; **272**: 1427–32.

164. Vann JC, Biddle AK, Daeschner CW et al. Health insurance access to young adult survivors of childhood cancer in North Carolina. *Med Pediatr Oncol* 1995; **25**: 389–95.

165. Kingma A, Rammeloo LA, van Der Does-van den Berg A et al. Academic career after treatment for acute lymphoblastic leukaemia. *Arch Dis Child* 2000; **82**: 353–7.

166. Rauck AM, Green DM, Yasui Y et al. Marriage in the survivors of childhood cancer: a preliminary description from the Childhood Cancer Survivor Study. *Med Pediatr Oncol* 1999; **33**: 60–3.

167. Teta MJ, Del Po MC, Kasl SV et al. Psychosocial consequences of childhood and adolescent cancer survival. *J Chronic Dis* 1986; **39**: 751–9.

168. Ross L, Johansen C, Dalton SO et al. Psychiatric hospitalisations among survivors of cancer in childhood or adolescence. *N Engl J Med* 2003; **349**: 650–7.

169. Chessells JM, Cox TC, Kendall B et al. Neurotoxicity in lymphoblastic leukaemia : comparison of oral and intramuscular methotrexate and two doses of radiation. *Arch Dis Child* 1990; **65**: 416–22.

170. Paakko E, Vainionpaa L, Lanning M et al. White matter changes in children treated for acute lymphoblastic leukemia. *Cancer* 1992; **70**: 2728–33.

171. Kingma A, Mooyaart EL, Kamps WA et al. Magnetic resonance imaging of the brain and neuropsychological evaluation in children treated for acute lymphoblastic leukemia at a young age. *Am J Pediatr Hematol Oncol* 1993; **15**: 231–8.

172. Paakko E, Talvensaari K, Pyhtinen J, Lanning M. Late cranial MRI after cranial irradiation in survivors of childhood cancer. *Neuroradiology* 1994; **36**: 652–5.

173. Laitt RD, Chambers EJ, Goddard PR et al. Magnetic resonance imaging and magnetic resonance angiography in long term survivors of acute lymphoblastic leukemia treated with cranial irradiation. *Cancer* 1995; **76**: 1846–52.

174. Matsumoto K, Takahashi S, Sato A et al. Leukoencephalopathy in childhood hematopoietic neoplasm caused by moderate-dose methotrexate and prophylactic cranial radiotherapy – an MR analysis. *Int J Radiat Oncol Biol Phys* 1995; **32**: 913–18.

175. Harila-Saari AH, Paakko EL, Vainionpaa LK et al. A longitudinal magnetic resonance imaging study of the brain in survivors in childhood acute lymphoblastic leukemia. *Cancer* 1998; **83**: 2608–17.

176. Asato R, Akiyama Y, Ito M et al. Nuclear magnetic resonance abnormalities of the cerebral white matter in children with acute lymphoblastic leukemia and malignant lymphoma during and after central nervous system prophylactic treatment with intrathecal methotrexate. *Cancer* 1992; **70**: 1997–2004.

177. Demopoulos A, DeAngelis LM. Neurologic complications of leukemia. *Curr Opin Neurol* 2002; **15**: 691–9.

178. Reddy AT, Witek K. Neurologic complications of chemotherapy for children with cancer. *Curr Neurol Neurosci Rep* 2003; **3**: 137–42.

179. Neglia JP, Meadows AT, Robison LL et al. Second neoplasms after acute lymphoblastic leukemia in childhood. *N Engl J Med* 1991; **325**: 1330–6.

180. Kimball Dalton VM, Gelber RD, Li F et al. Second malignancies in patients treated for childhood acute lymphoblastic leukemia. *J Clin Oncol* 1998; **16**: 2848–53.

181. Loning L, Zimmermann M, Reiter A et al. Secondary neoplasms subsequent to Berlin–Frankfurt–Münster therapy of acute lymphoblastic leukemia in childhood: significantly lower risk without cranial radiotherapy. *Blood* 2000; **95**: 2770–5.

182. Bhatia S, Sather HN, Pabustan OB et al. Low incidence of second neoplasms among children diagnosed with acute lymphoblastic leukemia after 1983. *Blood* 2002; **99**: 4257–64.

183. Pui CH, Cheng C, Leung W et al. Extended follow-up of long-term survivors of childhood acute lymphoblastic leukemia. *N Engl J Med* 2003; **349**: 640–9.

184. Hawkins MM, Draper GJ, Kingston JE. Incidence of second primary tumours among childhood cancer survivors. *Br J Cancer* 1987; **56**: 339–47.

185. Rimm IJ, Li FC, Tarbell NJ et al. Brain tumors after cranial irradiation for childhood lymphoblastic leukemia. A 13-year experience from the Dana-Faber Institute and the Children's Hospital. *Cancer* 1987; **59**: 1506–8.

186. Nygaard R, Garwicz S, Haldorsen T et al. Second malignant neoplasms in patients treated for childhood leukemia: a population-based cohort study from the Nordic countries. *Acta Paediatr Scand* 1991; **80**: 1220–8.

187. Rosso P, Terracini B, Fears TR et al. Second malignant tumors after elective end of therapy for a first cancer in childhood: a multicenter study in Italy. *Int J Cancer* 1994; **59**: 451–6.

188. Walter AW, Hancock ML, Pui CH et al. Secondary brain tumours in children treated for acute lymphoblastic leukemia at St Jude Children's Research Hospital. *J Clin Oncol* 1998; **16**: 3761–7.

189. de Vathaire F, Hawkins M, Campbell S et al. Second malignant neoplasms after a first cancer in childhood : temporal pattern of risk according to type of treatment. *Br J Cancer* 1999; **79**: 1884–93.

190. Socie G, Curtis RE, Deeg HJ et al. New malignant diseases after allogeneic marrow transplantation for childhood acute leukemia. *J Clin Oncol* 2000; **18**: 348–57.

191. Klein G, Michaelis J, Spix C et al. Second malignant neoplasms after treatment of childhood cancer. *Eur J Cancer* 2003; **39**: 808–17.

192. Pui CH, Ribeiro RC, Hancock ML et al. Acute myeloid leukemia in children treated with epipodophyllotoxins for acute lymphoblastic leukemia. *N Engl J Med* 1991; **325**: 1682–7.

193. Pedersen-Bjergaard J, Philip P, Larsen SO et al. Therapy-related myelodysplasia and acute myeloid leukemia. Cytogenetic characteristics of 115 consecutive cases and risk in seven cohorts of patients treated intensively for malignant disease in the Copenhagen series. *Leukemia* 1993; **7**: 1975–86.

194. Smith MA, Rubinstein L, Anderson JR et al. Secondary leukemia or myelodysplastic syndrome after treatment with epipodophyllotoxins. *J Clin Oncol* 1999; **17**: 569–77.

195. Eket H. Infinite follow-up? *Med Pediatr Oncol* 2002; **38**: 303.

# 45 Late effects following allogeneic stem cell transplantation

## Gérard Socié and Lionel Ades

## Introduction

Over the past two decades, large numbers of patients have survived for years after hematopoietic stem cell transplantation (SCT). Immediate survival as well as prevention of relapse are no longer the sole interest for long-term survivors. Thus, studies on late effects after SCT is a major concern in the 21st century. Malignant diseases are of particular clinical concern, as more patients survive the early phase after transplantation and remain free of their original disease.[1,2] They are closely related to the preparative regimens used before transplantation. These malignant complications have been previously reviewed[3] and recently updated.[4] Non-malignant late effects are heterogeneous delayed complications of multifactorial etiology. Although often not life-threatening, they may impair the quality of life of long-term survivors.[5] This chapter will cover both malignant and non-malignant late effects.

## Malignant complications

Secondary malignancies are a well recognized complication in patients with Hodgkin lymphoma (HL) or non-Hodgkin lymphoma (NHL) treated with chemotherapy or combined-modality treatment (see Chapter 43). However, it was only in the early 1990s that the risk of secondary malignant diseases was described after allogeneic SCT. Experiments in murine models in the 1960s and 1970s, and in rhesus monkeys, and dogs in the 1970s and 1980s, showed a significant increase in the incidence of malignancies relative to controls in animals irradiated with lethal doses of total body irradiation (TBI) and infused with allogeneic marrow cells. Thus, it should not be surprising that new malignancies occur in patients after allogeneic hematopoietic SCT where one or several of these risk factors are present.

According to the Seattle group, it has been usual to divide the problem of secondary malignancies following hematopoietic SCT into three groups: leukemia, lymphoma, and solid tumors. Chronologically, lymphoma, leukemia, and solid tumors have a typical time course: most lymphomas occur within the first months of transplant, while solid tumors and leukemia are mostly diagnosed years after transplant.

### Post-transplant lymphoproliferative disorders and lymphomas

Most cases of post-transplant lymphoproliferative disorders (PTLD) are best classified as B-cell PTLD rather than NHL. In addition, lymphomas with clinical and biological characteristics typical of NHL or HL as seen in non-transplanted patients have occurred following SCT.

#### B-cell PTLD

B-cell PTLD are clinically and morphologically heterogeneous; they are usually associated with T-cell dysfunction and the presence of Epstein–Barr virus (EBV). The mean interval from transplantation to the development of B-cell PTLD lies between 5 and 6 months, with most cases being diagnosed within 3 months. The diagnostic criteria may differ from one study to another. For example, a non-lethal 'infectious mononucleosis-like' syndrome may resolve spontaneously, and acute-onset extensive disease may be diagnosed only at autopsy. In the largest series, involving 18 014 patients, PTLD developed in 78 recipients, with 64 cases occurring less than a year after transplantation.[6] The cumulative incidence of PTLD was $1.0 \pm 0.3\%$ at 10 years. The incidence was highest 1–5 months post transplant (120 cases/ 10 000/year), followed by a steep decline to less than 5/10 000/year among 1 year-plus survivors.

The most frequent presenting findings of PTLD are fever and organomegaly. As with other lymphoproliferative disorders developing in the context of immunodeficiency patients, extrahematopoietic organ involvement, including lungs, kidneys, and the central nervous system (CNS), is frequent. The differential diagnosis should include PTLD a priori in high-risk situations. Today, the use of quantitative polymerase chain reaction (PCR) of EBV DNA has dramatically changed diagnostic criteria. Using EBV viral load, patients are now frequently diagnosed with 'PTLD' while they present only isolated fever with (or even without) low tumor burden and a monoclonal gammaglobulin. This became important in the late 1990s after the development of powerful therapeutic tools. It soon appeared that early diagnosis can be established and the effect of therapy can now be monitored by quantitative PCR of the EBV DNA.

PTLD occurring after allogeneic SCT are almost always of donor origin, and associated with EBV genomic DNA integration. Biopsies reveal monomorphic or polymorphic, diffuse large-cell lymphoma of B-cell origin. PTLD after SCT are pathologically similar to the polymorphic PTLD described in solid organ transplant recipients, but as many as half of the cases after SCT show aggressive features of immunoblastic lymphoma.[7] Also, in contrast to PTLD after organ transplantation, most B-cell PTLD occurring after SCT are oligo- or monoclonal.[7–11] PTLD express the full array of latent EBV antigens, including EBNA1, 2, 3, 4, 5, and 6, and LMP1.[7,12–16]

B-cell PTLD were the first post-transplant malignancies for which risk factors were identified[6,7,17–20] (Table 45.1). The largest study included 18 014 patients.[6] In multivariate analyses, the risk of early-onset PTLD (<1 year) was strongly associated with unrelated or HLA-mismatched related donors, T-cell depletion of donor marrow, and the use of antithymocyte globulin or an anti-CD3 monoclonal antibody. Methods of T-cell depletion that selectively targeted T cells or T and natural killer (NK) cells were associated with markedly higher risks of PTLD than methods that removed both T and B cells, such as the alemtuzumab monoclonal antibody or elutriation.

B-cell PTLD develop because of a combination of depressed EBV-specific cellular immunity and the inherent transforming capacities of EBV. The virus persists as a latent infection in certain epithelial cells, where reactivation and replication may occur intermittently, and in B lymphocytes.[21] Among the 80–100 EBV-encoded proteins, latent membrane protein 1 (LMP1) plays an essential role in B-cell immortalization. Deletions near the 3′ end of the LMP1 gene have been reported in some EBV-related lymphoproliferative disorders.[22,23] Infection of B cells by EBV also induces high levels of interleukin-1 (IL-1), IL-5, IL-6, IL-10, CD23, and tumor necrosis factor (TNF). Deficiencies in EBV-specific cellular immunity contribute to EBV-PTLD susceptibility.[24–26] Adoptive transfer of EBV-specific cytotoxic T lymphocytes offers effective therapy for B-cell PTLD.[27]

The diagnosis of PTLD in the 2000's has changed dramatically since the introduction of effective and highly sensitive techniques to measure EBV load and to estimate early EBV-specific immune reconstitution after allogeneic SCT.[28] Truly quantitative PCR techniques allow frequent monitoring of the DNA load to predict the development of PTLD. After allogeneic SCT, the utility of such monitoring was confirmed by the Rotterdam group.[29,30] Finally EBV-specific T lymphocytes can now be monitored through the tetramer technology, which allows the detection of minute numbers of antigen-specific T cells.[31] The relative frequencies of T cells specific for different EBV peptides in transplant recipients closely reflect those of their respective donors. Investigation of patients at monthly intervals following unmanipulated allogeneic peripheral blood (PB) SCT demonstrated that the frequency of EBV-specific T cells correlates with the number of EBV genome copies in the peripheral blood and that expansion of EBV-specific T-cell populations occurs even in the setting of immunosuppressive therapy. In contrast, patients undergoing T-cell-depleted or unrelated cord blood transplantation have undetectable EBV-specific T cells, even in the presence of Epstein–Barr viremia. Thus, the

## Table 45.1 Incidence and risk factors of post-transplant EBV-related B-cell lymphoma

|  | Witherspoon et al[101] | Bhatia et al[18] | Kernan et al[19] | Curtis et al[6] |
|---|---|---|---|---|
| Number of patients | 2246 | 2150 | 462 | 18 014 |
| Immune disease | — | RR=2.5 (p=0.06) | — | — |
| HLA mismatch | RR=3.8 | RR=8.9 (p<0.001) | — | RR=4.1 (p<0.0001) |
| Total body irradiation | RR=3.9 | — | — | RR=2.9 (p=0.02) |
| Anti-CD3 | RR=4.2 | — | — | RR=43.2 (p<0.0001) |
| Antithymocyte globulin | RR=13.6 | RR=5.9 (p<0.001) | — | RR=6.4 (p<0.0001) |
| Acute GVHD II–IV | — | — | — | RR=1.9 (p=0.02) |
| T-cell depletion of the graft | RR=12.4 | RR=11.9 (p<0.001) | 5% patients | RR=12.7 (p<0.0001) |

RR, relative risk; GVHD, graft-versus-host disease.

protective shield provided by EBV-specific CD8+ T cells seems to be rapidly established following unmanipulated matched sibling allogeneic PBSCT.

Complete regression of B-cell PTLD has been reported in 40% of patients following reduction or discontinuation of immunosuppressive drugs, particularly in renal transplant recipients. Immunosuppression is intrinsic to marrow transplantation, and discontinuation of immunosuppression is likely to result in flares of graft-versus-host disease (GVHD) and a further delay in recovery of T-cell-mediated immunity. EBV-transformed B cells contain a circular viral DNA that is not susceptible to inhibition with thymidine kinase (TK) inhibitors. Nevertheless, anecdotal reports suggest tumor regression with either acyclovir or ganciclovir therapy. Chemotherapy and irradiation generally have not proven useful. The use of monoclonal antibodies to treat PTLD was first reported by the Necker group in Paris.[32–34] However, the anti-CD21 and anti-CD24 antibodies used in these studies are no longer available for clinical us. Most recently, efficacy of the anti-CD20 monoclonal antibody rituximab in the treatment of PTLD after SCT has been reported, and rituximab seems to be highly effective in this setting[35,36] (Hôpital St Louis, unpublished data). In 1994, Papadopoulos and co-workers first reported the therapeutic efficacy of the infusion of donor leukocytes in five patients who developed a B-cell PTLD following T-cell-depleted allogeneic marrow transplantation. Subsequently, Rooney et al[27] reported on the use of gene-marked EBV-specific T lymphocytes to control or prevent B-cell PTLD in 10 patients. The St Jude group described the prophylactic use of EBV-specific T-cell clones in 25 patients, none of whom developed PTLD.[37] The use of EBV-specific cytotoxic T lymphocytes (CTL) still requires high-level biotechnology laboratories to provide EBV-specific CTL clones. The most readily available and most efficacious treatment seems to be rituximab, but this still needs further studies with larger numbers of patients before it can be considered as the gold standard treatment for allogeneic SCT recipients.

### Late-onset lymphomas

Some cases of late-occurring lymphomas have been reported in the literature (reviewed in reference 4). These cases presented like ordinary NHL. Among more than 18 000 patients, 14 late-onset NHL were reported.[6] The only risk factor identified for late-onset PTLD was extensive chronic GVHD. Eight patients were diagnosed with HL.[38] HL differed from PTLD in its later onset (>2.5 years), lack of established risk factors, and relatively good prognosis.

### Solid tumors

Observations in animal models suggested that post-transplant solid tumors occurred with considerable delay (median 8–11.5 years). Extrapolation to humans with a longer expected lifespan would suggest that solid tumors might develop a decade or more after transplantation. This appears to be borne out by the actual data,[3,39,40] since the median elapsed time from SCT to solid tumors lies between 5 and 6 years.

The largest series reporting solid tumors after SCT are summarized in Table 45.2.[17,41,42] In a collaborative study, Curtis et al[2] analyzed results in 19 220 patients. There were 80 solid tumors for an observed/expected (O/E) ratio of 2.7 ($p<0.001$). In patients surviving at least 10 years after transplantation, the risk was increased eightfold. The cumulative incidence of tumors was 2.2% at 10 years and 6.7% at 15 years. The risk was increased significantly for melanoma (O/E 5.0), cancers of the buccal cavity (11.1), liver (7.5), CNS (7.6), thyroid (6.6), bone (13.4), and connective tissue (8.0). The risk was highest for the youngest patients. Most striking was the link of squamous cell carcinoma with chronic GVHD and male gender. The underlying diagnosis was important insofar as the risk of solid tumors was higher for patients with leukemia and lower in patients with lymphoma or aplastic anemia. The risk associated with total body irradiation (TBI) declined if irradiation was given with a fractionation regimen but increased with the total cumulative dose administered. This analysis strongly suggests that reduced doses of TBI, the omission of limited-field irradiation, and the prevention of GVHD (in particular chronic GVHD) should reduce the risk of post-transplant solid tumors. Finally, since in this first study relatively few patients surviving more than 10 years post SCT were included, we have continued surveillance of these and other SCT survivors to determine whether the risk of solid tumors changed beyond 10 years after transplantation.[43] The preliminary results of this survey can be summarized as follows. New cancers were sought in 28 884 allogeneic SCT recipients. The cumulative incidence of invasive solid cancers for all patients was 5.0% at 15 years and 8.1% at 20 years. Compared with a matched general population, transplant recipients were at significantly higher risk of developing new invasive solid cancers (161 observed second cancers; O/E=2.3). The risk increased with time since transplantation; the O/E ratio was 4.8 among 10-year survivors. A new finding in this study, not seen in previous reports, is a significantly increased risk of breast cancer among 10-year survivors. These data indicate that SCT survivors face increasing risks of solid cancers with time after transplantation, supporting the need for lifelong surveillance. The main points concerning solid tumors are highlighted in Table 45.3.

### Myelodysplastic syndrome and acute leukemia

Already in the early 1970s, Thomas et al[44] reported on two patients with acute lymphoblastic leukemia

## Table 45.2  Incidence and risk factors of solid tumors after SCT

| | Witherspoon et al[101] | Deeg et al[42] | Bhatia et al[18] | Curtis et al[2] | Socié et al[102] |
|---|---|---|---|---|---|
| Number of patients | 2246 | 700 | 2150 | 19 226 | 3182 |
| Total solid tumors | 13 | 18 | 17 | 80 | 25 |
| Melanoma | 3 | | 3 | 9 | 3 |
| Squamous cell carcinoma | 3 | 17 | 1 | 22 | 3 |
| Mucoepidermoid carcinoma | | 1 | 3 | | 2 |
| Thyroid | | | 1 | 7 | 5 |
| Connective tissue sarcoma | | | 1 | 8 | 3 |
| Brain tumor | 3 | | 2 | 10 | 9 |
| Other | | | 6 | 24 | |
| Median time (range) | 1 year[a] (0.1–13.9 years) | 91 months (1.4–221 months) | 5.6% at 13 years | — | 6 years (0.3–14.3 years) |
| Risk factor: | | | | | |
| Irradiation | RR=3.9 | RR=3.9 | | RR=18.4[b] | RR=3.1 |
| aGVHD | | | | | |
| cGVHD | | | | RR=1.1 | |
| Azathioprine for cGVHD | | RR=7.5 | | | |
| T-cell depletion | | | | | |
| Antithymocyte globulin | RR=4.2 | | | | |
| Anti-CD3 | RR=13.6 | | | | |
| Male sex | | | | RR=1.2 | |
| Age | | RR=1.1 (older) | | | RR=3.7 (younger) |

RR, relative risk; a/cGVHD, acute/chronic graft-versus-host disease.
[a]Including PTLD. [b]Limited field.

## Table 45.3  Post-SCT solid tumors: main current points

- Cancer incidence continues to increase with prolonged follow-up, with no evidence of any plateau phase
- Irradiation is the strongest risk factor, but while chemotherapy alone must be used in patients with aplastic anemia, other diseases may need irradiation. Furthermore, recent data do suggest that solid cancers can occur after non-radiation-based conditioning regimens
- Chronic GVHD and/or its treatment is strongly associated with the occurrence of squamous cell carcinoma (SCC)
- Ongoing studies try to identify cancer-specific risk factors
- Biological data are needed to study oncogenetic process in SCT recipients.
- Most patients who underwent allogeneic SCT had received substantial amounts of chemotherapy and radiation before transplant. The role of those pretransplant treatments on the occurrence of solid tumors clearly needs evaluation
- How to treat patients with second solid tumors after SCT? There are very few data to answer this critical and practical question. In our experience, patients with SCC of the head and neck have a bad prognosis with conventional therapy. With this exception, patients with solid tumors can generally be treated safely with conventional treatment

(ALL) who developed leukemia in donor cells. Several similar cases were subsequently reported from other institutions (reviewed in reference 3). The mechanisms that lead to leukemia in previously healthy transplanted cells are not clear. More recent studies have employed variable-number tandem repeat (VNTR) analysis to determine the origin of cells in patients post transplant.[45]

## Conclusions

Second malignancies after allogeneic SCT have emerged as a significant complication. The development of highly immunosuppressive but non-myeloablative conditioning before transplantation from HLA-identical sibling and unrelated donors makes it likely that the incidence of PTLD will rise in these patients. The incidence rate of solid tumors shows an alarming slope, with increasing incidence with increased follow-up. For solid tumors, the only practical approach is to closely follow long-term survivors on an (at least) annual basis to allow early diagnosis and treatment.

## Non-malignant late effects

Chronic GVHD and associated immunodeficiency are the major causes of late complications following allogeneic SCT. Chronic GVHD is the prime cause of transplant-related mortality late after marrow grafting. This complication – by far the main one of allogeneic SCT – is reviewed in reference 46. In a large study the 5-year probability of transplant-related mortality following discharge home was 22% in patients with and 6% in patients without chronic GVHD.[47] Despite conventional and new therapies for the treatment of chronic GVHD, this syndrome continues to account for significant morbidity and mortality after allogeneic SCT. With the expanded use of allogeneic PBSCT using matched unrelated as well as mismatched related donors, there is an increased incidence of chronic GVHD that poses a new clinical challenge.[46,48,49] Although improvements have been made in the prevention of acute GVHD, these advances have not resulted in a concomitant decrease in the incidence of chronic GVHD.[46] This sustained incidence of chronic GVHD is likely related to changes in clinical SCT practice.

Whereas the prophylactic use of multiagent immunosuppression has reduced the incidence and severity of acute GVHD, the incidence of chronic GVHD remains unchanged. The incidence of chronic GVHD after sibling-matched related, unrelated, and PBSCT lies in the ranges 27–50%, 42–72%, and 54–57%, respectively.[50] Factors that increase the risk of development of chronic GVHD include increased donor and recipient ages, prior acute GVHD, the use of alloimmune female donors, the type of GVHD prophylaxis, and a history of recipient herpesvirus infection.

As will be summarized in this chapter, chronic GVHD and/or its treatment with glucocorticoids is the major risk factor leading to late non-malignant complications after allogeneic SCT. The other main risk factor for many non-malignant late complications is irradiation.

### Late infections and immune deficiency

Immune reconstitution plays a pivotal role in the long-term consequences of allogeneic SCT, not only because an immune defect is related to infectious morbidity post transplant, but also because it may influence the risk of relapse and the development of secondary malignancies after SCT. Several studies have characterized the immune reconstitution in the few months following allogeneic SCT, but data on large numbers of patients regarding long-term immune reconstitution are scarce.[51–54] A large number of variables related to patient or transplant characteristics, such as age of recipients, stem cell engineering, type and duration of disease, and conditioning regimen, may influence the recovery of immunity after SCT. Other post-transplant variables – in particular chronic GVHD and the consequent administration of immunosuppressive drugs – also have an impact. Chronic GVHD is the leading factor affecting immune reconstitution of CD4+ and CD8+ T cells and of B cells. Donor source (marrow versus peripheral blood), unrelated versus sibling transplant, and the degree of histocompatibility between donor and recipient also affect the pace of immune reconstitution. Low B-cell count, inverted CD4+/CD8+ ratio, and decreased IgA level are risk factors associated with late infections. Recent immunological methods such as repertoire analysis and the presence of recent thymic emigrants are currently being evaluated as tools to investigate immune reconstitution after SCT.[54]

Late bacterial and viral infections have been reviewed extensively, and guidelines for preventing these opportunistic infections after SCT have been proposed in a document published under the auspices of the US Centers for Disease Control (CDC), the Infectious Disease Society of America (IDSA), and the American Society of Blood and Marrow Transplantation (ASBMT).[55] Susceptibility to encapsulated bacteria (*Streptococcus pneumoniae, Haemophilus influenzae*, and *Neisseria meningitidis*) has been well documented, especially in patients with current or previous chronic GVHD. Late (>2 years) fungal or cytomegalovirus (CMV) diseases are rare, and almost invariably occur in patients with ongoing immune suppression for GVHD. Varicella zoster infections are, on the contrary, extremely frequent (even in patients without GVHD), but usually occur within months post SCT after discontinuation of acyclovir prophylaxis. Finally, among parasitic infections, late *Pneumocystis carinii* pneumonia (PCP) and *Toxoplasma gondii* infections usually occur in patients receiving active therapy for chronic GVHD.

### Late ocular effects

#### Microvascular retinopathy

Ischemic retinopathy, including cottonwool spots and optic disk edema, is the most frequent complication of the posterior ocular segment following transplantation.[56] Microvascular retinopathy is observed only after allogeneic transplantation, in patients conditioned with TBI and receiving cyclosporine for GVHD prophylaxis. Ocular lesions appear during the first 6 months after transplantation. Visual acuity decreases in most patients, but recovers in all patients with a follow-up of at least 12 months on withdrawal of cyclosporine.[57]

## Cataract

Cataract formation, particularly posterior subcapsular cataracts, has been recognized in transplant recipients as one of most frequent late complications of TBI. Single-dose TBI of 10 Gy or more causes cataract formation in all patients. Fractionation of the dose was attempted to reduce the side-effects on tissues and particularly on the lens.[58–60] The estimated incidence of cataract lies between 80% after single-dose TBI and 20% in non-irradiated recipients.[61] The only treatment for cataract is to surgically remove the opacified lens from the eye to restore transparency of the visual axis. Today, cataract surgery is less risky and improves visual acuity in 95% of eyes without pre-existing ocular comorbidity.

## Kerato conjunctivitis sicca syndrome

This complication is usually part of the more general sicca syndrome with xerostomia, vaginitis, and dryness of the skin.[62] All of these manifestations are closely related to chronic GVHD, which may lead in its most extensive forms to a Sjögren-like syndrome. The ocular manifestations include reduced tear flow, keratoconjunctivitis sicca, sterile conjunctivitis, corneal epithelial defects, and corneal ulceration. The incidence, time course, and risk factors associated with late-onset keratoconjunctivitis sicca syndrome after transplantation was evaluated in a retrospective cohort study of the European Group for Blood and Marrow Transplantation (EBMT) Working Party on Late Effects.[63] Of the 248 patients, 48 (19%), with a minimum follow-up of 5 years, developed a keratoconjunctivitis sicca syndrome between 3 and 127 months (median 13.8 months) after transplantation. The probability of developing keratoconjunctivitis sicca syndrome at 15 years was 38% for patients with and 10% for those without chronic GVHD. Factors associated with an increased risk of late-onset keratoconjunctivitis are chronic GVHD, female sex, age older than 20 years, single-dose irradiation for pretransplant preparation, and methotrexate for prevention of GVHD.

## Pulmonary late effects

Significant late toxicity involving both the airways and the lungs affects at least 15–40% of patients after SCT. Clinical syndromes are not well defined or definable because of overlapping of pathogenetic mechanisms and/or because they represent a continuum rather than a distinct disorder. Sensitivity to cytotoxic agents and irradiation, infections, and immune-mediated lung injury associated with GVHD are the most prominent among the multiple factors that contribute to late respiratory complications.[64] Respiratory abnormalities are a consequence of scarring and thickening of the interstitial space, leading to interference with gas exchange and respiratory dynamics. Impaired growth of both lung and chest can be an additional factor in children. Immune-mediated injury due to GVHD can play an important role in damaging the small airways.

## Chronic obstructive pulmonary disease

Chronic obstructive pulmonary disease can be evident in up to 20% of long-term survivors after SCT.[65–67] Airflow obstruction can be an indirect consequence of chronic GVHD (aspiration secondary to esophageal GVHD, sinobronchial sicca syndrome, abnormal mucociliary transport, and recurrent infections due to immunosuppression) or can be due to direct immune-mediated damage to the airway by donor T lymphocytes and cytokines. Mortality is high among these patients, particularly those with an earlier onset and rapid decline of $FEV_1$ (forced expiratory volume in 1 second). Symptoms consist of non-productive cough, wheezing, and dyspnea; the chest radiograph is normal in most cases. High-resolution computed tomography (CT) may show abnormalities similar to those reported in patients with bronchiolitis obliterans. Symptomatic relief can be obtained in some patients with bronchodilators; however, in most cases, obstructive abnormalities are not changed by this treatment. Patients with low IgG and IgA levels should receive immunoglobulin to prevent infections, which may further damage the airways. Immunosuppressive therapy leads to improvements in less than 50% of cases, probably because the damage has already become irreversible or because other pathogenetic factors still persist. Asymptomatic patients with abnormal pulmonary function tests (PFT) should be closely monitored for the development of respiratory symptoms – early recognition of airflow obstruction allows the initiation of treatment at a potentially reversible stage.

Obliterative bronchiolitis (OB) has been reported in 2–14% of allogeneic SCT recipients, with a mortality rate of 50%. It is strongly associated with chronic GVHD and a low level of immunoglobulin. GVHD is most likely responsible for the initial mucosal injury to the small airways,[68] with further damage being caused by repeated infections. The initial symptoms often resemble those of recurrent upper respiratory tract infections, and then persistent cough, wheezing, inspiratory rales and dyspnea appear. PFT gradually deteriorate, with severe and non-reversible obstructive abnormalities. Chest radiographs and CT reveal hyperinflation with or without infiltrates and vascular attenuation; however, radiological findings do not correlate with lung function. It is not clear to what extent combined immunosuppressive treatment can be effective in the treatment of this disease, which typically does not respond to conventional treatment with steroids.

## Late liver complications

When faced with a patient with liver dysfunction after SCT, it must be borne in mind that more than one cause of liver disease – of viral and/or non-viral origin – may coexist. The pattern of viral serology is often atypical, and, moreover, besides the most important hepatotropic viruses, other agents, such as herpesviruses (including CMV), adenoviruses, and EBV, may also be implicated, sometimes causing a life-threatening fulminant hepatitis, due to their cytopathic effect.[69] Useful tools for differential diagnosis are timing post transplant, the type of clinical and biochemical deterioration, previous evidence of liver complication (including veno-occlusive disease), acute or chronic GVHD, and infection. Histological examination can be very helpful in discriminating between acute exacerbation of a viral hepatitis or an acute onset of chronic GVHD.

Based on serum ferritin levels, a diagnosis of iron overload is made in up to 88% of long-term survivors of SCT.[70] Iron deposition begins before SCT, and other causes of iron accumulation (e.g. prolonged dyserythropoiesis and increased iron absorption) contribute to iron overload. Hepatic iron overload may worsen the natural course of chronic hepatitis, especially hepatitis C.[71] Iron overload spontaneously decreases in the years following SCT.

## Late complications of bone and joints

### Avascular necrosis of bone

The main reports on avascular necrosis (AVN) are summarized in Table 45.4.[72-75] Pain is usually the first sign, and often early diagnosis cannot be made by standard radiography, while magnetic resonance imaging (MRI) already shows extensive necrosis. While the hip is the most frequent location (in over 80% of cases, with bilateral involvement in over 60%), other locations have been described, including the knee (10% of patients with AVN). Symptomatic relief of pain and orthopedic measures to decrease the pressure on the joint can be helpful, but most adult patients with advanced damage will need surgery.[76,77] Studies on risk factors for AVN have clearly identified steroids (both total dose and duration) as the strongest risk factor. Thus, avoiding unnecessary low-dose steroids for months in non-active chronic GVHD is probably a good way to prevent AVN. The other important risk factor is TBI (with the highest risk being for 10 Gy single dose or >12 Gy fractionated), as demonstrated elegantly in a Seattle case–control study.[75]

### Osteoporosis

Transplantation-associated osteoporosis is a well-known side-effect of solid organ transplantation, but data for SCT are still few (reviewed in reference 78 and 79). SCT can induce bone loss and osteoporosis because of direct toxic effects of radiation therapy, chemotherapy, and gonadal and pituitary hormone secretion. The incidence and course of bone mineral density (BMD) abnormalities following SCT was studied in a series of 104 patients.[80] The cumulative dose and number of days of glucocorticoid therapy and the number of days of cyclosporine or tacrolimus therapy showed significant associations with loss of bone density. Non-traumatic fractures occurred in 10.6% of patients. In a prospective study from the Hôpital St Louis, 105 asymptomatic patients had BMD measurement 12–18 months post transplant.[81] By multivariate analysis, including also as cofactors hormonal replacement (in women) and peripheral gonadal deficiency in both sexes, only steroid treatment for chronic GVHD was associated with decreased BMD.

---

### Table 45.4 Avascular necrosis of bone following SCT

| Ref | Incidence (%) | Time to necrosis (months)[a] | Median age at diagnosis (years) | Risk factors |
|---|---|---|---|---|
| 72 | 10.4 | 12 (1–62) | 19 | GVHD/steroids |
| 73 | 8.1 | 13.2 (4–58) | 16 | GVHD/steroids Aplastic anemia ALL |
| 74 | 4.3 | 22 (2–132) | 16 | GVHD/steroids Male gender |
| 75 | 4.5 | 26.3 | — | Irradiation Steroid dose |

GVHD, graft-versus-host disease; ALL, acute lymphoblastic leukemia.
[a]Range in parentheses.

## Endocrine function after SCT

### Thyroid

Between 7% and 15.5% of patients will develop post-SCT subclinical hypothyroidism, a condition where slightly-high serum thyroid-stimulating hormone (TSH) and normal free thyroxine levels are found.[82] This condition is an early finding after transplantation. It has not yet been clarified whether patients who develop subclinical hypothyroidism should be treated with L-thyroxine, since the majority of these cases are mild, compensated, and resolve spontaneously.[83] Furthermore, treatment with L-thyroxine might induce early osteoporosis, especially if given to those women after SCT with gonadal failure who are already at risk for developing osteoporosis due to sex hormone deficiency. The great majority of overt hypothyroidism after SCT is due to a primary lesion to the thyroid gland. Secondary hypothyroidism, caused by pituitary damage, is rare in patients after SCT, but is frequently observed in brain tumor patients who receive high doses of cranial irradiation. Hypothyroidism is usually diagnosed after a median period of 50 months from transplant. The frequency of hypothyroidism requiring L-thyroxine replacement therapy is highly variable,[84,85] and depends to a large extent on the type of pretransplant conditioning applied.[61,84–87] Treatment with L-thyroxine is indicated in all cases with frank hypothyroidism (elevated TSH with low free thyroxine blood levels). An emerging condition of thyroid dysfunction in transplanted patients is that due to an autoimmune thyroiditis, presumably transferred by the affected donor cells.[88]

### Growth

Linear growth is an intricate process that depends on a number of factors, such as genetic (i.e. mid parental height), nutritional, hormonal, and psychological. Children who undergo SCT form an extremely heterogeneous group. Pretransplant conditioning differs significantly with regard to the modality of irradiation and of chemotherapy. In addition, GVHD and its treatment, especially steroids used for long periods, might also induce growth failure in childhood.[89–92] Growth deficiency is found in some patients who underwent SCT during childhood. The mean loss of height (as estimated by the standard deviation score SDS) is estimated to be of approximately 1 height-SDS (equivalent to 6 cm) compared with both the mean height at the time of transplant and the mean genetic height. A cohort study on 181 children conducted by the Late-Effect Working Party (LEWP) of the EBMT showed that 143 (79%) reached 'normal' adult height.[93] Growth deficiency is more pronounced in children transplanted at younger age (before 10 years old) and in those who received irradiation.[94] The reduction in growth observed in the irradiated group may be explained by the direct effect of radiation on the gonads, by damage to the thyroid gland, and/or by damage to the bone epiphyses.

### Puberty and gonadal failure

Gonadal failure (both testicular and ovarian) is a common long-term consequence of prior chemotherapy and intensive pretransplant conditioning. The major cause of gonadal damage, which will eventually result in hypergonadotropic hypogonadism, is irradiation.[95] Similar damage can be also caused by busulfan, which is often used in children because of its minor effect on growth.

In males, the testicular germinal epithelium (Sertoli cells), where spermatogenesis occurs, is more vulnerable to radio- and chemotherapy compared with the testicular Leydig cell component involved in sex hormone (testosterone) secretion. Therefore, reduced or absence spermatogenesis, increased follicle-stimulating hormone (FSH) serum levels, and elevated luteinizing hormone (LH) levels, with (usually) normal testosterone, are commonly observed in most patients. The great majority of these patients will therefore not require testosterone replacement treatment to guarantee sexual activity, libido, erection, and ejaculation.

In females, the ovaries are more vulnerable to radiation and chemotherapy compared with the testes, and hypergonadotropic hypogonadism is almost the rule. The age at transplant is of great importance, since the younger the patient, the better will be the chances for gonadal recovery. In fact, ovarian failure in adult women is usually irreversible, while in prepubertal girls, although uncommon, there is still a greater possibility for subsequent spontaneous recovery and achievement of spontaneous menarche. Fractionation of irradiation reduces the impact on the ovaries.[90,96] With the increasing utilization of non-irradiation-based protocols in pediatric pretransplnt conditioning, it has become clear that the majority of girls of any age at transplant develop ovarian failure.[97]

The majority of females will need sex hormone replacement therapy (SHRT), both for the induction of pubertal process in girls who received a transplant during childhood and for maintaining menstrual cycles and bone turnover and mineralization in adult women. In girls who were transplanted during childhood and who are without spontaneous onset of puberty, and who show clinical and hormonal signs of gonadal failure, estrogen treatment should be started at age 12–13 years in order to achieve increased breast size, uterus volume, and pubertal growth spurt. After 1–2 years of continuous estrogen treatment in gradually increasing doses, when the breast shape is satisfactory, combined cyclic estrogen–progesterone treatment is introduced to achieve menses and to reduce the risk of osteoporosis. SHRT can be interrupted once every 2–3 years, for a period of 6 months, to evaluate the possible spontaneous recovery of ovarian activity, which can occur in a minority of women. SHRT should be reconsidered in those patients who develop amenorrhea and high gonadotropin levels during the interruption period.

Infertility is common following SCT, but conception is possible both for male and for female recipients. Return of gonadal function following cyclophosphamide conditioning for aplastic anemia is well documented.[98] In patients with malignant diseases, recovery of gonadal function occurs in 10–14% of the women, although the incidence of pregnancy is less than 3%.[98,99] In men, recovery of gonadal function has been reported in less than 20% of patients, and the use of increasing doses of TBI may be associated with considerably lower recovery.[98] Parenting following the administration of TBI is a rare event in men.[98,99] Busulfan plus cyclophosphamide (BuCy) is also associated with a high incidence of gonadal failure in women, and there have been no pregnancies reported with the use of BuCy for patients with leukemia.[98,99] In men, this conditioning regimen appears to be associated with the return of gonadal function in approximately 17% of cases, which is similar to the recovery after TBI conditioning for malignancy. Few patients have subsequently fathered children naturally; however, 20 patients were identified by the EBMT LEWP[99] and 2 patients

out of a series of 46 men receiving TBI from Seattle.[98] Pregnancies have also been reported after high-dose melphalan plus cyclophosphamide conditioning for allogeneic SCT.[100] Post-transplant management should routinely include symptomatic and biochemical monitoring of gonadal function. While the patient should be prepared for infertility, the possible need for contraception soon after SCT must also be emphasized, particularly in women who resume menstruation or in patients who do not wish to become parents. Distressing vasomotor symptoms may commence acutely post SCT, but may be prevented by initiating hormone replacement therapy.

## Conclusions

Allogeneic SCT has been able to cure thousands of patients with otherwise-lethal diseases. In this century, we move to an aim that is not only to cure patients but also to provide them with as few late complications as possible and to give them the best quality of life that we can. The two main risk factors (conditioning and chronic GVHD) were, until recently, deemed to be poorly amenable to modifications. However, new hope in reduced-intensity conditioning and new immunosuppressive drugs has shed new light in the field, and opens the door for a curable procedure with, hopefully, few late effects.

## REFERENCES

1. Kolb HJ, Socié G, Duell T et al. Malignant neoplasms in long-term survivors of bone marrow transplantation. *Ann Intern Med* 1999; **131**: 738–44.
2. Curtis RE, Rowlings PA, Deeg HJ et al. Solid cancers after bone marrow transplantation. *N Engl J Med* 1997; **336**: 897–904.
3. Deeg HJ, Socié G. Malignancies after hematopoietic stem cell transplantation: many questions, some answers. *Blood* 1998; **91**: 1833–44.
4. Adès L, Guardiola P, Socié G. Second malignancies after allogeneic stem cell transplantation: new insight and current problems. *Blood Rev* 2002; **16**: 1–12.
5. Duell T, Vanlint MT, Ljungman P et al. Health and functional status of long-term survivors of bone marrow transplantation. *Ann Intern Med* 1997; **126**: 184–92.
6. Curtis RE, Travis LB, Rowlings PA et al. Risk of lymphoproliferative disorders after bone marrow transplantation: a multi-institutional study. *Blood* 1999; **94**: 2208–16.
7. O'Reilly RJ, Lacerda JF, Lucas KG et al. Adoptive cell therapy with donor lymphocytes for EBV-associated lymphomas developing after allogeneic marrow transplants. In: DeVita TD, Hellman S, Rosenberg SA (eds) *Important Advances in Oncology 1996.* Philadelphia: Lippincott-Raven, 1996: 149–66.
8. Seiden MV, Sklar J. Molecular genetic analysis of posttransplant lymphoproliferative disorders. *Hematol Oncol Clin North Am* 1993; **7**: 447–65.
9. Cleary ML, Nalesnik MA, Shearer WT et al. Clonal analysis of transplant-associated lymphoproliferations based on the structure of the genomic termini of Epstein–Barr virus. *Blood* 1988; **72**: 349–52.
10. Knowles DM, Cesarman E, Chadburn A et al. Correlative morphologic and molecular geneitc analysis demonstrates three distinct categories of posttransplantation lymphoproliferative disorders. *Blood* 1997; **85**: 552–65.
11. Chadburn A, Suciufoca N, Cesarman E et al. Post-transplantation lymphoproliferative disorders arising in solid organ transplant recipients are usually of recipient origin. *Am J Pathol* 1995; **147**: 1862–70.
12. Young L, Alfieri C, Hennessy K et al. Expression of Epstein–Barr virus transformation-associated genes in tissue of patients with EBV lymphoproliferative disease. *N Engl J Med* 1989; **321**: 1080–5.
13. Suhrbier A, Burrows SR, Fernan A et al. Peptide epitope induced apoptosis of human cytotoxic T-lymphocytes – implications for peripheral T-cell deletion and peptide vaccination. *J Immunol* 1993; **150**: 2169–78.
14. Cen H, Williams PA, Breinig MC et al. Evidence for restricted Epstein–Barr virus latent gene expression and anti-EBNA antibody response in solid organ transplant recipients with posttransplant lymphoproliferative disorders. *Blood* 1993; **81**: 1393–403.
15. Mcknight JLC, Chen H, Riddler SA et al. EBV gene expression, EBNA antibody responses and EBV+ peripheral

blood lymphocytes in post-transplant lymphoproliferative disease. *Leuk Lymphoma* 1994; **15**: 9–16.

16. Randhawa PS, Jaffe R, Demetris AJ et al. Expression of Epstein–Barr virus encoded small RNA (by the *EBER-1* gene) in liver specimens from transplant recipients with post-transplantation lymphoproliferative disease. *N Engl J Med* 1992; **327**: 1710–14.

17. Witherspoon RP, Fisher L, Schoch G et al. Secondary cancers after bone marrow transplantation for leukemia or aplastic anemia. *N Engl J Med* 1989; **321**: 784–9.

18. Bhatia S, Ramsay NKC, Steinbuch M et al. Malignant neoplasms following bone marrow transplantation. *Blood* 1996; **87**: 3633–9.

19. Kernan NA, Bartsch G, Ash RC et al. Analysis of 462 transplantations from unrelated donors facilitated by the National Marrow Donor Program. *N Engl J Med* 1993; **328**: 593–602.

20. Hale G, Wardman H. Risks of developing Epstein–Barr virus-related lymphoproliferative disorders after T-cell-depleted marrow transplants. *Blood* 1998; **91**: 3079–83.

21. Klein G. Epstein–Barr virus strategy in normal and neoplastic B cells. *Cell* 1997; **77**: 791–3.

22. Kingma DW, Weiss WB, Jaffe ES et al. Epstein–Barr virus latent membrane protein-1 oncogene deletions: correlations with malignacy in Epstein–Barr virus-associated lymphoproliferative disorders and malignant lymphomas. *Blood* 1996; **88**: 242–51.

23. Gottschalk S, Ng CY, Perez M et al. An Epstein–Barr virus deletion mutant associated with fatal lymphoproliferative disease unresponsive to therapy with virus-specific CTLs. *Blood* 2001; **97**: 835–43.

24. Lucas KG, Small TN, Heller G et al. The development of cellular immunity to Epstein–Barr virus after allogeneic bone marrow transplantation. *Blood* 1996; **87**: 2594–603.

25. Lacerda JF, Ladanyi M, Louie DC et al. Human Epstein–Barr virus (EBV)-specific cytotoxic T lymphocytes home preferentially to and induce selective regressions of autologous EBV-induced B cell lymphoproliferations in xenografted C.B-17 *scid/scid* mice. *J Exp Med* 1996; **183**: 1215–28.

26. Heslop H, Ng CYC, Smith CA et al. Long-term restoration of immunity against Epstein–Barr virus infection by adoptive transfer of gene-modified virus-specific T lymphocytes. *Nat Med* 1996; **2**: 551–5.

27. Rooney CM, Smith CA, Ng CYC et al. Use of gene-modified virus-specific T lymphocytes to control Epstein–Barr-virus-related lymphoproliferation. *Lancet* 1995; **345**: 9–13.

28. Gustafsson A, Levitsky V, Zou JZ et al. Epstein–Barr virus (EBV) load in bone marrow transplant recipients at risk to develop post-transplant lymphoproliferative disease: prophylactic infusion of EBV-specific cytotoxic T cells. *Blood* 2000; **95**: 807–14.

29. Van Esser JW, Van der HB, Meijer E et al. Epstein–Barr virus (EBV) reactivation is a frequent event after allogeneic stem cell transplantation (SCT) and quantitatively predicts EBV-lymphoproliferative disease following T-cell-depleted SCT. *Blood* 2001; **98**: 972–8.

30. Van Esser JW, Niesters HG, Thijsen SF et al. Molecular quantification of viral load in plasma allows for fast and accurate prediction of response to therapy of Epstein–Barr virus-associated lymphoproliferative disease after allogeneic stem cell transplantation. *Br J Haematol* 2001; **113**: 814–21.

31. Marshall NA, Howe JG, Formica R et al. Rapid reconstitution of Epstein–Barr virus-specific T lymphocytes following allogeneic stem cell transplantation. *Blood* 2000; **96**: 2814–21.

32. Fischer A, Blanche S, Le Bidois J et al. Anti-B-cell monoclonal antibodies in the treatment of severe B-cell lymphoproliferative syndrome following marrow and organ transplantation. *N Engl J Med* 1991; **324**: 1451–6.

33. Blanche S, Le Diest F, Veber F et al. Treatment of Epstein–Barr virus-induced polyclonal B-lymphocyte proliferation by anti-B-cell monoclonal antibodies. *Ann of Intern Med* 1997; **108**: 199–203.

34. Benkerrou M, Jais JP, Leblond V et al. Anti-B-cell monoclonal antibody treatment of severe posttransplant B-lymphoproliferative disorder: prognostic factors and long-term outcome. *Blood* 1998; **92**: 3137–47.

35. Kuehnle I, Huls MH, Liu Z et al. CD20 monoclonal antibody (rituximab) for therapy of Epstein–Barr virus lymphoma after hemopoietic stem-cell transplantation. *Blood* 2000; **95**: 1502–5.

36. Milpied N, Vasseur B, Parquet N et al. Humanized anti-CD20 monoclonal antibody (rituximab) in post-transplant B-lymphoproliferative disorder: a retrospective analysis on 32 patients. *Ann Oncol* 2000; **11**(Suppl 1): S113–16.

37. Heslop HE, Smith CA, Ng CYC et al. Efficacy of adoptively transferred virus specific cytotoxic lymphocytes for prophylaxis and treatment of EBV lymphoma. *Blood* 1996; **88**: 681a.

38. Rowlings PA, Curtis RE, Passweg JR. Increased incidence of Hodgkin's disease after allogeneic bone marrow transplantation. *J Clin Oncol* 1999; **17**: 3122–7.

39. Deeg HJ, Witherspoon RP. Risk factors for the development of secondary malignancies after marrow transplantation. *Hematol Oncol Clin North Am* 1993; **7**: 417–29.

40. Socie G, Kolb HJ. Malignant diseases after bone marrow transplantation: the case for tumor banking and continued reporting to registries. *Bone Marrow Transplant* 1995; **16**: 493–5.

41. Socie G, Henryamar M, Cosset JM et al. Increased incidence of solid malignant tumors after bone marrow transplantation for severe aplastic anemia. *Blood* 1991; **78**: 277–9.

42. Deeg HJ, Socie G et al. Malignancies after marrow transplantation for aplastic anemia and Fanconi anemia: a joint Seattle and Paris analysis of results in 700 patients. *Blood* 1996; **87**: 386–92.

43. Rizzo J, Curtis RE, Deeg H et al. Solid cancers in survivors of allogeneic bone marrow transplantation. *Blood* 2000; **96**: 557a.

44. Thomas ED, Bryant JI, Buckner CD et al. Leukaemic transformation of engrafted human marrow cells in vivo. *Lancet* 1972; **i**: 1310–13.

45. Browne PV, Lawler M, Humphries P et al. Donor-cell leukemia after bone marrow transplantation for severe aplastic anemia. *N Engl J Med* 1991; **325**: 710–13.

46. Vogelsang GB. How I treat chronic graft-versus-host disease. *Blood* 2001; **97**: 1196–201.

47. Sullivan KM, Agura E, Anasetti C et al. Chronic graft-versus-host disease and other late complications of bone marrow transplantation. *Semin Hematol* 1991; **28**: 250–9.

48. Akpek G, Zahurak ML, Piantadosi S et al. Development of a prognostic model for grading chronic graft-versus-host disease. *Blood* 2001; **97**: 1219–26.

49. Flowers ME, Parker PM et al. Comparison of chronic graft-

versus-host disease after transplantation of peripheral blood stem cells versus bone marrow in allogeneic recipients: long-term follow-up of a randomized trial. *Blood* 2002; **100**: 415–19.

50. Lee SJ, Klein JP, Barrett AJ et al. Severity of chronic graft-versus-host disease: association with treatment-related mortality and relapse. *Blood* 2002; **100**: 406–14.

51. Maury S, Mary JY, Rabian C et al. Prolonged immune deficiency following allogeneic stem cell transplantation: risk factors and complications in adult patients. *Br J Haematol* 2001; **115**: 630–41.

52. Small TN, Papadopoulos EB, Boulad F et al. Comparison of immune reconstitution after unrelated and related T-cell-depleted bone marrow transplantation: effect of patient age and donor leukocyte infusions. *Blood* 1999; **93**: 467–80.

53. Storek J, Espino G, Dawson MA et al. Low B-cell and monocyte counts on day 80 are associated with high infection rates between days 100 and 365 after allogeneic marrow transplantation. *Blood* 2000; **96**: 3290–3.

54. Storek J, Joseph A, Espino G et al. Immunity of patients surviving 20 to 30 years after allogeneic or syngeneic bone marrow transplantation. *Blood* 2001; **98**: 3505–12.

55. CDC/IDSA/ASBMT. Guidelines for preventing opportunistic infections among hematopoietc stem cell transplant recipients. *Biol Blood Marrow Transplant* 2000; **6**: 659–741.

56. Bernauer W, Gratwohl A, Keller A et al. Microvasculopathy in the ocular fundus after bone marrow transplantation. *Ann Intern Med* 1991; **115**: 925–30.

57. Coskuncan NM, Jabs DA, Dunn JP et al. The eye in bone marrow transplantation. VI. Retinal complications. *Arch Ophthalmol* 1994; **112**: 372–379.

58. Deeg HJ, Flournoy N, Sullivan KM et al. Cataracts after total body irradiation and marrow transplantation: a sparing effect of dose fractionation. *Int J Radiat Oncol Biol Phys* 1984; **10**: 957–64.

59. Tichelli A, Gratwohl A, Egger T et al. Cataract formation after bone marrow transplantation. *Ann Intern Med* 1993; **119**: 1175–80.

60. Benyunes MC, Sullivan KM, Deeg HJ et al. Cataracts after bone marrow transplantation: long-term follow-up of adults treated with fractionated total body irradiation. *Int J Radiat Oncol Biol Phys* 1995; **32**: 661–70.

61. Socie G, Clift RA, Blaise D et al. Busulfan plus cyclophosphamide compared with total-body irradiation plus cyclophosphamide before marrow transplantation for myeloid leukemia: long-term follow-up of 4 randomized studies. *Blood* 2001; **98**: 3569–74.

62. Janin-Mercier A, Devergie A, Arrago JP et al. Systemic evaluation of Sjögren-like syndrome after bone marrow transplantation in man. *Transplantation* 1987; **43**: 677–9.

63. Tichelli A, Duell T, Weiss M et al. Late-onset keratoconjunctivitis sicca syndrome after bone marrow transplantation: incidence and risk factors. European Group for Blood and Marrow Transplantation (EBMT) Working Party on Late Effects. *Bone Marrow Transplant* 1996; **17**: 1105–11.

64. Soubani AO, Miller KB, Hassoun PM. Pulmonary complications of bone marrow transplantation. *Chest* 1996; **109**: 1066–77.

65. Clark JG, Crawford SW, Madtes DK et al. Obstructive lung disease after allogeneic marrow transplantation. Clinical presentation and course. *Ann Intern Med* 1989; **111**: 368–76.

66. Curtis DJ, Smale A, Thien F et al. Chronic airflow obstruction in long-term survivors of allogeneic bone marrow transplantation. *Bone Marrow Transplant* 1995; **16**: 169–73.

67. Schultz KR, Green GJ, Wensley D et al. Obstructive lung disease in children after allogeneic bone marrow transplantation. *Blood* 1994; **84**: 3212–20.

68. Cooke KR, Krenger W, Hill G et al. Host reactive donor T cells are associated with lung injury after experimental allogeneic bone marrow transplantation. *Blood* 1998; **92**: 2571–80.

69. Locasciulli A, Nava S, Sparano P et al. Infections with hepatotropic viruses in children treated with allogeneic bone marrow transplantation. *Bone Marrow Transplant* 1998; **21**(Suppl 2): S75–7.

70. McKay PJ, Murphy JA, Cameron S et al. Iron overload and liver dysfunction after allogeneic or autologous bone marrow transplantation. *Bone Marrow Transplant* 1996; **17**: 63–6.

71. Bonkovsky HL, Banner BF, Rothman AL. Iron and chronic viral hepatitis. *Hepatology* 1997; **25**: 759–68.

72. Enright H, Haake R, Weisdorf D. Avascular necrosis of bone: a common serious complication of allogeneic bone marrow transplantation. *Am J Med* 1990; **89**: 733–8.

73. Socie G, Cahn JY, Carmelo J et al. Avascular necrosis of bone after allogeneic bone marrow transplantation: analysis of risk factors for 4388 patients by the Societé Française de Greffe de Moelle (SFGM). *Br J Haematol* 1997; **97**: 865–70.

74. Socie G, Selimi F, Sedel L et al. Avascular necrosis of bone after allogeneic bone marrow transplantation: clinical findings, incidence and risk factors. *Br J Haematol* 1994; **86**: 624–8.

75. Fink JC, Leisenring WM, Sullivan KM et al. Avascular necrosis following bone marrow transplantation: a case–control study. *Bone* 1998; **22**: 67–71.

76. Bizot P, Witvoet J, Sedel L. Avascular necrosis of the femoral head after allogenic bone-marrow transplantation – a retrospective study of 27 consecutive THAs with a minimal two-year follow-up. *J Bone Joint Surg [Br]* 1996; **78B**: 878–83.

77. Bizot P, Nizard R, Socie G et al. Femoral head osteonecrosis after bone marrow transplantation. *Clin Orthop* 1998; **357**: 127–34.

78. Weilbaecher KN. Mechanisms of osteoporosis after hematopoietic cell transplantation. *Biol Blood Marrow Transplant* 2000; **6**: 165–74.

79. Schimmer AD, Minden MD, Keating A. Osteoporosis after blood and marrow transplantation: clinical aspects. *Biol Blood Marrow Transplant* 2000; **6**: 175–81.

80. Stern JM, Sullivan KM, Ott SM et al. Bone density loss after allogeneic hematopoietic stem cell transplantation: a prospective study. *Biol Blood Marrow Transplant* 2001; **7**: 257–64.

81. Socie G, Mary JY, Esperou H et al. Health and functional status of adult recipients 1 year after allogeneic haematopoietic stem cell transplantation. *Br J Haematol* 2001; **113**: 194–201.

82. Al Fiar FZ, Colwill R, Lipton JH et al. Abnormal thyroid stimulating hormone (TSH) levels in adults following allogeneic bone marrow transplants. *Bone Marrow Transplant* 1997; **19**: 1019–22.

83. Katsanis E, Shapiro RS, Robison LL et al. Thyroid dysfunction following bone marrow transplantation: long-

term follow-up of 80 pediatric patients. *Bone Marrow Transplant* 1990; **5**: 335–40.

84. Keilholz U, Max R, Scheibenbogen C et al. Endocrine function and bone metabolism 5 years after autologous bone marrow/blood-derived progenitor cell transplantation. *Cancer* 1997; **79**: 1617–22.

85. Borgstrom B, Bolme P. Thyroid function in children after allogeneic bone marrow transplantation. *Bone Marrow Transplant* 1994; **13**: 59–64.

86. Boulad F, Bromley M, Black P et al. Thyroid dysfunction following bone marrow transplantation using hyperfractionated radiation. *Bone Marrow Transplant* 1995; **15**: 71–6.

87. Toubert ME, Socie G, Gluckman E et al. Short- and long-term follow-up of thyroid dysfunction after allogeneic bone marrow transplantation without the use of preparative total body irradiation. *Br J Haematol* 1997; **98**: 453–7.

88. Aldouri MA, Ruggier R, Epstein O et al. Adoptive transfer of hyperthyroidism and autoimmune thyroiditis following allogeneic bone marrow transplantation for chronic myeloid leukaemia. *Br J Haematol* 1990; **74**: 118–19.

89. Sanders JE, Pritchard S, Mahoney P et al. Growth and development following marrow transplantation for leukemia. *Blood* 1986; **68**: 1129–35.

90. Sanders JE. The impact of marrow transplant preparative regimens on subsequent growth and development. The Seattle Marrow Transplant Team. *Semin Hematol* 1991; **28**: 244–9.

91. Cohen A, Duell T, Socié G et al. Nutritional status and growth after bone marrow transplantation (BMT) during childhood: EBMT Late-Effects Working Party retrospective data. European Group for Blood and Marrow Transplantation. *Bone Marrow Transplant* 1999; **23**: 1043–7.

92. Michel G, Socie G, Gebhard F et al. Late effects of allogeneic bone marrow transplantation for children with acute myeloblastic leukemia in first complete remission: the impact of conditioning regimen without total-body irradiation – a report from the Societé Française de Greffe de Moelle. *J Clin Oncol* 1997; **15**: 2238–46.

93. Cohen A, Rovelli A, Bakker B et al. Final height of patients who underwent bone marrow transplantation for hematological disorders during childhood: a study by the Working Party for Late Effects–EBMT. *Blood* 1999; **93**: 4109–15.

94. Sklar C, Mertens A, Walter A et al. Final height after treatment for childhood acute lymphoblastic leukemia: comparison of no cranial irradiation with 1800 and 2400 centigrays of cranial irradiation. *J Pediatr* 1993; **123**: 59–64.

95. Mertens AC, Ramsay NK, Kouris S et al. Patterns of gonadal dysfunction following bone marrow transplantation. *Bone Marrow Transplant* 1998; **22**: 345–50.

96. Sanders JE, Buckner CD, Amos D et al. Ovarian function following marrow transplantation for aplastic anemia or leukemia. *J Clin Oncol* 1988; **6**: 813–18.

97. Afify Z, Shaw PJ, Clavano-Harding A et al. Growth and endocrine function in children with acute myeloid leukaemia after bone marrow transplantation using busulfan/cyclophosphamide. *Bone Marrow Transplant* 2000; **25**: 1087–92.

98. Sanders JE, Hawley J, Levy W et al. Pregnancies following high-dose cyclophosphamide with or without high-dose busulfan or total-body irradiation and bone marrow transplantation. *Blood* 1996; **87**: 3045–52.

99. Salooja N, Szydlo RM, Socié G et al. Pregnancy outcomes after peripheral blood or bone marrow transplantation: a retrospective survey. *Lancet* 2001; **358**: 271–6.

100. Singhal S, Powles R, Treleaven J et al. Melphalan alone prior to allogeneic bone marrow transplantation from HLA-identical sibling donors for hematologic malignancies: alloengraftment with potential preservation of fertility in women. *Bone Marrow Transplant* 1996; **18**: 1049–55.

101. Witherspoon RP, Deeg HJ, Storb R. Secondary malignancies after marrow transplantation for leukemia or aplastic anemia. *Transplantation* 1994; **57**: 1413–18.

102. Socié G, Curtis RE, Deeg HJ et al. New malignant diseases after allogeneic marrow transplantation for childhood acute leukemia. *J Clin Oncol* 2000; **18**: 348–57.

# 46 Hematopoietic growth factors

Stephen Devereux and Antonio Pagliuca

## Introduction

Over the last 20 years, numerous growth factors with activity on the hematopoietic system have been discovered. Although a considerable number were tested in phase I and II clinical trials, only granulocyte and granulocyte–macrophage colony-stimulating factors (G-CSF and GM-CSF), interleukin-11 (IL-11), and erythropoietin (EPO) have been licensed for clinical use. Growth factors with multilineage effects, such as IL-3 and IL-1 in the main proved too toxic, whilst others such as thrombopoietin (TPO) failed to produce sufficient clinical benefit to justify full development or had unexpected side-effects.[1] It is now some years since a new growth factor with major clinical potential was discovered, and the emphasis has instead been on the modification of existing agents to improve their pharmacokinetic properties.

The data supporting the clinical use of G-CSF and EPO are similarly now relatively mature, and although questions remain to be answered, it is unlikely that many of these will be addressed by further randomized trials. The evaluation of growth factor studies is notoriously difficult, and evidence-based guidelines have been produced by a number of bodies to assist with decision-making in this area. This chapter will review the biology and indications for the use of currently available factors, concentrating mainly on EPO and G-CSF, since these are the most widely used.

## Erythropoietin

### Biology of EPO

The existence of a soluble regulator of red cell development was postulated at the start of the last century[2] and confirmed in the 1950s by animal cross-circulation experiments[3] and by studies on the plasma of anemic rabbits.[4] The renal origin of EPO was demonstrated soon afterwards,[5] and it is now known that in adult humans EPO is secreted almost exclusively by renal cortical fibroblasts in response to tissue hypoxia.[6]

The cloning of the EPO cDNA was reported in 1985,[7,8] allowing the production of recombinant material, characterization of its in vitro and in vivo properties, and investigation of clinical applications. Recombinant human (rh)EPO has been reported to contain tetraacidic structures whilst native serum EPO has only mono-, di-, and triacidic oligosaccharides.[9] The two forms of rhEPO used clinically differ somewhat in their glycosylation pattern, with more basic sugars, more non-sialyated N-glycans, and higher in vivo : in vitro activity ratio in EPO-β compared with EPO-α.[10]

The effects of EPO on erythropoiesis include an expansion of the number of erythroid precursors and an increased rate of reticulocyte release. EPO has no major effects on erythroid cell cycle length or the number of mitotic divisions, and inhibition of progenitor apoptosis appears to be the major effect at the cellular level.[11] EPO receptor (EPOR) knockout mice fail to produce mature red blood cells,[12] although a few very early erythroid cells are seen, suggesting that the commitment to the erythroid lineage is EPO-independent. EPOR density increases between the erythroid burst-forming and colony-forming (BFU-E and CFU-E) compartments, which are dependent on EPO for survival.

Although the most important physiological effects of EPO are on erythropoiesis, EPOR have also been found in a number of other tissues including brain, ovary, oviduct, uterus, testis, and developing gastrointestinal (GI) mucosa and vasculature. In the embryonal forebrain, EPO stimulates the proliferation of neuronal progenitor cells,[13] and a protective effect in ischemic brain injury in rats has also been reported.[14] EPO also influences GI vascular growth in the neonatal rat, leading to the suggestion that EPO present in breast milk may be important in the normal development of this tissue[15] or that it might act as a growth factor in gastric cancer.[16] The precise biological and clinical significance of these intriguing observations remains to be determined.

## Clinical use of EPO

EPO has been used to augment erythropoiesis in situations of absolute or relative deficiency or in an effort to overcome bone marrow insensitivity. Therapy with EPO is now an important component of the supportive care of patients with end-stage renal failure; however, this is outside the scope of the present chapter and will not be discussed further. Cancer-associated anemia is more complex and the place of EPO in its management has yet to be fully defined. Contributory factors include bone marrow infiltration, myelosuppressive chemotherapy, anemia of chronic disease, iron, folate, or vitamin $B_{12}$ deficiency, as well as blood loss and hemolysis.[17] In addition, a study that compared EPO levels in iron deficiency and malignant disease showed that levels were lower for a given hemoglobin (Hb) value in the patients with cancer, suggesting that production may be impaired in these individuals.[18]

There are wide variations in the use of EPO in cancer-related anemia across and within different healthcare systems that relate to uncertainty over its cost-effectiveness. Concerns over the safety of blood products, their increasing cost, and the shrinking donor pool, along with quality of life (QoL) considerations and commercial pressures, have, however, resulted in a year-on-year increase in EPO use in this situation. The evidence supporting this is reviewed below.

## Evaluation of clinical trials with EPO

The endpoints of clinical trial of EPO therapy have included increment in Hb level, the effect on the requirement for blood transfusion as well as QoL. Evaluation of these trials is often problematic; for example, it is important to know whether factors such as hematinic deficiency are equally addressed in treatment and control groups and that there are clear triggers for blood transfusion that are equally adhered to. QoL assessment raises particular difficulties, since although appropriate questionnaires have been devised, whether patients participate in this aspect of the study might depend on how well they are feeling – thus biasing the result in favor of improved QoL. In addition, although many studies are double-blinded, patients are often not blinded to their Hb result, thus further confounding QoL assessment. A detailed discussion of the methodological aspects of these studies is provided in the American Societies of Hematology (ASH) and Clinical Oncology (ASCO) guidelines.[19]

## Use of EPO for anemia primarily due to hematological disease

### Myelodysplastic syndromes

The myelodysplastic syndromes (MDS) are acquired clonal disorders of the bone marrow characterized by bone marrow failure and a predisposition to develop acute myeloid leukemia (AML). Patients with less than 10% myeloblasts in the bone marrow at presentation have a relatively low risk of leukemic transformation, and up to 80% of these individuals will become dependent on red cell transfusion. In the new World Health Organization classification, such patients would be categorized as having refractory anemia (RA), RA with ringed sideroblast (RARS) with or without multilineage dysplasia, and RA with an excess (5–10%) of bone marrow blasts (RAEB-1).[20] Although such patients may have a relatively good prognosis, anemia is a major problem, leading to reduced QoL. Excessive apoptosis[21] and impaired erythroid colony growth[22] are frequent observations in bone marrow from low-risk MDS patients, and are thought to contribute to the anemia. The finding that the addition of higher concentrations of EPO and other growth factors[23,24] to in vitro cultures can reduce apoptosis led a number of groups to investigate whether this is also the case in vivo.

*EPO.* A randomized controlled trial of EPO at a dose of 150 iu/kg/day in 87 patients with low-risk MDS showed a complete or partial responses in the subgroup with RA.[25] A baseline EPO level of less than 200 iu/l predicted response, and the best outcome was observed in those patients who were untransfused prior to study entry. Two meta-analyses covering trials of EPO alone until late 1994 (205 patients from 17 trials and 115 patients from 11 trials) demonstrated response rates of 16% and 23.5%, respectively.[26] Longer-term follow-up shows that in some cases these responses can be maintained for a number of years.[27] No data on QoL is available from the published studies, although extrapolation from other studies suggests that it may be improved.

*EPO and G-CSF.* A number of non-randomized uncontrolled studies have suggested that the combination of G-CSF and EPO might be superior to EPO alone. A trial that randomized patients to receive either G-CSF followed by G-CSF plus EPO or EPO followed by the same combination showed an overall response rate of 38%, with more responses in the group with RARS. A scoring system based on the serum EPO level and transfusion requirement has been devised to predict the response to EPO plus G-CSF.[28] This has been validated in two non-randomized uncontrolled studies.[29,30] In the very best group of patients, a response rate of 61% accompanied by an improvement in QoL was reported. The ASH/ASCO guidelines concluded that a trial of 8 weeks of EPO in patients with low-risk MDS and a serum EPO level below 200 iu/l would be appropriate on the evidence available.[19] There are no randomized trials comparing EPO plus G-CSF with either EPO alone or best supportive care; however, uncontrolled studies look promising. There is a need for randomized trials incorporating QoL analysis to address this issue.

### Aplastic anemia

There is no convincing evidence that EPO has any place in the management of aplastic anemia (AA), and its use is not recommended.[31] This is in line with the observation that serum EPO levels are very high in AA[32] whilst the number of progenitors that are able to respond is very low.[33] EPO has also been used in combination with G-CSF in the treatment of AA. In a study in which patients were randomized to receive either G-CSF or G-CSF plus 200 or 400 iu/kg EPO, some response was observed at the higher dose; however, this was confined to those with non-severe disease and lower baseline EPO levels.[34]

### Stem cell transplantation

The results of clinical studies of EPO administration after autologous (auto) or allogeneic (allo) hematopoietic stem cell transplantation (HSCT) are in keeping with the observed changes in endogenous serum EPO level. In the early post-transplant period, a consistent increase in EPO level has been reported in both auto- and alloHSCT patients.[35–41] This is followed by a period in which EPO levels are inappropriately low in allograft patients whilst levels are mainly appropriate for the degree of anemia in autologous transplant recipients. Cyclosporine (cyclosporin A) is known to inhibit EPO secretion,[42] but graft-versus-host disease (GVHD) and cytomegalovirus (CMV) may also contribute to this phenomenon.[36,40,43,44]

In keeping with these observations, EPO administration has no effect on indices of red cell production or transfusion requirement after autoHSCT. As predicted from the data on serum levels, the effect of EPO administration in the allogeneic setting is most marked later in the post-transplant period when the relative deficiency is greatest. Although an effect of EPO on the reticulocyte count has been consistently observed in the early post-transplant period, this has required doses of 1000 iu/kg/week and the impact on red cell transfusion requirement has been variable in randomized controlled trials.[45–47] In contrast, EPO administration later in the post-transplant period at a dose of 500 iu/kg/week produced a major response in over 90% of patients;[48] however, there have been no randomized controlled trials to confirm this finding.

### Other hematological malignancies

A number of studies have been performed in anemic patients with chronic lymphocytic leukemia (CLL), multiple myeloma, and non-Hodgkin lymphoma (NHL).[49–52] All of the studies included patients who were also receiving chemotherapy, and compared the outcome of EPO therapy with conventional support with blood transfusion. EPO therapy was associated with an improvement in Hb level and a reduction in transfusion requirement that was especially evident in those patients with low endogenous EPO levels and good bone marrow function as evidenced by a normal platelet count. Based on the quality of the evidence, the ASH/ASCO guidelines recommend therapy of the underlying disorder in the first instance, with EPO being reserved for those who do not respond according to the guidance in chemotherapy-associated anemia.

### Use of EPO for chemotherapy-induced anemia

There is evidence from a number of randomized clinical trials that EPO administration is effective at increasing Hb level and reducing the requirement for blood transfusion in patients with a Hb of 10 g/dl or lower who are receiving chemotherapy for malignant disease.[53–58] It is also likely that this leads to symptomatic improvement; however, due to the methodological difficulties in assessing QoL outlined above, the evidence for this is less convincing. For patients with a baseline Hb level between 10 and 12 g/dl, the evidence supporting the use of EPO is also less strong. Any potential benefit of raising the Hb in this situation must relate to improvement in QoL, since few clinicians would transfuse such a patient. A recent study that assessed QoL at different Hb levels in cancer patients revealed a nonlinear relationship between the two over the range 8–14 g/dl, with the maximum benefit at 12 g/dl, suggesting that use of EPO in patients with a Hb level above 10 g/dl may be warranted.[59] The ASH/ASCO guidelines on EPO use are summarized in Table 46.1.

### Use of EPO in transfusion medicine

There are a number of possible applications of EPO therapy in blood transfusion medicine. In the main, these center around the avoidance of transfusion in patients scheduled for surgery. A variety of strategies have been proposed, including raising the preoperative Hb level to facilitate preoperative autologous blood donation or acute normovolemic hemodilution (in which autologous blood is deposited, with saline replacement immediately preoperatively) or simply to give the patient a higher baseline Hb. Appropriate iron supplementation is important in this situation if the maximum erythropoietic response is to be achieved. The contribution of EPO to transfusion medicine has recently been reviewed.[60,61]

### Side-effects of EPO

EPO is remarkably free of side-effects in patients with hematological malignancies, since the very rapid

**Table 46.1  Indications for the use of erythropoietin (EPO)[a]**

1. Chemotherapy-induced anemia where Hb ≤10 g/dl
2. Chemotherapy-induced anemia where the Hb >10 g/l but falling. Depends on clinical circumstances
3. EPO starting dose 150 iu/kg, 3 × weekly s.c. for 4 weeks. Consider increase to 300 iu/kg for 4–8 weeks in non-responders. Alternative regimen of 40 000 iu/week may be effective, but there is less evidence for this
4. If there is no response after 6–8 weeks, discontinue. Investigate for tumor progression plus iron deficiency
5. Titrate EPO dose to maintain Hb at around 12 g/dl
6. Measure serum iron, total iron-binding capacity, transferrin saturation, or ferritin at baseline and at intervals during therapy
7. There is some evidence to support EPO use in low-risk myelodysplasia in the absence of chemotherapy. Evidence in other disorders such as myeloma, lymphoma, and chronic lymphocytic leukemia is less convincing if patients are not receiving chemotherapy
8. Anemia associated with myeloma, lymphoma, and CLL should initially be treated with chemotherapy and corticosteroids. If there is no response in Hb, consider supplementing with EPO

[a] Summary of the main points in the ASH/ASCO guidelines,[19] which state that in all circumstances blood transfusion would be an acceptable alternative.

rises in Hb that may lead to hypertension in patients with renal failure do not occur. Similarly, thromboembolic events such as clotted arteriovenous shunts, pulmonary embolism, and myocardial infarction, which have been consistently reported in renal failure patients, have been less of a feature in hematological malignancies. A recent study in patients with cervical cancer undergoing combination chemotherapy did, however, show that EPO therapy was associated with a higher risk of venous thrombosis.[62] Possible reasons for the observed increased risk of thromboembolism during EPO therapy include changes in blood viscosity,[63] transient thrombocytosis, and direct effects on the vascular endothelium resulting in increased expression of tissue factor.[64]

A recently described adverse event of EPO therapy has been the development of neutralizing antibodies to EPO in a small number of renal failure patients treated with EPO-α over the last few years.[65] This has resulted in pure red cell aplasia (PRCA) due to cross-reactivity of the antibody with native EPO; in most cases, this has responded to EPO withdrawal and immunosuppression. So far, there have been no cases of EPO-associated PRCA outside of renal medicine; however, there is no reason in principle why this

might not happen, and it has led some physicians to avoid starting new patients on EPO-α.

## Newer agents derived from EPO

The relatively inconvenient schedule of thrice-weekly subcutaneous injection has led to the development of agents with modified pharmacokinetic properties. The first of these is darbepoietin-α, a hypersialated glycoform of EPO-α whose circulating half-life is prolonged because of reduced clearance by hepatic galactose receptors.[66] A randomized clinical trial in patients with chronic renal failure showed that a once or alternate weekly schedule of darbepoietin gives a similar response to thrice-weekly or weekly dosing with conventional EPO.[67] Randomized clinical trials in cancer patients have shown darbepoietin to be well tolerated and active on a weekly schedule.[68–70] A pegylated form of EPO is also in clinical trials and appears to have similar pharmacokinetics.[71] The place of these newer agents remains to be determined, and there will inevitably be a trade-off between cost and patient convenience, especially when generic EPO becomes available.

# G-CSF and GM-CSF

## Biology of G-CSF and GM-CSF

The colony-stimulating factors (CSFs) are a family of glycoproteins, initially identified using cell culture assays developed in the 1960s,[72] that control the survival, proliferation differentiation, and functional activity of myeloid cells. Cloning of the cDNAs for granulocyte CSF (G-CSF)[73,74] and granulocyte–macrophage CSF (GM-CSF)[75] in the mid 1980s allowed characterization of the biological properties of these molecules, and clinical trials with recombinant materials followed soon afterwards.

The physiological role of these factors was elucidated by gene deletion studies in mice and measurements of the levels of the factors during cytopenia. Mice with a disruption of the gene for either G-CSF[76] or its receptor[77] are neutropenic and cannot respond to infection. In contrast, mice with a similar disruption of GM-CSF signaling are hematologically normal and instead suffer from pulmonary alveolar proteinosis.[78–80] During neutropenia and infection in humans, G-CSF levels rise whilst GM-CSF levels remain unchanged.[81] These observations suggest that whilst G-CSF is important for both steady-state and stress hematopoiesis, GM-CSF is not.

G-CSF acts at all stages of neutrophil development[82] and causes the release of progenitors and mature neutrophils from bone marrow stores. Functional attributes such as phagocytic activity, killing of microorganisms, and antibody-dependent cell-mediated cytotoxicity (ADCC) are enhanced by G-CSF.[83,84] GM-CSF has similar effects on neutrophil, macrophage, and eosinophil production[85] and function. The differentiation of dendritic cells (DC) from CD34+ progenitors[86] and monocytes[87] is also induced by GM-CSF, whilst G-CSF mobilizes DC that cause T-helper type 2 (Th2) polarization of lymphocytes into the peripheral blood.[88]

Commercially available forms of G-CSF include filgrastim, a non-glycosylated *Escherichia coli*-derived recombinant protein, and lenograstim, a glycosylated form of G-CSF produced in Chinese hamster ovary cell lines.[89] An N-terminal mutated form of lenograstim, known as nartograstim, is also available commercially, but few data are available.[90,91] A long-acting filgrastim called pegfilgrastim will be discussed separately below.[92,93] Currently, only a non-glycosylated *E. coli*-derived preparation of recombinant GM-CSF (molgramostim) is available. There are potential differences in pharmacokinetics, potency, and immunogenicity of the various preparations; however, so far these do not appear to be clinically important and the preparations will therefore be considered together.

### Clinical use of G-CSF and GM-CSF: indications and evaluation of studies

Since the introduction of G-CSF and GM-CSF in the early 1990s, numerous studies have sought to define their place in hematological oncology. The specific aims have been:

- The prevention of neutropenic sepsis following conventional chemotherapy, thereby reducing treatment-associated mortality, morbidity, and the attendant cost, and improving QoL. Practically, this entails:
  - primary prophylaxis in which all patients are treated;
  - secondary prophylaxis, when only high-risk patients are treated (e.g. those who had an episode of neutropenic sepsis during a previous cycle of chemotherapy);
  - interventional therapy, when a growth factor is used as an adjunct to antibiotics in patients with established neutropenic sepsis.
- To accelerate hematopoietic reconstitution after auto- or alloHSCT.
- To induce proliferation of leukemic cells and increase sensitivity to chemotherapy.
- To facilitate the harvesting of peripheral blood stem cells and mature neutrophils.

The evaluation of clinical trials of growth factor support has been notoriously difficult and several points are worth bearing in mind. The duration of neutropenia is a valuable hard endpoint that is reported in all studies; however, unless it leads to a reduction in morbidity or mortality, its only clinical relevance is as

**Table 46.2 Summary of indications for granulocyte and granulocyte–macrophage colony-stimulating factors (G-CSF and GM-CSF)**

| Indication | Recommendation |
|---|---|
| Primary prophylaxis | Use if the expected risk of febrile neutropenia is greater than 40% |
| Secondary prophylaxis | Use when there is good evidence that treatment delay or dose reduction would compromise outcome |
| Established neutropenia | Use only in high-risk patients |
| Stem cell transplantation | CSFs are indicated following autologous and allogeneic hematopoietic stem cell transplantation |
| Progenitor mobilization | CSFs are indicated for progenitor mobilization |
| Neutrophil collection | Possible use. Clinical trials are required |

a reassurance to the clinician. The risk of death after chemotherapy is now so low after even the most intensive regimens that it has not been possible to demonstrate a survival benefit in patients treated with G-CSF or GM-CSF. Rates of infection are also difficult to assess accurately, and alternative endpoints such as 'days of febrile neutropenia' (FN) are completely dependent on the duration of neutropenia, which will always favor the growth factor-treated group. QoL and cost-effectiveness analyses are also complex and difficult to evaluate. A frequent flaw in pharmaco-economic studies, for example, is the fact that clinical trials are often performed in large centers, where costs may be quite different from the smaller centers in which the majority of patients are treated.

To address these difficulties, a number of well-researched guidelines, position papers, and Cochrane reviews of growth factor use have been published, and these are summarized below along with evidence supporting the use of these factors in particular disorders.[94–101] Guidance on the clinical use of CSFs is summarized in Tables 46.2 and 46.3. Although much of what can be said about G-CSF is also applicable to GM-CSF, the former is much more widely used, mainly because of its superior safety profile.

### Prophylactic and therapeutic use of G-CSF and GM-CSF

#### Primary prophylaxis

At present, the routine use of G-CSF as primary prophylaxis in previously untreated patients undergoing

## Table 46.3  Use of G-CSF and GM-CSF in specific disorders

| Disorder | Ref | Result | Recommendation |
|---|---|---|---|
| Acute myeloid leukemia (AML) induction | 190–200 | Reduced duration of neutropenia and/or hospital stay. Some studies show increased CR rate, OS, or DFS | Possible use if appropriate to reduce inpatient stay and antibiotic and antifungal costs |
| AML consolidation | 193, 201 | Reduced neutropenia and antibiotic use | Recommended |
| AML sensitization | 196–199, 202–207 | Generally a limited effect. One study showed an increased CR rate; another reduced relapse and improved OS | Not recommended. Clinical trial only |
| Acute lymphoblastic leukemia induction | 208–213 | | Recommended |
| Myelodysplastic syndrome | 28, 214–218 | | Possible use with chemotherapy or episodic infection. Chronic use not recommended |
| Congenital neutropenia | 84, 219–221 | | Recommended. Caution over leukemia risk in long-term use |
| Aplastic anemia | 222–224 | | Not recommended. Clinical trial only |
| Non-Hodgkin lymphoma | 225–231 | | Possible use if risk of infection is greater than 40% |
| Hodgkin lymphoma | 232, 233 | | Possible use |

CR, complete remission; OS, overall survival; DFS, disease-free survival.

induction chemotherapy is not recommended, since the proportion of patients who might benefit is small compared with the cost and inconvenience of G-CSF administration.[95] Moreover, it is possible that CSFs themselves may induce fever that may be interpreted as FN, leading to inappropriate use of empiric antibiotics. A pharmaco-economic analysis suggested that primary prophylaxis is worthwhile when the risk of FN exceeds 40%,[102] for example in patients with AIDS-related NHL or during dose-escalated treatment schedules for lymphoma. This has been incorporated into some guidelines, although there is so far no evidence for clinical benefit.[95,96] It has been suggested that if current US estimates of hospitalization costs and indirect 'societal' costs such as loss of productivity, and out-of-pocket patient expenses are included, routine primary prophylaxis is warranted if the risk of FN is 18% or greater.[103]

Recent efforts have focused on risk-adapted strategies that might be used to target growth factor prophylaxis to patients who are at greatest risk, especially the elderly. A retrospective study of patients with NHL showed that serum albumin, lactate dehydrogenase (LDH), and presence of bone marrow involvement may be used to predict the risk of FN.[104] Elderly patients are also at particular risk of FN and may warrant growth factor prophylaxis. If predisposing factors such as these can be defined and validated then they may provide the basis for more appropriate decisions about primary prophylaxis in individual patients.[105]

### Secondary prophylaxis

There is no published evidence of a survival advantage for patients treated in this way; however, as the alternative is usually treatment delay and since acceleration of treatment has been shown to be beneficial in lymphoma,[106] it seems reasonable to extrapolate a role for CSFs in this situation.[96,107]

### Treatment of established neutropenia

It is necessary to distinguish in this context between afebrile and febrile neutropenic patients. One randomized trial showed no clinical benefit for the routine use of CSFs in afebrile neutropenic patients,[108] whilst in febrile patients, the results of nine randomized trials were variable, with the expected reduction in the duration of neutropenia but different effects on clinical outcome and cost.[109–117] G-CSF is not currently recommended in this situation unless there are particular high risk factors such as neutropenia (absolute neutrophil count (ANC) $<0.1 \times 10^9/l$), hypotension, multiorgan failure, invasive fungal infection, or an elderly patient.

### Use of G-CSF and GM-CSF in specific disorders

Many studies have now been conducted to investigate the potential benefits of G-CSF and to a lesser extent GM-CSF in specific disorders. The data and key recommendations from these mainly randomized studies are summarized in Table 46.3.

## Use of G-CSF and GM-CSF for mobilization of peripheral blood progenitor cells

A marked rise in the number of circulating progenitor cells in the blood during recovery from myelosuppressive chemotherapy was first described by Richman and colleagues in 1976.[118] The clinical exploitation of this finding was, however, limited by the number of leukaphereses required to yield sufficient cells. Both G-CSF and GM-CSF also mobilize progenitor cells into the peripheral blood,[119,120] particularly when given after myelosuppressive chemotherapy, and autologous G-CSF mobilized peripheral blood progenitor cells (PBPC) are now routinely used to support high-dose chemotherapy.

A randomized study comparing transplants using autologous bone marrow and mobilized PBPC showed accelerated neutrophil and platelet recovery, fewer platelet transfusions, and less hospitalization in the PBPC group.[121] A randomized comparison between GM-CSF- and G-CSF-mobilized autologous PBPC in patients with Hodgkin lymphoma (HL)[122] showed no difference in outcome; however, superior tolerability has resulted in the almost exclusive use of the latter. Accelerated neutrophil and platelet recovery has also been reported with allogeneic PBPC.[123,124] The higher T-cell dose found in PBPC harvests has been associated with an increased risk of GVHD in some studies but not others, and this is still under investigation.

## Use of G-CSF for neutrophil mobilization

Neutrophils collected by steady-state apheresis of normal donors fell out of favor for the treatment of neutropenic sepsis as they had little clinical impact. More recently, however, several groups have begun to administer G-CSF, with or without dexamethasone, to mobilize peripheral blood neutrophils.[125–127] G-CSF (600 μg subcutaneously) and dexamethasone (8 mg orally) given 12 hours before standard leukapheresis routinely results in the collection of approximately 80 × 10$^9$ granulocytes. This number of cells is sufficient to increase the neutrophil count of a severely neutropenic patient to normal and restore the recipient's ability to develop a neutrophil response in tissues. Several trials are ongoing to establish the clinical benefit of this new approach to supportive care for neutropenic patients.

## Use of G-CSF and GM-CSF in stem cell transplantation

### Autologous PBPC transplantation

Most randomized trials employing CSFs after high-dose chemotherapy and autologous PBPC transplantation (PBPCT) have shown them to be valuable in terms of significantly shortening the duration of neutropenia and hospitalization[128–131] and possibly reducing costs.[121,128,132] In a UK study, for example, the clinical benefits of G-CSF started at day +5 after autologous PBPCT were shown to be associated with a mean cost saving of £1816 per patient, even taking into account the cost of the G-CSF.[128] One placebo-controlled trial showed no benefit for therapy with GM-CSF following transplantation of GM-CSF-mobilized PBPC, with significantly fewer febrile days with the placebo.[133]

The optimal timing of CSF administration after autologous PBPCT is still under investigation. Two randomized studies demonstrated no significant differences in efficacy between early or delayed G-CSF (day +1 versus day +7,[134] and day 0 versus day +3 versus day +5[135]), but both reported cost savings with the delayed treatment.[133,135] On the other hand, a non-randomized study showed significant benefits for early compared with delayed G-CSF (day +1 versus day +4) with regard to neutrophil recovery, length of hospital stay, and duration of non-prophylactic antibiotic use, together with an 11% reduction in costs.[136]

### Autologous and allogeneic BMT

There are fewer data on the role of CSFs following bone marrow transplantation (BMT), but those that are available are positive. In a randomized trial of G-CSF (0, 10, or 30 μg/kg/day) in 54 patients with HL or NHL undergoing autologous BMT, G-CSF treatment was well tolerated and associated with significant reductions in the duration of neutropenia (by up to 16 days) and days with FN (by up to 5 days).[137] There were no significant differences between the two doses of G-CSF in this study. In a non-randomized trial in 81 patients undergoing allogeneic BMT, G-CSF started on day +1 post transplant was found to result in a significantly decreased time to engraftment and time from marrow infusion to discharge, together with significantly lower median costs (a $3400 difference).[138] In a further randomized study, G-CSF compared with placebo following alloHSCT significantly shortened the time to neutrophil regeneration. [139]

### Pegfilgrastim

G-CSF has a short half-life necessitating daily administration. Recently, pegfilgrastim, a bioengineered form of filgrastim, was created by covalently binding a 20 kDa polyethylene glycol (PEG) molecule to the N-terminal methionine residue of filgrastim.[140] This modification reduces renal clearance and results in a sustained duration of action. The predominant route of elimination of pegfilgrastim is through binding to G-CSFR on neutrophils and their precursors, so that clearance is directly related to the ANC, and serum levels remain elevated during neutropenia and decrease as the ANC rises.

Pegfilgrastim is administered as a single subcutaneous injection per cycle of chemotherapy. Clinical trials in hematological and non-hematological malignancies have shown it to have similar efficacy to filgrastim in decreasing the incidence of febrile neutropenia following chemotherapy. The safety profile and tolerability of pegfilgrastim are similar to those of the parent molecule,[141–147] and it has now been licensed to reduce the duration of neutropenia and the incidence of febrile neutropenia following chemotherapy for malignant disease (chronic myeloid leukemia (CML) and MDS excluded). The once-per-cycle dosing is of benefit to the patient and carers, and may improve compliance and QoL. The cost and benefits of single-dose pegfilgrastim will need to be compared closely with daily G-CSF before it can be recommended for routine use.

# Interleukin-11

IL-11 is a member of the IL-6 hematopoietic growth factor family, with in vitro and in vivo effects on megakaryocytopoiesis[148] and synergy with factors acting on other lineages.[149] In mice, in vivo administration results in elevated platelet counts,[150] and there is acceleration of platelet recovery after both chemotherapy and BMT.[151] Multilineage effects are also evident in these systems, with acceleration of neutrophil and reticulocyte recovery. In addition to its effects on the hematopoietic system, IL-11 has a protective effect in models of chemotherapy-induced gastrointestinal mucosal damage.[152] Studies in IL-11-deficient mice have shown that it is required for the maintenence of female fertility and has no essential role in hematopoiesis.[153,154]

A number of phase I and II clinical trial with IL-11 (oprelvekin) have been reported, leading to its approval by the US Food and Drug Administration (FDA) for the prevention of chemotherapy-induced thrombocytopenia in non-myeloid malignancies. The first of these was a dose-finding study in which IL-11 was given to women with advanced breast cancer before and after combination chemotherapy.[155] The maximum tolerated dose was 75 µg/kg, with dose-limiting fatigue, arthralgia, and myalgia above this level in all patients. A dose-independent reduction in hematocrit (mean 20%), possibly due to the previously observed expansion in plasma volume,[156] was noted. Although there was an increase in acute phase proteins, the fever and capillary leak syndrome observed with some of the other pleiotropic cytokines did not occur. Dose-related increases in platelet count were seen when IL-11 was given alone, and at higher dose levels the severity of thrombocytopenia in the first two cycles of chemotherapy was reduced.

Further phase I/II studies in a variety of tumors confirmed the modest effect of IL-11 on platelet (and sometimes neutrophil) recovery after chemotherapy,[157,158] and a randomized study in which placebo or IL-11 was given to patients who required platelet transfusion after the first course of myelotoxic therapy showed a significant reduction in the frequency of platelet transfusion in the second cycle. IL-11 was reportedly well tolerated, with side-effects similar to those previously seen; however, atrial arrhythmias (7 fibrillation and 1 flutter) developed in 8 out of 55 patients receiving IL-11 but in none of the controls. These effects were thought to be due to plasma volume changes, and it was suggested that they might be prevented by diuretic treatment. The effects of IL-11 on the gastrointestinal tract have led to trials in inflammatory bowel disease and as a protective agent following chemotherapy. A subset of patients with active Crohn's disease showed improvement in a randomized clinical trial.[159] Based on encouraging data in a murine study,[160] a small randomized study of IL-11 in the prevention of mucositis and GVHD was performed; however, no beneficial effect was shown.[161] A pharmaco-economic study of IL-11 as secondary prophylaxis of thrombocytopenia in solid tumor patients receiving chemotherapy showed that although some platelet transfusions were prevented, the costs were significantly higher than for conventional supportive care.[162]

# Thrombopoietin

The identification of the cDNA for thrombopoietin (TPO) was reported by five different groups in 1994, a decade after the original colony-stimulating factors.[163] There is good evidence that TPO is the principal regulator of platelet production, since TPO levels rise during thrombocytopenia[164] and transgenic mice with disruption of either the *TPO* gene or its receptor *c-mpl* are constitutively thrombocytopenic.[165–167] TPO deficiency in knockout mice can be largely corrected by liver transplantation,[168] and in humans there is a correlation between the platelet count and TPO level prior to liver transplantation,[169] suggesting that this organ is the most important physiological source of TPO. Factors other than TPO must be involved in the control of platelet production, since although TPO-deficient mice are thrombocytopenic, some platelets are produced and there is no spontaneous bleeding.

In vitro studies confirmed that TPO induces megakaryocyte differentiation, and synergistic effects with other factors on earlier progenitors were also observed. The multilineage effects of TPO were confirmed by the finding that in addition to a reduction in megakaryocytic progenitors, TPO- or c-Mpl-deficient mice also have significantly reduced numbers of early erythroid and myeloid cells.[165,166] Unlike G-CSF and GM-CSF, TPO has relatively minor effects on the function of mature cells, and although there is in vitro priming of platelet aggregation to some agonists,[170] TPO itself has no effect on platelet aggregation.

Preclinical and clinical trials of TPO have been conducted both with a full-length glycosylated recombinant molecule (rTPO) synthesized in mammalian cells and with a non-glycosylated truncated *E. coli*-derived variant with a polyethylene glycol moiety (megakaryocyte growth and differentiation factor, PEG-rMGDF). Although biochemically distinct, these preparations have a similar receptor affinity and in vivo half-life[171] In healthy primates, TPO increased the platelet count and the ploidy of bone marrow megakaryocytes.[172] These effects take several days to occur, presumably because TPO acts on earlier progenitors and not mature cells. Studies in animals treated with chemotherapy or radiation[173–176] showed that TPO reduced the degree of thrombocytopenia, leukopenia, and anemia.

Clinical trials in humans have mainly used the PEG-rMGDF preparation. When given to patients with advanced malignancies prior to chemotherapy, a dose-dependent increase in platelet count was observed, without evidence of any effect on platelet function,[177] and similar findings were subsequently reported in normal platelet donors.[178] A number of randomized clinical trials subsequently showed that in the context of intensive but non-ablative chemotherapy, TPO induces an earlier and often less marked platelet nadir.[177,179–181] In some studies, the need for platelet transfusion was reduced, but this was confined to the early cycles of therapy. In contrast to animal studies, there was no effect on the recovery of other lineages. Following more intensive chemotherapy and HSCT, no significant effect of TPO on the duration of thrombocytopenia or need for platelet transfusion has been reported.[182–184]

TPO has also been studied as an adjunct to PBPC mobilization and in platelet apheresis from normal donors. In a large randomized study, the addition of TPO to G-CSF improved the yield of CD34+ cells obtained and reduced the number of patients who failed to mobilize over $2\times10^6$ CD34+ cells/kg.[185] When administered 10–14 days prior to platelet apheresis in normal donors, TPO improved the yield and reduced the number of transfusions required compared with standard collections.[178,186]

An unexpected adverse effect of PEG-rMGDF administration was the development of neutralizing anti-TPO antibodies associated with thrombocytopenia and in some cases neutropenia and anemia.[1,187] The highest frequency (8.9%) was observed in normal donors given three subcutaneous doses of PEG-rMGDF, although antibody formation also occurred at a lower rate in chemotherapy and HSCT patients. It is not known whether truncation, pegylation, lack of glycosylation, or route of administration of the agent were the primary cause of this phenomenon, which resulted in the suspension of clinical trials in 1998. The relatively modest efficacy observed in clinical trials combined with this severe side-effect have meant that no form of TPO has yet been licensed for clinical use. Alternative thrombopoietic agents such as peptide[188] and chemical[189] mimetics have been described and may prove clinically useful in the future.

## REFERENCES

1. Li J, Yang C, Xia Y et al. Thrombocytopenia caused by the development of antibodies to thrombopoietin. *Blood* 2001; **98**: 3241–8.
2. Carnot P, Deflandre C. Sur l'activité hématopoietique des serum au cours de la regeneration du sang. *Acad Med Sci* 1906; **3**: 384.
3. Reissmann K. Studies on the mechanism of erythropoietic stimulation in parabiotic rats during hypoxia. *Blood* 1950; **5**: 372.
4. Erslev A. Humoral regulation of red cell production. *Blood* 1953; **8**: 349.
5. Jacobson L, Goldwasser E, Fried W, Plzak L. Role of the kidney in erythropoiesis. *Nature* 1957; **179**: 633.
6. Koury ST, Koury MJ, Bondurant MC et al. Quantitation of erythropoietin-producing cells in kidneys of mice by in situ hybridization: correlation with hematocrit, renal erythropoietin mRNA, and serum erythropoietin concentration. *Blood* 1989; **74**: 645–51.
7. Lin FK, Suggs S, Lin CH et al. Cloning and expression of the human erythropoietin gene. *Proc Natl Acad Sci USA* 1985; **82**: 7580–4.
8. Jacobs K, Shoemaker C, Rudersdorf R et al. Isolation and characterization of genomic and cDNA clones of human erythropoietin. *Nature* 1985; **313**: 806–10.
9. Skibeli V, Nissen-Lie G, Torjesen P. Sugar profiling proves that human serum erythropoietin differs from recombinant human erythropoietin. *Blood* 2001; **98**: 3626–34.
10. Storring PL, Tiplady RJ, Gaines Das RE et al. Epoetin alfa and beta differ in their erythropoietin isoform compositions and biological properties. *Br J Hematol* 1998; **100**: 79–89.
11. Koury MJ, Bondurant MC. Erythropoietin retards DNA breakdown and prevents programmed death in erythroid progenitor cells. *Science* 1990; **248**: 378–81.
12. Lin CS, Lim SK, D'Agati V, Costantini F. Differential effects of an erythropoietin receptor gene disruption on primitive and definitive erythropoiesis. *Genes Dev* 1996; **10**: 154–64.
13. Shingo T, Sorokan ST, Shimazaki T, Weiss S. Erythropoietin regulates the in vitro and in vivo production of neuronal progenitors by mammalian forebrain neural stem cells. *J Neurosci* 2001; **21**: 9733–43.
14. Kumral A, Ozer E, Yilmaz O et al. Neuroprotective effect of erythropoietin on hypoxic-ischemic brain injury in neonatal rats. *Biol Neonate* 2003; **83**: 224–8.
15. Ashley RA, Dubuque SH, Dvorak B et al. Erythropoietin stimulates vasculogenesis in neonatal rat mesenteric microvascular endothelial cells. *Pediatr Res* 2002; **51**: 472–8.

16. Ribatti D, Marzullo A, Nico B et al. Erythropoietin as an angiogenic factor in gastric carcinoma. *Histopathology* 2003; **42**: 246–50.

17. Spivak JL. Recombinant human erythropoietin and the anemia of cancer. *Blood* 1994; **84**: 997–1004.

18. Miller CB, Jones RJ, Piantadosi S et al. Decreased erythropoietin response in patients with the anemia of cancer. *N Engl J Med* 1990; **322**: 1689–92.

19. Rizzo JD, Lichtin AE, Woolf SH et al. Use of epoetin in patients with cancer: evidence-based clinical practice guidelines of the American Society of Clinical Oncology and the American Society of Hematology. *Blood* 2002; **100**: 2303–20.

20. Brunning RD, Bennett JM, Flandrin G et al. Myelodysplastic syndromes. In: Jaffe E, Harris N, Stein H, Vardiman J (eds) *World Health Organization Classification of Tumours. Pathology and Genetics of Tumours of the Hematopoietic and Lymphoid Tissues.* Lyon: IARC Press, 2001: 61–73.

21. Parker JE, Mufti GJ, Rasool F et al. The role of apoptosis, proliferation, and the Bcl-2-related proteins in the myelodysplastic syndromes and acute myeloid leukemia secondary to MDS. *Blood* 2000; **96**: 3932–8.

22. Merchav S, Nagler A, Fleischer-Kurtz G, Tatarsky I. Regulatory abnormalities in the marrow of patients with myelodysplastic syndromes. *Br J Hematol* 1989; **73**: 158–64.

23. Backx B, Broeders L, Lowenberg B. Kit ligand improves in vitro erythropoiesis in myelodysplastic syndrome. *Blood* 1992; **80**: 1213–17.

24. Schmidt-Mende J, Tehranchi R, Forshlom AM et al. Granulocyte colony-stimulating factor inhibits Fas-triggered apoptosis in bone marrow cells isolated from patients with refractory anemia with ringed sideroblasts. *Leukemia* 2001; **15**: 742–51.

25. Italian Cooperative Study Group for rHuEpo in Myelodysplastic Syndromes. A randomized double-blind placebo-controlled study with subcutaneous recombinant human erythropoietin in patients with low-risk myelodysplastic syndromes. *Br J Hematol* 1998; **103**: 1070–4.

26. Hellstrom-Lindberg E. Efficacy of erythropoietin in the myelodysplastic syndromes: a meta-analysis of 205 patients from 17 studies. *Br J Hematol* 1995; **89**: 67–71.

27. Hast R, Wallvik J, Folin A et al. Long-term follow-up of 18 patients with myelodysplastic syndromes responding to recombinant erythropoietin treatment. *Leuk Res* 2001; **25**: 13–18.

28. Hellstrom-Lindberg E, Negrin R, Stein R et al. Erythroid response to treatment with G-CSF plus erythropoietin for the anemia of patients with myelodysplastic syndromes: proposal for a predictive model. *Br J Hematol* 1997; **99**: 344–51.

29. Remacha AF, Arrizabalaga B, Villegas A et al. Erythropoietin plus granulocyte colony-stimulating factor in the treatment of myelodysplastic syndromes. Identification of a subgroup of responders. The Spanish Erythropathology Group. *Hematologica* 1999; **84**: 1058–64.

30. Hellstrom-Lindberg E, Gulbrandsen N, Lindberg G et al. A validated decision model for treating the anemia of myelodysplastic syndromes with erythropoietin + granulocyte colony-stimulating factor: significant effects on quality of life. *Br J Hematol* 2003; **120**: 1037–46.

31. Marsh JC, Ball SE, Darbyshire P et al. Guidelines for the diagnosis and management of acquired aplastic anemia. *Br J Hematol* 2003; **123**: 782–801.

32. Das REG, Milne A, Rowley M et al. Serum immunoreactive erythropoietin in patients with idiopathic aplastic and Fanconi anemias. *Br J Hematol* 1992; **82**: 601–7.

33. Marsh JC, Chang J, Testa NG et al. The hematopoietic defect in aplastic anemia assessed by long-term marrow culture. *Blood* 1990; **76**: 1748–57.

34. Bessho M, Hirashima K, Asano S et al. Treatment of the anemia of aplastic anemia patients with recombinant human erythropoietin in combination with granulocyte colony-stimulating factor: a multicenter randomized controlled study. *Eur J Hematol* 1997; **58**: 265–72.

35. Birgegard G, Wide L, Simonsson B. Marked erythropoietin increase before fall in Hb after treatment with cytostatic drugs suggests mechanism other than anemia for stimulation. *Br J Hematol* 1989; **72**: 462–6.

36. Ireland RM, Atkinson K, Concannon A et al. Serum erythropoietin changes in autologous and allogeneic bone-marrow transplant patients. *Br J Hematol* 1990; **76**: 128–34.

37. Schapira L, Antin JH, Ransil BJ et al. Serum erythropoietin levels in patients receiving intensive chemotherapy and radiotherapy. *Blood* 1990; **76**: 2354–9.

38. Crown J, Jakubowski A, Kemeny N et al. A phase 1 trial of recombinant interleukin-1β alone and in combination with myelosuppressive doses of 5 flurouracil in patients with gastrointestinal cancer. *Blood* 1991; **78**: 1420–7.

39. Grace RJ, Kendall RG, Chapman C et al. Changes in serum erythropoietin levels during allogeneic bone marrow transplantation. *Eur J Hematol* 1991; **47**: 81–5.

40. Beguin Y, Clemons GK, Oris R, Fillet G. Circulating erythropoietin levels after bone marrow transplantation: inappropriate response to anemia in allogeneic transplants. *Blood* 1991; **77**: 868–73.

41. Miller CB, Jones RJ, Zahurak ML, et al. Impaired erythropoietin response to anemia after bone-marrow transplantation. *Blood* 1992; **80**: 2677–82.

42. Vannucchi AM, Grossi A, Bosi A et al. Impaired erythropoietin production in mice treated with cyclosporin A. *Blood* 1991; **78**: 1615–18.

43. Bosi A, Vannucchi AM, Grossi A et al. Serum erythropoietin levels in patients undergoing autologous bone-marrow transplantation. *Bone Marrow Transplant* 1991; **7**: 421–5.

44. Beguin Y, Oris R, Fillet G. Dynamics of erythropoietic recovery following bone-marrow transplantation – role of marrow proliferative capacity and erythropoietin production in autologous versus allogeneic transplants. *Bone Marrow Transplant* 1993; **11**: 285–92.

45. Link H, Boogaerts MA, Fauser AA et al. A controlled trial of recombinant human erythropoietin after bone marrow transplantation. *Blood* 1994; **84**: 3327–35.

46. Klaesson S, Ringden O, Ljungman P et al. Reduced blood-transfusions requirements after allogeneic bone-marrow transplantation – results of a randomized, double-blind study with high-dose erythropoietin. *Bone Marrow Transplant* 1994; **13**: 397–402.

47. Biggs JC, Atkinson KA, Booker V et al. Prospective randomized double-blind trial of the in vivo use of recombinant human-erythropoietin in bone-marrow transplantation from HLA-identical sibling donors. *Bone Marrow Transplant* 1995; **15**: 129–34.

48. Baron F, Sautois B, Baudoux E et al. Optimization of recombinant human erythropoietin therapy after allogeneic hematopoietic stem cell transplantation. *Exp Hematol* 2002; **30**: 546–54.

49. Garton JP, Gertz MA, Witzig TE et al. Epoetin alfa for the treatment of the anemia of multiple myeloma – a prospective, randomized, placebo-controlled, double-blind trial. *Arch Intern Med* 1995; **155**: 2069–74.

50. Cazzola M, Messinger D, Battistel V et al. Recombinant human erythropoietin in the anemia associated with multiple myeloma or non-Hodgkin's lymphoma – dose-finding and identification of predictors of response. *Blood* 1995; **86**: 4446–53.

51. Osterborg A, Boogaerts MA, Cimino R et al. Recombinant human erythropoietin in transfusion-dependent anemic patients with multiple myeloma and non-Hodgkin's lymphoma – a randomized multicenter study. *Blood* 1996; **87**: 2675–82.

52. Dammacco F, Silvestris F, Castoldi GL et al. The effectiveness and tolerability of epoetin alfa in patients with multiple myeloma refractory to chemotherapy. *Int J Clin Lab Res* 1998; **28**: 127–34.

53. Case DC Jr, Bukowski RM, Carey RW et al. Recombinant human erythropoietin therapy for anemic cancer patients on combination chemotherapy. *J Natl Cancer Inst* 1993; **85**: 801–6.

54. Cascinu S, Fedeli A, Delferro E et al. Recombinant human erythropoietin treatment in cisplatin-associated anemia – a randomized, double-blind trial with placebo. *J Clin Oncol* 1994; **12**: 1058–62.

55. Henry DH, Brooks BJ Jr, Case DC Jr et al. Recombinant human erythropoietin therapy for anemic cancer patients receiving cisplatin chemotherapy. *Cancer J Sci Am* 1995; **1**: 252.

56. Wurnig C, Windhager R, Schwameis E et al. Prevention of chemotherapy-induced anemia by the use of erythropoietin in patients with primary malignant bone tumors (a double-blind, randomized, phase I–II study). *Transfusion* 1996; **36**: 155–9.

57. Kurz C, Marth C, Windbichler G et al. Erythropoietin treatment under polychemotherapy in patients with gynecologic malignancies: a prospective, randomized, double-blind placebo-controlled multicenter study. *Gynecol Oncol* 1997; **65**: 461–6.

58. Littlewood TJ, Bajetta E, Nortier JW et al. Effects of epoetin alfa on hematologic parameters and quality of life in cancer patients receiving nonplatinum chemotherapy: results of a randomized, double-blind, placebo-controlled trial. *J Clin Oncol* 2001; **19**: 2865–74.

59. Crawford J, Cella D, Cleeland CS et al. Relationship between changes in hemoglobin level and quality of life during chemotherapy in anemic cancer patients receiving epoetin alfa therapy. *Cancer* 2002; **95**: 888–95.

60. Goodnough LT, Skikne B, Brugnara C. Erythropoietin, iron, and erythropoiesis. *Blood* 2000; **96**: 823–33.

61. Goodnough LT, Shander A, Spence R. Bloodless medicine: clinical care without allogeneic blood transfusion. *Transfusion* 2003; **43**: 668–76.

62. Wun T, Law L, Harvey D et al. Increased incidence of symptomatic venous thrombosis in patients with cervical carcinoma treated with concurrent chemotherapy, radiation, and erythropoietin. *Cancer* 2003; **98**: 1514–20.

63. Shand BI, Buttimore AL, Hurrell MA et al. Hemorheology and fistula function in home hemodialysis patients following erythropoietin treatment: a prospective placebo-controlled study. *Nephron* 1993; **64**: 53–7.

64. Fuste B, Serradell M, Escolar G et al. Erythropoietin triggers a signaling pathway in endothelial cells and increases the thrombogenicity of their extracellular matrices in vitro. *Thromb Haemost* 2002; **88**: 678–85.

65. Casadevall N, Nataf J, Viron B et al. Pure red-cell aplasia and antierythropoietin antibodies in patients treated with recombinant erythropoietin. *N Engl J Med* 2002; **346**: 469–75.

66. Egrie JC, Browne JK. Development and characterization of novel erythropoiesis stimulating protein (NESP). *Nephrol Dial Transplant* 2001; **16** (Suppl 3): 3–13.

67. Vanrenterghem Y, Barany P, Mann JF et al. Randomized trial of darbepoetin alfa for treatment of renal anemia at a reduced dose frequency compared with rHuEPO in dialysis patients. *Kidney Int* 2002; **62**: 2167–75.

68. Glaspy JA, Jadeja JS, Justice G et al. A randomized, active-control, pilot trial of front-loaded dosing regimens of darbepoetin-alfa for the treatment of patients with anemia during chemotherapy for malignant disease. *Cancer* 2003; **97**: 1312–20.

69. Hedenus M, Adriansson M, San Miguel J et al. Efficacy and safety of darbepoetin alfa in anaemic patients with lymphoproliferative malignancies: a randomized, double-blind, placebo-controlled study. *Br J Hematol* 2003; **122**: 394–403.

70. Vansteenkiste J, Pirker R, Massuti B et al. Double-blind, placebo-controlled, randomized phase III trial of darbepoetin alfa in lung cancer patients receiving chemotherapy. *J Natl Cancer Inst* 2002; **94**: 1211–20.

71. Dougherty F, Reigner B, Jordan P, Pannier A. CERA (continuous erythropoiesis receptor activator) demonstrates dose-dependent activity and is well tolerated in phase 1 multiple ascending dose studies. *Blood* 2003; **102**: 713a.

72. Bradley TR, Metcalf D. The growth of mouse bone marrow cells in vitro. *Aust J Exp Biol Med Sci* 1966; **44**: 287–99.

73. Nagata S, Tsuchiya M, Asano S et al. Molecular cloning and expression of cDNA for human granulocyte colony-stimulating factor. *Nature* 1986; **319**: 415–18.

74. Souza LM, Boone TC, Gabrilove J et al. Recombinant human granulocyte colony-stimulating factor: effects on normal and leukemic myeloid cells. *Science* 1986; **232**: 61–5.

75. Wong G, Witek J, Temple P et al. Human GM-CSF: molecular cloning of the complementary DNA and purification of the natural and recombinant proteins. *Science* 1985; **228**: 810.

76. Lieschke GJ, Grail D, Hodgson G et al. Mice lacking granulocyte colony-stimulating factor have chronic neutropenia, granulocyte and macrophage progenitor cell deficiency, and impaired neutrophil mobilization. *Blood* 1994; **84**: 1737–46.

77. Liu F, Wu HY, Wesselschmidt R et al. Impaired production and increased apoptosis of neutrophils in granulocyte colony-stimulating factor receptor-deficient mice. *Immunity* 1996; **5**: 491–501.

78. Dranoff G, Crawford AD, Sadelain M et al. Involvement of granulocyte-macrophage colony-stimulating factor in pulmonary homeostasis. *Science* 1994; **264**: 713–16.

79. Stanley E, Lieschke GJ, Grail D et al. Granulocyte/macrophage colony-stimulating factor-deficient mice show no major perturbation of hematopoiesis but develop

a characteristic pulmonary pathology. *Proc Natl Acad Sci USA* 1994; **91**: 5592–6.

80. Nishinakamura R, Nakayama N, Hirabayashi Y et al. Mice deficient for the IL-3/GM-CSF/IL-5 βc receptor exhibit lung pathology and impaired immune response, while β IL-3 receptor-deficient mice are normal. *Immunity* 1995; **2**: 211–22.

81. Cebon J, Layton JE, Maher D, Morstyn G. Endogenous hematopoietic growth factors in neutropenia and infection. *Br J Hematol* 1994; **86**: 265–74.

82. Lord BI, Bronchud MH, Owens S et al. The kinetics of human granulopoiesis following treatment with granulocyte colony-stimulating factor in vivo. *Proc Natl Acad Sci USA* 1989; **86**: 9499–503.

83. Demetri GD, Griffin JD. Granulocyte colony-stimulating factor and its receptor. *Blood* 1991; **78**: 2791–808.

84. Dale DC, Cottle TE, Fier CJ et al. Severe chronic neutropenia: treatment and follow-up of patients in the Severe Chronic Neutropenia International Registry. *Am J Hematol* 2003; **72**: 82–93.

85. Lord BI, Gurney H, Chang J et al. Hemopoietic cell kinetics in humans treated with rGM-CSF. *Int J Cancer* 1992; **50**: 26–31.

86. Reid CD, Stackpoole A, Meager A, Tikerpae J. Interactions of tumor necrosis factor with granulocyte–macrophage colony-stimulating factor and other cytokines in the regulation of dendritic cell growth in vitro from early bipotent CD34+ progenitors in human bone marrow. *J Immunol* 1992; **149**: 2681–8.

87. Romani N, Gruner S, Brang D et al. Proliferating dendritic cell progenitors in human blood. *J Exp Med* 1994; **180**: 83–93.

88. Arpinati M, Green CL, Heimfeld S et al. Granulocyte-colony stimulating factor mobilizes T helper 2-inducing dendritic cells. *Blood* 2000; **95**: 2484–90.

89. Hoglund M. Glycosylated and non-glycosylated recombinant human granulocyte colony-stimulating factor (rhG-CSF) – what is the difference? *Med Oncol* 1998; **15**: 229–33.

90. Kuwabara T, Kato Y, Kobayashi S et al. Nonlinear pharmacokinetics of a recombinant human granulocyte colony-stimulating factor derivative (nartograstim): species differences among rats, monkeys and humans. *J Pharmacol Exp Ther* 1994; **271**: 1535–43.

91. Takemoto Y, Wada H, Takatsuka H et al. Mobilization of peripheral blood stem cells by granulocyte-colony stimulating factors: comparison of a standard dose of glycosylated and mutated granulocyte-colony stimulating factor in non-Hodgkin's lymphoma patients following CHOP therapy. *Drugs Exp Clin Res* 2000; **26**: 1–5.

92. Crawford J. Pegfilgrastim: the promise of pegylation fulfilled. *Ann Oncol* 2003; **14**: 6–7.

93. Crawford J. Safety and efficacy of pegfilgrastim in patients receiving myelosuppressive chemotherapy. *Pharmacotherapy* 2003; **23**: 15S–19S.

94. Ozer H. American Society of Clinical Oncology guidelines for the use of hematopoietic colony-stimulating factors. *Curr Opin Hematol* 1996; **3**: 3–10.

95. Ozer H, Armitage JO, Bennett CL et al. 2000 update of recommendations for the use of hematopoietic colony-stimulating factors: evidence-based, clinical practice guidelines. American Society of Clinical Oncology Growth Factors Expert Panel. *J Clin Oncol* 2000; **18**: 3558–85.

96. Pagliuca A, Carrington PA, Pettengell R et al. Guidelines on the use of colony-stimulating factors in haematological malignancies. *Br J Haematol* 2003; **123**: 22–33.

97. Clark OA, Lyman G, Castro AA et al. Colony stimulating factors for chemotherapy induced febrile neutropenia. *Cochrane Database Syst Rev* 2003; **3**: CD003039.

98. Bohlius J, Reiser M, Schwarzer G, Engert A. Impact of granulocyte colony-stimulating factor (CSF) and granulocyte–macrophage CSF in patients with malignant lymphoma: a systematic review. *Br J Haematol* 2003; **122**: 413–23.

99. Croockewit AJ, Bronchud MH, Aapro MS et al. A European perspective on hematopoietic growth factors in hemato-oncology: report of an expert meeting of the EORTC. *Eur J Cancer* 1997; **33**: 1732–46.

100. Balducci L, Yates J. General guidelines for the management of older patients with cancer. *Oncology (Huntingt)* 2000; **14**: 221–7.

101. Repetto L, Biganzoli L, Koehne CH et al. EORTC Cancer in the Elderly Task Force guidelines for the use of colony-stimulating factors in elderly patients with cancer. *Eur J Cancer* 2003; **39**: 2264–72.

102. Lyman GH, Lyman CG, Sanderson RA, Balducci L. Decision analysis of hematopoietic growth factor use in patients receiving cancer chemotherapy. *J Natl Cancer Inst* 1993; **85**: 488–93.

103. Lyman GH. Balancing the benefits and costs of colony-stimulating factors: a current perspective. *Semin Oncol* 2003; **30**(4 Suppl 13): 10–17.

104. Intragumtornchai T, Sutheesophon J, Sutcharitchan P, Swasdikul D. A predictive model for life-threatening neutropenia and febrile neutropenia after the first course of CHOP chemotherapy in patients with aggressive non-Hodgkin's lymphoma. *Leuk Lymphoma* 2000; **37**: 351–60.

105. Lyman GH. Risk assessment in oncology clinical practice. From risk factors to risk models. *Oncology (Huntingt)* 2003; **17**(11 Suppl 11): 8–13.

106. Pfreundschuh M, Trumper l, Kloess M et al. 2 weekly CHOP (CHOP14): the new standard regimen for patients wiyh aggressive non-Hodgkin's lymphoma (NHL) >60 years of age. *Proc Am Soc Hematol* 2001; **98**: 725a.

107. Lepage E, Gisselbrecht C, Haioun C et al. Prognostic significance of received relative dose intensity in non-Hodgkin's lymphoma patients: application to LNH-87 protocol. The GELA (Groupe d'Etude des Lymphomes de l'Adulte). *Ann Oncol* 1993; **4**: 651–6.

108. Hartmann LC, Tschetter LK, Habermann TM et al. Granulocyte colony-stimulating factor in severe chemotherapy-induced afebrile neutropenia. *N Engl J Med* 1997; **336**: 1776–80.

109. Maher DW, Lieschke GJ, Green M et al. Filgrastim in patients with chemotherapy-induced febrile neutropenia. A double-blind, placebo-controlled trial. *Ann Intern Med* 1994; **121**: 492–501.

110. Mitchell PL, Morland B, Stevens MC et al. Granulocyte colony-stimulating factor in established febrile neutropenia: a randomized study of pediatric patients. *J Clin Oncol* 1997; **15**: 1163–70.

111. Vellenga E, Uyl-de Groot CA, de Wit R et al. Randomized placebo-controlled trial of granulocyte–macrophage colony-stimulating factor in patients with chemotherapy-related febrile neutropenia. *J Clin Oncol* 1996; **14**: 619–27.

112. Anaissie EJ, Vartivarian S, Bodey GP et al. Randomized comparison between antibiotics alone and antibiotics

plus granulocyte–macrophage colony-stimulating factor (*Escherichia coli*-derived) in cancer patients with fever and neutropenia. *Am J Med* 1996; **100**: 17–23.

113. Mayordomo JI, Rivera F, Diaz-Puente MT et al. Improving treatment of chemotherapy-induced neutropenic fever by administration of colony-stimulating factors. *J Natl Cancer Inst* 1995; **87**: 803–8.

114. Ravaud A, Chevreau C, Cany L et al. Granulocyte–macrophage colony-stimulating factor in patients with neutropenic fever is potent after low-risk but not after high-risk neutropenic chemotherapy regimens: results of a randomized phase III trial. *J Clin Oncol* 1998; **16**: 2930–6.

115. Riikonen P, Saarinen UM, Makipernaa A et al. Recombinant human granulocyte–macrophage colony-stimulating factor in the treatment of febrile neutropenia: a double blind placebo-controlled study in children. *Pediatr Infect Dis J* 1994; **13**: 197–202.

116. Biesma B, de Vries EG, Willemse PH et al. Efficacy and tolerability of recombinant human granulocyte-macrophage colony-stimulating factor in patients with chemotherapy-related leukopenia and fever. *Eur J Cancer* 1990; **26**(9): 932–6.

117. Garcia-Carbonero R, Mayordomo JI, Tornamira MV et al. Granulocyte colony-stimulating factor in the treatment of high-risk febrile neutropenia: a multicenter randomized trial. *J Natl Cancer Inst* 2001; **93**: 31–8.

118. Richman CM, Weiner RS, Yankee RA. Increase in circulating stem cells following chemotherapy in man. *Blood* 1976; **47**: 1031–9.

119. Duhrsen U, Villeval JL, Boyd J et al. Effects of recombinant human granulocyte colony-stimulating factor on hematopoietic progenitor cells in cancer patients. *Blood* 1988; **72**: 2074–81.

120. Socinski MA, Cannistra SA, Elias A et al. Granulocyte–macrophage colony stimulating factor expands the circulating hematopoietic progenitor cell compartment in man. *Lancet* 1988; **i**: 1194–8.

121. Schmitz N, Linch DC, Dreger P et al. Randomized trial of filgrastim-mobilised peripheral blood progenitor cell transplantation versus autologous bone-marrow transplantation in lymphoma patients. *Lancet* 1996; **347**: 353–7.

122. Hohaus S, Martin H, Wassmann B et al. Recombinant human granulocyte and granulocyte–macrophage colony-stimulating factor (G-CSF and GM-CSF) administered following cytotoxic chemotherapy have a similar ability to mobilize peripheral blood stem cells. *Bone Marrow Transplant* 1998; **22**: 625–30.

123. Bensinger WI, Martin PJ, Storer B et al. Transplantation of bone marrow as compared with peripheral-blood cells from HLA-identical relatives in patients with hematologic cancers. *N Engl J Med* 2001; **344**: 175–81.

124. Blaise D, Kuentz M, Fortanier C et al. Randomized trial of bone marrow versus lenograstim-primed blood cell allogeneic transplantation in patients with early-stage leukemia: a report from the Societé Française de Greffe de Moelle. *J Clin Oncol* 2000; **18**: 537–46.

125. Adkins D, Spitzer G, Johnston M et al. Transfusions of granulocyte-colony-stimulating factor-mobilized granulocyte components to allogeneic transplant recipients: analysis of kinetics and factors determining posttransfusion neutrophil and platelet counts. *Transfusion* 1997; **37**: 737–48.

126. Dale DC, Liles WC. Return of granulocyte transfusions. *Curr Opin Pediatr* 2000; **12**: 18–22.

127. Yeghen T, Devereux S. Granulocyte transfusion: a review. *Vox Sang* 2001; **81**: 87–92.

128. Lee SM, Radford JA, Dobson L et al. Recombinant human granulocyte colony-stimulating factor (filgrastim) following high-dose chemotherapy and peripheral blood progenitor cell rescue in high-grade non-Hodgkin's lymphoma: clinical benefits at no extra cost. *Br J Cancer* 1998; **77**: 1294–9.

129. Klumpp TR, Mangan KF, Goldberg SL et al. Granulocyte colony-stimulating factor accelerates neutrophil engraftment following peripheral-blood stem-cell transplantation: a prospective, randomized trial. *J Clin Oncol* 1995; **13**: 1323–7.

130. Linch DC, Milligan DW, Winfield DA et al. G-CSF after peripheral blood stem cell transplantation in lymphoma patients significantly accelerated neutrophil recovery and shortened time in hospital: results of a randomized BNLI trial. *Br J Haematol* 1997; **99**: 933–8.

131. Nademanee A, Sniecinski I, Schmidt GM et al. High-dose therapy followed by autologous peripheral-blood stem-cell transplantation for patients with Hodgkin's disease and non-Hodgkin's lymphoma using unprimed and granulocyte colony-stimulating factor-mobilized peripheral-blood stem cells. *J Clin Oncol* 1994; **12**: 2176–86.

132. Tarella C, Castellino C, Locatelli F et al. G-CSF administration following peripheral blood progenitor cell (PBPC) autograft in lymphoid malignancies: evidence for clinical benefits and reduction of treatment costs. *Bone Marrow Transplant* 1998; **21**: 401–17.

133. Legros M, Fleury J, Bay JO et al. rhGM-CSF vs placebo following rhGM-CSF-mobilized PBPC transplantation: a phase III double-blind randomized trial. *Bone Marrow Transplant* 1997; **19**: 209–13.

134. Bence-Bruckler I, Bredeson C, Atkins H et al. A randomized trial of granulocyte colony-stimulating factor (Neupogen) starting day 1 vs day 7 post-autologous stem cell transplantation. *Bone Marrow Transplant* 1998; **22**: 965–9.

135. Bolwell BJ, Pohlman B, Andresen S et al. Delayed G-CSF after autologous progenitor cell transplantation: a prospective randomized trial. *Bone Marrow Transplant* 1998; **21**: 369–73.

136. Colby C, McAfee SL, Finkelstein DM, Spitzer TR. Early vs delayed administration of G-CSF following autologous peripheral blood stem cell transplantation. *Bone Marrow Transplant* 1998; **21**: 1005–10.

137. Schmitz N, Dreger P, Zander AR et al. Results of a randomized, controlled, multicentre study of recombinant human granulocyte colony-stimulating factor (filgrastim) in patients with Hodgkin's disease and non-Hodgkin's lymphoma undergoing autologous bone marrow transplantation. *Bone Marrow Transplant* 1995; **15**: 261–6.

138. Lee SJ, Weller E, Alyea EP et al. Efficacy and costs of granulocyte colony-stimulating factor in allogeneic T-cell depleted bone marrow transplantation. *Blood* 1998; **92**: 2725–9.

139. Bishop MR, Tarantolo SR, Geller RB et al. A randomized, double-blind trial of filgrastim (granulocyte colony-stimulating factor) versus placebo following allogeneic blood stem cell transplantation. *Blood* 2000; **96**: 80–5.

140. Molineux G, Kinstler O, Briddell B et al. A new form of filgrastim with sustained duration in vivo and enhanced

ability to mobilize PBPC in both mice and humans. *Exp Hematol* 1999; **27**: 1724–34.

141. Crawford J. Once-per-cycle pegfilgrastim (Neulasta) for the management of chemotherapy-induced neutropenia. *Semin Oncol* 2003; **30**(4 Suppl 13): 24–30.

142. Grigg A, Solal-Celigny P, Hoskin P et al. Open-label, randomized study of pegfilgrastim vs. daily filgrastim as an adjunct to chemotherapy in elderly patients with non-Hodgkin's lymphoma. *Leuk Lymphoma* 2003; **44**: 1503–8.

143. Green MD, Koelbl H, Baselga J et al. A randomized double-blind multicenter phase III study of fixed-dose single-administration pegfilgrastim versus daily filgrastim in patients receiving myelosuppressive chemotherapy. *Ann Oncol* 2003; **14**: 29–35.

144. Holmes FA, O'Shaughnessy JA, Vukelja S et al. Blinded, randomized, multicenter study to evaluate single administration pegfilgrastim once per cycle versus daily filgrastim as an adjunct to chemotherapy in patients with high-risk stage II or stage III/IV breast cancer. *J Clin Oncol* 2002; **20**: 727–31.

145. Holmes FA, Jones SE, O'Shaughnessy J et al. Comparable efficacy and safety profiles of once-per-cycle pegfilgrastim and daily injection filgrastim in chemotherapy-induced neutropenia: a multicenter dose-finding study in women with breast cancer. *Ann Oncol* 2002; **13**: 903–9.

146. Siena S, Piccart MJ, Holmes FA et al. A combined analysis of two pivotal randomized trials of a single dose of pegfilgrastim per chemotherapy cycle and daily filgrastim in patients with stage II–IV breast cancer. *Oncol Rep* 2003; **10**: 715–24.

147. Vose JM, Crump M, Lazarus H et al. Randomized, multicenter, open-label study of pegfilgrastim compared with daily filgrastim after chemotherapy for lymphoma. *J Clin Oncol* 2003; **21**: 514–19.

148. Bruno E, Briddell RA, Cooper RJ, Hoffman R. Effects of recombinant interleukin-11 on human megakaryocyte progenitor cells. *Exp Hematol* 1991; **19**: 378–81.

149. Musashi M, Yang YC, Paul SR et al. Direct and synergistic effects of interleukin-11 on murine hematopoiesis in culture. *Proc Nat Acad Sci USA* 1991; **88**: 765–9.

150. Hangoc G, Yin TG, Cooper S et al. In vivo effects of recombinant interleukin-11 on myelopoiesis in mice. *Blood* 1993; **81**: 965–972.

151. Du XX, Neben T, Goldman S, Williams DA. Effects of recombinant human interleukin-11 on hematopoietic reconstitution in transplant mice – acceleration of recovery of peripheral-blood neutrophils and platelets. *Blood* 1993; **81**: 27–34.

152. Du XX, Doerschuk CM, Orazi A, Williams DA. A bone-marrow stromal-derived growth factor, interleukin-11, stimulates recovery of small-intestinal mucosal cells after cytoablative therapy. *Blood* 1994; **83**: 33–7.

153. Nandurkar HH, Robb L, Tarlinton D et al. Adult mice with targeted mutation of the interleukin-11 receptor (IL11Ra) display normal hematopoiesis. *Blood* 1997; **90**: 2148–59.

154. Robb L, Li R, Hartley L et al. Infertility in female mice lacking the receptor for interleukin 11 is due to a defective uterine response to implantation. *Nat Med* 1998; **4**: 303–8.

155. Gordon MS, McCaskill Stevens WJ, Battiato LA et al. Phase-I trial of recombinant human interleukin-11 (Neumega rhIL-11 growth factor) in women with breast cancer receiving chemotherapy. *Blood* 1996; **87**: 3615–24.

156. Ault KA, Mitchell J, Knowles C et al. Recombinant human interleukin-11 (Neumega rhIL-11 growth factor) increases

157. Champlin RE, Mehra R, Kaye JA et al. Recombinant human interleukin-11 (rhIL-11) following autologous BMT for breast cancer. *Blood* 1994; **84**(10 S1): A395.

158. Cairo MS, Davenport V, Reaman G et al. Accelerated hematopoietic recovery with rhIL-11 following ifosfamide, carboplatin, and etoposide administration in children with solid tumor or lymphoma – preliminary results of a phase I/II trial. *Exp Hematol* 1996; **24**: 432–4.

159. Sands BE, Winston BD, Salzberg B et al. Randomized, controlled trial of recombinant human interleukin-11 in patients with active Crohn's disease. *Aliment Pharmacol Ther* 2002; **16**: 399–406.

160. Teshima T, Hill GR, Pan L et al. IL-11 separates graft-versus-leukemia effects from graft-versus-host disease after bone marrow transplantation. *J Clin Invest* 1999; **104**: 317–25.

161. Antin JH, Lee SJ, Neuberg D et al. A phase I/II double-blind, placebo-controlled study of recombinant human interleukin-11 for mucositis and acute GVHD prevention in allogeneic stem cell transplantation. *Bone Marrow Transplant* 2002; **29**: 373–7.

162. Cantor SB, Elting LS, Hudson DV Jr, Rubenstein EB. Pharmacoeconomic analysis of oprelvekin (recombinant human interleukin-11) for secondary prophylaxis of thrombocytopenia in solid tumor patients receiving chemotherapy. *Cancer* 2003; **97**: 3099–100.

163. Kaushansky K. Thrombopoietin – the primary regulator of platelet production. *Trends Endocrinol Metab* 1997; **8**: 45–50.

164. Wendling F, Maraskovsky E, Debili N et al. c-Mpl ligand is a humoral regulator of megakaryocytopoiesis. *Nature* 1994; **369**: 571–4.

165. Alexander WS, Roberts AW, Nicola NA et al. Deficiencies in progenitor cells of multiple hematopoietic lineages and defective megakaryocytopoiesis in mice lacking the thrombopoietic receptor c-Mpl. *Blood* 1996; **87**: 2162–70.

166. Carver-Moore K, Broxmeyer HE, Luoh SM et al. Low levels of erythroid and myeloid progenitors in thrombopoietin- and c-Mpl-deficient mice. *Blood* 1996; **88**: 803–8.

167. Gurney AL, Carvermoore K, Desauvage FJ, Moore MW. Thrombocytopenia in c-Mpl-deficient mice. *Science* 1994; **265**: 1445–7.

168. Qian S, Fu F, Li W et al. Primary role of the liver in thrombopoietin production shown by tissue-specific knockout. *Blood* 1998; **92**: 2189–91.

169. Peck-Radosavljevic M, Zacherl J, Meng YG et al. Is inadequate thrombopoietin production a major cause of thrombocytopenia in cirrhosis of the liver? *J Hepatol* 1997; **27**: 127–31.

170. Oda A, Miyakawa Y, Druker BJ et al. Thrombopoietin primes human platelet aggregation induced by shear stress and by multiple agonists. *Blood* 1996; **87**: 4664–70.

171. Kuter DJ, Begley CG. Recombinant human thrombopoietin: basic biology and evaluation of clinical studies. *Blood* 2002; **100**: 3457–69.

172. Harker LA, Marzec UM, Hunt P et al. Dose–response effects of pegylated human megakaryocyte growth and development factor on platelet production and function in nonhuman primates. *Blood* 1996; **88**: 511–21.

173. Hokom MM, Lacey D, Kinstler OB et al. Pegylated megakaryocyte growth and development factor abrogates

plasma volume and decreases urine sodium excretion in normal human subjects. *Blood* 1994; **84**(10 S1): A276.

the lethal thrombocytopenia associated with carboplatin and irradiation in mice. *Blood* 1995; **86**: 4486–92.

174. Harker LA, Marzec UM, Kelly AB et al. Prevention of thrombocytopenia and neutropenia in a nonhuman primate model of marrow suppressive chemotherapy by combining pegylated recombinant human megakaryocyte growth and development factor and recombinant human granulocyte colony-stimulating factor. *Blood* 1997; **89**: 155–65.

175. Ulich TR, del Castillo J, Yin S et al. Megakaryocyte growth and development factor ameliorates carboplatin-induced thrombocytopenia in mice. *Blood* 1995; **86**: 971–6.

176. Neelis KJ, Hartong SC, Egeland T et al. The efficacy of single-dose administration of thrombopoietin with coadministration of either granulocyte/macrophage or granulocyte colony-stimulating factor in myelosuppressed rhesus monkeys. *Blood* 1997; **90**: 2565–73.

177. Basser RL, Rasko JEJ, Clarke K et al. Thrombopoietic effects of pegylated recombinant human megakaryocyte growth and development factor (PEG-rHuMGDF) in patients with advanced cancer. *Lancet* 1996; **348**: 1279–81.

178. Kuter DJ, Goodnough LT, Romo J et al. Thrombopoietin therapy increases platelet yields in healthy platelet donors. *Blood* 2001; **98**: 1339–45.

179. Fanucchi M, Glaspy J, Crawford J et al. Effects of polyethylene glycol-conjugated recombinant human megakaryocyte growth and development factor on platelet counts after chemotherapy for lung cancer. *N Engl J Med* 1997; **336**: 404–9.

180. Basser RL, Rasko JEJ, Clarke K et al. Randomized, blinded, placebo-controlled phase I trial of pegylated recombinant human megakaryocyte growth and development factor with filgrastim after dose-intensive chemotherapy in patients with advanced cancer. *Blood* 1997; **89**: 3118–28.

181. Basser RL, Underhill C, Davis I et al. Enhancement of platelet recovery after myelosuppressive chemotherapy by recombinant human megakaryocyte growth and development factor in patients with advanced cancer. *J Clin Oncol* 2000; **18**: 2852–61.

182. Archimbaud E, Ottmann OG, Yin JA et al. A randomized, double-blind, placebo-controlled study with pegylated recombinant human megakaryocyte growth and development factor (PEG-rHuMGDF) as an adjunct to chemotherapy for adults with de novo acute myeloid leukemia. *Blood* 1999; **94**: 3694–701.

183. Schiffer CA, Miller K, Larson RA et al. A double-blind, placebo-controlled trial of pegylated recombinant human megakaryocyte growth and development factor as an adjunct to induction and consolidation therapy for patients with acute myeloid leukemia. *Blood* 2000; **95**: 2530–5.

184. Nash RA, Kurzrock R, DiPersio J et al. A phase I trial of recombinant human thrombopoietin in patients with delayed platelet recovery after hematopoietic stem cell transplantation. *Biol Blood Marrow Transplant* 2000; **6**: 25–34.

185. Somlo G, Sniecinski I, ter Veer A et al. Recombinant human thrombopoietin in combination with granulocyte colony-stimulating factor enhances mobilization of peripheral blood progenitor cells, increases peripheral blood platelet concentration, and accelerates hematopoietic recovery following high-dose chemotherapy. *Blood* 1999; **93**: 2798–806.

186. Goodnough LT, Kuter DJ, McCullough J et al. Prophylactic platelet transfusions from healthy apheresis platelet donors undergoing treatment with thrombopoietin. *Blood* 2001; **98**: 1346–51.

187. Basser RL, O'Flaherty E, Green M et al. Development of pancytopenia with neutralizing antibodies to thrombopoietin after multicycle chemotherapy supported by megakaryocyte growth and development factor. *Blood* 2002; **99**: 2599–602.

188. Cwirla SE, Balasubramanian P, Duffin DJ et al. Peptide agonist of the thrombopoietin receptor as potent as the natural cytokine. *Science* 1997; **276**: 1696–9.

189. Duffy KJ, Darcy MG, Delorme E et al. Hydrazinonaphthalene and azonaphthalene thrombopoietin mimics are nonpeptidyl promoters of megakaryocytopoiesis. *J Med Chem* 2001; **44**: 3730–45.

190. Dombret H, Chastang C, Fenaux P et al. A controlled study of recombinant human granulocyte colony-stimulating factor in elderly patients after treatment for acute myelogenous leukemia. AML Cooperative Study Group. *N Engl J Med* 1995; **332**: 1678–83.

191. Rowe JM, Andersen JW, Mazza JJ et al. A randomized placebo-controlled phase III study of granulocyte–macrophage colony-stimulating factor in adult patients (>55 to 70 years of age) with acute myelogenous leukemia: a study of the Eastern Cooperative Oncology Group (E1490). *Blood* 1995; **86**: 457–62.

192. Stone RM, Berg DT, George SL et al. Granulocyte-macrophage colony-stimulating factor after initial chemotherapy for elderly patients with primary acute myelogenous leukemia. Cancer and Leukemia Group B. *N Engl J Med* 1995; **332**: 1671–7.

193. Heil G, Hoelzer D, Sanz MA et al. A randomized, double-blind, placebo-controlled, phase III study of filgrastim in remission induction and consolidation therapy for adults with de novo acute myeloid leukemia. The International Acute Myeloid Leukemia Study Group. *Blood* 1997; **90**: 4710–18.

194. Usuki K, Urabe A, Masaoka T et al. Efficacy of granulocyte colony-stimulating factor in the treatment of acute myelogenous leukaemia: a multicentre randomized study. *Br J Haematol* 2002; **116**: 103–12.

195. Godwin JE, Kopecky KJ, Head DR et al. A double-blind placebo-controlled trial of granulocyte colony-stimulating factor in elderly patients with previously untreated acute myeloid leukemia: a Southwest Oncology Group study (9031). *Blood* 1998; **91**: 3607–15.

196. Lowenberg B, Boogaerts MA, Daenen SM et al. Value of different modalities of granulocyte–macrophage colony-stimulating factor applied during or after induction therapy of acute myeloid leukemia. *J Clin Oncol* 1997; **15**: 3496–506.

197. Lowenberg B, Suciu S, Archimbaud E et al. Use of recombinant GM-CSF during and after remission induction chemotherapy in patients aged 61 years and older with acute myeloid leukemia: final report of AML-11, a phase III randomized study of the Leukemia Cooperative Group of European Organisation for the Research and Treatment of Cancer and the Dutch Belgian Hemato-Oncology Cooperative Group. *Blood* 1997; **90**: 2952–61.

198. Zittoun R, Suciu S, Mandelli F et al. Granulocyte–macrophage colony-stimulating factor associated with induction treatment of acute myelogenous leukemia: a randomized trial by the European

Organization for Research and Treatment of Cancer Leukemia Cooperative Group. *J Clin Oncol* 1996; **14**: 2150–9.

199. Witz F, Sadoun A, Perrin MC et al. A placebo-controlled study of recombinant human granulocyte–macrophage colony-stimulating factor administered during and after induction treatment for de novo acute myelogenous leukemia in elderly patients. Groupe Ouest Est Leucemies Aigues Myeloblastiques (GOELAM). *Blood* 1998; **91**: 2722–30.

200. Takeshita A, Ohno R, Hirashima K et al. A randomized double-blind controlled study of recombinant human granulocyte colony-stimulating factor in patients with neutropenia induced by consolidation chemotherapy for acute myeloid leukemia. (rG.CSF clinical study group). *Rinsho Ketsueki* 1995; **36**: 606–14.

201. Harousseau JL, Witz B, Lioure B et al. Granulocyte colony-stimulating factor after intensive consolidation chemotherapy in acute myeloid leukemia: results of a randomized trial of the Groupe Ouest–Est Leucemies Aigues Myeloblastiques. *J Clin Oncol* 2000; **18**: 780–7.

202. Thomas X, Fenaux P, Dombret H et al. Granulocyte–macrophage colony-stimulating factor (GM-CSF) to increase efficacy of intensive sequential chemotherapy with etoposide, mitoxantrone and cytarabine (EMA) in previously treated acute myeloid leukemia: a multicenter randomized placebo-controlled trial (EMA91 trial). *Leukemia* 1999; **13**: 1214–20.

203. Ohno R, Naoe T, Kanamaru A et al. A double-blind controlled study of granulocyte colony-stimulating factor started two days before induction chemotherapy in refractory acute myeloid leukemia. Kohseisho Leukemia Study Group. *Blood* 1994; **83**: 2086–92.

204. Hansen PB, Johnsen HE, Jensen L et al. Priming and treatment with molgramostim (rhGM-CSF) in adult high-risk acute myeloid leukemia during induction chemotherapy: a prospective, randomized pilot study. *Eur J Haematol* 1995; **54**: 296–303.

205. Uyl-de Groot CA, Löwenberg B, Vellenga E et al. Cost-effectiveness and quality-of-life assessment of GM-CSF as an adjunct to intensive remission induction chemotherapy in elderly patients with acute myeloid leukemia. *Br J Haematol* 1998; **100**: 629–36.

206. Löwenberg B, van Putten W, Theobald M et al. Effect of priming with granulocyte colony-stimulating factor on the outcome of chemotherapy for acute myeloid leukemia. *N Engl J Med* 2003; **349**: 743–52.

207. Estey EH, Thall PF, Pierce S et al. Randomized phase II study of fludarabine + cytosine arabinoside + idarubicin ± all-*trans* retinoic acid ± granulocyte colony-stimulating factor in poor prognosis newly diagnosed acute myeloid leukemia and myelodysplastic syndrome. *Blood* 1999; **93**: 2478–84.

208. Larson RA, Dodge RK, Linker CA et al. A randomized controlled trial of filgrastim during remission induction and consolidation chemotherapy for adults with acute lymphoblastic leukemia: CALGB study 9111. *Blood* 1998; **92**: 1556–64.

209. Ottmann OG, Hoelzer D, Gracien E et al. Concomitant granulocyte colony-stimulating factor and induction chemoradiotherapy in adult acute lymphoblastic leukemia: a randomized phase III trial. *Blood* 1995; **86**: 444–50.

210. Geissler K, Koller E, Hubmann E et al. Granulocyte colony-stimulating factor as an adjunct to induction chemotherapy for adult acute lymphoblastic leukemia – a randomized phase-III study. *Blood* 1997; **90**: 590–6.

211. Pui CH, Boyett JM, Hughes WT et al. Human granulocyte colony-stimulating factor after induction chemotherapy in children with acute lymphoblastic leukemia. *N Engl J Med* 1997; **336**: 1781–7.

212. Welte K, Reiter A, Mempel K et al. A randomized phase-III study of the efficacy of granulocyte colony-stimulating factor in children with high-risk acute lymphoblastic leukemia. Berlin–Frankfurt–Münster Study Group. *Blood* 1996; **87**: 3143–50.

213. Clarke V, Dunstan FD, Webb DK. Granulocyte colony-stimulating factor ameliorates toxicity of intensification chemotherapy for acute lymphoblastic leukemia. *Med Pediatr Oncol* 1999; **32**: 331–5.

214. Yoshida Y, Nakahata T, Shibata A et al. Effects of long-term treatment with recombinant human granulocyte–macrophage colony-stimulating factor in patients with myelodysplastic syndrome. *Leuk Lymphoma* 1995; **18**: 457–63.

215. Willemze R, van der Lely N, Zwierzina H et al. A randomized phase-I/II multicenter study of recombinant human granulocyte–macrophage colony-stimulating factor (GM-CSF) therapy for patients with myelodysplastic syndromes and a relatively low risk of acute leukemia. EORTC Leukemia Cooperative Group. *Ann Hematol* 1992; **64**: 173–80.

216. Ossenkoppele GJ, van der Holt B, Verhoef GE et al. A randomized study of granulocyte colony-stimulating factor applied during and after chemotherapy in patients with poor risk myelodysplastic syndromes: a report from the HOVON Cooperative Group. Dutch–Belgian Hemato-Oncology Cooperative Group. *Leukemia* 1999; **13**: 1207–13.

217. Bernasconi C, Alessandrino EP, Bernasconi P et al. Randomized clinical study comparing aggressive chemotherapy with or without G-CSF support for high-risk myelodysplastic syndromes or secondary acute myeloid leukaemia evolving from MDS. *Br J Haematol* 1998; **102**: 678–83.

218. Thompson JA, Gilliland DG, Prchal JT et al. Effect of recombinant human erythropoietin combined with granulocyte/macrophage colony-stimulating factor in the treatment of patients with myelodysplastic syndrome. GM/EPO MDS Study Group. *Blood* 2000; **95**: 1175–9.

219. Kumar M, Alter BP. Hematopoietic growth factors for the treatment of aplastic anemia. *Curr Opin Hematol* 1998; **5**: 226–34.

220. Dale DC. Hematopoietic growth factors for the treatment of severe chronic neutropenia. *Stem Cells* 1995; **13**: 94–100.

221. Ancliff PJ, Gale RE, Liesner R et al. Long-term follow-up of granulocyte colony-stimulating factor receptor mutations in patients with severe congenital neutropenia: implications for leukaemogenesis and therapy. *Br J Haematol* 2003; **120**(4): 685–90.

222. Kojima S. Use of granulocyte colony-stimulating factor for treatment of aplastic anemia. *Nagoya J Med Sci* 1999; **62**: 77–82.

223. Kojima S, Hibi S, Kosaka Y et al. Immunosuppressive therapy using antithymocyte globulin, cyclosporine, and danazol with or without human granulocyte colony-

stimulating factor in children with acquired aplastic anemia. *Blood* 2000; **96**: 2049–54.

224. Marsh JC. Hematopoietic growth factors in the pathogenesis and for the treatment of aplastic anemia. *Semin Hematol* 2000; **37**: 81–90.

225. Gisselbrecht C, Haioun C, Lepage E et al. Placebo-controlled phase III study of lenograstim (glycosylated recombinant human granulocyte colony-stimulating factor) in aggressive non-Hodgkin's lymphoma: factors influencing chemotherapy administration. Groupe d'Etude des Lymphomes de l'Adulte. *Leuk Lymphoma* 1997; **25**: 289–300.

226. Fridrik MA, Greil R, Hausmaninger H et al. Randomized open label phase III trial of CEOP/IMVP-Dexa alternating chemotherapy and filgrastim versus CEOP/IMVP-Dexa alternating chemotherapy for aggressive non-Hodgkin's lymphoma (NHL). A multicenter trial by the Austrian Working Group for Medical Tumor Therapy. *Ann Hematol* 1997; **75**: 135–40.

227. Zinzani PL, Pavone E, Storti S et al. Randomized trial with or without granulocyte colony-stimulating factor as adjunct to induction VNCOP-B treatment of elderly high-grade non-Hodgkin's lymphoma. *Blood* 1997; **89**: 3974–9.

228. Aviles A, Diaz-Maqueo JC, Talavera A et al. Effect of granulocyte colony-stimulating factor in patients with diffuse large cell lymphoma treated with intensive chemotherapy. *Leuk Lymphoma* 1994; **15**: 153–7.

229. Gerhartz HH, Engelhard M, Meusers P et al. Randomized, double-blind, placebo-controlled, phase III study of recombinant human granulocyte-macrophage colony-stimulating factor as adjunct to induction treatment of high-grade malignant non-Hodgkin's lymphomas. *Blood* 1993; **82**: 2329–39.

230. Pettengell R, Gurney H, Radford JA et al. Granulocyte colony-stimulating factor to prevent dose-limiting neutropenia in non-Hodgkin's lymphoma: a randomized controlled trial. *Blood* 1992; **80**: 1430–6.

231. Osby E, Hagberg H, Kvaloy S et al. CHOP is superior to CNOP in elderly patients with aggressive lymphoma while outcome is unaffected by filgrastim treatment: results of a Nordic Lymphoma Group randomized trial. *Blood* 2003; **101**: 3840–8.

232. Dunlop DJ, Eatock MM, Paul J et al. Randomized multicentre trial of filgrastim as an adjunct to combination chemotherapy for Hodgkin's disease. West of Scotland Lymphoma Group. *Clin Oncol (R Coll Radiol)* 1998; **10**: 107–14.

233. Gustavsson A. G-CSF (filgrastim) as an adjunct to MOPP/ABVD therapy in Hodgkin's disease. *Acta Oncol* 1997; **36**: 483–8.

# 47 Management of infectious complications in hematological patients

**Catherine Cordonnier**

## Introduction

Hematological malignancy is a field where significant progress has been made in therapeutic possibilities and prognosis. Some patients who would previously have succumbed can now aspire to a cure and a return to a normal, or almost normal, quality of life. However, these results are obtained with treatments that have side-effects and that increase the risk of opportunistic infections. This means that infections, which are already an inherent risk in some hematological diseases, are even more frequent when treatments increase immune deficiency.

A physician who individually decides a treatment for a patient must be aware of the infectious complications that may threaten that patient, and must know if special prophylactic measures are needed, and how to manage the patient if a complication occurs. On another level of decision, therapeutic groups who design a new protocol for a malignancy should always have data on the infectious complications, such as morbidity or mortality factors. Chemotherapy A may give similar results to chemotherapy B in disease-free survival. However, if patients die mainly from relapse in arm A and mainly from infection in arm B, an approach to prevention of the infections could improve the results for arm B. Therapy can also change the predisposition of a hematological disease for a particular infection. A good example is the association of hairy cell leukemia and legionellosis, which although common some 15 years ago, has almost disappeared since interferon-α has greatly improved the prognosis of the disease.

Finally, understanding the mechanisms predisposing to each kind of infection in each setting is the best way to propose a prophylactic policy. In that way, experimental models and in vitro data are valuable. However, many patients have multiple risk factors for infections (e.g. neutropenia and steroids), and this may make individual analysis difficult. Analysis of each case, taking simple parameters into account, should help in deciding a suitable diagnostic and therapeutic approach.

## The different factors that predispose to infections

### Host factors related to disease or treatment

The factors that predispose the 'compromised' host to infection are not completely understood. However, lessons drawn from clinical observations and from in vitro data and experimental models allow the proposition of reasonable hypotheses on the association of some infections and risk factors, and also on the specific mechanisms of predisposition. It is usual to consider three categories of compromising factors: neutropenia, cellular immune dysfunction, and humoral immune dysfunction.

### Neutropenia

Over 30 years ago, Bodey et al[1] showed that infection is related to the absolute level of circulating neutrophils (PMN), especially when granulocytes fall below $0.5 \times 10^9$/l. However, today, 'high-risk' neutropenia refers to patients with PMN$<0.1 \times 10^9$/l.

Neutropenia may be due to the primary disease (e.g. in acute leukemia) or to treatment. Most neutropenias are due to chemotherapy and are dose-related. More rarely, functional deficiencies of granulocytic functions, such as chemotaxis, phagocytosis, or microbial killing, may predispose to the same kind of complications. These functional deficiencies may be associated with quantitative deficiencies, as in some myelodysplastic syndromes (MDS).

Neutropenia predisposes to the occurrence of bacterial infection, and to the severity of infection if untreated. The first source of infection during neutropenia is the gut. Bacterial translocation through the gut barrier in the setting of neutropenia explains most bacteremias of gut origin.[2] This is the rationale for gut decontamination in severe and prolonged neutropenia. The strains that are most often found in this setting are enterobacteria, and more rarely *Pseudomonas* spp.; however, any strain colonizing the gut may be a source. Systemic bacterial infections may also come from any infected site. Any latent focus may, in the case of neutropenia, become symptomatic and life-threatening.

Neutropenia is also the main predisposing factor, with steroid administration, for fungal infections. Although reported, the occurrence of fungal infection during short-term neutropenia is extremely rare, and this is the basis for reserving antifungal prophylactic measures to, and developing pre-emptive antifungal strategies for, patients who are expected to have at least 10 days of neutropenia. Additionally, prolonged neutropenia consecutive to chemotherapy in hematological diseases is often associated with functional and quantitative deficiencies of the alveolar macrophage populations, which may be an additional factor in pulmonary fungal infections, mainly due to *Aspergillus*.

### Humoral immune deficiency

Because of the role of antibodies in opsonization, global hypogammaglobulinemia or specific deficiencies in classes or subclasses predispose to bacterial infections, and especially to infections with encapsulated bacteria, such as *Streptococcus pneumoniae* or *Haemophilus influenzae*. This may be encountered in particular in myeloma, other dysglobulinemias, chronic lymphocytic leukemia (CLL), and bone marrow transplantation (BMT).

### Cellular immune deficiency

This category involves the most complicated features of immune deficiencies. These deficiencies are more specific in certain diseases such as lymphomas, but are mostly induced by treatment, such as steroids, fludarabine or BMT/peripheral blood stem cell transplant (PBSCT) conditioning. The complexity of cellular immune function, the number of cells involved, the interactions between them, and the role of cytokines engaged in the infectious process probably explain the long list of potential pathogens in patients with cellular deficiencies. Most of these pathogens are infective through reactivation (i.e. *Toxoplasma gondii* or cytomegalovirus (CMV)), although others are newly acquired and responsible for primary infections. Most of them have an intracellular development, and include *Salmonella*, *Listeria*, mycobacteria, and *Legionella* for the bacteria, mainly *Pneumocystis carinii*, *Cryptococcus neoformans*, and coccid-

ioidomycosis for fungi, and *T. gondii*, *Strongyloides stercoralis*, and *Cryptosporidium* for protozoa.

### Other host factors

Any obstruction of natural orifices may lead to or favor infection. This may be the cause in lymphomas when mediastinal nodes are responsible for tracheobronchial obstruction. Moreover, any procedure leading to cutaneous or mucosal barrier disruption offers an opportunity for bacteria and fungi to colonize and then to infect the host. Long-term venous catheters have become routine practice, and are major sources for staphylococcal bacteremia and fungemia.[3–5] Also, certain treatments require bladder catheterization.

### Environmental factors

The natural or iatrogenic predisposition of hematological patients to infectious pathogens may favor the acquisition both of nosocomial and of community infections. However, because the periods of highest risk usually follow therapies given during hospitalization, most infections occur in the hospital and should be considered nosocomial. Some pathogens, such as *Aspergillus*, may, however, be acquired outside or inside the hospital. After allogeneic stem cell transplantation, it has been shown that there are two waves of onset of *Aspergillus* infection in this population, one during the neutropenic phase and acquired in the hospital, and a second one later, during the second or third month post transplant, this one being acquired either in or outside the hospital.[6, 7]

### Nosocomial infections

Hematological patients are subjected to multiple sources of pathogens through food, beverages, air, invasive procedures, and contact with staff. The potential role of food and beverages in the acquisition of enterobacteria, *Salmonella*, and *Pseudomonas* spp. has been documented.[8] This justifies regular quality-control procedures and makes it logical to use cooked food for high-risk patients, especially those with prolonged neutropenia and those receiving gut decontamination.

Although the environment is a reservoir for microorganisms, most nosocomial infections require a human vector.[9] Because of multiple patient contacts, hospital care workers are the second potential source of pathogens and the obligatory intermediary between patients, especially for methicillin-resistant staphylococci and for gram-negative nosocomial strains. Handwashing and simple measures of hygiene remain the most logical and economical procedures to avoid the transmission of most nosocomial bacterial and candidial infections.

In any hospitalized high-risk patient, colonization with bacterial and fungal pathogens usually precedes infection. Multiple routine microbiological samples (nose, ears, gingivae, axillae, etc.) are not generally helpful in predicting infection. Stool and, to a lesser degree, urine cultures are more useful in routine practice in neutropenic patients to isolate *Pseudomonas* spp., *Klebsiella,* or *Staphylococcus aureus.*[2] Colonization by bacteria, especially when resistant, should be taken into account in choosing empiric antibiotic therapy in cases of subsequent infections, and can lead to prophylactic measures of isolation to avoid dissemination to other patients. Colonization by *Candida* does not have the same predictive value, depending on the *Candida* sp.: this predictive value is usually poor for *C. albicans* and high for other species, such as *C. tropicalis* or *glabrata.*[10,11]

Other infections are airborne. The most important in hematological patients is aspergillosis, which can occur at any time and in any hospital. There are climatic and geographical variations in its incidence, and epidemics may be triggered by construction work, which increases the number of spores in suspension in the air.[12] This is also probably the mechanism of acquisition for more unusual filamentous airborne infections such as mucormycosis. Most cases occur after airway colonization or sinusitis. Although specific risk factors, such as neutropenia of long duration and steroid therapy, have been well established, hematologists should always maintain a high level of suspicion regarding this possibility and be aware that aspergillosis is difficult to diagnose and difficult to treat.

### Community-acquired infections

The distinction between nosocomial and community infections is to some extent artificial, since some pathogens may be acquired in both ways. This is the case for *Aspergillus*, especially in case of chronic graft-versus-host disease (GVHD).[7] *Legionella* spp. may be acquired through contaminated water and so may be also of concern to both in- and outpatients. In the same way, a patient susceptible to the acquisition of varicella zoster virus (VZV) may be in contact with infected persons both in and out of hospital. However, some pathogens are predominantly associated with community infections. This is the case for hypogammaglobulinemic patients, who are predisposed to *S. pneumoniae* and *H. influenzae* infections, but this risk will remain while the patient is hospitalized.

# Febrile neutropenia

Since the demonstration of the relationship between neutropenia and infection,[1] and the initial study showing that febrile neutropenia must be urgently and empirically treated with broad-spectrum antibiotics,[13,14] numerous epidemiological and therapeutic studies have been published. However, despite progressive modifications in the epidemiology of bacterial strains responsible for febrile neutropenia, little has changed in the general principles of first-intention therapy in this setting, except for a better recognition of low-risk patients, which allows a reduction in the antibiotic regimens of these patients whenever possible.

### Epidemiology of infections during neutropenia

As a result of multiple factors, including the increasing use of indwelling catheters and prophylactic measures that modify the incidence of some infections, the epidemiology of bacterial pathogens in neutropenic patients has changed. While 25 years ago, gram-negative bacteria were predominant, gram-positive bacteria now represent the most frequently isolated pathogens.[15,16] It is known that only 30–40% of febrile neutropenic patients have a microbiologically documented infection (MDI). This documentation comes in 85–90% of the cases from positive blood cultures. The documentation from other sites is rarer.

Among these 30–40% of patients with MDI, two-thirds will be gram-positive and one-third gram-negative. Coagulase-negative staphylococci are the most frequent pathogens isolated and, despite the lack of strong data supporting the rule, it is routine, at least in therapeutic trials, to consider that two positive blood cultures are necessary to consider these staphylococci responsible for the infection. Streptococci, especially oral strains, have become more frequent over the last 15 years. The main risk factors for oral streptococcal bacteremia in the setting of neutropenia have been studied in retrospective[17,18] and prospective studies,[19] and have been found to be profound neutropenia ($<0.1\times10^9$/l), presence of mucositis, prophylaxis with quinolone or cotrimoxazole or gut decontamination, anti-$H_2$ drugs, and high-dose cytarabine. Previous administration of antibiotics decreases the risk. The mortality rate from gram-negative bacteremia was reported to be similar to that from gram-positive bacteremia,[20] while that from streptococcal bacteremia appears to be slightly higher.[18] Strict anaerobes are very rare in neutropenic patients, and their occurrence is usually associated with severe buccopharyngeal mucositis or perineal cellulitis. Although *Pseudomonas* infections are found in less than 5% of patients during their first febrile neutropenic episode, their incidence increases with the duration of aplasia.

Although not restricted to the setting of neutropenia, candidiasis and aspergillosis are usual complications arising in bone marrow-suppressed patients, and have to be listed in the diagnostic possibilities complicating neutropenia, especially if it is of long duration. The incidence of candidemia depends on multiple factors, including underlying disease, therapy, degree of colonization, and antifungal prophylaxis.[11,20] What is clear, however, is that the *Candida* spp. isolated nowadays in hematological patients are not the same as 15 years ago. *C. albicans* has become less frequent, while an increasing number of cases due to non-*albicans* species, such as *C. tropicalis*, *C. glabrata*, *C. krusei* and *C. lusitaniae,* have been reported.[22,23]

## Management of febrile patients during aplasia

Febrile neutropenic patients must be treated emergently and empirically. One should not wait for results of cultures or procedures that may never reveal the likely source. This dogma is the cornerstone of management, and is based on the following points:

1.  Bacterial infections in neutropenic patients may kill the patient rapidly if antibiotics are not started very quickly after the occurrence of fever. This strategy, combined with the use of more and more potent antibiotics, has been mainly responsible for the dramatic decline in mortality rates during aplasia, especially from gram-negative bacteremia.
2.  The antibiotic regimen must offer an optimal coverage of the more frequently isolated strains, and also of the most dangerous. For this reason, it is strongly recommended in high-risk patients to give a synergistic combination of broad-spectrum antibiotics active against the more frequent enterobacteria (*Escherichia coli, Klebsiella pneumoniae,* and *Serratia*) and *Pseudomonas aeruginosa.* Some aspects of this approach can now be questioned, since the antibiotics and the epidemiology are different from 20 years ago, but the general principles of this rationale have to be kept in mind.
3.  Foci in neutropenic patients are less obvious than in any other septic condition, probably because the inflammatory process is minimal in neutropenia.[24] The absence of a visible focus does not mean that the patient is not infected, and should not delay or change the initiation of antibiotics. On the other hand, it has been shown that some foci, such as pneumonia, cellulitis, or intraabdominal infections, have a major impact on the prognosis of a bacteremic episode occurring during neutropenia, especially in terms of survival to aplasia.[25]

### Initial clinical evaluation

Each febrile neutropenic patient must be carefully evaluated by a very complete clinical examination before starting antibiotics:

*   because the severity of the septic process may require additional measures (e.g. haemodynamic monitoring or oxygen);
*   because the presence of certain clinical foci associated with particular pathogens may be important for the therapeutic choice of first intention;
*   because the decision to change the antibiotic treatment during aplasia will be based on the evolution of the initial manifestations of infection during treatment.

The multinational Association for Supportive Care in Cancer (MASCC) has proposed a scoring system in order to identify high-risk febrile neutropenic patients[26] (Table 47.1). More than 1000 patients were prospectively studied at presentation of febrile neutropenia to predict low-risk of fever resolution without serious medical complication development. Almost two-thirds of these patients were hematology patients. A score of 21 or higher identifies low-risk patients with a positive predictive value of 91%, a specificity of 68%, and a sensitivity of 71% (Table 47.1).

The findings of the clinical examination should be precisely recorded and the patient reevaluated at least daily.

### Minimal microbiological examinations

Neutropenic patients (PMN$<0.5\times10^9$/l), or patients who are expected to be at that count in the next 48 hours because of recent chemotherapy, should have at least two blood cultures from two different sites and a microbiological sample from any clinical focus, if easily accessible, as soon as they become febrile, so that the antibiotics may be started as soon as possible in the next few hours following the onset of fever.[14]

---

**Table 47.1 Scoring system proposed by the Multinational Association for Supportive Care in Cancer (MASCC) to identify low-risk febrile neutropenic cancer patients[26]**

| Characteristic | Weight |
| --- | --- |
| Burden of illness: no or mild symptoms[a] | 5 |
| No hypotension | 5 |
| No chronic obstructive pulmonary disease | 4 |
| Solid tumor or no previous fungal infection | 4 |
| No dehydration | 3 |
| Burden of illness: moderate symptoms[a] | 3 |
| Outpatient status | 3 |
| Age <60 years | 2 |

The maximal theoretical score is 26. A risk-index score of 21 or more identifies low-risk patients with a predictive value of 91%, a specificity of 68%, and a sensitivity of 71%.

[a] Points attributed to the variable 'burdens of illness' are not cumulative.

Hypothermia and hypotension represent an even more unfavorable situation, since these patients often evolve rapidly to septic shock and have to be treated without waiting.

### Empiric therapy for first intention

The first-intention empiric therapy has to consider at least

- the general rule of broad-spectrum antibiotic treatment, including the possibility of synergistic effects between two drugs in the more at-risk patients;
- the risk status of the patient;
- the most common strains isolated in the particular setting;
- the epidemiology of the ward in the case of nosocomial infection;
- the presence of special foci that may add other microbiological possibilities to the list of pathogens usually found;
- the risk of adverse effects from the drug(s).

Ideally, the choice should also preserve the epidemiology of the ward by avoiding the empiric use of antibiotics able to induce a significant risk of multidrug resistance and superinfections.

A broad-spectrum antibiotic treatment is an antibiotic or a combination of antibiotics that are active against the most frequently isolated gram-negative and gram-positive strains. Beta-lactams are actually the sole class of antibiotics satisfying all the criteria cited above.[14] Most of them, except aztreonam, are active against both gram-positive and gram-negative strains. However, because of differences in activity and, to a lesser degree, in safety, all are not equal, and the choice should be determined both on their respective biological activities and on the results of clinical trials.

Moreover, it is usual to consider at least two groups of patients – mainly according to the duration and depth of neutropenia, but also other risk factors as those identified in the MASCC score[26] (Table 47.1). The first group (standard-risk or low-risk patients: PMN$<0.5\times10^9$/l for less than 5 days) are usually those who received sequential chemotherapy, often as outpatients, such as low- or intermediate-grade lymphoma patients. This population is very similar to solid tumor patients. They often have community infection, so that the fear of a multiresistant pathogen is low, since they did not receive previous systemic prophylaxis before or were not colonized with hospital strains.

The second group includes usually those already hospitalized when fever occurs, such as acute leukemia patients in the induction or consolidation phases of treatment, or stem cell transplant patients. They have neutropenia that lasts for more than 10 days, and frequently reach a nadir PMN$<0.1\times10^9$/l. In Europe, these patients often receive prophylactic gut decontamination, including at least colimycin and an aminoglycoside. Because of special risk factors and therapeutic approaches, the epidemiology of these patients is often different from that of the first group: they have more streptococci, more coagulase-negative staphylococci, and sometimes more multiresistant gram-negative hospital strains than the first group.

For the low-risk group, two options are recommended:[14] either the oral administration of ciprofloxacin plus amoxicillin–clavulanic acid, or the intravenous administration of a beta-lactam. Monotherapy with an intravenous beta-lactam is the standard in hematology patients, because the benefit from the addition of an aminoglycoside in this population is not clearly supported by clinical trials. Although intravenous antibiotic therapy was until recently the standard, two large randomized trials have shown that in a low-risk inpatient population with short-term neutropenia and no initial morbidity or complication, the oral association of amoxicillin/ clavunamic acid and ciprofloxacin has the same efficacy as an intravenous cephalosporin.[27,28] It should be emphasized that the term 'low-risk patients' should not let one forget that these patients may die from an uncontrolled infectious process, especially when the hematological disease is not controlled – even if they are treated without delay. They require very careful management in the first hours and days of treatment. It is likely that in the future such patients will be managed as outpatients, as has been done in clinical trials for patients with solid tumors.[14,29]

For the other groups (standard or high-risk patients), and for reasons of toxicity and cost, efforts are also being made to restrict the use of combinations, and if possible to replace them with monotherapy. It is clear, however, that the choice of monotherapy should restrict the choice of the drug to very potent ones, active on *Pseudomonas* spp. and on most multiresistant gram-negative bacteria. Three options are possible:[14]

1. In the absence of first-line glycopeptide indication, either monotherapy with, for example, ceftazidime,[15] cefepime,[30] imipenem, or the newer meropenem, which was found to be as effective as the ceftazidime–amikacin combination in high-risk patients.[20] Piperacillin–tazobactam is another alternative, which was shown to be more active than ceftazidime plus amikacin in a large trial.[16]

2. A combination of a beta-lactam and an aminoglycoside. It is true that there are now antibiotics that, even without the addition of an aminoglycoside, have bactericidal activities comparable to or better than those obtained 10–15 years ago only with combinations. Therefore, the combination

beta-lactam–aminoglycoside is becoming more and more restricted to high-risk patients, such as where there is suspicion of *Pseudomonas* sp. infections, or to clinically documented infections with severe foci. Those teams who add to the beta-lactam an aminoglycoside usually stop it at 48 hours if blood cultures are negative or if a pathogen is isolated that is resistant to aminoglycosides. It is clear, however, that patients with enterobacterial or *Pseudomonas* bacteremia benefit from the administration of a long course (7 days) of aminoglycoside, both in terms of efficacy and of superinfections.[31]

3.  When there is suspicion of gram-positive infections, such as patients colonized with penicillin- or cephalosporin-resistant pneumococci or methicillin-resistant *S. aureus* (MRSA), patients with clinically suspected severe catheter-related infections, patients with severe mucositis, or patients receiving high-dose cytarabine or quinolone prophylaxis, a glycopeptide (usually vancomycin) is recommended as first-line therapy, in combination with a broad-spectrum beta-lactam, with or without an aminoglycoside. However, the glycopeptide should be stopped after 48–72 hours in the absence of documentation of gram-positive infection.

Even in large cohorts of patients, it is very difficult to demonstrate that the difference in any microbiological activity between any two of these drugs has any clinical consequences as determined by response rates in neutropenic patients. All of these drugs have very similar clinical efficacy, and the choice should be based on the epidemiology in a given center and the potential risk of selection of resistant mutants, especially when monotherapy is chosen.

The routine empiric addition of glycopeptides to initial therapy is more controversial. It has been clearly demonstrated to be unnecessary in terms of time to defervescence and survival from aplasia when compared with delayed administration at day 3 in the case of persistent fever or documented methicillin-resistant gram-positive infection. This applies to both vancomycin and teicoplanin.[32–34] However, their empiric use may be justified in centers with a high incidence of MRSA, or in the case of suspicion of beta-lactam-resistant gram-positive infection. The problems that have already been encountered with vancomycin-resistant enterococci (VRE) could be encountered in the near future with coagulase-negative staphylococci. That possibility could have major implications, and physicians on hematological wards should be more and more restrictive with the empiric use of glycopeptides.

The addition of an antibiotic active against strict anaerobes (e.g. imipenem, clindamycin or metronidazole) is needed in patients with severe buccopharyngeal or perineal cellulitis or in any case of perianal or perirectal infection. In the case of ulcerative mucositis suggestive of herpes simplex infection, the administration of acyclovir is also needed, especially in high-risk patients (acute leukemia or BMT/PBSCT), if possible after a virological or cytological documentation.

Because mycotic infections are not usually early complications of the first febrile episode of aplasia, empiric antifungal treatment is rarely warranted in first-line therapy, except in high-risk patients with particular presentations. These include those with colonization due to a non-*albicans Candida* sp. (which is also unusual at the beginning of aplasia in previously untreated patients) or a history of *Candida* septicemia or aspergillosis during a previous aplastic phase.

### Reconsidering therapy during aplasia

In clinical trials, it has been routinely recommended to evaluate patients on day 3 of antibiotics and to reconsider the treatment then. However, in most recent clinical trials in high-risk patients, roughly 50% of the patients did not defervesce before day 5, even if no antibiotic change was made until the end of aplasia, suggesting that day 3 is perhaps too early to observe a defervescence even in favorable cases.

However, it is clear that, whatever the requirements of therapeutic trials, these patients must be routinely evaluated daily, because the occurrence of a new focus, or the deterioration of the clinical condition, may justify earlier therapeutic changes.

If an MDI has been found, the choice of strategy will depend on the susceptibility of the isolated strain(s), always keeping in mind the necessity of a broad-spectrum treatment. If glycopeptides had been given initially and are found to be unnecessary because a gram-negative strain only has been documented, the glycopeptide should be stopped.

In most cases, microbiological samples are negative. If the patient has defervesced and is clinically stable or better, then the same regimen must be continued until the end of aplasia, and the aminoglycoside, if initially given, may be stopped at day 3.[31] In low-risk adult patients who have defervesced between days 3 and 5, and without microbiological documentation, the intravenous regimen may be changed to oral ciprofloxacin plus amoxicillin–clavulanic acid.[14] In other cases, several strategies may be adopted, none of which can really be recommended more than another.

1.  The first is to change the beta-lactam or the beta-lactam–aminoglycoside combination to a more potent treatment. However, if the initial treatment was already very broad, the benefit of changing such a treatment is unclear when given empirically in the absence of a new

clinical focus guiding the choice, and most teams will continue to perform periodic sampling for microbiological documentation before making changes.

2.  The second is to empirically add a glycopeptide to the initial combination, which was routine practice in high-risk patients in Europe until recently. However, a trial by the International Antimicrobial Therapy Cooperative Group of the European Organization for Research and Treatment of Cancer (EORTC-IATCG) shows that patients do not benefit from the addition of vancomycin to tazocillin when they have only unexplained fever, with no microbiological documentation of gram-positive infection.[35]

3.  The third option, which may be combined with the first two, is to add an antifungal drug. It has been shown that adding intravenous amphotericin B (0.5–1 mg/kg/day) in patients remaining febrile despite 5–7 days of broad-spectrum antibiotics could be beneficial for those with severe and persistent neutropenia.[36,37] However, because the standard antifungal, deoxycholate amphotericin B, is highly toxic, this approach has been evaluated using other antifungal drugs, especially with intravenous azole compounds and the various forms of liposomal amphotericin B.[38–42] Among azoles, fluconazole has been found to have comparable efficacy to amphotericin B in the empiric indication.[40] However, due to its lack of efficacy on mold infections, it is not widely used. Itraconazole[41] and voriconazole[42] have both been compared with amphotericin B in its deoxycholate form[41] or its liposomal formulation.[42] Although the methodology of these trials have been widely debated, it can be concluded from both that azoles have comparable efficacy to amphotericin B, with fewer adverse events, especially less renal failure with azoles than with polyenes. Due to its broad spectrum and its safety profile, liposomal amphotericin B is recommended for empiric treatment of persistent febrile neutropenia in high-risk patients – those who have renal failure of any cause before first-line antibiotic therapy, those who develop renal failure under deoxycholate amphotericin B, or those who concomitantly receive other nephrotoxic drugs, especially the allogeneic stem cell transplant population who receive cyclosporine.

## The place of growth factors

Both granulocyte colony-stimulating factor (G-CSF) and granulocyte–macrophage colony-stimulating factor (GM-CSF) diminish the duration of neutropenia and fever, and generally the length of hospital stay (see Chapter 46). However, few randomized trials have been performed on the treatment of febrile neutropenia. Although no trial has clearly shown that the administration of growth factors, begun after the occurrence of the fever, decreases the mortality of aplasia, it seems logical to give one of them each time a documented infection is life-threatening, when the prognosis depends on the duration of neutropenia, and when the spontaneous recovery from neutropenia is not expected for several days.[43–45] Theoretically, GM-CSF should be preferable to G-CSF in cases of fungal infection because of its activity on the monocyte–macrophage system, although there are no clinical data to support this.

# Infections according to the site of infection

## Pneumonia

Pneumonia occurring in an immunocompromised host represents a major dilemma for the clinician.[46] First, the lung is by far the most common site of infection. Second, the chest X-ray may be normal, especially in neutropenic patients, despite a pulmonary infection.[24] Third, even without neutropenia, the main problem is whether to risk invasive procedures to have a reasonable chance of finding the etiological agent while weighing the risks of the morbidity and mortality of the procedure.

In hematological patients, pneumonia may be very difficult to diagnose (Table 47.2). Sputum culture is rarely useful in determining the true etiology of the pneumonia, and presents the risk of identifying an agent that is not finally responsible for the pneumonia. Therefore sputum is not recommended, except to look for strains that do not normally inhabit the oropharynx, such as *Legionella*, mycobacteria, and certain fungi.

The standard for diagnosis is bronchoscopic sampling with bronchoalveolar lavage (BAL): in neutropenic patients, this procedure should be considered urgently and specimens sent as described below. Empiric antibiotics against the likely organisms must be started without delay. Consideration should be given to the likelihood of fungus in patients with prolonged neutropenia and on steroid therapy. In nonneutropenic patients who are clinically stable and not asplenic or severely immunocompromised, one may sometimes be able to await the results of laboratory investigations before initiating treatment. In all patients with pneumonia, it is crucial to consider the following:

*   the type of immune deficiency, underlying disease and previous treatments;
*   the recent environment of the patient and exposure to nosocomial or any community-transmissible disease;
*   clinical and radiological pattern and rapidity of evolution;

- association of pneumonia with other infectious lesions (especially skin and brain).

The possibility of non-infectious processes (fluid overload, alveolar hemorrhage, pulmonary embolism, or tumor) should be considered rapidly. Non-invasive procedures should be performed, depending on the clinical setting: blood cultures, microbiological samples of any easily accessible focus (skin, cerebrospinal fluid), and a first set of serologies (*Legionella* and mycoplasmas) and antigenemia (*Aspergillus*, *Candida*, and CMV). Then, one should consider fibroscopy with BAL. A routine BAL protocol should include:

### Table 47.2 Main etiologies of pneumonia in hematological patients

| Etiology | Pathogens | Relationship to neutropenia | Main population at risk |
|---|---|---|---|
| **Infectious** | **Bacteria** | | |
| | • *Streptococcus pneumoniae* and *Haemophilus influenzae* | – | Allo BMT/PBSCT, myeloma, splenectomized patients, |
| | • Other gram-positive bacteria | + | Ig deficiencies |
| | • Other gram-negative bacteria | +/– | |
| | • Mycobacteria | – | |
| | • *Nocardia* | +/– | |
| | • *Legionella pneumophila* | – | Hairy cell leukemia |
| | **Fungi** | | |
| | • *Aspergillus* and mucorales | + | Acute leukemia, high-grade NHL and alloBMT/PBSCT |
| | • *Candida* spp. | + | Acute leukemia |
| | • *Cryptococcus* | – | CLL |
| | • *Pneumocystis jirovecii (carinii)* | – | Acute leukemia, high-grade NHL, alloBMT/PBSCT, any patient receiving steroids for more than 4 weeks |
| | **Viruses** | | |
| | • Herpes simplex virus (HSV) | +/– | |
| | • Varicella zoster virus (VZV) | – | Children, CLL, BMT/PBSCT |
| | • Cytomegalovirus (CMV) | – | AlloBMT/PBSCT |
| | • Adenovirus and respiratory syncytial virus (RSV) | – | BMT/PBSCT |
| | **Protozoa** | | |
| | • *Toxoplasma gondii* | – | Seropositive alloBMT/PBSCT recipient, HL |
| | **Helminths** | | |
| | • *Strongyloides stercoralis* | – | Patients originally from endemic countries |
| **Non-infectious** | | | |
| Vascular and embolic complications | • Alveolar hemorrhage | | |
| | • Pulmonary embolism | | |
| | • Intrathoracic bleeding post procedure | | |
| | • Pulmonary veno-occlusive disease | | |
| Inflammatory and/or immune diseases | • Hypersensitivity drug reaction | | |
| | • Radiation pneumonitis | | |
| | • Idiopathic interstitial pneumonia | | |
| | • Bronchiolitis obliterans | | |
| Others | • Fluid overload | | |
| | • Pulmonary edema | | |
| | • Alveolar proteinosis | | |
| | • Leukoagglutinin reaction | | |

(allo)BMT/PBSCT, (allogeneic) bone marrow/peripheral blood stem cell transplantation; Ig, immunoglobulin; NHL, non-Hodgkin lymphoma; CLL, chronic lymphocytic leukemia; HL, Hodgkin lymphoma.

- total and differential cell counts on cytocentrifuge preparations using May–Grünwald–Giemsa (MGG) stain;
- a cell pellet obtained by centrifugation and cytocentrifugation, stained by MGG, Papanicolaou, Perls–Prussian blue,[47] and Gomori–Crocott methods, and examined for cytological evidence of viral, fungal, and parasitic infections and for the detection of siderophages.

A sample of fluid should be reserved for bacteriological, viral, and fungal cultures. Aspiration rather than BAL fluid should be examined for *Legionella pneumophilia* by direct immunofluorescence and cultures. The choice of viruses to be detected by immunological assay should be determined with the laboratory according to the clinical setting. Some populations are at high risk of viral pneumonia, such as allogeneic BMT/PBSCT patients, and the panel of viruses to seek in these cases must include at least herpes simplex virus (HSV) and CMV, and adenovirus and respiratory viruses (influenza, parainfluenza virus, and respiratory syncytial virus (RSV)). However, in most patients who are less immunosuppressed, where the probability of the virus is low, given the cost of the procedure and the absence of effective treatment in most cases, the systematic use of a large panel of antiviral antibodies on first assessment is probably not justified, based on the data in the literature up to now. In the same way, periodic acid–Schiff (PAS) staining on BAL fluid is mandatory if there is a suspicion of alveolar proteinosis,[48] but its systematic use cannot be yet recommended in all hematological patients. A protected bacteriological sample should be considered with BAL – at least each time the patient has not been on broad-spectrum antibiotics and the clinical pattern is consistent with a bacterial pneumonia. This sample may be obtained either by protected specimen brush or by plugged telescoping catheter,[49] and processed by quantitative culture techniques. These samples should be considered positive if they show over $10^3$ cfu/ml.

Empiric treatment should then be discussed, especially in the case of acute occurrence of pneumonia. In hematological patients, BAL will give the diagnosis in approximately two-thirds of patients.[50,51] However, in one-third, the etiology of the pneumonia will not be revealed through BAL, because, despite identification of a pathogen, there is no diagnostic criterion clearly established in that case with that tool (e.g. *Candida* pneumonia), or because the cause or the responsible pathogen is difficult to reach (e.g. peripheral lesions), or because the alveolar lesions are non-specific.

In cases where bronchoscopy does not yield the diagnosis, other procedures may be considered, such as a second BAL, and/or a transbronchial biopsy (TBB), or transthoracic needle puncture under computed tomography (CT) scan in the case of peripheral dense lesions. The final decision between lung biopsy (through open or video-assisted thoracoscopy) or empiric treatment against the most likely organisms should be made between at least the hematologist and the lung specialist after consideration of the risk of the surgical procedure, the iatrogenic risk of each empiric treatment and the consequences, for the whole management of the patient, of not having a definite diagnosis for the pneumonia. Lung biopsy is more helpful in a prolonged clinical course, and in nodular or cavitary patterns, than in acute and/or non-nodular diseases, and also more helpful in hematological than in solid tumor patients.[52,53]

## Dermatological manifestations

Skin is both the first line of defense against the environment and also a warning system for the diagnosis of infectious complications in immunocompromised hosts, both through systemic and local development. We shall not discuss here the obvious importance of preserving its integrity and of keeping the skin as clean as possible to avoid colonization and infection by this route.

Numerous types of cutaneous infectious manifestations may be observed in hematological patients. They may occur from hematogenous diffusion or from local infection. They are sometimes the sole visible and accessible manifestation of the infectious process, and so have to be investigated carefully. Biopsies should be performed urgently and processed for both histological and microbiological examinations. The most frequent pathogens and their usual manifestations are listed in Table 47.3. However, not all of them are attributable to direct invasion of the skin by the pathogen, but may also be the consequence of immune or non-specific inflammatory reactions.

## Central nervous system infections

Few data are available in the literature on the incidence of central nervous system (CNS) infections in hematological patients. It is likely that this incidence is lower than 3%.[54] However, though infrequent, the diagnosis of these cases is always quite difficult when the cerebrospinal fluid (CSF) examination is not immediately helpful or the CSF cannot be sampled because of a contraindication to lumbar puncture, and when CNS involvement is not associated with another more accessible focus.

In non-neutropenic patients, and especially in patients with cellular immune deficiencies such as lymphomas, the most frequent infections are due to *Listeria monocytogenes*, which causes meningitis or meningo-encephalitis, with or without cerebritis. Where this is a possibility, once the CSF has been

**Table 47.3  Most frequent dermatological infectious manifestations observed in hematological patients**

| Pathogen | Main types of lesion |
|---|---|
| **Bacteria** | |
| • Streptococci, staphylococci | Erysipelas, rash, abscess, cellulitis |
| • Enterobacteria, *Pseudomonas* | Nodules, vesicules, ecthyma gangrenosum, cellulitis |
| • Strict anaerobes | Cellulitis, gangrene |
| • *Nocardia* | Abscess, cellulitis |
| • *Legionella* | Abscess, cellulitis, panniculitis |
| • Mycobacteria | Nodules, papules, abscess, panniculitis |
| **Fungi** | |
| • *Candida* | Macules, nodules, papules, cellulitis |
| • *Aspergillus* and mucorales | Abscess, cellulitis, macules, hemorrhagic nodules, pustules |
| **Viruses** | |
| • Herpesviruses | Vesicles, bullae, rash, papules, perineal ulcers |
| • Parvovirus B19, others | Rash, vesiculopustules |
| • Papillomavirus | Extensive warts, condylomata |
| **Parasites** | |
| • *Strongyloides stercolaris* | Papules |
| • Crusted (Norwegian) scabies | Crusted erythematous lesions |

examined in the laboratory, empiric treatment with intravenous ampicillin (200 mg/kg/day), with or without an aminoglycoside, should be begun urgently. Patients with meningitis and who have been splenectomized or those with hypogammaglobulinemia should be considered at high risk of *S. pneumoniae*, *H. influenzae* and *N. meningitidis* infection. *Nocardia asteroides* may be responsible for brain abscess, but may also involve subcutaneous tissues, liver, and lungs.[54] Toxoplasmosis has been mainly reported in Hodgkin lymphoma and, more recently, after allogeneic BMT, where non-invasive procedures such as blood polymerase chain reaction (PCR) may be useful.[55,56] The viruses that affect hematological patients, especially herpesviruses, may be responsible for meningitis or meningoencephalitis.

In neutropenic patients, fungi, especially *Aspergillus*, are the most frequent pathogens involved in neurological processes, and are usually – but not always – associated with pulmonary involvement, while *Candida* abscesses are more often associated with fungemia.[57] The incidence of neurological involvement during invasive candidiasis in hematological patients has been reported to be about 10%.[58] Bacteria causing meningitis during aplasia are usually those encountered in other kinds of infections in neutropenic patients, such as *E. coli*, *P. aeruginosa*, and streptococci. One should emphasize that in cases of meningitis occurring in profoundly neutropenic patients, the inflammatory reaction in the CSF is usually poor and the number of cells in the CSF may be very low or even normal.

The approach to a patient suspected of having CNS infection must be very cautious. Some of these CNS infections are easily identified by routine examination of CSF. Routine bedside ophthalmological examinations should be performed. They may be very useful in detecting signs of toxoplasmosis or *Candida* infections. However, these are uncommon, and it is very important to consider the likely causes according to the clinical presentation and the pattern of immune deficiency, and then to discuss with the laboratory what kind of additional techniques should be employed on an individual basis. For example, the diagnosis of cryptococcal meningitis should combine an Indian ink preparation and serological methods. CT scan and magnetic resonance imaging (MRI) can detect asymptomatic lesions, and these are especially helpful in making an etiological diagnosis by showing the localization and pattern and localizations of involvement. When the CSF is normal or non-contributory despite the use of specific procedures, and where there is no accessible focus due to the same pathogen, empiric treatment should be balanced with invasive procedures and, especially if lesions are visible on CT scan or MRI, with brain biopsy. The advantages and risks of the procedure should be weighed carefully. If the clinical status of the patient and the risk/benefit ratio of the procedure permit, everything should be done to optimize the processing of the samples in the pathology, microbiology, and mycology laboratories according to a written protocol established prior to the procedure.

# Diagnosis and treatment of fungal infections

Fungal infections have become the main infectious concern of hematologists in all populations of patients experiencing prolonged neutropenic phases. The incidence and mortality of fungal infections increase significantly over years, especially in stem cell transplant patients.[59,60] The incidence of *Aspergillus* infection varies greatly according mainly to the underlying disease and the therapeutic approach to the disease, but is roughly estimated at around 4–8% by episode of aplasia in Europe in patients receiving induction or consolidation phases of chemotherapy, and at up to 20–25% in adult allogeneic stem cell transplant recipients from an unrelated donor.[60] It is the principle infectious cause of death following allogeneic stem cell transplantation. The lung is the main target organ. A non-specific pulmonary focus or thoracic pain usually reveal the disease. Due to the low diagnostic yield of fibroscopy for the early diagnosis of *Aspergillus*, new diagnostic tests have been developed. These include detection of *Aspergillus* galactomannan by an enzyme-linked immunosorbent assay (ELISA). Early results show good sensitivity during neutropenia and after stem cell transplantation, but the test has a false-positive rate of 10–15%.[61] Nucleic acid detection is also currently being explored.[62,63] However, due to the lack of standardization, and to discrepancies between antigenemia and PCR results,[64] there is currently no consensus on the use of these new tests in clinical practice, and, despite its limitations, galactomannan is currently the most reliable test in neutropenic patients for the early diagnosis of *Aspergillus* infections. A CT scan may also help in the early diagnosis of *Aspergillus*, and has been shown to improve the prognosis of the disease[65] in neutropenic patients, where a halo sign can be seen on lung CT scan at the very early phase of development of the disease. The addition of such approaches, and the development of additional, more sensitive, diagnostic tests should finally decrease the mortality of the disease. However, for now, the recommendation is to consider the possibility of *Aspergillus* infection in any patient at risk (i.e. those with neutropenia of more than 10 days duration, especially in cases of concommitant steroid therapy), and to give antifungals active against *Aspergillus* until the suspicion has been confirmed. In a large prospective trial of first-line treatment,[66] voriconazole has been shown to improve the survival at 12 weeks in patients with *Aspergillus* infection, compared with amphotericin B. There is no randomized study of voriconazole versus liposomal amphotericin B. However, the latter has shown similar efficacy to voriconazole in previous trials versus conventional amphotericin B, and is therefore another option for first-line treatment. Micafungin has been shown to be efficacious in salvage treatment of aspergillosis.[67] Prospective trials are running to study the effect of echinocandins in combination either with amphotericin B compounds or with azoles.

*Candida* infections have also been increasing in frequency, and are now more and more often due to non-*albicans Candida* spp.[23] A rare manifestation of *Candida* infection is hepatosplenic candidiasis, which is usually misdiagnosed during the neutropenic phase, and is mostly diagnosed after the patient has recovered a normal granulocyte count. The early signs are fever and an increase in phosphatases.

A major progress in clinical research in this field has come with the publication of a consensus text from the EORTC-IFICG and the MSG for definitions of invasive fungal infections in cancer patients.[68]

# Special considerations for allogeneic BMT/PBSCT recipients

Allogeneic BMT/PBSCT offers a unique model of gradual immune reconstitution, and illustrate perfectly the relationship between the type of immune deficiency and infection by specific pathogens. This is also a setting where the impact of therapy may erase the importance of the underlying disease. It is usual to assume that after allogeneic BMT/PBSCT, immunodepression is often so profound that the post-transplant infectious complications are roughly the same whatever the previous underlying disease.

The description of the three classical phases of immune reconstitution has been the subject of a large literature describing how the donor cells are able to proliferate, mature, and differentiate in the recipient until they are capable of attaining the full functions of immune cells.[69] However, it is known most patients with severe GVHD will never regain normal immune function. After allogeneic BMT/PBSCT, it is usually considered that the sequence of infections may be classified into three periods (Table 47.4).[70]

1.  The first is the conditioning period and the aplastic phase until neutrophil recovery from the donated marrow. This phase is characterized by neutropenia and thrombocytopenia, and the infectious complications of BMT/PBSCT patients are not very different at this time from those encountered in other profoundly neutropenic patients such as acute leukemia patients, except that the conditioning regimen (especially total body irradiation (TBI)) usually induces more

**Table 47.4 Main pathogens responsible for infectious complications after allogeneic geno-identical bone marrow or peripheral blood stem cell transplantation**

|  | First phase (from conditioning regimen to the end of the 1st month) | Second phase (2nd–4th month) | Third phase (5th month and after) |
|---|---|---|---|
| **Bacteria** | Gram-positive:<br>• Oral streptococci<br>• Coagulase-negative staphylococci<br><br><br>Gram-negative enterobacteria | Nosocomial bacteria for patients staying in the unit because of graft-versus-host disease or rejection (*Pseudomonas aeruginosa*, enterococci, etc.) | *Streptococcus pneumoniae*<br>*Haemophilus influenzae*<br>Unusually:<br>• *Nocardia*<br>• Mycobacteria<br>• *Legionella*<br>• *Listeria monocytogenes* |
| **Fungi** | *Candida* spp.<br>*Aspergillus* spp. | *Aspergillus* spp.<br>*Pneumocystis carinii* | Fungi are observed only in severely immunosuppressed patients |
| **Viruses** | Herpes simplex virus 1 and 2 (HSV1 and HSV2) | Cytomegalovirus, human herpesvirus 6 (HHV6)<br>Varicella zoster virus<br>Epstein–Barr virus (EBV)<br>Adenovirus | Varicella zoster virus (VZV)<br>Adenovirus<br>Respiratory viruses |
| **Parasites** |  | Toxoplasmosis | Toxoplasmosis |

severe mucosal damage than chemotherapy given outside this setting. It has also been found that allogeneic BMT/PBSCT patients have a higher risk of aspergillosis than other hematological patients, even though it is also known that the aplastic phase of BMT/PBSCT is not the sole period at risk, since many cases have occurred during the second or third month of the graft when steroids are being administered.

2. The second phase corresponds to the period from initial marrow engraftment to at least the third or fourth month, and is characterized by cell-mediated immune deficiency with decreased number and function of specific and non-specific cytotoxic cells. CMV infection, which is mainly due to reactivation, was the most disquieting problem in this setting until improved therapy and the routine practice of early diagnosis through PCR or antigenemia and of preemptive therapy, which finally decreased the mortality due to CMV disease. Other viral diseases, less frequent than CMV, have been described during this phase, especially those due to adenovirus and enteric and respiratory viruses. The occurrence and severity of GVHD is the main factor delaying immune recovery and favoring infections. Although most investigations have focused on lymphocytic reconstitution, it is known that these patients also have phagocytic deficiencies of both neutrophils and macrophages, responsible for defects in bactericidal and fungicidal activities that may sometimes last for more than a year.

3. The third phase, beginning after the fourth month, is considered to be the late post-transplantation period. Here again, immune reconstitution is mainly influenced by the presence and severity of chronic GVHD. Most patients have immunoglobulin deficiency, particularly of IgG2, which is responsible for a decrease in the response to polysaccharide antigens. Mainly in this way, patients are threatened with encapsulated bacteria (e.g. *S. pneumoniae* and *H. influenzae*), which should be considered particularly in cases of pneumonia occurring after 3 months and should be treated urgently. In the absence of chronic GVHD, this deficiency will often be transient and will resolve over time. In other cases, it may persist indefinitely. However, even in these cases, active immunization may be beneficial, especially with conjugate vaccines.[71]

Although immune reconstitution after geno-identical allogeneic BMT/PBSCT is well known, it must be noted that each time a new approach in BMT/PBSCT is undertaken, new infectious complications can be observed. Mismatched transplants, for example, or pheno-identical transplants, are followed by more severe and protracted immune deficiency, and the best prophylactic and therapeutic approaches to these patients for infection have not been yet determined, since the characterization of immune reconstitution in these patients is currently poorly understood.

**Table 47.5  Main anti-infectious prophylactic measures for nosocomial infections that should be proposed in hematology departments**

| Pathogen | Main sources of acquisition | Prophylactic measure | Medical prophylaxis |
|---|---|---|---|
| **Bacteria** | | Total protective environment (debated) | Gut decontamination (debated) |
| • *Pseudomonas* spp. | | | |
| • Gram-negative strains | Food | Regular quality control of food and beverages | |
| • *Salmonella* spp. | | | |
| | Staff | Education of patients and staff Isolation of colonized or infected patients Labeling of colonized or infected patients | |
| • *Staphylococcus aureus* | Nasal portage Staff–patient contact Cutaneous colonization | Isolation of patient if methicillin-resistant Handwashing | Mupirocin for nasal portage (debated) |
| • Coagulase-negative staphylococci | Intravenous catheters | Written procedures for care of central lines Periodic removal (every 2–3 days) of peripheral intravenous lines if possible | None demonstrated to be efficacious |
| **Fungi** | | | |
| • *Candida* spp. | Food Staff Central intravenous lines | Food quality control Handwashing Written procedures for care of central lines | Antifungals (polyenes or azoles) through oral or systemic route |
| | Plastic devices (urinary, etc.) | Use urinary catheter only if essential, and manage according to written protocols | |
| • *Aspergillus* spp. | Air Increased risk in construction | HEPA filters (laminar-airflow rooms, units at positive pressure) | Debated or not demonstrated: • Local amphotericin B (sprays, aerosols) |
| | | Staff education about air circulation Room cleaning | • Systemic antifungals active against *Aspergillus* |
| • *Pneumocystis carinii* | Reactivation? Interhuman transmission? | Isolation of patients infected (debated) | Trimethoprim–sulfamethoxazole Pentamidine isethionate aerosols |
| **Viruses** | | | |
| • Cytomegalovirus (CMV) | Reactivation +++ Blood transfusions containing leukocytes Marrow graft from a seropositive donor | Blood products from seronegative donors or leukocyte-depleted products Selection of a CMV-seronegative donor for BMT if possible | Established: preemptive therapy Antivirals active against CMV: value not established for systematic prophylaxis in BMT/PBSCT |
| • Varicella zoster virus (VZV) | Reactivation for zoster Reinfection from infected persons for varicella | Patient and staff education to avoid direct contacts with infected persons Isolation of infected patients in the hematology ward | Active immunization during complete remission for children with acute lymphoblastic leukemia Passive immunization by IVIG during the first 48 h after contact in patients at risk Acyclovir (not established as prophylaxis) |
| • Respiratory syncytial virus (RSV), adenovirus | Air Saliva | Isolation of patients infected Exclusion of infected staff members | Ribavirin (not established) IVIG (not established) |
| **Parasite** | | | |
| *Strongyloides stercoralis* | Reactivation | Isolation of infected patients | Thiabendazole or mebendazole |

# Prophylactic measures

The main reason for having an in-depth knowledge of the infectious complications of a hematological disease is to be able to employ an individually based prophylactic approach. Much has been achieved in the understanding of risk factors for infection and consequently in the protection of these patients from the most common infectious risks. Among the measures summarized in Table 47.5, some are simply obvious and logical proposals for the organization of care in hematology wards to decrease infections, and especially the nosocomial risk, while others have been shown to be effective in controlled trials.

# Conclusions

Most treatments used in hematology are intensive and given in repeated cycles. Obviously, the morbidity and mortality due to infection in a given hematological disease are influenced by the therapy and its effect on the underlying disease, and also by the specific mechanisms of immune dysfunction induced and by the necessity for the use of foreign devices. Although the role of infection as a cause of death is difficult to assess in cases of refractory disease, it is more common to die from infection than from the disease. It is therefore mandatory that the hematologists who understand the malignancy also understand the specific infections, the need to follow a prophylactic approach, and the need to be aware of the urgency of treating certain infections.

## REFERENCES

1. Bodey GP, Buckley M, Sathe YS, Freireich EJ. Quantitative relationships between circulating leukocytes and infections in patients with acute leukemia. *Ann Intern Med* 1966; **39**: 1403–8.

2. Tancrede C, Andremont A. Bacterial translocation and gram-negative bacteraemia in patients with haematological malignancies. *J Infect Dis* 1985; **151**: 99–103.

3. Lecciones JA, Lee JW, Navarro EE. Vascular catheter associated fungemia in patients with cancer: analysis of 155 episodes. *Clin Infect Dis* 1992; **14**: 875–83.

4. Voss A, Hollis RJ, Pfaller M et al. Investigation of the sequence of colonization and candidemia in nonneutropenic patients. *J Clin Microbiol* 1994; **32**: 975–80.

5. Rex JH, Bennett JE, Sugar A et al. Intravascular catheter exchange and duration of candidemia. *Clin Infect Dis* 1995; **21**: 994–6.

6. Ribaud P, Chastang C, Latge JP et al. Survival and prognostic factors of invasive aspergillosis after allogeneic bone marrow transplantation. *Clin Infect Dis* 1999; **28**: 322–30.

7. Alangaden GJ, Wahiduzzaman M, Chandrasekar PH. Aspergillosis: the most common community-acquired pneumonia with gram-negative bacilli as copathogens in stem cell transplant recipients with graft-versus-host disease. *Clin Infect Dis* 2002: **35**: 659–64.

8. Pizzo PA, Purvis DS, Waters C. Microbiological evaluation of food items for patients undergoing gastrointestinal decontamination and protected isolation. *J Am Diet Assoc* 1982; **81**: 272–9.

9. Maki DG, Aluarado CJ, Hessewer CA, Zil Z. Relation of the inanimate hospital environment to endemic nosocomial infection. *N Engl J Med* 1982; **307**: 1562–6.

10. Martino P, Girmenia C, Venditti M et al. *Candida* colonization and systemic infection in cancer patients: a retrospective study. *Cancer* 1989; **64**: 2030–4.

11. Pfaller MA. Nosocomial candidiasis: emerging species, reservoirs, and modes of transmission. *Clin Infect Dis* 1996; **22**(Suppl 2): S89–94.

12. Weems JJ, Davis BJ, Tablan OC et al. Construction activity: an independent risk factor for invasive aspergillosis and zygomycosis in patients with hematologic malignancy. *Infect Control* 1987; **8**: 71–5.

13. Pizzo PA. Management of fever in patients with cancer and treatment-induced neutropenia. *N Engl J Med* 1993; **328**: 1323–30.

14. Hughes WT, Armstrong DA, Bodey GP et al. Guidelines for the use of antimicrobial agents in neutropenic patients with unexplained fever. *J Infect Dis* 1990; **161**: 381–96.

15. De Pauw BE, Deresinski SC, Feld R et al, for the Intercontinental Antimicrobial Study Group. Ceftazidime compared with piperacillin and tobramycin for the empiric treatment of fever in neutropenic patients with cancer. *Ann Intern Med* 1994; **120**: 834–44.

16. Cometta A, Zinne S, De Bock R et al. Piperacillin–tazobactam plus amikacin versus ceftazidime plus amikacin as empiric therapy for fever in granulocytopenic patients with cancer. *Antimicrob Agents Chemother* 1995; **39**: 445–52.

17. Elting LS, Bodey GP, Keefe BH. Septicemia and shock syndrome due to viridans streptococci: a case-control study of predisposing factors. *Clin Infect Dis* 1992; **14**: 1201–7.

18. Bochud PY, Calandra T, Francioli P. Bacteremia due to *Streptococcus viridans* in neutropenic patients: review of the literature. *Am J Med* 1994; **97**: 256–64.

19. Cordonnier C, Buzyn-Lévy A, Leverger G et al. Epidemiology and risk factors for gram-positive cocci infections in neutropenia : toward a more targeted antibiotic strategy. *Clin Infect Dis*, in press.

20. Cometta A, Calandra T, Gaya H et al. Monotherapy with meropenem versus combination therapy with ceftazidime plus amikacin as empiric therapy for fever in granulocytopenic patients with cancer. *Antimicrob Agents Chemother* 1996; **40**: 1108–15.

21. Swerdloff JN, Filler SG, Edwards JE. Severe candidal infections in neutropenic patients. *Clin Infect Dis* 1993; **17**(Suppl 2): S457–67.

22. Wingard JR. Importance of *Candida* species other than *C. albicans* as pathogens in oncology patients. *Clin Infect Dis* 1995; **20**: 115–25.

23. Viscoli C, Girmenia C, Marinus A et al. Candidemia in

cancer patients: a prospective, multicenter surveillance study by the Invasive Fungal Infection Group of the European Organization for Research and Treatment of Cancer. *Clin Infect Dis* 1999; **28**: 1071–9.

24. Sickles EA, Greene WH, Wiernick PH. Clinical presentation of infection in granulocytopenic patients. *Arch Intern Med* 1975; **135**: 715–19.

25. Elting LS, Rubenstein EB, Rolston KVI, Bodey GP. Outcomes of bacteremia in patients with cancer and neutropenia: observations from two decades of epidemiological and clinical trials. *Clin Infect Dis* 1997; **25**: 247–59.

26. Klastersky J, Paesmans M, Rubenstein EB et al. The multinational association for supportive care in cancer risk index: a multinational scoring system for identifying low-risk febrile neutropenic cancer patients. *J Clin Oncol* 2000; **18**: 3038–51.

27. Freifeld A, Marchigiani D, Walsh T et al. A double-blind comparison of empirical oral and intravenous antibiotic therapy for low-risk febrile patients with neutropenia during cancer chemotherapy. *N Engl J Med* 1999; **341**: 305–11.

28. Kern WV, Cometta A, De Bock R et al. Oral versus intravenous empirical antimicrobial therapy for fever in patients with granulocytopenia who are receiving cancer chemotherapy. International Antimicrobial Therapy Cooperative Group of the European Organization for Research and Treatment of Cancer. *N Engl J Med* 1999; **341**: 312–18.

29. Rubenstein EB, Rolston K, Benjamin RS et al. Outpatient treatment of febrile episodes in low risk neutropenic patients with cancer. *Cancer* 1993; **71**: 3640–6.

30. Cordonnier C, Herbrecht R, Pico JL et al. Cefepime/amikacin versus ceftazidime/amikacin as empirical therapy for febrile episodes in neutropenic patients: a comparative study. *Clin Infect Dis* 1997; **24**: 41–51.

31. The EORTC International Antimicrobial Therapy Cooperative Group. Ceftazidime combined with a short or long course of amikacin for empirical therapy of gram-negative bacteremia in cancer patients with granulocytopenia. *N Engl J Med* 1987; **317**: 1692–8.

32. The EORTC International Antimicrobial Therapy Cooperative Group. Vancomycin added to empirical combination antibiotic therapy for fever in granulocytopenic cancer patients. *J Infect Dis* 1991; **163**: 951–8.

33. Ramphal R, Bolger M, Oblon D et al. Vancomycin is not an essential component of the initial empiric treatment regimen for febrile neutropenic patients receiving ceftazidime: a randomized prospective study. *Antimicrob Agents Chemother* 1992; **36**: 1062–7.

34. Martino P, Micozzi A, Gentile G et al. Piperacillin plus amikacin vs. piperacillin plus amikacin plus teicoplanin for empirical treatment of febrile episodes in neutropenic patients receiving quinolone prophylaxis. *Clin Infect Dis* 1992; **15**: 290–4.

35. Cometta A, Kern WV, Debock R et al. Vancomycin versus placebo for treating persistent fever in patients with neutropenic cancer receiving piperacillin-tazobactum monotherapy. *Clin Infect Dis* 2003; **37**: 382–9.)

36. Pizzo PA, Robichaud KJ, Gill FA, Witebsky FG. Empiric antibiotic and antifungal therapy for cancer patients with prolonged fever and granulocytopenia. *Am J Med* 1982; **72**: 101–11.

37. EORTC International Antimicrobial Therapy Cooperative Group. Empiric antifungal therapy in febrile granulocytopenic patients. *Am J Med* 1989; **86**: 668–72.

38. Walsh TJ, Lee J, Lecciones J et al. Empiric therapy with amphotericin B in febrile granulocytopenic patients. *Rev Infect Dis* 1991; **13**: 496–503.

39. Hiemenz JW, Walsh TJ. Lipid formulations of amphotericin B: recent progress and future directions. *Clin Infect Dis* 1996; **22**(Suppl2): S133–44.

40. Winston DJ, Hathorn JW et al. A multicenter, randomized trial of fluconazole versus amphotericin B for empiric antifungal therapy of febrile neutropenic patients with cancer. *Am J Med* 2000; **108**: 282–9.

41. Boogaerts M, Winston DJ et al. Intravenous and oral itraconazole versus intravenous amphotericin B deoxycholate as empirical antifungal therapy for persistent fever in neutropenic patients with cancer who are receiving broad-spectrum antibacterial therapy. A randomized, controlled trial. *Ann Intern Med* 2001; **135**: 412–22.

42. Walsh TJ, Pappas P et al. Voriconazole compared with liposomal amphotericin B for empirical antifungal therapy in patients with neutropenia and persistent fever. *N Engl J Med* 2002; **346**: 225–34.

43. Bodey GP, Anaissie E, Gutterman J, Vadhan-Raj S. Role of granulocyte–macrophage colony-stimulating factor as adjuvant treatment in neutropenic patients with bacterial and fungal infection. *Eur J Clin Microbiol Infect Dis* 1994; **13**(Suppl2): S18–22.

44. Mather DW, Lieschke GJ, Green M. Filgrastim in patients with chemotherapy-induced febrile neutropenia. *Ann Intern Med* 1994; **121**: 492–6.

45. Schimpff SC. Growth factors and empiric therapy with antibiotics: Should they be used concurrently? *Ann Intern Med* 1994; **121**: 538–40.

46. White DA. Pulmonary infection in the immunocompromised patient. *Semin Thoracic Cardiovasc Surg* 1995; **7**: 78–87.

47. De Lassence A, Fleury-Feith J, Escudier E et al. Alveolar hemorrhage: diagnostic criteria and results in 194 immunocompromised hosts. *Am J Respir Crit Care Med* 1995; **151**: 157–63.

48. Cordonnier C, Fleury-Feith J, Escudier E et al. Secondary alveolar proteinosis is a reversible cause of respiratory failure in leukemic patients. *Am J Respir Crit Care Med* 1994; **149**: 788–94.

49. Pham LH, Brun-Buisson C, Legrand P et al. Diagnosis of nosocomial pneumonia in mechanically ventilated patients. *Am Rev Respir Dis* 1991; **143**: 1055–61.

50. Stover DE, Zaman MB, Hadju SI et al. Bronchoalveolar lavage in the diagnosis of diffuse pulmonary infiltrates in the immunosuppressed host. *Ann Intern Med* 1984; **101**: 1–7.

51. Cordonnier C, Bernaudin JF, Fleury-Feith J et al. Diagnostic yield of bronchoalveolar lavage in pneumonitis occurring after allogeneic bone marrow transplantation. *Am Rev Respir Dis* 1985; **132**: 1118–23.

52. Travis WD, Roth DB. Histopathologic evaluation of lung biopsy specimens. In: Shelhamer JPP, Parrillo JE (eds) *Respiratory Disease in the Immunosuppressed Host*. Philadelphia: Lippincott, 1991: 182–217.

53. Haverkos HW, Dowling JN, Pasculle AW et al. Diagnosis of pneumonitis in immunocompromised patients by open lung biopsy. *Cancer* 1983; **52**: 1093–7.

54. Singh N, Husain S. Infections of the central nervous system in transplant patients. *Transplant Infect Dis* 2000; **2**: 101–11.

55. Bretagne S, Costa JM, Kuentz M et al. Late toxoplasmosis evidenced by PCR in a marrow transplant recipient. *Bone Marrow Transplant* 1995; **15**: 809–11.

56. Martino R, Maertens J, Bretagne S et al. Toxoplasmosis after hematopoietic stem cell transplantation. A study by the European Group for Blood and Marrow Transplantation Infectious Diseases Working Party. *Clin Infect Dis* 2000; **31**: 1188–94.

57. Hagensee ME, Bauwens J, Kjos B, Bowden R. Brain abscess following marrow transplantation: experience at the Fred Hutchinson Cancer Research Center, 1984–1992. *Clin Infect Dis* 1994; **19**: 402–8.

58. Luna MA, Tortoledo ME. Histologic identification and pathological patterns of disease due to *Candida*. In: Bodey GP, Fainstein V (eds) *Candidiasis*. New York: Raven Press, 1985: 13–27.

59. McNeil M, Nash SL, Hajjeh RA et al. Trends in mortality due to invasive mycotic diseases in the United States, 1980–1997. *Clin Infect Dis* 2001; **33**: 641–7.

60. Marr KA. Epidemiology and outcome of mold infections in hematopoietic stem cell transplant recipients. *Clin Infect Dis* 2002; **34**: 909–17.

61. Maertens J, Verhaegen J, Lagrou K et al. Screening for circulating galactomannan as a noninvasive diagnostic tool for invasive aspergillosis in prolonged neutropenic patients and stem cell transplantation recipients: a prospective validation. *Blood* 2001; **97**: 1604–10.

62. Hebart H, Loffler J, Meisner C et al. Early detection of aspergillus infection after allogeneic stem cell transplantation by polymerase chain reaction screening. *J Infect Dis* 2000; **181**: 1713–19.

63. Costa C, Costa JM, Desterke C et al. Real time PCR coupled with automated DNA extraction and galactomannan antigen ELISA detection for diagnosis of invasive aspergillosis in serum. *J Clin Microbiol* 2002; **40**: 2224–7.

64. Bretagne S, Costa J-M, Bart-Delabesse E et al. Comparison of serum galactomannan antigen detection and competitive polymerase chain reaction in diagnosing invasive aspergillosis. *Clin Infect Dis* 1998; **26**: 1407–12.

65. Caillot D, Casasnovas O, Bernard A et al. Improved management of invasive pulmonary aspergillosis in neutropenic patients using early thoracic computed tomographic scan and surgery. *J Clin Oncol* 1997; **15**: 139–47.

66. Herbrecht R, Denning DW, Patterson TF et al. Voriconazole versus amphotericin B for primary therapy of invasive aspergillosis. *N Engl J Med* 2002; **347**: 408–15.

67. Maertens J, Raad I, Petrikkos G et al. Update of the multicenter noncomparative study of caspofungin in adults with invasive aspergillosis refractory or intolerant to other antifungal agents: analysis of 90 patients. In: *Proceedings of the 42nd Interscience Conference on Antimicrobial Agents and Chemotherapy, San Diego, CA, September 27–30, 2002.*

68. Ascioglu S, Rex JH et al. Defining opportunistic invasive fungal infections in immunocompromised patients with cancer and hematopoietic stem cell transplants: an international consensus. *Clin Infect Dis* 2002; **34**: 7–14.

69. Maury S, Mary JY, Rabian C et al. Prolonged immune deficiency following allogeneic stem cell transplantation: risk factors and complications in adult patients. *Br J Haematol*, 2001; 115: 630–41.

70. Sable CA, Donowitz GR. Infections in bone marrow transplant recipients. *Clin Infect Dis* 1994; **18**: 273–84.

71. Ljungman P, Cordonnier C, De Bock R et al. Immunisations after bone marrow transplantation: results of a European survey and recommendations from the Infectious Diseases Working Party of the European Group for Blood and Marrow Transplantation. *Bone Marrow Transplant* 1995; **15**: 455–60.

# Appendices

# Appendix I: Selected lineage-associated antigens in hematopoietic cells: CD nomenclature*

## B cells

| Antigen | Distribution | Structure | Function and comments |
|---|---|---|---|
| CD5 | Subset of mature B cells, mature T cells, thymocytes | 67 kDa transmembrane protein | Unknown function in B cells, but CD5+ B cells (B-1) cells are implicated in autoimmune disease. Co-stimulates T-cells |
| CD9 | Early B cells, activated B cells, activated T cells, platelets, eosinophils, basophils and endothelial cells | 22–27 kDa tetraspan protein that can form complexes with CD63, CD81 and CD82 | Platelet activation and aggregation; pre-B-cell adhesion; possible role in signaling mediated by interaction with GTP-binding proteins |
| CD10 (CALLA) | Widely expressed, including early T- and B-cell precursors, neutrophils, fibroblasts, and epithelial cells | 100 kDa integral membrane protein | Zinc metalloprotease. May act to limit activity of fMLP and peptide hormones. Possible role in B-cell development |
| CD19 | All B cells and B-cell precursors, FDC | 95 kDa protein of Ig superfamily | Regulation of B-cell activation and proliferation. Part of signal transduction complex that includes CD81, CD21 and Leu-13 |
| CD20 | All mature B cells, and pre-B cells, but not plasma cells | 33–37 kDa tetraspan protein: overall structure similar to 'channel-forming' proteins | Can generate intracellular $Ca^{2+}$ signal. May be involved in regulation of B-cell activation and proliferation. Used in treatment of B-cell NHL |
| CD21 (CR2R) | Mature sIg+ B cells (lost on activation), FDC, subset of normal thymocytes | 145 kDa transmembrane protein | Receptor for C3d and EBV. Involved in B-cell activation as part of signalling complex that includes CD19, CD81 and Leu-13. Binds CD23 and is implicated in regulation of IgE production |

*Adapted from *Immunology Today, Vol 18, Immune Receptor Supplement, 2nd edn* (Ager A, Callard R, Ezine S, eds), 1997, with permission from Elsevier Science. The reader is referred to this publication for a more complete listing.

| Antigen | Distribution | Structure | Function and comments |
|---------|--------------|-----------|----------------------|
| CD22 | Surface expression on mature B cells, cytoplasmic expression in late pro- and early pre-B cells Lost prior to plasma cell stage | α form (130 kDa) has five extracellular Ig-like domains; β form (140 kDa) has seven Ig-like domains | Mediates adhesion to erythrocytes T cells, B cells, monocytes and neutrophils. Probably limits B-cell receptor signaling |
| CD23 (FcεRII) | FcεRIIa form expressed on mature B cells and monocytes, FcεRIIb on monocytes, IL-4-activated macrophages, eosinophils, platelets, DC and FDC | 45 kDa type II membrane protein | Low-affinity IgE receptor with a role in IgE regulation. Binds CD21 and has role in B-cell activation, and may also prevent apoptosis of germinal-center B cells |
| CD24 | Expressed throughout B-cell development. Decreased on activation and lost on plasma cells. Expressed on immature thymocytes and activated T cells. Also found on mature granulocytes and a variety of epithelial cells | 35–70 kDa GPI-linked sialoglycoprotein | Crosslinking can induce a rise in intracellular Ca$^{2+}$ in mature B cells. May play a role in regulation of B-cell growth and antibody production. Co-stimulatory molecule for T-cell growth |
| CD25 | See under T cells | | |
| CD32 | FcγRIIB form present on B cells, FcγRIIA and C forms expressed on neutrophils; all forms are found on monocytes FcγRII proteins are also on Langerhans cells and some endothelial cells | 40 kDa. The different isoforms are encoded by three closely related genes: A, E, and C | Low-affinity receptor for aggregated IgG. Mediates endocytosis, activation of secretion and cytotoxicity. Binding to FcγRII on B cells can deliver a negative signal |
| CD38 | See under T cells | | |

| Antigen | Distribution | Structure | Function and comments |
|---|---|---|---|
| CD40 | Normal and neoplastic B cells, FDC, IDC, endothelial cells, thymic epithelium, macrophages, basal epithelia | 48–50 kDa transmembrane protein of the TNF superfamily | Binds CD40L (CD154) on activated T cells. Key signal for B-cell activation, proliferation and differentiation, formation of germinal centres, isotype switching, rescue from apoptosis, and differentiation into memory or plasma cells |
| CD74 | B cells, activated T cells, monocytes, activated endothelial and epithelial cells | 33, 35, and 41 kDa isoforms | Intracellular sorting of MHC class II molecules. Associates with α and β chains of MHC class II |
| CDw75 | Mature sIg+ B cells, small subset of blood T cells and erythrocytes | Carbohydrate NeuAc α2,6 Gal β1,4 GlcNac core epitope | Ligand for CD22, mediates B–B interactions |
| CD79 (α and β) | All B cells. Expressed early during B-cell ontogeny – probably before expression of cytoplasmic μ, and still present in cytoplasm of plasma cells | 33 kDa (CD79α) and 39 kDa (CD79β) transmembrane proteins | CD79 forms non-covalent association with sIg and is important for B-cell receptor signal transduction. CD79 may also mediate transport of IgM to cell surface |
| CD85 | Mature circulating B cells, many B-cell malignancies, especially hairy-cell leukemias (HCL), monocytes | Unknown | Unknown. Has diagnostic value for HCL |
| CD95 (Fas, Apo-1) | See under T cells | | |
| CD122 (IL-2Rβ, IL-15Rβ) | See under T cells | | |

| Antigen | Distribution | Structure | Function and comments |
|---------|-------------|-----------|----------------------|
| CD124 (IL-4R, gp140) | Mature B and T cells, hematopoietic precursors, fibroblasts, epithelial and endothelial cells. | 130–150 kDa transmembrane protein. Associates with 64 kDa $\gamma_c$ (CD132) to form higher-affinity IL-4 receptor complex. Also associates with IL-13Rα to form the IL-13R complex | Activates B cells, causing increased expression of surface CD23 and IgM. Switch factor involved in IgE regulation. Stimulates proliferative activity in pre-activated B and T cells. Induces differentiation of Th2 cells and stimulates development of CTL |
| CDw125 (IL-5Rα) | See under myeloid cells | | |
| CD126 (IL-6Rα) | Highly promiscuous. Activated B cells, plasma cells T cells, monocytes, epithelial cells, fibroblasts, hepatocytes, and neural cells | 80 kDa transmembrane protein that associates with gp130 (CDw130) to form high-affinity IL-6R | Promotes growth of myelomas, B-cell hybridomas, activated and EBV-transformed B cells and T-cell lines. Synergistic factor for early hematopoietic progenitor cells. Mediates acute-phase response of hepatic cells |
| CD127 (IL-7α) | Thymocytes, T-cell and B-cell progenitors, mature T cells, monocytes, some lymphoid and myeloid cell lines | 68 kDa transmembrane protein that associates with 64 kDa $\gamma_c$ (CD132) to form high-affinity IL-7R | Stimulates proliferation of pro- and pre-B cells, thymocytes and mature T cells, and induces monocyte activation |
| CD130 (gp130) | Widespread on hematopoietic cells and many other cell types | 130–140 kDa type I membrane glycoprotein | Signaling chain for receptors for oncostatin M, IL-6, IL-11, LIF, CNTF and cardiotropin |
| CD132 (IL-2Rγ, $\gamma_c$) | B cells, T cells, NK cells, monocytes, macrophages, neutrophils | 65–70 kDa. Subunit of IL-2R, IL-4R, IL-7R, IL-9R, IL-15R and IL-15R | Signaling component of receptors for IL-2R, IL-4R, IL-7R, IL-9R, IL-15R |

## T cells

| Antigen | Distribution | Structure | Function and comments |
|---|---|---|---|
| CD1 | Cortical thymocytes | 50–55 kDa heavy chain associated with a light chain of 12 kDa ($\beta$2-m). Different isotypes exist: CD1a,b,c,d, and e | Peptide presentation (CD1d). Lipid presentation (CD1b). Interacts with CD4⁻ CD8⁻ T cells |
| CD2 | Thymocytes, mature T cells, some NK cells | 55–60 kDa transmembrane glycoprotein. Binds CD58. Physically associated with CD3 $\epsilon$ and $\zeta$ chains | Adhesion: CTL to target cells, T cells to endothelium, and monocytes and thymocytes to TEC. Signal transductions: T-cell activation. Interaction with tubulin and regulation of energy |
| CD3 | All T cells | Three chains; $\gamma$ (25–28 kDa), $\delta$ (21 kDa), $\epsilon$ (20 kDa) associated with $\zeta$ (16 kDa) and $\eta$ (22 kDa) by disulfide bridges and with the T-cell receptor $\alpha\beta$ chains | T-cell activation and function |
| CD4 | Thymocytes, Th cells, monocytes | 60 kDa transmembrane protein of Ig superfamily. Interacts with p56$^{lck}$ | Helper activity, co-receptor with the TCR and signalling in association with p56$^{lck}$; adhesion (stabilizes TCR–MHC class II interaction) |
| CD5 | See under B cells | | |
| CD7 | Fetal liver stem/progenitor cells, thymocytes, mature T cells | 40 kDa transmembrane glycoprotein | Signal transduction |
| CD8 | Thymocytes, CTL, IEL (CD8$\alpha\alpha$), some DC | Disulfide-linked dimer $\alpha\beta$ or $\alpha\alpha$ of 34 kDa each. The short cytoplasmic tail interacts with p56$^{lck}$ ($\alpha$ chain only) | Maturation and positive selection of MHC class I restricted CTL. Stabilizes TCR–MHC class I interaction |
| CD10 | See under B cells | | |
| CD24 | See under B cells | | |

| Antigen | Distribution | Structure | Function and comments |
|---------|--------------|-----------|------------------------|
| CD25 (IL-2Rα) | Some thymocytes, and activated T cells, pre-B cells, NK cells and monocytes | 55 kDa chain (low-affinity receptor). Binds IL-2 with low affinity. Associates with IL-2R β and γ chains to form the high-affinity receptor | Induces activation and proliferation of T cells, B cells, thymocytes, NK cells, and macrophages |
| CD28 | T cells, plasma cells | 44 kDa homodimeric glycoprotein | Co-stimulatory molecule initiating signal transduction; events distinct from those initiated by TCR |
| CD30 | Activated T and B cells, Hodgkin's and Reed–Sternberg cells | 105 kDa membrane-bound glycoprotein of the TNF superfamily | Transduction of a death signal. Useful in diagnosis of Hodgkin disease and anaplastic large-cell lymphoma (ALCL) |
| CD38 | Early B cells and T cells, including thymocytes and pre-B cells. NK and DC precursors. Activated B and T cells, germinal-center B cells, plasma cells. Early but not most-primitive, myeloid stem cells | 45 kDa transmembrane protein | Probably gives a proliferative signal to T and B cells, and is involved in adhesion. Extracellular domain has ADP ribosyl cyclase activity |
| CD43 (leukosialin) | T cells, induced on activated CD4+ T cells, pre-B cells | 115 kDa sialylated mucin-like molecule | Role in T-cell proliferation, co-stimulation and adhesion. Role in HPC proliferation, apoptosis, and cell–cell interaction |
| CD44 | B and T cells, monocytes, neutrophils, epithelial cells, glial cells, fibroblasts and myocytes. Variant isoforms expressed widely and differentially in human tissues | 85 kDa hematopoietic form, CD44H lacks alternative exons. 110–250 kDa variant forms, vCD44, result from alternative splicing of 10 exons. V3 exon contains motifs for heparin and chondroitin sulfate addition | CD44H binds hyaluronic acid. Ligands for vCD44 unknown. Cell–cell and cell–ECM adhesion, T- and NK-cell activation. Can mediate lymphocyte rolling on endothelial cells, cell migration, and support of hematopoietic differentiation. Role for vCD44 in DC migration. Binding and presentation of chemokines and growth factors via proteoglycan forms |

| Antigen | Distribution | Structure | Function and comments |
|---|---|---|---|
| CD45 (leukocyte common antigen) | All hematopoietic cells except nucleated red cells – high levels on lymphocytes. CD45RO isoform expressed on naive T cells and CD45RA on memory T cells | Transmembrane glycoprotein of variable size (180–220 kDa). Different isoforms generated by alternative splicing | Protein tyrosine phosphatase. Role in thymocyte development, selection and TCR-mediated signal transduction. Can induce cell death under some circumstances |
| CD56 (NCAM) | T cells, NK cells | 200–220 kDa glycoprotein of Ig superfamily | Induces killer activity and MHC non-restricted cytotoxicity |
| CD57 (HNK-1) | Mature T cells, and CD16$^+$ NK cells | 110 kDa glycoprotein. | Mediates MHC non-restricted cytotoxicity after activation. Has low NK-cell activity |
| CD90 (Thy-1) | T-cell lineage, hematopoietic stem cells, and some progenitor cells and pre-B cells | 25–35 kDa membrane protein involved in transmembrane signaling via CD45 and p56$^{lck}$ | Role in lymphocyte recirculation, adherence, T-cell activation, cellular recognition |
| CD95 (Fas, Apo-1) | Thymocytes, mature T cells, activated lymphocytes | 36–45 kDa transmembrane protein of TNFR superfamily | Induces apoptosis signal when triggered by FasL or anti-Fas Ab. Role in clonal deletion of peripheral T cells and activation-induced cell death of mature cells. |
| CD122 (IL-2Rβ, IL-15Rβ) | B cells, T cells, NK cells, monocytes, macrophages | 70–75 kDa transmembrane glycoprotein | Signaling subunit of IL-2R and IL-15R. Associates with CD25 and CD132 (γ$_c$) to form high-affinity IL-2R, and with IL-15Rα and CD132 to form high-affinity IL-15R |
| CD124 | See under B cells | | |
| CD127 | See under B cells | | |

## Myeloid/monocyte

| Antigen | Distribution | Structure | Function and comments |
|---|---|---|---|
| CD10 | See under B cells | | |
| CD11a | Widespread on hematopoietic cells, lymphocytes, monocytes, macrophages, neutrophils, and eosinophils | 180 kDa $\alpha$ subunit (CD11a; $\alpha_L$), which non-covalently associates with 95 kDa (CD18; $\beta_2$) subunit to form LFA-1 | Mediates leukocyte adhesion to endothelium via ICAM-1 and ICAM-2 during migration and inflammation; homotypic and heterotypic adhesion between T cells, B cells and monocytes; neutrophil homotypic aggregation via ICAM-3 |
| CD11b | Monocytes, macrophages, NK cells, neutrophils | 170 kDa $\alpha$ subunit (CD11b; $\alpha_M$), which associates with the $\beta_2$ subunit to form MAC-1/CR3 | Mediates adhesion of monocytes and neutrophils to vascular endothelium via ICAM-1, fibrinogen and subsequent extravasation via ICAM-1. Opsonization of complement-coated particles by macrophages via iC3b |
| CD11c | Monocytes, macrophages, NK cells, neutrophils, activated lymphocytes | 150 kDa $\alpha$ subunit (CD11b; $\alpha_X$), which non-covalently associates with the $\beta_2$ subunit to form CR4 | Binds fibrinogen and iC3b. Mediates adhesion of monocytes and granulocytes to inflamed endothelium. Phagocytic receptor. Involved in T-cell aggregation |
| CD13 | Granulocytes, monocytes and their precursors; endothelial cells, renal epithelial cells, bone marrow stromal cells, osteoclasts, subset of large granular lymphocytes | 150 kDa integral membrane protein expressed on the cell surface as a homodimer | Aminopeptidase N. Receptor for coronavirus and involved in interaction with cytomegalovirus |
| CD14 | Monocytes and granulocytes | 55 kDa $N$-glycosylated GPI-anchored glycoprotein; 48 kDa soluble form | Membrane-bound form is a high-affinity receptor for LPS–LBP complexes on granulocytes, monocytes and macrophages. Soluble form also binds LPS, and is required for LPS-induced activation of endothelial cells |

| Antigen | Distribution | Structure | Function and comments |
|---|---|---|---|
| CD15 (Lewis X) | Monocytes, granulocytes and their precursors; Langerhans cells. Many cancer cells | Carbohydrate antigen with a terminal structure of Gal $\beta 1,4$ (Fuc $\alpha 1,3$) GlcNA $\beta 1,3$ Gal $\beta 1,R$ | Possible ligand for selectins |
| CD16 (FcγRIII) | NK cells, granulocytes, macrophages, subset of T cells | 50–65 kDa glycoprotein of the Ig superfamily | Low-affinity IgG receptor, main receptor for ADCC; activation of cytotoxicity, cytokine production, and receptor expression |
| CD18 | Lymphocytes, monocytes, neutrophils, and eosinophils | 95 kDa $\beta_2$ subunit non-covalently associated with an $\alpha$ subunit (e.g. CD11a) | See under CD11a, CD11b and CD11c |
| CD23 | See under B cells | | |
| CD31 (PECAM-1) | Monocytes, platelets, neutrophils, naive T cells, NK cells, endothelial cells (lateral surfaces) | 130 kDa integral membrane glycoprotein of the Ig superfamily. Multiple isoforms produced by alternative splicing | Homophilic (CD31–CD31) and heterophilic (CD31–$\alpha_v\beta_3$ integrin) adhesion. Implicated in transendothelial migration of monocytes, neutrophils, NK cells and activated T cells |
| CD32 | See under B cells | | |
| CD33 | Monocytes, macrophages granulocytes, myeloid progenitor cells | 67 kDa glycoprotein expressed as a homodimer | Not known |
| CD34 | Hematopoietic stem/ progenitor cells. Widespread distribution on vascular endothelium | 90 kDa glycosylated protein; nature of glycosylation depends on the site of expression. | Mediates L-selectin-independent binding of leukocytes to high endothelial venules and L-selectin-independent binding of hematopoietic stem cells to stromal elements of bone marrow |

| Antigen | Distribution | Structure | Function and comments |
|---|---|---|---|
| CD35 (CR1) | Neutrophils, monocytes, eosinophils, B cells, subset of T cells, erythrocytes, FDC, glomerular podocytes and some astrocytes | Single-chain glycoprotein of variable length depending on allotype: 190 kDa (A), 220 kDa (B), 160 kDa (C), 250 kDa (D) | Receptor for C3b or C4b. Mediates adherence of C4b/C3b-coated particles prior to phagocytosis. Major role in removing and processing immune complexes of facilitating their localization to lymphoid follicles |
| CD36 | Monocytes, macrophages, platelets, microvascular endothelial cells, DC, mammary endothelial cells | 88 kDa single-chain glycoprotein | Receptor for thrombospondin; scavenger receptor for oxidized LDL; recognition and phagocytosis of apoptotic cells; cell adhesion molecule in platelet adhesion and aggregation, platelet–monocyte and platelet–tumor cell interactions |
| CD64 (FcγRI) | Monocytes, macrophages, blood DC, activated neutrophils, early myeloid-lineage cells | 72 kDa transmembrane glycoprotein encoded by three related genes | High-affinity receptor for monomeric IgG promoting phagocytosis, ADCC, superoxide and cytokine release in macrophage activation |
| CD66a | Granulocytes and epithelial cells | 140–180 kDa transmembrane heavily N-glycosylated glycoprotein | Capable of homophilic and heterophilic adhesion, E-selectin binding. Role in signaling and regulates adhesion activity of β₂ integrins in neutrophils |
| CD66b | Granulocytes | 95–100 kDa GPI-anchored glycoprotein | Uncertain, but capable of heterophilic adhesion and transmembrane signaling; capable of activating neutrophils |
| CD66c | Granulocytes and epithelial cells | 90 kDa GPI-anchored glycoprotein, heavily N-glycosylated | Unclear, but capable of homophilic and heterophilic adhesion, E-selectin binding, galectin binding; capable of activating neutrophils |
| CD66d | Granulocytes | 35 kDa heavily N-glycosylated transmembrane glycoprotein | Unclear, but capable of activating neutrophils |
| CD71 (transferrin receptor) | Macrophages and proliferating cells, including hematopoietic progenitor cells – high levels on erythroid progenitors | 95 kDa disulfide-linked homodimeric transmembrane molecule | Receptor for transferrin; important in iron metabolism and cell growth |

| Antigen | Distribution | Structure | Function and comments |
|---|---|---|---|
| CD87 (uPAR) | Activated monocytes, neutrophils, activated T cells, NK cells, vascular endothelial cells, fibroblasts, smooth muscle cells, keratinocytes, placental trophoblasts, hepatocytes. Wide variety of tumor cells | 35–59 kDa heavily glycosylated GPI-anchored glycoprotein | Cellular receptor for pro-uPA and uPA; implicated in the process of inflammatory cell invasion and tumor cell metastasis; binds to vitronectin; may contribute to integrin-dependent adherence and chemotaxis |
| CD114 (G-CSFR) | Granulocytes, monocytes granulocyte precursors, trophoblast cells | 130 kDa single-chain transmembrane glycoprotein | Receptor for G-CSF |
| CD115 (M-CSFR, c-Fms) | Monocytes, macrophages, and their progenitors. Osteoclasts, trophoblasts, and certain carcinomas | 150 kDa transmembrane glycoprotein | Receptor for M-CSF |
| CD116 (GM-CSFRα) | Myeloid progenitors and precursors. Macrophages, neutrophils, eosinophils, DC | 80 kDa type I transmembrane glycoprotein; associated with CDw131 | Binds GM-CSF with low affinity when expressed alone. Binds GM-CSF with high affinity when co-expressed with $\beta_c$ (CDw131) |
| CD117 (SCFR, c-Kit) | Hematopoietic stem and progenitor cells, tissue mast cells, early thymocytes | 145–150 kDa transmembrane glycoprotein | Growth factor receptor that binds SCF (c-Kit ligand) |
| CDw119 (IFN-γRα) | Macrophages and most leukocytes | 95 kDa transmembrane glycoprotein which associates with the IFN-γRII (β chain) | IFN-γ receptor α chain, which transduces IFN-γ-dependent signals |

| Antigen | Distribution | Structure | Function and comments |
|---|---|---|---|
| CD120a (TNFRI) | Some granulocytes, FDC and endothelial cells; soluble type I (30 kDa form) released from activated granulocytes and monocytes | 55 kDa transmembrane molecule | Receptor for TNF; mediates antitumor effects; induces and primes inflammatory response; upregulates leukocyte adhesion molecules and MHC class I |
| CD120b (TNFRII) | Monocytes and macrophages; soluble form released from activated granulocytes and monocytes | 75 kDa transmembrane molecule | Receptor for TNF; functions similarly to TNFR type I (CD120a) |
| CD121a (IL-1R) | Macrophages and virtually all leukocytes | 75–85 kDa single-chain transmembrane molecule | Binds biologically active IL-1 $\alpha$ and $\beta$, and the biologically inactive IL-1ra |
| CDw123 (IL-3R$\alpha$) | Most myeloid cells and their progenitors, lymphocytes, neutrophils, eosinophils | 70 kDa transmembrane protein | Binds IL-3 with low affinity when expressed alone. Binds IL-3 with high affinity when co-expressed with $\beta_c$ (CDw131) |
| CDw125 (IL-5R$\alpha$) | Eosinophils and B cells | 60 kDa transmembrane protein with homology to $\alpha$ chains of IL-3R and GM-CSFR | Binds IL-5 with low affinity when expressed alone. Binds IL-5 with high affinity when co-expressed with $\beta_c$ (CDw131). Stimulates growth and differentiation of eosinophils B cells (mouse) |
| CD126 (IL-6R$\alpha$) | See under B cells | | |

| Antigen | Distribution | Structure | Function and comments |
|---|---|---|---|
| CDw128 (IL-8R) | Neutrophils, monocytes, subset of NK cells, astrocytes, microglia CD8+ T cells | Two variants: IL-8RA, 44–59 kDa glycoprotein; IL-8RB, 67–70 kDa glycoprotein. Both contain seven transmembrane domains | IL-8RA binds IL-8; IL-8RB binds IL-8, gro, NAP-2 and ENA78. Critical regulators of IL-8-mediated neutrophil chemotaxis and activation |
| CD130 (gp130) | See under B cells | | |
| CDw131 (βc) | Most myeloid cells, including early progenitors, early B cells | 120–140 kDa transmembrane protein | Functions as a β subunit that associates with the α subunits of IL-3R (CDw123), IL-5R (CDw125) and GM-CSFR (CD116) |
| CD135 (Flt-3) | Multipotential myelo-monocytic and primitive B-cell progenitors | 130 kDa receptor of the tyrosine kinase family | Growth factor receptor for early hematopoietic progenitors |
| CD141 (thrombo-modulin) | Monocytes, neutrophils, endothelial cells, platelets, megakaryocytes, keratinocytes, smooth muscle cells, synovial lining cells | 75 kDa single-chain membrane glycoprotein | Cofactor for thrombin-mediated activation of protein C |
| CD142 (tissue factor, thromboplastin) | Activated monocytes, vascular endothelial cells and fibroblasts; epidermal keratinocytes, glomerular epithelial cells and stromal cells | 45–47 kDa single-chain transmembrane glycoprotein | Procoagulant molecule that binds factor VIIa and zymogen factor VII. It is the major initiator of clotting in normal haemostasis |
| CD153 | Activated macrophages, neutrophils, activated T cells and B cells | 75 kDa transmembrane glycoprotein of the TNF superfamily | CD30 ligand. Physiological role unclear |

| Antigen | Distribution | Structure | Function and comments |
|---|---|---|---|
| CD156 (ADAM 8) | Neutrophils and monocytes | 69 kDa transmembrane protein | Disintegrin and metalloproteinase. May be involved in leukocyte extravasation |
| CD164 | Monocytes, bone marrow stromal cells. Normal and neoplastic epithelial cells | 80 kDa integral membrane glycoprotein expressed as a homodimer | Possibly mediates adhesion between bone marrow stromal cells and hematopoietic progenitor cells |

*Acronyms*: ADCC, antibody-dependent cellular cytotoxicity; CKR-SF, cytokine receptor superfamily; CNTF, ciliary neurotrophic factor; CTL, cytotoxic T lymphocyte; DC, dendritic cell; EBV, Epstein–Barr virus; ECM, extracellular matrix; FDC, follicular dendritic cell; G-CSF, granulocyte colony-stimulating factor; GM-CSF, granulocyte–macrophage colony-stimulating factor; GPI, glycosyl-phosphatidylinositol; HPC, hematopoietic precursor cell; ICAM, intercellular adhesion molecule; IDC, interdigitating dendritic cell; IEL, intraepithelial lymphocyte; IFN, interferon; IL, interleukin; LBP, lipopolysaccharide-binding protein; LDL, low-density lipoprotein; LIF, leukemia inhibitory factor; LPS, lipopolysaccharide; M-CSF, macrophage colony-stimulating factor; NK, natural killer; SCF, stem cell factor; TCR, T-cell receptor; TEC, thymic epithelial cell; Th, T helper; TNF, tumor necrosis factor.

## Appendix II:  Concise summary of the cytokines involved in human hematopoiesis

| Cytokine* | Cellular source in hematopoietic tissues† | Main target cells†,‡ | Chromosomal location |
|---|---|---|---|
| IL-1 | End, F, T, B, NK, Mo, Mf | SC+, PC+, B+, T+, Mo+ | 2q12–21 |
| IL-2 | T | T+, B+, NK+, Mo, Mf | 4q26–27 |
| IL-3 | T, Ma, Eo | SC+, PC+, E+, G+, Meg+, PL+ | 5q23–31 |
| IL-4 | T, Ma, PC, F, G | | 5q31 |
| IL-5 | Ma, T, Eo, PC | Eo+ | 5q23–31 |
| IL-6 | End, F, T, B, Mo, Mf, PC | SC+, PC+ | 7p21–14 |
| IL-7 | F | B+, T+ | 8q12–13 |
| IL-8 | End, F, T, B, Mo, G | Ne+, Ba+, T+ | 4q12–21 |
| IL-9 | T | T+, Ma+, E+ | 5q31.1 |
| IL-10 | T | T+/−, Mo−, NK−, B+, Ma+ | 1q31–q32 |
| IL-11 | End, F | SC+, PC+, Meg, Mf | 19q13.3–13.4 |
| IL-12 | B, Mo, Mf | SC+, PC+, T+, NK+ | 19p13.1 and 1p31.2 |
| IL-13 | T | Mo−, B+ | 5q31 |
| IL-14 | T | B−/+ | – |
| IL-15 | Mo, G, T, B | T+ | 4q25–35 |
| IL-16 | Ma | T+ | – |
| M-CSF | End, F, T, Mo | Mo+, Mf+ | 5q33.1 |
| G-CSF | End, F, Mo, Mf | SC+, PC+, G+ | 17q21–22 |
| GM-CSF | F, End, T, Mf, G | G+, Mo+, Mf+ | 5q21–32 |
| Flt-3L | F | SC+, PC+, Mo+ | – |
| EPO | Mf | E+, Meg+ | 7pter–q22 |
| TPO | F | SC+, PC+, Meg+, E+ | 3q26–27 |
| bFGF | End, Mo | Mf+, End+, SC+, PC+ | 4q25–q27 |
| IFN-γ | T, NK | T+, B+, Mf+, NK+, End+, F+, SC+, PC− | 12q24.1 |
| LIF | F, T, Mo, G | SC+, Mf+, Pl+ | 22q14 |

| Cytokine* | Cellular source in hematopoietic tissues† | Main target cells†,‡ | Chromosomal location |
|---|---|---|---|
| MIP-1α | T, B, Ne, Mf | Mf⁺, PC⁻, B⁺, Eo⁺ | 17q11–21 |
| OSM | T, Mo | SC | 22q12 |
| SCF | F | SC⁺, PC⁺, E⁺, G⁺, Pl⁺ | 12q22–24 |
| TNF-α | F, B, T, Mo, Mf | M⁻, PC⁻ | 6p21.3 |
| TGF-β1 | End, F, Lymf, Mo, G, PC, | SC⁻, PC⁻, Mc⁺ | 19q13 |
| | Mf, Pl | | |

* *Cytokine acronyms:* IL, interleukin; CSF, colony-stimulating factor; Flt-3L, ligand for stem cell tyrosine kinase 1 (STK-1, gene symbol *Flt-3*); EPO, erythropoietin; TPO, thrombopoietin; bFGF, basic fibroblast growth factor; IFN, interferon; LIF, leukemia inhibitory factor; MIP, macrophage inflammatory protein; OSM, oncostatin M; SCF, stem cell factor (c-Kit ligand, Steel factor); TNF, tumor necrosis factor; TGF, transforming growth factor.
† *Cellular sources and activities:* B, B lymphocyte; Ba, basophil; E, erythrocytic; End, endothelium; Eo, eosinophil; F, stromal fibroblastic cells; G, granulocytic; Lymf, lymphoid; Ma, mast cells; Meg, megakaryocytic; Mf, macrophage; Mo, monocytic; Ne, neutrophil; NK, natural killer cells; PC, progenitor cells; Pl, platelet; SC, stem cells; T, T lymphocyte.
‡ Activities on target cells represent a diversity of effects, including stimulation or inhibition of survival, proliferation, differentiation, cycle induction, activation, maturation, cytokine production or elaboration, chemotaxis, and antitumor effects.

# Index